TRAVELL, SIMONS & SIMONS'
Myofascial Pain and Dysfunction
THE TRIGGER POINT MANUAL

THIRD EDITION

Editor in Chief

Joseph M. Donnelly, PT, DHS
Board-Certified Clinical Specialist in Orthopaedic Physical Therapy (OCS)
Fellow of the American Academy of Orthopaedic Manual Physical Therapists (Honorary)
Clinical Professor and Director of Postprofessional Education
Department of Physical Therapy, College of Health Professions, Mercer University
Atlanta, Georgia

Editorial Board

César Fernández de las Peñas, PT, MSc, PhD
Head Division of the Department of Physical Therapy, Occupational Therapy, Rehabilitation and Physical Medicine
Cátedra de Investigación y Docencia en Fisioterapia: Terapia Manual y Punción Seca
Universidad Rey Juan Carlos
Alcorcón, Madrid, Spain

Michelle Finnegan, PT, DPT
Board-Certified Clinical Specialist in Orthopaedic Physical Therapy (OCS)
Fellow of the American Academy of Orthopaedic Manual Physical Therapists
Certified Cervical and Temporomandibular Therapist
Senior Instructor, Myopain Seminars
Bethesda, Maryland

Jennifer L. Freeman, PT, DPT
Board-Certified Clinical Specialist in Orthopaedic Physical Therapy (OCS)
Intown Physical Therapy, LLC
Adjunct Clinical Assistant Professor
Department of Physical Therapy, College of Health professions, Mercer University
Atlanta, Georgia

Photography by Christynne Helfrich, PT, DPT
Board-Certified Clinical Specialist in Orthopaedic Physical Therapy (OCS)

Illustrations by Barbara D Cummings

TRAVELL, SIMONS & SIMONS'
Myofascial Pain and Dysfunction
THE TRIGGER POINT MANUAL

THIRD EDITION

Joseph M. Donnelly

César Fernández de las Peñas
Michelle Finnegan
Jennifer L. Freeman

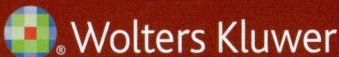

Philadelphia · Baltimore · New York · London
Buenos Aires · Hong Kong · Sydney · Tokyo

Acquisitions Editor: Michael Nobel
Product Development Editor: Amy Millholen
Editorial Coordinator: John Larkin
Marketing Manager: Shauna Kelley
Production Project Manager: David Saltzberg
Design Coordinator: Terry Mallon
Manufacturing Coordinator: Margie Orzech-Zeranko
Prepress Vendor: S4Carlisle Publishing Services

Third edition

Copyright © 2019 Wolters Kluwer.

All rights reserved. This book is protected by copyright. No part of this book may be reproduced or transmitted in any form or by any means, including as photocopies or scanned-in or other electronic copies, or utilized by any information storage and retrieval system without written permission from the copyright owner, except for brief quotations embodied in critical articles and reviews. Materials appearing in this book prepared by individuals as part of their official duties as U.S. government employees are not covered by the above-mentioned copyright. To request permission, please contact Wolters Kluwer at Two Commerce Square, 2001 Market Street, Philadelphia, PA 19103, via e-mail at permissions@lww.com, or via our website at lww.com (products and services).

9 8 7 6 5 4 3

Printed in China

Library of Congress Cataloging-in-Publication Data

Names: Donnelly, Joseph M., editor. | Preceded by (work): Simons, David G. Travell & Simons' myofascial pain and dysfunction.
Title: Travell, Simons & Simons' myofascial pain and dysfunction: the trigger point manual / [edited by] Joseph M. Donnelly; editorial board, César Fernández-de-las-Peñas, Michelle Finnegan, Jennifer L. Freeman; photography by Christynne Helfrich; illustrations by Barbara D. Cummings.
Other titles: Travell, Simons and Simons' myofascial pain and dysfunction | Myofascial pain and dysfunction
Description: Third edition. | Philadelphia: Wolters Kluwer Health, [2019] | Preceded by: Travell & Simons' myofascial pain and dysfunction: the trigger point manual / David G. Simons, Janet G. Travell, Lois S. Simons; illustrations by Barbara D. Cummings, with contributions by Diane Abeloff and Jason Lee. 2nd ed. 1999- | Includes bibliographical references and index.
Identifiers: LCCN 2018024798 | ISBN 9780781755603 (hardback)
Subjects: | MESH: Myofascial Pain Syndromes
Classification: LCC RC925.5 | NLM WE 550 | DDC 616.7/4—dc23 LC record available at https://lccn.loc.gov/2018024798

This work is provided "as is," and the publisher disclaims any and all warranties, express or implied, including any warranties as to accuracy, comprehensiveness, or currency of the content of this work.

This work is no substitute for individual patient assessment based upon healthcare professionals' examination of each patient and consideration of, among other things, age, weight, gender, current or prior medical conditions, medication history, laboratory data, and other factors unique to the patient. The publisher does not provide medical advice or guidance, and this work is merely a reference tool. Healthcare professionals, and not the publisher, are solely responsible for the use of this work, including all medical judgments and for any resulting diagnosis and treatments.

Given continuous, rapid advances in medical science and health information, independent professional verification of medical diagnoses, indications, appropriate pharmaceutical selections and dosages, and treatment options should be made and healthcare professionals should consult a variety of sources. When prescribing medication, healthcare professionals are advised to consult the product information sheet (the manufacturer's package insert) accompanying each drug to verify, among other things, conditions of use, warnings and side effects and identify any changes in dosage schedule or contraindications, particularly if the medication to be administered is new, infrequently used or has a narrow therapeutic range. To the maximum extent permitted under applicable law, no responsibility is assumed by the publisher for any injury and/or damage to persons or property, as a matter of products liability, negligence law or otherwise, or from any reference to or use by any person of this work.

LWW.com

To
David G. Simons (June 7, 1922-April 5, 2010)
and
Lois S. Simons (March 6, 1934-July 3, 2004), whose guiding spirits are ever with us.

This third edition of **The Trigger Point Manual** has been a labor of love and is dedicated to the memory of David G. Simons, who devoted his post-military medical career to advancing myofascial pain and trigger point scientific and clinical research. His passion, commitment, and dedication to expanding the scientific body of knowledge of muscle pain in order to help decrease the pain and suffering of human beings was unparalleled. David G. Simons was a true pioneer, both as one of the most highly respected scientists in the field of myofascial pain and in the treatment of patients with chronic pain. His wife and coauthor, Lois S. Simons, used her expertise in muscle anatomy and kinesiology as well as her outstanding clinical skills to build on the solid physician-oriented clinical foundation laid by Janet G. Travell (1901-1997) in the first edition.

For those of us who knew David and Lois, we have tried to respect their goals for this third edition and are pleased to have had the opportunity to complete the task they were unable to finish.

Contributors

Ingrid Allstrom Anderson, PT, DPT
Board-Certified Clinical Specialist in Orthopaedic Physical Therapy
Principal, Intown Physical Therapy, LLC
Atlanta, Georgia

José L. Arias-Buría, PT, MSc, PhD
Department of Physiotherapy, Occupational Therapy, Rehabilitation, and Physical Medicine
Cátedra de Investigación y Docencia en Fisioterapia: Terapia Manual y Punción Seca
Universidad Rey Juan Carlos
Alcorcón, Madrid, Spain

Amanda Blackmon, PT, DPT
Board-Certified Clinical Specialist in Orthopaedic Physical Therapy
Clinical Assistant Professor
Department of Physical Therapy
College of Health Professions, Mercer University
Series Instructor, Myopain Seminars
Atlanta, Georgia

Deanna Hortman Camilo, PT, DPT
Board-Certified Clinical Specialist in Orthopaedic Physical Therapy
Motion Stability Physical Therapy Group
Atlanta, Georgia

Thomas L. Christ, MS, DPT
Department of Physical Therapy
College of Health Professions, Mercer University
Atlanta, Georgia

Corine S. Cicchetti, MD
Board-Certified in Physical Medicine and Rehabilitation
Buffalo Spine and Sports Medicine, PLLC
Buffalo, New York

Derek Clewley, PT, DPT, PhD
Board-Certified Clinical Specialist in Orthopaedic Physical Therapists
Fellow of the American Academy of Orthopaedic Manual Physical Therapists
Assistant Professor
Doctor of Physical Therapy Division, Duke University School of Medicine
Durham, NC

N. Beth Collier, PT, DPT
Board-Certified Clinical Specialist in Orthopaedic Physical Therapy
Fellow of the American Academy of Orthopaedic Manual Physical Therapists
Clinical Assistant Professor
Department of Physical Therapy
College of Health Professions, Mercer University
Atlanta, Georgia

Carol A. Courtney, PT, PhD, ATC
Fellow of the American Academy of Orthopaedic Manual Physical Therapists
Professor
Department of Physical Therapy
Department of Rehabilitation Sciences
College of Applied Health Sciences, University of Illinois at Chicago
Chicago, Illinois

Ana I. de-la-Llave-Rincón, PT, MSc, PhD
Department of Physiotherapy, Occupational Therapy, Rehabilitation, and Physical Medicine
Cátedra de Investigación y Docencia en Fisioterapia: Terapia Manual y Punción Seca
Universidad Rey Juan Carlos
Alcorcón, Madrid, Spain

Jan Dommerholt, PT, DPT, MPS, DAAPM
President
Myopain Seminars
President and Owner
Bethesda Physiocare
Bethesda, Maryland

Thomas Eberle, PT, DPT
Fellow of the American Academy of Orthopaedic Manual Physical Therapists
Director, Florida Physical Therapy Association
Assistant Professor
University of St. Augustine for Health Sciences
Miami, Florida

Jeffrey Gervais Ebert, PT, DPT
Board-Certified Clinical Specialist in Orthopaedic Physical Therapy
Clinical Assistant Professor
Department of Physical Therapy
College of Health Professions, Mercer University
Atlanta, Georgia

Seth Jason Fibraio, PT, DPT, MTC, CSCS
Certified Cervical and Temporomandibular Therapist
Owner/Chief Executive Officer
Cornerstone Physical Therapy, Inc
Asheville, North Carolina

Timothy Flynn, PT, PhD
Board-Certified Clinical Specialist in Orthopaedic Physical Therapy
Fellow of the American Academy of Orthopaedic Manual Physical Therapists
Fellow of the American Physical Therapy Association
Owner, Colorado in Motion
Principle, Evidence in Motion
Professor, Doctor of Physical Therapy Program, South College, Nashville, TN

Lynne M. Fries, PA-C, MPAS, DPT
Doctor of Physical Therapy
Physician Assistant
UBMD Internal Medicine
Buffalo Spine and Sports Medicine, PLLC
Buffalo, New York

Stella Fuensalida-Novo, PT, MSc
Department of Physiotherapy, Occupational Therapy, Rehabilitation, and Physical Medicine
Cátedra de Investigación y Docencia en Fisioterapia: Terapia Manual y Punción Seca
Universidad Rey Juan Carlos
Alcorcón, Madrid, Spain

Margaret M. Gebhardt, PT, DPT
Board-Certified Clinical Specialist in Orthopaedic Physical Therapy
Fellow of the American Academy of Orthopaedic Manual Physical Therapists
Fit Core Physical Therapy
Adjunct Clinical Assistant Professor
Department of Physical Therapy
College of Health Professions, Mercer University
Lab Instructor
Myopain Seminars
Atlanta, Georgia

Kathleen Geist, PT, DPT
Board-Certified Clinical Specialist in Orthopaedic Physical Therapists
Fellow of the American Academy of Orthopaedic Manual Physical Therapists
Assistant Professor
Department of Rehabilitation Medicine
Emory University School of Medicine
Atlanta, Georgia

Robert D. Gerwin, MD, FAAN
Associate Professor of Neurology
School of Medicine, Johns Hopkins University
Baltimore, Maryland

Enrique Lluch Girbés, PT, PhD
Associate Professor
Department of Physical Therapy
Faculty of Physiotherapy
University of Valencia, Valencia, Spain

Laura Gold, PT, DPT
Board-Certified Clinical Specialist in Orthopaedic Physical Therapy
Adjunct Clinical Assistant Professor
Department of Physical Therapy
College of Health Professions, Mercer University
Atlanta, Georgia

Blake A. Hampton, PT, DPT, CSCS
Owner/Chief Executive Officer
Practical Pain Solutions, LLC
Adjunct Faculty
Department of Physical Therapy
College of Health Professions, Mercer University
Atlanta, Georgia

Dhinu J. Jayaseelan, DPT
Board-Certified Clinical Specialist in Orthopaedic Physical Therapy
Fellow of the American Academy of Orthopaedic Manual Physical Therapists
Assistant Professor
Program in Physical Therapy, School of Medicine and Health Sciences, The George Washington University
Washington, District of Columbia

Michael Karegeannes, PT, MHSc, LAT, MTC
Certified Cranio-Facial Specialty
Certified Cervical and Temporomandibular Therapist
Owner, Freedom Physical Therapy Services, S.C.
Fox Point, Wisconsin

Visnja King, PT, DPT, MTC, CSCS
Board-Certified Clinical Specialist in Orthopaedic Physical Therapy
Research Physical Therapist and Adjunct Instructor–Musculoskeletal Curriculum
Department of Physical Therapy
University of Pittsburgh
Pittsburgh, Pennsylvania
Owner/President/Clinical Director
King Physical Therapy North Huntingdon
North Huntingdon, Pennsylvania

Savas Koutsantonis, PT, DPT
One on One Physical Therapy
Series Instructor
Myopain Seminars
Atlanta, Georgia

Joshua J. Lee, PT, DPT
Orthopaedic Physical Therapy Resident
Department of Physical Therapy
College of Health Professions, Mercer University
Atlanta, Georgia

Ann M. Lucado, PT, PhD, CHT
Board-Certified Hand Therapist
Associate Professor
Department of Physical Therapy
College of Health Professions, Mercer University
Atlanta, Georgia

Sophia Maines, PT, DPT, CSCS
Board-Certified Clinical Specialist in Orthopaedic Physical Therapy
Owner, Sun Physical Therapy
Austin, Texas

Orlando Mayoral del Moral, PT, PhD
Physical Therapist
Hospital Provincial de Toledo
Academic Director
Seminarios Travell y Simons
Toledo, Spain

Johnson McEvoy, BSc, MSc, DPT, MISCP, PT
Chartered Physiotherapist
United Physiotherapy Clinic
Limerick, Ireland
David G Simons Academy
Winterthur, Switzerland
Myopain Seminars
Bethesda, Maryland

Timothy J. McMahon, PT, DPT
Board-Certified Clinical Specialist in Orthopaedic Physical Therapy
Fellow of the American Academy of Orthopaedic Manual Physical Therapists
Clinical Assistant Professor and Director, Mercer Physical Therapy Clinic
Department of Physical Therapy
College of Health Professions, Mercer University
Atlanta, Georgia

Carolyn McMakin, MA, DC
Fibromyalgia and Myofascial Pain Clinic of Portland
Portland, Oregon

Óscar Sánchez Méndez, PT, MSc
Physical Therapist and Professor
Seminarios Travell y Simons
Madrid, Spain

Amir Minerbi, MD, PhD
Board-Certified in Pain Medicine and Family Medicine
Institute for Pain Medicine, Rambam Health Care Campus
Bruce Rappaport Faculty of Medicine, Technion
Haifa, Israel
Department of Family Medicine, Clalit Health Services
Haifa and Western Galilee District, Israel

Jennifer Marie Nelson, PT, DPT, DScPT
Fellow of the American Academy of Orthopaedic Manual Physical Therapists
Myopain Seminars
PhysioPartners
Chicago, Illinois

Ricardo Ortega-Santiago, PT, MSc, PhD
Department of Physiotherapy, Occupational Therapy, Rehabilitation, and Physical Medicine
Cátedra de Investigación y Docencia en Fisioterapia: Terapia Manual y Punción Seca, Universidad Rey Juan Carlos
Alcorcón, Madrid, Spain

María Palacios-Ceña, PT, MSc, PhD
Department of Physiotherapy, Occupational Therapy, Rehabilitation, and Physical Medicine
Cátedra de Investigación y Docencia en Fisioterapia: Terapia Manual y Punción Seca
Universidad Rey Juan Carlos
Alcorcón, Madrid, Spain

Leigh E. Palubinskas, PT, DPT
Board-Certified Clinical Specialist in Orthopaedic Physical Therapy
Performance Physical Therapy
Stockbridge, Georgia

Gustavo Plaza-Manzano, PT, PhD
Department of Radiology, Rehabilitation and Physiotherapy
Universidad Complutense de Madrid
Instituto de Investigación Sanitaria del Hospital Clínico San Carlos
Madrid, Spain

Ryan Reed, PT, DPT
Board-Certified Clinical Specialist in Orthopaedic Physical Therapy
Fellow of the American Academy of Orthopaedic Manual Physical Therapists
Instructor, DPT Program
University of St. Augustine for Health Sciences
Miami, Florida

Susan H. Rightnour, PT, MTC
Certified Cranio-Facial Specialty
NovaCare Rehabilitation
Bowie, Maryland

Jaime Salom-Moreno, PT, PhD
Department of Physiotherapy, Occupational Therapy, Rehabilitation, and Physical Medicine
Cátedra de Investigación y Docencia en Fisioterapia: Terapia Manual y Punción Seca
Universidad Rey Juan Carlos
Alcorcón, Madrid, Spain

Isabel Salvat, PT, PhD
Full Professor
Department of Medicine and Surgery, Faculty of Medicine and Health Sciences
Rovira i Virgili University
Reus, Spain

Timothy Douglas Sawyer, BSPT
National Center for Pelvic Pain
Pelvic Pain Technologies
Stanford Urology Research Team
Owner, Sawyer Physical Therapy
Los Gatos, California

John Sharkey, MSc
Clinical Anatomist (BACA), Exercise Physiologist (BASES)
Senior Lecturer
Medicine, Dentistry and Life Sciences
University of Chester/National Training Centre
Dublin, Ireland

Gabriel Somarriba, PT, DPT
Assistant Professor
Assistant Program Director
Campus Director
University of St. Augustine for Health Sciences
Miami, Florida

Leslie F. Taylor, PT, PhD, MS
Associate Dean and Professor
Department of Physical Therapy
College of Health Professions, Mercer University
Atlanta, Georgia

Paul Thomas, PT, DPT
Board-Certified Clinical Specialist in Orthopaedic Physical Therapy
Fellow of the American Academy of Orthopaedic Manual Physical Therapists
Impact Physical Therapy
Chicago, Illinois

María Torres-Lacomba, PT, PhD
Full Professor
Head of the "Physiotherapy in Women's Health Research Group"
Physical Therapy Department
University of Alcalá
Alcalá de Henares, Madrid, Spain

Derek L. Vraa, PT, DPT, CSCS
Board-Certified Clinical Specialist in Orthopaedic Physical Therapy
Fellow of the American Academy of Orthopaedic Manual Physical Therapists
Senior Faculty, United States Air Force Tactical Sports and Orthopaedic Manual Physical Therapy Fellowship Program
United States Air Force Academy
Colorado Springs, Colorado

Matthew Vraa, PT, DPT, MBA
Board-Certified Clinical Specialist in Orthopaedic Physical Therapy
Fellow of the American Academy of Orthopaedic Manual Physical Therapists
Program Director
Physical Therapist Assistant Department
Rasmussen College
Brooklyn Park/Maple Grove, Minnesota
Physical Therapist, Orthology, Inc
Maple Grove, Minnesota

Simon Vulfsons, MD
Board-Certified Specialist in Internal Medicine
Board-Certified Specialist in Pain Medicine
President, The International Federation of Musculoskeletal Medicine
Director, The Institute for Pain Medicine and the Rambam School for Pain Medicine
Rambam Health Care Campus, the Bruce Rappaport Faculty of Medicine
Technion–Israel Institute for Technology
Haifa, Israel

Wesley J. Wedewer, PT, DPT, CSCS
Board-Certified Clinical Specialist in Orthopaedic Physical Therapy
Board-Certified Clinical Specialist in Sports Physical Therapy
Fellow of the American Academy of Orthopaedic Manual Physical Therapists
Athletico Physical Therapy
Chicago, Illinois

Deborah M. Wendland, PT, DPT, PhD, CPed
Associate Professor
Department of Physical Therapy
College of Health Professions, Mercer University
Atlanta, Georgia

Brian Yee, PT, DPT, MPhty
Board-Certified Clinical Specialist in Orthopaedic Physical Therapy
Fellow of the American Academy of Orthopaedic Manual Physical Therapists
Owner, Motion Stability Physical Therapy Group
Adjunct Clinical Assistant Professor
Department of Physical Therapy
College of Health Professions, Mercer University
Atlanta, Georgia

Foreword

The publication of Travell & Simons' first volume of *Myofascial Pain and Dysfunction: The Trigger Point Manual*, in 1982, followed 10 years later by the second volume, and in 1999 the second edition of volume one, created a revolution in the understanding and management of musculoskeletal pain, but also caused an eruption of critical comments of volcanic proportions. The revolution amounted to a new way of looking at musculoskeletal pain via the concept of the myofascial trigger point, a concept introduced and expanded upon over the preceding three decades by Dr Janet G. Travell, later joined by Dr David G. Simons, but never before presented in a comprehensive text. Travell's unique insight that was detailed in the first volume was the appreciation that muscle pain could present as pain referred to a distant site. Referred pain, now known to be mediated through the central nervous system and associated with visceral organs and joints as well as with muscle, was neither well understood at the time nor widely accepted. Moreover, Dr Travell identified the myofascial trigger point as the cause of local pain in muscle and the cause of pain referred to distant sites. She identified the trigger point on physical examination by manual palpation. There was no objective way to identify the trigger point by laboratory test, for example, by imaging or by electrodiagnostic examination. The idea that pain could be referred from one place to another was ridiculed at national medical meetings and dismissed as fantastical thinking. The storm that Travell created was largely due to the inability of the mainstream medical profession to understand the concept of referred pain from muscle, coupled with an inability to examine muscle as carefully and as well as she could. Lacking in the texts by Travell and Simons, however, was a critical, evidence-based approach to the descriptions of trigger point pain and their referred pain patterns. Dr Travell's description of referred pain patterns was based on decades of meticulous record-keeping of patient's reports and the drawings that Dr Travell made of her patient's descriptions of their pain, but all of her descriptions were qualitative, not quantitative. Neither was the science of pain medicine advanced enough to understand referred pain. The pathophysiology of peripheral and central pain mechanisms had barely begun to be revealed by the time the single volume of the second edition appeared in 1999, and objective markers of the myofascial trigger point were only starting to appear, most notably an electrophysiologic change in the muscle of the trigger point that is now called endplate noise. Even that was controversial for decades, claimed by many to be nothing more than normal endplate electrical activity. Despite these shortcomings, the texts by Travell and Simons were eagerly read by those who treated musculoskeletal pain. With the passage of time, and more knowledge of the pathophysiology of muscle pain, the texts achieved an iconic status.

Almost 20 years have passed since the publication of the last edition of *Myofascial Pain and Dysfunction: The Trigger Point Manual, 2nd edition*, and medicine has advanced and changed greatly since then. Much more is known about the development of pain, about peripheral and central sensitization as it applies to muscle, with major contributions by Siegfried Mense and his colleagues, and central pain modulation is now an accepted phenomenon, thanks to the work of David Yarnitsky and others. Nociception is now understood to be a complex matter involving integration of multimodal sensory input, interconnectedness of cerebral centers, and functional coordination with the motor system. Furthermore, much more is known about myofascial trigger point anatomy and physiology through the studies using microdialysis analysis of the trigger point milieu performed at the National Institutes of Health by Jay Shah and his associates, the ultrasound appearance of the trigger point that has been detailed by Sikdar and his colleagues in Northern Virginia, and the work done by Hubbard and his associates, and Hong and his colleagues on the electrodiagnostic features of the trigger point. The importance of fascia in pain of myofascial origin is undergoing its own revolution. Knowledge of fascial anatomy and physiology is rapidly increasing, though how fascia and muscle interact to produce pain is still not well explicated. In addition, and most importantly, medicine has moved progressively toward an evidence-based, scientifically supported, practice, rather than so much an art that we used to emphasize, although this is not to denigrate the role of history and physical examination in defining a patient's pain problem. There is still a need for an educated, intuitive evaluation of the patient that we call the art of medicine, both in diagnosis and in treatment. It is at this time of great change and expansion of knowledge that this new edition of *Myofascial Pain and Dysfunction: The Trigger Point Manual* appears.

The present volume, the third edition of Simons, Travell, and Simons' text, brings the previous editions of this popular resource up to date. It is an evidence-based text where evidence is available. The references to muscle function and anatomy are updated. The initial chapters in the text are a general introduction to myofascial pain, written by Jan Dommerholt, who is both clinically well acquainted with myofascial pain syndromes and extremely well versed in the current literature, having authored regular reviews of the literature in this field for over a decade. Dommerholt provides the background of pain science, reviews what is currently known about the trigger point, and provides the basis for a proper understanding of the later chapters that detail diagnosis and treatment of particular muscle trigger points and of regional trigger point syndromes. He has also introduced for the first time in this text a detailed discussion of the anatomy and of the role of the fascia in myofascial pain. Of great importance is that the treatment modalities used in the management of myofascial pain that are described in the text, most importantly the technique of dry needling, are supported by the citation of randomized, controlled trials and by systematic reviews and meta-analyses. Gone are the detailed instructions of spray and stretch in favor of dry needling as a treatment of trigger points. In keeping with David Simons' inquisitive mind and drive to understand what underlies myofascial trigger points, a chapter is included that expands on Simons' Integrated Hypothesis of the Trigger Point and presents new and novel hypotheses about the origin of the trigger point, but based on firm evidence of trigger point characteristics. Likewise, a chapter on perpetuating factors is included in recognition of treatment of a trigger point as being the beginning of management of myofascial pain syndromes, not the end. The chapter on perpetuating factors includes material that was not included in previous editions, such as gonadal hormone and sex effects on pain, and integrated postural considerations involving motor control.

The text has, of necessity, many contributing authors. In this respect, it differs greatly from the first two editions, which spoke in the unique voices of Janet G. Travell and David G. Simons, with only six additional contributors in the second edition. In the previous editions, one can hear Travell's admonitions and gems regarding the patient's history that truly expressed the art of medicine, while Simons' voice was grounded meticulously in the scientific literature. This volume, written by many authors, maintains a consistent approach as each chapter about a specific muscle follows a similar format that includes anatomy, function, pain presentation, referred pain patterns, and perpetuating factors and conditions that are specific to a given muscle. The detailed reviews of the literature regarding these topics is left to the previous volumes, perhaps out of the recognition that a single volume of 77 chapters would otherwise become too unwieldy. The presence of many contributors means that each chapter reflects the interest and voice of the author(s) of that chapter. The chapters by César Fernández de las Peñas and Orlando Mayoral del Moral are models of detailed and well-documented discussions of their subjects, for example, which is not to say that others do not also achieve their level of distinction. The editors and publishers have elected to keep the illustrations made by Barbara Cummings from the previous editions, a wise choice as they were made in close consultation with David G. Simons, who went to the anatomy laboratory in order to ensure accuracy in the illustrations. These illustrations are unequaled in their clarity and usefulness. Moreover, the X's that Travell and Simons added, to signify the major sites in each muscle where trigger points can be found, have been removed from the figures in recognition of the fact that trigger points can be found elsewhere in the muscle, and the muscle must be systematically examined. It must be said, however, in recognition of the need to keep this volume to a usable size and affordable cost, that the previous editions of this text should be kept on the shelf as a reference for the greater detail of description that the previous format permitted, as well as for the unique voice of its authors, which is not found in this edition.

Finally, recognition and thanks must be given to Joseph M. Donnelly, who gamely undertook this rather daunting project. David G. Simons had planned to edit a third edition himself, but was unable to do so during his lifetime. Donnelly accepted the arduous work of assembling a team of associate editors and a stable of writers, wringing the chapters out of them, writing chapters himself, shepherding the project with all of the delays, procrastination, and frustrations associated with such a project, and doing so for the first time in his career. This project has been an arduous task, one that I hope will be recognized as a labor of love, for the welfare of all of our patients everywhere, but most importantly for the love of David G. Simons, a man who taught us, cajoled us, nursed us, urged us to think clearly, and who was indeed responsible for getting the first two editions published. It is truly in gratitude to David G. Simons, and to Janet G. Travell, that Joe Donnelly and all of us associated with this project have worked together to produce this text, which we hope will serve as an indispensable guide for the next generation of myofascial pain practitioners.

Robert D. Gerwin, MD, FAAN

Preface

This third edition of *The Trigger Point Manual* is presented at a time of exponential growth of knowledge, rapid advancements in technology, immediate access to information, and constant change. As each professional is required to learn more and more to practice in smaller and smaller specialties, we can only cope by collaborating with others whose expertise lies in adjacent fields of knowledge. This new edition of *The Trigger Point Manual* has evolved to meet the needs of this environment. Dr Janet G. Travell authored Volume I of the first edition of *The Trigger Point Manual*, which David G. Simons wrote for and with her. In turn, informed by his Veteran's Administration clinical experience, he authored and wrote practically all of Volume II with significant help from Lois S. Simons. The second edition of Volume I was truly coauthored by David G. Simons and Lois S. Simons with significant help from clinicians in multiple disciplines. This third edition is the combined effort of many more people, each representing expertise in one or more of the many aspects of myofascial pain and trigger points (TrPs).

This third edition of *The Trigger Point Manual* is a transitional work. It continues the discussion of the TrP conceptual model that took form out of a syndrome of unknown etiology and then evolved into an experimentally established neurophysiologic disease entity. Improvements in technology have enabled the empirical identification of signs of myofascial pain and dysfunction, including electrophysiologic markers formerly known as "endplate noise," which was first established by David G. Simons; histopathophysiologic markers such as contractures of sarcomeres; and histochemical changes such as decreased pH and elevated levels of neuropeptides and cytokines. There have been significant scientific advancements in regard to TrPs and myofascial pain since the second edition of Volume I was published in 1999; however, many important details remain to be resolved in regard to the TrP conceptual model. This third edition aims to be not the final answer to the questions that remain regarding myofascial dysfunction and TrPs, but, instead, like the seminal works that preceded it, another touchstone to mark a new era of discovery.

CHANGES IN THIS EDITION

In alignment with the vision of David G. Simons and Lois S. Simons, the third edition of *The Trigger Point Manual* evolved from a two-volume reference text written mainly by two individuals to a singular volume written by numerous individuals with clinical expertise in the examination and treatment of myofascial pain and dysfunction. This is a multidisciplinary effort aimed at presenting the depth and breadth of TrPs and myofascial pain concepts. This edition presents the major progress made in our understanding of the pathophysiologic basis for many of the clinical phenomena associated with TrPs, including the role of muscle pain and TrPs in peripheral nociceptive drive to the central nervous system, as well as the role that TrPs play in perpetuating peripheral and/or central sensitization. This text is an evidence-informed review based on clinical and scientific research.

The book is organized into eight sections. The first section introduces the TrP conceptual model and general concepts related to pain and myofascial dysfunction. Psychosocial considerations in myofascial pain syndrome and chronic pain are discussed in Chapter 5 of the first section of the book. Each muscle or muscle group is considered in Sections 2 to 7. A major change to these sections was the merging of the lower torso pain section from Volume II with the upper torso pain section from Volume I to create a new section called "Trunk and Pelvic Pain." Other changes include merging of the pectineus muscle chapter into the chapter that addresses the adductor muscle group, pulling the tensor fasciae latae muscle into the gluteus minimus muscle chapter, adding the sartorius muscles to the quadriceps muscle group chapter, and combining the superficial and deep foot intrinsic muscle chapters to better reflect current anatomical organizational concepts of the foot. Also new in Sections 2 to 7 is a Clinical Considerations chapter for each section that discusses myofascial factors relevant to common neuromusculoskeletal and medical conditions of each region from a holistic perspective. Section 8 of the book presents a comprehensive summary of treatment options for muscle dysfunction and TrPs. Deviating from the previous editions' redundant and cumbersome treatment discussions placed within each muscle chapter, this edition gives an overview of each treatment option that can be applied to any muscle in the body with TrPs or in patients presenting with myofascial pain syndrome. The treatment section includes chapters on injection/dry needling, manual therapy, therapeutic exercise, therapeutic modalities, and postural and footwear considerations.

Each of the muscle chapters in Sections 2 to 7 is consistently organized throughout the book with the following sections and subsections: Introduction; Anatomical Considerations, which includes Innervation and Vascularization, Function, and the Functional Unit; Clinical Considerations, which includes Referred Pain Pattern, Symptoms, Patient Examination, and Trigger Point Examination; Differential Diagnosis, including Activation and Perpetuation of Trigger Points, Associated Trigger Points, and Associated Pathology; and Corrective Actions. This new layout includes both clinician-centric and patient-friendly additions as well as a streamlined look for ease of use.

Several new features within the new organizational layout merit note. The introduction of each chapter serves as an overview of all the sections that follow it as an abstract does for the journal articles that have become the staple of research consumption. Vascularization, which was previously omitted, has been included in the anatomical section along with innervation. The new tabular format of the functional unit allows for easier clinical application with additional functional relationships noted in the text below the functional unit boxes. The corrective actions section is written in patient-friendly language and gives the layperson simple self-treatment techniques, as well as signs that warrant seeking professional guidance.

Some changes are reflected in the above organizational theme, but owing to their substantive nature, require further explanation. One such change is replacement of the terms "satellite" and "secondary" TrPs with "associated" TrP (discussed in each muscle chapter in the Differential Diagnosis section, under the subsection titled "Associated Trigger Points") to more accurately describe pathophysiologic relationships between TrPs. To enhance this edition's focus on muscle dysfunction and TrPs, discussions of articular dysfunctions, postural deviations, bony alignment issues, and other related musculoskeletal concerns that were lengthy in the previous editions have been truncated. With widespread availability of and access to comprehensive resources on the examination and treatment of articular dysfunctions and the like, clinicians are encouraged to seek out other texts for more information on those topics.

Trigger point palpation techniques for each muscle, as well as some examination techniques and special tests, are presented with new full-color digital photographs to give the entire text a more modern feel, while the classic anatomy and pain pattern illustrations have been preserved and updated. Lastly, and of special importance, this edition eliminates the "X's" from the illustrations of referred symptom (pain) patterns. Current evidence supports the need to examine the entire muscle for the presence of a taut band, spot tenderness, and referred symptoms (pain) in order to diagnose the presence of TrPs. It is also known that these referred symptom illustrations are guidelines and that any portion of the muscle can create all or part of the featured referred symptom (pain) patterns.

The third edition of *The Trigger Point Manual* is a testament to the groundbreaking work of Janet G. Travell, David G. Simons, and Lois S. Simons in the realm of TrPs and myofascial pain. This comprehensive *Trigger Point Manual* was designed and written with the patients we serve at the forefront of every decision. The intent of this edition of *The Trigger Point Manual* is to facilitate practice, support education, and inspire clinical and scientific research in the area of TrPs, myofascial pain, and other musculoskeletal syndromal diagnoses. This *Trigger Point Manual* is also designed to assist clinicians with clinical decision making and with the management of patients and individuals presenting with painful and nonpainful conditions resulting in activity limitations and participation restrictions.

Acknowledgments

The editors would like to thank all of the contributing authors of this third edition of *The Trigger Point Manual*. This book was a massive project and could not have been completed without their passion, dedication, and commitment. We appreciate the time they took out of their busy clinical, teaching, and research schedules, and we are indebted to these individuals for sharing their expertise in the area of TrPs and myofascial pain. Special thanks to Jan Dommerholt for his significant clinical and research contributions in the area of TrPs and myofascial pain syndrome. His vast knowledge of the scientific and clinical evidence is apparent in his evidence-informed review in Section 1. Thanks also to John Lyftogt, MD for his input on use of dextrose in the treatment of myofascial pain and to Blair Green, PT for her contribution to the pelvic floor section of the trigger point injection (TrPI) and dry needling (DN) material. Lastly, many thanks to Shantel Phillips, PT for helping confirm postural deviations for Chapter 76.

This book represents years of planning and dedicated effort, and it could not have been finished without the assistance of Sharon Barker and Samantha Pierce. Their rich historical perspective and administrative experience from working with David G. Simons, MD and Lois S. Simons PT was pivotal in achieving the goals of this new edition.

We also want to thank Susan and Norris Ganstrom and the Simons family for their support and encouragement to finish the work their father had set out to accomplish prior to his passing. Thanks to Carolyn McMakin, DC who had the foresight to push the initiative forward with the publisher and wisdom to keep the ball rolling so the project would finally be set in motion.

We would like to thank Christynne Helfrich, PT for her willingness to be our photographer for the entire project. Her clinical expertise and her optimistic perspective made photo shoots seamless and enjoyable. To all the Mercer University Doctor of Physical Therapy students (and their loved ones) who modeled for the photo shoots on Saturdays, we thank you for your enthusiasm and patience. Additionally, we would like to thank Cody Klein, Taylor Smith, Tom Christ, and Rebecca Goldberg, our graduate research assistants, who performed countless literature searches and organizational tasks, always with a smile.

The Editor in Chief, Joseph M. Donnelly, would like to personally thank Leslie F. Taylor, PT, PhD, Associate Dean at Mercer University, for her unwavering support and contributions to the third edition of *The Trigger Point Manual*. I also want to thank my faculty colleagues and staff for their support and encouragement over the past four years. Without their commitment and dedication to teaching and scholarship, this project would never have been completed.

Finally, we would like to acknowledge the support of our respective families and friends. We thank them for their continued support of our professional endeavors and owe them an incalculable debt of gratitude. May this book be a valuable resource for clinicians and patients, worthy of their sacrifice.

Contents

Foreword ix
Preface xi
Acknowledgments xiii
Pain Pattern Quick Reference Guide xvi

Section 1 Introduction to Myofascial Pain and Dysfunction

1. Pain Sciences and Myofascial Pain — 2
2. Trigger Point Neurophysiology — 29
3. The Role of Muscles and Fascia in Myofascial Pain Syndrome — 44
4. Perpetuating Factors for Myofascial Pain Syndrome — 55
5. Psychosocial Considerations — 67

Section 2 Head and Neck Pain

6. Trapezius Muscle — 80
7. Sternocleidomastoid Muscle — 94
8. Masseter Muscle — 103
9. Temporalis Muscle — 113
10. Medial Pterygoid Muscle — 120
11. Lateral Pterygoid Muscle — 127
12. Digastric Muscle and Anterior Neck Muscles — 135
13. Cutaneous I: Facial Muscles — 148
14. Cutaneous II: Occipitofrontalis — 156
15. Splenius Capitis and Splenius Cervicis Muscles — 161
16. Posterior Cervical Muscles: Semispinalis Capitis, Longissimus Capitis, Semispinalis Cervicis, Multifidus, and Rotatores — 168
17. Suboccipital Muscles — 178
18. Clinical Considerations of Head and Neck Pain — 187

Section 3 Upper Back, Shoulder, and Arm Pain

19. Levator Scapulae Muscle — 199
20. Scalene Muscles — 208
21. Supraspinatus Muscle — 222
22. Infraspinatus Muscle — 231
23. Teres Minor Muscle — 241
24. Latissimus Dorsi Muscle — 247
25. Teres Major Muscle — 254
26. Subscapularis Muscle — 259
27. Rhomboid Minor and Major Muscles — 268
28. Deltoid Muscle — 276
29. Coracobrachialis Muscle — 285
30. Biceps Brachii Muscle — 292
31. Brachialis Muscle — 301
32. Triceps Brachii and Anconeus Muscles — 306
33. Clinical Considerations of Upper Back Shoulder and Arm Pain — 318

Section 4 Forearm, Wrist, and Hand Pain

34. Wrist Extensor and Brachioradialis Muscles — 329
35. Extensor Digitorum and Extensor Indicis Muscles — 343
36. Supinator Muscle — 352
37. Palmaris Longus Muscle — 360
38. Wrist and Finger Flexors in the Forearm — 366
39. Adductor and Opponens Pollicis Muscles — 378
40. Interosseous, Lumbrical, and Abductor Digiti Minimi Muscles — 386
41. Clinical Considerations of Elbow, Wrist, and Hand Pain — 395

Section 5 Trunk and Pelvis Pain

42. Pectoralis Major and Subclavius Muscles — 407
43. Sternalis Muscle — 421
44. Pectoralis Minor Muscle — 426
45. Intercostal and Diaphragm Muscles — 435
46. Serratus Anterior Muscle — 453
47. Serratus Posterior Superior and Inferior Muscles — 460
48. Thoracolumbar Paraspinal Muscles — 469
49. Abdominal Muscles — 483
50. Quadratus Lumborum Muscle — 497
51. Psoas Major, Psoas Minor, and Iliacus Muscles — 513
52. Pelvic Floor Muscles — 523
53. Clinical Considerations of Trunk and Pelvic Pain — 540

Section 6 Hip, Thigh, and Knee Pain

54. Gluteus Maximus Muscle — 554
55. Gluteus Medius Muscle — 566

56	Gluteus Minimus and Tensor Fasciae Latae Muscles	577
57	Piriformis, Obturator Internus, Gemelli, Obturator Externus, and Quadratus Femoris Muscles	589
58	Quadriceps Femoris and Sartorius Muscles	604
59	Adductor Longus, Adductor Brevis, Adductor Magnus, Pectineus, and Gracilis Muscles	621
60	Hamstring Muscles	635
61	Popliteus Muscle	647
62	Clinical Considerations of Hip, Thigh, and Knee Pain	655

Section 7 Leg, Ankle, and Foot Pain

63	Tibialis Anterior Muscle	666
64	Fibularis Longus, Brevis, and Tertius Muscles	674
65	Gastrocnemius Muscle	687
66	Soleus and Plantaris Muscles	697
67	Tibialis Posterior Muscle	709
68	Long Toe Extensor Muscles	718
69	Long Toe Flexor Muscles	726
70	Intrinsic Muscles of the Foot	734
71	Clinical Considerations of Leg, Ankle, and Foot Pain	748

Section 8 Treatment Considerations for Myofascial Pain and Dysfunction

72	Trigger Point Injection and Dry Needling	757
73	Manual Therapy Considerations	833
74	Therapeutic Exercise Considerations	843
75	Therapeutic Modality Considerations	850
76	Postural Considerations	867
77	Footwear Considerations	891

Index   897

Section 2 | Head and Neck Pain

Pain Pattern Quick Reference Guide

Forehead Pain
- Sternocleidomastoid (clavicular) (7)
- Sternocleidomastoid (sternal) (7)
- Semispinalis capitis (16)
- Frontalis (14)
- Zygomaticus major (13)

Eye and Eyebrow Pain
- Sternocleidomastoid (sternal) (7)
- Temporalis (9)
- Splenius cervicis (15)
- Masseter (superficial) (8)
- Suboccipital group (17)
- Occipitalis (14)
- Orbicularis oculi (13)
- Trapezius (6)

Teeth Pain
- Temporalis (9)
- Masseter (superficial) (8)
- Digastric (anterior) (12)

Cheek and Jaw Pain
- Sternocleidomastoid (sternal) (7)
- Masseter (superficial) (8)
- Lateral pterygoid (11)
- Trapezius (6)
- Masseter (deep) (8)
- Digastric (12)
- Medial pterygoid (10)
- Buccinator (13)
- Platysma (13)
- Orbicularis oculi (13)
- Zygomaticus major (13)

Ear and TMJ Pain
- Lateral pterygoid (11)
- Masseter (deep) (8)
- Sternocleidomastoid (clavicular) (7)
- Medial pterygoid (10)

Top of Head Pain
- Sternocleidomastoid (sternal) (7)
- Splenius capitis (15)

Side of Head Pain
- Trapezius (6)
- Sternocleidomastoid (sternal) (7)
- Temporalis (9)
- Splenius cervicis (15)
- Suboccipital group (17)
- Semispinalis capitis (16)

Back of Head Pain
- Trapezius (6)
- Sternocleidomastoid (sternal) (7)
- Sternocleidomastoid (clavicular) (7)
- Semispinalis capitis (16)
- Semispinalis cervicis (16)
- Splenius cervicis (15)
- Suboccipital group (17)
- Occipitalis (14)
- Digastric (12)
- Temporalis (9)

Back of Neck Pain
- Trapezius (6)
- Cervical multifidi (16)
- Levator scapulae (19)
- Splenius cervicis (15)
- Infraspinatus (22)

Throat and Front of Neck Pain
- Sternocleidomastoid (sternal) (7)
- Digastric (12)
- Longus capitus and longus colli (12)
- Medial pterygoid (10)

Section 2 Head and Neck Pain

Trapezius
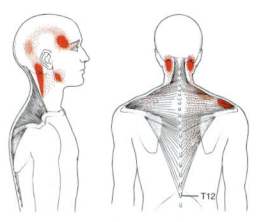

Sternocleidomastoid
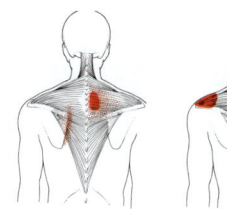

Sternal division   Clavicular division

Masseter
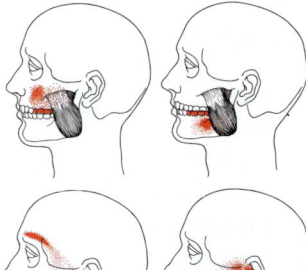

Temporalis
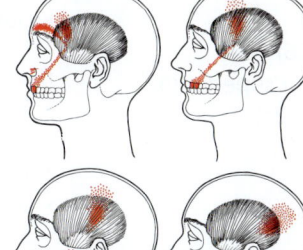

Medial pterygoid
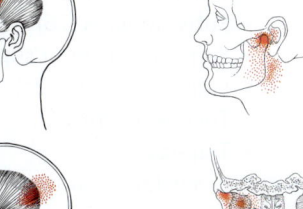

Lateral pterygoid
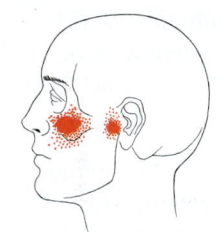

Digastric
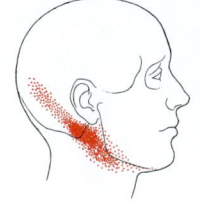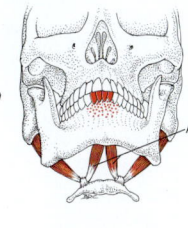

Posterior belly   Anterior belly

longus colli
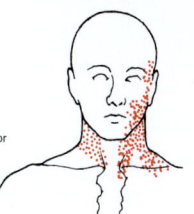

Buccinator
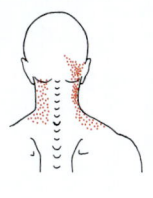

Occipitofrontalis
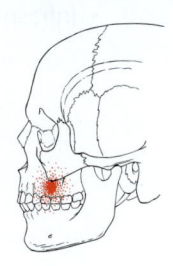

Splenius capitis and splenius cervicis
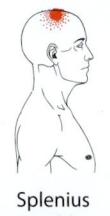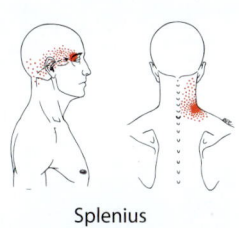

Splenius capitis   Splenius cervicis

Posterior cervical muscles
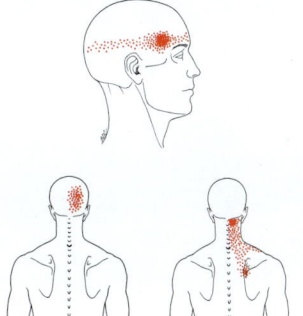

Suboccipital muscles
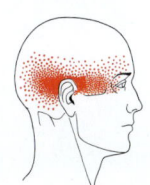

xvii

Section 3: Upper Back, Shoulder, and Arm Pain

Pain Pattern Quick Reference Guide

Upper Back Pain
- Scalene (20)
- Levator scapulae (19)
- Trapezius (6)
- Thoracic multifidi (48)
- Rhomboids (27)
- Splenius cervicis (15)
- Triceps brachii (32)
- Biceps brachii (30)

Front of Shoulder Pain
- Infraspinatus (22)
- Deltoid (anterior) (28)
- Scalene (20)
- Supraspinatus (21)
- Pectoralis major (42)
- Pectoralis minor (44)
- Biceps brachii (30)
- Coracobrachialis (29)
- Sternalis (43)
- Subclavius (42)
- Latissimus dorsi (24)

Back of Shoulder Pain
- Deltoid (posterior) (28)
- Levator scapulae (19)
- Scalene (20)
- Supraspinatus (21)
- Teres major (25)
- Teres minor (23)
- Subscapularis (26)
- Serratus posterior superior (47)
- Latissimus dorsi (24)
- Triceps brachii (32)
- Trapezius (6)
- Iliocostalis thoracis (48)

Outside of shoulder Pain
- Deltoid (middle) (28)
- Supraspinatus (21)
- Scalene (20)

Front of Arm Pain
- Scalene (20)
- Infraspinatus (22)

- Biceps brachii (30)
- Brachialis (31)
- Triceps brachii (32)
- Supraspinatus (21)
- Deltoid (28)
- Sternalis (43)
- Subclavius (42)

Back of Arm Pain
- Scalene (20)
- Triceps brachii (32)
- Deltoid (posterior) (28)
- Subscapularis (26)
- Supraspinatus (21)
- Teres major (25)
- Teres minor (23)
- Latissimus dorsi (24)
- Serratus posterior superior (47)
- Coracobrachialis (29)

Section 3 Upper Back, Shoulder, and Arm Pain

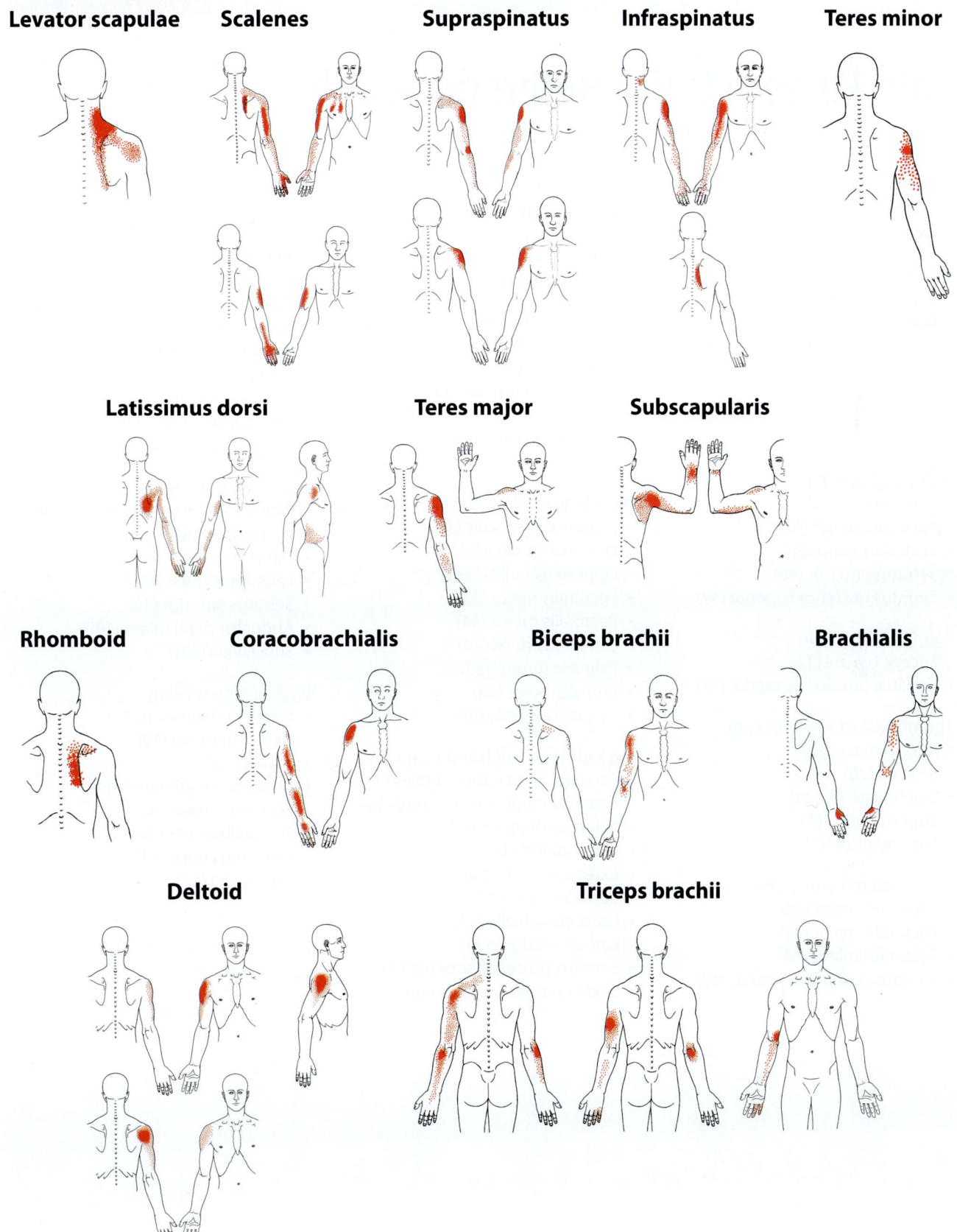

Section 4: Forearm, Wrist, and Hand Pain

Pain Pattern Quick Reference Guide

Front of Elbow Pain
- Brachialis (31)
- Biceps brachii (30)

Outside of Elbow Pain
- Supinator (36)
- Brachioradialis (34)
- Extensor carpi radialis longus (34)
- Triceps brachii (32)
- Supraspinatus (21)
- Fourth and fifth finger extensors (35)
- Anconeus (32)

Inside of Elbow Pain
- Triceps brachii (32)
- Pectoralis major (42)
- Pectoralis minor (44)
- Serratus anterior (46)
- Serratus posterior superior (47)

Point of Elbow Pain
- Triceps brachii (32)
- Serratus posterior superior (47)

Thumb side of Forearm Pain
- Infraspinatus (22)
- Scalene (20)
- Brachioradialis (34)
- Supraspinatus (21)
- Subclavius (42)

Pinky Side of Forearm Pain
- Latissimus dorsi (24)
- Pectoralis major (42)
- Pectoralis minor (44)
- Serratus posterior superior (47)

Palm side of Forearm Pain
- Palmaris longus (37)
- Pronator teres (38)
- Serratus anterior (46)
- Triceps brachii (32)

Back of Forearm Pain
- Triceps brachii (32)
- Teres major (25)
- Extensores carpi radialis longus and brevis (34)
- Coracobrachialis (29)
- Scalene (20)

Palm Side of Wrist and Hand Pain
- Flexor carpi radialis (38)
- Flexor carpi ulnaris (38)
- Opponens pollicis (39)
- Pectoralis major (42)
- Pectoralis minor (44)
- Latissimus dorsi (24)
- Palmaris longus (37)
- Pronator teres (38)
- Serratus anterior (46)

Back of Wrist and Hand Pain
- Extensor carpi radialis brevis (34)
- Extensor carpi radialis longus (34)
- Extensor digitorum (35)
- Extensor indicis (35)
- Extensor carpi ulnaris (34)
- Subscapularis (26)
- Coracobrachialis (29)
- Latissimus dorsi (24)
- Serratus posterior superior (47)
- First dorsal interosseus (40)

Thumb and Base of Thumb Pain
- Supinator (36)
- Scalene (20)
- Brachialis (31)
- Infraspinatus (22)
- Extensor carpi radialis longus (34)
- Brachioradialis (34)
- Opponens pollicis (39)
- Adductor pollicis (39)
- Subclavius (42)
- First dorsal interosseus (40)
- Flexor pollicis longus (38)

Palm Side of Fingers Pain
- Flexors digitorum superficialis and profundus (38)
- Hand interossei (40)
- Latissimus dorsi (24)
- Serratus anterior (46)
- Abductor digiti minimi (40)
- Subclavius (42)

Back of Fingers Pain
- Extensor digitorum (35)
- Hand interossei (40)
- Scalene (20)
- Abductor digiti minimi (40)
- Pectoralis major (42)
- Pectoralis minor (44)
- Latissimus dorsi (24)
- Subclavius (42)

Section 4 Forearm, Wrist, and Hand Pain

Extensor carpi ulnaris
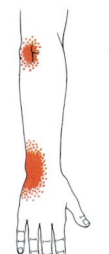

Extensor carpi radialis brevis
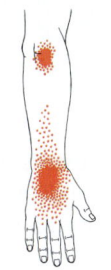

Extensor carpi radialis longus
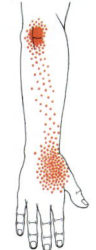

brachioradialis
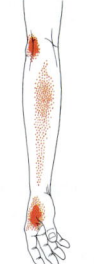

Extensor digitorum and indicis
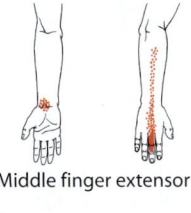
Middle finger extensor

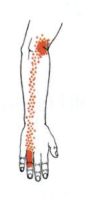
Ring finger extensor

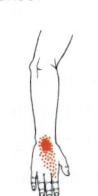
Extensor indicis

Supinator
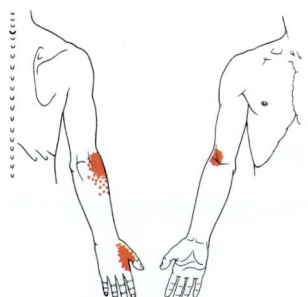

Palmaris Longus
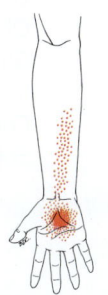

Flexor carpi radialis
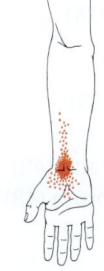

Flexor carpi ulnaris
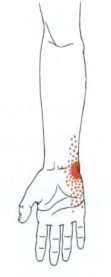

Flexor pollicis longus
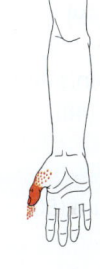

Pronator quadratus
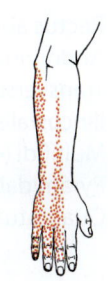

Flexor digitorum superficialis and profundus muscles
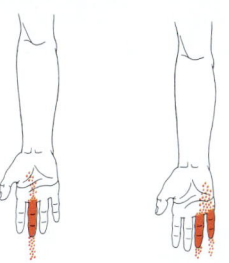
Radial head   Humeral head

Pronator teres
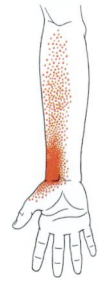

Adductor pollicis
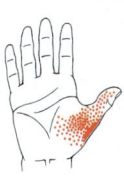

Opponens pollicis
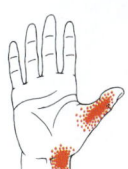

First dorsal interosseous
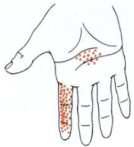

Abductor digiti minimi
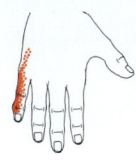

Second dorsal interosseous
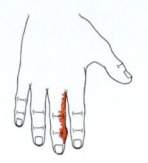

xxi

Section 5: Trunk and Pelvis Pain

Pain Pattern Quick Reference Guide

Chest Pain
- Pectoralis major (42)
- Pectoralis minor (44)
- Scalene (20)
- Sternocleidomastoid (sternal) (7)
- Sternalis (43)
- Intercostals (45)
- Iliocostalis cervicis (48)
- Subclavius (42)
- External abdominal oblique (49)
- Diaphragm (45)

Abdominal Pain
- Rectus abdominis (49)
- Abdominal obliques (49)
- Transversus abdominis (49)
- Iliocostalis thoracis (48)
- Multifidi (48)
- Pyramidalis (49)
- Quadratus lumborum (50)

Flank Pain
- Serratus anterior (46)
- Intercostals (45)
- Latissimus dorsi (24)
- Diaphragm (45)

Mid Back Pain
- Iliopsoas muscle group (51)
- Iliocostalis thoracis (48)
- Multifidi (48)
- Serratus posterior inferior (47)
- Rectus abdominis (49)
- Intercostals (45)
- Latissimus dorsi (24)

Low Back Pain
- Gluteus medius (55)
- Iliopsoas (51)
- Longissimus thoracis (48)
- Iliocostalis lumborum (48)

- Iliocostalis thoracis (48)
- Multifidi (48)
- Rectus abdominis (49)

Sacral and Buttock Pain
- Longissimus thoracis (48)
- Iliocostalis lumborum (48)
- Multifidi (48)
- Quadratus lumborum (50)
- Piriformis (57)
- Gluteus medius (55)
- Gluteus maximus (54)
- Levator ani and coccygeus (52)
- Obturator internus (52)
- Gluteus minimus (56)
- Sphincter ani (52)
- Coccygeus (52)
- Soleus (66)

Section 5 Trunk and Pelvis Pain

Pectoralis major
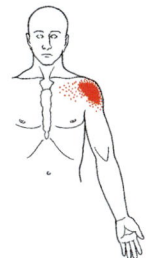 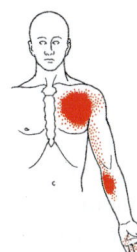 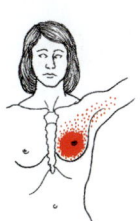 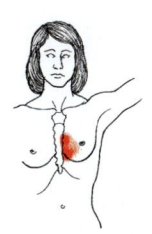

Sternalis
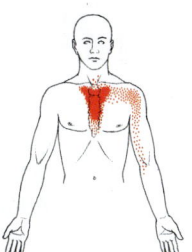

Pectoralis minor
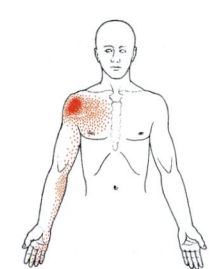

Intercostals
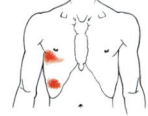

Diaphragm
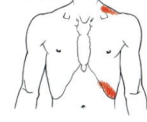

Serratus posterior interior
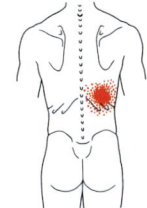

Serratus anterior
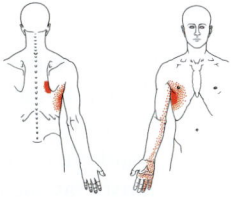 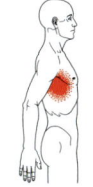

Serratus posterior superior
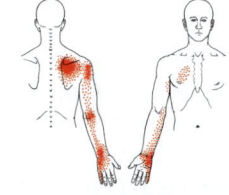

Erector spinae
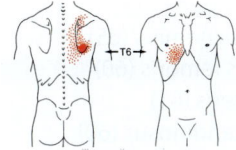 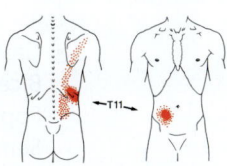 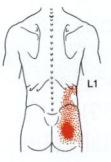 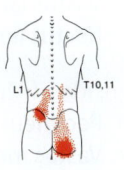

Iliocostalis thoracis Iliocostalis thoracis Iliocostalis lumborum Longissimus thoracis

Deep paraspinal
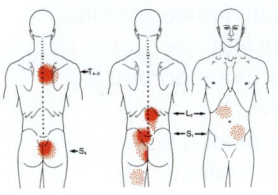

Internal and external oblique abdominis
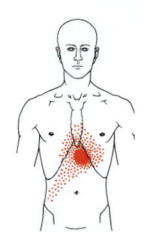 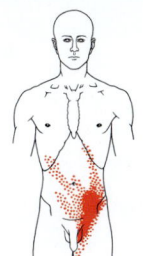 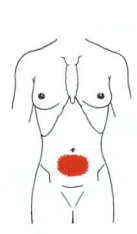

Rectus abdominis
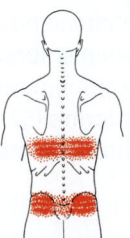 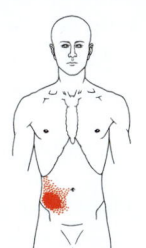 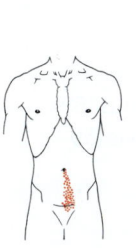

Quadratus lumborum
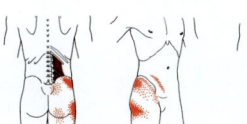 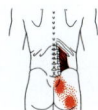

Iliopsoas
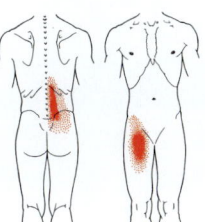

Pelvic floor muscles
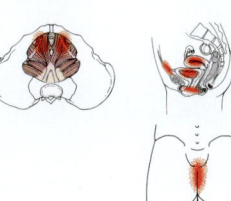

Obturator Internus
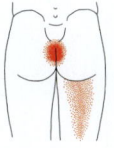

xxiii

Section 6: Hip, Thigh, and Knee Pain

Pain Pattern Quick Reference Guide

Pelvic Pain
- Coccygeus (52)
- Levator ani (52)
- Obturator internus (52)
- Adductor magnus (59)
- Piriformis (57)
- Internal abdominal oblique (49)

Hip and Groin Pain
- Vastus intermedius (58)
- Adductor magnus (59)
- Adductor longus (59)
- Adductor brevis (59)
- Pectineus (59)

Sacral and Buttock Pain
- Longissimus thoracis (48)
- Iliocostalis lumborum (48)
- Multifidi (48)
- Quadratus lumborum (50)
- Piriformis (10)
- Gluteus medius (55)
- Gluteus maximus (54)
- Levator ani (52)
- Obturator internus (52)
- Gluteus minimus (56)
- Sphincter ani (52)
- Coccygeus (52)
- Soleus (66)

Front of Thigh Pain
- Adductor longus (59)
- Adductor brevis (59
- Iliopsoas group (51)
- Adductor magnus (59)
- Vastus intermedius (58)
- Pectineus (59)
- Sartorius (58)
- Quadratus lumborum (50)
- Rectus femoris (58)

Outside of Thigh and Hip Pain
- Gluteus minimus (56)
- Vastus lateralis (58)
- Piriformis (57)
- Quadratus lumborum (50)
- Tensor fasciae latae (56)
- Vastus intermedius (58)
- Gluteus maximus (54)
- Vastus lateralis (58)
- Rectus femoris (58)

Inside of Thigh Pain
- Pectineus (59)
- Vastus medialis (58)
- Gracilis (59)
- Adductor magnus (59)
- Sartorius (58)

Back of Thigh Pain
- Gluteus minimus (56)
- Semitendinosus (60)
- Semimembranosus (60)
- Biceps femoris (60)
- Piriformis (57)
- Obturator internus (52)

Font of Knee Pain
- Rectus femoris (58)
- Vastus medialis (58)
- Adductor longus (59)
- Adductor brevis (59)

Outside of Knee Pain
- Vastus lateralis (58)

Inside of Knee Pain
- Vastus medialis (58)
- Gracilis (59)
- Rectus femoris (58)
- Sartorius (58)
- Adductor longus (59)
- Adductor brevis (59)

Back of Knee Pain
- Gastrocnemius (65)
- Biceps femoris (60)
- Popliteus (61)
- Semitendinosus (60)
- Semimembranosus (60)
- Gastrocnemius (65)
- Soleus (66)
- Plantaris (66)

Section 6 Hip, Thigh, and Knee Pain

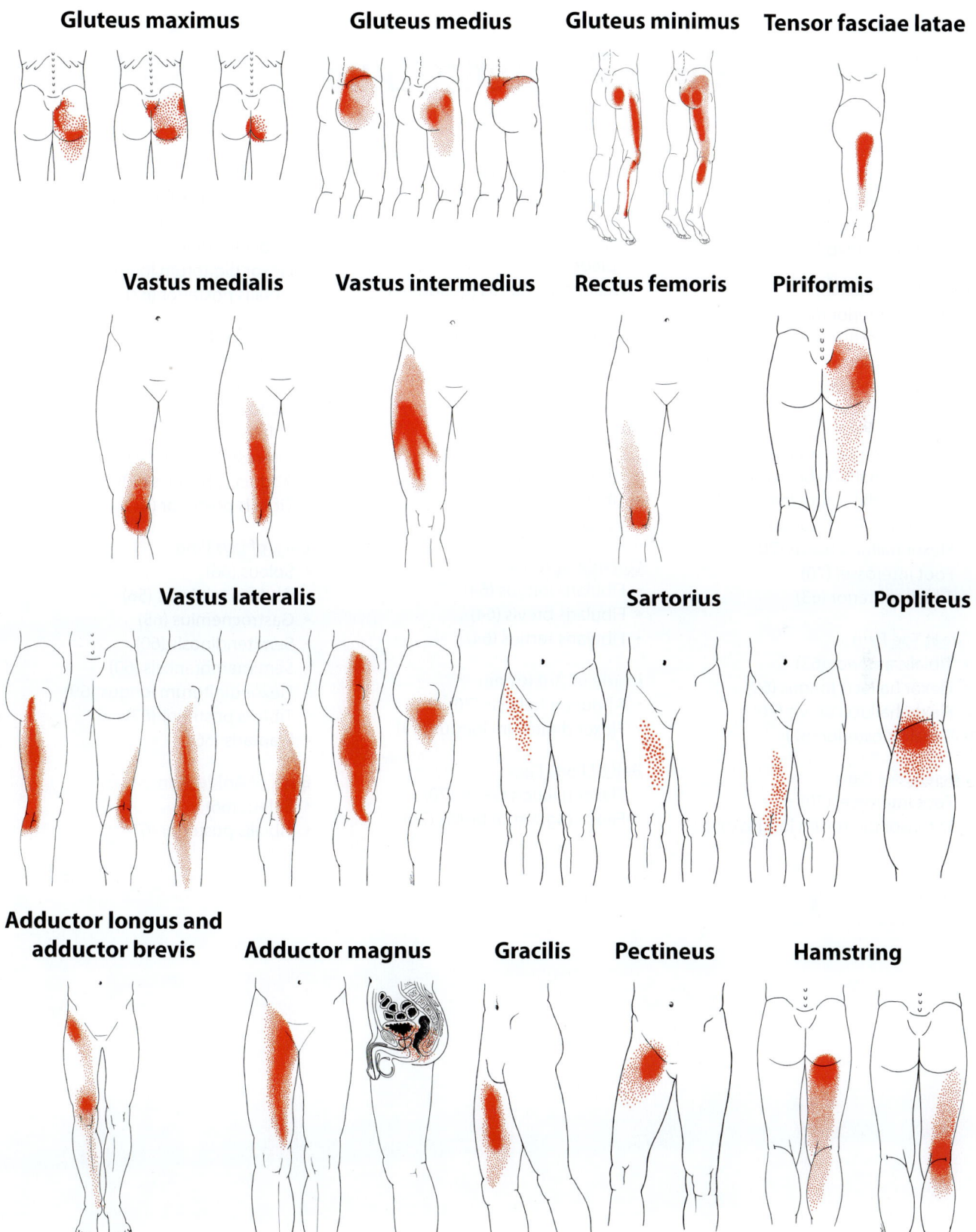

Section 7: Leg, Ankle, and Foot Pain

Pain Pattern Quick Reference Guide

Anterior Leg Pain
- Tibialis anterior (63)
- Adductor longus (59)
- Adductor brevis (59)

Anterior Ankle Pain
- Tibialis anterior (63)
- Fibularis tertius (64)
- Extensor digitorum longus (68)
- Extensor hallucis longus (68)

Top of Foot Pain
- Extensor digitorum brevis (70)
- Extensor hallucis brevis (70)
- Extensor digitorum longus (68)
- Extensor hallucis longus (68)
- Flexor hallucis brevis (70)
- Foot interossei (70)
- Tibialis anterior (63)

Great Toe Pain
- Tibialis anterior (63)
- Flexor hallucis longus (69)
- Flexor hallucis brevis (70)
- Tibialis posterior (67)

Lesser Toes Pain
- Foot interossei (70)
- Extensor digitorum longus (68)

- Flexor digitorum longus (69)
- Tibialis posterior (67)

Heel Pain
- Soleus (66)
- Flexor accessorius (quadratus plantae) (70)
- Abductor hallucis (70)
- Tibialis posterior (67)

Outside of Leg Pain
- Gastrocnemius (65)
- Gluteus minimus (56)
- Fibularis longus (64)
- Fibularis brevis (64)
- Vastus lateralis (58)

Outside of Ankle Pain
- Fibularis longus (64)
- Fibularis brevis (64)
- Fibularis tertius (64)

Inside of Ankle Pain
- Abductor hallucis (70)
- Flexor digitorum longus (69)

Ball of Foot Pain
- Flexor hallucis brevis (70)
- Flexor digitorum brevis (70)

- Adductor hallucis (70)
- Flexor hallucis longus (69)
- Interossei of foot (70)
- Abductor digiti minimi (70)
- Flexor digitorum longus (69)
- Tibialis posterior (67)

Arch of Foot Pain
- Gastrocnemius (65)
- Flexor digitorum longus (69)
- Adductor hallucis (70)
- Soleus (66)
- Interossei of foot (70)
- Abductor hallucis (70)
- Tibialis posterior (67)

Back of Leg Pain
- Soleus (66)
- Gluteus minimus (56)
- Gastrocnemius (65)
- Semitendinosis (60)
- Semimembranosis (60)
- Flexor digitorum longus (69)
- Tibialis posterior (67)
- Plantaris (66)

Back of Ankle Pain
- Soleus (66)
- Tibialis posterior (67

Section 7 Leg, Ankle, and Foot Pain

Tibialis anterior

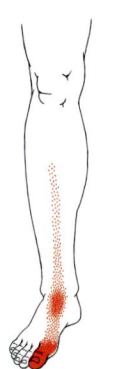

Fibularis

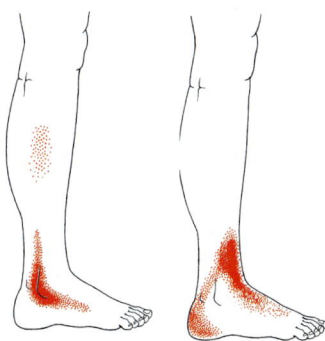

Gastrocnemius

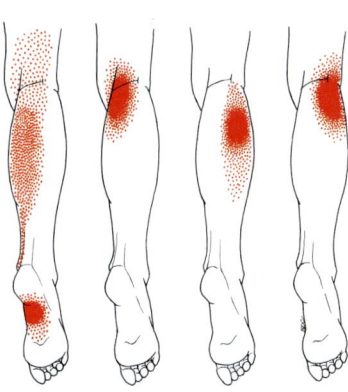

Soleus

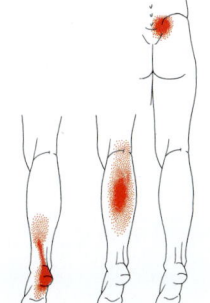

Plantaris

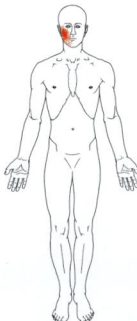

Tibialis posterior

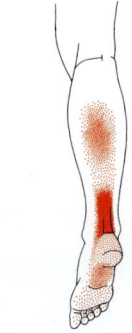

Extensor digitorum longus

Extensor hallucis longus

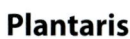
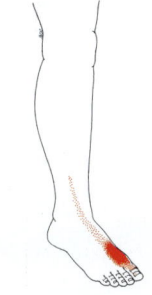

Flexor hallucis longus

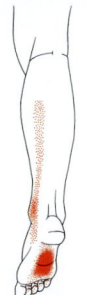

Flexor digitorum longus

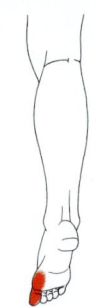

Abductor hallucis

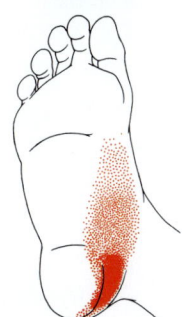

Abductor digiti minimi

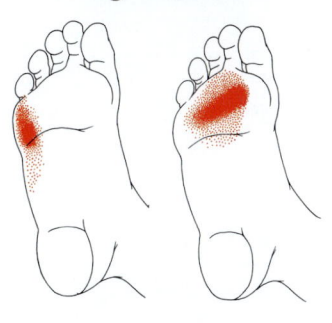

Flexor accessorius

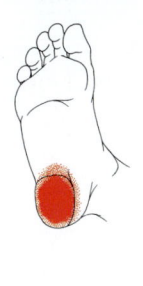

Adductor hallucis and flexor hallucis brevis

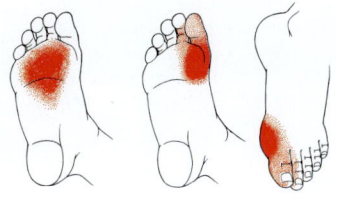

First dorsal interosseous

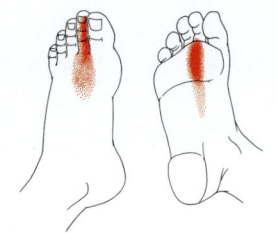

Extensor digitorum brevis and extensor hallucis brevis

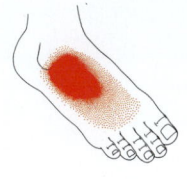

xxvii

Section 1: Introduction to Myofascial Pain and Dysfunction

Chapter 1

Pain Sciences and Myofascial Pain

Jan Dommerholt, Robert D. Gerwin, and Carol A. Courtney

1. INTRODUCTION

Chronic or persistent pain conditions are the most common cause of disability at an annual cost greater than $650 billion in healthcare and lost employment in the United States alone.[1] The economic costs associated with chronic pain outpace the combined costs from diabetes, cancer, and heart disease. Chronic pain leads to more deaths than motor vehicle accidents. In spite of the staggering economic costs and overwhelming personal impact, there are few efforts to prevent chronic (persistent) pain conditions and to develop evidence-informed management strategies.[2]

Chronic (persistent) pain is often defined as pain lasting for more than 3 or 6 months, but length of time as the main criterion is not based on any specific mechanism that separates acute from chronic pain. Reichling et al proposed that there are at least two distinct types of chronic pain.[3] Type I is acute pain that persists for a prolonged period of time, whereas Type II involves a mechanistic transition from acute to chronic, involving the disconnection of the generation of pain by the initial tissue injury, or the loss of responsiveness to therapies that are successful for acute pain. Myofascial pain takes a prominent place in the spectrum of acute and chronic pain syndromes. In the original volumes of the Trigger Point Manual, Travell and Simons maintained that most people will experience painful myofascial trigger points (TrPs) at one time or another.[4,5] Recent prevalence and incidence studies have confirmed that TrPs are indeed very common in a wide variety of conditions.[6-22]

Myofascial pain, unfortunately, is often overlooked as a potential contributing or causative factor to other pain problems.[23] Trigger points commonly constitute a primary dysfunction, and they may occur in the absence of any underlying medical condition or tissue damage.[24] As such, TrPs can function as sources of persistent peripheral nociceptive input independent of tissue damage.[25-27] They can be associated with other conditions such as whiplash injuries or osteoarthritis.[8,28,29] Trigger points in the upper trapezius correlate with cervical spine dysfunction at the C3 and C4 segmental levels without necessarily having a causal relationship.[30] A single spinal manipulation induced changes in pressure pain sensitivity in latent TrPs in the upper trapezius muscle.[31] Trigger points may compound the symptoms of other conditions and persist long after the original initiating condition has been resolved. They can be associated with visceral conditions and dysfunctions, including endometriosis, interstitial cystitis, irritable bowel syndrome, dysmenorrhea, and prostatitis.[32-39] Myofascial pain can mimic other pain diagnoses such as neuropathic pain, complex regional pain syndrome, systemic diseases, tinnitus, and certain metabolic, parasitic, and nutritional disorders, among others.[40-48] Although different definitions of TrPs are used among different disciplines, the most commonly accepted definition maintains that "a TrP is a hyperirritable spot in a taut band of a skeletal muscle that is painful on compression, stretch, overload or contraction of the tissue which usually responds with a referred pain that is perceived distant from the spot."[49] Although Travell and Simons distinguished different types of TrPs, including active, latent, satellite, and primary and secondary TrPs, in the current thinking, only active and latent TrPs are considered in research and clinical practice.

In the previous edition of the Trigger Point Manual, Simons et al defined an active TrP as "a myofascial TrP that causes a clinical pain complaint. It is always tender, prevents full lengthening of the muscle, weakens the muscle, refers a patient-recognized pain on direct compression, mediates a local twitch response (LTR) of muscle fibers when adequately stimulated, and, when compressed within the patient's pain tolerance, produces referred motor phenomena and often autonomic phenomena, generally in its pain reference zone, and causes tenderness in the pain reference zone."[49] Similarly, a latent TrP was defined as "a myofascial TrP that is clinically quiescent with respect to spontaneous pain; it is painful only when palpated. A latent TrP may have all the other clinical characteristics of an active TrP and always has a taut band that increases muscle tension and restricts range of motion".[49] Members of the International Association for the Study of Pain and the American Academy of Pain Medicine considered the presence of tender spots causing local pain and a re-creation of a patient's symptoms as essential diagnostic components of myofascial pain syndrome (MPS).[50] Tough et al found that the most commonly applied criteria in research included a tender spot within a taut band of a skeletal muscle, the patient's pain recognition, a predictable pain referral pattern, and an LTR.[51]

Latent TrPs, characterized by motor dysfunction, including stiffness and restricted range of motion, and the presence of referred pain, are far more common than active TrPs, which also feature spontaneous local pain. It has now been established that latent TrPs contribute to the process of nociception, but without reaching the threshold to activate ascending pathways from the dorsal horn (DH) to the brain.[53-55] Mense suggested that referred pain from latent TrPs may occur when normally ineffective synapses to DH neurons are being sensitized.[56] A panel of 60 experts from 12 countries agreed through a Delphi study process that the reproduction of symptoms experienced by patients and the recognition of pain are the main clinical differences between active and latent TrPs.[52] Box 1-1 identifies the clinical characteristics of TrPs identified by Simons, Simons and Travell,[49] and by expert opinion from the Delphi study. In addition, active TrPs feature larger referred pain areas and higher pain intensities than latent TrPs,[57] and their overlying cutaneous and subcutaneous tissues are usually more sensitive to pressure and electrical stimulation.[58,59] The degree of irritability of TrPs is correlated with the prevalence of endplate noise, which is more pronounced at active TrPs.[60]

Since 1999, when the last volume of the TrP Manual was published,[49] much has changed in the scientific understanding of TrPs. Where in the past myofascial pain was commonly attributed to tissue injury, especially damage to the sarcoplasmic reticulum, tissue damage is no longer the prevailing model. The energy crisis hypothesis and subsequent integrated TrP hypothesis were the first attempts to consider MPS in a broader context.[61] Although the integrated TrP hypothesis is still the prevailing model, it is indeed time for a revision of the myofascial pain construct

> **Box 1-1 Clinical characteristics of trigger points**

	Common Findings of TrPs	
Simons, Simons and Travell[49]	■ Palpable taut band with cross-fiber flat or pincer palpation ■ Hypersensitive spot within the taut band ■ Local twitch response when adequately stimulated ■ May produce motor and autonomic phenomena ■ May prevent full lengthening of the muscle (restricts range of motion) ■ May cause inhibition weakness of the muscle	
	Active TrPs	**Latent TrPs**
	■ Refers or produces a patient's recognized pain ■ Spontaneous local or referred pain	■ Local or referred unrecognized pain ■ Painful only when palpated or needled
Expert opinion Delphi study[52]	■ Reproduce any symptom(s), not just pain, experienced by the patient ■ Patient recognizes the symptom as familiar ■ The symptom(s) may be absent at the moment of the examination, but will appear during manual palpation	■ Do not reproduce symptoms experienced by the patient ■ Patient does not recognize symptoms caused by cross-fiber flat or pincer palpation

considering current knowledge and evidence of pain science combined with new clinical insights.[26,61] It is encouraging that the quality of myofascial pain research has improved consistently over the past decades.[62] Although several new hypothetical models have been developed in an effort to better describe myofascial pain,[63-72] most are still lacking adequate experimental support. To better understand myofascial pain, it is necessary to become familiar with the basics of contemporary pain science and pain mechanisms. This chapter provides a comprehensive review of various pain models and pertinent aspects of nociception, and peripheral and central sensitization.

2. PAIN MODELS

The International Association for the Study of Pain defines pain as "an unpleasant sensory and emotional experience associated with actual or potential tissue damage, or described in terms of such damage".[73] In 2018, Cohen et al offered an alternate definition of pain: "Pain is a mutually recognizable somatic experience that reflects a person's apprehension of threat to their bodily or existential integrity."[74] In a commentary, Treede critiqued the interpretation by Cohen et al for not considering the multidimensional nature of the pain experience, for broadening the scope from threat to bodily integrity, which is a poorly defined term, and for suggesting that pain recognition requires an outside observer.[75] The discussion about the optimal definition of pain will likely continue. What is clear is that pain does not necessarily reflect injury, as previously suggested by proponents of a now outdated strict structural-pathology model, and pain, including myofascial pain, can occur without a specific tissue lesion.

A recent study showed that 96% of asymptomatic 80-year-old individuals and 37% of 20-year olds had demonstrable disk degeneration.[76] Nakashima et al found that in 1211 asymptomatic individuals in their twenties, 73.3% of males and 78.0% of females had bulging disks.[77] Battie et al showed that spinal degeneration is not the result of aging and excessive wear and tear.[78] In another study of 393 subjects with a symptomatic a-traumatic full-thickness rotator cuff tear, the symptoms of pain did not correlate with the severity of the injury.[79] Degenerative changes of the rotator cuff muscles are not a primary source of pain.[80] These and other studies clearly illustrate that spine and shoulder degeneration are not necessarily correlated to low back and shoulder pain, and in a broader sense, they confirm that a strict biomedical approach is inadequate to understand pain conditions.[81,82] On the other hand, another study showed that disk bulges, degeneration, extrusions, protrusions, Modic 1 changes, and spondylolysis were more prevalent in adults 50 years of age or younger with back pain compared with asymptomatic individuals.[83] Interpreting imaging studies without clinical correlations can be rather misleading and may result in unnecessary interventions and extensive medical treatments such as surgery, polypharmacy, including an excessive use of opioids, immobilization and bedrest, and increased disability and pain.[2,84,85] In spite of much progress, pain continues to be a poorly understood phenomenon, although multiple pain models have emerged since the publication of the gate control theory.[86]

Historically, many researchers and clinicians, including Travell and Simons, thought that muscle pain would cause spasms of the same muscle, which, in turn, would cause more pain leading to more spasms.[87] This vicious cycle hypothesis, known as the pain–spasm–pain cycle, was based on the assumption that pain would excite alpha-motor neurons and possibly even gamma motor neurons. More recent experimental and human evidence has demonstrated that alpha and gamma motor neurons generally are inhibited by nociceptive input from the same muscle.[88-92] A change in muscle spindle sensitivity may alter proprioceptive functioning, but there is no convincing evidence of facilitation of spindle activity,[93] which means that muscle pain does not appear to cause an increase in fusimotor drive.[94] Nevertheless, proponents of this concept have suggested that TrPs are the result of dysfunctional muscle spindle activation.[71] Although the pain–spasm–pain cycle is frequently referenced, it is a refuted concept based on an outdated and simplified understanding of the structure and function of alpha and gamma motor neurons.[95,96]

The updated pain-adaptation model provided new insights.[97] According to this model, muscle pain inhibits alpha-motor neurons, leading to the activation of antagonists and an overall reduction in motor function. These patterns are, however, not universally applicable either, as Martin et al demonstrated that muscle nociception resulted in excitation of both elbow flexor and extensor muscles.[98] Activity of motor neurons is not necessarily uniformly reduced.[96]

Hodges and Tucker proposed a new motor adaptation model, realizing that the vicious pain cycle and pain-adaptation hypotheses are inadequate models of motor adaptation.[99] Instead, they proposed that a redistribution of activity within and between muscles must occur. Pain will likely change the mechanical behavior of muscles by creating modified movements and stiffness, leading to improved protection from further pain or injury, or from threatened pain or injury. Inhibition or facilitation of select agonist and antagonists may occur. They maintained that simple changes in excitability do not explain motor adaptation, but complementary, additive, or competitive changes at multiple levels of the motor system are more likely to be involved.

Combining Hodges and Tucker's motor adaptation model with the TrP model, TrPs change muscle activity. Lucas et al found altered movement activation patterns in shoulder abduction in subjects with latent TrPs in their shoulder musculature.[100,101] Bohlooli et al confirmed the findings by Lucas et al, and expanded the concept to faster movements in all movement planes of the shoulder.[102] In a recent study, Schneider et al showed that active TrPs also alter muscle activation patterns.[103] The characteristic taut bands found in myofascial pain can be considered to be functional adaptations of motor activity within muscles.[104] Muscles with TrPs result in restrictions in range of motion.[105-110] Trigger points inhibit overall muscle function, leading to muscle weakness without atrophy, or perhaps more accurately, to motor inhibition.[111]

As new data and facts become available, pain theories will evolve. Following the publication of the gate theory in 1965,[86] which in itself was conceived out of preceding pain models,[112] several new models have been formulated. Although the gate control theory provided a strong impulse to take pain seriously and foster research into pain mechanisms, the model is not perfect and has been modified multiple times since its publication.[113,114] In 1998, Gifford introduced the mature organism model, which considered the interactions between the periphery and the central nervous system.[115,116] He maintained that the combination of tissue health, environmental factors, past experiences, and personal beliefs are processed by the central nervous system, leading to specific output mechanisms that involve the motor, neuroendocrine, autonomic, immune, and descending control systems.[115,116] Melzack also recognized the multidimensional nature of pain when he formulated the neuromatrix model, which, like the mature organism model, aimed to develop a better understanding of the role of the brain.[112,114,117,118] Melzack specifically included TrPs as sources of peripheral nociceptive input, among many other possible inputs. The neuromatrix and mature organism model are examples of biopsychosocial models of care, which are very much in line with how Travell practiced as a physician. According to Travell, "in this age of specialization, few clinicians are broad enough to see the whole patient and his/her problem . . . understanding with the delicate interplay between the patient's mind, body, environment is a paramount importance in helping a patient overcome an illness."[119]

Although the brain is actively involved in the processing of sensory input and the experience of pain, pain is much more than just a linear process initiated by tissue injury and inflammation. Pain involves the integration of sensory, emotional, and cognitive dimensions. According to Melzack, pain experiences reflect the cultural background of the individual, the context of the circumstances triggering a pain experience and other environmental impacts, psychological variables, stress responses, past experiences, and personal aspects, including genetics.[112,120] In persistent pain, however, the correlation between pain and tissue injury becomes less pronounced and may even be nonexisting.[121] It has been established that nociception is not necessary for the perception of pain.[122,123] In persistent pain conditions, the experience and degree of pain do not provide meaningful information about the state of the tissues, but this should not be interpreted to mean that peripheral nociceptive input from specific tissues or regions would never be irrelevant.[26,124]

Nijs et al have proposed guidelines to differentiate low back pain disorders with predominant nociceptive pain, neuropathic pain, and central sensitization.[125] They defined nociceptive pain as pain arising from actual or threatening damage to nonneural tissue due to the activation of nociceptors, or as pain attributable to the activation of the peripheral receptive terminals of primary afferent neurons in response to noxious chemical, mechanical, or thermal stimuli, which may include myofascial pain. Neuropathic pain was defined as "pain caused by a primary lesion or disease of the somatosensory nervous system," such as a lumbar radiculopathy. Central sensitization was defined as "an amplification of neural signaling within the central nervous system that elicits pain hypersensitivity," "increased responsiveness of nociceptive neurons in the central nervous system to their normal or subthreshold afferent input," or "an augmentation of responsiveness of central neurons to input from unimodal and polymodal receptors."[125] Nijs et al consider TrPs as peripheral sources of nociception in patients with low back pain in line with Moseley' findings that "elimination of myofascial TrPs is an important component of the management of chronic musculoskeletal pain."[126]

A common theme in the various pain models is that clinicians would need to identify which pain mechanisms are dominant in a given patient to determine the optimal treatment parameters. In Gifford's mature organism model, exercise and manual therapies are thought to be most effective when the pain is primarily input-dominant or nociceptive, meaning that tissue injury or abnormal peripheral nerve input are the most important causative factors. Even under those circumstances, Gifford recognized that psychological dysfunction, such as anxiety, or a poor understanding of the problem would require a different approach emphasizing the inclusion of cognitive and affective aspects.[115] In cases where the output-dominant processes are prevailing, advocates of this model emphasize that the focus of therapy should be on therapeutic pain science education, gentle exercise, and pain-free interventions to avoid further sensitization.[127-129] Pain science education should not be offered as a stand-alone intervention.[130] Furthermore, even when pain science education is included in the care, developing a therapeutic alliance with the patient is essential, as is listening to the patient without restricting time constraints.[131,132] See Chapter 5 for more on the therapeutic alliance.

Following that thought process, some clinicians and researchers have concluded that considering TrPs in the clinical thought process would reflect an antiquated model in the context of modern pain sciences, based on the assumption that "the issues are not in the tissues," and that pain is produced by the brain or by other mechanisms.[72,133,134] Quite to the contrary, the manual examination of peripheral joints, muscles, skin, and fascia continues to be important, especially within a contemporary pain science and neuromatrix perspective.[135] There is much evidence that both active and latent TrPs provide a mechanism of peripheral nociceptive input that can contribute to both peripheral and central sensitization.[25-27,126,136] Referred pain, or secondary hyperalgesia, is a characteristic of central sensitization.[137] Experts reached agreement that referred pain from TrPs can include different sensory sensations, including pain, a dull ache, tingling, or burning pain.[52] In the aforementioned Delphi study, the experts proposed the term "referred sensation" instead of referred pain because of the variety of symptoms associated to TrP stimulation.[52]

3. NOCICEPTION

Peripheral and central sensitization are important aspects of myofascial pain and other clinical pain syndromes.[27,138] There are three distinct parts of the nervous system responsible for the perception of pain, including afferent pathways from the periphery to the DH and from the DH to higher centers in the central nervous system; integration centers in the brainstem, midbrain, and cortex, among others; and efferent pathways from the brain to the spinal cord.[139] Sensitization is characterized by a reduction in pain thresholds and an increase in responsiveness of peripheral nociceptors and plays a critical role in pain syndromes,[3] including MPS.[6,26,27,140] There is emerging evidence that as persistent sources of nociceptive input, TrPs contribute to the propagation and maintenance of pain and central sensitization.[26,27,141,142] Ongoing, strong, and sustained peripheral nociceptive input leads to profound neuroplastic and even anatomic changes, including changes in gray matter.[123,143-146] Anatomic volume changes may include the brainstem, the right anterior thalamus, the dorsolateral prefrontal cortex, the somatosensory cortex, and the posterior parietal cortex.[147] Treatments aimed at reducing pain may reverse the anatomic changes.[148,149] Of interest is that mechanical stimuli do not contribute as much to peripheral stimulation as thermal and chemical stimuli do.[114,150] Central nociceptive neurons respond to the synaptic input from peripheral nociceptors.[143] Because the latter have a primary warning function, they can generate signals before tissue injury occurs. Central sensitization is commonly maintained by ongoing peripheral nociceptive input, which has been described for fibromyalgia,[151] musculoskeletal pain,[152] neuropathic pain,[153] and myofascial pain,[137] among others. Reichling et al wrote an exceptionally lucid and thorough review that is the basis for many of the concepts referred to in this section along with several other informative reviews.[3,154,155]

There are four stages of nociception, namely transduction, transmission, perception, and modulation (Box 1-2).

Nociception is the process of perception of painful sensations, which starts with the detection of potentially painful stimuli by the peripheral terminals or nerve endings of afferent nerve axons, called primary afferent fibers with cell bodies located in the dorsal root ganglion (DRG) for the body and in the trigeminal ganglion for the face. The main afferent nerve fiber types are the small-diameter, myelinated, faster-conducting Aδ (group IV) fibers that mediate localized pain sensations and the small-diameter unmyelinated, slower conducting C (group IV) fibers that mediate more dull, poorly localized, and delayed pain. It is important to understand that not all small-diameter, slowly conducting fibers are nociceptive. Skeletal muscle and cutaneous nerves feature low-threshold group IV mechanoreceptors. Cutaneous nerves also include thermoreceptors (Figure 1-1).[156,157]

Aδ nociceptors are divided into two main classes. Type I or high threshold mechanical nociceptors are polymodal receptors that respond to both mechanical and chemical stimuli. Normally, type I receptors have a high thermal threshold, but with prolonged heat stimulation, their threshold is reduced and they can become sensitized. Type II Aδ nociceptors have a high mechanical threshold, but a low thermal threshold.[158,159] C fibers have either mechanothermal nociceptors, cold nociceptors, or polymodal nociceptors (Figure 1-2).[160]

Noxious stimuli can be located outside the body, such as exogenous mechanical stimuli, or can arise internally from injured and inflamed tissues, referred to as endogenous stimuli. Both exogenous and endogenous noxious stimuli produce a variety of algesic and proalgesic mediators, including lipid mediators, cytokines, protons, and neurotransmitters. Both activate ionotropic (ligand-gated ion) channels and metabotropic (G-protein-coupled) receptors in the cell membrane.[161] Ionotropic receptors are transmembrane molecules that can "open" or "close" a channel to transport smaller particles, such as K^+, Na^+, Cl, and Ca^{2+} ions, across the cell membrane. Ionotropic receptors are closed until a specific ligand binds to the receptor, such as substance P, protons, adenosine triphosphate (ATP), or glutamate. Metabotropic receptors do not feature an ion channel. They are linked to a "G-protein" and have a guanine nucleotide-binding. After activating a G-protein, the protein activates another molecule, referred to as the "secondary messenger." The activation of secondary messengers, particularly the protein kinases, involves phosphorylation of ion channels, which increases the opening time or opening probability of an ionotropic channel. As an example, bradykinin (BK) and prostaglandins (PG) act on metabotropic receptors.[162-164] Metabotropic channels are always slower than ionotropic channels. Capsaicin, ATP, nerve growth factor (NGF), and protons are common stimulants for muscle nociceptors by activating such receptors.[156,165]

Many substances have multiple receptors. For example, there are six families of human glutamate receptors, including three types of ionotropic receptors, namely AMPA (α-amino-3-hydroxy-5-methyl-4-isoxazolepropionic acid), NMDA (N-methyl-D-aspartate), and kainate receptors, and three types of metabotropic receptors (Groups I-III),[166] which shows that glutamate plays a key role in many processes.[154] In experimental studies, different substances, such as glutamate or capsaicin, are commonly used to elicit local and referred muscle pain (Figure 1-3).[167-170]

The first neurotrophic factor implicated in producing pain was NGF. Injections of NGF into low back musculature induced prolonged hypersensitivity in rats.[171] Other studies demonstrated that peripheral administration of NGF caused thermal and mechanical hyperalgesia.[172,173] Injections of NGF in the tibialis anterior muscle and its overlaying fascia triggered significantly greater hyperalgesia in the fascia.[174] The thoracolumbar fascia was more sensitive than the tibial fascia.[174] Increased levels of NGF have been shown in the cerebrospinal fluid of patients with multiple sclerosis and central neuropathic pain,[175] diabetic neuropathy,[176] chronic arthritis,[177] and rheumatoid arthritis.[178] NGF acts at the high-affinity NGF tropomyosin receptor kinase A (TrkA) receptor and at the low-affinity p75 receptor. The NGF-activated TrkA receptor selectively triggers several intracellular signaling pathways via the binding of specific effector proteins to phosphorylated docking sites. The activation of the p75 receptor also activates several intracellular pathways. The two receptors function together: p75 improves the binding at the TrkA receptor. A loss of function of the TrkA receptor causes insensitivity to pain, which illustrates its important role in pain perception.[179] NGF is part of a family of growth factors referred to as neurotrophins, which also includes brain-derived neurotrophic factor (BDNF) and neurotrophin-3 (NT-3), among others.[180] BDNF acts at the TrkB receptor and NT-3 at the TrKC receptor.[181]

Neuropeptides like substance P and calcitonin gene-related peptide (CGRP) act at peptidergic nociceptors. Substance P is released from peripheral nerve endings of DRG neurons, causing neurogenic inflammation, and in the DH where it binds to neurokinin type 1 receptors.[182] CGRP is well known for its role as a vasodilator, especially in the cardiovascular system and with migraine headaches,[183] but it also plays a major role in muscle physiology, especially in skeletal muscles excitation-contraction coupling.[184] In addition, CGRP enhances the expression of dihydropyridine receptors,[185] which is relevant for TrPs and myofascial pain (see Chapter 2). Motor endplates and sensory nerves feature CGRP immunoreactivity.[186] CGRP is released from motor neurons following electrical stimulation[187] and binds to membrane receptors of the skeletal muscle.[188,189] NGF regulates the expression of substance P and CGRP within the spinal cord.[190] When NGF antibodies are administered, the upregulation of CGRP and mechanical hyperalgesia are suppressed.[191]

3.1. Nociception and Transduction

Transduction is the molecular process by which thermal, chemical, and mechanical stimuli are converted to electrical impulses or electrical energy in the form of an action potential. Transduction takes place at the cell membrane of the peripheral nerve ending. The electrical impulses or action potentials are transmitted centrally along primary afferent nerve fibers to DRG neurons. Action potentials from the first-order DRG neurons travel centrally through short afferent fibers to spinal DH neurons. Different fiber types synapse to second-order neurons in the DH in specific laminae: Aδ and C fibers terminate in Rexed laminae I and II. The substantia gelatinosa (lamina II) is an important region with many synaptic connections between primary sensory afferent neurons, interneurons, and ascending and descending fibers allowing modulation of the pain signal transmission,[154]

Box 1-2 Stages of nociception

Transduction
Transmission
Perception
Modulation

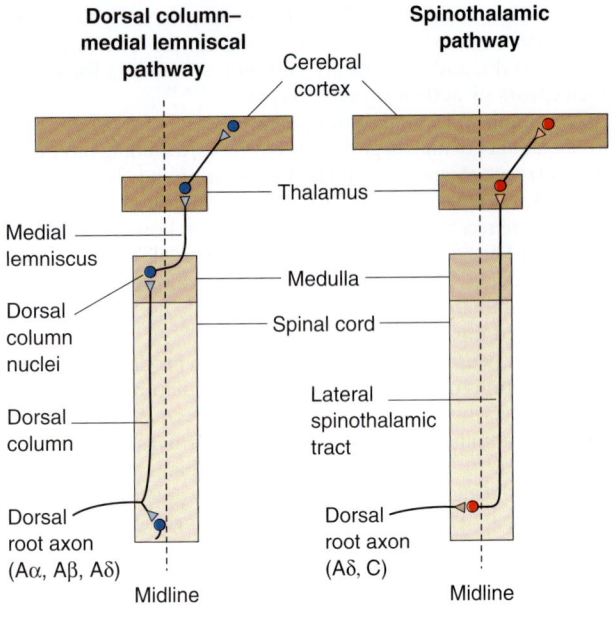

Figure 1-1. Overview of somatosensory input and two ascending pathways of somatic sensation. (From Bear MF, Connors BW, Paradiso MA. *Neuroscience: Exploring the Brain*. 4th ed. Philadelphia, PA: Wolters Kluwer; 2016.)

which is a key aspect of the gate control theory.[114] Aδ fibers also terminate in lamina V. The distribution of Aδ and C fiber terminations in the DH is determined to a large degree by the type of receptor that is activated, and therefore, the process is receptor and stimulus specific (Figure 1-4).[159]

Signal transduction is usually considered as a process of information transfer mediated by neurotransmitters, hormones, or cytokines that bind to transmembrane receptors at the cell surface, such as substance P, somatostatin, glutamate, dynorphin, and cholecystokinin (CCK), among others.[192] Transduction is enhanced by intracellular processes mediated by second-messenger pathways such as G-protein membrane receptors; however, there are many other possible signal transduction pathways. Berridge identified as many as 19 different signal transduction cascades.[193] Transduction can be modulated downward (inhibited) by receptor antagonists, such as the acid-sensing ion channels (ASICs) receptor antagonists oxytocin and arginine vasopressin,[194] and by the transient receptor potential cation channel subfamily V member 1 (TRPV1) channel antagonist ARA 290.[195] Some transducers reside on nonneuronal cells, which, when stimulated, release mediators that signal to the nociceptor, such as the keratinocyte and the satellite glial cell.

3.2. Nociception and Transmission

Nociceptive impulses from the DH are transmitted primarily via the ascending neospinothalamic tract to the thalamus, the contralateral parietal somatosensory cortex, and other cortical centers, to provide the accurate location of pain. The neospinothalamic tract is a fast-conducting discriminative tract (Figure 1-5). On the other hand, the paleospinothalamic tract is a slower

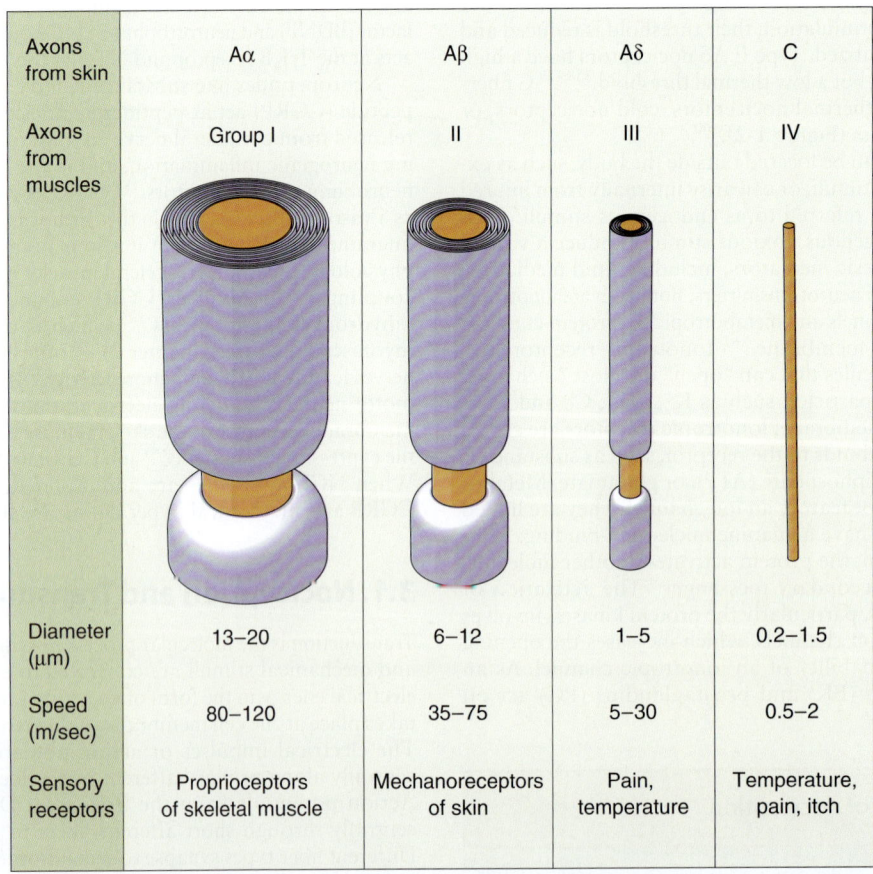

Figure 1-2. Various sizes of primary afferent axons. The axons are drawn to scale, but they are shown 2000 times larger than life size. The diameter of an axon is correlated with its conduction velocity and with the type of sensory receptor to which it is connected. (From Bear MF, Connors BW, Paradiso MA. *Neuroscience: Exploring the Brain*. 4th ed. Philadelphia, PA: Wolters Kluwer; 2016.)

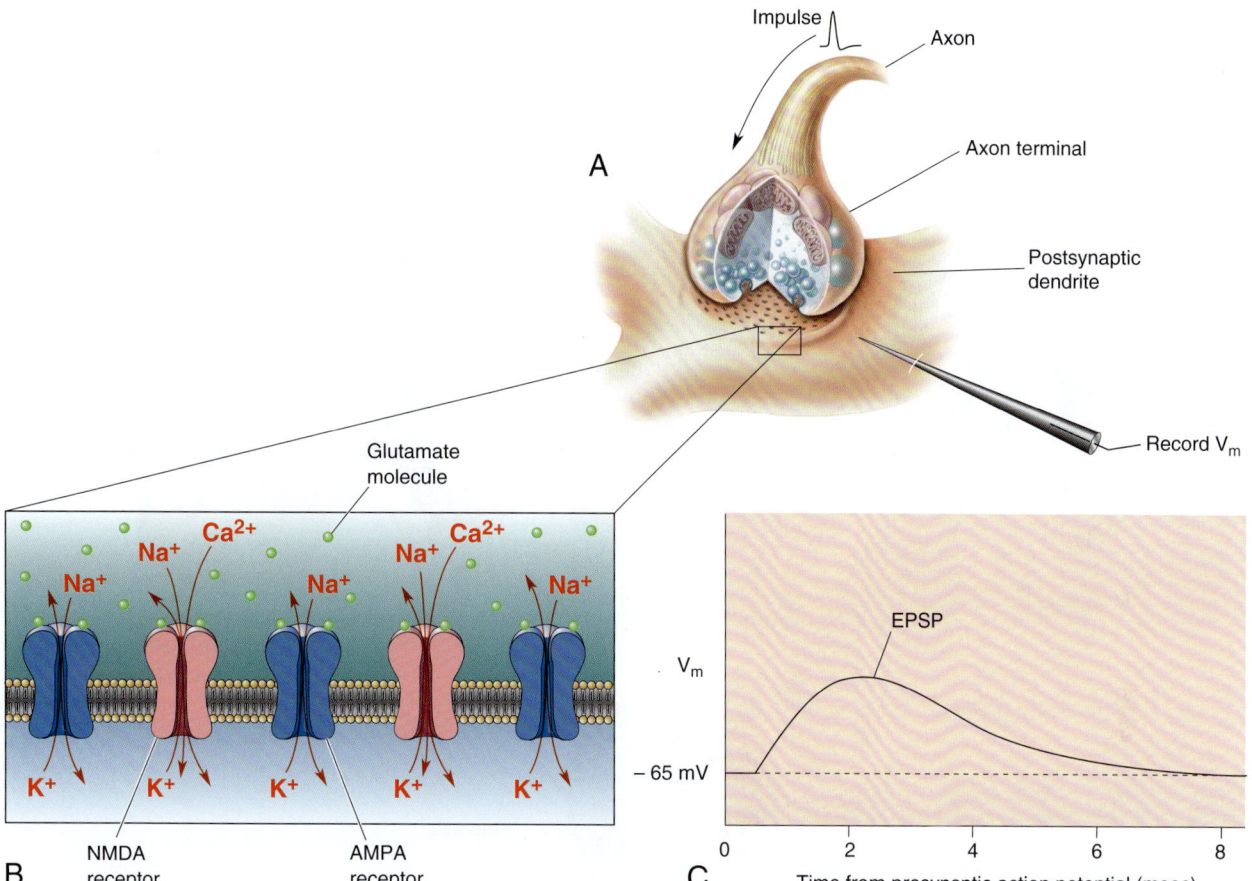

Figure 1-3. The coexistence of NMDA (*N*-methyl-D-aspartate) and AMPA (α-amino-3-hydroxy-5-methyl-4-isoxazolepropionic acid) receptors in the postsynaptic membrane of a central nervous system synapse. (A) An action potential arriving in the presynaptic terminal causes the release of glutamate. (B) Glutamate binds to AMPA receptor channels and NMDA receptor channels in the postsynaptic membrane. (C) The entry of Na through the AMPA channels, and Na and Ca^2 through the NMDA channels, causes an EPSP. (From Bear MF, Connors BW, Paradiso MA. *Neuroscience: Exploring the Brain*. 4th ed. Philadelphia, PA: Wolters Kluwer; 2016.)

conducting tact, corresponding to the spinomesencephalic, the spinoreticulothalamic, and spinoparabachial projections (Figure 1-1). The cortical representation of pain involves the anterior cingular cortex and the posterior operculo-insular cortex for C-afferent stimulation. The contralateral somatosensory cerebral cortex in the parietal lobe for nociceptive Aδ afferent stimulation and in associated areas such as the amygdala, the thalamus, the insula, and the prefrontal and posterior parietal cortices.[139,196,197] During a pain experience, these areas appear to communicate with each other.[128] Modulation that amplifies or inhibits the response to nociceptive stimulation occurs at all levels of transduction and transmission. Box 1-3 summarizes the stages of peripheral nociception.

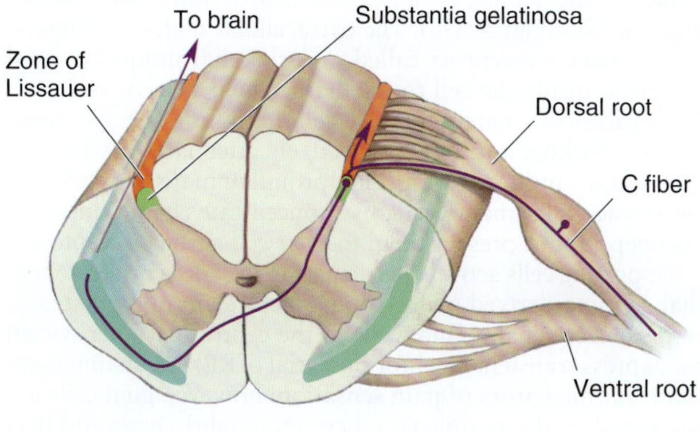

3.3. Nociception and Sex Differences

As a side note, many studies suggest that women are more sensitive to noxious stimuli and have greater pain sensitivity.[198,199] The mechanisms underlying these sex differences are poorly understood,[200] but it is likely that psychological, cultural, and biological factors all contribute to these differences. Biological factors may include hormonal, genetic, behavioral, and environmental aspects.[201-206] Total sleep deprivation triggered significant alterations in the descending pain inhibition in women but not in men.[207] In general, women had greater pain responses with electrical and thermal stimuli than men,[208] but when comparing older men and women, there were no differences in pain sensitivity or brain activation.[209] Most women display a lower threshold to painful stimuli and more brain activity in regions associated with affective pain.[210] However, when anxiety was better controlled, the differences between men and women were less pronounced.[211] Intolerance of uncertainty was relevant in both sexes and increased the pain intensity.[212] Women with shoulder pain exhibited a lower mechanical and thermal pain threshold than men.[213,214] Brain studies have confirmed that women have a greater activation of the anterior cingular cortex.[215]

Differential sex responses to nociceptive stimuli suggest that there is hormonal modulation of transduction or transmission to the cerebral cortex. Hormones are likely to influence the

Figure 1-4. Spinal connections of nociceptive axons. (From Bear MF, Connors BW, Paradiso MA. *Neuroscience: Exploring the Brain*. 4th ed. Philadelphia, PA: Wolters Kluwer; 2016.)

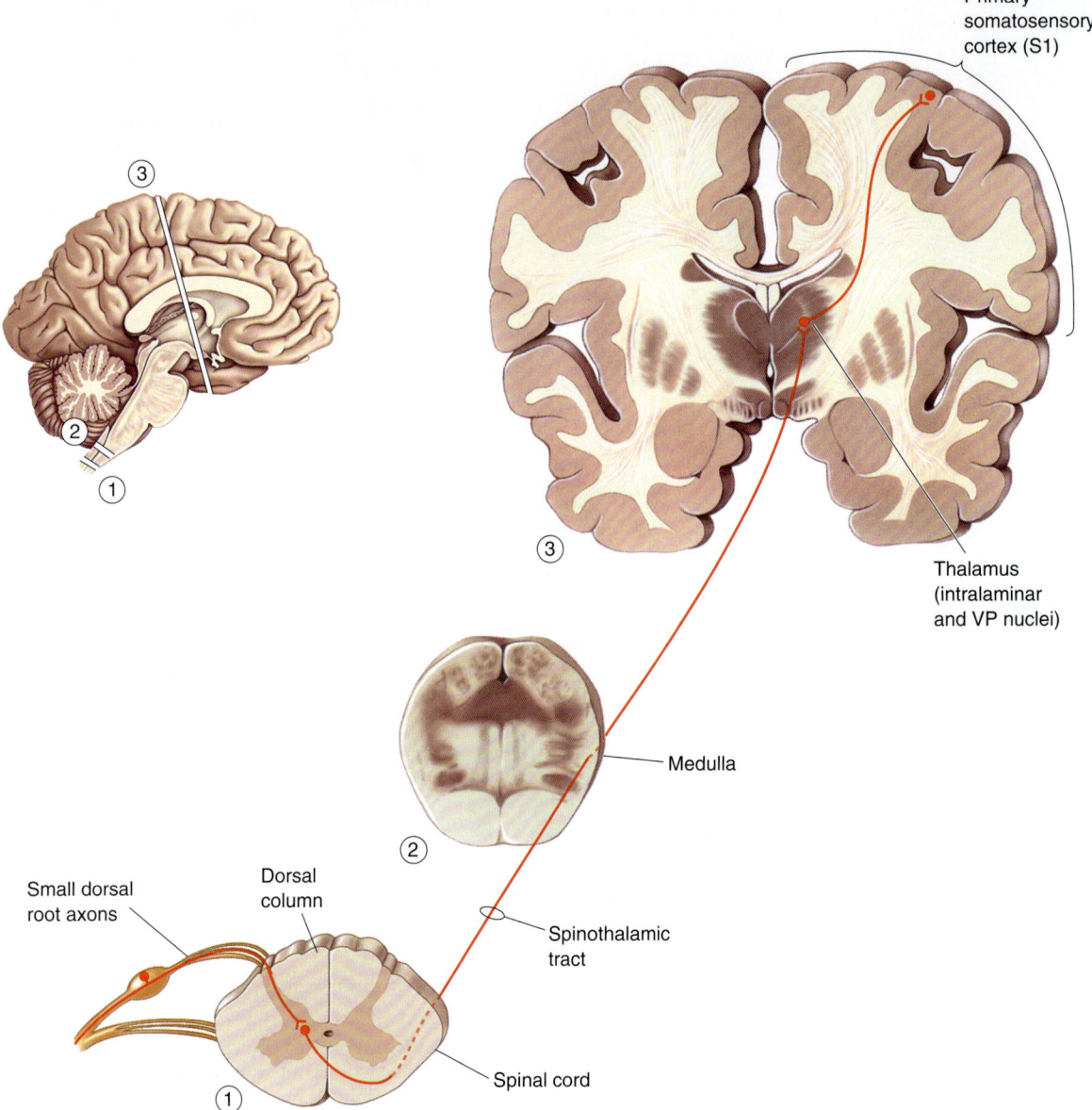

Figure 1-5. The spinothalamic pathway. This is the major route by which pain and temperature information ascend to the cerebral cortex. (From Bear MF, Connors BW, Paradiso MA. *Neuroscience: Exploring the Brain.* 4th ed. Philadelphia, PA: Wolters Kluwer; 2016.)

efficacy of endogenous pain-control systems and the integration of nociceptive input.[216,217] For example, estradiol potentiates ASICs function and also BK signaling, accounting for at least some of the observed sex difference in responsiveness to nociceptive stimuli, with females being more sensitive.[218,219] One method of potentiation is the increase in the density of cell-surface receptors by the method of transcription, or the synthesis of more receptor molecules, which are moved to the cell surface by a process of exocytosis. The action of estrogen is rapid, however, occurring over a matter of seconds, indicating a different mechanism of action than gene transcription.[220] Second-messenger signaling pathways for the induction of mechanical hyperalgesia are estrogen-dependent. This topic is discussed in greater detail in Chapter 4 on perpetuating factors.

3.4. The Extracellular Milieu

The extracellular milieu contains inflammatory mediators and chemokines produced by immune system cells. Immune cells act on cell-surface receptors through these mediators. Individual neurotrophic factors released by immune system cells act on different subpopulations of nociceptors, contributing to specific pain syndromes. These mediators are the current or potential targets of therapeutic agents, such as nonsteroidal anti-inflammatory drugs, for PG (Figure 1-6). The extracellular matrix is a ligand for cell surface receptors called integrins that uniquely signal both from inside the cell to the extracellular matrix and from the extracellular matrix into the cell. Inhibiting specific integrins, eg, blocking antibodies, selectively attenuates mechanical hyperalgesia induced by specific proinflammatory cytokines. The extracellular matrix can also concentrate chemokines and neuropeptides to present them to their cell-surface receptors.

Supporting cells actively participate in the nociceptive process. Glial cell-line-derived neurotrophic factors are upregulated in the presence of pain. Glial cells in the central nervous system that express transient receptor potential (TRP) ion channels are important mediators of pain sensation; however, glial cells are also found in the periphery, where they tightly enwrap DRG neurons. Glial cells in the peripheral nervous system are referred to as satellite glial cells.[221] They have the potential for regulating neuronal excitability through the release of mediators such as

Box 1-3 The stages of peripheral nociception

Stimuli	Extracorporeal
	  Thermal
	  Mechanical
	  Chemical
	Endogenous (Extracellular Milieu)
	  Injury
	  Inflammation

Cell-surface detection	Receptors
	  Voltage-gated ion channels
	  G-Protein-coupled receptors

Transduction	Conversion of stimuli to action potentials

Modulation	Satellite glial cells
	Facilitation or inhibition
	  Cell membrane
	  Intracellular
	  Dorsal horn
	Estrogen
	Descending inhibitory system

Transmission	Afferent nerve fiber to
	  Dorsal root ganglion neuron
	Dorsal root ganglion neuron to dorsal
	  Horn neuron

Sensitization	Neuroplastic changes (transcription)
Chronic pain	Transcription Sensitization

interleulkin-1β and other cytokines, and ATP that bind to purinergic receptors on the cell membrane.[221-224] Of interest is that a release of ATP and the activation of purinergic P2 receptors, specifically $P2X_7$, recruits phagocytes, including neutrophils, macrophages, and dendritic cells (DCs) to the site of injury. The activation of $P2X_7$ receptors increased the motility of DCs, which was further amplified by pannexin 1 channels. In addition, pannexin 1 increased the permeability of the plasma membrane, leading to an additional ATP release.[225]

As mentioned previously, the detection of nociceptive stimuli begins at the cell-surface membrane of the peripheral nerve ending, where a variety of receptors are located. These receptor families, which respond to one or more potentially noxious mechanical, thermal, and chemical stimuli, are critical to the process not only of nociception, but also to the process of sensitization wherein nociceptive impulses are amplified and prolonged, resulting in hyperalgesia and allodynia, and chronic pain states. Key to the excitation of the peripheral nerve ending is the binding of ligands or other mediators like protons to specific cell-surface or ionotropic receptors. Different receptor types contribute to different types of pain, and excite discrete groups of neurons in laminae I, II, and V in the DH (Figure 1-4).

Peripheral primary afferent nociceptors have a particular ability to be sensitized. Repeated input of nociceptive stimuli lowers the threshold to excitation and thus enhances and prolongs the response to stimulation, a function relevant to both inflammatory and neuropathic pain syndromes. However, nociceptors that transduce pressure (and touch and special senses such as vision, taste, and smell) desensitize with repeated stimulation. Nociceptor sensitization involves second-messenger signaling pathways like cyclic adenosine monophosphate (cAMP)/protein kinase A and protein kinase C. Sodium, potassium, and calcium ion channel families are all involved in sensitization.

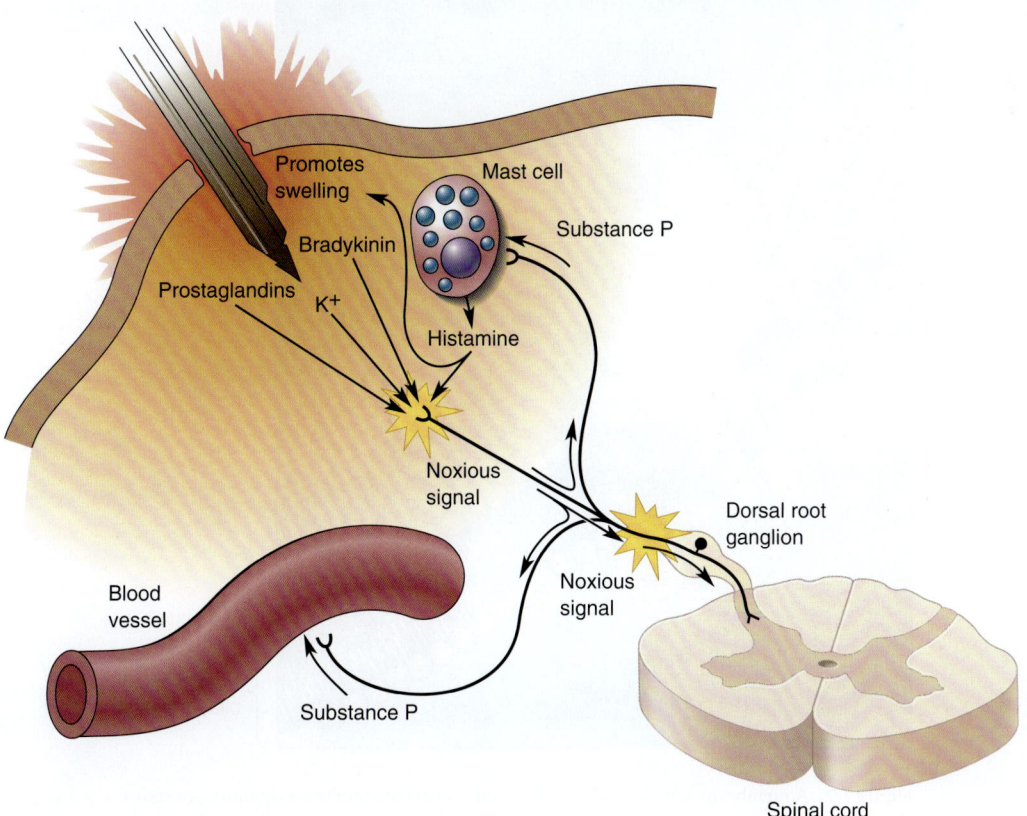

Figure 1-6. Peripheral chemical mediators of pain and hyperalgesia. (From Bear MF, Connors BW, Paradiso MA. *Neuroscience: Exploring the Brain*. 4th ed. Philadelphia, PA: Wolters Kluwer; 2016.)

The mechanisms include phosphorylation of the channels, a process that is faster than transcription, which requires new protein synthesis, and transcription that inserts a newly synthesized ion or other channel receptor molecule into the plasma membrane. A calcium-dependent exocytotic insertion of TRPV1 receptors to the neuronal plasma membrane is one such mechanism that increases the neuronal excitability.[226] Additionally, there are nociceptors that become responsive only to mechanical stimulation when exposed to inflammatory mediators.[227,228] Modulation of nociceptive input occurs not only at the peripheral terminal of the afferent neuron, but also at the neuronal level in the DRG.[229]

There are categorized nociceptors in various tissues that are based on their responses to different ligands. The skin, for example, has two main subtypes of nociceptors. One subtype consists of peptidergic afferents that operate via neuropeptides like substance P and CGRP, and respond to painful heat stimuli. The other subtype consists of nonpeptidergic afferents that are primarily mechanoreceptors. Both use L-glutamate as their primary excitatory neurotransmitter in their DH synaptic connections to second-order neurons and interneurons.

Families of membrane receptors respond to one or more types of stimuli. When activated, a receptor will be open to the passage of certain ions, like sodium or potassium, resulting in the generation of an action potential. One such family of membrane receptors is the ligand-gated TRP nonselective ion channel family that detects all three types of potential nociceptive stimuli and are therefore called polymodal receptors.[230,231] They play a crucial role in pathologic pain perception and were first described as the receptors of capsaicin.[232] They are only one of many types of ion channels (Figure 1-7) that convert sensory stimuli into nociceptive signals. There are 6 TRP subfamilies and 28 nonselective cation channels (TRPV1–6, TRPM1–8, TRPC1–7, TRPA1, TRPP1–3, and TRPML1–3).[233] TRP ion channels are also involved in the transduction of chemical stimuli. TRPV1 is expressed in trigeminal and dorsal root sensory ganglia, and also outside the nervous system, for example, in the gastrointestinal tract and the kidneys.[234] Of interest is that oxytocin can reduce pain via TRPV1 receptors, which implies that TRPV1 is also an ionotropic oxytocin receptor.[235]

Other such membrane receptors include the ASIC family that detects protons in the extracellular milieu,[236,237] and Piezo cation channels that detect mechanical stimuli.[238] There are six known ASIC receptors, namely, ASIC1a and ASIC1b, ASIC2a and ASIC2b, ASIC3, and ASIC4.[239] TRPV1 ion channels and ASIC3 are likely to participate in the development and maintenance of prolonged secondary allodynia and hyperalgesia.[240] Neuroimmune interactions, critical for the development of chronic pain, also play a role in the development of both peripheral and central sensitization. ASIC receptors are activated where the pH in the extracellular milieu drops below normal, even in the absence of tissue damage.

Piezo channels sense light touch, proprioception, and vascular blood flow, and they open in response to mechanical stimuli, although many aspects of their channel function remain unknown.[238,241] There are two types of Piezo channels. Piezo 1 channels are activated by fluid pressure and primarily expressed in nonsensory tissues such as the kidneys and red blood cells. They are involved in red blood cell homeostasis.[241] Piezo 2 channels are located in sensory tissues, such as DRG sensory neurons and Merkel cells, and are involved with light touch and proprioception (Figure 1-8).[238,241] The Piezo channels are sensitized by G protein-coupled pathways, linked to the BK receptor and the cAMP receptor likely through the activation of protein kinase A and protein kinase C. They are excitatory channels that allow Ca^{2+} to enter the cell, which may lead to activating intracellular Ca^{2+} signaling pathways.[241] There are other ligand-gated ion and G-protein-coupled receptors that are also involved in nociceptive sensory perception. They respond to a variety of chemical stimuli, including purines and PG.[242] The activation of these cell-surface receptors converts nociceptive stimuli to nerve impulses.

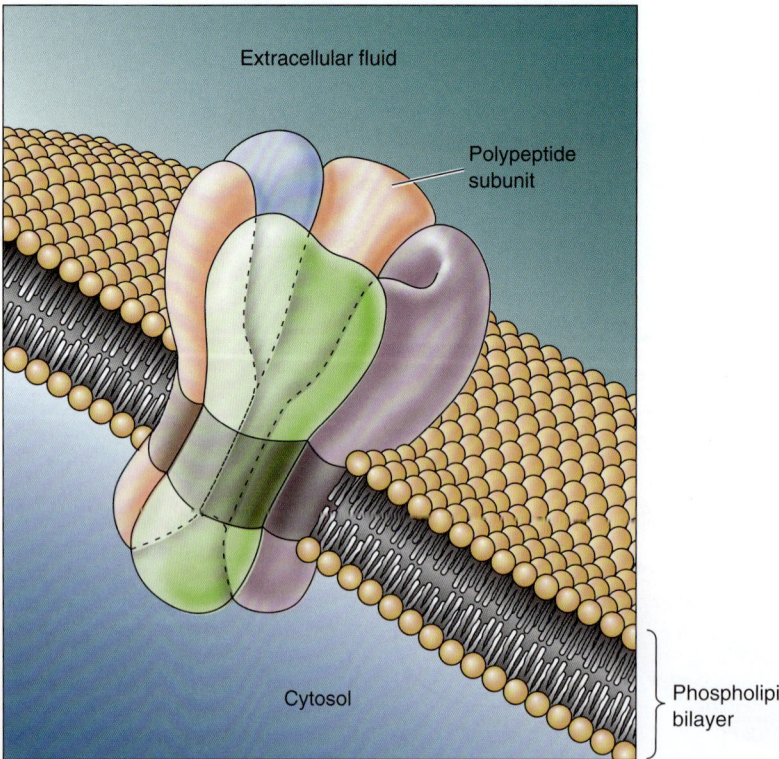

Figure 1-7. A membrane ion channel. Ion channels consist of membrane-spanning proteins that assemble to form a pore. In this example, the channel protein has five polypeptide subunits. Each subunit has a hydrophobic surface region (shaded) that readily associates with the phospholipid bilayer. (From Bear MF, Connors BW, Paradiso MA. *Neuroscience: Exploring the Brain.* 4th ed. Philadelphia, PA: Wolters Kluwer; 2016.)

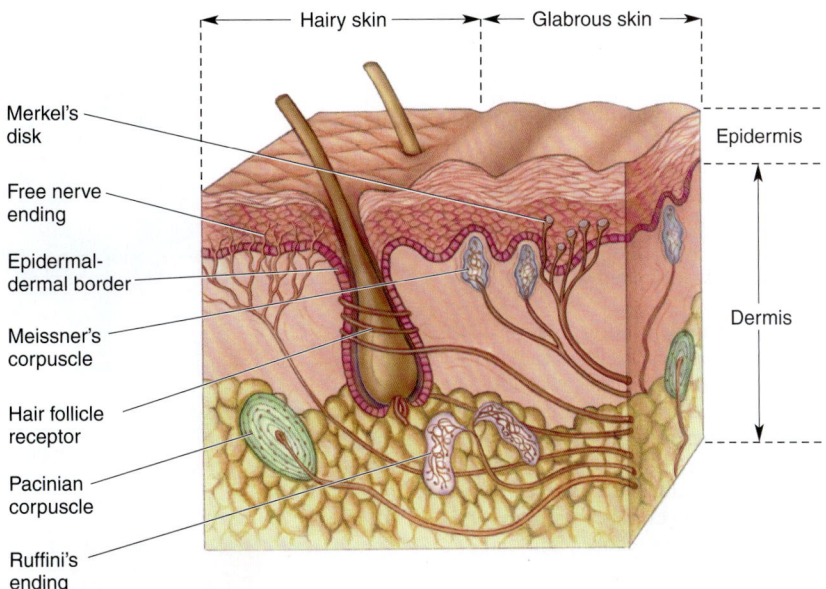

Figure 1-8. Somatic sensory receptors in the skin. Hairy skin and glabrous skin have a variety of sensory receptors within the dermal and epidermal layers. Each receptor has an axon and, except for free nerve endings, all of them have associated nonneural tissues. (From Bear MF, Connors BW, Paradiso MA. *Neuroscience: Exploring the Brain*. 4th ed. Philadelphia, PA: Wolters Kluwer; 2016.)

The activation of specific ion channels is not a simple, one-step process. The state or availability of such cell-surface receptors as TRP ion channels or ASICs is enhanced or inhibited by interaction with other ion channels that can be activated by extracellular stimuli or intracellular calcium.[243-245] Different receptors respond to different stimuli or at different thresholds:
- Piezo receptors are relevant to the functioning of mechanoreceptors.[246,247]
- TRPV1 responds to heat, low pH, to capsaicin, and probably also to mechanical stimuli. NGF promotes chronic pain in humans and its effect is mediated through TRPV1 receptors.[248]
- Serotonin receptors exist on peripheral nerve terminals as well as the central nervous system, where they activate inhibitory interneurons. The activation of peripheral 5-HT1B, 5-HT2A, and 5-HT3 receptors inhibits mechanical hyperalgesia.[249]
- The P2Y receptor agonist uridine-5″ triphosphate enhances the activity of the ASICs, which sense extracellular protons.[250]

3.5. Nociception and Modulation

Modulation at the Cellular Level

Modulation either amplifies or inhibits the response to nociceptive stimulation, which occurs at all levels of transduction and transmission. With respect to intracellular modulation, cAMP was the first intracellular signaling molecule implicated in nociceptor sensitization. The pathway is activated by a G-protein-couples receptor. When coupled to a stimulatory G-protein, it activates adenyl cyclase, leading to the production of cAMP and the downstream activation of protein kinase A (PKA). PKA, in turn, phosphorylates voltage-gated ion channels and thereby regulates neuronal excitability (Figure 1-9). There are a number of such second-messenger families. One particular second-messenger family is mediated by the epsilon isoform of protein kinase C (PKC) that is found on almost all DRG

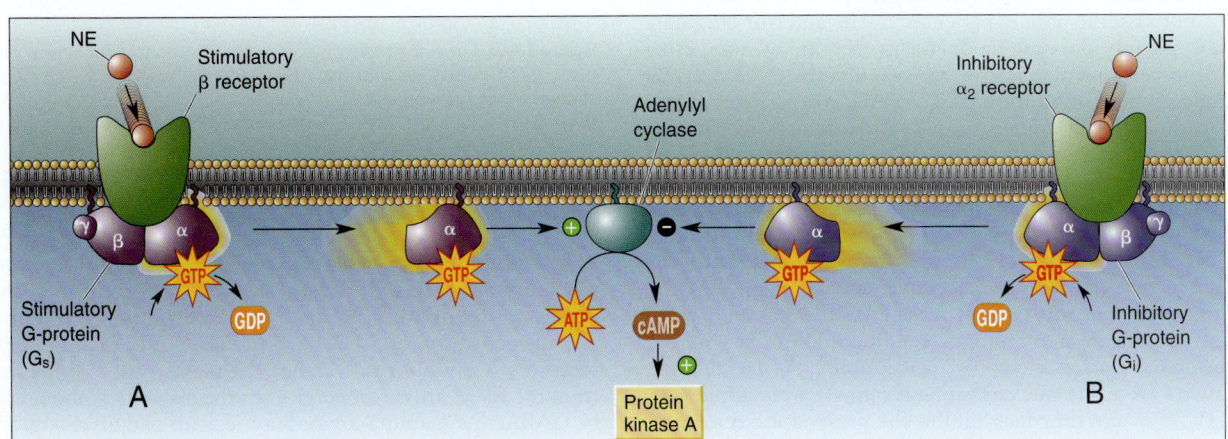

Figure 1-9. The stimulation and inhibition of adenylyl cyclase by different G-proteins. (A) Binding of norepinephrine (NE) to the receptor activates G_s, which, in turn, activates adenylyl cyclase. Adenylyl cyclase generates cyclic adenosine monophosphate, which activates the downstream enzyme protein kinase A. (B) Binding of NE to the 2 receptor activates G_i, which inhibits adenylyl cyclase. (From Bear MF, Connors BW, Paradiso MA. *Neuroscience: Exploring the Brain*. 4th ed. Philadelphia, PA: Wolters Kluwer; 2016.)

neurons, but only a subpopulation of DRG neurons is activated by it in pain. Reichling et al described a potential mechanism of neuronal plasticity in peripheral neurons in response to the exposure of primary afferent nerve fibers that have been exposed to an acute inflammatory insult followed by a low concentration of an inflammatory mediator.[3] They called this "hyperalgesic priming." It is also dependent on the activation of the epsilon isoform of PKC and a switch in intracellular signaling pathways from PKA alone to PKA and PKC together. The activation of other intracellular protein kinases may also play a role, for example in the neuroplastic changes associated with late-phase long-term potentiation.

Intracellular organelles, such as mitochondria (Figure 1-10), play a role in nociceptor sensitization, especially in the peripheral terminal, which is at a far distance from the cell body. The peripheral terminal has a high concentration of mitochondria that regulate intracellular calcium, aerobic energy metabolism, generation of reactive oxygen species (ROS), and apoptosis. There are five mitochondrial electron transport chain complexes and the inhibition of any of these reduces pain in a number of pain syndromes, including HIV syndrome, cancer, and diabetic neuropathic pain models.[251]

Higher-level organization at the cellular level plays an important part in nociceptor excitation, by increasing the likelihood of depolarizing the membrane and initiating an action potential. This includes multimolecular complexes in the plasma membrane, intracellular organelles in the cytoplasm, such as the mitochondria, Golgi apparatus, endoplasmic reticulum, and cytoskeleton (Figure 1-11A and B). Micro-domains in the plasma membrane extend the effect of a single ion channel being activated by phosphorylation. A small depolarization produced by a transducer can be amplified, for example, in response to a specific stimulus that leads to single ion channel activation. A micro-domain acts by bringing molecular elements of a signaling pathway together, excludes elements of other pathways, and thereby produces a very efficient signaling complex, also known as a "signalosome." There are about 200 different types of these signalosome components with extensive interconnectivity pathways, which is why the signalosome complex is more accurately described as "a non-linear network of interacting circuits."[192]

Top-Down Modulation

Throughout the central nervous system are many opportunities to modify nociception and pain messages. Modulation can be facilitatory or inhibitory.[252] The main control system from higher brain areas to the DH, commonly referred to as the descending inhibitory system, influences not only pain levels but also the pain experience.[253] The anterior cingulate cortex and amygdala can modulate nociception by interacting with the periaqueductal gray (PAG) to activate descending opioidergic pain inhibition.[254] The PAG, rostral ventral medial medulla (RVM), nucleus raphe, and interactions between these systems play a key role in the inhibition of pain from the brain to the spinal cord.[255-257] The PAG does express mu-opiate receptors, enkephalin and beta-endorphin, which appear to contribute to the PAG's endogenous antinociceptive capability (Figure 1-12).[258] CCK, a peptide found in the PAG, can reduce the antinociceptive activity of the PAG.[259] Of interest is that substance P in the PAG also has an antinociceptive effect by activating descending inhibition, whereas in the spinal cord, it increases nociception.[260,261] Descending pathways from the nucleus raphe terminate in laminae I, II, and IV,[262] where they may inhibit the presynaptic release of substance P, among others.[154]

The control of pain transmission is a bidirectional process.[263] For example, descending excitatory pathways from the brain can activate serotonin receptors, which may exacerbate spinal mechanisms of pain through the activation of spinal TRPV1 terminals.[264-268] However, serotonergic projections can also

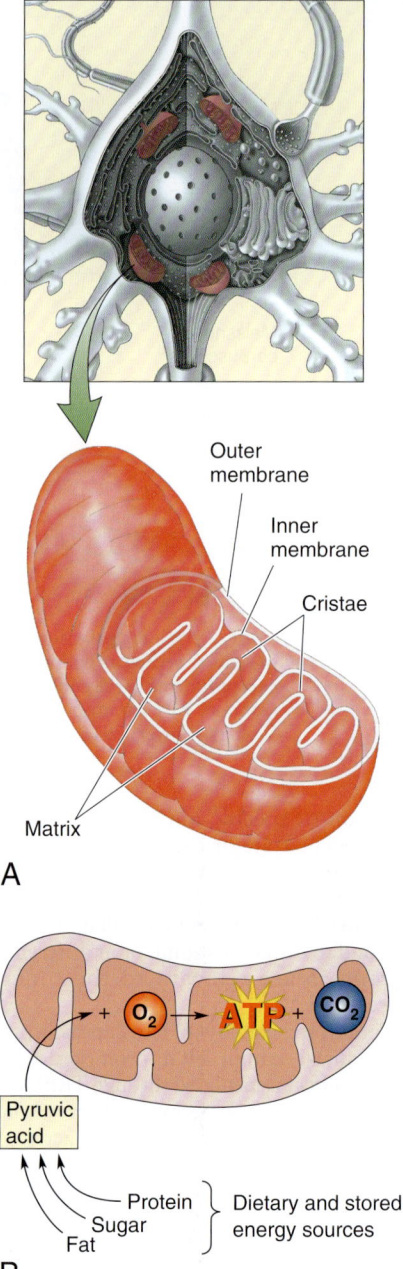

Figure 1-10. The role of mitochondria. (A) Components of a mitochondrion. (B) Cellular respiration. Adenosine triphosphate is the energy currency that fuels biochemical reactions in neurons. (From Bear MF, Connors BW, Paradiso MA. *Neuroscience: Exploring the Brain.* 4th ed. Philadelphia, PA: Wolters Kluwer; 2016.)

trigger inhibition, dependent upon which subtypes of serotonin receptors are targeted. Several studies have confirmed that the activation of 5-HT2A and 5-HT3 receptors is facilitatory, and the activation of 5-HT1A, 5-HT1B, 5-HT1D, and 5-HT7 receptors is inhibitory.[269-272] Approximately 20% of neurons from the RVM are serotonergic, but the majority is thought to be GABAergic (gamma-aminobutyric acid) and glycinergic.[273] It is not yet known how the RVM modulates the spinal levels of serotonin. When the descending inhibitory system is inhibited, pain may become chronic.[274-276]

Characteristic of chronic pain conditions, such as central neuropathic pain, MPS, fibromyalgia, and complex regional pain syndrome, is a dysfunction of the descending inhibitory system

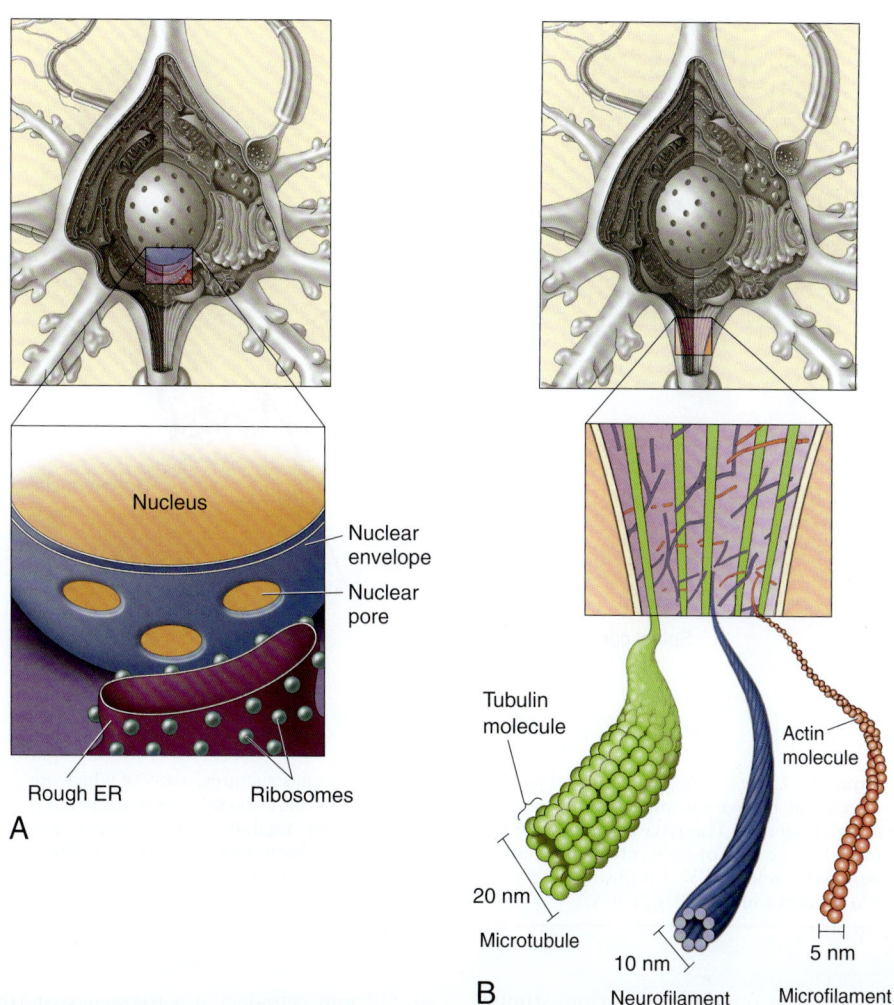

Figure 1-11. A, Rough endoplasmic reticulum. B, Components of the cytoskeleton. The arrangement of microtubules, neurofilaments, and microfilaments gives the neuron its characteristic shape. (From Bear MF, Connors BW, Paradiso MA. *Neuroscience: Exploring the Brain.* 4th ed. Philadelphia, PA: Wolters Kluwer; 2016.)

to modulate pain, which has a profound impact on the degree of chronic pain an individual will experience.[277,278] Bannister and Dickenson emphasized that top-down processing pathways do exert significant controls over spinal neuronal processes, mostly through the actions of norepinephrine (NE) and 5-HT.[279] NE reuptake inhibitors such as tramadol, tapentadol, or duloxetine can be helpful in reducing pain. Nuseir and Proudfit confirmed that noradrenergic descending projections can also exert a bidirectional control of nociceptive inputs.[280]

A specific mechanism of top-down inhibition is referred to as diffuse noxious inhibitory controls (DNICs), which require a noxious input that can modulate spinal wide dynamic neurons through the subnucleus reticularis dorsalis, caudal medulla, and nucleus raphe magnus.[281-286] It is conceivable that the therapeutic pain-reducing effect of TrP dry needling, which is often perceived as a noxious stimulus, may activate the DNIC system. Of interest is that there are genetic differences in DNIC. For example, non-Hispanic white individuals experienced a significantly greater reduction in pain than African Americans.[287] Furthermore, a systematic review demonstrated that male subjects may have a more efficient DNIC than females,[288] although individual studies do not always confirm this observation.[289] In conclusion, altered neurophysiologic processing is a major factor in persistent pain problems. How to assess this altered processing will be reviewed in the next section.

QUANTITATIVE SENSORY TESTING

Carol A. Courtney

Establishing the relevance of altered somatosensory findings during patient examination may be challenging, particularly when a condition has progressed from acute to chronic stages (Figure 1-13). Quantitative sensory testing (QST) refers to a set of neurologic assessments that expands upon the classic neurologic examination, providing objective or "quantitative" measures of various sensory modalities for the purpose of identifying altered neurophysiologic processing.[290] Although QST is not considered a diagnostic test for a particular disease entity, this set of tools may be valuable in the mechanism-based diagnosis of pain.[291] Diagnosis, by definition, directs treatment. Therefore, identifying aberrant pain mechanisms and applying interventions accordingly may allow for more effective management strategies for acute and chronic painful conditions. QST may identify both "negative" (diminished neural function) and "positive" (heightened neural function) signs.[292] Standardized QST performed by trained examiners has been found to have good test–retest (>75%) and interobserver reliability over 2 days.[293] The German Research Network on Neuropathic Pain (DFNS) has developed a standardized battery of tests for the identification of neuropathic pain.[290] This protocol, as well as others, provides a reference for the continuing development of

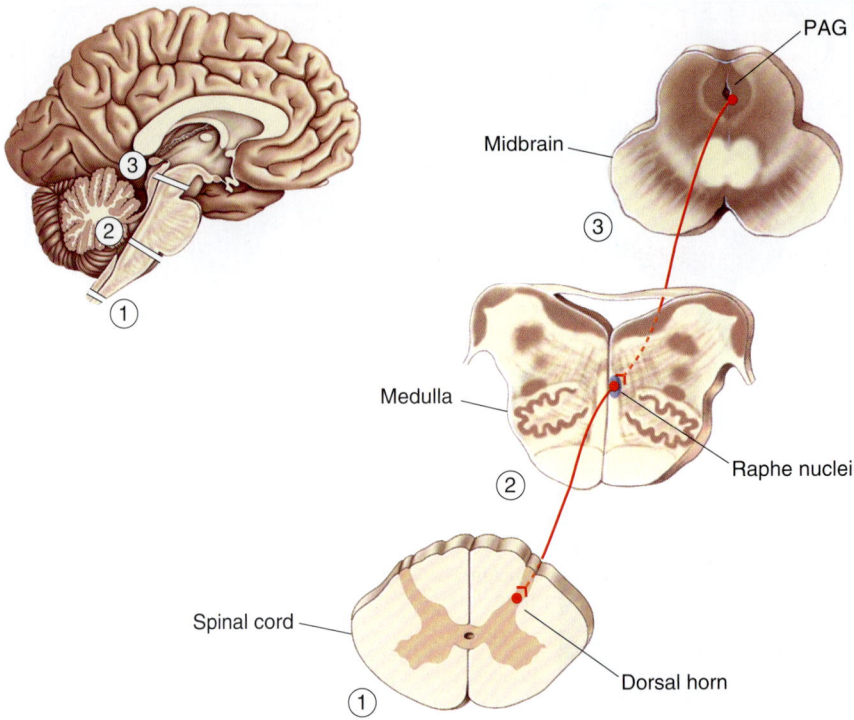

Figure 1-12. Descending pain-control pathways. A variety of brain structures, many of which are affected by behavioral state, can influence activity within the periaqueductal gray matter (PAG) of the midbrain. The PAG can influence the raphe nuclei of the medulla, which, in turn, can modulate the flow of nociceptive information through the dorsal horns of the spinal cord. (From Bear MF, Connors BW, Paradiso MA. *Neuroscience: Exploring the Brain.* 4th ed. Philadelphia, PA: Wolters Kluwer; 2016.)

QST tools. These tools apply noxious and nonnoxious stimuli to assess the function of cutaneous and deep tissue neural receptors. Measures can be considered "static," representing the present, nonprovoked state of the nervous system, or "dynamic," where a painful stimulus is applied in a specific manner to facilitate nociceptive processing. QST measures can be grouped as follows:

1. MECHANICAL OR TACTILE DETECTION THRESHOLD

Cutaneous mechanical or tactile detection threshold is usually assessed with Von Frey hairs or Semmes-Weinstein monofilaments, which are gradated in pliability such that known quantities of varying degrees of force (commonly 0.07-0.4 g of force) are applied through the tips of the monofilaments (rounded tip, 0.5 mm in diameter). The monofilament is applied slowly until the filament bows slightly. The stimulus is maintained for approximately 1.5 seconds (Figure 1-14). The most common form of testing used is the method of limits: different threshold determinations are made with a series of ascending and descending stimulus intensities. The subject is instructed to close the eyes during the test procedure and to indicate a stimulus in the test site is perceived. By calculating the geometric mean of these series (usually 5), the mean threshold value is determined.[290]

2. VIBRATION DETECTION THRESHOLD

The ability to perceive vibration is assessed either by applying an increasing or decreasing amplitude of vibratory stimulus. The biothesiometer delivers vibration via an oscillating vibratory tip (13 mm cylinder) at a frequency of 100 Hz at the site of application, which typically is a bony prominence. Vibration amplitude is increased by 1 V/s at the site until the participant perceives the vibration sensation.[294] Excellent intrarater and test–retest reliability has been reported.[295] The DFNS protocol suggests the use of a Rydel–Seiffer tuning fork (64 Hz, 8/8 scale) placed over a bony prominence (Figure 1-15). Vibration threshold is determined when the perception of vibration is extinguished as the vibratory amplitude diminishes.[290] The Rydel–Seiffer tuning fork has been found to be reliable and valid.[296]

3. THERMAL DETECTION AND PAIN THRESHOLD

Thermal quantitative sensory measures, such as heat or cold detection thresholds, or heat pain/cold pain detection thresholds, have been used to identify lesions in somatosensory pathways. Thermal QST is commonly used in the assessment of neuropathic pain.[297] Increased expression of cold sensing ion channels, the TRPM8 channels, has been demonstrated in an animal model of chronic nerve injury, and is believed to be a source of cold hypersensitivity.[298] Similarly, heat hypersensitivity is thought to be mediated, in part, by increased expression of the TRPV1 channel.[299] Warm detection threshold is defined as the first sensation of warmth, and cold detection threshold as the first sensation of cold. Heat and cold pain thresholds are defined as the change in sensation from warmth or cold to one of heat or cold pain, respectively. The most commonly used tools for thermal QST are TSA-II (MEDOC, Israel) or MSA (SOMEDIC, Sweden) equipment; however, clinicians have used an inexpensive alternative by applying the end of warm or cold objects such as test tubes to the skin. These measures, however, provide only a gross assessment of thermal sensitivity.

Chapter 1: Pain Sciences and Myofascial Pain 15

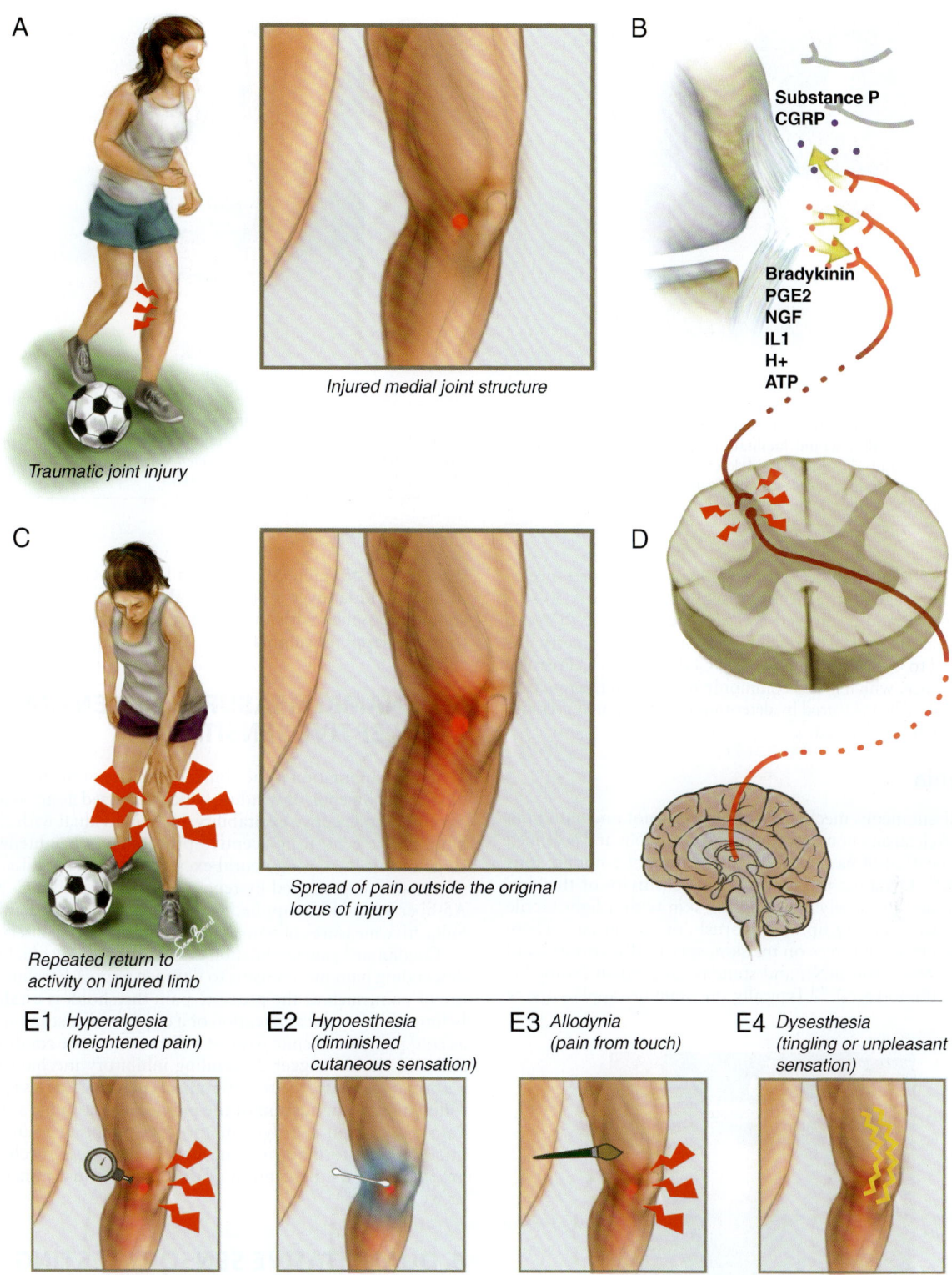

Figure 1-13. Peripheral and central sensitization. A, Injury to the knee joint. B, Nociceptive response to the injury. C, Peripheral sensitization. D, Secondary hyperalgesia. E1-E4, Quantitative sensory testing to differentiate peripheral and central sensitization.

4. MECHANICAL PAIN THRESHOLD

Cutaneous mechanical pain threshold is assessed using custom-made weighted pinprick stimuli as a set of different pinprick mechanical stimulators with fixed stimulus intensities (flat contact area: 0.2 mm diameter). The stimulators are usually applied at a rate of 2 seconds on, 2 seconds off in an ascending and descending order, determining which of the stimuli are perceived as painful. The final threshold is the geometric mean of five series of ascending and descending stimuli.

4.1. Mechanical Pain Sensitivity

Deep tissue mechanical pain sensitivity is commonly assessed via pressure pain thresholds, measured with an algometer (Figure 1-16). Pressure is applied with the algometer typically via a 1-cm^2 probe, which preferentially stimulates deep tissue, such as muscle, tendon or joints, rather than cutaneous receptors.[300] The algometer is applied perpendicular to the tissue at a constant rate of approximately 30 kPa/s. Subjects are instructed

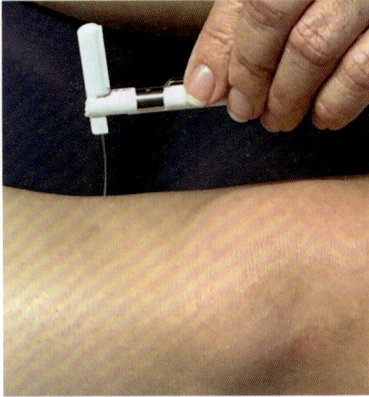

Figure 1-14. Mechanical detection threshold is measured with a standardized set of monofilaments that exert forces upon bending between 0.25 and 512 mN. The contact area of monofilaments is rounded to avoid sharp edges that would facilitate nociceptor activation. Using the "method of limits," five threshold determinations were made, each with a series of ascending and descending stimulus intensities. The final threshold was the geometric mean of these five series.

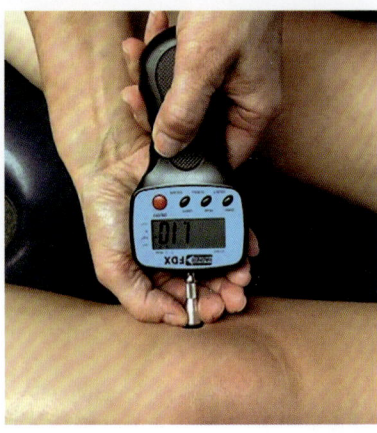

Figure 1-16. Pressure pain threshold is determined using an algometer with a probe area of 1 cm². Three trials of ascending stimulus intensity are applied with a slowly increasing ramp of 50 kPa/s. (From Bear MF, Connors BW, Paradiso MA. *Neuroscience: Exploring the Brain*. 4th ed. Philadelphia, PA: Wolters Kluwer; 2016.)

to press a switch when the sensation changes from pressure to pain. The average of three trials is usually calculated. A 30-second resting period is allowed between each measure to avoid temporal summation. The reliability of pressure algometry has been found to be high (ICC 0.91, 95% CI 0.82-0.97).[301] Pressure pain tolerance, which is less commonly reported in the research literature, may be measured by determining the maximal pressure stimulus that is tolerated.[302]

Allodynia

Tactile or cutaneous mechanical allodynia is not uncommon in musculoskeletal and nonmusculoskeletal conditions and is defined as the evocation of pain with the application of a nonnoxious stimulus.[303] Dynamic mechanical pain sensitivity of the skin is determined by slowly brushing the skin with a light tactile stimulus, such as a Q-tip, a soft brush, or cotton ball. These devices exert small forces on the skin, specifically, cotton wool (3 mN), Q-tip (100 mN), and standardized brush (Somedic, Sweden: 200-400 mN).[304] Typically, the examiner applies one of three tactile stimuli to an area of at least a 2-cm-long skin area of an individual over a period of about 2 seconds. All stimuli should be applied with an interstimulus interval of 10 seconds, to avoid temporal summation.

5. DYNAMIC MEASURES OF CENTRAL NOCICEPTIVE SENSITIVITY

Temporal summation is the clinical correlate of the neurophysiologic phenomenon of windup, which is defined as an escalation of central nociceptive excitability. In an individual with chronic pain, where central nociceptive processing is heightened, the slope of this increasing neural excitability is steeper. Temporal summation is produced by repetitive high threshold C- and/or Aδ-fiber stimulation applied at a frequency of less than 3 Hz. Subjective measures of pain are collected at specific intervals.[303]

Conditioned pain modulation examines the ability of inhibitory descending pain mechanisms to dampen pain. A baseline measure of pain, such as the pressure pain threshold, is established before and after the application of a conditioning stimulus, such as cold pain or ischemic pain, at a distant site. The conditioning stimulus should trigger descending inhibitory mechanisms. In a normal response, the test stimulus is perceived as less painful following the application of the painful conditioning stimulus. Pain modulation is a dynamic process, adapting to incoming nociceptive information as needed. When these mechanisms are impaired, the perception of the test stimulus is unchanged or worsened.[303]

6. QUANTITATIVE SENSORY TESTING AND TRIGGER POINTS

As an example, a recent study compared several QST, including thermal detection threshold, thermal pain thresholds, mechanical detection thresholds, mechanical pain thresholds, vibration detection thresholds, and pressure pain thresholds between latent TrPs and its referred pain area in the extensor radialis carpi brevis muscle and contralateral mirror sites.[305] This study found that latent TrPs showed mechanical hyperesthesia, pressure pain hyperalgesia, and vibration hypoesthesia when compared with a contralateral mirror non-TrP, whereas the referred pain area showed pinprick and vibration hypoesthesia compared with the contralateral mirror nonreferred pain area. Interestingly, thermal pain and detection thresholds were not different between

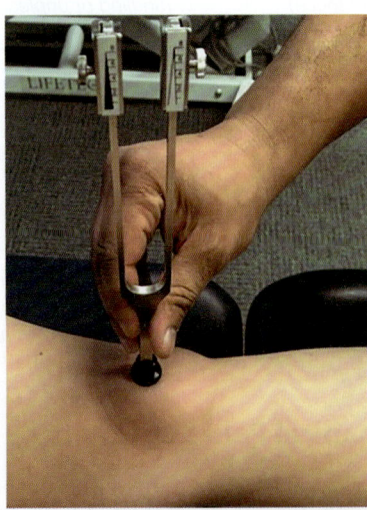

Figure 1-15. Vibration is initiated by squeezing and quickly releasing the tines. The tuning fork is then placed on a bony prominence. Vibration Perception Threshold is determined as a disappearance threshold with three stimulus repetitions.

TrP/contralateral mirror point and their respectively referred pain areas, suggesting that myofascial pain is mostly related to hyperalgesia to pressure pain.

MYOFASCIAL PAIN

Jan Dommerholt

As Wall and Woolf established, muscle nociceptive afferents are very effective in inducing neuroplastic changes in the spinal DH.[306] Similar to other pain syndromes, myofascial pain activates specific cortical structures, including the anterior cingulate gyrus.[307,308] In chronic pain conditions, many parts of the brain are involved, and it has been suggested that "the brain is enslaved by pain."[128] Many of the pain mechanisms described in this chapter apply to myofascial pain, but in addition to contributing to pain, TrPs have significant implications for motor function, movement patterns, and range of motion.[101,102] In clinical practice, pain science, biomechanics, and clinical reasoning should be combined to achieve the optimal outcome.[309]

1. A BRIEF HISTORICAL REVIEW

Travell is commonly considered as the first physician to focus on myofascial pain and TrPs, although several others had already described similar phenomena many years earlier as reported by Simons and by Baldry.[310-314] In 1940, Steindler introduced the term "trigger point,"[315] which Travell and Rinzler modified into "myofascial trigger point."[316] Travell was strongly influenced by the work of Kellgren, a British rheumatologist affiliated with the University College Hospital in London, who published a series of papers on referred pain from muscles.[317-320] In 1952, Travell and Rinzler described typical referred pain patterns from 32 muscles,[316] followed by many other papers,[321-333] and eventually, the publication of the Trigger Point Manual, coauthored by Simons.[4,5,49] The Trigger Point Manual has been translated into many other languages.

In 1981, Simons and Travell conceptualized the "energy crisis hypothesis," which assumed that trauma and subsequent damage to the sarcoplasmic reticulum or the muscle cell membrane were ultimately responsible for the development of TrPs.[321] Damage would lead to an increase in intracellular Ca^{2+} concentration, increased activation of actin and myosin, a relative shortage of ATP, and an impaired calcium pump, which, in turn, would increase the intracellular calcium concentration even more, perpetuating the cycle. The energy crisis hypothesis was later incorporated into the integrated TrP hypothesis, which remains the most accepted and often cited hypothesis. As with most scientific explorations, the hypothesis has been modified and expanded several times and new hypotheses have been suggested.[63-72,140] This chapter introduces components of the integrated TrP hypothesis. Considering the complexity of this information, it will be extensively reviewed in more detail in Chapter 2.

2. IDENTIFYING TAUT BANDS AND TRIGGER POINTS

By definition, TrPs are located within taut bands, which are discrete bands of contractured muscle fibers that can be palpated, and visualized with sonography and magnetic resonance imaging, especially when combined with elastography.[334-345] Older studies did not show great inter- and intrarater reliability[346-349]; however, recent studies have demonstrated that taut bands and TrPs can be palpated reliably.[20,350-360]

When comparing the TrP region with the surrounding tissue, vibration amplitudes assessed with spectral Doppler were on average 27% lower,[337] which implies a greater than normal degree of stiffness compared with normal muscle tissue.[336]

The mechanism for the formation of muscle taut band is not yet completely explained, but it is likely that when a muscle is overloaded, in other words, when an applied load exceeds the capability of the muscle to respond adequately, taut bands may develop, particularly following unusual or excessive eccentric or concentric loading.[63,140] The formation of TrPs has been documented in computer operators and musicians, among others,[361-363] where submaximal contractions cause smaller motor units to be recruited before larger motor units and derecruited last without any substitution.[361,362] This has been described as the Cinderella Hypothesis with the additional application of Henneman's size principle.[364-367]

3. THE INTEGRATED HYPOTHESIS

3.1. Introduction

According to the integrated TrP hypothesis, abnormal depolarization of the postjunctional membrane of motor endplates may cause a localized hypoxic energy crisis associated with sensory and autonomic reflex arcs sustained by complex sensitization mechanisms.[65] Qerama et al described higher pain intensities and pain features similar to TrPs when noxious stimuli were applied to motor endplate areas compared with silent muscle sites.[368]

The Role of the Motor Endplate

The integrated TrP hypothesis postulates that TrPs are linked to dysfunctional motor endplates. Normally, when a nerve impulse from an alpha-motor neuron reaches the motor nerve terminal orthodromically, it will open voltage-gated Na^+ channels, which triggers an influx of Na^+ that depolarizes the terminal membrane and opens voltage-gated P-type Ca^{2+} channels. After Ca^{2+} enters the cell, a quantal, but graded, release occurs from the nerve terminal into the synaptic cleft of approximately 100 acetylcholine(ACh)-containing synaptic vesicles, ATP, 5HT, glutamate, and CGRP, among others (Figure 1-17).[369,370] Inhibitory neuronal receptors, including muscarinic, alpha 2- and beta-adrenoceptors, nitric oxide (NO) receptors, and purinergic P2Y receptors, among others, prevent an excessive release of ACh release,[369] and under normal circumstances, these inhibitory mechanisms should prevent the development of persistent contractures as seen in myofascial pain. The quantal ACh release

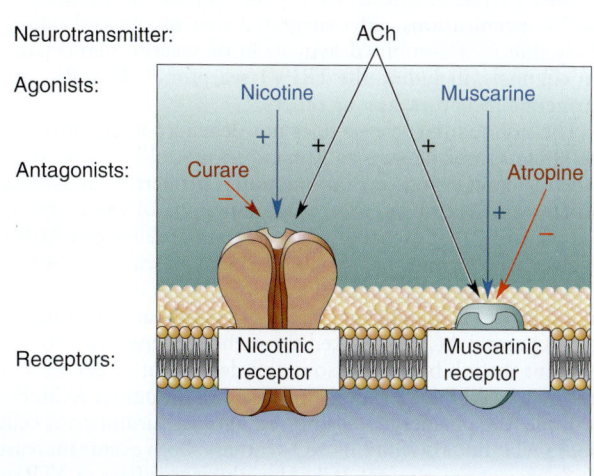

Figure 1-17. The neuropharmacology of cholinergic synaptic transmission. Sites on transmitter receptors can bind either the transmitter itself (ACh), an agonist that mimics the transmitter, or an antagonist that blocks the effects of the transmitter and agonists. (From Bear MF, Connors BW, Paradiso MA. *Neuroscience: Exploring the Brain*. 4th ed. Philadelphia, PA: Wolters Kluwer; 2016.)

is also modulated through second-messenger systems involving PKA and PKC. The neurotransmitter adenosine synchronizes the release of quantal release of ACh. A product of the breakdown of adenosine 5′ triphosphate, it acts at the inhibitory adenosine A1 and facilitatory A2a receptors. The activation of A1 receptors reduces the number of ACh molecules released in each quantum. An increase of intracellular Ca^{2+} in the nerve terminal activates the exocytotic process that is mediated by A2a receptors.

With a quantal release, ACh crosses the synaptic cleft following exocytosis and binds to acetylcholine receptors (AChRs) on the motor endplate. Acetylcholine is almost immediately partially diffused and partially hydrolyzed by acetylcholine esterase (AChE) into acetate and choline. The latter is reabsorbed into the nerve terminal, where, by combining choline and acetyl co-enzyme A from the mitochondria, it is synthesized into ACh via acetyltransferase. The release of ACh is modulated by the concentration of AChE (Figure 1-17). A soluble form of AChE prevents ACh from reaching the receptors and a second source, found within the synaptic clefts, removes ACh from the receptors binding sites. The inhibition of AChE will cause an accumulation of ACh in the synaptic cleft, which may stimulate motor nerve endings and tonically activate nAChRs (Figure 1-18). CGRP and an acidic environment also inhibit AChE. Following stimulation by ACh, nAChRs are temporarily inhibited.[371] The synthesis of AChE and nAChR involves ATP through P2Y1 nucleotide receptors.[372] The inhibition of AChE may also cause an increase of intracellular levels of Ca^{2+}, which likely contributes to the formation of taut bands. When Ca^{2+} is not removed from the cytosol, actin–myosin cross-bridges would remain. Removing Ca^{2+} by reuptake into the sarcoplasmic reticulum is an energy demanding process, which occurs via the Na^+/K^+-ATPase (sarcoendoplasmic reticulum ATPase) system.

Jafri speculated that ROS may be intricately involved in the TrP etiology.[66] He maintains that the role of Ca^{2+} has been undervalued. Although this will be discussed in more detail in Chapter 2, Jafri hypothesized that mechanical stress can trigger an excessive release of Ca^{2+} in muscles through so-called X-ROS signaling. Mechanical deformation of the microtubule network can activate NOX_2, which would produce ROS. The ROS oxidizes ryanodine receptors, leading to increases in Ca^{2+} release from the sarcoplasmic reticulum. The Ca^{2+} mobilization resulting from mechanical stretch through this pathway is referred to as X-ROS signaling. In skeletal muscles, X-ROS sensitizes Ca^{2+}-permeable sarcolemmal TRP channels, which may be a source of nociceptive input and inflammatory pain. Activating the TRPV1 receptor leads to a quick increase in intracellular Ca^{2+} concentrations. Jafri suggested that myofascial pain is likely due to a combined activation of several ligand-gated ion channels, including the TRPV1 receptor, ASIC3, BK, and purinergic receptors, among others.[66]

The nonquantal release does not depend on activation via the alpha-motor neuron and functions more like a fine regulator in maintaining several functional properties of skeletal muscles and various neurotrophic functions of the endplate. It is plausible that especially the nonquantal release of ACh is involved with creating taut bands seen in myofascial pain. Several neurotransmitters play a role in the regulation of ACh release. Presynaptic ATP blocks the release of quantal and nonquantal ACh. Quantal ACh is blocked through purinergic P2Y receptors, but the inhibition is also redox-dependent. A decrease in presynaptic ATP increases the release of nonquantal ACh. For example, the purinergic receptor antagonist suramin not only blocks ATP, but also inhibits NO synthase. Both events increase the release of nonquantal ACh. The inhibitory effect of ATP on the nonquantal release of ACh occurs through phospholipase C via metabotropic P2Y purinergic receptors.[373] Noteworthy is a recent rodent study that demonstrated that dry needling does reduce the levels of ACh and AChR, while increasing AChE.[374]

There are many possible mechanisms leading to an excessive quantal or nonquantal release of ACh, such as increased muscle tension, an increased sensitivity of nAChR, AChE insufficiency,

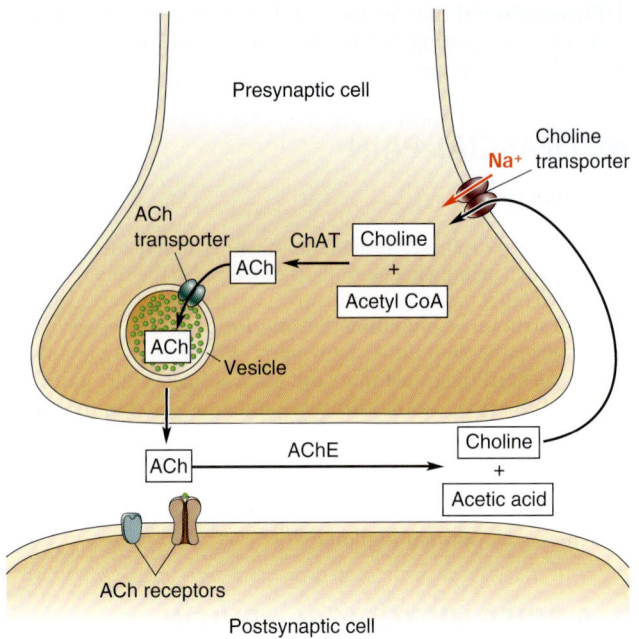

Figure 1-18. The life cycle of acetylcholine (ACh).

hypoxia, a low pH, a shortage of ATP, certain genetic mutations, drugs, increased levels of CGRP and diisopropyl fluorophosphate, or organophosphate pesticides.[63,64,375-377] CGRP plays a key role in the regulation of ACh at the motor endplate in addition to its many other functions, such as microvascular vasodilation in wound healing, prevention of ischemia, and several autonomic and immune functions.[378] CGRP and its receptors are widely expressed in the central and peripheral nervous system. CGRP is released from the trigeminal ganglion and from trigeminal nerves within the dura and contributes to peripheral sensitization.[379] CGRP Type I is also produced in the cell body of motor neurons in the ventral horn of the spinal cord and is excreted via an axoplasmatic transport mechanism. It stimulates the phosphorylation of ACh receptors, which prolongs their sensitivity to ACh.[380] Furthermore, it promotes the release of ACh and inhibits AChE. CGRP is found in higher concentrations in the immediate vicinity of active TrP.[381-383] A2a receptors near motor endplates also contribute to the facilitatory effect of CGRP on the release of ACh.

According to the integrated TrP hypothesis, the excessive amount of ACh in the synaptic cleft will cause constant depolarizations of the postsynaptic cell, trigger miniature endplate potentials, and produce action potentials, that travels along the T-tubules toward the sarcoplasmic reticulum. Persistent contractures are likely to compromise local blood vessels, reduce the local oxygen supply, cause hypoxia, a lowered pH, and hypoperfusion, which, in turn, reinforce the excessive release of ACh and contribute to muscle pain and dysfunction.[140,384] Trigger point hypoxia has been confirmed in German and American research studies.[385,386] The combination of hypoxia and an increased metabolic demand results in a local energy shortage and a local shortage of ATP,[65] in addition to triggering an increased release of ACh at the neuromuscular junction and a decrease in the tissue pH, which, once again, will activate TRPV channels and ASICs and trigger pain, hyperalgesia, and central sensitization without inflammation or any damage or trauma to the muscle.[236,237,387-392]

A 1993 paper by Hubbard et al of spontaneous electromyographic (EMG) activity in the vicinity of TrPs triggered a new line of research into the role of motor endplates.[393] Hubbard et al described a low-amplitude constant background EMG activity of 50 µV and an intermittent higher-amplitude spike-like of

100 to 700 μV. They assumed a pertinent role for muscle spindles, but subsequent human and animal research demonstrated that the observed EMG activity was, in fact, endplate noise caused by an excess of ACh at the neuromuscular junction.[60,61,394-402] In fact, the prevalence of endplate noise elicited from a TrP was directly correlated with irritability, pain intensity, and pressure pain thresholds.[60] Nevertheless, TrPs feature a reduced reflex threshold and a higher reflex amplitude, which could be related to a greater density or excitability of muscle spindle afferents.[53] It appears that TrP pain and tenderness are closely associated with sustained focal ischemia and muscle cramps within muscle taut bands, possibly because cramps may induce intramuscular hypoxia, increased concentrations of algogenic mediators, direct mechanical stimulation of nociceptors, and eventually, the experience of pain.[402] The intramuscular and surface EMG activity recorded from a TrP showed that the electrical signal was similar to a muscle cramp potential.[54] Dry needling, laser, calcium blockers, and botulinum toxin injections were found to be able to reduce the degree of endplate noise.[374,398,403-407]

The Biochemical Milieu of Trigger Points

Human studies at the US National Institutes of Health have identified a unique biochemical milieu of active TrPs with elevated levels of CGRP, substance P, 5-HT, NE, BK, PG, tumor necrosing factor-alpha (TNF-alpha), interleukins IL-1β, IL-6, and IL-8, as well as a significantly lowered pH.[381,383,408] Hsieh et al studied the biochemical environment in rabbits and confirmed elevated levels of multiple other chemicals, such as beta-endorphin, substance P, TNF-alpha, cyclo-oxygenase-2 (COX-2), hypoxia-inducible factor 1-alpha, inducible nitric oxide synthase, and vascular endothelial growth factor.[409,410] The elevated levels of many of these substances near active TrPs are consistent with biochemical pathways involved in tissue injury and inflammation.[382,383]

The orthodromic and antidromic release of these chemicals is enhanced in response to nociceptor activation, for example by protons and BK.[411] It should come as no surprise that each of these chemicals has specific receptors and that their increased concentrations will have a potential impact on pain and function. The low pH, which often is the result of ischemia and hypoxia, will activate ASIC and TRPV receptors, as discussed previously. A further complicating factor is that many of these substances reinforce each other. BK stimulates the release of TNF-alpha, which, in turn, facilitates the release of IL-1β and IL-6. The interleukins stimulate the COX nociceptive pathway, which leads to the production of PGs.[412,413] TNF-alpha produces a time- and dose-dependent muscle hyperalgesia, which is completely reversed by systemic treatment with the nonopioid analgesic metamizol.[414] BK, 5-HT, and PG interact at many levels at the vanilloid receptors and synergistically may cause local muscle pain.[415] An injection of the combination of BK and 5-HT into the temporalis muscle of healthy volunteers caused more pain than when each stimulant was injected alone.[416]

Substance P causes mast cell degranulation with the subsequent release of histamine, 5-HT, and upregulation of proinflammatory cytokines, including TNF-alpha and IL-6, and anti-inflammatory cytokines, including IL-4 and IL-10. TNF-alpha is the only cytokine restored in the mast cell and is released immediately following mast cell degranulation.[417,418] Increased levels of NE suggest involvement of the autonomic nervous system in myofascial pain, as suggested by Ge et al.[419] The local or systemic administration of the alpha-adrenergic antagonist phentolamine to TrPs caused an immediate reduction in endplate noise.[420,421] In other studies, sympathetic blockers reduced TrP and tender point pain sensitivity.[422-424] The specific pathway is not known, but perhaps alpha- and beta-adrenergic receptors at the endplate provide a potential mechanism.[63,425,426] TNF-alpha can also contribute to an autonomic pathway by stimulating the release of IL-8,[427] which can induce a dose- and time-dependent mechanical hypernociception.[428] Hence, elevated levels of IL-8 may mediate inflammatory hypernociception, muscle tenderness, and pain in active TrPs. It is conceivable that the increased concentration of chemical substances near active TrPs may contribute to an increased static fusimotor drive to muscle spindles or to increased muscle spindle sensitivity.[429]

Dry needling and laser can reduce the levels of the substances found in the immediate TrP environment, especially after eliciting LTRs with dry needling, but excessive treatment increased the concentrations.[409,410,430] An LTR is thought to be a spinal cord reflex, and can perhaps best be described as a sudden contraction of muscle fibers within a taut band.[431,432] There is some preliminary evidence that the number of LTRs may be related to the irritability of a TrP,[57] likely due to sensitization of muscle nociceptors by BL, 5-HT, and PG, among others. Recently, several authors have questioned whether eliciting LTRs is necessary or even desirable,[433-435] whereas others have strongly advocated in favor of eliciting LTRs.[431]

Pain and Trigger Points

One of the most important contributions of Travell was her attention to referred pain from TrPs.[5,49,316,328] Familiarity with common referred pain patterns is critical in clinical practice, and a lack of awareness may lead to an incorrect diagnosis, a less than optimal treatment approach, unnecessary surgery, immobilization, bedrest, and medicalization. Referred pain, also known as secondary hyperalgesia, is a common phenomenon whereby pain is experienced in a different region than the source of pain.[436,437] Referred pain associated with TrPs is very common and seen with nearly all myofascial pain problems.[13,27,57,70,152,170,438-457] Referred pain can be elicited from many different structures and can be perceived in any region of the body. The size of the referred pain area is variable and is dependent upon pain-induced changes in central somatosensory maps.[318,458] As mentioned before, active TrPs have larger referred pain areas than latent TrPs.[57] Latent TrPs provide nociceptive input into the DH, and as such, they also feature referred pain.[55,459-463] The size of the referred pain area is correlated with the intensity and duration of muscle pain, which supports the presence of a central sensitization phenomenon maintained by peripheral sensitization input.[452]

Muscle referred pain occurs usually in a central to peripheral direction, but some muscles have referred pain patterns that may develop in a caudal and cranial direction (Figure 1-19). Muscle referred pain is often described as deep, diffuse, burning, tightening, or pressing pain, which differentiates it from neuropathic or cutaneous pain. Other symptoms, such as numbness, coldness, stiffness, weakness, fatigue, or musculoskeletal motor dysfunction, may also be associated with muscle pain, which suggests that perhaps the term "referred sensation" would be more appropriate.[52] Muscle referred pain patterns are similar to joint referred pain patterns. Historically, several models of referred pain have been developed, including the convergent-projection theory, the convergence-facilitation theory, the axon-reflex theory, the thalamic-convergence theory, and the central hyperexcitability theory.[464-467]

The exact mechanisms of referred pain are still not completely understood, but there is enough data to support that "muscle referred pain is a process of central sensitization, which is mediated by a peripheral activity and sensitization, and which can be facilitated by sympathetic activity and dysfunctional descending inhibition."[419,468] The central hyperexcitability theory is consistent with most of the characteristics of muscle and fascia referred pain. The degree of referred pain is dependent on the stimulus. Often, the onset of referred pain is more delayed following a stimulus than the onset of local pain. Animal models have shown that muscle referred pain, which can appear within minutes, features an expansion of receptive fields and sensitization.[467,469,470] Mense suggested that the appearance of new receptive fields may indicate that latent convergent afferents on the DH neuron are opened by noxious stimuli from muscle

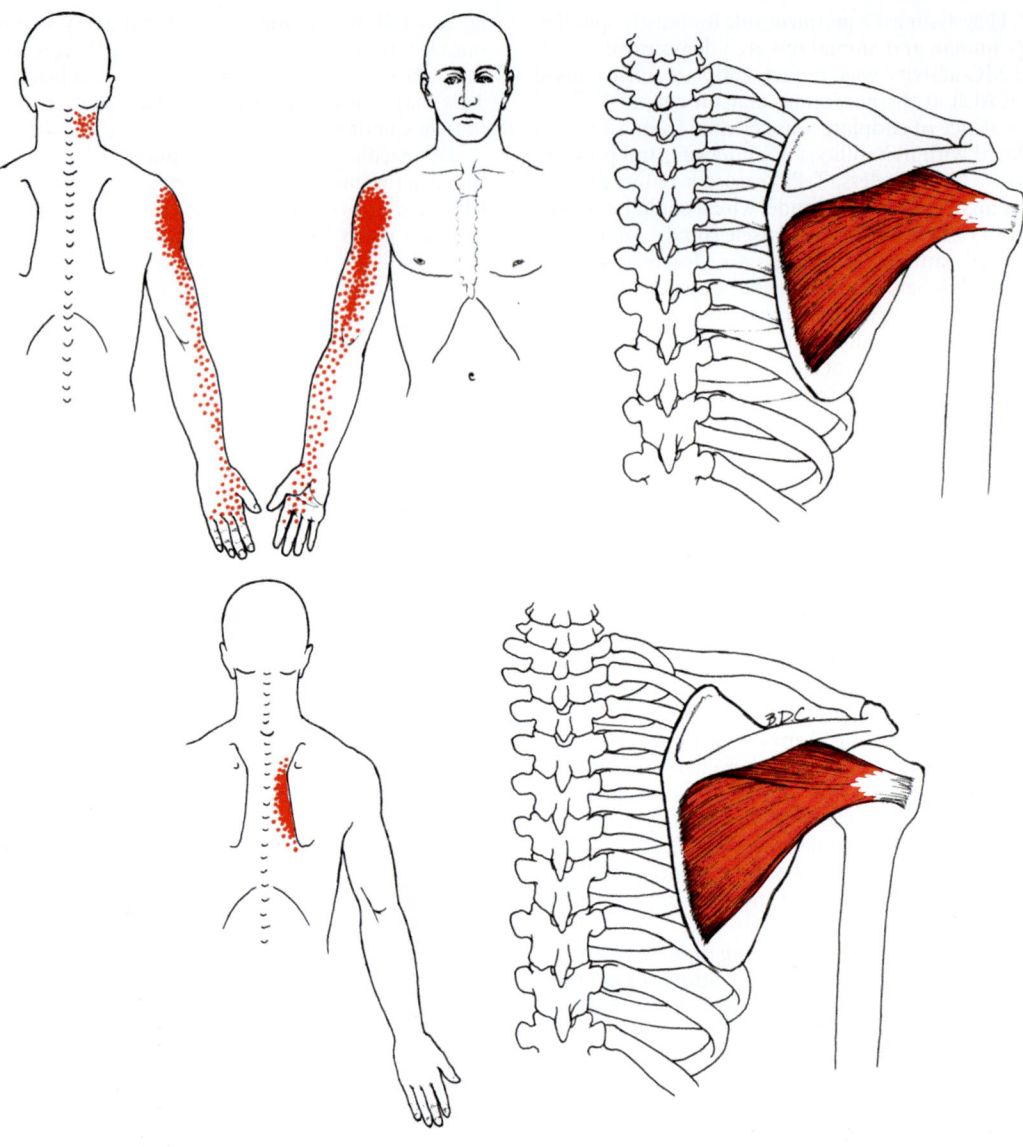

Figure 1-19. Infraspinatus pain referral pattern.

tissues, which could induce the referred pain.[437] Trigger points are more effective in inducing referred pain and other neuroplastic changes in the DH neurons than non-TrPs regions.[471]

Considering the available evidence, TrPs function as persistent sources of nociceptive input and contribute to peripheral and central sensitization.[26,27] Arendt-Nielsen et al provided evidence that experimentally induced muscle pain is able to impair DNIC mechanisms, supporting an important role of muscle tissues in chronic pain.[472] Mechanical stimulation of latent TrPs can induce central sensitization in healthy subjects leading to pressure hypersensitivity in extrasegmental tissues.[55] There is also some evidence that central sensitization can increase the sensitivity of TrPs,[67,68,473] but it is more likely that TrPs induce sensitization, as latent TrPs are present in healthy individuals without evidence of central sensitization. Persistent pain, for example, in patients with fibromyalgia or in experimental conditions, is frequently maintained by persistent nociceptive input from muscles.[151,152,441,474,475] The pain associated with TrPs and TrP therapies, such as manual compression and dry needling, is not related to particular anatomic lesions, but is the result of physiologic changes and peripheral and central sensitization.[27] Treatments directed at TrPs seem to reverse peripheral and central sensitization.[28,136,476,477] The underlying mechanisms of myofascial pain and TrPs will be further explored in Chapter 2.

References

1. Institute of Medicine (US). *Committee on Advancing Pain Research Care and Education. Relieving Pain in America: A Blueprint for Transforming Prevention, Care, Education, and Research.* Washington, DC: National Academies Press; 2011.
2. Fricton J. The need for preventing chronic pain: the "big elephant in the room" of healthcare. *Glob Adv Health Med.* 2015;4(1):6-7.
3. Reichling DB, Green PG, Levine JD. The fundamental unit of pain is the cell. *Pain.* 2013;154 suppl 1:S2-S9.
4. Travell JG, Simons DG. *Myofascial Pain and Dysfunction: The Trigger Point Manual.* Vol 1. Baltimore, MD: Williams & Wilkins; 1983.
5. Travell J, Simons DG. *Myofascial Pain and Dysfunction: The Trigger Point Manual.* Vol 2. Baltimore, MD: Williams & Wilkins; 1992.
6. Lluch E, Nijs J, De Kooning M, et al. Prevalence, incidence, localization, and pathophysiology of myofascial trigger points in patients with spinal pain: a systematic literature review. *J Manipulative Physiol Ther.* 2015;38(8):587-600.

7. Chiarotto A, Clijsen R, Fernández-de-Las-Peñas C, Barbero M. Prevalence of myofascial trigger points in spinal disorders: a systematic review and meta-analysis. *Arch Phys Med Rehabil.* 2016;97(2):316-337.
8. Castaldo M, Ge HY, Chiarotto A, Villafane JH, Arendt-Nielsen L. Myofascial trigger points in patients with whiplash-associated disorders and mechanical neck pain. *Pain Med.* 2014;15(5):842-849.
9. Cerezo-Tellez E, Torres-Lacomba M, Mayoral-Del Moral O, Sanchez-Sanchez B, Dommerholt J, Gutierrez-Ortega C. Prevalence of myofascial pain syndrome in chronic non-specific neck pain: a population-based cross-sectional descriptive study. *Pain Med.* 2016;17:2369-2377.
10. Chen CK, Nizar AJ. Myofascial pain syndrome in chronic back pain patients. *Korean J Pain.* 2011;24(2):100-104.
11. Donnelly JM, Palubinskas L. Prevalence and inter-rater reliability of trigger points. *J Musculoskelet Pain.* 2007;15(suppl 13):16.
12. Ettlin T, Schuster C, Stoffel R, Bruderlin A, Kischka U. A distinct pattern of myofascial findings in patients after whiplash injury. *Arch Phys Med Rehabil.* 2008;89(7):1290-1293.
13. Fernandez-Carnero J, Fernández-de-Las-Peñas C, de la Llave-Rincon AI, Ge HY, Arendt-Nielsen L. Prevalence of and referred pain from myofascial trigger points in the forearm muscles in patients with lateral epicondylalgia. *Clin J Pain.* 2007;23(4):353-360.
14. Fernandez-Perez AM, Villaverde-Gutierrez C, Mora-Sanchez A, Alonso-Blanco C, Sterling M, Fernández-de-Las-Peñas C. Muscle trigger points, pressure pain threshold, and cervical range of motion in patients with high level of disability related to acute whiplash injury. *J Orthop Sports Phys Ther.* 2012;42(7):634-641.
15. Fleckenstein J, Zaps D, Ruger LJ, et al. Discrepancy between prevalence and perceived effectiveness of treatment methods in myofascial pain syndrome: results of a cross-sectional, nationwide survey. *BMC Musculoskelet Disord.* 2010;11:32.
16. Granges G, Littlejohn G. Prevalence of myofascial pain syndrome in fibromyalgia syndrome and regional pain syndrome: a comparative study. *J Musculoskelet Pain.* 1993;1(2):19-35.
17. Grieve R, Barnett S, Coghill N, Cramp F. The prevalence of latent myofascial trigger points and diagnostic criteria of the triceps surae and upper trapezius: a cross sectional study. *Physiotherapy.* 2013;99(4):278-284.
18. Hayden RJ, Louis DS, Doro C. Fibromyalgia and myofascial pain syndromes and the workers' compensation environment: an update. *Clin Occup Environ Med.* 2006;5(2):455-469, x-xi.
19. Skootsky SA, Jaeger B, Oye RK. Prevalence of myofascial pain in general internal medicine practice. *West J Med.* 1989;151(2):157-160.
20. Zuil-Escobar JC, Martínez-Cepa CB, Martín-Urrialde JA, Gómez-Conesa A. Prevalence of myofascial trigger points and diagnostic criteria of different muscles in function of the medial longitudinal arch. *Arch Phys Med Rehabil.* 2015;96(6):1123-1130.
21. Zuil-Escobar JC, Martinez-Cepa CB, Martin-Urrialde JA, Gomez-Conesa A. The prevalence of latent trigger points in lower limb muscles in asymptomatic subjects. *PM R.* 2016;8(11):1055-1064.
22. Azadeh H, Dehghani M, Zarezadeh A. Incidence of trapezius myofascial trigger points in patients with the possible carpal tunnel syndrome. *J Res Med Sci.* 2010;15(5):250-255.
23. Hendler NH, Kozikowski JG. Overlooked physical diagnoses in chronic pain patients involved in litigation. *Psychosomatics.* 1993;34(6):494-501.
24. Mense S. Functional anatomy of muscle: muscle, nociceptors and afferent fibers. In: Mense S, Gerwin RD, eds. *Muscle Pain: Understanding the Mechanisms.* Berlin, Germany: Springer; 2010:17-48.
25. Arendt-Nielsen L, Castaldo M. MTPs are a peripheral source of nociception. *Pain Med.* 2015;16(4):625-627.
26. Dommerholt J. Dry needling—peripheral and central considerations. *J Man Manip Ther.* 2011;19(4):223-227.
27. Fernández-de-las-Peñas C, Dommerholt J. Myofascial trigger points: peripheral or central phenomenon? *Curr Rheumatol Rep.* 2014;16(1):395.
28. Freeman MD, Nystrom A, Centeno C. Chronic whiplash and central sensitization; an evaluation of the role of a myofascial trigger points in pain modulation. *J Brachial Plex Peripher Nerve Inj.* 2009;4:2.
29. Bajaj P, Bajaj P, Graven-Nielsen T, Arendt-Nielsen L. Trigger points in patients with lower limb osteoarthritis. *J Musculoskelet Pain.* 2001;9(3):17-33.
30. Fernández-de-Las-Peñas C, Fernandez-Carnero J, Miangolarra-Page J. Musculoskeletal disorders in mechanical neck pain: myofascial trigger points versus cervical joint dysfunction—a clinical study. *J Musculoskelet Pain.* 2005;13(1):27-35.
31. Ruiz-Saez M, Fernández-de-las-Peñas C, Blanco CR, Martinez-Segura R, Garcia-Leon R. Changes in pressure pain sensitivity in latent myofascial trigger points in the upper trapezius muscle after a cervical spine manipulation in pain-free subjects. *J Manipulative Physiol Ther.* 2007;30(8):578-583.
32. Jarrell J. Myofascial pain in the adolescent. *Curr Opin Obstet Gynecol.* 2010;22(5):393-398.
33. Jarrell J. Endometriosis and abdominal myofascial pain in adults and adolescents. *Curr Pain Headache Rep.* 2011;15(5):368-376.
34. Weiss JM. Pelvic floor myofascial trigger points: manual therapy for interstitial cystitis and the urgency-frequency syndrome. *J Urol.* 2001;166(6):2226-2231.
35. Anderson RU. Management of chronic prostatitis-chronic pelvic pain syndrome. *Urol Clin North Am.* 2002;29(1):235-239.
36. Anderson RU, Sawyer T, Wise D, Morey A, Nathanson BH. Painful myofascial trigger points and pain sites in men with chronic prostatitis/chronic pelvic pain syndrome. *J Urol.* 2009;182(6):2753-2758.
37. Anderson RU, Wise D, Sawyer T, Glowe P, Orenberg EK. 6-Day intensive treatment protocol for refractory chronic prostatitis/chronic pelvic pain syndrome using myofascial release and paradoxical relaxation training. *J Urol.* 2011;185(4):1294-1299.
38. Doggweiler-Wiygul R. Urologic myofascial pain syndromes. *Curr Pain Headache Rep.* 2004;8(6):445-451.
39. Fuentes-Marquez P, Valenza MC, Cabrera-Martos I, Rios-Sanchez A, Ocon-Hernandez O. Trigger points, pressure pain hyperalgesia, and mechanosensitivity of neural tissue in women with chronic pelvic pain. *Pain Med.* 2017. doi:10.1093/pm/pnx206.
40. Hightower JM, Dalessandri KM, Pope K, Hernandez GT. Low 25-hydroxyvitamin D and myofascial pain: association of cancer, colon polyps, and tendon rupture. *J Am Coll Nutr.* 2017;36(6):455-461.
41. Cardoso LR, Rizzo CC, de Oliveira CZ, dos Santos CR, Carvalho AL. Myofascial pain syndrome after head and neck cancer treatment: prevalence, risk factors, and influence on quality of life. *Head Neck.* 2015;37(12):1733-1737.
42. Crawford JS, Simpson J, Crawford P. Myofascial release provides symptomatic relief from chest wall tenderness occasionally seen following lumpectomy and radiation in breast cancer patients. *Int J Radiat Oncol Biol Phys.* 1996;34(5):1188-1189.
43. Torres Lacomba M, Mayoral del Moral O, Coperias Zazo JL, Gerwin RD, Goni AZ. Incidence of myofascial pain syndrome in breast cancer surgery: a prospective study. *Clin J Pain.* 2010;26(4):320-325.
44. Dommerholt J, Gerwin RD. Nutritional and metabolic perpetuating factors in myofascial pain. In: Dommerholt J, Huijbregts PA, eds. *Myofascial Trigger Points: Pathophysiology and Evidence-Informed Diagnosis And Management.* Boston, MA: Jones & Bartlett; 2011.
45. Gerwin RD. A review of myofascial pain and fibromyalgia—factors that promote their persistence. *Acupunct Med.* 2005;23(3):121-134.
46. Waldock C. Myofascial pain masquerading as neuropathic pain. *Acupunct Physiother.* 2017;29:1.
47. Chang SH. Complex regional pain syndrome is a manifestation of the worsened myofascial pain syndrome: case review. *J Pain Relief.* 2017;6:294.
48. Bezerra Rocha CA, Sanchez TG. Myofascial trigger points: another way of modulating tinnitus. In: Langguth B, Hajak G, Kleinjung T, Cacace A, Moller AR, eds. *Progress in Brain Research.* Vol 166. Amsterdam, The Netherlands: Elsevier; 2007:209-214.
49. Simons DG, Travell J, Simons L. *Travell & Simon's Myofascial Pain and Dysfunction: The Trigger Point Manual.* Vol 1. 2nd ed. Baltimore, MD: Williams & Wilkins; 1999.
50. Rivers WE, Garrigues D, Graciosa J, Harden RN. Signs and symptoms of myofascial pain: an international survey of pain management providers and proposed preliminary set of diagnostic criteria. *Pain Med.* 2015;16(9):1794-1805.
51. Tough EA, White AR, Richards S, Campbell J. Variability of criteria used to diagnose myofascial trigger point pain syndrome—evidence from a review of the literature. *Clin J Pain.* 2007;23(3):278-286.
52. Fernández-de-Las-Peñas C, Dommerholt J. International consensus on diagnostic criteria and clinical considerations of myofascial trigger points: a delphi study. *Pain Med.* 2018;19(1):142-150.
53. Ge HY, Serrao M, Andersen OK, Graven-Nielsen T, Arendt-Nielsen L. Increased H-reflex response induced by intramuscular electrical stimulation of latent myofascial trigger points. *Acupunct Med.* 2009;27(4):150-154.
54. Ge HY, Zhang Y, Boudreau S, Yue SW, Arendt-Nielsen L. Induction of muscle cramps by nociceptive stimulation of latent myofascial trigger points. *Exp Brain Res.* 2008;187(4):623-629.
55. Xu YM, Ge HY, Arendt-Nielsen L. Sustained nociceptive mechanical stimulation of latent myofascial trigger point induces central sensitization in healthy subjects. *J Pain.* 2010;11(12):1348-1355.
56. Mense S. How do muscle lesions such as latent and active trigger points influence central nociceptive neurons? *J Musculoskelet Pain.* 2010;18(4):348-353.
57. Hong C-Z, Kuan TS, Chen JT, Chen SM. Referred pain elicited by palpation and by needling of myofascial trigger points: a comparison. *Arch Phys Med Rehabil.* 1997;78(9):957-960.
58. Vecchiet L, Giamberardino MA, Dragani L, De Bigontina P, Albe-Fessard D. Latent myofascial trigger points: changes in muscular and subcutaneous pain thresholds at trigger point and target level. *J Man Med.* 1990;5:151-154.
59. Vecchiet L, Giamberardino MA, De Bigontina P, Dragani L. Chapter 13, Comparative sensory evaluation of parietal tissues in painful and nonpainful areas in fibromyalgia and myofascial pain syndrome. Paper presented at: Proceedings of the 7th World Congress on Pain, Progress in Pain Research and Management1994; Seattle.
60. Kuan TS, Hsieh YL, Chen SM, Chen JT, Yen WC, Hong CZ. The myofascial trigger point region: correlation between the degree of irritability and the prevalence of endplate noise. *Am J Phys Med Rehabil.* 2007;86(3):183-189.
61. Simons DG. Review of enigmatic MTrPs as a common cause of enigmatic musculoskeletal pain and dysfunction. *J Electromyogr Kinesiol.* 2004;14(1):95-107.
62. Stoop R, Clijsen R, Leoni D, et al. Evolution of the methodological quality of controlled clinical trials for myofascial trigger point treatments for the period 1978-2015: a systematic review. *Musculoskelet Sci Pract.* 2017;30:1-9.
63. Gerwin RD, Dommerholt J, Shah JP. An expansion of Simons' integrated hypothesis of trigger point formation. *Curr Pain Headache Rep.* 2004;8(6):468-475.
64. McPartland JM. Travell trigger points—molecular and osteopathic perspectives. *J Am Osteopath Assoc.* 2004;104(6):244-249.
65. McPartland JM, Simons DG. Myofascial trigger points: translating molecular theory into manual therapy. *J Manual Manipulative Ther.* 2006;14(4):232-239.
66. Jafri MS. Mechanisms of myofascial pain. *Int Sch Res Notices.* 2014;2014.
67. Srbely JZ. New trends in the treatment and management of myofascial pain syndrome. *Curr Pain Headache Rep.* 2010;14(5):346-352.

68. Hocking MJ. Exploring the central modulation hypothesis: do ancient memory mechanisms underlie the pathophysiology of trigger points? *Curr Pain Headache Rep.* 2013;17(7):347.
69. Hocking MJ. Trigger points and central modulation—a new hypothesis. *J Musculoskelet Pain.* 2010;18(2):186-203.
70. Farasyn A. Referred muscle pain is primarily peripheral in origin: the "barrier-dam" theory. *Med Hypotheses.* 2007;68(1):144-150.
71. Partanen JV, Ojala TA, Arokoski JP. Myofascial syndrome and pain: a neurophysiological approach. *Pathophysiology.* 2010;17(1):19-28.
72. Quintner JL, Bove GM, Cohen ML. A critical evaluation of the trigger point phenomenon. *Rheumatology (Oxford).* 2015;54(3):392-399.
73. IASP. IASP Taxonomy. http://www.iasp-pain.org/Taxonomy. Accessed March 10, 2018.
74. Cohen M, Quintner J, van Rysewyk S. Reconsidering the International Association for the study of pain definition of pain. *Pain Rep.* 2018;3(2):e634.
75. Treede RD. The International Association for the study of pain definition of pain: as valid in 2018 as in 1979, but in need of regularly updated footnotes. *Pain Rep.* 2018;3(2):e643.
76. Brinjikji W, Luetmer PH, Comstock B, et al. Systematic literature review of imaging features of spinal degeneration in asymptomatic populations. *AJNR Am J Neuroradiol.* 2015;36(4):811-816.
77. Nakashima H, Yukawa Y, Suda K, Yamagata M, Ueta T, Kato F. Abnormal findings on magnetic resonance images of the cervical spines in 1211 asymptomatic subjects. *Spine (Phila Pa 1976).* 2015;40(6):392-398.
78. Battie MC, Videman T, Kaprio J, et al. The Twin Spine Study: contributions to a changing view of disc degeneration. *Spine J.* 2009;9(1):47-59.
79. Dunn WR, Kuhn JE, Sanders R, et al. Symptoms of pain do not correlate with rotator cuff tear severity: a cross-sectional study of 393 patients with a symptomatic atraumatic full-thickness rotator cuff tear. *J Bone Joint Surg Am.* 2014;96(10):793-800.
80. Vincent K, Leboeuf-Yde C, Gagey O. Are degenerative rotator cuff disorders a cause of shoulder pain? Comparison of prevalence of degenerative rotator cuff disease to prevalence of nontraumatic shoulder pain through three systematic and critical reviews. *J Shoulder Elbow Surg.* 2017;26(5):766-773.
81. Foster NE, Pincus T, Underwood MR, Vogel S, Breen A, Harding G. Understanding the process of care for musculoskeletal conditions—why a biomedical approach is inadequate. *Rheumatology (Oxford).* 2003;42(3):401-404.
82. Pelletier R, Bourbonnais D, Higgins J. Nociception, pain, neuroplasticity and the practice of osteopathic manipulative medicine. *Int J Osteopath Med.* 2018;27:34-44.
83. Brinjikji W, Diehn FE, Jarvik JG, et al. MRI findings of disc degeneration are more prevalent in adults with low back pain than in asymptomatic controls: a systematic review and meta-analysis. *AJNR Am J Neuroradiol.* 2015;36(12):2394-2399.
84. Epstein NE, Hood DC. "Unnecessary" spinal surgery: a prospective 1-year study of one surgeon's experience. *Surg Neurol Int.* 2011;2:83.
85. Sakaura H, Hosono N, Mukai Y, Fujii R, Iwasaki M, Yoshikawa H. Persistent local pain after posterior spine surgery for thoracic lesions. *J Spinal Disord Tech.* 2007;20(3):226-228.
86. Melzack R, Wall PD. Pain mechanisms: a new theory. *Science.* 1965;150(3699):971-979.
87. Mandel LM, Berlin SJ. Myofascial pain syndromes and their effect on the lower extremities. *J Foot Surg.* 1982;21(1):74-79.
88. Mense S, Skeppar P. Discharge behaviour of feline gamma-motoneurones following induction of an artificial myositis. *Pain.* 1991;46(2):201-210.
89. Simons DG, Mense S. Understanding and measurement of muscle tone as related to clinical muscle pain. *Pain.* 1998;75(1):1-17.
90. Burke D. Critical examination of the case for or against fusimotor involvement in disorders of muscle tone. *Adv Neurol.* 1983;39:133-150.
91. Kniffki KD, Schomburg ED, Steffens H. Synaptic effects from chemically activated fine muscle afferents upon alpha-motoneurones in decerebrate and spinal cats. *Brain Res.* 1981;206(2):361-370.
92. Le Pera D, Graven-Nielsen T, Valeriani M, et al. Inhibition of motor system excitability at cortical and spinal level by tonic muscle pain. *Clin Neurophysiol.* 2001;112(9):1633-1641.
93. Masri R, Ro JY, Capra N. The effect of experimental muscle pain on the amplitude and velocity sensitivity of jaw closing muscle spindle afferents. *Brain Res.* 2005;1050(1-2):138-147.
94. Birznieks I, Burton AR, Macefield VG. The effects of experimental muscle and skin pain on the static stretch sensitivity of human muscle spindles in relaxed leg muscles. *J Physiol.* 2008;586(11):2713-2723.
95. Mense S, Masi AT. Increased muscle tone as a cause of muscle pain. In: Mense S, Gerwin R, eds. *Muscle Pain: Understanding the Mechanisms.* Vol 1. Heidelberg, Germany: Springer; 2011:207-249.
96. Hodges PW. Pain and motor control: from the laboratory to rehabilitation. *J Electromyogr Kinesiol.* 2011;21(2):220-228.
97. Lund JP, Donga R, Widmer CG, Stohler CS. The pain-adaptation model: a discussion of the relationship between chronic musculoskeletal pain and motor activity. *Can J Physiol Pharmacol.* 1991;69(5):683-694.
98. Martin PG, Weerakkody N, Gandevia SC, Taylor JL. Group III and IV muscle afferents differentially affect the motor cortex and motoneurones in humans. *J Physiol.* 2008;586(5):1277-1289.
99. Hodges PW, Tucker K. Moving differently in pain: a new theory to explain the adaptation to pain. *Pain.* 2011;152(3 suppl):S90-S98.
100. Lucas KR, Polus PA, Rich J. Latent myofascial trigger points: their effect on muscle activation and movement efficiency. *J Bodyw Mov Ther.* 2004;8:160-166.
101. Lucas KR, Rich PA, Polus BI. Muscle activation patterns in the scapular positioning muscles during loaded scapular plane elevation: the effects of Latent Myofascial Trigger Points. *Clin Biomech.* 2010;25(8):765-770.
102. Bohlooli N, Ahmadi A, Maroufi N, Sarrafzadeh J, Jaberzadeh S. Differential activation of scapular muscles, during arm elevation, with and without trigger points. *J Bodyw Mov Ther.* 2016;20(1):26-34.
103. Schneider K, Sohn S, Licht G, Dommerholt J, von Piekartz H. Do active myofascial trigger points alter the muscle activation pattern of five select shoulder muscles during controlled arm abduction? Short-term effects of placebo-controlled myofascial therapy on muscle activation patterns. (in press)
104. Chaitow L, DeLany J. Neuromuscular techniques in orthopedics. *Tech Orthop.* 2003;18(1):74-86.
105. Fernández-de-Las Peñas C, Cuadrado ML, Pareja JA. Myofascial trigger points, neck mobility and forward head posture in unilateral migraine. *Cephalalgia.* 2006;26(9):1061-1070.
106. Fernández-de-Las-Peñas C, Cuadrado ML, Pareja JA. Myofascial trigger points, neck mobility, and forward head posture in episodic tension-type headache. *Headache.* 2007;47(5):662-672.
107. Grieve R, Clark J, Pearson E, Bullock S, Boyer C, Jarrett A. The immediate effect of soleus trigger point pressure release on restricted ankle joint dorsiflexion: a pilot randomised controlled trial. *J Bodyw Mov Ther.* 2011;15(1):42-49.
108. Grieve R, Cranston A, Henderson A, John R, Malone G, Mayall C. The immediate effect of triceps surae myofascial trigger point therapy on restricted active ankle joint dorsiflexion in recreational runners: a crossover randomised controlled trial. *J Bodyw Mov Ther.* 2013;17(4):453-461.
109. Grieve R, Goodwin F, Alfaki M, Bourton AJ, Jeffries C, Scott H. The immediate effect of bilateral self myofascial release on the plantar surface of the feet on hamstring and lumbar spine flexibility: a pilot randomised controlled trial. *J Bodyw Mov Ther.* 2015;19(3):544-552.
110. Stuner A, Delafontaine A. Compression ischemique des points gachettes du trapeze superieur chez la personne agee. *Kinesitherapie, la Revue.* 2016;16(170):17-22.
111. Sohn MK, Graven-Nielsen T, Arendt-Nielsen L, Svensson P. Inhibition of motor unit firing during experimental muscle pain in humans. *Muscle Nerve.* 2000;23(8):1219-1226.
112. Melzack R, Katz J. Pain. *Wiley Interdiscip Rev Cogn Sci.* 2013;4(1):1-15.
113. Mendell LM. Constructing and deconstructing the gate theory of pain. *Pain.* 2014;155(2):210-216.
114. Treede RD. Gain control mechanisms in the nociceptive system. *Pain.* 2016;157(6):1199-1204.
115. Jones M, Edwards I, Gifford L. Conceptual models for implementing biopsychosocial theory in clinical practice. *Man Ther.* 2002;7(1):2-9.
116. Gifford L. *Topical Issues in Pain 2.* Vol 2. Falmouth, England: CNS Press; 1998.
117. Melzack R. Pain—an overview. *Acta Anaesthesiol Scand.* 1999;43(9):880-884.
118. Melzack R. Pain and the neuromatrix in the brain. *J Dent Educ.* 2001;65(12):1378-1382.
119. Travell J. *Office Hours: Day and Night.* New York, NY: The World Publishing Company; 1968.
120. Moseley GL, Arntz A. The context of a noxious stimulus affects the pain it evokes. *Pain.* 2007;133(1-3):64-71.
121. Moseley GL. Reconceptualising pain according to modern pain science. *Phys Ther Rev.* 2007;12(3):169-178.
122. Acerra NE, Moseley GL. Dysynchiria: watching the mirror image of the unaffected limb elicits pain on the affected side. *Neurology.* 2005;65(5):751-753.
123. Woolf CJ. Central sensitization: implications for the diagnosis and treatment of pain. *Pain.* 2011;152(3 suppl):S2-S15.
124. Moseley GL, Butler DS. Fifteen years of explaining pain: the past, present, and future. *J Pain.* 2015;16(9):807-813.
125. Nijs J, Apeldoorn A, Hallegraeff H, et al. Low back pain: guidelines for the clinical classification of predominant neuropathic, nociceptive, or central sensitization pain. *Pain Physician.* 2015;18(3):E333-E346.
126. Moseley GL. Pain: why and how does it hurt? In: Brukner P, Khan K, eds. *Brukner & Kohn's Clinical Sports Medicine.* Vol 4. North Ryde, Australia: McGraw-Hill; 2012:41-53.
127. Jull GA. Management of cervical spine disorders: where to now? *J Orthop Sports Phys Ther.* 2012;42(10):A1-A83.
128. Louw A. Treating the brain in chronic pain. In: Fernández-de-Las Peñas C, Cleland J, Dommerholt J, eds. *Manual Therapy for Musculoskeletal Pain Syndromes—An Evidenced and Clinical-Informed Approach.* Edinburgh, Scotland: Churchill Livingstone (Elsevier); 2016.
129. Tellez-Garcia M, de-la-Llave-Rincon AI, Salom-Moreno J, Palacios-Cena M, Ortega-Santiago R, Fernández-de-Las-Peñas C. Neuroscience education in addition to trigger point dry needling for the management of patients with mechanical chronic low back pain: a preliminary clinical trial. *J Bodyw Mov Ther.* 2015;19(3):464-472.
130. Geneen LJ, Martin DJ, Adams N, et al. Effects of education to facilitate knowledge about chronic pain for adults: a systematic review with meta-analysis. *Syst Rev.* 2015;4:132.
131. Wijma AJ, Speksnijder CM, Crom-Ottens AF, et al. What is important in transdisciplinary pain neuroscience education? A qualitative study. *Disabil Rehabil.* 2017:1-11.
132. Diener I, Kargela M, Louw A. Listening is therapy: patient interviewing from a pain science perspective. *Physiother Theory Pract.* 2016;32(5):356-367.
133. Meakins A. Soft tissue sore spots of an unknown origin. *Br J Sports Med.* 2015;49(6):348.
134. Jacobs DF, Silvernail JL. Therapist as operator or interactor? Moving beyond the technique. *J Man Manip Ther.* 2011;19(2):120-121.
135. Rabey M, Hall T, Hebron C, Palsson TS, Christensen SW, Moloney N. Reconceptualising manual therapy skills in contemporary practice. *Musculoskelet Sci Pract.* 2017;29:28-32.
136. Giamberardino MA, Tafuri E, Savini A, et al. Contribution of myofascial trigger points to migraine symptoms. *J Pain.* 2007;8(11):869-878.

137. Mense S. Muscle pain: mechanisms and clinical significance. *Dtsch Arztebl Int.* 2008;105(12):214-219.
138. Arendt-Nielsen L, Morlion B, Perrot S, et al. Assessment and manifestation of central sensitisation across different chronic pain conditions. *Eur J Pain.* 2018;22(2):216-241.
139. Apkarian AV, Bushnell MC, Treede RD, Zubieta JK. Human brain mechanisms of pain perception and regulation in health and disease. *Eur J Pain.* 2005;9(4):463-484.
140. Bron C, Dommerholt JD. Etiology of myofascial trigger points. *Curr Pain Headache Rep.* 2012;16(5):439-444.
141. Calandre EP, Hidalgo J, Garcia-Leiva JM, Rico-Villademoros F. Trigger point evaluation in migraine patients: an indication of peripheral sensitization linked to migraine predisposition? *Eur J Neurol.* 2006;13(3):244-249.
142. Fernández-de-Las-Peñas C, Cuadrado ML, Arendt-Nielsen L, Simons DG, Pareja JA. Myofascial trigger points and sensitization: an updated pain model for tension-type headache. *Cephalalgia.* 2007;27(5):383-393.
143. Latremoliere A, Woolf CJ. Central sensitization: a generator of pain hypersensitivity by central neural plasticity. *J Pain.* 2009;10(9):895-926.
144. Obermann M, Rodriguez-Raecke R, Naegel S, et al. Gray matter volume reduction reflects chronic pain in trigeminal neuralgia. *Neuroimage.* 2013;74:352-358.
145. Rodriguez-Raecke R, Niemeier A, Ihle K, Ruether W, May A. Brain gray matter decrease in chronic pain is the consequence and not the cause of pain. *J Neurosci.* 2009;29(44):13746-13750.
146. Rodriguez-Raecke R, Niemeier A, Ihle K, Ruether W, May A. Structural brain changes in chronic pain reflect probably neither damage nor atrophy. *PLoS One.* 2013;8(2):e54475.
147. Apkarian AV, Sosa Y, Sonty S, et al. Chronic back pain is associated with decreased prefrontal and thalamic gray matter density. *J Neurosci.* 2004;24(46):10410-10415.
148. Ceko M, Shir Y, Ouellet JA, Ware MA, Stone LS, Seminowicz DA. Partial recovery of abnormal insula and dorsolateral prefrontal connectivity to cognitive networks in chronic low back pain after treatment. *Hum Brain Mapp.* 2015;36(6):2075-2092.
149. Seminowicz DA, Wideman TH, Naso L, et al. Effective treatment of chronic low back pain in humans reverses abnormal brain anatomy and function. *J Neurosci.* 2011;31(20):7540-7550.
150. Treede RD, Meyer RA, Raja SN, Campbell JN. Peripheral and central mechanisms of cutaneous hyperalgesia. *Prog Neurobiol.* 1992;38(4):397-421.
151. Staud R, Nagel S, Robinson ME, Price DD. Enhanced central pain processing of fibromyalgia patients is maintained by muscle afferent input: a randomized, double-blind, placebo-controlled study. *Pain.* 2009;145(1-2):96-104.
152. Rubin TK, Henderson LA, Macefield VG. Changes in the spatiotemporal expression of local and referred pain following repeated intramuscular injections of hypertonic saline: a longitudinal study. *J Pain.* 2010;11(8):737-745.
153. Samineni VK, Premkumar LS, Faingold CL. Neuropathic pain-induced enhancement of spontaneous and pain-evoked neuronal activity in the periaqueductal gray that is attenuated by gabapentin. *Pain.* 2017;158(7):1241-1253.
154. Mertens P, Blond S, David R, Rigoard P. Anatomy, physiology and neurobiology of the nociception: a focus on low back pain (Part A). *Neurochirurgie.* 2015;61 suppl 1:S22-S34.
155. Fong A, Schug SA. Pathophysiology of pain: a practical primer. *Plast Reconstr Surg.* 2014;134(4 suppl 2):8S-14S.
156. Hoheisel U, Unger T, Mense S. Excitatory and modulatory effects of inflammatory cytokines and neurotrophins on mechanosensitive group IV muscle afferents in the rat. *Pain.* 2005;114(1-2):168-176.
157. Light AR, Perl ER. Unmyelinated afferent fibers are not only for pain anymore. *J Comp Neurol.* 2003;461(2):137-139.
158. Millan MJ. The induction of pain: an integrative review. *Prog Neurobiol.* 1999;57(1):1-164.
159. Basbaum AI, Bautista DM, Scherrer G, Julius D. Cellular and molecular mechanisms of pain. *Cell.* 2009;139(2):267-284.
160. Mense S. Anatomy of nociceptors. In: Bushnell MC, Basbaum AI, eds. *The Senses: A Comprehensive Reference.* Vol 5. Oxford, England: Elsevier; 2008:11-41.
161. Piomelli D, Hohmann AG, Seybold V, Hammock BD. A lipid gate for the peripheral control of pain. *J Neurosci.* 2014;34(46):15184-15191.
162. Ferreira SH, Nakamura M, de Abreu Castro MS. The hyperalgesic effects of prostacyclin and prostaglandin E2. *Prostaglandins.* 1978;16(1):31-37.
163. Burch RM, Farmer SG, Steranka LR. Bradykinin receptor antagonists. *Med Res Rev.* 1990;10(2):237-269.
164. Steranka LR, Manning DC, DeHaas CJ, et al. Bradykinin as a pain mediator: receptors are localized to sensory neurons, and antagonists have analgesic actions. *Proc Natl Acad Sci U S A.* 1988;85(9):3245-3249.
165. Hoheisel U, Reinohl J, Unger T, Mense S. Acidic pH and capsaicin activate mechanosensitive group IV muscle receptors in the rat. *Pain.* 2004;110(1-2):149-157.
166. Dwyer TM. Chemical signaling in the nervous system. In: Haines DE, Mihailoff GA, eds. *Fundamental Neuroscience for Basic and Clinical Applications.* 5th ed. Philadelphia, PA: Elsevier; 2018:54-71.
167. Babenko VV, Graven-Nielsen T, Svensson P, Drewes AM, Jensen TS, Arendt-Nielsen L. Experimental human muscle pain induced by intramuscular injections of bradykinin, serotonin, and substance P. *Eur J Pain.* 1999;3(2):93-102.
168. Babenko V, Graven-Nielsen T, Svensson P, Drewes AM, Jensen TS, Arendt-Nielsen L. Experimental human muscle pain and muscular hyperalgesia induced by combinations of serotonin and bradykinin. *Pain.* 1999;82(1):1-8.
169. Graven-Nielsen T, Babenko V, Svensson P, Arendt-Nielsen L. Experimentally induced muscle pain induces hypoalgesia in heterotopic deep tissues, but not in homotopic deep tissues. *Brain Res.* 1998;787(2-3):203-210.
170. Gibson W, Arendt-Nielsen L, Graven-Nielsen T. Referred pain and hyperalgesia in human tendon and muscle belly tissue. *Pain.* 2006;120(1-2):113-123.
171. Hoheisel U, Reuter R, de Freitas MF, Treede RD, Mense S. Injection of nerve growth factor into a low back muscle induces long-lasting latent hypersensitivity in rat dorsal horn neurons. *Pain.* 2013;154(10):1953-1960.
172. Obreja O, Rukwied R, Nagler L, Schmidt M, Schmelz M, Namer B. Nerve growth factor locally sensitizes nociceptors in human skin. *Pain.* 2018;159(3):416-426.
173. Rukwied R, Schley M, Forsch E, Obreja O, Dusch M, Schmelz M. Nerve growth factor-evoked nociceptor sensitization in pig skin in vivo. *J Neurosci Res.* 2010;88(9):2066-2072.
174. Weinkauf B, Deising S, Obreja O, et al. Comparison of nerve growth factor-induced sensitization pattern in lumbar and tibial muscle and fascia. *Muscle Nerve.* 2015;52(2):265-272.
175. Monteleone F, Nicoletti CG, Stampanoni Bassi M, et al. Nerve growth factor is elevated in the CSF of patients with multiple sclerosis and central neuropathic pain. *J Neuroimmunol.* 2018;314:89-93.
176. Cheng HT, Dauch JR, Hayes JM, Hong Y, Feldman EL. Nerve growth factor mediates mechanical allodynia in a mouse model of type 2 diabetes. *J Neuropathol Exp Neurol.* 2009;68(11):1229-1243.
177. Aloe L, Tuveri MA, Carcassi U, Levi-Montalcini R. Nerve growth factor in the synovial fluid of patients with chronic arthritis. *Arthritis Rheum.* 1992;35(3):351-355.
178. del Porto F, Aloe L, Lagana B, Triaca V, Nofroni I, D'Amelio R. Nerve growth factor and brain-derived neurotrophic factor levels in patients with rheumatoid arthritis treated with TNF-alpha blockers. *Ann N Y Acad Sci.* 2006;1069:438-443.
179. Indo Y. Nerve growth factor and the physiology of pain: lessons from congenital insensitivity to pain with anhidrosis. *Clin Genet.* 2012;82(4):341-350.
180. Petruska JC. Nerve growth factor. In; *Reference Module in Neuroscience and Biobehavioral Psychology.* New York, NY: Elsevier; 2017.
181. Ichikawa H, Matsuo S, Silos-Santiago I, Jacquin MF, Sugimoto T. The development of myelinated nociceptors is dependent upon trks in the trigeminal ganglion. *Acta Histochem.* 2004;106(5):337-343.
182. Gautam M, Prasoon P, Kumar R, Reeta KH, Kaler S, Ray SB. Role of neurokinin type 1 receptor in nociception at the periphery and the spinal level in the rat. *Spinal Cord.* 2016;54(3):172-182.
183. Durham PL. Calcitonin gene-related peptide (CGRP) and migraine. *Headache.* 2006;46 suppl 1:S3-S8.
184. Vega AV, Ramos-Mondragon R, Calderon-Rivera A, Zarain-Herzberg A, Avila G. Calcitonin gene-related peptide restores disrupted excitation-contraction coupling in myotubes expressing central core disease mutations in RyR1. *J Physiol.* 2011;589(pt 19):4649-4669.
185. Vega AV, Avila G. CGRP, a vasodilator neuropeptide that stimulates neuromuscular transmission and EC coupling. *Curr Vasc Pharmacol.* 2010;8(3):394-403.
186. Rodrigo J, Polak JM, Terenghi G, et al. Calcitonin gene-related peptide (CGRP)-immunoreactive sensory and motor nerves of the mammalian palate. *Histochemistry.* 1985;82(1):67-74.
187. Tarabal O, Caldero J, Ribera J, et al. Regulation of motoneuronal calcitonin gene-related peptide (CGRP) during axonal growth and neuromuscular synaptic plasticity induced by botulinum toxin in rats. *Eur J Neurosci.* 1996;8(4):829-836.
188. Fernandez HL, Chen M, Nadelhaft I, Durr JA. Calcitonin gene-related peptides: their binding sites and receptor accessory proteins in adult mammalian skeletal muscles. *Neuroscience.* 2003;119(2):335-345.
189. Rossi SG, Dickerson IM, Rotundo RL. Localization of the calcitonin gene-related peptide receptor complex at the vertebrate neuromuscular junction and its role in regulating acetylcholinesterase expression. *J Biol Chem.* 2003;278(27):24994-25000.
190. Lindsay RM, Harmar AJ. Nerve growth factor regulates expression of neuropeptide genes in adult sensory neurons. *Nature.* 1989;337(6205):362-364.
191. Gwak YS, Nam TS, Paik KS, Hulsebosch CE, Leem JW. Attenuation of mechanical hyperalgesia following spinal cord injury by administration of antibodies to nerve growth factor in the rat. *Neurosci Lett.* 2003;336(2):117-120.
192. Hofer AM. Signal transduction and second messengers. In: Sperelakis N, ed. *Cell Physiology Source Book.* 4th ed. London, England: Academic Press; 2012:85-98.
193. Berridge MJ, Bootman MD, Roderick HL. Calcium signalling: dynamics, homeostasis and remodelling. *Nat Rev Mol Cell Biol.* 2003;4(7):517-529.
194. Qiu F, Qiu CY, Cai H, et al. Oxytocin inhibits the activity of acid-sensing ion channels through the vasopressin, V1A receptor in primary sensory neurons. *Br J Pharmacol.* 2014;171(12):3065-3076.
195. Zhang W, Yu G, Zhang M. ARA 290 relieves pathophysiological pain by targeting TRPV1 channel: integration between immune system and nociception. *Peptides.* 2016;76:73-79.
196. Treede RD, Apkarian AV, Bromm B, Greenspan JD, Lenz FA. Cortical representation of pain: functional characterization of nociceptive areas near the lateral sulcus. *Pain.* 2000;87(2):113-119.
197. Flor H. The functional organization of the brain in chronic pain. *Prog Brain Res.* 2000;129:313-322.
198. Riley JL III, Gilbert GH, Heft MW. Orofacial pain symptom prevalence: selective sex differences in the elderly? *Pain.* 1998;76(1-2):97-104.
199. Fillingim RB. *Sex, Gender and Pain.* Vol 17. Seattle, WA: IASP Press; 2000.
200. Rhudy JL, Bartley EJ, Williams AE, et al. Are there sex differences in affective modulation of spinal nociception and pain? *J Pain.* 2010;11(12):1429-1441.
201. Yunus MB. Psychological factors in fibromyalgia syndrome. *J Musculoskelet Pain.* 1994;2(1):87-91.
202. Yunus MB. Genetic factors in fibromyalgia syndrome. *Z Rheumatol.* 1998;57 suppl 2:61-62.
203. Ablin JN, Buskila D. Update on the genetics of the fibromyalgia syndrome. *Best Pract Res Clin Rheumatol.* 2015;29(1):20-28.

204. Albrecht PJ, Rice FL. Fibromyalgia syndrome pathology and environmental influences on afflictions with medically unexplained symptoms. *Rev Environ Health.* 2016;31(2):281-294.
205. Neeck G, Crofford LJ. Neuroendocrine perturbations in fibromyalgia and chronic fatigue syndrome. *Rheum Dis Clin North Am.* 2000;26(4):989-1002.
206. Loke H, Harley V, Lee J. Biological factors underlying sex differences in neurological disorders. *Int J Biochem Cell Biol.* 2015;65:139-150.
207. Eichhorn N, Treede RD, Schuh-Hofer S. The role of sex in sleep deprivation related changes of nociception and conditioned pain modulation. *Neuroscience.* 2017. doi:10.1016/j.neuroscience.2017.09.044.
208. Fillingim RB, King CD, Ribeiro-Dasilva MC, Rahim-Williams B, Riley JL III. Sex, gender, and pain: a review of recent clinical and experimental findings. *J Pain.* 2009;10(5):447-485.
209. Monroe TB, Fillingim RB, Bruehl SP, et al. Sex differences in brain regions modulating pain among older adults: a cross-sectional resting state functional connectivity study. *Pain Med.* 2017. doi:10.1093/pm/pnx084.
210. Paulson PE, Minoshima S, Morrow TJ, Casey KL. Gender differences in pain perception and patterns of cerebral activation during noxious heat stimulation in humans. *Pain.* 1998;76(1-2):223-229.
211. Goffaux P, Michaud K, Gaudreau J, Chalaye P, Rainville P, Marchand S. Sex differences in perceived pain are affected by an anxious brain. *Pain.* 2011;152(9):2065-2073.
212. Belanger C, Blais Morin B, Brousseau A, et al. Unpredictable pain timings lead to greater pain when people are highly intolerant of uncertainty. *Scand J Pain.* 2017;17:367-372.
213. Kindler LL, Valencia C, Fillingim RB, George SZ. Sex differences in experimental and clinical pain sensitivity for patients with shoulder pain. *Eur J Pain.* 2011;15(2):118-123.
214. Valencia C, Kindler LL, Fillingim RB, George SZ. Stability of conditioned pain modulation in two musculoskeletal pain models: investigating the influence of shoulder pain intensity and gender. *BMC Musculoskelet Disord.* 2013;14:182.
215. Traub RJ, Ji Y. Sex differences and hormonal modulation of deep tissue pain. *Front Neuroendocrinol.* 2013;34(4):350-366.
216. Gaumond I, Arsenault P, Marchand S. Specificity of female and male sex hormones on excitatory and inhibitory phases of formalin-induced nociceptive responses. *Brain Res.* 2005;1052(1):105-111.
217. Melchior M, Poisbeau P, Gaumond I, Marchand S. Insights into the mechanisms and the emergence of sex-differences in pain. *Neuroscience.* 2016;338:63-80.
218. Qu ZW, Liu TT, Ren C, et al. 17Beta-estradiol enhances ASIC activity in primary sensory neurons to produce sex difference in acidosis-induced nociception. *Endocrinology.* 2015;156(12):4660-4671.
219. Rowan MP, Berg KA, Roberts JL, Hargreaves KM, Clarke WP. Activation of estrogen receptor alpha enhances bradykinin signaling in peripheral sensory neurons of female rats. *J Pharmacol Exp Ther.* 2014;349(3):526-532.
220. Ralya A, McCarson KE. Acute estrogen surge enhances inflammatory nociception without altering spinal Fos expression. *Neurosci Lett.* 2014;575:91-95.
221. Gu Y, Chen Y, Zhang X, Li GW, Wang C, Huang LY. Neuronal soma-satellite glial cell interactions in sensory ganglia and the participation of purinergic receptors. *Neuron Glia Biol.* 2010;6(1):53-62.
222. Rajasekhar P, Poole DP, Liedtke W, Bunnett NW, Veldhuis NA. P2Y1 receptor activation of the TRPV4 ion channel enhances purinergic signaling in satellite glial cells. *J Biol Chem.* 2015;290(48):29051-29062.
223. Magni G, Ceruti S. The purinergic system and glial cells: emerging costars in nociception. *Biomed Res Int.* 2014;2014:495789.
224. Magni G, Riccio D, Ceruti S. Tackling chronic pain and inflammation through the purinergic system. *Curr Med Chem.* 2017. doi:10.2174/0929 867324666170710110630.
225. Saez PJ, Vargas P, Shoji KF, Harcha PA, Lennon-Dumenil AM, Saez JC. ATP promotes the fast migration of dendritic cells through the activity of pannexin 1 channels and P2X7 receptors. *Sci Signal.* 2017;10(506).
226. Devesa I, Ferrandiz-Huertas C, Mathivanan S, et al. alphaCGRP is essential for algesic exocytotic mobilization of TRPV1 channels in peptidergic nociceptors. *Proc Natl Acad Sci U S A.* 2014;111(51):18345-18350.
227. Rollman GB, Lautenbacher S. Sex differences in musculoskeletal pain. *Clin J Pain.* 2001;17(1):20-24.
228. Roza C, Reeh PW. Substance P, calcitonin gene related peptide and PGE2 co-released from the mouse colon: a new model to study nociceptive and inflammatory responses in viscera, in vitro. *Pain.* 2001;93(3):213-219.
229. Joca HC, Vieira DC, Vasconcelos AP, Araujo DA, Cruz JS. Carvacrol modulates voltage-gated sodium channels kinetics in dorsal root ganglia. *Eur J Pharmacol.* 2015;756:22-29.
230. Dai Y. TRPs and pain. *Semin Immunopathol.* 2016;38(3):277-291.
231. Caterina MJ. Transient receptor potential ion channels as participants in thermosensation and thermoregulation. *Am J Physiol Regul Integr Comp Physiol.* 2007;292(1):R64-R76.
232. Caterina MJ, Schumacher MA, Tominaga M, Rosen TA, Levine JD, Julius D. The capsaicin receptor: a heat-activated ion channel in the pain pathway. *Nature.* 1997;389(6653):816-824.
233. Roohbakhsh A, Shamsizadeh A. Opioids and TRPV1 receptors. In: Preedy VR, ed. *Neuropathology of Drug Addictions and Substance Misuse.* Vol 1. London, England: Academic Press; 2016:433-442.
234. Backes TM, Rossler OG, Hui X, Grotzinger C, Lipp P, Thiel G. Stimulation of TRPV1 channels activates the AP-1 transcription factor. *Biochem Pharmacol.* 2018;150:160-169.
235. Nersesyan Y, Demirkhanyan L, Cabezas-Bratesco D, et al. Oxytocin modulates nociception as an agonist of pain-sensing TRPV1. *Cell Rep.* 2017;21(6):1681-1691.
236. Deval E, Lingueglia E. Acid-sensing ion channels and nociception in the peripheral and central nervous systems. *Neuropharmacology.* 2015;94:49-57.
237. Walder RY, Rasmussen LA, Rainier JD, Light AR, Wemmie JA, Sluka KA. ASIC1 and ASIC3 play different roles in the development of Hyperalgesia after inflammatory muscle injury. *J Pain.* 2010;11(3):210-218.
238. Wu J, Lewis AH, Grandl J. Touch, tension, and transduction—the function and regulation of piezo ion channels. *Trends Biochem Sci.* 2017;42(1):57-71.
239. Vick JS, Askwith CC. ASICs and neuropeptides. *Neuropharmacology.* 2015;94:36-41.
240. Martinez-Rojas VA, Barragan-Iglesias P, Rocha-Gonzalez HI, Murbartian J, Granados-Soto V. Role of TRPV1 and ASIC3 in formalin-induced secondary allodynia and hyperalgesia. *Pharmacol Rep.* 2014;66(6):964-971.
241. Parpaite T, Coste B. Piezo channels. *Curr Biol.* 2017;27(7):R250-R252.
242. Pereira V, Busserolles J, Christin M, et al. Role of the TREK2 potassium channel in cold and warm thermosensation and in pain perception. *Pain.* 2014;155(12):2534-2544.
243. Deba F, Bessac BF. Anoctamin-1 Cl(-) channels in nociception: activation by an N-aroylaminothiazole and capsaicin and inhibition by T16A[inh]-A01. *Mol Pain.* 2015;11:55.
244. Kwon SG, Roh DH, Yoon SY, et al. Role of peripheral sigma-1 receptors in ischaemic pain: potential interactions with ASIC and P2X receptors. *Eur J Pain.* 2016;20(4):594-606.
245. Huang D, Huang S, Peers C, Du X, Zhang H, Gamper N. GABAB receptors inhibit low-voltage activated and high-voltage activated Ca(2+) channels in sensory neurons via distinct mechanisms. *Biochem Biophys Res Commun.* 2015;465(2):188-193.
246. Coste B, Mathur J, Schmidt M, et al. Piezo1 and Piezo2 are essential components of distinct mechanically activated cation channels. *Science.* 2010;330(6000):55-60.
247. Lolignier S, Eijkelkamp N, Wood JN. Mechanical allodynia. *Pflugers Arch.* 2015;467(1):133-139.
248. Eskander MA, Ruparel S, Green DP, et al. Persistent nociception triggered by nerve growth factor (NGF) is mediated by TRPV1 and oxidative mechanisms. *J Neurosci.* 2015;35(22):8593-8603.
249. Diniz DA, Petrocchi JA, Navarro LC, et al. Serotonin induces peripheral mechanical antihyperalgesic effects in mice. *Eur J Pharmacol.* 2015;767:94-97.
250. Ren C, Gan X, Wu J, Qiu CY, Hu WP. Enhancement of acid-sensing ion channel activity by metabotropic P2Y UTP receptors in primary sensory neurons. *Purinergic Signal.* 2016;12(1):69-78.
251. Letts JA, Sazanov LA. Clarifying the supercomplex: the higher-order organization of the mitochondrial electron transport chain. *Nat Struct Mol Biol.* 2017;24(10):800-808.
252. Yarnitsky D, Granot M, Granovsky Y. Pain modulation profile and pain therapy: between pro- and antinociception. *Pain.* 2014;155(4):663-665.
253. Giesecke T, Gracely RH, Clauw DJ, et al. Central pain processing in chronic low back pain. Evidence for reduced pain inhibition [in German]. *Schmerz.* 2006;20(5):411-414, 416-417.
254. Eippert F, Bingel U, Schoell ED, et al. Activation of the opioidergic descending pain control system underlies placebo analgesia. *Neuron.* 2009;63(4):533-543.
255. Behbehani MM. Functional characteristics of the midbrain periaqueductal gray. *Prog Neurobiol.* 1995;46(6):575-605.
256. Ennis M, Behbehani M, Shipley MT, Van Bockstaele EJ, Aston-Jones G. Projections from the periaqueductal gray to the rostromedial pericoerulear region and nucleus locus coeruleus: anatomic and physiologic studies. *J Comp Neurol.* 1991;306(3):480-494.
257. Murphy AZ, Behbehani MM. Role of norepinephrine in the interaction between the lateral reticular nucleus and the nucleus raphe magnus: an electrophysiological and behavioral study. *Pain.* 1993;54(2):183-193.
258. De Felice M, Ossipov MH. Cortical and subcortical modulation of pain. *Pain Manag.* 2016;6(2):111-120.
259. Tang NM, Dong HW, Wang XM, Tsui ZC, Han JS. Cholecystokinin antisense RNA increases the analgesic effect induced by electroacupuncture or low dose morphine: conversion of low responder rats into high responders. *Pain.* 1997;71(1):71-80.
260. Rosen A, Zhang YX, Lund I, Lundeberg T, Yu LC. Substance P microinjected into the periaqueductal gray matter induces antinociception and is released following morphine administration. *Brain Res.* 2004;1001(1-2):87-94.
261. Drew GM, Lau BK, Vaughan CW. Substance P drives endocannabinoid-mediated disinhibition in a midbrain descending analgesic pathway. *J Neurosci.* 2009;29(22):7220-7229.
262. Rigoard P, Blond S, David R, Mertens P. Pathophysiological characterisation of back pain generators in failed back surgery syndrome (part B). *Neurochirurgie.* 2015;61 suppl 1:S35-S44.
263. McMahon SB, Wall PD. Descending excitation and inhibition of spinal cord lamina I projection neurons. *J Neurophysiol.* 1988;59(4):1204-1219.
264. Rahman W, Sikandar S, Suzuki R, Hunt SP, Dickenson AH. Superficial NK1 expressing spinal dorsal horn neurones modulate inhibitory neurotransmission mediated by spinal GABA(A) receptors. *Neurosci Lett.* 2007;419(3):278-283.
265. Rahman W, Suzuki R, Hunt SP, Dickenson AH. Selective ablation of dorsal horn NK1 expressing cells reveals a modulation of spinal alpha2-adrenergic inhibition of dorsal horn neurones. *Neuropharmacology.* 2008;54(8):1208-1214.
266. Porreca F, Ossipov MH, Gebhart GF. Chronic pain and medullary descending facilitation. *Trends Neurosci.* 2002;25(6):319-325.
267. Guo W, Miyoshi K, Dubner R, et al. Spinal 5-HT3 receptors mediate descending facilitation and contribute to behavioral hypersensitivity via a reciprocal neuron-glial signaling cascade. *Mol Pain.* 2014;10:35.

268. Tian B, Wang XL, Huang Y, et al. Peripheral and spinal 5-HT receptors participate in cholestatic itch and antinociception induced by bile duct ligation in rats. *Sci Rep.* 2016;6:36286.
269. Bannister K, Bee LA, Dickenson AH. Preclinical and early clinical investigations related to monoaminergic pain modulation. *Neurotherapeutics.* 2009;6(4):703-712.
270. Green GM, Scarth J, Dickenson A. An excitatory role for 5-HT in spinal inflammatory nociceptive transmission; state-dependent actions via dorsal horn 5-HT(3) receptors in the anaesthetized rat. *Pain.* 2000;89(1):81-88.
271. Rahman W, Bauer CS, Bannister K, Vonsy JL, Dolphin AC, Dickenson AH. Descending serotonergic facilitation and the antinociceptive effects of pregabalin in a rat model of osteoarthritic pain. *Mol Pain.* 2009;5:45.
272. Dogrul A, Ossipov MH, Porreca F. Differential mediation of descending pain facilitation and inhibition by spinal 5HT-3 and 5HT-7 receptors. *Brain Res.* 2009;1280:52-59.
273. Kato G, Yasaka T, Katafuchi T, et al. Direct GABAergic and glycinergic inhibition of the substantia gelatinosa from the rostral ventromedial medulla revealed by in vivo patch-clamp analysis in rats. *J Neurosci.* 2006;26(6):1787-1794.
274. Ossipov MH, Morimura K, Porreca F. Descending pain modulation and chronification of pain. *Curr Opin Support Palliat Care.* 2014;8(2):143-151.
275. Pielsticker A, Haag G, Zaudig M, Lautenbacher S. Impairment of pain inhibition in chronic tension-type headache. *Pain.* 2005;118(1-2):215-223.
276. Daenen L, Nijs J, Roussel N, Wouters K, Van Loo M, Cras P. Dysfunctional pain inhibition in patients with chronic whiplash-associated disorders: an experimental study. *Clin Rheumatol.* 2013;32(1):23-31.
277. Gruener H, Zeilig G, Laufer Y, Blumen N, Defrin R. Differential pain modulation properties in central neuropathic pain after spinal cord injury. *Pain.* 2016;157(7):1415-1424.
278. Mense S. Descending antinociception and fibromyalgia. *Z Rheumatol.* 1998;57 suppl 2:23-26.
279. Bannister K, Dickenson AH. What the brain tells the spinal cord. *Pain.* 2016;157(10):2148-2151.
280. Nuseir K, Proudfit HK. Bidirectional modulation of nociception by GABA neurons in the dorsolateral pontine tegmentum that tonically inhibit spinally projecting noradrenergic A7 neurons. *Neuroscience.* 2000;96(4):773-783.
281. Gall O, Villanueva L, Bouhassira D, Le Bars D. Spatial encoding properties of subnucleus reticularis dorsalis neurons in the rat medulla. *Brain Res.* 2000;873(1):131-134.
282. Villanueva L. Diffuse Noxious Inhibitory Control (DNIC) as a tool for exploring dysfunction of endogenous pain modulatory systems. *Pain.* 2009;143(3):161-162.
283. Villanueva L, Cadden SW, Le Bars D. Diffuse noxious inhibitory controls (DNIC): evidence for post-synaptic inhibition of trigeminal nucleus caudalis convergent neurones. *Brain Res.* 1984;321(1):165-168.
284. Villanueva L, Cadden SW, Le Bars D. Evidence that diffuse noxious inhibitory controls (DNIC) are medicated by a final post-synaptic inhibitory mechanism. *Brain Res.* 1984;298(1):67-74.
285. Villanueva L, Peschanski M, Calvino B, Le Bars D. Ascending pathways in the spinal cord involved in triggering of diffuse noxious inhibitory controls in the rat. *J Neurophysiol.* 1986;55(1):34-55.
286. Chebbi R, Boyer N, Monconduit L, Artola A, Luccarini P, Dallel R. The nucleus raphe magnus OFF-cells are involved in diffuse noxious inhibitory controls. *Exp Neurol.* 2014;256:39-45.
287. Campbell CM, France CR, Robinson ME, Logan HL, Geffken GR, Fillingim RB. Ethnic differences in diffuse noxious inhibitory controls. *J Pain.* 2008;9(8):759-766.
288. Popescu A, LeResche L, Truelove EL, Drangsholt MT. Gender differences in pain modulation by diffuse noxious inhibitory controls: a systematic review. *Pain.* 2010;150(2):309-318.
289. France CR, Suchowiecki S. A comparison of diffuse noxious inhibitory controls in men and women. *Pain.* 1999;81(1-2):77-84.
290. Rolke R, Magerl W, Campbell KA, et al. Quantitative sensory testing: a comprehensive protocol for clinical trials. *Eur J Pain.* 2006;10(1):77-88.
291. Jensen TS, Baron R. Translation of symptoms and signs into mechanisms in neuropathic pain. *Pain.* 2003;102(1-2):1-8.
292. Arendt-Nielsen L, Yarnitsky D. Experimental and clinical applications of quantitative sensory testing applied to skin, muscles and viscera. *J Pain.* 2009;10(6):556-572.
293. Geber C, Klein T, Azad S, et al. Test-retest and interobserver reliability of quantitative sensory testing according to the protocol of the German Research Network on Neuropathic Pain (DFNS): a multi-centre study. *Pain.* 2011;152(3):548-556.
294. Shakoor N, Agrawal A, Block JA. Reduced lower extremity vibratory perception in osteoarthritis of the knee. *Arthritis Rheum.* 2008;59(1):117-121.
295. van Deursen RW, Sanchez MM, Derr JA, Becker MB, Ulbrecht JS, Cavanagh PR. Vibration perception threshold testing in patients with diabetic neuropathy: ceiling effects and reliability. *Diabet Med.* 2001;18(6):469-475.
296. Pestronk A, Florence J, Levine T, et al. Sensory exam with a quantitative tuning fork: rapid, sensitive and predictive of SNAP amplitude. *Neurology.* 2004;62(3):461-464.
297. Hansson P, Backonja M, Bouhassira D. Usefulness and limitations of quantitative sensory testing: clinical and research application in neuropathic pain states. *Pain.* 2007;129(3):256-259.
298. Xing H, Chen M, Ling J, Tan W, Gu JG. TRPM8 mechanism of cold allodynia after chronic nerve injury. *J Neurosci.* 2007;27(50):13680-13690.
299. Bevan S, Quallo T, Andersson DA. Trpv1. *Handb Exp Pharmacol.* 2014;222:207-245.
300. Courtney CA, Kavchak AE, Lowry CD, O'Hearn MA. Interpreting joint pain: quantitative sensory testing in musculoskeletal management. *J Orthop Sports Phys Ther.* 2010;40(12):818-825.
301. Chesterton LS, Sim J, Wright CC, Foster NE. Interrater reliability of algometry in measuring pressure pain thresholds in healthy humans, using multiple raters. *Clin J Pain.* 2007;23(9):760-766.
302. Vanderweeen L, Oostendorp RA, Vaes P, Duquet W. Pressure algometry in manual therapy. *Man Ther.* 1996;1(5):258-265.
303. Courtney CA, Fernández-de-Las-Peñas C, Bond S. Mechanisms of chronic pain—key considerations for appropriate physical therapy management. *J Man Manip Ther.* 2017;25(3):118-127.
304. Mucke M, Cuhls H, Radbruch L, et al. Quantitative Sensory Testing (QST). *Schmerz.* 2016. doi:10.1007/s00482-015-0093-2.
305. Ambite-Quesada S, Arias-Buria JL, Courtney CA, Arendt-Nielsen L, Fernández-de-Las-Peñas C. Exploration of quantitative sensory testing in latent trigger points and referred pain areas. *Clin J Pain.* 2018;34(5):409-414.
306. Wall PD, Woolf CJ. Muscle but not cutaneous C-afferent input produces prolonged increases in the excitability of the flexion reflex in the rat. *J Physiol.* 1984;356:443-458.
307. Niddam DM, Chan RC, Lee SH, Yeh TC, Hsieh JC. Central modulation of pain evoked from myofascial trigger point. *Clin J Pain.* 2007;23(5):440-448.
308. Niddam DM, Chan RC, Lee SH, Yeh TC, Hsieh JC. Central representation of hyperalgesia from myofascial trigger point. *Neuroimage.* 2008;39(3):1299-1306.
309. Bialosky JE, Bishop MD, Price DD, Robinson ME, George SZ. The mechanisms of manual therapy in the treatment of musculoskeletal pain: a comprehensive model. *Man Ther.* 2009;14(5):531-538.
310. Simons DG. Muscle pain syndromes—part I. *Am J Phys Med.* 1975;54(6):289-311.
311. Simons DG. Muscle pain syndromes—part II. *Am J Phys Med.* 1976;55(1):15-42.
312. Simons DG. Cardiology and myofascial trigger points: Janet G. Travell's contribution. *Tex Heart Inst J.* 2003;30(1):3-7.
313. Baldry PE. *Acupuncture, Trigger Points and Musculoskeletal Pain. A Scientific Approach to Acupuncture for Use by Doctors and Physiotherapists in the Diagnosis and Management of Myofascial Trigger Point Pain.* 3rd ed. Edinburgh, Scotland: Elsevier Churchill Livingstone; 2005.
314. Baldry P, Yunus M, Inanici F, Hazelman B. *Myofascial Pain and Fibromyalgia Syndromes.* Edinburgh, Scotland: Churchill Livingstone; 2001.
315. Steindler A. The interpretation of sciatic radiation and the syndrome of low-back pain. *J Bone Joint Surg Am.* 1940;22:28-34.
316. Travell J, Rinzler SH. The myofascial genesis of pain. *Postgrad Med.* 1952;11(5):425-434.
317. Kellgren JH. Observations on referred pain arising from muscle. *Clin Sci.* 1938;3:175-190.
318. Kellgren JH. A preliminary account of referred pains arising from muscle. *Br Med J.* 1938;1:325-327.
319. Kellgren JH. Deep pain sensibility. *Lancet.* 1949;1(6562):943-949.
320. Lewis T, Kellgren JH. Observations relating to referred pain, visceromotor reflexes and other associated phenomena. *Clin Sci.* 1939;4:47-71.
321. Simons DG, Travell J. Myofascial trigger points, a possible explanation. *Pain.* 1981;10(1):106-109.
322. Simons DG, Travell JG. Myofascial origins of low back pain. 3. Pelvic and lower extremity muscles. *Postgrad Med.* 1983;73(2):99-105, 108.
323. Simons DG, Travell JG. Myofascial origins of low back pain. 2. Torso muscles. *Postgrad Med.* 1983;73(2):81-92.
324. Simons DG, Travell JG. Myofascial origins of low back pain. 1. Principles of diagnosis and treatment. *Postgrad Med.* 1983;73(2):66, 68-70, 73 passim.
325. Simons DG, Travell J. Chapter 2.A.7, Myofascial pain syndromes. In: Wall PD, Melzack R, eds. *Textbook of Pain.* Edinburgh, Scotland: Churchill Livingstone; 1984:263-276.
326. Travell J. Pain mechanisms in connective tissue. Paper presented at: Connective tissues transactions of the second conference1952; New York.
327. Travell J. Ethyl chloride spray for painful muscle spasm. *Arch Phys Med Rehabil.* 1952;33(5):291-298.
328. Travell J. Referred pain from skeletal muscle; the pectoralis major syndrome of breast pain and soreness and the sternomastoid syndrome of headache and dizziness. *N Y State J Med.* 1955;55(3):331-340.
329. Travell J. Temporomandibular joint pain referred from muscles of the head and neck. *J Prosthet Dent.* 1960;10:745-763.
330. Travell J. Mechanical headache. *Headache.* 1967;7(1):23-29.
331. Travell J. Myofascial trigger points: clinical view. In: Bonica JJ, Albe-Fessard D, eds. *Advances in Pain Research and Therapy.* Vol 1. New York, NY: Raven Press; 1976:919-926.
332. Travell J. Identification of myofascial trigger point syndromes: a case of atypical facial neuralgia. *Arch Phys Med Rehabil.* 1981;62(3):100-106.
333. Weeks VD, Travell J. *How to Give Painless Injections.* AMA Scientific Exhibits. New York, NY: Grune & Stratton; 1957:318-322.
334. Chen Q, Basford JR, An KN. Ability of magnetic resonance elastography to assess taut bands. *Clin Biomech (Bristol, Avon).* 2008;23(5):623-629.
335. Chen Q, Bensamoun S, Basford JR, Thompson JM, An KN. Identification and quantification of myofascial taut bands with magnetic resonance elastography. *Arch Phys Med Rehabil.* 2007;88(12):1658-1661.
336. Chen Q, Wang HJ, Gay RE, et al. Quantification of myofascial taut bands. *Arch Phys Med Rehabil.* 2016;97(1):67-73.
337. Sikdar S, Shah JP, Gebreab T, et al. Novel applications of ultrasound technology to visualize and characterize myofascial trigger points and surrounding soft tissue. *Arch Phys Med Rehabil.* 2009;90(11):1829-1838.

338. Turo D, Otto P, Egorov V, Sarvazyan A, Gerber LH, Sikdar S. Elastography and tactile imaging for mechanical characterization of superficial muscles. *J Acoust Soc Am.* 2012;132(3):1983.
339. Turo D, Otto P, Hossain M, et al. Novel use of ultrasound elastography to quantify muscle tissue changes after dry needling of myofascial trigger points in patients with chronic myofascial pain. *J Ultrasound Med.* 2015;34(12):2149-2161.
340. Turo D, Otto P, Shah JP, et al. Ultrasonic characterization of the upper trapezius muscle in patients with chronic neck pain. *Ultrason Imaging.* 2013;35(2):173-187.
341. Bubnov RV. The use of trigger point "dry" needling under ultrasound guidance for the treatment of myofascial pain (technological innovation and literature review). *Lik Sprava.* 2010(5-6):56-64.
342. Rha DW, Shin JC, Kim YK, Jung JH, Kim YU, Lee SC. Detecting local twitch responses of myofascial trigger points in the lower-back muscles using ultrasonography. *Arch Phys Med Rehabil.* 2011;92(10):1576.e1-1580.e1.
343. Maher RM, Hayes DM, Shinohara M. Quantification of dry needling and posture effects on myofascial trigger points using ultrasound shear-wave elastography. *Arch Phys Med Rehabil.* 2013;94(11):2146-2150.
344. Muller CE, Aranha MF, Gaviao MB. Two-dimensional ultrasound and ultrasound elastography imaging of trigger points in women with myofascial pain syndrome treated by acupuncture and electroacupuncture: a double-blinded randomized controlled pilot study. *Ultrason Imaging.* 2015;37(2):152-167.
345. Gerwin RD, Duranleau D. Ultrasound identification of the myofascial trigger point. *Muscle Nerve.* 1997;20(6):767-768.
346. Wolfe F, Simons DG, Fricton J, et al. The fibromyalgia and myofascial pain syndromes: a preliminary study of tender points and trigger points in persons with fibromyalgia, myofascial pain syndrome and no disease. *J Rheumatol.* 1992;19(6):944-951.
347. Nice DA, Riddle DL, Lamb RL, Mayhew TP, Rucker K. Intertester reliability of judgments of the presence of trigger points in patients with low back pain. *Arch Phys Med Rehabil.* 1992;73(10):893-898.
348. Lucas N, Macaskill P, Irwig L, Moran R, Bogduk N. Reliability of physical examination for diagnosis of myofascial trigger points: a systematic review of the literature. *Clin J Pain.* 2009;25(1):80-89.
349. Lew PC, Lewis J, Story I. Inter-therapist reliability in locating latent myofascial trigger points using palpation. *Man Ther.* 1997;2(2):87-90.
350. Gerwin RD, Shannon S, Hong C-Z, Hubbard DR, Gevirtz R. Interrater reliability in myofascial trigger point examination. *Pain.* 1997;69:65-73.
351. Bron C, Franssen J, Wensing M, Oostendorp RA. Interrater reliability of palpation of myofascial trigger points in three shoulder muscles. *J Man Manip Ther.* 2007;15(4):203-215.
352. Barbero M, Bertoli P, Cescon C, Macmillan R, Coutts F, Gatti R. Intra-rater reliability of an experienced physiotherapist in locating myofascial trigger points in upper trapezius muscle. *J Man Manip Ther.* 2012;20(4):171-177.
353. De Groef A, Van Kampen M, Dieltjens E, et al. Identification of myofascial trigger points in breast cancer survivors with upper limb pain: interrater reliability. *Pain Med.* 2017. doi:10.1093/pm/pnx299.
354. Mayoral del Moral O, Torres Lacomba M, Russell IJ, Sanchez Mendez AO, Sanchez Sanchez B. Validity and reliability of clinical examination in the diagnosis of myofascial pain syndrome and myofascial trigger points in upper quarter muscles. *Pain Med.* 2017. doi:10.1093/pm/pnx315.
355. Mora-Relucio R, Nunez-Nagy S, Gallego-Izquierdo T, et al. Experienced versus inexperienced interexaminer reliability on location and classification of myofascial trigger point palpation to diagnose lateral epicondylalgia: an observational cross-sectional study. *Evid Based Complement Alternat Med.* 2016;2016:6059719.
356. Al-Shenqiti AM, Oldham JA. Test-retest reliability of myofascial trigger point detection in patients with rotator cuff tendonitis. *Clin Rehabil.* 2005;19(5):482-487.
357. Anders HL, Corrie M, Jan H, et al. Standardized simulated palpation training—development of a palpation trainer and assessment of palpatory skills in experienced and inexperienced clinicians. *Man Ther.* 2010;15(3):254-260.
358. Myburgh C, Lauridsen HH, Larsen AH, Hartvigsen J. Standardized manual palpation of myofascial trigger points in relation to neck/shoulder pain; the influence of clinical experience on inter-examiner reproducibility. *Man Ther.* 2011;16(2):136-140.
359. McEvoy J, Huijbregts PA. Reliability of myofascial trigger point palpation: a systematic review. In: Dommerholt J, Huijbregts PA, eds. *Myofascial Trigger Points. Pathophysiology and Evidence-Informed Diagnosis and Management.* Boston, MA: Jones & Bartlett; 2011:65-88.
360. Rozenfeld E, Finestone AS, Moran U, Damri E, Kalichman L. Test-retest reliability of myofascial trigger point detection in hip and thigh areas. *J Bodyw Mov Ther.* 2017;21(4):914-919.
361. Hoyle JA, Marras WS, Sheedy JE, Hart DE. Effects of postural and visual stressors on myofascial trigger point development and motor unit rotation during computer work. *J Electromyogr Kinesiol.* 2011;21(1):41-48.
362. Treaster D, Marras WS, Burr D, Sheedy JE, Hart D. Myofascial trigger point development from visual and postural stressors during computer work. *J Electromyogr Kinesiol.* 2006;16(2):115-124.
363. Chen S-M, Chen JT, Kuan T-S, Hong J, Hong C-Z. Decrease in pressure pain thresholds of latent myofascial trigger points in the middle finger extensors immediately after continuous piano practice. *J Musculoskelet Pain.* 2000;8(3):83-92.
364. Hagg GM. Static work and myalgia-a new explanation model. In: Andersson PA, Hobart DJ, Danoff JV, eds. *Electromyographical Kinesiology.* Amsterdam, The Netherlands: Elsevier; 1991:115-199.
365. Hagg GM. The Cinderella hypothesis. In: Johansson H, Windhorst U, Djupsjobacka M, Passotore M, eds. *Chronic Work-Related Myalgia.* Gavle, Sweden: University Press; 2003:127-132.
366. Forsman M, Kadefors R, Zhang Q, Birch L, Palmerud G. Motor-unit recruitment in the trapezius muscle during arm movements and in VDU precision work. *Int J Ind Ergon.* 1999;24:619-630.
367. Zennaro D, Laubli T, Krebs D, Klipstein A, Krueger H. Continuous, intermitted and sporadic motor unit activity in the trapezius muscle during prolonged computer work. *J Electromyogr Kinesiol.* 2003;13(2):113-124.
368. Qerama E, Fuglsang-Frederiksen A, Kasch H, Bach FW, Jensen TS. Evoked pain in the motor endplate region of the brachial biceps muscle: an experimental study. *Muscle Nerve.* 2004;29(3):393-400.
369. Wessler I. Acetylcholine release at motor endplates and autonomic neuroeffector junctions: a comparison. *Pharmacol Res.* 1996;33(2):81-94.
370. Malomouzh AI, Mukhtarov MR, Nikolsky EE, Vyskocil F. Muscarinic M1 acetylcholine receptors regulate the non-quantal release of acetylcholine in the rat neuromuscular junction via NO-dependent mechanism. *J Neurochem.* 2007;102(6):2110-2117.
371. Magleby KL, Pallotta BS. A study of desensitization of acetylcholine receptors using nerve-released transmitter in the frog. *J Physiol.* 1981;316:225-250.
372. Choi RC, Siow NL, Cheng AW, et al. ATP acts via P2Y1 receptors to stimulate acetylcholinesterase and acetylcholine receptor expression: transduction and transcription control. *J Neurosci.* 2003;23(11):4445-4456.
373. Malomouzh AI, Nikolsky EE, Vyskocil F. Purine P2Y receptors in ATP-mediated regulation of non-quantal acetylcholine release from motor nerve endings of rat diaphragm. *Neurosci Res.* 2011;71(3):219-225.
374. Liu QG, Liu L, Huang QM, Nguyen TT, Ma YT, Zhao JM. Decreased spontaneous electrical activity and acetylcholine at myofascial trigger spots after dry needling treatment: a pilot study. *Evid Based Complement Alternat Med.* 2017;2017:3938191.
375. Bukharaeva EA, Salakhutdinov RI, Vyskocil F, Nikolsky EE. Spontaneous quantal and non-quantal release of acetylcholine at mouse endplate during onset of hypoxia. *Physiol Res.* 2005;54(2):251-255.
376. Grinnell AD, Chen BM, Kashani A, Lin J, Suzuki K, Kidokoro Y. The role of integrins in the modulation of neurotransmitter release from motor nerve terminals by stretch and hypertonicity. *J Neurocytol.* 2003;32(5-8):489-503.
377. Chen BM, Grinnell AD. Kinetics, Ca2+ dependence, and biophysical properties of integrin-mediated mechanical modulation of transmitter release from frog motor nerve terminals. *J Neurosci.* 1997;17(3):904-916.
378. Smillie SJ, Brain SD. Calcitonin gene-related peptide (CGRP) and its role in hypertension. *Neuropeptides.* 2011;45(2):93-104.
379. Durham PL, Vause CV. Calcitonin gene-related peptide (CGRP) receptor antagonists in the treatment of migraine. *CNS Drugs.* 2010;24(7):539-548.
380. Hodges-Savola CA, Fernandez HL. A role for calcitonin gene-related peptide in the regulation of rat skeletal muscle G4 acetylcholinesterase. *Neurosci Lett.* 1995;190(2):117-120.
381. Shah JP. A novel microanalytical technique for assaying soft tissue demonstrates significant quantitative biochemical differences in 3 clinically distinct groups: normal, latent, and active (Abstract). *Arch Phys Med Rehabil.* 2003;84(9):A4.
382. Shah JP, Danoff JV, Desai MJ, et al. Biochemicals associated with pain and inflammation are elevated in sites near to and remote from active myofascial trigger points. *Arch Phys Med Rehabil.* 2008;89(1):16-23.
383. Shah JP, Gilliams EA. Uncovering the biochemical milieu of myofascial trigger points using in vivo microdialysis: an application of muscle pain concepts to myofascial pain syndrome. *J Bodyw Mov Ther.* 2008;12(4):371-384.
384. Dommerholt J, Bron C, Franssen J. Myofascial trigger points; an evidence-informed review. *J Manual Manipulative Ther.* 2006;14(4):203-221.
385. Bruckle W, Suckfull M, Fleckenstein W, Weiss C, Muller W. Gewebe-p02-Messung in der verspannten Ruckenmuskulatur (m. erector spinae). [Tissue pO2 measurement in taut back musculature (m. erector spinae)]. *Z Rheumatol.* 1990;49(4):208-216.
386. Ballyns JJ, Shah JP, Hammond J, Gebreab T, Gerber LH, Sikdar S. Objective sonographic measures for characterizing myofascial trigger points associated with cervical pain. *J Ultrasound Med.* 2011;30(10):1331-1340.
387. Deval E, Gasull X, Noel J, et al. Acid-sensing ion channels (ASICs): pharmacology and implication in pain. *Pharmacol Ther.* 2010;128(3):549-558.
388. Sluka KA, Gregory NS. The dichotomized role for acid sensing ion channels in musculoskeletal pain and inflammation. *Neuropharmacology.* 2015;94:58-63.
389. Sluka KA, Kalra A, Moore SA. Unilateral intramuscular injections of acidic saline produce a bilateral, long-lasting hyperalgesia. *Muscle Nerve.* 2001;24(1):37-46.
390. Sluka KA, Price MP, Breese NM, Stucky CL, Wemmie JA, Welsh MJ. Chronic hyperalgesia induced by repeated acid injections in muscle is abolished by the loss of ASIC3, but not ASIC1. *Pain.* 2003;106(3):229-239.
391. Sluka KA, Radhakrishnan R, Benson CJ, et al. ASIC3 in muscle mediates mechanical, but not heat, hyperalgesia associated with muscle inflammation. *Pain.* 2007;129(1-2):102-112.
392. Sluka KA, Rohlwing JJ, Bussey RA, Eikenberry SA, Wilken JM. Chronic muscle pain induced by repeated acid injection is reversed by spinally administered mu- and delta-, but not kappa-, opioid receptor agonists. *J Pharmacol Exp Ther.* 2002;302(3):1146-1150.
393. Hubbard DR, Berkoff GM. Myofascial trigger points show spontaneous needle EMG activity. *Spine.* 1993;18(13):1803-1807.
394. Simons DG. Do endplate noise and spikes arise from normal motor endplates? *Am J Phys Med Rehabil.* 2001;80(2):134-140.
395. Simons DG. New views of myofascial trigger points: etiology and diagnosis. *Arch Phys Med Rehabil.* 2008;89(1):157-159.

396. Simons DG, Hong CZ, Simons LS. Endplate potentials are common to midfiber myofascial trigger points. *Am J Phys Med Rehabil.* 2002;81(3):212-222.
397. Chen JT, Chen SM, Kuan TS, Chung KC, Hong CZ. Phentolamine effect on the spontaneous electrical activity of active loci in a myofascial trigger spot of rabbit skeletal muscle. *Arch Phys Med Rehabil.* 1998;79(7):790-794.
398. Tsai CT, Hsieh LF, Kuan TS, Kao MJ, Chou LW, Hong CZ. Remote effects of dry needling on the irritability of the myofascial trigger point in the upper trapezius muscle. *Am J Phys Med Rehabil.* 2009;89(2):133-140.
399. Kuan T-A, Lin T-S, Chen JT, Chen S-M, Hong C-Z. No increased neuromuscular jitter at rabbit skeletal muscle trigger spot spontaneous electrical activity sites. *J Musculoskelet Pain.* 2000;8(3):69-82.
400. Couppe C, Midttun A, Hilden J, Jorgensen U, Oxholm P, Fuglsang-Frederiksen A. Spontaneous needle electromyographic activity in myofascial trigger points in the infraspinatus muscle: a blinded assessment. *J Musculoskelet Pain.* 2001;9(3):7-16.
401. Macgregor J, Graf von Schweinitz D. Needle electromyographic activity of myofascial trigger points and control sites in equine cleidobrachialis muscle—an observational study. *Acupunct Med.* 2006;24(2):61-70.
402. Ge HY, Fernández-de-Las-Peñas C, Yue SW. Myofascial trigger points: spontaneous electrical activity and its consequences for pain induction and propagation. *Chin Med.* 2011;6:13.
403. Chen JT, Chung KC, Hou CR, Kuan TS, Chen SM, Hong CZ. Inhibitory effect of dry needling on the spontaneous electrical activity recorded from myofascial trigger spots of rabbit skeletal muscle. *Am J Phys Med Rehabil.* 2001;80(10):729-735.
404. Chen JT, Kuan T-S, Hong C-Z. Inhibitory effect of calcium channel blocker on the spontaneous electrical activity of myofascial trigger point (Abstract). *J Musculoskelet Pain.* 1998;6(suppl 2):24.
405. Kuan TS, Chen JT, Chen SM, Chien CH, Hong CZ. Effect of botulinum toxin on endplate noise in myofascial trigger spots of rabbit skeletal muscle. *Am J Phys Med Rehabil.* 2002;81(7):512-520; quiz 521-513.
406. Chen S-M, Chen JT, Kuan T-S, Hong C-Z. Effect of neuromuscular blocking agent on the spontaneous activity of active loci in a myofascial trigger spot of rabbit skeletal muscle (Abstract). *J Musculoskelet Pain.* 1998;6(suppl 2):25.
407. Chen KH, Hong CZ, Kuo FC, Hsu HC, Hsieh YL. Electrophysiologic effects of a therapeutic laser on myofascial trigger spots of rabbit skeletal muscles. *Am J Phys Med Rehabil.* 2008;87(12):1006-1014.
408. Shah JP, Phillips TM, Danoff JV, Gerber LH. An in vivo microanalytical technique for measuring the local biochemical milieu of human skeletal muscle. *J Appl Physiol.* 2005;99(5):1977-1984.
409. Hsieh YL, Yang SA, Yang CC, Chou LW. Dry needling at myofascial trigger spots of rabbit skeletal muscles modulates the biochemicals associated with pain, inflammation, and hypoxia. *Evid Based Complement Alternat Med.* 2012;2012:342165.
410. Hsieh YL, Hong CZ, Chou LW, Yang SA, Yang CC. Fluence-dependent effects of low-level laser therapy in myofascial trigger spots on modulation of biochemicals associated with pain in a rabbit model. *Lasers Med Sci.* 2015;30(1):209-216.
411. Willis WD. Retrograde signaling in the nervous system: dorsal root reflexes. In: Bradshaw RA, Dennis EA, eds. *Handbook of Cell Signaling.* Vol 3. San Diego, CA: Academic/Elsevier Press; 2004.
412. Zeilhofer HU, Brune K. Analgesic strategies beyond the inhibition of cyclo-oxygenases. *Trends Pharmacol Sci.* 2006;27(9):467-474.
413. Verri WA Jr, Cunha TM, Parada CA, Poole S, Cunha FQ, Ferreira SH. Hypernociceptive role of cytokines and chemokines: targets for analgesic drug development? *Pharmacol Ther.* 2006;112(1):116-138.
414. Schafers M, Sorkin LS, Sommer C. Intramuscular injection of tumor necrosis factor-alpha induces muscle hyperalgesia in rats. *Pain.* 2003;104(3):579-588.
415. Vyklicky L, Knotkova-Urbancova H, Vitaskova Z, Vlachova V, Kress M, Reeh PW. Inflammatory mediators at acidic pH activate capsaicin receptors in cultured sensory neurons from newborn rats. *J Neurophysiol.* 1998;79(2):670-676.
416. Jensen K, Tuxen C, Pedersen-Bjergaard U, Jansen I, Edvinsson L, Olesen J. Pain and tenderness in human temporal muscle induced by bradykinin and 5-hydroxytryptamine. *Peptides.* 1990;11(6):1127-1132.
417. Gordon JR, Galli SJ. Mast cells as a source of both preformed and immunologically inducible TNF-alpha/cachectin. *Nature.* 1990;346(6281):274-276.
418. Iuvone T, Den Bossche RV, D'Acquisto F, Carnuccio R, Herman AG. Evidence that mast cell degranulation, histamine and tumour necrosis factor alpha release occur in LPS-induced plasma leakage in rat skin. *Br J Pharmacol.* 1999;128(3):700-704.
419. Ge HY, Fernández-de-las-Peñas C, Arendt-Nielsen L. Sympathetic facilitation of hyperalgesia evoked from myofascial tender and trigger points in patients with unilateral shoulder pain. *Clin Neurophysiol.* 2006;117(7):1545-1550.
420. Banks S, Jacobs D, Gevirtz R, Hubbard D. Effects of autogenic relaxation training on electromyographic activity in active myofascial trigger points. *J Musculoskelet Pain.* 1998;6(4):23-32.
421. Lewis C, Gevirtz R, Hubbard DR, et al. Needle trigger point and surface frontal EMG measurements of psychophysiological responses in tension-type headache patients. *Biofeedback Self Regul.* 1994;19(3):274-275.
422. Backman E, Bengtsson A, Bengtsson M, Lennmarken C, Henriksson KG. Skeletal muscle function in primary fibromyalgia. Effect of regional sympathetic blockade with guanethidine. *Acta Neurol Scand.* 1988;77(3):187-191.
423. Bengtsson A, Bengtsson M. Regional sympathetic blockade in primary fibromyalgia. *Pain.* 1988;33(2):161-167.
424. Martinez-Lavin M. Fibromyalgia as a sympathetically maintained pain syndrome. *Curr Pain Headache Rep.* 2004;8(5):385-389.
425. Maekawa K, Clark GT, Kuboki T. Intramuscular hypoperfusion, adrenergic receptors, and chronic muscle pain. *J Pain.* 2002;3(4):251-260.
426. Bowman WC, Marshall IG, Gibb AJ, Harborne AJ. Feedback control of transmitter release at the neuromuscular junction. *Trends Pharmacol Sci.* 1988;9(1):16-20.
427. Lund T, Osterud B. The effect of TNF-alpha, PMA, and LPS on plasma and cell-associated IL-8 in human leukocytes. *Thromb Res.* 2004;113(1):75-83.
428. Loram LC, Fuller A, Fick LG, Cartmell T, Poole S, Mitchell D. Cytokine profiles during carrageenan-induced inflammatory hyperalgesia in rat muscle and hind paw. *J Pain.* 2007;8(2):127-136.
429. Thunberg J, Ljubisavljevic M, Djupsjobacka M, Johansson H. Effects on the fusimotor-muscle spindle system induced by intramuscular injections of hypertonic saline. *Exp Brain Res.* 2002;142(3):319-326.
430. Chen KH, Hong CZ, Hsu HC, Wu SK, Kuo FC, Hsieh YL. Dose-dependent and ceiling effects of therapeutic laser on myofascial trigger spots in rabbit skeletal muscles. *J Musculoskelet Pain.* 2010;18(3):235-245.
431. Hong C-Z, Torigoe Y. Electrophysiological characteristics of localized twitch responses in responsive taut bands of rabbit skeletal muscle. *J Musculoskelet Pain.* 1994;2(2):17-43.
432. Hong CZ, Simons DG. Pathophysiologic and electrophysiologic mechanisms of myofascial trigger points. *Arch Phys Med Rehabil.* 1998;79(7):863-872.
433. Koppenhaver SL, Walker MJ, Rettig C, et al. The association between dry needling-induced twitch response and change in pain and muscle function in patients with low back pain: a quasi-experimental study. *Physiotherapy.* 2017;103(2):131-137.
434. Perreault T, Dunning J, Butts R. The local twitch response during trigger point dry needling: is it necessary for successful outcomes? *J Bodyw Mov Ther.* 2017;21(4):940-947.
435. Dunning J, Butts R, Mourad F, Young I, Flannagan S, Perreault T. Dry needling: a literature review with implications for clinical practice guidelines. *Phys Ther Rev.* 2014;19(4):252-265.
436. Ballantyne JC, Rathmell JP, Fishman SM. *Bonica's Management of Pain.* Baltimore, MD: Lippincott Williams & Williams; 2010.
437. Mense S. Referral of muscle pain: new aspects. *Amer Pain Soc J.* 1994;3(1):1-9.
438. Vecchiet L, Dragani L, De Bigontina P, Obletter G, Giamberardino MA. Chapter 19, Experimental referred pain and hyperalgesia from muscles in humans. In: Vecchiet L, Albe-Fessard D, Lindblom U, Giamberardino MA, eds. *New Trends in Referred Pain and Hyperalgesia.* Vol 27. Amsterdam, The Netherlands: Elsevier Science Publishers; 1993:239-249.
439. Vecchiet L, Giamberardino MA. Referred pain: clinical significance, pathophysiology and treatment. In: Fischer AA, ed. *Myofascial Pain: Update in Diagnosis and Treatment.* Vol 8. Philadelphia, PA: W.B. Saunders Company; 1997:119-136.
440. Vecchiet L, Vecchiet J, Giamberardino MA. Referred muscle pain: clinical and pathophysiologic aspects. *Curr Rev Pain.* 1999;3(6):489-498.
441. Rubin TK, Lake S, van der Kooi S, et al. Predicting the spatiotemporal expression of local and referred acute muscle pain in individual subjects. *Exp Brain Res.* 2012;223(1):11-18.
442. Hooshmand H. Referred pain and trigger point. In: Hooshmand H, ed. *Chronic Pain: Reflex Sympathetic Dystrophy, Prevention and Management.* Boca Raton, FL: CRC Press; 1993:83-90.
443. Hwang M, Kang YK, Kim DH. Referred pain pattern of the pronator quadratus muscle. *Pain.* 2005;116(3):238-242.
444. Hwang M, Kang YK, Shin JY, Kim DH. Referred pain pattern of the abductor pollicis longus muscle. *Am J Phys Med Rehabil.* 2005;84(8):593-597.
445. Jaeger B. Myofascial referred pain patterns: the role of trigger points. *CDA J.* 1985;13(3):27-32.
446. Kleier DJ. Referred pain from a myofascial trigger point mimicking pain of endodontic origin. *J Endod.* 1985;11(9):408-411.
447. Koelbaek Johansen M, Graven-Nielsen T, Schou Olesen A, Arendt-Nielsen L. Generalised muscular hyperalgesia in chronic whiplash syndrome. *Pain.* 1999;83(2):229-234.
448. Fernández-de-Las-Peñas C, Galan-Del-Rio F, Alonso-Blanco C, Jimenez-Garcia R, Arendt-Nielsen L, Svensson P. Referred pain from muscle trigger points in the masticatory and neck-shoulder musculature in women with temporomandibular disorders. *J Pain.* 2010;11(12):1295-1304.
449. Fernández-de-Las-Peñas C, Ge HY, Alonso-Blanco C, Gonzalez-Iglesias J, Arendt-Nielsen L. Referred pain areas of active myofascial trigger points in head, neck, and shoulder muscles, in chronic tension type headache. *J Bodyw Mov Ther.* 2010;14(4):391-396.
450. Fernández-de-Las-Peñas C, Grobli C, Ortega-Santiago R, et al. Referred pain from myofascial trigger points in head, neck, shoulder, and arm muscles reproduces pain symptoms in blue-collar (manual) and white-collar (office) workers. *Clin J Pain.* 2012;28(6):511-518.
451. Giamberardino MA, Affaitati G, Iezzi S, Vecchiet L. Referred muscle pain and hyperalgesia from viscera. *J Musculoskelet Pain.* 1999;7(1/2):61-69.
452. Graven-Nielsen T, Arendt-Nielsen L, Svensson P, Jensen TS. Quantification of local and referred muscle pain in humans after sequential i.m. injections of hypertonic saline. *Pain.* 1997;69(1-2):111-117.
453. Hong C-Z, Chen Y-N, Twehous D, Hong DH. Pressure threshold for referred pain by compression on the trigger point and adjacent areas. *J Musculoskelet Pain.* 1996;4(3):61-79.
454. Fernández-de-Las-Peñas C, Ge HY, Arendt-Nielsen L, Cuadrado ML, Pareja JA. Referred pain from trapezius muscle trigger points shares similar characteristics with chronic tension type headache. *Eur J Pain.* 2007;11(4):475-482.
455. Fernández-de-Las-Peñas C, Ge HY, Arendt-Nielsen L, Cuadrado ML, Pareja JA. The local and referred pain from myofascial trigger points in

the temporalis muscle contributes to pain profile in chronic tension-type headache. *Clin J Pain.* 2007;23(9):786-792.
456. Alonso-Blanco C, Fernández-de-Las-Peñas C, de-la-Llave-Rincon AI, Zarco-Moreno P, Galan-Del-Rio F, Svensson P. Characteristics of referred muscle pain to the head from active trigger points in women with myofascial temporomandibular pain and fibromyalgia syndrome. *J Headache Pain.* 2012;13(8):625-637.
457. Choi TW, Park HJ, Lee AR, Kang YK. Referred pain patterns of the third and fourth dorsal interosseous muscles. *Pain Physician.* 2015;18(3):299-304.
458. Gandevia SC, Phegan CM. Perceptual distortions of the human body image produced by local anaesthesia, pain and cutaneous stimulation. *J Physiol.* 1999;514 (pt 2):609-616.
459. Zhang Y, Ge HY, Yue SW, Kimura Y, Arendt-Nielsen L. Attenuated skin blood flow response to nociceptive stimulation of latent myofascial trigger points. *Arch Phys Med Rehabil.* 2009;90(2):325-332.
460. Ge HY, Arendt-Nielsen L. Latent myofascial trigger points. *Curr Pain Headache Rep.* 2011;15(5):386-392.
461. Ge HY, Nie H, Madeleine P, Danneskiold-Samsoe B, Graven-Nielsen T, Arendt-Nielsen L. Contribution of the local and referred pain from active myofascial trigger points in fibromyalgia syndrome. *Pain.* 2009;147(1-3):233-240.
462. Li LT, Ge HY, Yue SW, Arendt-Nielsen L. Nociceptive and non-nociceptive hypersensitivity at latent myofascial trigger points. *Clin J Pain.* 2009;25(2):132-137.
463. Wang C, Ge HY, Ibarra JM, Yue SW, Madeleine P, Arendt-Nielsen L. Spatial pain propagation over time following painful glutamate activation of latent myofascial trigger points in humans. *J Pain.* 2012;13(6):537-545.
464. Ruch TC. Pathophysiology of pain. In: Ruch TC, Patton HD, eds. *Physiology and Biophysics: The Brain and Neural Function.* Philadelphia, PA: W.B. Saunders Company; 1979:272-324.
465. Sinclair DC, Weddell G, Feindel WH. Referred pain and associated phenomena. *Brain.* 1948;71(2):184-211.
466. Theobald GW. The relief and prevention of referred pain. *J Obstet Gynaecol Br Emp.* 1949;56(3):447-460.
467. Hoheisel U, Mense S, Simons DG, Yu XM. Appearance of new receptive fields in rat dorsal horn neurons following noxious stimulation of skeletal muscle: a model for referral of muscle pain? *Neurosci Lett.* 1993;153(1):9-12.
468. Arendt-Nielsen L, Ge HY. Patho-physiology of referred muscle pain. In: Fernández-de-Las Peñas C, Arendt-Nielsen L, Gerwin R, eds. *Tension-Type and Cervicogenic Headache: Patho-Physiology, Diagnosis and Treatment.* Boston, MA: Jones & Bartlett Publishers; 2009:51-59.
469. Mense S, Hoheisel U. New developments in the understanding of the pathophysiology of muscle pain. *J Musculoskelet Pain.* 1999;7(1/2):13-24.
470. Taguchi T, Hoheisel U, Mense S. Dorsal horn neurons having input from low back structures in rats. *Pain.* 2008;138(1):119-129.
471. Kuan TS, Hong CZ, Chen JT, Chen SM, Chien CH. The spinal cord connections of the myofascial trigger spots. *Eur J Pain.* 2007;11(6):624-634.
472. Arendt-Nielsen L, Sluka KA, Nie HL. Experimental muscle pain impairs descending inhibition. *Pain.* 2008;140(3):465-471.
473. Srbely JZ, Dickey JP, Lee D, Lowerison M. Dry needle stimulation of myofascial trigger points evokes segmental anti-nociceptive effects. *J Rehabil Med.* 2010;42(5):463-468.
474. Staud R. Peripheral pain mechanisms in chronic widespread pain. *Best Pract Res Clin Rheumatol.* 2011;25(2):155-164.
475. Rubin TK, Gandevia SC, Henderson LA, Macefield VG. Effects of intramuscular anesthesia on the expression of primary and referred pain induced by intramuscular injection of hypertonic saline. *J Pain.* 2009;10(8):829-835.
476. Mellick GA, Mellick LB. Regional head and face pain relief following lower cervical intramuscular anesthetic injection. *Headache.* 2003;43(10):1109-1111.
477. Affaitati G, Costantini R, Fabrizio A, Lapenna D, Tafuri E, Giamberardino MA. Effects of treatment of peripheral pain generators in fibromyalgia patients. *Eur J Pain.* 2011;15(1):61-69.

Chapter 2

Trigger Point Neurophysiology

Robert D. Gerwin

1. INTRODUCTION

The myofascial trigger point (TrP) is the accepted basis for the local and referred pain of the myofascial pain syndrome (MPS). Despite recent studies of the TrP, the actual mechanisms of the development and resolution of the TrP remain speculative. Simons' Integrated Hypothesis painted a broad picture of the mechanism by which the TrP taut band and TrP-induced pain developed, but left out the necessary details by which the TrP actually occurs.[1] More details were offered by Gerwin et al,[2] but many details of the taut band, the TrP, and the MPS remain obscure. Since then, others have summarized or added to these hypotheses, particularly Bron and Dommerholt.[3] However, these proposals have been accompanied in recent years by new studies that have confirmed some aspects of the hypotheses, whereas others remain completely speculative. Among unanswered questions are the mechanism(s) by which the sympathetic nervous system (SNS) influences the taut band, the mechanism by which the taut band develops and is maintained, the mechanism leading to endplate noise, the mechanism of the local twitch response, and the mechanism by which the TrP is resolved. Moreover, the role that the fascia tissue plays in the creation and maintenance of TrPs remains to be explicated, which is addressed in Chapter 3. Finally, the question as to why the TrP is transient in some people, and persists in others, has not been adequately explored. Many of the premises have been introduced in Chapter 1. There will be some overlap, but the combination of the two chapters will provide a comprehensive review of the current thinking.

This discussion will briefly review what is known about the development of the TrP taut band, as that seems to be the first clinical sign of the TrP. Then, the role of functional changes in the neuromuscular junction (NMJ) will be explored. The role of the alpha-adrenergic SNS will also be considered. Calcium (Ca^{2+}) is required for cross-bridging to occur between actin and myosin molecules to produce muscle contraction. Therefore, perturbations in the excitation-contraction coupling (ECC) mechanism will be discussed, in particular the possibility that a polymorphism affecting a major calcium ion channel could play a role in the maintenance of the taut band (TB). As adenosine triphosphate (ATP) is required for the removal of Ca^{2+} from the cytosol to reverse actin–myosin cross-bridging, the effect of changes in ATP concentration will be reviewed, especially in relationship to another ion channel polymorphism. Furthermore, the beta-adrenergic SNS also modulates cytosolic Ca^{2+} levels, and its role must be explored. In the end, mutations leading to polymorphism associated with ion channel function, important in regulating cytosolic Ca^{2+} concentrations ($[Ca^{2+}]c$), are considered a major possibility for the development and maintenance of the taut band in certain individuals.

2. EVIDENCE-BASED PRESENT UNDERSTANDING OF THE TRIGGER POINT

Segmental Sarcomere Contraction

The observation that discrete, tender, muscle bands develop led to the concept that there is an underlying localized intense contraction of sarcomeres that can be felt as a discrete knot in the muscle. This concept was given impetus by the reexamination of a photomicrograph published by Simons and Stolov of canine muscle showing a region of intense sarcomere contraction under a structure that could possibly be an NMJ[4] (Figure 2-1). This observation led to efforts to replicate focal zones of sarcomere contraction in the experimental animal, primarily by using an anticholinesterase (AChE) inhibitor, an effort that has not been wholly successful.[5] Nevertheless, the concept of segmental sarcomere contraction has given rise to a search for mechanisms that will cause sustained sarcomere contraction and that are consistent with clinical observations. There has not been a published study showing that zones of intense sarcomere contraction occur at TrP sites in either humans or animals.

Trigger Point Electrophysiology

There is a characteristic electromyographic (EMG) signature of the active TrP that is used as a marker for the TrP. It is a combination of low-amplitude fast activity consistent with miniature endplate potentials (MEPPs), though of higher frequency than is usually seen with MEPPs, and intermittent, higher-amplitude spike activity called endplate spikes (EPSs) that generally have an initial electrical negativity. These characteristic discharges were first reported by Hubbard and Berkoff,[6] and subsequently studied in detail by Simons et al,[7,8] and also by Couppé et al.[9] The spontaneous electrical activity (SEA) of the TrP (Figure 2-2) described by Hubbard and Berkoff was confined to a 1 to 2 mm diameter locus, and was of a rather constant low-amplitude discharge of about 50 μm or less, punctuated by higher-amplitude spikes that were about 50 to 100 μm. The SEA is present in the resting muscle as shown by EMG recording of adjacent muscle outside the taut band. Couppé et al reported the TrP electrical discharges to be characteristic of endplate noise with both MEPPs of low voltage, monophasic, negative potentials, and EPS of up to 600 μV amplitude, initially negative and irregular in nature. These authors associated the electrical activity with motor endplate activity. Ojala et al reported EPS at TrPs, but also found complex repetitive discharges (CRDs) in some TrPs.[10] Moreover, they reported that EPSs were not confined to TrPs. SEA is most prominent in the taut band at the TrP zone, has a restricted range in the taut band, and is long-lasting and persistent.

The mechanism of TrP SEA is still unknown but has been attributed to a dysfunctional NMJ and motor endplate,[1] although Hubbard and Berkoff[6] and later Partanen et al[11] were of the opinion that the source of the activity was the muscle spindle,

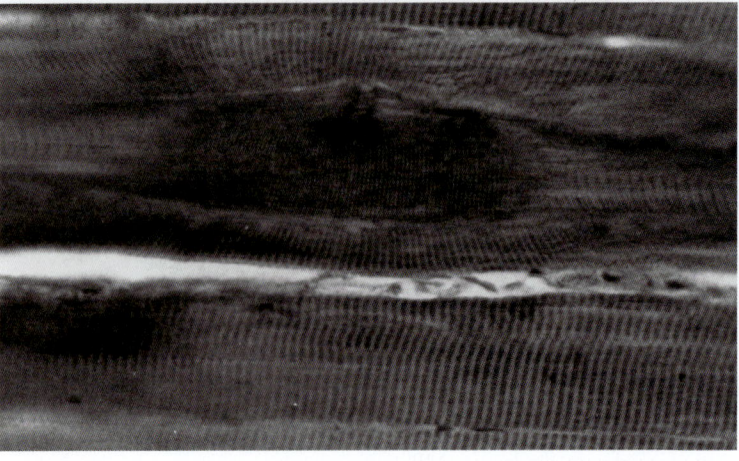

Figure 2-1. Longitudinal section of an example of the contraction knots seen in biopsies of canine muscles, in this case the gracilis. An exquisitely tender spot in a taut band of the muscle was selected as the biopsy site. These are two essential TrP criteria. The striations (corresponding to sarcomere length) indicate severe contracture of the approximately 100 sarcomeres in the knot section of the muscle fiber. The sarcomeres on both sides of the knot show compensatory elongation compared with the normally spaced sarcomeres in the muscle fibers running across the bottom of the figure. The fiber diameter is markedly increased in the region of the knot and abnormally decreased on either side of it. The irregularity of the sarcolemma along the upper border of the fiber (in the center of the contraction knot) may represent an endplate. The distortion of the sarcomere alignment in adjacent muscle fibers represents sheer stresses in those fibers that may, in time, play a part in the propagation of this dysfunction to neighboring muscle fibers.

and that the spindle was the anatomic site of the dysfunction causing the TrP and the taut band itself. This will be discussed in detail later in this section. In any event, the high frequency of the MEPP-like activity begs explanation.

3. THE NEUROMUSCULAR JUNCTION

Trigger Point Taut Band

The discrete TrP taut band in muscle is a dense band of muscle that was demonstrated on ultrasound by Gerwin and Duranleau in 1997,[12] and then later with modern techniques and in much greater clarity by Sikdar et al.[13] Increased synaptic efficiency at the NMJ could cause greater motor endplate activation, but should not lead to persistent contraction because of other regulatory mechanisms that stop excessive acetylcholine (ACh) release from the motor nerve. Concentration of ACh at the motor endplate, the key factor in determining motor endplate activity, can be modulated by any one of several mechanisms. A brief review of the way in which ACh is released and then binds with the acetylcholine receptor (AChR) will form the basis for understanding the regulatory mechanisms that control ACh at the motor endplate.

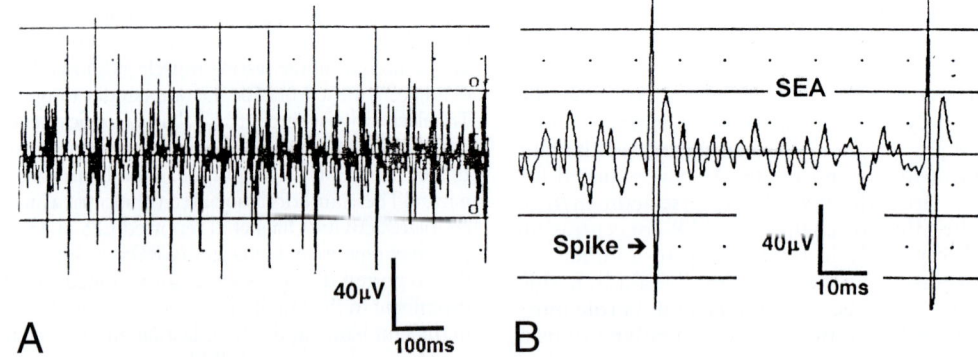

Figure 2-2. Typical recording of the spontaneous electrical activity and spikes recorded from an active locus of a TrP at two different sweep speeds. A, Recording at the same slow sweep speed of 100 msec/div used by Hubbard and Berkoff[6] to report this electrical activity. Only spikes of unknown initial polarity are identifiable. B, A similar amplification but a 10-times higher sweep speed of 10 msec/div that was used in subsequent studies by others[7,8] who also have observed the low-amplitude noise component as well as the polarity of initial deflection of the spikes from active loci. This additional information is of critical importance for understanding the source and nature of these potentials.

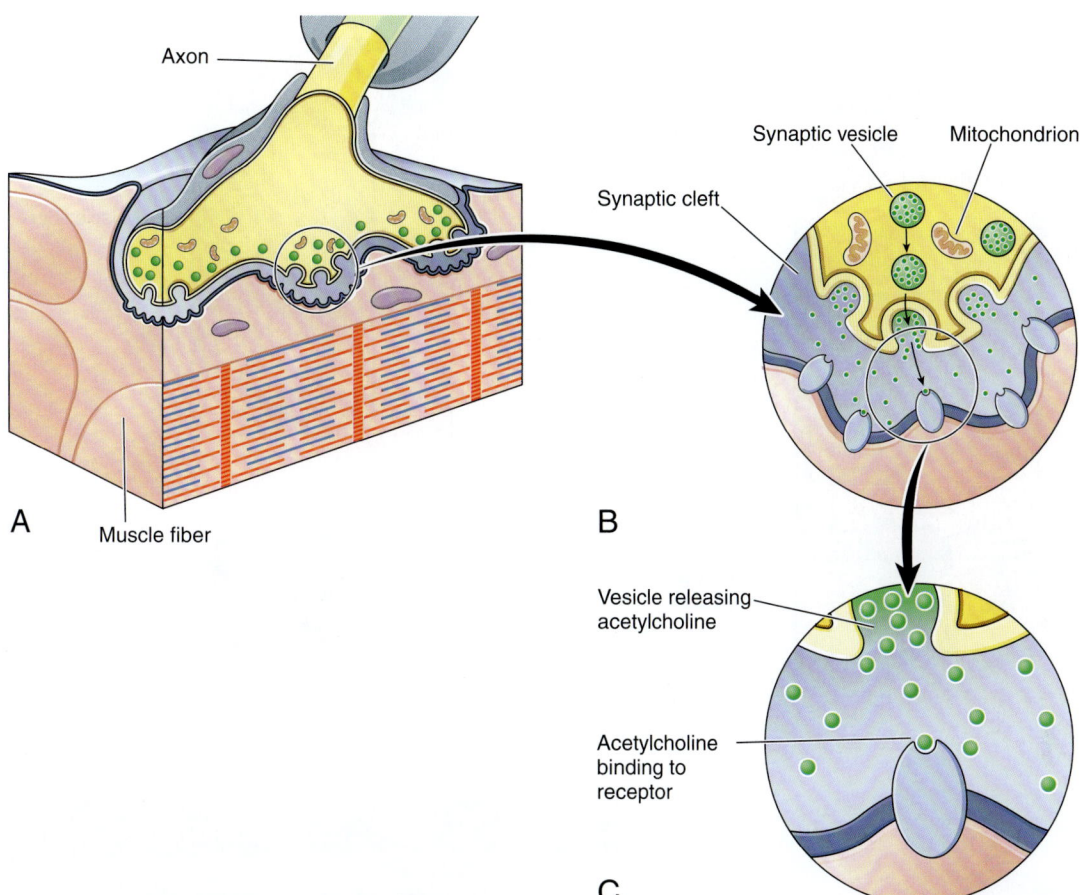

Figure 2-3. Neuromuscular junction. A, Neurons and muscle fibers communicate at the neuromuscular junction. B, Electrical signals travel along the axon and stimulate synaptic vesicles at its end to release acetylcholine, a neurotransmitter, into the synaptic cleft. C, Acetylcholine crosses the synaptic cleft and binds to receptors in the sarcolemma of muscle fibers, causing changes within the muscle cell that initiate muscle contraction.

Orthodromic Axon-Stimulus-Evoked Release

Orthodromic axon-stimulus-evoked release of ACh at the NMJ is a quantal but graded (not an "all-or-none") release that results in muscle contraction through depolarization of the muscle membrane at the motor endplate. Acetylcholine, released from the motor nerve terminal, crosses the synaptic cleft and binds to AChR on the motor endplate (Figure 2-3). A sufficient number of ACh molecules binding to AChR on the motor endplate will depolarize the muscle membrane, generating an action potential that travels down membrane invaginations called T-tubules to the dihydropyridine receptor (DHPR) that is located in the T-tubule membrane (Figure 2-4A and B). The intermolecular signal is transmitted from L-type Ca^{2+} channels in the plasma membrane to a ryanodine receptor (RyR) calcium channel that is situated 10/nm away.[14] The DHPR physically blocks the RyR calcium channel situated in the sarcoplasmic reticulum (SR). Membrane depolarization disengages DHPRs from RyRs, opening the channels and allowing the transit of Ca^{2+} from the SR into the cytosol, thus increasing the concentration of cytosolic calcium ($[Ca^{2+}]c$).[15]

Cytosolic Ca^{2+} Requirement for Muscle Contraction

Cytosolic Ca^{2+} interacts with actin and myosin to produce sarcomere shortening through cross-bridge formation, leading to contraction and shortening of the sarcomere. Actin-binding sites on myosin heads, blocked by tropomyosin (Figure 2-5A), are displaced by Ca^{2+} that binds to troponin, thereby displacing tropomyosin to expose myosin-head binding sites (Figure 2-5B). Cross-bridging links then form between actin and myosin (Figures 2-5B and 2.6). A configurational change occurs bending the myosin heads. Repeated binding, and then release, of Ca^{2+} to troponin leads to a progressive "walking" of actin molecules overlapping myosin, resulting in an increasing overlap of the two molecules. Actin, attached to sarcomere Z lines by titin, contracts the sarcomere as the actin–myosin complex is shortened (Figure 2-7). The process is terminated by the removal and reuptake of Ca^{2+} into the SR, an energy-requiring process mediated by CaATPase and ATP dependent.[16]

Subthreshold Depolarization

Acetylcholine molecules binding at the motor endplate in insufficient quantities to produce an AP are still able to produce a subthreshold, local, depolarization that does not result in a propagated membrane depolarization. However, a sufficient subthreshold depolarization has been shown to cause localized sarcomere contraction in cardiac muscle at regions with high concentrations of cytosolic Ca^{2+} ($[Ca^{2+}]c$). The local cardiac myocyte contraction results in a wave of focal sarcomere contraction that travels along the muscle membrane.[17] Thus, it is known that a sufficient number of

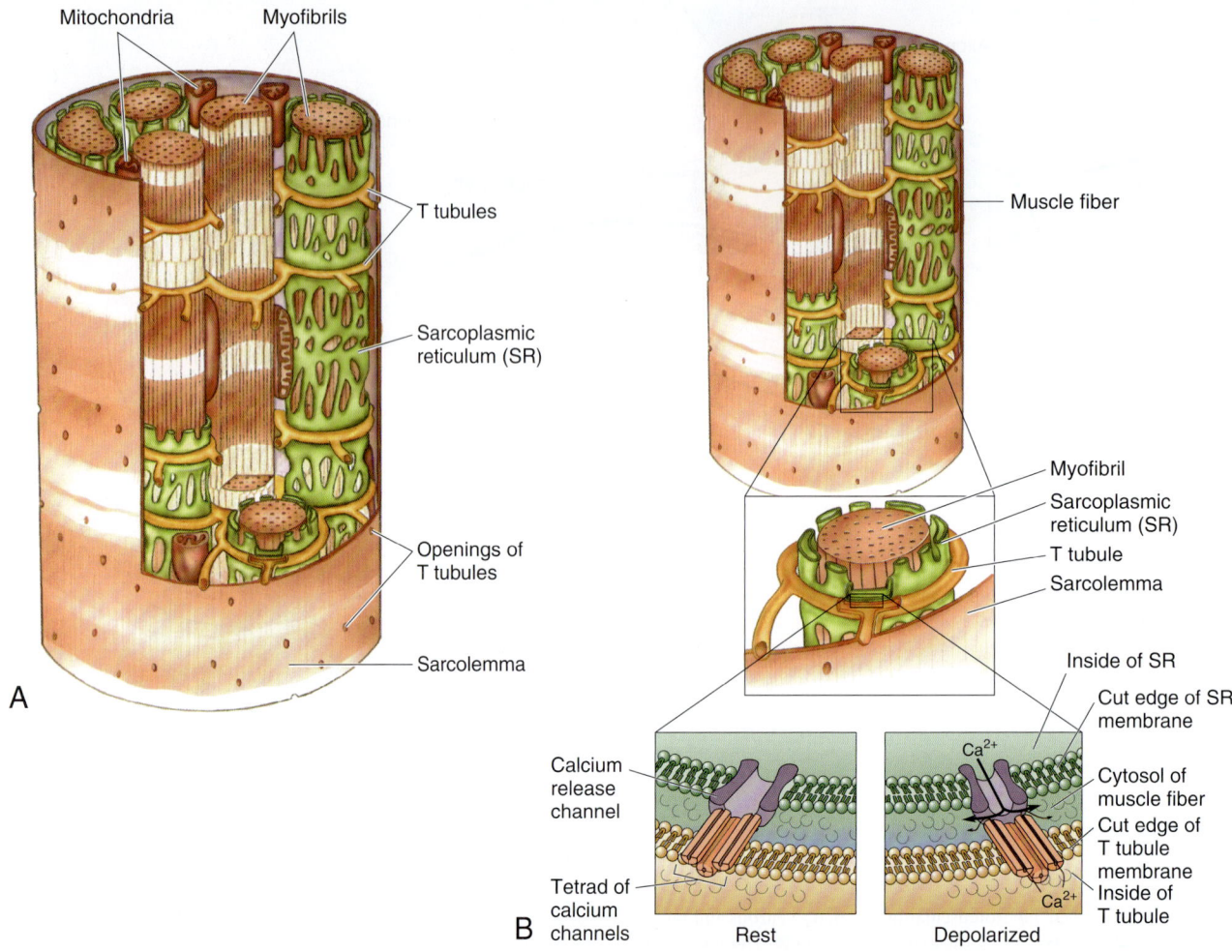

Figure 2-4. A, The structure of a muscle fiber. T-tubules conduct electrical activity from the surface membrane into the depths of the muscle fiber. B, The release of Ca^2 from the sarcoplasmic reticulum (SR). Depolarization of the T-tubule membrane causes conformational changes in proteins that are linked to calcium channels in the SR, releasing stored Ca^2 into the cytosol of the muscle fiber.

ACh molecules at the motor endplate will generate an action potential that depolarizes the muscle membrane, and an insufficient number of ACh molecules can cause a localized membrane depolarization.

4. HISTOPATHOLOGY OF THE TRIGGER POINT

There is no definitive histopathologic study of TrPs. The Integrated Hypothesis presupposes a dysfunctional NMJ, giving rise to multiple, local foci of hypercontractured sarcomeres.[1] The TrP in this model is envisioned as a locus of multiple localized sarcomere contractions, more appropriately considered to be contractures (Figure 2-8). Excessive muscle work resulting in muscle overload, such as excessive eccentric contraction, is one suggested mechanism leading to TrPs. However, muscle subjected to eccentric contraction and muscle subjected to delayed onset muscle soreness syndrome, another candidate thought possibly to produce TrPs, shows disruption of sarcomeres with loss of structure, decreased or lost alpha-actinin, titin, and nebulin, and Z-disc streaming,[18,19] but no contracture knots. Contractured sarcomeres have been found in the rat adductor longus muscle subjected to unloaded eccentric lengthening,[20] but only a few sarcomeres in succession were shortened, and none to the degree postulated by Simons and Travell,[1] and none with increased muscle fiber widening at the site of hypercontracted sarcomeres as seen in the one canine muscle microphotograph that has become the paradigm of the TrP.[4] Thus, the hypothesis that there are contracture knots in muscle TrPs has not been confirmed by morphologic studies in some of the conditions thought likely to produce TrPs. The limitation of the morphologic studies is that we do not know where samples were taken from in the muscle, or whether sections were taken from TrP sites or not.

4.1. Neurotransmitters

Presynaptic Neurotransmitters

Multiple neurotransmitters are coreleased from the motor nerve ending along with ACh, substances such as ATP, calcitonin gene-related peptide (CGRP), and serotonin (5 HT). ATP is the main neurotransmitter released along with ACh.[21] It inhibits nerve-evoked, quantal release of ACh from the nerve terminal.

Nonquantal release (NQR) of ACh is not nerve-evoked, but is a spontaneous and variable release of ACh directly through the nerve terminal membrane rather than by vesicle exocytosis. It is thought to maintain the integrity of the skeletal muscle.[22] However, if nonquantal ACh increases beyond a certain level, it is postulated that it could produce local membrane depolarization and sarcomere contraction under the motor endplate, and thus initiate the changes that result in the TrP. ATP also inhibits NQR of ACh from the motor neuron. The regulation of quantal release

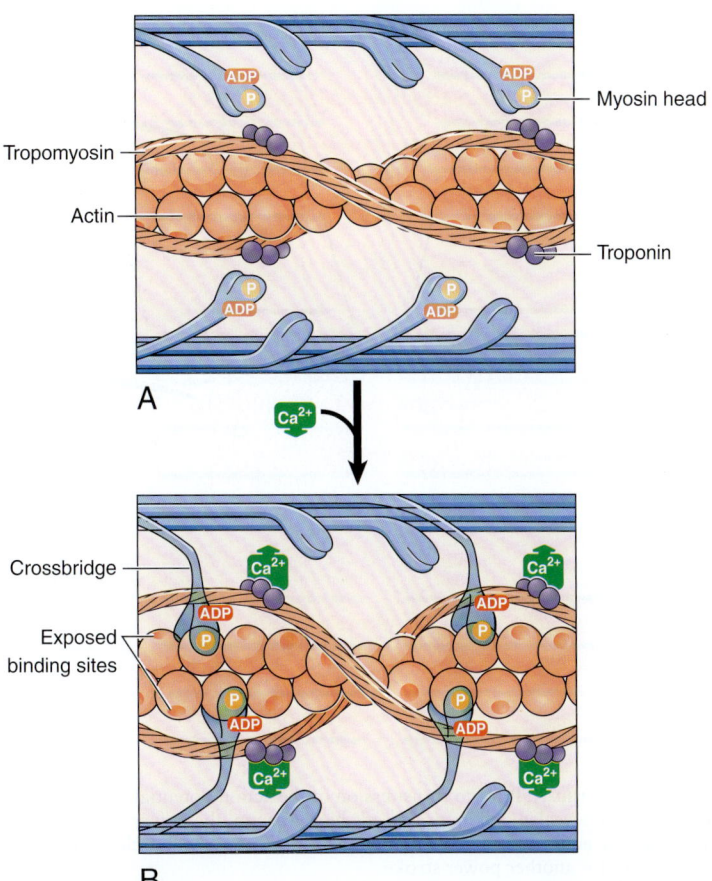

Figure 2-5. The events of muscle contraction. A, At rest, strands of tropomyosin proteins cover binding sites on actin and prevent interaction between actin and myosin. B, Action potentials release calcium into the sarcoplasm, which bind to troponin. The bound calcium deforms the tropomyosin protein, exposing actin-binding sites and allowing cross-bridges to form between the myosin heads and actin.

is mediated through Ca^{2+} influx into the motor nerve terminal through presynaptic voltage-gated calcium channels. Nonquantal regulation of ACh release is inhibited by Mg^{2+} through nitric oxide (NO) and purine pathways. However, intensive muscle contraction depletes ATP, thereby diminishing its inhibitory effect on ACh release from the nerve terminal.

4.2. Adenosine Triphosphate and the Energy Crisis Theory of Simons

The effect of ATP on the development of the TrP has been attributed to its role in Ca^{2+} reuptake into the SR.[1] However, ATP has a profound effect on NQR of ACh that may be important in TrP formation. The role of ATP and of NQR of ACh has been reviewed in detail by Vyskočil et al.[23] In a series of studies performed over almost 30 years, Vyskočil et al studied the release of ACh from nerve in muscle. They found that NQR of ACh from nerve endings provides about 90% to 98% of ACh release in the resting muscle. Nonquantal ACh release occurs directly through the nerve terminal membrane and not through vesicles as quantal release does. NQR of ACh produces MEPPs that increase in frequency directly related to an increase in nonquantal ACh release. ATP depresses nonquantal ACh release independently of $[Ca^{2+}]$. Severe muscle fatigue and hypoxia both reduce ATP concentrations and increase both nonquantal ACh release and MEPP frequency. Nonquantal ACh release occurs at the endplate region but also in the peri-endplate zone where there is less AChE. The current model for TrP formation is that local areas of muscle hypoxia occur in the TrP zone. Thus, ATP concentrations fall, and the regulatory, inhibitory effect of ATP on NQR of ACh in the resting muscle is diminished, and ACh levels in the endplate and peri-endplate regions increase, causing localized muscle membrane depolarization and localized sarcomere contraction. In other words, a fall in ATP levels increases the spontaneous release of ACh, increases the likelihood of localized sarcomere contraction, and increases the frequency of MEPPs, all of which are seen in the TrP.

4.3. Postsynaptic Effects: Acetylcholine Effects at the Motor Endplate

The MEPPs, persistent low-amplitude activity with an initial negativity, interspersed with high-amplitude discharges, EPS, found at the active TrP zone and highly localized within the taut band, has been interpreted as motor endplate activity by Simons and others.[7,8,24] SEA found at the TrP, also called endplate noise, is caused by ACh binding at the motor endplate. Several possible causes of an excess of ACh at the motor end plate were summarized by Gerwin et al and others,[2,3] refer to Box 2-1. CGRP, coreleased with ACh, is known to facilitate the release of ACh and inhibit AChE. It also induces AChR synthesis, thus increasing the number of receptor sites at and beyond the

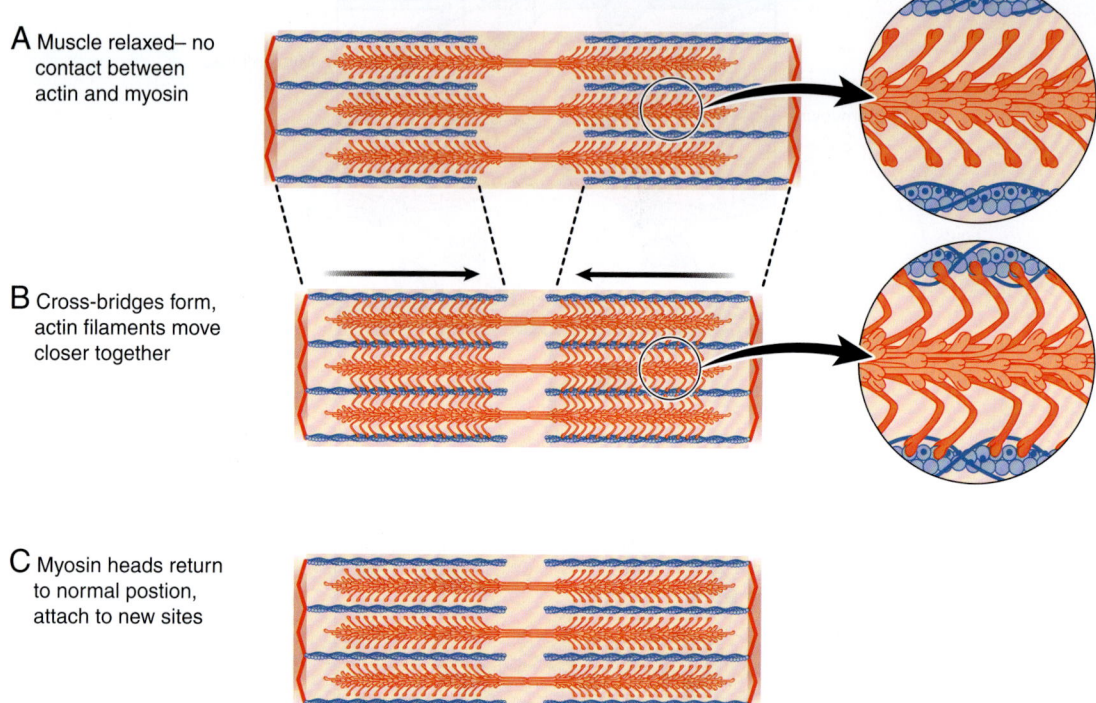

Figure 2-6. Sliding-filament mechanism. A, Prior to transmission of the action potential, no cross-bridges connect actin and myosin. B, Once the active sites are revealed and myosin heads bind to actin, the power stroke occurs. Synchronized movement of the myosin heads pulls the ends of the sarcomere together, shortening the muscle. C, Energy from ATP releases the myosin heads and positions them for another power stroke.

endplate region. Additionally, protons (H$^+$) that are increased in the TrP milieu inhibit AChE.[25]

4.4. Regulation of Acetylcholine Release From Motor Nerve Terminals by ATP

Release of ACh from the motor nerve terminal is highly regulated. Some examples will be discussed to illustrate the degree of complexity of regulatory mechanisms. A feedback mechanism involving NO reduces ACh release when the frequency of repetitive APs is too high,[26] thereby preventing hypercontracted muscle and cell damage. The corelease of ATP with ACh provides one such mechanism for this feedback regulation by inhibiting the release of ACh from the motor nerve terminal. The neurotransmitter adenosine, generated by the breakdown of ATP, is a modulator of presynaptic release in both peripheral and central synapses.[16] Adenosine acts at adenosine receptors on the motor nerve terminal surface. The adenosine receptor A1 is inhibitory and the adenosine receptor A2a is facilitatory for the release of ACh. Adenosine synchronizes the quantal release of ACh, thereby improving synaptic efficiency. This is mediated by purinergic A1 receptors on the presynaptic nerve terminal.[16,27] Activation of A1 receptors reduces ACh molecules released in each quantum. Adenosine receptor activity that modulates both evoked and spontaneous ACh release is dependent on the coactivity of muscarinic AChRs.[28] In this way, ATP has a direct inhibitory action on the release of ACh. The breakdown of ATP and decreased synthesis of ATP increases adenosine levels. Thus, lower ATP levels may correlate with higher adenosine levels. The inhibitory effect of ATP via adenosine generated by ATP breakdown is also redox dependent. Thus, the effect of ATP may be amplified by oxidative stress.[29]

Increasing intracellular Ca^{2+} in the nerve terminal also activates the exocytotic process that is mediated by A2a receptors, further facilitating the ACh release.[30] In these ways, the corelease of ATP with ACh from the motor nerve terminal serves to modulate the release of ACh, preventing excess muscle contraction by a feedback loop mechanism, through inhibitory and facilitatory influences that are rate dependent.

4.5. Adenosine Receptor Activation Effect on ACh Release

Presynaptic adenosine receptors are key ACh release modulators. A1 receptor activation inhibits ACh release, and A2a receptors facilitate ACh release.[31,32] Activation of A2a is essential for the facilitatory effect of CGRP on ACh release. A2a facilitatory effect is mediated via an external Ca^{2+}-independent mechanism that involves mobilization of Ca^{2+} from ryanidine-sensitive internal stores, and, at high [K$^+$], probably by modulating the L-type VDCCs which may cause the opening of the RyR, and thereby activating the exocytotic machinery, thus facilitating ACh release.

The importance of purigenic adenosine receptors is further shown by a study using mice deficient in the P$_2$X$_2$ receptor subunit which have their motor nerve terminals displaced from AChR sites, reduced density of postsynaptic junctional folds, endplate fragmentation, and muscle fiber atrophy.[27] Further modulation of ACh release occurs through second messenger systems involving protein kinase A and C (PKA and PKC).[33,34] Acetylcholine release from the motor nerve terminal is both facilitated and inhibited by various mechanisms. The exact role that any of one factor plays in the development of the TP taut band remains a fertile area for research.

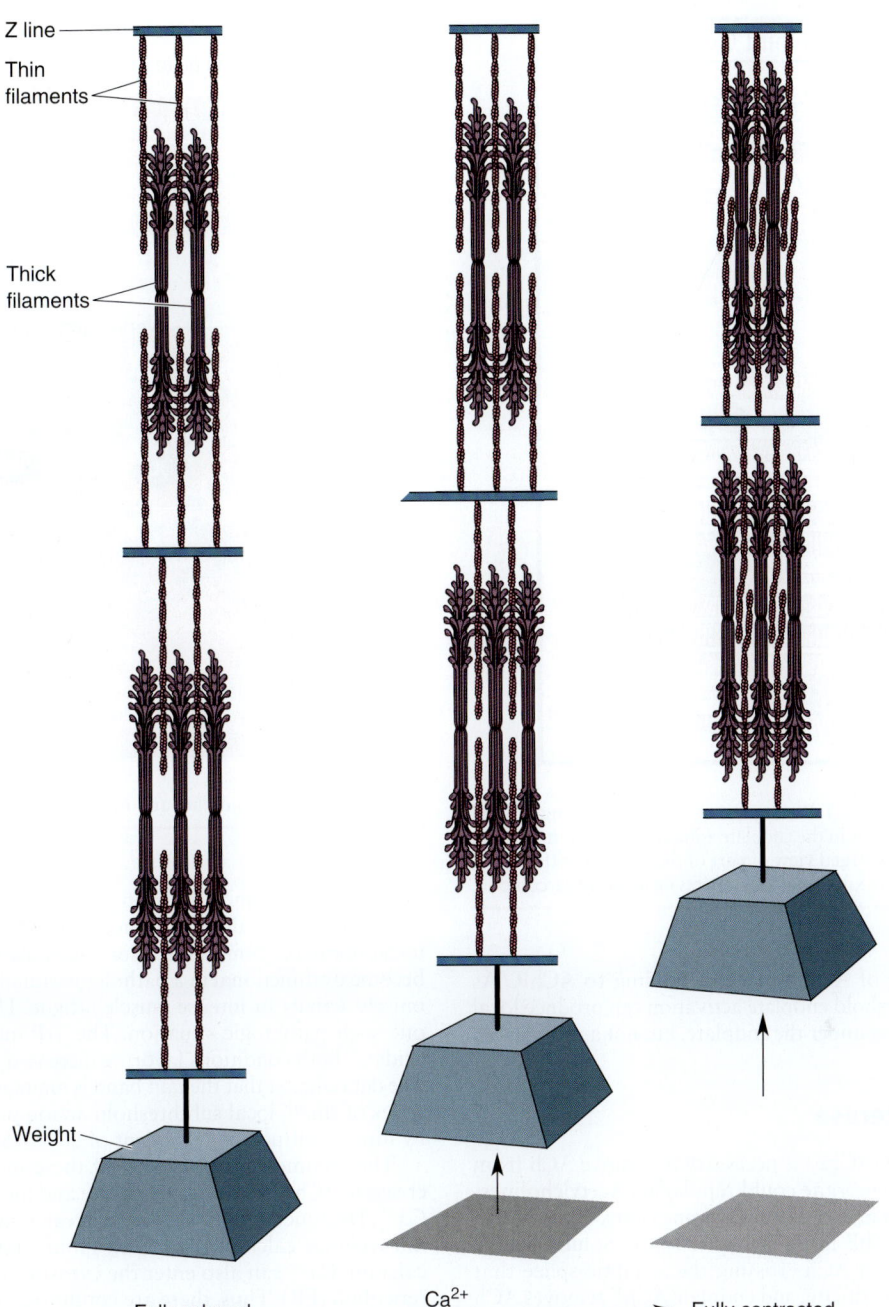

Figure 2-7. The sliding-filament model of muscle contraction. Myofibrils shorten when the thin filaments slide toward one another on the thick filaments.

Box 2-1   Causes of excessive ACh at the motor endplate
1. Increased release of ACh from the motor nerve terminal
2. Decreased breakdown of ACh in the synaptic cleft extracellular fluid
3. Increased numbers of AChR providing binding sites for ACh
4. Decreased removal of ACh from AChRs on the motor endplate

5. THE MOTOR ENDPLATE

5.1. Excitation-Contraction Coupling

The contraction of muscle fibers at the NMJ is dependent on membrane depolarization and conversion of electrical activity to molecular cross-bridging and conformation change. This is accomplished through membrane invaginations called T-tubules (Figure 2-4A). Depolarization activates the DHPR that blocks the RyR and causes it to disengage from the RyR to allow the efflux of Ca^{2+} from the SR into the cytoplasm (Figure 2-4B). This process is called ECC. Membrane depolarization requires

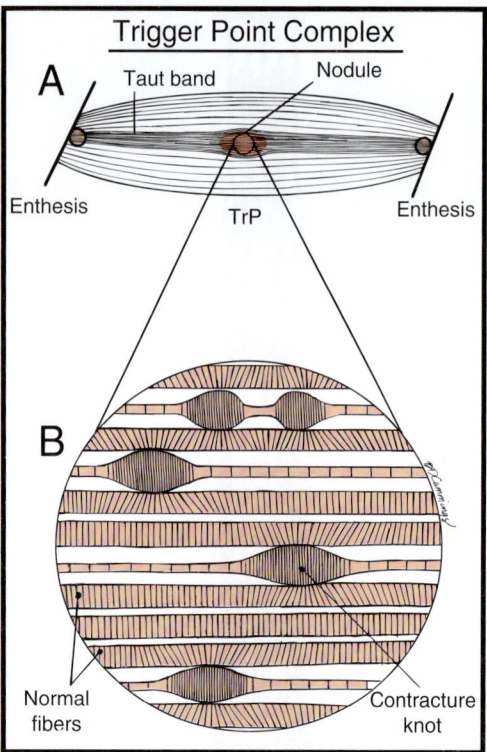

Figure 2-8. Schematic of a TrP complex of a muscle in longitudinal section. A, The TrP which is in the endplate zone and contains numerous contracture knots. B, Enlarged view of part of the TrP shows the distribution of five contracture knots and their effects on adjacent sarcomeres.

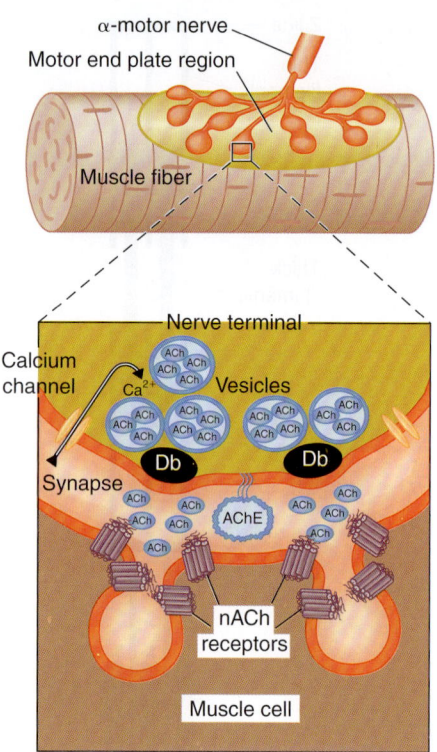

Figure 2-9. Motor endplate and neuromuscular junction.

a sufficient number of ACh molecules binding to AChR. As noted earlier, subthreshold endplate activation can produce local sarcomere contraction under the endplate, but not a propagated action potential.

Acetylcholinesterase

Acetylcholinesterase (AChE) is necessary to remove ACh from AChR so that the membrane could repolarize. Acetylcholinesterase is located deep in endplate membrane clefts. There is also a soluble form of AChE in the synaptic space. Soluble AChE reduces the amount of ACh crossing the synaptic space that reach AChRs on the endplate, and endplate AChE removes ACh from the endplate binding sites (Figure 2-9). Acetylcholinesterase activity is inhibited in an acidic environment, such as that found in the TrP milieu, and by CGRP. Acetylcholinesterase inhibition increases the efficiency of ACh binding at the motor endplate, but may be deleterious, increasing intracellular $[Ca^{2+}]$ to damaging levels. It may also be one reason why the taut band forms and why TP endplate noise (EPS) are more frequent and persistent than normal endplate activity.

5.2. Other Neurotransmitter Feedback Control Mechanisms

Adenosine triphosphate, coreleased from the motor nerve terminal with ACh, is also active at the endplate. Adenosine triphosphate stimulates, via the P_2Y_1 nucleotide receptor, the transcription genes that synthesize AChE, and the transcription genes for AChR, thus increasing the endplate expression of both AChE and AChR.[35] CGRP, also coreleased from the motor nerve terminal with ACh, increases the number and expands the domain of AChRs at the motor endplate. Thus, both ATP and CGRP increase the binding sites on the motor endplate, increasing the efficiency of ACh

binding. The balance between the release of ACh, binding to AChR, and removal by AChE acts to control muscle contraction under normal circumstances. Normal regulatory mechanisms may become dysfunctional in a pathologic situation such as excessive muscle activity or intense muscle fatigue. The TrP is likely to be one such pathologic situation. The TrP milieu is hypoxic and acidic,[25] both conditions favoring increased ACh at the endplate. The data suggest that the taut band is maintained by a continuous series of small, local subthreshold action potentials rather than by muscle stiffness independent of electrical activity.

The common feature in all of these mechanisms is the increase in ACh at the motor endplate and the increase in cytosolic Ca^{2+}. Dysfunctional RyRs can leak calcium, thereby increasing intracellular calcium, and "sick" mitochondria can also leak calcium. Ca^{2+} can also enter the cytosol from the endoplasmic reticulum (ER). Thus, there are conditions in which $[Ca^{2+}]$ may be increased that are unrelated to the evoked stimulus release of ACh, and that may serve to initiate or maintain muscle contraction. The role that these mechanisms may play in TP genesis remains speculative. One model for the role of inappropriate release of calcium through RyRs within muscle cells is malignant hyperthermia, a condition that is also characterized by persistent muscle contraction.

6. TRIGGER POINT HYPOTHESES

6.1. The Integrated Hypothesis and the Muscle Spindle Hypothesis

Simons' Integrated Hypothesis

A theory of persistent sarcomere contraction underlying the TrP phenomena that we see clinically occurring from ACh excess at endplates has some limitations. Simons' Integrated Hypothesis (Figure 2-10) postulated an energy crisis such that Ca^{2+} is not removed from the cytosol, so that muscle actin and myosin

Chapter 2: Trigger Point Neurophysiology   37

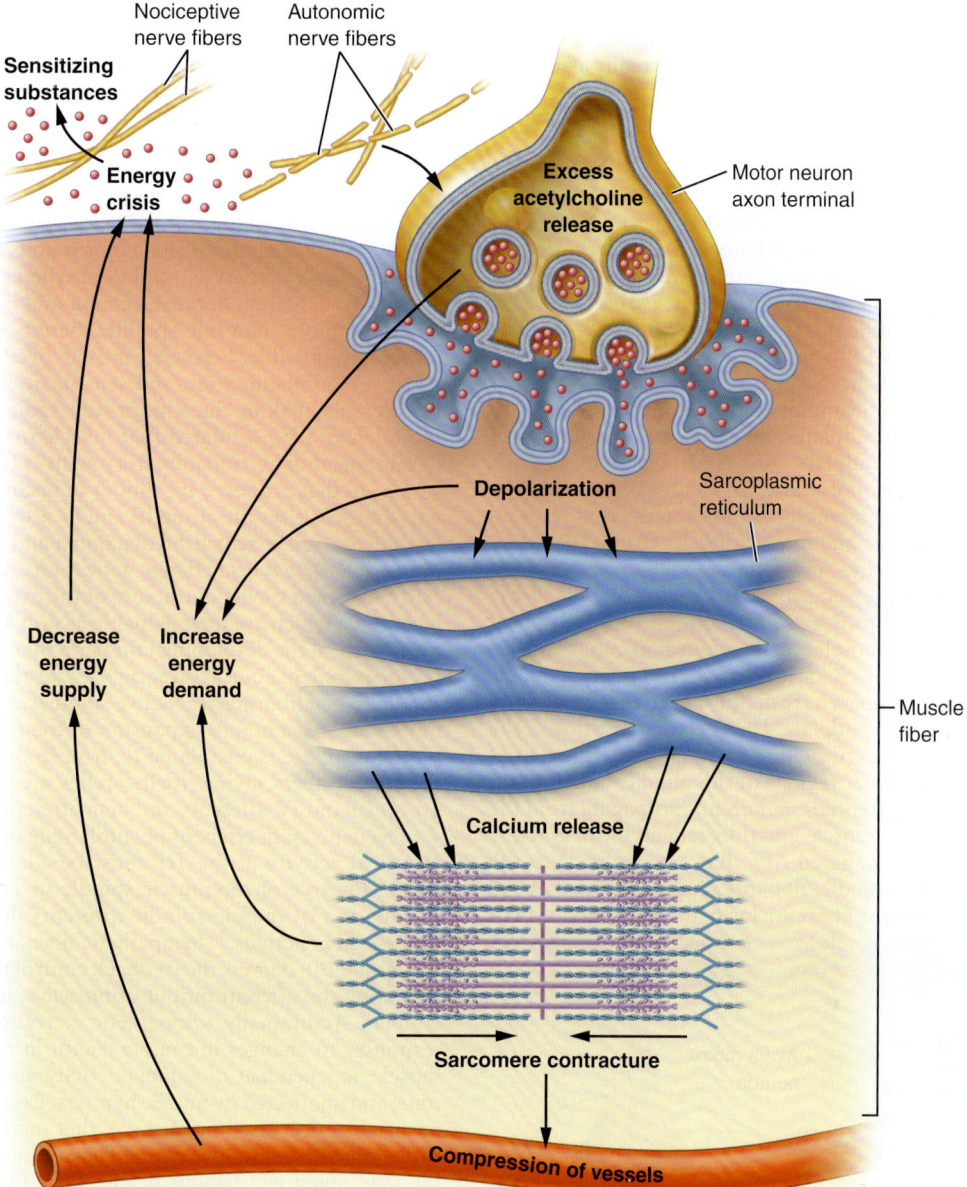

Figure 2-10. Integrated hypothesis. The primary dysfunction hypothesized here is an abnormal increase (by several orders of magnitude) in the production and release of acetylcholine packets from the motor nerve terminal under resting conditions. The greatly increased number of miniature endplate potentials produces endplate noise and sustained depolarization of the postjunctional membrane of the muscle fiber. This sustained depolarization could cause a continuous release and uptake of calcium ions from local sarcoplasmic reticulum and produce sustained shortening (contracture) of sarcomeres. Each of these four highlighted changes would increase energy demand. The sustained muscle fiber shortening compresses local blood vessels, thereby reducing the nutrient and oxygen supplies that normally meet the energy demands of this region. The increased energy demand in the face of an impaired energy supply would produce a local energy crisis, which leads to the release of sensitizing substances that could interact with autonomic and sensory (some nociceptive) nerves traversing that region. Subsequent release of neuroactive substances could in turn contribute to excessive acetylcholine release from the nerve terminal, completing what then becomes a self-sustaining vicious cycle.

cross-bridging persist; muscle fibers, therefore, would not relax. Release of actin–myosin cross-bridging requires that Ca^{2+} is removed from the cytosol, primarily by reuptake into the SR. This energy-requiring process occurs via the Na^+/K^+-ATPase (sarcoendoplasmic reticulum ATPase [SERCA]) system that supports influx of Ca^{2+} into the SR, thereby lowering the $[Ca^{2+}]c$. The theory is based on several observations, refer to Box 2-2.

However, problems of interpretation and lack of evidence remain. There is controversy over the origin of endplate noise/spikes. Elevated levels of ACh at trigger sites in the resting muscle

Box 2-2 Theory of persistent sarcomere contractures

1. SEA or EPS at the TrP zone
2. The TrP zone is ischemic
3. The single photomicrograph of the canine muscle (Figure 2-1) showing contracted sarcomeres

have never been measured, and so have never been found to be increased. There has never been a definitive histologic demonstration that hypercontracted sarcomeres are actually associated with TPs, or even that they are found in human muscle.

The Muscle Spindle Hypothesis

The argument supporting the role of the muscle spindle in the generation of TrPs is summarized by Partanen et al,[11] and expands on the argument of Hubbard and Berkoff cited earlier.[6] Partanen's et al argument is summarized here. EPSs are derived from intrafusal chain and bag fibers. MEPPs can also be recorded from spindle intrafusal fibers (Figure 2-11). The two types of activity, MEPPs and EPS, are usually seen together near the NMJ. MEPPs have been recorded at the NMJ and close to motor nerve terminals. EPS can be recorded both inside and outside the endplate zone. The electrical activity of active TrPs defined as endplate noise is identical with the EPS of muscle spindles. Fusimotor afferent (sensory) fibers include type IA and II muscle afferent mechanoreceptors that respond to muscle length change and rate of change. Group III and IV afferents are both mechano- and chemoresponders, and respond to acidosis and to algogesic substances such as kinins, 5-hydroxytryptamine, and prostaglandins. Group IA and II fibers respond to changes in muscle length, whereas group III and IV afferents respond to the chemical changes of muscle damage. Activated nuclear bag fibers have nonpropagating local activity in the area of the motor endplate. The efferent activation of the spindle is selective, occurring either at the equatorial region of the spindle or at the polar regions of the spindle. Nuclear bag fibers have junction potentials that do not propagate from the endplate region of the muscle and thus remain local. Nuclear chain fibers have propagated APs that are confined to the polar regions of the spindle, not spreading to the equatorial region where IA afferent fibers are located. The innervation of the spindle, therefore, is selective, confined either to the polar region of the spindle or to the equatorial region. A single axon will generally innervate just one spindle pole. Spindle electrical activity, therefore, is highly localized. However, in contrast to the spindle theory, two-thirds of the EPS discharges have a negative onset, consistent with an endplate origin, but not spindle origin. Moreover, spontaneous fusimotor activity does not occur in the relaxed muscle, at a time when SEA is present. Partanen et al further observe that group III and IV afferent activity increases with persistent muscle contraction and fatigue, whereas the firing rate of alpha motor units decreases.[11] Alpha motor neuron activity is inhibited, whereas gamma efferent activity is increased. Because gamma and beta efferent nerves innervate more than one spindle, there is some local spread of activity possible. Persistent muscle overload may result in neurogenic inflammation and sensitization of group III and IV afferents, making them more vulnerable to work overload. Partanen et al[11] postulated that muscle overload leads to the development of an "inflammatory soup" of algesic substances, similar to that proposed by Simons in his Integrated Hypothesis,[1] that sensitizes the group III and IV afferent sensory nerves, leading to a reflex activation of gamma and beta efferent drive. He postulates that beta efferent activation causes fatigue, energy crisis, and then silent contracture of the extrafusal fibers of the beta units, which are then palpable as taut bands. CRDs occur transiently in the developing taut band that finally fatigues and becomes a silent contracture (rigor). The aberrant activity may spread to neighboring, less active spindles, activating their beta motor units, leading to expansion of the taut band. The local twitch response is postulated to arise from the stimulation of IA afferent fibers, giving rise to a reflex arc involving intrafusal group III and IV afferents and beta efferent fibers.

The depressant effect of phentolamine on the characteristic electrical activity at the TrP must be considered when evaluating the role of the muscle spindle in TrP formation. SNS stimulation of muscle spindle afferents depresses IA and II afferent-fiber activity.[36] Sympathetic fibers innervate intrafusal fibers, and can depress the feedback control of muscle length by inhibiting the afferent output of muscle spindle group IA and II fibers. Additionally, sympathetic activation reduces spindle responses to changes in muscle length in rabbit jaw elevator muscle, independent of gamma activity and intrafusal muscle tone, and unaffected by muscle hypoxia. Resting spindle activity is variable, decreased in IA and either increased or decreased rather equally in group II fibers. The SNS acts on the spindle at the extrajunctional regions of intrafusal fibers, at the sensory endings of group IA and group II afferents, and at the encoder site, but not at gamma fibers.[36,37] An alpha-adrenergic blocking agent should not depress EPS activity in the resting muscle if it arose from muscle spindles.

The muscle spindle hypothesis of TrP formation has been critiqued explicitly by Simons et al.[1] The electrical activity characteristic of the TrP is consistent with studies that localize the electrically active loci to the endplate region. The electrically active loci are chiefly found in the TrP region, somewhat in the endplate zone but not specifically at TrPs, and not found outside the endplate region. The low-amplitude endplate noise that looks like greater frequency and higher amplitude MEPPs is highly localized to the TrP region, found only within a 1 to 2 mm wide locus. Muscle spindles are distributed more extensively in muscle than just in endplate zones, and outside the region where endplate noise is found. The morphology of TrP electrical activity is the same as endplate waveform morphology. EPSs are also found at the TrP zone, but they can be seen propagated up to 2.6 cm from the TrP along the taut band. Spindle intrafusal fibers are not that long, so that the spike activity must be propagated by extrafusal fibers. The EMG needle would not be able to penetrate the spindle capsule to record intrafusal fiber activity.

The problem has not been studied adequately pharmacologically. The systemic administration of curare should block cholinergic activity at the motor endplate and gamma activity,

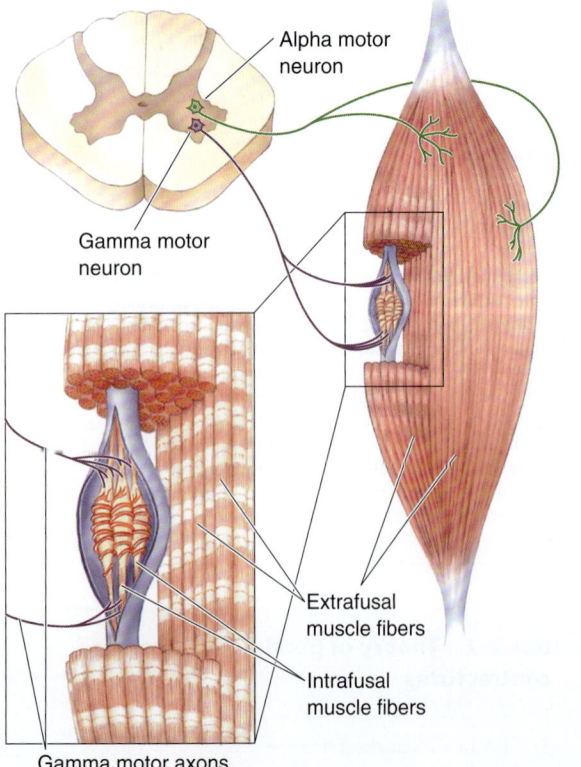

Figure 2-11. Alpha motor neurons, gamma motor neurons, and the muscle fibers they innervate.

but not the adrenergic activity of group IA and group II afferent spindle fibers. This has not been adequately studied in TrPs, and no information regarding the selective effect of curare-like drugs on cholinergic activity in TrPs is available.

6.2. The Sympathetic Nervous System in Myofascial Pain

Implications of the Effect of Phentolamine on Endplate Noise

No currently published hypothesis adequately explains the observed depressant effect of phentolamine on the electrical activity at the TrP. Sympathetic nerve stimulation suppresses group IA activity and produces a mixed response among group II fibers. However, spindle responses to sympathetic nerve stimulation vary from one muscle to another, and among species. Nevertheless, on the basis of these studies, one would expect that blocking or decreasing SNS would increase both muscle spindle and motor endplate activity, not inhibit it. Moreover, the studies of SNS modulation of both muscle spindle activity and of motor endplate activity are done either by SNS stimulation or by examining the effects of beta-adrenergic blockade. The effect of alpha-adrenergic inhibitors has been little studied. However, there is one study of the effect of the alpha-adrenergic blocking agent clonidine that shows markedly suppressed EPPs and MEPPs, but no suppression of the quantal release of motor nerve terminal ACh.[38] The mechanism was thought to be a noncompetitive blockade of AChR, but not via an alpha-2-adrenoreceptor pathway on the motor nerve terminal. A possible postsynaptic effect of phentolamine on TrP formation will be discussed in the section on the role of K_{ATP} channels in muscle contraction later in this section.

Sympathetic Nervous System Effects on Calcium Flux

The alpha-1&2-adrenergic blocking agent phentolamine significantly depresses endplate noise, indicating that the electrical activity generated at the TrP zone is driven in part by the SNS.[39] The mechanism remains unproven. The mean average integrated signal (AIS) of TrP SEA was reported to be of 9.89 µV compared with 7.92 µV in the phentolamine group ($P < 0.05$), a significant decrease. However, the depression of electrical activity at the TrP represents a presynaptic site of action where ACh is released, especially because most postsynaptic sympathetic modulation is via beta-adrenergic pathways. One potential target of sympathetic modulation is the regulation of calcium concentration within the muscle fiber, which may be related to the maintenance of the taut band. Muscle contraction requires an increase in ($[Ca^{2+}]c$). The force of muscle contraction is directly related to $[Ca^{2+}]c$. Mechanisms that affect muscle cell $[Ca^{2+}]c$ can be summarized as those mechanisms that are mediated primarily by the RyR1-SR system or mechanisms mediated through other systems such as those involving second messenger systems. Ca^{2+} is also released from mitochondria. Dysfunctional mitochondria will release more Ca^{2+} than normal mitochondria, for example. Furthermore, Ca^{2+} itself induces the release of Ca^{2+} from the SR via RyR1 channels, a process known as Ca^{2+}-induced Ca^{2+} release.[40]

Beta-Adrenergic Effects on Ca^{2+} Levels

Thus, there may be two broad categories of effects of the SNS on muscle contraction: (1) regulation of the excitation phase of ECC through the modulation of the AP, most likely by controlling the effective concentration of ACh at the NMJ. This has been discussed earlier. (2) Modulation of $[Ca^{2+}]c$. There is good evidence that the SNS modulates $[Ca^{2+}]c$. The force of contraction can be enhanced in the skeletal muscle by beta-adrenergic agonists.[41] Ca^{2+} levels are modulated through beta-adrenergic effects on second messenger systems. One such pathway is mediated through cyclic adenosine monophosphate (cAMP). Beta-adrenergic stimulation increases cAMP levels, leading to increased basal levels of $[Ca^{2+}]$ and decreased concentration of Ca^{2+} in the SR ($[Ca^{2+}]sr$) during contraction, and increased fiber contraction and efficacy of the Ca^{2+} release/uptake cycle during motor nerve stimulation.[42] Under normal conditions, Ca^{2+} is released from the SR as described earlier, reducing $[Ca^{2+}]sr$ after tetanic stimulation and even after a single stimulus-evoked fast twitch.[42] The mechanism involves PKA-dependent phosphorylation of DHPR and possibly RyR1 as well. Beta-adrenergic stimulation increases cAMP levels and improves Ca^{2+} uptake in the SR after contraction. Complete SERCA inhibition allows muscle to contract only a few times but with greater contraction intensity, whereas resting $[Ca^{2+}]sr$ is lower than in controls.[42] $[Ca^{2+}]c$ increase in the presence of SERCA inhibitors may be due to a reduced SR uptake of Ca^{2+} after contraction, or that a constant influx of Ca^{2+} into the cytosol from the SR that is normally masked by SERCA activity, but that is unmasked when SERCA is inhibited. In the case of myofascial TrPs, there may be a partial inhibition of SERCA by an "energy crisis" as postulated by Simons, because of a lack of ATP, or there could be a higher "leak" or influx of Ca^{2+} into the cytosol by leaky RyR1 or from "sick" mitochondria.

Second Messenger System Regulation of $[Ca^{2+}]c$

Another mechanism for the increase in $[Ca^{2+}]c$ upon beta-adrenergic stimulation may be PKA activation of glycogen metabolism, providing more glucose and therefore more ATP to explain higher Ca^{2+} loading of the SR. Both release from and uptake into the SR of Ca^{2+} are amplified in the mouse anterior tibialis muscle under beta-adrenergic stimulation.[42,43] Beta-adrenergic agonists augment peak contraction force (positive inotropic effect) and shorten the relaxation of slow-twitch muscles (positive lusitropic effect), except that under some circumstances a peak force reduction is induced in slow-twitch muscles.

Summary of Beta-Adrenergic Effects

Beta-adrenergic stimulation activates beta 2 adrenoceptors that are coupled to G proteins, thereby activating adenylate cyclase that converts ATP to adenosine 7' 5' cAMP. Cyclic AMP-dependent protein kinases phosphorylate certain target proteins, including DHPR, thereby altering receptor activity and ion flux.[43] They modulate sarcolemmal processes by increasing the resting membrane potential and increasing the action potential amplitude via enhanced Na^+-K^+ pump and Na^+-K^+-$2Cl^-$ cotransporter function. Myofibril Ca^{2+} sensitivity and maximum Ca^{2+}-activated force are unchanged. Increase in contractile force is mediated through the phosphorylation of SR-RyR1 channels, which sensitize the Ca^{2+}-induced Ca^{2+} release mechanism. Greater Ca^{2+} loading may then contribute to force potentiation seen in fast-twitch muscles. However, some studies in humans show no force potentiation, which seems to be related to the low beta-adrenergic concentration used. High-dose beta-adrenergic agonists, however, enhance $[Ca^{2+}]sr$ release rates and increase maximum voluntary strength in humans.[43] Beta-adrenergic effects on peak force and on relaxation do not involve myofilament processes, in contrast to cardiac muscle. Ca^{2+} sensitivity and Ca^{2+}-activated maximum force reflecting maximum cross-bridging activity are unchanged in the skeletal muscle. The positive inotropic effect is fully accounted for by ECC processes. Cairns and Borrani state that the beta-adrenergic effects on Ca^{2+} processing involve the following proteins: voltage-gated L-type CaV1.1 channel, the DHPR in the T-tubule membrane, phospholamban (PLB), a protein in slow-twitch fibers associated with SERCA, and RyR1.[43] PLB does not mediate the beta-adrenergic potentiation of force in the skeletal muscle, but it is involved in shortening the relaxation time in the slow-twitch muscle by a PKA-phosphorylation-related increase in SR Ca^{2+} uptake. The force of contraction in a given muscle, enhanced or decreased, may ultimately depend on the relative rates of Ca^{2+} release and uptake from and to the SR in that muscle, and that force will be affected by alpha-adrenergic presynaptic activity and beta-adrenergic postsynaptic activity.

Alpha-Adrenergic Effects on Muscle Function and $[Ca^{2+}]c$

SEA endplate noise that looks like increased amplitude MEPPs and higher-amplitude EPS is decreased by the mixed alpha 1- and 2-antagonist phentolamine. MEPPs were discovered in 1950 by Bernard Katz.[44] They were first recorded intracellularly. MEPP is highly localized to the endplate region. Its activity is greatly attenuated even millimeters from the endplate region.[45] The fact that it could be recorded by extracellular electrodes led Simons to think that it was an amplified MEPP activity that was part of the endplate activity. Catecholamine activity is mediated through the presynaptic alpha-adrenergic receptors and the postsynaptic beta-adrenergic receptors.[46] Epinephrine and norepinephrine each can increase the size of MEPPs by modulating the release of ACh. Epinephrine acts at both pre- and postsynaptic receptors, at both alpha- and beta-adrenergic receptors. Norepinephrine, however, is active primarily at alpha 1- and alpha 2-adrenergic receptors. Isoproterenol, a beta-adrenergic agonist, does not affect MEPPs or EPPs. Catecholamine modulation of TrP endpoint noise has not been reported. However, knowledge of the origin of endplate noise could be useful in developing pharmacologic approaches to the treatment of MPS. Norepinephrine increases MEPP frequency and EPP amplitude. The inhibitory effect of phentolamine on EPS, and the lack of effect on MEPPs and EPPs by isoproterenol, indicates that the control of MEPP frequency and EPS amplitude are alpha-adrenergic-modulated functions. Furthermore, because it is the high-amplitude EPS discharges that are abolished by phentolamine, it may not be the NQR release of ACh that drives MEPP that is critical in reducing the AIS of endplate noise, but rather the loss of EPS. Control of catecholamine expression in humans through such modalities as meditation and mindfulness practices may, therefore, be a useful focus of clinical research.

7. ION CHANNEL POLYMORPHISMS AS A CAUSE OF INCREASED CYTOSOLIC Ca^{2+}

Ion Channel Control of Ca^{2+} Influx

Hong and Simons had already come to the conclusion by 1998 that endplate noise was caused by the leakage of ACh from the motor nerve terminal.[45] They hypothesized that the effect of a localized increase in ACh would cause excessive release of calcium from the SR (and from the ER and other sources of Ca^{2+}), causing localized sarcomere contraction, but also requiring more ATP to remove Ca^{2+}, thus causing a hypermetabolic state in the muscle, and, abetted by capillary constriction from muscle contraction, an energy crisis whereby excess Ca^{2+} remained in the cytosol, facilitating prolonged or chronic contractile interaction between actin and myosin. These ideas were embodied in the Integrated Trigger Point Hypothesis referred to earlier (Figure 2-10).

The Problem of Excessive Cytosolic Ca^{2+}: The Case of Malignant Hyperthermia

Any explanation for taut band formation and maintenance must include a process for increasing $[Ca^{2+}]c$, because Ca^{2+} is required for the actin–myosin interaction described previously. Two mechanisms to consider are those that cause malignant hyperthermia on the one hand and those that cause the stiffness of rigor mortis on the other hand. In malignant hyperthermia, the cytosol is flooded with excessive Ca^{2+} that overwhelms the processes that remove it from the cytosol.[47] The problem of excessive cytosolic Ca^{2+} in malignant hyperthermia is that a mutation in an RyR1 subunit allows it to stay open longer than it normally does, allowing more Ca^{2+} to leave the SR and enter the cytosol. There are over 100 known mutations of this receptor. Gain of function mutations causes the ion channel to be open for prolonged periods. Thus, there is uncontrolled entry of Ca^{2+} into the cytosol where it interacts with tropinin to allow actin and myosin cross-bridging to occur.

Ca^{2+} must be removed from actin in order to reverse cross-bridge formation and allow the muscle to relax, and the sarcomere to lengthen. Reuptake of Ca^{2+} into the SR is an ATP-dependent energy-requiring process. The process releases energy in the form of heat, which is why persons with malignant hyperthermia develop high fevers. In malignant hyperthermia, ATP is depleted, Ca^{2+} is not removed from the cytosol, and muscle contraction is prolonged.

Rigor Mortis: The Ultimate Depletion of ATP

A different situation occurs in rigor mortis, where there is increased permeability of cell membranes to Ca^{2+} and an accumulation of Ca^{2+} in the cytosol. ATP cannot be regenerated, so that Ca^{2+} is not removed from the cytosol. Cross-bridges remain, and the muscle is stiff. A third mechanism not involving $[Ca^{2+}]c$ is static stiffness, discussed subsequently.

The Role of ATP

If the mechanism for taut band development involves excessive $[Ca^{2+}]c$, then we must have a mechanism to explain this. One mechanism of increasing $[Ca^{2+}]c$ is by increased NQR of ACh from the motor nerve terminal. That possibility has been discussed in conjunction with MEPPs, EPPs, and endplate noise. We still do not know if reduction in EPS is accompanied by reduction in hardness or stiffness of the taut band. We also do not know if the presumed increase in the NQR of ACh is sufficient to cause focal sarcomere contraction as it is hypothesized, or if it is sufficient to cause the formation of taut bands. Mense et al showed that the inhibition of AChE caused focal muscle fiber contraction, but they were distributed along the muscle fiber and were not located precisely at endpoint regions.[5] Nevertheless, they showed focal sarcomere contractions, although they looked more like disks and differed in appearance from the hypothesized TrP contraction knots. Second, the development of the taut band may be unrelated to the NQR of ACh. It may instead be related to the relative ischemia secondary to capillary compression that excessive muscle contraction may produce, resulting in a decrease in ATP availability. Lack of sufficient ATP may affect the concentration of Ca^{2+} in a way that has not previously been considered. This will be discussed in more detail subsequently.

8. REACTIVE OXYGEN SPECIES AND MUSCLE DYSFUNCTION: JAFRI'S HYPOTHESIS

An interesting and novel hypothesis for TrP formation and maintenance has been proposed by Jafri and described in detail in his discussion on the nature of TrPs.[48] Jafri's concern is that the current theories of TrP formation do not adequately explain what we currently know about the TrP. In particular, he addresses the question of the persistent hypercontraction of the taut band. He suggests a mechanism that would sustain an elevated level of [Ca^{2+}]c to drive the process. Jafri's theory is based on the observation that increased muscle activity generates reactive oxygen species (ROS). ROS are overproduced by excessive striated muscle activity (muscle overload). Ischemia at the TrP region decreases the mitochondrial membrane potential and leads to excessive extramitochondrial proton (H^+) accumulation, thereby lowering intracellular pH, reducing the ability of the mitochondria to remove ROS. ROS are normally removed by superoxide dismutase, which converts superoxide to hydrogen peroxide (H_2O_2) and ultimately to oxygen and water through catalase or glutathione peroxidase pathways. Repetitive muscle contraction results in the generation of ROS through phospholipase A2, xanthine oxidase, or NADPH oxidase (NOX) pathways. Mechanical deformation of the T-tubule system acts as a mechanotransducer that activates NOX2, which also results in the production of ROS. Activated ROS also deform the T-tubule, increasing their density, and contributing to the hypoechoic appearance on ultrasound of the TrP. Furthermore, ROS oxidize RyRs, opening them to Ca^{2+} influx from the SR. The sarcolemma "transient receptor potential" channels become sensitized; these are essential for maintaining the integrity of the SR during repetitive muscle contractions. The ROS signaling cascade in the skeletal muscle just described is maladaptive, because it maintains excessively high levels of [Ca^{2+}]c. The great excess of [Ca^{2+}]c in TrPs is thought to lead to focal muscle contraction and regions of increased sarcomere lengthening, or muscle stretch, further activating ROS. The result is a persistent increase in [Ca^{2+}]c and muscle fiber contraction. This mechanism, Jafri proposes, acting through microtubule cytoskeletal elements and activation of NOX, produces ROS, causes excessive Ca^{2+} to enter the cytosol through RyRs, and causes local sarcomere contraction.

Jafri's hypothesis addresses the issue of energy depletion or a decreased concentration of ATP generated by mitochondria, proposed in the Integrated Hypothesis of the TrP as the increase in ROS concentrations is associated with mitochondrial dysfunction.[1,22] It addresses the development of the TrP from muscle overuse and also the muscle weakness associated with the TrP. It does not address the role of the SNS in the formation of the taut band but neither does it exclude a role of the SNS. Jafri's model offers a credible explanation for the development and maintenance of the TrP taut band that is compatible with other possible mechanisms, and that fills in some of the details of Simons' Integrated Theory.

9. A NEW HYPOTHESIS: K_{ATP} RECEPTOR CHANNEL POLYMORPHISMS

9.1. K_{ATP} Activation and Trigger Points: A New Construct

The key to the answer of how the taut band is formed and maintained may be found in the K_{ATP} channel. The K_{ATP} channel is a potassium channel that is ATP sensitive. The K_{ATP} channel is kept closed when ATP is at physiologic levels. An open or active K_{ATP} channel inhibits Ca^{2+} influx into the cytosol from the SR and the ER. A fall in ATP levels, as occurs in hypoxia or ischemia, opens the K_{ATP} channels. Open K_{ATP} channels lead to membrane hyperpolarization, shortening of the AP, and inhibition of voltage-gated Ca^{2+} channels. Ca^{2+} influx into the cytosol is decreased, particularly that from the SR. Reducing [Ca^{2+}]c minimizes the risk of Ca^{2+} overload and also reduces the likelihood of developing excessive ROS. Protons (H^+) also open K_{ATP} channels. Phentolamine, shown to decrease the EPS as described earlier, has the additional effect of blocking ATP release, thereby lowering ATP levels, which can lead to K_{ATP} activation. Hence, the action of phentolamine on TrPs may be both presynaptic at alpha1-adrenergic receptors, and postsynaptic, activating K_{ATP} channels. In cardiac muscle, phentolamine also reduced the frequency and amplitude of pacemaker currents.[49] The relevance of this modulation of cardiac currents on TrPs has not been examined.

K_{ATP} channels are energy sensors in that they respond to ATP levels. Boudreault et al link the energy state of the muscle fiber to the electrical activity of the cell membrane, regulating K^+ ion efflux.[50] Activation of K_{ATP} channels results in lower-amplitude action potentials, which may be reflected in the effect of phentolamine on EPS that in turn reduce Ca^{2+} release from the SR, and thereby decrease force generation. Activation of K_{ATP} channels results in faster onset of fatigue.

K_{ATP} Channel Deficiency

K_{ATP}-deficient mice develop supercontracted single muscle fibers, greater increases in unstimulated (not the result of a nerve stimulus) [Ca^{2+}]c, greater unstimulated force, and lower force recovery.[51] Impaired K_{ATP} function alters muscle response during fatiguing exercise. Downregulation of K_{ATP} activity in the fast-twitch muscle is associated with weakness.[52] Contractility is dysfunctional, actin–myosin cross-bridge formation is depressed, and force generation is impaired.

K_{ATP} Polymorphisms

There are four K_{ATP} subunits, SUR-1, 2A, 2B, and Kir6.2.[53] Subunit mutations can occur that can lead to a loss of function and loss of the regulation of [Ca^{2+}] at the time of intensive or repetitive exercise, thereby resulting in muscle fiber damage and in the development of prolonged actin–myosin interaction, leading to prolonged muscle contractility. Lack of functional K_{ATP} channels results in impaired energy metabolism in muscle fatigue such that CO_2 generation is decreased and lactate production is increased, despite an increase in the production of ATP to try to meet the energy demands associated with muscle fatigue.[54] Muscle fiber damage can lead to the cascade of events that lead to nociception and pain.

9.2. Implications of Polymorphisms and Channelopathies: A New TrP Construct

The current model of TrP formation is that acute or chronic muscle overload initiates a chain of events, resulting in the development of the taut band and of pain. The mechanism of injury that initiates the cascade of events is not known, but is thought to be focal muscle fiber damage, ischemia, and hypoxia. One possible mechanism is that excessive or intensive muscle activity reduces intracellular ATP, resulting in the activation of K_{ATP} channels. This reduces the amount of Ca^{2+} released from the SR as well as decreasing the reuptake of Ca^{2+} into the SR. This results in lower action potential amplitude, decreasing the force of contraction that can be generated, and ultimately leading to muscle damage that can occur in ischemia-reperfusion-induced apoptosis that K_{ATP} channel activation ordinarily modulates.[55] Moreover, if the K_{ATP} channel is not fully functional, focal supercontracted regions occur in single muscle fibers, suggesting that the long-considered role of excessive local concentration of ACh at the motor endpoint is not the sole or necessarily the primary cause of hyperintense sarcomere contraction. Clinically, we find that some persons with acute muscle overload recover well, and others do not. It could be that mutations in the RyR1 Ca^{2+} channel or in the genes coding the subunits for the K_{ATP} channel result in or contribute to the features of the TrP, or contribute to them.

10. STATIC STIFFNESS

10.1. Static Stiffness: An Additional Muscle Stiffening Mechanism

The first mechanical change that occurs with muscle contraction is an increase in stiffness before contraction, when there is zero active force.[56] Cross-bridging is one means that brings this about and is Ca^{2+} dependent. Some stiffness is not related to cross-bridging. Stiffness increases throughout the whole rise in tension during a muscle twitch because of the formation of cross-bridges between actin and myosin in the overlap region of the sarcomere. Static stiffness occurs in response to muscle fiber stretching. An increase in calcium-dependent static tension occurs before cross-bridging can take place. Static stiffness is dependent on sarcomere length and is independent of stretching amplitude and stretching velocity. Stiffening first occurs during the latent period between muscle fiber stimulation and active cross-bridging between actin and myosin molecules. The peak occurs shortly after activation. It is related to the length of the sarcomere, increasing as sarcomere length increases, peaking, but then decreasing as sarcomere length is further increased, exceeding the length at which actin and myosin no longer overlap.[57]

Titin

Titin is the most likely candidate for the component of the sarcomere that contributes to passive stiffness. Titin regulates passive force in the myofibril and stabilizes the ordered arrangement of myofilaments in the latent and early phases of contraction.[56] Titin spans half of the sarcomere and is anchored to the Z-line and to the M-line (Figure 2-12). Titin helps to center myosin in the middle of the sarcomere. The I-band portion of titin contains a highly elastic PEVK segment that changes conformation and shortens when combined with Ca^{2+}.[58] Titin attaches to the thin actin filament, so that the shortened flexible region of titin + Ca^{2+} effectively shortens, stiffening the thin filament.[57,59] Nocella et al comment, however, that PEVK segments stiffen without change in length and therefore without effect on force and therefore would not necessarily cause fiber stiffening.[57,58] Slow muscle fibers like those in the soleus muscle have larger titin isoforms, and their stress–strain relation is shifted to longer sarcomere length.[57,60] Static stiffness is greater and develops faster in fast muscle such as the extensor digitorum longus muscle.[58] There are no studies looking at differences between taut bands in slow and in fast muscle in human subjects or in animal models.

Summary of Static Stiffness

We have concentrated on the concept of intense sarcomere contracture as the heart of the TrP in recent years, considering that to be the underlying morphologic change in muscle. However, the sarcomeres on either side of the so-called contracture knots are stretched. The work from the lab of Bagni et al and others suggests that there may be increased static stiffness in the elongated sarcomeres, and that static stiffness may contribute to the persistent muscle contraction that we see in the taut band.[58,59] Moreover, static stiffness increases up to a point with stretching of the sarcomere, but stretch beyond the overlap region of actin and myosin reduces static stiffness. This may explain why stretching exercises as used therapeutically in the treatment of TrPs may reduce the degree of hardness in the taut band as well as tenderness.

11. CONCLUSION

All credible theories of TrP formation address the issue of excessive muscle activity and of persistent muscle contraction. Some hypotheses, like Jafri's, address one particular part of the puzzle, the development of the contracted, taut band, whereas others are more comprehensive, or combine several aspects, such as the role of the alpha-adrenergic and beta-adrenergic SNS activity and aspects of control of $[Ca^{2+}]c$. It is likely that the dysfunction caused by excessive muscle activity is multifaceted, and involves multiple pathways, including possible RyR1 mutations, K_{ATP} channel mutations, SNS regulation of both presynaptic ACh release and of postsynaptic Ca^{2+} flux, of ROS overproduction, stiffness produced by altered titin function, and an increase in NQR ACh caused by lowered concentrations of ATP. Thus, we are presented with a fruitful field for investigation to try to better characterize the processes that lead to the TrP taut band. Research needs to be undertaken to evaluate the response of the TrP SEA to various catecholamine agonists and antagonists to better understand the role of the SNS in TrPs, to explore the fatigability and recovery times of muscles with TrPs to better understand the role of ROS and of K_{ATP} in TrP muscle function, to see if substances like caffeine affect the TrP, giving information about RyR1 function, and to see if passive stretch affects SEA, to explore the role of the muscle spindle. Studies of the muscle histology of animals with trigger zones could expand our knowledge of the morphology of the TrP and allow further exploration of pharmacologic manipulation of the TrP to be studied. There is much yet to be done in TrP research. It is hoped that this discussion has opened new areas to consider in this very common condition.

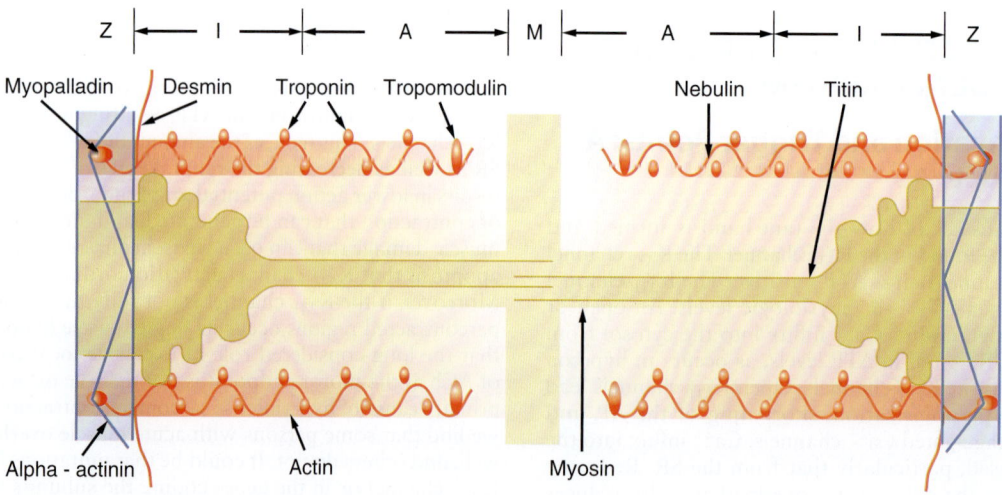

Figure 2-12. Sarcomere.

References

1. Simons DG, Travell JG, Simons LS. *Myofascial Pain and Dysfunction: The Trigger Point Manual.* Vol 1. Baltimore, MD: Williams & Wilkins; 1999.
2. Gerwin RD, Dommerholt JD, Shah J. An expansion of Simons' integrated hypothesis of trigger point formation. *Curr Pain Headache Rep.* 2004;8:468-475.
3. Bron C, Dommerholt J. Etiology of myofascial trigger points. *Curr Pain Headache Rep.* 2012;16(5):439-444.
4. Simons DG, Stolov WC. Microscopic features and transient contraction of palpable bands in canine muscle. *Am J Phys Med.* 1976;55(2):65-68.
5. Mense S, Simons DG, Hoheisel U, Quenzer B. Lesions of rat skeletal muscle after local block of acetylcholinesterase and neuromuscular stimulation. *J Appl Physiol.* 2003;94:2494-2501.
6. Hubbard DR, Berkoff GM. Myofascial trigger points show spontaneous needle-EMG activity. *Spine.* 1993;18(13):1803-1807.
7. Simons DG, Hong CZ, Simons LS. Prevalence of spontaneous electrical activity at trigger points and at control sites in rabbit skeletal muscle. *J Musculoskel Pain.* 1995;3(1):35-48.
8. Simons DG, Hong CZ, Simons LS. Endplate potentials are common to midfiber myofascial trigger points. *Am J Phys Med Rehabil.* 2002;81:212-222.
9. Couppé C, Midttun A, Hilden J, Jørgensen U, Oxholm P, Fuglsang-Frederiksen A. Spontaneous needle electromyographic activity in myofascial trigger points in the infraspinatus muscle: a blinded assessment. *J Musculoskelet Pain.* 2001;9(3):7-16.
10. Ojala TA, Arokoski JPA, Partanen JV. Needle electromyography findings of trigger points in neck-shoulder area before and after injection treatment. *J Musculoskelet Pain.* 2006;14(1):5-14.
11. Partanen JV, Ojala TA, Arokoski JP. Myofascial syndrome and pain: a neurophysiological approach. *Pathophysiology.* 2010;17(1):19-28.
12. Gerwin RD, Duranleau D. Ultrasound identification of the myofascial trigger point. *Muscle Nerve.* 1997;20(6):767-768.
13. Sikdar S, Shah JP, Gebreab T, Yen RH, Gilliams E, Danoff J, Gerber LH. Novel applications of ultrasound technology to visualize and characterize myofascial trigger points and surrounding soft tissue. *Arch Phys Med Rehabil.* 2009;90(11):1829-1838.
14. Bannister RA. Bridging the myoplasmic gap II: more recent advances in skeletal muscle excitation-contraction coupling. *J Exp Biol.* 2016;219(pt 2):175-182.
15. Pitake S, Ochs RS. Membrane depolarization increases ryanodine sensitivity to Ca2+ release to the cytosol in L6 skeletal muscle cells: implications for excitation-contraction coupling. *Exp Biol Med (Maywood).* 2016;241(8):854-862.
16. Tsentsevitsky A, Kovyazina I, Nikolsky E, Bukharaeva E, Giniatullin R. Redox-sensitive synchronizing action of adenosine on transmitter release at the neuromuscular junction. *Neuroscience.* 2013;248:699-707. doi:10.1016/j.neuroscience.2013.065.
17. Capogrossi MC, Houser ST, Bahinski A, Lakatta EG. Synchronous occurrence of spontaneous localized calcium release from the sarcoplasmic reticulum generates action potentials in rat cardiac ventricular myocytes at normal resting membrane potential. *Circ Res.* 1987;61:498-503.
18. Yu JG, Fürst DO, Thornell LE. The mode of myofibril remodelling in human skeletal muscle affected by DOMS induced by eccentric contractions. *Histochem Cell Biol.* 2003;119(5):383-393.
19. Balnave CD, Davey DF, Allen DG. Distribution of sarcomere length and intracellular calcium in mouse skeletal muscle following stretch-induced injury. *J Physiol.* 1997;502(pt 3):649-659.
20. Thompson JL, Balog EM, Fitts RH, Riley DA. Five myofibrillar lesion types in eccentrically challenged, unloaded rat adductor longus muscle—a test model. *Anat Rec.* 1999;254(1):39-52.
21. Malomouzh A, Nikolsky EE, Vyskočil F. Purine P2Y receptors in ATP-mediated regulation of non-quantal acetylcholine release from motor nerve endings of rat diaphragm. *Neurosci Res.* 2011;71(3):219-225.
22. Tintignac LA, Brenner HR, Rüegg MA. Mechanisms regulating neuromuscular junction development and function and causes of muscle wasting. *Physiol Rev.* 2015;95:809-852.
23. Vyskočil F, Malomouzh AI, Nikolsky EE. Non-quantal acetylcholine release at the neuromuscular junction. *Physiol Res.* 2009;58(6):763-784.
24. Simons DG. Do endplate noise and spikes arise from normal trigger points? *Am J Phys Med Rehabil.* 2001;80:134-140.
25. Shah JP, Phillips TM, Danoff JV, Gerber LH. An in vivo microanalytic technique for measuring the local biochemical milieu of human skeletal muscle. *J Appl Physiol.* 2005;99:1977-1984.
26. Malomouzh A, Mukhtarov MR, Nikolsky EE, Vyskočil F. Muscarinic M1 acetylcholine receptors regulate the non-quantal release of acetylcholine in the rat neuromuscular junction via NO-dependent mechanism. *J Neurochem.* 2007;102(6):2110-2117.
27. Ryten M, Koshi R, Knight GE, et al. Abnormalities in neuromuscular junction structure and skeletal muscle function in mice lacking the P2X2 nucleotide receptor. *Neuroscience.* 2007;148(3):700-711.
28. Santafé MM, Priego M, Obis T, et al. Adenosine receptors and muscarinic receptors cooperate in acetylcholine release modulation in the neuromuscular synapse. *Eur J Neurosci.* 2015;42(2):1775-1787.
29. Giniatullin A, Petrov M, Giniatullin R. The involvement of P2YK12 receptors, NADPH oxidase, and lipid rafts in the action of extracellular ATP on synaptic transmission at the fog neuromuscular synapse. *Neuroscience.* 2015;285:324-332.
30. Palma AG, Muchnik S, Losavio AS. Excitatory effect of the A2A adenosine receptor agonist CGS-21680 on spontaneous and K+-evoked acetylcholine release at the mouse neuromuscular junction. *Neuroscience.* 2011;172:164-176.
31. Ribeiro JA, Cunha RA, Correia-de-Sá P, Sebastião AM. Purinergic regulation of acetylcholine release. *Prog Brain Res.* 1996;109:231-241.
32. Oliveira L, Timóteo MA, Correia-de-Sá P. Modulation by adenosine of both muscarinic M1-facilitation and M2-inhibition of [3H]-acetylcholine release from the rat motor nerve terminals. *Eur J Neurosci.* 2002;15(11):1728-1736.
33. Obis T, Hurtado E, Nadal L, et al. The novel protein kinase C epsilon isoform modulates acetylcholine release in the rat neuromuscular junction. *Mol Brain.* 2015;8(1):80. doi:10.1186/s13041-015-0171-5.
34. Santafé MM, Garcia N, Lanuza MA, Tomàs M, Tomàs J. Interaction between protein kinase C and protein kinase A can modulate transmitter release at the rat neuromuscular synapse. *J Neurosci Res.* 2009;87(3):683-690.
35. Choi RC, Siow NL, Cheng AW, et al. ATP acts via P2Y1 receptors to stimulate acetylcholinesterase and acetylcholine receptor expression: transduction and transcription control. *J Neurosci.* 2003;23(11):4445-4456.
36. Hellström F, Roatta S, Thunberg J, Passatore M, Djupsjö M. Responses of muscle spindles in feline dorsal neck muscles to electrical stimulation of the cervical sympathetic nerve. *Exp Brain Res.* 2005;165:328-342.
37. Roatta S, Windhorst U, Ljubisavljevic M, Johansson H, Passatore M. Sympathetic modulation of muscle spindle afferent sensitivity to stretch in rabbit jaw closing muscles. *J Physiol.* 2002;540(pt 1):237-248.
38. Chiou LC, Chang CC. Effect of clonidine on neuromuscular transmission and the nicotinic receptor. *Proc Natl Sci Counc Repub China B.* 1984;8(2):148-154.
39. Chen JT, Chen SM, Kuan TS, Chung KC, Hong CZ. Phentolamine effect on the spontaneous electrical activity of active loci in a myofascial trigger spot of rabbit skeletal muscle. *Arch Phys Med Rehab.* 1998;79:790-794.
40. Endo M. Calcium release from the sarcoplasmic reticulum. *Physiol Rev.* 1977;57(1):71-108.
41. Cairns SP, Dulhunty AF. The effects of beta-adrenoceptor activation on contraction in isolated fast- and slow-twitch skeletal muscle fibers of the rat. *Br J Pharmacol.* 1993;110:1133-1141.
42. Rudolf R, Magalhães PJ, Pozzan T. Direct in vivo monitoring of sarcoplasmic reticulum Ca2+ and cytosolic cAMP dynamics in mouse skeletal muscle. *J Cell Biol.* 2006;173(2):187-193.
43. Cairns S, Borrani F. β-adrenergic modulation of skeletal muscle contraction: key role of excitation-contraction coupling. *J Physiol.* 2015;593(21):4713-4727.
44. Katz B. Neural transmitter release: from quantal secretion to exocytosis and beyond. The Fenn Lecture. *J Neurocytol.* 1996;25(12):677-688.
45. Hong CZ, Simons DG. Pathophysiologic and electrophysiologic mechanisms of myofascial trigger points. *Arch Phys Med Rehab.* 1998;79:863-872.
46. Vizi ES. Evidence that catecholamines increase acetylcholine release from neuromuscular junction through stimulation of alpha-1-adrenoceptors. *Naunyn Schmmiedebergs Arch Pharmacol.* 1991;343(5):435-438.
47. Correia AC, Silva PC, da Silva BA. Malignant hyperthermia: clinical and molecular aspects. *Rev Bras Anestesiol.* 2012;62(6):820-837.
48. Jafri MS. Nature of trigger points. *Int Sch Res Notices.* 2014;2014:523924.
49. Ahn SW, Kim SH, Kim JH, et al. Phentolamine inhibits the pacemaker activity of mouse interstitial cells of Cajal by activating ATP-sensitive K+ channels. *Arch Pharm Res.* 2010;33(3):479-489.
50. Boudreault L, Cifelli, Bourassa F, Scott K, Renaud JM. Fatigue preconditioning increases fatigue resistance in mouse flexor digitorum brevis muscles with non-functioning KATP channels. *J Physiol.* 2010;588(pt 22):4549-4562.
51. Cifelli C, Bourassa F, Gariépy L, Banas K, Benkhalti M, Renaus JM. KATP channel deficiency in mouse flexor digitorum brevis causes fibre damage and impairs Ca2+ release and force development during fatigue in vitro. *J Physiol.* 2007;582(pt 2):843-857.
52. Tricarico D, Selvaggi M, Passantino G, et al. ATP sensitive potassium channels in the skeletal muscle function: involvement of the KCNJ11(Kir6.2) gene in the determination of mechanical Warner Bratzer shear force. *Front Physiol.* 2016;7:167. doi:10.3389/fphys.2016.00167.
53. Mele A, Camerino GM, Cannone M, Conte D, Tricarico D. Dual response of the KATP channels to staurosporine: a novel role of SUR2B, SUR1 and Kir6.2 subunits in the regulation of the atrophy in different skeletal muscle phenotypes. *Biochem Pharmacol.* 2014;91(2):266-275.
54. Scott K, Benkhalti M, Calvert ND, et al. KATP channel deficiency in mouse FDB causes an impairment of energy metabolism during fatigue. *Am J Physiol Cell Physiol.* 2016;311(4):C559-C571.
55. Farahiini H, Haabibey R, Ajami M, et al. Late anti-apoptotic effect of K(ATP) channel opening in skeletal muscle. *Clin Exp Pharmacol Physiol.* 2012;39(11):909-916.
56. Colombini B, Nocella M, Bagni MA. Non-crossbridge stiffness in active muscles. *J Exp Biol.* 2016;219(pt 2):1533-160.
57. Pinniger GJ, Ranatunga KW, Offer GW. Crossbridge and non-crossbridge contributions to tension in lengthening rat muscle: force-induced reversal of the power stroke. *J Physiol.* 2006;573(pt 2):627-643.
58. Nocella M, Colombini B, Bagni MA, Burton J, Cecchi G. Non-crossbridge calcium-dependent stiffness in slow and fast skeletal fibers from mouse muscle. *J Muscle Res Cell Motil.* 2012;32:403. doi:10.1007/s10974-oll-9274-5.
59. Bagni MA, Cecchi G, Colombini B, Colomo F. A non-cross-bridge stiffness in activated frog muscle fibers. *Biophys J.* 2002;83:3118-3127.
60. Wang K, McCarter R, Wright J, Beverly J, Ramirez-Mitchell R. Regulation of skeletal muscle stiffness and elasticity by titin isoforms: a test of the segmental extension model of resting tension. *Proc Natl Acad Sci U S A.* 1991;88:7101-7105.

Chapter 3

The Role of Muscles and Fascia in Myofascial Pain Syndrome

Jan Dommerholt

1. INTRODUCTION

Travell and Simons defined myofascial pain syndrome (MPS) as "the sensory, motor, and autonomic symptoms caused by myofascial trigger points," with the additional comment that a clinician would need to identify the specific muscle or muscle group that causes the problem.[1] They defined a myofascial trigger point (TrP) from a clinical and an etiological perspective. According to the clinical definition, a TrP is "a hyperirritable spot in skeletal muscle that is associated with a hypersensitive palpable nodule in a taut band. The spot is painful on compression and can give rise to characteristic referred pain, (or other symptoms) referred tenderness, motor dysfunction, and autonomic phenomena." The etiologic definition of a TrP is "a cluster of electrically active loci each of which is associated with a contraction knot and a dysfunctional motor endplate in skeletal muscle." In an overview chapter in the previous edition of this book, the authors devoted several pages to the anatomy, structure, and function of muscles with detailed descriptions of the neuromuscular junction, motor unit, and motor endplate zone.[1] Although Travell opted to use the term "myofascial," the previous editions of the Trigger Point Manual contain practically no information about fascia or about the interactions between muscle and fascia. In fact, the indices of the two-volume book did not include an entry of the word "fascia," other than in the context of "trigger points in fascia."[2]

Nevertheless, muscles and fascia are strongly related to each other and it is not really possible to discuss MPS and TrPs without considering what role fascia may play in their etiology and in the symptoms commonly attributed to muscles and TrPs. The contributions of fascia are undervalued. Although Travell was probably one of the early physicians to recognize the importance of fascia in myofascial pain conditions, the knowledge about fascia was in its infancy when she defined the terms. This chapter aims to provide a review of the anatomy and functions of muscles and fascia in the context of myofascial pain. In the current thinking, only muscular TrPs are recognized, whereas Travell and Simons also considered cutaneous, ligamentous, periosteal, and nonmuscular TrPs.[1]

2. MUSCLES

Skeletal muscles represent approximately 42% to 47% of the human body mass. They are crucial for human movement, balance, breathing, eating (activities of daily living), regulating homeostasis and metabolism, and in the widest sense, for survival.[3] Most muscles attach to bones via their tendons, but some muscles attach to another muscle's tendon, such as the flexor accessorius muscle, which attaches to the tendons of the flexor digitorum longus muscle. In a few cases, muscles attach to another muscle(s), such as the zygomaticus muscles, the risorius, and the buccinator muscles attaching to the orbicularis oris muscle. Muscles actively generate forces when they contract and passively, they can be lengthened and stretched.

Muscles can be classified on the basis of their predominant type of fibers. Type I fibers are slow oxidative fibers with a slow contraction speed and a low myosin ATPase activity. They are designed for aerobic metabolism. Type IIa fibers are fast oxidative-glycolytic fibers and have a fast contraction speed and a high myosin ATPase activity. Typically, they are recruited when additional activity is required. Type I and IIa fibers are resistant to fatigue and are rich in mitochondria and myoglobin. Type IIb fibers are fast glycolytic fibers with a fast contraction speed and a high myosin ATPase activity. They are easily fatigued and have few mitochondria and little myoglobin. They generate adenosine triphosphate (ATP) by the anaerobic fermentation of glucose to lactic acid. Type I fibers correspond to the "dark meat" muscles of a chicken and mostly involved with posture and endurance sports, whereas type IIb fibers are found in "white meat" muscles and are better suited for short-term muscle contraction.

2.1. Muscle Anatomy and Physiology

Muscles are made of groups of fascicles, consisting of muscle fibers and myofibrils. A muscle fiber encloses approximately 1000 to 2000 myofibrils in most skeletal muscles. Each myofibril is approximately 1 to 2 μm in diameter and is separated from surrounding myofibrils by the mitochondria, the sarcoplasmic reticulum, and the transverse tubular systems or T-tubules (Figure 3-1). Each fibril consists of a chain of sarcomeres, which are the muscle smallest contractile elements. Muscles tend to have more sarcomeres, when the force-generating axis is parallel to the direction of the muscle fibers.[4] When skeletal muscle fibers are activated, the length of various sarcomeres can vary substantially, and it has been suggested that this nonuniformity would contribute to mechanical instability[5]; however, when muscles are contracted isometrically, the nonuniformity has no impact on stability.[6]

A sarcomere has contractile and structural proteins that together form a highly organized and structured network or lattice. Individual myofilaments have more or less fixed lengths and do not change much during contractions. A sarcomere consists of thin actin filaments, which are double-stranded helical polymers attached to the Z-line, and thick myosin filaments in the center of the sarcomere. Myosin features cross-bridges with ATPase and actin-binding sites. Titin, the largest known vertebrate protein, connects the myosin filament to the Z-line (Figure 3-2). It has established cross-links with titin molecules of adjacent sarcomeres. Titin filaments generate passive tension when sarcomeres are stretched and provide muscle stiffness. It keeps the myosin filaments positioned in the center of the sarcomere.[7,8] A small section of titin, the PEVK segment, interacts

Chapter 3: The Role of Muscles and Fascia in Myofascial Pain Syndrome   45

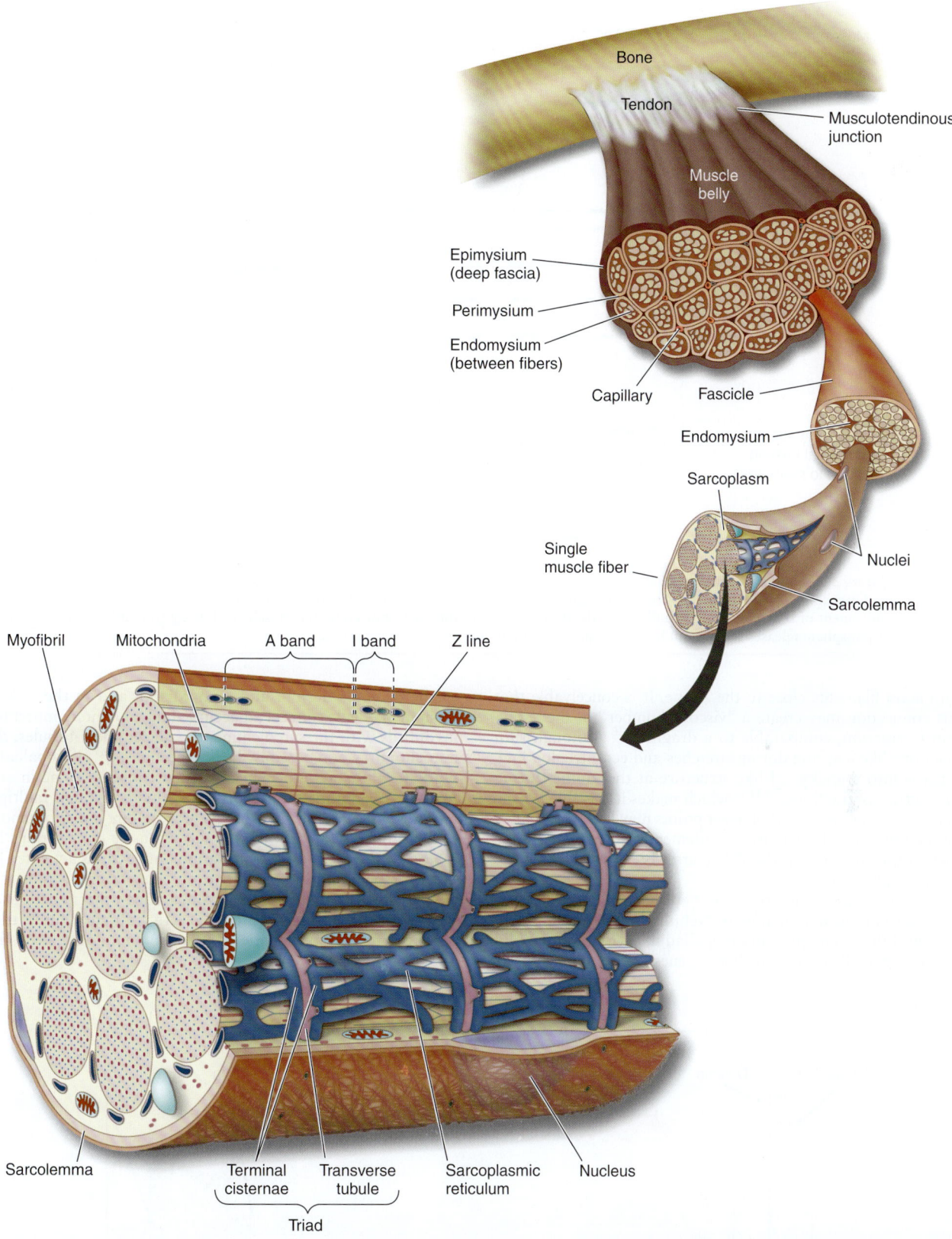

Figure 3-1. Macroscopic anatomy of the skeletal muscle. Muscle fibers are organized into muscles by successive layers of connective tissue, including the epimysium, perimysium, and endomysium. This arrangement separates and protects fragile muscle fibers while directing forces toward the bone. The sarcolemma envelops the nucleus, mitochondria, and myofibrils. Myofibrils contain well-organized proteins that overlap and form Z-lines, I bands, and A bands. The sarcoplasmic reticulum houses calcium and the transverse tubules transmit electrical signals from the sarcolemma inside the cell, both critical to muscle function.

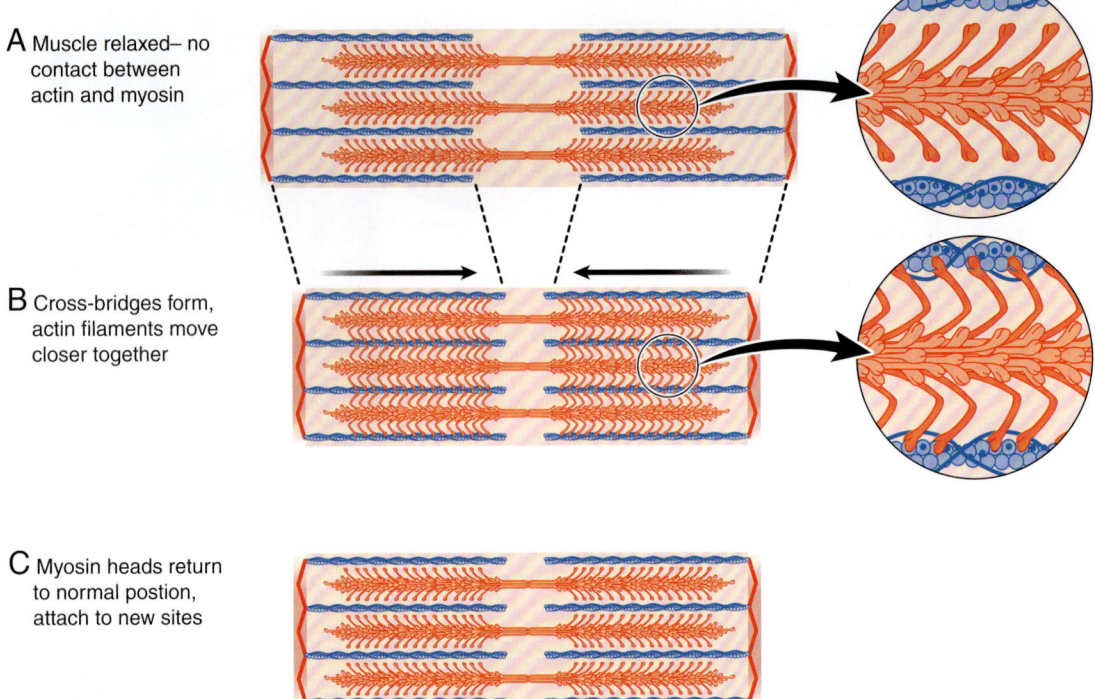

Figure 3-2. Sliding filament mechanism. A, Prior to transmission of the action potential, no cross-bridges connect actin and myosin. B, Once the active sites are revealed and myosin heads bind to actin, the power stroke occurs. Synchronized movement of the myosin heads pulls the ends of the sarcomere together, shortening the muscle. C, Energy from adenosine triphosphate releases the myosin heads and positions them for another power stroke.

with actin filaments close to the Z-line. It is conceivable that this connection may create a "viscous bumper" of the actin–titin interaction, comparable to a dragnet.[9,10] Although titin functions like a spring during stretches and eccentric loading, it turns into a sticky gel-like structure at the Z-line during concentric contractions,[7,8,11,12] which makes it possible for the muscle to generate force.[13] Trigger points may have a damaged sarcomere assembly, with myosin filaments getting stuck in the sticky titin substance at the Z-line after breaking through the actin–titin barrier.

Another important protein is nebulin, which covers the full length of the actin filaments. Nebulin interacts with actin, titin, and the Z-line protein myopalladin.[14] Titin and nebulin interact especially during myofibrillogenesis.[15] Nebulin connects to the proteins desmin and myopalladin and in the Z-line. Desmin filaments connect adjacent Z-lines and interconnect the myofibrils with the sarcolemma, the nuclei, the T-tubules, the mitochondria, and possibly the microtubules.[16,17] Myopalladin binds to alpha-actinin, which in turn connects to actin and to titin.[17] Nebulin stabilizes the sarcomere through multiple binding sites at actin, tropomyosin, troponin, and tropomodulin (Figure 3-3).[15,16,18-20] It regulates muscle contractions by inhibiting the cross-bridge formation until actin is activated by Ca^{2+}.[21] Troponin, a Ca^{2+} receptive protein, sensitizes actomyosin to Ca^{2+} together with tropomyosin, among other functions.[22] Tropomyosin and tropomodulin can influence molecular processes related to synaptic signaling and modulate neuronal morphology (Figure 3-4).[23]

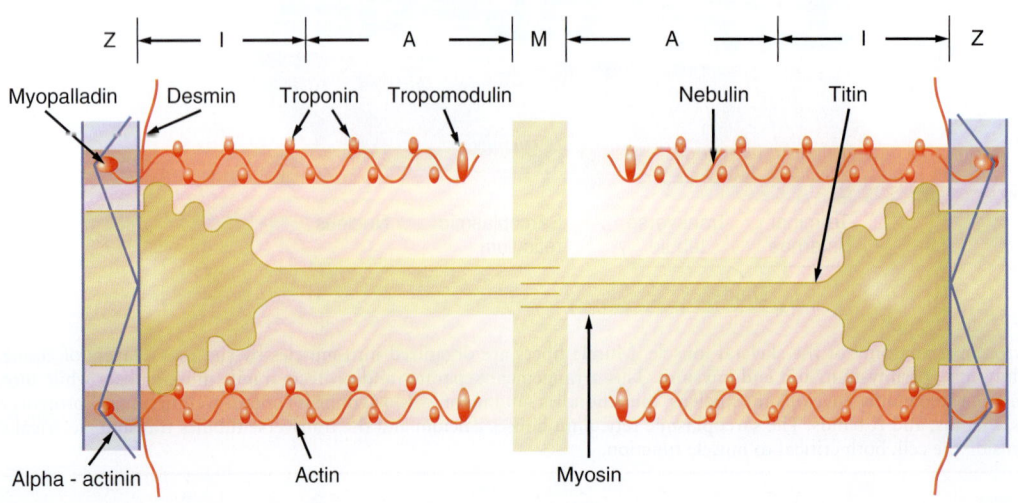

Figure 3-3. Sarcomere.

Chapter 3: The Role of Muscles and Fascia in Myofascial Pain Syndrome   47

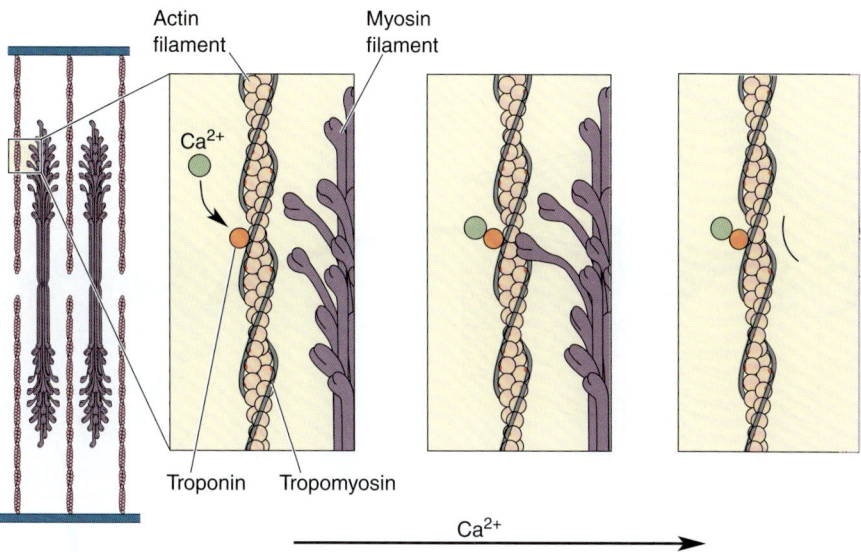

Figure 3-4. The molecular basis of muscle contraction. The binding of Ca^{2+} to troponin shifts tropomyosin and allows the myosin heads to bind to the actin filament. Then the myosin heads pivot, causing the filaments to slide with respect to one another.

Each muscle fiber is innervated by a single axon from an alpha-motor neuron in the spinal cord. An alpha-motor neuron with all the muscles fibers it innervates is referred to as a motor unit. There are considerable size differences between alpha-motor neurons and differences in excitability. Smaller motor neurons are more excitable than larger neurons. Similarly, smaller motor units feature a smaller alpha-motor neuron cell body, smaller axons, and fewer target muscle fibers than larger motor units (Figure 3-5). They supply in between 300 and 1500 muscle fibers and are involved in maintaining posture and activities such as walking (type I fibers), whereas larger motor units are activated with activities that require faster responses (type IIb fibers).

When the cell body of a motor neuron in the anterior horn initiates an action potential, the potential propagates along the axon through each of its arborizations to the specialized nerve terminal that helps form the neuromuscular junction (motor endplate) on each muscle fiber. On arrival at the nerve terminal, the electrical action potential is relayed chemically across the synaptic cleft of the neuromuscular junction to the postjunctional membrane of the muscle fiber (Figure 3-6). T-tubules, located perpendicular to the long axis of the muscle fiber with two zones of transverse tubules to each sarcomere, conduct impulses from the exterior to the interior of the muscle fiber and activate voltage-dependent L-type calcium channels

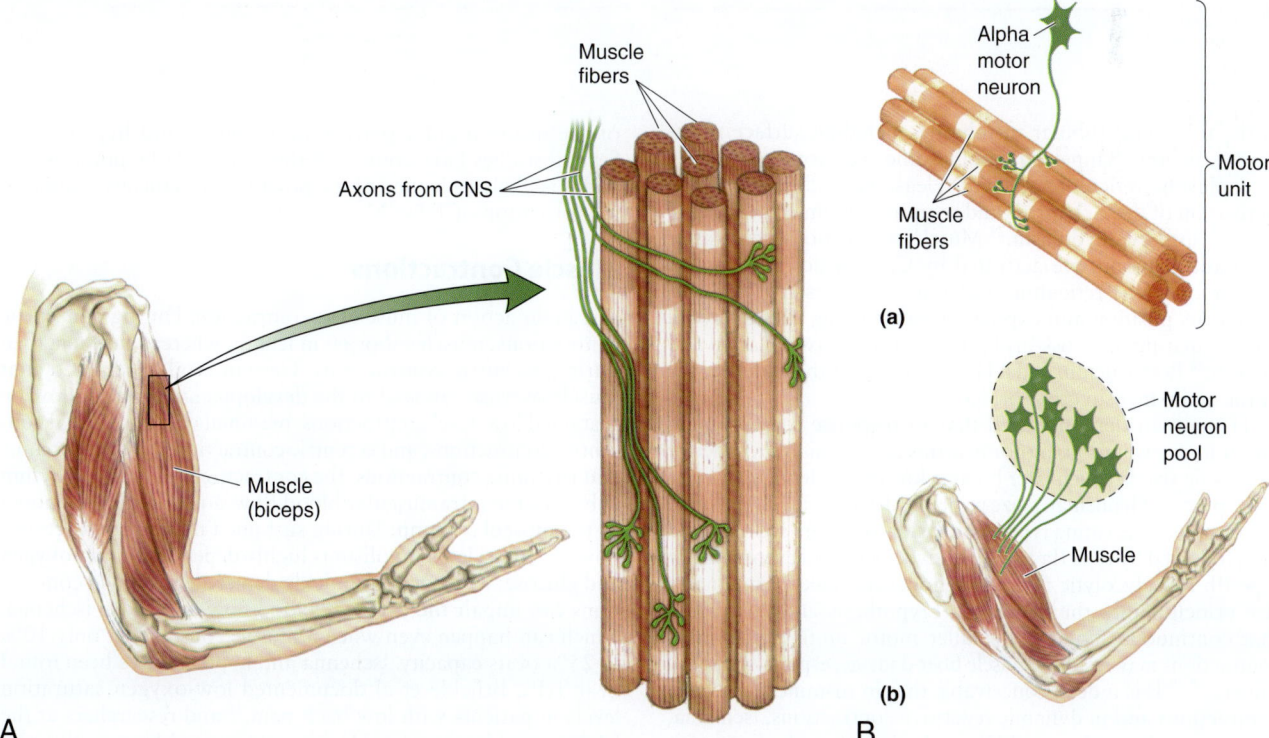

Figure 3-5. The structure of the skeletal muscle. A, Each muscle fiber is innervated by a single axon. B, A motor unit and motor neuron pool. (a), A motor unit is an alpha-motor neuron and all the muscle fibers it innervates. (b), A motor neuron pool is all the alpha-motor neurons that innervate one muscle.

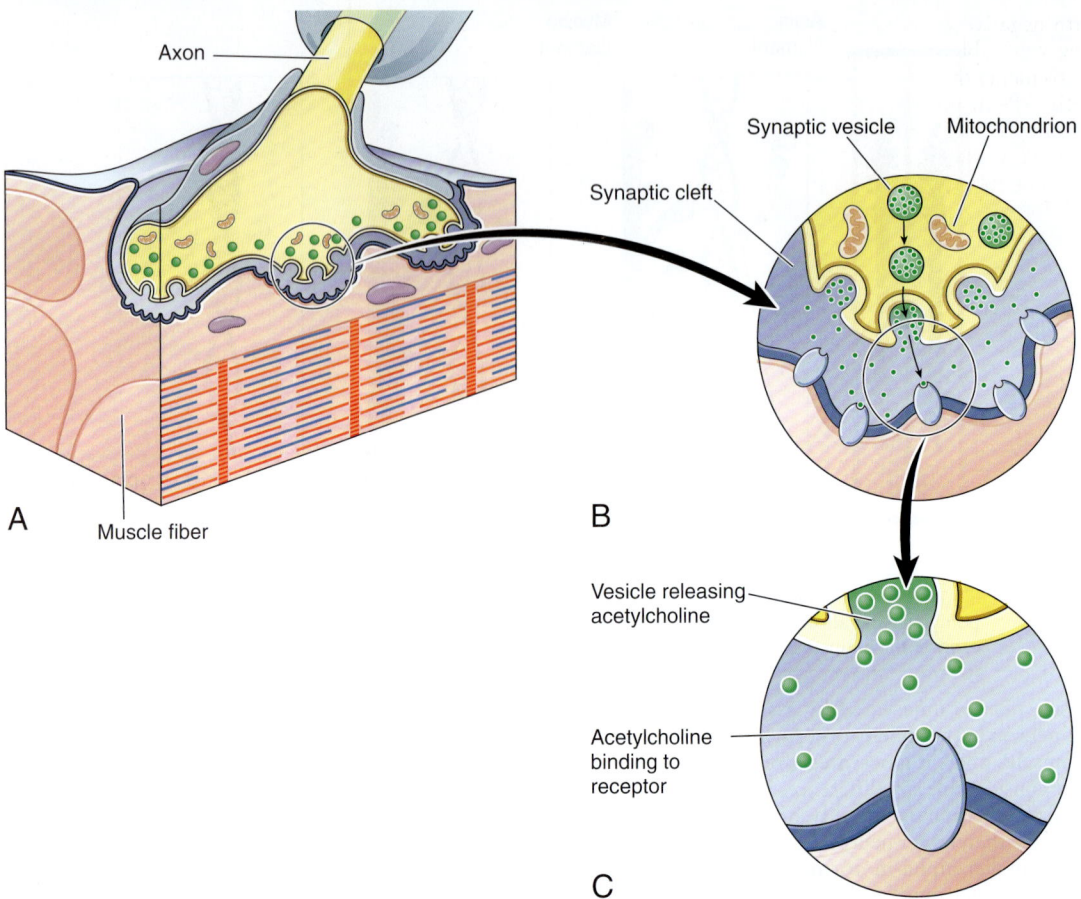

Figure 3-6. Neuromuscular junction. A, Neurons and muscle fibers communicate at the neuromuscular junction. B, Electrical signals travel along the axon and stimulate synaptic vesicles at its end to release acetylcholine, a neurotransmitter, into the synaptic cleft. C, Acetylcholine crosses the synaptic cleft and binds to receptors in the sarcolemma of muscle fibers, causing changes within the muscle cell that initiate muscle contraction.

in the transverse tubular membrane, including surface membrane calcium channel dihydropyridine receptors and type 1 sarcoplasmic reticulum calcium release ryanodine receptors. Activation of these channels and receptors results in the release of Ca^{2+} into the myoplasm.[24] Muscle contractions occur after actin and troponin are activated by Ca^{2+}, which is stored in the sarcoplasmic reticulum. Calcium facilitates tropomyosin to shift its position and expose myosin-binding sites on actin, thus regulating the cross-bridge interactions between actin and myosin.[16] Both calcium and ATP are critical for the maintenance of the actin–myosin cross-bridges.[25]

Henneman demonstrated that in response to increasing physiologic excitation, motor neurons are recruited in order of increasing size,[26] which later became known as Henneman's size principle.[27-29] Henneman's size principle demonstrated that small motor units innervating type I slow oxidative fibers are recruited first, followed by type IIa fast oxidative fibers, and eventually by type IIb fast glycolytic fibers. Hägg incorporated Henneman's size principle into the Cinderella Hypothesis and postulated that continuous activity of smaller motor units in sustained contractions may result in muscle fiber damage, especially to type I fibers.[30-32] It is indeed conceivable that in sustained low-level contractions and in dynamic repetitive contractions, ischemia, hypoxia, and insufficient ATP synthesis in type I motor unit fibers are responsible for increasing acidity, an accumulation of Ca^{2+}, and subsequently sarcomere contractures with a decrease of the intramuscular perfusion, ischemia, and hypoxia.[33-35] Several studies have confirmed the Cinderella Hypothesis,[36-40] and it is likely to be one of the possible mechanisms leading to the formation of TrPs.[34,35]

Muscle Contractions

The main action of muscles is contraction. During concentric contractions, muscles shorten in length, whereas they lengthen during eccentric contractions. Gerwin et al speculated that muscle overuse can lead to the development of TrPs following sustained low-level contractions, maximal or submaximal concentric contractions, and eccentric contractions.[41] With dynamic and rhythmic contractions, the contraction–relaxation rhythm enhances the intramuscular blood flow, a phenomenon known as the muscular pump. During sustained muscle contractions, however, muscle metabolism is highly dependent upon oxygen and glucose, which will be quickly depleted. Sustained contractions can impair the capillary blood flow and cause ischemia, which can happen even when a muscle contracts at only 10% to 25% of its capacity. Ischemia and hypoxia have been found near TrPs. Brückle et al documented low-oxygen saturation levels in patients with low back pain,[42] and researchers at the US National Institutes of Health and George Mason University documented a retrograde blood flow in the vicinity of active TrPs, characterized by increased systolic velocities and flow reversal with negative diastolic velocities.[43] A few sessions of dry needling were able to reverse this process with objective tissue improvements up to 8 weeks after the intervention.[44,45] Patients with TrPs in the upper trapezius muscle experienced a reduction of pain as much as 6 weeks after dry needling.[46,47]

An individual muscle's maximum voluntary contraction is highly dependent upon the architecture and shape of the muscle and the development of intramuscular pressure.[48-50] Not all muscles have the same shape and architecture, and depending on the pattern of the muscle fascicles, they are classified as parallel (eg, the rectus abdominis muscle), pennate (eg, the deltoid muscle), convergent (eg, the pectoralis major muscle), or circular (eg, the orbicularis oris muscle). Parallel muscles are by far the most common type accounting for about 85% of all muscles, and they are useful especially when speed is important. Pennate muscles are better designed to develop strength.

Muscle Contractions, Mitochondria, and the Ca^{2+} Pump

Increased pressure gradients during sustained low-level exertions may contribute to the development of pain and eventually to the formation of TrPs.[51] Ischemia, or the lack of blood flow, quickly leads to hypoxia, which in turn will cause a drop in tissue pH, a release of protons, and the suspension of the production of ATP by mitochondria. Mitochondria produce ATP through the process of respiration and oxidative phosphorylation (OXPHOS), which occurs via protein complexes of the electron transport chain (ETC).

Mitochondrial function in the skeletal muscle is quite complex. It is required for muscle homeostasis and is regulated by ATP Citrate Lyase (ACL). Citrate lyase is a cytosolic enzyme that catalyzes mitochondria-derived citrate into oxaloacetate and acetyl-coenzyme A (acetyl-CoA).[52-54] Acetyl-CoA is oxidized to carbon dioxide and water through the tricarboxylic acid cycle, which generates reduced nicotinamide adenine dinucleotide (NADH). The ETC oxidizes reducing equivalents NADH and a reduced form of flavin adenine dinucleotide, which creates a H^+ gradient across the mitochondrial membrane. The gradient facilitates the phosphorylation of adenosine diphosphate (ADP) to ATP by mitochondrial ATP synthase.[4] The ATP synthesis is the most prevalent biochemical process in the human body. Active individuals produce their own body weight of ATP every day.

Exercise provides one mechanism of improving mitochondrial function, in addition to increasing the contractile function of the skeletal muscle and improving muscle strength, endurance, and aerobic capacity.[55] Muscle strengthening improves muscle functioning by increasing its metabolic capacity.

Some of these effects are mediated by insulin growth factor 1, an anabolic growth factor that induces the activation of ACL,[52,55] and stimulates muscle hypertrophy, fatty acid uptake, and glucose metabolism.[56] Citrate Lyase also stimulates cardiolipin synthesis and mitochondrial supercomplex activity, which further improve mitochondrial function.[52] Cardiolipin is an important component of the mitochondrial membrane.[57] The term "mitochondrial supercomplex activity" suggests that the ETC is not a static entity in the inner mitochondrial membrane, but a complex dynamic entity. There are two concurrent OXPHOS models. According to the fluid state model, OXPHOS complexes diffuse freely in the mitochondrial inner membrane, whereas the solid-state model maintains that OXPHOS complexes are organized in rigid higher-order assemblies known as supercomplexes or respirasomes.[58,59] They consist of a combination of four complexes in the ETC that are still poorly understood.[60]

As already mentioned in Chapter 2, ATP is required for the removal of Ca^{2+} from the cytosol to reverse actin–myosin coupling. When ATP is attached to the myosin molecule, the link between myosin and actin weakens, and the myosin head detaches from actin. At the same time Ca^{2+} ion detaches from the troponin molecule, which blocks tropomyosin. Under normal physiologic circumstances, large quantities of free Ca^{2+} will reenter the sarcoplasmic reticulum by a functioning sarcoplasmic/endoplasmic reticulum Ca^{2+} ATPase (SERCA) pump. When energy is depleted, sarcomeres may stay contracted, until enough ATP is again available to resolve the intracellular Ca^{2+} accumulation. High concentrations of intracellular Ca^{2+} are associated with sustained sarcomere contraction and damage of the mitochondria and the muscle, which may have a causative role in the development of muscle disorders and TrPs.[61,62] Although SERCA abnormalities have been hypothesized to contribute to the dysregulation of intracellular Ca^{2+} homeostasis and signaling in the muscles of patients with myotonic dystrophy and hypothyroid myopathy, Guglielmi et al concluded that the SERCA function was not altered in these patient populations.[63]

Trigger points can develop without muscle damage, but increased levels of intracellular Ca^{2+} can cause a disruption of the cell membrane, damage to the sarcoplasmic reticulum, which will trigger an even greater influx of Ca^{2+}, and a disruption of cytoskeletal proteins, including titin, desmin, and dystrophin. A dysfunctional SERCA pump was an integral component of the original energy crisis hypothesis,[64] but has not yet been demonstrated in patients with myofascial pain. Nevertheless, many patients with myalgia present with ragged red fibers and increased numbers of cytochrome-c-oxidase (COX) negative fibers, which are indicative of a dysfunction of the mitochondrial OXPHOS.[65] Ragged red fibers are also observed in MERFF syndrome (Myoclonic Epilepsy with Ragged Red Fibers), but not always,[66,67] and in a wide variety of other disorders, such as hypothyroid myopathy, progressive external ophthalmoplegia, Leigh syndrome, adult-onset Pompe disease, and other mitochondrial myopathies.[68-71] Aging is associated with an increase in mitochondrial abnormalities, and healthy older adults can present with ragged red and COX-negative fibers.[72]

During sustained contractions, a muscle may switch quickly to anaerobic glycolysis in an effort to guarantee an adequate supply of ATP. Glycolysis involves splitting a glucose molecule into two pyruvic molecules, a process associated with the release of just enough energy to form two ATP molecules. Under aerobic circumstances, the reaction between oxygen and pyruvic acid can produce as many as 16 ATP molecules per pyruvic acid molecule, carbon dioxide, and water. Under anaerobic circumstances, however, the majority of glycolytic pyruvic acid is converted into lactic acid, which will further lower the intramuscular pH. When the capillary circulation is restricted, as in sustained low-level contractions, lactic acid may not diffuse out of the muscle as normally happens after exertions.[33]

Muscle Contractions and ATP

Submaximal and maximal concentric contractions require much ATP, which initially is released from internal storage units in the muscle. After 4 to 6 seconds, the muscle will need to rely on direct phosphorylation of ADP by creatine phosphate (CP). Phosphorylation produces ATP by coupling a phosphate group to an ADP molecule catalyzed by the enzyme creatine kinase. Stored ATP and CP provide enough energy for maximum muscle power for approximately 14 to 16 seconds. Hereafter, a short period of rest is needed to replenish the exhausted reserves of intracellular ATP and CP. When ongoing ATP demands are within the capacity of the aerobic pathway, muscular activity can continue for hours in well-conditioned individuals. However, when the demands of exercise begin to exceed the ability of the muscle cells to carry out the necessary reactions quickly enough, anaerobe glycolysis will contribute more and more of the total generated ATP. Finally, the muscle will run out of ATP and sustained sarcomere contractions may occur, starting the development of TrPs.

3. FASCIA

When an athlete suffers from some kind of overload injury, it is conceivable that fascia or connective tissues, such as tendons, ligaments, and joint capsules, are loaded more beyond their capacity than muscles or bones.[73,74] Although muscles are the main contractile tissue in the body, almost 40% of muscle force is transmitted to the fascia.[75] Each individual muscle has specific connections to the fascia,[76-81] and there is evidence that the angle at which muscle fibers connect to the intramuscular connective tissue and the connections between the deep fascia and the epimysium contribute to the patterns of force transmission.[82] As an example, the perimysium contributes to the lateral force transmission in the skeletal muscle.[83-85] Perimysium has a high density of fibroblasts.[86]

When muscles connect to other muscle fibers or to intramuscular connective tissue, epimuscular myofascial force transmission is directed toward connective tissues outside the muscle parameters.[87,88] Findley reported that this mechanism does not only facilitate complicated movement patterns involving adjacent muscles, but also contributes to increased joint stability.[89] The shape of the muscle determines the angle the muscle fibers can connect to the intramuscular fascia (Figure 3-7). Awareness of the continuity of muscles and their fascial connections and their potential implications for clinical practice are important to understand along with the nature of TrPs and biomechanical considerations. At this point in time, there are only a few studies and case reports in the myofascial and dry needling literature that consider the interconnections between muscles and fascia,[90-93] but the number of studies on fascia has grown exponentially during the past decade.[94-105] Fascia may play a significant role in muscle contractibility and possibly in the formation of TrPs.[106,107]

3.1. Definitions

During the 2015 fourth Fascia Research Congress in Washington, DC, USA, fascia was defined anatomically as "a sheath, a sheet or any number of other dissectible aggregations of connective tissue that forms beneath the skin to attach, enclose, separate muscles and internal organs."[108] This new definition was not necessarily acceptable to clinicians and researchers,[109] and a new committee was formed to define "the fascial system," which in 2017, was described as follows:

"The fascial system consists of the three-dimensional continuum of soft, collagen-containing, loose and dense fibrous connective tissues that permeate the body. It incorporates elements such as adipose tissue, adventitia and neurovascular sheaths, aponeuroses, deep and superficial fasciae, epineurium, joint capsules, ligaments, membranes, meninges, myofascial expansions, periostea, retinacula, septa, tendons, visceral fasciae, and all the intramuscular and intermuscular connective tissues including endo-/peri-/epimysium.

The fascial system interpenetrates and surrounds all organs, muscles, bones and nerve fibers, endowing the body with a functional structure, and providing an environment that enables all body systems to operate in an integrated manner."[105]

Muscles and fascia are intimately intertwined and connected. All muscles are enveloped by the epimysium. Individual muscle fiber bundles are situated within the perimysium and individual muscle fibers are contained within the endomysium. The endomysium, perimysium, and epimysium are components of the deep fascia,[86,97] not to be confused with the visceral and superficial fascia.[110] Stecco's Functional Atlas of the Human Fascial System gives an outstanding overview of fascial connections in the human body.[111]

3.2. Some Biomechanical Considerations

The importance of the interconnections between muscles and the epimysium, perimysium, and endomysium are slowly being realized. Each muscle has specific connections with the fascia,[77,80,81,112] and these connections allow force transmissions to take place from muscles to bones and to deeper fascial layers. It is truly impossible to separate the fascia from other structures, such as the skin, ligaments, and muscles (Figure 3-8).[82,113] Muscle fibers frequently connect to other muscles or to the connective tissue and these interconnections allow muscles to exert force on the fascia and connective tissues outside the muscle parameters.[88] A decline in flexibility and mobility with aging can be ascribed to changes in the fascia, such as decreased flexibility of the epimysium. Dense epimysium often restricts muscle function[76]; for example, the perimysium can increase muscle stiffness and is sensitive to changes in mechanical tension.[85]

Changes in fascial pliability can lead to altered movement patterns, local overuse, and a loss of strength and coordination. Stecco et al speculated that decreased viscoelasticity is due to a lack of hyaluronan (HA), which determines the viscosity between the deep fascia and the muscle.[76,114] Hyaluronan is a glycosaminoglycan polymer of the extracellular matrix (ECM) and is found between muscle fibers, nerves, and the fascial layers.[115,116] Decreased mobility between the layers of the aponeurotic fascia, such as the thoracolumbar fascia, will lead to

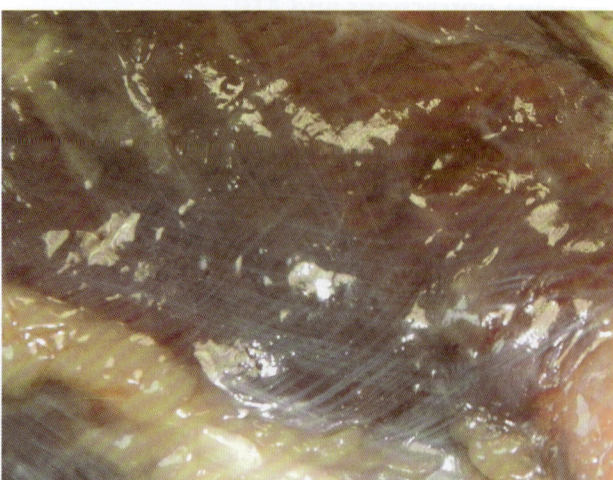

Figure 3-7. Tridimensional direction of the fascia.

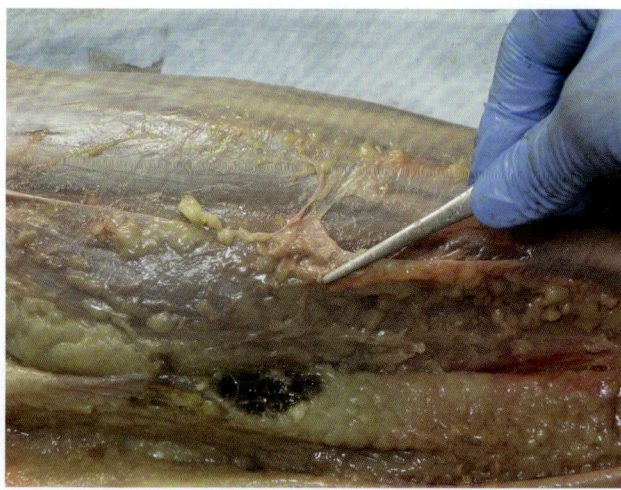

Figure 3-8. Fascial connections to the skin, muscles, and nerve.

stiffness and limited mobility. The aponeurotic fascia consists of two or three layers of parallel collagen fiber bundles oriented in different directions and is directly connected to muscles and tendons.[76,104,117] It transmits forces over greater distances than the epimysial fascia.[100] The deep fascia contains multiple mechanoreceptors,[118] and the ability of the fascia to process mechanoreceptive input is entirely dependent upon its structural relationship with bone tissue and muscles.[119]

Fibroblasts are located within the ECM and they play a significant role in the synthesis of collagen, ground substance, elastin, and reticulin. As a side note, the ECM consists of collagen, elastic fibers, proteoglycans, laminins, matricellular proteins, and fibronectin.[120-125] Fibroblasts register force-induced deformations in their ECM, and the mechanical stretching of fibroblasts regulates key ECM genes by stimulating the release of multiple substances, such as paracrine growth factor.[86] Fibroblasts feature integrins, which are critical for mechanical force patterning,[126] and they can register strain in response to changes in mechanical stress.[127] Under high tension, fibroblasts feature stress fibers and focal adhesions, and appear lamellar in shape, whereas under low stress, they are more or less rounded structures.[128-130] Lamellar fibroblasts can differentiate into myofibroblasts complete with a contractile apparatus of actin microfilaments and nonmuscle myosin.[131] In other words, the fascia is not just a passive structure; it can engage in very slow contractions.[132]

Fibroblasts are involved in wound closure, muscle contractions, and adhesions of scars.[133,134] Wound healing involves controlled remodeling of the ECM, which typically happens in three distinct phases (inflammation, proliferation, and remodeling). Following tissue injury, fibroblasts differentiate into myofibroblasts and deposit collagen, fibronectin, and glycosaminoglycans.[135] Fibrin and fibronectin are matrix proteins that prevent excessive blood loss. Fibronectin is relatively elastic, which makes it suitable for collagen assembly. Collagens are the major structural components of the ECM.[125] Fibrosis occurs when collagen being deposited by fibroblasts and myofibroblasts causes an increase in myofibroblasts with excessive matrix deposition and a disruption of matrix remodeling.[136]

Empirically, adhesions of the scar tissue can be treated effectively with manual techniques or with dry needling by placing a needle directly into each adhesion or densification and rotating the needle unidirectionally as much as possible to the pain tolerance level of the patient.[93,137] When the needle releases, periodic tightening is indicated until the adhesion has been diminished or even resolved (Figure 3-9). Langevin et al have shown that the effects of acupuncture and dry needling can at least partially be explained by the mechanical stimulation of fibroblasts.[138,139] Rotating the needle creates a bond between the contracted fascial tissues and the needle, causing mechanical stress over fibroblasts, cytoskeletal force patterns, intracellular signaling pathways, and mechanically induced gene activation, which in turn will restore the scar's mobility and pliability, and immediately reduce the subject's hyperalgesia and allodynia.[137] The torque increases exponentially with rotating the needle, which can be objectively measured up to several centimeters from the needle location.[140] Persistent adhesions are likely due to dysregulation of ECM proteins. Rotating the needle inhibits Rho-dependent kinase and suppresses the induction of the tenascin-C gene. One of the best approaches to accomplish the transcription of the tenascin-C gene and to positively impact fibronectin and collagen XII is to cyclically stretch fibroblasts in the ECM. Because of the nearly immediate response, it is debatable whether adhesions found near the scar tissue are in fact examples of fibrotic tissue as is often assumed. Perhaps the adhesions reflect contractures of the fascial tissue and not fibrosis.

3.3. Some Sensory Aspects of Fascia

To be a source of pain, fascia must contain sensory fibers and nociceptors.[141] A rodent study showed that nociceptors were three times more common in the thoracolumbar fascia than in back muscles.[142] Other studies have confirmed that lumbar dorsal horn neurons receive input not only from muscles but also from the thoracolumbar fascia.[143-146] Because most of these neurons feature a high mechanical threshold, they are probably nociceptive neurons.[147] Deising et al suggested that the sensitization of fascial nociceptors following mechanical and chemical stimulation may contribute to persistent myofascial pain, especially when the fascia is being stretched, for example, as occurs during muscle contractions.[148] Injections of nerve growth factor, a chemical that induces severe hyperalgesia, in the fascia of the erector spinae muscles caused significant hyperalgesia, exercise-induced pain, and a decreased pressure threshold for about seven days and ongoing sensitization to mechanical and chemical stimuli for two weeks.[148] Injections of hypertonic saline caused more delayed onset of muscle pain when targeting the tibial anterior fascia than when injecting directly into the muscle.[149] Hypertonic saline injections into the fascia resulted in significantly more pain than injections in the subcutis and the muscle.[150] Weinkauf et al had similar findings when they injected nerve growth factor into the anterior tibialis and erector spinae muscles and their fascia.[151] Mechanical hyperalgesia was more pronounced in the tibial fascia than in the muscle, and the thoracodorsal fascia appeared to be more sensitive than the tibial fascia.[151] Danielson et al found peptidergic sensory nerve endings with antibodies for calcitonin gene-related peptide and substance P in the loose connective tissue of the patellar tendon.[152] Of interest is also that under pathologic conditions, fascia is able to establish new nociceptive fibers that are immunoreactive to substance P.[153] The nerve endings in the fascia are located in the outer layer of the fascia, which is more or less continuous with the subcutaneous tissue. As the middle fascial layer is primarily involved with mechanical force transmissions, it makes sense that there are no nerve endings; otherwise movement would cause pain. Tesarz et al confirmed the presence of nociceptive sP endings in the subcutaneous tissue and the outer layer of the thoracolumbar fascia, which implies again that the fascia may play a significant role in low back pain.[154] Ruffini, Pacini receptors, and free nerve endings have been identified in the deep fascia.[134,155] There is also some evidence that Pacinian receptors may be involved in high-velocity manipulation,[156] but there are no studies that have explored whether manual TrP therapy or dry needling specifically target Pacinian receptors. Simmonds et al hypothesized what the role of the fascia in manual therapy could entail, but they did not reach any significant conclusions.[157]

3.4. Summary

Given the intricate connections between fascia and muscles, it is likely that the current explanatory models of myofascial pain and TrPs will continue to evolve as the knowledge and understanding

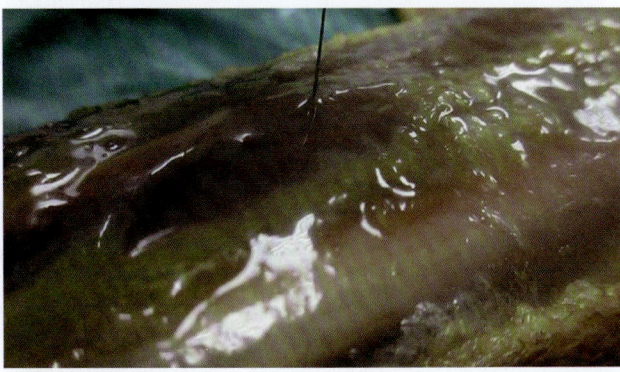

Figure 3-9. Filiform needle in the fascia.

increases. Schleip suggested that pain sensations from TrPs may originate from sensitized fascial nociceptors.[158] Treatment approaches for TrPs, scar tissue, and adhesions must involve manipulation of fascia. Manual stretching techniques will cause slow adaptations, but dry needling of the scar tissue alters the contractile elements almost immediately. The mechanisms of this phenomenon are not yet known and deserve further exploration.

References

1. Simons DG, Travell JG, Simons LS. *Travell and Simons' Myofascial Pain and Dysfunction: The Trigger Point Manual.* Vol 1. 2nd ed. Baltimore, MD: Williams & Wilkins; 1999.
2. Travell JG, Simons DG. *Myofascial Pain and Dysfunction: The Trigger Point Manual.* Vol 2. Baltimore, MD: Williams & Wilkins; 1992.
3. Baghdadia MB, Tajbakhsh S. Regulation and phylogeny of skeletal muscle regeneration. *Dev Biol.* 2018;433:200-209.
4. Miller MS, Palmer BM, Toth MJ, Warshaw DM. Muscle: anatomy, physiology, and biochemistry. In: Firestein GS, Budd RC, Gabriel SE, McInnes IB, O'Dell JR, eds. *Kelley and Firestein's Textbook of Rheumatology.* Vol 1. 10th ed. Philadelphia, PA: Elsevier; 2017:66-77.
5. Morgan DL, Mochon S, Julian FJ. A quantitative model of intersarcomere dynamics during fixed-end contractions of single frog muscle fibers. *Biophys J.* 1982;39(2):189-196.
6. Joumaa V, Leonard TR, Herzog W. Residual force enhancement in myofibrils and sarcomeres. *Proc Biol Sci.* 2008;275(1641):1411-1419.
7. Lindstedt SL, Reich TE, Keim P, LaStayo PC. Do muscles function as adaptable locomotor springs? *J Exp Biol.* 2002;205(Pt 15):2211-2216.
8. Wang K, McCarter R, Wright J, Beverly J, Ramirez MR. Viscoelasticity of the sarcomere matrix in skeletal muscles. The titin-myosin composite filament is a dual-stage molecular spring. *Biophys J.* 1993;64:1161-1177.
9. Nagy A, Cacciafesta P, Grama L, Kengyel A, Malnasi-Csizmadia A, Kellermayer MS. Differential actin binding along the PEVK domain of skeletal muscle titin. *J Cell Sci.* 2004;117(Pt 24):5781-5789.
10. Niederlander N, Raynaud F, Astier C, Chaussepied P. Regulation of the actin-myosin interaction by titin. *Eur J Biochem.* 2004;271(22):4572-4581.
11. Wang K. Titin/connectin and nebulin: giant protein rulers of muscle structure and function. *Adv Biophys.* 1996;33:123-134.
12. Gregorio CC, Granzier H, Sorimachi H, Labeit S. Muscle assembly: a titanic achievement? *Curr Opin Cell Biol.* 1999;11(1):18-25.
13. Rivas-Pardo JA, Eckels EC, Popa I, Kosuri P, Linke WA, Fernandez JM. Work done by titin protein folding assists muscle contraction. *Cell Rep.* 2016;14(6):1339-1347.
14. Ma K, Wang K. Interaction of nebulin SH3 domain with titin PEVK and myopalladin: implications for the signaling and assembly role of titin and nebulin. *FEBS Lett.* 2002;532(3):273-278.
15. McElhinny AS, Kazmierski ST, Labeit S, Gregorio CC. Nebulin: the nebulous, multifunctional giant of striated muscle. *Trends Cardiovasc Med.* 2003;13(5):195-201.
16. Clark KA, McElhinny AS, Beckerle MC, Gregorio CC. Striated muscle cytoarchitecture: an intricate web of form and function. *Annu Rev Cell Dev Biol.* 2002;18:637-706.
17. Bang ML, Gregorio C, Labeit S. Molecular dissection of the interaction of desmin with the C-terminal region of nebulin. *J Struct Biol.* 2002;137(1-2):119-127.
18. Jin JP, Wang K. Nebulin as a giant actin-binding template protein in skeletal muscle sarcomere. Interaction of actin and cloned human nebulin fragments. *FEBS Lett.* 1991;281(1-2):93-96.
19. Chu M, Gregorio CC, Pappas CT. Nebulin, a multi-functional giant. *J Exp Biol.* 2016;219(Pt 2):146-152.
20. Pappas CT, Bliss KT, Zieseniss A, Gregorio CC. The Nebulin family: an actin support group. *Trends Cell Biol.* 2011;21(1):29-37.
21. McElhinny AS, Schwach C, Valichnac M, Mount-Patrick S, Gregorio CC. Nebulin regulates the assembly and lengths of the thin filaments in striated muscle. *J Cell Biol.* 2005;170(6):947-957.
22. Ohtsuki I, Morimoto S. Troponin: regulatory function and disorders. *Biochem Biophys Res Commun.* 2008;369(1):62-73.
23. Gray KT, Kostyukova AS, Fath T. Actin regulation by tropomodulin and tropomyosin in neuronal morphogenesis and function. *Mol Cell Neurosci.* 2017;84:48-57.
24. Capes EM, Loaiza R, Valdivia HH. Ryanodine receptors. *Skelet Muscle.* 2011;1(1):18.
25. Houdusse A, Sweeney HL. How myosin generates force on actin filaments. *Trends Biochem Sci.* 2016;41(12):989-997.
26. Henneman E, Somjen G, Carpenter DO. Excitability and inhibitability of motoneurons of different sizes. *J Neurophysiol.* 1965;28(3):599-620.
27. De Luca CJ, Contessa P. Hierarchical control of motor units in voluntary contractions. *J Neurophysiol.* 2012;107(1):178-195.
28. Duchateau J, Enoka RM. Human motor unit recordings: origins and insight into the integrated motor system. *Brain Res.* 2011;1409:42-61.
29. Conwit RA, Stashuk D, Tracy B, McHugh M, Brown WF, Metter EJ. The relationship of motor unit size, firing rate and force. *Clin Neurophysiol.* 1999;110(7):1270-1275.
30. Hägg GM. The cinderella hypothesis. In: Johansson H, Windhorst U, Djupsjöbacka M, Passotore M, eds. *Chronic Work-related Myalgia.* Gävle, Sweden: Gävle University Press; 2003:127-132.
31. Hägg GM. Static work and myalgia—a new explanation model. In: Andersson PA, Hobart DJ, Danoff JV, eds. *Electromyographical Kinesiology.* Amsterdam, The Netherlands: Elsevier; 1991:115-199.
32. Hägg GM. Ny förklaringsmodell för muskelskador vid statisk belastning i skuldra och nacke. *Arbete Människa Miljö.* 1988;4:260-262.
33. Bron C, Dommerholt J. Etiology of myofascial trigger points. *Curr Pain Headache Rep.* 2012;16(5):439-444.
34. Treaster D, Marras WS, Burr D, Sheedy JE, Hart D. Myofascial trigger point development from visual and postural stressors during computer work. *J Electromyogr Kinesiol.* 2006;16(2):115-124.
35. Hoyle JA, Marras WS, Sheedy JE, Hart DE. Effects of postural and visual stressors on myofascial trigger point development and motor unit rotation during computer work. *J Electromyogr Kinesiol.* 2011;21(1):41-48.
36. Zennaro D, Laubli T, Krebs D, Krueger H, Klipstein A. Trapezius muscle motor unit activity in symptomatic participants during finger tapping using properly and improperly adjusted desks. *Hum Factors.* 2004;46(2):252-266.
37. Zennaro D, Laubli T, Krebs D, Klipstein A, Krueger H. Continuous, intermitted and sporadic motor unit activity in the trapezius muscle during prolonged computer work. *J Electromyogr Kinesiol.* 2003;13(2):113-124.
38. Forsman M, Birch L, Zhang Q, Kadefors R. Motor unit recruitment in the trapezius muscle with special reference to coarse arm movements. *J Electromyogr Kinesiol.* 2001;11:207-216.
39. Forsman M, Kadefors R, Zhang Q, Birch L, Palmerud G. Motor-unit recruitment in the trapezius muscle during arm movements and in VDU precision work. *Int J Ind Ergon.* 1999;24:619-630.
40. Forsman M, Taoda K, Thorn S, Zhang Q. Motor-unit recruitment during long-term isometric and wrist motion contractions: a study concerning muscular pain development in computer operators. *Int J Ind Ergon.* 2002;30:237-250.
41. Gerwin RD, Dommerholt J, Shah JP. An expansion of Simons' integrated hypothesis of trigger point formation. *Curr Pain Headache Rep.* 2004;8(6):468-475.
42. Brückle W, Sückfull M, Fleckenstein W, Weiss C, Müller W. Gewebe-pO2-Messung in der verspannten Rückenmuskulatur (m. erector spinae). *Z Rheumatol.* 1990;49:208-216.
43. Ballyns JJ, Shah JP, Hammond J, Gebreab T, Gerber LH, Sikdar S. Objective sonographic measures for characterizing myofascial trigger points associated with cervical pain. *J Ultrasound Med.* 2011;30(10):1331-1340.
44. Turo D, Otto P, Shah JP, et al. Ultrasonic characterization of the upper trapezius muscle in patients with chronic neck pain. *Ultrason Imaging.* 2013;35(2):173-187.
45. Turo D, Otto P, Hossain M, et al. Novel use of ultrasound elastography to quantify muscle tissue changes after dry needling of myofascial trigger points in patients with chronic myofascial pain. *J Ultrasound Med.* 2015;34(12):2149-2161.
46. Gerber LH, Sikdar S, Aredo JV, et al. Beneficial effects of dry needling for treatment of chronic myofascial pain persist for 6 weeks after treatment completion. *PM R.* 2017;9(2):105-112.
47. Gerber LH, Shah J, Rosenberger W, et al. Dry needling alters trigger points in the upper trapezius muscle and reduces pain in subjects with chronic myofascial pain. *PM R.* 2015;7(7):711-718.
48. Jarvholm U, Palmerud G, Karlsson D, Herberts P, Kadefors R. Intramuscular pressure and electromyography in four shoulder muscles. *J Orthop Res.* 1991;9(4):609-619.
49. Jarvholm U, Palmerud G, Styf J, Herberts P, Kadefors R. Intramuscular pressure in the supraspinatus muscle. *J Orthop Res.* 1988;6(2):230-238.
50. Palmerud G, Forsman M, Sporrong H, Herberts P, Kadefors R. Intramuscular pressure of the infra- and supraspinatus muscles in relation to hand load and arm posture. *Eur J Appl Physiol.* 2000;83(2-3):223-230.
51. Otten E. Concepts and models of functional architecture in skeletal muscle. *Exerc Sport Sci Rev.* 1988;16:89-137.
52. Das S, Morvan F, Jourde B, et al. ATP citrate lyase improves mitochondrial function in skeletal muscle. *Cell Metab.* 2015;21(6):868-876.
53. Das S, Morvan F, Morozzi G, et al. ATP citrate lyase regulates myofiber differentiation and increases regeneration by altering histone acetylation. *Cell Rep.* 2017;21(11):3003-3011.
54. Choudhary C, Weinert BT, Nishida Y, Verdin E, Mann M. The growing landscape of lysine acetylation links metabolism and cell signalling. *Nat Rev Mol Cell Biol.* 2014;15(8):536-550.
55. Egerman MA, Glass DJ. Signaling pathways controlling skeletal muscle mass. *Crit Rev Biochem Mol Biol.* 2014;49(1):59-68.
56. Clemmons DR. Metabolic actions of insulin-like growth factor-I in normal physiology and diabetes. *Endocrinol Metab Clin North Am.* 2012;41(2):425-443, vii-viii.
57. Li H, Sartorelli V. ATP citrate lyase: a new player linking skeletal muscle metabolism and epigenetics. *Trends Endocrinol Metab.* 2018;29(4):202-204.
58. Jha P, Wang X, Auwerx J. Analysis of mitochondrial respiratory chain supercomplexes using blue native polyacrylamide gel electrophoresis (BN-PAGE). *Curr Protoc Mouse Biol.* 2016;6(1):1-14.
59. Mourier A, Matic S, Ruzzenente B, Larsson NG, Milenkovic D. The respiratory chain supercomplex organization is independent of COX7a2l isoforms. *Cell Metab.* 2014;20(6):1069-1075.
60. Acin-Perez R, Fernandez-Silva P, Peleato ML, Perez-Martos A, Enriquez JA. Respiratory active mitochondrial supercomplexes. *Mol Cell.* 2008;32(4):529-539.
61. Gissel H, Clausen T. Excitation-induced Ca(2+) influx in rat soleus and EDL muscle: mechanisms and effects on cellular integrity. *Am J Physiol Regul Integr Comp Physiol.* 2000;279(3):R917-R924.
62. Jafri MS. Mechanisms of myofascial pain. *Int Sch Res Notices.* 2014;2014.
63. Guglielmi V, Oosterhof A, Voermans NC, et al. Characterization of sarcoplasmic reticulum Ca(2+) ATPase pumps in muscle of patients with myotonic dystrophy and with hypothyroid myopathy. *Neuromuscul Disord.* 2016;26(6):378-385.

64. Simons DG, Travell J. Myofascial trigger points, a possible explanation. *Pain.* 1981;10(1):106-109.
65. Larsson B, Bjork J, Henriksson KG, Gerdle B, Lindman R. The prevalences of cytochrome c oxidase negative and superpositive fibres and ragged-red fibres in the trapezius muscle of female cleaners with and without myalgia and of female healthy controls. *Pain.* 2000;84(2-3):379-387.
66. Mancuso M, Petrozzi L, Filosto M, et al. MERRF syndrome without ragged-red fibers: the need for molecular diagnosis. *Biochem Biophys Res Commun.* 2007;354(4):1058-1060.
67. Matsuoka T, Goto Y, Yoneda M, Nonaka I. Muscle histopathology in myoclonus epilepsy with ragged-red fibers (MERRF). *J Neurol Sci.* 1991;106(2):193-198.
68. Black JT, Judge D, Demers L, Gordon S. Ragged-red fibers. A biochemical and morphological study. *J Neurol Sci.* 1975;26(4):479-488.
69. Ching CK, Mak CM, Au KM, et al. A patient with congenital hyperlactataemia and Leigh syndrome: an uncommon mitochondrial variant. *Hong Kong Med J.* 2013;19(4):357-361.
70. Mak SC, Chi CS, Tsai CR. Mitochondrial DNA 8993 T > C mutation presenting as juvenile Leigh syndrome with respiratory failure. *J Child Neurol.* 1998;13(7):349-351.
71. Laforêt P, Lombès A, Eymard B, et al. Chronic progressive external ophthalmoplegia with ragged-red fibers: clinical, morphological and genetic investigations in 43 patients. *Neuromuscul Disord.* 1995;5(5):399-413.
72. Bourgeois JM, Tarnopolsky MA. Pathology of skeletal muscle in mitochondrial disorders. *Mitochondrion.* 2004;4(5-6):441-452.
73. Schleip R, Muller DG. Training principles for fascial connective tissues: scientific foundation and suggested practical applications. *J Bodyw Mov Ther.* 2013;17(1):103-115.
74. Counsel P, Breidahl W. Muscle injuries of the lower leg. *Semin Musculoskelet Radiol.* 2010;14(2):162-175.
75. Smeulders MJ, Kreulen M, Hage JJ, Huijing PA, van der Horst CM. Spastic muscle properties are affected by length changes of adjacent structures. *Muscle Nerve.* 2005;32(2):208-215.
76. Stecco A, Gesi M, Stecco C, Stern R. Fascial components of the myofascial pain syndrome. *Curr Pain Headache Rep.* 2013;17(8):352.
77. Stecco A, Gilliar W, Hill R, Fullerton B, Stecco C. The anatomical and functional relation between gluteus maximus and fascia lata. *J Bodyw Mov Ther.* 2013;17(4):512-517.
78. Stecco A, Macchi V, Masiero S, et al. Pectoral and femoral fasciae: common aspects and regional specializations. *Surg Radiol Anat.* 2009;31(1):35-42.
79. Stecco A, Macchi V, Stecco C, et al. Anatomical study of myofascial continuity in the anterior region of the upper limb. *J Bodyw Mov Ther.* 2009;13(1):53-62.
80. Stecco C, Gagey O, Macchi V, et al. Tendinous muscular insertions onto the deep fascia of the upper limb. First part: anatomical study. *Morphologie.* 2007;91(292):29-37.
81. Wilke J, Engeroff T, Nurnberger F, Vogt L, Banzer W. Anatomical study of the morphological continuity between iliotibial tract and the fibularis longus fascia. *Surg Radiol Anat.* 2016;38(3):349-352.
82. Turrina A, Martinez-Gonzalez MA, Stecco C. The muscular force transmission system: role of the intramuscular connective tissue. *J Bodyw Mov Ther.* 2013;17(1):95-102.
83. Passerieux E, Rossignol R, Chopard A, et al. Structural organization of the perimysium in bovine skeletal muscle: junctional plates and associated intracellular subdomains. *J Struct Biol.* 2006;154(2):206-216.
84. Passerieux E, Rossignol R, Chopard A, et al. Structural organization of the perimysium in bovine skeletal muscle: junctional plates and associated intracellular subdomains. In: Huijing PA, Hollander P, Findley T, Schleip R, eds. *Fascia Research II: Basic Science and Implications for Conventional and Complementary Health Care.* Munich, Germany: Urban & Fischer; 2009:186-196.
85. Passerieux E, Rossignol R, Letellier T, Delage JP. Physical continuity of the perimysium from myofibers to tendons: involvement in lateral force transmission in skeletal muscle. *J Struct Biol.* 2007;159(1):19-28.
86. Schleip R, Naylor IL, Ursu D, et al. Passive muscle stiffness may be influenced by active contractility of intramuscular connective tissue. *Med Hypotheses.* 2006;66(1):66-71.
87. Hijikata T, Ishikawa H. Functional morphology of serially linked skeletal muscle fibers. *Acta Anat (Basel).* 1997;159(2-3):99-107.
88. Huijing PA, Jaspers RT. Adaptation of muscle size and myofascial force transmission: a review and some new experimental results. *Scand J Med Sci Sports.* 2005;15(6):349-380.
89. Findley TW. Fascia research from a clinician/scientist's perspective. *Int J Ther Massage Bodywork.* 2011;4(4):1-6.
90. Finnoff JT, Rajasekaran S. Ultrasound-guided, percutaneous needle fascial fenestration for the treatment of chronic exertional compartment syndrome: a case report. *PM R.* 2016;8(3):286-290.
91. Anandkumar SM, Manivasagam M. Effect of fascia dry needling on non-specific thoracic pain—a proposed dry needling grading system. *Physiother Theory Pract.* 2017;33(5):420-428.
92. Lewit K. The needle effect in the relief of myofascial pain. *Pain.* 1979;6:83-90.
93. Lewit K, Olsanska S. Clinical importance of active scars: abnormal scars as a cause of myofascial pain. *J Manipulative Physiol Ther.* 2004;27(6):399-402.
94. Chaudhry H, Huang C-Y, Schleip R, Ji Z, Bukiet B, Findley T. Viscoelastic behavior of human fasciae under extension in manual therapy. *J Bodyw Mov Ther.* 2007;11(2):159-167.
95. Chaudhry H, Max R, Antonio S, Findley T. Mathematical model of fiber orientation in anisotropic fascia layers at large displacements. *J Bodyw Mov Ther.* 2012;16(2):158-164.
96. Chaudhry H, Schleip R, Ji Z, Bukiet B, Maney M, Findley T. Three-dimensional mathematical model for deformation of human fasciae in manual therapy. *J Am Osteopath Assoc.* 2008;108(8):379-390.
97. Roman M, Chaudhry H, Bukiet B, Stecco A, Findley TW. Mathematical analysis of the flow of hyaluronic acid around fascia during manual therapy motions. *J Am Osteopath Assoc.* 2013;113(8):600-610.
98. Huijing PA. Epimuscular myofascial force transmission: a historical review and implications for new research. International Society of Biomechanics Muybridge Award Lecture, Taipei, 2007. *J Biomech.* 2009;42(1):9-21.
99. Huijing PA. Epimuscular myofascial force transmission between antagonistic and synergistic muscles can explain movement limitation in spastic paresis. In: Huijing PA, Hollander P, Findley T, Schleip R, eds. *Fascia Research II: Basic Science and Implications for Conventional and Complementary Health Care.* Munich, Germany: Urban & Fischer; 2009.
100. Huijing PA, Baan GC. Myofascial force transmission via extramuscular pathways occurs between antagonistic muscles. *Cells Tissues Organs.* 2008;188(4):400-414.
101. Langevin HM, Huijing PA. Communicating about fascia: history, pitfalls, and recommendations. *Int J Ther Massage Bodywork.* 2009;2(4):3-8.
102. Schleip R, Findley TW, Chaitow L, Huijing P. *Fascia: The Tensional Network of the Human Body.* London, England: Churchill Livingstone; 2012.
103. Schuenke MD, Vleeming A, Van Hoof T, Willard FH. A description of the lumbar interfascial triangle and its relation with the lateral raphe: anatomical constituents of load transfer through the lateral margin of the thoracolumbar fascia. *J Anat.* 2012;221(6):568-576.
104. Willard FH, Vleeming A, Schuenke MD, Danneels L, Schleip R. The thoracolumbar fascia: anatomy, function and clinical considerations. *J Anat.* 2012;221(6):507-536.
105. Adstrum S, Hedley G, Schleip R, Stecco C, Yucesoy CA. Defining the fascial system. *J Bodyw Mov Ther.* 2017;21(1):173-177.
106. Schleip R, Klingler W, Lehmann-Horn F. Active fascial contractility: fascia may be able to contract in a smooth muscle-like manner and thereby influence musculoskeletal dynamics. *Med Hypotheses.* 2005;65(2):273-277.
107. Schleip R, Klingler W, Lehmann-Horn F. Fascia is able to contract in a smooth muscle-like manner and thereby influence musculoskeletal mechanics. *J Biomech.* 2006;39(S1):S488.
108. Stecco C, Schleip R. A fascia and the fascial system. *J Bodyw Mov Ther.* 2016;20(1):139-140.
109. Scarr G. Comment on 'Defining the fascial system'. *J Bodyw Mov Ther.* 2017;21(1):178.
110. Stecco A, Stern R, Fantoni I, De Caro R, Stecco C. Fascial disorders: implications for treatment. *PM R.* 2016;8(2):161-168.
111. Stecco C. *Functional Atlas of the Human Fascial System.* Edinburgh, Scotland: Churchill Livingstone; 2015.
112. Stecco C, Macchi V, Porzionato A, et al. The ankle retinacula: morphological evidence of the proprioceptive role of the fascial system. *Cells Tissues Organs.* 2010;192(3):200-210.
113. Saiz-Llamosas JR, Fernandez-Perez AM, Fajardo-Rodriguez MF, Pilat A, Valenza-Demet G, Fernández-de-Las-Peñas C. Changes in neck mobility and pressure pain threshold levels following a cervical myofascial induction technique in pain-free healthy subjects. *J Manipulative Physiol Ther.* 2009;32(5):352-357.
114. Stecco C, Stern R, Porzionato A, et al. Hyaluronan within fascia in the etiology of myofascial pain. *Surg Radiol Anat.* 2011;33(10):891-896.
115. Laurent C, Johnson-Wells G, Hellstrom S, Engstrom-Laurent A, Wells AF. Localization of hyaluronan in various muscular tissues. A morphological study in the rat. *Cell Tissue Res.* 1991;263(2):201-205.
116. Piehl-Aulin K, Laurent C, Engstrom-Laurent A, Hellstrom S, Henriksson J. Hyaluronan in human skeletal muscle of lower extremity: concentration, distribution, and effect of exercise. *J Appl Physiol.* 1991;71(6):2493-2498.
117. Vleeming A, Schuenke MD, Danneels L, Willard FH. The functional coupling of the deep abdominal and paraspinal muscles: the effects of simulated paraspinal muscle contraction on force transfer to the middle and posterior layer of the thoracolumbar fascia. *J Anat.* 2014;225(4):447-462.
118. Langevin HM. Connective tissue: a body-wide signaling network? *Med Hypotheses.* 2006;66(6):1074-1077.
119. van der Wal J. The architecture of the connective tissue in the musculoskeletal system—an often overlooked functional parameter as to proprioception in the locomotor apparatus. *Int J Ther Massage Bodywork.* 2009;2(4):9-23.
120. Iozzo RV, Schaefer L. Proteoglycan form and function: a comprehensive nomenclature of proteoglycans. *Matrix Biol.* 2015;42:11-55.
121. Jensen SA, Handford PA. New insights into the structure, assembly and biological roles of 10-12 nm connective tissue microfibrils from fibrillin-1 studies. *Biochem J.* 2016;473:827-838.
122. Zollinger AJ, Smith ML. Fibronectin, the extracellular glue. *Matrix Biol.* 2017;60-61:27-37.
123. Rogers RS, Nishimune H. The role of laminins in the organization and function of neuromuscular junctions. *Matrix Biol.* 2017;57-58:86-105.
124. Viloria K, Hill NJ. Embracing the complexity of matricellular proteins: the functional and clinical significance of splice variation. *Biomol Concepts.* 2016;7(2):117-132.
125. Ricard-Blum S, Baffet G, Theret N. Molecular and tissue alterations of collagens in fibrosis. *Matrix Biol.* 2018. doi:10.1016/j.matbio.2018.02.004.
126. Chiquet M, Renedo AS, Huber F, Fluck M. How do fibroblasts translate mechanical signals into changes in extracellular matrix production? *Matrix Biol.* 2003;22(1):73-80.
127. Lee DJ, Rosenfeldt H, Grinnell F. Activation of ERK and p38 MAP kinases in human fibroblasts during collagen matrix contraction. *Exp Cell Res.* 2000;257(1):190-197.
128. Grinnell F. Fibroblast biology in three-dimensional collagen matrices. *Trends Cell Biol.* 2003;13(5):264-269.

129. Langevin HM, Storch KN, Snapp RR, et al. Tissue stretch induces nuclear remodeling in connective tissue fibroblasts. *Histochem Cell Biol.* 2010;133(4):405-415.
130. Miron-Mendoza M, Seemann J, Grinnell F. Collagen fibril flow and tissue translocation coupled to fibroblast migration in 3D collagen matrices. *Mol Biol Cell.* 2008;19(5):2051-2058.
131. Tomasek JJ, Gabbiani G, Hinz B, Chaponnier C, Brown RA. Myofibroblasts and mechano-regulation of connective tissue remodelling. *Nat Rev Mol Cell Biol.* 2002;3(5):349-363.
132. Schleip R, Klingler W, Lehmann-Horn F. Faszien besitzen eine der glatten Muskulatur vergleichbare Kontraktionsfähigkeit und können so die muskuloskeletale Mechanik beeinflussen. *Osteopathische Medizin, Zeitschrift für ganzheitliche Heilverfahren.* 2008;9(4):19-21.
133. Yahia L, Rhalmi S, Newman N, Isler M. Sensory innervation of human thoracolumbar fascia. An immunohistochemical study. *Acta Orthop Scand.* 1992;63(2):195-197.
134. Yahia LH, Pigeon P, DesRosiers EA. Viscoelastic properties of the human lumbodorsal fascia. *J Biomed Eng.* 1993;15(5):425-429.
135. Keane TJ, Horejs CM, Stevens MM. Scarring vs. functional healing: matrix-based strategies to regulate tissue repair. *Adv Drug Deliv Rev.* 2018. doi:10.1016/j.addr.2018.02.002.
136. Rhett JM, Ghatnekar GS, Palatinus JA, O'Quinn M, Yost MJ, Gourdie RG. Novel therapies for scar reduction and regenerative healing of skin wounds. *Trends Biotechnol.* 2008;26(4):173-180.
137. Fernández de las Peñas C, Arias-Buría JL, Dommerholt J. Dry needling for fascia, scar and tendon. In: Dommerholt J, Fernández de las Peñas C, eds. *Trigger Point Dry Needling—An Evidence-based Approach.* Vol 2. Edinburgh, Scotland: Elsevier; 2018:in press.
138. Langevin HM, Churchill DL, Cipolla MJ. Mechanical signaling through connective tissue: a mechanism for the therapeutic effect of acupuncture. *FASEB J.* 2001;15(12):2275-2282.
139. Langevin HM, Churchill DL, Fox JR, Badger GJ, Garra BS, Krag MH. Biomechanical response to acupuncture needling in humans. *J Appl Physiol.* 2001;91(6):2471-2478.
140. Langevin HM, Konofagou EE, Badger GJ, et al. Tissue displacements during acupuncture using ultrasound elastography techniques. *Ultrasound Med Biol.* 2004;30(9):1173-1183.
141. Tesarz J. Die Fascia thoracolumbalis als potenzielle Ursache für Rückenschmerzen: anatomische Grundlagen und klinische Aspekte. *Osteopathische Medizin.* 2010;11(1):28-34.
142. Barry CM, Kestell G, Gillan M, Haberberger RV, Gibbins IL. Sensory nerve fibers containing calcitonin gene-related peptide in gastrocnemius, latissimus dorsi and erector spinae muscles and thoracolumbar fascia in mice. *Neuroscience.* 2015;291:106-117.
143. Taguchi T, Hoheisel U, Mense S. Dorsal horn neurons having input from low back structures in rats. *Pain.* 2008;138(1):119-129.
144. Gillette RG, Kramis RC, Roberts WJ. Characterization of spinal somatosensory neurons having receptive fields in lumbar tissues of cats. *Pain.* 1993;54(1):85-98.
145. Grant G. Projection patterns of primary sensory neurons studied by transganglionic methods: somatotopy and target-related organization. *Brain Res Bull.* 1993;30(3-4):199-208.
146. Mense S, Hoheisel U. Evidence for the existence of nociceptors in rat thoracolumbar fascia. *J Bodyw Mov Ther.* 2016;20(3):623-628.
147. Hoheisel U, Unger T, Mense S. A block of spinal nitric oxide synthesis leads to increased background activity predominantly in nociceptive dorsal horn neurones in the rat. *Pain.* 2000;88(3):249-257.
148. Deising S, Weinkauf B, Blunk J, Obreja O, Schmelz M, Rukwied R. NGF-evoked sensitization of muscle fascia nociceptors in humans. *Pain.* 2012;153(8):1673-1679.
149. Gibson W, Arendt-Nielsen L, Taguchi T, Mizumura K, Graven-Nielsen T. Increased pain from muscle fascia following eccentric exercise: animal and human findings. *Exp Brain Res.* 2009;194(2):299-308.
150. Schilder A, Hoheisel U, Magerl W, Benrath J, Klein T, Treede RD. Sensory findings after stimulation of the thoracolumbar fascia with hypertonic saline suggest its contribution to low back pain. *Pain.* 2014;155(2):222-231.
151. Weinkauf B, Deising S, Obreja O, et al. Comparison of nerve growth factor-induced sensitization pattern in lumbar and tibial muscle and fascia. *Muscle Nerve.* 2015;52(2):265-272.
152. Danielson P, Alfredson H, Forsgren S. Distribution of general (PGP 9.5) and sensory (substance P/CGRP) innervations in the human patellar tendon. *Knee Surg Sports Traumatol Arthrosc.* 2006;14(2):125-132.
153. Sanchis-Alfonso V, Rosello-Sastre E. Immunohistochemical analysis for neural markers of the lateral retinaculum in patients with isolated symptomatic patellofemoral malalignment. A neuroanatomic basis for anterior knee pain in the active young patient. *Am J Sports Med.* 2000;28(5):725-731.
154. Tesarz J, Hoheisel U, Wiedenhofer B, Mense S. Sensory innervation of the thoracolumbar fascia in rats and humans. *Neuroscience.* 2011;194:302-308.
155. Stecco C, Porzionato A, Lancerotto L, et al. Histological study of the deep fasciae of the limbs. *J Bodyw Mov Ther.* 2008;12(3):225-230.
156. Schleip R. Fascial plasticity—a new neurobiological explanation: Part 1. *J Bodyw Mov Ther.* 2003;7(1):11-19.
157. Simmonds N, Miller P, Gemmell H. A theoretical framework for the role of fascia in manual therapy. *J Bodyw Mov Ther.* 2012;16(1):83-93.
158. Schleip R. Myofascial trigger points and fascia. In: Irnich D, ed. *Myofascial Trigger Points: Comprehensive Diagnosis and Treatment.* Edinburgh, Scotland: Churchill Livingstone; 2013:49-51.

Chapter 4

Perpetuating Factors for Myofascial Pain Syndrome

Robert D. Gerwin

1. INTRODUCTION

The current concept regarding the origin of myofascial trigger points (MTrPs) states that muscle overload or excessive muscle activity, acutely or chronically, precipitates the cascade of events that leads to the development of the taut band, spot tenderness (TrP), and pain. Whether acute or chronic, repetitive or persistent, the term used to describe these conditions in this chapter is "muscle overload." Perpetuating factors are those elements that predispose individuals to the development, or contribute to the maintenance, of myofascial pain. Perpetuating factors can be classified into those causes that are mechanical and those that are metabolic, including hormonal, nutritional, or infectious. In a broader sense, these perpetuating factors impair the ability of a muscle to respond appropriately so that the muscle becomes overloaded when attempting to perform an action. It is muscle overload that is thought to lead to the development of trigger points (TrPs) through the final common pathway of an energy crisis as proposed by Simons[1] and expanded on by others.[2] Mechanical stresses producing muscle overload can be further classified as postural or structural, and as static or dynamic (repetitive). Metabolic effects include hypometabolic states, hormonal effects, adverse effects of drugs, infection, and nutritional insufficiency. Finally, there are neuroplastic changes in the central nervous system (CNS) that can maintain nociception and amplify the perception of pain, such as the inhibition or facilitation of descending nociceptive modulating factors and central sensitization, that are now being approached therapeutically, and therefore should be considered in people with chronic myofascial pain syndrome.

Many articles and book chapters have been written about perpetuating factors, hence this chapter will focus on those factors that have not been previously well covered or discussed.[3] This chapter will focus on hormonal conditions including the gonadal hormone conditions, estrogen or testosterone deficiency, and subclinical hypothyroidism; three nutritional factors, B vitamins (briefly) and vitamin D deficiency (VDD) and magnesium deficiency; and three mechanical factors, Joint hypermobility syndrome (Ehlers-Danlos syndrome), maladaptive movement patterns in chronic pain, and forward head posture. Furthermore, the focus is on evidence-based studies and on the physiology and biochemistry underlying the effect, appropriate for the understanding needed for the clinical management of people with myofascial pain syndrome.

2. HORMONAL FACTORS

2.1. Gonadal Hormones: Estrogen

Nociception and antinociception are sexually dimorphic, modulated differently in men and women, in both humans and in laboratory animals. Women have lower pain thresholds, lower pain tolerance, and higher pain scale ratings than men as reported in many studies, although there is some variance in the reports.[4-6] Nevertheless, the predominant finding of epidemiologic studies worldwide show that women have more chronic pain conditions such as irritable bowel syndrome, painful bladder, migraine headache, back pain, widespread pain and fibromyalgia, abdominal pain, and musculoskeletal disorders than men. Women show a greater prevalence of pain over all body sites, and a greater prevalence of inflammatory or nociceptive pain, and of neuropathic pain.[4,5,7] Studies in pain responses in healthy women showed greater temporal summation to nociceptive stimuli than in men. Central pain modulation (CPM), ie, the ability of descending influences to inhibit pain following a conditioning nociceptive stimulus, is less effective in women in suppressing pain than in men, in most studies.[8,9] Likewise, imaging studies show a significant difference between men and women in the activation of brain centers concerned with pain, men showing a greater responsiveness to peripheral nociceptive stimuli than women.[10] Recent research focused on neuroimmune mechanisms of pain have shown that the immune system plays a major role in nociception, particularly glial cells in the CNS, as well as mast cells, macrophages and T cells that can release proinflammatory cytokines.[11] Estrogen even affects glial cells by increasing proinflammatory cytokines including prostaglandins and cyclooxygenase (COX). The issue of sex differences and the role of gonadal hormones have been extensively considered in the past.[12]

The difference in pain responsiveness between women and men may in large part be due to hormonal effects on the nociceptive system. Pain tends to vary over the menstrual cycle and with the level of estrogen. In addition, the effects of gonadal hormones are different peripherally and centrally. For example, women show lower pain thresholds to most experimental pain modalities than men, the exception being ischemic pain.[5] Estrogen affects most body organs, including the CNS. The modulatory effects of estrogen are not easily described, as they differ from organ to organ. Most studies of estrogen effects on visceral pain have shown it to be pronociceptive, whereas most studies on deep somatic pain show that estrogen is antinociceptive.[7] Pain perception and nociceptive-input suppression vary over the reproductive cycle in women.[13] There is, therefore, great interest in the role of estrogen as a modulator of nociception.

Estrogen and testosterone are both synthesized from cholesterol. Estrone and estradiol are derived from testosterone and androstenedione through the action of the P450 aromatase monooxygenase enzyme complex,[14] primarily in the ovaries, but aromatase is also found in other tissues, and in particular for our discussion, in the brain and spinal cord. There are both positive and negative feedback loops that modulate the synthesis and release of estrogen throughout the menstrual cycle, accounting, to a great extent, for the pronociceptive and antinociceptive influences of the different phases of the estrous cycle (see Amandusson and Blomqvist[14] for a review of estrogen effects on pain). The effects of estrogen associated with different phases of the estrous cycle are slow and prolonged, whereas the effects of estrogen on neuronal function can be quick in response to the rapid changes of estrogen levels in the brain and nerve tissue. Estrogen effects are both genomic, acting through transcription pathways in cell nuclei for protein synthesis, and nongenomic, acting on membrane estrogen receptors that have a rapid onset of action.

Two primary theories of pain transmission must be reviewed in order to understand the action of estrogens on pain. One is that nociceptive input travels along specific pathways made up of distinct, modality-specific neurons. The other view is that the nociceptive system is comprised of multimodal neurons that, when activated, react to other sensory stimuli. Recent investigations have shown that nociceptive pathways are not solely within the somatosensory system, but are part of a homeostatic system that monitors the body status and interacts with the autonomic system, the hypothalamic–pituitary–adrenal axis, and other neuroendocrine systems, thus modulating nociceptive input and transmission.[14] Nociceptive input can be magnified or diminished by facilitatory or inhibitory influences, such as estrogens, that may in part be mediated by dorsal horn interneurons that make up about 95% of dorsal horn neurons, of which about 70% are excitatory and 30% are inhibitory. The interneurons, located primarily in lamina II where C-fibers terminate, release neuromodulating substances such as substance P and calcitonin gene-related peptide. Estrogen acting on estrogen receptors in the CNS acts as a modulating factor on nociceptive transmission. Blocking of dorsal horn inhibitory interneurons results in hyperalgesia and allodynia. Secondary- and tertiary-level neurons in the thalamus, in the anterior cingulate gyrus, and in the somatosensory cortex are likewise connected to other centers such as the amygdala, hypothalamus, and prefrontal cortex. These connections are integrative and give rise to the affective responses to pain. Thus, the nociceptive pathway is interactive and integrated with other sensory centers, and with those centers related to emotion and volition.

Nociceptive input is further modulated by descending supraspinal influences that are either facilitatory or inhibitory. The predominant descending nociceptive inhibition system is the endogenous opioid system that includes enkephalin and dynorphin as mediators. Additionally, thyroid hormones and glucocorticoids may regulate the transcription of the enkephalin gene. Estrogens also have that ability in certain regions of the brain. Hence, the action of estrogen on the nociceptive system is consistent with the concept that the nociceptive system is a homeostatic system with multimodal inputs, including gonadal hormones that help regulate and maintain basal body functions.

The role of estrogens in modulating the nociceptive system is seen in animal studies where low estrogen levels are associated with increased visceral and trigeminal neuronal sensitivity to painful stimuli.[14,15] Estrogen modulates opioid analgesia as well as endogenous opioid effects. Estrogen increases endogenous opioid production in both the brain and spinal cord of ovariectomized rats. Estrogen also modulates the expression and activity of opioid receptors in pain-related brain regions, affecting responses to both exogenous and endogenous opioids. The relevance of estrogen to pain in humans is suggested by studies that show that women given hormone replacement therapy (HRT) have higher levels of orofacial pain and lower pain thresholds and tolerances.[16] However, the effects are complex because estrogen also affects the levels of pro- and antinociceptive substances in the dorsal horn and has varying effects on pain, with no change in pain in women with fibromyalgia syndrome (FMS) taking HRT, but reduced levels of musculoskeletal pain compared with control subjects.

The estrogen effect may be direct, acting on estrogen receptors in the nervous system, or indirect, mediated through other systems such as the endorphin system.[13] Estradiol (17-β-estradiol) can be both pronociceptive and antinociceptive in female rats. A direct effect on transcription is mediated through nuclear estrogen receptors, through a genomic effect, and through G-protein-coupled estrogen receptors (GPER) on the plasma membrane where they activate signaling cascades of second messenger systems, affecting intracellular processes by modulating ion channel activity. These two mechanisms differ in their time courses. Activation of cell membrane GPER alters ion channel function in seconds to minutes, as opposed to genomic effects on transcription that occur over hours to days. GPER, activated by endomorphins (mu-opioid receptor ligands), may be related to the varied response in females of high analgesic responsiveness during proestrus and reduced responsiveness during diestrus. Intrathecal Endomorphin 2 i(EM2)s actively suppressed in diestrus in rats; spinally synthesized estrogens are required for this suppression. Suppression of spinal EM2 during diestrus results from locally synthesized estrogens activating spinal estrogen receptors that inhibit aromatase. There is a significant spinal antinociceptive response to EM2 during proestrus that is likely to be related to the loss of diestrus-associated membrane estrogen receptor suppression.[13] Nevertheless, the mechanism by which estrogen modulates pain perception remains imperfectly understood. One study looked at the effect of estrogen on the hypothalamic–pituitary–adrenal axis as the mechanism for suppression of nociceptive responsiveness and found that antinociception was independent of COX and hypothalamic–pituitary–adrenal activity.[17]

Estrogen is present systemically, produced by the ovaries, but it is also synthesized in the brain, particularly in the hypothalamus, amygdala, and periaqueductal gray matter, and in the integral part of the descending nociceptive modulation system. Aromatase, the enzyme that converts testosterone and androstenedione to estrogen, is also present in the rostral ventromedial medulla (RVM) of the rat.[18] The RVM is also an integral part of the descending nociceptive modulatory system and is involved both in nociceptive facilitation and inhibition. The upregulation of aromatase has been found in certain visceral pain conditions. It is now thought that the upregulation of aromatase activity in the RVM may be a factor in chronic visceral pain states.

The application of animal models to human clinical practice is fraught with uncertainty. Human and rodent hormonal cycles differ, for example, and rodents lack the thalamocortical nociceptive-transmitting pathways present in primates that play such a prominent role in human chronic pain conditions. Moreover, the results of HRT effects on pain are mixed, with some studies showing that painful conditions are more prevalent, and other studies showing that painful musculoskeletal disorders are less common in women taking HRT. The contradictory results of studies of estrogen effects may stem from the complex nature of estrogen's relationship to body homeostatic mechanisms, so that in addition to the nature and location of nociceptive origin, the menstrual cycle stage, estrogen dosage, other drugs with which it may be given, especially progesterone, and other factors that affect body homeostasis may all play a role in the effect estrogens have on pain.[14]

The role of estrogen on muscle function has been studied to a limited extent. Estrogen receptor alpha mRNA is found in the human skeletal muscle, which could indicate that there is a direct action of estrogen on the muscle. The conflicting results of studies on estrogen's effect on muscle strength is not clear. One mechanism may be the regulatory effect of estrogen on the utilization of muscle glycogen used as an energy source in the muscle.[19] There is a negative correlation between estrogen levels and the rate of force production and musculotendinous stiffness.[20] However, an earlier study from the same group showed no changes in these properties across the menstrual cycle.[21] Male and female castrated mice had reduced maximal muscle forces, though neuromuscular transmission was intact. Muscle weight gain was diminished in female castrated mice. Thus, female gonadal hormones promote muscle activity, but the mechanisms remain unclear.[22]

2.2. Gonadal Hormones: Testosterone

Testosterone also has an antinociceptive effect,[23] though it has not been as intensively studied as estradiol. The protective effect of testosterone on temporomandibular joint pain in male rats is thought to be centrally mediated through the activation of opioid receptors.[24] Aromatase is present in the brain and subcortical structures concerned with nociception, and can convert testosterone to estradiol. Testosterone downregulates CYP2D activity in the brain, thereby slowing the metabolism of certain opioid or opioid-related drugs centrally.[25] On the contrary, daily opioid use can result in androgen deficiency.[26,27] Hence, the role of testosterone itself in pain modulation is not clear.[4] However, gonadectomized male rats that had a drastic lowering of testosterone showed significantly more pain behavior to repetitive nociceptive stimulation than intact rats.[28] However, the gonadectomized rats with low testosterone had increased levels of estradiol. A pilot study of the treatment of pain in patients with FMS with testosterone reported a reduction in muscle pain, stiffness, and fatigue, and increased libido.[29] A study of patients with a variety of chronic, unresponsive, pain conditions (though none listed as having musculoskeletal pain) showed 32% with testosterone deficiency, including 16% of the women.[30] This finding is considered to be the result of the effect of chronic pain on the hypothalamic–pituitary–adrenal–gonad axis that renders it unable to meet the demands of pain-induced stress. This deficiency is compounded by the gonadal hormone depressant effect of opioid treatment on testosterone. Treatment effect could not be ascertained from this study. However, there is a randomized controlled study in which males with opioid-induced testosterone were treated with testosterone gel for 14 weeks. The testosterone-treated group had greater improvement in pressure and mechanical hyperalgesia and body composition, in addition to greater sexual desire and improvement in role limitation due to emotional problems.[31]

There is a sexual dimorphism in the skeletal muscle in humans and in other mammals. The anabolic effect of androgens is well known. Male muscle mass is androgen dependent. Androgen receptors are present on myocytes and on muscle fiber.[32] However, the effect on the muscle of male gonad-related factors that include testosterone, and that increased maximal force and improved muscle contractility, is independent of muscle growth or mass, and was found related only to male gonadal hormones and not to female gonadal hormones.[22] Thus, muscle effort or maximal force is hormone dependent. It may be that the muscle that operates at a submaximal level of function is more likely to be in overload in both males and females, and therefore is more likely to develop and maintain TrPs.

The role of gonadal hormones in antinociception is complex. The effect of gonadal hormones on TrP pain is largely unknown because it has not been studied systematically, and it may be part of a general effect mediated through central nociceptive modulating pathways, perhaps in part due to the direct effect of gonadal hormones on the muscle, rather than a specific role on the TrP. The role of gonadal hormones on TrPs or on myofascial pain itself has not been studied. However, testosterone replacement in male patients with chronic myofascial pain who have low testosterone levels could be beneficial. The issue with estrogen replacement in women is more difficult to discern, but even in women who have chronic myofascial pain and where definite estrogen deficiency is established, a trial of estrogen replacement therapy may be warranted. However, if hormone replacement is undertaken, in both men and in women, a clear understanding of potential adverse effects and close monitoring of the patient are paramount. Where possible, HRT for chronic myofascial pain should be undertaken in the setting of a clinical trial.

2.3. Subclinical Hypothyroidism

Hypothyroidism has long been thought to be associated with the development and persistence of TrP pain. Dr Janet Travell often emphasized this connection in her discussions of the etiology of TrPs. She made a particular point of the effect of what we now call subclinical hypothyroidism, ie, hypothyroidism that is not overt and that is not associated with a level of the thyroid hormone (TH) that is below the limits of the range of normal. In particular, she never accepted the thyroid-stimulating hormone (TSH) level as a sufficient indicator or the metabolic state of the individual, but instead preferred to use the basal metabolic rate (BMR) test that reflected the overall metabolic state of the individual. In truth, the first generation of the TSH assay was of low sensitivity and low specificity. The BMR was a sensitive but not specific test of thyroid function, sensitive because hypothyroidism depresses the metabolic rate, but not specific because many things alter the metabolic rate. For instance, infection and pregnancy can increase the metabolic rate and some drugs may either increase or decrease the metabolic rate. When the BMR test was no longer available, Dr Travell advocated using the basal morning temperature (taken before getting out of bed in the morning) as a surrogate for the BMR, cautioning us to beware that the use of a heating blanket could raise the basal morning temperature that would otherwise be low in subjects with hypothyroidism.[33] The current third-generation TSH assay is both sensitive and specific, except in the presence of thyroid peroxidase antibodies, which alter the correlation between free T4 and the TSH level by the current assay method.[34]

Both TSH and TH regulate many metabolic processes in the skeletal muscle, myogenesis and muscle fiber regeneration, and the contraction–relaxation actions of the muscle. The TSH and the TH are incorporated into muscle cells or myocytes via cell membrane and nuclear receptors that facilitate their transport across the respective membranes. Mitochondrial activity and the rate of calcium release and reuptake from the sarcoplasmic reticulum and through other means like those mediated by cyclic adenosine monophosphate (cAMP) and protein kinase A (PKA) are regulated on a rapid time basis, whereas genomic transcription affecting protein synthesis takes place over a longer time frame. Myocyte phenotype and phenotype plasticity is also regulated by the TH. Detailed reviews of the effect of the TH on skeletal muscle physiology outline these effects that are described in some further detail below.[35,36] TSHR are present on the skeletal muscle. Therefore, the TSH may have a direct effect on the muscle distinct from that of the TH itself, and therefore may be relevant in subclinical hypothyroidism where the TSH is elevated but free TH levels are normal. TSHR mRNA and protein are found in the skeletal muscle as well as other extra thyroidal tissues.[37] The THS improves insulin sensitivity in mouse skeletal muscle cells, activates cAMP and secondarily PKA.[37] The TH itself affects muscle cell regeneration and fiber type (eg, fast or slow-twitch fibers).[38] The active form of the TH, T3, is present in the muscle fiber cell, the myocyte, and helps maintain muscle homeostasis, muscle development and muscle regeneration, through binding to TH nuclear receptors. These subjects are reviewed in detail by Bloise et al[36] and by Salvatore et al[35] Three deiodinase enzymes in the myocyte regulate TH levels in the skeletal muscle. D1 removes one iodine molecule from T4, activating the TH, D2 also converts T4 to T3, activating the TH, whereas D3 converts T4 to reverse T3, allowing for another level of control of thyroid activity. Contraction and relaxation of muscle, the result of the interaction of actin and myosin, requires calcium. Ionized calcium (Ca^{2+}) levels are regulated both in the increase and the lowering of Ca^{2+} cytosolic concentrations, by TH. The expression of sarco/endoplasmic reticulum Ca^{2+} (SERCA), a group of proteins associated with adenosine triphosphate (ATP)–associated reuptake of Ca^{2+} into the sarcoplasmic reticulum, is regulated by the effect of T3 on gene transcription. Contraction and relaxation are energy-requiring actions of the muscle that utilize glucose. Glucose utilization is likewise regulated by the TH.

The TH plays a major role in regulating muscle metabolism. Muscle constitutes about 40% of the body mass, and is a major contributor to the BMR. The genomic transcription effects of T3, the active form of the TH, are mediated through nuclear TH receptors, similar to the manner in which TSH nuclear receptors mediate a genomic role for the TSH. The genomic effects of TSH and TH result in the upregulation and downregulation of over 600 genes in the skeletal muscle.[39] Moreover, T3-regulated gene transcription plays a role in the determination of fiber type through the transcriptional stimulation of myosin isoforms. The TH also affects the contraction–relaxation cycle of the muscle, resulting in the well-known slow recovery phase of the muscle tendon reflex in hypothyroidism. The TH also stimulates mitochondrial activity and glycolysis in the muscle.[35,36] Metabolic activity in the muscle is modulated by altering metabolic efficiency in the muscle or by uncoupling mitochondrial ATP synthesis in the muscle.

Gerwin[3] reviewed the information known about the relationship of thyroid function to myofascial pain, at which time there was little clinical experience that was published, and indeed, the literature was scant on the topic.[3] A major point that was made in this review, and that is still an important fact today, is that the TSH level has a rather broad range for the healthy population, but that each individual within the healthy normal range has a rather narrow range of euthyroid function. The TSH is part of the feedback mechanism that regulates the production of the TH in the thyroid gland. When the TH is insufficient, the TSH level rises, stimulating the thyroid gland to produce more TH. The importance of this relationship was evident in the treatment of a patient referred for consideration of the diagnosis of postpolio amyotrophy. Her medical records showed that 3 years prior to the referral her TSH was below 1, 2 years prior to the referral her TSH was about 2.5, 1 year before referral her TSH was about 3.5, and at the time of referral her TSH was over 4. All of the values were within the reference range for the laboratory. Because her widespread pain, and her TrP pain, subsided with thyroid supplementation treatment, the diagnosis of postpolio amyotrophy was likely erroneous.

Overt hypothyroidism clearly has an effect on an individual's level of activity, fatigue, and cardiac status, and it is recognized to be a cause of muscle cramps and pain (although the role of overt hypothyroidism in producing myofascial pain syndrome has been suspected but never actually established). Subclinical hypothyroidism is a subtler condition, but may also be symptomatic with neuromuscular manifestations relevant to our subject. Subclinical hypothyroidism occurs in up to 18% of the population in some studies, more commonly in women than in men, probably because it may occur as the result of autoimmune thyroiditis. It is defined as an elevated TSH in the face of normal free TH levels, TSH levels in the range of 4.5 to 20 mIU/L. Many subjects are said to be asymptomatic. There is a progression in some patients, particularly those with thyroid autoantibodies, to overt hypothyroidism. Subclinical hypothyroidism is not really subclinical at all in some patients, in the sense that it is not free of clinical manifestations. It is perhaps better called "mild hypothyroidism" in those patients who are symptomatic, even if the thyroid function tests are compatible with a diagnosis of subclinical hypothyroidism. In terms of muscle function, neuromuscular symptoms are common in subclinical hypothyroidism as shown by Reuters et al[40] Cramps occurred in 54.8% compared with 25.0% in controls ($P < 0.05$), weakness in 42.2% compared with 12.6% ($P < 0.05$), myalgia in 47.6% compared with 25.0% ($P = 0.07$), and altered manual muscle testing in 30.98% compared with 8.3% ($P = 0.04$). Quadriceps strength measured by a chair dynamometer was not impaired. A more recent study of the effect of overt and subclinical hypothyroidism on the musculoskeletal system showed that there was a slight but significant elevation of creatine phosphokinase in patients with subclinical hypothyroid, as well as cramps, myalgia, and impaired physical activity (impaired 6-minute walking test), all improved with thyroid replacement.[41]

Studies of the treatment of subclinical hypothyroidism have shown a mild improvement in tiredness in middle-aged individuals, but no improvement compared with placebo in older individuals.[42] However, these studies were done on large groups of subjects that included asymptomatic and mildly symptomatic subjects whose response may be quite different from the response of symptomatic patients. Treatment of subclinical hypothyroidism in the elderly with levothyroxine must be done with careful monitoring, as they are susceptible to atrial fibrillation and femoral fractures, and have a higher mortality rate than people without levothyroxine treatment.[43] Hypothyroidism itself, with depressed free TH levels, is associated with muscle fatigue and impaired exercise tolerance, muscle pain, cramps, and tenderness, stiffness, and loss of muscle mass. Extreme cases may present with rhabdomyolysis. The symptoms are not specific for hypothyroid myopathy, however. In hypothyroid myopathy, there is a change in muscle fiber type, with an increase in type I slow-twitch fibers and a loss of type II fast-twitch fibers, a change that may conserve energy in a hypometabolic disorder. Myofascial TrPs are not mentioned in a recent review of thyroid myopathies,[44] although hypothyroidism was present in about 10% of patients seen clinically with myofascial pain syndrome (Gerwin, unpublished data), an incidence that is not far from that found in the general population. Treatment of these patients with levothyroxine usually reduced or eliminated the myofascial pain, or noticeably facilitated the response to physical therapy treatment of TrP pain. Unfortunately, there are no adequate studies of this relationship.

Finally, insufficient levels of vitamin D (<25 ng/mL) are associated with an increased risk of autoimmune thyroiditis, and, perhaps of equal or greater significance, with elevated TSH,[45] providing another pathway to the development of muscle pain and an altered muscle fiber phenotype, with a shift away from type II fast-twitch fibers and toward slow-twitch type I fibers. This observation validates the need to consider multiple metabolic disorders coexisting in one patient. VDD, to be discussed below, is prevalent at latitudes far from the equator, but is common even close to the equator. Failure to respond to thyroid supplementation alone should raise the question of multiple metabolic disorders whether from drug usage, nutritional deficiency, parasitic infestation, or coexisting mechanical dysfunction. For this reason, a comprehensive evaluation at the outset is always recommended.

3. NUTRITIONAL FACTORS

3.1. B vitamins

B vitamins have not been shown to play a particular role in myofascial pain, although treating vitamin B_{12} deficiency in some individuals in my practice who also had chronic widespread myofascial pain, relieved their pain. Travell, furthermore, emphasized that low vitamin B_1, thiamine, could interfere with the action of TH, producing a TH insufficiency. An attempt, in collaboration with colleagues to see if there was an association between low vitamin B_{12} levels and myofascial pain, showed no difference in vitamin B_{12} levels between persons with myofascial pain and healthy normal controls, though there were only 36 subjects in that study (Gerwin, unpublished data). However, B vitamins have been shown to reduce neuropathic pain.[46-52] Furthermore, B-vitamin complex consisting of thiamine, pyridoxine, and cyanocobalamin, injected intrathecally into mice, potentiates acute morphine antinociception and attenuates antinociceptive tolerance, inhibits morphine-induced microglial activation, and suppresses the phosphorylation of the N-methyl-D-aspartate receptor-NR1 (NMDAR-NR1) to make NMDAR-NR1 subunit and protein kinase C (PKC) following chronic morphine treatment.[53] The NMDA receptor plays a critical role in the development of morphine tolerance.[54,55] Protein kinase C modulates NMDA receptor activation and contributes to morphine tolerance. Phosphorylation activates the NMDA receptor, an action that is augmented by morphine. Suppression of the phosphorylation of the NMDA receptor and of PKC will reduce the activity of the NMDA and attenuate its ability to promote tolerance to morphine antinociception. Microglia also play a role in the development of morphine tolerance.[56] The proinflammatory cytokine IL-β is increased with microglial activation, and has the potential for activating the NMDAR. Thus, the B vitamins thiamin, pyridoxine, and cyanocobalamin given together may play a role in the management of chronic pain treated with morphine.

3.2. Vitamin D

Vitamin D is a prohormone that contributes to the regulation of calcium and phosphorus in bone. It is synthesized in the skin in the presence of sunlight (ultraviolet B light) and converted to 25OH-vitamin D in the liver. The ability of the skin to synthesize vitamin D diminishes with age. Ceglia[57] has reviewed the role of vitamin D in muscle function. Vitamin D receptors are present in muscle tissue, providing a means for vitamin D to play a role in muscle function. VDD produces a type II, fast-twitch, muscle fiber atrophy. These type II, fast-twitch fibers are contained in the muscles that are first recruited to prevent falls. Vitamin D receptors on the muscle are nuclear transcription factors that affect muscle cell proliferation and differentiation.[57] There are also nongenomic effects of cell surface vitamin D receptors that act on calcium entry in the muscle cytosol that affect contraction and relaxation of the muscle, as well as myogenesis and muscle type differentiation. Vitamin D polymorphisms have been associated with reduced muscle strength. Vitamin D is also associated with a reduction in the release of proinflammatory cytokines, and it suppresses T cell responses. It inhibits the synthesis of prostaglandin E_2.[58] Thus, vitamin D can influence muscle pain and myofascial pain both by its direct effect on the muscle and by its indirect effect on nociceptive mechanisms.

VDD is a global epidemic. The 2001 to 2006 National Health and Nutrition Examination Study found that about 20% of children aged 1 to 11 years were vitamin D deficient. VDD in children was directly correlated with obesity.[59] Vitamin D levels may be low in northern and southern latitudes away from the equator, where the angle of the sun is below 45° for prolonged periods of the year, but VDD can be endemic in equatorial lands because cultural dress codes may lead to covering the body, and because the use of sunscreen blocks the ultraviolet B frequency needed for vitamin D synthesis in the skin. Powanda,[60] in a discussion of the relationship of vitamin D levels to chronic pain, notes that the racial discrepancy of vitamin D serum levels and pain between black and white people is not necessarily true, because black people have lower levels of vitamin D–binding protein, so that there is nearly equivalent bioavailability of vitamin D between white and black people. Hence, the observational studies that report an association between chronic pain and low vitamin D may be misleading, because polymorphisms of vitamin D receptors may mean that vitamin D levels may not give an adequate picture of bioavailable vitamin D. That said, there are good reasons to consider the surveys showing very low levels in vitamin D to be significant, as the levels can be very low, and they correlate with levels of pain. Studies of serum levels of vitamin D across populations and across various chronic musculoskeletal pain disorders show a consistent decrease in vitamin D levels, ranging from 26% to 93% of subjects with pain, but most studies show that the percent of persons with chronic pain and low vitamin D levels hovers about 60% to 70%. However, there are other studies that found no lower levels of vitamin D in subjects with chronic pain. Studies that show a correlation or an association of vitamin D with pain do not constitute evidence of causation. Moreover, studies of patients with chronic pain treated with vitamin D have not demonstrated a benefit with vitamin D supplementation.[61] VDD is associated with a wide variety of nonskeletal disorders as noted in many observational studies. Yet, supplementation with vitamin D does not reduce the occurrence of these conditions or reverse them. This result has led to the consideration that low vitamin D may not be a causal factor in these conditions, but may occur as a result of them. In particular, conditions associated with an elevation of inflammatory mediators may be associated with a reduction in vitamin D levels. As stated, it is impossible with observational studies to make a causal relationship that inflammatory mediators result in lower vitamin D levels.[62] Indeed, a single high-dose bolus of cholecalciferol significantly reduced TNFα and IL-6, but not other inflammatory mediators, indicating that vitamin D may regulate these cytokines rather than be regulated by them.[63]

Vitamin D has been studied in chronic widespread pain. An association between VDD and chronic widespread pain, including FMS, has been shown, with an odds ratio 1.63; 95% confidence interval (CI), 1.20 to 2.23 ($P = 0.117$), based on a review of 12 studies. There was no difference between genders, despite the predominance of women with chronic widespread pain. The odds ratio was higher when lower levels of vitamin D, 8 to 10 ng/mL were evaluated.[64] As with all observational studies, no causal relationship can be made from this data.

In other musculoskeletal disorders (which were not looking at myofascial pain, but in which TrPs could reasonably play a role), VDD was associated with knee pain and impaired knee function, and a nonsignificant reduction in lower extremity strength.[65] VDD has been shown to be directly correlated with chronic low back pain (LBP),[66] the pooled odds ratio = 1.60; the 95% CI 1.20 to 2.12; $P = 0.001$, the number of studies, nine. However, the correlation was significant only for women, and only for women in the Middle East and Mediterranean regions. This correlation was thought to be related to dietary habits and particularly to dress customs (veiling), sun exposure, physical activity, and obesity, although issues of osteoporosis, muscle weakness, and a bias in the articles reviewed could have skewed the findings. The authors considered that low vitamin D could be causal for LBP, but did not consider the possibility that people with LBP might be less active, more likely to be homebound, more prone to develop osteoporosis through reduced activity, and less likely to be exposed to sunlight.

Treatment effects from vitamin D supplementation have been varied and inconsistent. The association of chronic pain, especially musculoskeletal pain, and VDD is observational, and therefore no causal relationship can be inferred. Attempts to determine cause and effect in humans have been based on showing improvement with vitamin D supplementation in subjects with VDD. Attempts to demonstrate benefit from vitamin D supplementation have had mixed results. Further compounding the problem is that no suitable dose of vitamin D has been identified, and we do not know if different disorders require different doses. One goal would be to bring up the serum vitamin D level to between 50 and 70 ng/mL, but that is often not achieved when treating with 1000 IU vitamin D_3 per day. Some will treat with 2000 IU/d, and some will treat with 5000 IU/d. Treatment is compounded because if a pill is used, it must be taken with some fat, because vitamin D is poorly water soluble. A tablet taken with water, juice, or fat-free milk will not be well absorbed. Vitamin D in the form of a gel cap with oil is a better form to use. The results of treatment have been disappointing. No significant improvement in muscle strength, as measured by hand grip strength or in timed-up and -go (a common functional measure of lower body strength and balance), was seen with vitamin D supplementation.[67] The use of vitamin D supplementation for the prevention of falls and fractures is not supported by the literature, though the studies on this relationship are scant.[68] However, some randomized controlled studies do indeed show a significant reduction in falls risk, especially in individuals less than 75 years of age.[57] A nonsignificant trend toward pain reduction was found in one meta-analysis of over 3000 subjects of mixed pain etiologies, hospitalized and nonhospitalized, about half of whom were treated with vitamin D and about half were given placebo.[69]

There is no evidence in the literature that vitamin D supplements are beneficial for the treatment of TrPs in persons with vitamin D serum levels that are normal (50 ng/mL or higher), and no evidence that they are beneficial for mild insufficiency down to about 30 ng/mL. Moreover, there is scant evidence of benefit for persons with levels as low as 20 ng/mL. Below 20 ng/mL, there is an increased risk of secondary hyperparathyroidism and there is reason enough to treat individuals with severe VDD (certainly for levels below 15 ng/mL). However, most if not all of the studies that have shown failure to improve with vitamin D supplementation reported only on treatment with vitamin D, and did not take into account that the subjects in the studies might have mixed deficiency states, including other nutritional deficiencies and other disorders, such as hypothyroidism. Patients with VDD seen in clinical practice, commonly may have mixed deficiency states that include iron deficiency, vitamin B_{12} deficiency, and hormonal deficiency, ie, hypothyroidism. Moreover, vitamin D improves magnesium absorption in the jejunum, so that VDD may result in magnesium deficiency or inadequacy.[70] Replacement of vitamin D alone may leave an individual's magnesium deficient if dietary magnesium is inadequate. Magnesium deficiency may have consequences for muscle, including muscle weakness. The same is true for vitamin D and hypothyroidism (another condition made more likely in individuals deficient in vitamin D). Hence, treatment of the VDD alone can reasonably be considered as insufficient, so that it would not be surprising that there was little benefit for a cohort so treated. Clinically, some patients who had widespread myofascial pain and only VDD, responded quite well to vitamin D supplementation alone. In conclusion, a patient who has chronic myofascial pain syndrome of longer than 3 months duration should be evaluated for multiple deficiency states, and all deficiency states found should be corrected. In addition, treatment with vitamin D supplementation alone in a patient with normal vitamin D levels (30 ng/mL or higher) or with mild insufficiency, say 25 ng/mL or higher, should not be regarded as likely to be of benefit.

3.3. Magnesium

Magnesium (Mg^{2+}) supplementation has been a favorite of people with chronic widespread pain or FMS, either taken alone or taken in combination with other substances, sometimes injected as nutritional supplemental "cocktail." How much of this treatment is based on modern medical folklore is hard to determine, but Mg^{2+} supplementation has been a popular treatment in the FMS community for years, so much so that much of the literature of Mg^{2+} effect on pain is in the FMS literature. Given that many individuals with FMS have widespread MTrP pain, it is reasonable to consider the pain aspect of FMS, if not the fatigue, cognitive impairment, and the sleep disorder, as a MTrP pain issue, at least in part. Likewise, many of the comorbid disorders of FMS like temporomandibular joint dysfunction, migraine headache, and visceral pain syndromes have MTrPs as a significant component. Indeed, for those individuals with chronic and widespread MTrP-related pain, central sensitization has most certainly occurred, contributing to widespread pain, hypersensitivity, and allodynia. CPM and the supraspinal descending nociceptive modulation inhibitory and facilitatory pathways have been less intensively studied than central and peripheral sensitization. The data on peripheral nociceptive input from TrPs in FMS are so strong,[71,72] and the parallel underlying central sensitization of chronic MTrP pain to that of FMS is so great, that we may look carefully at the studies of Mg^{2+} in relationship to FMS pain and expect that we will learn something useful about MTrP pain.

Magnesium plays an essential role in a wide range of physiologic functions, including those in skeletal muscle. It is a cation that is second only to potassium in abundance in the body. It is involved in most metabolic and biochemical processes. It is a cofactor in an estimated 600 enzymatic reactions in the body. It is required for protein and DNA synthesis. It is estimated that as many as 60% of Americans do not consume enough magnesium and have some degree of magnesium insufficiency. Serum magnesium represents just 1% of the body's Mg^{2+} as magnesium is stored in other body tissues, including muscle, so that the estimate of inadequate magnesium levels in the general population may be understated. Moreover, most intracellular magnesium is bound to ribosomes, polynucleotides, and ATP, so that free magnesium levels are relatively low. Measurements of serum magnesium may not reflect tissue levels.[73] Magnesium is abundant in many foods, but processed foods are low in magnesium and boiling foods deplete magnesium. Hence, magnesium may not be plentiful in the diets of many people.

Magnesium is an antagonist to calcium (Ca^{2+}) in muscle. It is present in concentrations that are 10 000 times as great as Ca^{2+} concentrations in the resting muscle. Magnesium is bound to all of the Ca^{2+} binding sites on troponin C and myosin, and is displaced by Ca^{2+} after the latter is released from the sarcoplasmic reticulum. When there is too little magnesium in muscle, less Ca^{2+} is required to replace Mg^{2+} in the troponin-myosin complex, leading more easily to muscle contraction, and predisposing muscle to cramps.

Magnesium molecules block the NMDAR channel and prevent its activation, a critical step for the establishment of central sensitization and persistent (chronic) pain. Glutamate, an excitatory amino acid, displaces or removes Mg^{2+} from the NMDAR channel, thereby activating the NMDAR channel leading to the chain of events supporting pain chronicity.[74] It would seem logical that if Mg^{2+} were not displaced from the NMDAR, then pain might be alleviated. This thought may be behind the idea of using Mg^{2+} supplements in the treatment of chronic musculoskeletal pain.

Magnesium is required for the conformational change of myosin that takes place during contraction and relaxation. Myosin utilizes Mg ATP to produce the conformational change from straight to bent, the recovery stroke in the cycle. After the recovery stroke, myosin undergoes another conformational change back to straight. These changes constitute a pre- and postpower stroke process. Magnesium ATP binds to myosin in a process that releases phosphate and results in the hydrolysis of ATP. Mg^{2+} is thought to position the nucleotide within the active site of myosin for subsequent hydrolysis.[75]

Magnesium levels in clinical studies were found to be significantly lower in patients with FMS than in control subjects in an analysis of elements in hair, along with lower levels of calcium, manganese, and iron.[76] Serum levels of magnesium have also been found to be lower in subjects with FMS than in controls,[77] but are not reliable as indicators of tissue levels of Mg^{2+}. Romano[78] found lower than normal serum levels of Mg^{2+} in patients with FMS and/or myofascial pain than in controls, and advocated magnesium supplementation. Okumus et al[48] reported that the total myalgic score correlated inversely with serum magnesium in myofascial pain patients. However, serum magnesium levels correlate poorly with total body magnesium because magnesium levels are tightly controlled with only 1% of magnesium in the extracellular fluid and only 0.3% in serum.[79] These levels may be maintained in Mg^{2+} deficiency. These findings raise the question as to whether hypomagnesemia is actually underreported. On the contrary, serum Mg^{2+} levels may not reflect muscle Mg levels, which may be maintained even if serum levels are low.

Magnesium supplementation in patients with FMS using Mg^{2+} citrate 300 mg/d improved the tender point index, the Fibromyalgia Impact Questionnaire (FIQ) score, and the beck depression index score. Additional improvement in most of FMS symptoms was found when magnesium citrate was given along with amitriptyline 10 mg/d.[80] Magnesium is commonly included in intravenous micronutrient therapeutic infusions, including Myers Cocktail among others. These infusions have been popular for years in treating FMS and chronic widespread pain. However, a randomized, placebo-controlled study showed significant improvement in both the placebo arm and the intravenous micronutrient arm when intravenous infusions were given weekly over 8 weeks. The tender point index improved in both arms of the study; there was no statistical difference between the outcomes of the micronutrient infusion and the infusion of Ringer's lactate.[81] No other randomized, controlled, blinded, trials using Mg^{2+} to treat FMS were found by searching PubMed. Despite the interest in Mg as a treatment for FMS and musculoskeletal pain, no convincing data exist to support its use. The few studies that exist are small studies. There are no studies of magnesium supplementation for the treatment of MTrP.

Magnesium may play a role in muscle cramps as mentioned previously. However, studies of this relationship have shown mixed results. Magnesium supplementation was not shown to reduce the number of cramps except possibly in women who are pregnant.[73] A more recent study showed that muscle cramps were reduced from 90% to 10% in a cohort of pregnant woman who were Mg^{2+} deficient when given a supplement of 300 mg of magnesium daily (100 mg of a multimineral tablet plus 200 mg effervescent magnesium in the treated group to just the multimineral tablet in the control group).[82]

Magnesium may play a role in preventing age-related loss of muscle mass, but the studies that support this suggestion are mostly observational rather than randomized controlled studies.[83] Mg^{2+} was associated with improved physical performance in older adults in one randomized controlled trial, and was associated with the prevalence of age-related sarcopenia.[84] Mg^{2+} supplementation of elderly individuals whose Mg^{2+} intake was below the recommended daily allowance showed a significant improvement in the Short Physical Performance Battery, but not in isometric or isokinetic strength, in body composition, or in physical activity over the 12-week course of a randomized controlled trial in which the treated subjects were given magnesium oxide (equivalent to 300 mg bioavailable magnesium). There was no benefit in any of the outcome measures from supplementation in individuals considered to have an adequate magnesium intake.

Malignant hyperthermia is a condition in which there is a hypermetabolic response to volatile anesthetic agents, resulting in an elevation of temperature and muscular rigidity. The syndrome serves as a model for the persistent contraction of muscle fibers in the MTrP in some respects. Dantrolene, an effective treatment of malignant hyperthermia, is most effective when magnesium levels are above resting levels of magnesium. Higher levels of magnesium increase the binding of Mg^{2+} to the ryanodine receptor, thereby stabilizing the resting state of the muscle.[85] Thus, there is a rational for the use of Mg^{2+} in the treatment of MTrPs in that a return to the resting state of the muscle could relax the taut band without which the TrP does not exist. However, this has not been shown to occur in subjects with TrPs, or has never been looked at in patients with TrPs, perhaps because higher doses of magnesium act as a laxative, and adequate levels are not achieved in clinical practice.

Transdermal magnesium chloride administered as a spray, applied to the extremity was reported by patient responses on the Revised FIQ SF-36v2 to be effective in reducing symptoms at 2 and 4 weeks, but this study was open, unblinded, uncontrolled, and problematic in having no objective outcome measurement with a strong possibility of bias on the part of the subjects. Moreover, Mg^{2+} levels were not measured in this study.[86] Magnesium lactate 400 mg/d was given to 12 elite athletes during a full season of play. Measures of muscle damage were obtained four times, before and during the season. Creatine fell during the second-time period, but increased by the third- and fourth-time periods. No other parameters signifying muscle damage changed. The authors suggested that based on their results, Mg supplementation might prevent muscle damage.[87]

4. MECHANICAL PERPETUATING FACTORS

Mechanical stresses can be structural, postural, or the result of repetitive use. Structural stresses occur because of muscle overuse to compensate for muscle imbalances caused by body structure asymmetry. Structural asymmetries and joint laxity can be congenital or acquired, and postural mechanical stresses can occur as a result of stresses imposed on the body by ineffective body mechanics, whether the result of intrinsic body dysfunction or of extrinsic forces, such as poor workspace ergonomics. A few mechanical perpetuating factors discussed below illustrate these points.

4.1. Ehlers-Danlos Syndrome

Joint hypermobility is an important, yet often overlooked, cause of musculoskeletal pain. Generalized joint hypermobility is a manifestation of Ehlers-Danlos syndrome (EDS), a genetic collagen disorder or a heritable connective tissue disorder.[88] This discussion will not engage the issue of whether or not joint hypermobility is an entity distinct from EDS or not, nor whether there is such a condition as benign hypermobility syndrome. Suffice it to say that EDS may be an important cause of musculoskeletal pain, as well as pain and dysfunction from associated neurologic conditions like tethered cord syndrome, spinal cord compression, and posterior fossa abnormalities. A number of molecular defects are associated with this condition, among them defects in fibrillar collagen. The clinical expression or phenotype of EDS may vary, even within families. The variation of presentation extends to musculoskeletal pain as well, so that individuals with EDS and reports of pain may have family members with some degree of joint hypermobility, but who have no pain complaints. On the contrary, some individuals with EDS have reported that they thought that everyone had chronic pain; therefore, they never considered it something to report.

The prevalence of EDS ranges between 6% and 57% for females and 2% and 35% for males, occurring in 1:5000 to 1:10 000 persons, with great variability geographically and among different ethnic groups. There is also great variability based on different criteria for the diagnosis. In particular, the diagnosis has usually been based on the Beighton criteria[89] (Box 4-1) that assesses nine items. A score of 5 or more is commonly considered to be diagnostic of joint hypermobility, but some researchers have used a score of 4 or 3 to make the diagnosis, and some are stricter and use a score of 6 or more. The Beighton criteria emphasize findings in the large joints, and do not assess hypermobility in small- to medium-sized joints except for the 5th metacarpophalangeal joint. Furthermore, associated physical findings such as skin hyper-elasticity, and others mentioned below, are often required to confirm a suspected diagnosis. The Beighton criteria take these other manifestations of a connective tissue disorder into account and relate them to other connective tissue disorders.[90] The Beighton criteria are simple to use and can be done quickly, so that they are a useful screening tool. They can be supplemented by examining for additional features as is appropriate to a particular individual. There are nine types of EDS, though by the Villefranche nosology, they are collapsed into six subtypes, but type III, the hypermobile type, is by far the most common one, and is also most likely to present with pain. Pain is common in subjects with EDS, identified by means of the McGill Pain questionnaire in 90% of 273 subjects with confirmed EDS.[91]

4.2. Forward Head Posture

Forward head posture (FHP) is a significant risk factor for neck pain, temporal mandibular joint pain, and headache, as well as altered body mechanics. FHP drops the head, directing gaze toward the ground. The head must then be brought up to accomplish a horizontal gaze. This compensation has consequences for head and neck musculature that will be detailed below. Headache is

Box 4-1 Beighton criteria for joint hypermobility syndrome

Maneuver	Right Side	Left Side
Dorsiflexion and hyperextension of the 5th MCP beyond 90°	1	1
Apposition of the thumb to the volar aspect of the forearm	1	1
Hyperextension of the elbow beyond 10°	1	1
Hyperextension of the knee beyond 10°	1	1
Forward flexion of the trunk with the knees fully extended so that palms touch the floor		1

The first four maneuvers are passive, the last is active. The total score is X/9, where X represents the number of positive tests.
Adapted from Beighton P, De Paepe A, Steinmann B, Tsipouras P, Wenstrup RJ. Ehlers-Danlos syndromes: revised nosology, Villefranche, 1997. Ehlers-Danlos National Foundation (USA) and Ehlers-Danlos Support Group (UK). *Am J Med Genet.* 1998;77(1):31-37.

likely to be the consequence of referred pain from both neck muscles and orofacial muscles, the latter affected by the posterior displacement of the mandible that occurs in FHP.

FHP lengthens the ventral neck muscles, shortens posterior extensor muscles, weakens those muscles that are at a mechanical disadvantage, and places mechanical stress on the cervical zygapophyseal joints. As one would expect, thoracic kyphosis that would bring the head forward is associated with excessive cervical lordosis.[92] Flexion of the lower cervical vertebral segments is accompanied by hyperextension of suboccipital segments (OA-C1-C2) and shortening of the suboccipital musculature. Increased lower cervical flexion also increases the lower cervical neural foraminal areas, potentially relieving pressure on compressed cervical nerve roots.[93] Sternocleidomastoid muscle (SCM) thickness is increased, presumably because of tonic muscle contraction.[94] SCM activity is greatest in the fully flexed position, whereas middle trapezius muscle activity is reduced.[95] Rectus capitis posterior muscle activity is increased in FHP. These muscles are thought to stabilize the occipitoatlantal and the atlantoaxial joints,[96] but may also serve a proprioceptive function. Head position proprioception is impaired by FHP.[97] Static balance is also impaired by FHP, indicating that there is a more widespread effect of FHP on body balance mechanisms than just that affecting craniovertebral posture.[98] Postural balance has been shown to be altered in computer workers with FHP.[99] FHP and TrPs correlate positively with tension type headache (TTH).[100] Trigger points also correlate positively with FHP. This is an important aspect of TTH that needs to be included in the assessment of patients with TTH, as it affects treatment outcome. FHP is also associated with migraine headache.[101]

4.3. Other Mechanical Stresses Predisposing to Chronic MPS

Ergonomic factors have been well-documented as causes of muscle overuse and of MTrPs. These range from inappropriately designed work spaces to prolonged use of a keyboard (laptop or desktop computer). Prolonged, steady typing is clearly a precipitating factor, and shoulder muscle pain can start after as little as 30 minutes of typing.[102,103] Other occupational stresses are known, among which is the well-studied tendency of playing various musical instruments to overload muscle. Sitting in ill-fitting chairs can lead to neck, shoulder, and back pain. Eyeglasses with an inappropriate focal length cause neck muscle strain and overload. Carrying a backpack over one shoulder or a heavy bag in one arm will cause the ipsilateral shoulder to be elevated, a well-known cause of levator scapulae muscle overload and pain at the upper medial border of the scapula. Degenerative joint disease or osteoarthritis of the shoulder, the hip, and the knee is associated with painful TrPs in the muscles associated with the affected joint. Post total joint replacement recovery can be complicated by TrPs in the periarticular muscles. Pain can be reduced and active range of motion increased following inactivation of TrPs in these muscles. Finally, psychological factors, particularly kinesiophobia and catastrophizing, two potential responses to chronic pain, can impede recovery.

Clinical Presentation

Patients frequently present in the clinic with reports of pain, often not knowing that they were hypermobile. They often report, however, that they have unusual range of motion and that they knew this when they were small children. They often enjoyed ballet or gymnastics, activities suited to those persons who are hypermobile. However, they are otherwise generally less involved in sports than their nonhypermobile counterparts.[104] Pointed questions about their range of motion are often necessary because they have accepted their range of motion as typical. Questions about headache, numbness, tingling, and their voiding frequency must be included, as tethered cord syndrome appears to be more common in patients with EDS, and can cause neurologic impairments such as sensory abnormalities, bladder dysfunction, motor disturbances, and can be associated with the base of skull abnormalities. Hyperreflexia of deep tendon reflexes is a sign that there may be spinal cord dysfunction related to tethered cord in these patients. There are, moreover, protean manifestations of this connective tissue disorder in addition to joint laxity. The so-called classic type of EDS, types I/II, is characterized by significant skin involvement in addition to joint hypermobility. The hypermobile type III is characterized by joint hypermobility and mild skin involvement. The distinctions are not always clear clinically, but there are specific collagen and gene abnormalities for each type. The classic type of EDS is associated with an abnormality of type V procollagen, and genes COL5A1 and COL5A2. There is a decreased amount of type V collagen in tissues. The phenotype is caused by a disturbance in the regulatory function of type V collagen.[105] The diagnosis can be confirmed by genetic testing for COL5A1 and COL5A2. If genetic testing is negative or unavailable, the diagnosis can be confirmed by skin biopsy. The hypermobile type is associated with a defect in Tenascin X and a genetic abnormality in gene TNX-B. Both conditions are autosomal dominant. The clinical examination is usually sufficient for clinical management, and neither genetic testing nor skin biopsy is required. In hypermobility syndromes, molecular abnormalities exist in the constituents of the extracellular matrix (ECM) that result from defects in at least 19 different genes, in collagen types I, II, V, and therefore in connective tissue.[88] The term hypermobility spectrum disorder is currently used to describe a wide range of presenting symptoms and severity of involvement in people with EDS.

The physical findings of patients with EDS-hypermobile type, in addition to hypermobile joints, include skin stretch marks; velvety, soft skin (so-called "cigarette-paper"); widened, atrophic scars; translucent skin with prominent blue veins; high-arched palate; lack of a frenulum associated with the ability to touch the tip of the tongue to the nose; dysautonomia with unstable blood pressure and often postural orthostatic tachycardia (POTS); skin and vascular fragility; and evidence of cardiac conduction defects. Manifestations of joint hypermobility include a predilection for "popping" joints, recurvatum of the knees and elbows to 10° or more, unusual and excessive joint hypermobility such that an individual may be able to wrap an arm around the back and then be able to touch the umbilicus with that hand, and equal feats of hip and lower limb excessive joint mobility movement. Pectus excavatum may be present. There is often excessive lumbar lordosis and thoracic kyphosis, and scoliosis may be noted. Marfanoid features are common. Pes planus on weight bearing indicates collapse of the longitudinal arch when standing. Hyperactive deep tendon reflexes, and possibly clonus, suggest CNS involvement, such as tethered cord, posterior fossa abnormality, or cervical spinal cord compression from occipital-cervical spine instability. There may be patchy sensory loss throughout the body. Involvement of the brainstem may result in the absence of the gag reflex. Small fiber neuropathy causing moderate to severe pain was found in 95% of a cohort of 24 subjects with EDS.[106] Ulnar nerve subluxation was found frequently in the one study that looked at that issue.[107]

Pain is a common complaint in patients with EDS, although early studies of this association may have underestimated the prevalence of pain in EDS because hypermobility was often unrecognized and therefore underdiagnosed. Sacheti et al[108] published the first detailed study of pain in 51 subjects with EDS of different types. He found that musculoskeletal pain started in childhood or adolescence, progressively worsened to become chronic and then more widespread over time, primarily involved joints or joint regions, but also included the head and the abdomen. Later studies have confirmed these findings. Recent studies have shown that about 90% of individuals with the hypermobile type of EDS have chronic pain. Individuals with recurrent joint dislocation seem to have more pain. Ankle sprains are common with joint laxity and instability, leading to chronic ankle pain. Pain may be localized to one or more joints that have been repeatedly traumatized. However, there may be widespread joint pain as well. Myalgia, unrelated to specific joints, or perhaps more appropriately stated, relate to widespread joint laxity, occurs in addition to arthralgia. Pain tends to occur in three phases according to Rombaut et al[109]: an early phase of acute, local pain due to joint and soft tissue injuries, occurring in the first decade of life. A second phase occurring over the next three decades is one of widespread musculoskeletal pain, and the third phase, later in life, is characterized by what the authors call maladaptive cognition, ie, catastrophizing and related psychological responses to pain, which tend to increase disability. In other words, musculoskeletal pain tends to progress from being more acute and localized when patients are younger to being more constant and generalized, and therefore more disabling, as patients age. The most common pain report among patients with EDS is musculoskeletal pain. Joint pain, muscle cramps, tendinitis, headache, and fatigue are prominent symptoms.[104] Pain is both nociceptive and neuropathic, in almost equal proportions.[109]

Atlantoaxial instability and tethered cord syndrome are two structural abnormalities of the spine and CNS that are common in EDS more so than in the general population. The former may present with headache, and the latter with low back, leg, and feet pain among other symptoms. Tarlov cysts are seen in patients with EDS, presenting with sacral and pelvic region and lower extremity pain. The diagnosis of Tarlov cysts is made by imaging studies. The most effective treatment is surgical removal or ablation of the cyst(s).[110]

Fatigue is a commonly reported by patients with EDS. It may present in childhood as exercise intolerance, and in later life as delayed recovery from exercise. It is particularly associated with orthostatic intolerance that was present in almost 75% of subjects with EDS-hypermobile type.[111] Patients with reports of fatigue may be misdiagnosed with chronic fatigue syndrome before EDS is identified as an underlying condition. Sleep disturbances, muscle weakness, and medication may also contribute to the symptom of fatigue. POTS is a significant finding in patients who have EDS-related fatigue. Fatigue is positively correlated with pain.

The etiology of pain in patients with EDS is not always apparent, as Syx et al[88] point out. Gross joint trauma and microtrauma to joints that are unstable cause a nociceptive response that is certainly an accepted mechanism of injury. Myofascial pain syndromes, not mentioned in the literature about EDS pain, occur as muscles attempt to stabilize lax, unstable joints, and because of muscle stress resulting from muscle-imbalance scoliosis leading to muscle overuse syndromes. Injury to peripheral nerves from subluxation and small fiber neuropathy are other causes of neuropathic pain in patients with EDS.[106,112] Spinal cord compression in the neck or at the occipital-atlas junction results in instability of the cervical spine that can cause neck and back pain. Persistent or recurrent nociceptive and neuropathic pain results in peripheral and central sensitization with resultant hypersensitivity and allodynia. Kinesiophobia adds an additional pain augmenting factor.

Changes in the ECM resulting from defects in collagen, glycoproteins, and proteoglycans that cause connective tissue dysfunction can also be a major factor in the development of neuropathic pain.[88] In addition, some sequestered components of the ECM can act as damage-associated molecular patterns that are identified by pattern recognition receptors in the immune system. The release of proinflammatory cytokines that initiate or maintain nociceptive and neuropathic pain may then follow.

Management of EDS is mostly symptomatic and corrective of structural abnormalities wherever and to what extent is possible. Skin fragility requires skin protection. Bleeding abnormalities can be treated to minimize spontaneous hemorrhage. Physical therapy is useful to treat muscle hypotonia and delayed motor involvement, to treat musculoskeletal pain, and to guide individuals in strengthening programs designed to restore effective movement patterns. Ring splints are useful for unstable finger joints. Activities that can unduly stress joints are not advised. Functional movement modifications may help some individuals to more safely pursue certain sports activities. For example, if throwing a soccer ball overhead into plays risks shoulder dislocation, the ball should be thrown from the chest without raising the arms over the head. Cognitive behavioral therapy, dialectical behavioral therapy, or other psychological approaches can help avoid some of the problems of maladaptive psychological responses. Graded and progressive aerobic exercises can lead to effective strengthening that can support unstable joints. Treatment of TrPs can reduce muscle pain, and can also help reduce functional scoliosis.

5. CHRONIC PAIN, ALTERED CNS FUNCTION, AND MALADAPTIVE MOVEMENT PATTERNS

Patients who have chronic myofascial pain syndromes can develop altered movement patterns that compensate for restrictions or impairments of normal movement and that constitute maladaptive movement patterns. Maladaptive movement patterns have consequences that affect the CNS. Chronic or recurrent LBP induces changes in the primary motor cortex of the brain that are associated with increased pain and with altered sequencing of muscle activation patterns.[113] In healthy individuals, increasing lumbar lordosis activates the medial multifidi musculature to a greater extent than the iliocostalis muscles. In patients with LBP, the paraspinal muscles tend to be activated in toto as a group, rather than sequentially and discretely. Brain mapping with transcranial magnetic stimulation in patients with LBP shows reorganization of the motor cortex with loss of differential activation of selected paraspinal muscles, consistent with the observation of mass activation of lumbar paraspinal muscles instead of discrete activation of particular muscles.[114] This effect is directly related to increased severity of the LBP.[115] These results of neuroplastic changes in the CNS alter the responses to nociceptive input in the spinal cord, in subcortical structures, and in the somatosensory and motor cortices of the brain. As can be imagined in the situation of LBP, these changes may result in the persistence of pain by the development of hypersensitivity and by promoting maladaptive motor responses that could aggravate and amplify pain responses and thus lead to persistent (chronic) pain. These changes may persist even after the initial insult has passed, and despite healing of peripheral tissues, just as the TrP does. The importance of these changes lies in their potential contribution to the transition from acute to persistent pain, to amplification of pain, and to altered mechanical function. In short, the CNS changes may explain why therapies directed only at peripheral structural and pathophysiologic dysfunctions that cause acute musculoskeletal pain may not be beneficial in all patients.[116]

The primary motor cortex has a rich array of connections to cortical regions like the primary and secondary somatosensory cortices, the prefrontal cortex, and subcortical regions like the thalamus as well. These connections play a critical role, because the recovery of effective motor function is dependent on sensory input; eg, on input from the S1 sensory cortex.[113] These connections are important because effective motor function cannot take place except when motor cortex function is integrated with sensory input. Appropriate motor function requires proprioceptive input, and is integrated with auditory, visual, and vestibular input. Impaired sensory function results in ineffective motor control. The implication of sensorimotor integration is that sensory stimulation plays an important part in recovery from motor deficits, that continued nociceptive input degrades motor function, causing weakness among other impairments, and that rehabilitation that focuses solely on motor function is not as effective as rehabilitation that addresses both sensory and motor function.[117]

Silfies et al[113] postulate that chronic pain induces anxiety and hypervigilance about potentially painful movements, activates the parietal cortex that in turn amplifies the pain experience via its effect on the sensory cortex, producing abnormal patterns of movement. Moreover, the cortical mechanism of "attention switching" associated with fear of movement, which is a prefrontal cortical function, could lead to cognitive fatigue and a reduction in prefrontal cortical influence of sensorimotor integration. Depression, often associated with chronic pain, can increase the perception that nociceptive input is unpleasant and painful. Finally, the integration of altered sensory input with motor intention and movement leads to maladaptive motor patterns that may produce biomechanical stress and more nociceptive input from further muscle overload. These factors lead to the implication that rehabilitation of the patient with persistent musculoskeletal pain must include therapeutic modalities that target the disrupted and maladaptive sensorimotor communication. Conventional therapy directed primarily at strengthening muscle through exercise and through reducing local muscle pain, by, for example, TrP inactivation, will not correct the dysfunction of altered sensorimotor coordination, and therefore, may be ineffective in treating some patients with persistent pain. Specific treatments that target sensorimotor retraining, such as feedback-controlled movement activation exercises, or therapeutic or functional electrical stimulation,[117] can help restore the normal integration of sensory and motor information and function. Targeting fear avoidance, catastrophic thinking, and depression further help restore normal CNS functioning. These approaches go beyond the usual, conventional approaches of local treatment of painful conditions such as LBP and move therapy into the realm of addressing hitherto neglected factors that lead to the persistence of pain.

Altered muscle activation patterns are also seen in femoroacetabular impingement syndrome resulting in disturbed muscle synergy. Maladaptive muscle contraction of paraspinal muscles to "stabilize the spine" and minimize spinal movement and pain in people with chronic LBP is directly correlated with pain catastrophizing more than with pain intensity.[118] Experimentally produced LBP through the injection of hypertonic saline into low back paraspinal muscles resulted in greater muscle tightening (stabilizing the spine) in subjects who demonstrated pain catastrophizing compared with those who did not pain catastrophize, despite the lack of any difference in perceived pain intensity.[119] These studies show that in addition to the effects of persistent pain, the psychological response to acute and to persistent pain affects motor function and can lead to maladaptive motor patterning. These studies, and others, demonstrate that muscle pain and joint pain directly and indirectly alter movement patterns, and that they can lead to more pain through muscle overload. Unfortunately, there are few studies of TrP pain syndromes in association with maladaptive movement patterns, but I think that it is likely and believe that many of my chronic, difficult-to-treat patients with myofascial pain suffered from this complication. One notable study is that of Lucas et al[120] that showed that latent TrPs in the shoulder girdle muscles alter the normal sequence of muscle activation pattern in arm abduction.

6. Other Perpetuating Factors

Three mechanical perpetuating factors have been presented that are not often discussed in the myofascial pain literature as well as five metabolic perpetuating factors. There are a number of other perpetuating factors that have been covered in great detail in the past,[3,121] but that need to be reviewed for effectively evaluating and treating patients.

6.1. Iron Deficiency

Iron is required for the production of energy, and iron deficiency is one predisposing cause of a hypometabolic state and of refractory TrPs. There is only one published study that looked at this issue,[48] and it found no difference in serum iron levels between patients with myofascial pain syndrome (MPS) and healthy control subjects. However, the criterion for entry into the study was simply one or more TrPs in a shoulder muscle. There were only 38 subjects with MPS of whom 34 were female. It is doubtful that this study was powered well enough to detect changes in chronic myofascial pain. Some striking examples of the effect of iron deficiency have been noted in patients with persistent MPS. One example is a woman with MPS refractory to all usual effective treatments who had no stainable iron on bone marrow examination. She recovered uneventfully after iron replacement treatment. Iron deficiency is common among women because of menstrual bleeding. Serum iron levels below 20 ng/mL should be considered suspect for deficiency. Men are not typically iron deficient except in cases of a malignancy, or GI tract blood loss. Vitamin C chemically reduces iron and thereby facilitates its absorption, so iron supplementation should be accompanied by vitamin C supplementation.

6.2. Protozoal Infestation

Infestation by amoeba and some other parasites like fluke can cause diffuse myalgia and TrP pain. Exposure occurs when swimming in infested ponds or streams. Diagnosis is suggested by a history of exposure and confirmed by stool testing for ova and parasites. Clinically, the author of this chapter has never seen MPS associated with giardia or tapeworm infestation.

6.2. Sleep Deprivation

Sleep deprivation has long been known to be associated with muscle pain. Sleep apnea and restless legs syndrome are two conditions associated with a predisposition to muscle pain and to refractory myofascial pain syndrome.

References

1. Simons DG. Review of enigmatic MTrPs as a common cause of enigmatic musculoskeletal pain and dysfunction. *J Electromyogr Kinesiol.* 2004;14(1):95-107.
2. Gerwin RD, Dommerholt J, Shah JP. An expansion of Simons' integrated hypothesis of trigger point formation. *Curr Pain Headache Rep.* 2004;8(6):468-475.
3. Gerwin RD. A review of myofascial pain and fibromyalgia—factors that promote their persistence. *Acupunct Med.* 2005;23(3):121-134.
4. Traub RJ, Ji Y. Sex differences and hormonal modulation of deep tissue pain. *Front Neuroendocrinol.* 2013;34(4):350-366.
5. Fillingim RB, King CD, Ribeiro-Dasilva MC, Rahim-Williams B, Riley JL III. Sex, gender, and pain: a review of recent clinical and experimental findings. *J Pain.* 2009;10(5):447-485.
6. George SZ, Wittmer VT, Fillingim RB, Robinson ME. Sex and pain-related psychological variables are associated with thermal pain sensitivity for patients with chronic low back pain. *J Pain.* 2007;8(1):2-10.
7. Lu CL, Herndon C. New roles for neuronal estrogen receptors. *Neurogastroenterol Motil.* 2017;29(7).
8. Ge HY, Madeleine P, Arendt-Nielsen L. Sex differences in temporal characteristics of descending inhibitory control: an evaluation using repeated bilateral experimental induction of muscle pain. *Pain.* 2004;110(1-2):72-78.
9. Ge HY, Madeleine P, Cairns BE, Arendt-Nielsen L. Hypoalgesia in the referred pain areas after bilateral injections of hypertonic saline into the trapezius muscles of men and women: a potential experimental model of gender-specific differences. *Clin J Pain.* 2006;22(1):37-44.
10. Derbyshire SW, Nichols TE, Firestone L, Townsend DW, Jones AK. Gender differences in patterns of cerebral activation during equal experience of painful laser stimulation. *J Pain.* 2002;3(5):401-411.
11. Grace PM, Hutchinson MR, Maier SF, Watkins LR. Pathological pain and the neuroimmune interface. *Nat Rev Immunol.* 2014;14(4):217-231.
12. Craft RM, Mogil JS, Aloisi AM. Sex differences in pain and analgesia: the role of gonadal hormones. *Eur J Pain.* 2004;8(5):397-411.
13. Liu NJ, Murugaiyan V, Storman EM, Schnell SA, Wessendorf MW, Gintzler AR. Estrogens synthesized and acting within a spinal oligomer suppress spinal endomorphin 2 antinociception: ebb and flow over the rat reproductive cycle. *Pain.* 2017;158(10):1903-1914.
14. Amandusson A, Blomqvist A. Estrogenic influences in pain processing. *Front Neuroendocrinol.* 2013;34(4):329-349.
15. Giamberardino MA, Affaitati G, Valente R, Iezzi S, Vecchiet L. Changes in visceral pain reactivity as a function of estrous cycle in female rats with artificial ureteral calculosis. *Brain Res.* 1997;774(1-2):234-238.
16. Fillingim RB, Edwards RR. The association of hormone replacement therapy with experimental pain responses in postmenopausal women. *Pain.* 2001;92(1-2):229-234.
17. Hunter DA, Barr GA, Amador N, et al. Estradiol-induced antinociceptive responses on formalin-induced nociception are independent of COX and HPA activation. *Synapse.* 2011;65(7):643-651.
18. Gao P, Ding XW, Dong L, Luo P, Zhang GH, Rong WF. Expression of aromatase in the rostral ventromedial medulla and its role in the regulation of visceral pain. *CNS Neurosci Ther.* 2017;23(12):980-989.
19. Lemoine S, Granier P, Tiffoche C, Rannou-Bekono F, Thieulant ML, Delamarche P. Estrogen receptor alpha mRNA in human skeletal muscles. *Med Sci Sports Exerc.* 2003;35(3):439-443.
20. Bell DR, Blackburn JT, Norcorss MF, et al. Estrogen and muscle stiffness have a negative relationship in females. *Knee Surg Sports Traumatol Arthrosc.* 2012;20(2):361-367.
21. Bell DR, Blackburn JT, Ondrak KS, et al. The effects of oral contraceptive use on muscle stiffness across the menstrual cycle. *Clin J Sport Med.* 2011;21(6):467-473.
22. Ueberschlag-Pitiot V, Stantzou A, Messeant J, et al. Gonad-related factors promote muscle performance gain during postnatal development in male and female mice. *Am J Physiol Endocrinol Metab.* 2017;313(1):E12-E25.
23. White HD, Robinson TD. A novel use for testosterone to treat central sensitization of chronic pain in fibromyalgia patients. *Int Immunopharmacol.* 2015;27(2):244-248.
24. Macedo CG, Fanton LE, Fischer L, Tambeli CH. Coactivation of mu- and kappa-opioid receptors may mediate the protective effect of testosterone on the development of temporomandibular joint nociception in male rats. *J Oral Facial Pain Headache.* 2016;30(1):61-67.
25. Li J, Xie M, Wang X, et al. Sex hormones regulate cerebral drug metabolism via brain miRNAs: down-regulation of brain CYP2D by androgens reduces the analgesic effects of tramadol. *Br J Pharmacol.* 2015;172(19):4639-4654.
26. Rubinstein AL, Carpenter DM. Association between commonly prescribed opioids and androgen deficiency in men: a retrospective cohort analysis. *Pain Med.* 2017;18(4):637-644.
27. O'Rourke TK Jr, Wosnitzer MS. Opioid-induced androgen deficiency (OPIAD): diagnosis, management, and literature review. *Curr Urol Rep.* 2016;17(10):76.
28. Aloisi AM, Ceccarelli I, Fiorenzani P. Gonadectomy affects hormonal and behavioral responses to repetitive nociceptive stimulation in male rats. *Ann N Y Acad Sci.* 2003;1007:232-237.
29. White HD, Brown LA, Gyurik RJ, et al. Treatment of pain in fibromyalgia patients with testosterone gel: pharmacokinetics and clinical response. *Int Immunopharmacol.* 2015;27(2):249-256.
30. Tennant F. Hormone abnormalities in patients with severe and chronic pain who fail standard treatments. *Postgrad Med.* 2015;127(1):1-4.
31. Basaria S, Travison TG, Alford D, et al. Effects of testosterone replacement in men with opioid-induced androgen deficiency: a randomized controlled trial. *Pain.* 2015;156(2):280-288.
32. Monks DA, Holmes MM. Androgen receptors and muscle: a key mechanism underlying life history trade-offs. *J Comp Physiol A Neuroethol Sens Neural Behav Physiol.* 2018;204(1):51-60.
33. Travell JG, Simons DG. *Myofascial Pain and Dysfunction: The Trigger Point Manual.* Vol 1. Baltimore, MD: Williams & Wilkins; 1983 (pp. 145-146).
34. da Silva VA, de Almeida RJ, Cavalcante MP, et al. Two Thyroid Stimulating Hormone assays correlated in clinical practice show disagreement in subclinical hypothyroidism patients. *Clin Biochem.* 2018;53:13-18.
35. Salvatore D, Simonides WS, Dentice M, Zavacki AM, Larsen PR. Thyroid hormones and skeletal muscle—new insights and potential implications. *Nat Rev Endocrinol.* 2014;10(4):206-214.
36. Bloise FF, Cordeiro A, Ortiga-Carvalho TM. Role of thyroid hormone in skeletal muscle physiology. *J Endocrinol.* 2018;236(1):R57-R68.
37. Moon MK, Kang GH, Kim HH, et al. Thyroid-stimulating hormone improves insulin sensitivity in skeletal muscle cells via cAMP/PKA/CREB pathway-dependent upregulation of insulin receptor substrate-1 expression. *Mol Cell Endocrinol.* 2016;436:50-58.
38. Kopecka K, Zacharova G, Smerdu V, Soukup T. Slow to fast muscle transformation following heterochronous isotransplantation is influenced by host thyroid hormone status. *Histochem Cell Biol.* 2014;142(6):677-684.
39. Visser WE, Heemstra KA, Swagemakers SM, et al. Physiological thyroid hormone levels regulate numerous skeletal muscle transcripts. *J Clin Endocrinol Metab.* 2009;94(9):3487-3496.
40. Reuters VS, Teixeira Pde F, Vigario PS, et al. Functional capacity and muscular abnormalities in subclinical hypothyroidism. *Am J Med Sci.* 2009;338(4):259-263.
41. Gallo D, Piantanida E, Veronesi G, et al. Physical performance in newly diagnosed hypothyroidism: a pilot study. *J Endocrinol Invest.* 2017;40(10):1099-1106.
42. Stott DJ, Rodondi N, Kearney PM, et al. Thyroid hormone therapy for older adults with subclinical hypothyroidism. *N Engl J Med.* 2017;376(26):2534-2544.
43. Grossman A, Feldhamer I, Meyerovitch J. Treatment with levothyroxin in subclinical hypothyroidism is associated with increased mortality in the elderly. *Eur J Intern Med.* 2017. doi:10.1016/j.ejim.2017.11.010
44. Sindoni A, Rodolico C, Pappalardo MA, Portaro S, Benvenga S. Hypothyroid myopathy: a peculiar clinical presentation of thyroid failure. Review of the literature. *Rev Endocr Metab Disord.* 2016;17(4):499-519.
45. Barchetta I, Baroni MG, Leonetti F, et al. TSH levels are associated with vitamin D status and seasonality in an adult population of euthyroid adults. *Clin Exp Med.* 2015;15(3):389-396.
46. Hamel J, Logigian EL. Acute nutritional axonal neuropathy. *Muscle Nerve.* 2018;57(1):33-39.
47. Mostacci B, Liguori R, Cicero AF. Nutraceutical approach to peripheral neuropathies: evidence from clinical trials. *Curr Drug Metab.* 2017. doi:10.2174/1389200218666171031145419
48. Okumus M, Ceceli E, Tuncay F, Kocaoglu S, Palulu N, Yorgancioglu ZR. The relationship between serum trace elements, vitamin B12, folic acid and clinical parameters in patients with myofascial pain syndrome. *J Back Musculoskelet Rehabil.* 2010;23(4):187-191.
49. Wang ZB, Gan Q, Rupert RL, Zeng YM, Song XJ. Thiamine, pyridoxine, cyanocobalamin and their combination inhibit thermal, but not mechanical hyperalgesia in rats with primary sensory neuron injury. *Pain.* 2005;114(1-2):266-277.
50. Song XS, Huang ZJ, Song XJ. Thiamine suppresses thermal hyperalgesia, inhibits hyperexcitability, and lessens alterations of sodium currents in injured, dorsal root ganglion neurons in rats. *Anesthesiology.* 2009;110(2):387-400.
51. Mader R, Deutsch H, Siebert GK, et al. Vitamin status of inpatients with chronic cephalgia and dysfunction pain syndrome and effects of a vitamin supplementation. *Int J Vitam Nutr Res.* 1988;58(4):436-441.
52. Yxfeldt A, Wallberg-Jonsson S, Hultdin J, Rantapaa-Dahlqvist S. Homocysteine in patients with rheumatoid arthritis in relation to inflammation and B-vitamin treatment. *Scand J Rheumatol.* 2003;32(4):205-210.
53. Deng XT, Han Y, Liu WT, Song XJ. B vitamins potentiate acute morphine antinociception and attenuate the development of tolerance to chronic morphine in mice. *Pain Med.* 2017;18(10):1961-1974.
54. Mao J, Price DD, Mayer DJ. Mechanisms of hyperalgesia and morphine tolerance: a current view of their possible interactions. *Pain.* 1995;62(3):259-274.
55. Lim G, Wang S, Zeng Q, Sung B, Yang L, Mao J. Expression of spinal NMDA receptor and PKCgamma after chronic morphine is regulated by spinal glucocorticoid receptor. *J Neurosci.* 2005;25(48):11145-11154.
56. Hutchinson MR, Bland ST, Johnson KW, Rice KC, Maier SF, Watkins LR. Opioid-induced glial activation: mechanisms of activation and implications for opioid analgesia, dependence, and reward. *Sci World J.* 2007;7:98-111.
57. Ceglia L. Vitamin D and skeletal muscle tissue and function. *Mol Aspects Med.* 2008;29(6):407-414.
58. Helde-Frankling M, Bjorkhem-Bergman L. Vitamin D in pain management. *Int J Mol Sci.* 2017;18(10).
59. Cheng L. The convergence of two epidemics: vitamin D deficiency in obese school-aged children. *J Pediatr Nurs.* 2018;38:20-26.
60. Powanda MC. Is there a role for vitamin D in the treatment of chronic pain? *Inflammopharmacology.* 2014;22(6):327-332.
61. Martin KR, Reid DM. Is there role for vitamin D in the treatment of chronic pain? *Ther Adv Musculoskelet Dis.* 2017;9(6):131-135.
62. Autier P, Boniol M, Pizot C, Mullie P. Vitamin D status and ill health: a systematic review. *Lancet Diabetes Endocrinol.* 2014;2(1):76-89.
63. Grossmann RE, Zughaier SM, Liu S, Lyles RH, Tangpricha V. Impact of vitamin D supplementation on markers of inflammation in adults with cystic fibrosis hospitalized for a pulmonary exacerbation. *Eur J Clin Nutr.* 2012;66(9):1072-1074.

64. Hsiao MY, Hung CY, Chang KV, Han DS, Wang TG. Is serum hypovitaminosis D associated with chronic widespread pain including fibromyalgia? A meta-analysis of observational studies. *Pain Physician.* 2015;18(5):E877-E887.
65. Levinger P, Begg R, Sanders KM, et al. The effect of vitamin D status on pain, lower limb strength and knee function during balance recovery in people with knee osteoarthritis: an exploratory study. *Arch Osteoporos.* 2017;12(1):83.
66. Zadro J, Shirley D, Ferreira M, et al. Mapping the association between vitamin D and low back pain: a systematic review and meta-analysis of observational studies. *Pain Physician.* 2017;20(7):611-640.
67. Rosendahl-Riise H, Spielau U, Ranhoff AH, Gudbrandsen OA, Dierkes J. Vitamin D supplementation and its influence on muscle strength and mobility in community-dwelling older persons: a systematic review and meta-analysis. *J Hum Nutr Diet.* 2017;30(1):3-15.
68. Jackson C, Gaugris S, Sen SS, Hosking D. The effect of cholecalciferol (vitamin D3) on the risk of fall and fracture: a meta-analysis. *QJM.* 2007;100(4):185-192.
69. Wu Z, Malihi Z, Stewart AW, Lawes CM, Scragg R. Effect of vitamin D supplementation on pain: a systematic review and meta-analysis. *Pain Physician.* 2016;19(7):415-427.
70. Krejs GJ, Nicar MJ, Zerwekh JE, Norman DA, Kane MG, Pak CY. Effect of 1,25-dihydroxyvitamin D3 on calcium and magnesium absorption in the healthy human jejunum and ileum. *Am J Med.* 1983;75(6):973-976.
71. Ge HY, Nie H, Madeleine P, Danneskiold-Samsoe B, Graven-Nielsen T, Arendt-Nielsen L. Contribution of the local and referred pain from active myofascial trigger points in fibromyalgia syndrome. *Pain.* 2009;147(1-3):233-240.
72. Alonso-Blanco C, Fernández de las Peñas C, Morales-Cabezas M, Zarco-Moreno P, Ge HY, Florez-Garcia M. Multiple active myofascial trigger points reproduce the overall spontaneous pain pattern in women with fibromyalgia and are related to widespread mechanical hypersensitivity. *Clin J Pain.* 2011;27(5):405-413.
73. de Baaij JH, Hoenderop JG, Bindels RJ. Magnesium in man: implications for health and disease. *Physiol Rev.* 2015;95(1):1-46.
74. Correa AMB, Guimaraes JDS, Dos Santos EAE, Kushmerick C. Control of neuronal excitability by Group I metabotropic glutamate receptors. *Biophys Rev.* 2017;9(5):835-845.
75. Ge J, Huang F, Nesmelov YE. Metal cation controls phosphate release in the myosin ATPase. *Protein Sci.* 2017;26(11):2181-2186.
76. Kim YS, Kim KM, Lee DJ, et al. Women with fibromyalgia have lower levels of calcium, magnesium, iron and manganese in hair mineral analysis. *J Korean Med Sci.* 2011;26(10):1253-1257.
77. Sendur OF, Tastaban E, Turan Y, Ulman C. The relationship between serum trace element levels and clinical parameters in patients with fibromyalgia. *Rheumatol Int.* 2008;28(11):1117-1121.
78. Romano TJ. Magnesium deficiency in patients with myofascial pain. *J Myofas Ther.* 1994;1(3):11-12.
79. Grober U, Schmidt J, Kisters K. Magnesium in prevention and therapy. *Nutrients.* 2015;7(9):8199-8226.
80. Bagis S, Karabiber M, As I, Tamer L, Erdogan C, Atalay A. Is magnesium citrate treatment effective on pain, clinical parameters and functional status in patients with fibromyalgia? *Rheumatol Int.* 2013;33(1):167-172.
81. Ali A, Njike VY, Northrup V, et al. Intravenous micronutrient therapy (Myers' Cocktail) for fibromyalgia: a placebo-controlled pilot study. *J Altern Complement Med.* 2009;15(3):247-257.
82. Zarean E, Tarjan A. Effect of magnesium supplement on pregnancy outcomes: a randomized control trial. *Adv Biomed Res.* 2017;6:109.
83. van Dronkelaar C, van Velzen A, Abdelrazek M, van der Steen A, Weijs PJM, Tieland M. Minerals and sarcopenia; the role of calcium, iron, magnesium, phosphorus, potassium, selenium, sodium, and zinc on muscle mass, muscle strength, and physical performance in older adults: a systematic review. *J Am Med Dir Assoc.* 2018;19(1):6.e3-11.e3.
84. Veronese N, Berton L, Carraro S, et al. Effect of oral magnesium supplementation on physical performance in healthy elderly women involved in a weekly exercise program: a randomized controlled trial. *Am J Clin Nutr.* 2014;100(3):974-981.
85. Cho J, Lee E, Lee S. Upper thoracic spine mobilization and mobility exercise versus upper cervical spine mobilization and stabilization exercise in individuals with forward head posture: a randomized clinical trial. *BMC Musculoskelet Disord.* 2017;18(1):525.
86. Engen DJ, McAllister SJ, Whipple MO, et al. Effects of transdermal magnesium chloride on quality of life for patients with fibromyalgia: a feasibility study. *J Integr Med.* 2015;13(5):306-313.
87. Cordova Martinez A, Fernandez-Lazaro D, Mielgo-Ayuso J, Seco Calvo J, Caballero Garcia A. Effect of magnesium supplementation on muscular damage markers in basketball players during a full season. *Magnes Res.* 2017;30(2):61-70.
88. Syx D, De Wandele I, Rombaut L, Malfait F. Hypermobility, the Ehlers-Danlos syndromes and chronic pain. *Clin Exp Rheumatol.* 2017;35, suppl 107(5):116-122.
89. Beighton P, De Paepe A, Steinmann B, Tsipouras P, Wenstrup RJ. Ehlers-Danlos syndromes: revised nosology, Villefranche, 1997. Ehlers-Danlos National Foundation (USA) and Ehlers-Danlos Support Group (UK). *Am J Med Genet.* 1998;77(1):31-37.
90. Grahame R, Bird HA, Child A. The revised (Brighton 1998) criteria for the diagnosis of benign joint hypermobility syndrome (BJHS). *J Rheumatol.* 2000;27(7):1777-1779.
91. Voermans NC, Knoop H, Bleijenberg G, van Engelen BG. Pain in Ehlers-Danlos syndrome is common, severe, and associated with functional impairment. *J Pain Symptom Manage.* 2010;40(3):370-378.
92. Singla D, Veqar Z. Association between forward head, rounded shoulders, and increased thoracic kyphosis: a review of the literature. *J Chiropr Med.* 2017;16(3):220-229.
93. Patwardhan AG, Khayatzadeh S, Havey RM, et al. Cervical sagittal balance: a biomechanical perspective can help clinical practice. *Eur Spine J.* 2018;27:25-38.
94. Bokaee F, Rezasoltani A, Manshadi FD, Naimi SS, Baghban AA, Azimi H. Comparison of cervical muscle thickness between asymptomatic women with and without forward head posture. *Braz J Phys Ther.* 2017;21(3):206-211.
95. Cheon S, Park S. Changes in neck and upper trunk muscle activities according to the angle of movement of the neck in subjects with forward head posture. *J Phys Ther Sci.* 2017;29(2):191-193.
96. Hallgren RC, Pierce SJ, Sharma DB, Rowan JJ. Forward head posture and activation of rectus capitis posterior muscles. *J Am Osteopath Assoc.* 2017;117(1):24-31.
97. Yong MS, Lee HY, Lee MY. Correlation between head posture and proprioceptive function in the cervical region. *J Phys Ther Sci.* 2016;28(3):857-860.
98. Lee JH. Effects of forward head posture on static and dynamic balance control. *J Phys Ther Sci.* 2016;28(1):274-277.
99. Kang JH, Park RY, Lee SJ, Kim JY, Yoon SR, Jung KI. The effect of the forward head posture on postural balance in long time computer based worker. *Ann Rehabil Med.* 2012;36(1):98-104.
100. Abboud J, Marchand AA, Sorra K, Descarreaux M. Musculoskeletal physical outcome measures in individuals with tension-type headache: a scoping review. *Cephalalgia.* 2013;33(16):1319-1336.
101. Fernández de las Peñas C, Cuadrado ML, Pareja JA. Myofascial trigger points, neck mobility and forward head posture in unilateral migraine. *Cephalalgia.* 2006;26(9):1061-1070.
102. Strom V, Knardahl S, Stanghelle JK, Roe C. Pain induced by a single simulated office-work session: time course and association with muscle blood flux and muscle activity. *Eur J Pain.* 2009;13(8):843-852.
103. Park SY, Yoo WG. Effect of sustained typing work on changes in scapular position, pressure pain sensitivity and upper trapezius activity. *J Occup Health.* 2013;55(3):167-172.
104. Rombaut L, Malfait F, Cools A, De Paepe A, Calders P. Musculoskeletal complaints, physical activity and health-related quality of life among patients with the Ehlers-Danlos syndrome hypermobility type. *Disabil Rehabil.* 2010;32(16):1339-1345.
105. Bowen JM, Sobey GJ, Burrows NP, et al. Ehlers-Danlos syndrome, classical type. *Am J Med Genet C Semin Med Genet.* 2017;175(1):27-39.
106. Cazzato D, Castori M, Lombardi R, et al. Small fiber neuropathy is a common feature of Ehlers-Danlos syndromes. *Neurology.* 2016;87(2):155-159.
107. Granata G, Padua L, Celletti C, Castori M, Saraceni VM, Camerota F. Entrapment neuropathies and polyneuropathies in joint hypermobility syndrome/Ehlers-Danlos syndrome. *Clin Neurophysiol.* 2013;124(8):1689-1694.
108. Sacheti A, Szemere J, Bernstein B, Tafas T, Schechter N, Tsipouras P. Chronic pain is a manifestation of the Ehlers-Danlos syndrome. *J Pain Symptom Manage.* 1997;14(2):88-93.
109. Rombaut L, Scheper M, De Wandele I, et al. Chronic pain in patients with the hypermobility type of Ehlers-Danlos syndrome: evidence for generalized hyperalgesia. *Clin Rheumatol.* 2015;34(6):1121-1129.
110. Henderson FC Sr, Austin C, Benzel E, et al. Neurological and spinal manifestations of the Ehlers-Danlos syndromes. *Am J Med Genet C Semin Med Genet.* 2017;175(1):195-211.
111. De Wandele I, Rombaut L, De Backer T, et al. Orthostatic intolerance and fatigue in the hypermobility type of Ehlers-Danlos Syndrome. *Rheumatology (Oxford).* 2016;55(8):1412-1420.
112. Camerota F, Celletti C, Castori M, Grammatico P, Padua L. Neuropathic pain is a common feature in Ehlers-Danlos syndrome. *J Pain Symptom Manage.* 2011;41(1):e2-e4.
113. Silfies SP, Vendemia JMC, Beattie PF, Stewart JC, Jordon M. Changes in brain structure and activation may augment abnormal movement patterns: an emerging challenge in musculoskeletal rehabilitation. *Pain Med.* 2017;18(11):2051-2054.
114. Tsao H, Danneels LA, Hodges PW. ISSLS prize winner: smudging the motor brain in young adults with recurrent low back pain. *Spine (Phila Pa 1976).* 2011;36(21):1721-1727.
115. Schabrun SM, Elgueta-Cancino EL, Hodges PW. Smudging of the motor cortex is related to the severity of low back pain. *Spine (Phila Pa 1976).* 2017;42(15):1172-1178.
116. Pelletier R, Higgins J, Bourbonnais D. Is neuroplasticity in the central nervous system the missing link to our understanding of chronic musculoskeletal disorders? *BMC Musculoskelet Disord.* 2015;16:25.
117. Bolognini N, Russo C, Edwards DJ. The sensory side of post-stroke motor rehabilitation. *Restor Neurol Neurosci.* 2016;34(4):571-586.
118. Pakzad M, Fung J, Preuss R. Pain catastrophizing and trunk muscle activation during walking in patients with chronic low back pain. *Gait Posture.* 2016;49:73-77.
119. Ross GB, Sheahan PJ, Mahoney B, Gurd BJ, Hodges PW, Graham RB. Pain catastrophizing moderates changes in spinal control in response to noxiously induced low back pain. *J Biomech.* 2017;58:64-70.
120. Lucas KR, Polus PA, Rich J. Latent myofascial trigger points: their effect on muscle activation and movement efficiency. *Bodyw Mov Ther.* 2004;8:160-166.
121. Gerwin RD. Factores perpetuadores en el sindrome de dolor miofascial. In: Mayoral del Moral O, Salvat IS, eds. *Fisioterapia Invasiva del Sindrome de Dolor Miofascial.* Madrid, Spain: Editorial Medica Panamericana; 2017:39-52.

Chapter 5

Psychosocial Considerations

Leslie F. Taylor and Jennifer L. Freeman

1. INTRODUCTION

Pain is a both an intensely personal experience shaped by life events and a universal human experience conceptualized by era-specific norms. In prior times and in other places, pain has been diagnosed as a spiritual problem and treated as such. In the modern Western world, the origins of and the treatments for pain were forced into a purely biomedical box. As science advanced and the bioanatomic origins of pain were identified, the biomedical model rightfully gained prominence. The pain experience was defined in physical terms and considered objective and measureable. Pain was considered directly proportional to tissue injury. One of the downsides of this scientific perspective was the compartmentalization of pain management: physical pain managed by one team, psychological pain by another. The social, spiritual, and mind-body aspects of the pain experience were deemphasized. Now, fueled by more refined testing instruments as well as the acceptance of the phenomenologic nature of pain, the most appropriate model for the diagnosis and treatment of painful conditions is a biopsychosocial one. Myofascial pain, especially when accompanied by other painful conditions or perpetuated by factors discussed in Chapter 4 of this text, can be complicated and sometimes even persistent. For any patient experiencing pain, and even more importantly for those experiencing persistent or unexplainable pain, clinicians must be sensitive to the thoughts, emotions, behaviors, and social interactions that can either improve or worsen outcomes.

In the mid-1960s, Melzack and Wall introduced a new theory on the mechanisms of pain, later named the gate-control theory, which led the way for advancing pain sciences research.[1,2] Concurrently, George Engel[3] pioneered efforts to respond to the pervasive state of dehumanized medical care that he attributed to the dualistic nature of separating the body and mind, the excessively reductionist orientation of medical thinking that viewed the body as a machine, and the lack of humanity afforded to both the practitioner (the detached observer) and the patient.[4] The biopsychosocial model, guided by sociology's Systems Theory,[5] resulted from Engel's work. Current culture and evidence supports this more integrated approach. Although many musculoskeletal clinicians consider pain from a broader biopsychosocial point of view, actually practicing from such a theoretical base remains challenging.

As demonstrated in the preceding chapters, tremendous gains have been made in understanding the biological initiators of pain, how to diagnose its source, and in many cases, successfully treat it. Clinicians, on average, are well educated and well prepared to assess and manage physical factors related to patient disability.[6] Some have evolved past a strict biomedical mind-set and apply—or at least aim to apply—a broader biopsychosocial view with regard to managing patients with persistent pain.[7] However, this evolution is confounded by the fact that the majority of practicing clinicians were educated and trained in the biomedical model, with the "softer skills" of considering psychosocial factors, communication, and facilitating rapport-based patient–client interactions receiving far less attention, and at times, far less respect. Although clinicians may acknowledge and endorse the role of psychosocial variables, many feel a true lack of preparedness to address these concerns. Professional education courses addressing psychosocial concerns are often truncated and are rarely integrated across curricula, and postprofessional courses are almost always skills focused. So, despite evidence supporting a biopsychosocial philosophy of practice, clinicians feel ill-equipped to effectively manage patients with complex or persistent experiences of pain.

Decades of research have attempted to clarify, measure, or explain various aspects of the biopsychosocial model.[4] Although applying a reductionist approach to this model is antithetical to its intent, efforts are rightfully focused on finding ways to determine and understand how different aspects of the biopsychosocial model contribute to pain, how they interact, and which treatment interventions may be most effective. It is far beyond the scope of this chapter to even come close to mentioning, much less addressing, all of the complexities of this topic. Rather, this chapter provides an overview of some psychological and sociological theories and themes foundational to the experience of pain that may help guide treatment and improve outcomes.

2. PSYCHOLOGICAL AND SOCIOLOGICAL OVERVIEW

Prior to considering biopsychosocial strategies for the comprehensive management of patients with pain, a brief review of several major psychological and sociological theories and constructs is in order.

2.1. Psychological and Sociological Frameworks

The relationship of human thought, emotion, and behavior with the outside world has been a topic of study for centuries. Early behaviorists discovered that responses can be modified by external events. Cognitive-behaviorists rejected a purist form of behaviorism and integrated with it the power of thought in human experience and its role in shaping behavior. Existential-humanist theories focused on whole-person care and the importance of subjective meaning. And third-wave behaviorism has seemingly attempted to reunite psychology with philosophy to outline strategies for navigating life's difficulties with realistic expectations. Modern healthcare professionals, cognizant of the need for biopsychosocial care, find it useful to combine what could be seen as aspects from many viewpoints with more nuanced and dynamic models of the interplay between emotion, thought, behavior, social interaction, and meaning. The following concepts are far from an exhaustive list of theories and themes that can impact the diagnosis and treatment of myofascial pain and dysfunction. For more on psychological frameworks and concepts, refer to additional resources.

2.2. Behavioral Learning Theories

Classical Conditioning

In 1889, while researching digestion in dogs, Ivan Pavlov formed the psychological theory of classical or respondent conditioning.[8] In the oft-cited experiment, a bell rung prior to feeding over time initiated an involuntary canine response to salivate prior to the arrival of food. When food regularly did not appear after the bell, the conditioned response waned and eventually ceased. This "learning" and "extinction" was thought to apply universally to human behavior. Research suggests that classical conditioning can amplify pain (associative learning), but conclusions about whether or not classical conditioning can elicit pain remain under consideration.[9]

Operant Conditioning

In the 1950s, B.F. Skinner's theory of operant conditioning supported the premise that behavior could be altered because of consequences as well as stimuli.[10] The theory states that behavior followed by positive or negative reinforcement increases the probability of that behavior, whereas punishment reduces it. Fordyce[11,12] and Fowler et al[13] applied this theory in a behavioral model of pain, highlighting the importance of the stimulus response of learning in developing and maintaining chronic pain. Fordyce began exploration of the now widely accepted distinction between the factors that initiate pain and the factors that perpetuate pain.[14] The intent of integrating operant conditioning theory into musculoskeletal therapeutic interventions is to increase the occurrences of healthy behaviors through positive reinforcement and reduce the frequency of pain behaviors by removing reinforcement.[14]

2.3. Cognitive-Behavioral Themes

Self-Efficacy and Locus of Control

Albert Bandura's theory of self-efficacy, part of social cognitive theory, is the belief in one's ability to influence events that affect one's life and the way these events are experienced.[15] In a systematic review of the role of self-efficacy on the prognosis of individuals with chronic musculoskeletal pain, higher self-efficacy was associated with greater physical function, physical activity, health and work status, and satisfaction. Likewise, higher self-efficacy is associated with lower levels of pain, disability, disease activity, depressive symptoms, the presence of fibromyalgia tender points, fatigue, and presenteeism (at work, but not functioning at top level).[16] Somewhat counter to a biomedical focus on limited capacity as a result of injury/disease, Bandura emphasizes human capacity rather than human failings and dysfunction. In the same way that physical strength or endurance can be trained and improved, Bandura proposes that self-efficacy can also be strengthened, which, in turn, can improve function.[17] Low self-efficacy is associated with greater reports of pain, anxiety, and reduced ability to distract attention away from symptoms. Higher self-efficacy is associated with lower reports of pain and anxiety, higher resilience, and an ability to distract attention from sensations and to shift the meaning of pain/change the interpretation.[18] More optimistic, the person who is motivated from this perspective is able to make more effective management choices.

In the mid-20th century, Julian Rotter[19] developed a social-learning theory of personality that included the concept of locus of control (LOC). LOC identifies the degree to which people believe they can control the events in their lives. Individuals with a strong internal LOC believe that they can effect change in their lives, whereas those with a strong external control LOC believe that something external to them is in charge of their lives. Rotter intended LOC to be considered as a continuum, not a static dichotomy, as a person's learning can influence their perceptions in various situations.[20]

The application of this conceptual frame to health behaviors led to the development of a health-focused locus of control (HLOC).[21] HLOC refers to an individual's expectations regarding whether health is controlled by one's own behaviors (Internal HLOC), or by external factors including chance, luck, and fate (Chance HLOC), or by powerful others, including healthcare providers (Powerful Others HLOC).[22] Within each of these loci, the individual demonstrates behavioral, cognitive, decisional, and informational control reinforcing each internal world view. Stronger Internal HLOC correlates with better mental and physical health and more proactive health behaviors.[23,24] An individual with stronger Chance HLOC believes that he or she has very little, if any, control over his or her musculoskeletal pain, and may adopt more pessimistic attitudes and approaches that lead to poorer choices and reinforce this belief state.

Self-efficacy is also related to HLOC, it and impacts how stress is perceived and managed. Lower self-efficacy, combined with low Internal HLOC, is correlated with higher illness-related psychological distress, higher levels of psychological and physical problems, and increased vulnerability to external influences, resulting in increased stress responses.[25] Multimodal interventions associated with increasing self-efficacy and Internal HLOC and lowering Chance HLOC have been shown to predict better outcomes for patients with chronic back pain.[22] Also, patients with chronic pain can increase their Internal HLOC while still maintaining their positive expectancies related to the impact of the practitioner on their pain. In fact, trust in the practitioner (Powerful Others HLOC) can support the adoption of effective pain management behaviors, and its absence can be detrimental.[26]

Meaning/Beliefs/Illness Perceptions

Developed in response to a particular event or over a lifetime, health beliefs and meanings are adopted on the basis of experience. They support the person's perceptions of (1) their own personal vulnerability to the health concern, (2) the medical and social consequences of being ill or having the health problem, (3) how effective behaviors can be in reducing the risks associated with it, and (4) how barriers can be overcome to adopt those helpful behaviors.[27,28] An individual's beliefs and perspectives about a health problem are learned and evolve from a myriad of sources. Past experiences with health problems, research on the Internet, prior healthcare interactions, and prior injury-related education combine to form a complex system of beliefs about health and pain. Additionally, the meaning the individual attributes to the pain, and the theories of the pain's origins and why it persists are foundational to illness perceptions.

Leventhal's Common-Sense Model of Self-Regulation, also known as the Self-Regulation Model of Illness, centers on the individual's beliefs about the illness threat.[29-31] In studies addressing chronic pain, strong associations exist between specific illness perceptions about pain, function, psychological morbidity, provider-focused frustrations, medication use, and health status.[32-34] Self-regulation, both helpful and hurtful, of illness beliefs is reinforced through every interaction. The ability to strengthen physical self-regulation is achieved through shifts in and refinement of the belief system through positive reinforcement.[35,36] Related to the pain experience, Sauer and colleagues identify four dimensions to address: nociception, pain perception, suffering, and pain behavior.[32] Self-regulatory strength and autonomic nervous system regulation are enhanced, and physical and psychological symptoms improved, through carefully ordered and managed biopsychosocial interventions.[31,32,37] Self-regulation is self-efficacy actualized and can be trained in patients with myofascial pain to improve outcomes.

Cognitive Distortions

Within the category of illness perceptions are cognitive distortions, a concept from Aaron Beck's Cognitive-Behavioral Therapy (CBT),[38] which refer to various biased, exaggerated, or irrational ways of thinking.[39,40] Ineffective thought patterns can lead to and perpetuate anxiety, low self-esteem, low self-efficacy, and depression. Cognitive distortions are experienced by all people and are particularly relevant in the lived experience of the person with persistent pain.[41] Building on meaning and beliefs, cognitive distortions such as somaticizing and catastrophizing are common thought or belief responses to pain that can increase pain behaviors. "Somaticizing tendency is the predisposition to be more aware of, and to worry about common somatic symptoms. It is characterized by (1) a constant scanning of the environment for threats (hypervigilance), (2) a tendency to focus on certain relatively weak and infrequent body sensations, and (3) a predisposition to intensify somatic sensations, making them more alarming, noxious, and disturbing."[27] Catastrophizing is fearing the worst possible outcome of the current concern. Catastrophizing can lead the individual to identify uncomfortable pain experiences as unbearable or impossible.[27] Overgeneralization, where a general conclusion is surmised from a single piece of evidence with the expectation that it will happen over and over again, is highly correlated with disability. Other examples of cognitive distortions include control fallacies (identification as a helpless victim of fate or responsible for everything), filtering (focusing only the negative aspects of a situation), and polarized thinking (the "I am perfect or I am failure" dichotomy with no middle ground to allow for life's complexities).[42,43] A person's maladaptive thinking, belief in, and reliance on cognitive distortions about pain may lead to poor coping, increased pain and suffering, and greater disability.[18]

2.4. Existential-Humanistic Themes

Another mid-century reaction to the impersonal nature of behaviorist learning theories (as well as the deterministic psychotherapy of Sigmund Freud), humanistic psychologists like Abraham Maslow and Carl Rogers stressed the importance of the subjective experience of life with all of its psychological concerns. For the modern clinician, aspects of this branch of psychology can promote a positive therapeutic interaction including patient effort toward growth and improvement and away from pathology and pain.[44]

Patient-Centered Care

Now considered a hallmark of Western biopsychosocial care,[4] the concept of person-centered or patient-centered care was introduced by Carl Rogers decades before Engle.[45,46] Person-centered care contrasts with the historical biomedical model of patriarchal healthcare in which the physician directs care, and the patient is expected to oblige. In person-centered care, healthcare professionals are encouraged to recognize the patients' perspectives, respect their choices, and continually consider their values and goals.[47] Person-centered approaches are not only important in clinical care but show promise for improving research and better-informing clinical education.[48] Person-centered care does, however, have its drawbacks. Patient definitions of successful treatment may be lofty and difficult to achieve.[49] In these cases, the management of expectations may be possible only with persistent education communicated with compassion and understanding.

Nonpathologic Approach

In seemingly stark contrast to the biomedical model, Freud's psychoanalysis, and even CBT to an extent, one humanistic approach to improving health outcomes is focusing on systems that support growth and performance instead of ones that treat or manage pathology. Recognizing the breadth of human experience, humanistic psychology argues for reducing the labeling of thoughts, emotions, and behaviors as pathologic in a healthcare setting.[44,47] Patients worried about clinician judgment of their actions or internal experiences may understandably respond defensively to being told that their thoughts are irrational, that their emotions are exaggerated, and that their behaviors are keeping them in pain. Alternatively, they may also disengage from treatment. Instead, demonstrating understanding that many responses to pain are reasonable, given the situation, a clinician can gently guide patients to focusing on the most helpful responses. Even normalizing the fact that pain is a universal experience of the human condition and that ineffective responses to it are typical can be helpful in reducing the perceived threat of pathology for some patients. Validation and acceptance (see below) can also be helpful tools for applying a nonpathologic approach to helping patients in pain.

Values and Meaning

Personal growth and existential meaning can play a positive role in some patients with painful conditions. Similar to cognitive-behavioral theories, humanistic and existential psychology describe and explore the personal existential philosophies that provide meaning to individuals' lives.[44] Depending on the meaning patients ascribe to their pain, they can experience more distress or improved resilience, even posttraumatic growth.[50] Patients who successfully improve their self-awareness and self-knowledge, who adopt or move toward an internal LOC, and who adapt their behavior to maximize actions that align with their values may experience more personal meaning in their treatment than patients who do not.

2.5. Third-Wave Behavioral Themes

More recently, several other behavioral therapies, born out of the perceived deficiencies of pure behaviorism and CBT, could hold promise in improving outcomes for people with both psychological and physical pain.[51] These newer approaches, including Acceptance and Commitment Therapy,[52] Dialectical Behavioral Therapy,[53,54] and others, depart from classical CBT in that they accept distortive thoughts and negative emotions as a universal part of the human experience, not a departure from mental health that must be corrected to improve outcomes. Integrating many person-centered concepts from a humanist perspective with the effective strategies of CBT, these methods are usually quite palatable to even highly sensitive patients.[55] From this theoretical acceptance of difficult emotions and thoughts, patients are encouraged to note the realities of their internal experiences, allow them, and shift their behaviors toward those that support autonomy and effective navigation of life's inevitable difficulties. Applied to physical pain (and the psychological and emotional pain that so often accompanies physical pain), the following concepts have been shown to help disrupt the connection between fear and avoidance, mitigate catastrophizing, and improve symptoms of depression associated with chronic pain.[51] More research is needed to explore the potential benefits of these psychological approaches in treating patients with painful conditions, including myofascial pain.

Mindfulness and Meditation

A common theme of many third-wave behavioral therapies is the inclusion of a mindfulness and/or meditation component. Both mindfulness and meditation can be effective strategies for improving outcomes for people experiencing myofascial pain. Although related and often used interchangeably, mindfulness is the focus of attention on the present moment, whereas meditation is typically a more formal practice used to train the mind to witness thoughts, emotions, and sensations without attachment or aversion. A variety of methods exist for each, which allows patients to choose one that suits their preferences. Mindfulness training and meditation have been shown to improve pain modulation, reduce perceived pain intensity and unpleasantness, reduce patient reliance on opioids, and reduce sympathetic arousal; both can be effective for assisting in short- and long-term acute and chronic pain management.[56-60] Even when practiced for only 4 days, meditation has been shown to reduce perceived pain intensity by 40% and perceived unpleasantness by 57%.[56]

Acceptance

Psychological acceptance of the experience of pain can be key in both tolerating pain and improving pain and disability outcomes. Furthermore, acceptance as a strategy to improve emotion regulation in response to pain can reduce self and social stigma.[61] Acceptance, like many psychosocial strategies for managing painful conditions, can be easily misunderstood and dismissed. Acceptance is only the acknowledgment of the reality of pain and its consequences.[62-64] It is not submission or surrender to pain, but rather, it is a willingness to integrate it into adaptive and effective behavioral decision-making processes.[64,65] Acceptance strategies can mitigate perceived discomfort and unpleasantness with painful stimulus,[66] and it has been shown to be a helpful psychological tool in the management of chronic pain as well.[67] An outcome measure (the Chronic Pain Acceptance Questionnaire) has been created to help clinicians assess progress toward pain acceptance.[65,68] Curiosity about the particulars of a pain experience (eg, location, quality, timing) and an individual's responses to them is one way to engage an attitude of acceptance in a clinical setting. Gentle curiosity, by nature, focuses attention on the object of interest in a pleasantly anticipatory way (as opposed to anxiety, which is negatively anticipatory) that may reduce urges to ignore, control, or fight the discomfort.

Validation

Validation is more than empathy[69] and is key to developing a therapeutic alliance by creating safety of information sharing by the patient. Superficial validation is simple interest and active listening. Deeper validation happens when clinicians demonstrate that they can see the positive intent behind even ineffective responses to pain (eg, "It makes sense that you wouldn't want to go for walks anymore now that your back hurts so much—your body is just trying to protect itself."). Full validation, coupled with unconditional positive regard and person-centered care, communicates the message that the clinician truly believes that the patient is doing the best he or she can, given the circumstances.[62,63,69] Validation is best used early in establishing a therapeutic alliance to avoid the resistance and patient defensiveness that may occur when strategies focusing on behavioral change are used before establishing validation and mutual understanding.[70,71] From the solid ground of feeling totally understood and accepted as they are, patients can take the first steps toward change. Of course, the level of validation that a clinician can offer during any specific patient interaction is dependent on the clinician's ability to remain grounded in authenticity and genuine compassion while doing so (see Self-Care).[69]

2.6. Sociological Theories

Stigma

Stigma, the disapproval of a person or group based on social characteristics perceived to differentiate them from other members of society, was first considered by Emile Durkheim in the 1890s,[72] and it was further conceptualized as a phenomenon by Erving Goffman in the mid-20th century.[73] Goffman's theory of social stigma laid the groundwork for medical sociology, which supported the labeling of patients with persistent pain as "deviant."[74] This "deviance paradigm" (shame) was confronted by an "oppression paradigm" (blame),[74,75] which rightfully placed attention on those who stigmatized and labeled others, including healthcare providers. Link and Phelan[76] continued the conversation by focusing on power. Power differentials are particularly strong across all aspects of the healthcare experience and are reinforced on macro (health system), meso (organizational), and micro (individual) levels.[77] Stigmatization of illness is a matter of social injustice on a societal level,[78] and it can reduce help-seeking behavior on an individual level.[79] Disease and disability stigma is harmful, distressing, and marginalizing to individuals living with pain and leads to negative outcomes, including distress and social isolation.[80,81]

Attribution Theory

As previously noted, a negative consequence of the biomedical paradigm is that individuals with unexplainable or persistent pain are often stigmatized by clinicians whose care they seek. The stigma in this case may result from blaming patients for their experience, known formally as attribution theory.[82-84] Attribution theory describes how a clinician forms causal judgments on the basis of the assessment of the patient.[85] The practitioner can assign blame and attribute the onset and continued impacts of symptoms to something caused and controlled by the patient. Attributing causation to the patient has been associated with the practitioner demonstrating greater anger and less sensitivity to the patient, which can lead to missed diagnoses, undertreatment, or ineffective treatment protocols, severely damaging the therapeutic relationship and putting the patient at risk.[82,86]

2.7. Complexity of the Psychosocial Experience of Pain

Clearly, no one model or set of psychological concepts is sufficiently broad enough to manage all psychosocial factors associated with painful conditions of any kind. For a century, behavioral therapies have expanded to account for more and more of the human experience of the interplay between inner and outer perception, and they continue to evolve today. Operating from a biopsychosocial perspective requires a genuine understanding of each patient's personal experience, beliefs, and habitual emotional and behavioral responses to pain. Combining this understanding with knowledge of the above concepts can help clinicians understand and address the psychosocial factors of patients' pain that may affect the plan of care or clinical outcomes.

3. PATIENTS LIVING WITH PAIN

3.1. Common Affective Responses to Pain

Individuals living with pain experience a myriad of emotions and emotional responses that can impact their health trajectory. In considering mood, causal pathways have yet to be fully explained. However, low mood is correlated with the occurrence and persistence of pain symptoms, and its impact on the disability that follows appears to be even greater.[27,87] Depression significantly reduces the success of a multidisciplinary treatment of patients with chronic myofascial pain.[88] Emotional depressive symptoms vary from a sense of demoralization and sadness to suicidal tendencies. Differentiation is critical, because treatment varies from support and validation, to talk therapy, to pharmacologic and medical interventions, or a combination of all.

Apart from clinical depression, patients in pain often experience sadness and grief. Sadness is thought to occur after a perceived loss or when life's events deviate from expectations in a negative way.[62,63] In that sense, it is completely rational for the person with unexplained or persistent pain to experience sadness and even grief. Grieving for the loss of past and/or current abilities and activities and anticipatory grieving for the loss of future abilities and dreams should be recognized and honored.

Fear and anxiety are part of the emotional experiences of the majority of patients with persistent pain and are associated with the predisposition to develop trigger points (TrPs).[89] Anxiety and fear are closely related.[90] Fear is a response to a perceived threat and anxiety is future-projected fear.[62,63] Pain itself is a type of danger signal.[91] Patients can fear the effects their pain will have on work performance and expectations, home obligations, hobbies, and future events of all kinds. Kinesiophobia is the specific fear of movement and physical activity, and it is correlated with increased pain and vulnerability. Kinesiophobia can also contribute to fear-avoidant behaviors if it is not addressed.[92]

State and trait anxiety may also play a role for patients with painful conditions. State anxiety is related to an event, whereas trait anxiety is a lifelong pattern, such as generalized anxiety disorder.[89] Symptom presentation of both includes feelings of apprehension, tension, being alarmed/on alert, and physical manifestations including increased muscle tension, pain severity, and the constitutional changes associated with the stress response.[93,94] Unlike depression, Sorrell et al[88] found that patients with chronic musculoskeletal pain and anxiety did as well in a multidisciplinary treatment as those without anxiety.

Anger is an emotional response to an unjust situation or event, which can include the perceived injustice of living with persistent pain.[95] It can be a way of seeking control over feelings of fear and anxiety. Anger plays an important (modifiable) role in the feedback loop of thoughts, emotions, and behaviors. Healthy expression of anger can be an important part of a biopsychosocial treatment plan because inhibition of anger has been associated with higher pain intensity, increased pain behaviors, and lower activity level.[96,97]

Shame can also accompany physical pain in some patients. Shame, known as the "master emotion" due to its profound influence on social interaction, is the intensely uncomfortable feeling of not being enough.[98] Different from guilt ("I did something bad"), shame ("I am bad") is connected not to actions but to personhood.[99,100] The difference between "I'm a terrible person" and "I acted rudely" is that the former represents shame and the latter, guilt. Guilt can be useful in that it motivates reparation. Shame, however, is unproductive and is correlated with addiction, violence, and abuse[99,101,102] and should, therefore, be noted and addressed in any healthcare setting. A common shame verbalization in response to the experience of physical pain is, "I am broken." Reframing shame statements like this one can be helpful in increasing motivation to change and hope in improvement.

Of course, every person who experiences emotions associated with pain will do so in a personal manner. Some patients are more uncomfortable with some negative emotions than others. Some emotions may even be shame-bound for an individual.[99,100] A patient who is ashamed of feeling sad may turn to anger, or even rage, to avoid feeling sadness. Conversely, a patient who perceives anger as intolerably uncomfortable or socially inappropriate may display signs of sadness, even when another person would verbalize righteous indignation at the same event. Identifying and understanding emotions related to pain can be an important part of healing, and incorporating emotion regulation considerations within a treatment plan shows promise in improving outcomes with chronically painful conditions.[103]

3.2. Common Behavioral Responses to Pain

Behaviors are thought to be the conscious and unconscious responses to thoughts and feelings.[35,90,104] Individuals approach medical and health events with personal outlooks, predispositions, and memories. Albert Ellis' Rational Emotive Behavior Therapy demonstrates the connection between the thoughts and emotions of the (a) activating event and the (b) beliefs and behaviors that lead to (c) consequences.[105] The fear-avoidance behavior paradigm posits that thoughts and feelings about pain can lead to maladaptive behaviors and reinforce negative consequences. Pain perceived as nonthreatening may not inhibit engagement in daily activities, whereas thoughts of pain as threatening and harmful often lead to pain-related fear and safety-seeking behaviors. This model has been used to explain why some patients with acute low back pain develop chronic low back pain with associated disability.[90] The fear-avoidance model of musculoskeletal pain has evolved since its inception[92] to include pain severity, pain catastrophizing, attention to pain, escape/avoidance behavior, disability, disuse, and vulnerabilities.[90]

Similarly, patients' behaviors around exercise adherence can be linked to past experiences. Blaming or stigmatizing patients who appear reticent to engage in "active" therapy interventions is unwarranted and ineffective. Humans learn through experience. Reduction in pain-related anxiety predicts improvement in function and adoption of active behaviors. In their study of patients with central sensitization, Wijma and colleagues[106] presented three groupings of behavioral responses of patients with persistent pain: (1) healthy behaviors as defined by the pain experience with no or little fear, with constructive use of techniques (pain acceptance), (2) avoidant behaviors, with greater fear and nonconstructive techniques, and (3) persistence behaviors, defined as pushing through activities to completion despite the perception that the activity is too hard. The second and third groups display overactivity and underactivity responses, respectively.

Support and accountability, or lack thereof, can also impact behavioral responses to painful conditions. Just like the temporary use of a brace can be helpful in healing after an ankle sprain, so too can social bracing improve adherence to, and positive outcomes with, treatment strategies (see below on the therapeutic alliance). In contrast, patients without social support and who feel like no one cares if they get better may become overwhelmed and demotivated to take steps to improve their situation. Motivation and readiness-to-change are paramount to behavioral outcomes and are not static.[106,107] The interrelated components of many psychological and sociological theories within a single pain experience is often quite evident.

3.3. The Experience of Living With Pain

Individuals living with pain (especially when persistent and/or unexplainable) face daily hardships that are often compounded by interactions within the healthcare arena. Practicing within the boundaries of the biomedical model, stigmatization, discrimination, and disrespect of the individual with persistent pain are all disturbingly common. Frequently considered as "baggage" by clinicians, the psychosocial factors that accompany the patient are as significant as the physical ones, and the patient can often perceive the clinician's discomfort with those concerns.

Fragmented treatment episodes are common; chaotic and haphazard treatment experiences are the norm. Sometimes, desperate pleas for help and explanations can elicit labels like "high maintenance," "psych overlay," and "problem patient." These labels, and even the more modern, medicalized words, such as "catastrophizing," "fear-avoidant behaviors," and "somatization," can further alienate the patient and worsen feelings of shame. Intake forms with these words emblazoned on the top can trigger emotional response that may be ineffective in establishing a therapeutic alliance or hope in a new episode of care.

The complexity of relatively nonmodifiable psychosocial variables (eg, the individual's personality, the individual's diagnosed disordered personality),[106] and potentially modifiable variables (eg, access to healthcare, employment responsibilities, financial stressors, life stressors), are interactive. Negative effects on life roles are challenging and include role strain (inconsistencies within a role), role conflict (incompatible requirements between roles), role ambiguity (lack of clarity about expected behavior), and role insufficiency (the inability to fulfill role expectations, obligations, or goals).[108] These stresses compound and can increase pain when perceived task and role demands exceed perceived coping capabilities and abilities.[94] Conversely, underload stress may also occur—feeling unable to make full use of talents and skills because of the limiting force persistent pain and the accompanying loss of time and energy its management requires.

Many patients who feel distressed by, or even incapable of, tolerating a painful condition accrue a laundry list of diagnoses, both mental and physical. The psychology of diagnosis is extremely personal and official medical labels may be helpful or ineffective in a process of recovery, depending on the patient. Despite historical norms of many varied diagnoses under a general category of somatoform disorders, or the newer trend to lump any psychosocial concern into a catch-all of "Somatic Symptom Disorder," adjustment disorder remains the most appropriate, accurate, and acceptable diagnosis for people who are hyperconcerned about their pain.[109]

4. CLINICIANS WHO TREAT PATIENTS LIVING WITH PAIN

4.1. Current Challenges to Practicing Within a Biopsychosocial Model

Many clinicians feel a lack of preparedness to address social and behavioral concerns, and rightly so, because more often than not, neither their entry-level education nor their postprofessional development has equipped them to do so in any concrete way.[7] Others may feel that by asking questions on an intake form about living situations and a question or two about mood, that they are already practicing from as close to a biopsychosocial vantage point as they are willing to go. Some may not want to engage in a more holistic approach after rigorous biomedically specific training, and their practice reflects that.[110-112] Focusing on anatomic concerns and aggressively controlling the human interaction to minimize the patient's thoughts, emotions, and behaviors certainly can be "simpler." The practitioner may feel truly vulnerable and ill-prepared for his or her own emotional responses to a patient's expression of sorrow and suffering. External variables provide even more barriers—healthcare plans, productivity standards, lack of access to care, attempts to "streamline" care—all have the potential to weaken or limit clinicians' abilities to practice from a biopsychosocial perspective.

The biopsychosocially conscious practitioner acknowledges and embraces what can appear to be competing approaches to providing comprehensive care.[113] There is the linear structural causality of the biomedical piece (eg, the presence of myofascial TrPs) and the complexity and recursive aspects of the psychosocial pieces (eg, fear and anxiety, the lack of family support, "failed" prior efforts). The biopsychosocially aware practitioner links the two and designs and manages a treatment plan to support the trajectory of healing and function with the awareness of the often "three steps forward, two steps back" course of care.[4,106] It is often a fine line to tread. The clinician must have the knowledge and working framework of how, and how far, to delve into the patient's psychosocial experiences and the skills to provide an integrated treatment, to know which patients would benefit from referral for psychological or other specialized care, and when, how, and to whom to refer.[114] The clinician is obligated to know his or her own professional limitations and boundaries, and to refer appropriately.

Staying in the biomedical box is no longer an option, because there is ample evidence that clinicians' views are subsumed by patients, and that practicing from a purely biomedical model "teaches" fear-avoidant behaviors.[7,115,116] Given that patients likely come with strong biomedical views based on prior experiences, it is imperative that practitioners understand that their continued focus on that paradigm "is likely to result in poor compliance with evidence-based treatment guidelines, less treatment adherence, and poorer treatment outcomes" especially in terms of functional recovery.[7]

4.2. Clinician Self-Awareness

Poor clinician self-awareness lends itself to poor patient relationships. Behaving differently toward the person with a persistent pain problem may be secondary to the clinician's own prejudice, fear, or indifference.[117] The need to depersonalize, and efforts to evade or circumvent (consciously or not) patients' feelings by interrupting, shifting topics, or disallowing opportunities for broaching sensitive subjects may be rooted in the clinicians' need to distance themselves because of feeling powerless or may simply be a symptom of compassion fatigue.[117,118]

Improving self-awareness is a process and must be practiced. In her text aptly entitled, "Patient Practitioner Interaction: An Experiential Manual for Developing the Art of Health Care," Carol Davis addresses the underlying values practitioners may have that detract from a therapeutic interaction. She includes personal assessment tools for the reader to consider his or her own values to allow for the exploration of personal biases that may affect patient care. Nijs et al[7] present an approach toward effective and evidence-based care for clinicians treating patients with persistent pain. The clinician's first step is self-reflection. Just as patients must acknowledge and address their illness beliefs, clinicians must also address their own perceptions of biomedical versus biopsychosocial interventions. Because evidence demonstrates that clinicians' beliefs about musculoskeletal pain are predictive of treatment recommendations,[119] and that previous treatment by a biomedically oriented clinician is a risk factor for patients with low back pain on long-term leave from work,[120] clinicians must consider their own ineffective beliefs.[7] After self-assessment and adjustments in attitudes and beliefs regarding persistent pain, the clinician can better consider the patient's illness beliefs.[7] Ongoing self-audit is necessary because professional performance is never the same moment to moment.[121] Constant vigilance is a fundamental requirement for professionals who require high reliability in the face of unexpected events.[121] For clinicians who treat patients in pain within a biopsychosocial framework, this professional self-awareness must occur in an emotional realm as well as in the domains of skills and knowledge.

Countertransference

Countertransference refers to the reactions or feelings—positive or negative—that occur when the practitioner unconsciously transfers his or her own needs, desires, fears, or frustrations onto the patient. Engaging in regular self-reflection is needed with all patient interactions, not just the negative ones. The practitioner should consider why some interactions with patients are "good" and others "irritating." Instead of using any insight, or therapeutically helpful reactions, the practitioner may be using responses to label or find fault with the patient. Similarly, stigma and attribution occur in context.[122] Factors that intensify stigma include lower socioeconomic status, living in rural areas, race, gender, and preexisting ideas about a group.[82] As such, stigma and the associated blame ascribed to individuals with pain must also be simultaneously considered with stigma from other "labels."[123] Clinicians can take Internet-based tests to determine their own implicit bias against certain groups of people based on race, age, ability, gender, sexual orientation, and body type. Knowing one's own areas of bias is key to improving and practicing consistent care for all patients. The impact is cumulative or even exponential. Clinicians need to question their own perceptions regarding the attribution or stigma they may be applying to their patients with myofascial pain syndrome.

Discomfort With Negative Emotions

Clinicians who treat patients in pain must practice allowing patients to express negative emotions and to have complex, and sometimes paradoxical, thoughts and feelings about their pain experience.[113,114] According to Jung, "only paradox ... comes anywhere near to comprehending the fullness of life."[124] Painful emotions often accompany physical pain. Unfortunately, in attempts to improve a patient's outlook, clinicians can dismiss and invalidate the expression of difficult emotions from patients ("Oh, don't feel bad, you'll get better!"). Clinicians may even be unaware of their own discomfort with certain emotions. For example, a clinician who values strength and associates the expression of sadness or vulnerability with weakness may implicitly or explicitly require that the patient withhold his or her expression of these feelings, thus jeopardizing the therapeutic alliance and reducing patient motivation to actively engage in treatment. Conversely, a patient's negative reactions, well managed, can actually be used to strengthen the patient–clinician relationship.[125]

4.3. Psychosocial Strategies for Clinical Practice

Focusing on the Sphere of Influence

The challenge for many clinicians is where to start and how to begin this process of managing all of the varied biopsychosocial aspects that may emerge from the initial evaluation of a patient in pain. A variation of Stephen Covey's concept of "circle of concern/circle of influence" can be helpful for organizing and managing the various aspects of patients with complex presentations. Covey introduces this concept in his book, "7 Habits of Highly Effective People."[126] Although it is intended for the application for proactive personal change, a similar approach can be advantageous in helping clinicians develop a conceptual biopsychosocial framework.

In this context, the concept can be depicted with two overlaid objects. The larger, outer one is the Red Zone and includes those aspects of the patient's experience on which the clinician has no direct impact. The smaller, inner area, the green zone, includes those aspects upon which treatment has direct influence. Just as Covey posits that time and energy focused on the inner circle allows for personal growth and development, a clinician should focus time and energy on the aspects of patient's problems that can be affected with available treatment strategies to best effect change across the biopsychosocial continuum. For example, treating myofascial TrPs and postural issues, addressing cognitive distortions and erroneous thoughts, providing strategies for sleep positions and sleep hygiene, and addressing kinesiophobia and fear-avoidance behaviors could all be put into the inner green zone. Focusing interventions on these items enhances the patient's self-efficacy and HLOC. The outer realm includes those things that are outside of the clinician's ability to directly effect change, such as the patient's job situation, grief over an unhappy marriage, and the fact that the patient has had multiple back surgeries. The clinician can and should validate these concerns, empathize, and refer to other professionals as appropriate. Although no concern should be ignored or minimized, attention is best given to those things that can be influenced.

Coupled with the International Classification of Functioning, Disability, and Health model that considers the patient from structure and function (diseases/disorders and impairments), activity (limitations), and participation (restrictions) within the contextual factors of the environment and on a personal level, the clinician can develop a plan of care that has at its forefront the patient's goals, with pathways that include and link the biopsychosocial aspects of care.[127]

Developing an Effective Therapeutic Alliance

The evolution from the paternalistic model of decision-making to the shared decision-making model, and the more appropriately and comprehensively named, patient-centered care model, depends on facilitated therapeutic communication and the clinician's abilities to establish a therapeutic alliance with the patient.[128] Patient-centered care involves "taking into account the patient's desire for information and for sharing decision making and responding appropriately."[113] Founded on the clinician's ability to demonstrate the facilitative behaviors of acceptance ("I care"), genuineness (self-awareness), and empathy (an impartial, but caring understanding of the client's feelings and experiences),[46,129] it requires authenticity from the provider. Development and demonstration depend on the clinician and is clinician-specific. Clinicians with different personalities and communication styles use different approaches to establish an authentic client-centered atmosphere. Effective helpers must have a clear sense of self and their own personal boundaries. Their purpose is to facilitate and assist rather than control, and to be process-oriented and committed to working out solutions, rather than working toward preconceived goals or notions.[117,130]

Boundaries

Boundaries are extremely important for the maintenance of an effective therapeutic alliance between clinician and patient. It is up to the clinician to define his or her limits regarding things like communication, scheduling of appointments, and clinical interaction norms. For example, some clinicians find the use of e-mail or texting between appointments helpful, whereas others find this kind of communication oppressive. One clinician may not mind a patient's expressive use of curse words within the therapeutic interaction, whereas another may be offended. Oftentimes, clinicians learn their limits through trial and error. Resentment or social disgust felt by the clinician is a good signal that a boundary has been breached. Clinicians must stay mindful of internal cues such as resentment, dread, blame, or judgment around any particular patient. If these emotions arise, curious exploration will often elucidate a triggering event. After this event has been identified, communication with the patient to reaffirm the limits of the therapeutic relationship may or may not be necessary. When clinicians fail to set and honor their own personal boundaries with a particular patient or client, the therapeutic alliance will be jeopardized. When clinicians fail to set any clinical boundaries at all, professional burnout is likely.[131] Because boundaries are extremely personal, each clinician must practice self-awareness to establish and reestablish them, because what the clinician may be able to offer can change along with his or her own life circumstances.

Unconditional Positive Regard

Carl Rogers developed the concept of unconditional positive regard as part of his humanist client-centered therapy model.[45,46] Adapted for use in modern healthcare of many varieties,[47] unconditional positive regard may be understood as separating patients from the behaviors they demonstrate, or put colloquially, always "giving the patient the benefit of the doubt." As described above, patients with painful conditions can exhibit frustration, anger, distrust, and other emotions and behaviors that can be challenging in a fast-paced healthcare setting. Verbalizing that these emotional states and ineffective actions are self-protective and, given the circumstances of the patient's situation, completely understandable, can honor the hope of change and improvement. Labeling an individual as a "problem patient" or worse, negatively affects all aspects of the therapeutic relationship. Unconditional positive regard is a powerful antidote against the shame that many people feel when their emotional responses to pain cause further suffering.

Validation

Validation is a key component in establishing the trust that allows for the easy flow of information between patient and clinician. Patients with low back pain have been shown to respond negatively to the invalidation of pain by primary care physicians.[70] One strategy for using validation to respond to patients' verbalized pain reports, thoughts, or emotions may be summed up in two words: "Of course . . ." For example, a patient may verbalize frustration at not being able to lift his toddler due to shoulder pain. The reply, "Of course, you are frustrated by that. You love your daughter and want to be able to soothe her, hold her, and when needed, keep her safe" can be extremely effective in making the patient feel heard and understood. In contrast, the reply, "Don't worry about that—she's a big girl now and you'll be able to lift her again after this treatment" may be perceived as dismissive and pejorative, rather than optimistic and motivational, as intended.

The validation of a patient's feelings, thoughts, and past actions have been seen, clinically, to be invaluable in managing psychosocial distress related to physical pain. Verbalizing understanding that a patient is doing the best he or she can, given the circumstances, can be especially effective for patients who demonstrate a Powerful Others HLOC to increase their willingness to engage in effective pain behaviors. Lastly, recognizing the pervasive use of hyperbolic language in some cultures, clinicians may find that validating the feeling beneath an exaggerated statement more helpful than encouraging the patient to immediately reframe it. A statement like "I just can't take this pain anymore. It's killing me!" could be validated by saying, "It sounds like your pain is really intense and hard to even tolerate." Some patients who mark their pain as a 10/10 on a form are attempting to legitimize their suffering and may just need to feel heard and understood.

Self-Care

Self-care transcends basic hygiene and life-sustaining activities to include tending to the enjoyable aspects of an individual's personal life including creativity, spirituality, pleasure, and recreation, among others. Self-care outside of the clinic is important for both the patient and the clinician. Patient self-care may help mitigate physiologic distress. And because it is an opposing action to self-loathing and helplessness, it can also help reduce feelings of shame, while improving autonomy and strengthening an internal LOC. Clinicians may even instruct patients in basic self-care as part of a home exercise prescription. Tailoring specific self-care strategies to the needs, preferences, and values of the patient are more likely to garner adherence. One starting point for helping a patient craft a self-care plan is to instruct him or her to engage the five senses. Pleasant sensations can help soothe the autonomic nervous system and lift one's mood. Another way to consider self-care is to adopt strategies to improve physical wellness (eg, exercise or stretching), mental wellness (eg, meditation), emotional wellness (eg, practicing gratitude), spiritual wellness (eg, prayer), and social wellness (eg, volunteering). These strategies should align with the individual's values and vary in the amount and type of resource investment required (eg, time, energy, money, social support). For patients who prefer simple mantras, self-care can be described as anything that makes them feel "happy, safe, and good."

Self-care for the clinician is equally important and can improve the ability to empathize with and validate the negative emotions of patients. Because empathy has been shown to reduce with patient exposure,[132] clinicians must be persistent in their efforts to maintain the ability to do the exhausting emotional work of patient care.[118,133] Finally, clinicians who establish healthy boundaries, demonstrate unconditional positive regard, validate emotions, and practice effective self-care model the kinds of healthy behaviors that patients may use to improve distress tolerance, accept pain, and adopt values-based coping strategies.

First Impressions

The importance of the initial evaluation cannot be overstated. Developing the therapeutic alliance is the obligation of the clinician. Using a systematic approach to patient interactions such as the one described by Lyles and colleagues,[134] and introduced by Smith,[135] can be helpful. A 5-step approach to initial encounters with patients begins with (1) setting the stage—meeting the patient and introductions and is followed by (2) setting the agenda—letting the patient know what is going to happen, including the amount of time of that visit. These seemingly obvious steps take only a minute or two, but are often overlooked. Step 3 is nonfocused interviewing, where the patient has an opportunity to respond to an open-ended beginning question. Considering that patients are generally interrupted within the first 12 to 18 seconds of speaking during a medical appointment,[136,137] being provided an opportunity to speak might be a novel, and hopefully positive, experience. Active and focused listening during the nonfocused interview is key. Much can be learned during this time about patients' pain journeys and their prior episodes of care. Aspects of their personality and values can also be noted as well as their thoughts, feelings, and beliefs about their pain experiences. All of these impact the episode of care. Threats and vulnerability may be felt by the patient with regard to the ability to be autonomous, to fulfill roles, to retain life and work goals, and to economic well-being, to name but a few.[138] A comprehensive view of quality of life is subjective, and treatment must be founded on the patient's definition of quality and his or her goals.[139] Step 4 is focused interviewing, during which the clinician asks specific questions to guide the evaluation. And finally Step 5 is a clear transition to the physical examination and assessment. Simple additions to the initial evaluation, such as letting the patient know how much time he or she will have with the clinician and how long the appointment will last, enhance a sense of security and mutual respect.

Clinician as Educator

In addition to the goal of reducing and managing pain, another goal of any episode of care based on biopsychosocial principles should include carefully expanding patients' knowledge of their own body and the pain they experience—including the role of thoughts, emotions, and behaviors. The literature has yet to identify a single accepted term for this education, with therapeutic/pain neuroscience education (TNE and PNE) being most commonly cited. Moseley and Butler introduced the term "curriculum" to more fully capture the comprehensive education that occurs in biopsychosocial management and includes the learner, the deliverer, the message, and the context.[91] The clinician—the deliverer of the information—must be competent to do so. Similar to the practitioners' abilities to demonstrate intervention-based competence, abilities to demonstrate education-based competence is equally critical.[70,91]

Education along with CBT has been shown to be effective, but is not always well received by patients.[140] How and when the information is delivered is critical. Earnest efforts in relaying the concepts of operant conditioning or cognitive distortions can trigger a patient's all-too-familiar feelings of shame and stigma, where they only hear that they are causing their own pain. Education is most effectively initiated through lessons on physiology[37] with an emphasis on first validating the patient's experiences and decisions up to this point in time. Prior to incorporating education, it is vital that the clinician's and patient's attitudes and beliefs must be aligned.[141] Basing initial education on the consequences model, which distinguishes itself by its labeling of psychosocial distress in terms of consequences rather than as causes of physical symptoms, as Zonneveld and colleagues recommend, could be significant in a patient's receptiveness to embrace interventions that include aspects other than the expected physical ones like manual therapy and exercise. As such, clinicians need a basic understanding of a variety of cognitive and behavioral interventions, as well as the ability to incorporate at least a few with some level of comfort and expertise. These strategies are as important as knowledge and resources to refer out when appropriate. Learning how to teach, motivate, and support is a key component of success within a biopsychosocial healthcare model.

Intentional and Therapeutic Communication

Throughout all aspects of an episode of care, and especially during education, clinicians should choose their words carefully and with a goal of reducing fear and anxiety and improving the efficacy of therapeutic communication. Words matter. Most clinicians use metaphors to explain complex medical realities. These explanations can either increase the sense of danger for a patient or quell it.[91,142] Unfortunately, medical terms and the words clinicians use to describe and explain their patient's pain can add to misconceptions and confusion for the patient. Patients are constantly crafting stories about their pain and what is happening to them.[91] The patient who describes his pain as feeling "like I'm being stabbed in the back" not only needs relief from pain, but also needs the knife taken out of his pain story. Medical terms such as "degeneration," "herniation," and "pinched" may trigger fear and danger in a patient depending on his or her previous exposure to such terms. As noted above, even historical terms rooted in psychology and cited in this chapter (eg, cognitive distortions, catastrophizing) can sound judgmental and harsh to a patient. When in doubt, choosing the most accurate and least alarming words when describing a patient's condition ("crowded nerve" instead of "pinched nerve") may be the most effective way in reducing pain and improving functional outcomes related to pain behaviors.

Effective clinical education delivers a message that describes reality, encourages proactivity, and minimizes the patient's anxiety.[71,91,142] The wise clinician modifies language in response to the signs of increased distress during educational explanations. Because a patient's pain story is dynamic and ever evolving, the clinician's role is to help the former develop adaptive beliefs about the relationships between pain, movement, anxiety, and protective behaviors.[71] Individually tailored education programs must be constantly assessed and reassessed on the basis of patient response.

Another important communication strategy to employ is patient-first language when considering patients with persistent pain. Language that identifies patients by pathology or painful body part typifies the detached biomedical paradigm. Referring to an individual as "a fibromyalgia patient," "a chronic pain patient," or "a knee patient" is a counter to person-centered care and can reduce the efficacy of the therapeutic alliance. Clinicians should monitor the language they use to label patients, for labels prioritize the disease over the individual.[143]

5. CLINICAL REASONING

Clinical reasoning is grounded in human perception[71] and must address the complexity of the human experience. A biopsychosocial model should not be used as a reason to ignore biomedical matters. Clinical reasoning must include the reconceptualization of the clinician's and patient's attitudes and beliefs to narrow the gap and allow for alignment of beliefs between the two prior to incorporating education.[7] Several models exist to conceptualize both clinical reasoning processes and development and include the whole patient. Collier et al[144] presented a new model of clinical reasoning development demonstrating the trajectory from novice to expert clinician across the three areas of logic (diagnostic, contextual, and management thinking), performance (skill, time, and efficiency), and presence (rapport, confidence, therapist identity). This model supports the development of the interrelated clinical reasoning aspects of thinking, doing, and being as part of the biopsychosocial evaluation.

Edwards et al separated clinical reasoning into two major clinical strategies: diagnosis and management. They discuss the aspects of diagnostic reasoning strategy, narrative (inductive) reasoning, that is most focused on the patient's experience and beliefs, contextualized by social and environmental factors and combined with diagnostic (deductive) reasoning around physical impairments, symptoms, and physiologic mechanisms.[145] The management strategy is made up of interactive reasoning, collaborative reasoning, reasoning about procedures, reasoning about teaching, predictive reasoning, and ethical reasoning.

Biopsychosocial assessments incorporate somatic (bottom up) and psychosocial (top down) factors.[89,106] Speckens and vanRood[146] presented the SCEBS model for treating patients with unexplained physical symptoms. On the basis of CBT, the model addressed the following five factors for consideration: S: somatic and medical, C: cognitive (pain perceptions and beliefs), E: emotional (anxiety, fear of movement, anger, depressive feeling, stress), B: behavioral (operant conditioning, focusing on effective behaviors), and S: social. Wijma and colleagues added two factors to this model in 2016—identifying the type of pain (nociceptive, neuropathic, or nonneuropathic central sensitization) and motivation for change (Type of Pain + SCEBS model + Motivation).

Within the realm of clinical reasoning and persistent pain, stereotype-based bias must be addressed. Burgess and colleagues[147] identified two sets of cognitive processes that contribute to clinical judgment including evidence-based processes that are situation-specific, conscious, logical, effortful, and intuitive that are less situation-bound, almost automatic, affect-laden, and include clinicians' explicit and implicit biases. Intuition can be an excellent tool but is best utilized by the expert clinician because effective intuition is developed with experience and repeated exposure to large numbers of patients.[148] Biases, however, often hidden or minimized by colleagues, impact decision-making about pain[149] and can lead to negative outcomes. Bias is often perceptible to patients and serves as a barrier to quality care, increasing vulnerability to alienation and shame.[150]

The Use of Outcome Measures

Accurate evaluation of the biopsychosocial elements of a patient's pain presentation is important for any medical encounter. The use of validated surveys and questionnaires to garner more information to guide treatment and assess outcomes is helpful and recommended. One consideration, apart from the appropriate selection of these tools, is how a form appears from the patient's perspective when given with no context, sometimes even prior to meeting a clinician. The Pain Catastrophizing Scale,[151] although useful, is one example of a questionnaire with a title that may trigger a patient's real or perceived discrimination from the "powerful other" healthcare provider and may, therefore, exacerbate the internalized feelings of being burdensome, incapacitated, or powerless. It reduces the likelihood that the patient will follow through with suggested options for emotional or medical support, resulting in poorer long-term psychological and physical health problems for people with persistent pain.[152] Omitting the title(s) from these questionnaires can help avoid these challenges.[106]

5.1. Multimodal Treatment Strategies

Interventions that target single domains—physical only, psychological only—are less effective than multimodal ones.[153,154] Mind and body practices are a large and diverse group of techniques (National Center for Complementary and Alternative Medicine for the NIH). Combining manual therapy and exercise with PNE is more effective than when education is presented alone.[155,156] Integrating education pieces with active, movement-based strategies can be beneficial because they can reinforce each other; however, inconsistent messages between the two may adversely impact movement.[37] "Pain neuroscience education (PNE) alters the threat value of movement, while subsequent movement confirms or refutes this new belief while providing repeated sensory inputs required for creating enduring shifts in the autonomic movement and stress response."[37] In their review, Puentedura and Flynn[156] stated, "providing manual therapy within a PNE context can be seen as meeting or perhaps enhancing patient expectations, and also refreshing or sharpening body schema maps within the brain. Ideally, all of this should lead to better outcomes in patients".

Practitioner education, training, and mentoring for how to combine and deliver optimal physical and psychosocial interventions is needed and is paramount to the success of delivering integrated care models.[113,157,158] In a systematic review of the efficacy of PNE on musculoskeletal pain, Louw and colleagues[155] identified the benefits of reduced pain, improved patient knowledge of pain, improved function, lower disability, reduced impact of psychosocial factors, enhanced movement, and less healthcare utilization. Models of intervention varied from Physical Therapy-delivered one-on-one sessions to group sessions to patient-read options. There were no instances of the treatment group faring worse than the control group, which supports a risk-benefit ratio in favor of integrated models.[155] CBT-based techniques include distraction, imagery, motivational self-talk, relaxation training, biofeedback, the development of coping strategies, goal setting, and changing maladaptive beliefs about pain. CBT interventions are based on the view that an individual's beliefs, evaluation, and interpretation about his or her health condition, in addition to pain, disability, and coping abilities, impact the degree of both physical and emotional disability of the pain condition.

An understandable challenge to assessing the effectiveness of integrated interventions is the requirement that they be standardized, mandatory, and prescriptive, with home practice "dosage" (ie, the practice of skills like progressive muscle relaxation or distraction techniques) also standardized. Although necessary for measuring outcomes, it is antithetical to the biopsychosocial focus of individually tailored plans of care.

5.2. The Role of Referral

Referral is an important tool for any musculoskeletal clinician who practices from a biopsychosocial perspective. Just like any clinical strategy, referral can be both under- and overutilized. Many orthopedic clinicians are reticent to implement any psychosocial strategies for fear of overstepping professional margins. But evidence supports musculoskeletal clinician-delivered psychological interventions within the practice context.[155,157-161] Of course, swift referral is the most appropriate action for patients with high levels of psychological or emotional distress that feel unmanageable for either patient or clinician or that might result in harm to the patient or others. And patients with diagnosed psychological disorders should be monitored and managed by a mental health professional or team. Suggesting referral at the patient's first mention of psychological distress, however, can damage the therapeutic alliance and deter further divulgence of information related to a patient's experience that could impact the plan of care. Referral simply to reduce the risk of clinician liability does not necessarily produce the most effective patient outcomes. Clinically, it has been seen that effective referrals occur after the establishment of a sound therapeutic alliance and after the patient has acknowledged an interest in, and willingness toward, further treatment as presented by the clinician.

6. CONCLUSION

Clearly, the topic of psychosocial considerations for treating patients with painful conditions is too broad for a single chapter or book. This chapter merely highlights a few potentially helpful concepts and strategies. Because no psychosocial treatment intervention will work for every patient, clinical reasoning must be applied to each individual patient case to select strategies, assess outcomes, and modify the plan of care as needed. The biopsychosocially oriented clinician fosters seven key psychosocial aspects in daily practice: developing self-awareness as a result of ongoing self-audits, creating trust and minimizing countertransference, cultivating empathic curiosity, recognizing bias and attribution, educating emotions and tolerating uncertainty, using informed intuition, and effectively communicating the clinical plan and evidence.[4] Increasing patients' self-regulatory strengths should underpin all treatment interventions. For patients living with persistent pain, "It is exceedingly difficult to maintain hope and optimism if one is plagued by self-doubt in one's ability to influence events and convinced of the futility of effort."[162]

Providing an environment of support and accountability that fosters strengthening self-efficacy and healthy behaviors, and providing opportunities to redirect attention toward education and empowerment can all help improve pain and functional outcomes. Activities and beliefs are mutually positively reinforcing. Whether using physical, cognitive, motivational, or emotional strategies to augment the treatment of myofascial pain and dysfunction, clinicians should strive to maintain a positive therapeutic alliance, stay in the circle of influence, and increase patients' self-regulatory strength to improve progress toward functional goals and overall quality of life.

References

1. Melzack R, Wall PD. Pain mechanisms: a new theory. *Science.* 1965;150(3699):971-979.
2. Melzack R, Wall PD. The gate control theory of pain. *Br Med J.* 1978;2(6137):586-587.
3. Engel GL. The need for a new medical model: a challenge for biomedicine. *Science.* 1977;196(4286):129-136.
4. Borrell-Carrio F, Suchman AL, Epstein RM. The biopsychosocial model 25 years later: principles, practice, and scientific inquiry. *Ann Fam Med.* 2004;2(6):576-582.
5. von Bertalanffy L. *Perspectives on General Systems Theory.* New York, NY: George Braziller Inc; 1975.
6. Morris TH, Zadow M, Watts ER, Hewitt A. The knowledge: practice gap in physiotherapy practice: a clinical audit of the assessment and management of chronic low back pain within outpatient physiotherapy practice. *Int J Ther Rehabil Res.* 2015;4(4):61-66.
7. Nijs J, Roussel N, Paul van Wilgen C, Koke A, Smeets R. Thinking beyond muscles and joints: therapists' and patients' attitudes and beliefs regarding chronic musculoskeletal pain are key to applying effective treatment. *Man Ther.* 2013;18(2):96-102.
8. Dewsbury DA. In celebration of the centennial of Ivan P. Pavlov's (1897/1902) The Work of the Digestive Glands. *Am Psychol.* 1997;52(9):933-935.
9. Madden VJ, Harvie DS, Parker R, et al. Can pain or hyperalgesia be a classically conditioned response in humans? A systematic review and meta-analysis. *Pain Med.* 2016;17(6):1094-1111.
10. Skinner BF. *Science and Human Behavior.* New York, NY: Macmillan; 1953.
11. Fordyce WE. *Behavioral Methods for Chronic Pain and Illness.* St. Louis, MO: Mosby; 1976.
12. Fordyce WE. Psychological factors in the failed back. *Int Disabil Stud.* 1988;10(1):29-31.
13. Fowler RS, Fordyce WE, Berni R. Operant conditioning in chronic illness. *Am J Nurs.* 1969;69(6):1226-1228.
14. Gatzounis R, Schrooten MG, Crombez G, Vlaeyen JW. Operant learning theory in pain and chronic pain rehabilitation. *Curr Pain Headache Rep.* 2012;16(2):117-126.
15. Bandura A. *Self-Efficacy in Changing Societies.* Cambridge, NY: Cambridge University Press; 1997.
16. Martinez-Calderon J, Zamora-Campos C, Navarro-Ledesma S, Luque-Suarez A. The role of self-efficacy on the prognosis of chronic musculoskeletal pain: a systematic review. *J Pain.* 2018;19(1):10-34.
17. Bandura A. *Self-Efficacy: The Exercise of Control.* New York, NY: Freeman; 1997.
18. Turk DC, Monarch ES. Biopsychosocial perspective on chronic pain. In: Turk DC, Gatche RJ, eds. *Psychological Approaches to Pain Management: A Practitioner's Handbook.* 2nd ed. New York, NY: Guilford Press; 2002:3-30.
19. Rotter JB. Generalized expectancies for internal versus external control of reinforcement. *Psychol Monogr.* 1966;80(1):1-28.
20. Rotter JB. Some problems and misconceptions related to the construct of internal versus external control of reinforcement. *J Consult Clin Psychol.* 1975;43(1):56-67.
21. Walston KA, Walston BS. Who is responsible for your health: the construct of health locus of control. In: Sanders G, Suis J, eds. *Social Psychology of Health and Illness.* Hillsdale, NJ: Lawrence Erlbaum and Associates; 1982:65-95.
22. Keedy NH, Keffala VJ, Altmaier EM, Chen JJ. Health locus of control and self-efficacy predict back pain rehabilitation outcomes. *Iowa Orthop J.* 2014;34:158-165.
23. Bonetti D, Johnstone M, Rodriguez-Marin J, et al. Dimensions of perceived control: a factor analysis of three measures and an examination of their

23. relation to activity level and mood in a student and cross-cultural patient sample. *Psychol Health*. 2001;16(6):655-674.
24. Pucheu S, Consoli SM, D'Auzac C, Francais P, Issad B. Do health causal attributions and coping strategies act as moderators of quality of life in peritoneal dialysis patients? *J Psychosom Res*. 2004;56(3):317-322.
25. Bollini AM, Walker EF, Hamann S, Kestler L. The influence of perceived control and locus of control on the cortisol and subjective responses to stress. *Biol Psychol*. 2004;67(3):245-260.
26. Brincks AM, Feaster DJ, Burns MJ, Mitrani VB. The influence of health locus of control on the patient-provider relationship. *Psychol Health Med*. 2010;15(6):720-728.
27. Vargas-Prada S, Coggon D. Psychological and psychosocial determinants of musculoskeletal pain and associated disability. *Best Pract Res Clin Rheumatol*. 2015;29(3):374-390.
28. Janz NK, Becker MH. The Health Belief Model: a decade later. *Health Educ Q*. 1984;11(1):1-47.
29. Leventhal H, Cameron L. Behavioral theories and the problems of compliance. *Patient Educ Couns*. 1987;10(2):117-138.
30. Cameron LD, Leventhal H. Self-regulation, health, and illness: an overview. In: Cameron LD, Leventhal H, eds. *The Self-Regulation of Health and Illness Behaviour*. London, England: Routledge; 2003:1-14.
31. Cameron LD, Jago L. Emotion regulation interventions: a common-sense model approach. *Br J Health Psychol*. 2008;13(pt 2):215-221.
32. Sauer SE, Burris JL, Carlson CR. New directions in the management of chronic pain: self-regulation theory as a model for integrative clinical psychology practice. *Clin Psychol Rev*. 2010;30(6):805-814.
33. Hill S, Dziedzic K, Thomas E, Baker SR, Croft P. The illness perceptions associated with health and behavioural outcomes in people with musculoskeletal hand problems: findings from the North Staffordshire Osteoarthritis Project (NorStOP). *Rheumatology (Oxford)*. 2007;46(6):944-951.
34. Hale ED, Treharne GJ, Kitas GD. The common-sense model of self-regulation of health and illness: how can we use it to understand and respond to our patients' needs? *Rheumatology (Oxford)*. 2007;46(6):904-906.
35. Cameron LD, Moss-Morris R. Illness-related cognitions and behaviour. In: French D, Vedhara K, Kaptein AA, Weinman JA, eds. *Health Psychology*. 2nd ed. Oxford, England: Blackwell; 2010.
36. Leventhal H, Bodnar-Deren S, Breland JY, et al. Modeling health and illness behavior: the approach of the common-sense model. In: Baum A, Revenson T, Singer J, eds. *Handbook of Health Psychology*. 2nd ed. New York, NY: Erlbaum; 2011.
37. Blickenstaff C, Pearson N. Reconciling movement and exercise with pain neuroscience education: a case for consistent education. *Physiother Theory Pract*. 2016;32(5):396-407.
38. Beck AT. *Cognitive Therapy and the Emotional Disorders*. Madison, CT: International University Press Inc; 1975.
39. Bowie CR, Gupta M. Addressing cognitive distortions, dysfunctional attitudes, and low engagement in cognitive remediation. In: Medalia A, Bowie CR, eds. *Cognitive Remediation to Improve Functional Outcomes*. New York, NY: Oxford University Press; 2016:138-154.
40. Smith TW, Follick MJ, Ahern DK, Adams A. Cognitive distortion and disability in chronic low back pain. *Cognit Ther Res*. 1986;10(2):201-210.
41. Winterowd C, Beck AT, Gruener D. *Cognitive Therapy With Chronic Pain Patients*. New York, NY: Springer Publishing Company; 2003.
42. Leahy R. *Cognitive Therapy Techniques: A Practitioner's Guide*. 2nd ed. New York, NY: Guilford Press; 2017.
43. McKay M, Fanning P. *Self-Esteem: A Proven Program of Cognitive Techniques for Assessing, Improving, and Maintaining Your Self-Esteem*. New York, NY: New Harbinger Publications; 2016.
44. Schneider KT, Pierson JF, Bugental JF. *The Handbook of Humanistic Psychology: Theory, Research, and Practice*. 2nd ed. Thousand Oaks, CA: Sage Publications; 2015.
45. Rogers C, Kramer PD. *On Becoming a Person: A Therapist's view of Psychotherapy*. 2nd ed. Wilmington, DE: Mariner Books; 1995.
46. Rogers CR, Stevens B, Gendlin ET, Shlien JM, Van Dusen W. *Person to Person: The Problem of Being Human: A New Trend in Psychology*. Lafayette, CA: Real People Press; 1967.
47. Nay R. *Person Centered Care. Older People: Issues and Innovations in Care*. Australia: Elsevier; 2009.
48. Masi AT, White KP, Pilcher JJ. Person-centered approach to care, teaching, and research in fibromyalgia syndrome: justification from biopsychosocial perspectives in populations. *Semin Arthritis Rheum*. 2002;32(2):71-93.
49. O'Brien EM, Staud RM, Hassinger AD, et al. Patient-centered perspective on treatment outcomes in chronic pain. *Pain Med*. 2010;11(1):6-15.
50. Barskova T, Oesterreich R. Post-traumatic growth in people living with a serious medical condition and its relations to physical and mental health: a systematic review. *Disabil Rehabil*. 2009;31(21):1709-1733.
51. Linton SJ. Applying dialectical behavior therapy to chronic pain: a case study. *Scand J Pain*. 2010;1(1):50-54.
52. Hayes SC, Strosahl KD, Wilson KG. *Acceptance and Commitment Therapy: The Process and Practice of Mindful Change*. 2nd ed. New York, NY: The Guilford Press; 2016.
53. Linehan MM. *DBT® Skills Training Manual*. 2nd ed. New York, NY: The Guilford Press; 2014.
54. Dijk SV. *Calming the Emotional Storm: Using Dialectical Behavior Therapy Skills to Manage Your Emotions and Balance Your Life*. Oakland, CA: New Harbinger Publications; 2012.
55. Aron EN. *Psychotherapy and the Highly Sensitive Person: Improving Outcomes for That Minority of People Who Are the Majority of Clients*. 1st ed. London, England: Routledge; 2010.
56. Zeidan F, Martucci KT, Kraft RA, Gordon NS, McHaffie JG, Coghill RC. Brain mechanisms supporting the modulation of pain by mindfulness meditation. *J Neurosci*. 2011;31(14):5540-5548.
57. Zgierska AE, Burzinski CA, Cox J, et al. Mindfulness meditation and cognitive behavioral therapy intervention reduces pain severity and sensitivity in opioid-treated chronic low back pain: pilot findings from a randomized controlled trial. *Pain Med*. 2016;17(10):1865-1881.
58. Hilton L, Hempel S, Ewing BA, et al. Mindfulness meditation for chronic pain: systematic review and meta-analysis. *Ann Behav Med*. 2017;51(2):199-213.
59. Tang YY, Ma Y, Fan Y, et al. Central and autonomic nervous system interaction is altered by short-term meditation. *Proc Natl Acad Sci U S A*. 2009;106(22):8865-8870.
60. Panta P. The possible role of meditation in myofascial pain syndrome: a new hypothesis. *Indian J Palliat Care*. 2017;23(2):180-187.
61. Lamar S, Wiatrowski S, Lewis-Driver S. Acceptance & commitment therapy: an overview of techniques and applications. *JSSM*. 2014;7(3):216-221.
62. Linehan M. *Cognitive-Behavioral Treatment of Borderline Personality Disorder*. New York, NY: The Guildord Press; 1993.
63. Linehan MM. *Skills Training Manual for Treating Borderline Personality Disorder*. New York, NY: The Guilford Press; 1993.
64. Hayes SC, Jacobson NS, Follette VM, Dougher MJ. *Acceptance and Change: Content and Context in Psychotherapy*. Reno, NV: Context Press; 1994.
65. McCracken LM, Vowles KE, Eccleston C. Acceptance of chronic pain: component analysis and a revised assessment method. *Pain*. 2004;107(1-2):159-166.
66. Gutierrez O, Luciano C, Rodriguez M, Fink B. Comparison between an acceptance-based and a cognitive-control-based protocol for coping with pain. *Behav Ther*. 2004;35(4):767-784.
67. McCracken LM, Eccleston C. Coping or acceptance: what to do about chronic pain? *Pain*. 2003;105(1-2):197-204.
68. McCracken LM, Vowles KE, Eccleston C. Acceptance-based treatment for persons with complex, long standing chronic pain: a preliminary analysis of treatment outcome in comparison to a waiting phase. *Behav Res Ther*. 2005;43(10):1335-1346.
69. Linehan MM. Validation and psychotherapy. In: Bohart A, Greenber L, eds. *Empathy Reconsidered: New Directions in Psychotherapy*. Washington, DC: American Psychological Association; 1997:353-392.
70. Evers S, Hsu C, Sherman KJ, et al. Patient perspectives on communication with primary care physicians about chronic low back pain. *Perm J*. 2017;21:16-177.
71. Darlow B, Dowell A, Baxter GD, Mathieson F, Perry M, Dean S. The enduring impact of what clinicians say to people with low back pain. *Ann Fam Med*. 2013;11(6):527-534.
72. Durkheim E. *Rules of Sociological Method*. New York, NY: The Free Press; 1982.
73. Goffman E. *Notes on Management of a Spoiled Identity*. New York, NY: Simon and Schuster; 1963.
74. Scambler G. Health-related stigma. *Sociol Health Illn*. 2009;31(3):441-455.
75. Thomas C. *Sociologics of Disability and Illness: Contested Ideas in Disability Studies and Medical Sociology*. Basingstoke, England: Palgrave Macmillan; 2007.
76. Link BG, Phelan JC. Conceptualizing stigma. *Ann Rev Sociol*. 2001;27:363-385.
77. Pescosolido BA, Martin JK, Lang A, Olafsdottir S. Rethinking theoretical approaches to stigma: a Framework Integrating Normative Influences on Stigma (FINIS). *Soc Sci Med*. 2008;67(3):431-440.
78. Corrigan PW. Beating stigma? Augment good intentions with the critical eye. *Stigma Health*. 2016;1(1):1-2.
79. Clement S, Schauman O, Graham T, et al. What is the impact of mental health-related stigma on help-seeking? A systematic review of quantitative and qualitative studies. *Psychol Med*. 2015;45(1):11-27.
80. Corrigan PW, Kosylук KA. Mental illness stigma: types, constructs, and vehicles for change. In: Corrigan PW, ed. *The Stigma of Disease and Disability: Understanding Causes and Overcoming Injustices*. Washington, DC: American Psychological Association; 2014:35-56.
81. Goldberg DS. On stigma & health. *J Law Med Ethics*. 2017;45:475-486.
82. Cronan SB, Key KD, Vaughn AA. Beyond the dichotomy: modernizing stigma categorization. *Stigma Health*. 2016;1(4):225-243.
83. Weiner B. An attributional theory of achievement motivation and emotion. *Psychol Rev*. 1985;92(4):548-573.
84. Weiner B, Perry RP, Magnusson J. An attributional analysis of reactions to stigmas. *J Pers Soc Psychol*. 1988;55(5):738-748.
85. Fiske ST, Taylor SE. *Social Cognition*. 2nd ed. New York, NY: McGraw-Hill; 1991.
86. Stump TK, LaPergola CC, Cross NA, Else-Quest NM. The measure of disease-related stigma: construction, validation, and application across three disease contexts. *Stigma Health*. 2016;1(2):87-100.
87. Pincus T, Vogel S, Burton AK, Santos R, Field AP. Fear avoidance and prognosis in back pain: a systematic review and synthesis of current evidence. *Arthritis Rheum*. 2006;54(12):3999-4010.
88. Sorrell M, Flanagan W, McCall J. The effect of depression and anxiety on the success of multidisciplinary treatment of chronic resistant myofascial pain. *J Musculoskelet Pain*. 2003;11(1):17-20.
89. Vidor LP, Torres IL, Medeiros LF, et al. Association of anxiety with intracortical inhibition and descending pain modulation in chronic myofascial pain syndrome. *BMC Neurosci*. 2014;15:42.
90. Leeuw M, Goossens ME, Linton SJ, Crombez G, Boersma K, Vlaeyen JW. The fear-avoidance model of musculoskeletal pain: current state of scientific evidence. *J Behav Med*. 2007;30(1):77-94.
91. Butler D, Moseley L. *Explain Pain Super Charged*. Adelaide, Australia: NOI Group; 2017.
92. Vlaeyen JW, Linton SJ. Fear-avoidance and its consequences in chronic musculoskeletal pain: a state of the art. *Pain*. 2000;85(3):317-332.

93. Vedolin GM, Lobato VV, Conti PC, Lauris JR. The impact of stress and anxiety on the pressure pain threshold of myofascial pain patients. *J Oral Rehabil.* 2009;36(5):313-321.
94. Selye H. *The Stress of Life.* New York, NY: McGraw-Hill; 1984.
95. Kerns RD, Rosenberg R, Jacob MC. Anger expression and chronic pain. *J Behav Med.* 1994;17(1):57-67.
96. Burns JW, Gerhart JI, Bruehl S, et al. Anger arousal and behavioral anger regulation in everyday life among patients with chronic low back pain: relationships to patient pain and function. *Health Psychol.* 2015;34(5):547-555.
97. Burns JW, Quartana P, Gilliam W, et al. Effects of anger suppression on pain severity and pain behaviors among chronic pain patients: evaluation of an ironic process model. *Health Psychol.* 2008;27(5):645-652.
98. Scheff TJ, Retzinger S. Shame as the master emotion of everyday life; 2000. https://www.researchgate.net/publication/286785601_Shame_as_the_master_emotion_of_everyday_life
99. Brown B. *Men, Women and Worthiness: The Experience of Shame and the Power of Being Enough.* Sounds True; 2012.
100. Brown B. *The Gifts of Imperfection.* Center City, MN: Hazeldon; 2010.
101. Dearing RL, Stuewig J, Tangney JP. On the importance of distinguishing shame from guilt: relations to problematic alcohol and drug use. *Addict Behav.* 2005;30(7):1392-1404.
102. Violence: Our deadly epidemic and its causes. National Criminal Justice Reference Service; 1996. https://www.ncjrs.gov/App/Publications/abstract.aspx?ID=162700
103. Ben-Ami N. Outcomes in distressed patients with chronic low back pain: subgroup analysis of a clinical trial. *J Orthop Sports Phys Ther.* 2018;0(0):1-5.
104. Leventhal H, Brissette I, Leventhal EA. The common-sense model of self-regulation of health and illness. In: Cameron LD, Leventhal H, eds. *The Self-Regulation of Health and Illness Behaviour.* London, England: Routledge; 2003:42-65.
105. Ellis A, Harper RA, Powers M. *A Guide to Rational Living.* 3rd ed. North Hollywood, CA: Wilshire Book Company; 1975.
106. Wijma AJ, van Wilgen CP, Meeus M, Nijs J. Clinical biopsychosocial physiotherapy assessment of patients with chronic pain: the first step in pain neuroscience education. *Physiother Theory Pract.* 2016;32(5):368-384.
107. Fair SE. *Wellness and Physical Therapy.* Sudbury, MA: Jones & Bartlett Learning; 2009.
108. Macionis J. *Sociology.* 4th ed. Englewood Cliffs, NJ: Prentice Hall; 1993.
109. Katz J, Rosenbloom BN, Fashler S. Chronic pain, psychopathology, and DSM-5 somatic symptom disorder. *Can J Psychiatry.* 2015;60(4):160-167.
110. Daykin AR, Richardson B. Physiotherapists' pain beliefs and their influence on the management of patients with chronic low back pain. *Spine (Phila Pa 1976).* 2004;29(7):783-795.
111. LE Laekeman MA, Sitter H, Basler HD. The pain attitudes and beliefs scale for physiotherapists: psychometric properties of the German version. *Clin Rehabil.* 2008;22(6):564-575.
112. Oostendorp RA, Elvers H, Mikolajewska E, et al. Manual physical therapists' use of biopsychosocial history taking in the management of patients with back or neck pain in clinical practice. *Sci World J.* 2015;2015:170463.
113. Sanders T, Foster NE, Bishop A, Ong BN. Biopsychosocial care and the physiotherapy encounter: physiotherapists' accounts of back pain consultations. *BMC Musculoskelet Disord.* 2013;14:65.
114. Afrell M, Rudebeck CE. 'We got the whole story all at once': physiotherapists' use of key questions when meeting patients with long-standing pain. *Scand J Caring Sci.* 2010;24(2):281-289.
115. Cottrell E, Roddy E, Foster NE. The attitudes, beliefs and behaviours of GPs regarding exercise for chronic knee pain: a systematic review. *BMC Fam Pract.* 2010;11:4.
116. Darlow B, Fullen BM, Dean S, Hurley DA, Baxter GD, Dowell A. The association between health care professional attitudes and beliefs and the attitudes and beliefs, clinical management, and outcomes of patients with low back pain: a systematic review. *Eur J Pain.* 2012;16(1):3-17.
117. Davis C. *Patient Practitioner Interaction: An Experiential Manual for Developing the Art of Health Care.* 5th ed. Thorofare, NJ: SLACK; 2011.
118. Figley CR. Compassion fatigue: psychotherapists' chronic lack of self care. *J Clin Psychol.* 2002;58(11):1433-1441.
119. Houben RM, Gijsen A, Peterson J, de Jong PJ, Vlaeyen JW. Do health care providers' attitudes towards back pain predict their treatment recommendations? Differential predictive validity of implicit and explicit attitude measures. *Pain.* 2005;114(3):491-498.
120. Reme SE, Hagen EM, Eriksen HR. Expectations, perceptions, and physiotherapy predict prolonged sick leave in subacute low back pain. *BMC Musculoskelet Disord.* 2009;10:139.
121. Weick KE, Sutcliffe KM. *Managing the Unexpected: Assuring High Performance in the Age of Complexity.* San Francisco, CA: Jossey-Bass; 2008.
122. Tummula A, Roberts LW. Ethics conflicts in rural communities: stigma and illness. In: Nelson WA, ed. *Handbook for Rural Healthcare Ethics: A Practical Guide for Professionals.* Lebanon, NH: Dartmouth College Press; 2009.
123. Brown RL. Functional limitation and depressive symptomatology: considering perceived stigma and discrimination within a stress and coping framework. *Stigma Health.* 2017;2(2):98-109.
124. Jung CG. *The Collected Works of C.G. Jung: Aion.* Vol 9ii. Princeton, NJ: Princeton University Press; 1959.
125. Epstein RM. Mindful practice. *JAMA.* 1999;282(9):833-839.
126. Covey SR. *The 7 Habits of Highly Effective People: Powerful Lessons in Personal Change.* New York, NY: Simon & Schuster; 1989.
127. Escorpizo R, Stucki G, Cieza A, Davis K, Stumbo T, Riddle DL. Creating an interface between the International Classification of Functioning, Disability and Health and physical therapist practice. *Phys Ther.* 2010;90(7):1053-1063.
128. Vranceanu AM, Cooper C, Ring D. Integrating patient values into evidence-based practice: effective communication for shared decision-making. *Hand Clin.* 2009;25(1):83-96, vii.
129. Csillik AS. Understanding motivational interviewing effectiveness: contributions from Rogers' client-centered approach. *Humanist Psychol.* 2013;41(4):350-363.
130. Coombs AW. *Florida Studies in the Helping Professions.* Gainesville, FL: University of Florida Press; 1969.
131. Patti A. Fired up or burned out? Understanding the importance of professional boundaries in home healthcare and hospice. *Home Healthcare Now.* 2009;27(10):590-597.
132. Sherman JJ, Cramer A. Measurement of changes in empathy during dental school. *J Dent Educ.* 2005;69(3):338-345.
133. Barnett JE, Baker EK, Elman NS, Schoener GR. In pursuit of wellness: the self-care imperative. *Prof Psychol Res Pract.* 2007;38(6):603-612.
134. Lyles JS, Dwamena FC, Lein C, Smith RC. Evidence-based patient-centered interviewing. *J Clin Outcomes Manage.* 2001;8(7):28-34.
135. Smith R. *The Patient's Story: Integrated Patient-Doctor Interviewing.* Boston, MA: Little, Brown; 1996.
136. Beckman HB, Frankel RM. The effect of physician behavior on the collection of data. *Ann Intern Med.* 1984;101(5):692-696.
137. Rhoades DR, McFarland KF, Finch WH, Johnson AO. Speaking and interruptions during primary care office visits. *Fam Med.* 2001;33(7):528-532.
138. Larsen PD, Ludkin IM. *Chronic Illness: Impact and Intervention.* 7th ed. Boston, MA: Jones and Bartlett Publishers; 2009.
139. Schmidt SG. Recognizing potential barriers to setting and achieving effective rehabilitation goals for patients with persistent pain. *Physiother Theory Pract.* 2016;32(5):415-426.
140. Zonneveld LN, van 't Spijker A, Passchier J, van Busschbach JJ, Duivenvoorden HJ. The effectiveness of a training for patients with unexplained physical symptoms: protocol of a cognitive behavioral group training and randomized controlled trial. *BMC Public Health.* 2009;9:251.
141. Nijs J, Torres-Cueco R, van Wilgen CP, et al. Applying modern pain neuroscience in clinical practice: criteria for the classification of central sensitization pain. *Pain Physician.* 2014;17(5):447-457.
142. Butler D. *Explain Pain.* 2nd ed. Adelaide, Australia: NOI Group; 2013.
143. Mackelprang R. Cultural competence with persons with disabilities. In: Lum D, ed. *Culturally Competent Practice: A Framework for Understanding Diverse Groups and Justice Issues.* 4th ed. Belmont, CA: Brooks Cole; 2011:437-465.
144. Collier, Gebhardt, Ryn V. 3-dimensional model for developing clinical reasoning across the continuum of physical therapy education. In: Jensen G, Musolino G, eds. *Clinical Reasoning and Decision-Making in Physical Therapy: Facilitation, Assessment, and Implementation.* Thorofare, NJ: SLACK; in press.
145. Edwards I, Jones M, Carr J, Braunack-Mayer A, Jensen GM. Clinical reasoning strategies in physical therapy. *Phys Ther.* 2004;84(4):312-330; discussion 331-315.
146. Speckens AE, van Rood YR. Protocollaire behandeling van patiënten met onverklaarde klachten: cognitieve gedragstherapie. In: Keijsers GP, van Minnen AV, eds. *Protocollaire Behandelingen in de Ambulante Geestelijke Gezondheidszorg.* Netherlands: Houten, Bohn Stafleu Van Loghum; 2004:183-218 (182e herziene druk).
147. Burgess DJ, van Ryn M, Crowley-Matoka M, Malat J. Understanding the provider contribution to race/ethnicity disparities in pain treatment: insights from dual process models of stereotyping. *Pain Med.* 2006;7(2):119-134.
148. Pearson H. Science and intuition: do both have a place in clinical decision making? *Br J Nurs.* 2013;22(4):212-215.
149. Hirsh AT, Jensen MP, Robinson ME. Evaluation of nurses' self-insight into their pain assessment and treatment decisions. *J Pain.* 2010;11(5):454-461.
150. Macrae CN, Bodenhausen GV. Social cognition: categorical person perception. *Br J Psychol.* 2001;92 pt 1:239-255.
151. The Pain Catastrophizing Scale. 2009. http://www.aci.health.nsw.gov.au/__data/assets/pdf_file/0004/257422/Pain_Catastrophizing_Scale_Manual.pdf
152. Brewster ME, Esposito J. Chronic illness rejection and discrimination scale: an instrument modification and confirmatory factor analysis. *Stigma Health.* 2017;2(1):16-22.
153. Gerdle B, Molander P, Stenberg G, Stalnacke BM, Enthoven P. Weak outcome predictors of multimodal rehabilitation at one-year follow-up in patients with chronic pain-a practice based evidence study from two SQRP centres. *BMC Musculoskelet Disord.* 2016;17(1):490.
154. Kamper SJ, Apeldoorn AT, Chiarotto A, et al. Multidisciplinary biopsychosocial rehabilitation for chronic low back pain: cochrane systematic review and meta-analysis. *BMJ.* 2015;350:h444.
155. Louw A, Zimney K, Puentedura EJ, Diener I. The efficacy of pain neuroscience education on musculoskeletal pain: a systematic review of the literature. *Physiother Theory Pract.* 2016;32(5):332-355.
156. Puentedura EJ, Flynn T. Combining manual therapy with pain neuroscience education in the treatment of chronic low back pain: a narrative review of the literature. *Physiother Theory Pract.* 2016;32(5):408-414.
157. Birch S, Stilling M, Mechlenburg I, Hansen TB. Effectiveness of a physiotherapist delivered cognitive-behavioral patient education for patients who undergoes operation for total knee arthroplasty: a protocol of a randomized controlled trial. *BMC Musculoskelet Disord.* 2017;18(1):116.
158. Nielsen M, Keefe FJ, Bennell K, Jull GA. Physical therapist-delivered cognitive-behavioral therapy: a qualitative study of physical therapists' perceptions and experiences. *Phys Ther.* 2014;94(2):197-209.
159. Bennell KL, Ahamed Y, Jull G, et al. Physical therapist-delivered pain coping skills training and exercise for knee osteoarthritis: randomized controlled trial. *Arthritis Care Res (Hoboken).* 2016;68(5):590-602.
160. Diener I, Kargela M, Louw A. Listening is therapy: patient interviewing from a pain science perspective. *Physiother Theory Pract.* 2016;32(5):356-367.
161. Louw A, Diener I, Butler DS, Puentedura EJ. The effect of neuroscience education on pain, disability, anxiety, and stress in chronic musculoskeletal pain. *Arch Phys Med Rehabil.* 2011;92(12):2041-2056.
162. Bandura A. An agentic perspective on positive psychology. In: Lopez SJ, ed. *Positive Psychology: Expecting the Best in People.* Vol 1. New York, NY: Praeger; 2008.

Section 2: Head and Neck Pain

Chapter 6

Trapezius Muscle

"Stress Headache Producer"

Michelle Finnegan and César Fernández de las Peñas

1. INTRODUCTION

The trapezius muscle is one of the main muscles of the cervical spine, consisting of three portions: upper, middle, and lower. It is mainly involved in movements of the neck and shoulder region (upper portion), although the middle and lower portions are also involved in the thoracic spine. The trapezius muscle is probably the muscle most often affected by trigger points (TrPs) seen in common clinical practice. The upper portion of the muscle refers pain unilaterally upward along the posterolateral aspect of the neck and extends to the temple and the back of the orbit, mimicking tension-type headache; the middle portion of the muscle refers pain to the shoulder, and the lower portion of the muscle usually refers pain to the neck or suprascapular region, contributing to mechanical neck pain. Symptoms reported by patients may include reports of a "stiff neck," headache, "shivers running up and down my spine," and neck and shoulder pain. Activation and perpetuation of TrPs in the trapezius muscle usually result from sudden trauma, whiplash from a motor vehicle accident, a fall, or improper work station setup. Differential diagnosis should include tension type and migrainous headache, temperomandibular joint dysfunction, intervertebral joint dysfunction, occipital neuralgia, and interscapular pain as well as subacromial pain syndrome (shoulder impingement). Corrective actions include postural and ergonomic education, proper sleep positioning, avoiding activities that overload the trapezius muscle, self-pressure release of TrPs, and self-stretch exercises.

2. ANATOMIC CONSIDERATIONS

The upper, middle, and lower portions of the trapezius muscle have different fiber directions and often have different functions. In this chapter, the three parts are frequently identified as if they were three different muscles. Clinically, the boundary between any two parts is frequently indistinguishable by palpation and is defined only by the location of the attachment of fibers in relation to the spinous processes, scapular spine, acromion, and clavicle. When the right and left trapezius muscles are viewed together from the rear, they appear to have a large diamond shape. Together, the fibers of both upper trapezii muscles are shaped like a coat hanger.

Upper Trapezius Fibers

The upper (superior) fibers arise from the medial third of the superior nuchal line. In the midline, they arise from the ligamentum nuchae (Figure 6-1). The fibers converge laterally and forward and attach to the posterior border of the lateral third of the clavicle (Figure 6-2).[1]

A careful anatomic analysis of the direction of fibers in the upper trapezius muscle revealed that, contrary to the impression given by most authors on the subject, none of the superior (upper) trapezius fibers are in a position to exert a direct upward force

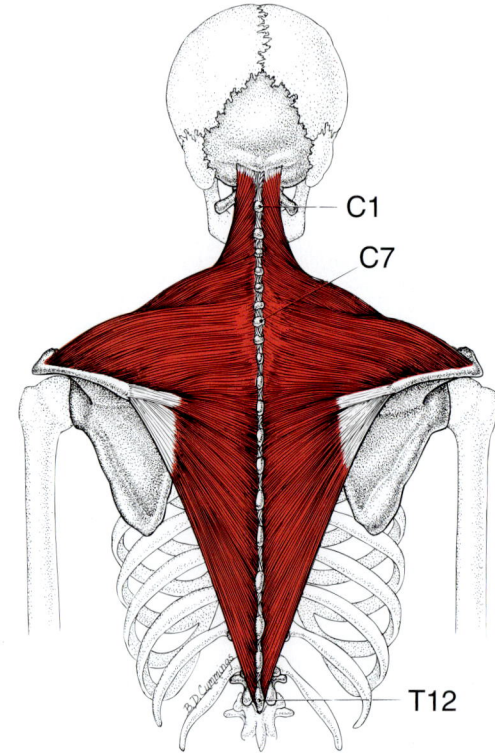

Figure 6-1. Attachments of the right and left trapezius muscles, rear view. The midline trapezius attachments extend from the occiput to the T12 spinous process.

on the clavicle or the scapula.[2] A few thin fibers that have a vertical orientation from the superior nuchal line swing around the neck and pass almost horizontally, only slightly downward, before attaching to the clavicle.

Johnson et al[2] reported the transversely oriented fascicles in this superior part of the trapezius muscle as arising from the lower half of the ligamentum nuchae and inserting into the lateral third of the clavicle. The larger fascicles of upper trapezius fibers run nearly horizontal (at an elevation of >20°) and are in a position to draw the lateral end of the clavicle medially and upward by swinging it around its attachment at the sternoclavicular joint. Through this rotation of the clavicle about the sternoclavicular joint, these fibers of the upper trapezius can raise the clavicle and (indirectly through the acromioclavicular joint) the scapula.

The greater occipital nerve can be compressed by the vertical fibers of the upper trapezius muscle.[3-5] The greater occipital nerve is the medial branch of the dorsal primary division of the second cervical nerve and supplies sensory branches to the scalp end of the scapular spine, and is attach to a tubercle at its lateral apex (Figure 6-1).[1] Johnson et al[2] considered the lower part of the trapezius muscle those fascicles arising from spinous processes starting at T2. The fascicles from T2 to T5 converge to a common aponeurotic tendon that attach on the scapula at the deltoid tubercle. When present, fascicles from T6 to of the scapula T10 insert into the medial border of the deltoid tubercle. Lower fascicles, when present, insert into the lower edge of the deltoid muscle.

2.1. Innervation and Vascularization

The trapezius muscle is innervated by the spinal (external) portion of the accessory nerve (cranial nerve XI). This nerve originates in the spinal nucleus of the spinal cord of the upper five[7] or six[8,9] cervical segments. The fibers from the cervical segments merge to form a trunk. The spinal root enters the posterior fossa of the cranium through the foramen magnum. Here the spinal root joins briefly with the cranial (internal) root to form a single nerve trunk (accessory nerve). The accessory nerve exits the jugular foramen, heading toward the retrostyloid space.[8] From here the nerve divides into the cranial and spinal portions of the accessory nerve. The spinal accessory nerve typically passes laterally to the internal jugular vein.[10-12] Although less frequent, the nerve can also pass medial,[12] through,[12,13] or split around[12] the internal jugular vein. The nerve then descends in an oblique manner, staying medial to the styloid process and stylohyoid and digastric muscles.[7] From here the nerve more commonly travels through the two heads of the sternocleidomastoid muscle,[8] but could also travel between the muscle's two heads.[14] In this region, the nerve forms an anastomosis with fibers from C2 to C4.[8,15-17] Then the nerve travels obliquely through the posterior triangle, toward the deep cervical fascia and the trapezius muscle, staying in a fat layer between the trapezius and levator scapulae muscles.[7,14]

It is thought that the C2-C4 connections carry sensory (mostly proprioceptive) information. Contrary to this thought, electromyographic[18,19] and histochemical[18] data show that the nerves have both sensory and motor functions, thereby contributing to some degree of contraction to the three portions of the trapezius muscle. However, the motor input from C2 to C4 nerves is not consistently present or is irregularly innervated to the three parts of the muscle when it is present.[19]

Although lesions to the spinal accessory nerve are rare, iatrogenic injury contributes to most of the insults to the spinal accessory nerve. Injury often occurs during radical neck dissection, modified radical neck dissection, or functional neck dissection for removal of cervical lymph node metastases from head and neck cancer.[16,20-23]

The vascularization of the upper portion of the trapezius muscle is supplied by a transverse muscular branch arising from the occipital artery at the level of the mastoid process.[24] The vascularization of the middle portion of the trapezius muscle is supplied by the superficial cervical artery or by a superficial branch of the transverse cervical artery.[24] Finally, the lower third of the trapezius muscle is supplied by a muscular branch from the dorsal scapular artery, passing medial to the medial border of the scapula.[24]

2.2. Function

To summarize descriptions of trapezius muscle effects on scapular motions (see Figure 6-3 for definitions), elevation of the scapula activates both upper and middle trapezius fibers; adduction activates all of its fibers but depends primarily on middle trapezius fibers[3]; and rotation of the glenoid cavity upward involves the upper, middle, and lower fibers.

Johnson et al,[2] in a report of a biomechanical and anatomic analysis of the trapezius muscle, state that the transverse orientation of the upper and middle trapezius fibers allows them to draw the clavicle, acromion, and spine of the scapula backward and

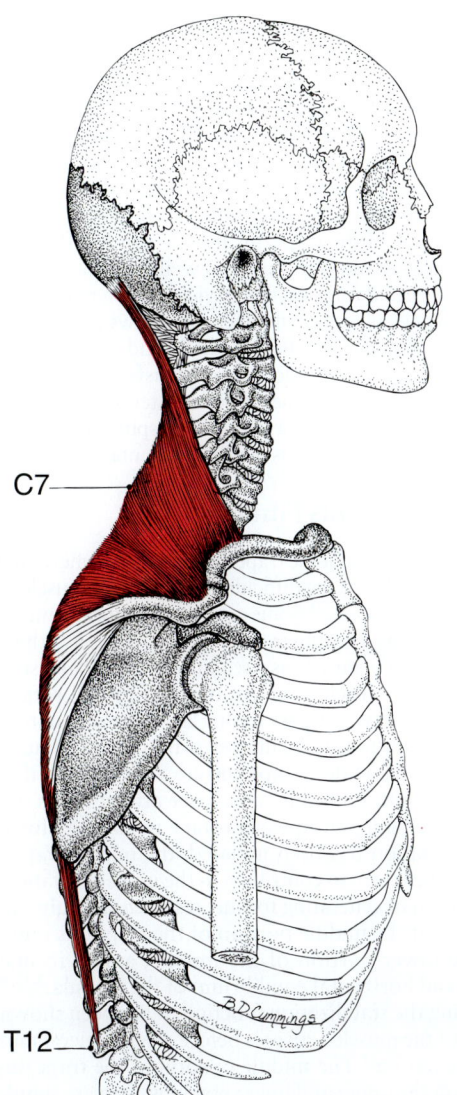

Figure 6-2. Attachments of the right trapezius muscle, side view. The longest, most vertical fibers (ones that cross the greatest number of joints) are the fibers most likely to develop trigger points.

over the vertex. This cervical nerve emerges below the posterior arch of the atlas above the lamina of the axis, and then it curves around the lower border of the oblique capitis inferior muscle, which it crosses before penetrating the semispinalis capitis and trapezius muscles near their attachments to the occipital bone.[3]

Middle Trapezius Fibers

According to Simons et al,[6] the middle portion of the trapezius muscle originates from the spinous processes and supraspinous ligaments from C7 to T3 vertebrae and inserts to the medial margin of the acromion and superior lip of the spine of the scapula (Figure 6-1).[1] Johnson et al[2] considered the middle part of the trapezius muscle those fascicles arising from C7 and T1, with the C7 fascicle attaching to the acromion and the T1 fascicle attaching to the scapular spine.

Lower Trapezius Fibers

According to Simons et al,[6] fibers from this fan-shaped part of the trapezius muscle originate in the spinous processes and supraspinous ligaments from T4 to T12 vertebrae, pass into an aponeurosis gliding over a smooth triangular surface at the medial

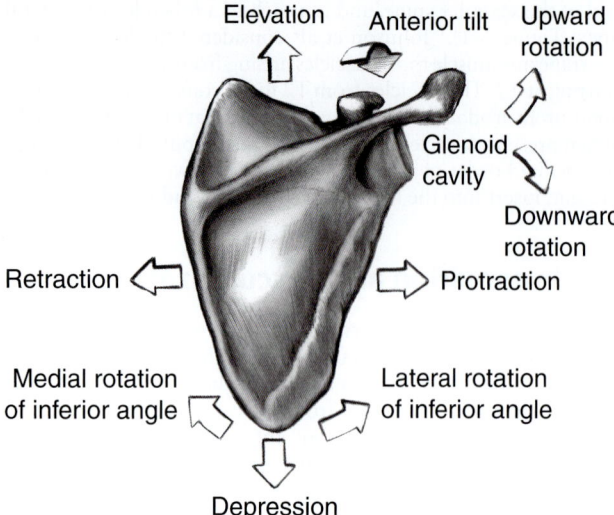

Figure 6-3. Illustration of terms used to describe movements of the right scapula, as seen from behind. Anterior tilt applies to the upper border of the scapula. Upward and downward rotation refers to direction of movement of the glenoid fossa. Medial and lateral rotation refers to direction of movement of the inferior angle. Retraction is scapular movement in a medial direction (toward the vertebral column), and protraction is movement of the scapula as a whole in a lateral direction (away from the vertebral column). Adapted and redrawn from Kendall FP, McCreary EK, Provance PG, et al. *Muscles, Testing and Function*. 5th ed. Baltimore, MD: Williams & Wilkins; 2005:303.

medially (aided by the lower, or thoracic fibers) and propose that any upward action of the thin superior (nuchal) portion would be dissipated in the cervical fascia before these muscle fibers reached the clavicle (which they approach in almost a horizontal plane). These authors suggest that, in regard to upward rotation of the scapula, the upper and lower fibers participate in different ways in conjunction with the serratus anterior muscle. They state that the lower fibers maintain the position of the deltoid tubercle, which becomes the axis of rotation, while the upper fibers exert an upward rotation moment about the axis to complement that of the serratus anterior muscle. Furthermore, they explain that the upper fibers of the muscle raise the scapula (indirectly) by rotating the clavicle about the sternoclavicular joint and exert no upward force on the scapula. This hypothesis was also supported by Guazzelli Filho et al,[25] who observed that the three portions of the trapezius muscle show increasing activity during abduction, adduction, and flexion-extension of the upper extremity. Nevertheless, electromyographic activity of the trapezius muscle is minimal when the upper extremity is unloaded, and heavy loads can be just suspended with a small contribution from the upper portion.[24]

Entire Muscle

Acting bilaterally, the entire muscle assists extension of the cervical and thoracic spine.

Upper Trapezius Fibers

Acting unilaterally, the upper portion of the trapezius muscle extends and laterally flexes the head and the neck toward the same side and aids in extreme rotation of the head so that the face turns to the opposite side. It can draw the clavicle bone (and *indirectly* the scapula) backward and can raise them by rotating the clavicle at the sternoclavicular joint.[2] It usually helps (but can be trained not) to carry the weight of the upper extremity (indirectly through the shoulder girdle) during standing, or to support a weight in the hand with the arm hanging. In conjunction with the levator scapulae muscle and upper digitations of the serratus anterior muscle, the upper trapezius muscle provides the upper component

of the force couple necessary to rotate the glenoid fossa upward. Ito[26] showed that during both flexion and abduction of the arm, the electromyographic activity of the upper trapezius increased progressively and became vigorous. In another study, when the arm was actively maintained in 90° of abduction, all subjects showed significant electromyographic evidence of fatigue within 1 minute, and, on average, in less than 30 seconds.[27]

The mechanism by which the nearly horizontally oriented upper portion of the trapezius muscle can be effective in assisting the serratus anterior muscle is well explained.[2] By exerting a medially directed force on the clavicle, which must rotate around the sternoclavicular joint, it effectively draws the lateral end of the clavicle (to which it attaches) medially and upward. The resulting elevated position of the acromion transfers much of the weight being carried by the humerus to the sternoclavicular joint as a compressive force relieving the cervical spine of compression. The orientation of these fibers is nearly horizontal rather than vertical.

Middle Trapezius Fibers

The function of the middle trapezius muscle is somewhat debatable. This is in part due to the difficulty to isolate the muscle specifically with specific exercises.[28] Some authors describe the middle portion of the muscle as a scapular retractor,[2,29] whereas others describe this portion of the muscle as a scapular retractor and stabilizer.[24,30] Although this muscle is active during upward rotation of the scapula, that is, when performing an upward rotation shrug,[31] the muscle cannot specifically perform upward rotation because the fibers of the middle trapezius are very close to the scapula's axis of rotation. With this short lever arm, it limits the muscle's ability to generate an upward rotary moment.[2] However, once upward rotation has been initiated, the middle trapezius has a better moment arm to contribute to the upward rotation motion.[2]

Rather than generating torque, research strongly supports the concept that the middle portion of the trapezius muscle, along with the lower portion of the muscle, assists in maintaining vertical and horizontal equilibrium of the scapula.[2,32-34] Further supporting the stabilization function, it has been shown that this portion of the muscle activates before glenohumeral muscles with specific exercise.[5] The middle portion of the trapezius muscle, along with the upper and lower portions, activate simultaneously in response to sudden movements.[35]

Lower Trapezius Fibers

The function of the lower trapezius muscle is also somewhat debatable. This is in part due to the challenge of isolating the muscle to determine its functions.[28] In addition, some authors consider the muscle to produce scapular adduction, depression, and rotation,[30] whereas others suggest the muscle is an important stabilizer of the scapula,[2,5,35] which helps maintain vertical and horizontal equilibrium of the scapula.[2] On the basis of attachments of the lower trapezius muscle to the deltoid tubercle and the fact that the muscle fibers do not change length with upward rotation of the scapula, it would be a challenge for this muscle to generate any net torque for upward rotation.[2] This portion of the muscle assists with upward rotation, but more to resist the displacement of the serratus anterior muscle drawing the scapula laterally. With the stabilization component of the lower and upper portions of the trapezius (and serratus anterior) muscles exerting an upward rotation moment, upward rotation of the scapula is achieved.[2] Electromyographic studies support that this portion of the trapezius muscle is active, along with the upper and middle trapezius muscles, during upward rotation.[10,31]

2.3. Functional Unit

The functional unit to which a muscle belongs includes the muscles that reinforce and counter its actions as well as the joints that the muscle crosses. The interdependence of these structures functionally is reflected in the organization and neural connections of the sensory motor cortex. The functional unit is emphasized because the presence of a TrP in one muscle of the unit increases the likelihood that the other muscles of the unit will also develop TrPs. When inactivating TrPs in a muscle, one must be concerned about TrPs that may develop in muscles that are functionally interdependent. Box 6.1 grossly represents the functional unit of the trapezius muscle.[6] The trapezius, levator scapulae, rhomboids, and serratus anterior muscle combine in producing a variety of scapular rotations.[24]

Upper Trapezius Fibers

The upper part of the trapezius muscle acts synergistically with the sternocleidomastoid muscle for head and neck motions, extension of the head, ipsilateral side bending, and contralateral rotation. Acting with the levator scapulae muscle, the upper portion of the trapezius muscle elevates the scapula and the point of the shoulder; when acting with the serratus anterior muscle, the trapezius muscle rotates the scapula forward (upward) so that the arm can be raised above the head; and acting with the rhomboid muscles, the upper trapezius muscle retracts the scapula, bracing back the shoulder. With the shoulder fixed, the trapezius muscle may bend the head and neck backward and laterally.

Middle Trapezius Fibers

Middle fibers of the trapezius muscle are synergistic to the rhomboid muscles for adduction of the scapula and antagonistic to the serratus anterior and pectoralis major muscles. For upward rotation, the muscle is synergistic to the upper and lower trapezius and serratus anterior muscles.[2] The muscle is synergistic to the upper and lower portions of the trapezius muscle for scapular stabilization.[2,5,32-35] Because of the stabilization component, the middle trapezius is also synergistic to the deltoid, rotator cuff, and long head of the biceps brachii muscles for elevation of the arm.

Lower Trapezius Fibers

In stabilizing the axis of rotation of the scapula muscle, these lower fibers are synergistic with the serratus anterior and upper and middle fibers of the trapezius muscle for upward rotation of the glenoid fossa of the scapula. These fibers are synergistic to the upper and middle trapezius fibers for scapular stabilization and with the deltoid, rotator cuff, and long head of the biceps brachii muscles for elevation of the arm.

3. CLINICAL PRESENTATION

3.1. Referred Pain Pattern

Upper Trapezius Fibers

The upper portion of the trapezius muscle is one of the most common areas affected by TrPs. The upper portion of the trapezius muscle can exhibit TrPs in any fiber of the muscle belly. A common place, clinically observed, where TrPs can be mostly found is the anterior border of the muscle and involves the most vertical fibers that attach anteriorly to the clavicle. Based on clinical experience, TrPs in this area consistently refer pain unilaterally upward along the posterolateral aspect of the neck to the mastoid process. The referred pain, when intense, extends to the side of the head, centering in the temple and back of the orbit (Figure 6-4). It may also include the angle of the jaw,[36] also described as the region of the masseter.[37] Occasionally, pain extends to the occiput, and rarely some pain is referred to the lower molar teeth. Referred pain from TrPs in the upper portion of the trapezius muscle is a major source of tension-type headache.[38]

The upper portion of the trapezius muscle can also exhibit TrPs in the posterior border of the muscle, in the most horizontal fibers that attach to the spinous processes of the cervical spine. The referred pain of TrPs in this portion of the muscle

---

Box 6-1 Functional unit of the trapezius muscle

Action	Synergists	Antagonists
Head and neck extension	Sternocleidomastoid Posterior cervical muscle group Semispinalis capitis Semispinalis cervicis	Rectus capitis anterior Longus capitis Longus colli Hyoid muscles
Head and neck side bending (ipsilateral)	Ipsilateral sternocleidomastoid Ipsilateral scalenes Ipsilateral rectus capitis Posterior major/minor Ipsilateral obliquus capitis superior	Contralateral sternocleidomastoid Contralateral scalenes Contralateral upper trapezius Contralateral rectus capitis Posterior major/minor Contralateral obliquus capitis superior
Head and neck rotation (contralateral)	Ipsilateral sternocleidomastoid Contralateral splenius capitis Contralateral rectus capitis Posterior major/minor Contralateral obliquus capitis inferior	Contralateral sternocleidomastoid Ipsilateral splenius capitis Ipsilateral rectus capitis Posterior major/minor Ipsilateral obliquus capitis inferior
Scapular elevation	Levator scapulae	Latissimus dorsi Pectoralis minor Subclavius Serratus anterior
Scapular upward rotation	Serratus anterior	Levator scapula Rhomboid minor Rhomboid major
Scapular retraction	Rhomboid minor Rhomboid major	Pectoralis major Serratus anterior

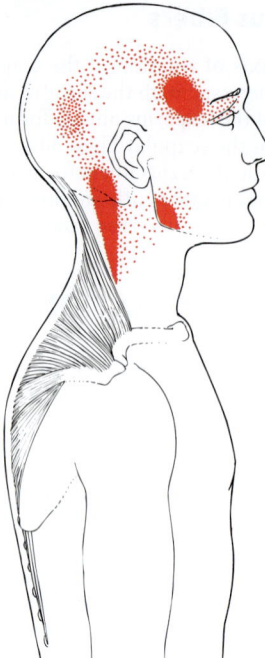

Figure 6-4. Referred pain pattern from trigger points located in the most vertical fibers of the upper portion of the trapezius muscle. Solid red shows the essential referred pain zone whereas the stippling maps the spillover zone.

is perceived in the posterior part of the cervical spine, with an abnormal sensation of tightness in the occipital region (Figure 6-5, pattern on left of figure). This TrP is highly frequent in patients with mechanical neck pain.[39]

Middle Trapezius Fibers

Trigger points in the middle trapezius muscle can refer superficial burning pain between the medial scapular border and the spinous processes of C7-T3 vertebrae (Figure 6-6, pattern on right of figure). This reported burning sensation should not be confused with pain of cervical origin, which can also refer to this area.[1,9,40] Trigger points can also refer an aching pain to the top of the shoulder by the acromion (Figure 6-7, pattern on left of figure). This pattern overlaps with the pain referral pattern of the lower portion of the trapezius muscle (Figure 6-5,

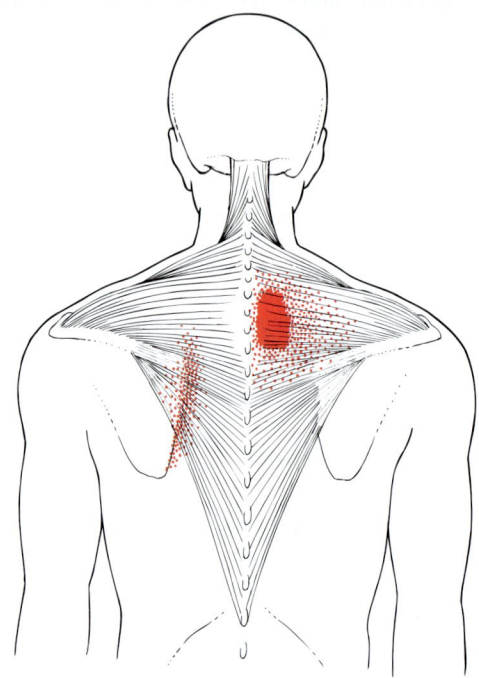

Figure 6-6. Left side of figure shows referred pain pattern of TrP in the region of lateral attachment of the left lower trapezius. Right side of figure shows referred pain pattern of TrP region in the midfiber region of the middle portion of the trapezius muscle.

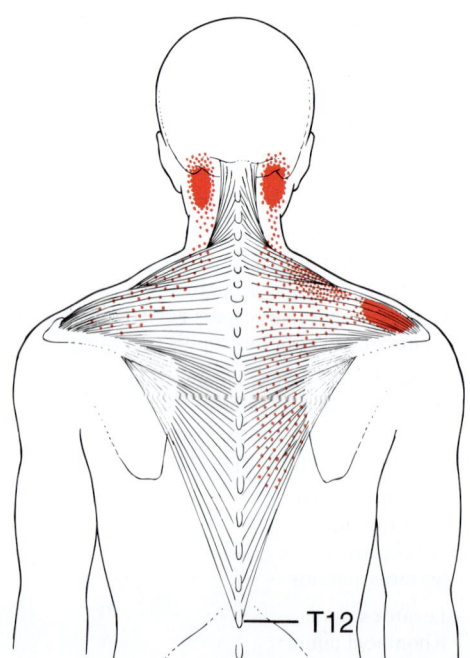

Figure 6-5. Left side of figure shows the referred pain pattern of TrPs in the posterior and more horizontal fibers of the upper portion of left trapezius muscle. Right side of figure shows the referred pain pattern of TrPs in a right lower trapezius muscle.

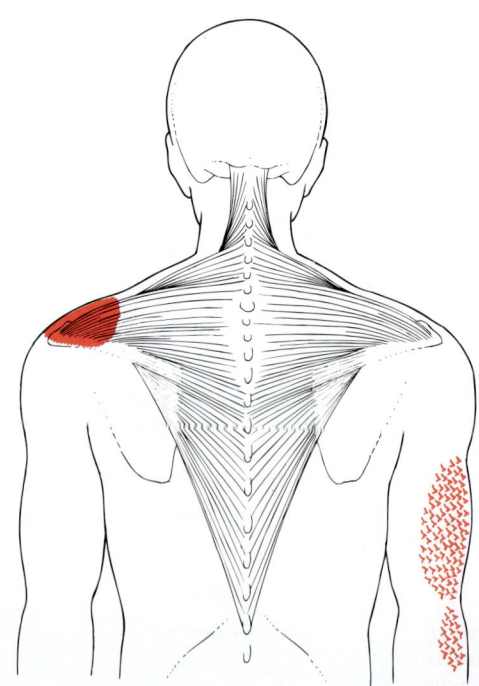

Figure 6-7. Referred pain pattern of TrPs at the lateral attachment region of the left middle trapezius muscle. Trigger points in the middle trapezius muscle can refer pilomotor activity, or "gooseflesh," as identified on the right upper limb by red ">" symbols.

pattern on right of figure). The middle portion of the muscle can also produce an autonomic sensation whereby the patient reports a "shivery" sensation with associated pilomotor erection on the lateral aspect of the ipsilateral arm (Figure 6-7, pattern on right of figure).

Lower Trapezius Fibers

Trigger points in the lower portion of the trapezius, although common, are frequently overlooked as a source of cervical pain. They have been shown to refer pain to the high cervical region of the paraspinal muscles, adjacent to the mastoid area (Figure 6-5, pattern on right of figure).[41,42] The muscle can also refer pain to the acromion[41] and over the suprascapular region.[43] Trigger points in the muscle closer to the attachment on the scapula (Figure 6-6, pattern on left of figure) can refer a burning pain along and medial to the medial border of the scapula. This reported burning sensation should not be confused with pain of cervical origin, which can refer to the same area.[1,9,40]

3.2. Symptoms

Upper Trapezius Fibers

Patients with TrPs in the trapezius muscle can exhibit pain in the head, cervical spine, or the back, depending on the affected portion of the muscle. It seems that TrPs in the upper portion of the trapezius can contribute to tension-type headache,[38] migraine[44] or neck pain.[13,39] In patients with chronic neck and head pain symptoms, the pain pattern is likely to be a composite of referred pain from several neck and masticatory muscles. Patients with TrPs in the upper portion of the trapezius muscle can exhibit restricted neck range of motion, or pain on motion, but this usually occurs when the head and neck are almost fully rotated actively to the opposite side, which contracts the muscle in a shortened position. The most restricted movement is usually lateral flexion of the head and neck away from the involved upper trapezius muscle. If a TrP in trapezius muscle is combined with the presence of other muscles including the levator scapulae or splenius cervicis, the patient may develop an acute "stiff neck."[45] This painfully limits rotation of the head toward the same side, which elongates the upper trapezius muscle.

With entrapment of the greater occipital nerve as a sequela to prolonged activation of upper trapezius muscle TrPs, patients report numbness, tingling and burning pain in the scalp over the ipsilateral occipital region ("occipital neuralgia") in addition to headache. It is interesting to observe that the referred pain from TrPs in the upper portion of the trapezius muscle resembles the topographical pain pattern of greater occipital nerve compression, so careful examination of both muscle and nerve tissues is highly relevant. Patients with nerve entrapment usually prefer cold rather than heat. Entrapment symptoms of the greater occipital nerve apparently develop when TrP activity in one of the muscles that it penetrates (the semispinalis capitis or the upper trapezius muscles) produces taut bands of muscle fibers that compress the nerve as it penetrates the muscle.

Middle Trapezius Fibers

Patients with TrPs in the middle trapezius muscle can report deep burning interscapular pain. Similar symptoms can also originate from the cervical or upper thoracic spine and should be ruled out. Therefore, in addition to examining the middle trapezius muscle for TrPs, clinicians should examine the cervical/thoracic zygapophyseal joints. Trigger points referring to the acromion area create pain and tenderness in the region. Patients will report that they have intolerance to pressure from bags on their shoulders[46] or discomfort with wearing heavy coats. Trigger points can also produce a referred autonomic response that is described like "shivers running up and down the spine" when a fingernail scrapes across the blackboard.

Lower Trapezius Fibers

Trigger points in this muscle can cause neck,[42] suprascapular, interscapular, or acromial pain with little, if any, restriction of motion. Trigger points often induce associated TrPs in the upper back and neck muscles. This muscle is often forgotten about as a source of upper neck pain, which can contribute to less-than-optimal treatment results until TrPs in this muscle are treated.[42] Clinicians should consider the presence of TrPs in the lower portion of the trapezius muscle in patients with neck pain exhibiting a rounded shoulder position and a thoracic kyphosis because the lower fibers of the trapezius muscle are stretched in this position.

3.3. Patient Examination

After a thorough subjective examination, the clinician should make a detailed drawing representing the pain pattern that the patient has described. This depiction will assist in planning the physical examination and can be useful in monitoring the progression of the patient as symptoms improve or change. For proper assessment and examination of the trapezius muscle, the clinician should assess accessory motion of the sternoclavicular, acromioclavicular, and glenohumeral joints because hypomobility in all or some of these joints can contribute to scapular dyskinesia.[47]

Upper Trapezius Fibers

Trigger points in the upper fibers of the trapezius muscle typically do not contribute to weakness of the muscle.[7] This is likely because the upper trapezius muscle typically tends to be hyperactive and tense.[48] In fact, patients typically present with an elevated shoulder on the side of the tense upper trapezius muscle with a slight tilt of the neck toward the affected side. Trigger points in this muscle can also contribute to reduced cervical range of motion,[49,50] neck pain,[15,50,51] and shoulder impairment.[52] Cervical range of motion is particularly affected in lateral flexion of the head and neck away from the involved upper trapezius. Active rotation of the head to the opposite side is usually painful at the extreme range of motion because the muscle contracts strongly in this most shortened position. Active rotation to the same side is usually pain free, unless either the levator scapulae muscle on the same side, or the opposite upper trapezius muscle, also have TrPs. In addition, the increased intramuscular electromyographic activity of latent TrPs in the upper trapezius muscle is significantly greater with shoulder abduction, suggesting that it can impair the synergies of muscles during osteokinematic motions.[14] Other studies also support the theory of alteration in muscle activation patterns from TrPs.[53,54]

Middle Trapezius Fibers

The patient with pain arising from the middle trapezius muscle is likely to have a rounded shoulder posture secondary to shortening and/or TrPs of the antagonistic pectoralis muscles. A shortened pectoralis major muscle maintains the humerus in internal rotation and adduction, which causes the scapula to abduct away from the spine and alter the length tension relationship of the muscle.[48] As a result, this forward-head posture can reduce the muscle's ability to fire properly.[55] Although not specific to the pectoralis major and middle trapezius muscles, research has shown that latent TrPs affect reciprocal inhibition.[54] Resultantly, TrPs in the pectoralis muscles could influence how the middle trapezius muscle fires.

Lower Trapezius Fibers

The fibers of the lower trapezius muscle are often more susceptible to inhibition than the upper trapezius muscle. This weakness can be due to a structural lesion or adaptive changes.[48] Tightness of the pectoralis minor muscle can be one factor contributing to the inhibition of lower portion of the trapezius muscle. The pectoralis minor muscle is known to contribute to altered scapular kinematics[47,56]; as a result, this can impair firing of the scapular muscles, including the lower trapezius muscle.[57] Weakness of this muscle can also be associated with neck pain.[58] It is known that TrPs can contribute to altered muscle firing.[14,53,54] Trigger points can also contribute to inhibition of muscles, as it has been shown that utilizing dry needling immediately improves the firing of scapular muscles with latent TrPs.[53]

Trigger points in the lower fibers of the trapezius muscle may affect upward rotation of the scapula because of impairment of the stabilization function. If the lower trapezius muscle is inhibited and weak from the activity of TrPs, the scapula may be elevated and the upper part tilted forward (coracoid process tilted forward and downward), and the patient will exhibit a rounded shoulder posture.

3.4. Trigger Point Examination

Manual examination of TrPs requires adequate manual skills, training, and clinical practice to develop a high degree of reliability in the examination. To determine the most useful diagnostic criteria for TrPs, Gerwin et al[59] tested the reliability with four experienced physicians and could identify five characteristics of TrPs in five pairs of muscles (one was the upper trapezius muscle). Four criteria are highly reliable in this muscle: the detection of spot tenderness, palpation of a taut band, the presence of referred pain, and reproduction of the subject's symptomatic pain (agreement 90% to perfect and kappa 0.61-0.84). Identification of a local twitch response by manual palpation was unreliable in this muscle. When present, however, a local twitch response is a strong confirmatory finding and is especially valuable when needling TrPs therapeutically. A more recent study found a moderate to high intrarater reliability (ICC ranging from 0.62 to 0.81) for the diagnosis of TrPs in the upper trapezius muscle with a limit of agreement around 26 mm.[60] No reliability studies have been performed on the middle and lower portions of the trapezius muscle.

Upper Trapezius Fibers

Although no exact location of TrPs should be considered when clinicians examine the upper trapezius muscle, a recent cadaver study has shown that some locations may be more susceptible for TrP development because these are the areas where the spinal accessory nerve innervates the muscle.[61]

For clinical examination of the anterior and most vertical fibers of the upper trapezius muscle, the patient is supine, or possibly prone. Supine is preferred because the upper trapezius muscle is more relaxed. The upper portion of the trapezius muscle is placed on moderate slack by bringing the ear slightly toward the shoulder on the same side. In a pincer grasp, the entire mass of the free margin of the upper trapezius muscle is lifted off the underlying supraspinatus muscle and apex of the lung (Figure 6-8A and B). Then the muscle is firmly rolled between the fingers and thumb to palpate the taut bands. With this cross-fiber pincer palpation, a local twitch response can be easily provoked with snapping palpation and strumming of the taut band. In fact, the local twitch response can be easily appreciated by the clinician. After identifying the taut band, these fibers should be searched for a spot eliciting local and referred pain to the neck or the head.

For clinical examination of the posterior and horizontal fibers of the upper trapezius muscle, the patient is prone (image not shown). Trigger points are identified by a similar pincer technique as for the anterior fibers. Patients with firmer tissue require cross-fiber flat palpation.

Middle Trapezius Fibers

Prone positioning is one option for examination of the middle portions of the trapezius muscle (Figure 6-8C). Alternatively, the patient can sit with the arms folded across the front of the body to abduct the scapulae and flex the thoracic spine. Cross-fiber flat palpation identifies taut bands in the muscle by rolling them against the underlying ribs. The firm bands usually exhibit visible local twitch responses to snapping palpation of the TrP. A preferred way to palpate the muscle is in the prone position. In the prone position, the muscle is more relaxed. Research shows that the seated versus prone position influence the stiffness of the muscle.[62] In the prone position, the muscle can be palpated in a cross-fiber pincer palpation or with a flat cross-fiber palpation similar to the seated position. The type of palpation would be determined in part by which part of the muscle is being assessed and the muscle thickness of the patient.

There are three common areas that TrPs can be found in the middle trapezius muscle. These areas have recently been supported by a cadaver study showing that they are the same locations where the spinal accessory nerve innervates the muscle.[61] The first area is about 1 cm (½ in) medial to the scapular attachment of the levator scapulae muscle (Figure 6-8C). The second area is in the lateral attachment region of the middle trapezius (Figure 6-6, left side). A cross-fiber flat palpation is necessary in this area. The third area is over the midmuscle region of the middle trapezius muscle (Figure 6-6, right side), which can be palpated with either a cross-fiber flat or pincer palpation.

Lower Trapezius Fibers

The patient is positioned prone for examination of the lower trapezius muscle (Figure 6-8D). Alternatively, the patient can sit with the arms folded across the front of the body. According to Simons et al,[6] this position takes up the tissue slack, preventing the TrP within the taut band from being missed. Cross-fiber flat palpation is performed across the muscle. The preferred way to palpate the muscle is in the prone position. In the prone position, the muscle is more relaxed. Research shows that the seated versus prone position influence the stiffness of the muscle.[62] In the prone position, the muscle can be palpated in a cross-fiber pincer palpation, or similarly as in the seated position with a cross-fiber flat palpation. In either position, the entire muscle should be examined for TrPs.

There are two common areas that TrPs can be found in the lower trapezius muscle. These areas have recently been supported by a cadaver study showing that they are the same locations where the spinal accessory nerve innervates the muscle.[61] The first is close to where the fibers cross the medial border of the scapula, or sometimes at or below the level of the inferior angle of the scapula (Figure 6-5, right side). The second is close to the lateral musculo-tendinous junction where the lower trapezius muscle attaches to the deltoid tubercle of the spine of the scapula (Figure 6-5, left side). Here TrPs have been noted to feel like thicker bands within the tissue.

4. DIFFERENTIAL DIAGNOSIS

4.1. Activation and Perpetuation of Trigger Points

Any posture or activity that activates a TrP, if not corrected, can also perpetuate it. In any part of the trapezius muscle, TrPs may be activated by unaccustomed eccentric loading, eccentric exercise in an unconditioned muscle, or maximal or submaximal concentric loading (Gerwin et al. 2004). Trigger points may also be activated or aggravated when the muscle is placed in a shortened and/or lengthened position for an extended period of time. In addition, sudden trauma, such as whiplash in an auto accident,[13,64] falling off a horse, or falling down from steps can also cause TrP formation.

Upper Trapezius Fibers

The upper trapezius fibers' function of neck stabilization is commonly overloaded by tilting of the shoulder girdle axis due to a lower limb-length inequality or small hemipelvis (body asymmetry). The limb asymmetry tilts the pelvis laterally, which bows the spine into

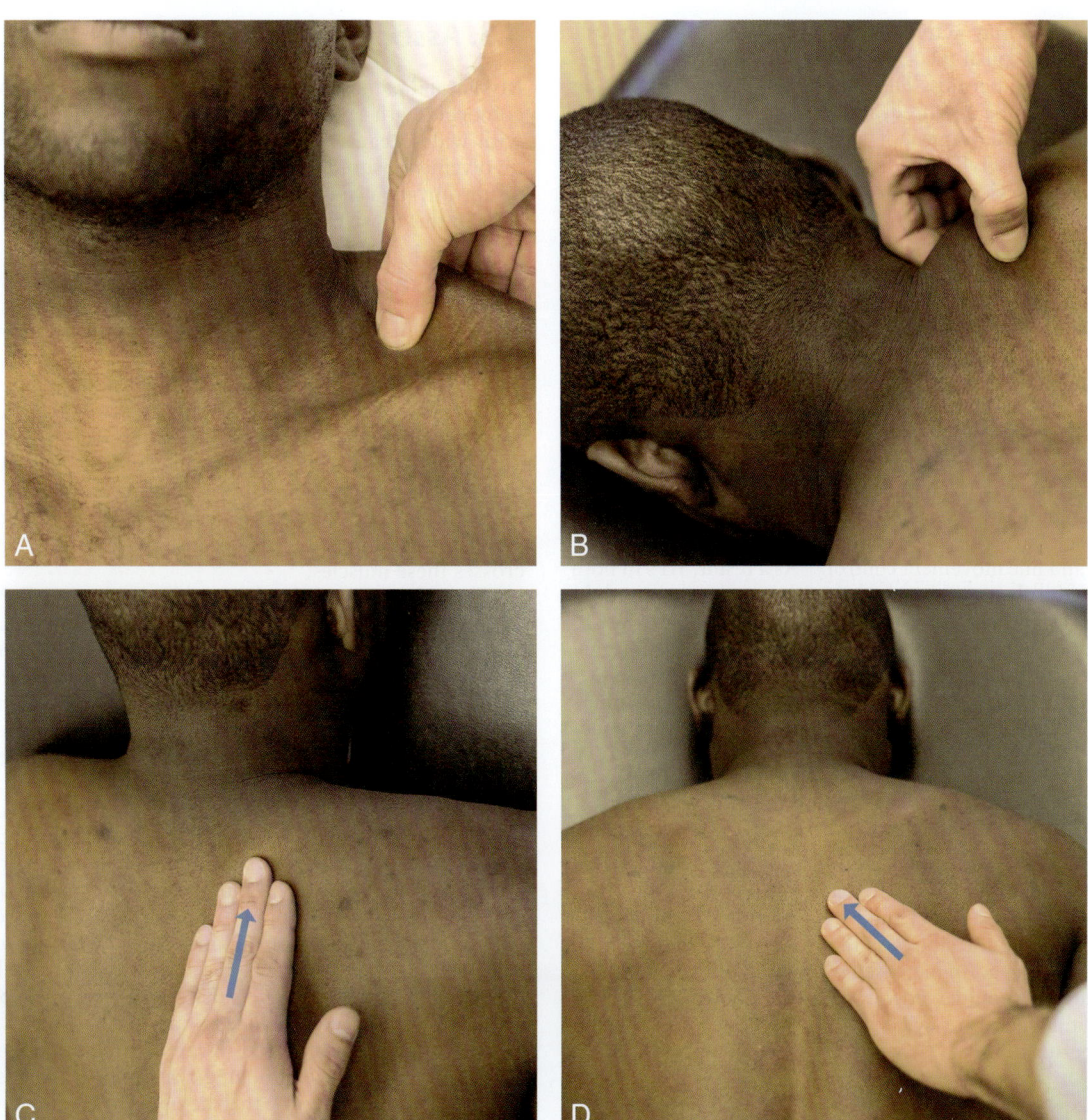

Figure 6-8. Positioning of the patient and technique for examining TrPs in the trapezius muscle: A, Cross-fiber pincer palpation for TrPs in the left upper trapezius muscle, patient supine. B, Cross-fiber pincer palpation for TrPs in the right upper trapezius muscle, patient prone. C, Cross-fiber flat palpation for TrPs in the midfiber portion of the right middle trapezius muscle, patient prone. D, Cross-fiber flat palpation for TrPs in the right lower trapezius muscle, patient prone.

a functional scoliotic curve and, in turn, tilts the shoulders, causing one to sag. The upper trapezius muscle must work constantly to keep the head and neck vertical and the eyes level.

The normally minimal antigravity function of the upper trapezius muscle is overstressed by any position or activity in which the muscle helps to carry the weight of the arm for a prolonged period: using the phone or sitting without armrest support, particularly when the upper arms are congenitally short; holding the arms elevated to reach a high keyboard or a high drawing board; or working with sewing material on the lap with the elbows unsupported. In fact, trapezius myalgia is usually considered a work-related disorder.[11,65-67]

The upper trapezius muscle may be strained by obvious acute gross trauma, but more often it is strained by chronic injury due to overload or microtrauma that may not be so obvious. Such injury can be caused by clothing and accessories, by pressure from tight narrow bra straps supporting large breasts, by the shoulder strap of a ponderous purse,[46] a heavy backpack, or by a heavy coat. It may also be caused by a sustained load in habitual elevation of the shoulders, as an expression of anxiety or other emotional distress, during long telephone calls, playing the violin, or by rotation of the head *far* to one side in a fixed position (holding the head turned to converse with a person seated at the side, or sleeping prone with the head strongly rotated).

Occupational overload is receiving increasingly serious attention; however, the important contribution of TrPs as a major cause of the pain is not yet generally recognized. In a prospective study of employees,[65] the authors recorded the electromyographic activity of the upper (acromial) fibers of the middle trapezius muscle doing repetitive tasks. Elevated static and mean electromyographic activity levels and fewer electromyographic gaps of at least 0.6 second duration correlated significantly with future reports of neck and shoulder pain. These subjects, were not examined for TrPs, but chronic overload such as this without adequate periods of relief, activates TrPs. A similar prospective 1-year study of 30 female packers doing repetitive light work[66] revealed that within 1 year, 17 of the 30 developed sufficient work-related trapezius myalgia to be classified as patients, with a median time of onset of 26 weeks. The authors did not address the cause of the pain, which was likely TrPs in many subjects. A more recent study by Hoyle and colleagues[68] showed that TrPs develop in subjects after 1 hour of typing regardless of the high or low visual and postural stresses placed on each individual.

Other factors may activate upper trapezius TrPs. Armrests that are too *high* push the scapulae up and shorten the upper trapezius for long periods. The muscle's accessory function of head rotation can be overused, and the muscle overstressed, by the quick repetitive movement of flicking long hair out of the eyes.

Upper trapezius TrPs may also be activated by, and remain as sequelae to, cervical radicular pain.[69]

Middle Trapezius Fibers

This part of the muscle can be overloaded eccentrically with upright row exercises,[70] so caution should be considered when considering this exercise and the amount of weight used. The fibers of the middle trapezius muscle also becomes overloaded when the arm is held up and forward for a long time, that is, prolonged reaching activities or when the driver of a car holds the hands on top of the steering wheel. Sustaining this position overloads the pectoralis major fibers, which are prone to develop TrPs, which increases their tension. Trigger points in the antagonistic muscles are known to contribute to unbalanced muscle activation and fine movement control.[54] As a result, TrPs in both muscles need to be considered when either one is impaired. In addition, TrPs in the pectoralis major muscle can contribute to shortening of the muscle. This maintains the humerus in internal rotation and adduction, which causes the scapula to abduct away from the spine.[48] Resultantly, the middle trapezius fibers may be lengthened and weak, contributing to the development of TrPs and associated pain.

Lower Trapezius Fibers

The lower fibers are strained during prolonged bending and reaching forward while sitting (to reach the desk when the knees lack space under its surface) and by supporting the chin on the hand, while resting the elbow on the front of the chest because armrests are missing. An increased thoracic kyphosis combined with a rounded shoulder posture is also a good perpetuating and promoting factor for TrP development in the lower portion of the trapezius muscle.

4.2. Associated Trigger Points

It has been shown that associated TrPs can develop in the referred pain areas caused by TrPs[71]; therefore, muscles in the referred pain areas for each muscle should also be considered. In the presence of TrPs in the upper portion of the trapezius muscle, associated TrPs are likely to develop in the functionally related levator scapulae, sternocleidomastoid, and contralateral trapezius muscles, and also in the ipsilateral supraspinatus and rhomboid muscles. Associated TrPs may appear in the temporalis and occipital muscles, which lie within the zones of pain referred from TrPs in the upper trapezius muscle. Hong[72] identified a number of associated TrPs that were inactivated by inactivating TrPs in the upper trapezius muscle. The associated TrPs appeared in the temporalis, masseter, splenius, semispinalis, levator scapulae, and rhomboid minor muscles.

When the middle trapezius muscle is involved, associated TrPs can develop in the rhomboids, serratus posterior superior, thoracic paraspinals at the levels of T1-T6, and the supraspinatus muscles. Outside of the referred pain areas, other muscles that could also be involved include the antagonistic pectoralis major and pectoralis minor muscles.

Trigger points in the lower portion of the trapezius muscle are prone to induce associated TrPs in the upper trapezius, supraspinatus, and sometimes in the levator scapulae and the posterior cervical muscles. For this reason, one should routinely check the lower trapezius muscle for TrPs, especially when the upper trapezius TrPs responds poorly to treatment.[42] Keep in mind, however, that a TrP in the lower trapezius muscle may itself be an associated TrP of a TrP in the latissimus dorsi muscle.

4.3. Associated Pathology

Myofascial pain in the trapezius muscle is highly prevalent and comorbid with several underlying medical conditions. Patients with widespread chronic pain that includes multiple regional involvements should be clinically examined for the diagnosis of fibromyalgia since these patients exhibit a higher number of TrPs in this muscle.[73]

Upper Trapezius Fibers

Trigger points in the upper portion of the trapezius muscle are associated with medical conditions such as neck pain, temporomandibular pain disorders, or headaches. Shoulder pain has also been associated with a high prevalence of TrPs in the upper trapezius muscle.[74] A common cause of upper trapezius muscle (and other muscles) TrPs is the impact stress from a whiplash injury.[13,64] Furthermore, pain originating from TrPs in the upper trapezius and the splenius capitis muscles can confusingly simulate occipital neuralgia because the greater occipital nerve crosses these muscles.[75]

The symptoms caused by upper trapezius TrPs may be closely associated with, and confusingly similar to, somatic or articular dysfunctions from C2 to C4. Commonly, one or more of these restricting articular dysfunctions and upper trapezius TrPs coexist, and both must be treated. In fact, Fernández de las Peña et al[76] found a clinical association between the presence of TrPs in the upper trapezius muscle and intervertebral joint dysfunctions at C3-C4 levels.

Hypermobility of the C4 segment has been observed clinically to be associated with the upper trapezius muscle dysfunction. Joint stress that causes referred pain can involve the upper trapezius muscle secondarily, and this muscle often becomes hyperirritable and develops TrPs. An upper trapezius muscle source of pain may be differentiated from a joint source by testing for pain on side bending of the cervical spine and then (1) passively support the patient's upper limb and side-bend the cervical spine again; if the pain is markedly reduced or absent, the problem may be in the trapezius muscle; and (2) apply pressure downward on the shoulder (as in lengthening the upper trapezius muscle); if there is an increase in pain, the upper trapezius muscle may be the source of the problem. If *neither* of these tests changes the pain, the cervical joints (perhaps C4) may be the problem. In addition, different manual testing of joint mobility are generally applied in these cases.

Trigger point involvement of the upper trapezius, splenius capitis and cervicis, levator scapulae, and sternocleidomastoid muscles must be distinguished from spasmodic torticollis (cervical dystonia), which is a neurologic condition characterized by involuntary dystonic movements of the head[77,78] that can be genetic, acquired, or idiopathic.[79] The muscles most commonly involved in this condition include the sternocleidomastoid, trapezius, scalenes, and platysma,[80] thus making the differential diagnosis of this condition (versus TrPs) essential to ensure proper care. With spasmodic torticollis, hypertrophy of the muscles may develop.[77] In contrast, the apparent shortening of a muscle due to TrPs does not cause hypertrophy, nor does it cause involuntary movements of the head.

Middle Trapezius Fibers

The main underlying medical conditions related to dysfunction of the middle portion of the trapezius muscle are related to changes in thoracic curvature, for example, scoliosis or kyphosis, osteoporosis, tumors, fractures, and the like. The cervicothoracic junction is a troublesome transitional vertebral area that commonly develops dysfunctions, primarily of C6, C7, T1, and occasionally T2. Commonly, these dysfunctions are associated with adduction of the scapulae and elevation of the first rib on the same side.

Lower Trapezius Fibers

Articular dysfunctions associated with interscapular pain and lower trapezius TrPs[81] may extend from T4 to T12. There is usually a central painful segment near T6 or T7, which is the primary structural dysfunction that must be treated along with inactivation of the TrPs. The dorsal scapular nerve[82] and cervical spine[1,9,40,83] should also be considered in patients with interscapular pain.

5. CORRECTIVE ACTIONS

Correction of poor posture (particularly rounded shoulder posture with an excessive forward head posture) and maintenance of good posture are primary in any treatment approach, both for initial relief of pain and for lasting relief. Refer to Chapter 72 for discussions of posture and body mechanics.

The upper trapezius muscle is generally recognized as prone to hyperactivity and increased tension, whereas the middle and lower trapezius muscles tends to be just the opposite, inhibited, weak, and overstretched.[48] Self-treatment that depends primarily on stretch can be counterproductive in muscles prone to inhibition and weakness and are not recommended. Therefore, we emphasize for the middle and lower portions of the trapezius muscle the application of massage to the taut band, TrP pressure release, and other techniques, carefully avoiding excessive stretch. The use of TrP self-pressure release tools can be useful for treatment of these muscles. Specific corrective actions for each portion of the trapezius muscle are described below.

Upper Trapezius Fibers

Patients with TrPs in the upper trapezius muscle should not sleep on a foam pillow; its springiness can aggravate TrP symptoms. Antigravity stress on the upper trapezius muscle in normally proportioned individuals is corrected by selecting chairs with armrests of the correct height to provide elbow support or by building up the height of the armrests, if they were designed too low (refer to Chapter 79).[84] Every seated person benefits by learning to distinguish between chairs that fit and chairs that enforce poor posture, which can aggravate the muscles.[85]

Patients who are intensely preoccupied with what they are doing are susceptible to lose track of time and maintain an undesirable posture. This can happen while engrossed at a computer or leaning forward over a desk for a prolonged period while writing. Trigger points have been shown to develop with 1 hour of typing.[68] These individuals can relieve muscle tension every 20 or 30 minute, without interrupting the train of thought, by setting an interval-timer for that length of time and placing it across the room. Then they must get up and can stretch while they walk to turn off the buzzer and reset the timer. Downloadable applications from the Internet can be set on a computer as well for break reminders.

Muscles are more tolerant of prolonged activity if they have frequent short breaks permitting relaxation. A few cycles of active range of motion makes the break more effective. In the case of the upper trapezius muscle, this may be achieved by slowly rotating the shoulders in a full circle several times, first in one direction and then in the other.

For office workers, a common source of stress to the upper trapezius muscle is a keyboard set so high that the shoulders are maintained in an elevated position. Lowering the keyboard eliminates excessive sustained electromyographic activity of the upper trapezius muscle.[86] The keyboard should be placed at an appropriate height. If the keyboard height is properly adjusted but the subject leans forward away from the backrest, the upper trapezius muscles may still be overloaded (refer to Chapter 76). Leaning back against the backrest of a chair so that it supports the scapulae can provide much relief. The individual must lean back and allow the shoulders to drop down so the backrest supports them. In most chairs, a small cushion for lumbar support facilitates good posture. If modification of sitting postures is insufficient, using an adjustable standing desk is an alternative. Refer to Chapter 76 for additional suggestions regarding the correction of poor posture and ergonomics.

For patients who have long conversations on the telephone or cellphone, a head set or hands-free setting relieves the neck and arm muscles from the strain of holding a phone.

When conversing with someone, the patient should turn his or her chair to face the other person or turn the entire body and not just the head.

It is best to try to avoid sleeping prone when the upper portion of the trapezius muscle has TrPs. If one does sleep prone, a pillow placed under the shoulder and chest on the same side to which the face is turned helps to reduce rotation of the neck. A semiprone position, achieved by flexing the knee and hip of the side toward which the face is turned, also helps by partly rotating the torso.

Objectionable pressure on the trapezius muscle by a thin, tight bra strap should be relieved by wearing a wider, nonelastic bra strap, and/or by slipping a soft shield under the strap to distribute the pressure. Sliding the strap laterally to rest on the acromion relieves pressure on the muscle. A professional bra fitting may be indicated if TrPs in the upper trapezius muscle are resistant to treatment. A strapless bra that constricts too tightly around the ribs may cause comparable pressure activation of TrPs in the latissimus dorsi, serratus anterior, or serratus posterior inferior muscles.

Supporting and/or offloading the upper trapezius muscle during seated activities may be beneficial for decreasing TrP activity (Figure 6-9). A recent study also demonstrated that tensioned and nontensioned taping across the upper portion of the trapezius muscle reduces its activity during a typing task.[87]

Middle Trapezius Fibers

When the arm must be held out in front of the body for long periods of time, some form of elbow rest should be devised. The middle trapezius exercise (Figure 6-10) is tailored to maintain full active range of motion in both the middle and lower trapezius muscles. The patient is instructed to lie supine on the floor. To reduce strain on the lower back, the knees should be bent so the feet are on the floor. The core muscles should also be activated to prevent arching of the back as the arms move. Place the elbows, forearms, and palms of the hands together in front of the abdomen (Figure 6-10A). Keep the elbows tightly together as long as possible while raising the forearms over the face (Figure 6-10B). Then, drop the forearms past the ears to the floor (Figure 6-10C). Keeping the back of the elbows and wrists in contact with the floor, swing the arms down against the sides of the body (Figure 6-10D and E). Pause and relax, while taking several slow deep breaths. Repeat the cycle.

The importance of checking both pectoral muscles for tightness (and TrPs) cannot be overemphasized. Most commonly, middle trapezius weakness and TrPs are from overload and are secondary to other causes. Unless the tightness of the thoracic anterior muscles causing the problem is effectively addressed, the patient will continue to have trouble. The pectoral fibers can be stretched by performing the doorway stretch exercise (refer to Figure 49.10). The middle hand position of this exercise specifically stretches the sternal division of the pectoralis major muscle, which most directly opposes the middle trapezius muscle. An alternative to the doorway stretch exercise is to lie on a foam roller in the supine position with the arms elevated to different positions (refer to Figure 42-11). To treat TrPs of the pectoralis muscle, TrP self-pressure release tools can be used. Each release procedure is followed promptly by full active range of motion and moist heat to the treated region.

The middle trapezius muscle responds well to TrP pressure release by the operator or self-release by the patient using a cold tennis ball (Figure 6-11) or other types of TrP self-pressure release tools. Each release procedure is followed promptly by full active range of motion and moist heat to the treated region.

Section 2: Head and Neck Pain

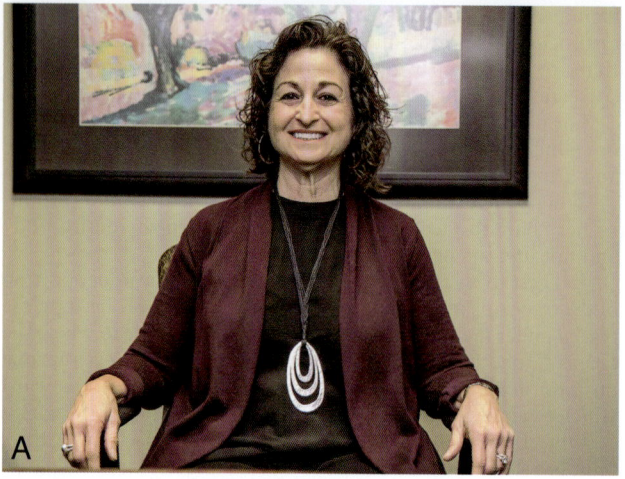
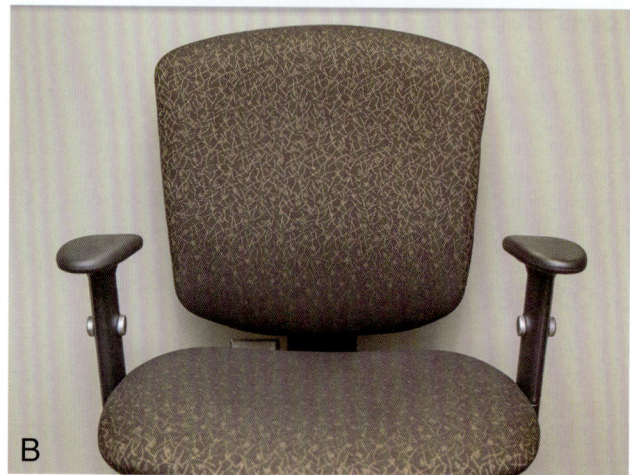
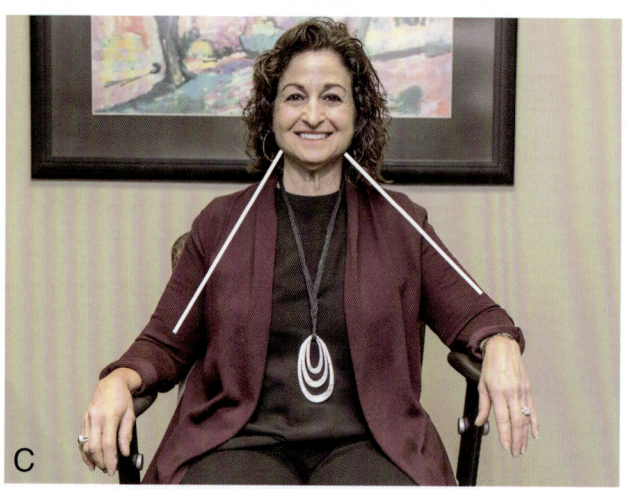
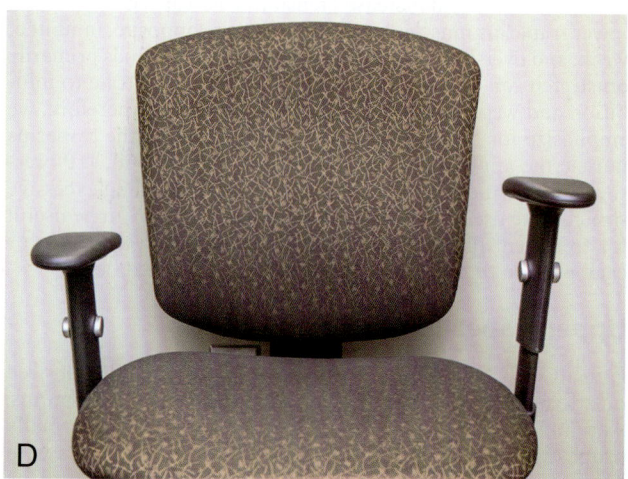

Figure 6-9. Ergonomic solutions for the upper trapezius muscle. A, Effective support of the arms by armrests of a desk chair. B, Desk chair with adjustable armrests at an appropriate height to support the upper extremities during desk tasks. C, Offloading the left upper extremity by raising the left armrest. D, Desk chair with left armrest raised to offload the left upper trapezius muscle.

Lower Trapezius Fibers

Proper workstation posture can reduce symptoms arising from TrPs in the lower trapezius muscle. Every patient should arrange seated workspace to provide adequate room for the knees underneath the desk or table. The chair should be pulled close enough to the workspace so that the patient can lean back firmly against the backrest; both elbows should rest on the work surface or on short armrests of about the same height as the desk surface. The middle trapezius exercise (Figure 6-10) is also helpful for at-home maintenance of full range of motion in the lower trapezius muscle.

The lower portion of the trapezius muscle is often the key to successful treatment of the upper trapezius, levator scapulae, and

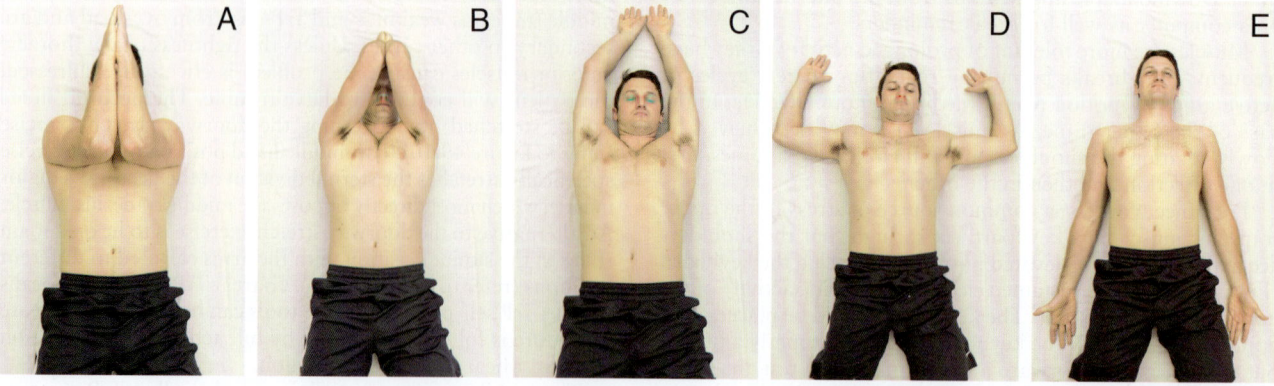

Figure 6-10. The middle trapezius exercise helps to maintain full range of motion in the middle and lower parts of the trapezius muscle by abducting and rotating the scapulae. Movements progress from (A) through (E). When completed, the patient pauses, breathes deeply to relax, and repeats the sequence.

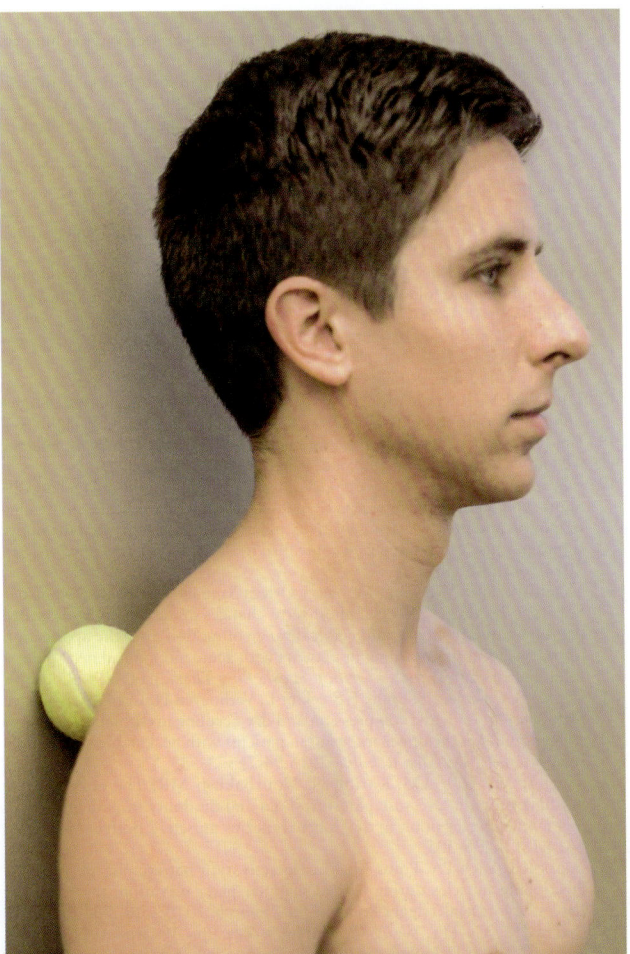

Figure 6-11. Trigger point self-pressure release of the middle trapezius muscle with a cold tennis ball.

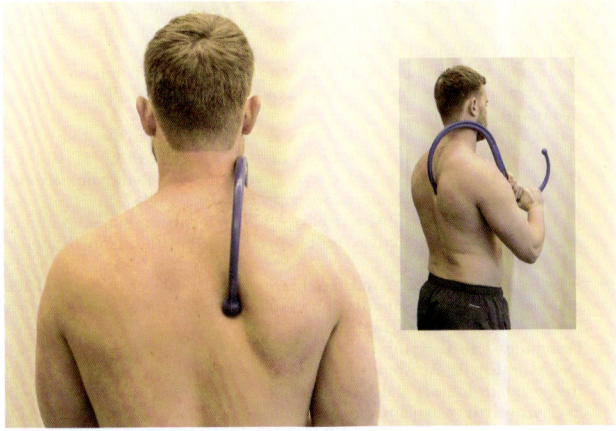

Figure 6-12. Trigger point self-pressure release of the lower trapezius muscle using a TrP release tool.

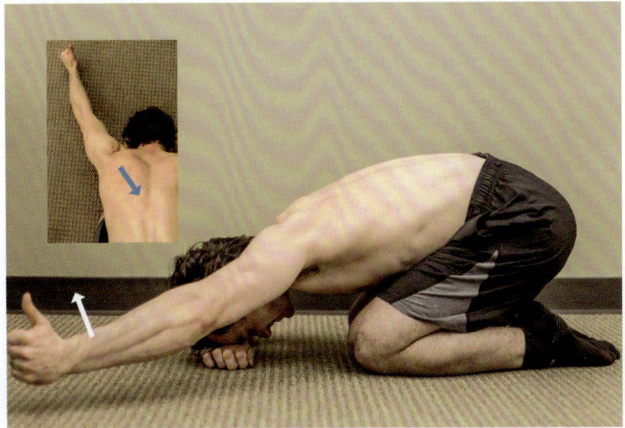

Figure 6-13. Scapular posterior tilting. The patient starts in the quadruped position and rocks back slowly to sit on his heels. With the arm elevated to approximately 145°, elbow extended, and the thumb side of the wrist facing upward, the arm is actively lifted until it is lifted to the level of the ear. The position is held for 5 seconds before lowering the arm back down to the starting position.

some neck extensor muscles; these muscles lie in the referred pain zone of the lower trapezius muscle and may develop satellite TrPs to the key lower trapezius TrP. The lower trapezius muscle itself (and by extension the above-mentioned muscles) may develop pain and TrPs because of TrP tension in the antagonistic pectoralis major (refer to Chapter 42) and pectoralis minor muscles (refer to Chapter 43). When the pectoral muscles are involved, their full normal resting length must be restored in order for the lower trapezius muscle to be relieved of overload. The pectoral fibers can be stretched by performing the in-doorway stretch exercise (refer to Figure 42-10) or lying supine on a foam roller (refer to Figure 42-11). To treat TrPs of the pectoralis muscles, TrP self-pressure release tools can be used. Each release procedure is followed promptly by full active range of motion to the treated region.

Because the lower trapezius muscle is often weak, the aim is not primarily stretch but rather release of tension in the taut band. Toward this aim, the patient can apply self-TrP pressure release by lying on a tennis ball that is positioned to press on the TrPs. Other types of TrP self-pressure release tools can also be used to apply pressure to the TrPs (Figure 6-12). Each release procedure is followed promptly by full active range of motion and moist heat to the treated region.

Performing a scapular posterior tilting motion (Figure 6-13) in conjunction with assisted pectoralis minor stretching has also been shown to be effective to improve activation of the lower trapezius muscle.[57]

When using a moist heating pad or hot pack for relief of pain referred from TrPs in the lower fibers of the trapezius muscle, the patient should apply the heat to the mid back area where the TrPs are located, rather than solely to the suprascapular region and neck where pain is felt. The patient should never lie on the pad; instead the pad should be placed on the back while the patient is semiprone.

Women should consider wearing a brassiere with crossed versus parallel straps as this has been shown to improve activity of the lower trapezius muscle and reduce activity of the upper trapezius muscle.[88]

References

1. Cooper G, Bailey B, Bogduk N. Cervical zygapophysial joint pain maps. *Pain Med.* 2007;8(4):344-353.
2. Johnson G, Bogduk N, Nowitzke A, House D. Anatomy and actions of the trapezius muscle. *Clin Biomech.* 1994;9:44-50.
3. de Freitas V, Vitti M. Electromyographic study of the trapezius (middle portion) and rhomboideus major muscles in free circumduction and pendular movements of the arm. *Anat Anz.* 1981;149(3):265-269.
4. Bovim G, Bonamico L, Fredriksen TA, Lindboe CF, Stolt-Nielsen A, Sjaastad O. Topographic variations in the peripheral course of the greater occipital nerve. Autopsy study with clinical correlations. *Spine.* 1991;16(4):475-478.
5. De Mey K, Cagnie B, Danneels LA, Cools AM, Van de Velde A. Trapezius muscle timing during selected shoulder rehabilitation exercises. *J Orthop Sports Phys Ther.* 2009;39(10):743-752.

6. Simons DG, Travell J, Simons L. *Travell & Simon's Myofascial Pain and Dysfunction: The Trigger Point Manual.* Vol 1. 2nd ed. Baltimore, MD: Williams & Wilkins; 1999.
7. Doraisamy MA, Anshul. Effect of latent myofascial trigger points on strength measurements of the upper trapezius: a case-controlled trial. *Physiother Can.* 2011;63(4):405-409.
8. Caliot P, Bousquet V, Midy D, Cabanie P. A contribution to the study of the accessory nerve: surgical implications. *Surg Radiol Anat.* 1989;11(1):11-15.
9. Dwyer A, Aprill C, Bogduk N. Cervical zygapophyseal joint pain patterns. I: A study in normal volunteers. *Spine.* 1990;15(6):453-457.
10. Ebaugh DD, McClure PW, Karduna AR. Three-dimensional scapulothoracic motion during active and passive arm elevation. *Clin Biomech.* 2005;20(7):700-709.
11. Feng B, Liang Q, Wang Y, Andersen LL, Szeto G. Prevalence of work-related musculoskeletal symptoms of the neck and upper extremity among dentists in China. *BMJ Open.* 2014;4(12):e006451.
12. Fernandez-Lao C, Cantarero-Villanueva I, Fernández de las Peñas C, Del-Moral-Avila R, Arendt-Nielsen L, Arroyo-Morales M. Myofascial trigger points in neck and shoulder muscles and widespread pressure pain hypersensitivtiy in patients with postmastectomy pain: evidence of peripheral and central sensitization. *Clin J Pain.* 2010;26(9):798-806.
13. Fernandez-Perez AM, Villaverde-Gutierrez C, Mora-Sanchez A, Alonso-Blanco C, Sterling M, Fernández de las Peñas C. Muscle trigger points, pressure pain threshold, and cervical range of motion in patients with high level of disability related to acute whiplash injury. *J Orthop Sports Phys Ther.* 2012;42(7):634-641.
14. Ge HY, Monterde S, Graven-Nielsen T, Arendt-Nielsen L. Latent myofascial trigger points are associated with an increased intramuscular electromyographic activity during synergistic muscle activation. *J Pain.* 2014;15(2):181-187.
15. Gerber LH, Shah J, Rosenberger W, et al. Dry needling alters trigger points in the upper trapezius muscle and reduces pain in subjects with chronic myofascial pain. *PM & R.* 2015;7(7):711-718.
16. Glenn JA, Yen TW, Fareau GG, Carr AA, Evans DB, Wang TS. Institutional experience with lateral neck dissections for thyroid cancer. *Surgery.* 2015;158(4):972-978; discussion 978-980.
17. Brennan PA, St J Blythe J, Alam P, Green B, Parry D. Division of the spinal accessory nerve in the anterior triangle: a prospective clinical study. *Br J Oral Maxillofac Surg.* 2015;53(7):633-636.
18. Pu YM, Tang EY, Yang XD. Trapezius muscle innervation from the spinal accessory nerve and branches of the cervical plexus. *Int J Oral Maxillofac Surg.* 2008;37(6):567-572.
19. Kim JH, Choi KY, Lee KH, Lee DJ, Park BJ, Rho YS. Motor innervation of the trapezius muscle: Intraoperative motor conduction study during neck dissection. *ORL J Otorhinolaryngol Relat Spec.* 2014;76(1):8-12.
20. Orhan KS, Demirel T, Baslo B, et al. Spinal accessory nerve function after neck dissections. *J Laryngol Otol.* 2007;121(1):44-48.
21. Gun K, Uludag M, Delil S, et al. Spinal accessory nerve injury: eight cases and review of the literature. *Clin Ter.* 2014;165(4):211-216.
22. Cesmebasi A, Spinner RJ. An anatomic-based approach to the iatrogenic spinal accessory nerve injury in the posterior cervical triangle: how to avoid and treat it. *Clin Anat.* 2015;28(6):761-766.
23. Park SH, Esquenazi Y, Kline DG, Kim DH. Surgical outcomes of 156 spinal accessory nerve injuries caused by lymph node biopsy procedures. *J Neurosurg Spine.* 2015;23(4):518-525.
24. Standring S. *Gray's Anatomy: The Anatomical Basis of Clinical Practice.* 41st ed. London, UK: Elsevier; 2015.
25. Guazzelli Filho J, Furlani J, De Freitas V. Electromyographic study of the trapezius muscle in free movements of the arm. *Electromyogr Clin Neurophysiol.* 1991;31(2):93-98.
26. Ito N. Electromyographic study of shoulder joint. *Nihon Seikeigeka Gakkai Zasshi.* 1980;54(11):1529-1540.
27. Hagberg M. Electromyographic signs of shoulder muscular fatigue in two elevated arm positions. *Am J Phys Med.* 1981;60(3):111-121.
28. Arlotta M, Lovasco G, McLean L. Selective recruitment of the lower fibers of the trapezius muscle. *J Electromyogr Kinesiol.* 2011;21(3):403-410.
29. Moore KL, Agur AMR, Dalley AF. *Clinically Oriented Anatomy.* Baltimore, MD: Lippincott Williams & Wilkins; 2014.
30. Kendall FP, McCreary EK. *Muscles: Testing and Function, with Posture and Pain.* Baltimore, MD: Lippincott Williams & Wilkins; 2005.
31. Pizzari T, Wickham J, Balster S, Ganderton C, Watson L. Modifying a shrug exercise can facilitate the upward rotator muscles of the scapula. *Clin Biomech.* 2014;29(2):201-205.
32. Mottram SL. Dynamic stability of the scapula. *Man Ther.* 1997;2(3):123-131.
33. Wadsworth DJ, Bullock-Saxton JE. Recruitment patterns of the scapular rotator muscles in freestyle swimmers with subacromial impingement. *Int J Sports Med.* 1997;18(8):618-624.
34. Kibler WB. The role of the scapula in athletic shoulder function. *Am J Sports Med.* 1998;26(2):325-337.
35. Cools AM, Witvrouw EE, Declercq GA, Danneels LA, Cambier DC. Scapular muscle recruitment patterns: trapezius muscle latency with and without impingement symptoms. *Am J Sports Med.* 2003;31(4):542-549.
36. Travell J. Mechanical headache. *Headache.* 1967;7(1):23-29.
37. Carlson CR, Okeson JP, Falace DA, Nitz AJ, Lindroth JE. Reduction of pain and EMG activity in the masseter region by trapezius trigger point injection. *Pain.* 1993;55(3):397-400.
38. Fernández de las Peñas C, Ge HY, Arendt-Nielsen L, Cuadrado ML, Pareja JA. Referred pain from trapezius muscle trigger points shares similar characteristics with chronic tension type headache. *Eur J Pain.* 2007;11(4):475-482.
39. Fernández de las Peñas C, Alonso-Blanco C, Miangolarra JC. Myofascial trigger points in subjects presenting with mechanical neck pain: a blinded, controlled study. *Man Ther.* 2007;12(1):29-33.
40. Fukui S, Ohseto K, Shiotani M, et al. Referred pain distribution of the cervical zygapophyseal joints and cervical dorsal rami. *Pain.* 1996;68(1):79-83.
41. Travell J. Symposium on mechanism and management of pain syndromes. *Proc Rudolf Virchow Med Soc.* 1957;16:126-136.
42. Pecos-Martin D, Montanez-Aguilera FJ, Gallego-Izquierdo T, et al. Effectiveness of dry needling on the lower trapezius in patients with mechanical neck pain: a randomized controlled trial. *Arch Phys Med Rehabil.* 2015;96(5):775-781.
43. Wyant GM. Chronic pain syndromes and their treatment. II. Trigger points. *Can Anaesth Soc J.* 1979;26(3):216-219.
44. Fernández de las Peñas C, Cuadrado ML, Pareja JA. Myofascial trigger points, neck mobility and forward head posture in unilateral migraine. *Cephalalgia.* 2006;26(9):1061-1070.
45. Travell J. Rapid relief of acute stiff neck by ethyl chloride spray. *J Am Med Womens Assoc.* 1949;4(3):89-95.
46. Engle WK. Ponderous-purse disease. *N Engl J Med.* 1978;299:557.
47. Ludewig PM, Reynolds JF. The association of scapular kinematics and glenohumeral joint pathologies. *J Orthop Sports Phys Ther.* 2009;39(2):90-104.
48. Page P, Frank C, Lardner R. *Assessment and Treatment of Muscle Imbalance: The Janda Approach.* Champaign, IL: Human Kinetics; 2009.
49. Oliveira-Campelo NM, de Melo CA, Alburquerque-Sendin F, Machado JP. Short- and medium-term effects of manual therapy on cervical active range of motion and pressure pain sensitivity in latent myofascial pain of the upper trapezius muscle: a randomized controlled trial. *J Manipulative Physiol Ther.* 2013;36(5):300-309.
50. Mejuto-Vazquez MJ, Salom-Moreno J, Ortega-Santiago R, Truyols-Dominguez S, Fernández de las Peñas C. Short-term changes in neck pain, widespread pressure pain sensitivity, and cervical range of motion after the application of trigger point dry needling in patients with acute mechanical neck pain: a randomized clinical trial. *J Orthop Sports Phys Ther.* 2014;44(4):252-260.
51. Cagnie B, Castelein B, Pollie F, Steelant L, Verhoeyen H, Cools A. Evidence for the use of ischemic compression and dry needling in the management of trigger points of the upper trapezius in patients with neck pain: a systematic review. *Am J Phys Med Rehabil.* 2015;94(7):573-583.
52. Ziaeifar M, Arab AM, Karimi N, Nourbakhsh MR. The effect of dry needling on pain, pressure pain threshold and disability in patients with a myofascial trigger point in the upper trapezius muscle. *J Bodyw Mov Ther.* 2014;18(2):298-305.
53. Lucas KR, Rich PA, Polus BI. Muscle activation patterns in the scapular positioning muscles during loaded scapular plane elevation: the effects of Latent Myofascial Trigger Points. *Clin Biomech.* 2010;25(8):765-770.
54. Ibarra JM, Ge HY, Wang C, Martinez Vizcaino V, Graven-Nielsen T, Arendt-Nielsen L. Latent myofascial trigger points are associated with an increased antagonistic muscle activity during agonist muscle contraction. *J Pain.* 2011;12(12):1282-1288.
55. Lee KJ, Han HY, Cheon SH, Park SH, Yong MS. The effect of forward head posture on muscle activity during neck protraction and retraction. *J Phys Ther Sci.* 2015;27(3):977-979.
56. Borstad JD, Ludewig PM. The effect of long versus short pectoralis minor resting length on scapular kinematics in healthy individuals. *J Orthop Sports Phys Ther.* 2005;35(4):227-238.
57. Lee JH, Cynn HS, Yoon TL, et al. Comparison of scapular posterior tilting exercise alone and scapular posterior tilting exercise after pectoralis minor stretching on scapular alignment and scapular upward rotators activity in subjects with short pectoralis minor. *Phys Ther Sport.* 2015;16(3):255-261.
58. Petersen SM, Wyatt SN. Lower trapezius muscle strength in individuals with unilateral neck pain. *J Orthop Sports Phys Ther.* 2011;41(4):260-265.
59. Gerwin RD, Shannon S, Hong C-Z, Hubbard DR, Gevirtz R. Interrater reliability in myofascial trigger point examination. *Pain.* 1997;69:65-73.
60. Barbero M, Bertoli P, Cescon C, Macmillan F, Coutts F, Gatti R. Intra-rater reliability of an experienced physiotherapist in locating myofascial trigger points in upper trapezius muscle. *J Man Manip Ther.* 2012;20(4):171-177.
61. Akamatsu FE, Ayres BR, Saleh SO, et al. Trigger points: an anatomical substratum. *Biomed Res Int.* 2015;2015:623287.
62. Maher RM, Hayes DM, Shinohara M. Quantification of dry needling and posture effects on myofascial trigger points using ultrasound shear-wave elastography. *Arch Phys Med Rehabil.* 2013;94(11):2146-2150.
63. Gerwin RD, Dommerholt J, Shah JP. An expansion of Simons' integrated hypothesis of trigger point formation. *Curr Pain Headache Rep.* 2004;8(6):468-475.
64. Castaldo M, Ge HY, Chiarotto A, Villafane JH, Arendt-Nielsen L. Myofascial trigger points in patients with whiplash-associated disorders and mechanical neck pain. *Pain Med.* 2014;15(5):842-849.
65. Veiersted KB, Westgaard RH, Andersen P. Electromyographic evaluation of muscular work pattern as a predictor of trapezius myalgia. *Scand J Work Environ Health.* 1993;19(4):284-290.
66. Veiersted KB, Westgaard RH. Development of trapezius myalgia among female workers performing light manual work. *Scand J Work Environ Health.* 1993;19(4):277-283.
67. Memarpour M, Badakhsh S, Khosroshahi SS, Vossoughi M. Work-related musculoskeletal disorders among Iranian dentists. *Work.* 2013;45(4):465-474.
68. Hoyle JA, Marras WS, Sheedy JE, Hart DE. Effects of postural and visual stressors on myofascial trigger point development and motor unit rotation during computer work. *J Electromyogr Kinesiol.* 2011;21(1):41-48.
69. Sari H, Akarirmak U, Uludag M. Active myofascial trigger points might be more frequent in patients with cervical radiculopathy. *Eur J Phys Rehabil Med.* 2012;48(2):237-244.

70. McAllister MJ, Schilling BK, Hammond KG, Weiss LW, Farney TM. Effect of grip width on electromyographic activity during the upright row. *J Strength Cond Res*. 2013;27(1):181-187.
71. Hsieh YL, Kao MJ, Kuan TS, Chen SM, Chen JT, Hong CZ. Dry needling to a key myofascial trigger point may reduce the irritability of satellite MTrPs. *Am J Phys Med Rehabil*. 2007;86(5):397-403.
72. Hong CZ. Considerations and recommendations regarding myofascial trigger point injection. *J Musculoskelet Pain*. 1994;2(1):29-59.
73. Alonso-Blanco C, Fernández de las Peñas C, Morales-Cabezas M, Zarco-Moreno P, Ge HY, Florez-Garcia M. Multiple active myofascial trigger points reproduce the overall spontaneous pain pattern in women with fibromyalgia and are related to widespread mechanical hypersensitivity. *Clin J Pain*. 2011;27(5):405-413.
74. Bron C, Dommerholt J, Stegenga B, Wensing M, Oostendorp RA. High prevalence of shoulder girdle muscles with myofascial trigger points in patients with shoulder pain. *BMC Musculoskelet Diso*. 2011;12(1):139-151.
75. Tubbs RS, Watanabe K, Loukas M, Cohen-Gadol AA. The intramuscular course of the greater occipital nerve: novel findings with potential implications for operative interventions and occipital neuralgia. *Surg Neurol Int*. 2014;5:155.
76. Fernández de las Peñas C, Fernandez-Carnero J, Miangolarra-Page J. Musculoskeletal disorders in mechanical neck pain: myofascial trigger points versus cervical joint dysfunction: a clinical study. *J Musculoskelet Pain*. 2005;13(1):27-35.
77. Waldman SD. *Atlas of Uncommon Pain Syndromes*. 3rd ed. Philadelphia, PA: Elsevier Saunders; 2014.
78. Mills RR, Pagan FL. Patient considerations in the treatment of cervical dystonia: focus on botulinum toxin type A. *Patient Prefer Adherence*. 2015;9:725-731.
79. Albanese A, Bhatia K, Bressman SB, et al. Phenomenology and classification of dystonia: a consensus update. *Mov Disord*. 2013;28(7):863-873.
80. Jankovic J, Leder S, Warner D, Schwartz K. Cervical dystonia: clinical findings and associated movement disorders. *Neurology*. 1991;41(7):1088-1091.
81. Lewit K. *Manipulative Therapy in Rehabilitation of the Locomotor System*. 2nd ed. Oxford, England: Butterworth Heinemann; 1991.
82. Sultan HE, Younis El-Tantawi GA. Role of dorsal scapular nerve entrapment in unilateral interscapular pain. *Arch Phys Med Rehabil*. 2013;94(6):1118-1125.
83. Mizutamari M, Sei A, Tokiyoshi A, et al. Corresponding scapular pain with the nerve root involved in cervical radiculopathy. *J Orthop Surg (Hong Kong)*. 2010;18(3):356-360.
84. Madeleine P. On functional motor adaptations: from the quantification of motor strategies to the prevention of musculoskeletal disorders in the neck-shoulder region. *Acta Physiol*. 2010;199 suppl 679:1-46.
85. Travell J. Chairs are a personal thing. *House Beautiful*. 1955;97:190-193.
86. Cook C, Burgess-Limerick R, Papalia S. The effect of upper extremity support on upper extremity posture and muscle activity during keyboard use. *Appl Ergon*. 2004;35(3):285-292.
87. Takasaki H, Delbridge BM, Johnston V. Taping across the upper trapezius muscle reduces activity during a standardized typing task: an assessor-blinded randomized cross-over study. *J Electromyogr Kinesiol*. 2015;25(1):115-120.
88. Kang MH, Choi JY, Oh JS. Effects of crossed brassiere straps on pain, range of motion, and electromyographic activity of scapular upward rotators in women with scapular downward rotation syndrome. *PM & R*. 2015;7(12):1261-1268.

Chapter 7

Sternocleidomastoid Muscle

"Migraine and Sinus Headache Imposter"

Michelle Finnegan and Susan H. Rightnour

1. INTRODUCTION

The sternocleidomastoid (SCM) muscle is an important muscle of the neck for posture and control of head movement and is commonly seen in clinical practice to have trigger points (TrPs). It is composed of two heads, sternal and clavicular, which both originate from the mastoid process. The sternal division inserts onto the manubrium of the sternum, whereas the clavicular division inserts along the medial third of the clavicle. The muscle is innervated by the spinal accessory nerve and receives vascularization from branches of the occipital and posterior auricular arteries for the upper portion of the muscle, while the middle portion is supplied by the superior thyroid artery and the lower portion is supplied by the suprascapular artery. Bilaterally, the muscle functions to flex the head against gravity. It also assists with forced inspiration when the head is fixed. Unilaterally, the muscle functions to side bend the head ipsilaterally and rotate the head contralaterally. The pain referral of the sternal division of the muscle is distributed over the upper portion of the sternum, throughout the face, the pharynx and the back of the throat, the chin, the occipital area, and the vertex of the head. The clavicular division of the muscle refers to both the sides of the frontal region of the head, unilaterally deep in the ear, and the posterior auricular region. Trigger points in this muscle are associated with many different conditions including temporomandibular dysfunction whiplash-associated disorders, mechanical neck pain, episodic migraine, cervicogenic headache, and tension-type headache. Corrective actions for this muscle include avoiding prolonged positions with the head turned to one side, sleeping with proper pillow support, stretching of the muscle by turning the head toward the restricted side with a chin retraction, or passively stretching the muscle in supine over a pillow.

2. ANATOMIC CONSIDERATIONS

As stated earlier, the SCM muscle has two divisions with differing caudal attachments. They are separated near their attachments by a triangular interval, the lesser supraclavicular fossa. This muscle divides the neck into anterior and posterior triangles. Its central region is narrow and dense becoming broader and thinner at each end. It acts as a protective barrier to the vital structures that lie beneath it, including the common carotid artery, accessory nerve, brachial plexus roots, cervical plexus nerves, and cervical lymph nodes.[1] Cephalad, the two divisions blend to form a common attachment on the mastoid process (Figure 7-1). The relative size of the two divisions and the space between them at the clavicle are variable. Due to each head of the muscle having a different direction of pull, it may be classified as "cruciate" and slightly "spiralizer."[1] Anomalies of the SCM attachments have been reported in the literature including the presence of a third accessory head that lies between the sternal

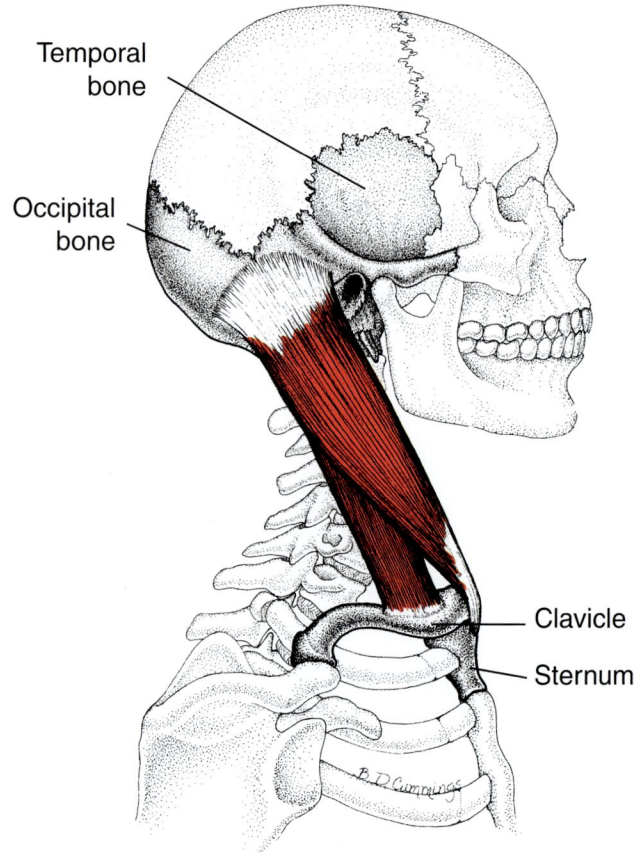

Figure 7-1. Attachments of the two divisions of the sternocleidomastoid muscle (dark red). The sternal division is more anterior, more diagonal, and more superficial than the clavicular division. The bones to which the muscle attaches show darker stipples.

and clavicular heads,[2,3] the absence of the SCM muscle,[4] and a blending of the SCM muscle with the platysma muscle.[5]

Sternal Division

The sternal fibers are the more medial, diagonal, and superficial fibers of the two heads of the SCM muscle, attaching to the anterior surface of the manubrium sterni. They ascend posterolaterally and attach above by a strong tendon to the lateral surface of the mastoid process and by a thin aponeurosis to the lateral half of the superior nuchal line of the occipital bone (Figure 7-1). The sternalis muscle may extend downward over the anterior chest, appearing like a continuation of the sternal division of the SCM muscle (see Chapter 43).

Clavicular Division

The clavicular fibers are the more lateral and deeper of the two heads of the SCM muscle distally. This portion of the muscle is variable in width and attaches below to the superior border of the anterior surface of the clavicle, along its medial third. It ascends almost vertically, attaching above to the same bony structures, as does the sternal division (Figure 7-1).[1]

The clavicular fibers are mainly directed to the mastoid process, whereas the sternal fibers are more oblique and superficial extending to the occiput. The thick, round belly of this muscle is formed by the blending of the two heads as the clavicular portion spirals behind the sternal head.[1]

2.1. Innervation and Vascularization

The fibers of the SCM muscle (and some of the trapezius muscle) have an unusually close association with the brain stem, which helps to account for its remarkable functional concomitants. The SCM muscle is innervated by the spinal (external) portion of the accessory nerve (cranial nerve XI). This nerve originates in the spinal nucleus of the spinal cord of the upper five[6] or six[7,8] cervical segments. The fibers from the cervical segments merge to form a trunk. The spinal root enters the posterior fossa of the cranium through the foramen magnum. Here, the spinal root briefly joins the cranial (internal) root to form a single nerve trunk, the accessory nerve. The accessory nerve exits the jugular foramen, heading toward the retrostyloid space.[7] From here the nerve divides into the cranial and spinal portions of the accessory nerve. The spinal accessory nerve typically passes laterally to the internal jugular vein.[9-11] Although less frequent, the nerve can also pass medially,[11] through,[11,12] or split around[11] the internal jugular vein. The nerve then descends in an oblique manner, staying medial to the styloid process, stylohyoid, and digastric muscles.[6] From here the nerve most commonly travels through the two heads of the SCM muscle,[7] but could also travel between the two heads of the muscle.[13] In this region, the nerve merges with fibers from C2 to C4.[7,14-16] Then, the nerve travels obliquely through the posterior triangle toward the deep cervical fascia and trapezius muscle, staying in a fat layer in between the trapezius and levator scapulae muscles.[6,13]

The second, third, and sometimes the fourth cervical spinal nerves of the ventral rami also enter the muscle.[1] It is thought that the C2-C4 connections carry sensory (mostly proprioceptive) information.[1] Contrary to this thought, electromyographic[15,17] and histochemical[17] data show that the nerves have both sensory and motor functions.

Several authors have also demonstrated variations of innervation of this muscle including the hypoglossal nerve,[18] ansa cervicalis,[19-21] facial nerve,[22] and aberrant rami of the transverse cervical nerve.[20]

Although lesions to the spinal accessory nerve are rare, iatrogenic injury contributes to most of the insults to the spinal accessory nerve. Injury often occurs during radical neck dissection, modified radical neck dissection, or functional neck dissection for the removal of cervical lymph node metastases from head and neck cancer.[23-27]

The blood supply to the upper portion of the SCM muscle comes from branches of the occipital and posterior auricular arteries. The superior thyroid artery supplies the middle portion of the muscle and the suprascapular artery supplies the lower portion of the muscle.[1]

2.2. Function

Both Muscles Bilaterally

The SCM muscles have several important functions while working together bilaterally. When in the upright position with the muscles acting from below, they bring the head forward, assisting the longus colli muscle to flex the cervical spine. When working against gravity, as in the supine position, the muscles work to lift the head up. When the head is fixed, the muscles assist in the elevation of the thorax with forced inspiration.[1]

With an upward gaze, the muscles function bilaterally as a checkrein to control hyperextension of the neck. They can also resist forceful backward movement of the head, which can occur when a passenger is riding in a vehicle that is struck from the rear.[28]

The two SCM muscles are coactivated with mandibular movements such as chewing[29-32] and swallowing.[33,34] Coactivation can also contribute to spatial orientation, weight perception, and motor coordination.[28]

One Muscle Unilaterally

Acting unilaterally, the SCM muscle can side bend the head to the ipsilateral side or rotate the head to the contralateral side. When combined together, these motions allow for an upward sideways glance.[1]

2.3. Functional Unit

The functional unit to which a muscle belongs includes the muscles that reinforce and counter its actions as well as the joints that the muscle crosses. The functional interdependence of these structures is reflected in the organization and neural

---

Box 7-1 Functional unit of the sternocleidomastoid muscle

Action	Synergists	Antagonist
Head and cervical spine rotation (contralateral)	Ipsilateral upper trapezius Contralateral splenius capitis Contralateral rectus capitis posterior major Contralateral rectus capitis posterior minor Contralateral obliquus capitis inferior	Contralateral upper trapezius Ipsilateral splenius capitis Ipsilateral rectus capitis posterior major Ipsilateral rectus capitis posterior minor Ipsilateral obliquus capitis inferior
Head and cervical spine side bending (ipsilateral)	Ipsilateral upper trapezius Ipsilateral scalenes Ipsilateral rectus capitis posterior major Ipsilateral rectus capitis posterior minor Ipsilateral obliquus capitis superior	Contralateral upper trapezius Contralateral scalenes Contralateral rectus capitis posterior major/minor Contralateral obliquus capitis superior
Cervical spine flexion	Longus colli Longus capitis Scalenes	Splenii capitis Splenii cervicis Semispinalis capitis Semispinalis cervicis

connections of the sensory motor cortex. The functional unit is emphasized because the presence of a TrP in one muscle of the unit increases the likelihood that the other muscles of the unit also develop TrPs. When inactivating TrPs in a muscle, one should be concerned about TrPs that may develop in muscles that are functionally interdependent. **Box 7-1** grossly represents the functional unit of the SCM muscle.[28]

Together, both SCM muscles are synergistic in controlling hyperextension of the head and neck with a checkrein function. Likewise, they are synergistic with the scalene muscles bilaterally during vigorous chest breathing (inhalation).

Acting with the ipsilateral scalene and trapezius muscles, the SCM helps compensate for the head tilt that is due to tilting of the shoulder girdle axis, which, in turn, is often caused by the functional scoliosis associated with a length discrepancy (LLD), small hemipelvis, and/or quadratus lumborum TrPs (Refer to Chapter 50).

Both SCM muscles are also synergistic to the muscles of mastication (masseter, temporalis, and medial and lateral pterygoid) and the supra- and infrahyoid muscles because they are activated with chewing and swallowing, respectively.

3. CLINICAL PRESENTATION

3.1. Referred Pain Pattern

The sternal and clavicular divisions of SCM have their own characteristic referred pain patterns.[35-38] Face pain referred from TrPs in this muscle is frequently the basis for the diagnoses of "atypical facial neuralgia."[37] Trigger points in this muscle can also be the source of pain and associated symptoms related to the ears, nose, and throat.[39]

Sternal Division

The sternal division of the SCM muscle can exhibit TrPs in any part of the muscle. Commonly, TrPs found in the lower portion of the sternal division refer pain to the upper portion of the sternum (Figure 7-2A). This presentation is the only downward reference of pain from this muscle.[35,37] Trigger points in this lower portion have also been seen to contribute to a paroxysmal dry cough.

In the midportion of the sternal division, TrPs refer a deep aching pain ipsilaterally across the cheek (often in finger-like projections) and into the maxilla, over the supraorbital ridge, and deep within the orbit (Figure 7-2A).[40] They can also refer pain to the pharynx and to the back of the tongue during swallowing[41] (which can be reported as a "sore throat") as well as to a small round area at the tip of the chin.[37] Marbach[42] shows a similar pattern that includes the cheek, temporomandibular joint, and mastoid areas. Trigger points in this region have also been reported to reproduce the crackling sound in one patient's ear.[28]

In the proximal end of the sternal division, TrPs commonly refer pain to the occipital ridge far behind the ear and to the vertex of the head with scalp tenderness in the pain reference zone.

Autonomic symptoms of TrPs in the sternal division relate to the ipsilateral eye and nose.[35,37] Eye symptoms may include excessive lacrimation, reddening of the conjunctiva, apparent "ptosis" (narrowing of the palpebral fissure) with normal pupillary size and reactions, and visual disturbances. This "ptosis" is not caused by weakness of the levator palpebrae muscle, but rather it is due to the spasm of the orbicularis oculi muscle, which is caused by referred increased excitability of the motor units of this muscle. The patient may have to tilt the head backward to look up, because of the inability to raise the upper eyelid. Visual disturbances can include not only blurred vision,[35,43] but also perceived dimming of light intensity.[44] Sometimes coryza and maxillary sinus congestion develop on the affected side.

Trigger points in SCM muscle have also been linked with unilateral deafness in a few patients with no associated reports of tinnitus.[28] Wyant[40] attributed tinnitus in one patient to TrPs in either the upper trapezius, or the cervical paraspinal muscles. More recently, Teachey[39] has reported similar symptoms of TrPs in the SCM including visual blurring, light sensitivity, reddening of the conjunctiva, tearing of the eyes, and "sinusitis" symptoms.

Clavicular Division

The clavicular division of the SCM muscle can exhibit TrPs in any part of the muscle. Commonly, TrPs in the midfiber part of this division commonly refer pain to the frontal area of the head and when severe, the pain extends across the forehead to the other side,[35,44] which is very unusual for TrPs. The upper part of this division is likely to refer pain deep into the ipsilateral ear and to the posterior auricular region (Figure 7-2B). Recently, Min et al[45] reported similar findings of the clavicular head of the SCM muscle referring to the posterior auricular region in a patient. Travell has even reported poorly localized pain to the cheek and molar teeth on the same side with this division of the muscle.[37]

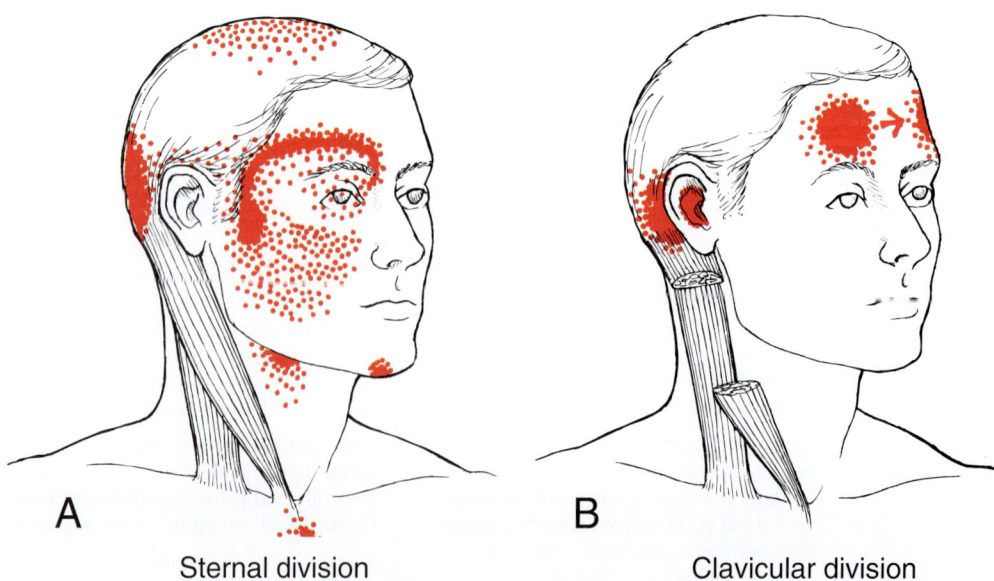

Figure 7-2. Referred pain patterns (solid red shows essential zones and stippling shows the spillover areas) of the right SCM muscle. A, The sternal (more anterior and more superficial) division. B, The clavicular (more posterior and deeper) division.

Trigger points in the clavicular division can also contribute to spatial disorientation.[43,46] The reported dizziness is more of a sensation within the head, and less often, a true sensation of vertigo.[43,46] Weeks and Travell[46] found that during severe attacks, syncope following sudden turning of the head may be due to stretch-stimulation of TrPs in the clavicular division. Episodes of dizziness lasting from seconds to hours are induced by a change of position that require contraction of the SCM muscle, or that places it on a sudden stretch. Disequilibrium may occur separately from, or be associated with, postural dizziness and may cause sudden falls when bending or stooping, or ataxia (unintentional veering to one side while walking with the eyes open).[38] Good[47] attributed symptoms of dizziness to TrPs in either the SCM or the upper trapezius muscles; however, Simons et al[28] have only observed this symptom from the former, despite both muscles being commonly involved. More recently, Teachey[39] has reported dizziness, hearing loss, hyperacusis, hypoacusis, and the sensation of blocked ears with TrPs in the clavicular division of the SCM muscle.

Trigger points in the clavicular division can also cause the autonomic phenomena of localized sweating and vasoconstriction (blanching and thermographic cooling) to the frontal area of the head where pain is commonly referred.

3.2. Symptoms

Contrary to expectation, neck pain and stiffness are generally not the most common reports with SCM TrPs,[48] although this muscle may add an additional component to the "stiff neck" syndrome,[48] which is primarily due to TrP activity in the levator scapulae, posterior cervical, and trapezius muscles. Trigger points in this muscle may cause tilting of the head to the ipsilateral side, because holding the head upright causes pain.[49]

The patient may report "soreness" in the neck when rubbing these muscles, but the symptom is often mistakenly attributed to lymphadenopathy. Surprisingly, the patient with SCM TrPs prefers to lie on the side of the sore muscle if a pillow is adjusted to support the head, so that the area of referred tenderness in the face does not bear weight.

Sternal Division

Pain referred from the sternal division may occur independently of pain referred from the clavicular division.[37] Patients with TrPs in the sternal division can report pain in the cheek, temple, and orbit. Pressure behind the eye is a very common complaint. Patients with cheek pain may seek medical attention for a suspected sinus infection. However, on evaluation, no other signs or symptoms are found to support the diagnosis of "sinus infection."

The patient may report ipsilateral sweating of the forehead, reddening of the conjunctiva, and tearing of the eye, rhinitis, and apparent "ptosis" (narrowing of the palpebral fissure). Blurred or double vision is sometimes reported, yet the pupils react normally to stimuli. Patients likely report this symptom more when viewing strongly contrasting parallel lines such as Venetian blinds. With the report of visual blurring and light sensitivity patients may be misdiagnosed of suffering migraines, yet the symptoms may arise solely from TrPs in the SCM muscle. Patients with bilateral TrPs may report a persistent dry, tickling cough.

Clavicular Division

Patients with TrPs in the clavicular division of the SCM muscle may report deep pressure and pain, localized sweating, and/or cooling sensations on one or both sides of the frontal region of the head.

Patients may report dizziness with hyperextension of the neck and overstretching of the muscle, for example, when lying without a pillow on a hard examination table, or with turning over in bed at night. During the day, transient loss of equilibrium is likely to follow quick vigorous rotation of the head and neck. During an acute attack of this postural dizziness, a person suddenly has serious difficulty performing a task at hand. Postural responses are also exaggerated in some patients; when looking up, they feel as if they will "pitch over backward," and when glancing down, they tend to fall forward. Patients may even report difficulty walking in a straight line across the room.

Nausea is common, but vomiting is infrequent. Dimenhydrinate (Dramamine) may relieve the nausea, but not the dizziness. Patients may even complain of a "sick stomach" with nausea resulting in anorexia that could lead to a poor diet. Reports of seasickness or carsickness could also be related to TrPs in this muscle.

Loss of equilibrium may also follow sustained tilting of the head to one side, as when holding a phone to the ear, or bird-watching with binoculars. The disturbed proprioception causing postural dizziness may be more disabling than the head pain coming from this muscle. These symptoms may appear in any combination, or all can appear together.

It has been reported in a few patients that hearing was impaired unilaterally. Although less common, tinnitus can originate from TrPs in the SCM muscle, but is more likely to originate in TrPs of the deep division of the masseter muscle.

3.3. Patient Examination

After a thorough subjective examination, the clinician should make a detailed drawing representing the pain pattern that the patient has described. This depiction will assist in planning the physical examination and can be useful in monitoring the progression of the patient as symptoms improve or change. For proper assessment and examination of the SCM muscle, the clinician should assess head and neck posture, range of motion, and joint accessory motion of the occiput-C1 and C1-C2 segments. Testing of the C1-C2 segment should be assessed with locking of the mid and lower cervical spine in side bending and then rotating the head on the neck in the side-bent position. Many times "restrictions" of this segment are normalized with the treatment of the SCM muscle. Observation of posture typically reveals a forward head position with an extended upper cervical spine, and a flexed lower cervical spine. A lateral tilt of the head may also be observed. A patient with headache primarily due to SCM TrPs has minimal restriction of the active range of head and neck motion. Active flexion may be slightly restricted as noted by the lack of about one fingerbreadth distance between the chin and the sternum.

When examining the patient with SCM TrPs in standing, one may observe a leg length discrepancy. If the discrepancy is less than 6 mm (0.25 in), the shoulder opposite to the short leg usually sags, whereas in a patient with 1.2 cm (0.5 in) or more of leg length discrepancy, the shoulder is more likely to droop on the same side as the short leg.[28,50]

The patient with dizziness and disequilibrium due to TrPs in the clavicular division typically has a negative Romberg sign and nystagmus. With myofascial disequilibrium, the patient cannot walk in a straight line toward a point across the room where he or she fixes the gaze. The patient's path instead veers to one side, usually to the side of active TrPs in the clavicular division. With any symptoms related to dizziness or disequilibrium, a thorough examination of the vestibular system should be performed to rule out other potential disorders. Refer to other sources for a thorough examination of the vestibular system.

When objects of equal weight are placed in the hands of a patient with unilateral TrPs of the clavicular division, an abnormal Weight Test may be positive.[28] When asked to determine which of the two objects is heavier, the patient demonstrates baragnosia by underestimating the weight of the object held in the hand on the same side as the affected SCM muscle. If TrPs are present bilaterally, the baragnosia is difficult to observe.

3.4. Trigger Point Examination

Currently, there are no reliability studies specific to the examination of the SCM muscle for TrPs; however, in other muscles

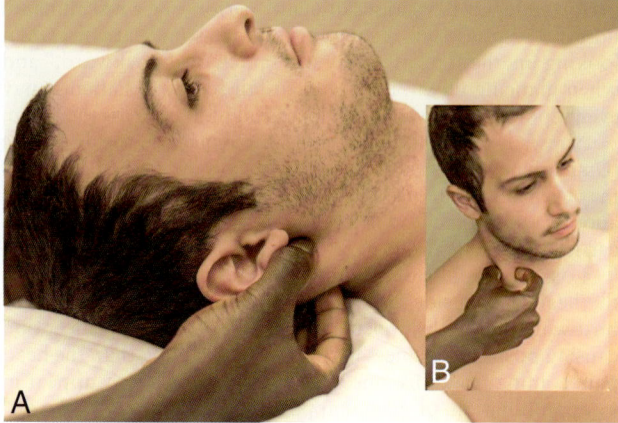

Figure 7-3. Examination of the SCM muscle is most effective using pincer palpation for both divisions and may be done with the patient supine or seated. A, Examination of the deeper clavicular division, with the patient supine and the head tilted toward the same side to slacken the muscle and permit the clinician's fingers to reach between it and underlying structures. B, Examination of the lower end of the sternal division, with the patient seated.

Gerwin et al[51] found that the most reliable examination criteria for making the diagnosis of TrPs were the identification of a taut band by palpation, the presence of spot tenderness in the band, the presence of referred pain, and reproduction of the patient's symptomatic pain. Although identification of a local twitch response by palpation was unreliable, it is a valuable objective confirmatory finding when present.

For examination of the SCM muscle, a cross-fiber pincer palpation is utilized with the muscle held between the thumb and the fingers, separating it from the underlying structures in the neck. The patient is positioned supine, preferably (Figure 7-3A), or may be seated (Figure 7-3B). Supine position is the most effective because the muscle is more relaxed. The muscle is slackened somewhat by tilting the patient's head toward the ipsilateral shoulder on the symptomatic side (Figure 7-3B) and, if necessary, by turning the face slightly away from the muscle to be examined. Snapping a band between the fingers at the TrP regularly produces a visible twitch response, which may be seen as a slight jerk of the head. The entire muscle should be examined for TrPs because TrPs may lie close to the upper or lower attachments, or at the midlevel of either division. Both divisions should be examined thoroughly. Trigger points close to the proximal and distal ends of this muscle may be more effectively examined using a cross-fiber flat palpation.

A prickling sensation over the mandible, which is the characteristic referred response of TrPs in the overlying platysma muscle, may inadvertently be triggered while palpating the SCM muscle. This may startle and concern the patient, especially if this unexpected sensation is not explained.

4. DIFFERENTIAL DIAGNOSIS

4.1. Activation and Perpetuation of Trigger Points

A posture or activity that activates a TrP, if not corrected, can also perpetuate it. In any part of the SCM muscle, TrPs may be activated by unaccustomed eccentric loading, eccentric exercise in an unconditioned muscle, or maximal or submaximal concentric loading.[52] Trigger points may also be activated or aggravated when the muscle is placed in a shortened and/or lengthened position for an extended period of time. For instance, maintaining a position of protracted neck extension places a significant amount of strain on the muscles, for example, painting a ceiling, hanging curtains, and sitting in a front-row seat in a theater with a high stage.

Paradoxical breathing, a chronic cough, emphysema, or asthma (COPD), can chronically overload this accessory muscle of respiration. An acute cough due to upper respiratory infection can activate SCM TrPs and cause an intense headache with every coughing spell.

Patients may acutely overstress the SCM muscles with the hauling and pulling associated with horseback riding, the handling of horses, and moving heavy equipment or furniture.

Trigger points may also be activated or aggravated when the muscle is placed in a shortened or lengthened position for an extended period of time. Reading in bed with your head turned to one side (Figure 7-4A) can activate and perpetuate SCM TrPs, because the muscle on one side is in a shortened position and the other side is in a lengthened position. This is corrected by placing the head and neck in a neutral supported position (Figure 7-4B). Similarly, cocking or tilting the head to avoid the reflection of overhead lights from corrective eyewear,[35] to accommodate for a short cord on a handheld electronic device, or to improve hearing in one-ear deafness, can stress the SCM muscle in some patients. Other postures that are problematic due to keeping the muscle in a shortened position include excessive forward head posture; sitting with the head turned to the side for prolonged periods, for example, when watching television or while talking to another person; or sleeping on too many pillows to improve "sinus drainage." If the head should have to be elevated, it is advisable to use a

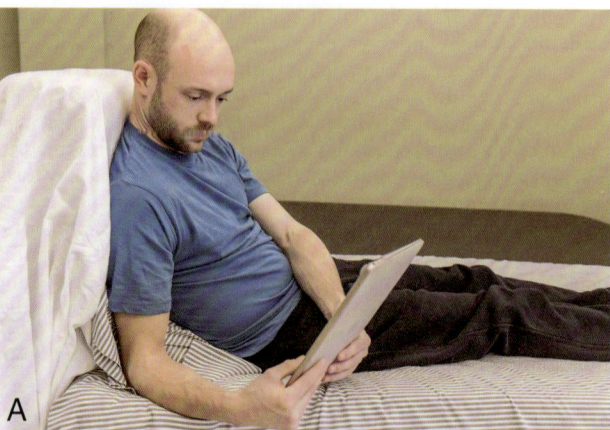
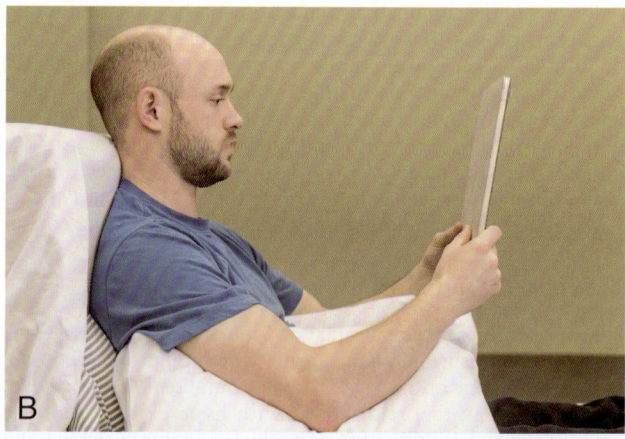

Figure 7-4. A, Undesirable head and neck position with head turned to one side and arms unsupported. This can activate and perpetuate TrPs due to sustained contraction and overload, particularly in the uppermost portion of the SCM muscle. B, Desirable head and neck position for reading in bed with arms supported and head forward.

wedge under the upper trunk and head, rather than to use extra pillows to only raise the head.

Another problem is a structural inadequacy, such as a leg length discrepancy or small hemipelvis, both of which produce a functional scoliosis and shoulder girdle tilting. The SCM muscles, in conjunction with the scalene muscles, are easily overloaded by maintaining normal head position to level the eyes in compensation for a tilted shoulder girdle axis.

The SCM muscle can be affected by anything that produces a severe deviation from the normal pattern of gait. Limping on a weight-bearing limb (with resultant torso adjustments) and lack of normal push-off at the end of the stance phase can activate TrPs in the SCM (and levator scapulae and scalene muscles), because those muscles contract excessively in their reflex attempt to "help the movement" and/or maintain equilibrium.

Sternocleidomastoid TrPs can be also be activated and/or perpetuated by a tight clavicular head of the pectoralis major muscle, pulling down and forward on the clavicle, thereby placing tension on the clavicular head of the SCM muscle.

The leakage of cerebrospinal fluid, which occasionally follows a spinal tap or myelogram, may cause irritation of brain stem structures and activate SCM TrPs.[53] These TrPs may then persist and cause chronic headache for weeks, months, or years, which, regardless of the duration, can be relieved by inactivating the responsible myofascial TrPs.

Finally, sudden trauma, such as sustaining a whiplash from an auto accident,[54,55] falling off a horse, or falling down steps can also contribute to TrP activation.

4.2. Associated Trigger Points

Associated TrPs can develop in the referred pain areas caused by TrPs.[56] Therefore, musculature in the referred pain areas for each muscle should also be considered. Muscles in the referred pain regions of the SCM muscle include the masseter, temporalis, orbicularis oculi, and occipitofrontalis muscles. These muscles, as well as a painful temporomandibular joint, may not respond to treatment completely until the SCM muscle is effectively released. Hong[57] demonstrated that SCM TrPs can contribute to the development of associated TrPs in the temporalis, masseter, and digastric muscles, and that inactivation of the SCM TrP inactivated its associated TrPs without any further treatment of them.

Commonly, when TrPs are present in one SCM muscle, they are usually found in the opposite muscle as well. The scalene muscles also tend to develop TrPs, especially if the SCM muscle has been affected for an extended period of time. If the neck rotation is "stiff," TrPs may be present in the levator scapulae, trapezius, splenius cervicis, and other posterior neck muscles.[48]

The sternalis muscle may also develop associated TrPs as a result of TrPs in the lower portion of the sternal division of the SCM muscle. Sternalis TrPs refer pain deep under the sternum and across the upper pectoral region to the arm on the same side (refer to Chapter 43). As a result of this referral pattern, the pectoral muscles may then develop associated TrPs.

Finally, the platysma muscle, a thin muscle that overlies the SCM muscle, may develop TrPs in relation to involvement of the SCM muscle.

4.3. Associated Pathology

Trigger points in this muscle are associated with or can mimic many different conditions; therefore, a thorough medical screening and examination are essential and a possible referral to another healthcare practitioner may be necessary.

Migraines,[58] tension-type headaches,[59-61] cervicogenic headaches,[62-64] temporomandibular dysfunction,[65] whiplash-associated disorder,[54,55] and mechanical neck pain[66] are all associated with TrPs in the SCM muscle.

Vertigo should be distinguished from postural dizziness; the latter is a nonspecific feeling of disorientation, reported by some patients as a "swimming in the head" sensation. The patient's imbalance and spatial disorientation due to myofascial TrPs may mimic ataxia.

Dizziness from conditions such as benign paroxysmal positional vertigo (BPPV) and Ménière disease should be ruled out. BPPV is a problem of the inner ear that is associated with nystagmus and vertigo while moving the head in specific directions, which depends on the canal involved. Clinical tests to help aid in the diagnosis include the Dix-Hallpike, and supine head roll test.[67]

Unlike Ménière disease, symptoms and signs arising from TrPs in the clavicular division are rarely associated with unilateral deafness. Vestibular evaluation reveals a normal calorimetric test, a negative Romberg sign, normal pupillary response, no nystagmus, and no neurologic deficit. Consciousness is unimpaired. These features distinguish the myofascial syndromes from more serious conditions such as trigeminal neuralgia, Ménière disease, cerebellopontine tumors, intracranial vascular lesions, inflammation of the labyrinth, hemorrhage into the pons, and petit mal epilepsy.[28]

Dizziness due to vestibular disease is identified by nystagmus and other tests of vestibular function as described above. The nonvestibular sources of dizziness include ear wax that touches the tympanic membrane; stenosis of the internal carotid artery, which may be detected by listening for a bruit over the bifurcation of the carotid artery or higher in the neck; hypertension; or intracranial aneurysm or tumor.

The pain from SCM TrPs can mimic true trigeminal neuralgia in distribution; however, the pain is described quite differently. First, the pain of trigeminal neuralgia is typically described as "shock-like." According to the International Headache Society,[68] the criteria for this diagnosis include at least three attacks of unilateral facial pain that meet the following criteria: (1) occurring in one or more divisions of the trigeminal nerve, with no radiation beyond the trigeminal distribution and (2) pain with at least three of the following four characteristics: (a) recurring pain in paroxysmal attacks lasting from a fraction of a second to 2 minutes; (b) severe intensity; (c) electric shock-like, shooting, stabbing, or sharp in quality; and (d) precipitated by innocuous stimuli to the affected side of the face. The facial grimace of trigeminal neuralgia clearly distinguishes this neurologic disease from atypical facial neuralgia and from pain due to TrPs in the sternal division of the SCM muscle.[37]

Trigger point involvement of the SCM, splenii capitis and cervicis, levator scapulae, and upper trapezius muscles should be distinguished from spasmodic torticollis (cervical dystonia), which is a neurologic condition characterized by involuntary dystonic movements of the head[69,70] that can be genetic, acquired, or idiopathic.[71] The muscles most commonly involved in this condition include the SCM, trapezius, scalenes, and platysma muscles,[72] making the differential diagnosis of this condition (versus TrPs) essential to ensure proper care. With spasmodic torticollis, hypertrophy of the muscles may develop.[69] In contrast, the apparent shortening of a muscle due to TrPs does not cause hypertrophy, nor does it cause involuntary movements of the head. Although physical therapy interventions can be effective for spasmodic torticollis,[73,74] botulinum toxin is the preferred treatment.[70,75-78]

Ocular torticollis may result in abnormal head positions to optimize visual acuity and maintain binocularity. In many of these ocular muscle conditions the patient presents in a chin up head position. With ocular muscle palsy's, the head usually tilts to the weak side and turns toward the uninvolved side, representing a functional torticollis.[79]

When the spinal accessory nerve (cranial nerve XI) penetrates the SCM muscle en route to the trapezius muscle, myogenic torticollis due to contracture of the SCM muscle can cause paresis of the ipsilateral trapezius muscle.[80]

Any local areas of chronic infection such as sinusitis or a dental abscess should be identified and resolved. Herpes simplex (oral) recurrent infection may be a stubborn perpetuator of TrPs in the neck and the masticatory muscles.

When autonomic symptoms are due to myofascial TrPs in the sternal division, the absence of miosis and enophthalmos, and the presence of a ciliospinal reflex rule out a Horner syndrome.[81] The eye symptoms should also be distinguished from paralysis of the extraocular muscles.

For further discussion on the differential diagnosis of "stiff neck" of myofascial origin,[48] refer to Chapter 18.

Intramuscular hemangiomas (IH) are rare benign vascular neoplasms, especially uncommon in the SCM muscle, but important to recognize.[82] They typically present as a localized, palpable mass with distinct edges and a rubbery consistency. Pain may or may not be present, but when present, it is due to nerve compression. Commonly, pulsations and bruits are absent.[82]

5. CORRECTIVE ACTIONS

An effective ergonomic workstation is essential for anyone who spends time at a desk with a computer. It is important to learn how to keep joints in a neutral position when possible, and to minimize excessive twisting and turning movements or prolonged positions with the head turned. For a lasting relief, mechanical perpetuating factors such as forward head posture and rounded shoulder posture should be corrected (see Chapter 76).

Patients who are intensely preoccupied with what they are doing are susceptible to lose track of time and maintain an undesirable posture. This can happen while engrossed at a computer or leaning forward over a desk for a prolonged period while writing. Trigger points have been shown to develop with 1 hour of typing.[83] Patients can relieve muscle tension every 20 or 30 minutes, without significantly interrupting work, by setting an interval-timer for that length of time and placing it across the room. Then, they should get up and stretch while they walk to turn off the buzzer and reset the timer. Computer or phone timers may also be used as effective tools for break reminders. Muscles are more tolerant of prolonged activity if they have frequent short breaks permitting relaxation. A few cycles of active range of motion makes the break more effective. For the SCM muscle, this is achieved by slowly rotating or side bending the head to the right and then the left.

A person with SCM TrPs should not sit with the body facing in one direction while looking in another direction for a prolonged period because this rotation leads to neck muscle problems. For example, when one needs to direct attention toward another person for an extended conversation or toward the television set for a prolonged time, either the chair or the person's body should be turned, not just the head.

When turning over in bed at night, the patient should roll the head on the pillow, not lift the head. When getting out of bed in the morning, the patient should roll onto one side and swing the legs off the bed to sit up instead of pulling the trunk straight up because this action places additional strain on the SCM muscles.

During nighttime sleep, because of the increased firmness and recoil, foam pillows tend to be more uncomfortable than softer pillows for patients with SCM TrPs. Pillows should not be placed under the shoulder, but instead behind the neck to allow for proper support. Depending on the amount of kyphosis a patient has and the thickness of his or her pillows, 1 to 2 pillows should be appropriate. In a supine position, proper thickness does not allow any extension of the head, but also does not place the head in excessive flexion, causes prolonged lengthening or shortening of the anterior neck muscles, respectively, during sleep. A small towel roll can be placed inside the pillowcase to support the neck in a neutral position, thus placing the face parallel to the bed. The patient can tuck the corner of the side pillow between the shoulder and the chin (Figure 7-5A), but NOT under the shoulder. For sleeping on the side, the pillow should be thick enough to keep the head and neck in a neutral position, so that the head is not bent excessively to either side

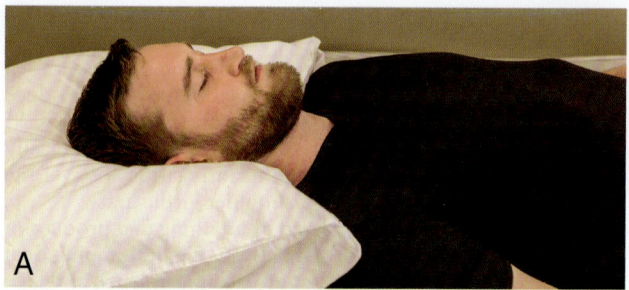
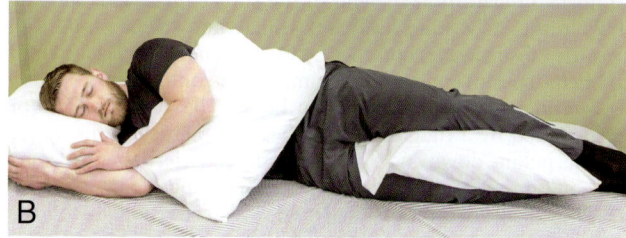
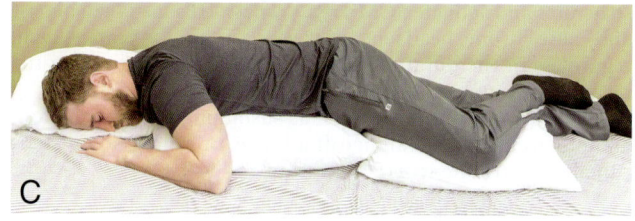

Figure 7-5. A, Correct position, patient supine with the corners of the pillow tucked between the chin and shoulders. B, Correct position, patient side lying, with the pillow between the head and shoulder. C, Effective position for stomach sleepers to decrease stress on the SCM muscle.

because this causes excessive lengthening of the muscle on the top side and excessive shortening of the muscle on the pillow side. The patient can tuck the corner of the pillow between the shoulder and the chin in side-lying position as well (Figure 7-5B), but not under the shoulder. It is recommended to avoid sleeping prone due to the excessive shorting of the muscle on one side and excessive lengthening of the muscle on the other side. If one does sleep prone, a pillow placed under the shoulder and chest on the same side to which the face is turned helps reduce rotation of the neck. A semiprone position can also be utilized, achieved by flexing the knee and hip of the side toward which the face is turned, which helps by partly rotating the torso (Figure 7-5C).

If reading in bed, the light should be located directly overhead, on the headboard, on the wall, or suspended from the ceiling. It should not illuminate only one side of the bed because this placement can place excessive strain on the SCM muscles, if the head is turned to maximize the light cast on reading material.

When using a phone, it should not be held between the head and the shoulder by tilting the head. Instead, a headset, headphones, or hands-free speaker function should be utilized.

An LLD or a small hemipelvis that tilts the shoulder girdle axis should be corrected by suitable lifts.

Pressure on the SCM muscles and activation of TrPs may be caused by tightness of a shirt collar. The clinician's finger should fit comfortably inside the collar, not only when the patient is looking straight ahead, but also when the head is turned, which increases the diameter of the neck inside the collar. Tying a necktie too tightly should be avoided.

To stretch the SCM muscle, the patient rotates the head toward the affected side and gently assists retraction of the head with two fingers of the opposite hand (Figure 7-6). This motion is also a good self-mobilization technique for the C1-C2 segment that is often found to be restricted in patients with SCM TrPs.

Missaghi[84] described a passive stretch technique that can improve symptoms associated with SCM TrPs when incorporated into a home program. In the supine position, the patient side bends the head toward the affected side, rotates the head away from the affected side, and then performs a chin tuck with cervical extension. This position is held for 5 to 45 seconds.

Lewit[50] illustrated and described a gravity-induced postisometric relaxation technique suitable for a home program for release of TrPs in the clavicular division of the SCM muscle. The supine patient rests the head at the edge of the bed and turns the face to one side, chin supported by the edge of the supporting surface acting as a fulcrum. The patient looks up with the eyes only, and takes in a slow, deep breath using diaphragmatic (abdominal) breathing. This effort lightly activates the uppermost SCM muscle. During slow exhalation, the patient looks down and relaxes, allowing the head to drop slightly, elongating the SCM muscle with each breath (Figure 7-7).

Because a tight clavicular head of the pectoralis major muscle can influence the SCM muscle, this muscle might also need to be addressed. Refer to Chapter 42, Figure 42-10, for a procedure on stretching of this muscle. It should be noted that while performing this stretch, the patient should not protrude the head forward or look down because this shortens the SCM muscles.

Proper diaphragmatic breathing should be established in all patients with SCM TrPs because this muscle is an accessory muscle of respiration. If proper breathing is not established, the SCM muscle can be overutilized, which can further perpetuate TrPs. For those who have asthma, allergies, or other respiratory conditions, this strategy is even more important. Proper pharmacologic management of respiratory symptoms related to these conditions should be encouraged as well.

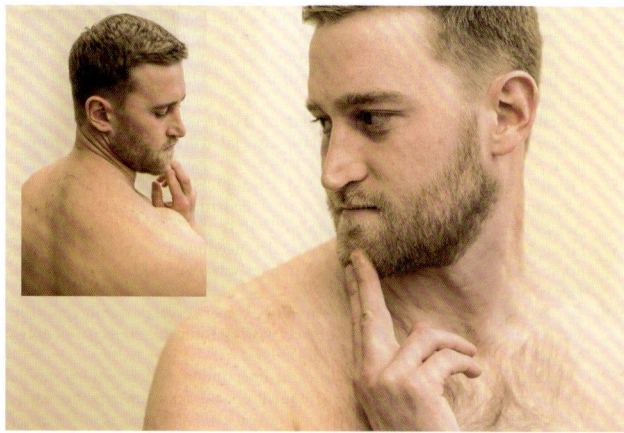

Figure 7-6. Stretching of the right SCM muscle in sitting. The patient rotates the head toward the side to be stretched. From this rotated position, the opposite hand (two fingers) is placed on the chin guiding the head and neck to retract, creating a gentle stretch along the SCM muscle.

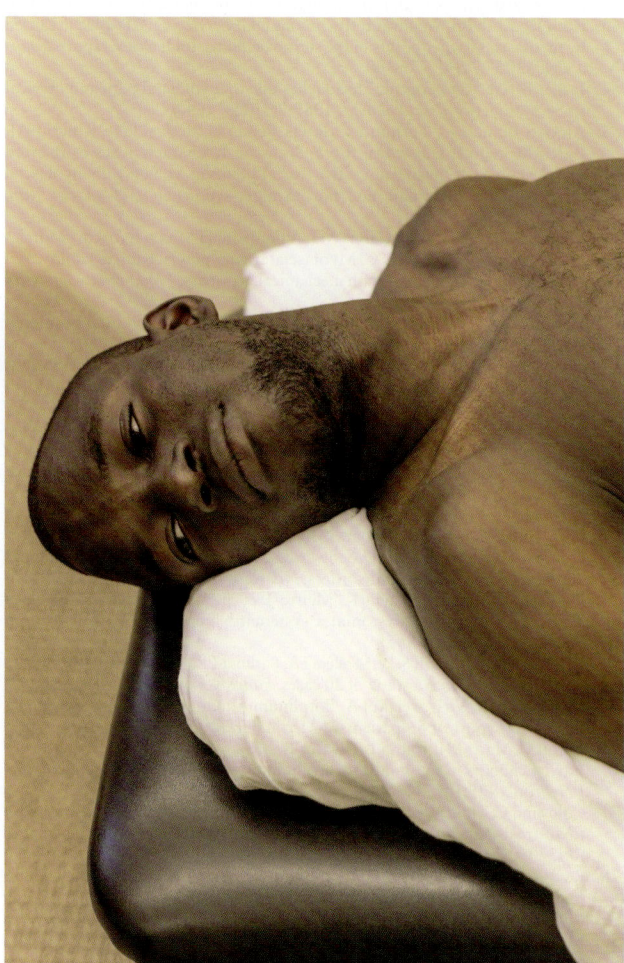

Figure 7-7. Postisometric relaxation for SCM muscle. The supine patient rests the head at the edge of the bed and turns the face to one side, chin supported by the edge of the supporting surface acting as a fulcrum. The patient looks up with the eyes only, and takes in a slow, deep breath using diaphragmatic (abdominal) breathing. This effort lightly activates the uppermost SCM muscle. During slow exhalation, the patient looks down and relaxes, allowing the head to drop slightly, elongating the SCM muscle with each breath.

References

1. Standring S. *Gray's Anatomy: The Anatomical Basis of Clinical Practice*. 41st ed. London, UK: Elsevier; 2015.
2. Goswami P, Yadav Y, Chakradharv V. Anatomical description and clinical significance of unilateral triheaded sternocleidomastoid muscle. *Int J Res Med Sci*. 2014;2(3):1161-1164.
3. Pushpa MS, Nandhini V. Unusual bilateral presence of third head of sternocleidomastoid muscle and its clinical significance—a case report. *Int J Recent Sci Res*. 2014;5(1):5-7.
4. Takahashi H, Umeda M, Sakakibara A, et al. Absence of the sternocleidomastoid muscle in a patient that underwent neck dissection for squamous cell carcinoma of the tongue. *Kobe J Med Sci*. 2014;59(5):E167-E171.
5. Kumar MS, Sundaram SM, Fenn A, et al. Cleido-occipital platysma muscle: a rare variant of sternocliedomastoid. *Int J Anat Variations*. 2009;2:9-10.
6. Lloyd S. Accessory nerve: anatomy and surgical identification. *J Laryngol Otol*. 2007;121(12):1118-1125.
7. Caliot P, Bousquet V, Midy D, Cabanie P. A contribution to the study of the accessory nerve: surgical implications. *Surg Radiol Anat*. 1989;11(1):11-15.
8. Tawfik EA, Walker FO, Cartwright MS. Neuromuscular ultrasound of cranial nerves. *J Clin Neurol*. 2015;11(2):109-121.
9. Hinsley ML, Hartig GK. Anatomic relationship between the spinal accessory nerve and internal jugular vein in the upper neck. *Otolaryngol Head Neck Surg*. 2010;143(2):239-241.
10. Saman M, Etebari P, Pakdaman MN, Urken ML. Anatomic relationship between the spinal accessory nerve and the jugular vein: a cadaveric study. *Surg Radiol Anat*. 2011;33(2):175-179.
11. Taylor CB, Boone JL, Schmalbach CE, Miller FR. Intraoperative relationship of the spinal accessory nerve to the internal jugular vein: variation from cadaver studies. *Am J Otolaryngol*. 2013;34(5):527-529.
12. Hashimoto Y, Otsuki N, Morimoto K, Saito M, Nibu K. Four cases of spinal accessory nerve passing through the fenestrated internal jugular vein. *Surg Radiol Anat*. 2012;34(4):373-375.
13. Hong MJ, Baek JH, Kim DY, et al. Spinal accessory nerve: ultrasound findings and correlations with neck lymph node levels. *Ultraschall Med*. 2016;37(5):487-491.
14. Lanisnik B, Zargi M, Rodi Z. Identification of three anatomical patterns of the spinal accessory nerve in the neck by neurophysiological mapping. *Radiol Oncol*. 2014;48(4):387-392.
15. Kim JH, Choi KY, Lee KH, Lee DJ, Park BJ, Rho YS. Motor innervation of the trapezius muscle: Intraoperative motor conduction study during neck dissection. *ORL J Otorhinolaryngol Relat Spec*. 2014;76(1):8-12.
16. Brennan PA, St J Blythe J, Alam P, Green B, Parry D. Division of the spinal accessory nerve in the anterior triangle: a prospective clinical study. *Br J Oral Maxillofac Surg*. 2015;53(7):633-636.

17. Pu YM, Tang EY, Yang XD. Trapezius muscle innervation from the spinal accessory nerve and branches of the cervical plexus. *Int J Oral Maxillofac Surg.* 2008;37(6):567-572.
18. Koizumi M, Horiguchi M, Sekiya S, Isogai S, Nakano M. A case of the human sternocleidomastoid muscle additionally innervated by the hypoglossal nerve. *Okajimas Folia Anat Jpn.* 1993;69(6):361-367.
19. Hegazy AMS. Anatomical study of the human ansa cervicalis nerve and its variations. *Int J Anat Physiol.* 2013;2(3):14-19.
20. Paraskevas GK, Natsis K, Nitsa Z, Mavrodi A, Kitsoulis P. Unusual morphological pattern and distribution of the ansa cervicalis: a case report. *Rom J Morphol Embryol.* 2014;55(3):993-996.
21. Blythe JN, Matharu J, Reuther WJ, Brennan PA. Innervation of the lower third of the sternocleidomastoid muscle by the ansa cervicalis through the C1 descendens hypoglossal branch: a previously unreported anatomical variant. *Br J Oral Maxillofac Surg.* 2015;53(5):470-471.
22. Cvetko E. Sternocleidomastoid muscle additionally innervated by the facial nerve: case report and review of the literature. *Anat Sci Int.* 2015;90(1):54-56.
23. Orhan KS, Demirel T, Baslo B, et al. Spinal accessory nerve function after neck dissections. *J Laryngol Otol.* 2007;121(1):44-48.
24. Gun K, Uludag M, Delil S, et al. Spinal accessory nerve injury: eight cases and review of the literature. *Clin Ter.* 2014;165(4):211-216.
25. Cesmebasi A, Spinner RJ. An anatomic-based approach to the iatrogenic spinal accessory nerve injury in the posterior cervical triangle: how to avoid and treat it. *Clin Anat.* 2015;28(6):761-766.
26. Glenn JA, Yen TW, Fareau GG, Carr AA, Evans DB, Wang TS. Institutional experience with lateral neck dissections for thyroid cancer. *Surgery.* 2015;158(4):972-978; discussion 978-980.
27. Park SH, Esquenazi Y, Kline DG, Kim DH. Surgical outcomes of 156 spinal accessory nerve injuries caused by lymph node biopsy procedures. *J Neurosurg Spine.* 2015;23(4):518-525.
28. Simons DG, Travell J, Simons L. *Travell & Simon's Myofascial Pain and Dysfunction: The Trigger Point Manual.* Vol 1. 2nd ed. Baltimore, MD: Williams & Wilkins; 1999:104.
29. Haggman-Henrikson B, Nordh E, Eriksson PO. Increased sternocleidomastoid, but not trapezius, muscle activity in response to increased chewing load. *Eur J Oral Sci.* 2013;121(5):443-449.
30. Ries LG, Alves MC, Berzin F. Asymmetric activation of temporalis, masseter, and sternocleidomastoid muscles in temporomandibular disorder patients. *Cranio.* 2008;26(1):59-64.
31. Shimazaki K, Matsubara N, Hisano M, Soma K. Functional relationships between the masseter and sternocleidomastoid muscle activities during gum chewing. *Angle Orthod.* 2006;76(3):452-458.
32. Giannakopoulos NN, Hellmann D, Schmitter M, Kruger B, Hauser T, Schindler HJ. Neuromuscular interaction of jaw and neck muscles during jaw clenching. *J Orofac Pain.* 2013;27(1):61-71.
33. Bazzotti L. Mandible position and head posture: electromyography of sternocleidomastoids. *Cranio.* 1998;16(2):100-108.
34. Monaco A, Cattaneo R, Spadaro A, Giannoni M. Surface electromyography pattern of human swallowing. *BMC Oral Health.* 2008;8:6.
35. Travell J. Temporomandibular joint pain referred from muscles of the head and neck. *J Prosthet Dent.* 1960;10:745-763.
36. Travell J. Mechanical headache. *Headache.* 1967;7(1):23-29.
37. Travell J. Identification of myofascial trigger point syndromes: a case of atypical facial neuralgia. *Arch Phys Med Rehabil.* 1981;62(3):100-106.
38. Travell J. Pain mechanisms in connective tissue. Paper presented at: Connective Tissues, Transactions of the Second Conference, 1951; New York.
39. Teachey WS. Otolaryngic myofascial pain syndromes. *Curr Pain Headache Rep.* 2004;8(6):457-462.
40. Wyant GM. Chronic pain syndromes and their treatment. II. Trigger points. *Can Anaesth Soc J.* 1979;26(3):216-219.
41. Brody SI. Sore throat of myofascial origin. *Mil Med.* 1964;129:9-19.
42. Marbach JJ. Arthritis of the temporomandibular joints. *Am Fam Physician.* 1979;19(2):131-139.
43. Travell J. Referred pain from skeletal muscle; the pectoralis major syndrome of breast pain and soreness and the sternomastoid syndrome of head and dizziness. *N Y State J Med.* 1955;55(3):331-340.
44. Travell J. Symposium on mechanism and management of pain syndromes. *Proc Rudolf Virchow Med Soc.* 1957;16:126-136.
45. Min SH, Chang SH, Jeon SK, Yoon SZ, Park JY, Shin HW. Posterior auricular pain caused by the trigger points in the sternocleidomastoid muscle aggravated by psychological factors -A case report. *Korean J Anesthesiol.* 2010;59 suppl:S229-S232.
46. Weeks VD, Travell J. Postural vertigo due to trigger areas in the sternocleidomastoid muscle. *J Pediatr.* 1955;47(3):315-327.
47. Good MG. Senile vertigo caused by a curable cervical myopathy. *J Am Geriatr Soc.* 1957;5(7):662-667.
48. Travell J. Rapid relief of acute stiff neck by ethyl chloride spray. *J Am Med Womens Assoc.* 1949;4(3):89-95.
49. Aftimos S. Myofascial pain in children. *N Z Med J.* 1989;102(874):440-441.
50. Lewit K. *Manipulative Therapy in Rehabilitation of the Locomotor System.* 3rd ed. Oxford, UK: Butterworth Heinemann; 1999.
51. Gerwin RD, Shannon S, Hong C-Z, Hubbard DR, Gevirtz R. Interrater reliability in myofascial trigger point examination. *Pain.* 1997;69:65-73.
52. Gerwin RD, Dommerholt J, Shah JP. An expansion of Simons' integrated hypothesis of trigger point formation. *Curr Pain Headache Rep.* 2004;8(6):468-475.
53. Dunteman E, Turner MS, Swarm R. Pseudo-spinal headache. *Reg Anesth.* 1996;21(4):358-360.

54. Fernandez-Perez AM, Villaverde-Gutierrez C, Mora-Sanchez A, Alonso-Blanco C, Sterling M, Fernández de las Peñas C. Muscle trigger points, pressure pain threshold, and cervical range of motion in patients with high level of disability related to acute whiplash injury. *J Orthop Sports Phys Ther.* 2012;42(7):634-641.
55. Castaldo M, Ge HY, Chiarotto A, Villafane JH, Arendt-Nielsen L. Myofascial trigger points in patients with whiplash-associated disorders and mechanical neck pain. *Pain Med.* 2014;15(5):842-849.
56. Hsieh YL, Kao MJ, Kuan TS, Chen SM, Chen JT, Hong CZ. Dry needling to a key myofascial trigger point may reduce the irritability of satellite MTrPs. *Am J Phys Med Rehabil.* 2007;86(5):397-403.
57. Hong CZ. Lidocaine injection versus dry needling to myofascial trigger point. The importance of the local twitch response. *Am J Phys Med Rehabil.* 1994;73(4):256-263.
58. Tali D, Menahem I, Vered E, Kalichman L. Upper cervical mobility, posture and myofascial trigger points in subjects with episodic migraine: case-control study. *J Bodyw Mov Ther.* 2014;18(4):569-575.
59. Karadas O, Gul HL, Inan LE. Lidocaine injection of pericranial myofascial trigger points in the treatment of frequent episodic tension-type headache. *J Headache Pain.* 2013;14:44.
60. Alonso-Blanco C, de-la-Llave-Rincon AI, Fernández de las Peñas C. Muscle trigger point therapy in tension-type headache. *Expert Rev Neurother.* 2012;12(3):315-322.
61. Alonso-Blanco C, Fernández de las Peñas C, Fernandez-Mayoralas DM, de-la-Llave-Rincon AI, Pareja JA, Svensson P. Prevalence and anatomical localization of muscle referred pain from active trigger points in head and neck musculature in adults and children with chronic tension-type headache. *Pain Med.* 2011;12(10):1453-1463.
62. Bodes-Pardo G, Pecos-Martin D, Gallego-Izquierdo T, Salom-Moreno J, Fernández de Las Peñas C, Ortega-Santiago R. Manual treatment for cervicogenic headache and active trigger point in the sternocleidomastoid muscle: a pilot randomized clinical trial. *J Manipulative Physiol Ther.* 2013;36(7):403-411.
63. Roth JK, Roth RS, Weintraub JR, Simons DG. Cervicogenic headache caused by myofascial trigger points in the sternocleidomastoid: a case report. *Cephalalgia.* 2007;27(4):375-380.
64. Jaeger B. Are "cervicogenic" headaches due to myofascial pain and cervical spine dysfunction? *Cephalalgia.* 1989;9(3):157-164.
65. Alonso-Blanco C, Fernández de las Peñas C, de-la-Llave-Rincon AI, Zarco-Moreno P, Galan-Del-Rio F, Svensson P. Characteristics of referred muscle pain to the head from active trigger points in women with myofascial temporomandibular pain and fibromyalgia syndrome. *J Headache Pain.* 2012;13(8):625-637.
66. Munoz-Munoz S, Munoz-Garcia MT, Alburquerque-Sendin F, Arroyo-Morales M, Fernández de las Peñas C. Myofascial trigger points, pain, disability, and sleep quality in individuals with mechanical neck pain. *J Manipulative Physiol Ther.* 2012;35(8):608-613.
67. Purnamasari PP. Diagnosis and management benign paroxysmal positional vertigo (BPPV). *E-Jurnal Medika Udayana.* 2013;2(6):1056-1080.
68. Headache Classification Committee of the International Headache Society. The International Classification of Headache Disorders, 3rd edition (beta version). *Cephalalgia.* 2013;33(9):629-808.
69. Waldman SD. *Atlas of Uncommon Pain Syndromes.* 3rd ed. Philadelphia, PA: Elsevier Saunders; 2014.
70. Mills RR, Pagan FL. Patient considerations in the treatment of cervical dystonia: focus on botulinum toxin type A. *Patient Prefer Adherence.* 2015;9:725-731.
71. Albanese A, Bhatia K, Bressman SB, et al. Phenomenology and classification of dystonia: a consensus update. *Mov Disord.* 2013;28(7):863-873.
72. Jankovic J, Leder S, Warner D, Schwartz K. Cervical dystonia: clinical findings and associated movement disorders. *Neurology.* 1991;41(7):1088-1091.
73. De Pauw J, Van der Velden K, Meirte J, et al. The effectiveness of physiotherapy for cervical dystonia: a systematic literature review. *J Neurol.* 2014;261(10):1857-1865.
74. Queiroz MA, Chien HF, Sekeff-Sallem FA, Barbosa ER. Physical therapy program for cervical dystonia: a study of 20 cases. *Funct Neurol.* 2012;27(3):187-192.
75. Poungvarin N, Viriyavejakul A. Botulinum A toxin treatment in spasmodic torticollis: report of 56 patients. *J Med Assoc Thai.* 1994;77(9):464-470.
76. Marin C, Marti MJ, Tolosa E, Alvarez R, Montserrat L, Santamaria J. Muscle activity changes in spasmodic torticollis after botulinum toxin treatment. *Eur J Neurol.* 1995;1(3):243-247.
77. Colosimo C, Tiple D, Berardelli A. Efficacy and safety of long-term botulinum toxin treatment in craniocervical dystonia: a systematic review. *Neurotox Res.* 2012;22(4):265-273.
78. Ramirez-Castaneda J, Jankovic J. Long-term efficacy and safety of botulinum toxin injections in dystonia. *Toxins (Basel).* 2013;5(2):249-266.
79. Rubin SE, Wagner RS. Ocular torticollis. *Surv Ophthalmol.* 1986;30(6):366-376.
80. Motta A, Trainiti G. Paralysis of the trapezius associated with myogenic torticollis. A report of 6 cases. *Ital J Orthop Traumatol.* 1977;3(2):207-213.
81. Dutton M. *Dutton's Orthopaedic Examination, Evaluation and Intervention.* 3rd ed. New York, NY: McGraw Hill; 2012.
82. Ferri E, Pavon I, Armato E. Intramuscular cavernous hemangioma of the sternocleidomastoid muscle: an unusual neck mass. *Otolaryngol Head Neck Surg.* 2007;137(4):682-683.
83. Hoyle JA, Marras WS, Sheedy JE, Hart DE. Effects of postural and visual stressors on myofascial trigger point development and motor unit rotation during computer work. *J Electromyogr Kinesiol.* 2011;21(1):41-48.
84. Missaghi B. Sternocleidomastoid syndrome: a case study. *J Can Chiropr Assoc.* 2004;48(3):201-205.

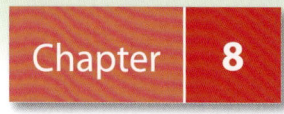

Masseter Muscle

"Dental Drama"

Seth Jason Fibraio and Michelle Finnegan

1. INTRODUCTION

The masseter muscle is one of the most common muscles involved with patients who have temporomandibular dysfunction (TMD) and oftentimes it restricts jaw opening. The muscle is comprised of three layers. The superficial and intermediate layers attach proximally to the anterior two-thirds of the zygomatic arch. The superficial layer inserts distally to the lower posterior half of the mandibular ramus. The middle layer of the muscle attaches to the central part of the ramus of the mandible. The deep layer of the masseter muscle attaches to the posterior one-third of the zygomatic arch and inserts distally to the lateral surface of the coronoid process of the mandible. The masseter muscle is innervated by the masseteric nerve and receives its vascularization from the masseteric branch of the maxillary artery, the transverse branch of the superficial temporal artery, and the facial artery. The primary function of the masseter muscle is mandibular elevation and it plays a small role in ipsilateral lateral excursion, protrusion, and retraction of the mandible. Trigger points (TrPs) in the masseter muscle commonly refer pain in the middle third of the zygomatic arch superiorly, to the lateral aspect of the mandible inferiorly and to the lateral aspect of the forehead. Symptoms are exacerbated with mouth opening, chewing, and lying on the affected side. Perpetuating factors include static activities such as clenching, dynamic activities such as nocturnal bruxism, and stretching activities such as yawning. Trigger points in the masseter muscle are associated with tension-type headaches (TTH), TMD, and unilateral tinnitus. Differential diagnosis should include screening to rule out TMD, trigeminal neuralgia, masseter hypertrophy, and/or neoplasms. Corrective actions for this muscle include maintaining an effective rest position of the tongue, correction of forward head posture, reducing/eliminating parafunctional behaviors, stress management, and self-release of the muscle, either intraorally or extraorally.

2. ANATOMIC CONSIDERATIONS

The masseter muscle is a pennate-shaped muscle, with thick aponeurotic layers. It is comprised of three layers, superficial, middle, and deep, which aide in creating a great amount of force needed for mastication. The superficial and intermediate portions of the masseter muscle are considered together as the superficial layer of the muscle, because they both attach proximally to the anterior two-thirds of the zygomatic arch and have a similar fiber direction. The superficial layer is the largest. Distally, the superficial layer attaches to the lower posterior half of the mandibular ramus externally (Figure 8-1). The middle layer of the masseter muscle attaches into the central part of the ramus of the mandible. The deep masseter muscle attaches proximally to the posterior one-third of the zygomatic arch and attaches distally to the lateral surface of the coronoid process of the mandible and to the superior half of the ramus (Figure 8-1).[1,2] This attachment may extend to the angle of the mandible.[1] There is debate on whether there are fibers that attach to the articular disc of the temporomandibular joint and whether it can influence the disc.[1,3] The deep fibers run more vertically than the superficial fibers and the most posterior of the deep fibers are considerably shorter than those in the rest of the muscle.[4]

The proximal tendon of the masseter muscle is referred to as a "tendinous digitation," which is longer and wider in men than in women, with men having three digitations and women having two. Fewer digitations lead to decreased bite force production in women as compared with that in men.[5] The thickness of the masseter muscle ranges from a relaxed thickness of 12.1 ± 1.4 mm to a contracted thickness of 14.2 ± 1.7 mm.[6]

In one study,[7] the anterior fibers of the masseter muscle (both superficial and deep) were nearly 87% type-I (slow twitch) fibers and nearly 7% type-II-B (fast twitch) fibers. The posterior muscle fibers were also predominantly type-I fibers (70% superficial and 77% deep), but the posterior portion had more type-II-B fibers (20% superficial and 15% deep) than the anterior portion. The large amount of type-I fibers facilitate fine control as the molar teeth approach occlusion during chewing.[7] A more recent study revealed a different composition of muscle fiber types. Rowlerson et al[8] suggest that the normal distribution of fibers is: Type-I fibers ~50%, Type-II fibers ~15% (smaller than normal diameter), Type-I/II hybrid fibers 20%, and neo-atrial fibers ~15%. Compared with most limb and trunk muscles, this is an unusually high proportion of slow twitch fibers, which indicates that the muscle is suited primarily for sustained workloads with few brief rapid adjustments. Patients with TMD tend to have an increased number of type-II fibers.[8,9] The number of intrafusal fibers per muscle spindle was found to be unusually high in this muscle (up to 36).[10] This finding supports the understanding that masseter muscle spindles have a strong proprioceptive influence on fine control of jaw closure.

2.1. Innervation and Vascularization

The masseter muscle is innervated by the masseteric nerve that arises from the anterior branch of the mandibular division of the trigeminal nerve (cranial nerve V).[1] The mandibular nerve descends through the foramen ovale into the infratemporal fossa proximally to the lateral pterygoid. The mandibular nerve is divided into a posterior and an anterior trunk. The anterior trunk contains the buccal, masseteric, and anterior deep temporal nerves. The masseteric nerve then passes laterally to the lateral pterygoid muscle near the base of the skull, then crosses the mandibular coronoid notch where it innervates the masseter muscle.[11] The masseteric nerve and artery travel together, with the nerve having 3 to 7 separate innervations to the superficial and deep portions of the masseter muscle.[5]

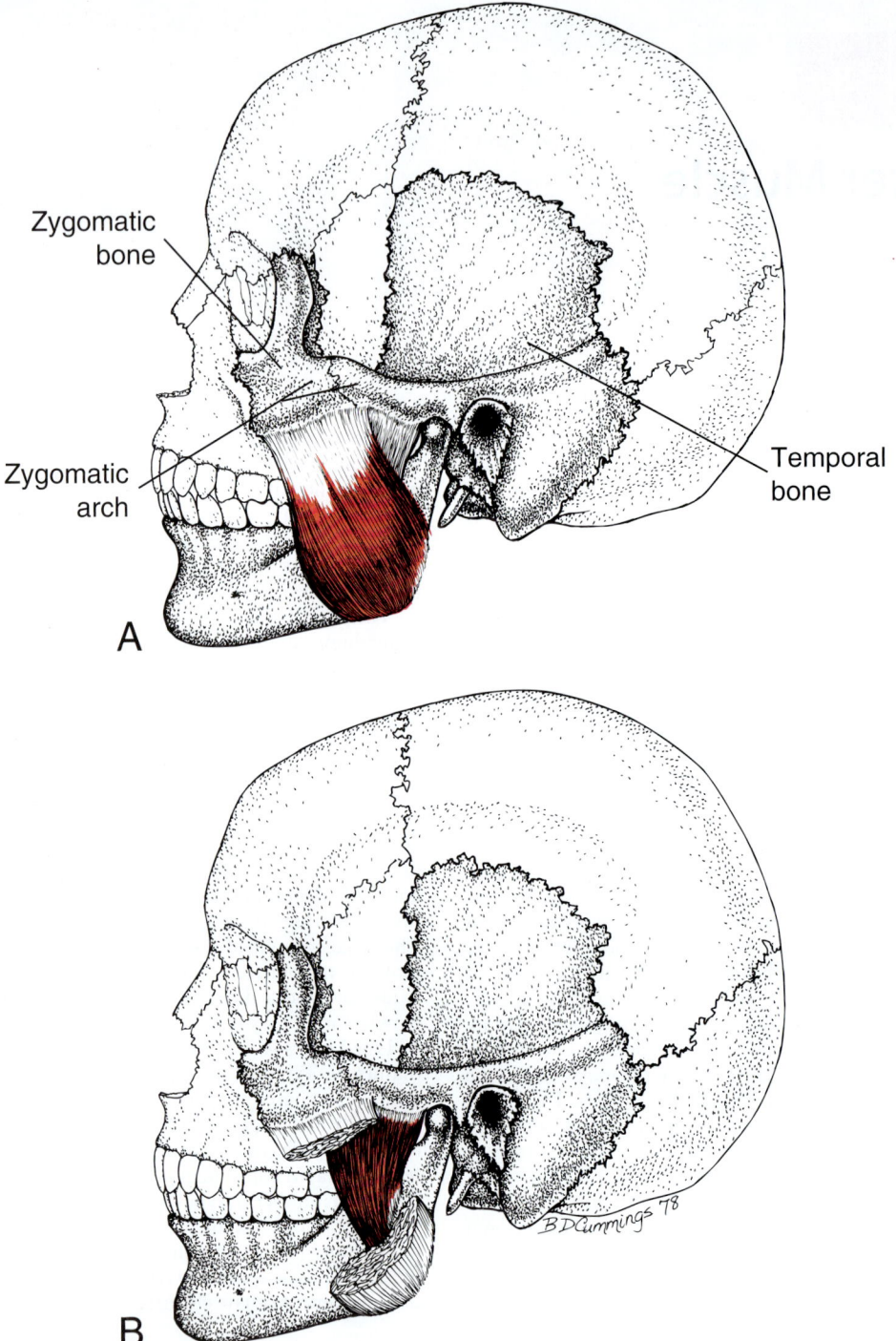

Figure 8-1. Masseter muscle attachments are from the maxillary process of the zygomatic bone and the anterior two-thirds of the inferior border of the zygomatic arch.

The vascular supply to the masseter muscle is via the masseteric branch of the maxillary artery, the transverse branch of the superficial temporal artery, and the facial artery.[1] The masseteric branch of the premasseteric artery, the masseteric branch of the transverse facial artery, the masseteric branch of the external carotid artery, and a muscular branch of the deep temporal artery have also been reported to supply blood to the masseter muscle.[12] The maxillary vein emerges between the masseter muscle and the mandible, causing it to be potentially entrapped by masseter TrPs. The pterygoid venous plexus, which empties primarily into the maxillary vein, lies between the temporalis and the lateral pterygoid muscles and between the two pterygoid muscles; the plexus drains the temporalis muscle via the deep temporal vein and drains the infraorbital region via the orbital vein.[1]

2.2. Function

The primary action of the masseter muscle is to elevate the mandible and close the jaw during clenching into centric occlusion.[1,13-16] The deep fibers also retract the mandible.[1,13] There is a small contribution of this muscle to lateral excursion without bite force.[17] Interestingly, clenching during left and right lateral excursion, results in a decrease in the electromyographic (EMG) activity of the masseter and temporalis muscles bilaterally.[18]

The masseter muscle contributes to the morphologic role of lower face contour (facial height and mandible size)[19] and functions in the biting down of food, drinking, swallowing, and speaking and nonfunctional activities such as clenching and grinding.[20,21] Normally, activity of the masseter muscle is not required to maintain the mandibular rest position (centric relation).[13]

With mouth opening and closing, it has been observed that simultaneous head flexion and extension occurs.[22] When the mouth opens, the cranium rotates posteriorly. During mouth closing (mandibular elevation), the cranium rotates anteriorly. This demonstrates a functional relationship between the trigeminal and craniocervical systems. Any disruption in normal mechanics in either system may alter movement patterns in the other system and increase risk for development of musculoskeletal pain in the head, neck, and jaw.[23]

The masseter muscle responds before the temporalis muscle during chewing[24] and is typically more active than the temporalis muscle.[25-27] Patients with TMD had asymmetry in the temporalis and masseter muscles during standard activity when compared with controls, with a greater amount of difficulty chewing hard foods.[28]

As long as the mandibular rest position is maintained, the masseter muscle showed little difference in electrical activity between sitting and supine postures.[29] Valdes et al[30] demonstrated no significant difference in EMG activity in the temporal and masseter muscles with the tongue elevated to the roof of the mouth or with the tongue on the floor of the mouth, but vertical dimension did increase with the tongue placed on the floor of the mouth.

2.3. Functional Unit

The functional unit to which a muscle belongs includes the muscles that reinforce and counter its actions as well as the joints that the muscle crosses. The interdependence of these structures is functionally reflected in the organization and neural connections of the sensory motor cortex. The functional unit is emphasized because the presence of a TrP in one muscle of the unit increases the likelihood that the other muscles of the unit will also develop TrPs. When inactivating TrPs in a muscle, one should be concerned about TrPs that may develop in muscles that are functionally interdependent. Box 8-1 grossly represents the functional unit of the masseter muscle.[31]

The masseter and temporalis muscles function together closely, with only minor differences in motor unit activity. The temporalis muscle is more likely to respond for mandibular balance and posture control, where the masseter muscle is used for greater closing force.[32]

Box 8-1 Functional unit of the masseter muscle[13,15,32–36]

Action	Synergists	Antagonist
Mandibular elevation	Contralateral masseter Temporalis (bilateral) Medial pterygoid (bilateral)	Lateral pterygoid (inferior division) Geniohyoid Digastric Mylohyoid
Mandibular retraction	Temporalis (posterior fibers more than anterior)	Medial pterygoid Lateral pterygoid Temporalis

3. CLINICAL PRESENTATION

3.1. Referred Pain Pattern

The masseter muscle is one of the most commonly involved muscles in patients with TMD,[33] and it has been found to be the most common muscle to elicit referred pain.[34] Fernández de Las Peñas et al[35] demonstrated that this muscle reproduces patients' familiar TMJ-related pain. In addition, referred pain from the masseter muscle indicates a 3-times greater risk for the presence of temporomandibular arthralgia.[36] Other conditions in which masseter TrPs play a contributing role include tension-type headache[37,38] and mechanical neck pain,[39] especially if TrPs in neck muscles contribute to the pain.[40,41]

Superficial Layer

Trigger points in the superficial layer of the masseter muscle commonly refer pain to the lower jaw, molar teeth, related gums, and the middle one-third of the zygomatic arch of the maxilla.[33,34,42,43] In addition to referring pain to the upper and lower teeth, TrPs in the superficial masseter muscle can also refer to the ear.[35] Oftentimes TrPs in the anterior border and superior part of this layer refer pain to the upper premolar[44] and molar teeth, adjacent gums, and maxilla (Figure 8-2A).[42,45] Trigger points located just below the midbelly of the muscle commonly refer pain to the lower molar teeth and mandible (Figure 8-2B).[33,42,46,47] Trigger points close to the angle of the mandible frequently refer pain in an arc that extends across the temple and over the eyebrow, as well to the lower jaw (Figure 8-2C).[48,33,39,42,43] Kellgren[48] experimentally induced referred pain from the masseter muscle in a normal subject by injecting 0.1 mL of 6% saline solution into its fibers just above the angle of the mandible. This procedure caused "toothache" of the upper jaw, pain in the region of the TMJ, and pain in the external auditory meatus.

Similar to TrPs in the temporalis muscle, masseter TrPs may also cause tooth hypersensitivity to any or all stimuli, including occlusal pressure, percussion, heat, and cold.[47]

Deep Layer

Trigger points in the underlying deep layer of the masseter muscle, over the ramus of the mandible, are likely to refer pain diffusely to the midcheek area in the region of the lateral pterygoid muscle and sometimes in the region of the TMJ. Oftentimes, TrPs close to the posterior zygomatic attachment of the deep portion of the masseter muscle refer pain deep into the ear (Figure 8-2D).[34,42,49-52] The deep layer may also cause tinnitus of the ipsilateral ear.[42,53] The tinnitus may be constant or may be set off by pressure on the TrP, even though the patient may be unaware of its presence, and therefore its link to his or her symptoms, until the TrP is deactivated.[42,54] A study by Saldanha et al[55] showed an association between TMD and subjective tinnitus with the masseter and anterior temporalis muscles having a lower pain pressure threshold compared with controls.

3.2. Symptoms

Patients with TrPs in the superficial layer of the masseter muscle often report pain in the zygomatic region as a "sinusitis." Frequently, patients seek medical care thinking they are sick, yet no other findings can confirm the patient is ill.

Similar to the temporalis muscle, pain referred to a tooth by superficial masseter TrPs can easily be misinterpreted as being of endodontic origin.[44] Patients go to the dentist thinking they have a cavity or some other tooth-related problem. Regrettably, at times, patients have had significant dental procedures for the "tooth" pain, only to find out the problem persists because it was actually nonodontogenic.[47]

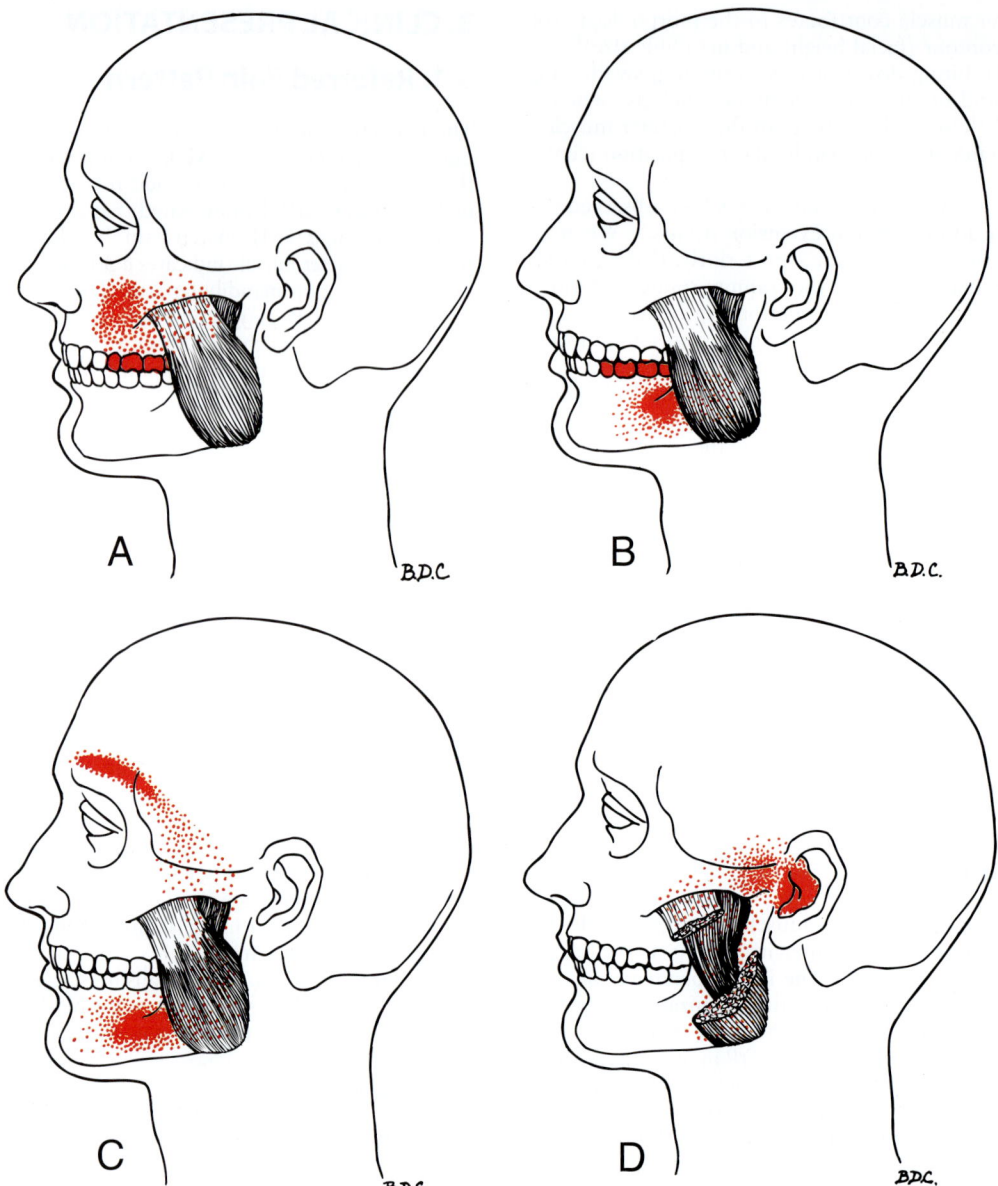

Figure 8-2. Referred pain patterns arising from TrPs in the masseter muscle. Solid red shows essential referred pain zones, and the stippled areas are spillover pain zones. A, Referral patterns from TrPs near the musculotendinous junction of the superficial layer, upper portion. B, Referral patterns from TrPs in midmuscle of the superficial layer. C, Referral patterns from TrPs of the lowest portion of the superficial layer, near its attachment. D, Referral patterns from TrP in the upper posterior part of the deep layer below the temporomandibular joint.

If tinnitus is present, patients might notice that stretching the jaw wide open may either activate or interrupt the tinnitus. The tinnitus is usually described as "low roaring" and is not associated with the deafness and vertigo that is common with a vestibular or central neurologic lesion. They may also report that applying pressure to the masseter muscle alters tinnitus.[54]

With TrPs in either or both layers of the masseter muscle, patients can report difficulty with full mouth opening.[56] It has also been seen clinically that TrPs can contribute to closing of the mandible in a quick, almost snapping-like, motion instead of a controlled movement.

In addition, TrPs in the masseter muscle might restrict venous flow from the infraorbital subcutaneous tissues. This engorgement of the orbital vein produces puffiness ("bags") beneath the eye on the affected side, and thus narrows the palpebral fissure. Narrowing of the fissure may also be caused by associated TrPs in the orbicularis oculi muscle, which lies in the pain reference zone of TrPs in the sternal division of the sternocleidomastoid muscle.

3.3. Patient Examination

The clinician should be aware that TrPs not only contribute to pain, but also decrease the jaw range of motion. Ipsilateral masseter myofascial pain has been correlated with the presence of TMD.[36] Before beginning the physical examination, the clinician should take a thorough patient history. After establishing the history of the condition, the clinician should create a detailed diagram representing the pain described by the patient.

A unilateral dysfunction, whether due to muscle problems or internal derangement of a TMJ, also has an effect on the contralateral side because the mandible spans the midline and attaches to both sides of the cranium. As a result, assessment should always include a bilateral visual and palpatory examination for musculoskeletal dysfunction.

The clinician should check specifically for forward head posture (loss of sternal/malar positioning). Although the relationship between TMD and head posture is somewhat controversial and unclear,[57] it is thought that forward head posture

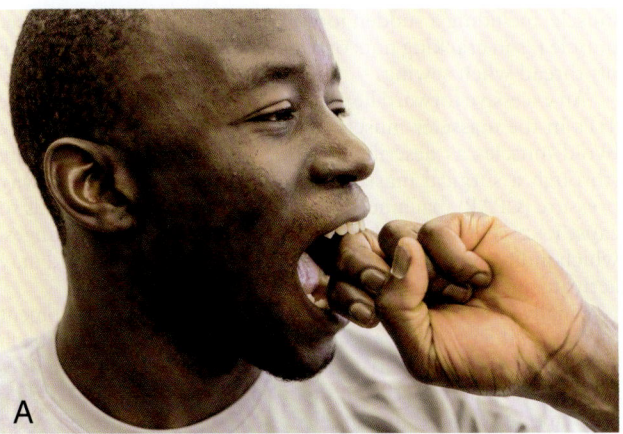
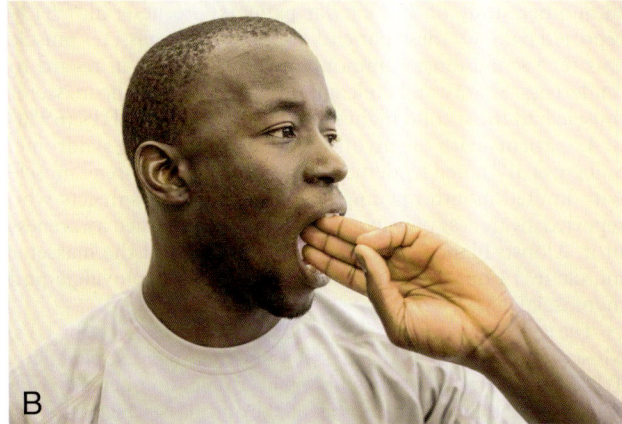

Figure 8-3. A, Two-knuckle test. B, Tiered three-finger test.

indirectly induces tension in the hyoid muscles, which in turn pulls downward to create light tensile forces on the mandible.[58] As a result, this causes the mandibular elevator muscles, such as the masseter muscle, to work harder, to contract to keep the mouth closed.

Masseter TrPs, whether unilateral or bilateral, may cause restriction of mouth opening,[56] which is evident on examination, although the patient may not be aware of it. Unilateral masseter TrPs tend to deviate the mandible toward the affected side, a deviation that is apparent when the patient slowly opens and closes the mouth. This should be differentiated from a unilateral TMJ internal derangement, which may also cause the mandible to deviate toward the affected side. Of course, with a history of painful joint derangement (localized TMJ pain, + joint sounds), both factors may be present and ultimately need treatment.

A convenient way to estimate interincisal opening that is adjusted to the size of the individual is with the "two-knuckle test" (see Figure 8-3A). Together, the first two knuckles (proximal interphalangeal joints of the second and third digits) should easily fit between the upper and lower incisor teeth. A more critical test is the insertion of a tier of the distal phalanges (not knuckles) of the first three fingers placed between the incisor teeth (Figure 8-3B). This was easily accomplished in an asymptomatic population of patients who were unscreened for masticatory symptoms and/or tender masticatory muscles.[59]

Individuals with TrPs in the mandibular elevator muscles are very unlikely to pass the more rigorous "three-knuckle test," which was first reported by Dorrance[60] in 1929. This test was found to be a reliable method in a follow-up study in 2008.[61] The patient places the first three knuckles (second, third, and fourth digits) of the nondominant hand between the upper and lower incisor teeth. This test is more demanding than the loose two-knuckle test and requires a degree of forcing for many individuals even when no TrPs are present. This forcing would be unwise for individuals who might have an internal derangement of the TMJ. If the three-knuckle test can be accomplished without forcing, the subject is very unlikely to have masseter (or temporalis) TrPs or significant TMJ dysfunction, but they could have a hypermobile joint.

A more standardized, objective way to measure mouth opening is with a vertical ruler to measure the distance between the upper and lower incisors.[62,63] Normal mouth opening for women is 41 to 45 mm and men is 43 to 45 mm.[64,65]

3.4. Trigger Point Examination

Among the masticatory muscles, the masseter muscle frequently has TrPs. In one study of 56 patients with myofascial pain dysfunction syndrome as defined by Laskin,[66] the superficial portion of the masseter muscle was the most commonly involved muscle, and the deep masseter muscle was the fifth most commonly involved.[67] In patients with temporomandibular arthralgia, 61.6% presented with pain from at least one masseter muscle.[36]

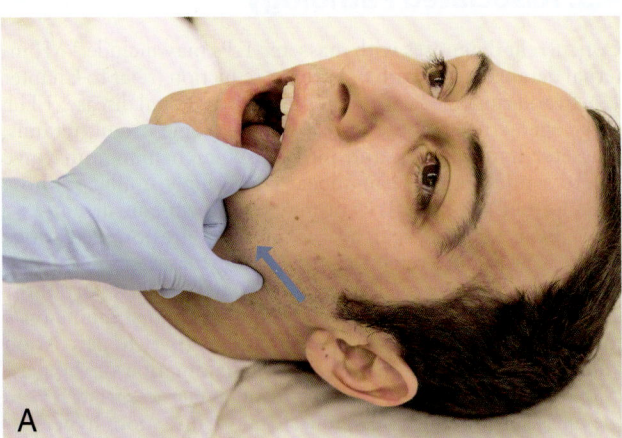
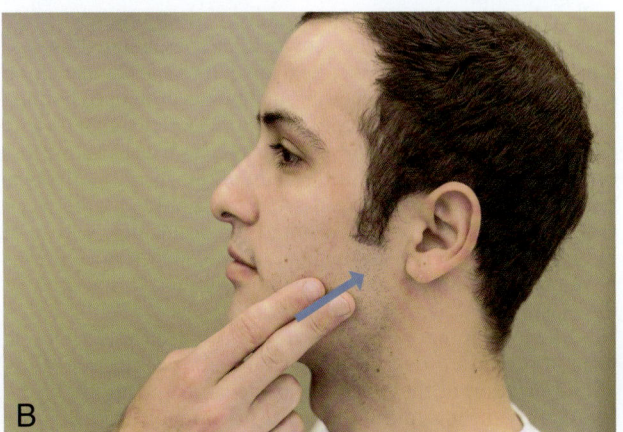

Figure 8-4. Pincer palpation method for locating TrPs in the masseter muscle. A, The clinician utilizes intraoral cross-fiber pincer palpation to detect TrPs in the masseter muscle. B, Extraoral cross-fiber flat palpation technique. Both techniques can be performed with the patient seated or in a supine position.

In another study of 277 similar patients Greene et al,[68] 81% reported pain. Of these patients with pain, the masseter muscle was the second most commonly involved muscle in regard to tenderness. Sharav and colleagues[69] observed that the masseter muscle had the second highest prevalence of active TrPs (69%) of 42 patients with the myofascial pain dysfunction syndrome. Solberg et al[70] noted tenderness in the superficial masseter muscle with limited mouth opening 4 times as often in subjects who reported awareness of bruxism as in those who denied awareness of it. Alonso-Blanco et al[33] found active TrPs of the masseter muscle in 14 out of 20 female patients with fibromyalgia and myofascial TMD.

The entire masseter muscle should be palpated to assess for TrPs. Most of the midbelly of the masseter muscle can be examined for TrPs effectively with a cross-fiber pincer palpation between one digit inside the cheek and another on the outside (see Figure 8-4A). The patient can be in the seated position or, more preferably, in the supine position to ensure adequate relaxation of the patient. Only a thin layer of mucosa separates the palpating finger and the midportion of the muscle. If the clinician has difficulty localizing the muscle itself, he can ask the patient to bite down gently so that he can confirm being on the muscle. Then, with the muscle relaxed, taut bands can be identified by rubbing the muscle fibers between the fingers. The tenderness of the TrP is increased if the patient opens the mouth far enough to take up most of the slack in the muscle (usually the width of a tongue depressor placed on its edge between the upper and lower incisors provides this slack). The finger inside the mouth can feel the muscle structure much more clearly than can the finger on the outside, because the parotid gland lies between the skin and much of the midfiber portion of the muscle where many masseter TrPs are located.

To assess the muscle near the angle of the mandible, a cross-fiber flat palpation is utilized extraorally (Figure 8-4B). The clinician can confirm accurate palpation of the muscle by asking the patient to bite down briefly and the clinician feels a contraction under the palpating finger.

4. DIFFERENTIAL DIAGNOSIS

4.1. Activation and Perpetuation of Trigger Points

A posture or activity that activates a TrP, if not corrected, can also perpetuate it. In any part of the masseter muscle, TrPs may be activated by unaccustomed eccentric loading, eccentric exercise in an unconditioned masseter muscle, overuse, or maximal or submaximal concentric loading.[71] Trigger points may also be activated or aggravated when the muscle is placed in a shortened or lengthened position for an extended period of time.

Specifically, TrPs may be activated and perpetuated by sustained or repetitive parafunctional jaw habits such as clenching or bruxing the teeth, gum chewing, nail biting, prolonged holding of the jaw on the mouthpiece of a pipe or cigarette holder,[72] late childhood thumb sucking, or significant occlusal disharmony loss of posterior teeth, worn denture teeth, or resorption of alveolar bone. A positive association has been demonstrated between excessive parafunctional habits and malocclusions, with nail biting found to be most common at 65.5%.[73] Malocclusions have been found to cause a variability of muscle activities of the masseter and temporalis muscles.[74]

Other events that might activate TrPs in the masseter muscle include prolonged over-stretching during a dental procedure, immobilization of the mandible in the closed position (by the head halter during continuous neck traction, or by wiring the jaw shut), direct trauma to the muscle, particularly with a blow to the side of the face, and overload of the masseter muscle following a motor vehicle accident causing a flexion–extension injury to the suprahyoid or infrahyoid muscles, which in turn produce tension on the jaw and thereby on the masseter muscle.[75] Acute overload situations can also activate TrPs in the masseter muscle, including a sudden forcible contraction of the masseter muscle (as in cracking nuts or ice between the teeth), and biting off thread when sewing.

An excessive forward head posture can activate or perpetuate TrPs in the masseter muscle by way of increased stress to the hyoid muscles as described earlier. Chronic mouth breathing (through a surgical mask, with a continuous positive airway pressure (CPAP) machine, or due to nasal obstruction) tends to cause excessive forward head positioning and postural changes, which indirectly add stress to the masticatory muscles and may activate and perpetuate TrPs in these muscles.[76]

Finally, emotional stressors can play a role in the development of TrPs in the masseter muscle. Schwartz et al[77] and Auerbach et al[78] observed the contribution of emotional stress to the development of active TrPs and pain in patients with TMD. The masseter muscles are among the first to contract in persons who are in a state of extreme emotional tension, intense determination, or desperation, and they often remain contracted for abnormally long periods of time.[46] Bell[79] presented case reports that indicate the contribution of life stress situations and bruxism to the development and perpetuation of TrP pain. People who engage in nocturnal bruxism have higher levels of salivary cortisol and perceived psychological stress,[80] which supports the idea that stress can contribute to the development of TrPs via excessive activation of the masseter muscle with bruxing.

4.2. Associated Trigger Points

Associated TrPs can develop in the referred pain areas of other TrPs.[81] Therefore, muscles in the referred pain areas for each muscle should also be considered. Facial muscles such as the corrugator supercilii and the buccinators muscles may have TrPs due to the involvement of the masseter muscle.

It is important to recognize that masseter TrPs are often associated TrPs from the sternocleidomastoid or upper trapezius muscles as a result of increased motor unit activity.[82,83] In this situation, treatment of the TrPs in those muscles often obviates treating the masseter TrPs directly. Masseter and other masticatory muscle TrPs often resolve sufficiently with appropriate treatment of the cervical muscles, making TrP release techniques for the masticatory muscles unnecessary.

Masseter TrPs are likely to be associated with TrPs in other masticatory muscles as well. The most frequent being the ipsilateral temporalis and the contralateral masseter muscles. Less commonly, either or both the medial and lateral pterygoid muscles might be involved, and sometimes bilaterally.

4.3. Associated Pathology

Concurrent diagnoses with masseter TrPs may include TMJ internal derangements with or without reduction (refer to Chapter 18). In addition, medical conditions such as dental disease, TTH, cervicogenic headache, tinnitus of neurologic origin, tetanus, masseter hypertrophy, and intramuscular hemangioma give rise to symptoms that can appear confusingly similar to those produced by masseter TrPs or may be present concurrently.

A diseased tooth, such as one with a nonrestorable carious lesion, can produce referred pain over the masseter muscle that closely emulates the referred pain from a TrP in that part of the muscle. Prolonged pain responses to a thermal stimulus on a tooth may indicate a pulpitis, whereas sensitivity to percussion and pressure can result from apical inflammation of the periodontal ligament.[84,85] Referred pain and tenderness from TrPs in the masseter (or temporalis) muscle may cause tooth hypersensitivity to any or all stimuli: occlusal pressure, percussion, heat, and cold. Appropriate treatments for pulpitis, inflammation of the periodontal ligament, and masseter TrPs are quite different, therefore making an accurate diagnosis essential.

Masseter TrPs are frequently associated with headaches. In patients with cervicogenic headache, TrPs can be a pain producing mechanism.[86] Similarly, masseter TrPs are associated with patients diagnosed with TTH.[37,38,41]

Tinnitus of neurologic origin should be distinguished from that of myofascial origin as presented earlier in this chapter. Interestingly, tinnitus associated with hearing loss was frequently responsive to B$_{12}$ therapy,[87] if the patient was low in this vitamin. Similarly, B$_{12}$ therapy would help tinnitus of myofascial origin. One vitamin-inadequacy cause of tinnitus may be relieved by supplements of both niacin amide and thiamine. Restoration of normal plasma melatonin and vitamin B$_{12}$ blood serum levels proved helpful in patients with tinnitus associated with hearing loss.[87,88]

Trismus is a firm closing of the jaw caused by spasms of the masticatory muscles. It can be due to spasms of the masseter muscle from cellulitis in adjacent tissues,[89] spasms of the medial pterygoid muscle from cellulitis in the pterygomandibular space,[89] spasms of the temporalis muscle from cellulitis in the infratemporal fossa,[89] infection of the masticatory space of an odontogenic origin,[90,91] local anesthetic injections,[90,91] surgical removal of teeth[91] (especially the third molar),[90] jaw or facial fractures,[90,91] or postradiation therapy to the facial area (radiation fibrosis).[91]

Although tetanus is uncommon in developed countries due to vaccinations, it is a serious medical condition that can also cause trismus and should be ruled out. As recently as 2012, in a case study by Fusetti et al,[92] a 78-year-old farmer was diagnosed with tetanus with progressive onset of lockjaw and muscular stiffness. In addition, a 31-year-old in another case study, who had proper levels of tetanus antibodies, was treated for tetanus symptoms after puncturing his hand with a rusty nail.[93]

Attempts to open the jaw are commonly painful with trismus. The pain is aggravated if the spastic muscles also have TrPs. Trigger points can be treated by injection, but only if there is no evidence of infection in the area. Mouth-opening exercises,[94] as well as the use of devices and medications, can help increase motion, decrease pain, and improve quality of life.[90,95]

Masseter hypertrophy can mistakenly be confused with pathology of the masseter muscle because limitation of motion is a clinical finding of both conditions.[96,97] Masseter hypertrophy is a painless swelling of the muscle at the parotid and posterior cheek area. With palpation, the masseter muscle is firm and solid with normal skin and mucosa. Magnetic resonance imaging (MRI) is positive for an increased size of muscle bundles in the masseter muscle.[98] The patient might present with limited mouth opening and occasional pain, but no fever or abnormal lab tests.[96,97]

An intramuscular hemangioma is a rare vascular tumor that, when present in the head region, is most commonly found in the masseter muscle.[99-101] It can be accelerated with a growth spurt or trauma to the muscular tissue and can spontaneously regress.[99] Pain is present in 50% to 60% of cases,[100] with a majority of the cases occurring before 30 years of age.[99-101] Diagnostic tests such as magnetic resonance imaging, ultrasonography, and color Doppler are commonly used to help determine what type of soft-tissue lesion is present.[99,101] Treatment is a surgical excision.[99-101]

Pathology of the masseter muscle, as mentioned earlier, is commonly associated with TMD. Refer to other texts for comprehensive information regarding examination and differential diagnosis for TMD.

5. CORRECTIVE ACTIONS

First, because TrPs in the masseter muscle can be due to pathology in other muscles such as the sternocleidomastoid and trapezius muscles, these muscles should be addressed first (refer to Chapters 6 and 7).

Forward head posture should be corrected to reduce the masseter muscle activity. This correction might require changes to ensure that the patient can breathe through the nose, rather than the mouth. In addition, the patient should develop awareness of the mandibular posture (sternal/malar position), and reduce clenching, nail biting, exhaustive chewing, or other parafunctional oral habits.[21,58,76] Correct tongue position, with the tongue against the roof of the mouth behind the upper incisor

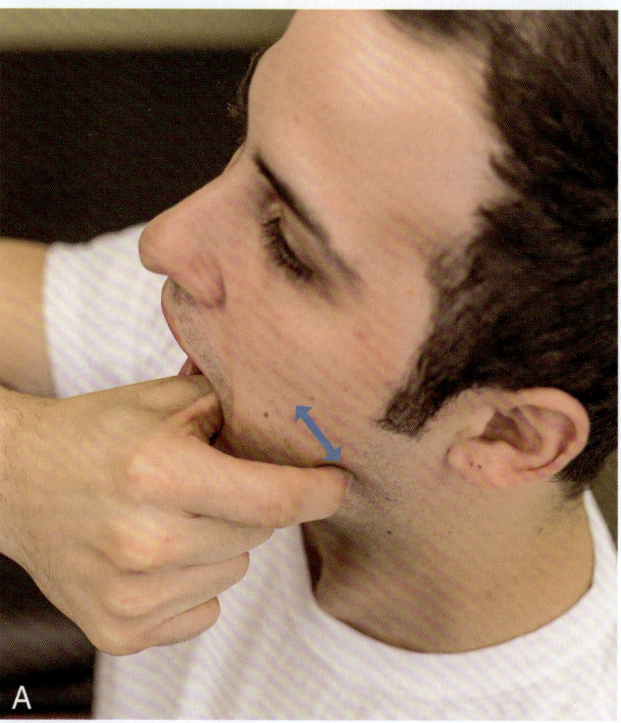 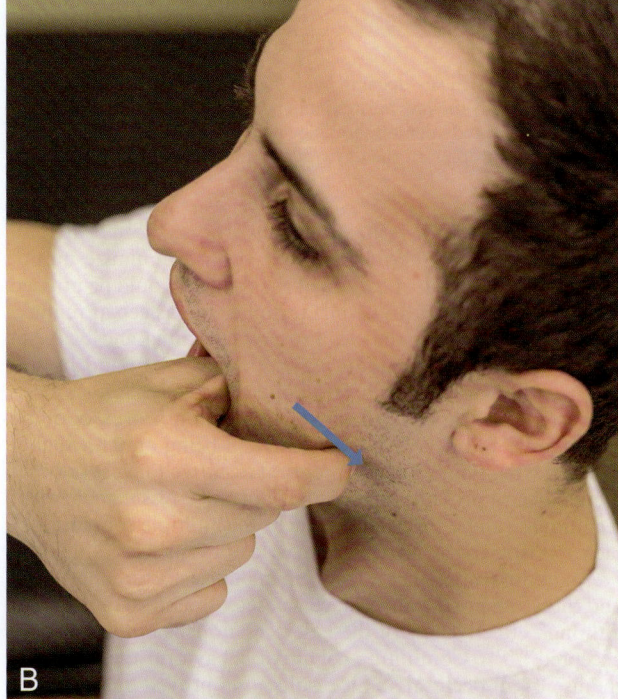

Figure 8-5. Self-intraoral release of the masseter muscle. The patient places the thumb on the inside of the cheek under the masseter muscle belly and the index finger is on the outside of the cheek (over the masseter muscle). A, The digits then apply a slight compression to the muscle. B, Or the thumb may push the masseter muscle further outward to stretch the muscle.

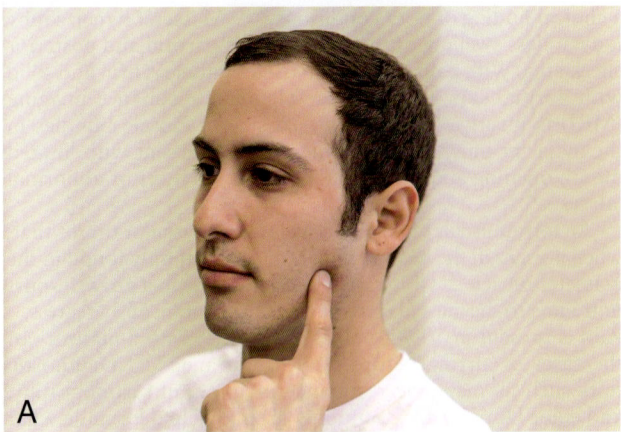 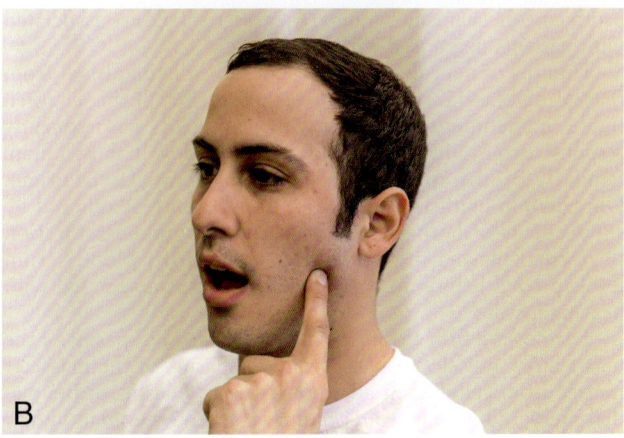

Figure 8-6. Extraoral active release of the masseter muscle. A, The patient identifies a TrP in the masseter muscle and applies pressure to tolerance for 30 seconds with a finger. This technique is repeated 3 to 5 times, and may be performed throughout the day as needed. B, Or, while maintaining pressure on the TrP, the patient very gently closes the jaw for 3 seconds then completely relaxes and opens the jaw to gently stretch the muscle. This technique may be repeated up to 3 to 5 times to reduce the pain and tenderness.

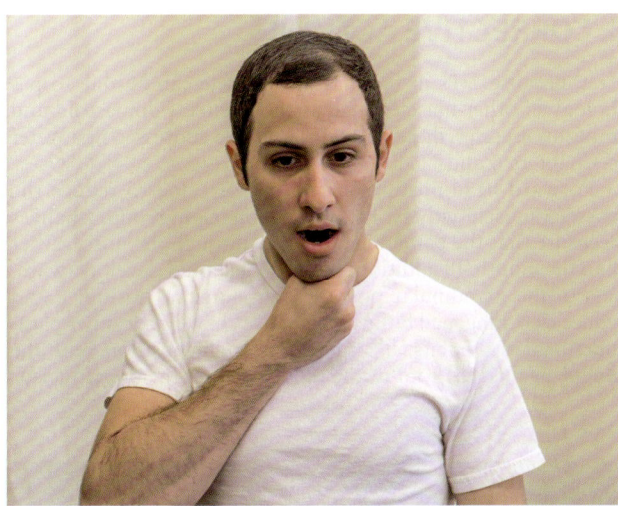

Figure 8-7. Resisted jaw opening. With the patient's fist under their chin, the patient opens the jaw approximately 1 in against the resistance of the fist. The resisted opening should be held for 5 seconds and repeated several times throughout the day when clenching is noted.

teeth (the "N" part of verbalizing the word "no") can be helpful to reduce stress to the masseter muscle and minimize mouth breathing. The correct position of the tongue should be utilized during waking hours and while trying to fall asleep at night.

Stress and anxiety that lead to jaw clenching and bruxism should be managed by reducing emotional strain and by improving the patient's ability to cope effectively. Studies have suggested that those with higher depression scores, somatic complaints, and decreased physical well-being are at a higher risk of having symptoms.[102] A referral to a psychologist or other mental health provider for specific pain and stress management techniques can be very helpful due to the multiple contributory factors associated with TrPs in masticatory muscles.[89]

An occlusal appliance might help minimize nocturnal bruxism and therefore potentially reduce masseter muscle activity,[103-105] although effectiveness of these devices alone is not universally accepted.[106,107] Combining cognitive behavioral therapy with the use of an occlusal splint results in improved outcomes,[108] and behavioral changes in conjunction with occlusal devices effectively reduce masticatory myofascial pain.[109]

The patient should also stop chewing gum, ice, or tough meat; eating caramels; biting pens, pencils, apples, or finger nails; cracking nuts with the teeth; or engaging in any other parafunctional oral behaviors that could increase the strain of the masseter muscle.

To improve mobility of the masseter muscle, the patient can perform an intraoral release (Figure 8-5) or an extraoral active release of the muscle (Figure 8-6).

For patients who clench their jaw during the day, performing repetitions of jaw opening against resistance (Figure 8-7) contributes to reciprocal inhibition of the masseter muscle, thereby reducing excessive activation of the muscle.

References

1. Standring S. *Gray's Anatomy: The Anatomical Basis of Clinical Practice*. 41st ed. London, UK: Elsevier; 2015.
2. Shore NA. *Temporomandibular Joint Dysfunction and Occlusal Equilibration*. Philadelphia, PA: J.B. Lippincott; 1976.
3. Schmolke C. The relationship between the temporomandibular joint capsule, articular disc and jaw muscles. *J Anat*. 1994;184(pt 2):335-345.
4. Hannam AG, McMillan AS. Internal organization in the human jaw muscles. *Crit Rev Oral Biol Med*. 1994;5(1):55-89.
5. Lee JY, Kim JN, Yoo JY, et al. Topographic anatomy of the masseter muscle focusing on the tendinous digitation. *Clin Anat*. 2012;25(7):889-892.
6. Strini PJ, Strini PJ, Barbosa Tde S, Gaviao MB. Assessment of thickness and function of masticatory and cervical muscles in adults with and without temporomandibular disorders. *Arch Oral Biol*. 2013;58(9):1100-1108.
7. Eriksson PO. Muscle fiber composition system. *Swed Dent J*. 1982;12(suppl):8-38.
8. Rowlerson A, Raoul G, Daniel Y, et al. Fiber-type differences in masseter muscle associated with different facial morphologies. *Am J Orthod Dentofacial Orthop*. 2005;127(1):37-46.
9. Sciote JJ, Raoul G, Ferri J, Close J, Horton MJ, Rowlerson A. Masseter function and skeletal malocclusion. *Rev Stomatol Chir Maxillofac Chir Orale*. 2013;114(2):79-85.
10. Eriksson PO, Butler-Browne GS, Thornell LE. Immunohistochemical characterization of human masseter muscle spindles. *Muscle Nerve*. 1994;17(1):31-41.
11. Johansson AS, Isberg A, Isacsson G. A radiographic and histologic study of the topographic relations in the temporomandibular joint region: implications for a nerve entrapment mechanism. *J Oral Maxillofac Surg*. 1990;48(9):953-961; discussion 962.
12. Won SY, Choi DY, Kwak HH, Kim ST, Kim HJ, Hu KS. Topography of the arteries supplying the masseter muscle: using dissection and Sihler's method. *Clin Anat*. 2012;25(3):308-313.
13. Basmajian J, Deluca C. *Muscles Alive*. 5th ed. Baltimore, MD: Williams & Wilkins; 1985.
14. Moyers RE. An electromyographic analysis of certain muscles involved in temporomandibular movement. *Am J Orthod*. 1950;36(7):481-515.
15. Woelfel JB, Hickey JC, Stacey RW, et al. Electromyographic analysis of jaw movements. *J Prosthet Dent*. 1960;10:688-697.
16. Yamaguchi S, Itoh S, Watanabe Y, Tsuboi A, Watanabe M. Quantitative analysis of masticatory activity during unilateral mastication using muscle fMRI. *Oral Dis*. 2011;17(4):407-413.
17. Yamaguchi S, Rikimaru H, Yamaguchi K, Itoh M, Watanabe M. Overall activity of all masticatory muscles during lateral excursion. *J Dent Res*. 2006;85(1):69-73.

18. Hugger S, Schindler HJ, Kordass B, Hugger A. Surface EMG of the masticatory muscles (Part 3): impact of changes to the dynamic occlusion. *Int J Comput Dent.* 2013;16(2):119-123.
19. Nakamura K, Hara A, Nakata S, Hyakutake H, Takahashi I. Relationship between the stability of muscle activity in the masseter muscle and craniofacial morphology. *Orthodontic Waves.* 2013;72(2):55-62.
20. Farella M, Palla S, Erni S, Michelotti A, Gallo LM. Masticatory muscle activity during deliberately performed oral tasks. *Physiol Meas.* 2008;29(12):1397-1410.
21. Michelotti A, Cioffi I, Festa P, Scala G, Farella M. Oral parafunctions as risk factors for diagnostic TMD subgroups. *J Oral Rehabil.* 2010;37(3):157-162.
22. Eriksson PO, Zafar H, Nordh E. Concomitant mandibular and head-neck movements during jaw opening-closing in man. *J Oral Rehabil.* 1998;25(11):859-870.
23. Wiesinger B, Haggman-Henrikson B, Hellstrom F, Wanman A. Experimental masseter muscle pain alters jaw-neck motor strategy. *Eur J Pain.* 2013;17(7):995-1004.
24. Steiner JE, Michman J, Litman A. Time sequence of the activity of the temporal and masseter muscles in healthy young human adults during habitual chewing of different test foods. *Arch Oral Biol.* 1974;19(1):29-34.
25. Mioche L, Bourdiol P, Martin JF, Noel Y. Variations in human masseter and temporalis muscle activity related to food texture during free and side-imposed mastication. *Arch Oral Biol.* 1999;44(12):1005-1012.
26. Fueki K, Yoshida E, Sugiura T, Igarashi Y. Comparison of electromyographic activity of jaw-closing muscles between mixing ability test and masticatory performance test. *J Prosthodont Restor.* 2009;53(2):72-77.
27. Miyawaki S, Ohkochi N, Kawakami T, Sugimura M. Changes in masticatory muscle activity according to food size in experimental human mastication. *J Oral Rehabil.* 2001;28(8):778-784.
28. De Felicio CM, Ferreira CL, Medeiros AP, Rodrigues Da Silva MA, Tartaglia GM, Sforza C. Electromyographic indices, orofacial myofunctional status and temporomandibular disorders severity: a correlation study. *J Electromyogr Kinesiol.* 2012;22(2):266-272.
29. Moller E, Sheik-Ol-Eslam A, Lous I. Deliberate relaxation of the temporal and masseter muscles in subjects with functional disorders of the chewing apparatus. *Scand J Dent Res.* 1971;79(7):478-482.
30. Valdes C, Gutierrez M, Falace D, Astaburuaga F, Manns A. The effect of tongue position and resulting vertical dimension on masticatory muscle activity. A cross-sectional study. *J Oral Rehabil.* 2013;40(9):650-656.
31. Simons DG, Travell J, Simons L. *Travell & Simon's Myofascial Pain and Dysfunction: The Trigger Point Manual.* Vol 1. 2nd ed. Baltimore, MD: Williams & Wilkins; 1999:104.
32. Staling LM, Fetchero P, Vorro J. Premature occlusal contact influence on mandibular kinesiology. In: Komi PV, ed. *Biomechanics.* Vol 1A. Baltimore, MD: University Park Press; 1976:280-288.
33. Alonso-Blanco C, Fernández de las Peñas C, de-la-Llave-Rincon AI, Zarco-Moreno P, Galan-Del-Rio F, Svensson P. Characteristics of referred muscle pain to the head from active trigger points in women with myofascial temporomandibular pain and fibromyalgia syndrome. *J Headache Pain.* 2012;13(8):625-637.
34. Sanches ML, Juliano Y, Novo NF, et al. Frequency and location of referred pain in patients with temporomandibular disorder. *Int J Odontostomat.* 2014;8(2):309-315.
35. Fernández de Las Peñas C, Galan-Del-Rio F, Alonso-Blanco C, Jimenez-Garcia R, Arendt-Nielsen L, Svensson P. Referred pain from muscle trigger points in the masticatory and neck-shoulder musculature in women with temporomandibular disorders. *J Pain.* 2010;11(12):1295-1304.
36. da Silva Parente Macedo LC, de Goffredo Filho GS, de Souza Tesch R, de Queiroz Farias Goes CP. Frequency of temporomandibular arthralgia among myofascial pain patients with pain on palpation of ipsilateral masseter. *Cranio.* 2015;33(3):206-210.
37. Karadaş Ö, Gul HL, Inan LE. Lidocaine injection of pericranial myofascial trigger points in the treatment of frequent episodic tension-type headache. *J Headache Pain.* 2013;14:44.
38. Fernández de las Peñas C, Fernandez-Mayoralas DM, Ortega-Santiago R, Ambite-Quesada S, Palacios-Cena D, Pareja JA. Referred pain from myofascial trigger points in head and neck-shoulder muscles reproduces head pain features in children with chronic tension type headache. *J Headache Pain.* 2011;12(1):35-43.
39. De-la-Llave-Rincon AI, Alonso-Blanco C, Gil-Crujera A, Ambite-Quesada S, Svensson P, Fernández de las Peñas C. Myofascial trigger points in the masticatory muscles in patients with and without chronic mechanical neck pain. *J Manipulative Physiol Ther.* 2012;35(9):678-684.
40. Jaeger B, Reeves JL, Graff-Radford SB. A psychophysiological investigation of myofascial trigger point sensitivity vs. EMG activity and tension headache. *Cephalalgia.* 1985;5(suppl 3):68-69.
41. Fernández de las Peñas C, Ge HY, Alonso-Blanco C, Gonzalez-Iglesias J, Arendt-Nielsen L. Referred pain areas of active myofascial trigger points in head, neck, and shoulder muscles, in chronic tension type headache. *J Bodyw Mov Ther.* 2010;14(4):391-396.
42. Travell J. Temporomandibular joint pain referred from muscles of the head and neck. *J Prosthet Dent.* 1960;10:745-763.
43. Travell J, Rinzler SH. The myofascial genesis of pain. *Postgrad Med.* 1952;11(5):425-434.
44. Kleier DJ. Referred pain from a myofascial trigger point mimicking pain of endodontic origin. *J Endod.* 1985;11(9):408-411.
45. Marbach JJ. Arthritis of the temporomandibular joints. *Am Fam Physician.* 1979;19(2):131-139.
46. Wolff HG. *Wolff's Headache and Other Head Pain.* 3rd ed. New York, NY: Oxford University Press; 1972.
47. Handa T, Fukuda K, Ichinohe T. Effect of combination of trigger point injection and stellate ganglion block on non-odontogenic mandibular molar pain referred from masseter muscle: a case report. *Bull Tokyo Dent Coll.* 2013;54(3):171-175.
48. Kellgren JH. Observations on referred pain arising from muscle. *Clin Sci.* 1938;3:175-190, 180.
49. Bell WE. *Orofacial Pains: Differential Diagnosis.* Dallas, TX: Denedco of Dallas; 1973.
50. Reynolds MD. Myofascial trigger point syndromes in the practice of rheumatology. *Arch Phys Med Rehabil.* 1981;62(3):111-114.
51. Schwartz LL. Ethyl chloride treatment of limited, painful mandibular movement. *J Am Dent Assoc.* 1954;48(5):497-507.
52. Travell J. Mechanical headache. *Headache.* 1967;7(1):23-29.
53. Wyant GM. Chronic pain syndromes and their treatment. II. Trigger points. *Can Anaesth Soc J.* 1979;26(3):216-219.
54. Bezerra Rocha CA, Sanchez TG, Tesseroli de Siqueira JT. Myofascial trigger point: a possible way of modulating tinnitus. *Audiol Neurootol.* 2008;13(3):153-160.
55. Saldanha AD, Hilgenberg PB, Pinto LM, Conti PC. Are temporomandibular disorders and tinnitus associated? *Cranio.* 2012;30(3):166-171.
56. Fernandez-Carnero J, La Touche R, Ortega-Santiago R, et al. Short-term effects of dry needling of active myofascial trigger points in the masseter muscle in patients with temporomandibular disorders. *J Orofac Pain.* 2010;24(1):106-112.
57. Rocha CP, Croci CS, Caria PH. Is there relationship between temporomandibular disorders and head and cervical posture? A systematic review. *J Oral Rehabil.* 2013;40(11):875-881.
58. Gonzalez HE, Manns A. Forward head posture: its structural and functional influence on the stomatognathic system, a conceptual study. *Cranio.* 1996;14(1):71-80.
59. Agerberg G, Osterberg T. Maximal mandibular movements and symptoms of mandibular dysfunction in 70-year old men and women. *Sven Tandlak Tidskr.* 1974;67(3):147-163.
60. Dorrance GM. New and useful surgical procedures: the mechanical treatment of trismus. *Pa Med J.* 1929;32:545-546.
61. Abou-Atme YS, Chedid N, Melis M, Zawawi KH. Clinical measurement of normal maximum mouth opening in children. *Cranio.* 2008;26(3):191-196.
62. Walker N, Bohannon RW, Cameron D. Discriminant validity of temporomandibular joint range of motion measurements obtained with a ruler. *J Orthop Sports Phys Ther.* 2000;30(8):484-492.
63. List T, John MT, Dworkin SF, Svensson P. Recalibration improves inter-examiner reliability of TMD examination. *Acta Odontol Scand.* 2006;64(3):146-152.
64. Gallagher C, Gallagher V, Whelton H, Cronin M. The normal range of mouth opening in an Irish population. *J Oral Rehabil.* 2004;31(2):110-116.
65. Muller L, van Waes H, Langerweger C, Molinari L, Saurenmann RK. Maximal mouth opening capacity: percentiles for healthy children 4-17 years of age. *Pediatr Rheumatol Online J.* 2013;11:17.
66. Laskin DM. Etiology of the pain-dysfunction syndrome. *J Am Dent Assoc.* 1969;79(1):147-153.
67. Butler JH, Folke LE, Bandt CL. A descriptive survey of signs and symptoms associated with the myofascial pain-dysfunction syndrome. *J Am Dent Assoc.* 1975;90(3):635-639.
68. Greene CS, Lerman MD, Sutcher HD, Laskin DM. The TMJ pain-dysfunction syndrome: heterogeneity of the patient population. *J Am Dent Assoc.* 1969;79(5):1168-1172.
69. Sharav Y, Tzukert A, Refaeli B. Muscle pain index in relation to pain, dysfunction, and dizziness associated with the myofascial pain-dysfunction syndrome. *Oral Surg Oral Med Oral Pathol.* 1978;46(6):742-747.
70. Solberg WK, Clark GT, Rugh JD. Nocturnal electromyographic evaluation of bruxism patients undergoing short term splint therapy. *J Oral Rehabil.* 1975;2(3):215-223.
71. Gerwin RD, Dommerholt J, Shah JP. An expansion of Simons' integrated hypothesis of trigger point formation. *Curr Pain Headache Rep.* 2004;8(6):468-475.
72. McInnes B. Jaw pain from cigarette holder. *N Engl J Med.* 1978;298(22):1263.
73. Giugliano D, Apuzzo F, Jamilian A, Perillo L. Relationship between malocclusion and oral habits. *Curr Res Dent.* 2014;5(2):17-21.
74. Wozniak K, Szyszka-Sommerfeld L, Lichota D. The electrical activity of the temporal and masseter muscles in patients with TMD and unilateral posterior crossbite. *Biomed Res Int.* 2015;2015:1-7.
75. Fernandez-Perez AM, Villaverde-Gutierrez C, Mora-Sanchez A, Alonso-Blanco C, Sterling M, Fernández de las Peñas C. Muscle trigger points, pressure pain threshold, and cervical range of motion in patients with high level of disability related to acute whiplash injury. *J Orthop Sports Phys Ther.* 2012;42(7):634-641.
76. La Touche R, Paris-Alemany A, von Piekartz H, Mannheimer JS, Fernandez-Carnero J, Rocabado M. The influence of cranio-cervical posture on maximal mouth opening and pressure pain threshold in patients with myofascial temporomandibular pain disorders. *Clin J Pain.* 2011;27(1):48-55.
77. Schwartz RA, Greene CS, Laskin DM. Personality characteristics of patients with myofascial pain-dysfunction (MPD) syndrome unresponsive to conventional therapy. *J Dent Res.* 1979;58(5):1435-1439.
78. Auerbach SM, Laskin DM, Frantsve LM, Orr T. Depression, pain, exposure to stressful life events, and long-term outcomes in temporomandibular disorder patients. *J Oral Maxillofac Surg.* 2001;59(6):628-633; discussion 634.
79. Bell WH. Nonsurgical management of the pain-dysfunction syndrome. *J Am Dent Assoc.* 1969;79(1):161-170.
80. Karakoulaki S, Tortopidis D, Andreadis D, Koidis P. Relationship between sleep bruxism and stress determined by saliva biomarkers. *Int J Prosthodont.* 2015;28(5):467-474.

81. Hsieh YL, Kao MJ, Kuan TS, Chen SM, Chen JT, Hong CZ. Dry needling to a key myofascial trigger point may reduce the irritability of satellite MTrPs. *Am J Phys Med Rehabil.* 2007;86(5):397-403.
82. Hong C-Z. Considerations and recommendations regarding myofascial trigger point injection. *J Musculoskelet Pain.* 1994;2(1):29-59.
83. Carlson CR, Okeson JP, Falace DA, Nitz AJ, Lindroth JE. Reduction of pain and EMG activity in the masseter region by trapezius trigger point injection. *Pain.* 1993;55(3):397-400.
84. Bellizzi R, Hartwell GR, Ingle JI, et al. Diagnostic procedures, Chapter 9. In: Ingle JI, Bakland LK, eds. *Endodontics.* 4th ed. Baltimore, MD: Williams & Wilkins; 1994:465-523.
85. Seltzer S. Dental conditions that cause head and neck pain, Chapter 7. *Pain Control in Dentistry: Diagnosis and Management.* Philadelphia, PA: J.B. Lippincott; 1978:105-136.
86. Jaeger B. Are "cervicogenic" headaches due to myofascial pain and cervical spine dysfunction? *Cephalalgia.* 1989;9(3):157-164.
87. Shemesh Z, Attias J, Ornan M, Shapira N, Shahar A. Vitamin B_{12} deficiency in patients with chronic-tinnitus and noise-induced hearing loss. *Am J Otolaryngol.* 1993;14(2):94-99.
88. Lasisi AO, Fehintola FA, Lasisi TJ. The role of plasma melatonin and vitamins C and B_{12} in the development of idiopathic tinnitus in the elderly. *Ghana Med J.* 2012;46(3):152-157.
89. Bell WE. *Orofacial Pains—Classification, Diagnosis, Management.* Chicago, IL: Year Book Medical Publishers, Inc; 1985.
90. Vaishali MR, Roopasri G, David MP, Indira AP. Trismus. *Indian J Dent Adv.* 2010;2(3):303-309.
91. Dhanrajani PJ, Jonaidel O. Trismus: aetiology, differential diagnosis and treatment. *Dent Update.* 2002;29(2):88-92, 94.
92. Fusetti S, Ghirotto C, Ferronato G. A case of cephalic tetanus in a developed country. *Int J Immunopathol Pharmacol.* 2013;26(1):273-277.
93. Vollman KE, Acquisto NM, Bodkin RP. A case of tetanus infection in an adult with a protective tetanus antibody level. *Am J Emerg Med.* 2014;32(4):392 e393-392 e394.
94. Lee LY, Chen SC, Chen WC, Huang BS, Lin CY. Postradiation trismus and its impact on quality of life in patients with head and neck cancer. *Oral Surg Oral Med Oral Pathol Oral Radiol.* 2015;119(2):187-195.
95. Dijkstra PU, Kalk WW, Roodenburg JL. Trismus in head and neck oncology: a systematic review. *Oral Oncol.* 2004;40(9):879-889.
96. Tabrizi R, Ozkan BT, Zare S. Correction of lower facial wideness due to masseter hypertrophy. *J Craniofac Surg.* 2010;21(4):1096-1097.
97. Ozkan BT, Tabrizi R, Cigerim L. Management of bilateral masseter muscle hypertrophy. *J Craniofac Surg.* 2012;23(1):e14-e16.
98. Andreadis D, Stylianou F, Link-Tsatsouli I, Markopoulos A. Bilateral masseter and internal pterygoid muscle hypertrophy: a diagnostic challenge. *Med Princ Pract.* 2014;23(3):286-288.
99. Lakshmi KC, Sankarapandiyan S, Mohanarangam VSP. Intramuscular hemangioma with diagnostic challenge: a cause for strange pain in the masseter muscle. *Case Rep Dent.* 2014:1-4.
100. Narayanan CD, Prakash P, Dhanasekaran CK. Intramuscular hemangioma of the masseter muscle: a case report. *Cases J.* 2009;2:7459.
101. Jolly SS, Rattan V, Rai S, Kaur K, Gupta A. Intramuscular cavernous haemangioma of masseter muscle—a case report of surgical excision. *J Clin Diagn Res.* 2015;9(4):ZD01-ZD02.
102. Dougall AL, Jimenez CA, Haggard RA, Stowell AW, Riggs RR, Gatchel RJ. Biopsychosocial factors associated with the subcategories of acute temporomandibular joint disorders. *J Orofac Pain.* 2012;26(1):7-16.
103. Matsumoto H, Tsukiyama Y, Kuwatsuru R, Koyano K. The effect of intermittent use of occlusal splint devices on sleep bruxism: a 4-week observation with a portable electromyographic recording device. *J Oral Rehabil.* 2015;42(4):251-258.
104. Landry ML, Rompre PH, Manzini C, Guitard F, de Grandmont P, Lavigne GJ. Reduction of sleep bruxism using a mandibular advancement device: an experimental controlled study. *Int J Prosthodont.* 2006;19(6):549-556.
105. Takahashi H, Masaki C, Makino M, et al. Management of sleep-time masticatory muscle activity using stabilisation splints affects psychological stress. *J Oral Rehabil.* 2013;40(12):892-899.
106. Suvinen TI, Kemppainen P. Review of clinical EMG studies related to muscle and occlusal factors in healthy and TMD subjects. *J Oral Rehabil.* 2007;34(9):631-644.
107. Sjoholm T, Kauko T, Kemppainen P, Rauhala E. Long-term use of occlusal appliance has impact on sleep structure. *J Oral Rehabil.* 2014;41(11):795-800.
108. Trindade M, Orestes-Cardoso S, de Siqueira TC. Interdisciplinary treatment of bruxism with an occlusal splint and cognitive behavioral therapy. *Gen Dent.* 2015;63(5):e1-e4.
109. Conti PC, de Alencar EN, da Mota Correa AS, Lauris JR, Porporatti AL, Costa YM. Behavioural changes and occlusal splints are effective in the management of masticatory myofascial pain: a short-term evaluation. *J Oral Rehabil.* 2012;39(10):754-760.

Chapter 9

Temporalis Muscle
"TMJ Train Wreck"

César Fernández de las Peñas and Ricardo Ortega-Santiago

1. INTRODUCTION

The temporalis muscle is one of the main muscles of the masticatory system consisting of three portions: anterior, middle, and posterior. It originates from the entire temporal fossa up to the inferior temporal line, excluding the part formed by the zygomatic bone and from the deep surface of the temporal fascia. It inserts onto the medial surface, apex, and anterior and posterior borders of the coronoid process of the mandible. It is innervated by the anterior and posterior deep temporal nerves, which branch from the anterior division of the mandibular portion of the trigeminal nerve (cranial nerve V). The vascularization of the temporalis muscle is supplied by the deep temporal branches from the second part of the maxillary artery. It is one of the main contributors to the dynamic stability of the temporomandibular joint by controlling the movement during mouth closing. Its primary function is closing the mouth, although the posterior fibers can assist in lateral movement to the same side, whereas the anterior fibers can contribute to the protrusion of the jaw. The referred pain from the temporalis muscle produces tooth pain or deep head pain, depending on the clinical presentation of the patient. This muscle is commonly involved in different pain syndromes of the craniocervical system, particularly in headaches, temporomandibular pain disorders, orofacial pain, and mechanical neck pain. In the last decade, there has been increasing evidence of the contribution of active trigger points (TrPs) in the temporalis muscle in symptoms associated with tension-type headache (TTH) and temporomandibular pain disorders (TMDs). Symptoms can spontaneously occur, and they may often be perpetuated by dysfunctional habits such as bruxism, chewing gum, biting fingernails, and chewing ice. It has been demonstrated that the temporalis muscle exhibits pressure pain hypersensitivity, expressed as lower pressure pain thresholds, in people with headache. Corrective actions include maintaining good postural alignment, proper tongue resting position in the mouth, stopping parafunctional habits, and passively stretching the muscle.

2. ANATOMIC CONSIDERATIONS

The temporalis muscle originates from the entire temporal fossa up to the inferior temporal line, excluding the part formed by the zygomatic bone, and from the deep surface of the temporal fascia. It inserts onto the medial surface, apex, and anterior and posterior borders of the coronoid process of the mandible (Figure 9-1).[1] A thick temporalis fascia, which splits into superficial and deep layers approximately 2 cm superior to the zygomatic arch, covers this muscle. Between the superficial and deep fascia lies the superficial temporal fat pad.

The temporalis muscle can be divided into three portions, depending on the orientation of the fibers: the anterior fibers that are nearly vertical, the middle fibers that are oblique, and the posterior fibers that are nearly horizontal.[1] With the different fiber directions, there is also a difference in the composition of fiber types of the muscle, which is due to specific portions of the muscle being more active than others portions of the muscle for a given task, that is, chewing. It is known that the muscle is comprised of both Type-I (slow twitch) and Type-II (fast twitch) fibers[2,3]; however, studies have shown discrepancies as to the percentage of Type-I fibers in different parts of the muscle.[2,4]

2.1. Innervation and Vascularization

The innervation of the temporalis muscle is supplied by the anterior and posterior deep temporal nerves, which branch from the anterior division of the mandibular portion of the trigeminal nerve (cranial nerve V). In addition, the vascularization of the temporalis muscle is supplied by the deep temporal branches from the second part of the maxillary artery.[1] In addition, the temporal arterial system provides reliable vascular anatomy for the temporalis muscle flap.[5]

2.2. Function

All the fibers of the temporalis muscle contribute to its primary function of elevation of the mandible (mouth closing). This movement requires both the upward pull of the anterior fibers and the backward pull of the posterior fibers.[1] When the mandible is closed and the jaw is clenched tightly in centric occlusion, the temporalis muscle is activated before the masseter muscle and all parts of the temporalis muscle are involved.[6,7] Interestingly, the temporalis muscle has demonstrated an antagonistic contraction during mouth opening in patients with masseter muscle contracture.[8,9]

The temporalis muscle also contributes to side-to-side movements of the mandible. Lateral movements of the mandible to the same side consistently activate the temporalis muscle, with the posterior fibers activated more than its anterior fibers.[10,11] Cecílio et al[7] reported similar findings; however, the portion of the temporalis muscle was not specified in their study.

Finally, this muscle is also involved in retrusion and protrusion of the mandible. For retrusion, all fibers of the temporalis muscle are active; however, the posterior fibers have demonstrated higher electromyographic (EMG) peak activity than the anterior fibers with this motion.[11] This supports earlier studies that reported similar findings.[12-14] Research in this area has not been done of late. For protrusion, the muscle is active, although not as strongly as during retrusion[7] and it is thought that the anterior fibers are more active with this motion.[10]

In the mandibular rest position, the anterior fibers of the temporalis muscle are active.[15] Other studies, however, have conflicting opinions—one study reported that that the posterior fibers are more active than the anterior fibers,[16] whereas another found no activity in repeated recordings of three temporalis muscles in seated subjects at rest with the head and trunk erect.[17]

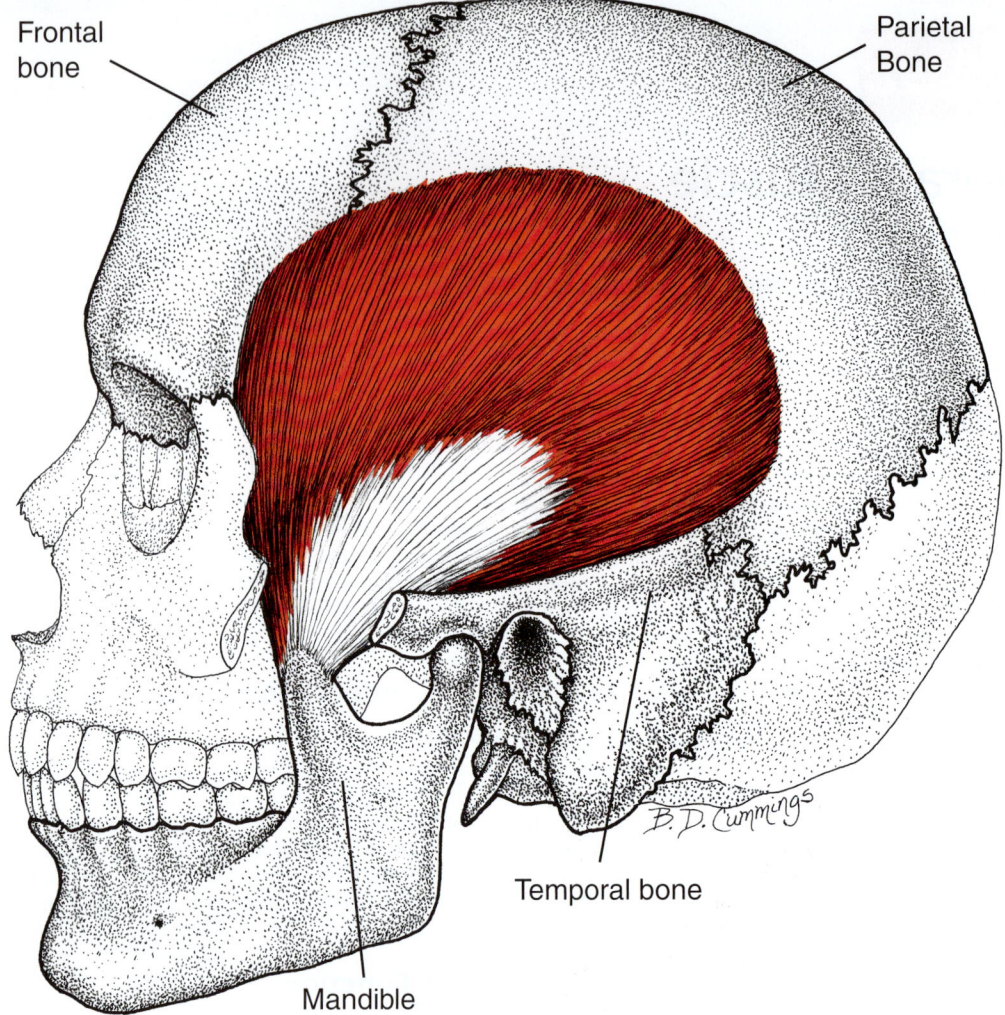

Figure 9-1. Attachments of the temporalis muscle, inferiorly, are chiefly to the coronoid process of the mandible and, superiorly, to the temporal fossa. The anterior fibers of this fan-shaped muscle are nearly vertical, and the posterior fibers are nearly horizontal but change direction and exert a mostly upward pull. The zygomatic arch, which has been partly removed, covers much of the tendinous attachment of the muscle to the coronoid process unless the mouth is opened.

These differing conclusions could result from the variation in the rest position, differences in the degree of anxiety-induced muscle tension, variations in electrode technique, head position, and the presence of latent TrPs in the masticatory musculature.

2.3. Functional Unit

The functional unit to which a muscle belongs includes the muscles that reinforce and counter its actions as well as the joints that the muscle crosses. The interdependence of these structures functionally is reflected in the organization and neural connections of the sensory motor cortex. The functional unit is emphasized because the presence of a TrP in one muscle of the unit increases the likelihood that the other muscles of the unit will also develop TrPs. When inactivating TrPs in a muscle, one should be concerned about TrPs that may develop in muscles that are functionally interdependent. Box 9-1 grossly represents the functional unit of the temporalis muscle.[18]

In addition to its primary function of mandibular elevation, the temporalis muscle can assist with ipsilateral mandibular elevation. The role of the superior division of the lateral pterygoid muscle during mandibular elevation (mouth closing) is under debate, although it is claimed that this muscle acts in eccentric contraction to recapture the disc during the movement.[19]

Box 9-1 Functional unit of the temporalis muscle

Action	Synergists	Antagonist
Mandibular elevation	Masseter Medial pterygoid	Lateral pterygoid (inferior division) Digastric Omohyoid Mylohyoid

3. CLINICAL PRESENTATION

3.1. Referred Pain Pattern

The temporalis muscle is commonly involved in patients with TTH[20-22] or TMD.[23] Interestingly, the temporalis muscle is also highly involved in children with TTH.[24] The referred pain elicited by TrPs in the temporalis muscle is described as pain felt widely throughout the temple, along the eyebrow, retro-orbitally, and in any or all the upper teeth.[25] Temporalis TrPs might also cause hypersensitivity to percussion and to moderate temperature changes that appears in any or all the upper teeth on the same side, depending on the TrP location.[25] Trigger points can be located in any portion of the temporalis muscle. It has been clinically observed that the anterior portion of the temporalis muscle can refer pain forward along the supraorbital ridge and downward to the upper incisor teeth[25] (Figure 9-2A). Trigger points in the middle portion of the muscle can refer pain upward in finger-like projections to the midtemple area and downward to the intermediate maxillary teeth on the same side (Figure 9-2B and C). Finally, TrPs located in the posterior portion of the muscle can refer pain backward and upward inside to the head, mimicking headache features (Figure 9-2D).[25] Other studies have also examined the referred pain patterns of the temporalis muscle with injections of hypertonic saline. Jensen and Norup[26] found that the muscle referred to the jaw. Schmidt-Hansen et al[27] reported referred pain to trigeminal innervated dermatomes, particularly to the ophthalmic and mandibular areas. The differences in the reported pain patterns highlight clinicians should consider that any portion of the temporalis muscle can refer pain to any part of the head or the teeth.

More recent studies have tried to represent the anatomic location of the referred pain from TrPs located in the temporalis muscle in individuals with TMD or TTH. Alonso-Blanco et al[28] observed that women with TMD exhibited more active TrPs in the temporalis and masseter muscles than women with fibromyalgia syndrome. In addition, the referred pain was located more posteriorly in TMD women. In another study, the same authors found that children with TTH had larger referred pain areas than adults for the temporalis muscle, but the referred pain area of temporalis muscle was located more inferiorly in adults with TTH than in children with TTH.[29] Finally, a clinical study investigating topographical distribution of TrPs in the temporalis muscle in patients with TTH observed two important findings for clinical practice: (1) the temporalis muscle usually exhibits multiple active TrPs in the same patient; (2) TrPs are mainly located in the anterior and the middle portions of the muscle belly.[30]

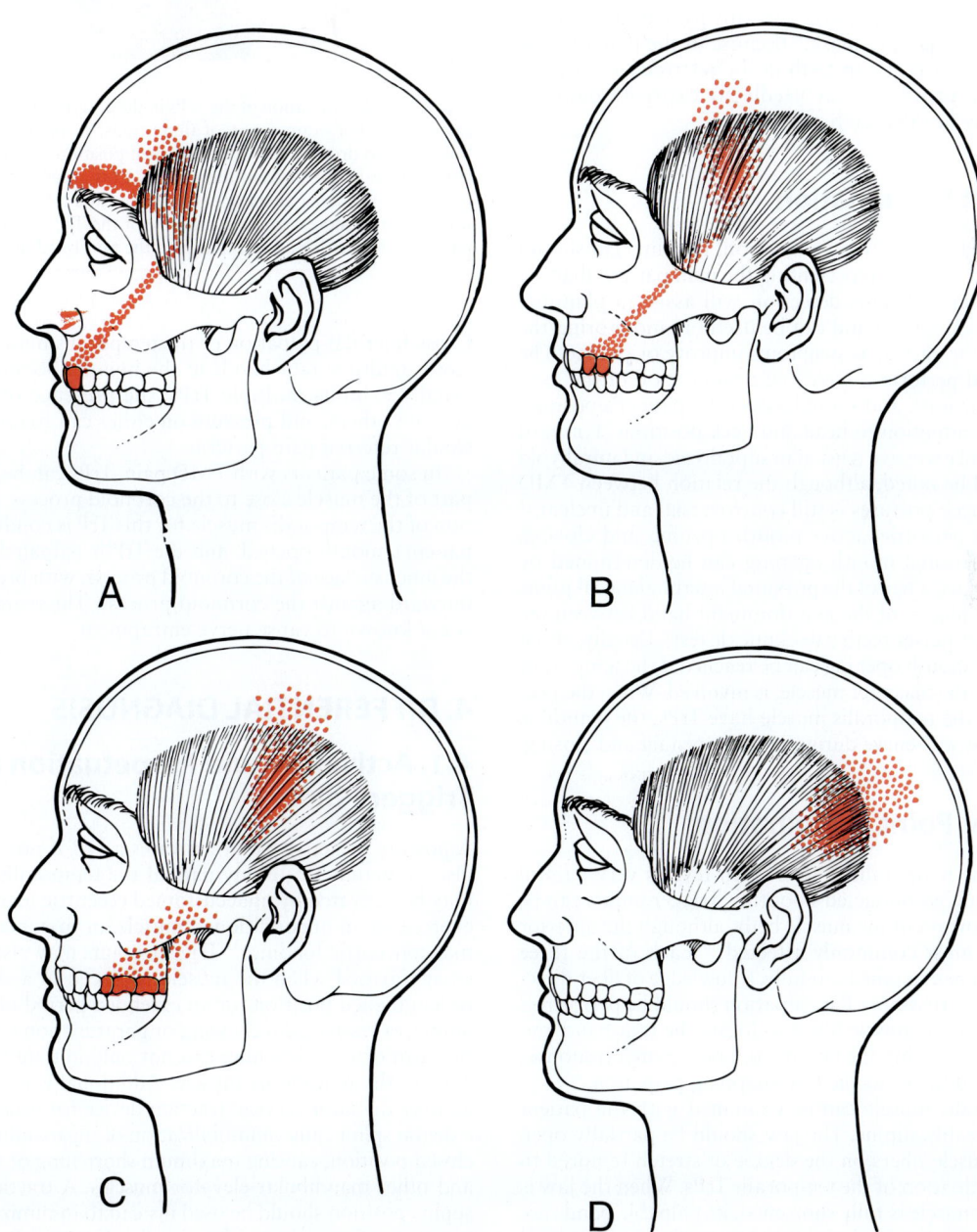

Figure 9-2. Patterns of pain and tenderness referred from trigger points (TrPs) in the left temporalis muscle (essential zone solid red, spillover zone stippled). A, referred pain from TrPs in the anterior portion of the temporalis muscle; B and C, represent referred pain arising from TrPs in the middle portion of the temporalis muscle; D, referred pain from TrPs in the posterior portion of the muscle.

3.2. Symptoms

Patients with temporalis TrPs might report having a headache, either TTH or migraine, toothache or tooth site pain, as previously described, but they are rarely aware of any restriction of jaw opening, which is usually reduced only by 5 to 10 mm (about 3/8 in). It is the masseter muscle that more frequently induces limitation of jaw opening (refer to Chapter 8). Thus, ordinary mandibular movement does not usually cause pain with TrPs in the temporalis muscle. It seems that a common phenotypic hyperalgesic response in the temporalis muscle in people with headache is expressed as lower pressure pain thresholds.[31] It is interesting to note that in clinical practice, the referred pain elicited by TrPs in the temporalis muscle adopts the phenotypic symptoms of the patient, that is, in a patient with TMD, the temporalis muscle refers pain to the teeth or the mouth, but not to the head, whereas in a patient with TTH, the referred pain is perceived deep into the head, but not into the teeth. Patients with TMD might say, "My teeth don't meet right," whereas patients with TTH or migraine might say, "I feel my pain inside the head or into the eye like an eye mask." Because of the potential for attendant hypersensitivity in teeth in the referred site of pain, unaware dental providers may needlessly extirpate pulps or extract perfectly healthy teeth.[25]

3.3. Patient Examination

After a thorough subjective examination, the clinician should make a detailed drawing representing the pain pattern that the patient has described. This depiction will assist in planning the physical examination and can be useful in monitoring the progression of the patient as symptoms improve or change. The clinician should perform a screening examination of the temporomandibular joint and should assess the patient's posture, with particular attention to head and neck positions. Forward head posture and excessive tension in suprahyoid and infrahyoid muscles should be noted, although the relation between TMD and head and neck postures is still controversial and unclear.[32]

The patient performs active mouth opening and closing. Normal or functional mouth opening can be determined by attempting to place a tier of the proximal interphalangeal joints of the first two fingers of the non-dominant hand between the upper and lower incisor teeth (two-knuckle test). Usually, about 2½ knuckles of mouth opening can be reached if the temporalis muscle, but not the masseter muscle, is involved. When the posterior fibers of the temporalis muscle have TrPs, the mandible is likely to show a C-curve during mouth opening and closing.

3.4. Trigger Point Examination

Palpation of the temporalis muscle often reveals very painful TrPs even when it is conducted smoothly. Trigger points can be found in any portion of the muscle belly, although the anterior portion is the most commonly affected.[30] Each of the three portions should be examined carefully. Knowledge of fiber direction is critical as cross-fiber flat palpation should be performed perpendicular to the muscle fibers to locate the taut band and then identify TrPs within the taut band. Local twitch responses are moderately difficult to elicit by snapping palpation.

The temporalis muscle can be examined with the patient sitting or preferably supine. The jaw should be partially open to place the muscle fibers on the degree of stretch required to optimize the palpation of the temporalis TrPs. When the jaw is closed and the muscle is fully shortened, its palpable bands are can be more difficult to feel; they are less tender, and the local twitch response to cross-fiber palpation may be unobtainable. When the patient allows the jaw to drop in the relaxed open position while keeping the lips gently closed or just slightly apart, it takes up the slack for examination of this muscle (Figure 9-3).

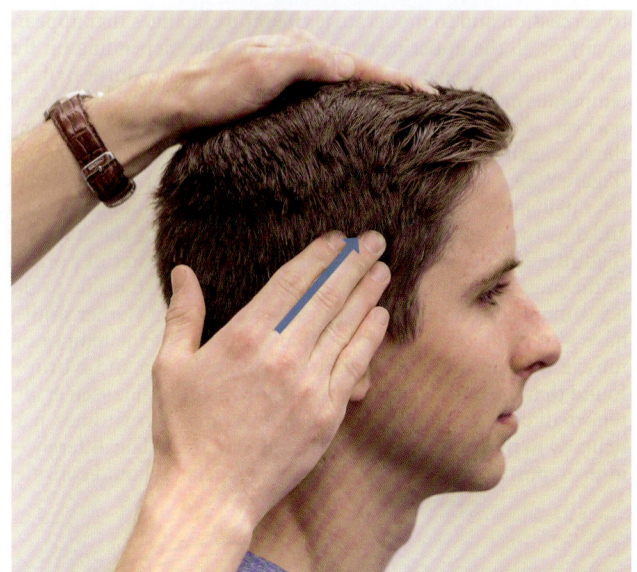

Figure 9-3. Examination of the TrPs in the anterior portion of the temporalis muscle. For examination of all portions, the patient should allow the lower jaw to drop into the relaxed open position (lips remaining gently closed) to take up slack in the muscle. This accentuates firm bands of muscle fibers, increases the spot tenderness and referred pain of a TrP to pressure, and increases the sensitivity of the TrP response to snapping palpation to test for a local twitch of the taut band fibers.

Cross-fiber flat palpation of the temporalis muscle usually discloses multiple taut bands in the muscle. Because this muscle usually exhibits multiple TrPs, the presence of one tends to activate others, and pressure on either can frequently produce similar referred pain patterns.

In some patients with TMD pain, TrPs can be located in the part of the muscle close to the coronoid process. The examination of the temporalis muscle for this TrP is conducted with the patient's mouth opened, and the TrP is palpated internally on the inner surface of the coronoid process, with pressure directed outward against the coronoid process. The temporalis muscle is not known to cause nerve entrapment.

4. DIFFERENTIAL DIAGNOSIS

4.1. Activation and Perpetuation of Trigger Points

A posture or activity that activates a TrP, if not corrected, can also perpetuate it. In any part of the temporalis muscle, TrPs may be activated by unaccustomed eccentric loading, eccentric exercise in an unconditioned muscle, or maximal or submaximal concentric loading.[33] Trigger points may also be activated or aggravated when the muscle is placed in a shortened and/or lengthened position for an extended period of time. For example, excessive gum chewing or parafunctional habits such as bruxism or jaw clenching can not only initiate but perpetuate TrPs in the temporalis muscle. Additionally, patients who use an over the door cervical traction device for neck pain without a dental splint cause immobilization of the mandible in the fully closed position, causing maximum shortening of the temporalis and other mandibular elevator muscles. A traction unit in the supine position should be used instead to minimize undue strain to the jaw. For patients who visit the dentist, TrPs in the temporalis muscle can develop when the mouth has been kept in an open position for a prolonged period of time. This situation can be considered as an iatrogenic activation of temporalis muscle TrPs. Iatrogenic temporalis TrPs might then add the symptoms of facial pain, toothache, and possibly altered occlusion to the initial complaint.

Sudden trauma such as whiplash in an auto accident,[34,35] or direct trauma to the muscle, as from a fall on the head, blow to the face, impact from a golf ball or baseball, or impact of the head against the side of the car in a motor vehicle accident can also cause TrP formation.

An anteriorly displaced disc of the TMJ might cause the patient to experience a feeling of pressure. In an attempt to do something to relieve the sense of pressure, the patient might bite down, which does not correct the disc problem and only perpetuates temporalis (and masseter) TrPs.

Often overlooked or forgotten is the reflex muscle contraction occurring with chronic infection or inflammation. When prolonged, this is believed to contribute to the development of TrPs. Thus, true painful pulpal pathology or an inflamed TMJ, if protracted, may cause temporalis (or other masticatory muscle) TrPs to develop. These TrPs become self-sustaining, and even after resolution of the pulpal pathology or inflamed joint, may continue to cause intermittent or constant pain, typically referred back to the original site of pain. The unaware clinician, unfortunately, continues to treat the tooth or the joint instead of the TrPs, with potentially negative results.

The mandibular position induced by a forward head posture can produce increased activity in the temporalis muscle and can activate and/or perpetuate TrPs. Excessive tension in the suprahyoid and infrahyoid muscles can create light tensile forces, which pull down on the mandible and require the temporalis and masseter muscles to contract to counteract the pull and keep the mouth closed, resulting in the activation or perpetuation of TrPs in these muscles.[36]

Especially when the patient is fatigued, temporalis TrPs may be activated by a cold draft over the muscle (eg, a blast of cold air from an air conditioner or wind through an open car window).[25] Persons with low-normal serum levels of thyroid hormones (T3 and T4 by radioimmunoassay), as well as people with hypothyroidism, are particularly vulnerable to such muscle cooling.

Temporalis TrPs might be activated by associated TrPs when they lie within the pain reference zone of TrPs in the upper trapezius and sternocleidomastoid muscles. Trigger points in leg muscles have also been observed to indirectly cause a reduction of maximal interincisal opening, and thus may influence masticatory muscle function.[37,38] This phenomenon is an example of dysfunction set up by dynamic and static postural asymmetries, in this instance originating in a weight-bearing limb.

4.2. Associated Trigger Points

Associated TrPs can develop in the referred pain areas caused by TrPs (Hsieh et al., 2007). Therefore, musculature in the referred pain areas for the temporalis muscle should also be considered. Muscles in the referred pain areas of the temporalis muscle include the corrugator and masseter. Temporalis TrPs are also likely to be associated with TrPs in the other masticatory muscles. The most frequent being the ipsilateral masseter and the contralateral temporalis muscles. Less commonly, either or both the medial and lateral pterygoid muscles might be involved, sometimes bilaterally.

Associated TrPs often develop in the temporalis muscle from TrPs in the commonly involved upper trapezius[39] and sternocleidomastoid muscles. In fact, TrPs in the masticatory muscles are also highly prevalent in individuals with mechanical neck pain.[40]

4.3. Associated Pathology

Some medical conditions give rise to symptoms that can appear confusingly similar to those produced by temporalis TrPs or may be present concurrently. Concurrent diagnosis may include TMJ internal derangements. Other medical conditions include dental disease, TTH, cervicogenic headache, migraine, polymyalgia rheumatica, temporal arteritis, and temporal tendinitis. One of the main medical diagnoses that should be excluded before treating temporalis TrPs is temporal arteritis.

A diseased tooth, such as one with a non-restorable carious lesion, can produce referred pain over the temporalis muscle that closely emulates the referred pain from a TrP in that part of the muscle.

The head pain of polymyalgia rheumatica is distinguished from that due to temporalis TrPs in several ways. First, by the more extensive distribution of the *bilateral* pain of polymyalgia that usually includes the shoulders, and often the neck, back, upper arms, and thighs. Second, the erythrocyte sedimentation rate is increased. Third, morning stiffness commonly lasts more than 45 minutes, and finally, the age of the patient is more than 50 years.[41,42]

The diagnosis of temporal tendinitis can be based on tendon-attachment enthesopathy that results from TrPs in the temporalis muscle. The clinician should examine for that possibility before proceeding with palliative care or steroid injections, or worse, a more drastic surgical procedure such as excising the condylar attachment of the muscle.[43] If temporalis TrPs are responsible for the symptoms, inactivating them is much simpler, less invasive, less painful, and less expensive.

An important differential diagnosis is giant cell arteritis or temporal arteritis, a systemic inflammatory vasculitis of unknown etiology occurring in older persons and can result in a wide variety of medical complications. Common signs and symptoms of temporal arteritis include visual disturbances, headache, jaw claudication, neck pain, and scalp tenderness. Therefore, some of these symptoms can overlap those originated in temporalis muscle TrPs. This is important because a recent study has observed that the temporalis muscle is also affected in around 20% of patients with temporal arteritis.[44]

5. CORRECTIVE ACTIONS

The patient should be instructed to maintain good head and neck postures and effective resting jaw and tongue position to correct the problems of forward head posture and aberrant tongue position. Instructions on body mechanics and ergonomics are also essential. In addition, most patients need to learn general neck stretching exercises to help inactivate any TrPs in the cervical muscles that may be perpetuating the temporalis TrPs. In fact, in some patients, TrPs resolve following correction of these two powerful perpetuating factors alone.

Body asymmetry and the resultant functional scoliosis should be corrected by appropriate lifts, because this postural stress may activate TrPs in the neck muscles that cause associated TrPs in the masticatory muscles. If the habit of mouth breathing produces forward head posture, mouth breathing should be corrected by eliminating contributory factors such as nasal obstruction.

When the temporalis muscle has shortened in association with an occlusal abnormality, the muscle should be stretched to its normal resting length prior to being fitted for dental appliances, so that they can be adjusted to work properly. Correct neutral head position is also critical during adjustment of any appliances. If the head is in extension in the dental chair, the occlusion will be different from that when the patient is sitting or standing with correct head and neck alignment. Goldstein et al[45] found that a forward head posture alters the forces of the path of mandibular closure by increasing the activity of the masticatory muscles in maximal intercuspal position at rest.

The activation of TrPs during a prolonged dental procedure may be prevented by taking breaks for the patient to go through several cycles of active range of motion.

Prolonged maximal shortening of the muscle during sleep may be prevented by a "night guard" or occlusal splint with a flat occlusal plane, which keeps the upper and lower teeth a few millimeters apart and can relieve bruxism.[46-48] This is especially helpful during periods of high stress.[49] For more significant benefit, cognitive behavioral therapy can be undergone in addition to the use of an occlusal splint because this has been shown be more effective than splint use alone.[50]

The patient should be persuaded to stop chewing gum, ice, or tough meat; eating caramels; biting pens, pencils, apples, or their finger nails; cracking nuts with the teeth; or engaging in any other parafunctional behaviors of the teeth or mouth. The patient should avoid cold drafts that blow directly on the temple by wearing a nightcap, protective hood, or scarf.

The patient should learn how to passively stretch the temporalis in the seated position by doing the temporalis self-stretch exercise daily (Figure 9-4). Caution should be exercised not to overstretch this muscle, because this will place abnormal forces on joint structures. Before this exercise is done, the patient might apply moist heat over the temporalis muscle, covering the side of the head and face for 10 to 15 minutes before retiring at night.

When the patient is comfortable with the passive exercise described above, the next step is initiating an active-resistive mouth-opening exercise, which helps overcome restricted motion through reciprocal inhibition. The patient can release the muscle by lightly resisting opening of the mouth (with two fingers below the chin) for a few seconds, followed by active opening of the mouth to take up slack in the muscle. The amount of opening can be controlled with correct tongue position on the hard palate behind the upper teeth. This protective maneuver is recommended for patients with TMJ inflammation or painful TMJ derangements (ie, disc displacement with reduction), so that they will stretch within the nonpainful limits or avoid the painful click.

If the posterior fibers of the temporalis muscle are involved, causing the mandible to deviate on opening, the patient should modify the above exercise: the patient opens the jaw to stretch while first placing one hand against the opposite maxilla (contralateral to the involved temporalis) and the other hand against the ipsilateral side of the mandible. The lower jaw is pushed away from the side toward which it deviates during opening, while the patient actively assists the motion with the jaw muscles for the most effective stretch. The mandible is gently restored to the starting position before the pressure is fully released. Placing the tongue in its resting position during this exercise also promotes symmetrical mouth opening. When full relief is obtained, the exercises might be reduced to 2 or 3 times weekly as a health maintenance measure and be incorporated into a regular postexercise muscle stretching routine.

If there is no articular dysfunction, the patient is encouraged to induce a wide-open yawn as a regular exercise. The addition of this reflex inhibition helps obtain full normal stretch length of the temporalis muscle (and other mandibular elevator muscles).

Finally, the patient should be checked for evidence of reduced thyroid function, other metabolic disorders, and nutritional deficiencies, any of which might increase neuromuscular irritability, as described in Chapter 4.

References

1. Standring S. *Gray's Anatomy: The Anatomical Basis of Clinical Practice*. 41st ed. London, UK: Elsevier; 2015.
2. Korfage JA, Van Eijden TM. Regional differences in fibre type composition in the human temporalis muscle. *J Anat*. 1999;194(pt 3):355-362.
3. Korfage JA, Koolstra JH, Langenbach GE, van Eijden TM. Fiber-type composition of the human jaw muscles—(part 2) role of hybrid fibers and factors responsible for inter-individual variation. *J Dent Res*. 2005;84(9):784-793.
4. Eriksson PO. Muscle fiber composition system. *Swed Dent J*. 1982;12(suppl):8-38.
5. Lam D, Carlson ER. The temporalis muscle flap and temporoparietal fascial flap. *Oral Maxillofac Surg Clin North Am*. 2014;26(3):359-369.
6. Kimoto K, Fushima K, Tamaki K, Toyoda M, Sato S, Uchimura N. Asymmetry of masticatory muscle activity during the closing phase of mastication. *Cranio*. 2000;18(4):257-263.
7. Cecilio FA, Regalo SC, Palinkas M, et al. Ageing and surface EMG activity patterns of masticatory muscles. *J Oral Rehabil*. 2010;37(4):248-255.
8. Yamaguchi T, Satoh K, Komatsu K, Inoue N, Minowa K, Totsuka Y. Electromyographic activity of the jaw-closing muscles during jaw opening in patients with masseter muscle contracture. *Cranio*. 2002;20(1):48-54.
9. Yamaguchi T, Satoh K, Komatsu K, et al. Electromyographic activity of the jaw-closing muscles during jaw opening—comparison of cases of masseter muscle contracture and TMJ closed lock. *J Oral Rehabil*. 2002;29(11):1063-1068.
10. Woelfel JB, Hickey JC, Stacey RW, et al. Electromyographic analysis of jaw movements. *J Prosthet Dent*. 1960;10:688-697.
11. Blanksma NG, van Eijden TM, van Ruijven LJ, Weijs WA. Electromyographic heterogeneity in the human temporalis and masseter muscles during dynamic tasks guided by visual feedback. *J Dent Res*. 1997;76(1):542-551.
12. McDougall JDB, Andrew BL. An electromyographic study of the temporalis and masseter muscles. *J Anat*. 1953;87:37-45.
13. Greenfield BE, Wyke BD. Electromyographic studies of some of the muscles of mastication. *Br Dent J*. 1956;100:129-143.
14. Vitti M, Basmajian JV. Integrated actions of masticatory muscles: simultaneous EMG from eight intramuscular electrodes. *Anat Rec*. 1977;187(2):173-189.
15. Yilmaz G, Ugincius P, Sebik O, Turker KS. Tonic activity of the human temporalis muscle at mandibular rest position. *Arch Oral Biol*. 2015;60(11):1645-1649.
16. Vitti M, Basmajian JV. Muscles of mastication in small children: an electromyographic analysis. *Am J Orthod*. 1975;68(4):412-419.
17. Yemm R. The question of "resting" tonic activity of motor units in the masseter and temporal muscles in man. *Arch Oral Biol*. 1977;22(5):349-351.
18. Simons DG, Travell J, Simons L. *Travell & Simon's Myofascial Pain and Dysfunction: The Trigger Point Manual*. Vol 1. 2nd ed. Baltimore, MD: Williams & Wilkins; 1999:104.
19. Park JT, Lee JG, Won SY, Lee SH, Cha JY, Kim HJ. Realization of masticatory movement by 3-dimensional simulation of the temporomandibular joint and the masticatory muscles. *J Craniofac Surg*. 2013;24(4):e347-e351.
20. Fernández de las Peñas C, Ge HY, Arendt-Nielsen L, Cuadrado ML, Pareja JA. The local and referred pain from myofascial trigger points in the temporalis muscle contributes to pain profile in chronic tension-type headache. *Clin J Pain*. 2007;23(9):786-792.
21. Alonso-Blanco C, de-la-Llave-Rincon AI, Fernández de las Peñas C. Muscle trigger point therapy in tension-type headache. *Expert Rev Neurother*. 2012;12(3):315-322.
22. Karadas O, Gul HL, Inan LE. Lidocaine injection of pericranial myofascial trigger points in the treatment of frequent episodic tension-type headache. *J Headache Pain*. 2013;14:44.
23. Fernández de las Peñas C, Galan-Del-Rio F, Alonso-Blanco C, Jimenez-Garcia R, Arendt-Nielsen L, Svensson P. Referred pain from muscle trigger points in the masticatory and neck-shoulder musculature in women with temporomandibular disorders. *J Pain*. 2010;11(12):1295-1304.

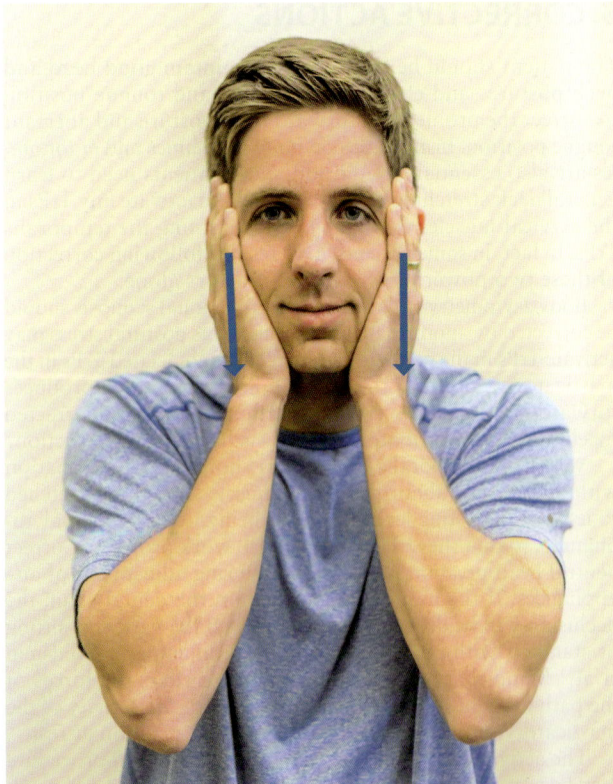

Figure 9-4. Self-stretch of the temporalis muscle. The jaw elevator muscles are elongated by pulling down firmly with broad pressure of the hands on the side of the head and face, stretching the temporalis muscle while taking in a long full breath to augment muscle relaxation.

24. Fernández de las Peñas C, Fernandez-Mayoralas DM, Ortega-Santiago R, Ambite-Quesada S, Palacios-Cena D, Pareja JA. Referred pain from myofascial trigger points in head and neck-shoulder muscles reproduces head pain features in children with chronic tension type headache. *J Headache Pain.* 2011;12(1):35-43.
25. Travell J. Temporomandibular joint pain referred from muscles of the head and neck. *J Prosthet Dent.* 1960;10:745-763.
26. Jensen K, Norup M. Experimental pain in human temporal muscle induced by hypertonic saline, potassium and acidity. *Cephalalgia.* 1992;12(2):101-106.
27. Schmidt-Hansen PT, Svensson P, Jensen TS, Graven-Nielsen T, Bach FW. Patterns of experimentally induced pain in pericranial muscles. *Cephalalgia.* 2006;26(5):568-577.
28. Alonso-Blanco C, Fernández de las Peñas C, de-la-Llave-Rincon AI, Zarco-Moreno P, Galan-Del-Rio F, Svensson P. Characteristics of referred muscle pain to the head from active trigger points in women with myofascial temporomandibular pain and fibromyalgia syndrome. *J Headache Pain.* 2012;13(8):625-637.
29. Alonso-Blanco C, Fernández de las Peñas C, Fernandez-Mayoralas DM, de-la-Llave-Rincon AI, Pareja JA, Svensson P. Prevalence and anatomical localization of muscle referred pain from active trigger points in head and neck musculature in adults and children with chronic tension-type headache. *Pain Med.* 2011;12(10):1453-1463.
30. Fernández de las Peñas C, Caminero AB, Madeleine P, et al. Multiple active myofascial trigger points and pressure pain sensitivity maps in the temporalis muscle are related in women with chronic tension type headache. *Clin J Pain.* 2009;25(6):506-512.
31. Andersen S, Petersen MW, Svendsen AS, Gazerani P. Pressure pain thresholds assessed over temporalis, masseter, and frontalis muscles in healthy individuals, patients with tension-type headache, and those with migraine—a systematic review. *Pain.* 2015;156(8):1409-1423.
32. Rocha CP, Croci CS, Caria PH. Is there relationship between temporomandibular disorders and head and cervical posture? A systematic review. *J Oral Rehabil.* 2013;40(11):875-881.
33. Gerwin RD, Dommerholt J, Shah JP. An expansion of Simons' integrated hypothesis of trigger point formation. *Curr Pain Headache Rep.* 2004;8(6):468-475.
34. Fernandez-Perez AM, Villaverde-Gutierrez C, Mora-Sanchez A, Alonso-Blanco C, Sterling M, Fernández de las Peñas C. Muscle trigger points, pressure pain threshold, and cervical range of motion in patients with high level of disability related to acute whiplash injury. *J Orthop Sports Phys Ther.* 2012;42(7):634-641.
35. Castaldo M, Ge HY, Chiarotto A, Villafane JH, Arendt-Nielsen L. Myofascial trigger points in patients with whiplash-associated disorders and mechanical neck pain. *Pain Med.* 2014;15(5):842-849.
36. Darling DW, Kraus S, Glasheen-Wray MB. Relationship of head posture and the rest position of the mandible. *J Prosthet Dent.* 1984;52(1):111-115.
37. Fernández de las Peñas C, Carratalá-Tejada M, Luna-Oliva L, Miangolarra-Page JC. The immediate effects of hamstring muscle stretching in subjects' trigger points in the masseter muscle. *J Musculoske Pain.* 2006;14(1):27-35.
38. Bretischwerdt C, Rivas-Cano L, Palomeque-del-Cerro L, Fernández de las Peñas C, Alburquerque-Sendin F. Immediate effects of hamstring muscle stretching on pressure pain sensitivity and active mouth opening in healthy subjects. *J Manipulative Physiol Ther.* 2010;33(1):42-47.
39. Hong C-Z. Considerations and recommendations regarding myofascial trigger point injection. *J Musculoskelet Pain.* 1994;2(1):29-59.
40. De-la-Llave-Rincon AI, Alonso-Blanco C, Gil-Crujera A, Ambite-Quesada S, Svensson P, Fernández de las Peñas C. Myofascial trigger points in the masticatory muscles in patients with and without chronic mechanical neck pain. *J Manipulative Physiol Ther.* 2012;35(9):678-684.
41. De Bandt M. Current diagnosis and treatment of polymyalgia rheumatica. *Joint Bone Spine.* 2014;81(3):203-208.
42. Nesher G. Polymyalgia rheumatica—diagnosis and classification. *J Autoimmun.* 2014;48-49:76-78.
43. Ernest EA III, Martinez ME, Rydzewski DB, Salter EG. Photomicrographic evidence of insertion tendonosis: the etiologic factor in pain for temporal tendonitis. *J Prosthet Dent.* 1991;65(1):127-131.
44. Veldhoen S, Klink T, Geiger J, et al. MRI displays involvement of the temporalis muscle and the deep temporal artery in patients with giant cell arteritis. *Eur Radiol.* 2014;24(11):2971-2979.
45. Goldstein DF, Kraus SL, Williams WB, Glasheen-Wray M. Influence of cervical posture on mandibular movement. *J Prosthet Dent.* 1984;52(3):421-426.
46. Matsumoto H, Tsukiyama Y, Kuwatsuru R, Koyano K. The effect of intermittent use of occlusal splint devices on sleep bruxism: a 4-week observation with a portable electromyographic recording device. *J Oral Rehabil.* 2015;42(4):251-258.
47. Hugger S, Schindler HJ, Kordass B, Hugger A. Surface EMG of the masticatory muscles (Part 4): effects of occlusal splints and other treatment modalities. *Int J Comput Dent.* 2013;16(3):225-239.
48. Zhang FY, Wang XG, Dong J, Zhang JF, Lu YL. Effect of occlusal splints for the management of patients with myofascial pain: a randomized, controlled, double-blind study. *Chin Med J (Engl).* 2013;126(12):2270-2275.
49. Rugh JD, Solberg WK. Electromyographic studies of bruxist behavior before and during treatment. *J Calif Dent Assoc.* 1975;3(9):56-59.
50. Trindade M, Orestes-Cardoso S, de Siqueira TC. Interdisciplinary treatment of bruxism with an occlusal splint and cognitive behavioral therapy. *Gen Dent.* 2015;63(5):e1-e4.

Chapter 10

Medial Pterygoid Muscle

"Deep Deceiver"

Michelle Finnegan and Joseph M. Donnelly

1. INTRODUCTION

The medial pterygoid muscle is an important muscle of mastication that lies deep to the mandible. It is comprised of two heads, the superficial and deep, that work together closely to support the jaw along with the masseter and lateral pterygoid muscles. The deep head originates from the inner surface of the lateral pterygoid plate of the sphenoid bone, just deep to the lateral pterygoid muscle. The superficial head attaches to the maxillary tuberosity just above the third molar and to the pyramidal process of the palatine bone. Both heads insert to the medial surface of the lower border of the ramus and angle of the mandible. The muscle is innervated by the medial pterygoid branch of the mandibular division of the trigeminal nerve. It receives vascularization from the pterygoid branches of the maxillary artery. The muscle functions bilaterally to close the mandible, whereas unilaterally it deviates the jaw to the contralateral side. Trigger points (TrPs) in this muscle can refer to the temporomandibular joint (TMJ), ear, and parts of the mouth. They can also contribute to many different otolaryngic symptoms and pain in the teeth, making differential diagnosis essential for proper treatment. Medial pterygoid TrPs can be perpetuated by parafunctional habits, forced contraction of the muscle like when biting down hard on food, mouth breathing, and stress. Although not researched as extensively as other muscles influencing the TMJ, this muscle can be involved in temporomandibular dysfunction (TMD). Pathologies associated with this muscle include entrapment of the lingual nerve, facial asymmetry due to muscle hypertrophy, trismus, myositis ossificans, and oromandibular dystonia. Corrective actions include addressing posture and tongue positioning, eliminating parafunctional habits, eliminating TrPs in cervical muscles that can refer to the region of the medial pterygoid, stress management, and resisted jaw opening exercises.

2. ANATOMIC CONSIDERATIONS

The medial pterygoid muscle is a thick quadrilateral muscle that consists of two heads (deep and superficial) (Figure 10-1A and B). The larger, deep head of the medial pterygoid muscle commonly originates from above to the medial (inner) surface of the lateral pterygoid plate of the sphenoid bone, just deep to the inferior head of the lateral pterygoid muscle[1,2]; however, variations with attachments to the pterygoid fossa have been reported.[3]

The smaller superficial head of the medial pterygoid muscle attaches to the maxillary tuberosity just above the third molar[4] and to the pyramidal process of the palatine bone by a strong tendinous cone,[3] passing over the lateral surface of the lateral pterygoid plate, and covering the lower end of the inferior head of the lateral pterygoid muscle.[1] Sakamoto and Akita[2] reported that this portion of the muscle is only attached to the lateral surface of the pyramidal process of the palatine bone.

Both heads of the medial pterygoid muscle descend posterolaterally almost in parallel with the masseter muscle, inserting by a short aponeurosis to the medial surface of the lower border of the ramus and the angle of the mandible (Figure 10-1B).[1,3] Variations in its insertion can be as far posterior as the mandibular fossa and as far anterior as the mylohyoid groove of the mandible.[1] Variations in these attachments are likely due to the insertions' composition of alternating tendinous sheets and fleshy fibers that partly cover themselves as they attach to the ramus and angle of the mandible. Seven layers of this muscle have been reported, all with slightly different insertions.[3]

An accessory bundle of the medial pterygoid muscle may be present, inserting just superior to the mylohyoid line. It can also be identified as a part of the posterior region of the mylohyoid muscle.[2]

Along with the medial pterygoid muscle, the inferior division of the lateral pterygoid muscle (Figure 10-1A, light red) on the inside of the mandible and the masseter muscle on the outside suspend the angle of the mandible like a sling.

The anterior and lateral parts of the medial pterygoid muscle has a high percentage of Type-I (slow twitch) fibers (reported as high as 79%) whereas the posterior and medial portions have, as in most skeletal muscles, approximately half Type-I fibers (52%).[5,6] Also, the medial pterygoid muscle has a high percentage of hybrid fibers, as well as a small percentage of Type-IIA and -IIX fibers[2,6-8] compared with muscles that open the jaw. Differences in the studies of fiber type are likely due to the way the fiber types were assessed.

2.1. Innervation and Vascularization

Typically, the medial pterygoid muscle is supplied by the medial pterygoid branch of the mandibular division of the trigeminal nerve (cranial nerve V),[1,2] though a small branch from the lingual nerve can innervate the posterolateral portion of the muscle.[2] When present, the accessory muscle bundle is innervated by a small branch of the lingual nerve.[2]

Vascularization of the medial pterygoid muscle is supplied via the pterygoid branches of the maxillary artery.[1,9]

2.2. Function

Acting unilaterally, the medial pterygoid muscle deviates the mandible toward the contralateral side.[1,9,10] This lateral motion is especially important during the grinding motions of chewing, which require fine control.

Bilaterally, the medial pterygoid muscles help elevate the mandible (close the jaw) along with the masseter and temporalis

Chapter 10: Medial Pterygoid Muscle

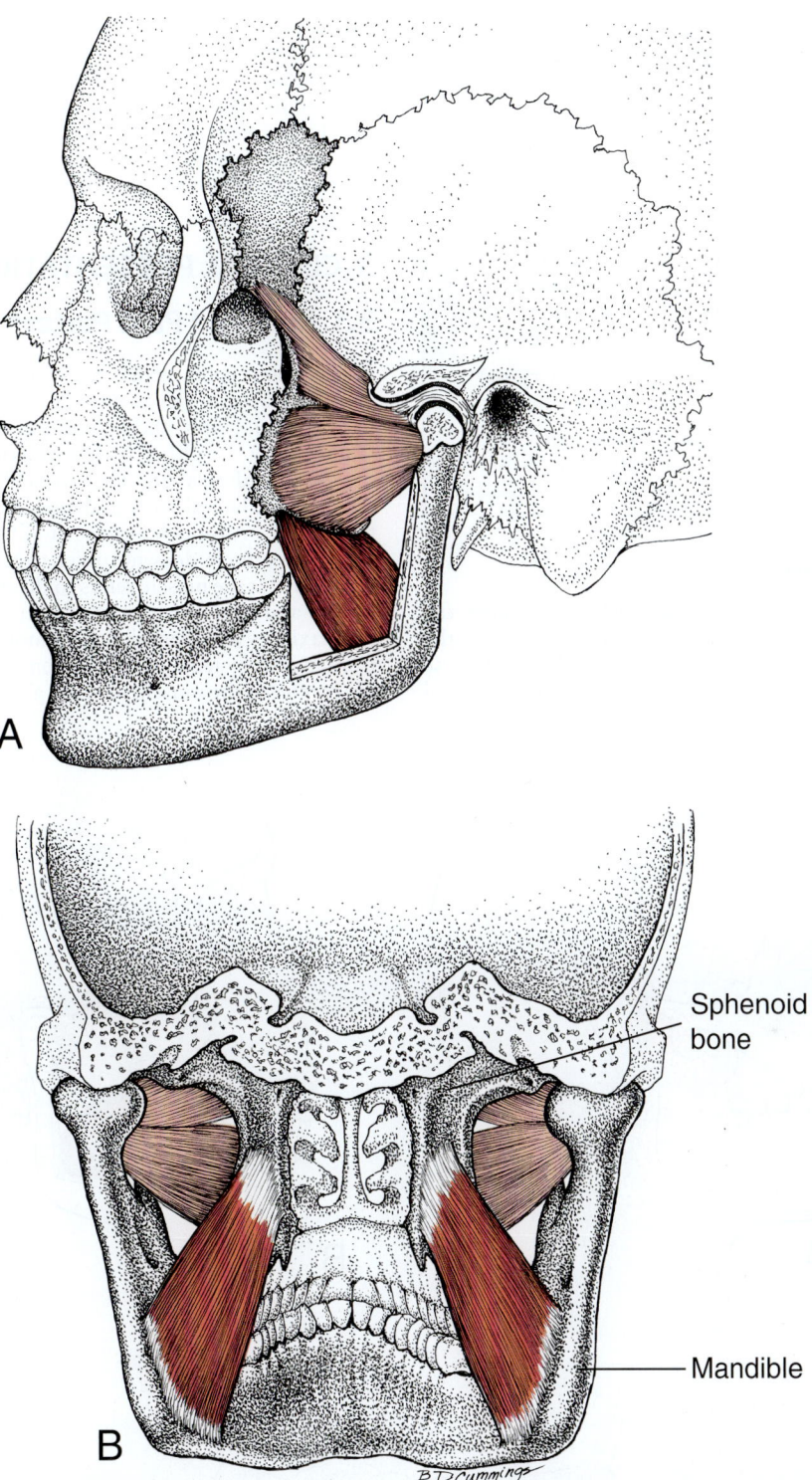

Figure 10-1. Attachments of the medial pterygoid muscle (dark red) and its relation to the lateral pterygoid muscle (light red). A, Lateral view showing the medial pterygoid muscle on the inner side of the mandible. Part of the mandible and the zygomatic arch have been removed. B, Coronal section of the skull just behind the temporomandibular joint, looking forward inside the mouth. The medial pterygoid muscle attaches, above, to the medial (inner) surface of the lateral pterygoid plate of the sphenoid bone and, below, to the medial surface of the mandible near its angle.

muscles.[1,9] The activity of the medial pterygoid muscle is increased if the mandible is protruded while it is being elevated.[9] Together, these muscles also have a minor contributory role in protrusion of the mandible.[9-11]

The medial pterygoid muscle is active bilaterally with chewing; however, the activity is higher on the side that the chewing occurs on.[12-14] Similar to the lateral pterygoid muscle, this muscle has also demonstrated heterogeneous activation,[15] with the anterior and posterior portions of the muscle being active during different clenching tasks. The posterior portion demonstrates greater activity during anterior and anterolateral clenching, whereas the anterior region showed greater activity with anteromedial, medial, and posterolateral clenching.

Box 10-1 Functional unit of the medial pterygoid muscle

Action	Synergists	Antagonist
Contralateral mandibular deviation	Ipsilateral lateral pterygoid Contralateral masseter Contralateral temporalis	Contralateral lateral pterygoid Contralateral medial pterygoid
Mandibular elevation	Masseter Temporalis	Lateral pterygoid Digastric muscles
Mandibular protrusion	Lateral pterygoid	Temporalis Masseter

2.3. Functional Unit

The functional unit to which a muscle belongs includes the muscles that reinforce and counter its actions as well as the joints that the muscle crosses. The interdependence of these structures functionally is reflected in the organization and neural connections of the sensory motor cortex. The functional unit is emphasized because the presence of a TrP in one muscle of the unit increases the likelihood that the other muscles of the unit will also develop TrPs. When inactivating TrPs in a muscle, one should be concerned about TrPs that may develop in muscles that are functionally interdependent. Box 10-1 grossly represents the functional unit of the medial pterygoid muscle.[16]

3. CLINICAL PRESENTATION

3.1. Referred Pain Pattern

Trigger points in the medial pterygoid muscle refer pain in poorly demarcated regions related to the mouth (tongue, pharynx, and hard palate), below and behind the TMJ, and deep in the ear (Figure 10-2).[17-19] Others have found that pain can be referred to the retromandibular and infra-auricular area,[19,20] including the region of the lateral pterygoid muscle, the floor of the nose, and the throat.[21] Although Simons et al[16] reported that the medial pterygoid muscle does not refer to the teeth, Svensson et al[22] reported that the muscle refers to the maxillary and mandibular molars and gingiva, the mandibular premolars, the gingiva of the maxillary and mandibular premolars, and the gingiva of the front maxillary teeth with injections of hypertonic saline. They also reported the muscle referred along the entire length of the

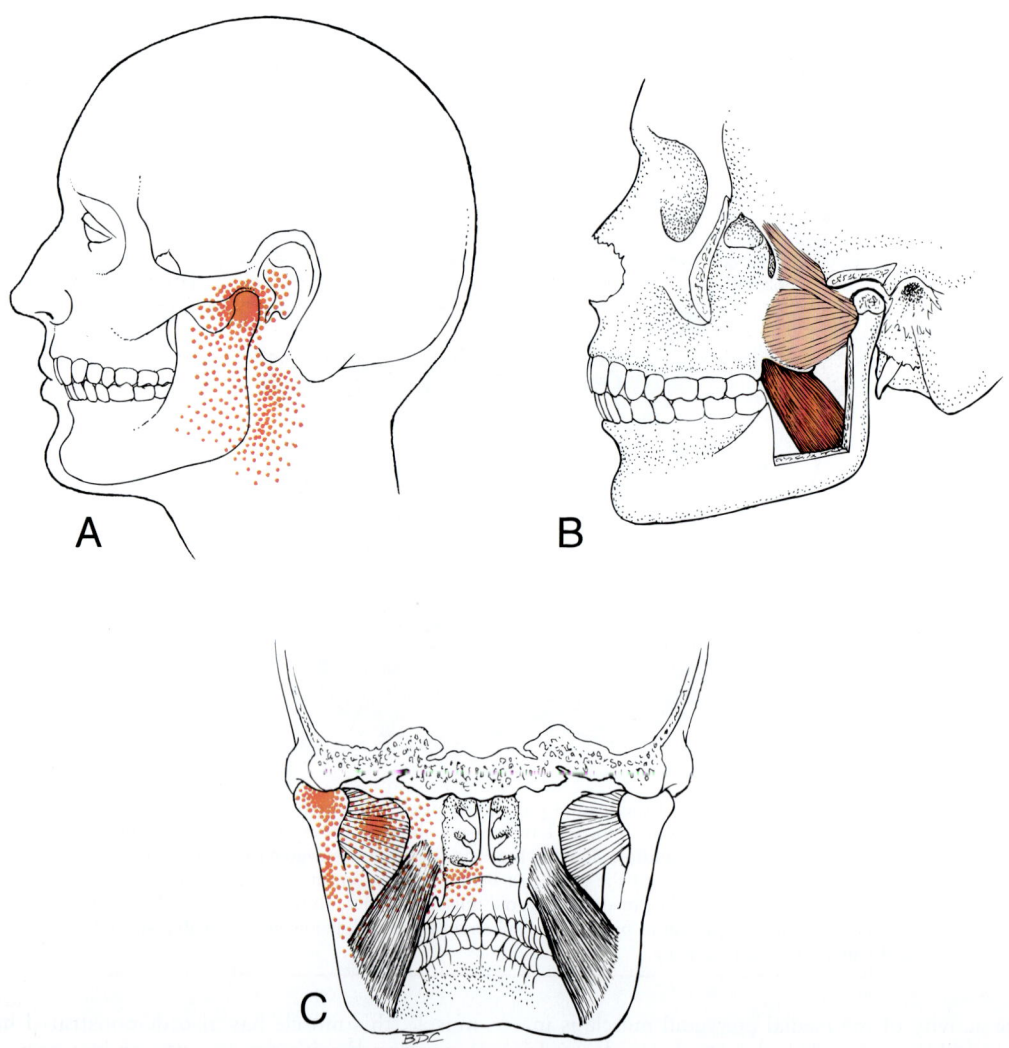

Figure 10-2. Referred pain pattern (red) in the left medial pterygoid muscle. A, Referral pattern to temporomandibular joint (red) and lateral neck (stippled). B, Anatomic cut-away to show the location of the TrP area in the muscle, which lies on the inner side of the mandible. C, Posterior to anterior view of a coronal section of the head through the temporomandibular joint. Internal areas of pain also appear as stippled red.

ipsilateral mandible, more extensively throughout the ear, as well as into the anterior neck, just below the mandible.

Stuffiness of the ear may also be a symptom of medial pterygoid TrPs. For the tensor veli palatini muscle to dilate the Eustachian tube, it should push the adjacent medial pterygoid muscle and interposed fascia aside. In the resting state, the presence of the medial pterygoid muscle helps to keep the Eustachian tube closed. Tense TrP bands in the medial pterygoid muscle might block the opening action of the tensor veli palatini muscle on the Eustachian tube producing baro hypoacusis (ear stuffiness).[16]

3.2. Symptoms

Patients with TrPs in the medial pterygoid muscle report that pain increases with attempts to open the mouth wide, with chewing food, or with clenching the teeth. Jaw-opening is usually restricted as well.

Patients describe pain from the medial pterygoid muscle as being more diffuse than the pain referred from TrPs in the lateral pterygoid muscle. Svensson et al[22] reported that the most common descriptors with involvement of this muscle included boring, shooting, hot, and aching. Those less commonly used were taut, spreading, tight, intense, sharp, and pressing.

Teachey[23] has reported several different symptoms of the nose, sinus, ears, throat/neck, mouth, and teeth/gums with medial pterygoid TrPs. Symptoms specific to the nose include nasal pain, congestion, "obstruction," or pressure. Patients may be given the diagnosis of paradoxical nasal obstruction. Although the lateral pterygoid muscle is more frequently associated with sinus pain and "sinusitis," the medial pterygoid muscle has been shown to contribute to these symptoms as well. Symptoms specific to the ear include ear pain, clogging, foreign body sensation, "blocked" ears, hyperacusis, hypoacusis, hearing loss, tinnitus, and dizziness. When otolaryngic studies are normal, including an audiometric evaluation, TrPs should be considered as a cause of these symptoms. Symptoms related to the throat/neck may include chronic/recurrent discomfort, sore throat, or tonsillitis; dysphagia; odynophagia; burning sensations; throat "congestion"; throat "drainage"; and voice irregularities. Medial pterygoid TrPs may also cause pain or burning of the mouth or pain to the teeth and/or gums.

Finally, TrPs in this muscle might be the cause of a patient's report of stuffiness of the ears, especially if a medical examination is unremarkable.

3.3. Patient Examination

After a thorough subjective examination, the clinician should make a detailed drawing representing the pain pattern that the patient has described. This depiction will assist in planning the physical examination and can be useful in monitoring the progression of the patient as symptoms improve or change. The clinician should perform a screening examination of the TMJ and should assess the patient's posture, with particular attention to head and neck position. Although the relationship between TMD and the head posture is somewhat controversial and unclear,[24] it is thought that forward head posture indirectly induces tension in the supra- and infrahyoid muscles, which in turn pulls downward to create light tensile forces on the mandible.[25] As a result, this tension causes the mandibular elevator muscles such as the medial pterygoid (and masseter) muscle to contract to keep the mouth closed.

Mandibular opening is usually restricted in patients with medial pterygoid TrPs. A quick functional screen to assess the opening is with the two-knuckle test (refer to Chapter 8). Patients are usually not able to pass this test when TrPs in the medial pterygoid muscle are present. If preferred, a standardized way to objectively measure mouth opening is with a disposable vertical ruler to measure the distance between the upper and lower incisors.[26,27] Normal opening for women is 41 to 45 mm and 43 to 45 mm is typical for men.[28,29]

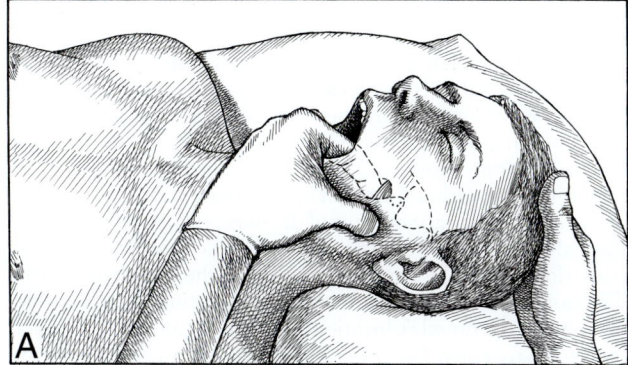

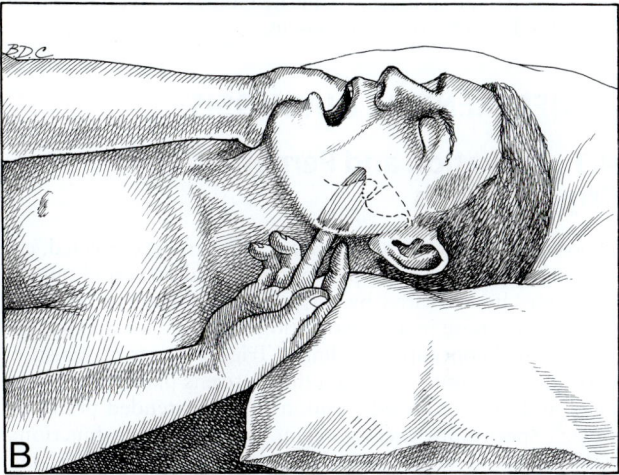

Figure 10-3. Examination of the medial pterygoid muscle for TrPs. A, Intraoral palpation (with a gloved hand) of TrPs behind the last molar tooth, with the muscle and the ramus of the mandible between the palpating digits. The mouth is opened wide enough for the finger to be placed between the molar teeth. The clinician may wish to prop the mouth open with a cork to protect the finger and help the patient to relax. B, Extraoral palpation of TrPs in the region of the attachment of the muscle to the inner surface of the mandible, at its angle.

3.4. Trigger Point Examination

For examination of the medial pterygoid muscle, the patient should be in supine position with the jaw open as far as is comfortable to take up any slack in the muscle. A cross-fiber flat palpation for TrPs in the midmuscle region is performed with the mouth open, intraorally with gloved fingers (Figure 10-3A). The pad of the palpating index finger faces outward and slides over the molar teeth until it encounters the bony anterior edge of the ramus of the mandible, which lies behind and lateral to the last molar tooth. The belly of the medial pterygoid muscle lies immediately beyond (posterior to) this bony edge. The muscle can be identified by having the patient alternately clench and relax against a block or cork placed between the teeth while the operator palpates for the changes in tissue tension. The orientation and texture of this muscle are readily palpable because only a thin layer of mucosa separates the palpating finger from the muscle. Palpation will elicit exquisite tenderness in the patient with medial pterygoid TrPs.

If there is concern for the safety of the examining finger in the mouth, the block or cork can be left in place between the patient's teeth throughout the TrP examination.

Palpating this muscle through the pharyngeal mucosa may make the patient gag, therefore palpation should always be done slowly and cautiously. One way to reduce the gag reflex is to tap the ipsilateral temporalis muscle to provide sensory distraction during the examination. Another technique is to have the patient curl the tip of the tongue as far as possible down the throat behind the molar teeth on the opposite side. The harder the patient forces the tongue backward and down the throat, the less sensitive the reflex becomes.

To palpate for TrPs extraorally, the head is tilted slightly toward the side to be palpated to slacken tissues and improve access to the muscle. One finger examines the inner (medial) surface of the mandible by pressing upward at its angle (Figure 10-3B). The firm mass, approximately 1 cm (3/8 in) above the angle of the mandible, just within the reach of the finger, is the inferior part of the mandibular attachment of the muscle. Pressure is exerted inward to the muscle to assess for TrPs. The specific cross-fiber palpation cannot be performed to assess the muscle from this direction because only the attachment of the muscle is accessible. To confirm the muscle's location, the patient can actively clench their teeth together. The clinician feels the contraction under the tip of the palpating finger. Exquisite tenderness with palpation indicates TrP activity in the muscle.

4. DIFFERENTIAL DIAGNOSIS

4.1. Activation and Perpetuation of Trigger Points

A posture or activity that activates a TrP, if not corrected, can also perpetuate it. In any part of the medial pterygoid muscle, TrPs may be activated by unaccustomed eccentric loading, eccentric exercise in an unconditioned muscle, or maximal or submaximal concentric loading.[30] Trigger points may also be activated or aggravated when the muscle is placed in a shortened and/or lengthened position for an extended period of time.[30] Specifically, excessive gum chewing or parafunctional habits such as bruxism, jaw clenching, nail biting, or persistent thumb-sucking by a child can not only initiate but perpetuate TrPs in the medial pterygoid muscle. Excessive chewing on one side contributes to overload in the ipsilateral medial pterygoid muscle.[12]

Acute overload situations can also activate TrPs in the medial pterygoid muscle, including a sudden forcible contraction of the muscle (as in cracking nuts, chewing ice, or using the teeth to tear thread).

Trigger points in the medial pterygoid muscle may be activated by excessive forward head posture that places mild but persistent stress on the medial pterygoid (along with the masseter and temporalis) muscle by way of increased stress to the hyoid muscles, as described earlier.

Chronic mouth breathing (as through a continuous positive airway pressure [CPAP] machine, or due to nasal obstruction) also tends to cause excessive forward head positioning and postural changes that indirectly add stress to the masticatory muscles and may activate and perpetuate TrPs in these muscles.[31]

The medial pterygoid muscle on one side may develop and retain TrPs because of the increased stress imposed on it by TrP activity and distorted function of the muscle on the opposite side. Activation and perpetuation of medial pterygoid TrPs can also be secondary to the muscular dysfunction that results from TrPs in the lateral pterygoid muscle.

In the past, occlusal imbalance was considered one cause for the activation of medial pterygoid TrPs. It is now thought that the abnormal muscle tension caused by TrPs in masticatory muscles, including the medial pterygoid muscle, can cause the occlusal abnormalities. Masticatory muscle myofascial TrPs should be inactivated prior to initiating any prosthodontic treatment.

Other factors that can contribute to the development of TrPs in the medial pterygoid muscle include anxiety and stress.

4.2. Associated Trigger Points

Associated TrPs can develop in muscles within the referred pain areas of other TrPs.[32] Therefore, musculature in the referred pain areas for each muscle should also be considered. Muscles such as the sternocleidomastoid and masseter muscles can contribute to the development of TrPs in the medial pterygoid muscle. Trigger points of the medial pterygoid muscle can also contribute to the associated TrPs in other muscles including the masseter, lateral pterygoid, and posterior digastric muscles.

The medial pterygoid muscle usually develops TrPs in association with functionally related muscles, including the lateral pterygoid, masseter, and temporalis muscles.

If the patient continues to have difficulty in swallowing following the inactivation of the medial pterygoid TrPs, the sternocleidomastoid (see Chapter 7), the digastric, and possibly the longus capitis and longus colli muscles (see Chapter 12) should be examined.

4.3. Associated Pathology

Some medical conditions give rise to symptoms that can appear confusingly similar to those produced by medial pterygoid TrPs or may be present concurrently. Concurrent diagnosis may include TMD (refer to Chapter 18). Other medical conditions include dental disease, nerve entrapment, myositis ossificans, trismus, otolaryngic symptoms, and oromandibular dystonia.

Because this muscle refers to the TMJ, misdiagnosis of joint involvement can easily be mistaken for pain associated with TrPs of the medial pterygoid muscle; therefore, a thorough examination of all the structures related to the TMJ is essential. In patients with TMJ ankylosis, the medial pterygoid muscle (along with the masseter muscle) has been shown to be significantly larger compared with the controls, suggesting that hyperactivity of these muscles can be a factor in patients with this diagnosis.[33] Interestingly, no changes in the thickness of the medial pterygoid (or masseter and temporalis) muscle have been seen in patients with rheumatoid arthritis.[34] Other literature on how this muscle relates to TMD is limited.

Pain in the teeth or gums could easily be mistaken for a true dental problem if a thorough examination is not done that includes muscle assessment. As mentioned, the medial pterygoid muscle can refer to the teeth and gums[22,23] and should be considered in the differential diagnosis, especially if a dental examination does not show carious lesions or inflammation of the gums.

The medial pterygoid muscle can be a site of entrapment of the lingual nerve that can penetrate the muscle[2,35] and become entrapped between the medial pterygoid muscle and an ossified pterygospinous ligament.[36,37] If entrapped, symptoms such as altered sensation to the floor of the mouth, mucosa, lingual gingiva, and the mucosa of the anterior two thirds of the tongue can occur.[38]

Trismus is a firm closing of the jaw due to spasm of masticatory muscles that, for example, is characteristic of tetanus. Differential diagnosis of the cause of trismus is essential. Tetanus may also result from dental sepsis, injury, surgery, needle abscess, and the Morgagni syndrome caused by a malignant tumor. As recently as 2012, in a case study by Fusetti et al,[39] a 78-year-old farmer was diagnosed with tetanus with progressive onset of lockjaw and muscular stiffness. Furthermore, a 31-year-old patient in another case study who had proper levels of tetanus antibodies was treated for tetanus symptoms after puncturing his hand with a rusty nail.[40] Trismus can also be due to spasm of the medial pterygoid muscle from cellulitis in the pterygomandibular space, spasm of the masseter muscle from cellulitis in adjacent tissues, or spasm of the temporalis muscle from cellulitis in the infratemporal fossa.[41] Trismus in the medial pterygoid muscle can also occur after an inferior alveolar nerve block.[42] Attempts to open the jaw are painful and limited because of the spasm. Trigger points can be treated by injection only if there is no evidence of infection in the region to be treated. Mouth-opening exercises, heat, muscle relaxants, and physical therapy are beneficial for treatment of patients for whom injections are not recommended.[42]

Hypertrophy of the medial pterygoid muscle is a very rare condition that is more often asymptomatic than not. More commonly, the masseter muscle is involved than the medial pterygoid muscle. The most common report with this condition is of facial asymmetry. A recent case report highlights a rare case of hypertrophy of the medial pterygoid and masseter muscles together. The patient reported facial asymmetry from swelling on the posterior lower left tooth region for 4 years.[43]

Myositis ossificans is a rare condition wherein heterotropic bone forms in muscle or soft tissue, usually after some type of trauma or injury. It is not very common to occur in muscles of the masticatory system. From 2001 to 2014, only 11 cases (of the 20 in the masticatory system) have been reported in the medial pterygoid muscle.[44] Although rare, this diagnosis should be considered as a possibility if there is loss of jaw range of motion after facial trauma or invasive medical or dental procedures.[45,46] In addition, this condition can occur idiopathically, so even without trauma, this condition should be considered in the differential diagnosis.

As stated previously, TrPs in the medial pterygoid muscle can mimic otolaryngic symptoms including sinusitis, hearing changes, ear pain and clogging, throat pain and congestion, and tonsillitis.[23] When diagnostic testing does not yield significant findings for the cause of symptoms, TrPs in the medial pterygoid muscle should be considered.[23]

Oromandibular dystonia is a focal neurologic disorder that can affect the face and the jaw. Typically, involuntary facial grimacing and jaw or tongue movements occur. Those with jaw-closing dystonia more frequently have orobuccolingual involvement than those with jaw-opening dystonia.[47] The cause of the dystonia is more frequently idiopathic,[48,49] but can also be secondary to neurologic diseases,[48,49] infections,[49] or antipsychotic drugs.[50] The masseter and temporalis muscles are the most commonly involved for jaw-closing dystonia/myospasm[48]; however, the medial pterygoid muscle can be involved as well.[51-53] Knowledge of this condition is essential because it can easily be misdiagnosed as TMD or bruxism.[48]

5. CORRECTIVE ACTIONS

First, because TrPs in the medial pterygoid muscle may develop as a result of dysfunction in other muscles such as the sternocleidomastoid and masseter muscles, these should be addressed first (refer to Chapters 7 and 8).

Forward head posture should be corrected to reduce muscle activity in the medial pterygoid muscle and other jaw elevator muscles. Mouth breathing as compared with naso-diaphragmatic breathing has a negative impact on posture,[54-59] and should therefore be corrected. Performing strengthening and flexibility exercises in conjunction with naso-diaphragmatic breathing can help improve posture.[57]

Effective resting jaw position (with the tongue on the hard palate behind the top teeth, lips together, and teeth slightly separated) can be helpful to reduce stress on the muscle and minimize open mouth breathing during waking hours and attempts to fall asleep.

Parafunctional habits such as clenching, nail biting, and exhaustive chewing should be identified and discontinued immediately to reduce strain on the medial pterygoid muscle.

If the patient sleeps on the side, proper pillow positioning can prevent increased muscle activity caused by the jaw dropping down to one side during the night. A corner of the pillow should be tucked between the side of the face and the shoulder so that the pillow supports the jaw in a neutral position.

In addition to inactivating masticatory muscle TrPs, bruxism should be identified and treated. Use of an intraoral orthosis may be required. For a more significant benefit, cognitive behavioral therapy concurrent with use of an occlusal splint may be advised.[60] Conti et al[61] demonstrated that behavioral changes in conjunction with occlusal devices were effective in treating masticatory myofascial pain.

Factors that increase anxiety and emotional stress should be identified and alleviated, if possible. Studies have suggested

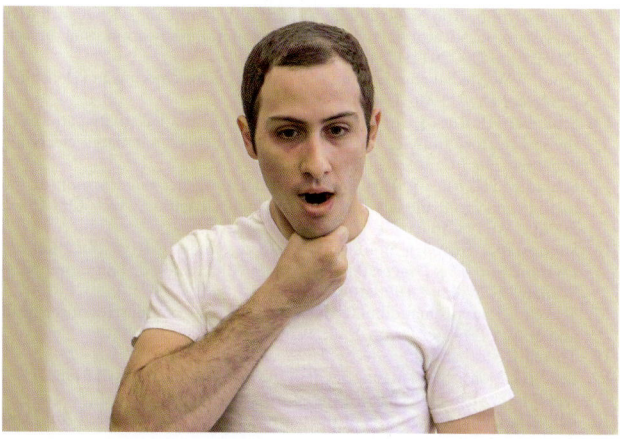

Figure 10-4. With the patient in a seated or standing position, the jaw is pressed into the fist underneath to activate the muscles that open the jaw. This reciprocally inhibits the medial pterygoid muscle (and other jaw-closing muscles).

that those with individuals with depression scores, somatic complaints, and decreased physical well-being are at a higher risk of suffering symptoms.[62] Referral to a psychologist or other mental health provider for specific pain and stress management techniques can be very helpful due to the importance of dealing with multiple contributory factors.[41]

Once dysphagia due to TrPs has been resolved, swallowing a tablet or capsule is facilitated by placing the medication underneath the tip of the tongue, behind the lower front teeth, where it can follow the bolus of liquid when the head is erect.[63] When the tablet is placed on top of the tongue, as is customary, the tongue presses it against the roof of the mouth where it tends to stick during swallowing.

Resisted jaw-opening is an augmented stretch technique based on reciprocal inhibition (Figure 10-4). Patients are instructed to open the jaw slowly against light resistance of their fist. The activation of the jaw depressors (digastric, suprahyoid, and infrahyoid muscles) inhibits the elevation function of the medial pterygoid muscle (and all other jaw elevators), providing a useful technique for releasing all the jaw elevator muscles simultaneously.

Activation of TrPs during a prolonged dental procedure may be prevented by taking breaks to allow the patient to perform several cycles of active range of motion.

References

1. Standring S. *Gray's Anatomy: The Anatomical Basis of Clinical Practice*. 41st ed. London, UK: Elsevier; 2015.
2. Sakamoto Y, Akita K. Spatial relationships between masticatory muscles and their innervating nerves in man with special reference to the medial pterygoid muscle and its accessory muscle bundle. *Surg Radiol Anat*. 2004;26(2):122-127.
3. El Haddioui A, Bravetti P, Gaudy JF. Anatomical study of the arrangement and attachments of the human medial pterygoid muscle. *Surg Radiol Anat*. 2007;29(2):115-124.
4. Drake RL, Wayne V, Mitchell AWM. *Gray's Anatomy for Students*. St. Louis, MO: Churchill Livingstone; 2005.
5. Eriksson PO. Muscle fiber composition system. *Swed Dent J*. 1982;12(suppl):8-38.
6. Korfage JA, Van Eijden TM. Myosin isoform composition of the human medial and lateral pterygoid muscles. *J Dent Res*. 2000;79(8):1618-1625.
7. Korfage JA, Koolstra JH, Langenbach GE, van Eijden TM. Fiber-type composition of the human jaw muscles—(part 1) origin and functional significance of fiber-type diversity. *J Dent Res*. 2005;84(9):774-783.
8. Korfage JA, Koolstra JH, Langenbach GE, van Eijden TM. Fiber-type composition of the human jaw muscles—(part 2) role of hybrid fibers and factors responsible for inter-individual variation. *J Dent Res*. 2005;84(9):784-793.
9. Moyers RE. An electromyographic analysis of certain muscles involved in temporomandibular movement. *Am J Orthod*. 1950;36(7):481-515.
10. Friedman MH. Pterygoid muscle function in excursive jaw movements: a clinical report. *J Prosthet Dent*. 1995;73(4):329-332.
11. Neumann DA. *Kinesiology of the Musculoskeletal System: Foundations for Rehabilitaion*. 2nd ed. St. Louis, MO: Mosby; 2010.

12. Yamaguchi S, Itoh S, Watanabe Y, Tsuboi A, Watanabe M. Quantitative analysis of masticatory activity during unilateral mastication using muscle fMRI. *Oral Dis.* 2011;17(4):407-413.
13. Wood WW. Medial pterygoid muscle activity during chewing and clenching. *J Prosthet Dent.* 1986;55(5):615-621.
14. Schindler HJ, Rues S, Turp JC, Schweizerhof K, Lenz J. Activity patterns of the masticatory muscles during feedback-controlled simulated clenching activities. *Eur J Oral Sci.* 2005;113(6):469-478.
15. Schindler HJ, Rues S, Turp JC, Lenz J. Heterogeneous activation of the medial pterygoid muscle during simulated clenching. *Arch Oral Biol.* 2006;51(6):498-504.
16. Simons DG, Travell J, Simons L. *Travell & Simon's Myofascial Pain and Dysfunction: The Trigger Point Manual.* Vol 1. 2nd ed. Baltimore, MD: Williams & Wilkins; 1999:104.
17. Travell J. Temporomandibular joint pain referred from muscles of the head and neck. *J Prosthet Dent.* 1960;10:745-763.
18. Travell J. Mechanical headache. *Headache.* 1967;7(1):23-29.
19. Bell WH. Nonsurgical management of the pain-dysfunction syndrome. *J Am Dent Assoc.* 1969;79(1):161-170.
20. Bell WE. Clinical diagnosis of the pain-dysfunction syndrome. *J Am Dent Assoc.* 1969;79(1):154-160.
21. Shaber EP. Consideration in the treatment of muscle spasm. In: Morgan DH, Hall WP, Vamvas SJ, eds. *Diseases of the Temporomandibular Apparatus.* St. Louis, MO: C.V. Mosby; 1977.
22. Svensson P, Bak J, Troest T. Spread and referral of experimental pain in different jaw muscles. *J Orofac Pain.* 2003;17(3):214-223.
23. Teachy WS. Otolaryngic myofascial pain syndromes. *Curr Pain Headache Rep.* 2004;8(6):457-462.
24. Rocha CP, Croci CS, Caria PH. Is there relationship between temporomandibular disorders and head and cervical posture? A systematic review. *J Oral Rehabil.* 2013;40(11):875-881.
25. Gonzalez HE, Manns A. Forward head posture: its structural and functional influence on the stomatognathic system, a conceptual study. *Cranio.* 1996;14(1):71-80.
26. Walker N, Bohannon RW, Cameron D. Discriminant validity of temporomandibular joint range of motion measurements obtained with a ruler. *J Orthop Sports Phys Ther.* 2000;30(8):484-492.
27. List T, John MT, Dworkin SF, Svensson P. Recalibration improves inter-examiner reliability of TMD examination. *Acta Odontol Scand.* 2006;64(3):146-152.
28. Gallagher C, Gallagher V, Whelton H, Cronin M. The normal range of mouth opening in an Irish population. *J Oral Rehabil.* 2004;31(2):110-116.
29. Muller L, van Waes H, Langerweger R, Molinari L, Saurenmann RK. Maximal mouth opening capacity: percentiles for healthy children 4-17 years of age. *Pediatr Rheumatol Online J.* 2013;11:17.
30. Gerwin RD, Dommerholt J, Shah JP. An expansion of Simons' integrated hypothesis of trigger point formation. *Curr Pain Headache Rep.* 2004;8(6):468-475.
31. La Touche R, Paris-Alemany A, von Piekartz H, Mannheimer JS, Fernandez-Carnero J, Rocabado M. The influence of cranio-cervical posture on maximal mouth opening and pressure pain threshold in patients with myofascial temporomandibular pain disorders. *Clin J Pain.* 2011;27(1):48-55.
32. Hsieh YL, Kao MJ, Kuan TS, Chen SM, Chen JT, Hong CZ. Dry needling to a key myofascial trigger point may reduce the irritability of satellite MTrPs. *Am J Phys Med Rehabil.* 2007;86(5):397-403.
33. Kumar VV, Malik NA, Visscher CM, Ebenezer S, Sagheb K, Lobbezoo F. Comparative evaluation of thickness of jaw-closing muscles in patients with long-standing bilateral temporomandibular joint ankylosis: a retrospective case-controlled study. *Clin Oral Investig.* 2015;19(2):421-427.
34. Yilmaz HH, Yildirim D, Ugan Y, et al. Clinical and magnetic resonance imaging findings of the temporomandibular joint and masticatory muscles in patients with rheumatoid arthritis. *Rheumatol Int.* 2012;32(5):1171-1178.
35. Shimokawa T, Akita K, Sato T, Ru F, Yi SQ, Tanaka S. Penetration of muscles by branches of the mandibular nerve: a possible cause of neuropathy. *Clin Anat.* 2004;17(1):2-5.
36. Nayak SR, Rai R, Krishnamurthy A, et al. An unusual course and entrapment of the lingual nerve in the infratemporal fossa. *Bratisl Lek Listy.* 2008;109(11):525-527.
37. Peuker ET, Fischer G, Filler TJ. Entrapment of the lingual nerve due to an ossified pterygospinous ligament. *Clin Anat.* 2001;14(4):282-284.
38. Rusu MC, Nimigean V, Podoleanu L, Ivascu RV, Niculescu MC. Details of the intralingual topography and morphology of the lingual nerve. *Int J Oral Maxillofac Surg.* 2008;37(9):835-839.
39. Fusetti S, Ghirotto C, Ferronato G. A case of cephalic tetanus in a developed country. *Int J Immunopathol Pharmacol.* 2013;26(1):273-277.
40. Vollman KE, Acquisto NM, Bodkin RP. A case of tetanus infection in an adult with a protective tetanus antibody level. *Am J Emerg Med.* 2014;32(4):392 e393-e394.
41. Bell WE. *Orofacial Pains—Classification, Diagnosis, Management.* Chicago, IL: Year Book Medical Publishers, Inc; 1985.
42. Wright EF. Medial pterygoid trismus (myospasm) following inferior alveolar nerve block: case report and literature review. *Gen Dent.* 2011;59(1):64-67.
43. Guruprasad R, Rishi S, Nair PP, Thomas S. Masseter and medial pterygoid muscle hypertrophy. *BMJ Case Rep.* 2011:pii: bcr0720114557.
44. Jiang Q, Chen MJ, Yang C, et al. Post-infectious myositis ossificans in medial, lateral pterygoid muscles: a case report and review of the literature. *Oncol Lett.* 2015;9(2):920-926.
45. Reddy SP, Prakash AP, Keerthi M, Rao BJ. Myositis ossificans traumatica of temporalis and medial pterygoid muscle. *J Oral Maxillofac Pathol.* 2014;18(2):271-275.
46. Torres AM, Nardis AC, da Silva RA, Savioli C. Myositis ossificans traumatica of the medial pterygoid muscle following a third molar extraction. *Int J Oral Maxillofac Surg.* 2015;44(4):488-490.
47. Singer C, Papapetropoulos S. A comparison of jaw-closing and jaw-opening idiopathic oromandibular dystonia. *Parkinsonism Relat Disord.* 2006;12(2):115-118.
48. Cao Y, Zhang W, Yap AU, Xie QF, Fu KY. Clinical characteristics of lateral pterygoid myospasm: a retrospective study of 18 patients. *Oral Surg Oral Med Oral Pathol Oral Radiol.* 2012;113(6):762-765.
49. Bakke M, Larsen BM, Dalager T, Moller E. Oromandibular dystonia—functional and clinical characteristics: a report on 21 cases. *Oral Surg Oral Med Oral Pathol Oral Radiol.* 2013;115(1):e21-e26.
50. Burke RE, Fahn S, Jankovic J, et al. Tardive dystonia: late-onset and persistent dystonia caused by antipsychotic drugs. *Neurology.* 1982;32(12):1335-1346.
51. Sinclair CF, Gurey LE, Blitzer A. Oromandibular dystonia: long-term management with botulinum toxin. *Laryngoscope.* 2013;123(12):3078-3083.
52. Dressler D. Botulinum toxin for treatment of dystonia. *Eur J Neurol.* 2010;17 suppl 1:88-96.
53. Tintner R, Jankovic J. Botulinum toxin type A in the management of oromandibular dystonia and bruxism. In: Brin MF, Hallett M, Jankovic J, eds. *Scientific and Therapeutic: Aspects of Botulinum Toxin.* Philadelphia, PA: Lippincott Williams & Wilkins; 2002:343-350.
54. Milanesi JM, Borin G, Correa EC, da Silva AM, Bortoluzzi DC, Souza JA. Impact of the mouth breathing occurred during childhood in the adult age: biophotogrammetric postural analysis. *Int J Pediatr Otorhinolaryngol.* 2011;75(8):999-1004.
55. Cuccia AM, Lotti M, Caradonna D. Oral breathing and head posture. *Angle Orthod.* 2008;78(1):77-82.
56. Sforza C, Colombo A, Turci M, Grassi G, Ferrario VF. Induced oral breathing and craniocervical postural relations: an experimental study in healthy young adults. *Cranio.* 2004;22(1):21-26.
57. Correa EC, Berzin F. Efficacy of physical therapy on cervical muscle activity and on body posture in school-age mouth breathing children. *Int J Pediatr Otorhinolaryngol.* 2007;71(10):1527-1535.
58. Neiva PD, Kirkwood RN, Godinho R. Orientation and position of head posture, scapula and thoracic spine in mouth-breathing children. *Int J Pediatr Otorhinolaryngol.* 2009;73(2):227-236.
59. Vig PS, Showfety KJ, Phillips C. Experimental manipulation of head posture. *Am J Orthod.* 1980;77(3):258-268.
60. Trindade M, Orestes-Cardoso S, de Siqueira TC. Interdisciplinary treatment of bruxism with an occlusal splint and cognitive behavioral therapy. *Gen Dent.* 2015;63(5):e1-e4.
61. Conti PC, de Alencar EN, da Mota Correa AS, Lauris JR, Porporatti AL, Costa YM. Behavioural changes and occlusal splints are effective in the management of masticatory myofascial pain: a short-term evaluation. *J Oral Rehabil.* 2012;39(10):754-760.
62. Dougall AL, Jimenez CA, Haggard RA, Stowell AW, Riggs RR, Gatchel RJ. Biopsychosocial factors associated with the subcategories of acute temporomandibular joint disorders. *J Orofac Pain.* 2012;26(1):7-16.
63. Travell J. Nonstick trick for pill swallowing. *Patient Care.* 1975;9:17.

Chapter 11

Lateral Pterygoid Muscle
"TMD Disaster"

Michelle Finnegan, Amanda Blackmon, and Joseph M. Donnelly

1. INTRODUCTION

The lateral pterygoid muscle is an important muscle for movement and control of the jaw that is comprised of two divisions: superior and inferior. The superior division of the lateral pterygoid muscle originates from the infratemporal crest and infratemporal surface of the greater wing of the sphenoid bone, while the inferior division of the lateral pterygoid muscle originates from the lateral surface of the lateral pterygoid plate. The two divisions converge to insert onto the pterygoid fovea, a depression on the front of the neck of the mandible. A branch of the buccal nerve innervates the superior division and the lateral part of the inferior division of the lateral pterygoid muscle. The medial part of the inferior division of the lateral pterygoid muscle is innervated by a branch directly from the anterior trunk of the mandibular nerve. The lateral pterygoid muscle receives its vascularization from the pterygoid branches of the maxillary artery. Bilaterally, the muscle functions to open and protrude the mandible, and unilaterally it functions to deviate the mandible to the opposite side. It also assists in approximating the structures of the temporomandibular joint (TMJ) during mouth closing. Trigger points (TrPs) in the lateral pterygoid muscle may refer pain in and around the maxillary sinus and near the TMJ. They can also contribute to increased secretion of the maxillary sinus, tinnitus, and limitations in range of the motion of the TMJ. Trigger points in this muscle are perpetuated by excessive gum chewing, parafunctional habits, strain to the mandible when playing instruments, and by TrPs in cervical muscles that refer to the lateral pterygoid region. Differential diagnosis is of utmost importance due to the variety of symptoms this muscle can engender. This muscle is associated with temporomandibular disorders (TMD), TMD with migraine, infection, nerve entrapments, myositis ossificans, otolaryngic symptoms, and oromandibular dystonia. Corrective actions for the lateral pterygoid muscle include correction of posture, proper tongue and jaw position, elimination of parafunctional habits, nasal breathing, and inactivation of cervical muscle TrPs that refer to the lateral pterygoid muscle.

2. ANATOMIC CONSIDERATIONS

The lateral pterygoid muscle is a short, thick muscle that lies deep into, and largely behind, the zygomatic arch and the coronoid process of the mandible. The superior division of the lateral pterygoid muscle originates from the infratemporal crest and infratemporal surface of the greater wing of the sphenoid bone[1] and travels in an inferior, lateral, and posterior direction toward its insertion.[2] The inferior division of the lateral pterygoid muscle originates from the lateral surface of the lateral pterygoid plate[1] and travels in an upward, lateral, and posterior direction toward its insertion[2] (Figures 11-1 and 11-2A). The fibers of the two divisions converge to insert onto the pterygoid fovea, a depression on the front of the neck of the mandible (Figures 11-1 and 11-2A).[1] The insertion for the superior division, however, is controversial. The superior division has been shown to have attachments to the condyle only,[2] disc–capsule complex only,[2-5] and to both the disc–capsule complex and the condyle.[2-5] Of these, the attachments to both the disc–capsule complex and the condyle are the most common and the disc–capsule complex only attachment is the least common. Usui et al[6] reported different anatomic attachments from others, with fibers of the lateral pterygoid originating from the posterior half of the lateral pterygoid plate inserting onto the medial surface of the condylar process of the mandible. They also found that only a superficial layer of the fibers in the horizontal portion of the muscle originated from the inferior part of the greater wing of the sphenoid and attached to the inferior surface of the disc in all specimens.

In addition to variations in the attachments of this muscle, Sugisaki et al[7] reported variations in the number of heads of this muscle including one head; three heads; medial and lateral heads; superior and inferior heads; and superior, inferior, and medial heads. Recently, others have also reported the lateral pterygoid muscle having three heads.[3,8]

Interestingly, an aberrant muscle located between the temporalis and lateral pterygoid muscles named the pterygoideus proprius muscle has also been reported. Akita et al[9] described this muscle as originating from the medial surface of the anteromedial muscle bundle of the temporalis muscle and running in an inferomedial direction, with one of the specimens also originating from the infratemporal crest of the greater wing of the sphenoid bone. From this origin, the muscle attached to the inferolateral surface of the lower head of the lateral pterygoid muscle in one specimen, and in two specimens the insertion also continued to insert on the inferior margin of the lateral pterygoid plate of the sphenoid bone.

The lateral pterygoid muscle changes its fiber composition with aging. Older adults have a large proportion of type-IIA fibers compared with young adults who rarely, if ever, exhibit this fiber type in the lateral pterygoid muscle.[10,11] Interestingly, only the inferior division of the muscle showed atrophy with aging.

2.1. Innervation and Vascularization

A branch of the buccal nerve innervates the superior division and the lateral part of the inferior division of the lateral pterygoid muscle. The medial part of the inferior division of the lateral pterygoid muscle is innervated by a branch directly from the anterior trunk of the mandibular nerve.[1] Kim et al reported that the buccal nerve penetrates the inferior lateral pterygoid muscle in 12.5% of cases.[12] This muscle, particularly the inferior division, has several different reported innervation variations including innervation from ansa pterygoidea,[12] anterior deep temporal nerve,[12,13] and mandibular nerve trunk.[12] Various combinations of the above-listed nerves may innervate the muscle.

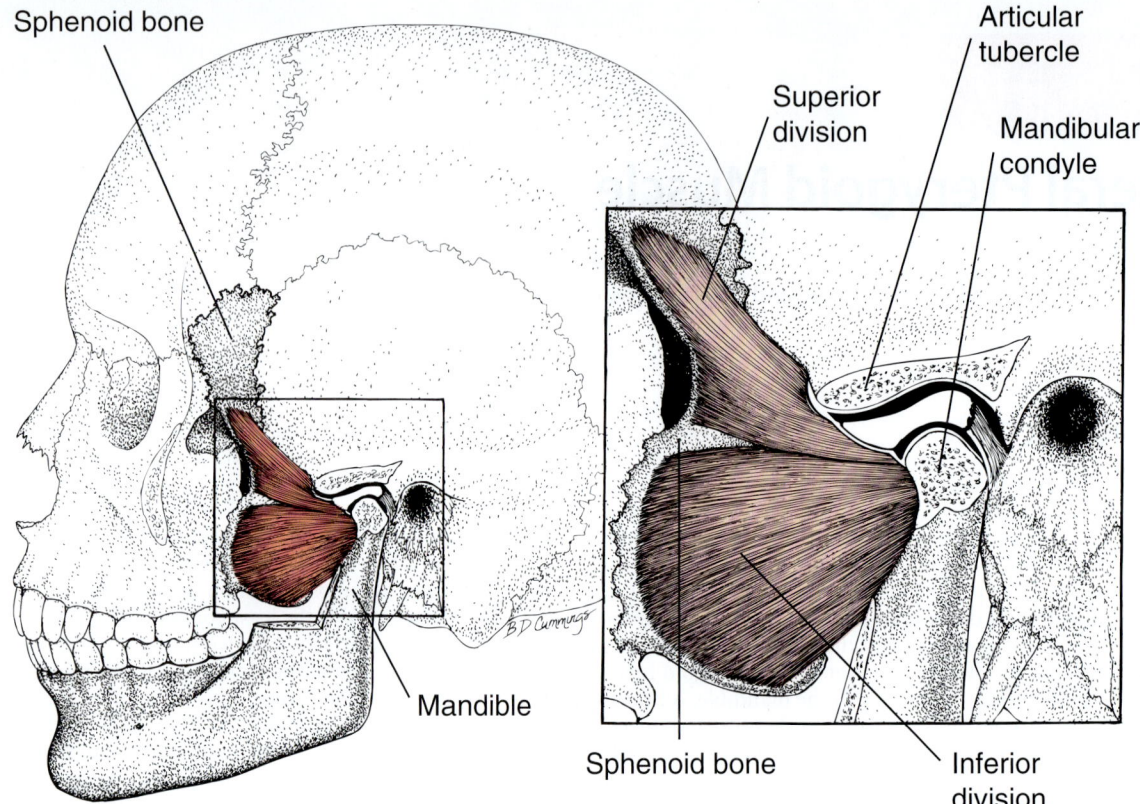

Figure 11-1. Anatomy and muscle attachments of the lateral pterygoid muscle. The zygomatic arch and superficial portion of the temporomandibular joint have been removed. Both divisions of the muscle attach to the neck of the mandibular condyle. The condyle normally articulates with the posterior surface of the articular tubercle of the temporal bone in this position until the mouth is opened wide as in a yawn.

The superior division can receive innervation from the mandibular nerve trunk (middle deep temporal nerve),[12,13] anterior deep temporal nerve,[12,13] and mandibular nerve trunk.[12] A recurrent branch of the inferior alveolar nerve[14,15] and a branch from the auriculotemporal nerve have been reported to innervate the lateral pterygoid muscle as well,[16] although it was not specific to which division of the muscle.

Vascularization of the lateral pterygoid muscle is supplied by the pterygoid branches of the maxillary artery. These branches are given off as the artery crosses the muscle, and from the ascending palatine branch of the facial artery.[1] The artery frequently courses superficial to the inferior division of the lateral pterygoid muscle, and less often it courses deep to the inferior division.[17,18]

2.2. Function

The function of the lateral pterygoid muscle remains controversial in the literature. Some investigators believe that the lateral pterygoid muscle is two distinctly different muscles with very unique actions[19] whereas others think the muscle is made up of two heads that have alternating functions at different times during mouth opening, closing, and chewing.[20,21] Most authors agree that the primary function of the lateral pterygoid muscle is that of mandibular depression (mouth opening) and contralateral excursion (lateral deviation), especially during chewing.[1,22,23]

Classically, the function of the inferior head of the lateral pterygoid (IHLP) muscle includes mandibular depression (mouth opening) and protrusion of the mandible with the muscles on both sides acting together, and lateral deviation of the mandible to the opposite side by one muscle acting unilaterally (contralateral excursion).[1,20] The superior head of the lateral pterygoid (SHLP) muscle is active during mandibular elevation (mouth closing), retrusion, and ipsilateral excursion. Other functions of the SHLP muscle were to decrease tension in the disc by contracting eccentrically during mouth closing, keeping the disc positioned beneath the condyle by creating a forward tension on the disc and neck of the mandible.[20]

Electromyographic (EMG) studies utilizing computerized tomography and functional magnetic resonance imaging (MRI) have provided evidence for functional heterogeneity in both the SHLP and IHLP muscles.[20] Functional heterogeneity is described as the ability of different regions in a muscle to exhibit different actions during the same task.[21] Electromyographic activity of single motor units was recorded from multiple sites in the SHLP and IHLP muscles, and was then confirmed with computerized tomography. The EMG data from the SHLP muscle shows that it has an important role in mandibular depression (mouth opening), contralateral excursion, and protrusion of the mandible.[21,24] The EMG data for the IHLP muscle are consistent with the classical description of its function in mandibular depression (mouth opening), contralateral excursion, and protrusion of the mandible.[23-26]

Ipsilaterally, the medial pterygoid and both divisions of the lateral pterygoid muscles, along with the contralateral masseter and temporalis muscles, participate in the lateral and closing movements of the jaw during grinding of food between the molar teeth.[27]

The lateral pterygoid muscle contributes to the creation and fine motor control of mandibular forces in protrusion and contralateral excursion.[28] Electromyographic studies investigating the function of the lateral pterygoid muscle[23-26] indicate a complex physiology with multifaceted muscle activation patterns in the layers of the SHLP and IHLP muscles during mastication. This may be attributed to selective sequencing of single motor units

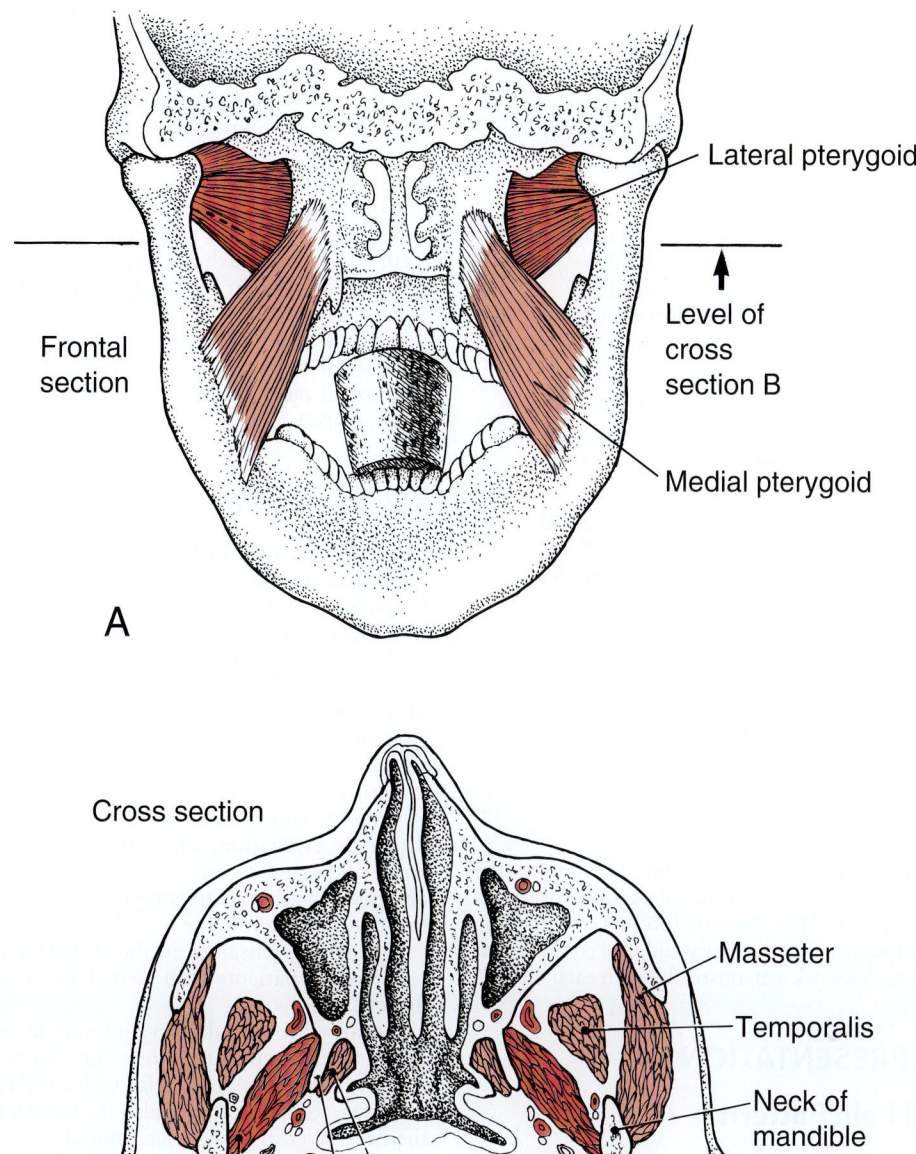

Figure 11-2. A, Frontal section of the head (level of cross section shown in B). This view looks forward through the open mouth. The condylar neck of the mandible obscures part of the needle, which penetrates the inferior division of the muscle. The medial pterygoid muscle (light red) lies in the foreground and attaches to the inner surface of the pterygoid plate. B, Cross section showing the masseter muscle and then the temporalis muscle (light red) as it passes in front of the condylar neck of the mandible above the mandibular notch (level of cross section is shown in A). The needles reach the anterior and posterior portions of the inferior division of the lateral pterygoid muscle (dark red).

as a result of central pattern generators highlighting the role of the reticular formation in oral function.[22]

2.3. Functional Unit

The functional unit to which a muscle belongs includes the muscles that reinforce and counter its actions as well as the joints that the muscle crosses. The interdependence of these structures is functionally reflected in the organization and neural connections of the sensory motor cortex. The functional unit is emphasized because the presence of a TrP in one muscle of the unit increases the likelihood that the other muscles of the unit will also develop TrPs. When inactivating TrPs in a muscle, one should be concerned about TrPs that may develop in muscles that are functionally interdependent. Box 11-1 grossly represents the functional unit of the lateral pterygoid muscle.[29]

Despite the variation in the literature regarding the specific functions of each part of the lateral pterygoid muscle, in general the lateral pterygoid muscle plays a role in mouth opening,

Box 11-1 Functional unit of the lateral pterygoid muscle

Action	Synergists	Antagonist
Mandibular depression	Digastric Suprahyoid muscles Contralateral lateral pterygoid	Masseter (bilaterally) Temporalis (bilaterally) Medial pterygoid (bilaterally)
Mandibular protrusion	Contralateral lateral pterygoid Medial pterygoid (bilaterally)	Temporalis Deep head of the masseter
Mandibular lateral deviation	Contralateral lateral pterygoid Contralateral medial pterygoid Ipsilateral temporalis Ipsilateral masseter	Ipsilateral lateral pterygoid Ipsilateral medial pterygoid Contralateral temporalis

protrusion, and lateral deviation of the jaw. The temporalis muscle is active during protrusion, although it does not fire as strongly as with retrusion.[30] For chewing food on one side, the ipsilateral masseter, ipsilateral medial pterygoid, and contralateral lateral pterygoid muscles work synergistically with each other.[27]

3. CLINICAL PRESENTATION

3.1. Referred Pain Pattern

To date, no distinction between the pain patterns of the two divisions of this muscle have been recorded. The lateral pterygoid muscle refers pain deep into the TMJ and to the region of the maxillary sinus (Figure 11-3).[31-33] Injections of hypertonic saline into the lateral pterygoid muscle refer pain throughout the entire lateral mandible, cheek, ear, and anterior temporal regions, with pain described as shooting, boring, sharp, pressing, hot, aching, taut, intense, spreading, and tight.[34] Interestingly, Svensson et al[34] also reported referred pain to the teeth and gingiva from the lateral pterygoid muscle, although this was not observed by Simons et al.[29] Teachey[35] reported similar findings of the lateral pterygoid muscle referring pain to the teeth and gums. Teachey[35] also described multiple otolaryngic symptoms related to TrPs in the lateral pterygoid muscle, which is described below.

Simons et al[29] believe that TrPs in this muscle are the chief myofascial source of referred pain felt in the TMJ area. The myofascial pain syndrome is easily mistaken for the pain of TMJ arthritis.[36]

3.2. Symptoms

Patients with TrPs in the lateral pterygoid muscle often describe pain in the maxillary area as "sinus pain." They report frequent or recurrent "sinusitis," however, the pain does not respond to medications. Chronic or recurrent throat and/or neck symptoms including discomfort/drainage/congestion, sore throat, and "tonsillitis," may be reported as well as nasal obstruction, nasal congestion, nasal pressure, ear pain, and clogging.[35] As a result, patients may think that they are sick when they are not, and they may be prescribed unnecessary medications.

Patients with normal otolaryngic studies, including an audiometric evaluation, who have changes in hearing including either increased sensitivity to sounds (hyperacusis) or slight decreased sensitivity to sounds (hypoacusis), or even hearing loss may have TrPs in the lateral (or medial) pterygoid muscle.[35]

A burning sensation in the throat or mouth may also be reported by patients who have TrPs in the lateral pterygoid muscle.[35]

Because the lateral pterygoid muscle can refer to the TMJ, patients often report that their "jaw hurts." Severe pain in the TMJ region is commonly referred from TrPs not only in the lateral pterygoid muscle, but also the medial pterygoid muscle or the deep layer of the masseter muscle.

Loss of jaw movement or difficulty with jaw movement is common,[37,38] as well as reports of "stiffness" that can resultantly contribute to patients having difficulty eating foods that require

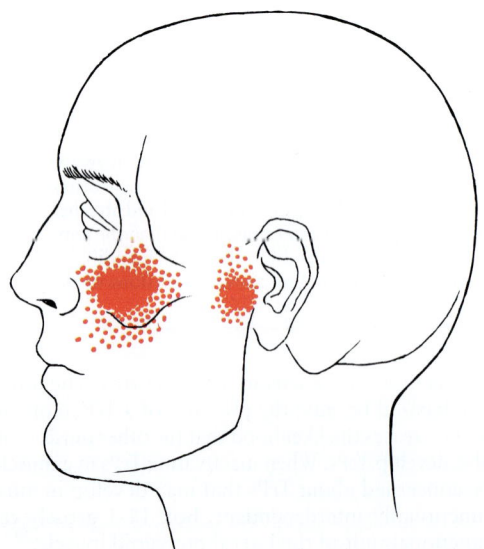
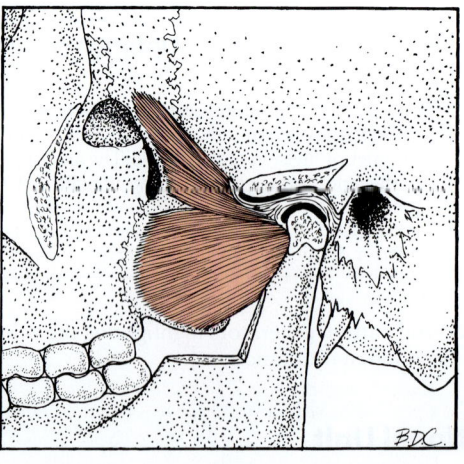

Figure 11-3. The referred pain pattern (dark red) of TrPs in the left lateral pterygoid muscle (pink).

wide mouth opening. In addition to having difficulty opening the mouth when eating, patients may also report difficulty swallowing (dysphagia) or pain with swallowing (odynophagia).[35]

Patients may report that their teeth do not contact evenly anymore, or their bite "feels different," oftentimes despite extensive work to the teeth or TMJ, and/or use of appliances.[36]

Although not common, tinnitus may be due to TrPs in the lateral pterygoid muscle in some patients.[35,39]

3.3. Patient Examination

After a thorough subjective examination, the clinician should make a detailed drawing representing the pain pattern that the patient has described. This depiction will assist in planning the physical examination and can be useful in monitoring the progression of the patient as symptoms improve or change. The clinician should perform a brief examination of the TMJ and should also assess the patient's posture, with particular attention to head and neck positions. Forward head posture and excessive tension in suprahyoid and infrahyoid muscles should be noted, although the relation between TMD and head and neck posture is still controversial and unclear.[40]

Normal or functional mouth opening can be determined by attempting to place stacked proximal interphalangeal joints of the first two fingers of the nondominant hand between the upper and lower incisor teeth (Figure 8-3, two-knuckle test). Usually, about 2½ knuckles of mouth opening is functional. When the inferior division of the lateral pterygoid muscle is affected, there will likely be a decrease in jaw-opening that prevents the entry of two knuckles between the incisor teeth. Lateral excursion of the mandible is reduced toward the same side because of the increased muscle tension. When the patient slowly opens and closes the jaw, the midline incisal path of the mandible deviates in an S-curve. The most marked deviation from the midline during the movement is usually away from the side of the more affected lateral pterygoid muscle, but this is not a reliable sign because TrP involvement of other masticatory muscles, especially the medial pterygoid muscle, can produce or alter this finding.

A more standardized, objective way to measure mouth opening is with a vertical ruler to measure the distance between the upper and lower incisors.[41,42] Normal opening for women is 41 to 45 mm and for men is 43 to 45 mm.[43,44]

3.4. Trigger Point Examination

Of all the masticatory muscles, the lateral pterygoid muscle seems to be the one to most likely have TrPs. As a result, palpation of this muscle is of utmost importance; however, the specificity and reliability of palpating the lateral pterygoid muscle is controversial. Several authors report it cannot be dependably palpated[45,46] because the reliability and validity are so poor[47-49]; others more recently report that it can be palpated accurately with confirmation through MRI.[50,51] Reasons for this extreme difference of opinion are that the space where the finger needs to access part of the lateral pterygoid muscle is reportedly smaller than the average finger,[45] and even if the finger can access the area, oftentimes what is actually being palpated is part of the superficial head of the medial pterygoid muscle, not the lateral pterygoid muscle.[45-47] Even when the superficial medial pterygoid muscle was absent, the lateral pterygoid muscle was only able to be accessed 50% of the time.[46] Another reason for inaccurate palpation of this muscle is the high percentage of control patients who feel very tender in this region.[49] More recently, Conti et al[48] reported similar findings that 66.7% of controls and 79.5% of those with myofascial pain felt tender in this muscle; whereas palpation of other muscles examined, the control group did not feel tender in as many areas. Since this region is painful in a large percentage of controls, patients can be misdiagnosed as experiencing myofascial pain or involvement of the lateral pterygoid muscle.

Despite the controversy in palpating this muscle, the technique that is commonly used to access the region of the lateral pterygoid muscle is described. Clinicians should interpret the information from this palpation technique with caution for reasons stated above. To examine intraorally for TrP tenderness in the region of the anterior attachment of the inferior division of the lateral pterygoid muscle, the mouth is opened about 2 cm (3/4 in) while the index or little finger presses posteriorly as far as possible along the vestibule that forms the roof of the cheek pouch. The finger goes a little past the maxillary tuberosity and the finger should squeeze between the maxilla and the coronoid process as it does this. This area can be small and difficult to move the finger through; lateral deviation of the jaw to the ipsilateral side can be done to increase the space slightly.[29,51] Interestingly, others who describe accurate palpation of this muscle do not report using lateral deviation to increase accessibility of this muscle.[48,50] Once reaching the softer area behind the maxillary tuberosity, the direction of palpation varies among those who report that the muscle can be palpated. Directions described include the finger pressing medially toward the lateral pterygoid plate[29]; in a posterior, superior, and medial direction[48]; the finger hooking medially to[50]; or going in a craniomedial direction[51] (Figure 11-4B). Stelzenmueller et al[51] also reported utilizing opening and closing of the mouth with palpation to confirm the location of the muscle.

The handle end of a dental mirror or other blunt instrument has been reported by others to substitute for the finger if the space is too restricted,[45] but this may produce a more concentrated pressure stimulus and may be ineffective for precise identification of structures.

It would be expected with TrPs that this area would be very tender to palpation; however, as stated previously, this area can also be very tender in those who have no pain in the craniofacial region.[48,49] With the high incidence of false positives, caution is warranted in using pain with palpation to diagnose TrPs.

Tenderness of temporalis fibers attaching to the medial aspect of the coronoid process, lateral to the palpating finger (or probe), is distinguished from tenderness of lateral pterygoid fibers, medial to the finger (or probe), by the patient's response to the direction of pressure.[45]

It is possible that the posterior attachment region of both divisions is accessible to external palpation at the neck of the mandibular condyle just below the TMJ. Both muscle bellies can, with proper precautions, be examined externally through the masseter muscle for tenderness and referred pain.

Accessing the lateral pterygoid muscle by external palpation has not been confirmed or validated in the literature at this time. Simons et al[29] reported the muscle can be palpated, but not if the jaw is closed because the superior division lies deep to the zygomatic arch and the inferior division lies deep to the ramus of the mandible. With the jaw separated about 3 cm (1 1/8 in), a posterior portion of the inferior division and of the superior division may be approached externally through masseter fibers at the opening between the mandibular notch and the zygomatic arch (Figure 11-4A).

Because the lateral pterygoid muscle can only be palpated through the masseter muscle, one should first identify and inactivate any TrPs in the masseter fibers of the area to be examined. When TrP tenderness is present in the masseter muscle, its taut bands are readily palpable, but TrP bands in the underlying lateral pterygoid muscle are too deep to be distinguished by more than their local tenderness and by their referred pain response to pressure. Trigger points in either the temporalis or the masseter muscle can prevent sufficient mouth opening for satisfactory examination of the lateral pterygoid muscle bellies for tenderness. Unless the temporalis and masseter TrPs are successfully inactivated, only the posterior attachment region can be examined for any involvement.

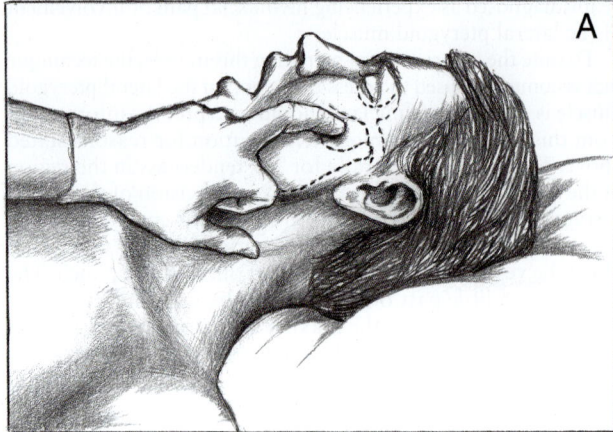

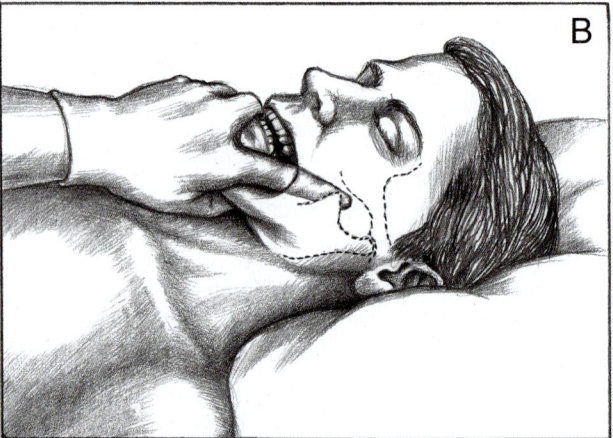

Figure 11-4. A and B, External and intraoral examination of the left lateral pterygoid muscle. A, External palpation of the posterior part of the muscle bellies of both divisions of the lateral pterygoid through the masseter muscle. The mouth is voluntarily held open by the patient to relax the masseter muscle and permit palpation through that muscle and through the aperture between the mandibular notch and the zygomatic process (dotted lines). External examination permits indirect palpation for tenderness of the posterior parts of both divisions of the muscle because they approach their attachments to the neck of the condyle inferior to the temporomandibular joint. B, intraoral palpation permits more direct examination of the region of the anterior attachment of the inferior division. With a gloved hand, the operator slips a finger into the uppermost rear corner of the cheek pouch toward the head of the mandible and then presses medially toward the pterygoid plate. The jaws should be open about 5 to 8 mm (about ¼ in) to allow room for the fingertip to squeeze into the space deep to the coronoid process. See text for additional comments regarding examination.

4. DIFFERENTIAL DIAGNOSIS

4.1. Activation and Perpetuation of Trigger Points

A posture or activity that activates a TrP, if not corrected, can also perpetuate it. In any part of the lateral pterygoid muscle, TrPs may be activated by unaccustomed eccentric loading, eccentric exercise in an unconditioned muscle, or maximal or submaximal concentric loading.[52] Trigger points may also be activated or aggravated when the muscle is placed in a shortened and/or lengthened position for an extended period of time. Specifically, excessive gum chewing or parafunctional habits such as bruxism, jaw clenching, nail biting, or persistent thumb-sucking by a child can not only initiate but also perpetuate TrPs in the lateral pterygoid muscle. Excessive chewing on one side contributes to overload in the contralateral lateral pterygoid muscle.[27]

In addition, playing a wind instrument with the mandible fixed in protrusion or by maintaining mandibular side pressure to hold a violin in playing position can also contribute to the development of TrPs in this muscle.

Lateral pterygoid TrPs may develop in response to TrP activity of the neck muscles, especially the sternocleidomastoid muscle, which, in turn, may be activated by the mechanical stress caused by a leg length discrepancy, a small hemipelvis, or other lower-body postural abnormalities. As a result, TrPs in the lateral pterygoid muscle are not fully resolved until the sternocleidomastoid muscle or other structural impairments are addressed.

4.2. Associated Trigger Points

Associated TrPs can develop in the referred pain areas caused by TrPs.[53] Therefore, musculature in the referred pain areas for each muscle should also be considered. Trigger points in the lateral pterygoid muscle can be due to TrPs in the sternocleidomastoid muscle. Additionally, TrPs in the lateral pterygoid muscle can contribute to associated TrPs in other muscles including the masseter, medial pterygoid, orbicularis oculi, and zygomaticus major and minor muscles.

When the inferior division of the lateral pterygoid muscle has TrPs, its antagonists are likely to develop associated TrPs, including the contralateral medial and lateral pterygoid muscles, and ipsilateral deep masseter muscle, and posterior fibers of the temporalis muscle.

4.3. Associated Pathology

Some medical conditions give rise to symptoms that can appear confusingly similar to those produced by lateral pterygoid TrPs or may be present concurrently. Involvement of the lateral pterygoid muscle can be associated with TMJ internal derangements (Chapter 18). Some report that due to the attachment of the lateral pterygoid muscle to the disc, either completely or partially,[2-5] it can have an influence on disc dysfunction[54-56]; others report that it is unlikely.[3,5,57] Many studies have found lateral pterygoid muscle involvement in patients with TMD.[37,38,58,59] Patients with TMD and migraine can also have associated involvement of the lateral pterygoid muscle.[60] Lateral pterygoid TrPs can produce referred pain that is likely to be interpreted as coming from the TMJ. Refer to Chapter 18 for a description of TMJ clinical considerations. The referred tenderness from TrPs has neither the sharp localization nor the intensity of tenderness that is more characteristic of joint inflammation.

The lateral pterygoid muscle can also be a source of potential nerve entrapments; several different anatomic variations of the surrounding nerves have been reported. The auriculotemporal,[16,61] mandibular,[62] recurrent branch of the inferior alveolaor,[14] inferior alveolar,[61] buccal,[12] lingual,[61,63-65] and mylohyoid[61] nerves can all pierce through the IHLP muscle, which place the nerve at risk for compression. Only the anterior deep temporal nerve has been shown to pierce through the SHLP muscle.[13,61] The buccal nerve runs between the two heads of the lateral pterygoid muscle,[62] which can be a problem if the muscle is hypertrophied and/or in spasm.

The facial pain caused by TrPs from the lateral pterygoid muscle should not be mistakenly diagnosed as the paroxysmal electric-type pain of trigeminal neuralgia, because the symptoms are typically quite different. Ceneviz et al[66] reported a single case wherein TrPs in the lateral pterygoid muscle did mimic pain features of trigeminal neuralgia and initially met the criteria for a diagnosis of trigeminal neuralgia according to the criteria established by the International Association for the Study of Pain.

Pyomyositis is a rare infection of the striated muscle most frequently observed in the lower extremities. It is a life-threatening condition that, if misdiagnosed, can cause death. Involvement of the lateral pterygoid muscle has been reported, initially presenting with symptoms such as trigeminal neuralgia.[67] Knowledge of this condition is essential to ensure proper treatment and care.

Myositis ossificans is a rare condition in which heterotropic bone forms in muscle or soft tissue, usually after some type of trauma or injury. It does not commonly occur in muscles of the masticatory system, especially the lateral pterygoid muscle. From 2001 to 2014, only six cases (of the 20 in the masticatory system) occurred in the lateral pterygoid muscle.[68] Although rare, this diagnosis should be considered as a possibility if there is loss of jaw range of movement after trauma or injections to the face. In addition, this condition can occur idiopathically, even without trauma.

As stated previously, TrPs in the lateral pterygoid muscle can mimic otolaryngic symptoms including sinusitis, hearing changes, throat pain and congestion, and tonsillitis.[35,69] When diagnostic testing does not yield significant findings for the cause of symptoms, TrPs in the lateral pterygoid muscle should be considered.[35]

Oromandibular dystonia is a focal neurologic disorder that can affect the face and the jaw. Typical symptoms include involuntary facial grimace, jaw, or tongue movements. The cause of the dystonia is more frequently idiopathic[70-72] but can also be secondary to neurologic diseases,[70,71] infections,[71] or antipsychotic drugs.[73] The masseter and temporalis muscles are the most commonly involved, but the lateral pterygoid muscle can be affected as well.[70-72] Because the lateral pterygoid muscle is significantly deeper than the masseter and temporalis muscles, the diagnosis of lateral pterygoid involvement is more difficult. Three signs and symptoms that are characteristic of this condition include difficulty in jaw-closing after wide opening, jaw function disabilities, and involuntary jaw movements.[70] Knowledge of this condition is essential because it can easily be misdiagnosed as TMD or bruxism.[70,72]

5. CORRECTIVE ACTIONS

Excessive forward head posture should be addressed and the patient should be taught correct resting position of the jaw (tongue on the roof of the mouth on the hard palate behind the top teeth, lips together, and teeth slightly separated). The patient should also be instructed in good body mechanics and should learn how to maintain normal head and neck posture. Clenching, gum chewing, nail biting, and other parafunctional jaw habits should be identified and discontinued.

Mouth breathing, as compared with naso-diaphragmatic breathing, has also been shown to have a negative impact on posture[74-79] and should therefore be corrected. Performing strengthening exercises on an exercise ball and stretches, in conjunction with naso-diaphragmatic breathing, have been shown to improve the posture.[78]

Patients need to learn general neck stretching exercises to help inactivate any TrPs in the cervical muscles such as the sternocleidomastoid muscle that may be perpetuating lateral pterygoid TrPs. In fact, in some patients, TrPs resolve following correction of these two powerful perpetuating factors alone.

Body asymmetry and the resultant functional scoliosis should be corrected by appropriate lifts as this postural stress may activate TrPs in the neck muscles which can cause associated TrPs in the masticatory muscles. If the habit of mouth breathing produces forward head posture, mouth breathing should be corrected by eliminating contributory factors such as nasal obstruction.

The activation of TrPs during a prolonged dental procedure may be prevented by taking breaks for the patient to go through several cycles of active range of movement.

References

1. Standring S. *Gray's Anatomy: The Anatomical Basis of Clinical Practice*. 41st ed. London, UK: Elsevier; 2015.
2. Antonopoulou M, Iatrou I, Paraschos A, Anagnostopoulou S. Variations of the attachment of the superior head of human lateral pterygoid muscle. *J Craniomaxillofac Surg.* 2013;41(6):e91-e97.
3. Dergin G, Kilic C, Gozneli R, Yildirim D, Garip H, Moroglu S. Evaluating the correlation between the lateral pterygoid muscle attachment type and internal derangement of the temporomandibular joint with an emphasis on MR imaging findings. *J Craniomaxillofac Surg.* 2012;40(5):459-463.
4. Imanimoghaddam M, Madani AS, Hashemi EM. The evaluation of lateral pterygoid muscle pathologic changes and insertion patterns in temporomandibular joints with or without disc displacement using magnetic resonance imaging. *Int J Oral Maxillofac Surg.* 2013;42(9):1116-1120.
5. Omami G, Lurie A. Magnetic resonance imaging evaluation of discal attachment of superior head of lateral pterygoid muscle in individuals with symptomatic temporomandibular joint. *Oral Surg Oral Med Oral Pathol Oral Radiol.* 2012;114(5):650-657.
6. Usui A, Akita K, Yamaguchi K. An anatomic study of the divisions of the lateral pterygoid muscle based on the findings of the origins and insertions. *Surg Radiol Anat.* 2008;30(4):327-333.
7. Sugisaki M, Komori E, Nakazawa M, Tanabe H. Anatomical studies of the lateral pterygoid muscle by the superior approach and a review of the literature. *Jpn J Oral Maxillofacial Surg.* 1986;32:718-730.
8. Fujita S, Iizuka T, Dauber W. Variation of heads of lateral pterygoid muscle and morphology of articular disc of human temporomandibular joint—anatomical and histological analysis. *J Oral Rehabil.* 2001;28(6):560-571.
9. Akita K, Shimokawa T, Sato T. Aberrant muscle between the temporalis and the lateral pterygoid muscles: M. pterygoideus proprius (Henle). *Clin Anat.* 2001;14(4):288-291.
10. Monemi M, Thornell L, Eriksson P. Diverse changes in fibre type composition of the human lateral pterygoid and digastric muscles during aging. *J Neurol Sci.* 1999;171(1):38-48.
11. Eriksson PO, Eriksson A, Ringqvist M, Thornell LE. Special histochemical muscle-fibre characteristics of the human lateral pterygoid muscle. *Arch Oral Biol.* 1981;26(6):495-507.
12. Kim HJ, Kwak HH, Hu KS, et al. Topographic anatomy of the mandibular nerve branches distributed on the two heads of the lateral pterygoid. *Int J Oral Maxillofac Surg.* 2003;32(4):408-413.
13. Kwak HH, Ko SJ, Jung HS, Park HD, Chung IH, Kim HJ. Topographic anatomy of the deep temporal nerves, with references to the superior head of lateral pterygoid. *Surg Radiol Anat.* 2003;25(5-6):393-399.
14. Buch HA, Agnihotri RG. A recurrent variant branch of the inferior alveolar nerve: is it unique? *Clin Anat.* 2012;25(4):437-443.
15. Muraleedharan A, Veeramani R, Chand P. Variations in the branching pattern of posterior division of mandibular nerve: a case report. *Surg Radiol Anat.* 2014;36(9):947-950.
16. Shimokawa T, Akita K, Sato T, Ru F, Yi SQ, Tanaka S. Penetration of muscles by branches of the mandibular nerve: a possible cause of neuropathy. *Clin Anat.* 2004;17(1):2-5.
17. Gulses A, Oren C, Altug HA, Ilica T, Sencimen M. Radiologic assessment of the relationship between the maxillary artery and the lateral pterygoid muscle. *J Craniofac Surg.* 2012;23(5):1465-1467.
18. Hussain A, Binahmed A, Karim A, Sandor GK. Relationship of the maxillary artery and lateral pterygoid muscle in a caucasian sample. *Oral Surg Oral Med Oral Pathol Oral Radiol Endod.* 2008;105(1):32-36.
19. Okeson JP. *Management of Temporomandibular Disorders and Occlusion.* 6th ed. St Louis, MO: C.V. Mosby; 2005.
20. Murray GM. The lateral pterygoid: function and dysfunction. *Semin Orthod.* 2012;18(1):44-50.
21. Bhutada MK, Phanachet I, Whittle T, Peck CC, Murray GM. Regional properties of the superior head of human lateral pterygoid muscle. *Eur J Oral Sci.* 2008;116(6):518-524.
22. Desmons S, Graux F, Atassi M, Libersa P, Dupas PH. The lateral pterygoid muscle, a heterogeneous unit implicated in temporomandibular disorder: a literature review. *Cranio.* 2007;25(4):283-291.
23. Phanachet I, Whittle T, Wanigaratne K, Murray GM. Functional properties of single motor units in inferior head of human lateral pterygoid muscle: task relations and thresholds. *J Neurophysiol.* 2001;86(5):2204-2218.
24. Phanachet I, Whittle T, Wanigaratne K, Klineberg IJ, Sessle BJ, Murray GM. Functional heterogeneity in the superior head of the human lateral pterygoid. *J Dent Res.* 2003;82(2):106-111.
25. Bhutada MK, Phanachet I, Whittle T, Wanigaratne K, Peck CC, Murray GM. Threshold properties of single motor units in superior head of human lateral pterygoid muscle. *Arch Oral Biol.* 2007;52(6):552-561.
26. Bhutada MK, Phanachet I, Whittle T, Peck CC, Murray GM. Activity of superior head of human lateral pterygoid increases with increases in contralateral and protrusive jaw displacement. *Eur J Oral Sci.* 2007;115(4):257-264.
27. Yamaguchi S, Itoh S, Watanabe Y, Tsuboi A, Watanabe M. Quantitative analysis of masticatory activity during unilateral mastication using muscle fMRI. *Oral Dis.* 2011;17(4):407-413.
28. Uchida S, Whittle T, Wanigaratne K, Murray GM. Activity in the inferior head of the human lateral pterygoid muscle with different directions of isometric force. *Arch Oral Biol.* 2002;47(11):771-778.
29. Simons DG, Travell J, Simons L. *Travell & Simon's Myofascial Pain and Dysfunction: The Trigger Point Manual.* Vol 1. 2nd ed. Baltimore, MD: Williams & Wilkins; 1999:104.
30. Cecilio FA, Regalo SC, Palinkas M, et al. Ageing and surface EMG activity patterns of masticatory muscles. *J Oral Rehabil.* 2010;37(4):248-255.
31. Brechner VL. Myofascial pain syndrome of the lateral pterygoid muscle. *J Craniomandibular Pract.* 1982;1(1):42-45.
32. Travell J. Temporomandibular joint pain referred from muscles of the head and neck. *J Prosthet Dent.* 1960;10:745-763.
33. Travell J. Mechanical headache. *Headache.* 1967;7(1):23-29.

34. Svensson P, Bak J, Troest T. Spread and referral of experimental pain in different jaw muscles. *J Orofac Pain.* 2003;17(3):214-223.
35. Teachey WS. Otolaryngic myofascial pain syndromes. *Curr Pain Headache Rep.* 2004;8(6):457-462.
36. Reynolds MD. Myofascial trigger point syndromes in the practice of rheumatology. *Arch Phys Med Rehabil.* 1981;62(3):111-114.
37. Gonzalez-Perez LM, Infante-Cossio P, Granados-Nunez M, Urresti-Lopez FJ. Treatment of temporomandibular myofascial pain with deep dry needling. *Med Oral Patol Oral Cir Bucal.* 2012;17(5):e781-e785.
38. Gonzalez-Perez LM, Infante-Cossio P, Granados-Nunez M, Urresti-Lopez FJ, Lopez-Martos R, Ruiz-Canela-Mendez P. Deep dry needling of trigger points located in the lateral pterygoid muscle: efficacy and safety of treatment for management of myofascial pain and temporomandibular dysfunction. *Med Oral Patol Oral Cir Bucal.* 2015;20(3):e326-e333.
39. Bjorne A. Tinnitus aereum as an effect of increased tension in the lateral pterygoid muscle. *Otolaryngol Head Neck Surg.* 1993;109(5):969.
40. Rocha CP, Croci CS, Caria PH. Is there relationship between temporomandibular disorders and head and cervical posture? A systematic review. *J Oral Rehabil.* 2013;40(11):875-881.
41. Walker N, Bohannon RW, Cameron D. Discriminant validity of temporomandibular joint range of motion measurements obtained with a ruler. *J Orthop Sports Phys Ther.* 2000;30(8):484-492.
42. List T, John MT, Dworkin SF, Svensson P. Recalibration improves inter-examiner reliability of TMD examination. *Acta Odontol Scand.* 2006;64(3):146-152.
43. Gallagher C, Gallagher V, Whelton H, Cronin M. The normal range of mouth opening in an Irish population. *J Oral Rehabil.* 2004;31(2):110-116.
44. Muller L, van Waes H, Langerweger C, Molinari L, Saurenmann RK. Maximal mouth opening capacity: percentiles for healthy children 4-17 years of age. *Pediatr Rheumatol Online J.* 2013;11:17.
45. Johnstone DR, Templeton M. The feasibility of palpating the lateral pterygoid muscle. *J Prosthet Dent.* 1980;44(3):318-323.
46. Stratmann U, Mokrys K, Meyer U, et al. Clinical anatomy and palpability of the inferior lateral pterygoid muscle. *J Prosthet Dent.* 2000;83(5):548-554.
47. Turp JC, Minagi S. Palpation of the lateral pterygoid region in TMD—where is the evidence? *J Dent.* 2001;29(7):475-483.
48. Conti PC, Dos Santos Silva R, Rossetti LM, De Oliveira Ferreira Da Silva R, Do Valle AL, Gelmini M. Palpation of the lateral pterygoid area in the myofascial pain diagnosis. *Oral Surg Oral Med Oral Pathol Oral Radiol Endod.* 2008;105(3):e61-e66.
49. Thomas CA, Okeson JP. Evaluation of lateral pterygoid muscle symptoms using a common palpation technique and a method of functional manipulation. *Cranio.* 1987;5(2):125-129.
50. Barriere P, Lutz JC, Zamanian A, et al. MRI evidence of lateral pterygoid muscle palpation. *Int J Oral Maxillofac Surg.* 2009;38(10):1094-1095.
51. Stelzenmueller W, Umstadt H, Weber D, Goenner-Oezkan V, Kopp S, Lisson J. Evidence—the intraoral palpability of the lateral pterygoid muscle—a prospective study. *Ann Anat.* 2016;206:89-95.
52. Gerwin RD, Dommerholt J, Shah JP. An expansion of Simons' integrated hypothesis of trigger point formation. *Curr Pain Headache Rep.* 2004;8(6):468-475.
53. Hsieh YL, Kao MJ, Kuan TS, Chen SM, Chen JT, Hong CZ. Dry needling to a key myofascial trigger point may reduce the irritability of satellite MTrPs. *Am J Phys Med Rehabil.* 2007;86(5):397-403.
54. Taskaya-Yilmaz N, Ceylan G, Incesu L, Muglali M. A possible etiology of the internal derangement of the temporomandibular joint based on the MRI observations of the lateral pterygoid muscle. *Surg Radiol Anat.* 2005;27(1):19-24.
55. Tanaka E, Hirose M, Inubushi T, et al. Effect of hyperactivity of the lateral pterygoid muscle on the temporomandibular joint disk. *J Biomech Eng.* 2007;129(6):890-897.
56. Mazza D, Marini M, Impara L, et al. Anatomic examination of the upper head of the lateral pterygoid muscle using magnetic resonance imaging and clinical data. *J Craniofac Surg.* 2009;20(5):1508-1511.
57. Liu ZJ, Yamagata K, Kuroe K, Suenaga S, Noikura T, Ito G. Morphological and positional assessments of TMJ components and lateral pterygoid muscle in relation to symptoms and occlusion of patients with temporomandibular disorders. *J Oral Rehabil.* 2000;27(10):860-874.
58. Iwasaki LR, Liu H, Gonzalez YM, Marx DB, Nickel JC. Modeling of muscle forces in humans with and without temporomandibular joint disorders. *Orthod Craniofac Res.* 2015;18(suppl 1):170-179.
59. D'Ippolito SM, Borri Wolosker AM, D'Ippolito G, Herbert de Souza B, Fenyo-Pereira M. Evaluation of the lateral pterygoid muscle using magnetic resonance imaging. *Dentomaxillofac Radiol.* 2010;39(8):494-500.
60. Lopes SL, Costa AL, Gamba Tde O, Flores IL, Cruz AD, Min LL. Lateral pterygoid muscle volume and migraine in patients with temporomandibular disorders. *Imaging Sci Dent.* 2015;45(1):1-5.
61. Loughner BA, Larkin LH, Mahan PE. Nerve entrapment in the lateral pterygoid muscle. *Oral Surg Oral Med Oral Pathol.* 1990;69(3):299-306.
62. Piagkou M, Demesticha T, Skandalakis P, Johnson EO. Functional anatomy of the mandibular nerve: consequences of nerve injury and entrapment. *Clin Anat.* 2011;24(2):143-150.
63. Skrzat J, Walocha J, Srodek R. An anatomical study of the pterygoalar bar and the pterygoalar foramen. *Folia Morphol (Warsz).* 2005;64(2):92-96.
64. von Ludinghausen M, Kageyama I, Miura M, Alkhatib M. Morphological peculiarities of the deep infratemporal fossa in advanced age. *Surg Radiol Anat.* 2006;28(3):284-292.
65. Isberg AM, Isacsson G, Williams WN, Loughner BA. Lingual numbness and speech articulation deviation associated with temporomandibular joint disk displacement. *Oral Surg Oral Med Oral Pathol.* 1987;64(1):9-14.
66. Ceneviz C, Maloney G, Mehta N. Myofascial pain may mimic trigeminal neuralgia. *Cephalalgia.* 2006;26(7):899-901.
67. Kim KS. Facial pain induced by isolated lateral pterygoid pyomyositis misdiagnosed as trigeminal neuralgia. *Muscle Nerve.* 2013;47(4):611-612.
68. Jiang Q, Chen MJ, Yang C, et al. Post-infectious myositis ossificans in medial, lateral pterygoid muscles: a case report and review of the literature. *Oncol Lett.* 2015;9(2):920-926.
69. Alvarez-Arenal A, Gonzalez-Gonzalez I, Moradas Estrada M, deLlanos-Lanchares H, Costilla-Garcia S. Temporomandibular disorder or not? A case report. *Cranio.* 2015:1-6.
70. Cao Y, Zhang W, Yap AU, Xie QF, Fu KY. Clinical characteristics of lateral pterygoid myospasm: a retrospective study of 18 patients. *Oral Surg Oral Med Oral Pathol Oral Radiol.* 2012;113(6):762-765.
71. Bakke M, Larsen BM, Dalager T, Moller E. Oromandibular dystonia—functional and clinical characteristics: a report on 21 cases. *Oral Surg Oral Med Oral Pathol Oral Radiol.* 2013;115(1):e21-e26.
72. Moller E, Bakke M, Dalager T, Werdelin LM. Oromandibular dystonia involving the lateral pterygoid muscles: four cases with different complexity. *Mov Disord.* 2007;22(6):785-790.
73. Burke RE, Fahn S, Jankovic J, et al. Tardive dystonia: late-onset and persistent dystonia caused by antipsychotic drugs. *Neurology.* 1982;32(12):1335-1346.
74. Milanesi JM, Borin G, Correa EC, da Silva AM, Bortoluzzi DC, Souza JA. Impact of the mouth breathing occurred during childhood in the adult age: biophotogrammetric postural analysis. *Int J Pediatr Otorhinolaryngol.* 2011;75(8):999-1004.
75. Cuccia AM, Lotti M, Caradonna D. Oral breathing and head posture. *Angle Orthod.* 2008;78(1):77-82.
76. Sforza C, Colombo A, Turci M, Grassi G, Ferrario VF. Induced oral breathing and craniocervical postural relations: an experimental study in healthy young adults. *Cranio.* 2004;22(1):21-26.
77. Vig PS, Showfety KJ, Phillips C. Experimental manipulation of head posture. *Am J Orthod.* 1980;77(3):258-268.
78. Correa EC, Berzin F. Efficacy of physical therapy on cervical muscle activity and on body posture in school-age mouth breathing children. *Int J Pediatr Otorhinolaryngol.* 2007;71(10):1527-1535.
79. Neiva PD, Kirkwood RN, Godinho R. Orientation and position of head posture, scapula and thoracic spine in mouth-breathing children. *Int J Pediatr Otorhinolaryngol.* 2009;73(2):227-236.

Chapter 12

Digastric Muscle and Anterior Neck Muscles

"Tongue Pain Impersonator"

Seth Jason Fibraio, Jennifer Marie Nelson, Simon Vulfsons, Amir Minerbi, and Michelle Finnegan

1. INTRODUCTION

The anterior neck musculature is a dynamic collection of muscles that aid in the overall stability of the neck, participate in head and neck flexion, provide support for swallowing, aid in mastication, and participate in both vocalization and labored ventilation. This group includes the digastric, suprahyoid, infrahyoid, and the anterior vertebral muscles. The suprahyoid muscles are innervated by cranial nerves except for the geniohyoid muscle, which is innervated by C1 through the hypoglossal nerve. This nerve also supplies the thyrohyoid muscle. The ansa cervicalis innervates the sternohyoid, sternothyroid, and omohyoid muscles. The cervical nerves of C1 through C6 supply different parts of the anterior vertebral muscles. These muscles have various functions, including depression of the mandible, movement of the hyoid bone inferiorly and superiorly, and stabilization of the cervical spine. Although this area is not as commonly recognized and treated as a source of pain for craniocervical conditions, it should not be ignored. Trigger points (TrPs) in these muscles contribute to pain in multiple areas, including the anterior neck, larynx, tongue, and lower facial area. Some even refer pain as far as the ipsilateral eye and ear. After trauma and in the presence of pain, the longus colli muscle demonstrates decreased motor activation patterns. Activation and perpetuation of TrPs in the suprahyoid muscles, infrahyoid muscles, and longus colli and longus capitis muscles can be caused by trauma, such as those sustained in motor vehicle accidents, or mechanical trauma, such as choking or blunt trauma, or habitually poor posture. Differential diagnosis of this region is essential to rule out conditions such as infections or malignancies involving the cervical region, dystonia, Eagle syndrome, retropharyngeal calcific tendinitis, intramuscular hemangiomas, myositis ossificans, blood vessel entrapment, omohyoid muscle syndrome, and sternohyoid muscle syndrome. Corrective actions include correction of forward head posture and instruction in the resting position of the tongue. Instruction in good body mechanics and ergonomics is essential along with TrP self-pressure release and self-stretch exercises.

2. ANATOMIC CONSIDERATIONS

Digastric Muscle

The digastric muscle is one of the suprahyoid muscles comprised of two bellies. The posterior belly of the digastric muscle is longer than the anterior belly and arises from the mastoid notch of the mastoid process of the temporal bone (Figure 12-1). It is deep to the attachments of the longissimus capitis, splenius capitis, and sternocleidomastoid muscles. The anterior belly arises from the digastric fossa at the base of the mandible, close to its symphysis. The anterior belly travels posteriorly and inferiorly toward the hyoid; the posterior belly passes anteriorly and inferiorly to be united end-to-end by a common tendon that usually attaches indirectly to the hyoid bone (at the greater cornu) through a fibrous loop or sling, called the suprahyoid aponeurosis.[1-3] In some cases, the tendon can be lined by a synovial sheath or may lack an intermediate tendon. The common tendon may slide through the fibrous loop.[1,4] The tendon common to the two bellies of the digastric muscle perforates the stylohyoid muscle, which lies near the front half of the posterior belly of the digastric muscle.[2,5]

Anatomic variations of the anterior belly of the digastric muscle have been reported in the literature including atypical fibers,[5] bilateral superficial and deep heads of the muscle with associated accessory heads of the muscle arranged in a weave pattern,[6] and accessory heads fusing at midline without a weave pattern.[7]

Suprahyoid Muscles

The other suprahyoid muscles (Figure 12-2) include the stylohyoid, mylohyoid, geniohyoid, and hyoglossus muscles, all of which have their inferior attachment directly to the hyoid bone. The stylohyoid muscle attaches distally to the greater cornu of the hyoid bone[1] and attaches proximally to the styloid process of the temporal bone. The mylohyoid muscle attaches distally to the anterior lower border of hyoid bone and median raphe[3] and proximally to the entire length of the mylohyoid line of the mandible. The geniohyoid muscle attaches distally to the anterior surface of the body of the hyoid and proximally deep to the mylohyoid muscle at the inferior mental spine at the back of the symphysis menti.[1,2] Distally, the hyoglossus muscle attaches along the entire length of the inferior border of the hyoid bone over the greater cornu. It then passes almost vertically upward and enters the side of the tongue.[1,2]

Infrahyoid Muscles

The infrahyoid muscles (Figure 12-2) include the sternohyoid, thyrohyoid, sternothyroid, and omohyoid muscles, all of which have their proximal attachment to the hyoid bone, except the sternothyroid muscle. The sternohyoid muscle attaches to the posterior surface of the medial end of the clavicle, posterior sternoclavicular ligament, and upper posterior aspect of the manubrium distally. Proximally, it attaches to the inferior border of the hyoid bone on the posterior surface.[1,2,8]

The thyrohyoid muscle attaches distally to the oblique line on the lamina of the thyroid cartilage. It then passes upward, attaching along two-thirds of the lower border of the greater cornu of the hyoid bone.[1,2,8] This muscle has been regarded as a continuation of the sternothyroid muscle.[1]

The sternothyroid muscle attaches proximally to the oblique line of the thyroid cartilage. Inferiorly, it attaches to the sternum at the posterior surface of the manubrium[1,3] and to the posterior edge of the cartilage of the first rib.[1] It forms a continuum with the thyrohyoid muscle and lies deep and medial to the sternohyoid muscle.[1,8]

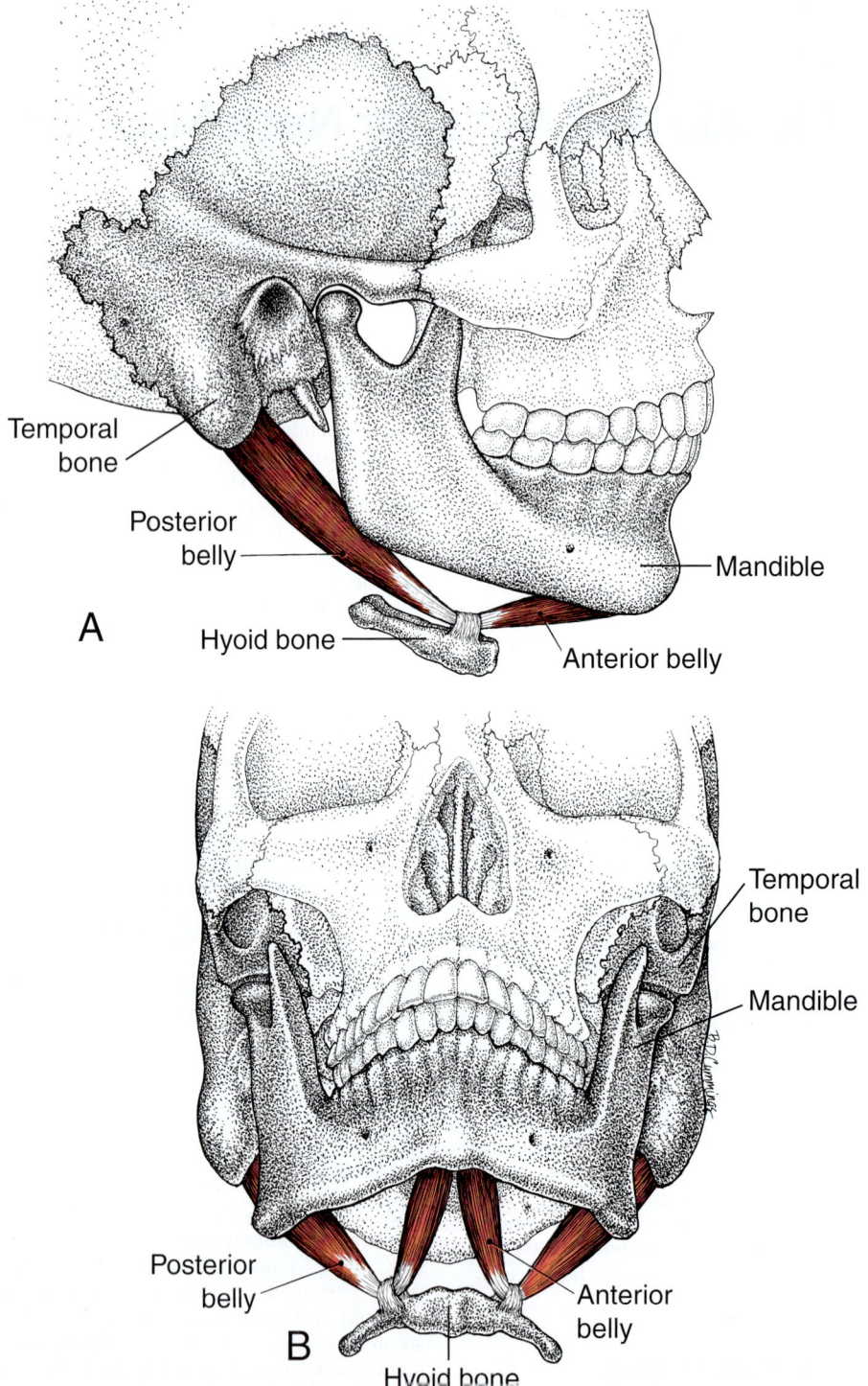

Figure 12-1. Attachments of the digastric muscle. A, Side view. B, Front view. The posterior belly attaches superiorly to the mastoid notch and inferiorly, at the muscle's common tendon, by fascial expansion indirectly to the hyoid bone. The anterior belly attaches superiorly to the mandible at the point of the chin and inferiorly, at the common tendon, by fascial expansion indirectly to the hyoid bone.

Finally, the omohyoid muscle has two bellies, superior and inferior. The superior belly attaches to the transverse process of C6, anterior to the scalenus medius muscle.[1,9] The inferior belly of the omohyoid muscle is separated from the superior belly by a central tendon (held in place by the deep cervical fascia; Figure 12-2). It attaches proximally on the hyoid bone near the border between the body and the greater cornu[2,3]; distally it attaches to the cranial border of the scapula near the scapular notch.[1,3,8] As the inferior belly passes forward and up to its attachment to the central tendon, it attaches to the clavicle by a fibrous expansion and passes diagonally over the middle and anterior scalene muscles but deep to the sternocleidomastoid muscle. The central tendon is held in position by a fibrous expansion of the deep cervical fascia that is prolonged caudally

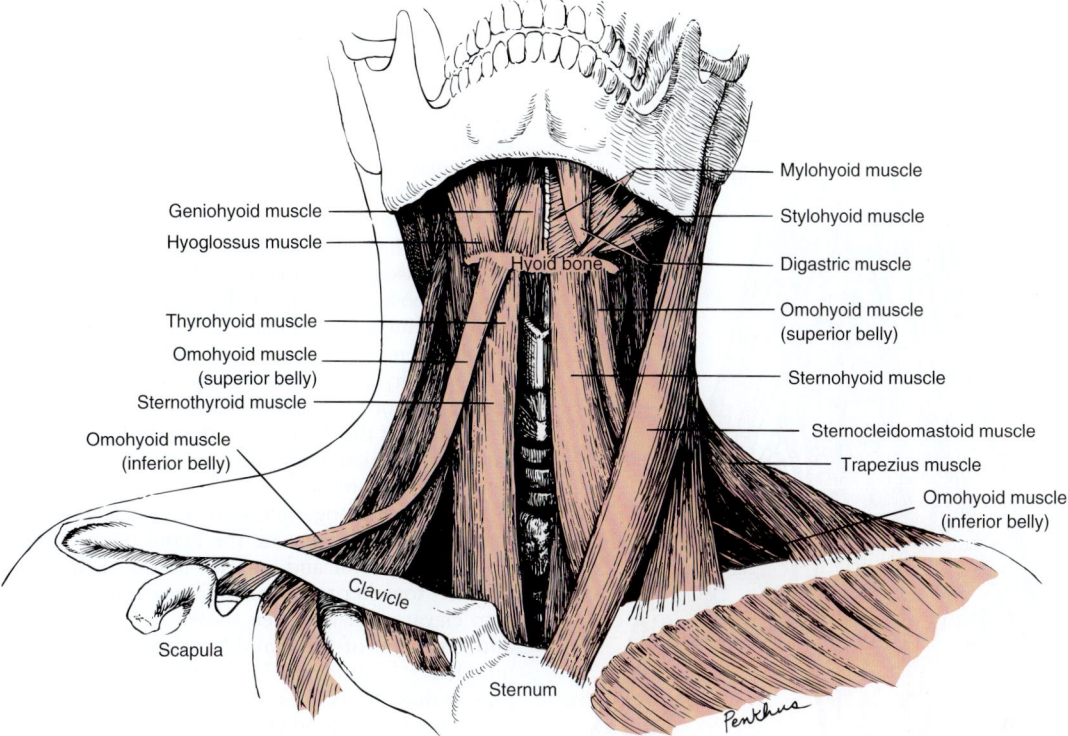

Figure 12-2. Relatively superficial muscles of the anterior neck including the suprahyoid and infrahyoid muscle groups. On the right side of the body, several of the most superficial muscles (the sternocleidomastoid, sternohyoid, and trapezius) have been removed. Reprinted with permission from Clemente CD. *Gray's Anatomy*. 30th ed. Philadelphia, PA: Lea & Febiger; 1985.

to attach to the clavicle and the first rib. From this attachment, the superior belly angles upward to attach to the hyoid bone (Figures 12-2 and 20-7).[1,2] There are three types of attachments of the omohyoid muscle according to its relationship with the sternohyoid muscle. In type 1, the muscle bundle is adjacent to the sternohyoid muscle, in type 2, it enters the sternohyoid muscle, and in type 3, the omohyoid muscle covers the sternohyoid muscle.[2] Anatomic anomalies of the omohyoid muscle have been reported, including the inferior belly of the omohyoid muscle originating directly from the clavicle, the superior belly merging with the stylohyoid muscle, and the presence of a double omohyoid muscle.[9]

Anterior Vertebral Muscles

The deeply placed anterior vertebral muscles are comprised of the longus colli, longus capitis, rectus capitis anterior, and rectus capitis lateralis muscles. They are situated along the anterior surface of the vertebral column (Figure 12-3) and lie directly deep to the posterior wall of the pharynx. The longus colli muscle is divided into three parts, a superior oblique portion, an inferior oblique portion, and a vertical portion. The inferior oblique portion arises from the 1st, 2nd, or 3rd thoracic vertebrae, ascends obliquely in a lateral inclination, and attaches to the anterior tubercles of the transverse process of the 5th and 6th cervical vertebrae. The superior oblique portion arises anteriorly from the transverse process of the 3rd, 4th, or 5th cervical vertebrae, ascends obliquely in a medial inclination, and attaches to the anterolateral surface of the anterior arch of the atlas.[1] The vertical intermediate portion arises from the body of the upper three thoracic and lower three cervical vertebrae and attaches to the body of the 2nd, 3rd, and 4th cervical vertebrae.[1,8] The average cross-sectional area of the longus colli muscle is 0.56 cm^2 ($\pm$0.12 cm).[10]

The longus capitis muscle is more lateral than the longus colli muscle, extending upward from the anterior tubercles of the transverse processes of C3-C6 to the basilar part of the occipital bone.[1,8]

The rectus capitis anterior muscle lies deep to the upper portion of the longus capitis muscle and passes upward and slightly medially from the lateral mass of the atlas to the basilar part of the occipital bone in front of the foramen magnum.[1,8]

The rectus capitis lateralis muscle arises from the superior surface of the transverse process of the atlas and angles laterally and upward to the lateral part of the jugular process of the occipital bone (Figure 12-3).[1,8]

2.1. Innervation and Vascularization

The geniohyoid muscle is innervated by C1 through the hypoglossal nerve.[3] All of the remaining suprahyoid muscles are innervated by cranial nerves. The mylohyoid muscle and the anterior belly of the digastric muscle are supplied by the mylohyoid nerve, a branch of the inferior alveolar nerve originating from the trigeminal (fifth cranial) nerve.[3,11] The stylohyoid muscle and the posterior belly of the digastric muscle are innervated by the facial (seventh cranial) nerve, which exits the skull through the stylomastoid foramen, close to where these muscles attach to the skull.[1] The hyoglossus muscle is innervated by the hypoglossal nerve.[1]

The ansa cervicalis nerves, which are derived from the first, second, and third cervical nerves, supply three of the infrahyoid muscles: the sternohyoid, sternothyroid, and both bellies of the omohyoid muscles.[3,12] The thyrohyoid muscle is innervated by fibers from the first cervical nerve via the hypoglossal nerve.[12]

The rectus capitis anterior and rectus capitis lateralis muscles are innervated by branches from a communicating loop formed between the first and second cervical nerves.[1,13] A secondary innervation for the rectus capitis lateralis and rectus capitis anterior muscles via the hypoglossal nerve has been reported.[14] The longus capitis muscle is innervated by the cervical ventral rami of C1, C2, and C3.[1,13] The longus colli muscle is innervated by the ventral rami of the second through sixth cervical nerves.[1,13]

The anterior digastric muscle receives its vascular supply via the submental branch of the facial artery; the posterior belly

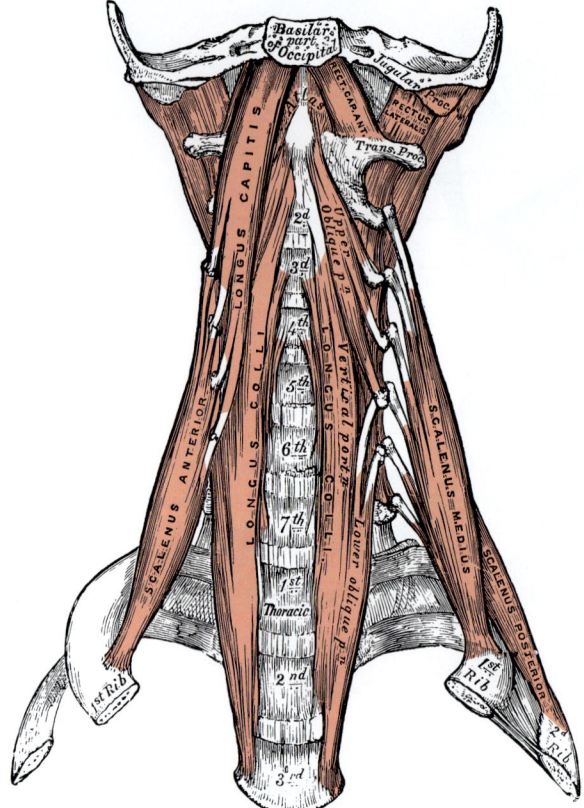

Figure 12-3. The deepest muscles of the anterior neck including the anterior and lateral vertebral muscles. Reprinted with permission from Clemente CD. *Gray's Anatomy*. 30th ed. Philadelphia, PA: Lea & Febiger; 1985.

of the digastric muscle receives its blood supply via the posterior auricular and occipital arteries.[1,3] The vascular supply of the geniohyoid muscle is the lingual artery.[1,15] The stylohyoid muscle receives its blood supply from branches of the occipital, posterior auricular, and facial arteries.[1] The sublingual branch of the lingual artery, the maxillary artery via the mylohyoid branch of the inferior alveolar artery, and the submental branch of the facial artery supply the mylohyoid muscle.[1] The sublingual branch of the lingual artery and the submental branch of the facial artery supply the hyoglossus muscle.[1]

For the infrahyoid muscles, the sternohyoid muscle receives its blood supply from the superior thyroid artery, whereas the sternothyroid, omohyoid, and thyrohyoid muscles receive their vascular supply from both the superior thyroid and lingual arteries.[1,3]

The longus colli muscle receives its vascular supply from the inferior thyroid, ascending pharyngeal, and vertebral arteries.[1] The longus capitis muscle is supplied by the ascending pharyngeal, the ascending cervical branch of the inferior thyroid, and the vertebral arteries.[1] The rectus capitis lateralis muscle receives its vascular supply from the occipital, vertebral, and ascending pharyngeal arteries, whereas the rectus capitis anterior muscle receives its vascular supply from the vertebral and ascending pharyngeal arteries.[1]

2.2. Function

Suprahyoid Muscles

The suprahyoid muscles are involved with jaw opening and are adapted mainly for velocity and displacement.[16] All four of the suprahyoid muscles (Figure 12-2) characteristically function in pairs and as a group to open the mouth.[17] They also work together to fix and elevate the tongue, hyoid bone, and thyroid cartilage[18] and are essential for swallowing.[19]

The digastric muscle functions with mandibular movements as well as with deglutition. The right and left digastric muscles nearly always contract together, not independently.[20] Together, the digastric muscles work to depress the mandible.[1,4] According to Basmajian and Deluca,[20] the anterior belly of the digastric muscle follows that of the inferior belly of the lateral pterygoid muscle. Although the digastric muscle appears to be less important than the lateral pterygoid muscle for initial opening of the jaw, it is essential for maximal depression or forced opening.[20] It is the posterior belly of the digastric muscle that is mainly active during jaw opening.[21] It works closely together with the stylohyoid muscle to open the mouth, but it can only be effective if the infrahyoid muscles contract and stabilize the position of the hyoid bone. Digastric muscle activity is inhibited during depression of the mandible if the mandible is protruded at the same time, which would be expected because of the retraction function of the muscle.

Contracting together, both digastric muscles retract the mandible[1,4,22] and elevate the hyoid bone.[1,4] During deglutition, the posterior and anterior bellies of the digastric muscle contract together to translate force to the hyoid bone, causing it to elevate.[23] It has been shown that coughing, swallowing, and retrusion of the mandible strongly recruit the digastric muscles,[20,24] but it may be the posterior belly of the digastric muscle that assists in oropharyngeal swallowing.[21]

Compared with other muscles of the jaw, the two bellies of the digastric muscle are unusual. The anterior and posterior bellies of the digastric muscle are practically devoid of muscle spindles.[25,26] The lack of muscle spindles in the jaw-opening muscles and the lack of evidence for control of the digastric muscle by the jaw-closing proprioceptors[27] suggest that functionally the jaw-opening muscles do not have a requirement for fine position control. The two bellies of the digastric muscle also have a low percentage of Type I fibers as compared with other muscles.[28] The anterior belly of the digastric muscle comprises a large number of Type IIX fibers, whereas the posterior belly comprises a greater number of Type IIA fibers.[29]

The stylohyoid muscle works to elevate and draw the hyoid bone backward, thereby elongating the floor of the mouth.[1]

The mylohyoid muscle raises the floor of the mouth during swallowing, and is active with mastication, sucking, and blowing. It elevates the hyoid bone anteriorly and superiorly and depresses the mandible.[1,23,30]

The geniohyoid muscle elevates the hyoid bone and draws it forward together with the digastric muscle.[1,20,23] It can also assist in retraction of the mandible, depression of the mandible, and protrusion of the tongue.[1,31]

As a group, the suprahyoid muscles have a larger percentage of Type IIA and IIX fibers (~57%) versus Type I fibers (34.7%). This difference in fibers is well adapted for the phasic activity needed for this muscle group.[32]

Infrahyoid Muscles

As a group, these muscles characteristically function in pairs to exert the essential depressive force on the hyoid bone that is required for the suprahyoid muscles to function normally. The omohyoid, sternothyroid, and sternohyoid muscles depress the larynx after it has been elevated during swallowing or vocal movements, whereas the thyrohyoid muscle elevates the larynx if the hyoid is fixed.[1] The sternohyoid and thyrohyoid muscles form a continuous unit (Figure 12-2) to depress the hyoid bone. The greatest intensity of contraction in the cricothyroid muscle occurs in swallowing.[1] Bilaterally, the omohyoid muscles are thought to be involved in prolonged inspiratory efforts because they tense the lower part of the cervical fascia and lessen the inward suction of soft parts.[1] The superior belly of the omohyoid muscle is also involved in movements of the tongue including placement of the tip of the tongue on soft and hard palates, placement of the tongue on the floor of the mouth, protrusion, and right and left lateral movements.[33]

When swallowing liquids, the anterior belly of the digastric, masseter, and geniohyoid muscles contracts together, whereas when swallowing solids, the masseter muscle contracts first, followed by the anterior belly of the digastric and geniohyoid muscles. When swallowing both solids and liquids, the sternohyoid muscle contracts last.[34] The geniohyoid muscle is primarily responsible for the anterior movement of the hyoid.[19]

The muscle fibers of the infrahyoid muscle group are similar to the suprahyoid muscles in that they are designed more for phasic activity, but the makeup of fiber type is slightly different, with approximately 47% of Type II (A and X fibers) versus 40.8% of Type I fibers.[32]

Anterior Vertebral Muscles

The anterior cervical muscles typically work in pairs to flex all or part of the neck. All portions of the longus colli muscle contribute to neck flexion. The oblique portion also contributes to ipsilateral lateral flexion and the inferior oblique portion rotates the neck to the contralateral side.[1] The longus capitis muscle flexes the head, whereas the rectus capitis lateralis muscle primarily tilts the head ipsilaterally. The rectus capitis anterior muscle flexes the head but does not contribute to ipsilateral tilting of the head. Both the rectus capitis lateralis and the rectus capitis anterior muscles assist in stabilization of the atlanto-occipital joint because of their fibers angling in opposite directions.[1]

The anterior vertebral muscles are thought to be postural in nature; however, recent evidence suggests that the longus colli and longus capitis muscles have both a postural and a phasic role. In elderly women, the average type 1 fiber was found to be 64.3% in the longus capitis and 55.7% in the longus colli muscle.[35] In elderly men, the longus capitis muscle had an average of 48.5% type 1 fibers and the longus colli muscle had 50%.[36] These percentages are notably lower than other known muscles that are tonic in nature, indicating both a tonic role as neck postural stabilizers and a phasic one as neck and head flexors.[37,38] The question whether these muscles are predominantly phasic or tonic is still debated.[39]

2.3. Functional Unit

The functional unit to which a muscle belongs includes the muscles that reinforce and counter their actions as well as the joints that the muscle crosses. The interdependence of these structures functionally is reflected in the organization and neural connections of the sensory motor cortex. The functional unit is emphasized because the presence of a TrP in one muscle of the unit increases the likelihood that the other muscles of the unit will also develop TrPs. When inactivating TrPs in a muscle, one must be concerned about TrPs that may develop in muscles that are functionally interdependent. Box 12-1 grossly represents the functional unit of the digastric and other anterior neck muscles.[40]

During mandibular depression, the infrahyoid muscles work to stabilize the hyoid bone.[41] The temporalis muscle, although a synergist for protrusion, is recruited more strongly with retrusion.[42]

3. CLINICAL PRESENTATIONS

3.1. Referred Pain Pattern

Digastric

There are distinctly different referred pain patterns for the two bellies of the digastric muscle. Trigger points in the posterior belly of the digastric muscle frequently refer pain into the upper portion of the sternocleidomastoid muscle[43] and to a lesser extent to the throat, under the chin, and the occipit[44,45]

Box 12-1 Functional unit of the digastric and other anterior neck muscles

Action	Synergists	Antagonist
Mandibular depression	Lateral pterygoid Stylohyoid Mylohyoid Geniohyoid	Masseter Temporalis Medial pterygoid
Mandibular retrusion	Masseter (deep portion) Temporalis	Lateral pterygoid Medial pterygoid
Hyoid elevation	Geniohyoid Mylohyoid Digastric (anterior belly)	Sternohyoid Sternothyroid Thyrohyoid Omohyoid
Head and neck flexion	Longus colli Longus capitis Rectus capitis anterior Sternocleidomastoid Hyoid muscles	Semispinalis capitis Semispinalis cervicis Splenii capitis Splenii cervicis Cervical multifidi Rectus capitis posterior major Rectus capitis posterior minor

(Figure 12-4A, B). The pain referred to the sternocleidomastoid muscle is sometimes mistaken as originating from that muscle, but when the sternocleidomastoid muscle is cleared of TrPs, the pain persists. The occipital component of pain is likely to be associated with referred "soreness" and tenderness. Trigger points in the posterior belly of the digastric muscle have also been shown to refer pain into the forehead, periorbital area, temple, postauricular area, ear, temporomandibular joint, cheek, mandibular teeth, and throat.[46-49]

Pain from TrPs in the anterior belly of the digastric muscle refers to the lower four incisor teeth (along the mandible), to the alveolar ridge below them (Figure 12-4C), and also to the tongue.[45,47,50] Pain from this belly may also refer to the periorbital area, temporomandibular joint, and cheek area.[47-49]

Clinically, this muscle has also been seen to refer pain along the mandible up toward the temporomandibular joint. Frequently, the TrPs are located in the muscle just under the tip of the chin and can be on either the left or the right side (Figure 12-4C).

Longus Colli

Pain referral patterns of the longus colli muscle have been explored in healthy individuals.[51] Eliciting pain in the longus colli muscle by either dry-needling or manual stimulation of the muscle provokes local pain mainly in the anterior cervical area (Figure 12-4D). Some patients report pain being referred to the posterior ipsilateral neck and around the ipsilateral ear and eye (Figure 12-4E). Interestingly, in some patients, pain originating in the longus colli muscle is referred to the contralateral anterior neck. Although being rather unusual, such contralateral referral has also been described in the adjacent sternocleidomastoid muscle (Figure 12-4D).

Other Anterior Cervical Musculature

The mylohyoid muscle can refer pain to the tongue.[50] In clinical practice, this muscle has also been seen to refer to the ipsilateral occipital region. Head and neck pain from the stylohyoid muscle is closely related to that arising from the posterior belly of the digastric muscle.[52] These two muscles lie close together, have

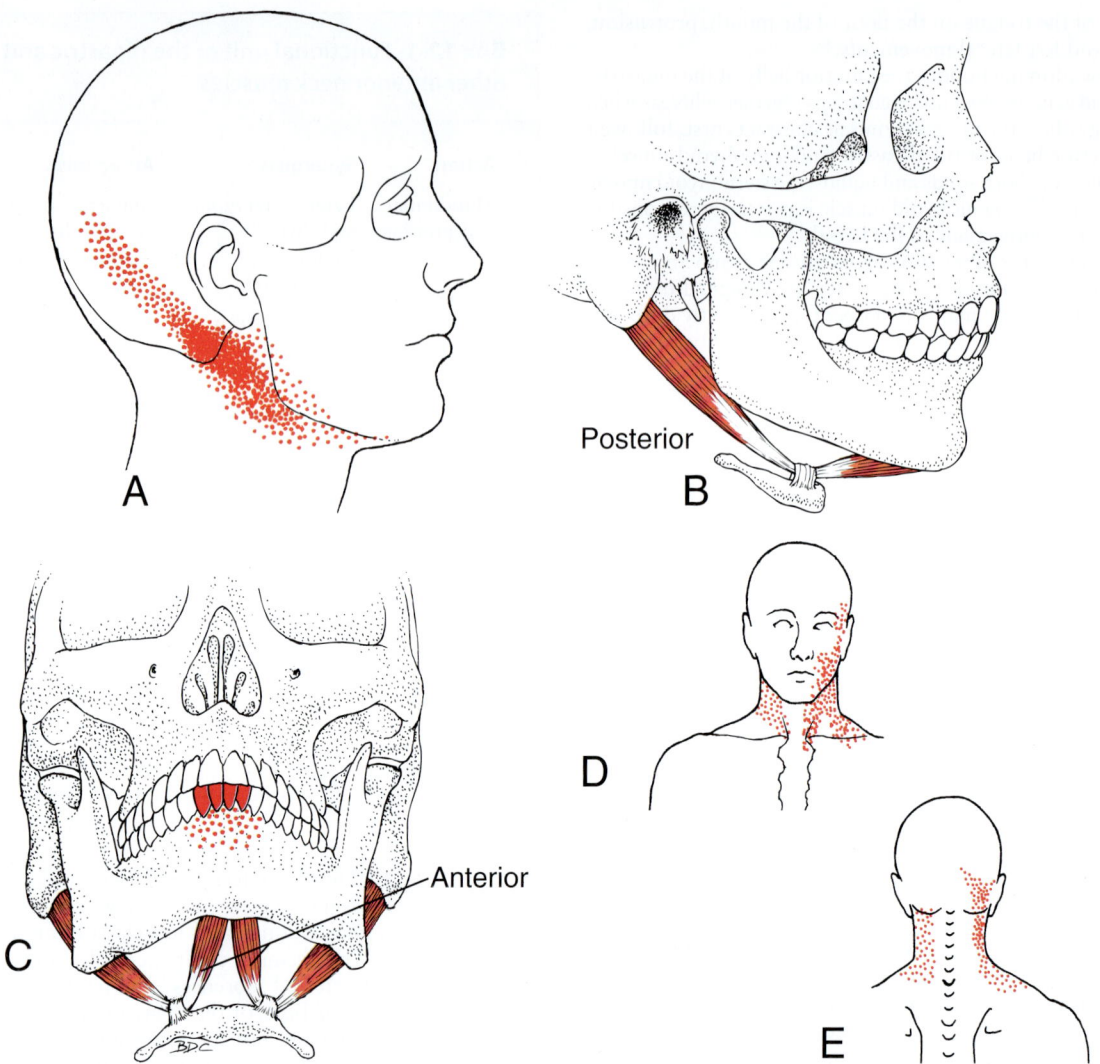

Figure 12-4. Referred pain patterns of TrPs in the digastric and longus colli muscles. A and B, Posterior belly of the digastric muscle. C, Anterior belly of the digastric muscle. D, Longus colli muscle, anterior view. E, Longus colli muscle, posterior view.

similar functions, are difficult to distinguish by palpation, and are presumed to have similar pain patterns.

The specific pain patterns of the remaining deep anterior neck muscles are not reported in the literature.[51] However, it has been demonstrated that the longus capitis and longus colli muscles have decreased activity when active nociception is present.[53] These muscles can refer pain to the laryngeal region, anterior neck, and sometimes into the mouth region.

3.2. Symptoms

It is hypothesized that unresolved posterior neck pain might result from sustained TrPs of the anterior neck muscles and tightening of their fasciae. If a patient has posterior digastric TrPs, the primary report may not be of pain but of difficulty swallowing, a sensation of a lump in the throat, and/or something being stuck in the throat and not going down. The patient is likely to palpate or point to the sternocleidomastoid muscle on the involved side. Although head rotation range of motion may not be reduced, the patient is likely to avoid turning the head to the involved side because the movement will elicit referred pain or aggravate the swallowing problem. The posterior digastric muscle referred pain pattern, as shown in Figure 12-4A, concentrates in the region of the superior part of the sternocleidomastoid muscle, as well as the cheek (closer to the angle of the mandible) and ear.[45] As a result of the overlap of the digastric muscle referred pain with other areas, the patient may not become aware of the digastric muscle referred pain component until after concurrent sternocleidomastoid TrPs on the same side have been inactivated, and the pain in that region still persists. This development can be very perplexing to the clinician unless the possibility of posterior digastric TrPs is investigated.

The chief symptom from TrPs in the anterior belly of the digastric muscle is pain in the region of the lower incisor teeth. The source of this tooth pain can also be confusing if the clinician considers only the teeth as the source of pain and does not consider the anterior digastric muscle. Patients with TrPs in the anterior digastric muscle may also report pain in the cheek and temporomandibular joint.[45]

There are no specific pain referral patterns reported in the literature for the omohyoid muscle; however, loosening of the intermediate tendon of the omohyoid muscle may lead to pseudodysphagia.[54] When the omohyoid muscle develops TrPs, it can act as a constricting band across the brachial plexus.[55] Adson[56] relieved pain and dysesthesia resulting from pressure on the brachial plexus because of abnormal tension in the omohyoid muscle by surgically sectioning the muscle. Rask[57] reported the diagnosis and treatment of four patients whose primary cause of pain was myofascial TrPs in this muscle.

Patients with TrPs in the longus capitis and/or longus colli muscles are likely to report difficulty with swallowing and/or having a lump in the throat. Patients with centralized posterior cervical pain should also be evaluated for TrPs in the longus colli muscle. When these symptoms occur in a person who has sustained a cervical flexion-extension injury ("whiplash") from a rear-end motor vehicle accident or any other head/neck trauma, longus colli TrPs are likely to be a contributing factor. Rocabado and Iglarsh[58] reported that patients with a "spasm" in the longus colli muscle reported symptoms of a dry mouth, a sore throat without infection, a persistent tickle in the throat, or a lump in the throat with swallowing. Further, recent studies that demonstrate an increase in fatty infiltrates of the longus colli and longus capitis muscles after whiplash injury may be a contributor of neck pain.[59] In cases of patients with temporomandibular dysfunction, vertical mandibular opening can be reduced in patients with decreased deep cervical flexor strength.[60]

3.3. Patient Examination

After a thorough subjective examination, the clinician should make a detailed drawing representing the pain pattern that the patient has described. This depiction will assist in planning the physical examination and can be useful in monitoring the progression of the patient as symptoms improve or change. Cervical range of motion assessment should include measurements in each direction and observation of the quality of motion, which can assist in determining range of motion restrictions at the atlanto-occipital and atlanto-axial region, mid and lower cervical spine. Any deviations in cervical flexion or extension, as well as any changes in C curvature into lateral flexion need to be further evaluated with assessment of the surrounding soft tissue and joint accessory mobility. A shortened longus colli muscle may present as a straightening of the physiologic cervical lordosis. Joint mobility and range of motion of the thoracic spine should also be examined.

The hyoid bone is a very important structure to evaluate as it may influence the curvature of the cervical spine,[61] movements of the mandible, swallowing, and sound formation in speech.[58] Trigger points in the suprahyoid and/or infrahyoid muscles can influence the position of the hyoid, creating dysfunction in the anterior neck musculature. The easiest and most clinically applicable way to evaluate the hyoid bone is with the clinician manually assessing the hyoid for free movement laterally in both directions. The hyoid can also be assessed with a cephalometric examination technique looking at the hyoid triangle.[62] With this measurement three lines are drawn: one from C3 to the most inferior/posterior portion of the symphysis menti (retrognathion, RGN), one from C3 to the hyoid, and one from the hyoid to the RGN. A normal vertical position of hyoid bone is below the line of the C3 and RGN.

Recognition of muscle balance is always important, especially between the suprahyoid and infrahyoid muscles because the hyoid bone is "floating" between them. The concept of inhibited and facilitated muscles contributing to imbalance[63] is widely accepted. The digastric muscle has been identified as being prone to weakness and inhibition[64]; as a result, this can have an effect on the antagonistic muscles, other suprahyoid muscles, and infrahyoid muscles.

Examination of the strength of the longus capitis and longus colli muscles is critical for all cervical spine and/or temporomandibular disorders. Research has demonstrated a high correlation between impaired activation of these muscles and neck pain, as well as impaired postural endurance.[65-67] The craniocervical flexion test assesses the strength of the longus colli, longus capitis, rectus capitis lateralis, and rectus capitis anterior muscles. This test has been shown to have moderate to good interrater reliability and good to excellent intrarater reliability.[68,69] The test has the patient perform a chin tuck and lift the head about 2.5 cm off the plinth. The patient is timed on how long they can hold the chin tuck position.[68] The average hold time for women is 38.43 seconds; men have an average hold time of 63.73 seconds.[68] The test can also be performed using a pressure sensor (blood pressure cuff/Chattanooga stabilizer). The patient starts at 20 mm Hg, holding a cranial nod for 5 to 10 seconds. The pressure is increased by 2 mm Hg (up to 30 mm Hg), with the cranial nod being repeated until the patient cannot perform the test without compensation that may be seen in either a loss of neutral position or increased activation of the scalene and/or sternocleidomastoid muscles.[70-72]

3.4. Trigger Point Examination

The muscles of the anterior cervical spine are particularly small, making it challenging to palpate for TrPs. A thorough understanding of the anatomy of this area is crucial to ensure the clinician is palpating tissues accurately.

The anterior and posterior bellies of the digastric muscle can be indirectly assessed by feeling for abnormal resistance when the hyoid bone is shifted from side to side. Oftentimes, decreased mobility of the hyoid bone to one side implicates involvement of the digastric muscle on the contralateral side.

The posterior belly of the digastric muscle is specifically examined with the patient supine and the head and chin tipped upward, in order to widen the area for palpation between the neck and the angle of the mandible (Figure 12-5A). The muscle is located behind the angle of the mandible[73] and is found by sliding the finger upward toward the ear lobe along the anterior border of the sternocleidomastoid muscle, pressing the finger inward against the underlying neck muscles.[45] To confirm identification of the muscle, light resistance of jaw opening is applied with the clinician's nonpalpating hand just under the chin. A thin, soft, rope-like muscle is felt with the contraction. A cross-fiber flat palpation technique with the tip of the finger is then performed to identify TrPs. Initial pressure on TrPs in the posterior belly elicits exquisite local tenderness, and sustained pressure may reproduce the patient's referred neck and head pain. The anterior belly of the digastric muscle is examined with the patient supine, the head tilted back, and the neck extended (Figure 12-5B). To identify the muscle, the clinician's finger is placed just beneath the point of the chin on either side medial to the inferior border of the mandible.[45] Again, light resistance of jaw opening is applied with the clinician's nonpalpating hand just under the chin. Under the palpating finger, a thin, soft, rope-like muscle is felt with the contraction. The muscle is then palpated from the mandible to the hyoid with a cross-fiber flat palpation to identify any TrPs.

One test for anterior digastric TrP involvement as a source of lower incisor tooth pain is to ask the patient to pull the corners of the mouth down vigorously enough to tense the anterior neck muscles. This "Anterior Digastric Test" activates the toothache when positive, indicating the likelihood of TrPs in the anterior belly of at least one digastric muscle.

The omohyoid muscle is easily mistaken for the upper trapezius muscle or a scalene muscle because the tense muscle stands out prominently when the head is tilted to the contralateral side. Because of blending of this muscle with other infrahyoid muscles, it is difficult to palpate and distinguish. General tenderness below the hyoid near the greater cornu and along the anterior/medial scalene muscle may be due to TrPs from the omohyoid muscle. If the inferior belly of the omohyoid muscle has a TrP, it can be mistaken for the anterior scalene muscle, although the two muscles have different fiber directions. The omohyoid muscle is more superficial than the scalene muscles, as it comes out from beneath the sternocleidomastoid muscle, and crosses diagonally over the anterior scalene muscle (see Figure 20-7). It can cross at about the same level as the location where scalene TrPs can be found, depending on which scalene muscle digitation is involved and the position of the head.

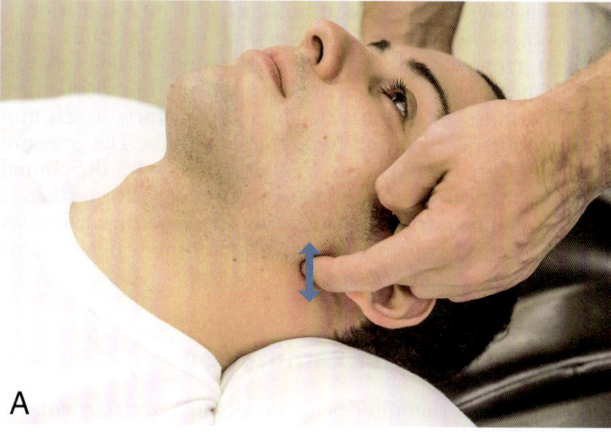
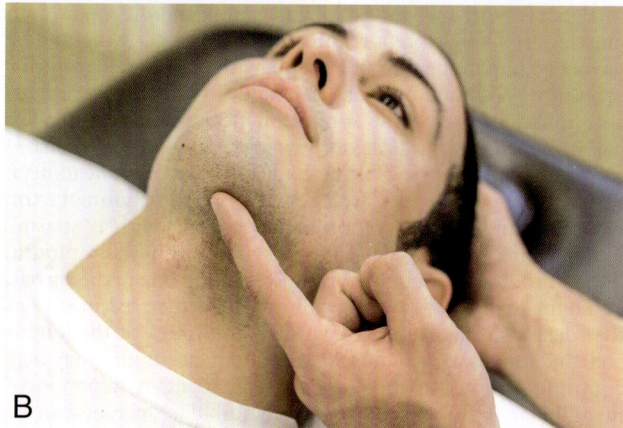
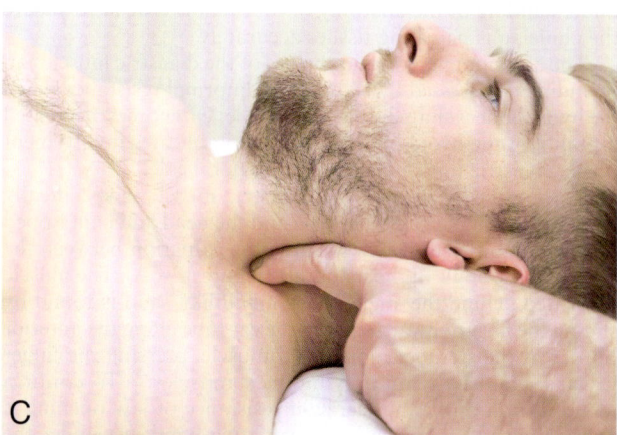

Figure 12-5. Examination of the digastric muscle. A, Posterior belly: palpated between the angle of the jaw and the mastoid process, against the underlying neck structures. B, Anterior belly: the head is tilted back and the neck extended, with the jaw closed, to stretch the muscle as it is palpated against the underlying soft tissues, as described in the text. C, Examination of the longus colli muscle using cross-fiber flat palpation.

Trigger points in the longus capitis muscle can be palpated behind the posterior pharyngeal wall through the open mouth. Trigger points in the longus colli muscle can be palpated by placing the examining finger along the lateral border of the trachea between the sternocleidomastoid muscle and the thyroid cartilage[58] and slowly advancing it by separating the musculature from the adjacent trachea by gentle rocking and wiggling motions of the finger. When the finger encounters the vertebral column, that region is explored for TrPs with a cross-fiber flat palpation. Another possible approach to palpation of the longus colli muscle is performed with the patient in the supine position; the 2nd and 3rd fingers of the clinician are slid posterior to the sternocleidomastoid and anterior to the easily palpable cervical transverse processes (Figure 12-5C). The muscle is then palpated in a cephalad-caudal direction.

4. DIFFERENTIAL DIAGNOSIS

4.1. Activation and Perpetuation of Trigger Points

A posture or activity that activates a TrP, if not corrected, can also perpetuate it. In any of the anterior neck muscles, TrPs may be activated by unaccustomed eccentric loading, eccentric exercise in an unconditioned muscle, or maximal or submaximal concentric loading.[74] Trigger points may also be activated or aggravated when the muscle is placed in a shortened and/or lengthened position for an extended period of time. Specifically, bruxing, gum chewing, and mandible retrusion can predispose the digastric muscles to activation of TrPs. Poor stabilization and control of the head and neck when performing abdominal exercises can also put excessive load on the anterior neck muscles.

Flexion-extension injuries, such as those sustained in motor vehicle accidents, or mechanical trauma, such as choking or blunt trauma, can activate TrPs in the suprahyoid, infrahyoid, longus colli, and longus capitis muscles. These injuries are typical in patients who have fallen backward.[51] Furthermore, forward head posture can then perpetuate these TrPs.[70] It has been demonstrated that the longus capitis and longus colli muscles exhibit larger amounts of fatty infiltrate in patients with whiplash-associated disorders[59] along with a decrease in muscle activity of the deep neck flexors and an increase in activity in the superficial neck flexors, such as the sternocleidomastoid muscle. Javanshir et al[75] found that the longus colli muscle exhibited smaller bilateral cross-sectional area in subjects with bilateral chronic neck pain as compared with healthy controls. It is unknown whether the changes are primary or secondary; however, fatty infiltration could be associated with muscle performance impairments,[76] whereas reduction in cross-sectional area could reduce the proprioception output of the neck flexors and contribute to the perpetuation of TrPs.[77,78]

Trigger points may also be activated when the muscle is placed in a shortened or lengthened position for an extended period of time (eg, excessive chin tuck position or forward head posture, respectively). Although it is thought that forward head posture indirectly induces tension in the supra- and infrahyoid muscles, which can create light tensile forces on the mandible,[79] recent studies report conflicting evidence regarding the activity of the suprahyoid muscles in this position. Song et al[80] demonstrated decreased EMG activity of the suprahyoid and infrahyoid muscles in those with a forward head posture compared to those with a normal head posture, whereas Ohmure et al[81] demonstrated that EMG activity of the digastric muscles is slightly increased with forward head posture.

Mouth breathing, versus nasal breathing, has also been shown to have a negative impact on posture,[82-87] which can resultantly contribute to a stretch weakness of the suprahyoid and infrahyoid muscles. Mouth breathing may result from mechanical blockage (such as nasal polyps), structural distortion of the nasal passages (deviated septum), sinusitis, or recurrent allergic rhinitis.

Sustained activation of the posterior belly of the digastric and stylohyoid muscles can overload, and therefore contribute to activation of TrPs in, the antagonistic fibers of the contralateral posterior temporalis muscle and the contralateral deep division of the masseter muscle. Tautness of these antagonists may potentially balance the mandibular deviation induced by the digastric muscles. If the contralateral muscles are cleared of TrPs, the mandible is then free to deviate to the side of the affected posterior belly of the digastric muscle. If deviation is due solely to posterior digastric TrPs, the mandible is pulled over as the jaw starts to separate, but with further opening, it returns to the midline.

4.2. Associated Trigger Points

Trigger points rarely appear in the anterior neck musculature alone. Commonly, patients will also have TrPs in the upper trapezius, temporalis, and semispinalis capitis muscles. Those with jaw pain will also have TrPs in the muscles of mastication and sternocleidomastoid muscle. In Eagle syndrome, because the posterior digastric and stylohyoid muscles are likely to have TrPs, the longus colli muscle will likely be involved. Those with neck pain will commonly have TrPs in the splenius capitis, splenius cervicis, suboccipitals, levator scapulae, sternocleidomastoid, upper trapezius, temporalis, and deep masseter muscles.

Trigger points can develop in the referred pain areas of primary TrPs[88]; therefore, TrPs in the digastric muscle can be due to primary TrPs in other muscles including the platysma, medial pterygoid, trapezius, and sternocleidomastoid muscles. Hong found that primary TrPs in the sternocleidomastoid muscle could induce associated TrPs in the digastric muscle.[89] Primary TrPs of the posterior digastric muscle may also contribute to associated TrPs in the occipital portion of the occipitofrontalis muscle and/or the sternocleidomastoid muscle.

4.3. Associated Pathology

Some medical conditions give rise to symptoms that can appear confusingly similar to those produced by TrPs of the anterior neck muscles or may be present concurrently. Additionally, several muscles of the anterior neck are susceptible to rare conditions, of which the examining clinician must be aware. One must bear in mind that although myofascial syndrome is a very common source of pain in the cervical area, in a minority of the cases it may be secondary to other pathologic processes, such as malignancy or infection. Secondary myofascial syndrome is common in patients suffering from head and neck tumors or infectious diseases involving the cervical lymph nodes. In patients with cancer, secondary myofascial pain may develop as a consequence of irritation or direct invasion of muscles by the tumor or as an iatrogenic side effect of irradiation, chemotherapy, or surgery.[90,91]

Dental disease, earaches, and glossodynia may be, or appear to be, a primary medical condition. However, if examination or diagnostic testing does not provide conclusive results, TrPs in the digastric muscles should be considered as a source of the symptoms because they can refer to the teeth, ear, and throat.[48,49]

Currently, no neurologic entrapments are attributed to TrP activity of the anterior neck musculature; however, Paraskevas et al[92] found one case where branches from the ansa cervicalis loop perforated the inferior belly of the omohyoid muscle. This could potentially contribute to symptoms associated with entrapment, if restrictions of the omohyoid muscle were present. Evidence of instances of blood vessel entrapment does exist. Loch et al[93] reported that among 85 anatomic specimens they found 7 cases of compression of the external carotid artery (in some cases including the posterior auricular artery) solely by the stylohyoid muscle without ossification of the styloid process. The omohyoid muscle has also been noted as a possible cause of internal jugular vein entrapment in two reported cases.[94,95]

There are two types of benign tumors that have been found in the anterior neck muscles, intramuscular hemangiomas and lipomas. Intramuscular hemangiomas are benign vascular tumors that occur in skeletal muscles. Compared to cutaneous hemangiomas, these are incredibly rare. Of those that occur, however, 13% to 15% develop in the head and neck region.[96,97] They vary in pain intensity, are nonmobile, nonpulsatile masses that can be difficult to diagnosis, and are best identified by magnetic resonance imaging.[98] Although they are most commonly seen in the masseter and upper trapezius muscles, a few cases have also been reported in the anterior neck muscles. There have been at least six cases of intramuscular hemangiomas in the digastric muscle[96,99-103]: two in the mylohyoid muscle[97,104] and one reported occurrence each in the geniohyoid, sternohyoid, and thyrohyoid muscles.[105-107] Lipomas are benign soft tissue tumors and have been found in the longus colli muscle at least twice.[108] If needed, these tumors are easily removed surgically.

Treatment for cancer of the head or neck, such as floor of the mouth cancer, can damage or change the tissue quality of the muscles in the anterior neck. Atrophy and soft tissue fibrosis of the omohyoid, digastric, sternohyoid, and sternothyroid muscles can occur after radiotherapy.[109]

Myositis ossificans is a rare condition where heterotopic bone or cartilage forms in muscle tissue after trauma or inflammation.[110,111] This condition rarely occurs in the head and neck region, with only 52 reported cases since 1924.[111] In the head and neck region, the masseter muscle is most commonly affected; however, one case involving the omohyoid muscle after physical trauma and one case involving the platysma muscle after a radical neck dissection have been reported.[110]

Myositis is benign inflammatory pseudotumor of the skeletal muscles that is painful and can limit movement.[112] When found in the upper neck it may also be called retropharyngeal calcific tendinitis.[113] In the anterior neck muscles, it can cause headaches, neck stiffness, and neck pain that can easily mimic TrPs. It is more common to find in the extremities, but Horowitz et al[114] found the rate of incidence to be 0.50 cases per 100,000 person-years for retropharyngeal calcific tendinitis of the longus colli muscle. There has also been one case reported in both the mylohyoid and sternohyoid muscles.[112,115]

Dystonia is a movement disorder characterized by intermittent or sustained muscle contractions that typically cause repetitive, abnormal movements and/or postures.[116] Oromandibular dystonia involves the masticatory, pharyngeal, and lingual muscles. Abnormal movements associated with this condition include jaw-closing, jaw-opening, jaw lateral deviation, or a combination of abnormal movements. The anterior belly of the digastric muscle is commonly involved with the jaw-opening form of oromandibular dystonia.[117] Three reported cases of this type of dystonia have been misdiagnosed in the literature as having temporomandibular joint dysfunction.[118,119] Hyoid dystonia is a subphenotype of craniocervical dystonia. With this condition, there is visible contraction of the hyoid muscles and inappropriate lowering or elevation of the larynx with speech or at rest. Commonly, it causes changes in speech, dysphagia, and tightness of the anterior neck instead of the typical abnormal movements and postures.[120] Cervical dystonia is the most common form of a primary focal dystonia.[121] There are several different types of cervical dystonia, of which a few can involve muscles of the anterior cervical spine. Anterocollis causes flexion of the cervical spine.[122] Although the sternocleidomastoid muscle is most frequently involved,[123] recently, the longus colli muscle has also been shown to be involved.[121,122,124] Anterocaput causes flexion of the head, with the longus capitis and longus colli muscles both being involved.[122] A posterior sagittal shift causes retraction of the chin, a posterior shift of the head in the sagittal plane, and can involve the longus colli and suprahyoid muscles.[125]

Omohyoid muscle syndrome is a rare condition where there is a protruding lateral neck mass when swallowing. Common reports include pseudodysphagia, neck discomfort, cosmetic problems, and concern for malignancy. Possible causes of this syndrome include failure of the omohyoid muscle to lengthen because of muscle fiber degeneration and failure of the facial-retaining mechanism of the muscle.[54]

Sternohyoid muscle syndrome can easily be confused with omohyoid muscle syndrome because the symptoms are very similar. Only two reported cases of this condition are in the literature, with symptoms including a lateral neck mass with swallowing, dysphagia with pain, and a sensation of a foreign body in the throat without aspiration or choking difficulties. Neck computed tomography confirmed abnormalities of the sternohyoid muscle.[126]

Eagle syndrome is a condition where the styloid process is elongated or there is calcification of the stylohyoid ligament. Signs and symptoms vary greatly but may include pain in the angle of the jaw, tongue pain, glossodynia, dysphagia, odynophagia, dysphonia, a sensation of increased salivation, foreign body sensation in the throat, voice changes, persistent pain radiating to the carotid artery, headache, neck pain, pain with turning of the head, pain radiating to the eye, blurring or decreased vision, ear pain, or vertigo.[127-130] The symptoms are related to irritation of cranial nerves V,[127,130] VII,[127,130] IX,[127,128,130] X,[127-130] XI,[129,130] and XII[128-130] because of their proximity of the styloid process or stylohyoid ligament. Diagnosis of this condition can be performed with intraoral palpation of the styloid process in the tonsillar fossa,[129-131] as well as three-dimensional computed tomography[128,129,131] or panoramic radiographs.[129,130] With this condition, involvement of the posterior belly of the digastric, stylohyoid, mylohyoid, sternocleidomastoid, and longus colli muscles should also be examined because they are commonly involved with this condition and can also contribute to some of the associated symptoms.

Other diagnoses may be present concurrently with digastric or anterior neck TrPs. For the digastric muscle, this may include headaches or temporomandibular joint internal derangements with or without reduction. For the anterior neck muscles, concurrent diagnoses include chronic or mechanical neck pain, tension-type headaches, whiplash-associated disorders, and upper quadrant pain. Trigger points in the splenii muscles have also been associated with these conditions,[132-137] and because the anterior neck muscles are antagonistic to the splenii muscles, these conditions should also be considered with the anterior neck muscles.

Understanding the clinical presentation of cervical pain is complicated by the similarity of symptoms arising from joint and muscle pathology. Trigger points in the longus colli, longus capitis, rectus capitis anterior, and rectus capitis lateralis muscles can mimic joint restrictions in the upper cervical spine. The interdependence of joint mobility and muscles makes it difficult to determine if it is a primary capsular problem or a muscle problem, but involvement of the upper neck flexors should be considered when range of motion of the upper cervical spine is restricted and/or painful.

5. CORRECTIVE ACTIONS

Similar to the other neck muscles, addressing posture is essential when anterior neck TrPs are present. Forward head posture and tongue position should always be corrected when identified as a problem. Instruction in good body mechanics and ergonomics is also essential (refer Chapter 76).

Care should be taken to find the proper corrective lenses to ensure the patient maintains a neutral head posture while viewing a digital screen. The use of bifocals or progressive lenses should be discouraged to reduce the repetitive motion used to try and focus on the information on the screen. If two or more computer monitors are being used simultaneously, they should be centered around the user so that the center of the whole viewing area is directly in front of the user instead of one monitor directly in front of the patient and the other to the side. It may also be helpful to angle the screens in a V or U shape to decrease the amount of cervical rotation and eye movement needed to see all screens. Chair size should also be evaluated because most

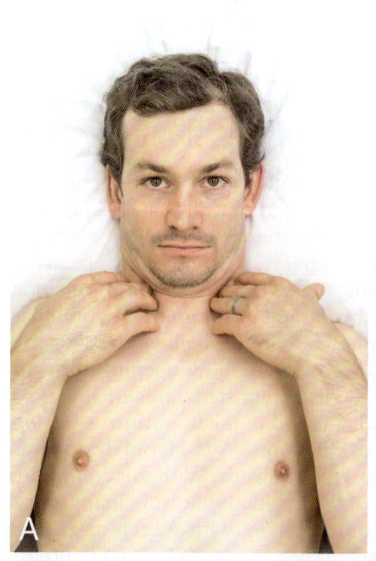
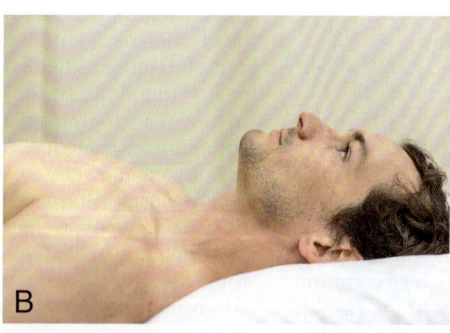
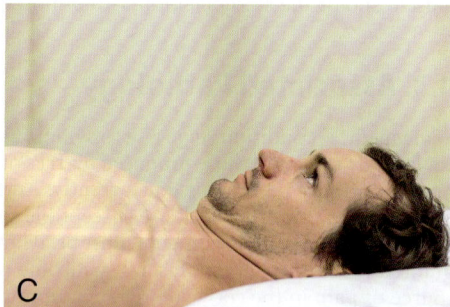
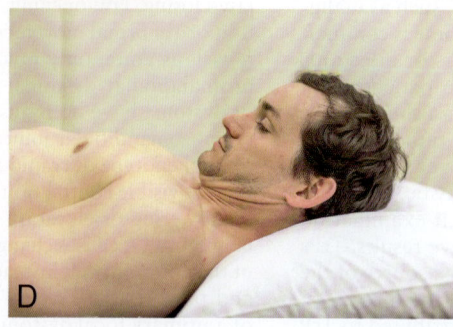

Figure 12-6. Activation of the deep neck flexors. A, To monitor the activity of the sternocleidomastoid muscle, the patient can place their fingers on the muscle to monitor activity. B and C, In the supine position, the patient performs a small forward nod of the head without initial or excessive activity of the sternocleidomastoid muscle. D, Exercise may be progressed to a head lift while maintaining the head nod.

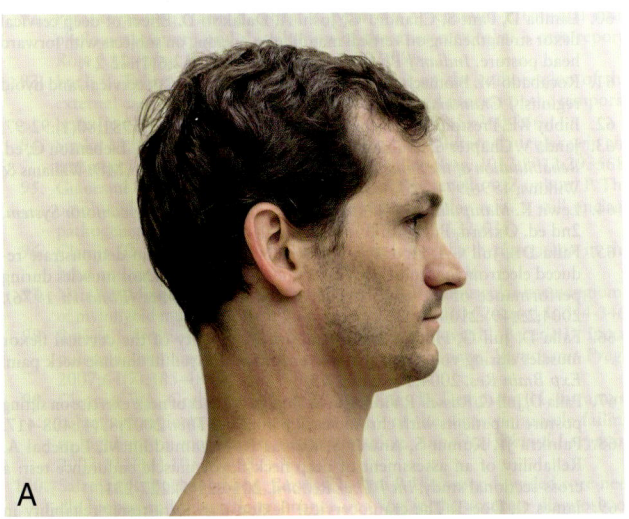 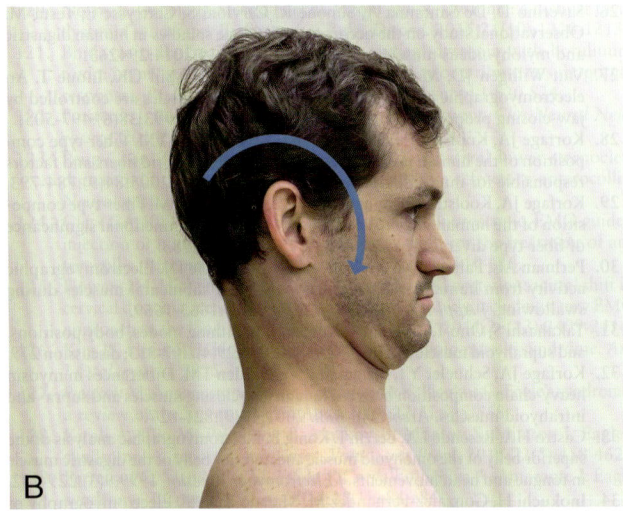

Figure 12-7. Activation of deep neck flexors in the seated position. A, Starting position. B, Ending position.

chairs are designed for an average sized man, thereby causing compensations in posture for individuals who are not this size.

Trigger points have been shown to develop with 1 hour of typing,[138] so short breaks every 20 or 30 minutes could help reduce TrP formation during computer work. Setting an interval timer or starting to integrate a quick stand break whenever a specific routine task is performed, such as answering the phone, can help to increase motion without interrupting the train of thought. Using a footrest or a standing desk can also encourage more movement.

Proper breathing is also important to assist with postural training, decrease bruxism, and help decrease muscle imbalances associated with those who have sleep apnea and dysphasia. Patients should be trained in naso-diaphragmatic breathing instead of mouth breathing because mouth breathing has a negative impact on posture.[82-87] Mouth breathing favors depression and retrusion of the mandible, causing activation and shortening of the digastric muscles. This can lead to malocclusion and an elevated hyoid bone position, changing the myoelectric properties of the hyoid musculature. Performing strengthening exercises on an exercise ball and stretches in conjunction with naso-diaphragmatic breathing has been shown to improve posture.[86]

Because decreased EMG activity and atrophy of the anterior neck muscles have been seen in a number of conditions including whiplash disorder and chronic neck pain, strengthening is appropriate. The patient should lie in the supine position while performing a forward nod of the head without excessive use of the sternocleidomastoid muscle (Figure 12-6). This exercise can be progressed to lifting the head while maintaining the nod and trying to hold that position for 5 to 10 seconds (Figure 12-6D). This exercise can also be performed in the seated position (Figure 12-7) during functional activities. Pain should be avoided with these exercises.[139-142]

To improve the tone of the suprahyoid muscles, the tip of the tongue can be pressed to the center of the hard palate, holding it for 2 seconds. This can be repeated for 3 sets of 10 repetitions.[143]

Chilling the skin of the neck, especially when the muscles are fatigued, often activates TrPs in anterior neck muscles. The patient should keep the neck warm, when possible, by sleeping in a high-necked sleep shirt, by wearing a turtleneck or scarf during the day, and by avoiding cold drafts.

References

1. Standring S. *Gray's Anatomy: The Anatomical Basis of Clinical Practice.* 41st ed: London, UK: Elsevier; 2015.
2. Sonoda N, Tamatsu Y. Observation on the attachment of muscles onto the hyoid bone in human adults. *Okajimas Folia Anat Jpn.* 2008;85(3):79-90.
3. Kohan EJ, Wirth GA. Anatomy of the neck. *Clin Plast Surg.* 2014;41(1):1-6.
4. Prendergast PM. *Facial Anatomy. Advanced Surgical Facial Rejuvenation.* Berlin, Heidelberg: Springer; 2012.
5. Ozgur Z, Govsa F, Celik S, Ozgur T. An unreported anatomical finding: unusual insertions of the stylohyoid and digastric muscles. *Surg Radiol Anat.* 2010;32(5):513-517.
6. Harvey JA, Call Z, Peterson K, Wisco JJ. Weave pattern of accessory heads to the anterior digastric muscle. *Surg Radiol Anat.* 2015;37(8):1001-1004.
7. Yamazaki Y, Shibata M, Ushiki T, Isokawa K, Sato N. Bilateral, asymmetric anomalies of the anterior bellies of digastric muscles. *J Oral Sci.* 2011;53(4):523-527.
8. Borst J, Forbes PA, Happee R, Veeger DH. Muscle parameters for musculoskeletal modelling of the human neck. *Clin Biomech (Bristol, Avon).* 2011;26(4):343-351.
9. Rai R, Ranade A, Nayak S, Vadgaonkar R, Mangala P, Krishnamurthy A. A study of anatomical variability of the omohyoid muscle and its clinical relevance. *Clinics (Sao Paulo).* 2008;63(4):521-524.
10. Mayoux-Benhamou MA, Revel M, Vallee C, Roudier R, Barbet JP, Bargy F. Longus colli has a postural function on cervical curvature. *Surg Radiol Anat.* 1994;16(4):367-371.
11. Thotakura B, Rajendran SS, Gnanasundaram V, Subramaniam A. Variations in the posterior division branches of the mandibular nerve in human cadavers. *Singapore Med J.* 2013;54(3):149-151.
12. Quadros LS, Bhat N, Babu A, D'souza AS. Anatomical variations in the ansa cervicalis and innervation of infrahyoid muscles. *Int J Anat Res.* 2013;1(2):69-74.
13. Sakamoto Y. Spatial relationships between the morphologies and innervations of the scalene and anterior vertebral muscles. *Ann Anat.* 2012;194(4):381-388.
14. Shimokawa T, Yi SQ, Tanaka A, et al. Contributions of the hypoglossal nerve to the innervations of the recti capiti laterals and anterior. *Clin Anat.* 2004;17(8):613-617.
15. Meguid EA, Agawany AE. An anatomical study of the arterial and nerve supply of the infrahyoid muscles. *Folia Morphol (Warsz).* 2009;68(4):233-243.
16. Van Eijden TM, Korfage JA, Brugman P. Architecture of the human jaw-closing and jaw-opening muscles. *Anat Rec.* 1997;248(3):464-474.
17. Carlsoo S. An electromyographic study of the activity of certain suprahyoid muscles (mainly the anterior belly of digastric muscle) and of the reciprocal innervation of the elevator and depressor musculature of the mandible. *Acta Anat (Basel).* 1956;26(2):81-93.
18. Tsukada T, Taniguchi H, Ootaki S, Yamada Y, Inoue M. Effects of food texture and head posture on oropharyngeal swallowing. *J Appl Physiol (1985).* 2009;106(6):1848-1857.
19. Pearson WG Jr, Hindson DF, Langmore SE, Zumwalt AC. Evaluating swallowing muscles essential for hyolaryngeal elevation by using muscle functional magnetic resonance imaging. *Int J Radiat Oncol Biol Phys.* 2013;85(3):735-740.
20. Basmajian J, Deluca C. *Muscles Alive.* 5th ed. Baltimore, MD: Williams & Wilkins; 1985.
21. Kurt T, Gurgor N, Secil Y, Yildiz N, Ertekin C. Electrophysiologic identification and evaluation of stylohyoid and posterior digastricus muscle complex. *J Electromyogr Kinesiol.* 2006;16(1):58-65.
22. Moyers RE. An electromyographic analysis of certain muscles involved in temporomandibular movement. *Am J Orthod.* 1950;36(7):481-515.
23. Pearson WG Jr, Langmore SE, Zumwalt AC. Evaluating the structural properties of suprahyoid muscles and their potential for moving the hyoid. *Dysphagia.* 2011;26(4):345-351.
24. Woelfel JB, Hickey JC, Stacey RW, Rinear L. Electromyographic analysis of jaw movements. *J Prosthet Dent.* 1960;10:688-697.
25. Eriksson PO. Muscle fiber composition system. *Swed Dent J.* 1982;12(suppl):8-38.

Chapter 13

Cutaneous I: Facial Muscles
Orbicularis Oculi, Zygomaticus Major, Platysma, Buccinator, Corrugator Supercilii and Procerus

"Wrinkle Wrecks"

Savas Koutsantonis

1. INTRODUCTION

The facial muscles lie in the subcutaneous tissue of the face. Most arise from the bones of the skull and insert into the skin. As flat, thin muscle sheets, they are distinct from other skeletal muscles in a morphologic aspect. The facial muscles serve as a sphincter or dilator of the facial orifices (orbit and mouth), and contraction of these muscles causes the skin of the face to move and wrinkle to form various emotional expressions. These movements are sensitive and do not demand significant force development. Facial muscles are not enveloped by definite fascia, and typical muscle bellies are never observed. The muscles vary considerably in their development among individuals, and there can be interlacing of fibers within adjacent facial muscles. They are innervated by different branches of the facial nerve. Pain patterns from facial muscle trigger points (TrPs) tend to be local. Activation and perpetuation of TrPs in these muscles frequently result from habitual facial expressions, dental appliances, or the playing of wind instruments. This group of muscles is also susceptible to the development of associated TrPs from active TrPs in larger muscle groups in the neck and the shoulder. Differential diagnosis of TrPs in these muscles includes blepharospasm. Corrective actions include self-stretching, treatment of active TrPs in the neck muscles that refer to the facial region, and breathing and relaxation exercises to decrease holding patterns within the face.

2. ANATOMIC CONSIDERATIONS

The facial muscles have distinct differences with regard to the fiber-type distribution and fiber size when compared with those of the limb muscles. The mean fiber diameter of the facial muscles (platysma, levator labii, zygomaticus major, and orbicularis oris) have been shown to be almost half that of normal limb muscles.[1]

The fiber-type composition of the orofacial muscles has been found to be qualitatively and quantitatively different from each other and from those of limb muscles. In general, the orofacial muscles contain a predominance of unusually high oxidative type II fibers. This composition is especially notable in the zygomatic minor, orbicularis oris, and orbicularis oculi muscles.[2,3] Exceptions include the buccinator and occipitofrontalis muscles, which are composed primarily of type I fibers for maintaining longer duration facial tone.[4]

Orbicularis Oculi

The orbicularis oculi muscle is a broad, flat, elliptical muscle surrounding the circumference of the orbit that spreads into adjacent regions of the eyelids, anterior temporal region, infraorbital cheek and superciliary region[5] (Figure 13-1). It is comprised of three parts (orbital, palpebral, and lacrimal) and a small ciliary bundle.[5]

The orbital part arises from the medial palpebral ligament, frontal process of the maxilla, and nasal component of the frontal bone. The fibers form complete ellipses, without interruption on the lateral side, with no bony attachment. The upper orbital fibers blend with fibers of the occipitofrontalis and corrugator supercilii muscles.

The palpebral part arises from the medial palpebral ligament and sweeps across the eyelids anterior to the orbital septum. The lacrimal portion arises from the upper part of the lacrimal crest, and the adjacent lateral surface, of the lacrimal bone. It passes laterally behind the nasolacrimal sac and divides into upper and lower slips. Some fibers are inserted into the tarsi of the eyelids close to the lacrimal canaliculi, but most continue across in front of the tarsi and interlace in the lateral palpebral raphe.[5] Lastly, the ciliary bundle is comprised of a small group of fine fibers, behind the eyelashes.[5]

Buccinator

The buccinator muscle (Figure 13-2B), meaning trumpet player in Latin, is the principal muscle of the cheek, occupying the space between the maxilla and the mandible. The posterior part of the buccinator muscle is deep, internal to the mandibular ramus and in the plane of the medial pterygoid plate, attaching to the anterior margin of the pterygomandibular raphe. The anterior component converges toward the angle of the mouth where fibers intersect with the orbicularis oris muscle. The highest and lowest fibers continue forward to enter their corresponding sides of the lips. As the buccinator muscles course through the cheek on each side, a substantial number of fibers are diverted internally to attach to submucosa. The parotid duct pierces the buccinator opposite the third molar, where it lies on the deep surface of the muscle before opening into the mouth.[5]

Zygomaticus Major

The zygomaticus major muscle occupies arises from the zygomatic bone, anterior to the zygomaticotemporal suture, and passes to the angle of the mouth, blending with fibers of levator anguli oris and orbicularis oris muscles[5,6] (Figure 13-1).

Platysma

The platysma muscle is a broad sheet of a muscle arising from the superficial pectoral and deltoid fascia; passing over the clavicle; and inserting into the inferior body of the mandible, skin

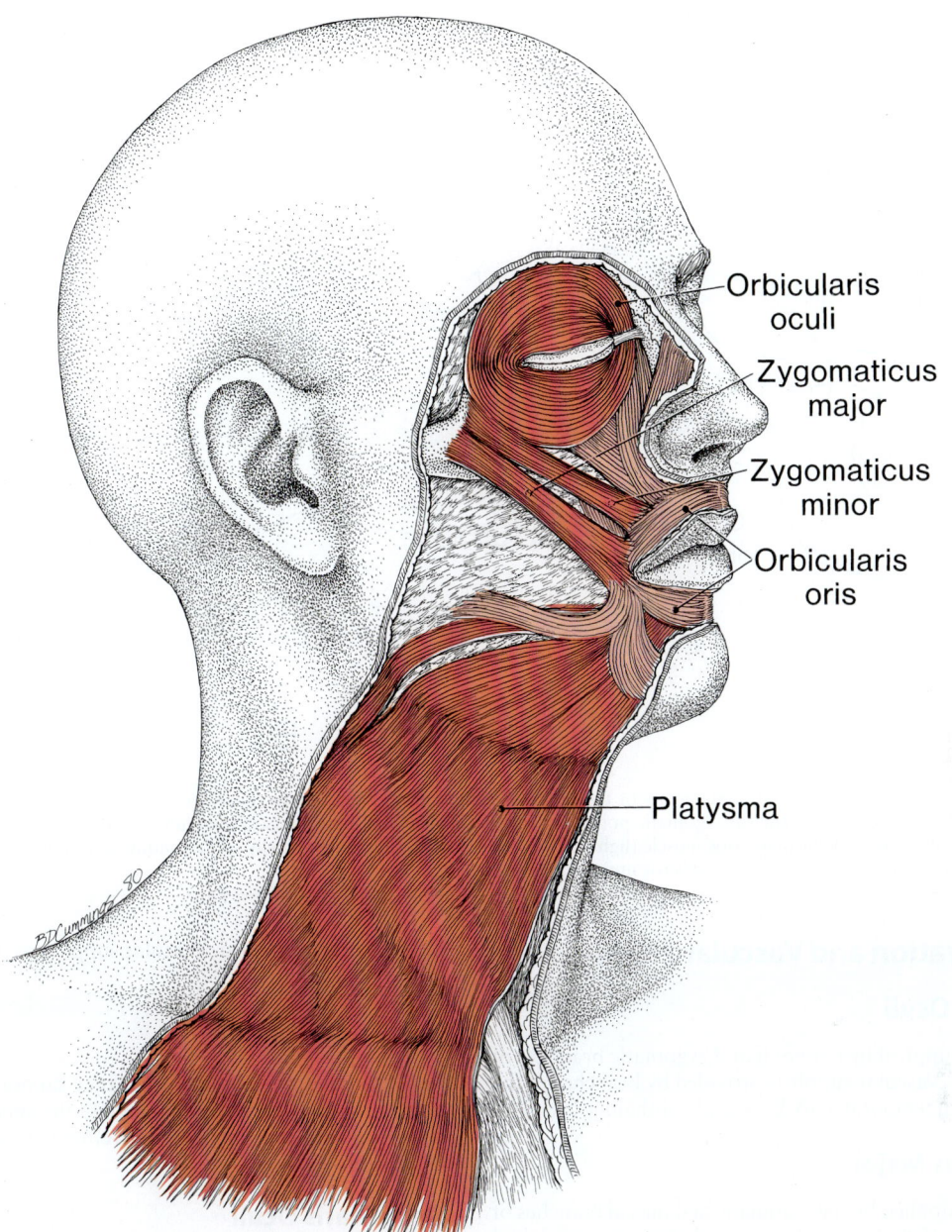

Figure 13-1. Attachments of selected facial muscles and face-related cutaneous muscles. The orbicularis oculi, the zygomaticus major, and the platysma muscles are dark red. The palpebral portion of the orbicularis oculi muscle covers only the eyelids; the remaining fibers are the orbital portion. The zygomaticus major muscle reaches from the zygoma to the corner of the mouth. The platysma muscle connects the skin muscles near the mouth to the subcutaneous fascia of the upper chest. The orbicularis oris muscle is light red.

and tissue of the lateral half of the lower lip[5,6] (Figure 13-1). Although the platysma muscle is described as a neck muscle, it is considered a contributor to the orbicularis oris complex since it has mandibular, labial, and modiolar portions, which are called the pars mandibularis, pars labialis, and pars modiolaris, respectively. The pars mandibularis attaches to the lower border of the body of the mandible; the pars labialis attaches to the tissue of the lateral half of the lower lip, as a direct labial retractor; while the pars modiolaris comprises all of the remaining bundles posterior to the pars labialis and attaches to the modiolus as one of the modiolar muscles.[5,7] In one study[5,7] 40.5% of cadaver specimens showed blending of the lateral deep slip of the platysma muscle into the inferior part of the buccinator muscle. Due to broad insertions of the platysma into the lower face, its connections with surrounding structures are important with respect to the formation of facial expressions.[5,7]

Corrugator Supercilii

The corrugator supercilii muscle is a small pyramidal muscle located at the medial end of each eyebrow, lying deep to the occipitofrontalis and orbicularis oculi muscles, with which it interdigitates. It arises from bone at the medial end of the superciliary arch and its fibers pass laterally and upward to exert traction on the skin above the middle of the supraorbital margin.[5]

Procerus

The procerus muscle arises from the fascia attached to the periosteum covering the lower part of the nasal bone and the upper parts of the lateral nasal cartilages. It inserts into the skin on the forehead between the eyebrows, interdigitating with the frontalis muscles on each side.[5]

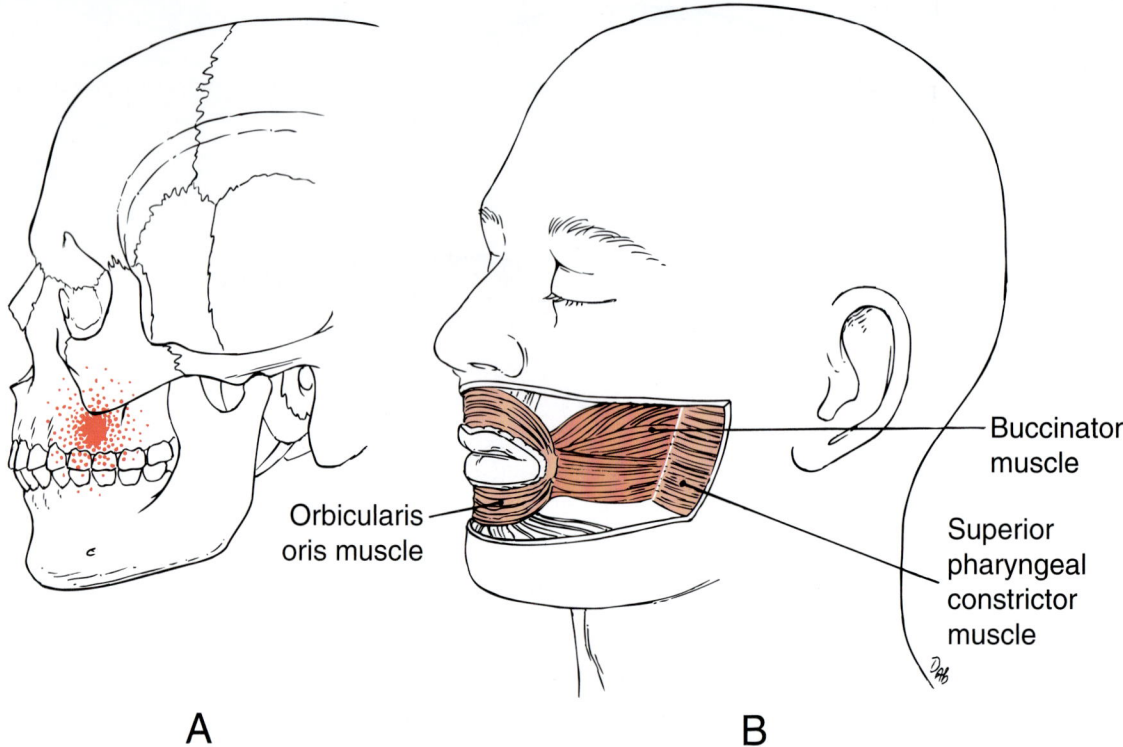

Figure 13-2. Pain pattern and attachments of the buccinator muscle. A, Pain pattern (dark red) showing location of pain in the cheek and deep to it in the subzygomatic portion of the jaw. B, The buccinator muscle (medium red) blends anteromedially with the fibers of the orbicularis oris muscle (light red). Posterolaterally, it attaches chiefly to the tendinous inscription that also anchors the superior pharyngeal constrictor muscle (light red).

2.1. Innervation and Vascularization

Orbicularis Oculi

Innervation is supplied by temporal and zygomatic branches of the facial nerve. Vascular supply is provided by branches of the facial, superficial temporal, maxillary, and ophthalmic arteries.[5]

Zygomaticus Major

Innervation is supplied by the zygomatic and buccal branches of the facial nerve. Vascular supply is provided by superior labial branch of the facial artery.[5]

Platysma

Innervation is supplied by the cervical branch of the facial nerve. Vascular supply is provided by the submental branch of the facial artery and by the suprascapular artery (from the thyrocervical trunk of the subclavian artery).[5]

Buccinator

Innervation is supplied by the buccal branch of the facial nerve. Vascular supply is provided by branches from the facial artery and the buccal branch of the maxillary artery.[5]

Corrugator Supercilii

Innervation is supplied by the temporal branches of the facial nerve. Vascular supply is provided by branches from adjacent arteries, mainly from the superficial temporal and ophthalmic arteries.[5]

Procerus

Innervation is supplied by the temporal and lower zygomatic branches of the facial nerve; a supply from buccal branches has also been described. Vascular supply provided by branches from the facial artery.[5]

2.2. Function

Facial muscles are unique in that they do not cross joints and they function to either open and close the apertures of the face or to tug skin into intricate movements that produce facial expressions.[8]

Orbicularis Oculi

The orbicularis oculi muscle is the sphincter muscle of the eyelids and plays important roles in both facial expression and protective blink reflexes.[5]

The orbital portion of the muscle produces vertical furrowing, narrowing of the palpebral fissure, and bunching or protrusion of the eyebrows.[5] This more forceful eyelid closure of the orbital portion can compress the lacrimal sac to produce tears into the nasolacrimal duct.[6] The palpebral portion performs light closure of the eyelids usually with sleep, or reflexively, as in blinking in a protective manner. When the entire orbicularis oculi muscle contracts, it causes folds that radiate from the lateral angle of the eye. With hyperactivity, this muscle causes wrinkles called "crow's feet."[5] Reduced or absent orbicularis oculi function (from palsies, trauma, or surgery) results in the inability to completely close the eyelid or to blink, exposing the cornea to break down, scarring, dry eye, and possible vision loss.[9]

Buccinator

Movement of food about the mouth depends on interplay between the tongue and the buccinator muscles. Contraction of the buccinator muscles compresses the cheek against the teeth and gums to decrease the size of the oral cavity.[5] When the cheeks have been distended with air, the buccinator muscles expel the air between the lips, as in whistling or playing a wind instrument. Cadaver studies have demonstrated that distinct muscle fibers from the buccinator muscle extend to and insert into the terminal portion of the carotid duct, giving it a physiologic role in salivary secretion.[10]

Zygomaticus Major

This muscle draws the angle of the mouth upward and laterally, as in smiling and laughing.[5]

Platysma

Contraction of the platysma muscle reduces the concavity between the jaw and the side of the neck, producing tense oblique ridges in the skin of the neck. It can also assist in depressing the mandible, by drawing down the lower lip and corners of the mouth, as with expressions of horror or surprise.[5] As confirmed by electromyography, the muscle is also active with large vertical jaw opening movements, but not during swallowing or neck movements.[11] Contraction of the lateral deep slip of the platysma muscle provides tension to the inferior part of the buccinator muscle, pulling it inferolaterally. In addition, the fibers of the slip that course longitudinally with the inferior fibers of the buccinator muscle may be involved in retraction of the lower lip, along with the buccinator muscles.[7]

Corrugator Supercilii

This muscle, in cooperation with the orbicularis oculi muscle, draws the eyebrow downward and medially to shield the eyes in bright light. It is also involved in frowning or deep concentration. The combined muscle action produces mainly vertical wrinkles on the supranasal strip of the forehead.[5]

Procerus

The procerus muscle draws down the medial angle of the eyebrows, producing transverse wrinkles over the bridge of the nose. As with the corrugator supercilii muscle, it is active during frowning and concentration and can help shield the eyes in bright sunlight.[5]

2.3. Functional Unit

Closure of the upper lid by the orbicularis oculi muscle is antagonized by the levator palpebrae muscle. The orbital portion of this muscle works synergistically with the corrugator supercilii and procerus muscles to create furrowing of the eyebrows.

The tongue works with the buccinator muscles to control the food during chewing. The muscles of exhalation work in close cooperation with the buccinator muscles when one is blowing a wind instrument. The orbicularis oris muscle frequently works in concert with the buccinator muscles for movements of the lips. The zygomaticus major muscle is assisted by the parallel-running fibers of the zygomaticus minor muscle, which also is known as the zygomatic head of the quadratus labii superioris muscle.[12]

3. CLINICAL PRESENTATION

3.1. Referred Pain Pattern

Orbicularis Oculi

This is one of the few muscles from which TrPs refer pain to the nose (Figure 13-3A). Currently, no other muscle is known to refer pain to the tip of the nose. Less intense pain may be felt in the cheek, close to the nose, and over the upper lip ipsilaterally.[13]

Zygomaticus Major

Trigger points in this muscle refer pain in an arc that extends along the side of the nose and then upward over the bridge of the nose to the mid-forehead (Figure 13-3B).[13]

Platysma

Trigger points in the platysma muscle usually overlie the sternocleidomastoid muscle and refer a prickling pain to the skin over the lateral surface of, and just below, the ipsilateral mandible (Figure 13-3C). A platysma TrP just above the clavicle may refer hot prickling pain across the front of the chest.

Buccinator

With TrPs in the buccinator muscle, the patient experiences pain locally in the cheek (Figure 13-2A) and pain referred deep to the cheek as a subzygomatic ache in the jaw.[14]

Corrugator Supercilii

Trigger points in this muscle project pain over the forehead and deep into the head, contributing to frontal headaches.

Procerus

As with the corrugator supercilii muscle, referred pain is projected over the forehead and deep into the head.

3.2. Symptoms

Individuals with myofascial dysfunction of the orbicularis oculi muscle may complain of "jumpy print" when reading. Eye strain and pain can be reported with visually demanding computer work.[15]

Patients with platysma TrPs will report a prickling pain that feels like multiple pinpricks in the area of referral. The sensation is not like the tingling caused by an electric current, a feature that usually denotes a neurologic origin.

Frontal headaches can be induced from corrugator supercilii and procerus TrPs and can mimic or combine with the TrP referral patterns of the sternocleidomastoid muscle.

When the buccinator muscle is involved, chewing may aggravate subzygomatic jaw pain. The patient may have a perception of difficulty in swallowing, although the swallowing movement appears normal.[14]

3.3. Patient Examination

After a thorough, subjective examination, the clinician should make a detailed drawing representing the pain pattern that the patient has described. This depiction will assist in planning the physical examination and can be useful in monitoring the progression of the patient as symptoms improve or change. A detailed medical history and screen of the cranial nerves are also essential to establish a proper diagnosis and plan of care. Activation of TrPs in the orbicularis oculi muscle may produce a unilateral narrowing of the palpebral fissure that resembles the ptosis of Horner's syndrome but without the change in pupillary size. When upward gaze is tested, these patients tilt the head backward because they cannot raise the upper eyelid sufficiently to look up.

Involvement of the zygomaticus major muscle may cause restriction of normal jaw opening by 10 or 20 mm; as a result this muscle should be assessed along with the masseter and temporalis muscles and the temporomandibular joint (TMJ) for restriction of mandibular opening. Patients presenting with frontal headaches are often found with TrPs in temporal, suboccipital and

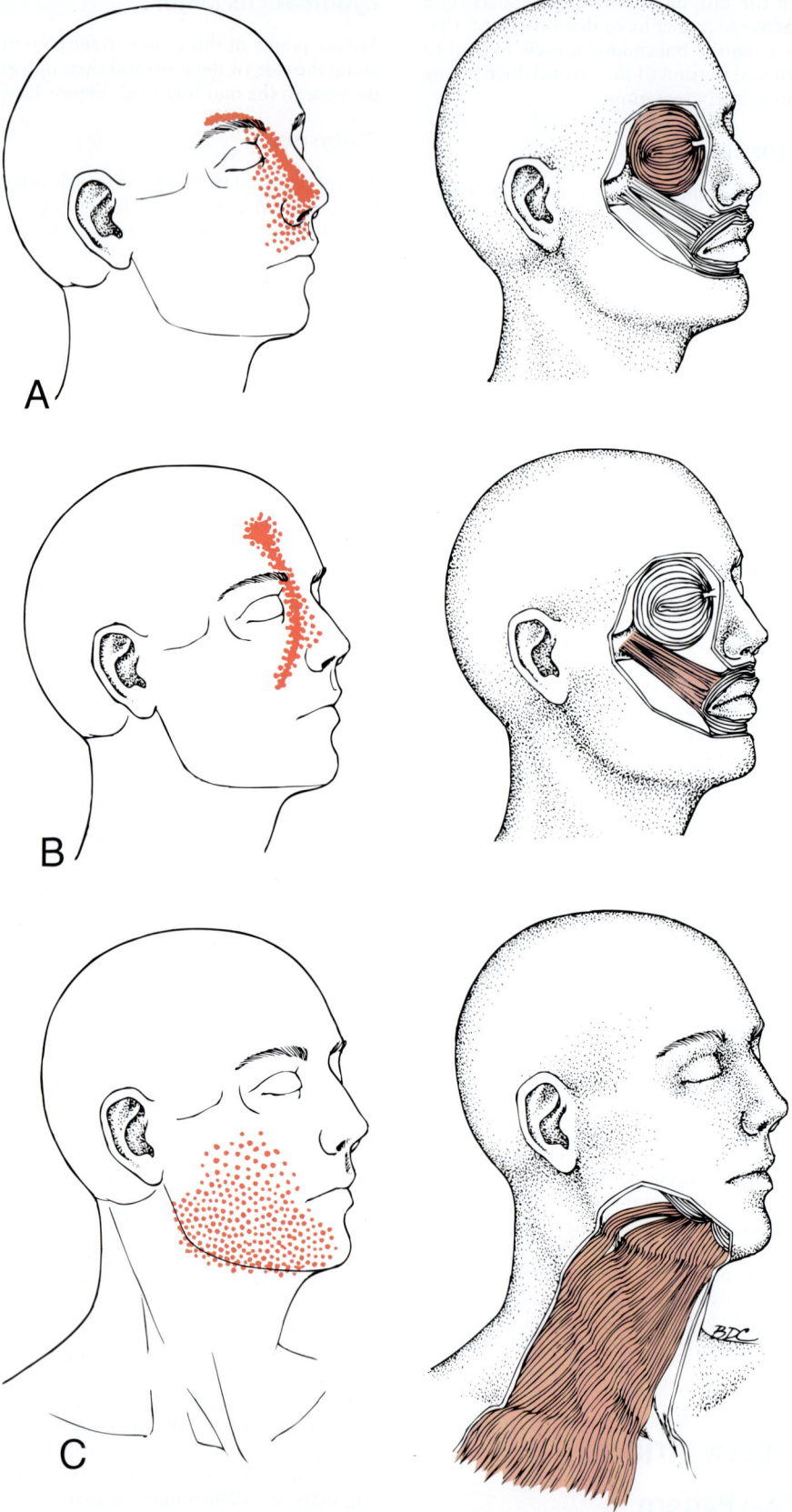

Figure 13-3. Pain patterns (dark red) and muscle (light red). A, Orbital portion of the right orbicularis oculi muscle. B, Right zygomaticus major muscle. C, Right platysma muscle.

shoulder musculature,[16,17] therefore, a thorough examination of these regions should be included along with local facial muscles.

3.4. Trigger Point Examination

Currently there are no reliability studies on the identification of TrPs in the cutaneous facial muscles.

Orbicularis Oculi

The TrPs in the upper orbital portion of this muscle are found by using a cross-fiber flat palpation to the muscle fibers that lie above the eyelid, just beneath the eyebrow and against the bone of the orbit. The lower portion can be palpated by rolling the muscle fibers and skin between the fingers to localize the TrP.

Buccinator

Trigger points in this muscle are commonly found mid-cheek, halfway between the angle of the mouth and the ramus of the mandible. The clinician uses a cross-fiber pincer palpation with one finger on the inside of the cheek and one finger outside. The band can be identified by sliding the inside finger up and down against the counterpressure of the outside finger, while squeezing gently. Tenderness of the TrP can be further increased by pulling the cheek outward, since this places the buccinator muscle on increased tension. Pulling and snapping the TrP in the taut band produces a painful, palpable, and usually visible local twitch response in this superficial muscle. See Figure 13-4 for a similar technique.

Zygomaticus Major

To examine the zygomaticus major muscle, the patient relaxes, either sitting or preferably supine, with the mouth open. Most of the length of the muscle can be palpated for spot tenderness by using a cross-fiber pincer palpation, with one finger inside the cheek and the other on the outside of the cheek, while pulling the muscle laterally taking up tissue slack (Figure 13-4). The palpable taut band is felt chiefly by the outside finger. External flat cross-fiber palpation may also be used for examination. Trigger points are commonly found in this muscle closer to the attachment of the muscle in the orbicularis oris muscle.

Platysma

Trigger points in the platysma muscle are assessed with the patient in sitting, or supine, tipping the head back far enough to take up the slack of the muscle. The clinician utilizes pincer palpation approximately 2 cm (1 in) above the clavicle to

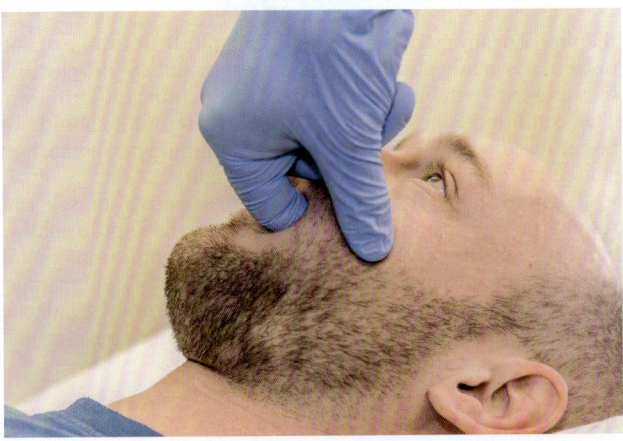

Figure 13-4. Palpation of the left zygomaticus major muscle, using pincer grasp to localize the TrPs between the digits.

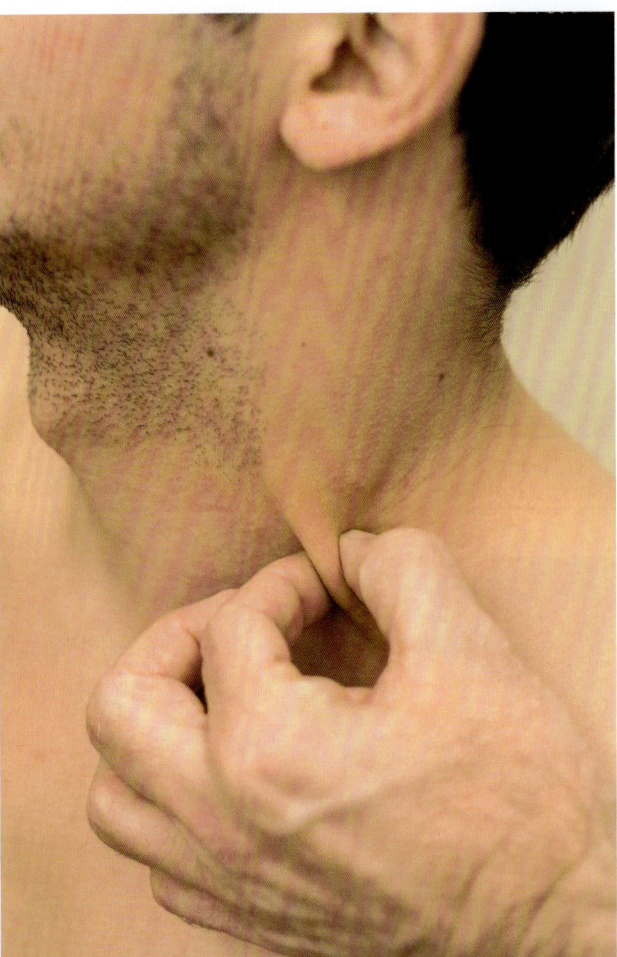

Figure 13-5. Examination of the platysma utilizing pincer palpation.

locate TrPs throughout the muscle (Figure 13-5). Patients will commonly complain of a prickling sensation in the face with pincer palpation of the platysma (Figure 13-3).

Corrugator Supercilii

Trigger points in the corrugator supercilii muscle are assessed by cross-fiber flat (Figure 13-6A) or pincer palpation (Figure 13-6B) with the patient in sitting or supine.

Procerus

As with the corrugator supercilii muscle, this muscle is assessed by using a cross-fiber flat (Figure 13-7A) or pincer palpation (Figure 13-7B) to identify taut bands and TrPs with the patient in sitting or supine.

4. DIFFERENTIAL DIAGNOSIS

4.1. Activation and Perpetuation of Trigger Points

A posture or activity that activates a TrP, if not corrected, can also perpetuate it. In any part of any of the facial muscles, TrPs may be activated by maximal or submaximal concentric loading,[18] as with habitual facial expressions. Trigger points may also be activated or aggravated when the muscle is placed in a shortened and/or lengthened position for an extended period of time. Habitual frowning, squinting (due to photophobia or

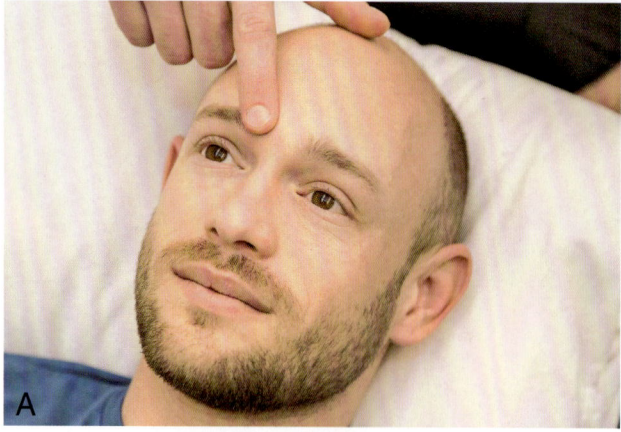
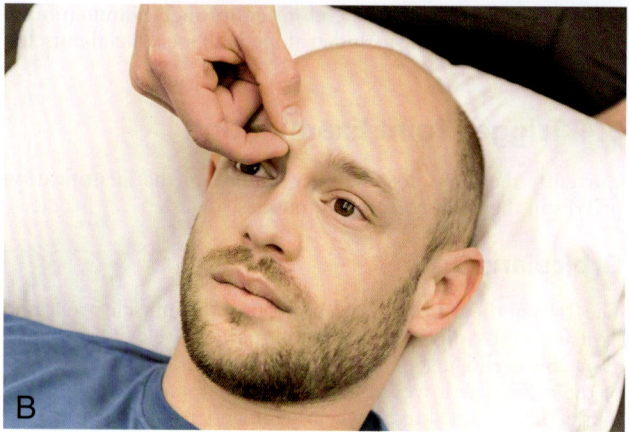

Figure 13-6. Examination of the corrugator supercilii muscle. A, Cross-fiber flat palpation. B, Pincer palpation.

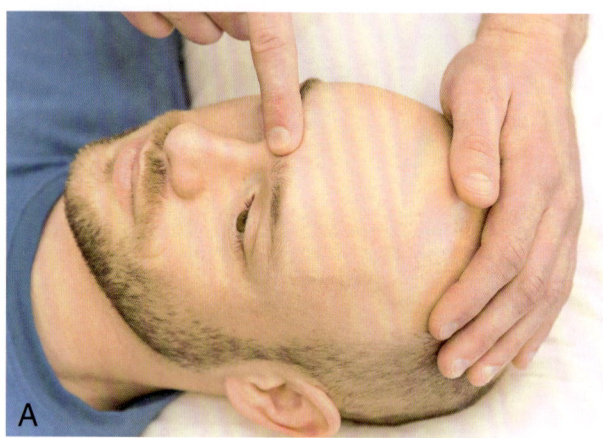
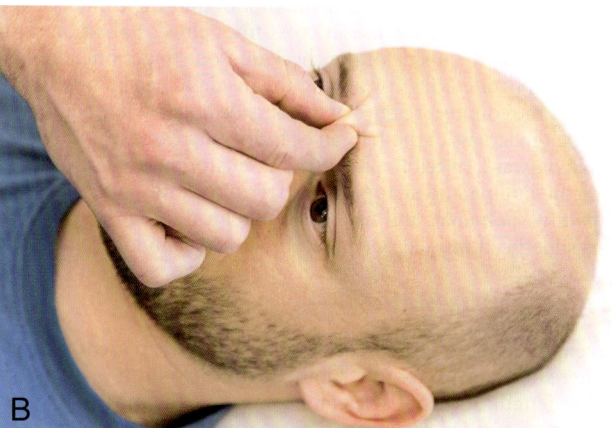

Figure 13-7. Examination of the procerus muscle. A, Cross-fiber flat palpation. B, Pincer palpation.

astigmatism), visual straining from computer work or TrPs in the sternal division of the sternocleidomastoid muscle (which refer pain to the orbit) may activate TrPs in the orbicularis oculi, corrugator supercilii and procerus muscles.[13] It is important to differentiate referred pain patterns of head, neck, and shoulder muscles in patients presenting with headache symptoms. Myofascial dysfunction of the masticatory muscles that is severe enough to cause trismus may activate TrPs in the zygomaticus major muscle. Stressful clenching of the jaw and even static bracing of orofacial muscles can lead to the development of facial muscle TrPs.

Platysma TrPs are typically associated with TrPs in the sternocleidomastoid and scalene muscles.

Buccinator TrPs may be activated by poorly fitted dental appliances or from the repetitive activation of muscles when playing wind instruments.

4.2. Associated Trigger Points

It has been shown that associated TrPs can develop in the referred pain areas of primary active TrPs,[19] therefore muscles that can refer to the facial region should be considered. Muscles such as the sternocleidomastoid, upper trapezius, masseter, temporalis and lateral pterygoid muscles can refer to different areas of the face, contributing to associated TrPs in the facial muscles. These associated TrPs will not improve with treatment until TrPs in the primary muscles are treated effectively.

Pain caused by TrPs in the orbicularis oculi, buccinator, and/or zygomaticus muscles is easily attributed erroneously to a form of tension headache. Patients with pain from buccinator TrPs are very likely to receive a misdiagnosis of TMJ dysfunction, especially since they have trouble chewing and swallowing, therefore TMJ dysfunction should be ruled out.

The sternocleidomastoid, scalene and masticatory muscles on the same side often contain active TrPs, and can produce associated TrPs in the platysma muscle which overlies this area.

4.3. Associated Pathology

Blepharospasm is a focal (usually bilateral) dystonia of the orbicularis oculi muscles causing abnormal eyelid closure, blinking, or twitching which can cause significant irritation. This condition is neurologically based, therefore it should not be confused with TrPs in this muscle. Botulinum toxin injection is used effectively in managing these symptoms.[20]

Tightness and TrPs in the corrugator supercilii muscle can result in nerve entrapment or pressure on the supratrochlear nerve causing frontal headache symptoms.[21] Compression or impingement of any branch of the trigeminal nerve (V1-ophthalmic, V2-maxillary, V3-mandibular) can mimic a frontal headache or orbital and facial pain patterns and should be considered.[22]

5. CORRECTIVE ACTIONS

The patient should be taught to palpate these facial muscles to locate taut bands and tender points and to appropriately apply sustained digital pressure to inactivate the identified TrPs.

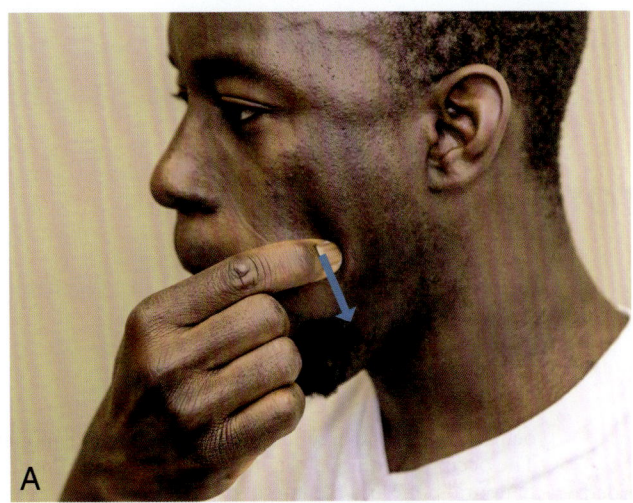
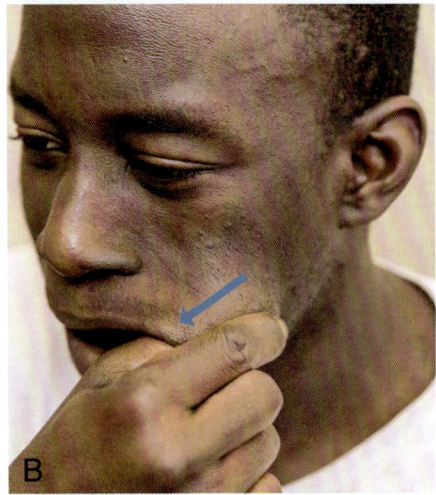

Figure 13-8. A, Self-stretching of the zygomaticus major muscle. B, Self-stretching of the buccinator muscle.

Self-stretching of the zygomaticus major (Figure 13-8A) and buccinator (Figure 13-8B) muscles can be performed with one finger in the mouth and one finger outside the mouth, holding and pulling the taut tissue outward.

Any TrPs in other muscles that are likely to refer pain to the same side of the face, such as the upper trapezius, sternocleidomastoid, and masticatory muscles, should be treated. Refer to Chapters 6, 7, 8, 9, and 11 for specific corrective actions for each of these muscles.

The patient should avoid excessive facial straining, this is especially important for those who work extensively at a desk and use a computer. Proper ergonomics and postures, along with wearing appropriate corrective lenses when needed to reduce visual strain, squinting, and facial stress can help to reduce this strain.

Hyperactivity of facial expression, holding patterns related to anxiety, tension, and visual stress (as with computer use) can lead to facial TrPs. A program of breathing, relaxation exercises, and self-awareness of habitual patterns can be helpful to minimize overuse of these muscles.

References

1. Schwarting S, Schroder M, Stennert E, Goebel HH. Enzyme histochemical and histographic data on normal human facial muscles. *ORL J Otorhinolaryngol Relat Spec*. 1982;44(1):51-59.
2. Stal P. Characterization of human oro-facial and masticatory muscles with respect to fibre types, myosins and capillaries. Morphological, enzyme-histochemical, immuno-histochemical and biochemical investigations. *Swed Dent J Suppl*. 1994;98:1-55.
3. Stal P, Eriksson PO, Eriksson A, Thornell LE. Enzyme-histochemical and morphological characteristics of muscle fibre types in the human buccinator and orbicularis oris. *Arch Oral Biol*. 1990;35(6):449-458.
4. Happak W, Burggasser G, Gruber H. Histochemical characteristics of human mimic muscles. *J Neurol Sci*. 1988;83(1):25-35.
5. Standring S. *Gray's Anatomy: The Anatomical Basis of Clinical Practice* (Procerus). 41st ed. London, UK: Elsevier; 2015.
6. Son E, Watts T, Quinn FJ, Quinn M. Superficial facial musculature. Grand Rounds Presentation: The University of Texas Medical Branch; March, 2012.
7. Hur MS, Bae JH, Kim HJ, Lee HB, Lee KS. Blending of the lateral deep slip of the platysma muscle into the buccinator muscle. *Surg Radiol Anat*. 2015;37(8):931-934.
8. Goodmurphy CW, Ovalle WK. Morphological study of two human facial muscles: orbicularis oculi and corrugator supercilii. *Clin Anat*. 1999;12(1):1-11.
9. Sohrab M, Abugo U, Grant M, Merbs S. Management of the eye in facial paralysis. *Facial Plast Surg*. 2015;31(2):140-144.
10. Kang HC, Kwak HH, Hu KS, et al. An anatomical study of the buccinator muscle fibres that extend to the terminal portion of the parotid duct, and their functional roles in salivary secretion. *J Anat*. 2006;208(5):601-607.
11. Widmalm SE, Nemeth PA, Ash MM Jr, Lillie JH. The anatomy and electrical activity of the platysma muscle. *J Oral Rehabil*. 1985;12(1):17-22.
12. Ito J, Moriyama H, Shimada K. Morphological evaluation of the human facial muscles. *Okajimas Folia Anat Jpn*. 2006;83(1):7-14.
13. Travell J. Identification of myofascial trigger point syndromes: a case of atypical facial neuralgia. *Arch Phys Med Rehabil*. 1981;62(3):100-106.
14. Curl DD. Discovery of a myofascial trigger point in the buccinator muscle: a case report. *Cranio*. 1989;7(4):339-345.
15. Thorud HM, Helland M, Aaras A, Kvikstad TM, Lindberg LG, Horgen G. Eye-related pain induced by visually demanding computer work. *Optom Vis Sci*. 2012;89(4):E452-E464.
16. Calandre EP, Hidalgo J, Garcia-Leiva JM, Rico-Villademoros F. Trigger point evaluation in migraine patients: an indication of peripheral sensitization linked to migraine predisposition? *Eur J Neurol*. 2006;13(3):244-249.
17. Fernández de las Peñas C, Ge HY, Alonso-Blanco C, Gonzalez-Iglesias J, Arendt-Nielsen L. Referred pain areas of active myofascial trigger points in head, neck, and shoulder muscles, in chronic tension type headache. *J Bodyw Mov Ther*. 2010;14(4):391-396.
18. Gerwin RD, Dommerholt J, Shah JP. An expansion of Simons' integrated hypothesis of trigger point formation. *Curr Pain Headache Rep*. 2004;8(6):468-475.
19. Hsieh YL, Kao MJ, Kuan TS, Chen SM, Chen JT, Hong CZ. Dry needling to a key myofascial trigger point may reduce the irritability of satellite MTrPs. *Am J Phys Med Rehabil*. 2007;86(5):397-403.
20. Hellman A, Torres-Russotto D. Botulinum toxin in the management of blepharospasm: current evidence and recent developments. *Ther Adv Neurol Disord*. 2015;8(2):82-91.
21. de Ru JA, Buwalda J. Botulinum toxin A injection into corrugator muscle for frontally localised chronic daily headache or chronic tension-type headache. *J Laryngol Otol*. 2009;123(4):412-417.
22. Magee DJ. *Orthopedic Physical Assessment*. 6th ed. St Louis, MO: Saunders Elsevier; 2014.

Chapter 14

Cutaneous II: Occipitofrontalis
"Head Tightness Twins"

Savas Koutsantonis and Jennifer L. Freeman

1. INTRODUCTION

The epicranius or occipitofrontalis muscle is generally regarded as one muscle composed of two distinct muscle bellies. It has a broad, musculofibrous layer that covers the vertex of the skull. The frontalis muscle adheres to the superficial fascia of the eyebrows and has no bony attachment. The occipitalis muscle originates at the mastoid process of the temporal bone and the lateral two-thirds of the superior nuchal line of the occipital bone. The muscle bellies of the frontalis and occipitalis are joined through the galea aponeurotica (epicranial aponeurosis), which covers the vertex of the skull. The temporal branch of the facial nerve innervates the frontalis muscle, and the posterior auricular branch innervates the occipitalis. Both muscle bellies work together for facial expressions. Frontalis trigger points (TrPs) refer pain on the ipsilateral forehead, whereas occipitalis TrPs refer diffusely over the back of the head and through the cranium, causing intense pain deep in the orbit. Trigger points in either muscle belly can be perpetuated by prolonged facial expressions or from TrPs in cervical muscles that refer to the head. Associated pathology may include nerve entrapment, tension-type headache (TTH), and migraine headache. Corrective actions include eliminating TrPs in cervical muscles and addressing factors that can contribute to excessive or prolonged facial expressions.

2. ANATOMIC CONSIDERATIONS

The occipitofrontalis muscle covers the dome of the skull from the eyebrows anteriorly, to the highest nuchal lines posteriorly. The frontal belly intertwines with the corrugator supercilii, procerus, and orbicularis oculi muscles, which act together to provide variations of facial expression. The occipital belly is, asymmetrical on both sides. The shape of this muscle varies greatly; cadaver studies show that irregular shapes are most common, followed by quadrangular, and then ellipse shapes. The occipital muscle bellies are often illustrated with muscle fibers angled in a straight line toward the frontal bellies with both sides close to each other. More recent studies not only suggest variations in shape but also fiber direction ranging in angles from 55° to 65° from the horizontal plane and variation in distance between the bellies.[1-3]

The muscle bellies of the frontalis and occipitalis are joined through the galea aponeurotica (epicranial aponeurosis),[2] which covers the vertex of the skull (Figure 14-1). Although the galea aponeurotica is firmly connected to the skin, it does slide over the periosteum[4] which allows both portions of the muscle to function with each other. The frontalis muscle adheres to the superficial fascia of the eyebrows and has no bony attachment.[4] Its fibers blend with those of the adjacent muscles; including the procerus, corrugator supercilii, and orbicularis oculi muscles; and ascend to join the epicranial aponeurosis.[4,5] The occipitalis muscle originates at the mastoid process of the temporal bone and the lateral two thirds of the superior nuchal line of the occipital bone. The superficial fascia overlying the occipital belly becomes the temporoparietal fascia and ends at the superior end of the frontal belly, creating a superficial musculoaponeurotic system. Underneath this superficial system, the occipital belly becomes the galea aponeurotica and enters into the underside of the frontal belly, creating a deep musculoaponeurotic system which pulls on the superficial system with activation.[1,2,4,5]

2.1. Innervation and Vascularization

The occipitofrontalis muscle is supplied by the facial nerve (cranial nerve VII), with the temporal branch innervating the frontalis and the posterior auricular branch innervating the occipitalis.[5] The posterior auricular nerve is the first extracranial branch of the facial nerve and although it is a delicate structure, it has clinical significance. This branch serves as a landmark when identifying the main trunk of the facial nerve. It is useful to surgeons to minimize damage to the facial nerve during surgeries such as a parotidectomy and mastoidectomy. This nerve also contributes cutaneous sensation from the skin over the mastoid process and parts of the auricle. It is most typically found as a single branch coming off the main trunk of the facial nerve, but it can also divide into two or three branches. These additional branches dive into the parotid gland.[1,6]

The vascular supply to the frontalis muscle is through the frontal branch of the superficial temporal and the ophthalmic arteries. The occipitalis is supplied by the posterior auricular and occipital arteries.[4]

2.2. Function

The frontalis muscle is voluntarily contracted when facial expressions are made. When acting from above, it raises the eyebrow and skin over the root of the nose as in expressions of surprise or horror.[7] Acting from below, it draws the scalp forward creating transverse wrinkles on the forehead.[4,5] It works with the corrugator supercilii and orbicularis oculi muscles during eye opening and closing (performed either smoothly or maximally) and with a straight gaze and frowning.[8] As several studies have shown, the frontalis muscle is also associated with increased muscle tension during stress or anxiety, as well as in individuals with TTH because electromyographic (EMG) activity is higher and pressure pain threshold (PPT) is lower when compared with control groups.[9-11]

The occipitalis muscle becomes the galea aponeurotica and enters into the underside of the frontalis muscle becoming the deep musculoaponeurotic system anchored to the occipital

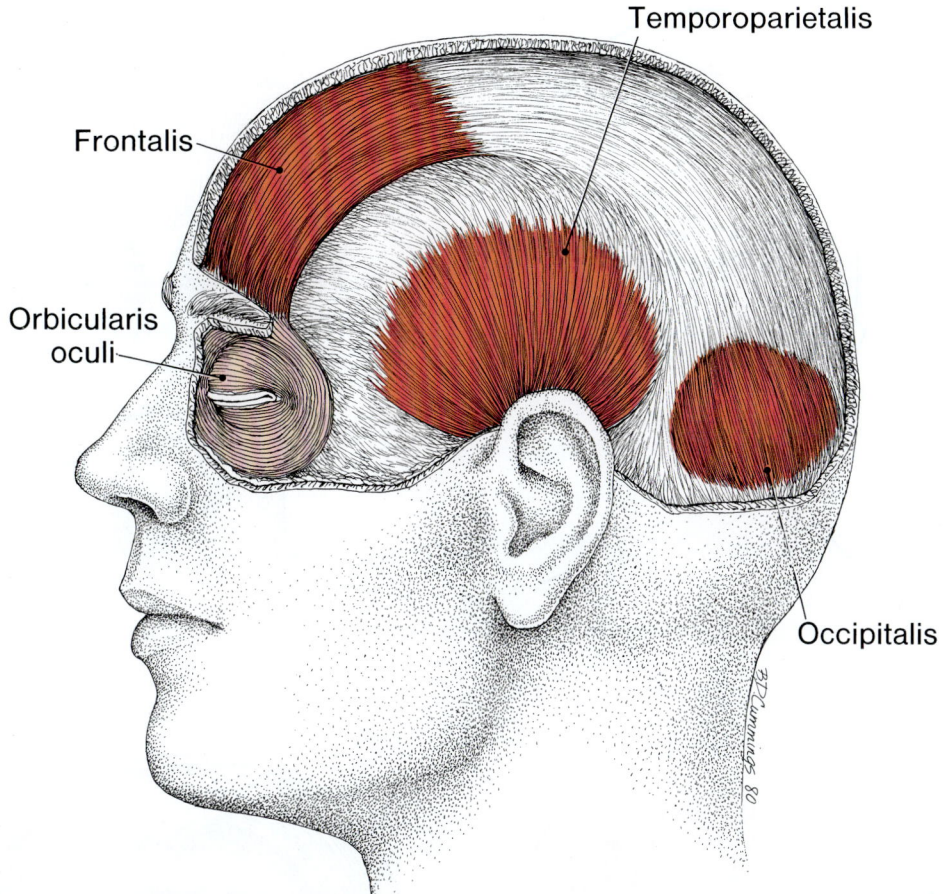

Figure 14-1. Attachments of the left epicranial muscles (*dark red*); the *frontalis* and *occipitalis* bellies of the occipitofrontalis muscle, and also the *temporoparietalis* muscle. Each connects above to the tendinous galea aponeurotica. Below and anteriorly, the frontalis muscle attaches to the skin near the eyebrow; the occipitalis muscle attaches to the bone along the superior nuchal line, and the temporoparietalis muscle to the skin above the ear. The cutaneous *orbicularis oculi* muscle is shown in light red.

bone. When activated, it draws the superficial musculoaponeurotic system backward with the scalp. When only the frontalis muscle contracts to lift the eyebrow and upper eyelid, it draws the scalp forward which results in wrinkling and narrowing of the forehead. When both the frontalis and occipitalis muscles contract to maximize the eyebrow and upper eyelid lifting, the galea aponeurotica draws the superficial musculoaponeurotic system backward with the frontalis muscle, resulting in a less-wrinkled forehead despite the contraction of the frontalis muscle.[2,4] Acting alternately, the frontalis and occipitalis muscles can move the entire scalp backward and forward.

The frontalis and occipitalis muscle bellies can also work together to lift the eyebrows to maintain a clear visual field. An upward gaze position up to 30° increases frontalis activity only, whereas a greater than 40° involves contraction of both the frontalis and occipitalis parts. Occipitalis EMG values increase significantly as the degree of gaze becomes higher.[2]

2.3. Functional Unit

The frontalis and occipitalis muscles function as synergists in tandem. The frontalis muscle may contract with, or independently of, the perpendicularly placed corrugator muscle which shortens the eyebrows in a frown.

The frontalis muscle works synergistically in a dynamic balance with the corrugator supercilii and the orbicularis oculi muscles during eye opening and closing as well as with straight gazing and frowning.[8] The frontalis muscle is an antagonist to the procerus muscle which pulls the medial end of the eyebrow down.[12]

3. CLINICAL PRESENTATION

3.1. Referred Pain Pattern

Frontalis

Trigger points in the frontalis muscle evoke pain that spreads upward and over the forehead on the same side (Figure 14-2A). The referred pain commonly remains local in the region of the muscle.[13]

Occipitalis

Trigger points in the occipitalis muscle are a recognized source of headache.[14] These TrPs often form secondarily to TrPs in the suboccipital muscles, which can refer pain over the occipital and temporal bones.[15] Commonly, TrPs in the occipitalis muscle refer pain laterally and anteriorly, diffusely over the back of the head and through the cranium, causing intense pain deep in the orbit (Figure 14-2B). This muscle also produced an "earache" sensation when injected with hypertonic saline.[16] Cyriax[7] found that injections into the galea aponeurotica referred pain ipsilaterally behind the eye, in the eyeball, and in the eyelids. These referred pain patterns were later confirmed clinically by Williams.[17]

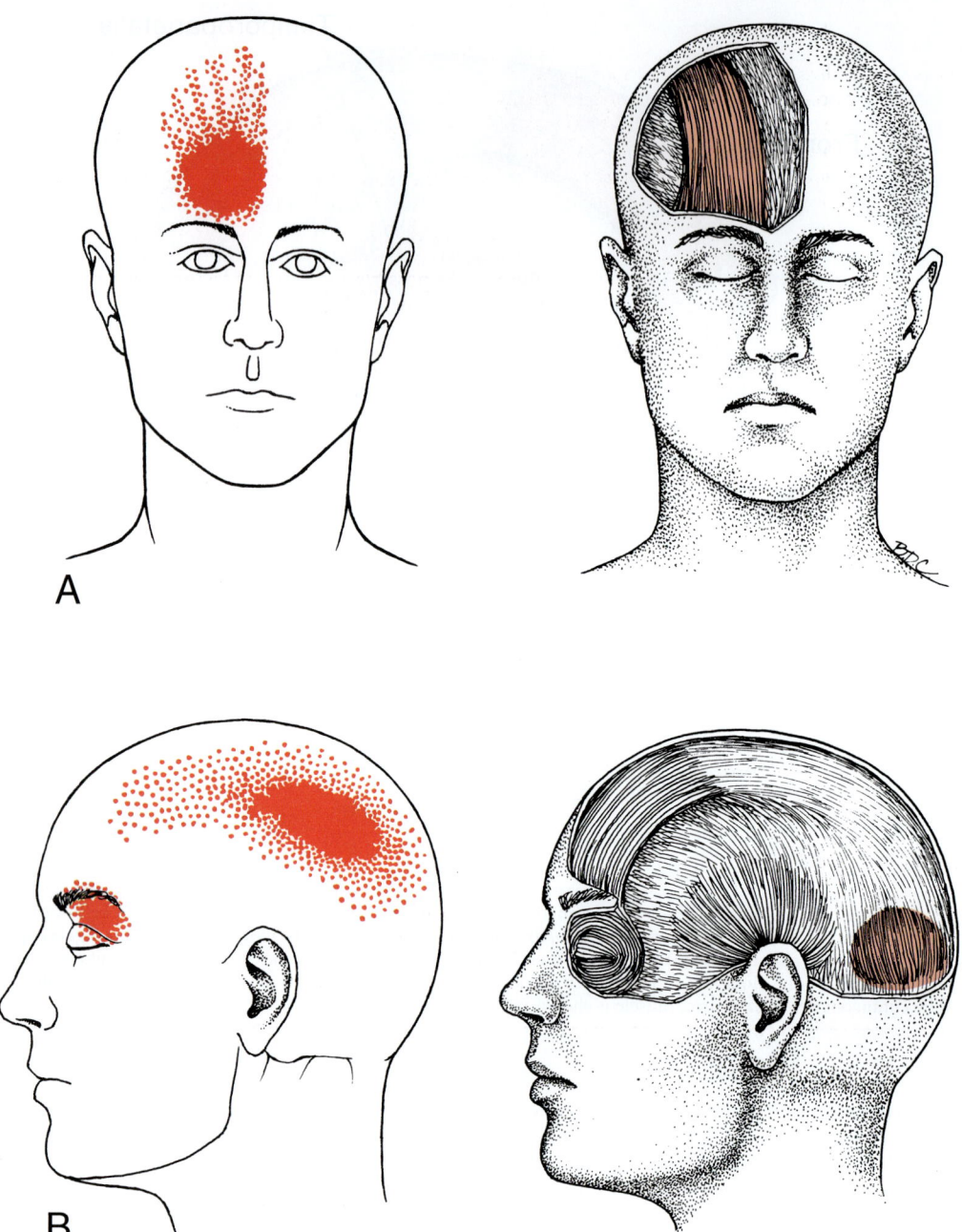

Figure 14-2. Pain patterns (*dark red*) referred from TrPs in the occipitofrontalis muscle (*medium red*). A, Right frontalis muscle belly. B, Left occipitalis muscle belly.

3.2. Symptoms

Patients with occipitalis TrPs typically report having to sleep on their side at night due to the inability to tolerate the back of the head on the pillow because of the pressure of the head compressing TrPs.

The deep-aching occipital pain caused by occipitalis TrPs should be distinguished from symptoms associated with the entrapment of the greater occipital nerve by the posterior cervical muscles; including the upper trapezius, oblique capitis inferior, and semispinalis capitis muscles;[18-20] and from referred pain by the head, neck, and shoulder musculature such as upper trapezius, sternocleidomastoid, splenius capitis, temporalis, masseter, levator scapulae, and superior oblique and suboccipital muscles.[9,21]

3.3. Patient Examination

After a thorough subjective examination, the clinician should make a detailed drawing representing the pain pattern that the patient has described. This depiction will assist in planning the physical examination and can be useful in monitoring the progression of the patient as symptoms improve or change. Additionally, patients presenting with frontal or occipital pain require more than a local examination. Several studies have demonstrated that the referred pain elicited by TrPs from neck, shoulder, and head muscles reproduces the headache pattern in patients with TTH, migraine, and cervicogenic headaches.[9,17,21,22] Therefore, a thorough examination is required of the suboccipital, the cervical, and the shoulder muscles to identify TrPs that can elicit familiar pain patterns.

Cervical zygapophyseal joints also need to be considered as a source for referred pain to the occipital region. Subjects who underwent cervical zygapophyseal injection and radiofrequency facet denervation reported occipital symptoms when performed at C0-C1 to C3-C4, with the highest percentage of reported occipital symptoms from C2 to C3. As a result, cervical facet joint disorders and accessory motion restrictions should be addressed as a possible source of occipital headaches.[23]

Sensitization from possible compression or entrapment of the ophthalmic branch (V1) of trigeminal cranial nerve (V) should also be considered. The sensory distribution of this nerve mimics the frontal headache (HA) symptoms.[24]

3.4. Trigger Point Examination

A TrP in the frontalis muscle is identified with cross-fiber flat palpation, commonly above the eyebrow, within the muscle fibers (Figure 14-2A). A very gentle pressure is necessary to ensure the clinician does not press through the TrP and miss it. A TrP in this muscle can feel like a small grain of rice.

A TrP in the occipitalis muscle is often found in the small hollow just above the superior nuchal line. A cross-fiber flat palpation is used to identify the TrP. Difficulty in properly localizing this muscle lies in the great variability in shape, size, and location; therefore, repeated contraction by elevation of the eyebrows with upward gaze may be necessary to isolate the proper location of this muscle.[1]

4. DIFFERENTIAL DIAGNOSIS

4.1. Activation and Perpetuation of Trigger Points

A posture or activity that activates a TrP, if not corrected, can also perpetuate it. In any part of the occipitofrontalis muscle, TrPs may be activated by maximal or submaximal concentric loading,[25] which for this muscle is frequently due to habitual facial expressions.[21]

The frontalis muscle may be activated by work overload, especially in anxious or tense people with great mobility of facial expression, and in people who persistently use the frontalis in an expression of attention with raised eyebrows and a wrinkled forehead. Excessive or prolonged gazing, along with maintained depressed eyebrows or frowning, also overactivates the frontalis muscle.[8]

Occipitalis TrPs are likely to occur in patients with decreased visual acuity due to persistent, strong contraction of the forehead and scalp muscles. Sustained eyebrow elevation in an effort to maintain an upward gaze significantly increases the activation of this muscle.[2]

4.2. Associated Trigger Points

Associated TrPs can develop in the referred pain areas caused by TrPs.[25] Therefore, musculature in the referred pain areas for each muscle should also be considered.[26] Because active TrPs in the frontalis muscle are often associated TrPs from long-standing TrPs in the clavicular division of the sternocleidomastoid muscle on the same side, this muscle should be examined. Lasting relief may also depend on inactivating associated TrPs in suboccipital, upper trapezius, sternocleidomastoid, and temporalis muscles that can refer symptoms to the frontal region of the head. Trigger points in the occipitalis can result from TrPs in the upper trapezius, sternal division of the sternocleidomastoid, and posterior cervical muscles, which refer pain and tenderness to the occipital region.[21] Additionally, the posterior digastric and levator scapulae muscles can refer to this region and contribute to associated TrPs of the occipitalis muscle.

4.3. Associated Pathology

Pain caused by TrPs in these muscles is likely to be diagnosed as TTH without any recognition of the treatable source. Mixed mechanisms such as neurovascular, neuropathic, myofascial, and cervicogenic may all contribute and should therefore be examined as possible contributing factors.[27] Peripheral nerve compression or entrapment should be considered when assessing for occipital or supraorbital neuralgias. The greater occipital nerve can be compressed as it courses through the inferior capitis oblique muscle, semispinalis capitis muscle, and cranial insertions of the upper trapezius muscle.[19,20] The supraorbital nerve can be entrapped by the facial muscles including the frontalis muscle.[28] This mechanical pressure on the peripheral nerve can be relieved by inactivating the TrP.

In cases of atypical history of pain, with no other signs and symptoms other than occipital headaches, further interdisciplinary referral and imaging may be necessary to exclude neurovascular pathology. One such case was reported of an internal carotid artery aneurysm presenting as orofacial pain and occipital headache.[29]

5. CORRECTIVE ACTIONS

When TrPs are found in the occipitofrontalis muscle, the patient should avoid persistent frowning and vigorous wrinkling of the forehead because this can continue to aggravate and/or perpetuate the development of TrPs.

Any associated TrPs in the clavicular division of the sternocleidomastoid and posterior neck muscles should be inactivated. Addressing perpetuating factors to the development of TrPs in the sternocleidomastoid and posterior neck muscles should also be done. (See Chapters 7, 15, and 16.) Correction of forward head posture is also necessary to reduce the strain on the sternocleidomastoid, splenii, and posterior cervical muscles that may have TrPs.

The frontalis muscle responds well to self-pressure release of TrPs (Figure 14-3). The same may be used for TrPs in the occipitalis muscle, with the patient using digital pressure to release the TrPs (Figure 14-4).

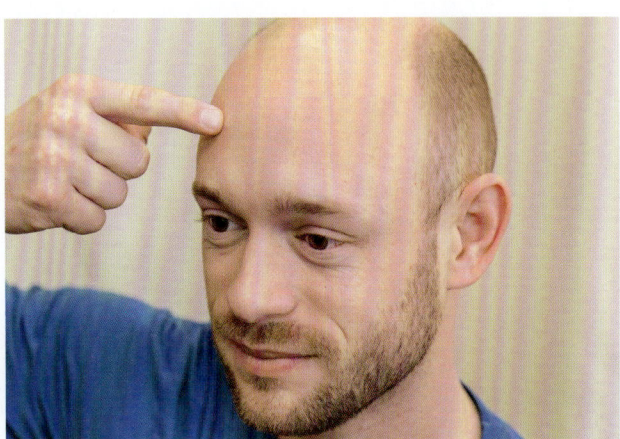

Figure 14-3. Self-pressure release of frontalis TrPs. In a sitting or standing position, the patient gently presses on the TrP in the muscle that is contributing to his or her pain.

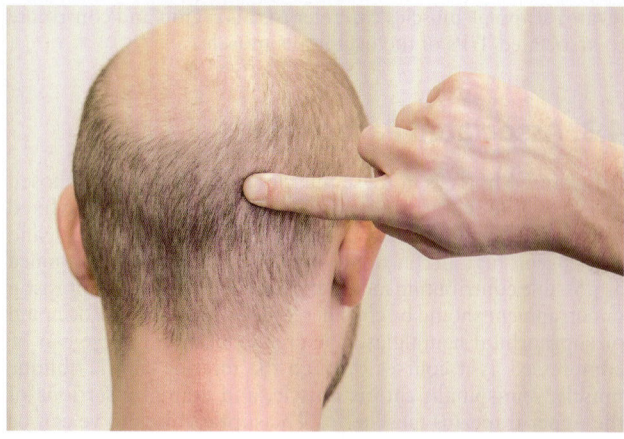

Figure 14-4. Self-pressure release of occipitalis TrPs. In a sitting or standing position, the patient gently presses on the TrP in the muscle that is contributing to his or her pain.

A program of self-awareness, breathing, and relaxation exercises may be helpful for patients with frontalis TrPs because decreased cognitive stress has been shown to increase resting activity of this muscle.[11]

References

1. Jeon A, Kim SD, Han SH. Morphological study of the occipital belly of the occipitofrontalis muscle and its innervation. *Surg Radiol Anat.* 2015;37(9):1087-1092.
2. Kushima H, Matsuo K, Yuzuriha S, Kitazawa T, Moriizumi T. The occipitofrontalis muscle is composed of two physiologically and anatomically different muscles separately affecting the positions of the eyebrow and hairline. *Br J Plast Surg.* 2005;58(5):681-687.
3. Spalteholz W. *Handatlas der Anatomie des Menschen*. Vol 2. 11th ed. Leipzig, Saxony: S. Hirzel; 1922.
4. Standring S. *Gray's Anatomy: The Anatomical Basis of Clinical Practice*. 41st ed. London, UK: Elsevier; 2015.
5. Son E, Watts T, Quinn FJ, Quinn M. Superficial facial musculature. Grand Rounds Presentation: The University of Texas Medical Branch; March, 2012.
6. Smith OJ, Ross GL. Variations in the anatomy of the posterior auricular nerve and its potential as a landmark for identification of the facial nerve trunk: a cadaveric study. *Anat Sci Int.* 2012;87(2):101-105.
7. Cyriax J. Rheumatic headache. *Br Med J (Clin Res Ed)*. 1938;2(4069):1367-1368.
8. Yun S, Son D, Yeo H, et al. Changes of eyebrow muscle activity with aging: functional analysis revealed by electromyography. *Plast Reconstr Surg.* 2014;133(4):455e-463e.
9. Alonso-Blanco C, de-la-Llave-Rincon AI, Fernández de las Peñas C. Muscle trigger point therapy in tension-type headache. *Expert Rev Neurother.* 2012;12(3):315-322.
10. Grossi DB, Chaves TC, Goncalves MC, et al. Pressure pain threshold in the craniocervical muscles of women with episodic and chronic migraine: a controlled study. *Arq Neuropsiquiatr.* 2011;69(4):607-612.
11. Leistad RB, Sand T, Westgaard RH, Nilsen KB, Stovner LJ. Stress-induced pain and muscle activity in patients with migraine and tension-type headache. *Cephalalgia.* 2006;26(1):64-73.
12. Basmajian J, Deluca C. *Muscles Alive*. 5th ed. Baltimore, MD: Williams & Wilkins; 1985.
13. Andersen S, Petersen MW, Svendsen AS, Gazerani P. Pressure pain thresholds assessed over temporalis, masseter, and frontalis muscles in healthy individuals, patients with tension-type headache, and those with migraine—a systematic review. *Pain.* 2015;156(8):1409-1423.
14. Pritchard DW, Wood MM. EMG levels in the occipitofrontalis muscles under an experimental stress condition. *Biofeedback Self Regul.* 1983;8(1):165-175.
15. Fernández de las Peñas C, Alonso-Blanco C, Cuadrado ML, Pareja JA. Myofascial trigger points in the suboccipital muscles in episodic tension-type headache. *Man Ther.* 2006;11(3):225-230.
16. Kellgren JH. Observations on referred pain arising from muscle. *Clin Sci.* 1938;3:175-190.
17. Williams HL. The syndrome of physical or intrinsic allergy of the head: myalgia of the head (sinus headache). *Proc Staff Meet Mayo Clin.* 1945;20(12):177-183.
18. Caviggioli F, Giannasi S, Vinci V, et al. Neurovascular compression of the greater occipital nerve: implications for migraine headaches. *Plast Reconstr Surg.* 2012;129(2):353e-354e.
19. Son BC, Kim DR, Lee SW. Intractable occipital neuralgia caused by an entrapment in the semispinalis capitis. *J Korean Neurosurg Soc.* 2013;54(3):268-271.
20. Tubbs RS, Watanabe K, Loukas M, Cohen-Gadol AA. The intramuscular course of the greater occipital nerve: novel findings with potential implications for operative interventions and occipital neuralgia. *Surg Neurol Int.* 2014;5:155.
21. Fernández de las Peñas C, Ge HY, Alonso-Blanco C, Gonzalez-Iglesias J, Arendt-Nielsen L. Referred pain areas of active myofascial trigger points in head, neck, and shoulder muscles, in chronic tension type headache. *J Bodyw Mov Ther.* 2010;14(4):391-396.
22. Fernández de las Peñas C. Myofascial head pain. *Curr Pain Headache Rep.* 2015;19(7):28.
23. Fukui S, Ohseto K, Shiotani M, et al. Referred pain distribution of the cervical zygapophyseal joints and cervical dorsal rami. *Pain.* 1996;68(1):79-83.
24. Magee DJ. *Orthopedic Physical Assessment*. 6th ed. St Louis, MO: Saunders Elsevier; 2014.
25. Gerwin RD, Dommerholt J, Shah JP. An expansion of Simons' integrated hypothesis of trigger point formation. *Curr Pain Headache Rep.* 2004;8(6):468-475.
26. Hsieh YL, Kao MJ, Kuan TS, Chen SM, Chen JT, Hong CZ. Dry needling to a key myofascial trigger point may reduce the irritability of satellite MTrPs. *Am J Phys Med Rehabil.* 2007;86(5):397-403.
27. Yi X, Cook AJ, Hamill-Ruth RJ, Rowlingson JC. Cervicogenic headache in patients with presumed migraine: missed diagnosis or misdiagnosis? *J Pain.* 2005;6(10):700-703.
28. Simons DG, Travell J, Simons L. *Travell & Simon's Myofascial Pain and Dysfunction: The Trigger Point Manual*. Vol 1. 2nd ed. Baltimore, MD: Williams & Wilkins; 1999.
29. Stone SJ, Paleri V, Staines KS. Internal carotid artery aneurysm presenting as orofacial pain. *J Laryngol Otol.* 2012;126(8):851-853.

Chapter 15

Splenius Capitis and Splenius Cervicis Muscles

"Corner of the Neck and Crown Complaints"

César Fernández de las Peñas, Jaime Salom-Moreno, and Michelle Finnegan

1. INTRODUCTION

The splenius capitis and cervicis muscles are the main posterior stabilizers of the cervical spine. The splenius capitis muscle originates from the mastoid process and occipital bone, just below the superior nuchal line. It inserts onto the spinous processes of the seventh cervical and upper three to four thoracic vertebrae and the supraspinous ligament. The splenius cervicis muscle originates from the transverse process of the atlas (C1) and axis (C2) as well as the posterior tubercle of the third cervical vertebra (C3). It inserts onto the third through sixth thoracic spinous processes (T3-T6). The splenius capitis muscle is innervated by the lateral branches of the second and third cervical dorsal rami (C2-C3), whereas the splenius cervicis muscle is innervated by the lateral branches of the lower cervical dorsal rami (C4-C6). Both muscles contribute to the dynamic stability of the neck by controlling movement during cervical extension. Furthermore, these muscles protect the neck during cervical flexion movements such as those during a whiplash injury. Their main function, when acting bilaterally, is extension of the cervical spine, whereas when they act unilaterally, they rotate the neck. Referred pain from splenius capitis trigger points (TrPs) can spread to the vertex of the head; splenius cervicis TrPs refer pain behind the eye and sometimes to the occiput. Activation and perpetuation of TrPs in these muscles include whiplash, poor posture when sitting at a desk, using a handheld electronic device, or playing musical instruments. Environmental or activity-based stresses can also play a role. These muscles can be implicated in different pain syndromes of the cervical spine, particularly mechanical neck pain and whiplash. In addition, TrPs in these muscles have been associated with individuals with cervical radicular pain or fibromyalgia syndrome. The main corrective actions include postural correction and education in ergonomics at work and home.

2. ANATOMIC CONSIDERATIONS

Splenius Capitis

The splenius capitis muscle originates from the mastoid process, underneath the attachment of the sternocleidomastoid muscle, and the rough surface on the occipital bone just below the lateral third of the superior nuchal line. It inserts onto the tips of the spinous processes of the seventh cervical vertebra, the upper three or four thoracic vertebrae, and the intervening supraspinous ligaments (Figure 15-1).[1] The tendons of the upper fibers of the splenius capitis muscle interlace at the midline with those of the contralateral splenius capitis muscle and with the upper trapezius and rhomboid minor muscles. This convergence point forms the dorsal raphe of the ligamentum nuchae in the lower half of the cervical region.[2]

Splenius Cervicis

The splenius cervicis muscle lies to the lateral side and caudal to the splenius capitis muscle. This muscle originates from the transverse process of the atlas (C1), the tip of the transverse process of the axis (C2), and the posterior tubercle of the third cervical vertebra (C3). It inserts onto the third through sixth thoracic spinous processes (T3-T6) (Figure 15-1).[1] On the cranial attachment of the muscle, the splenius cervicis muscle forms the most posterior of a triple attachment with the levator scapulae muscle in the middle and the scalenus medius muscle in front. Bilaterally, each of the paired splenius cervicis and splenius capitis muscles form a "V" shape.

2.1. Innervation and Vascularization

The splenius capitis muscle is innervated by the lateral branches of the second and third cervical dorsal rami (C2-C3), whereas the splenius cervicis muscle is innervated by the lateral branches of the lower cervical dorsal rami (C4-C6).[1] The dorsal muscles of the cervical spine receive their blood supply from the vertebral artery, deep cervical artery, superficial and deep descending branches of the occipital artery, and deep branch of the transverse cervical artery, when present.[1]

2.2. Function

Splenius Capitis

The splenius capitis muscle is active bilaterally during extension of the head and neck[3-5] and unilaterally during rotation of the face to the same side.[3] Takebe et al[6] has shown that the splenius capitis muscle demonstrates no activity at rest in the upright balanced position, and it does not become active during lateral flexion of the head and neck. Other authors have shown that the muscle is active, at least somewhat, during lateral flexion.[4,7,8] When the face is rotated to one side with the chin tilted upward, the splenius capitis muscles on *both* sides work vigorously. When in this rotated and extended position, the muscle on the same side rotates the head and neck; the opposite muscle helps extend the head and the neck.[6] The splenius capitis muscle also plays a subordinate role in ipsilateral tilting of the head.[9] More recent studies have observed that the activity of the splenius capitis muscle is not consistent during voluntary cervical motions depending on the initial position of the head.[10] This muscle is also active during cervical flexion,[11] most likely to assist in controlling the forward motion of the head.

Splenius Cervicis

Despite a lack of supportive electromyographic evidence, it is assumed that the splenius cervicis muscle rotates the upper cervical vertebrae when acting unilaterally and extends the cervical spine

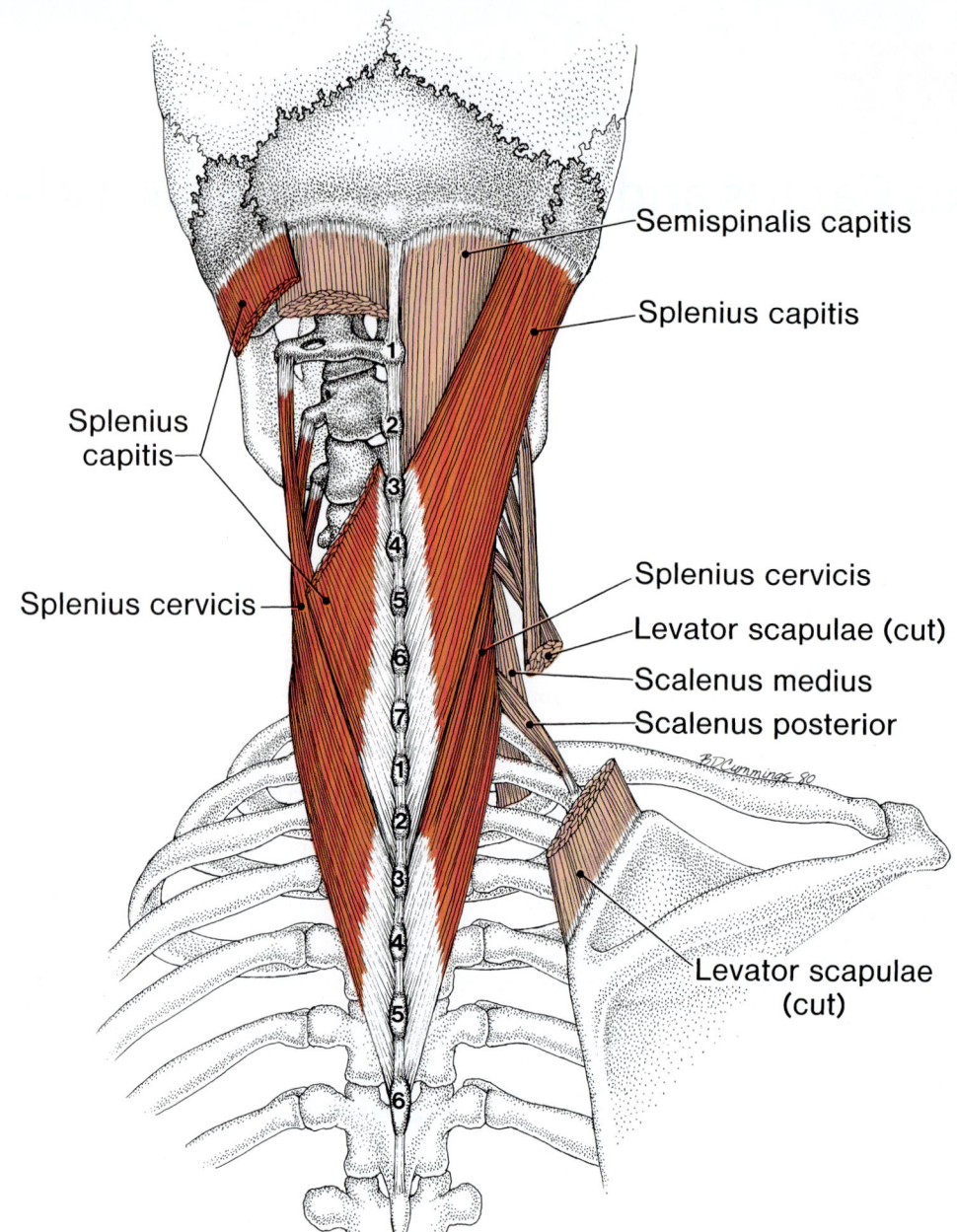

Figure 15-1. Attachments of the right splenius capitis muscle (upper dark red) and of the right splenius cervicis muscle (lower dark red). Adjacent muscles are shown in light red. The levator scapula muscle (right side, cut) crosses over the upper part of the splenius cervicis muscle, with which it has common attachments to the transverse processes of the upper cervical vertebrae. The trapezius muscle (not shown) covers much of both the splenii muscles.

when acting bilaterally. Its role during lateral flexion of the cervical spine is also questionable. However, it has been demonstrated that this muscle is active during cervical flexion,[11] most likely to assist in controlling the forward motion of the head and the neck.

2.3. Functional Unit

The functional unit to which a muscle belongs includes the muscles that reinforce and counter its actions as well as the joints that the muscle crosses. The interdependence of these structures is functionally reflected in the organization and neural connections of the sensory motor cortex. The functional unit is emphasized because the presence of a TrP in one muscle of the unit increases the likelihood that the other muscles of the unit

also develops TrPs. When inactivating TrPs in a muscle, one should be concerned about TrPs that may develop in muscles that are functionally interdependent. Box 15.1 grossly represents the functional unit of the splenii muscles.[12]

3. CLINICAL PRESENTATION

3.1. Referred Pain Pattern

Trigger points in the splenius capitis muscle usually refer pain to the vertex of the head on the same side (Figure 15-2A).[13] Schmidt-Hansen et al[14] observed that a hypertonic saline injection into the splenius capitis muscle induced referred pain to the trigeminal innervated dermatomes, particularly the ophthalmic area of the head (vertex).

Box 15-1 Functional unit of the splenius capitis and cervicis muscles

Action	Synergists	Antagonist
Head and neck extension	Posterior cervical muscle group Semispinalis capitis (bilaterally) Semispinalis cervicis (bilaterally)	Anterior vertebral cervical muscles Suprahyoid muscles Infrahyoid muscles Sternocleidomastoid (bilaterally)
Head rotation	Ipsilateral levator scapulae Contralateral upper trapezius Contralateral semispinalis cervicis Contralateral deep spinal rotator muscles Contralateral sternocleidomastoid	Contralateral levator scapulae Ipsilateral upper trapezius Ipsilateral semispinalis cervicis Ipsilateral deep spinal rotator muscles Ipsilateral sternocleidomastoid

Trigger points in the upper portion of the splenius cervicis (Figure 15-2B, pattern on far left of the figure) usually refer diffuse pain through the inside of the head that focuses strongly behind the eye on the same side and sometimes to the ipsilateral occiput. Trigger points in the lower portion of the splenius cervicis, at the angle of the neck (Figure 15-2B, middle figure) refer pain upward and to the base of the neck (Figure 15-2B, pattern on far right of the figure). This pattern generally lies within the upper part of the pain pattern of the levator scapula, but it can include pain spread more medially.

In addition to pain, a TrP in the upper portion of the splenius cervicis muscle may cause blurring of the vision in the ipsilateral eye without dizziness or conjunctivitis.

The referred pain patterns of TrPs in these muscles have mistakenly been diagnosed as occipital neuralgia in three patients as reported in Graff-Radford et al.[15] Prior to the diagnosis of myofascial pain, other treatments did not provide successful relief of symptoms. Once the correct diagnosis was made, two of the three patients were successfully treated. The third patient was not successfully treated due to inability to follow-up with care; however, the initial release of TrPs in the splenii capitis and cervicis muscles fully eliminated the pain for 2 days.

3.2. Symptoms

Patients with active splenius capitis TrPs usually present with a primary complaint of pain referred close to the vertex of the head, as described earlier in this chapter.

Patients with splenius cervicis TrPs primarily report pain in the neck, cranium, and eye; they may also report a "stiff neck,"[16] because active rotation of the head and neck is limited by pain.

Pain in the orbit and blurring of vision are disturbing symptoms that are occasionally referred unilaterally to the eye from TrPs in the upper part of the splenius cervicis muscle.

Patients with TrPs in the splenii capitis and cervicis muscles may also report a pressure-like pain in the occipital region, a pressure-like pain that radiates to the forehead, and/or numbness in the occipital region.[15]

3.3. Patient Examination

Observation of posture typically reveals a forward head position with an extended upper cervical spine and a flexed lower cervical spine. A lateral tilt of the head may also be observed. The patient oftentimes demonstrates painful and limited active cervical rotation to the same side and passive cervical rotation limited to the opposite side. Active cervical flexion may be limited by one or two finger widths.

Joint accessory motion testing of the upper cervical (C0-C1; C1-C2) joints is warranted if TrPs in the splenius capitis or cervicis muscles are suspected.[12] The most common joint dysfunction seems to be C1-C2, particularly when the splenius capitis muscle is involved. Another common accessory motion dysfunction relating to the splenius capitis muscle is an atlanto-occipital dysfunction (C0-C1). Joint accessory motion dysfunctions at C4 and C5 likely occur with splenius cervicis TrPs.

3.4. Trigger Point Examination

Splenius Capitis

Splenius capitis TrPs can be identified by flat cross-fiber palpation and are usually found near the region where the upper border of the upper trapezius muscle crosses the splenius capitis muscle. The clinician should know the direction of the muscle fibers (Figure 15-2A) and palpate perpendicular to the fibers to find a TrP within a taut band of the muscle tissue. This muscle can be palpated within the small muscular triangle bounded anteriorly by the sternocleidomastoid muscle, posteriorly by the upper trapezius muscle, and inferiorly by the levator scapulae muscle. To locate the splenius capitis muscle, palpate the mastoid process and the prominent sternocleidomastoid muscle. Place one finger posterior and medial to the sternocleidomastoid muscle below the occiput. Then palpate for a contraction of the diagonally directed splenius capitis fibers by asking the patient to turn the face toward the side being examined while extending and extend the head against light resistance provided by the clinician. Once the splenius capitis muscle is identified in this muscular triangle, it can be palpated for taut bands and TrPs. In some patients, the splenius capitis muscle may be taut enough to be clearly palpable without active movement from the patient (Figure 15-3).

Another way the muscle can be detected is by first identifying the upper border of the trapezius muscle (Figure 6-1) while the patient is supported in a reclined position with the muscles relaxed. The clinician then palpates for a muscle contraction in the splenius capitis muscle as the patient performs a sudden brief arm abduction movement against light resistance. The splenius capitis muscle is then palpated for taut bands and TrPs along and/or deep to the border of the upper trapezius muscle at approximately the level of the C2 spinous process.

Williams[17] described a splenius capitis TrP at the insertion of the muscle on the mastoid process and in the portion of the muscle just distal to this attachment. According to Simons et al,[12] the tenderness in this location is more likely to be caused by enthesopathy of the splenius capitis.

Splenius Cervicis

The splenius cervicis muscle is not readily palpable because the upper and middle trapezius muscles cover most of this muscle from behind. Only a small patch of the splenius cervicis muscle

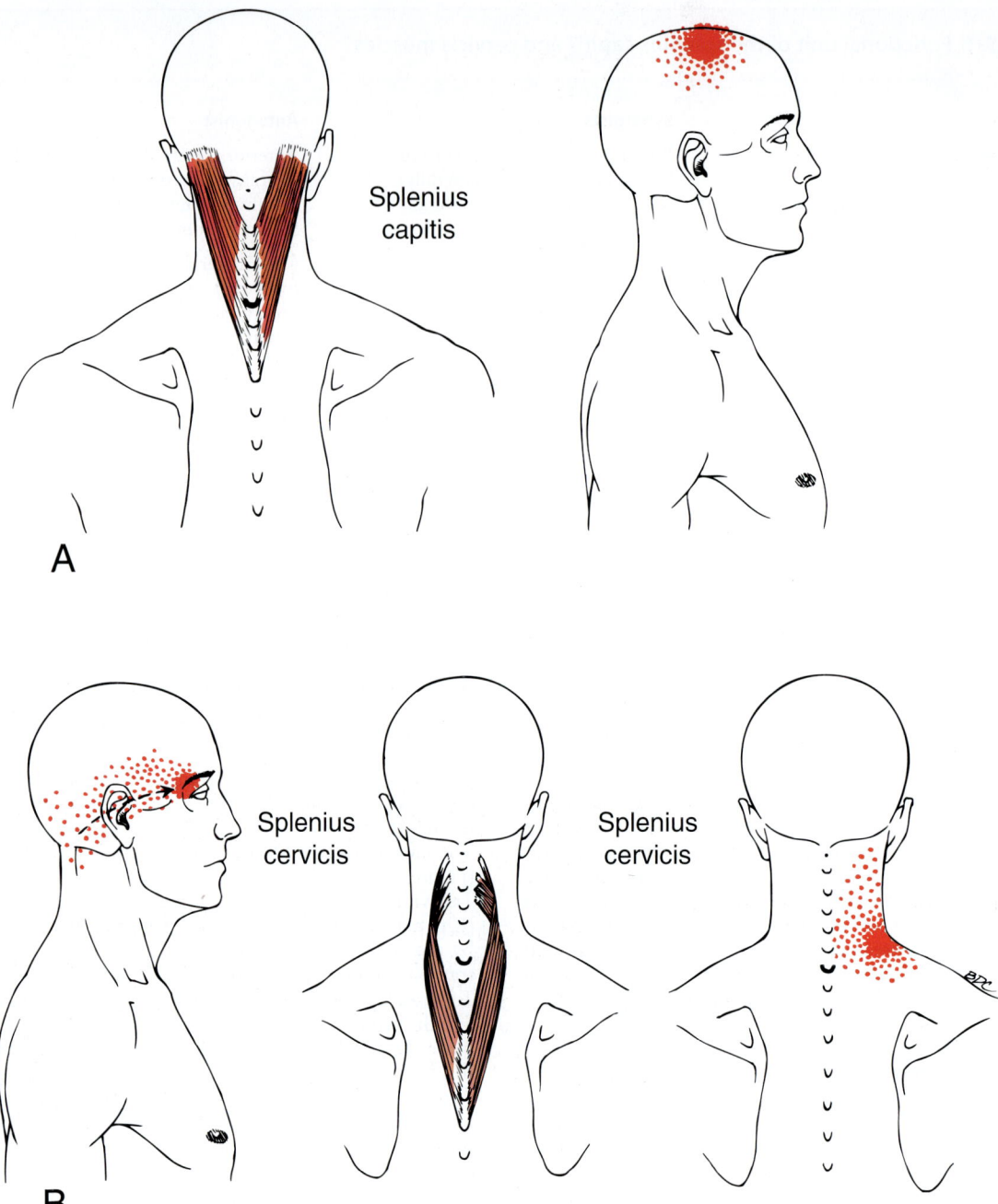

Figure 15-2. Referred pain patterns (dark red) for the right splenius capitis and splenius cervicis muscles (medium red). A, Referred pain from TrPs located in the upper portion of the splenius capitis, the only section of the muscle directly palpated. B, Trigger points in the splenius *cervicis* muscle refer pain to the orbit (pain figure on the left). The black dash line and arrow indicate that the pain seems to shoot through the inside of the head to the back of the eye. Splenius cervicis TrPs can also refer pain to the angle of the neck (figure on the right).

is not covered by the splenius capitis or the rhomboid minor muscles posteriorly or by the levator scapulae laterally.

The best method of eliciting tenderness from splenius cervicis TrPs is from the lateral side of the neck through or around the levator scapulae. If the skin and subcutaneous tissues are sufficiently mobile, the clinician slides the palpating finger anterior to the free border of the upper trapezius muscle at approximately the level of the C7 spinous process, toward and beyond the levator scapulae muscle. If the levator scapulae is not tender but additional pressure directed medially toward the spine is painful, it is likely a splenius cervicis TrP. In patients with mobile connective tissue, the taut bands may be palpable running caudally on a diagonal from lateral to medial. To differentiate palpation of the levator scapulae muscle from the splenius cervicis muscle, the levator scapulae muscle can be felt to contract with shoulder elevation, and in contrast, the splenius cervicis muscle contracts with neck extension.

Posteriorly, digital pressure to splenius cervicis TrPs is applied mid-muscle approximately 2 cm lateral to the spine at approximately the level of the C7 spinous process (Figure 15-3), which is just above the angle of the neck. Tenderness mid-muscle, just above the angle of the neck could also result from trapezius TrPs, however, trapezius taut bands are angled laterally, not medially, in the caudad direction. If the tenderness is deep to the trapezius muscle, it may be from either splenius cervicis or levator scapulae TrPs. If cervical flexion increases the sensitivity

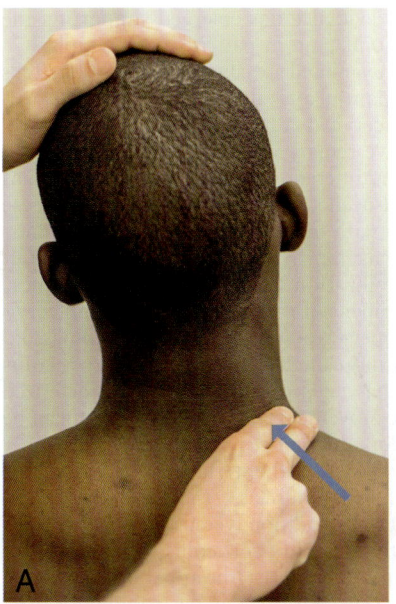
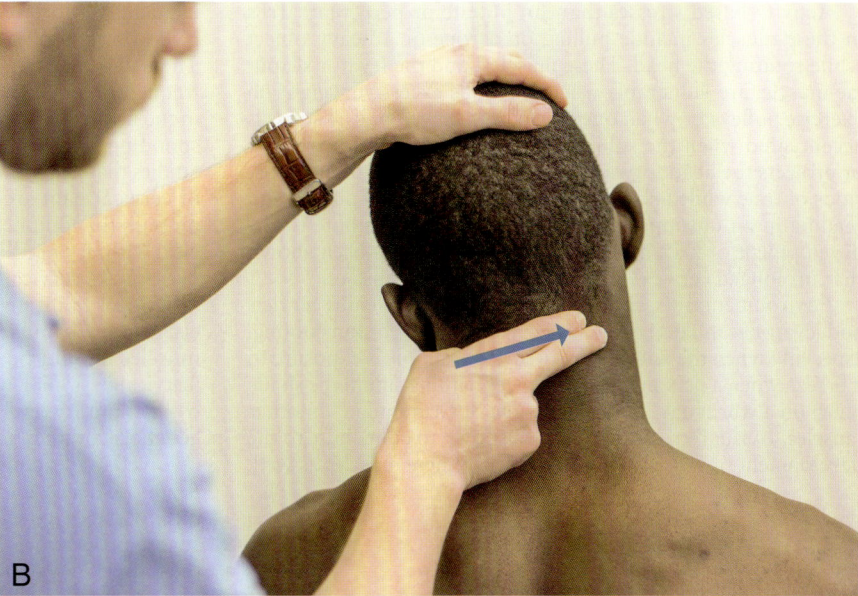

Figure 15-3. A, Examination for TrPs in the right splenius cervicis muscle. B, Examination for TrPs in the right splenius capitis muscle.

of the tenderness, it is more likely from splenius cervicis TrPs due to increasing tension on these fibers with flexion. Both the splenius capitis and splenius cervicis muscles are elongated by cervical flexion, but only the splenius capitis is further elongated by flexion of the head on the cervical spine.

In some patients, pressure applied from the lateral aspect of the neck directly toward the spine cephalad to the C7 level elicits tenderness in the region of the cephalad attachments of the splenius cervicis muscle. According to Simons et al,[12] this tenderness is thought to be due to enthesopathy.

4. DIFFERENTIAL DIAGNOSIS

4.1. Activation and Perpetuation of Trigger Points

A posture or activity that activates a TrP, if not corrected, can also perpetuate it. Trigger points may be activated by unaccustomed eccentric loading, eccentric exercise in unconditioned splenius muscle, and/or maximal or submaximal concentric loading.[18] Trigger points may also be activated or aggravated when the muscle is placed in a shortened or lengthened position for an extended period of time.

A common cause of splenius capitis TrPs is a whiplash injury.[19,20] These muscles are susceptible to injury due to the trauma of a rear-end collision in an automobile followed by a sudden stop,[21] especially if the head and neck are somewhat rotated at the time of the impact. Patients with a whiplash injury are known to develop refractory head and neck pain symptoms, probably due to joint injury and TrPs.[22] These patients are rarely examined properly and treated for the part of their pain that is of muscular origin. Baker[23] investigated 34 muscles for TrPs in each of 100 occupants (drivers or passengers) who sustained a single motor vehicle impact and identified the direction of the impact. The splenius capitis muscle was the second most frequently involved muscle: in 94% of the subjects in impacts from the front, in 77% of the subjects in impacts from behind, in 75% of the subjects when hit the broadside on the passenger side, and in 69% of the subjects when hit the broadside on the driver's side. In a review of the literature, Fernández de las Peñas et al[24] found that TrPs in the scalenes, splenius capitis, sternocleidomastoid,[23] upper trapezius, and pectoralis minor muscles[25] were the most affected following a whiplash injury.

Postural, activity-based, and environmental stresses can also activate or perpetuate TrPs in the splenius capitis or cervicis muscles.

Postural stresses include those that overload extension or rotation of the head and neck for prolonged periods of time. Clinical examples include working at a desk with the head turned to one side to view documents or a computer monitor while the body is facing forward; watching planes at an air show while seated in a poor position that extends the neck; using handheld electronic devices while lying prone on elbows (Figure 15-4); and playing musical instruments with poor head and neck positioning, as with the flute or violin. In addition, TrPs in either, or both, the splenius capitis and splenius cervicis muscles may be activated by falling asleep with the head and neck in a laterally flexed position as with the head on the armrest of a sofa without an adequate pillow for support. Cold air from an air conditioner or a cool draft blowing on the exposed neck, together with muscular fatigue, greatly increases the likelihood of activating TrPs in these muscles.[12]

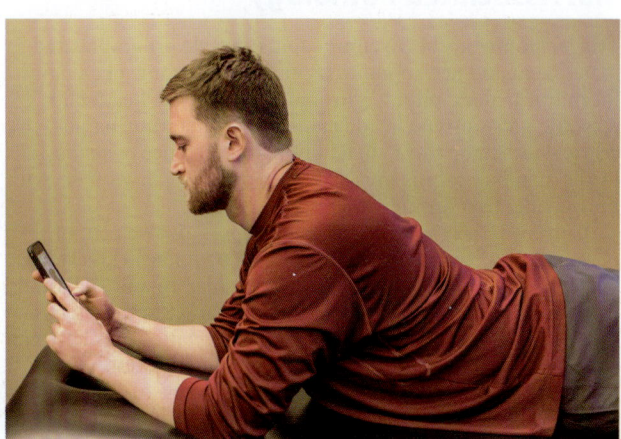

Figure 15-4. Postures that places the splenius cervicis muscles in sustained contraction should be avoided. These activities could include looking up at an air show, bird watching, watching TV from the floor in prone, or using handheld electronic devices while prone on elbows (shown in the figure).

Activity-based stresses that can initiate or perpetuate TrPs in these muscles include pulling on a rope or a heavy object while rotating the head. These muscles, and the levator scapulae muscle, are vulnerable when one pulls excessive weight on exercise pulleys or when one lifts excessive weight; the stress is accentuated when the subject rotates the head and neck and/or projects the head forward. Looking down for prolonged periods of time while texting, playing games on a cell phone, and reading in an unsupported posture can also contribute to the development of TrPs in the splenii muscles. It has been shown that prolonged cervical flexion activates these muscles.[11]

Environmental stress that can activate both splenius cervicis and levator scapulae TrPs may occur with marked skin cooling, especially when the muscles are tired. An example is exposure to a breeze when a person relaxes in a wet bathing suit in the shade (even on a warm day) after the fatigue of swimming.[12] In other muscles,[26] visual stressors have been shown to contribute to the development of TrPs and are plausible for these muscles as well.

4.2. Associated Trigger Points

Associated TrPs can develop in the referred pain areas of TrPs.[27] Therefore, musculature in the referred pain areas for each muscle should also be considered. Associated TrPs for the splenii muscles can develop in the occipitalis, temporalis, upper trapezius, levator scapulae, semispinalis capitis and cervicis, and suboccipital muscles.

Several other muscles have similar or overlapping pain patterns to the splenius capitis and splenius cervicis muscles, and therefore should be included in the examination and differential diagnosis. A thorough TrP examination should be performed for the semispinalis cervicis, suboccipitals, levator scapulae, sternocleidomastoid, upper trapezius, temporalis, and deep masseter muscles.

Trigger points rarely appear in the splenii muscles alone; usually, either or both the levator scapulae and other posterior cervical muscles are also involved. If the splenius cervicis muscle is involved without the levator scapulae muscle, cervical rotation is less restricted than when only the levator scapulae muscle is involved. Simultaneous TrP activity in both the levator and splenii muscles may almost completely block active head rotation to that side. Involvement of the splenius cervicis muscle may become apparent because of residual pain and stiffness following the elimination of TrP activity in the levator scapulae muscle.

4.3. Associated Pathology

Trigger points in the splenius capitis muscle are implicated in many head and neck conditions including chronic neck pain,[28] mechanical neck pain,[29] chronic tension-type headache,[30,31] episodic tension-type headache,[32] upper quadrant pain,[33] and cervical radiculopathy.[34] In addition, the presence of active TrPs in the splenius capitis muscle is also frequent in women with fibromyalgia syndrome.[35]

Currently, there is no research to support involvement of TrPs of the splenius cervicis muscle with other conditions. This evidence deficit is likely due to the difficulty of isolating and accurately palpating the muscle as it was described earlier in this chapter.

Research demonstrates that there is a relationship between TrPs in cervical muscles and cervical joint hypomobility;[36-38] evidence specifically outlining the involvement of the splenius capitis or splenius cervicis muscles is still needed. Nevertheless, Hsueh et al[39] observed that C4-C5 and C5-C6 disc lesions were associated with TrPs in the splenius capitis muscle.

Understanding the clinical presentation of cervical pain is complicated by the similarity of symptoms arising from joint and muscle pathology. A carefully controlled older study showed that painful zygapophyseal joints were present in 54% of 50 consecutive patients with chronic neck pain following a whiplash incident.[40] More recent evidence has emerged supporting the role of zygapophyseal joint pain in patients with whiplash.[41] These patients were not examined specifically for TrPs, but TrPs frequently coexist with painful articular dysfunctions. The TrPs in the neck muscles and cervical zygapophyseal joints, at corresponding levels, can have remarkably similar pain patterns.[42] Studies that help clinicians differentiate the cause of the symptoms of cervical pain are still needed. Clinically, treatment of these muscles (in conjunction with the other posterior cervical muscles) with dry needling has improved cervical mobility without performing cervical mobilization or manipulation techniques.

Trigger point involvement of the splenius capitis and cervicis, levator scapulae, upper trapezius and sternocleidomastoid muscles should be distinguished from spasmodic torticollis (cervical dystonia), which is a neurologic condition characterized by involuntary dystonic movements of the head[43,44] that can be genetic, acquired, or idiopathic.[45] The muscles most commonly involved in this condition include the sternocleidomastoid, trapezius, scalenes, and platysma muscles,[46] therefore making the differential diagnosis of this condition (versus TrPs) essential to ensure proper care. With spasmodic torticollis, hypertrophy of the muscles may develop.[43] In contrast, the apparent shortening of a muscle due to TrPs does not cause hypertrophy; nor does it cause involuntary movements of the head. Although physical therapy can be effective for spasmodic torticollis,[47,48] botulinum toxin is the preferred treatment[44] because studies have shown the effectiveness of this treatment.[49-52]

5. CORRECTIVE ACTIONS

Patients with TrPs in the splenii muscles should avoid postural strain by improving their posture. Correction of rounded shoulder posture and forward head position and maintenance of effective posture are primary in any treatment approach both for initial relief of pain and for lasting relief (Figure 6-9). Refer to Chapter 76 for discussions of posture and body mechanics.

Body asymmetry due to a leg length discrepancy or small hemipelvis should be corrected. An excessively long walking cane should be avoided. Neck strain is also avoided by sleeping with the head and neck in a neutral position with appropriate pillow support.

Good ergonomics at work are essential for anyone who spends time at a desk with a computer. It is important to learn how to keep joints in a neutral posture when possible and to minimize excessive twisting and turning movements or prolonged positions with the head turned. The computer screen should be directly in front of the body and at an angle that encourages erect posture while minimizing glare. Documents should be placed on a stand at the same level as the monitor (rather than flat on the desk to one side) for optimum viewing and to avoid excessive muscular strain. Reflections on eyeglasses and contact lenses can be managed by changing the relative position of the light source or by using anti-glare lenses. Patients receiving new progressive lenses should also be evaluated for proper workstation fitting.

Care should also be taken when pulling weights while using exercise equipment. Excessive weight should be avoided, and the patient should learn to pull the weight without rotating the head and neck or protruding the head forward.

Chilling the skin of the neck, especially when the muscles are fatigued, often activates TrPs in posterior neck muscles. The patient should keep the neck warm, when possible, by sleeping in a high-necked sleep shirt, by wearing a turtleneck or scarf during the day, and by avoiding cold drafts.

References

1. Standring S. *Gray's Anatomy: The Anatomical Basis of Clinical Practice*. 41st ed. London, UK: Elsevier; 2015.
2. Mercer SR, Bogduk N. Clinical anatomy of ligamentum nuchae. *Clin Anat*. 2003;16(6):484-493.

3. Mayoux-Benhamou MA, Revel M, Vallee C. Selective electromyography of dorsal neck muscles in humans. *Exp Brain Res.* 1997;113(2):353-360.
4. Gabriel DA, Matsumoto JY, Davis DH, Currier BL, An KN. Multidirectional neck strength and electromyographic activity for normal controls. *Clin Biomech (Bristol, Avon).* 2004;19(7):653-658.
5. Schomacher J, Erlenwein J, Dieterich A, Petzke F, Falla D. Can neck exercises enhance the activation of the semispinalis cervicis relative to the splenius capitis at specific spinal levels? *Man Ther.* 2015;20(5):694-702.
6. Takebe K, Vitti M, Basmajian JV. The functions of semispinalis capitis and splenius capitis muscles: an electromyographic study. *Anat Rec.* 1974;179(4):477-480.
7. Kumar S, Narayan Y, Amell T. EMG power spectra of cervical muscles in lateral flexion and comparison with sagittal and oblique plane activities. *Eur J Appl Physiol.* 2003;89(3-4):367-376.
8. Harrison MF, Neary JP, Albert WJ, et al. Measuring neuromuscular fatigue in cervical spinal musculature of military helicopter aircrew. *Mil Med.* 2009;174(11):1183-1189.
9. Benhamou MA, Revel M, Vallee C. Surface electrodes are not appropriate to record selective myoelectric activity of splenius capitis muscle in humans. *Exp Brain Res.* 1995;105(3):432-438.
10. Siegmund GP, Blouin JS, Brault JR, Hedensterna S, Inglis JT. Electromyography of superficial and deep neck muscles during isometric, voluntary, and reflex contractions. *J Biomech Eng.* 2007;129(1):66-77.
11. Lee TH, Lee JH, Lee YS, Kim MK, Kim SG. Changes in the activity of the muscles surrounding the neck according to the angles of movement of the neck in adults in their 20s. *J Phys Ther Sci.* 2015;27(3):973-975.
12. Simons DG, Travell J, Simons L. *Travell & Simon's Myofascial Pain and Dysfunction: The Trigger Point Manual.* Vol 1. 2nd ed. Baltimore, MD: Williams & Wilkins; 1999:104.
13. Travell J, Rinzler SH. The myofascial genesis of pain. *Postgrad Med.* 1952;11(5):425-434.
14. Schmidt-Hansen PT, Svensson P, Jensen TS, Graven-Nielsen T, Bach FW. Patterns of experimentally induced pain in pericranial muscles. *Cephalalgia.* 2006;26(5):568-577.
15. Graff-Radford SB, Jaeger B, Reeves JL. Myofascial pain may present clinically as occipital neuralgia. *Neurosurgery.* 1986;19(4):610-613.
16. Travell J. Rapid relief of acute stiff neck by ethyl chloride spray. *J Am Med Womens Assoc.* 1949;4(3):89-95.
17. Williams HL. The syndrome of physical or intrinsic allergy of the head: myalgia of the head (sinus headache). *Proc Staff Meet Mayo Clin.* 1945;20(12):177-183.
18. Gerwin RD, Dommerholt J, Shah JP. An expansion of Simons' integrated hypothesis of trigger point formation. *Curr Pain Headache Rep.* 2004;8(6):468-475.
19. Kumar S, Ferrari R, Narayan Y. Cervical muscle response to whiplash-type right anterolateral impacts. *Eur Spine J.* 2004;13(5):398-407.
20. Castaldo M, Ge HY, Chiarotto A, Villafane JH, Arendt-Nielsen L. Myofascial trigger points in patients with whiplash-associated disorders and mechanical neck pain. *Pain Med.* 2014;15(5):842-849.
21. Rubin D. An approach to the management of myofascial trigger point syndromes. *Arch Phys Med Rehabil.* 1981;62:107-110.
22. Dommerholt J. Persistent myalgia following whiplash. *Curr Pain Headache Rep.* 2005;9(5):326-330.
23. Baker B. The muscle trigger: evidence of overload injury. *J Neurol Orthop Med Surg.* 1986;7(1):35-44.
24. Fernández de las Peñas C, Fernandez-Carnero J, Alonso-Blanco C, Miangolarra-Page JC. Myofascial pain syndrome in whiplash injury. A critical review of the literature. International Whiplash Trauma Congress; October 9-10, 2003; Denver, USA.
25. Hong C-Z, Simons DG. Response to treatment for pectoralis minor myofascial pain syndrome after whiplash. *J Musculoskelet Pain.* 1993;1(1):89-131.
26. Hoyle JA, Marras WS, Sheedy JE, Hart DE. Effects of postural and visual stressors on myofascial trigger point development and motor unit rotation during computer work. *J Electromyogr Kinesiol.* 2011;21(1):41-48.
27. Hsieh YL, Kao MJ, Kuan TS, Chen SM, Chen JT, Hong CZ. Dry needling to a key myofascial trigger point may reduce the irritability of satellite MTrPs. *Am J Phys Med Rehabil.* 2007;86(5):397-403.
28. Lluch E, Arguisuelas MD, Coloma PS, Palma F, Rey A, Falla D. Effects of deep cervical flexor training on pressure pain thresholds over myofascial trigger points in patients with chronic neck pain. *J Manipulative Physiol Ther.* 2013;36(9):604-611.
29. Munoz-Munoz S, Munoz-Garcia MT, Alburquerque-Sendin F, Arroyo-Morales M, Fernández de las Peñas C. Myofascial trigger points, pain, disability, and sleep quality in individuals with mechanical neck pain. *J Manipulative Physiol Ther.* 2012;35(8):608-613.
30. Fernández de las Peñas C, Ge HY, Alonso-Blanco C, Gonzalez-Iglesias J, Arendt-Nielsen L. Referred pain areas of active myofascial trigger points in head, neck, and shoulder muscles, in chronic tension type headache. *J Bodyw Mov Ther.* 2010;14(4):391-396.
31. Martin-Herrero C, Rodrigues de Souza DP, Alburquerque-Sendin F, Ortega-Santiago R, Fernández de las Peñas C. Myofascial trigger points, pain, disability and quality of sleep in patients with chronic tension-type headache: a pilot study [in Spanish]. *Rev Neurol.* 2012;55(4):193-199.
32. Karadas O, Gul HL, Inan LE. Lidocaine injection of pericranial myofascial trigger points in the treatment of frequent episodic tension-type headache. *J Headache Pain.* 2013;14:44.
33. Fernández de las Peñas C, Grobli C, Ortega-Santiago R, et al. Referred pain from myofascial trigger points in head, neck, shoulder, and arm muscles reproduces pain symptoms in blue-collar (manual) and white-collar (office) workers. *Clin J Pain.* 2012;28(6):511-518.
34. Sari H, Akarirmak U, Uludag M. Active myofascial trigger points might be more frequent in patients with cervical radiculopathy. *Eur J Phys Rehabil Med.* 2012;48(2):237-244.
35. Alonso-Blanco C, Fernández de las Peñas C, Morales-Cabezas M, Zarco-Moreno P, Ge HY, Florez-Garcia M. Multiple active myofascial trigger points reproduce the overall spontaneous pain pattern in women with fibromyalgia and are related to widespread mechanical hypersensitivity. *Clin J Pain.* 2011;27(5):405-413.
36. Fernández de las Peñas C, Downey C, Miangolarra-Page JC. Validity of the lateral gliding test as a tool for the diagnosis of intervertebral joint dysfunction in the lower cervical spine. *J Manipulative Physiol Ther.* 2005;28(8):610-616.
37. Fernández de las Peñas C. Myofascial trigger points and postero-anterior joint hypomobility in the mid-cervical spine in subjects presenting with mechanical neck pain; a pilot study. *J Manual Manipulative Ther.* 2006;14(2):88-94.
38. Tali D, Menahem I, Vered E, Kalichman L. Upper cervical mobility, posture and myofascial trigger points in subjects with episodic migraine: case-control study. *J Bodyw Mov Ther.* 2014;18(4):569-575.
39. Hsueh TC, Yu S, Kuan TS, Hong CZ. Association of active myofascial trigger points and cervical disc lesions. *J Formos Med Assoc.* 1998;97(3):174-180.
40. Barnsley L, Lord SM, Wallis BJ, Bogduk N. The prevalence of chronic cervical zygapophysial joint pain after whiplash. *Spine.* 1995;20(1):20-25; discussion 26.
41. Bogduk N. On cervical zygapophysial joint pain after whiplash. *Spine (Phila Pa 1976).* 2011;36(25 suppl):S194-S199.
42. Bogduk N, Simons D. Neck pain: joint pain or trigger points? Chapter 20. In: Vaeroy H, Merskey H, eds. *Progress in Fibromyalgia and Myofascial Pain.* Vol 6 of Pain Research and Clinical Management. Amsterdam, Netherlands: Elsevier; 1993:267-273.
43. Waldman SD. *Atlas of Uncommon Pain Syndromes.* 3rd ed. Philadelphia, PA: Elsevier Saunders; 2014.
44. Mills RR, Pagan FL. Patient considerations in the treatment of cervical dystonia: focus on botulinum toxin type A. *Patient Prefer Adherence.* 2015;9:725-731.
45. Albanese A, Bhatia K, Bressman SB, et al. Phenomenology and classification of dystonia: a consensus update. *Mov Disord.* 2013;28(7):863-873.
46. Jankovic J, Leder S, Warner D, Schwartz K. Cervical dystonia: clinical findings and associated movement disorders. *Neurology.* 1991;41(7):1088-1091.
47. De Pauw J, Van der Velden K, Meirte J, et al. The effectiveness of physiotherapy for cervical dystonia: a systematic literature review. *J Neurol.* 2014;261(10):1857-1865.
48. Queiroz MA, Chien HF, Sekeff-Sallem FA, Barbosa ER. Physical therapy program for cervical dystonia: a study of 20 cases. *Funct Neurol.* 2012;27(3):187-192.
49. Poungvarin N, Viriyavejakul A. Botulinum A toxin treatment in spasmodic torticollis: report of 56 patients. *J Med Assoc Thai.* 1994;77(9):464-470.
50. Marin C, Marti MJ, Tolosa E, Alvarez R, Montserrat L, Santamaria J. Muscle activity changes in spasmodic torticollis after botulinum toxin treatment. *Eur J Neurol.* 1995;1(3):243-247.
51. Colosimo C, Tiple D, Berardelli A. Efficacy and safety of long-term botulinum toxin treatment in craniocervical dystonia: a systematic review. *Neurotox Res.* 2012;22(4):265-273.
52. Ramirez-Castaneda J, Jankovic J. Long-term efficacy and safety of botulinum toxin injections in dystonia. *Toxins (Basel).* 2013;5(2):249-266.

Chapter 16

Posterior Cervical Muscles: Semispinalis Capitis, Longissimus Capitis, Semispinalis Cervicis, Multifidus, and Rotatores

"Iron Man Helmet"

César Fernández de las Peñas and Ana I. de-la-Llave-Rincón

1. INTRODUCTION

The posterior cervical muscles include the middle layers of the cervical spine musculature and the deep cervical extensors. These muscles have attachments from the occiput down to T6. The semispinalis capitis muscle receives innervation from C1-C4, while the semispinalis cervicis receives its innervation from C3-C6. The deeper posterior cervical muscles are innervated by the medial branches of the dorsal rami of the adjacent cervical spinal nerves. These muscles contribute to segmental control of the zygapophyseal (facet) joints of the cervical spine. The main function of the more superficial muscles (ie, semispinalis capitis, longissimus capitis, and semispinalis cervicis) is extension of the cervical spine, whereas the main function of the deepest muscles (ie, multifidus and rotator muscles) is segmental extension and control of the cervical vertebrae. Pain from the semispinalis capitis and longissimus capitis trigger points (TrPs) refers to the head, whereas the multifidus refers pain deep to the cervical spine and sometimes cephalad to the suboccipital region. Activation and perpetuation of TrPs in these muscles can result from acute trauma, especially whiplash, activities that require sustained neck flexion, awkward posture, or positions that place the cervical spine in excessive extension. These muscles can be involved in pain syndromes of the cervical spine, particularly in mechanical neck pain or along with cervical radicular pain or radiculopathy. The semispinalis capitis muscle is more frequently affected by TrPs in patients with whiplash than in individuals with fibromyalgia syndrome. In addition, morphologic changes in these muscles have been observed in patients with cervical spine disorders. Specifically, fatty tissue infiltration of the multifidus muscles has been found in patients with whiplash-related neck pain. Also, patients with mechanical neck pain demonstrate reduced activation of the multifidus and semispinalis cervicis muscles as well as decreased cross-sectional areas of cervical multifidus. Corrective actions of this muscle group include optimizing posture to reduce gravitational stress and temporary use of a soft collar for support.

2. ANATOMIC CONSIDERATIONS

The posterior neck muscles are divided anatomically into four layers with fibers running in different directions at some levels,[1] suggesting the plies of a tire (Figure 16-1). The most superficial layer, the bilateral upper trapezius, converges above, tending to form a "^" or roof-top shape. The next deeper layer, the bilateral splenius fibers, converges below to form a "V" shape. The semispinalis capitis fibers of the third layer lie nearly vertical, parallel with the vertebral column. All the remaining innermost layers of fibers return to the "^" configuration. These include the more deeply placed semispinalis cervicis of the third layer and the multifidus and rotators fibers which constitute the fourth layer. Knowledge of this fiber arrangement is helpful to treat these muscles effectively. The erector spinae muscles of the cervical spine include the longissimus capitis and cervicis, iliocostalis cervicis, and the variable spinalis capitis and cervicis muscles.[2]

Functionally, these muscles can be categorized in two groups: four muscles that attach and control the movement of the head (upper trapezius, splenius capitis, semispinalis capitis, and longissimus capitis muscles), and three muscles that have only spinal vertebral attachments and do not act on the head (semispinalis cervicis, multifidus, and rotatores muscles). Digitations of the second group of muscles attach at each vertebral segmental level and analogous digitations extend throughout the thoracic region and into the lumbar region with basically the same arrangement. At successively greater depth, muscles of this group become shorter and more angulated.

The anatomic designation of the second functional group of muscles to three names, that is, semispinalis, multifidus, and rotatores, is quite arbitrary. In fact, there is a full and continuous

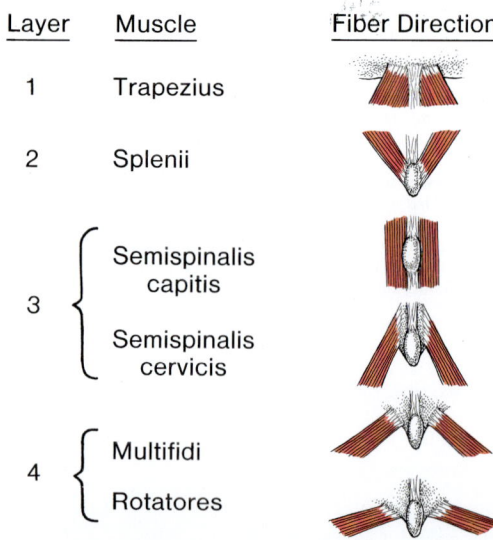

Figure 16-1. The changes in the directions of successively deeper fibers in the four layers of the posterior cervical muscles with layer 1 representing the most superficial muscle fibers and layer 4 the deepest fibers.

Chapter 16: Posterior Cervical Muscles: Semispinalis Capitis, Longissimus Capitis, Semispinalis Cervicis, Multifidus, and Rotatores **169**

transition of lengths at each spinal level. Digitations attaching at every vertebra span 0 to 5 vertebral segments.[2]

Semispinalis Capitis

The semispinalis capitis muscle lies superficial over the semispinalis cervicis muscle. This muscle originates on the medial aspect of the area between the superior and inferior nuchal lines of the occipital bone forming a thick muscle bundle in the suboccipital region and inserts onto the superior articular processes of C4-C7 and the tips of the transverse processes of T1 to T6 and sometimes T7 (Figure 16-2).[2] The semispinalis capitis muscle is usually divided by a tendinous inscription at the level of C6 vertebrae. These inscriptions divide the muscle into thirds, each with an endplate zone. The endplate zone of the upper third of the semispinalis capitis muscle is aligned nearly transversely at the suboccipital level. The endplate zone of the middle third is found at approximately the C3-C4 level.

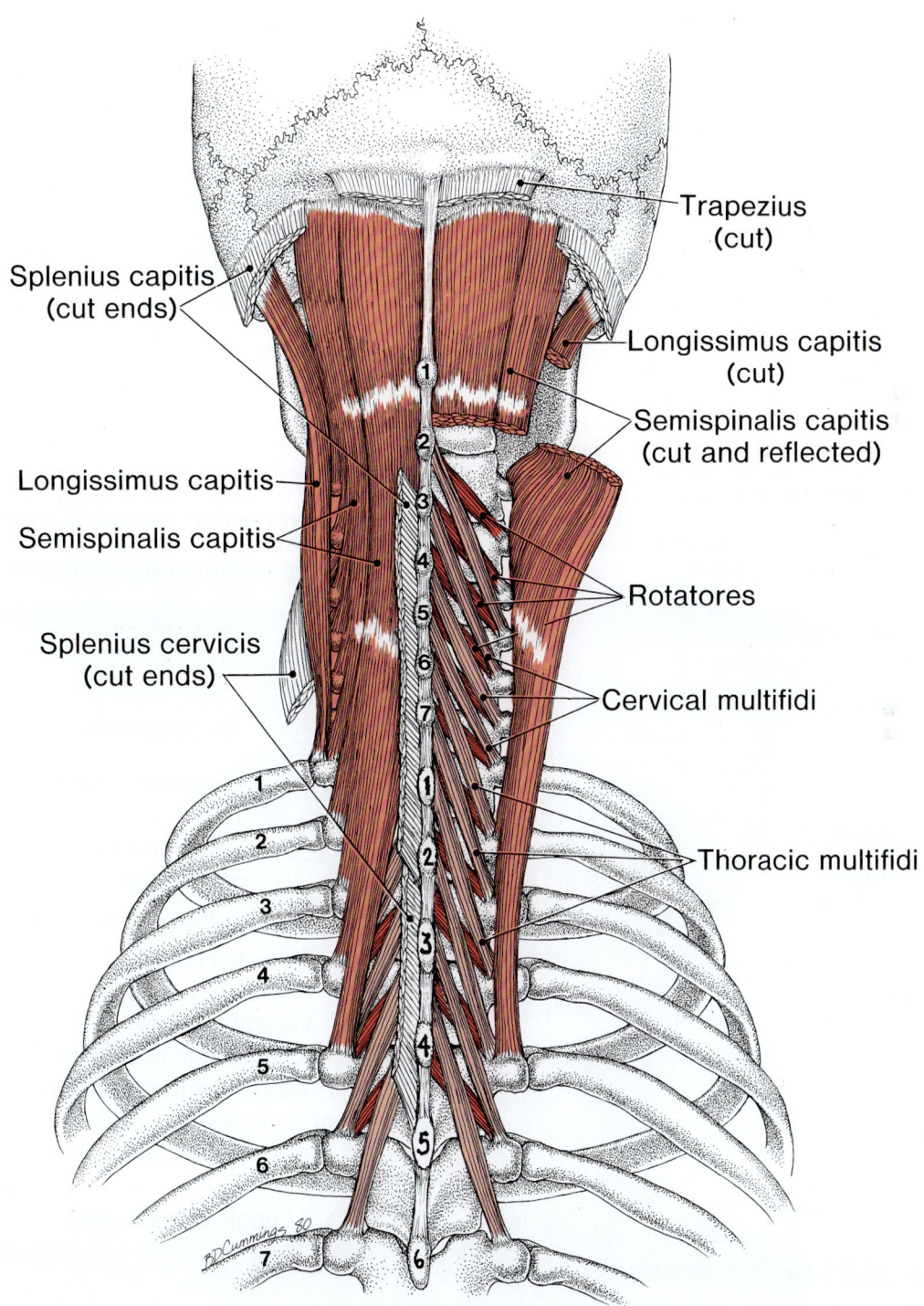

Figure 16-2. Attachments of the posterior cervical muscles. Left side, the fibers of the longissimus capitis and semispinalis capitis muscles (medium red) lie almost vertical, between the skull and the thoracic vertebrae. The semispinalis cervicis muscle is not shown here. It is intermediate between the semispinalis capitis and multifidus muscles in depth, fiber length, and angulation of fibers. Right side, the deepest layer, comprised of the multifidus (light red) and rotatores muscles (dark red). They travel diagonally to bilaterally form, the roof-top ∧ shape.

Due to the differing fiber lengths in the most inferior third of the muscle, this endplate zone is more variable.

The greater occipital nerve can be trapped by a tendinous band of the semispinalis capitis muscle, or as it passes through the semispinalis capitis muscle, traveling between its most medial fibers and the nuchal ligament (Figure 16-3).[3] The greater occipital nerve is the medial branch of the dorsal primary division of the second cervical nerve and supplies sensory branches to the scalp over the vertex as well as motor branches to the semispinalis capitis muscle. This cervical nerve emerges below the posterior arch of the atlas above the lamina of the axis (Figure 16-3). It then curves around the lower border of the oblique capitis inferior muscle which it crosses before penetrating the semispinalis capitis and trapezius muscles near their attachments to the occipital bone.

In an autopsy study of 20 cases (40 nerves) without a history of headache (according to hospital files), the greater occipital nerve penetrated the trapezius muscle in 45% of the cases, the semispinalis muscle in 90% of the cases, and the inferior oblique muscle in 7.5% of the cases.[4] Eleven of the 18 nerves that penetrated a trapezius muscle showed evidence of compression. This finding was unexpected because the selection was made on the basis of no established history of headache (according to hospital charts). Apparently, some degree of nerve compression at the point of a trapezius muscular penetration is common.[4]

Longissimus Capitis

The longissimus capitis muscle (Figure 16-2) originates at the posterior edge of the mastoid process, deep to the splenius capitis and sternocleidomastoid muscles, and inserts onto the transverse processes of C5-C7 and T1-T4 vertebrae.[2] It descends across the lateral surface of the semispinalis capitis muscle. The longissimus capitis muscle is often partially or completely divided into two muscle bellies by a tendinous inscription.

Semispinalis Cervicis

The semispinalis cervicis muscle (not illustrated here) lies deep to the semispinalis capitis muscle and originates from the spinous processes of C2 to C5 vertebrae and inserts into the transverse processes of T1 to T5.[2] Its fascicles span about six segments and cover the cervical and thoracic multifidus muscles. The diagonal orientation of the digitations of this muscle can be seen in Figure 16-1.

Multifidus and Rotatores

The cervical multifidus is formed by several fascicles originating from the caudal edge of the lateral surface of the spinous process and from the caudal end of the spinous process of C2 to C5 vertebrae and inserting onto the transverse process of vertebrae two, three, four, and five levels below (Figure 16-2).[2] The fascicles from a given segment are flanked and overlapped dorsolaterally by fascicles from successively higher segments, an arrangement that endows the intact muscle with a laminated structure. The cervical multifidus is the deepest muscle spanning the lamina of the vertebrae, and it directly attaches to the capsules of the cervical zygapophyseal joints.[5] These muscles, therefore, contribute to the segmental control of the zygapophyseal joints of the cervical spine.[6]

The cervical muscles, when present, also originate at C2 and extend downward segmentally. In each segment, a rotator brevis muscle originates from the lower border of the lateral surface of the lamina above and inserts onto the upper, posterior part of the transverse process of the vertebra immediately below. Additionally, a rotatores longus muscle connects the base of the spinous process above to the transverse process two levels below.[2] They are the shortest and deepest paraspinal muscles, connecting adjacent or alternate vertebrae, and therefore, are the most angulated (Figures 16-1 and 16-2). The degree of angulation of these muscles has important functional implications.

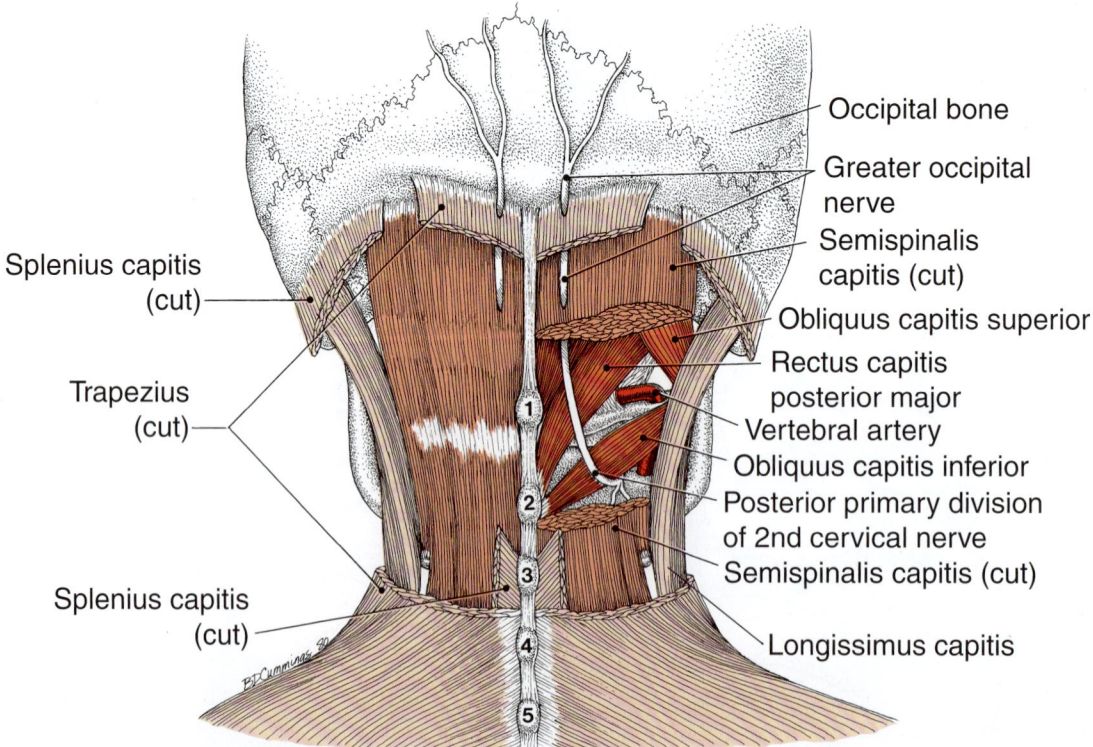

Figure 16-3. Course of the second cervical nerve which becomes the greater occipital nerve and then penetrates the semispinalis capitis (light medium red) and trapezius muscles (light red) to continue beneath the scalp. Entrapment can occur where the nerve passes through the semispinalis muscle. Note the vertebral artery (darkest red) in the suboccipital triangle which is bounded by the rectus capitis posterior major and the oblique capitis superior and inferior muscles (dark medium red).

2.1. Innervation and Vascularization

The semispinalis capitis muscle is supplied by branches of the posterior primary division of the first 4 or 5 cervical spinal nerves (C1-C4), and the semispinalis cervicis muscle is supplied by the third to sixth cervical spinal nerves (C3-C6). The longissimus capitis muscle and the deeper posterior cervical muscles are supplied by the medial branches of the dorsal rami of the adjacent cervical spinal nerves. The dorsal muscles of the cervical spine receive their blood supply from the vertebral artery, deep cervical artery, superficial and deep descending branches of the occipital artery, and deep branch of the transverse cervical artery, when present.[2]

2.2. Function

Functions of the semispinalis capitis muscle primarily relate to head movement; whereas the deeper intervertebral muscles are primarily concerned with stabilization and segmental movement of the cervical vertebrae.[7]

Semispinalis Capitis

The semispinalis capitis muscle has one main action, extension of the head, and it functions in antigravity control of the head when one leans forward. Electrical stimulation of the semispinalis capitis muscle produces head extension and slight inclination to the same side but not neck extension.[8] Nevertheless, the role of semispinalis capitis muscle in rotation is controversial because the assumption that all posterior muscles act synergistically as extensors is not clear.[8]

An older electromyographic (EMG) study using fine-wire electrodes in 15 subjects, reported that the semispinalis capitis muscle responded vigorously during the extension of the head and neck, but with training, electrical silence could be achieved while the head and neck were held in the erect, balanced position. Electrical activation of these muscles in support of the head appeared only during body activity that disturbed the balance of the head on the body.[9] Also, no EMG activity was observed in this muscle during lateral flexion of the head and during head rotation.

No study was found that specifically examined the slightly forward-flexed head posture commonly assumed for reading. The exercise data strongly suggests that the semispinalis capitis muscle consistently provides a checkrein function during even a slight flexion of the neck[9] which has been well demonstrated for the erector spinae muscles at the lumbar level. Abuse of this checkrein activity is a major cause of the frequently observed chronic strain of the posterior cervical muscles.

Longissimus Capitis

The longissimus capitis muscle is a head on neck extensor that is also reported to laterally flex the head to the same side and rotate it toward the same side.

Semispinalis Cervicis

The semispinalis cervicis muscle is reported to primarily extend the cervical spine and rotate it the opposite side.[8] The caudal insertion to the relatively immobile thoracic vertebrae serves primarily to stabilize the movement of the cervical spine. A study by Pauly[9] suggests that the semispinalis cervicis muscle, at times, provides a checkrein function during even a slight flexion of the neck.

Multifidus and Rotatores

Evidence clearly describing the functions of this group of muscles, specifically for the cervical area is lacking, but generally, when acting bilaterally, these deep muscles, extend the vertebral column. Acting unilaterally, they rotate the vertebrae to the opposite side. The multifidus muscles were identified as contributing to lateral flexion of the spine. Anderson et al[5] found that the total moment-generating capacity of the cervical multifidus muscles, in the neutral posture, was predicted to be approximately 0.7 Nm for extension and lateral bending and 0.3 Nm for axial rotation. However, these deeper muscles seem to be designed for control and are said to control positional adjustments between vertebrae, rather than movements of the spine as a whole.

2.3. Functional Unit

The functional unit to which a muscle belongs includes the muscles that reinforce and counter its actions as well as the joints that the muscle crosses. The interdependence of these structures functionally is reflected in the organization and neural connections of the sensory motor cortex. The functional unit is emphasized because the presence of a TrP in one muscle of the unit increases the likelihood that the other muscles of the unit will also develop TrPs. When inactivating TrPs in a muscle, one should be concerned about TrPs that may develop in muscles that are functionally interdependent. Box 16-1 grossly represents the functional unit of the posterior cervical muscles.[10]

For rotation of the neck, the semispinalis cervicis muscle functions synergistically with the contralateral splenius cervicis and levator scapulae muscles, and with the ipsilateral multifidus and rotatores muscles.

During combined extension and rotation of the neck, the multifidus and rotatores muscles act synergistically with the

---

Box 16-1 Functional unit of the posterior cervical muscles

Action	Synergists	Antagonist
Head extension (Semispinalis capitis and Longissimus capitis)	Suboccipital muscles (bilaterally) Upper trapezius Splenius capitis muscles	Cervical head flexors Rectus capitis anterior Sternocleidomastoid (bilaterally)
Neck extension (Semispinalis cervicis)	Splenius cervicis (bilaterally) Longissimus cervicis Semispinalis capitis Levator scapulae (bilaterally) Multifidus (bilaterally)	Anterior neck muscles Longus colli

semispinalis cervicis muscle. For each separate movement, synergists and antagonists are the same as those previously listed above for the semispinalis cervicis muscle.

3. CLINICAL PRESENTATION
3.1. Referred Pain Pattern

Semispinalis Capitis

Pain elicited from TrPs of the semispinalis capitis muscle refers to the head (Figure 16-4). Clinically, it has been observed that the upper portion of the muscle can refer pain to the skull traveling forward like a band and encircling the head halfway, reaching maximum intensity in the temporal region, and continuing forward over the eye (Figure 16-4B). The middle portion of the muscle can spread deep pain more posterior on the skull (Figure 16-4C). In fact, referred pain of the middle and lower parts of the semispinalis capitis muscle and the referred pain of the semispinalis cervicis muscle overlap with part of the pain distribution of the C2-C3 zygapophyseal joints.[11]

Longissimus Capitis

Pain from the longissimus capitis muscle (not illustrated) concentrates in the region of the ipsilateral ear or just behind and below it. The pain may extend a short distance down the neck and may also include pain in the periorbital region.

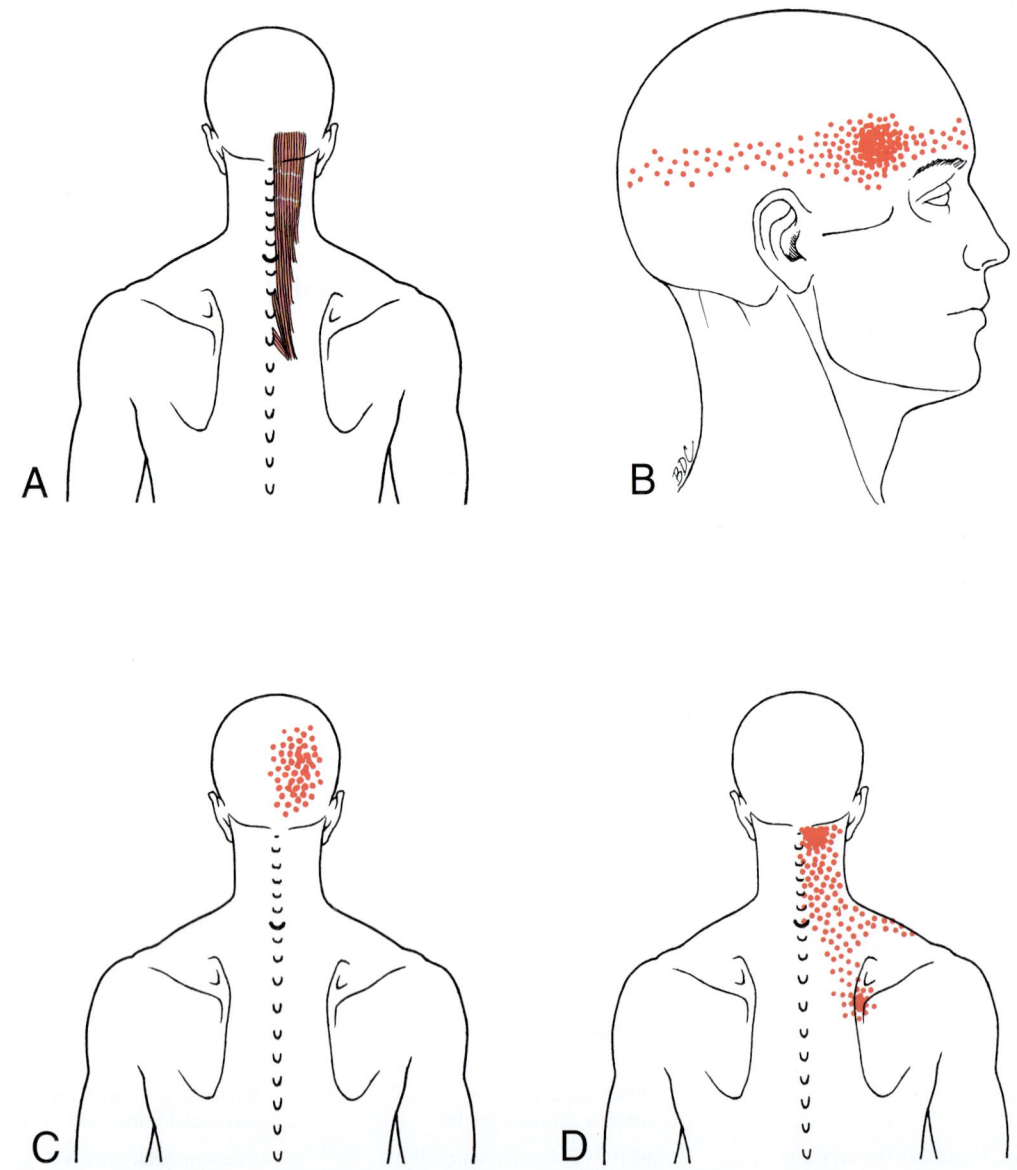

Figure 16-4. Referred pain patterns (red) from posterior cervical muscles. A, The semispinalis capitis muscle; B, Referred pain pattern from TrPs in the upper portion of the semispinalis capitis muscle. Trigger points in the upper third of the muscle can contribute to entrapment of the greater occipital nerve; C, Referred pain pattern of TrPs in the middle portion of semispinalis capitis muscle. The semispinalis cervicis muscle can also refer pain in a similar pattern; D, Referred pain pattern of the deeply placed cervical multifidus TrPs.

Semispinalis Cervicis

The referred pain from semispinalis cervicis TrPs is not illustrated separately because this muscle likely refers pain to the occipital region in a pattern similar to that shown in Figure 16-4 for the middle portion of semispinalis capitis muscle.

Cervical Multifidus

Trigger points from cervical multifidus muscles refer pain and tenderness cephalad to the suboccipital region and sometimes down the neck to the upper vertebral border of the scapula (Figure 16-4D).[12] Similar pain patterns have been produced by injection of hypertonic salt solution into the posterior cervical muscles.[13] The pain arising from the cervical multifidus muscles sometimes is related to cervical zygapophyseal joints on the same segment and can mimic deep localized pain around the spinous process.

Rotatores

When present, TrPs of cervical rotatores muscles produce midline pain and tenderness at the segmental level of the TrP. Pain is elicited by application of pressure or tapping on the spinous process of the vertebra to which the muscle attaches. This tenderness testing is also used to identify dysfunctional joints and differentiation can be difficult.

3.2. Symptoms

Patients reporting pain in the head elicited by cervical muscles are likely to be referred with the diagnosis of tension-type headache[14] or cervicogenic headache.[15] These muscles are also involved in individuals with whiplash-associated disorders[16] or mechanical neck pain.[17] With chronic headache sufferers, the pain pattern is likely to be a composite of referred pain from several neck and masticatory muscles (see Figure 17-1).

Patients are likely to be bothered by tenderness over the back of the head and neck so much so that pressure at that point from the weight of the head on a pillow at night may quickly become intolerable. Some degree of painfully restricted neck motion in one or more directions, especially head and neck flexion, is typical.

With entrapment of the greater occipital nerve as a sequela to prolonged activation of a semispinalis capitis or upper trapezius muscles, patients may report numbness, tingling, and burning pain in the scalp over the ipsilateral occipital region ("occipital neuralgia") in addition to headache. They may have received anesthetic blocks of the greater occipital nerve with relief only for the duration of the local anesthetic effect. Patients with nerve entrapment usually prefer cold rather than heat to relieve the burning neuropathic pain; this relief can also obscure the TrP pain. Entrapment symptoms of the greater occipital nerve may develop when TrP activity in one of the muscles that it penetrates (the semispinalis capitis or the upper trapezius muscles) produces taut bands of muscle fibers that compress the nerve.

The symptoms associated with entrapment of the greater occipital nerve are often relieved by the inactivation of TrPs in the semispinalis capitis and/or upper trapezius muscles.

3.3. Patient Examination

After a thorough subjective examination, the clinician should make a detailed drawing representing the pain pattern that the patient has described. This depiction will assist in planning the physical examination and can be useful in monitoring the progression of the patient as symptoms improve or change.

Patients with posterior cervical TrPs often hold the head and neck upright with the shoulders high and rounded; they may position the head with the face tilted up somewhat and tend to suppress the bobbing and nodding movements of the head that ordinarily accompany talking.

The patient usually demonstrates marked restriction of head and neck flexion, which can measure 5 cm short of the chin reaching the sternum. Altered segmental motion of the cervical spine with palpation is a common finding associated with muscular dysfunction. Marked restriction of head and neck rotation and cervical side-bending is usually due to the involvement of associated cervical muscles. In any one segment however, restriction in all directions likely indicates a capsular (or arthritic) pattern.

If involvement of the posterior cervical muscles is mainly unilateral and the head and neck are flexed, the muscles on the painful side may appear very prominent like a rope from the skull to the level of the shoulder girdle.

3.4. Trigger Point Examination

Semispinalis Capitis

Trigger point palpation of posterior cervical muscles is based on the proper knowledge of anatomy and the expected locations of the muscle because these muscles are not directly palpated. Slight flexion of the head and neck increases tension of the taut bands and the tenderness of TrPs in the posterior neck muscles. Trigger points are more easily identified by palpation if the posterior cervical musculature is relaxed by providing adequate head and body support for the patient in the seated or the side-lying position. All posterior cervical muscles are best examined using a flat cross-fiber palpation. It is often very difficult to elicit a detectable local twitch response by manual palpation of this muscle. However, if the upper trapezius muscle is relaxed, one may be able to palpate a taut band in the semispinalis capitis muscle that is distinguished by its vertical fiber direction.

Trigger points in the upper portion of the semispinalis muscle (Figure 16-4) are likely to feel indurated and often need to be pressed very firmly to elicit referred pain. Therefore, deep tenderness on examination is much less intense than would be expected from the severity of the patient's pain complaint. This region of tenderness is usually found at a distance of a centimeter or two from the midline at the base of the skull and is also in the region of one of the controversial tender point sites used to diagnose fibromyalgia syndrome, discussed in the following.[18]

Longissimus Capitis

The longissimus capitis muscle lies deep to the lateral part of the splenius capitis muscle near the level of the C3 vertebra. From the level of the C2 spinous process to the junction of C3-C4, clinicians can attempt to palpate TrPs and taut bands of the longissimus capitis muscle by locating the splenius capitis muscle (lateral to the trapezius muscle and posterior to the sternocleidomastoid muscle), and by pressing anteriorly and medially through the lateral part of the splenius capitis muscle. If the splenius capitis muscle has TrPs and taut bands they should be first released or the deeper tenderness of the longissimus capitis TrPs may not be distinguishable. If the longissimus capitis muscle has TrPs, it will present as prominent and firm, and its nearly vertical fibers will help distinguish it from the more diagonal fibers of the splenius capitis muscle. Superior to the level of C2 and inferior to the level of C4, the longissimus capitis muscle is too deep and covered by too many other muscles to be reliably identified, even indirectly.

Semispinalis Cervicis

Palpation for TrPs of this intermediate-to-deep posterior cervical muscle is possible 1 to 2 cm lateral to the spinous processes. Trigger points are commonly found at approximately the C4-C5 level, and deep pressure on the TrP may elicit referred pain over the

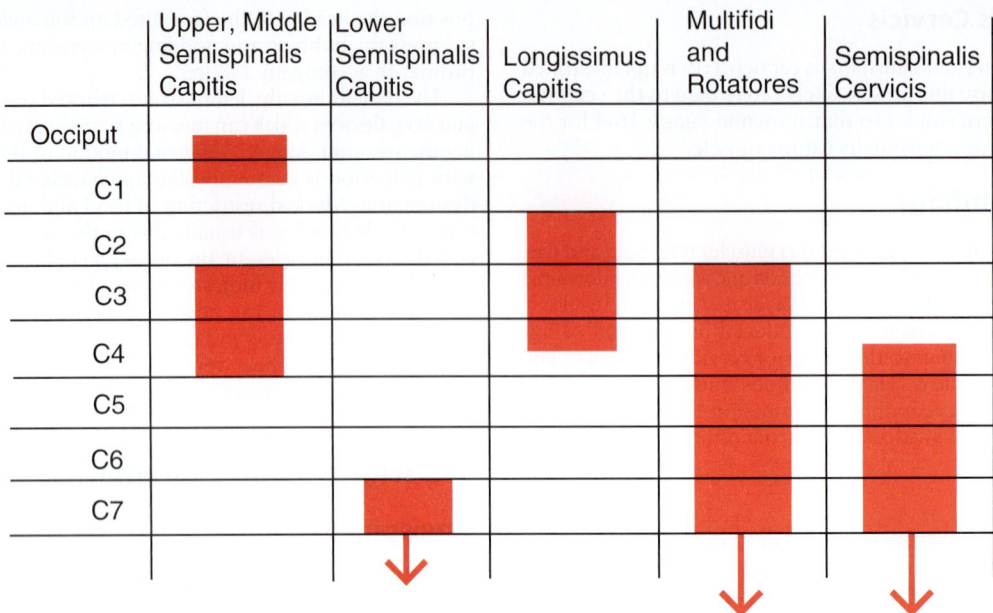

Figure 16-5. Possible locations (many may not be palpable) of TrPs in posterior cervical muscles based on clinical experience and expected locations of endplate zones for posterior cervical muscles. Segmental levels correspond to spinous processes (or the posterior tubercle of C1). All these locations should be considered as a guide, because the entire muscle belly should be searched for the presence of TrPs.

occipital region similar to the pattern shown in Figure 16-4. Only rarely can one distinguish taut bands in this relatively deep muscle.

Cervical Multifidus and Rotatores

Trigger points of cervical multifidus muscles can be located approximately halfway between a spinous process and a lower transverse process, usually 1 cm lateral to the spinous process. Because there are digitations of the cervical multifidus muscles for every segmental level from C2 inferiorly and because some digitations span more than one vertebra, TrPs in the cervical multifidus muscles could be found at any level between these processes starting at about the interface between spinous processes C3 and C4 and continuing inferiorly as thoracic multifidus. Manual palpation of this muscle, based on anatomic landmarks, may be limited because they form the deepest layer of the posterior cervical musculature.

The deepest muscles, the rotatores, are often not as fully developed in the cervical region as they are in the thoracic region. These muscles lie too deep for the fiber direction of their taut bands to be identified by palpation. They should be identified by characteristic deep tenderness to the pressure applied deep in the groove lateral to spinous processes and by tenderness to pressure or tapping at the spinous process. The pain distribution of the rotator muscles is essentially a midline pain at the segmental level and deep, simulating pain into the spinous process (bone pain).

Locations of TrPs in posterior cervical muscles are summarized in Figure 16-5. Because TrPs may form at any location throughout each muscle, a thorough examination is required for proper identification of TrPs.

4. DIFFERENTIAL DIAGNOSIS

4.1. Activation and Perpetuation of Trigger Points

A posture or activity that activates a TrP, if not corrected, can also perpetuate it. In any part of the posterior cervical muscles, TrPs may be activated by unaccustomed eccentric loading, eccentric exercise in an unconditioned muscle, or maximal or submaximal concentric loading.[19] Trigger points may also be activated or aggravated when the muscle is placed in a shortened and/or lengthened position for an extended period of time.

Many kinds of events can activate TrPs in the posterior cervical muscles, but other factors are required to perpetuate them. For instance, acute trauma can activate TrPs in these muscles. Falling on the head, experiencing forceful head movement in an automobile accident, or diving headfirst and hitting the head can produce forceful neck flexion and muscle strain which can activate TrPs in head and neck muscles even in the absence of fracture. Baker[20] examined 34 muscles bilaterally of 100 occupants (drivers or passengers) who sustained a single motor vehicle impact. All these patients complained of whiplash-associated disorders and all had active TrPs. The semispinalis capitis muscle was the third most frequently involved muscle with dysfunction present in 73% of subjects who reported impact from the front, in 69% of subjects who experienced impact on the passenger side, in 63% of subjects who experienced impact on the driver's side, and in 62% of subjects in vehicles struck from behind. Therefore, automobile impact from any direction is likely to activate semispinalis capitis TrPs.

Other factors can perpetuate the presence of TrPs in the posterior cervical muscles. A chronically activated stress response that eventually activates TrPs, if continued, also perpetuates them. Strain from ineffective posture, such as from reading or working at a desk while sitting with a forward head posture or with the neck in sustained flexion, commonly activates and perpetuates posterior cervical TrPs. Refer to Chapter 76 for proper posture and ergonomic set up to avoid activation and perpetuation of posterior cervical TrPs.

Excessive cervical extension at night tends to activate and perpetuate TrPs in the posterior cervical muscles by placing these muscles in a shortened position for a prolonged period. This posture occurs when a person lies supine without a pillow on a mattress that is too hard or when a too-hard, poorly fitted pillow is placed under the shoulders and neck. Sometimes young people (in particular) lie prone on the floor, propped up on elbows to support the head, while watching television. This position places the posterior cervical muscles in a shortened position for a prolonged period of time and may activate or perpetuate TrPs of the posterior cervical muscles.

Since the more longitudinal posterior cervical muscles commonly function bilaterally, TrP involvement of one side soon leads to at least some functional disturbance of the contralateral muscles which can activate TrPs in them also.

4.2. Associated Trigger Points

In addition to the bilateral posterior cervical muscles, the upper semispinalis thoracis and the erector spinae muscles that extend into the thorax may demonstrate TrPs associated with those found in the posterior cervical muscles. The segmental level of TrP involvement can be identified by a flattened spot in the normally smooth curvature of the thoracic region; when tested by voluntary forward flexion, at least one spinous process fails to stand out prominently as expected. Multiple bilateral deep short rotator muscles can look like the longer but less angulated multifidus muscle in this respect; however, multifidus muscle involvement would not cause as much restricted rotation as the rotator muscles do, and the multifidus muscle is less likely to cause a continuous series of pressure-sensitive vertebrae with restricted joint mobility. Manual techniques designed to improve both joint and muscle functions may be effective.

When the posterior cervical muscles have been treated and patients continue to complain of suboccipital pain and soreness, especially in the region of the mastoid process, the clinician should check for active TrPs in the trapezius muscle, in the posterior belly of the digastric muscle, and in the upper medial portion of the infraspinatus muscle on the same side as the pain. Trigger points in the latter two muscles cause little restriction of head motion and are easily overlooked.

Hong[21] pointed out that the semispinalis capitis muscle may develop associated TrPs in response to TrPs in either an upper trapezius or splenius capitis muscles. Elimination of TrPs in either of these two muscles usually inactivates the TrPs of the semispinalis capitis muscle without any specific treatment of the semispinalis capitis muscle itself. Conversely, inactivating only the associated TrP results in its reactivation and perpetuation by the TrP in the primarily involved muscle.

4.3. Associated Pathology

The location of the posterior neck muscles overlaps with "tender points" used for the diagnosis of fibromyalgia syndrome.[18] A brief examination of the designated tender points of fibromyalgia and associated widespread and fatigue-related symptoms assists in the exclusion or establishment of a correct diagnosis. Patients with fibromyalgia commonly have myofascial TrPs that contribute to their pain.[22] Finding a positive occipital tender point should alert the clinician to the possibility of an enthesopathy secondary to a semispinalis capitis TrPs.

Clinically, cervical radicular pain or radiculopathy can activate TrPs in the posterior cervical muscles that, following surgery, are then perpetuated by other factors. This is a common cause of cervical post-laminectomy pain syndromes.[23] Because the radicular pain and the TrPs can occur separately or concurrently, each condition should be diagnosed based on its own criteria.[24] Cervical radicular pain or radiculopathy from C4 to C8 rarely fails to cause upper extremity signs or symptoms. Posterior cervical TrPs alone do not produce upper extremity symptoms. Cervical radicular pain or radiculopathy is much more likely to show a positive Spurling test, pain elicited by spinal compression applied as a downward pressure on the head with the upright cervical spine slightly extended. Positive electrodiagnostic findings are helpful in identifying cervical radiculopathy.

One should distinguish between the local neurologically projected pain of a Tinel's sign (produced by tapping on the point of entrapment) and referred pain from a TrP. The shock-like tingling or "pins and needles" of the Tinel's sign is produced by pressure on a point of constriction, for example, where the greater occipital nerve passes through the semispinalis capitis muscle or upper trapezius muscle (Figure 16-3). Neural pain is usually projected along the distribution of the nerve. In comparison, TrP referred pain is usually described as a deep aching pain that is less well localized and has a nonneural distribution. Trigger points respond to snapping palpation with a local twitch response of the taut band. Injections at the point of neural entrapment should be avoided, whereas injection of the TrP in the muscle that contributes to the entrapment is an appropriate therapy.

Inflammatory disorders of the neck have the potential to cause erosions at the atlantoaxial (AA) articulation which can progress to lysis of the transverse ligament and subluxation of the odontoid process of C2. In addition to a careful history and clinical examination for systemic disease, a person suspected of having symptomatic arthritic involvement of the neck should have imaging confirmation. A pair of lateral neck radiographs, in voluntary flexion and extension, can help identify inappropriate motion (>4 mm) of the odontoid process away from the internal margin of the ring of C1. Imaging of subaxial disease requires computed tomography with contrast, magnetic resonance imaging, or even myelography. Halla and Hardin Jr[25] identified a distinctive clinical syndrome in 27 patients with C1-C2 facet joint osteoarthritis. Occipital TrPs were one of the major features of the syndrome. This syndrome was seen mainly in elderly women who also have osteoarthritis at other sites and who experienced occipital and post-auricular pain. Physical signs included limited head rotation, tender points or TrPs confined to the occipital area, palpable cervical crepitus, and abnormal head position to one side.[25] The crepitus of the C1-C2 arthritis and taut bands with recognition of pain on palpation of TrPs would be the two most clearly distinguishing characteristics. This strong association between cervical osteoarthritis and myofascial TrPs is compatible with the observation of Jaeger[15] who found the semispinalis capitis muscle to be one of the most frequently involved. Hence, cervical osteoarthritis is likely to activate and/or perpetuate cervical myofascial TrPs. In fact, Bogduk and Simons[11] have reported overlapping pain patterns of cervical zygapophyseal joints and posterior cervical muscles. The C2-C3 zygapophyseal joints in particular need to be considered in diagnosis when dealing with TrPs in the semispinalis capitis and semispinalis cervicis muscles. The C3-C4 and C4-C5 zygapophyseal joints refer pain in patterns that overlap partly with the pain distribution of cervical multifidus TrPs. It is possible that other arthritic conditions such as rheumatoid arthritis and seronegative spondyloarthropathies may have a similar influence on cervical TrPs.

The seronegative (meaning negative blood rheumatoid factor test) spondyloarthropathy disorders can include ankylosing spondylitis, Reiter's syndrome, reactive arthritis due to inflammatory bowel disease, or reactive arthritis associated with psoriasis.[26] A typical pathologic process in these patients is painful enthesopathy (inflammation at the site of attachment of ligament or tendon to bone) which tends to heal with diastrophic calcification. In ankylosing spondylitis, the spinal ligaments tend to calcify symmetrically from the sacroiliac joints upward until the entire spine is fused into what appears on x-rays like a vertical stick of bamboo (the so-called bamboo spine). In the other disorders such as Reiter's syndrome, the inflammatory involvement of the axial skeleton tends to be more asymmetric (skipping vertebral levels and involving only one side of some vertebrae). In any of these conditions, neck pain can be a prominent symptom, and involvement of the AA joint can place the spinal cord at a risk of serious injury. The presence of systemic symptoms, such as conjunctivitis and urethritis in Reiter's syndrome, can be helpful in establishing the correct diagnosis.

Two older studies reported palpatory spasm (or TrP contracture), tissue texture changes, and cervical restricted motion at C1-C3, assumed to be secondary to viscerosomatic reflexes from cardiac, upper gastrointestinal, and pulmonary disorders.[27,28]

4.4. Associated Cervical Joint Dysfunctions

When exploring the differential diagnosis of neck pain, one should consider a wide variety of cervical joint disorders that can cause symptoms in the cervical area but are usually diagnosed on the basis of patterns of involvement at other sites in the body. Fernández de las Peñas et al[29] observed a clinical association between the presence of TrPs in the neck muscles and cervical joint dysfunction in the innervation-related segment. Satisfactory management of head and neck pain of musculoskeletal origin often requires careful evaluation of posterior cervical muscles for TrPs and cervical joints for restricted mobility. Often both of these findings are present, and frequently both should be treated.

Jaeger[15] examined each of 11 patients, with symptoms of cervicogenic headache, for TrPs in seven head and neck muscles and for cervical spine dysfunction. All patients had at least three active myofascial TrPs. In eight patients, TrP palpation clearly reproduced the headache. Ten of the 11 patients (91%) had a specific segmental dysfunction of the atlanto-occipital (AO) joint or of the AA joint. The temporalis muscle was the one most likely to have TrPs (n = 7), and the semispinalis capitis muscle was the next most likely (n = 6). Trigger points were predominantly found on the most symptomatic side. Among the posterior cervical muscles, suboccipital articular dysfunction was most likely to be associated with TrPs in the semispinalis capitis muscle.

Semispinalis capitis TrPs are frequently associated with OA, C1, and C2 dysfunctions. Longissimus capitis TrPs can be associated with an apparent elevation of the first rib concurrent with T1 articular dysfunction. Part of this muscle spans the region from the mastoid process to the transverse process of T1, which allows it to *in*directly affect the first rib through its pull on the costotransverse junction. Resultant rotation of the vertebra produces the apparent rib elevation. The semispinalis cervicis, multifidus, and rotators muscle groups can form articular dysfunctions at various levels of the cervical and upper thoracic spine depending on the specific attachments.

A simple extension dysfunction of T1, T2, T3, and T4 segments is another important articular dysfunction associated with TrP involvement of bilateral posterior cervical muscles that attach to or span the upper thoracic vertebrae. This is particularly true of the semispinalis cervicis, multifidus, and rotator muscles with attachments in the upper thoracic region as well as the semispinalis thoracis digitations that extend to and cross these upper thoracic vertebral segments. The upper thoracic segments are particularly difficult to isolate. One should, however, treat these extension dysfunctions from T1 to T4 by using a manual stretch technique that also incorporates contract–relax and forward flexion progressing down the spine segment by segment.

5. CORRECTIVE ACTIONS

Chronic strain activates posterior cervical TrPs because these muscles control the weight of the head when it is held in partial flexion for prolonged periods. Optimizing posture to reduce gravitational stress[30] or improvement of biomechanical/ergonomic function reduces this strain. Refer to Chapter 76 for a full discussion of postural considerations. Corrections include the following:

1. Use of a reading stand or adjustable music stand to change the angle of, or to raise, the reading and work materials to approximate eye-level contact to avoid sustained flexion of the head and neck.
2. Elevation of the computer monitor when it requires a downward gaze and is used for prolonged periods.
3. Procurement of eyeglasses with adequate focal length, so that the patient can see clearly with the head held in a balanced upright position. Otherwise, a new prescription for longer focal length lenses ("card playing or computer glasses") should be obtained.
4. Selection of bifocal or transitional lenses that are large enough to allow for effective head posture for close work such as reading or sewing.
5. Adjustment of eyeglass frames so that the lower portion of the rim does not occlude the line of sight on looking down.
6. Alteration of exercise posture on a stationary bicycle by sitting upright with the arms swinging freely or placed on the hips and *not* hunched over holding low handlebars that do not steer the machine.
7. Addition of a cloth roll or pillow behind the thoracolumbar junction while sitting to maintain the normal lumbar lordotic curve and lift the sternum, improving the head and neck posture.
8. Inactivation of pectoralis major or minor TrPs (refer to Chapters 42 and 44) that induce rounded shoulder posture and a functional thoracic kyphosis.
9. Alteration of laptop behaviors. The use of laptops for on-the-go computer work can be problematic for maintaining balanced head posture. If the laptop is at the level of the eyes, the shoulders are likely to elevate to allow for typing. If the laptop is placed low so that the arms may be in contact with armrests or a table at the height of a bent elbow, the head and neck should flex to see the screen. Use of a portable keyboard to separate functions of the hands and eyes allow for improved posture of both the upper quadrants and the head and neck.

These last two corrections permit the erect head and neck to assume a balanced relaxed position over the thoracic spine. In summary, the patient should comfortably maintain a balanced head posture.

Another simple correction to promote erect balanced sitting posture is provided by placing a small pad under the ischial tuberosities. The pad should *not* extend under the upper thigh.

Excessive cervical extension at night is corrected by obtaining a slightly softer (nonsagging) mattress or by using a small soft neck pillow that comfortably supports the normal cervical curve. Chattopadhyay[31] described the rationale and importance of a well-fitting cervical pillow. A versatile and adaptable pillow that places the head and neck in a neutral position may be indicated.

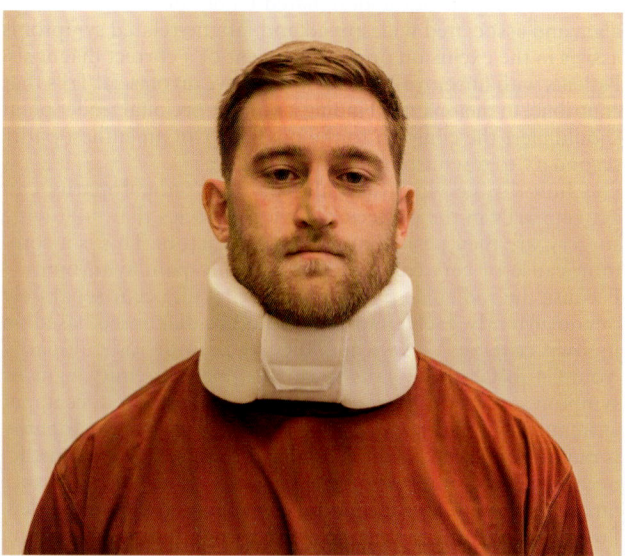

Figure 16-6. A soft collar may help relieve stress on posterior neck muscles when seated in the car or at a desk. It should be worn loosely as a chin rest and not for immobilization of the neck.

The neck muscles of patients with posterior cervical TrPs may be particularly vulnerable to chilling and if so, can be kept covered at night by a turtleneck sweater worn in bed or by a loose scarf draped around the neck. Similarly, the neck should be protected from cold drafts during the day. Long hair offers natural protection against this cold exposure.

To temporarily relieve neck strain after an acute exacerbation, one may prescribe a soft collar to be worn loosely as a chin rest when riding in a car or working at a desk (Figure 16-6). The collar is NOT tightly adjusted for immobilization of the neck but applied loosely. For instance, a Thomas plastic collar may be worn upside down and loose enough to allow space for head rotation and to look down at the sides, yet tight enough to support the chin so that the head is in the neutral position.

References

1. Wegley RS, Rumore AJ. Posterior cervical paraspinal musculature morphology: a cadaveric and CT scan study. *J Orthop Sports Phys Ther.* 1986;8(1):15-26.
2. Standring S. *Gray's Anatomy: The Anatomical Basis of Clinical Practice.* 41st ed. London, UK: Elsevier; 2015.
3. Tubbs RS, Watanabe K, Loukas M, Cohen-Gadol AA. The intramuscular course of the greater occipital nerve: novel findings with potential implications for operative interventions and occipital neuralgia. *Surg Neurol Int.* 2014;5:155.
4. Bovim G, Bonamico L, Fredriksen TA, Lindboe CF, Stolt-Nielsen A, Sjaastad O. Topographic variations in the peripheral course of the greater occipital nerve. Autopsy study with clinical correlations. *Spine.* 1991;16(4):475-478.
5. Anderson JS, Hsu AW, Vasavada AN. Morphology, architecture, and biomechanics of human cervical multifidus. *Spine.* 2005;30(4):E86-E91.
6. Schomacher J, Falla D. Function and structure of the deep cervical extensor muscles in patients with neck pain. *Man Ther.* 2013;18(5):360-366.
7. Blouin JS, Siegmund GP, Carpenter MG, Inglis JT. Neural control of superficial and deep neck muscles in humans. *J Neurophysiol.* 2007;98(2):920-928.
8. Siegmund GP, Blouin JS, Brault JR, Hedenstierna S, Inglis JT. Electromyography of superficial and deep neck muscles during isometric, voluntary, and reflex contractions. *J Biomech Eng.* 2007;129(1):66-77.
9. Pauly JE. An electromyographic analysis of certain movements and exercises. I. Some deep muscles of the back. *Anat Rec.* 1966;155(2):223-234.
10. Simons DG, Travell J, Simons L. *Travell & Simon's Myofascial Pain and Dysfunction: The Trigger Point Manual.* Vol 1. 2nd ed. Baltimore, MD: Williams & Wilkins; 1999:104.
11. Bogduk N, Simons D. Neck pain: joint pain or trigger points? Chapter 20. In: Vaeroy H, Merskey H, eds. *Progress in Fibromyalgia and Myofascial Pain.* Vol 6 of Pain research and Clinical Management. Amsterdam, Netherlands: Elsevier; 1993:267-273.
12. Travell J, Rinzler SH. The myofascial genesis of pain. *Postgrad Med.* 1952;11(5):425-434.
13. Cyriax J. Rheumatic headache. *Br Med J (Clin Res Ed).* 1938;2(4069):1367-1368.
14. Fernández de las Peñas C, Cuadrado ML, Arendt-Nielsen L, Simons DG, Pareja JA. Myofascial trigger points and sensitization: an updated pain model for tension-type headache. *Cephalalgia.* 2007;27(5):383-393.
15. Jaeger B. Are "cervicogenic" headaches due to myofascial pain and cervical spine dysfunction? *Cephalalgia.* 1989;9(3):157-164.
16. Ettlin T, Schuster C, Stoffel R, Bruderlin A, Kischka U. A distinct pattern of myofascial findings in patients after whiplash injury. *Arch Phys Med Rehabil.* 2008;89(7):1290-1293.
17. Munoz-Munoz S, Munoz-Garcia MT, Alburquerque-Sendin F, Arroyo-Morales M, Fernández de las Peñas C. Myofascial trigger points, pain, disability, and sleep quality in individuals with mechanical neck pain. *J Manipulative Physiol Ther.* 2012;35(8):608-613.
18. Wolfe F, Clauw DJ, Fitzcharles MA, et al. The American College of Rheumatology preliminary diagnostic criteria for fibromyalgia and measurement of symptom severity. *Arthritis Care Res (Hoboken).* 2010;62(5):600-610.
19. Gerwin R, Dommerholt J. Expansion of Simons' integrated trigger point hypothesis [Abstract]. Paper presented at: Myopain, Munich, Germany; 2004.
20. Baker B. The muscle trigger: evidence of overload injury. *J Neurol Orthop med Surg.* 1986;7(1):35-44.
21. Hong C-Z. Considerations and recommendations regarding myofascial trigger point injection. *J Musculoske Pain.* 1994;2(1):29-59.
22. Alonso-Blanco C, Fernández de las Peñas C, Morales-Cabezas M, Zarco-Moreno P, Ge HY, Florez-Garcia M. Multiple active myofascial trigger points reproduce the overall spontaneous pain pattern in women with fibromyalgia and are related to widespread mechanical hypersensitivity. *Clin J Pain.* 2011;27(5):405-413.
23. Reynolds MD. Myofascial trigger point syndromes in the practice of rheumatology. *Arch Phys Med Rehabil.* 1981;62(3):111-114.
24. Sari H, Akarirmak U, Uludag M. Active myofascial trigger points might be more frequent in patients with cervical radiculopathy. *Eur J Phys Rehabil Med.* 2012;48(2):237-244.
25. Halla JT, Hardin JG Jr. Atlantoaxial (C1-C2) facet joint osteoarthritis: a distinctive clinical syndrome. *Arthritis Rheum.* 1987;30(5):577-582.
26. Stucki G, Stoll T, Bruhlmann P, Michel BA. Construct validation of the ACR 1991 revised criteria for global functional status in rheumatoid arthritis. *Clin Exp Rheumatol.* 1995;13(3):349-352.
27. Beal MC, Morlock JW. Somatic dysfunction associated with pulmonary disease. *J Am Osteop Assoc.* 1984;84(2):179-183.
28. Beal MC. Viscerosomatic reflexes: a review. *J Am Osteop Assoc.* 1985;85(12):786-801.
29. Fernández de las Peñas C, Fernandez-Carnero J, Miangolarra-Page J. Musculoskeletal disorders in mechanical neck pain: myofascial trigger points versus cervical joint dysfunction: a clinical study. *J Musculoske Pain.* 2005;13(1):27-35.
30. Kuchera M. Gravitational stress, musculoligamentous strain and postural realignment. *Spine.* 1995;9(2):463-490.
31. Chattopadhyay A. The cervical pillow. *J Indian Med Assoc.* 1980;75(1):6-9.

Chapter 17

Suboccipital Muscles
"Mask of Zorro"

Michael Karegeannes, César Fernández de las Peñas, and Michelle Finnegan

1. INTRODUCTION

The suboccipital muscles include the rectus capitis posterior major, rectus capitis posterior minor, obliquus capitis superior, and obliquus capitis inferior muscles. They connect the occipital bone, atlas, and axis posteriorly. They are innervated by the branches of the dorsal primary division of the suboccipital (C1) nerve. These muscles contribute to dynamic stability of the upper cervical spine by assisting with proprioception of the head with a high muscle spindle count. They also contribute to small movements of the head on the neck. The referred pain from suboccipital trigger points (TrPs) is felt deep inside the head, to the occiput, temporal region, eye, and forehead. Activation and perpetuation of TrPs in this muscle group can result from awkward posture, improperly fitted eyeglasses, prolonged position of the head held in rotation to one side, and trauma. Trigger points in these muscles are commonly associated with tension-type headache, cervicogenic headache, occipital neuralgia, or chronic intractable benign pain. Corrective actions include postural correction, ergonomics assessment, strengthening, and self-stretching.

2. ANATOMIC CONSIDERATIONS

Rectus Capitis Posterior Minor

The rectus capitis posterior minor muscle originates by a narrow pointed tendon in the tubercle on the posterior arch of the atlas and attaches to the medial part of the inferior nuchal line and to the occipital bone between the inferior nuchal line and the foramen magnum[1] (Figure 17-1). Recently, this muscle was found to be absent in a subject bilaterally.[2] Hack et al[3] first reported the existence of a connective tissue bridge between the rectus capitis posterior minor muscle and the cervical dura at C0-C1 levels. Additional anatomic studies have confirmed the existence of the anatomic connection between this muscle and the cervical dura at C0-C1 vertebral level.[4-6] Histologic analysis revealed that this anatomic connection fuses with the posterior atlanto-occipital membrane, which ultimately coalesces with the cervical spinal dura.[5] In fact, it is one of the muscles with almost the highest number of muscle spindles.[7]

Rectus Capitis Posterior Major

The rectus capitis posterior major muscle originates from a pointed tendon to the spinous process of the axis and attaches to the lateral part of the inferior nuchal line and the occipital bone immediately below it[1] (Figure 17-1). Interestingly, in the same study described above, Nayak et al[2] found two of these muscles on each side of a subject when the rectus capitis posterior minor muscles were absent. Scali et al,[8] in an anatomic study, found a connective tissue bridge between the rectus capitis posterior major muscle and the cervical dura mater. The same authors conducted a histologic analysis of this connective tissue bridge between the rectus capitis posterior major muscle and the cervical dura observing proprioceptive and neural afferences in this tissue.[9]

Obliquus Capitis Superior

The obliquus capitis superior muscle originates from tendinous fibers in the upper surface of the transverse process of the atlas and attaches to the occipital bone between the superior and inferior nuchal lines, lateral to the semispinalis capitis muscle and overlapping the insertion of rectus capitis posterior major muscle[1] (Figure 17-1). A study by Pontell et al[10] has recently reported that the obliquus capitis superior muscle also attaches to the cervical dura by a connective tissue bridge such as the rectus capitis posterior minor and major muscles do. In fact, although this muscle and each of the rectus capitis posterior major muscles is independently connected to the dura mater, the proximity of their myodural connections leads to the appearance of a single atlantoaxial (AA) myodural bridge that links both suboccipital muscles to the dura mater.[10] Again, in a histologic study, the same authors observed that the connective tissue bridge of the obliquus capitis superior muscle also exhibited neuronal and proprioceptive afferences, similar to the connective tissue bridge of the rectus capitis posterior major muscle.[11] Interestingly, all these myodural connections have also been observed by magnetic resonance imaging.[12]

Obliquus Capitis Inferior

The obliquus capitis inferior muscle, the larger of the two oblique muscles, originates adjacent to the upper part of the lamina of the axis and attaches to the inferoposterior aspect of the transverse process of the atlas[1] (Figure 17-1). The greater occipital nerve can be compressed at the obliquus capitis inferior muscle, near the spinous process of the axis, because it passes in close proximity to this muscle.[13] In a small percentage of subjects this nerve travels through the muscle.[14-16]

Suboccipital Triangle

The suboccipital triangle is formed by the rectus capitis posterior major, the obliquus capitis superior, and the obliquus capitis inferior minor muscles. The triangular space is covered by the semispinalis capitis muscle and is filled largely with connective tissue. The posterior atlanto-occipital membrane and the posterior arch of the atlas form the floor of the triangle. The vertebral artery traverses the floor of this space in a groove on the surface of the posterior arch of the atlas. The greater occipital nerve crosses the ceiling of the suboccipital triangle.

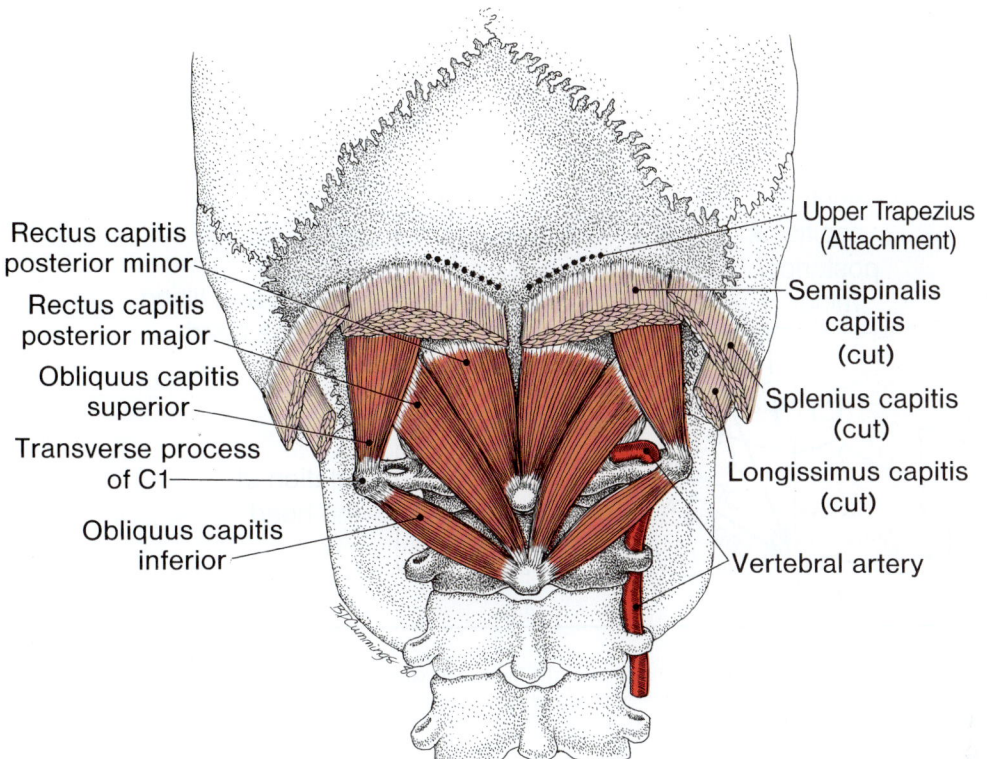

Figure 17-1. Attachments of the suboccipital muscles (medium red). The most lateral three of these four muscles define the suboccipital triangle. This triangle surrounds the transverse portion of the vertebral artery (dark red) and should be avoided when needling the posterior neck muscles. The more superficial overlying muscles are light red. The black dotted lines indicate the location of the attachment of the upper trapezius muscle, which is the most superficial posterior neck muscle.

2.1. Innervation and Vascularization

The suboccipital muscles are innervated by the branches of the dorsal primary division of the suboccipital (C1) nerve.[1] The C1 dorsal ramus passes dorsally and laterally through the suboccipital plexus of veins to enter the suboccipital triangle where it divides to form a branch for the rectus capitis posterior minor muscles.[17] One study showed that the dorsal rootlets of C1 had connections with the spinal accessory nerve 50% of the time.[18] The suboccipital muscles receive their blood supply from the vertebral artery and deep descending branches of the occipital artery.[1]

2.2. Function

The atlanto-occipital (C0-C1) and the AA (C1-C2) joints comprise the upper cervical region, which is the most mobile region within the entire vertebral column. These highly specialized joints facilitate precise positioning of the head and are involved in vision, hearing, smell, and equilibrium due to the function of the suboccipital muscles. Although the muscles do help to move the head on the neck, the main function of all suboccipital muscles is dynamic stability of upper cervical spine and proprioceptive feedback to the central nervous system.[19] The fact that the suboccipital muscles have a higher density of muscle spindles confirms their role in proprioception.[20]

Bilateral contraction of rectus capitis posterior minor and major muscles has been reported to contribute to the extension of the upper cervical spine, whereas a unilateral contraction of these two muscles contributes to ipsilateral rotation of the head.[1,2] Although both rectus capitis posterior muscles can be functionally classified as extensor muscles, due to their small size, these muscles are better suited for small movements of the head on the neck and to control cervical lordosis.[21] Their larger counterparts are better suited for the primary movement of the head and neck into extension.[22] The obliquus capitis superior muscle seems to have the best leverage to assist with side-bending (Figure 17-2); however, this muscle is likely more important for posture.[1] The obliquus capitis inferior muscle is the only one primarily active during upper cervical rotation of the atlas on the axis, helping to rotate the face to the ipsilateral side.[1] Figure 17-2 graphs the orientation of the suboccipital musculature and summarizes the action of each muscle. Independent of their theoretical function, the main function of the suboccipital musculature is to contribute significantly to the maintenance of a normal, neutral head posture as well as dynamic stability of the head during the performance of daily activities that require extension, rotation, and side-bending of the head on the neck.

In addition to these movements of the upper cervical spine, the head can also translate forward (protraction) and backward (retraction) within the sagittal plane. Typically, protraction of the head flexes the mid-lower cervical spine (C3-C7) and simultaneously extends the upper cervical spine (C0-C2). Retraction of the head, in contrast, extends or straightens the mid-lower cervical spine and simultaneously flexes the upper cervical region. Some recent studies have demonstrated that voluntary head retraction results in increased electromyographic activity in the rectus capitis posterior minor[23] and major[24] muscles. These studies concluded that head retraction results in eccentric contraction of both rectus capitis posterior muscles.

2.3. Functional Unit

The functional unit to which a muscle belongs includes the muscles that reinforce and counter its actions as well as the joints that the muscle crosses. The interdependence of these structures functionally is reflected in the organization and neural connections of the sensory motor cortex. The functional unit is

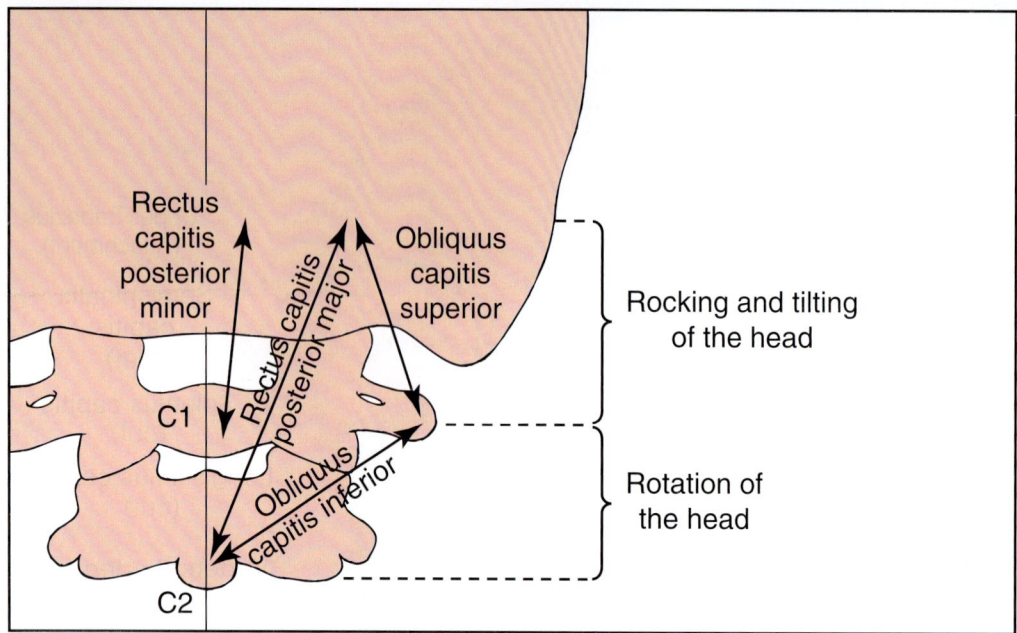

Figure 17-2. Graphic summary of the actions of the right suboccipital muscles.

Box 17-1 Functional unit of the suboccipital muscles

Action	Synergists	Antagonist
Upper cervical spine extension	Splenius capitis (bilaterally) Semispinalis capitis (bilaterally) Upper trapezius (bilaterally)	Longus capitis Rectus capitis anterior
Head rotation	Ipsilateral splenius capitis Contralateral sternocleidomastoid	Contralateral suboccipitals Contralateral splenius capitis Ipsilateral sternocleidomastoid

emphasized because the presence of a TrP in one muscle of the unit increases the likelihood that the other muscles of the unit will also develop TrPs. When inactivating TrPs in a muscle, one should be concerned about TrPs that may develop in muscles that are functionally interdependent. Box 17-1 grossly represents the functional unit of the suboccipital muscles.[25]

3. CLINICAL PRESENTATION

3.1. Referred Pain Pattern

Trigger points in these muscles commonly refer pain unilaterally from the occiput to the temporal region, eye, and the forehead (Figure 17-3). The pain seems to penetrate inside the skull and is difficult to localize; however, it does not have the straight-through-the-head quality of pain like what is referred by the splenius cervicis muscle. Trigger points in the suboccipital muscles are clearly associated with tension-type headache,[26] but they have also been found in patients with whiplash-associated disorders,[27] fibromyalgia syndrome,[28] and migraine.[29]

3.2. Symptoms

Patients with TrPs in the suboccipital muscles report headache (either tension-type headache [TTH] or migraine) or neck pain. In addition, patients with cervicogenic headache can also exhibit TrPs in these muscles. They are likely to describe the headache as pressing, hurting "all over," or more frequently like an eye mask.

When resting the head on a pillow in a supine position, patients often report a distressing headache that is of immediate onset. This pain is due to the weight of the occiput pressing against the pillow. Pain from the suboccipital muscles tends to be more deeply seated in the upper neck region and located more laterally than that experienced from the posterior cervical muscles. Patients often press with their fingers at the base of the skull, locating "a sore spot right here."

Because the greater occipital nerve passes close to the obliquus inferior capitis muscle, it is possible that patients with occipital neuralgia may also exhibit TrPs in the suboccipital muscles. Patients reporting pain radiating unilaterally from the occipital bone to the eye should be carefully examined for tenderness in the greater occipital nerve.

3.3. Patient Examination

After a thorough, subjective examination, the clinician should make a detailed drawing representing the pain pattern that the patient has described. This depiction will assist in planning the physical examination and can be useful in monitoring the progression of the patient as symptoms improve and/or change. For a proper assessment and examination related to the suboccipital muscles, the clinician should assess posture, accessory motion of the C0-C1 and C1-C2 vertebral segments, and breathing patterns.

Individuals with headache and suboccipital muscle TrPs usually exhibit a forward head posture and restricted range of motion.[30] In fact, forward head posture is one of the most common cervical posture abnormalities observed in clinical settings. Because a forward head posture includes extension of the upper cervical spine segments, this position induces a compression of the cranio-cervical structures, particularly the suboccipital and posterior neck musculature. Visual assessment is the most common way to assess the posture of an individual.

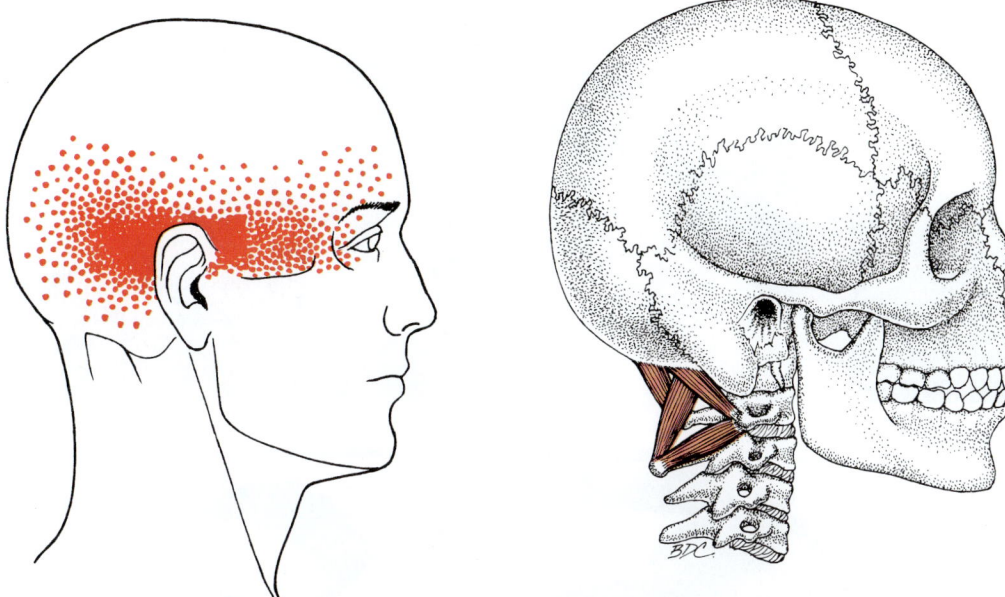

Figure 17-3. Referred pain pattern (dark red) of trigger points (TrPs) in the right suboccipital muscles (medium red).

Griegel-Morris et al[31] found a good intraexaminer ($\kappa = 0.825$) and a moderate interexaminer ($\kappa = 0.611$) reliability for postural visual assessment. Others have shown that the ability to detect a forward head posture is good as long as the differences are not subtle.[32,33] Other assessments such as photographs can be used for assessing a forward head posture in clinical practice[30] and have been shown to be reliable.[34,35]

In addition to head posture, suboccipital TrPs may be also be related to the presence of upper cervical spine joint dysfunctions, particularly OA or AA joints. These areas need to be clinically examined and treated, if considered to be a source of symptoms or a contributing factor to the patient's reports. In fact, suboccipital tightness due to TrPs can limit upper cervical flexion. This should be carefully assessed (Figure 17-4A). Upper cervical spine flexion combined with side-bending can help diagnose unilateral dysfunctions (Figure 17-4B). For specific details regarding the evaluation of upper cervical spine dysfunctions, refer to other texts on this topic.

Several studies have demonstrated that a manual assessment of upper cervical spine dysfunctions can help to diagnose patients with headache of cervical origin properly.[36,37] Proper manual assessment assists in the differential diagnosis between suboccipital muscle TrPs and upper cervical joint dysfunctions. In fact, both impairments can contribute to upper cervical joint restrictions. For instance, the cervical flexion–rotation test has been proposed as a proper tool for the diagnosis of upper cervical joint restriction. The cervical flexion–rotation test is conducted by placing the patient's neck in full flexion while passively rotating the head to one side (Figure 17-5A and B). The basis of the test is that cervical motion is more isolated to the C1-C2 (AA) level when the cervical spine is held in full flexion. It has been found that patients with cervicogenic headache have an average of 25° to 28° of AA rotation to the side of the headache as compared with an average rotation of 44° toward the asymptomatic side and as compared with healthy people (difference: 10°-15°). The cervical flexion–rotation test showed an overall diagnostic accuracy of 85% to 91%.[38] Frequently, a restriction in rotation toward one side is due to shortened suboccipital muscles, particularly the contralateral obliquus capitis inferior muscle. An alternative test for the AA joint is performed by placing the patient's neck in full lateral flexion while passively rotating the head to the opposite side (Figure 17-5C and D). Crepitus is a very common finding in patients with osteoarthritis of this joint.[39] In these patients, pain is often due to suboccipital TrPs.

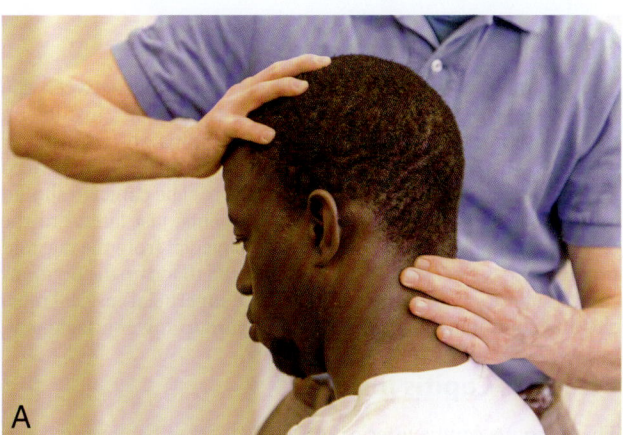
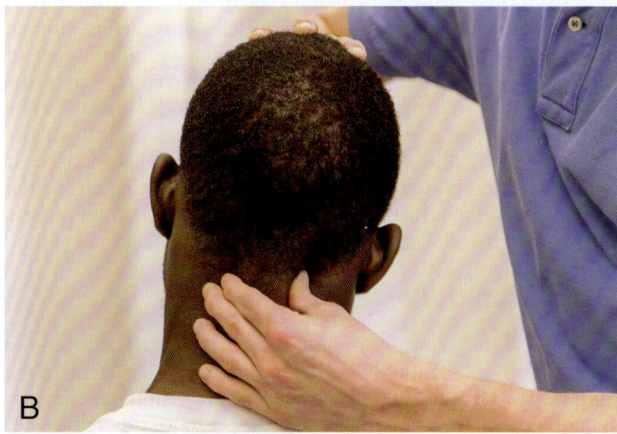

Figure 17-4. Tests for restricted motion due to tight suboccipital muscles. A, Restricted movement of the head on neck is found by flexing the atlanto-occipital joint (O-C1) and noting early motion between C2 and C3. B, Testing combined flexion of the atlanto-occipital joint (O-C1) with side-bending of the head on neck.

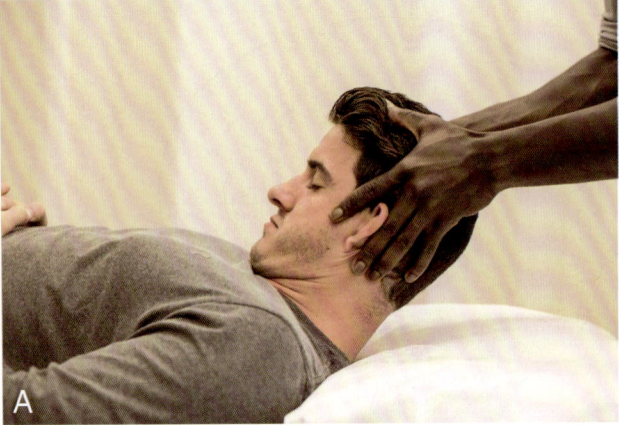
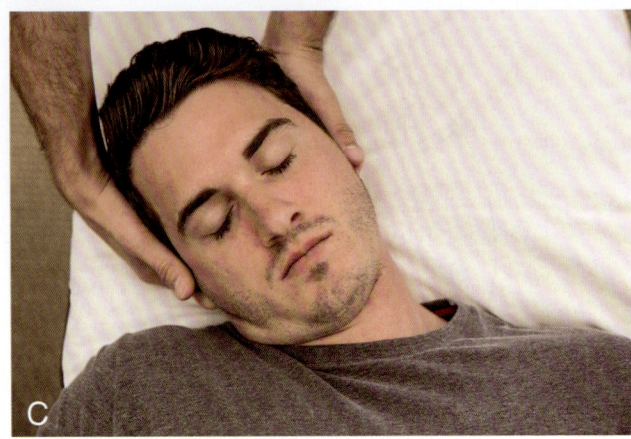
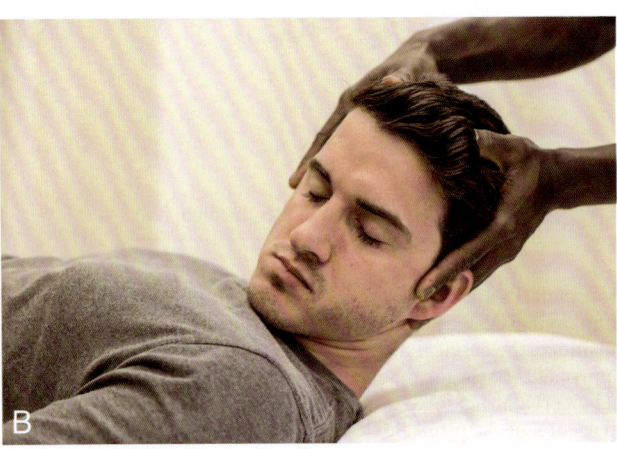
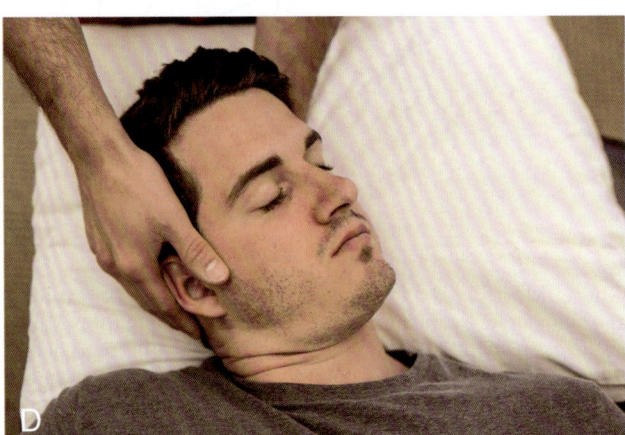

Figure 17-5. A and B, Cervical flexion–rotation test for isolated testing of the C1-C2 (AA) joint (left rotation) and right suboccipital muscle length. C and D, Cervical lateral flexion with contralateral rotation for isolated testing of the C1-C2 (AA) joint and right suboccipital muscle length. The same position can be used for treatment utilizing postisometric relaxation techniques.

3.4. Trigger Point Examination

Suboccipital muscles are the most deeply placed muscles just below the base of the skull. This region is also one of the most sensitive and tender areas of the body to palpate; thus, clinicians should be cognizant of the amount of pressure used with palpation in this area. These muscles are not directly palpable because the upper trapezius and other posterior neck muscles are more superficial. The application of pressure on the anatomic projection of each muscle, however, is able to elicit the referred pain from these muscles, which is clearly different from that of splenius capitis or upper trapezius muscles. It is seen in clinical practice that palpation of each of the suboccipital muscles, in some patients, can elicit slightly different referred pain patterns than that reported by Simons et al.[25] Fernández de las Peñas et al[26] developed a protocol for the diagnosis of TrPs in the suboccipital muscles. Although this has not been validated. It includes tenderness in the suboccipital area, referred pain elicited by maintained pressure, and increased referred pain on muscle contraction, specifically extension of the upper cervical spine.

Rectus Capitis Posterior Minor

The rectus capitis posterior minor muscle is located between the posterior tubercle of atlas (C1) and the occiput,[40] 1 cm lateral to the midline. For identification of its anatomic projection, the clinician starts palpating just superolateral to the posterior tubercle of C1. Another anatomic reference is the ligamentum nuchae. Utilizing cross-fiber flat palpation, the clinician should first locate the rectus capitis posterior minor region through the more superficial cervical muscles, then move toward the occipital attachment.

Rectus Capitis Posterior Major

The rectus capitis posterior major muscle is located between the spinous process of the axis (C2) and the occiput, just lateral to the rectus capitis posterior minor muscle.[40] For identification of its anatomic projection, the clinician starts palpating just to the spinous process of the axis. Cross-fiber flat palpation is utilized to locate the rectus capitis posterior major region through the more superficial muscles, continuing with assessment in the direction of the occipital attachment.

Obliquus Capitis Superior

The obliquus capitis superior muscle is located between the transverse process of the atlas (C1) and the occiput, just lateral to the superior attachment of the rectus capitis posterior major muscle.[40] This muscle is very challenging to palpate and to discern from superficial posterior neck musculature. The clinician should palpate starting on the occipital attachments, just lateral to the rectus capitis posterior major muscle and medial from the mastoid process. Cross-fiber flat palpation is utilized to locate the obliquus capitis superior region through the more superficial cervical muscles and continuing with assessment toward its lower attachment.

Obliquus Capitis Inferior

The obliquus capitis inferior muscle is located between the spinous process of C2 and the transverse process of C1, deep to the splenius capitis muscle.[40] Between these landmarks, the clinician palpates through the more superficial cervical muscles with a cross-fiber flat palpation technique to identify the obliquus capitis inferior region. The fiber direction of this muscle is typically more horizontal than what is depicted in anatomic pictures.

4. DIFFERENTIAL DIAGNOSIS

4.1. Activation and Perpetuation of Trigger Points

A posture or activity that activates a TrP, if not corrected, can also perpetuate it. In any portion of the suboccipital muscles, TrPs may be activated by unaccustomed eccentric loading, eccentric exercise in an unconditioned muscle, or maximal or sub-maximal concentric loading.[41] Trigger points may also be activated or aggravated when the muscle is placed in a shortened or lengthened position for an extended period of time. Because the suboccipital muscles are largely responsible for moving the head on top of the neck, they are likely to develop TrPs when working at either extreme range of motion. The checkrein function of the suboccipital extensors is overloaded by sustained forward flexion of the head and neck, which often occurs while using handheld electronic devices. If a person tips the head upward, the suboccipital musculature is strained by prolonged contraction (eg, when a person lies prone on the floor, propped up on the elbows to support the head while watching television).

Excessive forward head posture is usually accompanied by the extension of the upper cervical spine to accommodate for the line of vision, such as with excessive computer use. This position activates and perpetuates TrPs in the suboccipital muscles and other posterior cervical muscles. Mouth breathing as compared with nasal breathing has also been shown to have a negative impact on posture.[42-47]

Patients who are intensely preoccupied with desk or computer work are susceptible to losing track of time in an undesirable posture. In other muscles, TrPs have been shown to develop with 1 hour of typing, with visual and postural stressors,[48] and are plausible for these muscles as well.

Maladjusted eyeglass frames, uncorrected nearsightedness, lenses with too short a focal length, and the use of progressive lenses that require frequent or sustained fine adjustment of the head position can also activate and perpetuate TrPs in these muscles.

The rotation and head-tilt functions may be overused by sustained off-center head positions, as when the subject is talking to someone who is off to one side, sight-seeing to only one side from a vehicle, avoiding the glare from a strong light source that reflects off the inside of the eyeglass lenses, or by prolonged attention to work placed flat on the desk to the side of the keyboard.

Chilling the back of the neck, while tired neck muscles are being held in a fixed position, contributes to the activation of TrPs in these muscles.

Finally, any traumatic event with an impact on the cervical spine or the head, for example a whiplash injury, can activate TrPs in these muscles. Research supports the association of TrPs in other muscles and whiplash,[49,50] thus it is plausible that TrPs can develop in the suboccipitals as well. Patients with a whiplash injury are known to develop refractory head and neck pain symptoms, probably due to joint injury and TrPs.[51] Unfortunately these patients are rarely examined properly and treated for the part of their pain that is of a muscular origin.

4.2. Associated Trigger Points

Trigger points rarely appear in the suboccipital musculature alone; commonly those with a headache will have TrPs in the upper trapezius, temporalis, and semispinalis capitis muscles. They are also likely to be associated TrPs in the other masticatory muscles.

The referred pain from suboccipital TrPs may appear similar to, or overlap, the patterns of the temporalis, upper trapezius, sternocleidomastoid, splenius cervicis, and semispinalis capitis muscles; therefore, a thorough examination of each of these muscles is necessary.

Trigger points can also develop in the referred pain areas of TrPs,[52] therefore TrPs in the suboccipital muscles can be due to primary TrPs in other muscles including the upper trapezius, lower trapezius, splenius cervicis, and cervical multifidi muscles. Primary TrPs can also contribute to associated TrPs in other muscles including the occipitofrontalis, temporalis, orbicularis oculi, and corrugator muscles.

4.3. Associated Pathology

Patients with suboccipital TrPs are commonly diagnosed as having tension-type headache,[53] cervicogenic headache,[54] occipital neuralgia,[55] or chronic intractable benign pain. Chronic intractable benign pain is defined as "non-neoplastic pain of greater than 6 months duration without objective physical findings and known nociceptive peripheral input."[56] One study of patients with the "diagnosis" of chronic intractable benign pain of the neck reported TrPs or tender points in suboccipital muscles in 67.6% of 34 patients.[56] It is possible that patients with this diagnosis are today considered as suffering central sensitivity syndromes.[57]

Dural headache should be considered in the differential diagnosis of patients because of unique anatomic considerations with these muscles.[58] As Hack and Hallgren stated "The presence of a connective tissue bridge, attaching suboccipital muscles to the dura mater, is now recognized as a feature of normal human anatomy. The role that this myodural bridge may play in headache production is uncertain; however, a new conceptual model is emerging. Postsurgical myodural adhesions have been reported as a complication resulting from excision of acoustic tumors. Extensive research now exists implicating these myodural adhesions as a possible source of postoperative headache."[59] The authors report a case study of a single patient who experienced relief from chronic headache after a surgical procedure was performed to separate the suboccipital myodural bridge. Given this understanding of the connection between the suboccipital muscles to the dura, patients dealing with headache symptoms should be properly diagnosed before suboccipital TrP treatment is started. For instance, when a patient presents to the clinic with head pain but has not been previously examined by a physician, a thorough examination and medical screening should be conducted to rule out other underlying medical conditions. If warranted, referral to an appropriate medical practitioner for further diagnostic workup should be done.

Some studies have demonstrated that the suboccipital musculature, particularly the rectus capitis posterior minor and major muscles, exhibits larger amounts of fatty infiltrate in patients with whiplash-associated disorders[60] and decreased cross-sectional area in women with chronic tension-type headache.[61] Whether these muscle changes are a primary or secondary phenomenon remains unclear. In any case, fatty infiltration in these muscles could be associated with several mechanisms including generalized disuse, chronic denervation, motor-neuron lesions, metabolic disorders, or other muscle impairments.[60] Atrophy could possibly account for a reduction of proprioceptive output from the suboccipital musculature and thus contribute to the perpetuation of TrPs.[61,62]

Nerve entrapment has not been clinically observed as resulting from TrPs in the suboccipital muscles; however, TrPs in the obliquus capitis inferior muscle could potentially be a source of entrapment for the greater occipital nerve because this nerve has been shown in some instances to pierce the muscle.[14-16]

5. CORRECTIVE ACTIONS

For patients who develop TrPs in the suboccipital muscles, it is important to keep this part of the neck warm by wearing a turtleneck or a hood that covers the head and neck outdoors. Sleepwear rarely provides a collar high enough to cover the suboccipital area adequately; therefore, the patient should wear a soft hooded jacket or drape a scarf or bed covers in such a way as to keep the suboccipital region warm.

Sustained upward gaze, with the head tilted up, should be avoided for any activity by modifying or eliminating that activity. In a case seen by Dr Travell,[25] a stage director learned to direct the performance from farther back in the theater instead of from the front row where he had been at a level lower than that of the actors on the stage. This change allowed him to face the actors without looking up for prolonged periods.

Forward head posture and tongue position should always be corrected when identified as a problem. Instruction in good body mechanics is also essential (refer to Chapter 76).

To maximize the benefits of postural training, patients should be trained in naso-diaphragmatic breathing instead of mouth breathing, as mouth breathing has a negative impact on posture.[42-47] Performing strengthening exercises on a Swiss ball and stretches in conjunction with naso-diaphragmatic breathing has been shown to improve the posture[46] and decrease the activity of the suboccipital muscles.[46,63]

Sustained and strained positions of the head are reduced by (1) avoiding the use of trifocals; (2) using lenses with adequate focal length for the task at hand to allow the head to rest in a balanced upright position on top of the cervical spine; (3) rearranging the location of the patient or the room lighting to eliminate glare reflected from the inside of the lenses (or using antiglare lenses); (4) placing documents on a vertical stand; and (5) avoiding prolonged use of handheld electronic devices in the lap for lengthy tasks. Additional postural considerations are included in Chapter 76.

Intense preoccupation during desk tasks can result in a patient maintaining an undesirable posture for prolonged periods. Because TrPs have been shown to develop within 1 hour of typing,[48] desk workers should relieve muscle tension every 20 to 30 minutes by setting an interval-timer to remind them to take small breaks.

The rectus capitis posterior minor and major muscles can exhibit atrophy and fatty infiltration[60,62,64,65] similar to the posterior cervical muscles after whiplash[66,67] and therefore should be strengthened appropriately. Some recent studies have demonstrated that voluntary head retraction results in increased activity in the rectus capitis posterior minor[23] and major[24] muscles by inducing an eccentric contraction of both the muscles (Figure 17-6). Refer to supplementary texts on exercise prescription for more information.[68]

Finally, patients should learn how to relax the neck muscles and how to perform a passive self-stretch while seated on a stool or chair and, if possible, under a warm shower. The patient performs this stretch by manually assisting a nodding motion (flexion of the head on the neck) with the patient's fingers under the occiput (Figure 17-7). The patient uses his own fingers under the occiput to exert upward traction prior to directing the movement of the head. A comparable

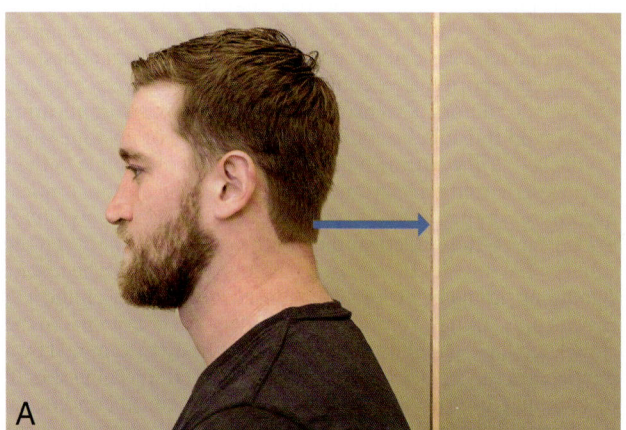
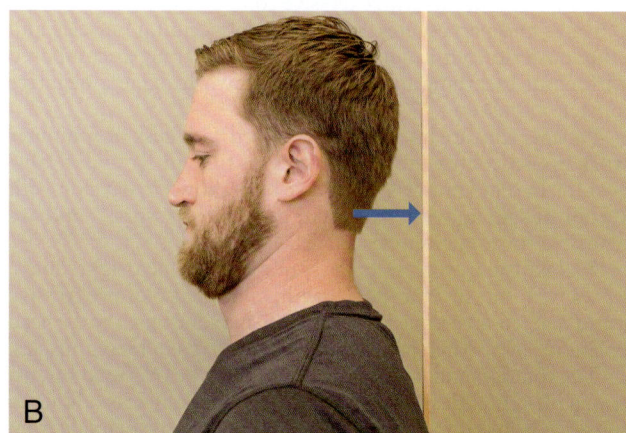

Figure 17-6. Active neck retraction from a neutral head position. A and B, In a seated or standing position, the patient actively retracts the head to bring the chin in line while the eyes stay level with the horizon. There should be no tipping of the head in a forward or backward direction.

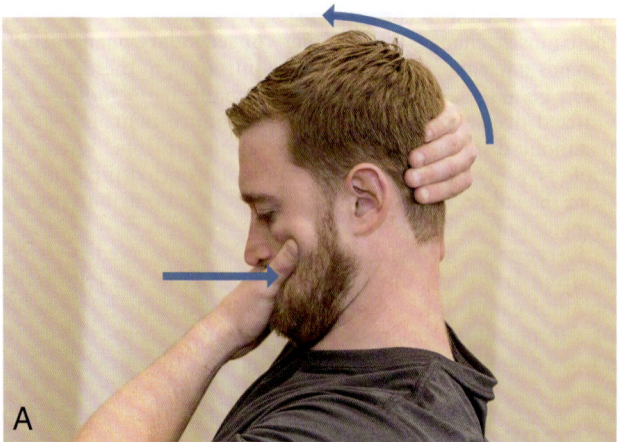
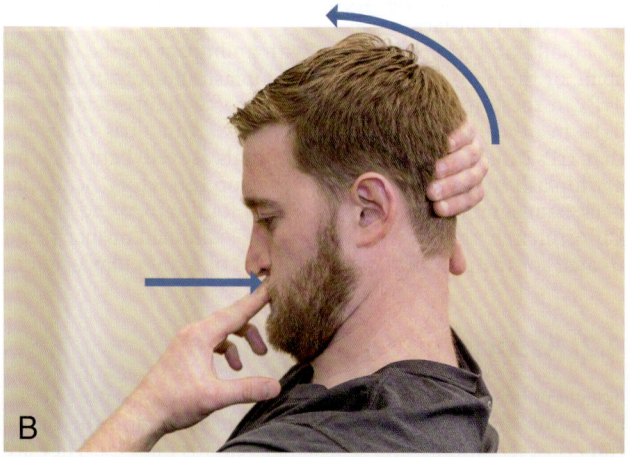

Figure 17.7. Self-stretching exercises of the suboccipital musculature. Stretch of the rectus capitis posterior major, minor, and obliquus capitis superior muscles. A and B, The patient flexes the head (by tucking the chin toward the chest) and nods the head forward.

self-stretch for the suboccipital muscles is described and illustrated by Lewit.[69] A series of passive stretches should be applied separately in unidirectional movements (no head rolling) with successive degrees of head rotation to fully stretch all the suboccipital muscles. Passive stretching should be followed by full active range of motion, contracting and stretching both agonists and antagonist muscles. This cycle of movements is repeated 3 to 5 times every couple of hours, slowly and without jerking.

References

1. Standring S. *Gray's Anatomy: The Anatomical Basis of Clinical Practice*. 41st ed. London, UK: Elsevier; 2015.
2. Nayak SR, Swamy R, Krishnamurthy A, Dasgupta H. Bilateral anomaly of rectus capitis posterior muscles in the suboccipital triangle and its clinical implication. *Clin Ter.* 2011;162(4):355-356.
3. Hack GD, Koritzer RT, Robinson WL, Hallgren RC, Greenman PE. Anatomic relation between the rectus capitis posterior minor muscle and the dura mater. *Spine*. 1995;20(23):2484-2486.
4. Humphreys BK, Kenin S, Hubbard BB, Cramer GD. Investigation of connective tissue attachments to the cervical spinal dura mater. *Clin Anat.* 2003;16(2):152-159.
5. Zumpano MP, Hartwell S, Jagos CS. Soft tissue connection between rectus capitus posterior minor and the posterior atlanto-occipital membrane: a cadaveric study. *Clin Anat.* 2006;19(6):522-527.
6. Kahkeshani K, Ward PJ. Connection between the spinal dura mater and suboccipital musculature: evidence for the myodural bridge and a route for its dissection: a review. *Clin Anat.* 2012;25(4):415-422.
7. McPartland JM, Brodeur RR. Rectus capitis posterior minor: a small but important suboccipital muscle. *J Bodyw Mov Ther.* 1999;3:30-35.
8. Scali F, Marsili ES, Pontell ME. Anatomical connection between the rectus capitis posterior major and the dura mater. *Spine*. 2011;36(25):E1612-E1614.
9. Scali F, Pontell ME, Enix DE, Marshall E. Histological analysis of the rectus capitis posterior major's myodural bridge. *Spine J.* 2013;13(5):558-563.
10. Pontell ME, Scali F, Marshall E, Enix D. The obliquus capitis inferior myodural bridge. *Clin Anat.* 2013;26(4):450-454.
11. Pontell ME, Scali F, Enix DE, Battaglia PJ, Marshall E. Histological examination of the human obliquus capitis inferior myodural bridge. *Ann Anat.* 2013;195(6):522-526.
12. Scali F, Pontell ME, Welk AB, Malmstrom TK, Marshall E, Kettner NW. Magnetic resonance imaging investigation of the atlanto-axial interspace. *Clin Anat.* 2013;26(4):444-449.
13. Janis JE, Hatef DA, Ducic I, et al. The anatomy of the greater occipital nerve: part II. Compression point topography. *Plast Reconstr Surg.* 2010;126(5):1563-1572.
14. Tubbs RS, Watanabe K, Loukas M, Cohen-Gadol AA. The intramuscular course of the greater occipital nerve: novel findings with potential implications for operative interventions and occipital neuralgia. *Surg Neurol Int.* 2014;5:155.
15. Natsis K, Baraliakos X, Appell HJ, Tsikaras P, Gigis I, Koebke J. The course of the greater occipital nerve in the suboccipital region: a proposal for setting landmarks for local anesthesia in patients with occipital neuralgia. *Clin Anat.* 2006;19(4):332-336.
16. Bovim G, Bonamico L, Fredriksen TA, Lindboe CF, Stolt-Nielsen A, Sjaastad O. Topographic variations in the peripheral course of the greater occipital nerve. Autopsy study with clinical correlations. *Spine*. 1991;16(4):475-478.
17. Bogduk N. The clinical anatomy of the cervical dorsal rami. *Spine*. 1982;7(4):319-330.
18. Tubbs RS, Loukas M, Slappey JB, Shoja MM, Oakes WJ, Salter EG. Clinical anatomy of the C1 dorsal root, ganglion, and ramus: a review and anatomical study. *Clin Anat.* 2007;20(6):624-627.
19. Liu JX, Thornell LE, Pedrosa-Domellof F. Muscle spindles in the deep muscles of the human neck: a morphological and immunocytochemical study. *J Histochem Cytochem.* 2003;51(2):175-186.
20. Peck D, Buxton DF, Nitz A. A comparison of spindle concentrations in large and small muscles acting in parallel combinations. *J Morphol.* 1984;180(3):243-252.
21. Jull G, Sterling M, Falia D, Treleaven J, O'Leary S. *Whiplash, Headache, and Neck Pain Research-Based Direction for Physical Therapies*. Philadelphia, PA: Churchhill Livingstone Elsevier; 2008.
22. Nolan JP Jr, Sherk HH. Biomechanical evaluation of the extensor musculature of the cervical spine. *Spine*. 1988;13(1):9-11.
23. Hallgren RC, Pierce SJ, Prokop LL, Rowan JJ, Lee AS. Electromyographic activity of rectus capitis posterior minor muscles associated with voluntary retraction of the head. *Spine J.* 2014;14(1):104-112.
24. Hallgren RC, Rowan JJ, Bai P, Pierce SJ, Shafer-Crane GA, Prokop LL. Activation of rectus capitis posterior major muscles during voluntary retraction of the head in asymptomatic subjects. *J Manipulative Physiol Ther.* 2014;37(6):433-440.
25. Simons DG, Travell J, Simons L. *Travell & Simon's Myofascial Pain and Dysfunction: The Trigger Point Manual*. Vol 1. 2nd ed. Baltimore, MD: Williams & Wilkins; 1999:104.
26. Fernández de las Peñas C, Alonso-Blanco C, Cuadrado ML, Gerwin R, Pareja J. Myofascial trigger points in the suboccipital muscles and forward head posture in chronic tension type headache. *Headache*. 2006;46:454-460.
27. Fernandez-Perez AM, Villaverde-Gutierrez C, Mora-Sanchez A, Alonso-Blanco C, Sterling M, Fernández de las Peñas C. Muscle trigger points, pressure pain threshold, and cervical range of motion in patients with high level of disability related to acute whiplash injury. *J Orthop Sports Phys Ther.* 2012;42(7):634-641.
28. Alonso-Blanco C, Fernández de las Peñas C, Morales-Cabezas M, Zarco-Moreno P, Ge HY, Florez-Garcia M. Multiple active myofascial trigger points reproduce the overall spontaneous pain pattern in women with fibromyalgia and are related to widespread mechanical hypersensitivity. *Clin J Pain*. 2011;27(5):405-413.
29. Fernández de las Peñas C, Cuadrado ML, Pareja JA. Myofascial trigger points, neck mobility and forward head posture in unilateral migraine. *Cephalalgia*. 2006;26(9):1061-1070.
30. Fernández de las Penas C, Blanco CR, Cuadrado ML, Pareja J. Forward head posture and neck mobility in chronic tension-type headache: a blinded, controlled study. *Cephalalgia*. 2006;26:314-319.
31. Griegel-Morris P, Larson K, Mueller-Klaus K, Oatis CA. Incidence of common postural abnormalities in the cervical, shoulder, and thoracic regions and their association with pain in two age groups of healthy subjects. *Phys Ther.* 1992;72(6):425-431.
32. Passier LN, Nasciemento MP, Gesch JM, Haines TP. Physiotherapist observation of head and neck alignment. *Physiother Theory Pract.* 2010;26(6):416-423.
33. Gadotti IC, Biasotto-Gonzalez DA. Sensitivity of clinical assessments of sagittal head posture. *J Eval Clin Pract.* 2010;16(1):141-144.
34. Ruivo RM, Pezarat-Correia P, Carita AI. Intrarater and interrater reliability of photographic measurement of upper-body standing posture of adolescents. *J Manipulative Physiol Ther.* 2015;38(1):74-80.
35. Dimitriadis Z, Podogyros G, Polyviou D, Tasopoulos I, Passa K. The reliability of lateral photography for the assessment of the forward head posture through four different angle-based analysis methods in healthy individuals. *Musculoskeletal Care*. 2015.
36. Jull G, Amiri M, Bullock-Saxton J, Darnell R, Lander C. Cervical musculoskeletal impairment in frequent intermittent headache. Part 1: subjects with single headaches. *Cephalalgia*. 2007;27(7):793-802.
37. Fernández de las Peñas C, Cuadrado ML. Therapeutic options for cervicogenic headache. *Expert Rev Neurother.* 2014;14(1):39-49.
38. Hall T, Briffa K, Hopper D, Robinson K. Reliability of manual examination and frequency of symptomatic cervical spine motion segment dysfunction in cervicogenic headache. *Man Ther.* 2010;15(6):542-546.
39. Halla JT, Hardin JG Jr. Atlantoaxial (C1-C2) facet joint osteoarthritis: a distinctive clinical syndrome. *Arthritis Rheum.* 1987;30(5):577-582.
40. Muscolino JE. *The Muscle and Bone Palpation Manual: With Trigger Points, Referral Patterns, and Stretching*. St. Louis, MO: Mosby; 2015.
41. Gerwin RD, Dommerholt J, Shah JP. An expansion of Simons' integrated hypothesis of trigger point formation. *Curr Pain Headache Rep.* 2004;8(6):468-475.
42. Milanesi JM, Borin G, Correa EC, da Silva AM, Bortoluzzi DC, Souza JA. Impact of the mouth breathing occurred during childhood in the adult age: biophotogrammetric postural analysis. *Int J Pediatr Otorhinolaryngol.* 2011;75(8):999-1004.
43. Cuccia AM, Lotti M, Caradonna D. Oral breathing and head posture. *Angle Orthod.* 2008;78(1):77-82.
44. Sforza C, Colombo A, Turci M, Grassi G, Ferrario VF. Induced oral breathing and craniocervical postural relations: an experimental study in healthy young adults. *Cranio*. 2004;22(1):21-26.
45. Vig PS, Showfety KJ, Phillips C. Experimental manipulation of head posture. *Am J Orthod.* 1980;77(3):258-268.
46. Correa EC, Berzin F. Efficacy of physical therapy on cervical muscle activity and on body posture in school-age mouth breathing children. *Int J Pediatr Otorhinolaryngol.* 2007;71(10):1527-1535.
47. Neiva PD, Kirkwood RN, Godinho R. Orientation and position of head posture, scapula and thoracic spine in mouth-breathing children. *Int J Pediatr Otorhinolaryngol.* 2009;73(2):227-236.
48. Hoyle JA, Marras WS, Sheedy JE, Hart DE. Effects of postural and visual stressors on myofascial trigger point development and motor unit rotation during computer work. *J Electromyography Kinesiology*. 2011;21(1):41-48.
49. Castaldo M, Ge HY, Chiarotto A, Villafane JH, Arendt-Nielsen L. Myofascial trigger points in patients with whiplash-associated disorders and mechanical neck pain. *Pain Med.* 2014;15(5):842-849.
50. Bismil Q, Bismil M. Myofascial-entheseal dysfunction in chronic whiplash injury: an observational study. *JRSM Short Rep.* 2012;3(8):57.
51. Dommerholt J. Persistent myalgia following whiplash. *Curr Pain Headache Rep.* 2005;9(5):326-330.
52. Hsieh YL, Kao MJ, Kuan TS, Chen SM, Chen JT, Hong CZ. Dry needling to a key myofascial trigger point may reduce the irritability of satellite MTrPs. *Am J Phys Med Rehabil.* 2007;86(5):397-403.
53. Fernández de las Peñas C, Cuadrado ML, Arendt-Nielsen L, Simons DG, Pareja JA. Myofascial trigger points and sensitization: an updated pain model for tension-type headache. *Cephalalgia*. 2007;27(5):383-393.
54. Jaeger B. Are "cervicogenic" headaches due to myofascial pain and cervical spine dysfunction? *Cephalalgia*. 1989;9(3):157-164.
55. Graff-Radford SB, Jaeger B, Reeves JL. Myofascial pain may present clinically as occipital neuralgia. *Neurosurgery*. 1986;19(4):610-613.
56. Rosomoff HL, Fishbain DA, Goldberg M, Santana R, Rosomoff RS. Physical findings in patients with chronic intractable benign pain of the neck and/or back. *Pain*. 1989;37(3):279-287.

57. Yunus MB. Central sensitivity syndromes: a new paradigm and group nosology for fibromyalgia and overlapping conditions, and the related issue of disease versus illness. *Semin Arthritis Rheum.* 2008;37(6):339-352.
58. Alix ME, Bates DK. A proposed etiology of cervicogenic headache: the neurophysiologic basis and anatomic relationship between the dura mater and the rectus posterior capitis minor muscle. *J Manipulative Physiol Ther.* 1999;22(8):534-539.
59. Hack GD, Hallgren RC. Chronic headache relief after section of suboccipital muscle dural connections: a case report. *Headache.* 2004;44(1):84-89.
60. Elliott J, Jull G, Noteboom JT, Darnell R, Galloway G, Gibbon WW. Fatty infiltration in the cervical extensor muscles in persistent whiplash-associated disorders: a magnetic resonance imaging analysis. *Spine.* 2006;31(22):E847-E855.
61. Fernández de las Peñas C, Bueno A, Ferrando J, Elliott JM, Cuadrado ML, Pareja JA. Magnetic resonance imaging study of the morphometry of cervical extensor muscles in chronic tension-type headache. *Cephalalgia.* 2007;27(4):355-362.
62. McPartland JM, Brodeur RR, Hallgren RC. Chronic neck pain, standing balance, and suboccipital muscle atrophy: a pilot study. *J Manipulative Physiol Ther.* 1997;20(1):24-29.
63. Correa EC, Berzin F. Mouth breathing syndrome: cervical muscles recruitment during nasal inspiration before and after respiratory and postural exercises on Swiss Ball. *Int J Pediatr Otorhinolaryngol.* 2008;72(9):1335-1343.
64. Andary MT, Hallgren RC, Greenman PE, Rechtien JJ. Neurogenic atrophy of suboccipital muscles after a cervical injury: a case study. *Am J Phys Med Rehabil.* 1998;77(6):545-549.
65. Hallgren RC, Greenman PE, Rechtien JJ. Atrophy of suboccipital muscles in patients with chronic pain: a pilot study. *J Am Osteopath Assoc.* 1994;94(12):1032-1038.
66. Elliott J, Sterling M, Noteboom JT, Treleaven J, Galloway G, Jull G. The clinical presentation of chronic whiplash and the relationship to findings of MRI fatty infiltrates in the cervical extensor musculature: a preliminary investigation. *Eur Spine J.* 2009;18(9):1371-1378.
67. Abbott R, Pedler A, Sterling M, et al. The geography of fatty infiltrates within the cervical multifidus and semispinalis cervicis in individuals with chronic whiplash-associated disorders. *J Orthop Sports Phys Ther.* 2015;45(4):281-288.
68. Fernández de las Peñas C, Huijbregts PA. Therapeutic exercise of the cervical spine for patients with headache. In: Fernández de las Peñas C, Arendt-Nielsen L, Gerwin R, eds. *Tension Type and Cervicogenic Headache: Patho-Physiology, Diagnosis and Treatment.* Boston, MA: Jones & Bartlett Publishers; 2009:379-391.
69. Lewit K. *Manipulative Therapy in Rehabilitation of the Locomotor System.* 2nd ed. Oxford, England: Butterworth Heinemann; 1991.

Chapter 18

Clinical Considerations of Head and Neck Pain

César Fernández de las Peñas and María Palacios-Ceña

Myofascial pain resulting from trigger points (TrPs) usually refers symptoms to both muscular and nonmuscular structures. In the head and neck regions, the patient may report having facial pain, headache, toothache, sinus pain, or temporomandibular joint (TMJ) pain. Clinical evaluation of these areas may not yield any evidence of local pathologic change. In fact, any undiagnosed pain, particularly but not exclusively deep, dull, and aching in character, may be of myofascial origin. If a patient describes two components to the pain or notes a dull aching quality in addition to other pain descriptors, pain from TrPs should be suspected as a contributing factor. The intensity of myofascial pain due to TrPs should not be underestimated because it has been rated by patients as equal to or greater than pain from other causes.[1] It is of paramount importance to distinguish between TrP origins and other pain syndromes in the head and neck.

1. TEMPOROMANDIBULAR DISORDER

1.1. Overview

Temporomandibular disorder (TMD) is a term including different conditions involving the TMJ, the masticatory muscles, and their associated tissues (eg, ligaments, disc, and connective tissues) that represent a clinical problem such as pain, limited jaw movements, and TMJ noises. There are several different TMDs; myofascial TMD and internal TMJ derangements are the most common subtypes. TMD pain is characterized by a classical triad of clinical features: muscle and/or joint pain; TMJ crepitus sounds, clicking, or popping (in the case or disc displacement or degenerative joint disorders); and restriction, limitation, or deviation of the mandible during mouth opening and closing movements.[2,3]

The lifetime prevalence of TMD is unclear, but some studies have shown prevalence rates ranging between 3% and 15% in the Western population, and incidence rates ranging between 2% and 4%.[4] Women are more frequently affected than men (ratio 2:1).[5] Myofascial TMD is the most frequent diagnosis (42%), followed by disc displacement with reduction (32.1%), and arthralgia (30%).[6]

This condition, particularly myofascial TMD, is commonly comorbid with other entities (eg, headaches). Gonçalves et al[7] found that subjects with myofascial TMD were significantly more likely to suffer from chronic daily headaches, migraine, and tension-type headache (TTH) than individuals without TMD pain.

One of the common clinical features of TMD includes spontaneous face pain or pain with mandibular motion. Patient-based drawings of their pain symptoms demonstrate a concentration around the masseter muscle and spreading to the temporalis muscle. The pain is felt deep and "spreading pain" is a descriptive phrase commonly used by patients. This presentation is a cardinal symptom in patients with a diagnosis of myofascial TMD pain, although not exclusive of this condition. The words describing the pain of patients suspected to have been dealing with myofascial TMD resemble the pain features of TrPs in general.

Another typical clinical sign of myofascial TMD is the tenderness or pain on palpation of muscle structures, particularly the masticatory musculature. Masticatory muscles are easily accessible to manual palpation and some authors have standardized the areas that should be explored as well as the pressure and time to be applied; however, no consensus has been achieved on this topic. Recommendations from the Diagnostic Criteria for TMD suggest 1 kg for 2 seconds to be applied to the masseter and temporalis muscles, and 0.5 kg to the TMJ.[8]

1.2. Initial Evaluation of Patients with Temporomandibular Disorder Pain

When a patient with TMD pain seeks treatment, a comprehensive initial evaluation is needed to determine if the patient would be a candidate for TrP management, referral to another professional (eg, Dentist), or a combination of treatment and referral. Clinicians should record the pain history including area and behavior, aggravating and alleviating features, and maneuvers or positions that increase or reduce symptoms. It is important that clinicians record and listen to the patient's description of their symptoms. Symptom descriptors such as deep, widespread, diffuse, pressure, or tight would indicate the presence and importance of referred pain from TrPs. Box 18-1 summarizes some pain features that may assist clinicians in identifying which TrPs to look for.

Regardless of the source of symptoms, a thorough examination and evaluation of the TMJ and cervical spine screening should be carried out. The examination should include examination

---

Box 18-1 Pain features that assist the clinician with examination of relevant TrPs

The McGill Pain Questionnaire may be useful to assess the quality of pain symptoms. During the subjective examination or patient interview, the clinician should note the following pain descriptions that may suggest the presence of TrPs.

- "It feels like my head or neck is burning."
- "My neck just feels so tight. My movement feels restricted."
- "It feels like a lot of pressure in my head, like it's being compressed."
- "My head feels really heavy. I feel like it is hard to hold up."

for TrPs that may be the source or contributing factor of the patient's presentation. The following sections summarize some common clinical aspects of the TMJ examination.

Joint Capsule Tenderness

Pain emanating from the TMJ itself is almost always associated with inflammation of the joint capsule or retrodiscal tissues, which results in the sensitization of these structures. Palpation of the TMJs often reveals tenderness if an acute inflammatory process is present. Palpation of the lateral poles, which are located just anterior to the tragus of the ear symptoms, may reveal tenderness or reproduce the patient's symptoms, indicating joint capsule involvement.[9] Firm palpation may be uncomfortable in healthy people but is only painful if the joint capsule is inflamed. Simultaneous palpation allows the patient to compare the sensations of one side to the other. Palpation of the lateral pole of the TMJ has shown fair to slight interrater agreement.[10,11] Palpation of the posterosuperior part of the joint can be accomplished by placing a finger in each external auditory meatus; here, potentially inflamed retrodiscal tissues can be identified as a source of the patient's symptoms.

An interesting observation is the report of persistent periarticular TMJ pain in the absence of joint inflammation. In this case, any tenderness to joint palpation is relatively mild compared with typical presentation of an acute inflammatory condition. This persistent periarticular tenderness may arise from masseter, pterygoid, and/or sternocleidomastoid TrPs that result in referred pain to the joint with associated secondary cutaneous and deep tissue hypersensitivity.[12]

Presence of acute inflammatory TMJ pain is clearly a reason to refer the individual to a dentist trained in orofacial pain and TMD. Resolution of joint inflammation is certainly essential for resolution of any concurrent masticatory muscle TrPs. The pain from an acutely inflamed joint restricts any masticatory muscle stretching and TrPs recur secondary to the central excitatory effects from the nociceptive source. Palliative care is essential to achieve resolution of the inflammatory process. One can start to manage any TrPs, while instituting palliative joint care, by simultaneously educating the patient in the resting position of the jaw, good posture and body mechanics, and reducing or eliminating parafunctional oral habits such as gum chewing, fingernail biting, and pen chewing. Once the joint inflammation is under control, masticatory TrPs can be thoroughly addressed if still necessary. Once acute inflammatory conditions have been ruled out, the remaining tests help determine the extent of TMJ internal derangement if present.

Joint Clicking Sounds

Although many TMJ disorders are accompanied by some variation of joint sounds, there is no reproducibly reliable clinical test to examine for these.[11,13] However, one study found that TMJ-related pain was correlated with TMJ-related magnetic resonance imaging diagnoses of internal derangement and osteoarthrosis.[14]

Palpation involves placing the pad of the index fingers over each TMJ (just anterior to the tragus of the ear) while the patient opens and closes the mouth. A normal joint is essentially silent and moves smoothly. Crepitation (rough, sandy, or diffuse noise or vibration) is usually a sign of degenerative joint changes (eg, osteoarthrosis). Discrete clicks and pops may represent a mechanical problem with the disc or more localized disc and articular surface abnormalities. The timing, quality, and intensity of joint noises help define the type and severity of joint involvement.[15] A loud discrete click on opening, followed by a quieter, less-intense click on closing (called a reciprocal click) is typical of an anteriorly displaced disc with reduction. The location of the opening click is usually at wider jaw opening than the closing click which often occurs just before the teeth come together. Discrete clicks that occur at the same point on opening and closing probably represent discrete disc and articular surface abnormalities. Not all intra-articular interferences with joint movement result in noise. Occasionally, only a brief lateral shift in the mandible or condyle is evident on examination. The presence of joint sounds alone, however, does not mean that the patient has a TMD. Many people have joint sounds without any sign of true joint disease.[15,16] Readers are referred to other texts for further info on TMJ examination.[3,17]

Auscultation using a stethoscope placed lightly over each TMJ while the patient opens and closes may be used to amplify joint sounds for clinical purposes. The technique is only moderately reliable (50%-65% agreement) when used by trained examiners, even when they were using a split stethoscope with two earpieces and one diaphragm.[18] Another study reported that the interexaminer reliability was moderate ($\kappa = 0.47$-0.59) for tests recording joint sounds.[19] Other studies have even less reliability when listening for joint sounds.[11]

Because the mandible connects the two TMJs, transfer of vibration and sound often makes it difficult to assess which joint, if only one, is causing the noise or irregular movement. Sometimes, the patient clearly senses which joint is involved; if not, another method involves continuing to palpate the lateral poles of the joints while the patient moves his or her jaw to the left and to the right without opening more than 1 or 2 mm. Although it is generally accepted that an involved right joint clicks or crepitates with jaw movements to the left and vice versa, this method of examination showed unacceptable between-examiner agreement for research purposes when studied.[15] Readers are referred to other texts for further info on TMJ examination.[3,17]

The presence of internal derangements is not a contraindication for treatment of TrPs. In fact, there is a widely accepted clinical opinion that the lateral pterygoid muscle may be dysfunctional in patients with TMD. The theory of internal derangement of the TMJ involves the anterior displacement of the disc as result of hyperactivity of the lateral pterygoid muscle. This hypothesis is based on the attachment of the superior head of the lateral pterygoid muscle which may pull the disc in an anterior and superomedial direction.[20]

Mandible Range of Motion

The mandible movements usually assessed in clinical practice include a maximum opening (passive/active), maximum bilateral excursions, and a maximum protrusion. However, restricted mandible movements do not provide relevant information for any specific diagnosis since multiple factors can be related to this impairment.

The normal minimum interincisal range of jaw opening is generally accepted to be between 36 and 44 mm with a maximum normal range of motion (ROM) of up to 60 mm. A quick screening test for normal jaw opening involves asking the patient whether he or she can fit the first two knuckles of the nondominant hand between the incisor teeth. In the absence of internal derangement and TrPs, all healthy people can accomplish this and some can fit three knuckles. For a reproducible numerical value, interincisal opening should be measured with a sterilized or linear disposable millimeter ruler. It is useful to use a ruler where zero is directly at one end of the ruler without any indentation space. Place the "0" end on top of one of the lower central incisors and measure to the incisal edge of the corresponding upper central incisor. The assessment should always be conducted between the same central incisors to be able to compare measurements from one time to the next. This is a very reliable and reproducible clinical measure and "represents the gold standard for evaluating mandible movement."[10,21,22] Readers are referred to other texts for further info on TMJ examination and assessment.[3,17]

Clinically, three vertical mandible measurements are useful: maximum comfortable opening, full unassisted opening (active ROM), and assisted opening (active assisted ROM). The pain-free ROM should be at least 36 to 44 mm. A normal joint has 1 to 2 mm of "give" at end range with manual assistance from the clinician. Restriction of oral opening due to muscle splinting may result in a relatively dramatic increase in jaw opening with the assisted range testing maneuver, although the patient may complain of pain. Muscular restriction may also cause tremor and reflex muscle guarding against the opening pressure. Restriction of the oral opening due to mechanical obstruction or ankylosis in the TMJ typically results in a hard end feel and no increased range.

Hypermobility of the TMJ (jaw opening greater than 60 mm) and history of open dislocations are indications for caution with assisted stretch of the masticatory muscles. This presentation contrasts starkly to one of restricted mouth opening which indicates internal derangement or ankylosis of the TMJs, tightness of the joint capsule, restriction due to muscular splinting, TrPs, or a combination of these factors. The mandible midline tends to deviate toward the side affected with the most pronounced joint and/or muscle restriction.

In general, restricted mandible ROM is an indication to institute jaw exercises and muscle treatment. Contraindications to opening exercises are limited and include:

1. True acute arthralgia, usually due to some inflammatory process, is a contraindication to muscle stretching due to pain and reflex muscle splinting. Once this has resolved, muscular stretching is permissible as needed.
2. Painful internal derangement.
3. Significant history of locking (frequent episodes of inability to open the mouth without any manipulation first).

If a patient exhibits a limited range of mandible motion and little is gained by muscle therapy, the TMJ capsule may be tight. Skilled joint mobilization would be the treatment of choice to improve mouth opening.[23] There are ample resources available to clinicians to learn these techniques.[24]

Mandible Path of Opening and Closing

The clinician should observe the path of mouth opening and closing, looking for S or C deviations from a straight path; these may be indicative of mechanical problems within the joint or muscle imbalances.

The jaw tends to deflect toward the side affected with an internal joint derangement or restricting mobility of the individual joint or to the side with masticatory muscle shortening or TrPs. Trigger points in the masseter or temporalis muscle can deviate the jaw to the same side, whereas TrPs in the medial or lateral pterygoid muscle deviate the jaw to the opposite side. The presence of jaw aberrant motion alone, in absence of inflammation or painful internal derangement, is not a contraindication for the treatment of TrPs. However, a significantly restricted mandible ROM (<36 mm) along with deviation to one side and a hard end feel may be indicative of either unilateral ankylosis or an anteriorly displaced disc without reduction. This joint situation merits an evaluation by a specialist in TMD although basic TrP pain management strategies such as specific TrP therapy, resting position of the jaw, good posture, and good body mechanics can be instituted immediately.

1.3. Trigger points and Temporomandibular Disorders

TMD diagnosis is mainly based on a combination of defined signs and symptoms. The most accepted worldwide diagnostic criteria are the Research Diagnostic Criteria for TMD, proposed in 1992[25] and currently being replaced by the validated Diagnostic Criteria for TMD (DC TMD).[8] Within the Research Diagnostic Criteria for TMD, axis I and axis II are mainly included. Three major diagnostic categories contemplated in axis I are myofascial pain, disc alterations, and arthralgia–arthritis–arthrosis.[25] Axis II contemplates the psychological aspects of TMD pain by including specific questionnaires assessing depression and anxiety, among other features.[25] The DC/TMD uses the same double-axes approach with three major groups related to axis I: muscle pain, TMJ disorders, and headache attributed to TMD.[8]

The term myofascial TMD clearly suggests that TrPs play a relevant role in the genesis of the pain. Of course, the most important part of any diagnostic effort is obtaining a good history; this is often enough to make a fairly accurate preliminary determination of the probable cause. Once it is clear that the patient may be suffering from either an articular disorder, TrPs, or a combination of both, the following examination techniques help delineate the extent of TMJ involvement. In clinical practice, it is highly common to see a combination of both muscle and joint imbalances independently of the main diagnosis.

Painless joint disorders are not typically associated with the development of TrPs. It is the acute, painful inflammatory process that may intermittently or persistently accompany chronic joint conditions that tend to herald the onset of TrPs. Acute inflammation intrinsic to the joint or acute stages of arthritis are the usual causes of pain emanating from the joint itself. In an older study conducted at the University of Minnesota TMJ and Facial Pain Clinic, doctors evaluated 296 consecutive patients with chronic head and neck pain complaints.[26] Only 21% of these patients had a TMD as the primary cause of pain. In all the 21% patients, the joint disorder included an inflammation of the TMJ capsule or the retrodiscal tissues. This type of pain is characteristically periarticular and aching in quality and will respond to acute pain management therapies; however, because these disorders are almost always accompanied by reflex muscle splinting, spasm, or pain, it is common to see the development of TrPs especially if the inflammation is prolonged or recurrent. Pain due to TrPs was the primary diagnosis in 55.4% of the patients in the Minnesota study, almost three times the incidence of primary joint pain. Painless internal derangements of the TMJs were felt to be a perpetuating factor of TrPs in 30.4% of the patients.[26] Therefore, it is important to make a distinction between true TMJ pain, pain due to TrPs alone, and pain due to TrPs that is being perpetuated by a noninflammatory or intermittently inflammatory joint condition. Treatment priorities are affected accordingly.

Scientific data from human pain models clearly support the notion that referred pain from masticatory muscles may be involved in myofascial TMD pain.[27] Nevertheless, clinical evidence is scarce. A nonblinded study revealed that the referred pain patterns following a manual stimulation of TrPs in the masticatory muscle was similar to the pain pattern experienced by individuals with TMD.[28] A blinded controlled study[29] demonstrated the existence of multiple active TrPs in the masticatory and neck–shoulder musculature in women with myofascial TMD. In this study, both local and referred pain elicited from manual palpation of active TrPs reproduced the pattern of pain symptoms in all TMD patients. It is suggested that different muscles may be involved in TMD and TTH. TMD pain is clinically more similar to the pain patterns produced by stimulation of the masseter muscle; in contrast, TTH is more similar to the pain patterns evoked by stimulation of cervical muscles, for example, upper trapezius.[30]

2. NECK PAIN SYNDROMES AND HEADACHES

2.1. Overview

Since headaches constitute a serious health problem, there has been an increasing interest in the pathogenic mechanisms of these pain disorders.[31] Among all the described headaches, attention from clinicians has focused on those three most prevalent: TTH, cervicogenic headache, and migraine. Population-based studies suggest a 1-year prevalence rate of 38.3% for the episodic form of TTH, and 2.2% for the chronic form,[32] making it the most common headache form. A more recent study reported that in the 21st century 42% of the patients suffer from TTH.[33] Although TTH is one of the most common headaches, it is also the most neglected.[34] Nillson reported the prevalence of approximately 16% of cervicogenic headache in a Scandinavian population.[35] The accepted prevalence for cervicogenic headache, using clinical criteria for the diagnosis, ranges from 1% to 4.1% of the general population.[36] Finally, an older population-based study estimated that 10% to 12% of adults have experienced migraine in the previous year making it the third most common.[37] More recent studies reported that the average lifetime prevalence of migraine seems to be 18% whereas the estimated average 1-year prevalence is around 13%.[38,39] A recent study observed that the prevalence of migraine increased in the first decade of the 21st century in Spain.[40]

Functional and work disability has been described by 60% of patients with headache and accounted for 64% of the reduction in working capacity due to head pain.[41] Importantly, quality of life is reduced by headache.[42,43] Recently, the Global Burden of Disease ranked migraine as the eighth most burdensome disease and as the first among neurologic conditions.[44]

Tension-Type Headache

Tension-type headache is characterized by attacks lasting from 30 minutes to 7 days with at least two of the following features: (a) bilateral location, (b) pressing and tightening pain quality, (c) mild or moderate pain intensity, and (d) lack of aggravation during routine physical activity. In addition, patients should not report photophobia, phonophobia, vomiting, or evident nausea during headache, although one of these features is sometimes permitted. Different versions of diagnostic criteria for headaches have been published in the last few decades by the International Headache Society[45,46] and more recently published in 2013.[47] No significant changes in the diagnostic criteria of TTH have been included.

Cervicogenic Headache

Cervicogenic headache is mainly characterized by the following: (a) generalized unilateral pain, (b) moderate to severe pain intensity, (c) nonthrobbing or nonlancinating pain quality, and (d) restriction of the range of neck motion. The required criteria for the diagnosis of this condition include head pain increased by head movement, maintained neck postures, or external pressure over the upper cervical joints.[48] Diagnostic criteria of this type of headache have been revised and modified in the third edition of the International Classification of the Headache Disorders (ICHD) (11.2. Headache attributed to disorders of the neck to 11.2.1 Cervicogenic headache).[47] There is a significant controversy regarding whether the signs and symptoms of neck involvement represent a true cervical source for head pain.

Migraine Headache Without Aura

Migraine headache without aura is characterized by attacks lasting from 4 to 72 hours with at least two of the following features: (a) unilateral location, (b) pulsating pain quality, (c) moderate or severe pain intensity, and (d) aggravation by routine activities. Furthermore, migraine attacks should be associated with phonophobia or photophobia.[47]

While some patients may present with two types of headaches simultaneously (TTH with migraine features, cervicogenic headache with TTH characteristics, etc.), it seems that the pain quality and features of these headaches are different. Differences in pain features may implicate different structures responsible for nociceptive irritation of the trigeminocervical nucleus caudalis.[49] For instance, pain features of cervicogenic headache suggest a peripheral nociceptive mechanism, for example, muscle or joint etiologic role of the pain; in contrast, pain features of migraine suggest the activation of the trigeminovascular system.[50,51] Nevertheless, from a theoretical and clinical viewpoint, muscle referred pain evoked by TrPs can contribute to pain perception in these headaches. Headaches that involve a significant component of pain referred from TrPs have been called myogenic headaches to indicate the role of muscle in the genesis of the headache.[52,53] Because nociceptive somatic afferents from muscles innervated by upper cervical roots (particularly C1-C3) and the trigeminal nerve (particularly V1 or ophthalmic and V3 or mandibular nerves) converge on the same relay second-order neurons (trigeminocervical nucleus caudalis), it is understandable that TrPs located in any head, neck, or shoulder muscle could refer pain to the head and contribute to pain perception in these headache disorders.

The pain features of TTH, cervicogenic headache, and migraine without aura resemble the descriptions of referred pain (steady, deep, aching pain) originating in TrPs. Because TrPs and other structures such as upper cervical joints or nerve tissues can contribute to head pain perception at the same time, clinicians should focus the differential diagnostic process on pain history, pain features, and pain provoking or relieving maneuvers to identify which TrPs are causing the patient's headache or neck pain complaint.

Several studies have reported increased tenderness to muscle palpation in patients with TTH or cervicogenic headache without identifying the presence of TrPs.[54-56] In addition, lower pressure pain thresholds (PPT) have been observed in both cephalic (eg, temporalis region) and extracephalic (eg, upper trapezius) regions when compared with healthy subjects.[57-59] However, latent TrPs constitute a different clinical entity than active TrPs. It has not been until the last decade that multiple studies have investigated the role of TrPs in head pain syndromes and even more recently that TrP studies distinguish active and latent TrPs. An exception is a study published more than three decades ago that demonstrated the role of pain referred from TrPs in the neck and shoulder muscles to the head, relevant to the pain of headache, and demonstrated that treatment of the TrPs by injection relieved the headache.[52]

It is also common that patients with headache have referred symptoms to and from the cervical spine. A recent study found a prevalence of neck pain of 89.3% in patients with migraine combined with TTH, 88.4% in those with TTH, and 76.2 in those with migraine.[60]

Neck Pain

Neck pain affects 45% to 54% of the general population at some time during their lives.[61] The lifetime prevalence of neck pain has been estimated to be between 67% and 71% indicating that approximately two-thirds of the general population experiences an episode of neck pain at some time during their life.[62] Neck pain can be classified as idiopathic or mechanical neck pain or neck pain associated with a rear-end motor vehicle accident (whiplash-associated disorders, WAD). Mechanical or idiopathic neck pain can be defined as generalized neck and/or shoulder pain with mechanical characteristics including symptoms provoked by awkward neck postures or movement or by palpation of the cervical muscles. Pain often has a gradual onset, without a clear cause for its origin. The pain profile in neck pain syndromes can be related to different anatomic structures: zygapophyseal joints, neural tissues, discs, muscles, or ligaments.[63] Nevertheless, in clinical practice it seems that TrPs are one of the main causes for neck pain symptoms.

Neck and head pain are common clinical manifestations of whiplash injuries.[64] According to the Quebec Task Force, "whiplash is an acceleration-deceleration mechanism of energy transfer to the neck. It may result from rear-end or side-impact motor vehicle collisions, but can also occur during diving or other mishaps. The impact may result in bony or soft tissue and neurologic injuries, which in turn may lead to a variety of clinical manifestations (whiplash associated disorders)."[65] Trigger points can contribute significantly to acute and/or chronic pain syndromes following vehicular impact which is a factor that is usually overlooked.[66] Cervical joint dysfunctions and TrPs are thought, by some authors, to be the most relevant sources of nociception in whiplash-related pain.[67]

2.2. Initial Evaluation of Patients with Headache and/or Neck Pain

When a patient with head or neck pain seeks treatment, a thorough initial evaluation is needed to determine if this patient would be a candidate for TrP management. First, clinicians should record the pain history, pain features, and pain provoking or relieving maneuvers that increase or reduce head and/or neck symptoms. It is very important that clinicians pay close attention to reported symptom descriptors such as a pressing or a tightening quality which would indicate the presence and importance of referred pain from TrPs (see Box 17-1).

Postural assessment should include the position of the head on neck along with any other postural deviations that are relevant. This visual exploration is focused on postural abnormalities that can promote or perpetuate TrP activity of this musculature. Forward head posture[68] and anteriorly rounded shoulders are the two postural impairments most commonly observed in individuals with neck and/or head pain syndromes. These two postural abnormalities can promote a biomechanical disadvantage for the cervical musculature that contributes to TrP activation.

Clinically, both TrPs and cervical joint hypomobility can contribute to head and neck pain syndromes. Clinicians should explore both inert and contractile structures in the initial evaluation. Muscles innervated by C1-C3 or the trigeminal nerve should be explored for the presence of TrPs. Specifically, the upper trapezius, sternocleidomastoid, masseter, splenius capitis and cervicis, semispinalis capitis, temporalis, levator scapulae, suboccipital, and superior oblique muscles should be examined for TrPs. Palpation of these muscles can be conducted by cross-fiber flat or cross-fiber pincer palpation (see specific muscle chapters for a description of these muscle-examinations) with the aim of finding TrPs. Clinicians should focus their examination on reproduction of neck or head symptoms with palpation of TrPs. In some patients TrPs could also affect cervical ROM, but this impairment is not always present. Figure 18-1 shows the overlapping and composite referred pain patterns from TrPs in masticatory and cervical musculature.

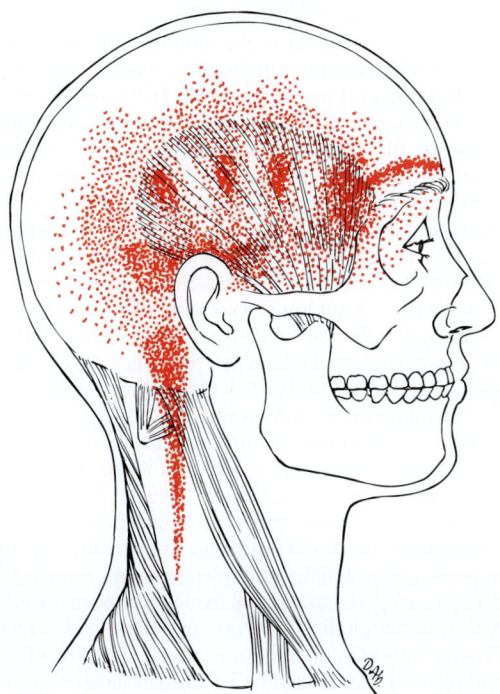

Figure 18-1. Overlapping pain referral patterns (red) from TrPs in masticatory and cervical muscles producing typical unilateral or bilateral migraine or tension-type headache symptoms.

Examination of the upper cervical joints for ROM impairments and accessory joint motion is very important to identify as a possible source of symptoms or a contributing factor to the patient's head or neck pain. Many manual examination techniques are used for evaluating passive accessory joint motion of the cervical zygapophyseal joints. One of the most widely used methods is described by Maitland.[69] Jull et al[70] reported that assessment using intersegmental tests, as described by Maitland, could identify the presence and location of painful zygapophyseal joints with 100% sensitivity and specificity compared with the gold standard of diagnostic joint blocks. These authors included the following signs of a symptomatic cervical zygapophyseal joint: abnormal end feel, abnormal quality of resistance, and reproduction of the patients' symptoms. Because reproduction of the patient's complaint is considered one of the most reliable signs of symptomatic joint hypomobility,[71] clinicians should focus the upper cervical joint examination on the reproduction of patient's symptoms. This is the same type of criterion used to clinically distinguish active from latent TrPs.

Based on the clinical signs found during the examination, management of a patient dealing with head or neck pain syndromes should focus on TrP management, cervical joint impairment, or both.

2.3. Trigger Points in Headache and Neck Pain

How Can Trigger Points Contribute to Headaches?

Several pain models explaining symptoms of headaches have been proposed. Olesen[72] proposed that headaches might be due to an excess of nociceptive inputs from peripheral structures (eg, muscle, joints, or arteries). The trigeminocervical nucleus caudalis would play a central role in this model because perceived headache intensity would result from the sum of nociceptive inputs from cranial and extracranial tissues converging on the neurons of the nucleus caudalis. Figure 18-2 depicts the headache model proposed by Olesen[72] where the roles of myofascial, supraspinal, and vascular inputs change depending on the headache.

In a posterior pain model, Bendtsen[73] suggested that the main problem in TTH is the sensitization of central pain pathways due to prolonged nociceptive inputs provoked by the liberation of algogenic substances and chemical mediator at the periphery from pericranial tender tissues. The presence of prolonged peripheral inputs can be of major importance for the conversion of episodic into chronic TTH. This model explains the sensitization of central pathways, the increased supraspinal sensitivity, the increased muscle activity and hardness, the chronic pain, and the absence of objective signs of peripheral pathology in patients with chronic TTH. However, these models do not account for what initiates the central sensitization that is the source of the pain from the periphery.[74]

Based on these pain models, the release of algogenic mediators in the peripheral tissues should be decisive for the sensitization mechanism. A recent study found no significant differences in change in interstitial concentrations of adenosine 5'-triphospate (ATP), glutamate, bradykinin, prostaglandin E2, glucose, pyruvate, and urea from baseline to exercise and postexercise periods between nonspecific tender spots of patients with chronic TTH and healthy patients. The study concludes that tender spots are not the peripheral structure responsible for the release of algogenic substances.[75] However, significantly higher levels of algogenic substances and lower pH levels have been recently found in active TrPs. Less significant levels have been found in latent TrPs or control spots (TrP-free muscle) demonstrating multiple reasons why active TrPs represent a peripheral sensitization focus.[76]

Fernández de las Peñas et al[77] have suggested, in an updated pain model, that TTH can at least partly be explained by referred

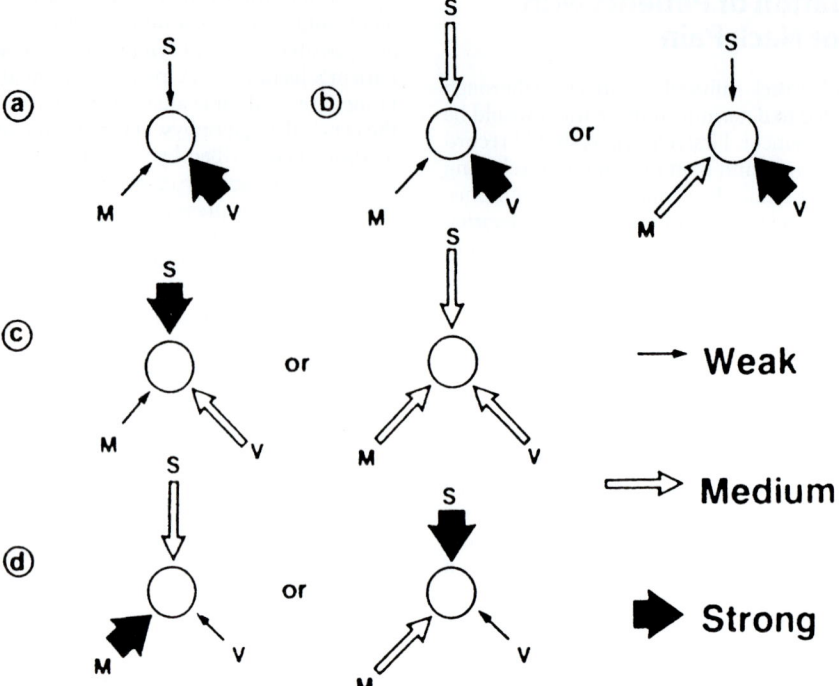

Figure 18-2. Predicted importance of supraspinal, vascular, and myofascial inputs to brain-stem neurons in migraine and TTH. Some examples of the innumerable modulations of the vascular/supra-spinal/myogenic model of migraine and other headaches. S, supraspinal net effect (usually facilitation during headache); M, myofascial nociceptive input; V, vascular nociceptive input. Thickness of arrows represents the relative intensity of input. a, migraine aura without headache: despite strong vascular input there is no pain because of small S and M; b, migraine with aura: because of stronger supra-spinal or myofascial input the subject now suffers from headache; c, migraine without aura: the vascular input is not as strong as in migraine with aura, but the headache is no less intense because of a stronger supra-spinal facilitation or the combined effects of V and M. The latter case is likely to suffer alternating migrainous or TTH depending on small shifts in the relative magnitude of M and V; d, TTH: M is greater than V, and S is medium or large. Reprinted with permission from Olesen J. Clinical and patho-physiologic observations in migraine and tension-type headache explained by integration of vascular, supra-spinal and myofascial inputs. *Pain*. 1991;46:125-132.

pain from active TrPs that is mediated through the spinal cord and the brainstem trigeminocervical nucleus caudalis.[77] Thus, active TrPs located in muscles innervated by C1-C3 or by the trigeminal nerve can be responsible for the peripheral nociceptive input and could produce a continuous afferent barrage into the trigeminal nerve nucleus caudalis. In fact, sensitization of nociceptive pain pathways in the central nervous system due to prolonged nociceptive stimuli from TrPs seems to be responsible for the conversion of episodic to chronic TTH.[78]

Trigger Points and Migraine

Many patients are mistakenly diagnosed as having migraine when the problem is entirely TrPs. In others, TrPs are the triggers for initiating headaches that are assumed to be migraine in nature. Current theories, for true migraine, postulate that sensory pain features of migraine attacks may be attributed to the activation of the trigeminovascular system,[50,51] probably provoked by the peripheral liberation of algogenic substances.[79] The link between TrPs and migraine attacks could be the activation of the trigeminocervical nucleus caudalis or the trigeminovascular system provoked by the liberation of algogenic substances (ie, bradykinin, substance P, calcitonin gene-related peptide, tumor necrosis factor-α, serotonin, etc.) in the periphery caused by active TrPs.[76] Therefore, TrPs located in any muscle innervated by the trigeminal nerve (ie, extraocular or masticator muscles) or the upper cervical nerves (ie, upper trapezius, suboccipital, splenius capitis, sternocleidomastoid, etc.) may be viewed as "hidden irritative thorns" that precipitate, perpetuate, or aggravate migraine. Other triggers for migraine could also exist that are not yet identified.

Trigger points in several neck, shoulder, and head muscles have been found in patients with both unilateral[80] and bilateral[81] migraine. In unilateral migraine, active TrPs were located ipsilateral to migraine attacks as compared with the asymptomatic side[80]; whereas in bilateral migraine without aura, active TrPs were located bilaterally.[81] Furthermore, referred pain elicited by manual palpation of the superior oblique muscle (an extraocular muscle) has also been found on the symptomatic side in patients with unilateral migraine.[82] These results have been confirmed in more recent studies where TrPs in neck muscles and hypomobility in the upper cervical facet joints were associated with migraine.[83] The referred pain elicited by active TrPs reproduced the pain features of migraine headache when patients were examined in a headache-free status. Table 18-1 details the muscles that had active TrPs in patients with migraine.

Another study demonstrated that patients with migraine who described having "imploding" (pain from inside to outside and pressing or tightening pain quality) or "ocular" (pain features in the ocular region) headache responded to injections of Botulinum Toxin A into several neck and head muscles (frontalis, upper trapezius, temporalis, semispinalis, and splenius capitis muscles).[84] The authors suggested that extracranial tissues may be involved in the pathogenesis of "imploding" or "ocular" migraine. Because pain features of patients with migraine are very similar to those characteristics of referred pain elicited by TrPs, others have suggested that TrPs are an etiologic factor for "imploding" or "ocular" migraine.[85]

Based on the aforementioned studies, it appears that inactivation of TrPs in patients with migraine could offer additional pain relief. Furthermore, it has been demonstrated that inactivation of TrPs can relieve head pain in patients with migraine.[86,87] These authors found that TrP inactivation was an effective palliative measure

Table 18-1 Percentages of Active TrPs Found in Patients With Migraine

Unilateral Migraine (Data Extracted From Fernández de las Peñas et al[80,82])

Suboccipital muscles	25% active trigger points (TrPs)
Upper trapezius	30% active TrPs on the symptomatic side
	5% active TrPs on the asymptomatic side
Sternocleidomastoid	45% active TrPs on the symptomatic side
	5% active TrPs on the asymptomatic side
Temporalis muscle	40% active TrPs on the symptomatic side
	0% active TrPs on the asymptomatic side
Superior oblique muscle	50% active TrPs on the symptomatic side
	0% active TrPs on the asymptomatic side

Bilateral Migraine (Data Extracted From Calandre et al[81])

Temporal area	42.6% active TrPs
Suboccipital muscles	33.4% active TrPs
Others (trapezius, masseter, etc)	24% active TrPs

Data for patients with unilateral migraine are based on a sample size of 20, and data for patients with bilateral migraine are based on a sample size of 98.

in the prophylactic management of severe refractory migraine and suggest that TrPs can be one of the hyperactive peripheral pain mechanisms linked to migraine predisposition. Therefore, TrP inactivation can reduce excitability of peripheral nociceptors and contribute to the amelioration of migraine attacks.[87]

Trigger Points and Cervicogenic Headache

Headache originating in the cervical spine (cervicogenic headache) is a common clinical situation. It should be noted that controversy exists in the research and in the clinical community about a proper classification of this condition. It has been established that any structure (eg, muscle, joints, ligament, or tendon) innervated by the trigeminocervical nucleus caudalis can elicit referred pain to the head.[88] Some authors support the concept that cervicogenic headache is mainly provoked by referred pain from upper cervical joints[89,90] rather than referred pain elicited by muscle tissues.[91] Several studies have found that cervicogenic headache is caused by the presence of upper cervical spine dysfunctions.[92,93] In these studies, head pain symptoms were reproduced by manual assessment of upper cervical joints (for clinical assessment of cervical joint dysfunctions see, Maitland[69]). Furthermore, the effectiveness of spinal manipulation or mobilization procedures aimed at correcting upper cervical joint dysfunctions supports the concept that upper cervical joint dysfunctions can be more relevant for the pathogenesis of cervicogenic headache than for other headaches.[67,94,95]

Features of this headache syndrome suggest that referred pain from TrPs can also contribute to the pain profile. Jaeger found, in a cohort of 11 cervicogenic headache sufferers, that all patients were found to have at least three TrPs on the symptomatic side.[96] The ipsilateral sternocleidomastoid and temporalis muscles were the muscles most affected by TrPs. Jaeger also found that those patients in whom TrPs were inactivated obtained a significant decrease in headache frequency and intensity, further supporting the role of TrPs in head pain perception in cervicogenic headache.[96] In addition, a case report found that referred pain from TrPs in the sternocleidomastoid muscle mimics the pain pattern of cervicogenic headache.[97] These authors demonstrated that the inactivation of TrPs in the sternocleidomastoid muscle was decisive for the relief of head symptoms in a patient in whom referred pain from other structures (eg, upper cervical joints) was not found. A pilot randomized controlled study found that manual therapy targeting sternocleidomastoid TrPs was effective in improving headache intensity, pressure sensitivity, cervical ROM, and motor performance of the deep cervical flexors in individuals with cervicogenic headache.[98]

Several theories on muscle–joint interactions have been proposed. Perhaps the increased tension of the taut bands and facilitation of motor activity can produce sustained, increased and displacement stresses on the joint by TrPs to provoke and maintain joint dysfunction.[99] The abnormal sensory input from the joint dysfunction may reflexively activate the TrP. Box 18-2 details some questions that may assist the clinician in determining whether head pain symptoms are related to upper cervical joint dysfunction or TrPs. Nevertheless, in some patients, pain from both joint dysfunctions and TrPs can occur simultaneously.

Motor control impairment in the deep cervical flexor muscles has been reported in patients presenting with cervicogenic headache.[100] Deep cervical flexor impairment is usually associated with higher EMG amplitudes in the superficial neck flexors such as the anterior scalene or sternocleidomastoid muscles.[101] An increase in EMG amplitude represents higher muscle activity during functional tasks of the cervical spine which would provoke muscle overload of these muscles. Therefore, motor control impairments of the deep cervical flexors may contribute to the development of TrPs in the superficial muscles from which referred pain can contribute to cervicogenic headache syndrome.

Trigger Points and Tension-Type Headache

Tension-type headache is the prototypical headache in which neck and/or shoulder muscles play an important role in the genesis of the pain.[102-104] Individuals suffering from TTH described their head pain as pressing, tightening, dull, or as a generalized soreness[105-107] which closely resembles the pain features of muscle referred pain elicited by TrPs.

Mercer et al found, in a non-controlled and nonblinded study, both active and latent TrPs in neck and shoulder muscles in individuals with TTH particularly in the splenius capitis or cervicis, semispinalis capitis or cervicis, levator scapulae, upper trapezius, and suboccipital muscles.[108] Marcus et al reported that individuals with TTH exhibit a greater number of either active or latent TrPs than healthy controls; these authors did not specify in which muscles TrPs were more frequently found.[109] Fernández de las Peñas et al found that either episodic or chronic TTH was associated with active TrPs in suboccipital,[110,111] upper trapezius,[112] superior oblique,[113] temporalis, and sternocleidomastoid

---

Box 18-2 Subjective questions to differentiate between neck pain arising from upper cervical joint dysfunction or trigger points (TrPs)

Does your pain change with neck movement?
Does your pain change with prolonged postures of the neck?
Does your pain change with passive movement of the neck?
Does the pain behind the eyes change with computer or TV use?
Does the pain change following or during active movement?
Does the pain change with muscle stretching?
Was the onset of the pain gradual or acute?
Does your pain feel superficial or deep?

muscles.[114,115] Table 18-2 summarizes which muscles were most commonly affected by TrPs in patients with TTH.

It has also been found that TrP activity was related to headache pain perception in chronic but not episodic TTH. Patients with chronic TTH and active TrPs exhibit greater headache intensity and frequency than those with latent TrPs. However, headache pain parameters did not differ between episodic TTH with either active or latent TrPs. The fact that patients with chronic, but not episodic, TTH with pain-producing active TrPs had more severe headache pain characteristics than those patients with latent TrPs could be considered as result of temporal integration of signals from TrPs.[116] Given that temporal summation of pain is centrally mediated,[117] this would suggest a temporal integration of nociceptive signals from TrPs by central nociceptive neurons leading to sensitization of central pathways in chronic TTH.[73,74] Finally, the fact that active TrPs are present in episodic TTH[111,115] to a degree similar to chronic TTH[110,112,114] does not support the hypothesis that active TrPs are the consequence of central sensitization.[118] Thus, it appears that, in addition to causing the well-known peripheral sensitization of nociceptive perception, TrPs can cause central sensitization, but central sensitization does not appear to cause TrPs. This is an important point because the two concepts are diametrically opposed and are central to two mutually exclusive ways of looking at the role of TrPs in TTH.[119]

Adoption of the term myogenic headache for headaches in which TrPs are etiologically important would underscore the importance of the concept of referred pain from active TrPs as a factor in headache development and emphasize the importance of treating these TrPs in the management of headache.

Mechanical Neck Pain

The presence of TrPs in patients with mechanical neck pain is often seen in clinical practice. Different studies have found that individuals with mechanical neck pain had active TrPs in neck–shoulder musculature, particularly the upper trapezius and levator scapulae muscles.[120,121] The presence of TrPs in the upper trapezius muscle has been associated with cervical joint dysfunction at C3 and C4 levels.[99] Several theories on muscle–joint interrelationship have been proposed. Perhaps the increased tension of the taut bands and facilitation of motor activity can maintain displacement stress on the joint such that a TrP provokes and maintains joint dysfunction. However, an abnormal sensory input from joint dysfunction may reflexively activate the TrP. The mutual positive feedback between the presence of TrPs in the cervical musculature and the presence of cervical joint hypomobility support the importance of a thorough examination of both muscles and joints when assessing patients with mechanical or idiopathic neck pain. Well-designed studies investigating the therapeutic effect of treating TrP and joint disorders, either sequentially or in combination, are needed.

Whiplash

In a review of the whiplash literature, Fernández de las Peñas et al[122] found that the most common muscles affected by TrPs were the scalene,[123] splenius capitis,[124] sternocleidomastoid,[125,126] upper trapezius, posterior neck muscles,[127] and pectoralis minor muscles.[128] Treatment strategies including both TrPs and spinal joint interventions have been advocated for in the management of posttraumatic head and neck pain.[129] McMakin et al[130] demonstrated that treatment with frequency-specific micro-current can also be very helpful in reducing symptoms. The investigators first treated the neurologic dysfunction caused by the initial bruising of the brainstem and the spinal cord caused by the trauma and then treated the remaining active TrPs responsible for some of the pain complaints.

The biomechanical analysis of a rear-end impact shows mechanisms for activating TrPs. The S-shaped cervical curvature occurring during a rear-end impact may result in a lengthening position of the sternocleidomastoid muscle which produces a lengthening contraction that overloads this muscle.[131] A 6% lengthening[132] or 179% of that produced by maximal voluntary contraction[124] of the sternocleidomastoid muscle has been described after rear-end impacts, a factor that readily explains TrPs in that muscle. Furthermore, deep cervical flexor impairment has also been found in patients with WAD.[133-135] This motor control disorder is usually related to higher EMG amplitudes in the sternocleidomastoid and anterior scalene muscles which may also induce overload of the cervical spine musculature. A recent study observed that patients with whiplash exhibited a greater number of active TrPs than those with mechanical neck pain.[136] The number of active TrPs was significantly associated with the area and intensity of pain symptoms in patients with WAD.[136] Fernández Pérez et al[137] demonstrated that the number of active TrPs was associated with higher pain intensity and the number of days following the accident in patients with acute whiplash. This study also found that the number of active TrPs was associated with a higher localized pressure pain sensitivity at the cervical spine in this group of patients.[137]

Several studies have demonstrated that patients with chronic whiplash pain develop more widespread hypersensitivity to mechanical pressure and thermal stimuli than those with chronic idiopathic neck pain[138] or healthy individuals.[139] These findings support the hypothesis that patients with WAD suffer from widespread hyperexcitability of the central nervous system.[140] Herren-Gerber et al found that central hypersensitivity was most likely dependent on local peripheral nociceptive input.[141] Therefore, nociceptive sensitization by active TrPs could perpetuate sensitization of central pathways in patients with chronic whiplash pain.[142] Nociceptive inputs from other structures (eg, zygapophyseal joint)[143] could also contribute to this central sensitization process. The results of the McMakin et al[130] study indicate that widespread pain hypersensitivity contributes to a central nervous system dysfunction initiated by the trauma. When these investigators normalized treatment of the central nervous system dysfunction, hypersensitivity disappeared.

Table 18-2	Active TrPs Found in Patients With Both Chronic and Frequent Episodic Tension-Type Headache (TTH)
Chronic TTH (Data Extracted From Fernández de las Peñas et al[110,114,129])	
Suboccipital muscles	65% active TrPs
Upper trapezius	24% active TrPs on the left side
	36% active TrPs on the right side
Sternocleidomastoid	20% active TrPs on the left side
	24% active TrPs on the right side
Temporalis muscle	32% active TrPs on the left side
	36% active TrPs on the right side
Superior oblique muscle	86% active TrPs on both sides
Frequent Episodic TTH (Data Extracted From Fernández de las Peñas et al[111,115])	
Suboccipital muscles	60% active TrPs
Upper trapezius	33% active TrPs on the left side
	14% active TrPs on the right side
Sternocleidomastoid	20% active TrPs on the left side
	14% active TrPs on the right side
Temporalis muscle	40% active TrPs on the left side
	46% active TrPs on the right side
Superior oblique muscle	15% active TrPs on both sides

They also noted that inactivation of active TrPs is essential to reducing central hypersensitivity.[130]

Based on the available data, it is postulated that the ongoing nociceptive input originated in active TrPs perpetuates or promotes sensitization of central pathways in head and neck syndromes. When this peripheral nociceptive input is identified and eliminated, the central sensitivity should be reduced. Because TrPs introduce ongoing peripheral nociceptive input,[76] inactivation of active TrPs should result in clinical improvement in patients with chronic TrPs[128] and in patients with acute, intractable TTH.

3. NEUROPATHIC PAIN SYNDROMES

From a clinical viewpoint, it is very important to distinguish between pain due to TrPs and that of neuropathic pain such as cranial or occipital neuralgias. Neuropathic pain is perceived as stabbing or shooting sensations occurring in paroxysms that follow the anatomic distribution of a nerve. In the head, the most common neuralgias are occipital and trigeminal neuralgia. Box 18-3 summarizes some common sources of head pain that are also common pain complaints from TrPs.

Some patients presenting with occipital neuralgia described their pain pattern as burning or aching sensations, suggesting that referred pain from TrPs can mimic occipital neuralgia.[144] In some patients, pain in the occipital region may have an exclusive TrP origin. The occipital nerve can cross or penetrate the semispinalis capitis or upper trapezius muscles[145,146] and taut bands associated with TrPs in these muscles may entrap the greater occipital nerve which could account for some aching and referred frontal pain. Therefore, it is important that clinicians differentiate between symptoms resulting from occipital neuralgia, referred pain from TrPs, and upper cervical zygapophyseal joints.

Several authors have documented the relevance of TrPs in several neuralgias. Chen et al found the presence of TrPs in the intercostal muscles following an acute episode of herpes zoster in the intercostal nerve which responded well to TrP injection.[147] Ceneviz et al found, in a case report, that TrPs in the lateral pterygoid muscle can mimic pain features of trigeminal neuralgia.[148] Future studies are needed to determine the relevance of TrPs in these conditions and if their treatment is necessary or helpful for relief of cranial neuralgias.

Finally, chronic medication-overuse headaches can be caused by excessive use of analgesic medications such as aspirin, acetaminophen, nonsteroidal anti-inflammatory drugs, or ergots. Clinical experience indicates that most patients with medication-overuse headache have active TrPs contributing to their head pain. Studies investigating TrP prevalence in this population are lacking and urgently needed.

References

1. Skootsky SA, Jaeger B, Oye RK. Prevalence of myofascial pain in general internal medicine practice. *West J Med*. 1989;151(2):157-160.
2. Poveda Roda R, Diaz Fernandez JM, Hernandez Bazan S, Jimenez Soriano Y, Margaix M, Sarrion G. A review of temporomandibular joint disease (TMJD). Part II: clinical and radiological semiology. Morbidity processes. *Med Oral Patol Oral Cir Bucal*. 2008;13(2):E102-E109.
3. Okeson JP. *Management of Temporomandibular Disorders and Occlusion*. 7th ed. London, England: Elsevier Mosby; 2013.
4. LeResche L. Epidemiology of temporomandibular disorders: implications for the investigation of etiologic factors. *Crit Rev Oral Biol Med*. 1997;8(3):291-305.
5. Isong U, Gansky SA, Plesh O. Temporomandibular joint and muscle disorder-type pain in U.S. adults: the National Health Interview Survey. *J Orofac Pain*. 2008;22(4):317-322.
6. Poveda-Roda R, Bagan JV, Sanchis JM, Carbonell E. Temporomandibular disorders. A case-control study. *Med Oral Patol Oral Cir Bucal*. 2012;17(5):e794-e800.
7. Goncalves DA, Camparis CM, Speciali JG, Franco AL, Castanharo SM, Bigal ME. Temporomandibular disorders are differentially associated with headache diagnoses: a controlled study. *Clin J Pain*. 2011;27(7):611-615.
8. Schiffman E, Ohrbach R, Truelove E, et al. Diagnostic Criteria for Temporomandibular Disorders (DC/TMD) for Clinical and Research Applications: recommendations of the International RDC/TMD Consortium Network* and Orofacial Pain Special Interest Group†. *J Oral Facial Pain Headache*. 2014;28(1):6-27.
9. Gray RJ, Davies SJ, Quayle AA. A clinical approach to temporomandibular disorders. 2. Examination of the articulatory system: the temporomandibular joints. *Br Dent J*. 1994;176(12):473-477.
10. Goulet JP, Clark GT, Flack VF, Liu C. The reproducibility of muscle and joint tenderness detection methods and maximum mandibular movement measurement for the temporomandibular system. *J Orofac Pain*. 1998;12(1):17-26.
11. Cleland JA, Koppenhaver S. *Netter's Orthopaedic Clinical Examination: An Evidence-Based Approach*. 2nd ed. Philadelphia, PA: Saunders Elsevier; 2011.
12. Mense S. Referral of muscle pain: new aspects. *Am Pain Soc J*. 1994;3(1):1-9.
13. Clark GT, Delcanho RE, Goulet JP. The utility and validity of current diagnostic procedures for defining temporomandibular disorder patients. *Adv Dent Res*. 1993;7(2):97-112.
14. Emshoff R, Innerhofer K, Rudisch A, Bertram S. The biological concept of "internal derangement and osteoarthrosis": a diagnostic approach in patients with temporomandibular joint pain? *Oral Surg Oral Med Oral Pathol Oral Radiol Endod*. 2002;93(1):39-44.
15. Dworkin SF, LeResche L, DeRouen T, Von Korff M. Assessing clinical signs of temporomandibular disorders: reliability of clinical examiners. *J Prosthet Dent*. 1991;63:574-579.
16. Lauriti L, Motta LJ, Silva PF, et al. Are occlusal characteristics, headache, parafunctional habits and clicking sounds associated with the signs and symptoms of temporomandibular disorder in adolescents? *J Phys Ther Sci*. 2013;25(10):1331-1334.
17. Leeuw R, Klasser GD. *Orofacial pain: Guidelines for Assessment, diagnosis and management*. 5th ed. Chicago, IL: Quintessence Publishing Co; 2013.
18. Dworkin SF, LeResche L, DeRouen T. Reliability of clinical measurement in temporomandibular disorders. *Clin J Pain*. 1988;4:89-99.
19. de Wijer A, Lobbezoo-Scholte AM, Steenks MH, Bosman F. Reliability of clinical findings in temporomandibular disorders. *J Orofac Pain*. 1995;9(2):181-191.
20. Fujita S, Iizuka T, Dauber W. Variation of heads of lateral pterygoid muscle and morphology of articular disc of human temporomandibular joint: anatomical and histological analysis. *J Oral Rehabil*. 2001;28(6):560-571.
21. Walker N, Bohannon RW, Cameron D. Discriminant validity of temporomandibular joint range of motion measurements obtained with a ruler. *J Orthop Sports Phys Ther*. 2000;30(8):484-492.
22. List T, John MT, Dworkin SF, Svensson P. Recalibration improves inter-examiner reliability of TMD examination. *Acta Odontol Scand*. 2006;64(3):146-152.
23. Cuccia AM, Caradonna C, Caradonna D. Manual therapy of the mandibular accessory ligaments for the management of temporomandibular joint disorders. *J Am Osteopath Assoc*. 2011;111(2):102-112.
24. Von Piekartz HJM. *Craniofacial Pain: Neuromuscular Assessment, Treatment and Management*. London, England: Butterworth Heinemann-Elsevier; 2007.
25. Dworkin SF, LeResche L. Research diagnostic criteria for temporomandibular disorders: review, criteria, examinations and specifications, critique. *J Craniomandib Disord*. 1992;6(4):301-355.
26. Fricton JR, Kroening R, Haley D, Siegert R. Myofascial pain syndrome of the head and neck: a review of clinical characteristics of 164 patients. *Oral Surg Oral Med Oral Pathol*. 1985;60(6):615-623.
27. Svensson P, Graven-Nielsen T. Craniofacial muscle pain: review of mechanisms and clinical manifestations. *J Orofac Pain*. 2001;15(2):117-145.
28. Wright EF. Referred craniofacial pain patterns in patients with temporomandibular disorder. *J Am Dent Assoc*. 2000;131(9):1307-1315.
29. Fernández de las Peñas C, Galan-Del-Rio F, Alonso-Blanco C, Jimenez-Garcia R, Arendt-Nielsen L, Svensson P. Referred pain from muscle trigger points in the masticatory and neck-shoulder musculature in women with temporomandibular disorders. *J Pain*. 2010;11(12):1295-1304.

Box 18-3 Trigger points can contribute to the following neuropathic pain syndromes

Trigeminal neuralgia is a unilateral disorder characterized by brief electric shock-like pain, abrupt in onset and termination, limited to the distribution of one or more divisions of the trigeminal nerve.

Supraorbital neuralgia is a disorder characterized by paroxysmal or constant pain in the region of the supraorbital notch and medial aspect of the forehead in the area supplied by the supraorbital nerve.

Occipital neuralgia is a paroxysmal jabbing pain in the distribution of the greater or lesser occipital nerves or of the third occipital nerve, sometimes accompanied by diminished sensation or dysesthesia in the affected area.

Herpes zoster is a viral infection that can affect the trigeminal nerve manifesting itself as head or facial pain.

These definitions are based on the International Classification of Headache Disorders done by Headache classification Subcommittee of the International Headache Society.[47]

30. Svensson P. Muscle pain in the head: overlap between temporomandibular disorders and tension-type headaches. *Curr Opin Neurol.* 2007;20(3):320-325.
31. Jensen R, Bendtsen L. Tension-type headache: why does this condition have to fight for its recognition? *Curr Pain Headache Rep.* 2006;10(6):454-458.
32. Schwartz BS, Stewart WF, Simon D, Lipton RB. Epidemiology of tension-type headache. *JAMA.* 1998;279(5):381-383.
33. Stovner L, Hagen K, Jensen R, et al. The global burden of headache: a documentation of headache prevalence and disability worldwide. *Cephalalgia.* 2007;27(3):193-210.
34. Bendtsen L, Jensen R. Tension-type headache: the most common, but also the most neglected, headache disorder. *Curr Opin Neurol.* 2006;19(3):305-309.
35. Nilsson N. The prevalence of cervicogenic headache in a random population sample of 20-59 year olds. *Spine.* 1995;20(17):1884-1888.
36. Sjaastad O, Bakketeig LS. Prevalence of cervicogenic headache: Vågå study of headache epidemiology. *Acta Neurol Scand.* 2008;117(3):173-180.
37. Stewart WF, Lipton RB, Celentano DD, Reed ML. Prevalence of migraine headache in the United States. Relation to age, income, race, and other sociodemographic factors. *JAMA.* 1992;267(1):64-69.
38. Jensen R, Stovner LJ. Epidemiology and comorbidity of headache. *Lancet Neurol.* 2008;7(4):354-361.
39. Stovner LJ, Andree C. Prevalence of headache in Europe: a review for the Eurolight project. *J Headache Pain.* 2010;11(4):289-299.
40. Fernández de las Peñas C, Palacios-Cena D, Salom-Moreno J, et al. Has the prevalence of migraine changed over the last decade (2003-2012)? A Spanish population-based survey. *PLoS One.* 2014;9(10):e110530.
41. Rasmussen BK. Epidemiology and socio-economic impact of headache. *Cephalalgia.* 1999;19 suppl 25:20-23.
42. van Suijlekom HA, Lame I, Stomp-van den Berg SG, Kessels AG, Weber WE. Quality of life of patients with cervicogenic headache: a comparison with control subjects and patients with migraine or tension-type headache. *Headache.* 2003;43(10):1034-1041.
43. Meletiche DM, Lofland JH, Young WB. Quality-of-life differences between patients with episodic and transformed migraine. *Headache.* 2001;41(6):573-578.
44. Leonardi M, Raggi A. Burden of migraine: international perspectives. *Neurol Sci.* 2013;34 suppl 1:S117-S118.
45. Headache Classification Committee of the International Headache Society. Classification and diagnostic criteria for headache disorders, cranial neuralgias and facial pain. Headache Classification Committee of the International Headache Society. *Cephalalgia.* 1988;8 suppl 7:1-96.
46. Headache Classification Subcommittee of the International Headache Society. The International Classification of Headache Disorders, 2nd edition. *Cephalalgia.* 2004;24:S9-S160.
47. Headache Classification Committee of the International Headache Society. The International Classification of Headache Disorders, 3rd edition (beta version). *Cephalalgia.* 2013;33(9):629-808.
48. Sjaastad O, Fredriksen TA, Pfaffenrath V. Cervicogenic headache: diagnostic criteria. The Cervicogenic Headache International Study Group. *Headache.* 1998;38(6):442-445.
49. Nilsson N, Bove G. Evidence that tension-type headache and cervicogenic headache are distinct disorders. *J Manipulative Physiol Ther.* 2000;23(4):288-289.
50. Edvinsson L. Aspects on the pathophysiology of migraine and cluster headache. *Pharmacol Toxicol.* 2001;89(2):65-73.
51. Goadsby PJ, Lipton RB, Ferrari MD. Migraine: current understanding and treatment. *N Engl J Med.* 2002;346(4):257-270.
52. Tfelt-Hansen P, Lous I, Olesen J. Prevalence and significance of muscle tenderness during common migraine attacks. *Headache.* 1981;21(2):49-54.
53. Gerwin R. Headache. In: Ferguson L, Gerwin R, eds. *Clinical Mastery in the Treatment of Myofascial Pain.* Philadelphia, PA: Lippincott Williams & Wilkins; 2005:1-29.
54. Jensen R, Rasmussen BK, Pedersen B, Olesen J. Muscle tenderness and pressure pain thresholds in headache. A population study. *Pain.* 1993;52(2):193-199.
55. Lipchik GL, Holroyd KA, Talbot F, Greer M. Pericranial muscle tenderness and exteroceptive suppression of temporalis muscle activity: a blind study of chronic tension-type headache. *Headache.* 1997;37(6):368-376.
56. Metsahonkala L, Anttila P, Laimi K, et al. Extracephalic tenderness and pressure pain threshold in children with headache. *Eur J Pain.* 2006;10(7):581-585.
57. Schoenen J, Bottin D, Hardy F, Gerard P. Cephalic and extracephalic pressure pain thresholds in chronic tension-type headache. *Pain.* 1991;47(2):145-149.
58. Bendtsen L, Jensen R, Olesen J. Decreased pain detection and tolerance thresholds in chronic tension-type headache. *Arch Neurol.* 1996;53(4):373-376.
59. Ashina S, Babenko L, Jensen R, Ashina M, Magerl W, Bendtsen L. Increased muscular and cutaneous pain sensitivity in cephalic region in patients with chronic tension-type headache. *Eur J Neurol.* 2005;12(7):543-549.
60. Ashina S, Bendtsen L, Lyngberg AC, Lipton RB, Hajiyeva N, Jensen R. Prevalence of neck pain in migraine and tension-type headache: a population study. *Cephalalgia.* 2015;35(3):211-219.
61. Cote P, Cassidy JD, Carroll L. The Saskatchewan Health and Back Pain Survey. The prevalence of neck pain and related disability in Saskatchewan adults. *Spine.* 1998;23(15):1689-1698.
62. Picavet HSJ, Van Gils HWV, Schouten JSAG. *Musculoskeletal Complaints in the Dutch Population [In Dutch: Klachten aan het bewegingsapparaat in de Nederlandse bevolking prevalenties, consequenties en risicogroepen].* The Netherlands: RIVM (National Institute of Public Health and the Environment; 2000.
63. Greenman PE. *Principles of Manual Medicine.* Baltimore, MD: Williams & Wilkins; 1989.
64. Drottning M, Staff PH, Sjaastad O. Cervicogenic headache (CEH) after whiplash injury. *Cephalalgia.* 2002;22(3):165-171.
65. Spitzer WO, Skovron ML, Salmi LR, et al. Scientific monograph of the Quebec Task Force on Whiplash-Associated Disorders: redefining "whiplash" and its management. *Spine.* 1995;20(8 suppl):1S-73S.
66. Dommerholt J, Royson MW, Whyte-Ferguson L. Neck pain and dysfunction following whiplash. In: Ferguson L, Gerwin R, eds. *Clinical Mastery in the Treatment of Myofascial Pain.* Philadelphia, PA: Lippincott Williams & Wilkins; 2005:57-89.
67. Fernández de las Peñas C, Alonso-Blanco C, Cuadrado ML, Pareja JA. Spinal manipulative therapy in the management of cervicogenic headache. *Headache.* 2005;45(9):1260-1263.
68. Fernández de las Peñas C, Blanco CR, Cuadrado ML, Pareja J. Forward head posture and neck mobility in chronic tension-type headache: a blinded, controlled study. *Cephalalgia.* 2006;26:314-319.
69. Maitland G, Hengeveld E, Banks K, English K. *Maitland's Vertebral Manipulation.* 6th ed. London, England: Butterworth Heinemann; 2001.
70. Jull G, Bogduk N, Marsland A. The accuracy of manual diagnosis for cervical zygapophysial joint pain syndromes. *Med J Aust.* 1988;148(5):233-236.
71. Jull G, Treleaven J, Versace G. Manual examination: is pain provocation a major cue for spinal dysfunction? *Aust J Physiother.* 1994;40(3):159-165.
72. Olesen J. Clinical and pathophysiological observations in migraine and tension-type headache explained by integration of vascular, supraspinal and myofascial inputs. *Pain.* 1991;46(2):125-132.
73. Bendtsen L. Central sensitization in tension-type headache: possible pathophysiological mechanisms. *Cephalalgia.* 2000;20(5):486-508.
74. Bendtsen L, Schoenen J. Synthesis of tension type headache mechanisms. In: Olesen J, Goasdby P, Ramdan NM, Tfelt-Hansen P, Welch K, eds. *The Headaches.* 3rd ed. Philadelphia, PA: Lippincott Williams & Wilkins; 2006.
75. Ashina M, Stallknecht B, Bendtsen L, et al. Tender points are not sites of ongoing inflammation -in vivo evidence in patients with chronic tension-type headache. *Cephalalgia.* 2003;23(2):109-116.
76. Shah JP, Phillips TM, Danoff JV, Gerber LH. An in vivo microanalytical technique for measuring the local biochemical milieu of human skeletal muscle. *J Appl Physiol.* 2005;99(5):1977-1984.
77. Fernández de las Peñas C, Cuadrado ML, Arendt-Nielsen L, Simons DG, Pareja JA. Myofascial trigger points and sensitization: an updated pain model for tension-type headache. *Cephalalgia.* 2007;27(5):383-393.
78. Fernández de las Peñas C. Myofascial head pain. *Curr Pain Headache Rep.* 2015;19(7):28.
79. Fusco M, D'Andrea G, Micciche F, Stecca A, Bernardini D, Cananzi AL. Neurogenic inflammation in primary headaches. *Neurol Sci.* 2003;24 suppl 2:S61-S64.
80. Fernández de las Peñas C, Cuadrado ML, Pareja JA. Myofascial trigger points, neck mobility and forward head posture in unilateral migraine. *Cephalalgia.* 2006;26(9):1061-1070.
81. Calandre EP, Hidalgo J, Garcia-Leiva JM, Rico-Villademoros F. Trigger point evaluation in migraine patients: an indication of peripheral sensitization linked to migraine predisposition? *Eur J Neurol.* 2006;13(3):244-249.
82. Fernández de las Peñas C, Cuadrado ML, Gerwin RD, Pareja JA. Myofascial disorders in the trochlear region in unilateral migraine: a possible initiating or perpetuating factor. *Clin J Pain.* 2006;22(6):548-553.
83. Tali D, Menahem I, Vered E, Kalichman L. Upper cervical mobility, posture and myofascial trigger points in subjects with episodic migraine: case-control study. *J Bodyw Mov Ther.* 2014;18(4):569-575.
84. Jakubowski M, McAllister PJ, Bajwa ZH, Ward TN, Smith P, Burstein R. Exploding vs. imploding headache in migraine prophylaxis with Botulinum Toxin A. *Pain.* 2006;125(3):286-295.
85. Fernández de las Peñas C, Arendt-Nielsen L, Simons DG. Exploding vs. imploding headache in migraine prophylaxis with Botulinum Toxin A. *Pain.* 2007;129(3):363-364; author reply 364-365.
86. Calandre EP, Hidalgo J, Garcia-Leiva JM, Rico-Villademoros F. Effectiveness of prophylactic trigger point inactivation in chronic migraine and chronic daily headache with migraine features [abstract]. *Cephalalgia.* 2003;23:713.
87. Garcia-Leiva JM, Hidalgo J, Rico-Villademoros F, Moreno V, Calandre EP. Effectiveness of ropivacaine trigger points inactivation in the prophylactic management of patients with severe migraine. *Pain Med.* 2007;8(1):65-70.
88. Bogduk N. The anatomical basis for cervicogenic headache. *J Manipulative Physiol Ther.* 1992;15(1):67-70.
89. Dreyfuss P, Michaelsen M, Fletcher D. Atlanto-occipital and lateral atlanto-axial joint pain patterns. *Spine.* 1994;19(10):1125-1131.
90. Aprill C, Axinn MJ, Bogduk N. Occipital headaches stemming from the lateral atlanto-axial (C1-2) joint. *Cephalalgia.* 2002;22(1):15-22.
91. Bogduk N. Cervicogenic headache: anatomic basis and pathophysiologic mechanisms. *Curr Pain Headache Rep.* 2001;5(4):382-386.
92. Hall T, Robinson K. The flexion-rotation test and active cervical mobility: a comparative measurement study in cervicogenic headache. *Man Ther.* 2004;9(4):197-202.
93. Zito G, Jull G, Story I. Clinical tests of musculoskeletal dysfunction in the diagnosis of cervicogenic headache. *Man Ther.* 2006;11(2):118-129.
94. Fernández de las Peñas C, Courtney CA. Clinical reasoning for manual therapy management of tension type and cervicogenic headache. *J Man Manip Ther.* 2014;22(1):44-50.
95. Bronfort G, Assendelft WJ, Evans R, Haas M, Bouter L. Efficacy of spinal manipulation for chronic headache: a systematic review. *J Manipulative Physiol Ther.* 2001;24(7):457-466.
96. Jaeger B. Are "cervicogenic" headaches due to myofascial pain and cervical spine dysfunction? *Cephalalgia.* 1989;9(3):157-164.
97. Roth JK, Roth RS, Weintraub JR, Simons DG. Cervicogenic headache caused by myofascial trigger points in the sternocleidomastoid: a case report. *Cephalalgia.* 2007;27(4):375-380.

98. Bodes-Pardo G, Pecos-Martin D, Gallego-Izquierdo T, Salom-Moreno J, Fernández de las Peñas C, Ortega-Santiago R. Manual treatment for cervicogenic headache and active trigger point in the sternocleidomastoid muscle: a pilot randomized clinical trial. *J Manipulative Physiol Ther.* 2013;36(7):403-411.

99. Fernández de las Peñas C, Fernandez-Carnero J, Miangolarra-Page J. Musculoskeletal disorders in mechanical neck pain: myofascial trigger points versus cervical joint dysfunction: a clinical study. *J Musculoskelet Pain.* 2005;13(1):27-35.

100. Jull G, Amiri M, Bullock-Saxton J, Darnell R, Lander C. Cervical musculoskeletal impairment in frequent intermittent headache. Part 1: subjects with single headaches. *Cephalalgia.* 2007;27(7):793-802.

101. Falla DL, Jull GA, Hodges PW. Patients with neck pain demonstrate reduced electromyographic activity of the deep cervical flexor muscles during performance of the craniocervical flexion test. *Spine.* 2004;29(19):2108-2114.

102. Jensen R, Bendtsen L, Olesen J. Muscular factors are of importance in tension-type headache. *Headache.* 1998;38(1):10-17.

103. Davidoff RA. Trigger points and myofascial pain: toward understanding how they affect headaches. *Cephalalgia.* 1998;18(7):436-448.

104. Arendt-Nielsen L, Castaldo M, Mechelli F, Fernández de las Peñas C. Muscle triggers as a possible source of pain in a sub-group of tension type headache patients? *Clin J Pain.* 2016;32(8):711-718.

105. Rasmussen BK, Jensen R, Schroll M, Olesen J. Epidemiology of headache in a general population: a prevalence study. *J Clin Epidemiol.* 1991;44(11):1147-1157.

106. Rasmussen BK, Jensen R, Schroll M, Olesen J. Interrelations between migraine and tension-type headache in the general population. *Arch Neurol.* 1992;49(9):914-918.

107. Chun WX. An approach to the nature of tension headache. *Headache.* 1985;25(4):188-189.

108. Mercer S, Marcus DA, Nash J. Cervical musculoskeletal disorders in migraine and tension type headache. Paper presented at: 68th Annual Meeting of the American Physical therapy Association; 1993; Cincinnati, Ohio.

109. Marcus DA, Scharff L, Mercer S, Turk DC. Musculoskeletal abnormalities in chronic headache: a controlled comparison of headache diagnostic groups. *Headache.* 1999;39(1):21-27.

110. Fernández de las Peñas C, Alonso-Blanco C, Cuadrado ML, Gerwin RD, Pareja JA. Trigger points in the suboccipital muscles and forward head posture in tension-type headache. *Headache.* 2006;46(3):454-460.

111. Fernández de las Peñas C, Alonso-Blanco C, Cuadrado ML, Pareja JA. Myofascial trigger points in the suboccipital muscles in episodic tension-type headache. *Man Ther.* 2006;11(3):225-230.

112. Fernández de las Peñas C, Ge HY, Arendt-Nielsen L, Cuadrado ML, Pareja JA. Referred pain from trapezius muscle trigger points shares similar characteristics with chronic tension type headache. *Eur J Pain.* 2007;11(4):475-482.

113. Fernández de las Peñas C, Cuadrado ML, Gerwin RD, Pareja JA. Referred pain from the trochlear region in tension-type headache: a myofascial trigger point from the superior oblique muscle. *Headache.* 2005;45(6):731-737.

114. Fernández de las Peñas C, Alonso-Blanco C, Quadrado ML, Gerwin R, Pareja JA. Myofascial trigger points and their relationship to headache clinical parameters in chronic tension-type headache. *Headache.* 2006;46(8):1264-1272.

115. Fernández de las Peñas C, Cuadrado ML, Pareja JA. Myofascial trigger points, neck mobility, and forward head posture in episodic tension-type headache. *Headache.* 2007;47(5):662-672.

116. Fernández de las Peñas C, Simons D, Cuadrado ML, Pareja J. The role of myofascial trigger points in musculoskeletal pain syndromes of the head and neck. *Curr Pain Headache Rep.* 2007;11(5):365-372.

117. Vierck CJ Jr, Cannon RL, Fry G, Maixner W, Whitsel BL. Characteristics of temporal summation of second pain sensations elicited by brief contact of glabrous skin by a preheated thermode. *J Neurophysiol.* 1997;78(2):992-1002.

118. Fernández de las Peñas C, Arendt-Nielsen L, Simons DG. Contributions of myofascial trigger points to chronic tension type headache. *J Manual Manipulative Ther.* 2006;14(4):222-231.

119. Gerwin RD. Chronic daily headache. *N Engl J Med.* 2006;354(18):1958; author reply 1958.

120. Fernández de las Peñas C, Alonso-Blanco C, Miangolarra JC. Myofascial trigger points in subjects presenting with mechanical neck pain: a blinded, controlled study. *Man Ther.* 2007;12(1):29-33.

121. Munoz-Munoz S, Munoz-Garcia MT, Alburquerque-Sendin F, Arroyo-Morales M, Fernández de las Peñas C. Myofascial trigger points, pain, disability, and sleep quality in individuals with mechanical neck pain. *J Manipulative Physiol Ther.* 2012;35(8):608-613.

122. Fernández de las Peñas C, Fernandez-Carnero J, Alonso-Blanco C, Miangolarra-Page JC. Myofascial pain syndrome in whiplash injury. A critical review of the literature. Paper presented at: International Whiplash Trauma Congress; October 9-10, 2003; Denver (USA).

123. Gerwin R, Dommerholt J. Myofascial trigger points in chronic cervical whiplash syndrome [Abstract]. *J Musculoskelet Pain.* 1998;6(suppl 2):28.

124. Kumar S, Narayan Y, Amell T. An electromyographic study of low-velocity rear-end impacts. *Spine.* 2002;27(10):1044-1055.

125. Baker B. The muscle trigger: evidence of overload injury. *J Neurol Orthop Med Surg.* 1986;7(1):35-44.

126. Schuller E, Eisenmenger W, Beier G. Whiplash Injury in Low Speed Car Accidents: Assessment of biomechanical cervical spine loading and injury prevention in a forensic sample. *J Musculoskelet Pain.* 2000;8(1/2):55-67.

127. Duffy MF, Stuberg W, DeJong S, Gold KV, Nystrom NA. Case report: whiplash-associated disorder from a low-velocity bumper car collision: history, evaluation, and surgery. *Spine.* 2004;29(17):1881-1884.

128. Hong C-Z, Simons DG. Response to treatment for pectoralis minor myofascial pain syndrome after whiplash. *J Musculoskelet Pain.* 1993;1(1):89-131.

129. Fernández de las Peñas C, Palomeque del Cerro L, Fernandez Carmero J. Manual Treatment of post-whiplash injury. *J Bodyw Mov Ther.* 2005;9(2):109-119.

130. McMakin C, Gregory WM, Philips TM. Cytokine changes with microcurrent treatment of fibromyalgia associated with cervical spine trauma. *J Bodyw Mov Ther.* 2005;9(3):169-176.

131. Panjabi MM, Nibu K, Cholewicki J. Whiplash injuries and the potential for mechanical instability. *Eur Spine J.* 1998;7(6):484-492.

132. Brault JR, Wheeler JB, Siegmund GP, Brault EJ. Clinical response of human subjects to rear-end automobile collisions. *Arch Phys Med Rehabil.* 1998;79(1):72-80.

133. Jull G. Deep cervical flexor muscle dysfunction in whiplash. *J Musculoskelet Pain.* 2000;8:143-154.

134. Sterling M, Jull G, Vicenzino B, Kenardy J, Darnell R. Development of motor system dysfunction following whiplash injury. *Pain.* 2003;103(1-2):65-73.

135. Jull G, Kristjansson E, Dall'Alba P. Impairment in the cervical flexors: a comparison of whiplash and insidious onset neck pain patients. *Man Ther.* 2004;9(2):89-94.

136. Castaldo M, Ge HY, Chiarotto A, Villafane JH, Arendt-Nielsen L. Myofascial trigger points in patients with whiplash-associated disorders and mechanical neck pain. *Pain Med.* 2014;15(5):842-849.

137. Fernandez-Perez AM, Villaverde-Gutierrez C, Mora-Sanchez A, Alonso-Blanco C, Sterling M, Fernández de las Peñas C. Muscle trigger points, pressure pain threshold, and cervical range of motion in patients with high level of disability related to acute whiplash injury. *J Orthop Sports Phys Ther.* 2012;42(7):634-641.

138. Scott D, Jull G, Sterling M. Widespread sensory hypersensitivity is a feature of chronic whiplash-associated disorder but not chronic idiopathic neck pain. *Clin J Pain.* 2005;21(2):175-181.

139. Sterling M, Jull G, Vicenzino B, Kenardy J. Sensory hypersensitivity occurs soon after whiplash injury and is associated with poor recovery. *Pain.* 2003;104(3):509-517.

140. Johansen MK, Graven-Nielsen T, Olesen AS, Arendt-Nielsen L. Generalized muscular hyperalgesia in chronic whiplash syndrome. *Pain.* 1999;83:229-234.

141. Herren-Gerber R, Weiss S, Arendt-Nielsen L, et al. Modulation of central hypersensitivity by nociceptive input in chronic pain after whiplash injury. *Pain Med.* 2004;5(4):366-376.

142. Dommerholt J. Persistent myalgia following whiplash. *Curr Pain Headache Rep.* 2005;9(5):326-330.

143. Lord S, Barnsley L, Wallis B, Bogduk N. Chronic cervical zygapophysial joint pain after whiplash: a placebo-controlled prevalence study. *Spine.* 1996;21(15):1737-1744.

144. Graff-Radford SB, Jaeger B, Reeves JL. Myofascial pain may present clinically as occipital neuralgia. *Neurosurgery.* 1986;19(4):610-613.

145. Natsis K, Baraliakos X, Appell HJ, Tsikaras P, Gigis I, Koebke J. The course of the greater occipital nerve in the suboccipital region: a proposal for setting landmarks for local anesthesia in patients with occipital neuralgia. *Clin Anat.* 2006;19(4):332-336.

146. Paluzzi A, Belli A, Lafuente J, Wasserberg J. Role of the C2 articular branches in occipital headache: an anatomical study. *Clin Anat.* 2006;19(6):497-502.

147. Chen S-M, Chen JT, Wu V-C, Kuan T-S, Hong C-Z. Myofascial Trigger points in intercostal muscles secondary to herpes zoster infection to the intercostal nerve [abstract]. *Arch Phys Med Rehabil.* 1996;77:961.

148. Ceneviz C, Maloney G, Mehta N. Myofascial pain may mimic trigeminal neuralgia. *Cephalalgia.* 2006;26(7):899-901.

Section 3   Upper Back, Shoulder, and Arm Pain

Chapter 19

Levator Scapulae Muscle
"Crick in the Neck"

Derek L. Vraa, Michelle Finnegan, and Joseph M. Donnelly

1. INTRODUCTION

The levator scapulae muscle is unique in its anatomic structure and attachments to the cervical spine and the scapula. The proximal fibers originate from the posterior tubercles of C1-C4. It descends inferiorly and posterolaterally with the distal fibers attaching to the medial scapular border from the superior angle of the scapula to the scapular spine. This muscle has a unique posterior twist from its origin to its insertion such that the anteriorly facing fibers at the origin become the posterior facing fibers on insertion. The muscle is innervated by branches of the C3 and C4 spinal nerves and from C5 via the dorsal scapular nerve. The primary functions of the levator scapulae muscle are downward rotation and elevation of the scapula and ipsilateral cervical rotation. Bilaterally, it also plays a key role in stabilizing the cervical spine during neck flexion. The pain referral pattern of the levator scapulae muscle is to the angle of the neck and the interscapular and posterior shoulder regions. Activation and perpetuation of trigger points (TrPs) in the levator scapulae muscle are typically caused by holding the shoulders in an elevated and shortened position, especially when fatigued or from prolonged exposure to a cold draft. Because TrPs can present anywhere in the muscle, it is important to examine the entire muscle for the presence of TrPs. The levator scapulae muscle is frequently involved in headaches, mechanical neck pain, whiplash-associated disorders, scapular dysfunction, fibromyalgia, as well as shoulder pain and impingement. In addition, consideration should be given to this muscle when treating patients with jaw pain, cervical radicular symptoms, and upper extremity dysfunctions due to its actions and involvement in postural syndromes. Corrective actions including postural counseling at work and home (including sleeping postures) are paramount for successful treatment of TrPs in the levator scapulae muscle. Trigger point self-pressure release and gentle self-stretching exercises are part of a comprehensive treatment program.

2. ANATOMIC CONSIDERATIONS

The levator scapulae muscle is located at the floor of the posterior cervical triangle. The proximal fibers originate from the posterior tubercles of C1-C4. It descends inferiorly and posterolaterally, with the distal fibers attaching to the medial scapular border from the superior angle of the scapula to the scapular spine (Figure 19-1).[1] In a cadaveric study of 10 human specimens, the average length of the levator scapulae muscle was 15.1 cm with an average cross-sectional area of 2.18 sq cm.[2] The angulation of descent from the origin to the insertion varied from 30° to 45°. Muscle fiber composition of the levator scapulae muscle has not been studied.

One of the nuances rarely appreciated in the levator scapulae muscle is the subtle posterior twist of the fiber orientation as the muscle travels from its origin to insertion (Figure 19-1). MacBeth and Martin[3] described the twist such that the superior fibers (C1) spiraled first laterally, then posteriorly, such that the anteriorly facing fibers at the origin become posteriorly facing on insertion. From C2 to C4, the fiber attachments originate posterior to the C1 fibers; however, as they spiral toward the insertion, the C2-C4 slips become deep to the C1 fibers. The biomechanical implications of this twist have not yet been fully studied.

Anatomic variations of the levator scapulae muscle are relatively uncommon, although some do exist. In a cadaveric study by Menachem et al,[4] the muscle inserted in two layers enveloping the medial border attachment in 63% (19/30) of the shoulders of individuals examined. Of those, 14 presented with a bursa in the areolar tissue between the two layers. In addition, the authors found that in 43% (13/30) of the shoulders of individuals examined, there existed a narrow band of the serratus anterior muscle attached over the medial border of the scapula around its upper angle, close to the attachment of the levator scapulae muscle. Furthermore, in 38% (5/13) another bursa was located between the serratus anterior muscle, the angle of the scapula, and the levator scapulae muscle. It is important to recognize that these bursae are potential sources of pain and tenderness in this region. More recently, one cadaveric dissection reported a single case where the levator scapulae muscle had an accessory head that inserted into the ligamentum nuchae, tendon of the rhomboid major muscle, and the superior aspect of the serratus posterior superior muscle by way of a flat aponeurotic band.[5]

Other anatomic variances have been documented including variable attachments to the cervical spine. Chotai et al[6] reported slips of the levator scapulae muscle attaching to the mastoid process. Bergman et al[7] reported myofascial slips extending to the mastoid process of the temporal bones, the occipital bone, ligamentum nuchae, the clavicle, the first and the second ribs, and spinous processes of the thoracic vertebrae. In addition, slips have extended to the rhomboids, serratus anterior, serratus posterior superior, and trapezius muscles.[7] MacBeth and Martin[3] observed that the superior fibers of origin inserted on to the inferior one half of the supraspinous portion of the vertebral border of the scapula in 63% (54/80) of the cases with more- and less-extensive insertions on the remaining specimens.

2.1. Innervation and Vascularization

The levator scapulae muscle is innervated from two sources. The first is via branches from the C3 and C4 spinal nerves. The other innervation is from the brachial plexus (C5) via the dorsal scapular nerve.[1]

Innervation of the levator scapulae muscle has consistent nerve pathways.[8] From C3 to C4, an average of 1.92 branches from the cervical plexus remain deep to prevertebral fascia. These branches then emerge from under the posterior border of

---

The views expressed herein are strictly those of the authors and do not represent the U.S. Air Force, the U.S. Department of Defense, or any other U.S. government entity.

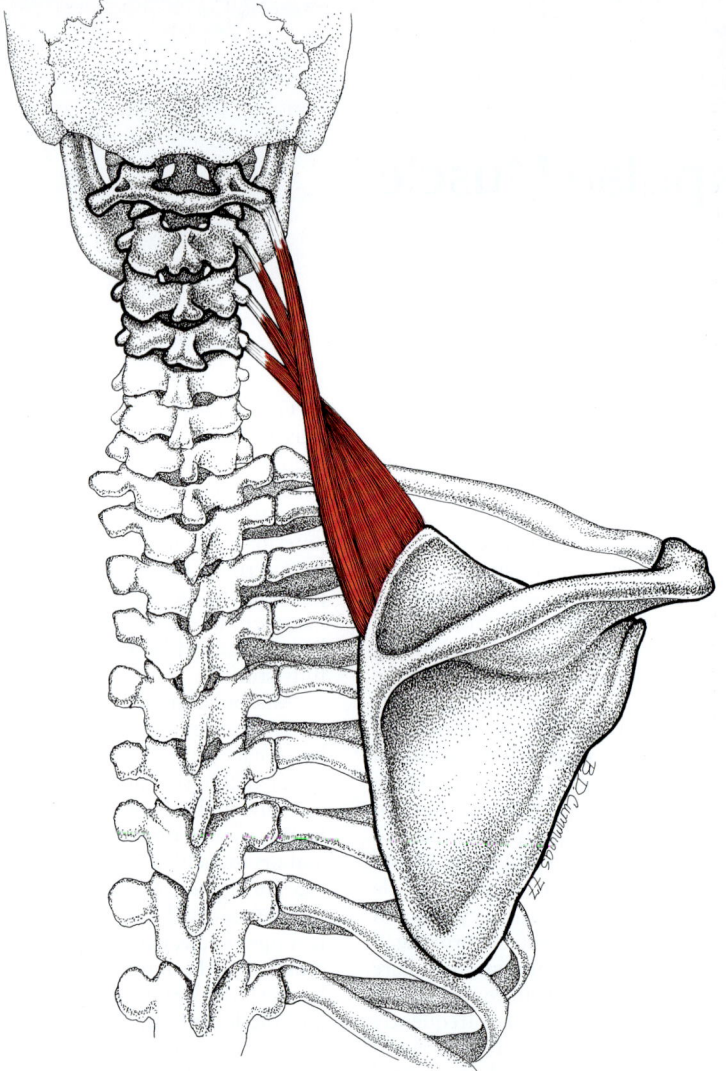

Figure 19-1. Attachments of the levator scapulae muscle. Note how the upper and lower digitations twist in their course from the superior attachment to the inferior attachment.

the sternocleidomastoid muscle, traveling in a cranial to caudal direction, to enter the posterior cervical triangle and innervate the levator scapulae muscle.

In the same cadaveric study, Frank et al[8] also documented the innervation of the levator scapula muscle by the dorsal scapular nerve. Originating from the ventral rami of C5, the dorsal scapular nerve pierces the middle scalene muscle, entering the inferior portion of the posterior triangle of the neck. As the nerve enters the posterior triangle of the neck, it travels a variable distance in a posteroinferior direction. Interestingly, in 24 of the 35 cervical spines examined, on the path toward the rhomboid muscle, the dorsal scapular nerve drove deep to the anterior border of the levator scapulae muscle without any contributing branches to the muscle. In only nine of the cadavers did the dorsal scapular nerve directly enter the levator scapulae muscle, with two specimens receiving small branches. In a different study of 20 dorsal scapular nerves, however, all instances resulted in a direct innervation of the levator scapulae muscle.[9] In a cadaveric study by Nguyen et al,[10] differences in origination from the spinal root level, as well as what muscles it innervated, were demonstrated. They reported that 70% of the dorsal scapular nerves examined originated from the spinal root of C5, 22% arose from C4, and 8% from C6. The levator scapulae, rhomboid major, and rhomboid minor muscles were all innervated in 52% specimens. The dorsal scapular nerve innervated only the levator scapulae muscle in 48% of the specimens.

The levator scapulae muscle receives its primary vascular supply from the dorsal scapular artery. The dorsal scapular artery itself has been shown to arise from the second or third part of the subclavian artery in 70% of individuals,[11] whereas 30% arise from branches from the transverse cervical and ascending cervical arteries. Secondarily, the superior aspect of the muscle is supplied by branches from the vertebral artery.[12] Of note, the dorsal scapular nerve can be intertwined with the dorsal scapular artery.[9]

2.2. Function

The levator scapulae muscle elevates the scapula and assists with scapular downward rotation. It also has a role in scapular retraction, ipsilateral rotation and side-bending of the cervical spine, and postural positioning of the head. It almost always acts synergistically with other muscles to influence scapular mobility. These synergistic relationships are discussed below.

Electromyography (EMG) studies of the levator scapula muscle have demonstrated increased activity in scapular elevation, with moderate activity during scapular retraction.[13] When moving the arm, the levator scapulae muscle assists scapular motion during shoulder elevation (abduction, flexion).[14] In an EMG study by Behrsin and Maguire,[15] the levator scapulae muscle was found to contract concentrically during the first 90° of shoulder abduction and eccentrically during the second 90°. Furthermore, it exerted more activity during end ranges of flexion and abduction of the shoulder. This finding is consistent with that of Ludewig et al[16] who demonstrated progressively increasing EMG activity of the levator scapulae muscle with increasing glenohumeral elevation as the scapula moves into upward rotation and posterior tilt. During sporting activities such as throwing or golf in which the shoulder is elevated, the levator scapulae muscle reaches a peak maximal voluntary isometric contraction (MVIC) of 33% to 72%.[17]

Magnusson[18] demonstrated that the levator scapulae muscle plays a role in postural stability of the head and neck during low-speed, rear-end collisions. It was one of the first muscles to react when the impact came from the sagittal plane. A more recent study found that the levator scapulae muscle played a limited role in the stabilization of the head and neck during multidirectional perturbations.[19]

With the scapula stabilized, the levator scapulae muscle offers a minor contribution to ipsilateral side-bending and rotation of the cervical spine and a larger contribution in maintaining head position because it becomes active during resisted ipsilateral side-bending.[20] It has a reduced EMG activity when correcting for habitual postures such as forward head positioning and slouched positions.[21]

Dr Vladimir Janda[22] described the Upper Crossed Syndrome (UCS) in which a patient presents with a classic forward head and rounded shoulder posture. In this syndrome, the levator scapulae muscle responds as tight and facilitated because it is a "postural muscle." With the prolonged presence of the UCS, there is an increase in muscle tension that may then increase the probability of TrP development within the muscle and can potentially contribute to a number of dysfunctions in the upper quarter.

2.3. Functional Unit

The functional unit to which a muscle belongs includes the muscles that reinforce and counter its actions as well as the joints that the muscle crosses. The interdependence of these structures functionally is reflected in the organization and neural connections of the sensory motor cortex. The functional unit is emphasized because the presence of a TrP in one muscle of the unit increases the likelihood that the other muscles of the unit will also develop TrPs. When inactivating TrPs in a muscle, one should be concerned about TrPs that may develop in muscles that are functionally interdependent. Box 19-1 grossly represents the functional unit of the levator scapulae muscle.[23]

Isometrically, the ipsilateral levator scapulae muscle becomes active with the ipsilateral upper trapezius and cervical spinal extensor muscles when resisting contralateral side-bending. The same muscles become active bilaterally, when acting isometrically, to retract and extend the head and neck.[24] With the scapulae stabilized, the muscle assists the sternocleidomastoid, splenius capitis and cervicis, scalenes, upper trapezius, and the erector spinae muscles with ipsilateral cervical side-bending.

Box 19-1 Functional unit of the levator scapulae muscle

Action	Synergists	Antagonists
Scapular elevation	Upper trapezius Rhomboid minor Rhomboid major	Latissimus dorsi Lower trapezius Serratus anterior (lower fibers) Pectoralis minor
Scapular downward rotation	Latissimus dorsi Rhomboid major Rhomboid minor	Upper trapezius Lower trapezius Serratus anterior

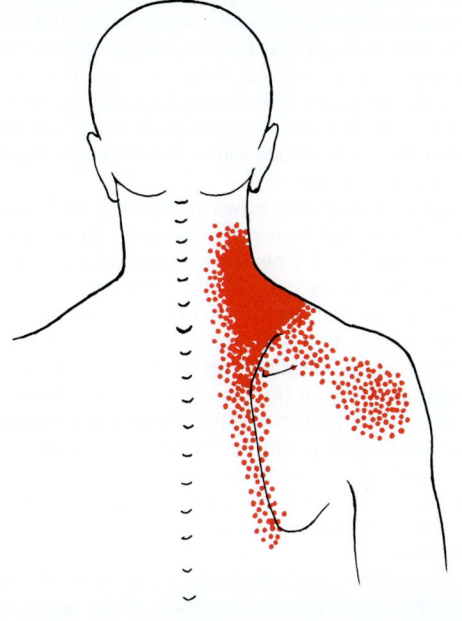
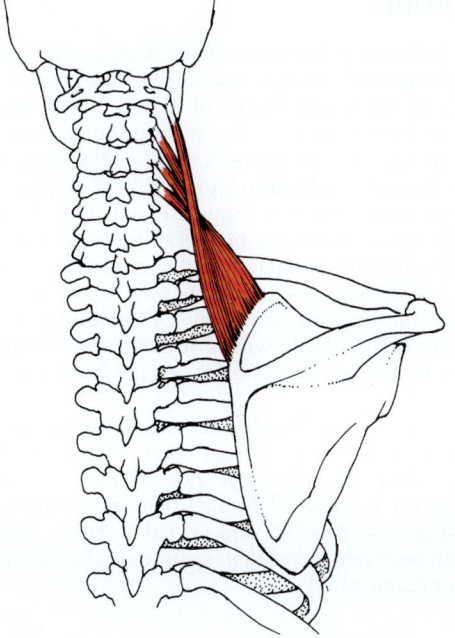

Figure 19-2. Consolidated referred pain pattern from TrPs in the right levator scapulae muscle. The essential pain pattern is solid red, and the spillover pattern is stippled red. The entire muscle should be palpated for the presences of TrPs. Trigger points may be present very close to the attachement of the muscle at the superior angle of the scapula.

3. CLINICAL PRESENTATION

3.1. Referred Pain Pattern

Trigger points can be found in any portion of the muscle, although frequently they are found in the midportion of the muscle or close to the insertion at the scapula. Both areas refer pain at the angle of the neck[25-27] with a spillover zone along the vertebral border of the scapula[25,27] and to the shoulder posteriorly[25,27-30] (Figure 19-2). If the TrPs are active, they can refer severe pain even at rest.

In clinical practice, the proximal half of the muscle often has TrPs relating to headaches and neck pain. In the distal half of the levator scapulae muscle, TrPs often produce pain in the posterior scapular region, often medial to the scapula but not crossing midline. In a study of 22 female patients with reports of shoulder pain over the superior medial angle of the scapula,[4] 95% of the patients had maximum tenderness within 2 cm of the superior angle of the scapula. Pressing on the tender spot reproduced or increased their typical pain. In 73% patients, small nodules or crepitation was palpable at the tender spot, which the authors identified as TrPs. In the same study, pressing on the tender point produced neck pain in the cervical spine in 73% of the patients. Shoulder pain was elicited with TrP palpation in 50%, and upper limb pain was elicited in 23%. In addition to pain, when the levator scapulae muscle is involved, it consistently limits neck rotation due to pain with movement.

Trigger points can contribute to neck pain[31] or shoulder pain[32] with the levator scapulae muscle being one of the most commonly involved shoulder girdle muscles. In an older study of shoulder girdle muscles of 200 young adults, Sola[33] found the frequency of TrPs in levator scapulae muscles was second only to the upper trapezius muscle. In a separate clinical study of active TrPs in the upper quarter,[34] the levator scapulae muscle was the most commonly involved shoulder girdle muscle. More recently, Fernández de las Peñas et al[35] identified TrPs in the levator scapulae muscle of white- and blue-collar workers as the third most prevalent. Cerezo-Téllez et al[36] reported that TrPs in the levator scapulae muscles were the second most prevalent in those with nonspecific neck pain.

3.2. Symptoms

Patients with TrPs in the levator scapulae muscle may report symptoms in the cranial, cervical, and/or scapular regions depending on the location and severity of the TrPs. With severe involvement of the levator scapulae muscle alone, patients describe pain at the angle of the neck or as a stiff neck. The diagnosis of stiff neck syndrome or torticollis[26,29] emphasizes the restriction of range of motion because tension in the levator scapulae muscle is a common cause of neck stiffness.[26,29] Patients with TrPs in the levator scapulae muscle are unable to turn the head fully to the same side because of pain on contraction and not fully to the opposite side because of painful increase in muscle tension. They likely will turn their entire body to look behind (refer to clinical considerations in Chapter 33 for more on stiff neck).

Patients with mechanical neck pain and levator scapulae TrPs report cervical pain and a limited range of motion. They also describe a "deep" scapular pain with TrP palpation near the insertion of the muscle.[37,38] Neoh[39] reported 75 patients describing a shortness of breath and nuchal soreness. Ninety percent of them were relieved of their symptoms after dry needling of levator scapulae TrPs.

3.3. Patient Examination

After a thorough subjective examination, the clinician should make a detailed drawing representing the pain pattern that the patient has described. This depiction will assist in planning the physical examination and can be useful in monitoring the progression of the patient as symptoms improve or change. Additionally, a complete medical screening should also be performed to rule out disease processes that can refer pain to the region of the levator scapulae muscle.[40]

Postural examination from anterior, posterior, and lateral views may give cues to problems in the levator scapulae muscle. In particular, the clinician should assess for asymmetries of the head, neck, and scapular positions. Forward head posture with excessive upper cervical extension, or lateral flexion to one side, may indicate bilateral or unilateral muscle dysfunction, respectively. In forward head or flexed neck positions, tightness or TrPs in the levator scapulae muscle has the potential to interfere with upward rotation and posterior tipping of the scapula that is a requirement of normal scapular movement during shoulder elevation.[41]

Assessment of the range of motion in the cervical spine and shoulder in all planes is also recommended. Active neck rotation is most restricted as the face turns toward the side of the pain. The degree of restriction depends on the severity of involvement. When both sides are involved, as it commonly occurs, rotation can be markedly restricted in both directions. Neck flexion is blocked only at the end (extreme range) of the movement, whereas extension is relatively unaffected. If rotation of the neck is unrestricted, TrPs in the levator scapulae muscle are unlikely.

There is usually only a minimal limitation of shoulder motion. Full abduction requires full upward rotation of the scapula, which can be painfully restricted by TrPs in the levator scapulae muscle. The Apley's Scratch Test (flexion, lateral rotation, and abduction) is normal (see Figure 21-3).

Assessment of the cervical spine for accessory joint motion restrictions is essential because TrPs or muscle length deficits in the levator scapulae muscle can restrict movement of the cervical spine. Utilizing methods described by Cook[42] have been shown to be valid and reliable.

It is also important to assess all joints of the shoulder complex. Because the muscle inserts onto the superior medial aspect of the scapula, it can directly affect scapulothoracic mobility, which can have an influence on the glenohumeral, acromioclavicular, and sternoclavicular joints. To accommodate for normal shoulder elevation and scapular motion, proper sternoclavicular and acromioclavicular coupling should occur.[43] Patients with shoulder pain demonstrate less sternoclavicular mobility.[43] Therefore, assessment of accessory joint mobility of the sternoclavicular and acromioclavicular joints should be incorporated into the examination process.

Loss of scapular upward rotation and anterior rotation has been noted as a potential contributor to shoulder impingement.[16,41,44] Upward rotation and posterior tipping are necessary for normal shoulder elevation to prevent rotator cuff impingement on the lateral aspects of the acromion.[45] Due to the line of action of the levator scapulae muscle, any TrPs, and even muscle tightening or muscle shortening, can have a potential effect on the scapular mobility. Increased tightening of the muscle pulls the scapula into a downward rotation and anteriorly tilted position. Therefore, shoulder pain could be a consequence of levator scapulae muscle dysfunction. Trigger points, as well as lowered pain pressure thresholds in the muscle, have been documented in patients with shoulder impingement syndrome.[46]

Considering the coordinated activation of muscles involved in scapular motion, examination of the antagonistic and synergistic muscles should be performed. Trigger points are often associated with a reduced efficiency of reciprocal inhibition that may contribute to delayed and impaired muscle activation, thus contributing to faulty scapular mobility and potential levator scapulae TrPs.[47] Elimination of associated TrPs may then improve scapular motor control and reduce of pain in the levator scapulae muscle and its associated areas.

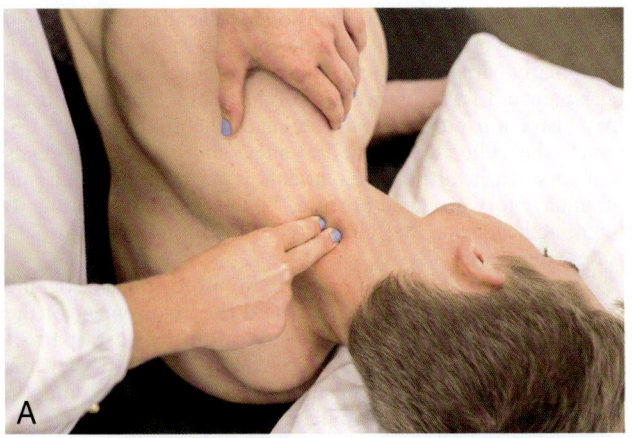
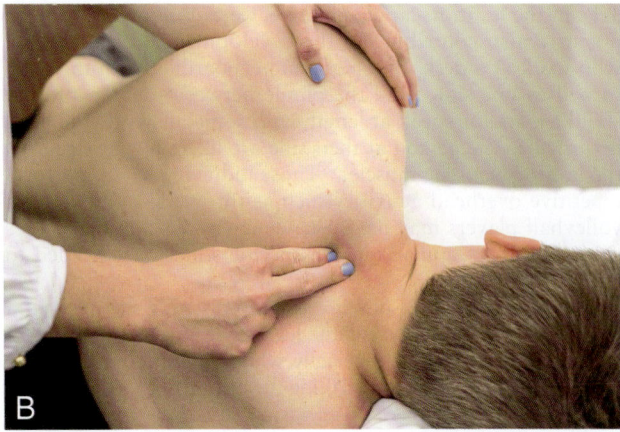
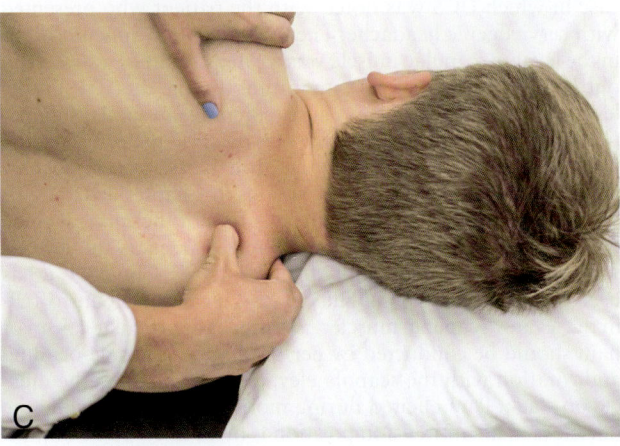

Figure 19-3. A, Cross-fiber flat palpation of the levator scapulae at mid-muscle belly. B, Cross-fiber flat palpation of the levator scapulae at the superior angle of the scapula. C, Alternative technique with affected side down, utilizing cross-fiber pincer palpation.

3.4. Trigger Point Examination

Examination of the levator scapulae muscle may be performed in side-lying with the symptomatic side upward, sitting, supine, or prone. However, side-lying or prone positioning is often more advantageous for the identification of TrPs as it allows for the relaxation of the head and neck, making identification easier.

The levator scapulae muscle commonly develops TrPs in two locations: a central area at the angle of the neck, where the muscle emerges from beneath the anterior border of the upper trapezius muscle,[29,48] and a much more readily identified secondary area close to where the muscle attaches to the superior angle of the scapula.[48-50]

Trigger points in the levator scapulae muscle at the angle of the neck can be palpated with the patient comfortably seated in a chair, or preferably, with the patient lying on the uninvolved side. When the patient is sitting, both the levator scapulae and upper trapezius muscles are slackened slightly by supporting the elbows on armrests, using a folded towel if needed. Supporting the patient's arms allows for the clinician's fingers to push the upper trapezius muscle posteriorly far enough to uncover and straddle the levator scapulae muscle (Figure 19-3A, with the patient lying on the uninvolved side). Once identified, a cross-fiber flat palpation is utilized to identify TrPs in this portion of the muscle. Successful palpation depends on slackening the upper trapezius muscle sufficiently to reach the TrPs within the belly of the levator scapulae muscle without tensing that whole muscle so much that the difference between the taut band and the adjacent uninvolved muscle tissue is obscured.

To locate TrPs closer to its attachment at the scapula, the patient may be seated or preferably lying on the opposite side (Figure 19-3B). The muscle is palpated with a cross-fiber flat palpation above the superior angle of the scapula. Pincer palpation may also be used with the patient lying on the affected side (Figure 19-3C). The TrPs in this region are exquisitely tender to pressure; however, local twitch responses and referred pain are not readily elicited from this area which is covered by the trapezius muscle. The attachment region frequently feels indurated and tender and it can be rocked back and forth between the fingers when they straddle it. When the attachment has been stressed for a period of time, the area may feel gritty (like gravel) or like scar tissue.

4. DIFFERENTIAL DIAGNOSIS

4.1. Activation and Perpetuation of Trigger Points

A posture or activity that activates a TrP, if not corrected, can also perpetuate it. In any part of the levator scapulae muscle, TrPs may be activated by unaccustomed eccentric loading, eccentric exercise in an unconditioned muscle, or maximal or submaximal concentric loading.[51] Trigger points may also be activated or aggravated when the muscle is placed in a shortened and/or lengthened position for an extended period of time, as in prolonged faulty postures or UCS (see Chapter 76). Patients who experience a whiplash injury are likely to develop TrPs in the levator scapulae and other cervical muscles. In separate studies on whiplash injuries by Ettlin et al,[52] Castaldo et al,[53] and Fernández-Pérez[54] researchers noted a high prevalence of

TrPs in the levator scapulae muscle. Certain faulty ergonomic postures also contribute to the development of TrPs. Those who work at a desk[4] and perform keyboarding with the head turned to one side, hold the phone between the ear and the shoulder, and/or speak at length with someone while the head is turned to the person at their side are likely to put stress on the levator scapulae muscle.[55] Those individuals who perform repetitive overhead activities such as throwers, swimmers, or volleyball players may have a tendency to develop more TrPs in the levator scapulae muscle; specific studies are needed to establish prevalence.

Another activating posture is sleeping with the neck in a tilted position that shortens the levator scapulae muscle, as in an uncomfortable seat, especially when the muscle is fatigued and exposed to a cold draft. Tilting the head while gazing fixedly at a stage, movie screen, or television can also precipitate the problem. Psychological stressors, which facilitate poor posture, may also be contributory.[55] Prolonged sitting in a chair with armrests that are too high elevates the scapulae and shortens the muscle bilaterally thus encouraging activation of TrPs. Walking with a cane that is too long, so that it forces unnatural elevation of one shoulder, tends to activate TrPs in the levator scapulae muscle on the same side.

The levator scapulae muscle can be overloaded and develop TrPs when the function of the serratus anterior muscle is inhibited by serratus anterior TrPs. Motor vehicle accidents and falls commonly activate levator scapulae TrPs due to acute overload stress.[56] Sometimes, TrPs in this muscle can arise secondarily from the activity of a primary TrP in the functionally related upper trapezius muscle.[57]

4.2. Associated Trigger Points

In a study by Hsieh and colleagues,[58] associated TrPs may develop in the referred pain area from other TrPs. As a result, with TrPs in the levator scapulae muscle, muscles such as the upper and middle trapezius, rhomboids, serratus posterior superior, infraspinatus, supraspinatus, posterior deltoid, posterior cervical, semispinalis thoracis, and iliocostalis thoracis muscles can develop associated TrPs.

Associated TrPs in the levator scapulae muscle can be due to primary TrPs in the splenius cervicis, cervical multifidi, scalenes, middle trapezius, and the long head of the triceps muscles. Identifying which muscle is the source of symptoms is imperative, as deactivating these TrPs may also inactivate associated TrPs.[57] Trigger points within the midsection of the muscle are frequently found in conjunction with TrPs within the upper fibers of the trapezius muscle.

4.3. Associated Pathology

Trigger points in this muscle are associated with, or can mimic, many different conditions; therefore, a thorough medical screening and examination are essential. Trigger point involvement of the levator scapulae, sternocleidomastoid, splenii capitis and cervicis, and upper trapezius muscles should be distinguished from spasmodic torticollis (cervical dystonia), which is a neurologic condition characterized by involuntary dystonic movements of the head[59,60] that can be genetic, acquired, or idiopathic.[61] Although the levator scapulae muscle is not as commonly involved as the sternocleidomastoid, trapezius, scalenes, and platysma muscles,[62] making the differential diagnosis of this condition (against TrPs) is essential to ensure proper care. With spasmodic torticollis, hypertrophy of the muscles may develop.[59] In contrast, the apparent shortening of a muscle due to TrPs does not cause hypertrophy, nor does it cause involuntary movements of the head.

The levator scapulae muscle can contribute to headaches. Fernández de las Peñas[63] noted a high prevalence of TrPs in this muscle in patients who have tension-type headaches. Although the muscle typically does not refer pain to the craniofacial region, many patients with tension-type headaches present with neck pain and TrPs. Involvement of the levator scapulae muscle may also contribute to a shortening of the muscle as in UCS, which alters the craniovertebral angle and places individuals in a forward head posture. Patients with unilateral migraine often have forward head posture,[64] potentially contributing to migraine headaches. See clinical considerations in Chapter 33 for greater detail.

The levator scapulae muscle is involved in cervicogenic headache as well. Bogduk[65] discussed the involvement of the cervical spine and the trigeminocervical nucleus as a part of cervicogenic headaches. Because of the origins of the levator scapulae muscle, myofascial involvement within the muscle can restrict upper cervical spine mobility and thereby has the potential to contribute to the headaches. Moore[66] described a case in which UCS was noted with the patient who presented with cervicogenic headache. The presence of documented TrPs in the levator scapulae muscle was treated as part of a successful outcome. Furthermore, it is important to note that TrPs in the levator scapulae muscle may cause temporal and spatial summation of nociceptive input into the nervous system decreasing the pain threshold and increasing the probability for cervicogenic headache[64] (see clinical considerations in Chapter 33).

Facet/zygapophyseal joint dysfunction of the cervical spine can also cause pain in the same referral areas as the levator scapulae muscle,[67] specifically from C4 to C7. Clinically, it has been observed that hypomobility at C2-C3 can contribute to TrPs in the levator scapulae muscle. Assessment of articular causes of pain should be conducted by performing passive side-bending and rotation with the scapula elevated, which places the muscle on slack. Pain elicited during motion assessment while the muscle is in an antitension position is more likely to be of joint origin. Examination of accessory joint motion should also be utilized to assess for specific joint mobility loss and correlation of patient symptoms.

The levator scapulae muscle is frequently involved in those who have a "SICK scapula" or Scapular malposition, Inferior medial border prominence, Coracoid pain and malposition, and dysKinesis of scapular movement as described by Burkhart and colleagues.[68] This condition is most prevalent in overhead throwers. A key feature in the SICK scapula is asymmetrical position and dyskinesis of the scapula, which in turn creates altered kinematics of the glenohumeral and acromioclavicular joints that affect the muscles that insert onto the scapula. As a result, the SICK scapula may play a role in a number of other diagnoses of the glenohumeral and acromioclavicular joints, including, but not limited to, subacromial impingement syndrome (SIS), superior labral anterior to posterior lesions, and instability. The levator scapulae muscle is frequently tender to palpation near its insertion. As a result, it is recommended to assess the scapula as described by Burkart and colleagues[68] and the levator scapulae muscle for TrP involvement in the SICK scapula. Furthermore, it is recommended that with this diagnosis all muscles attaching to the scapula be examined for TrPs as they will potentially affect scapular dyskinesis.[47]

Studies have demonstrated that individuals with SIS have impaired scapular mechanics,[69] specifically a loss of upward rotation. The levator scapulae muscle perpetuates downward rotation of the scapula; therefore, shortening of this muscle or the presence of TrPs is likely to contribute to the loss of scapular mobility in SIS patients. It is currently unknown if the presence of SIS perpetuates the loss of scapular mobility or the loss of scapular mobility leads to SIS.

The levator scapulae muscle is innervated by C3-C4 spinal nerves and the dorsal scapular nerve (C5); therefore, it is important to identify these differences when performing a differential diagnosis for patients with upper quadrant pain and injury. Currently, no primary nerve or vascular entrapments due to TrPs in the levator scapulae muscle are reported.

5. CORRECTIVE ACTIONS

The consistent use of computers or tablets in bed or in a chair is likely to facilitate suboptimal posture and head and neck positioning. Correction of faulty posture can reduce reports of pain originating from the levator scapulae muscle. For example, reduction in excessive EMG activity in the upper trapezius muscle has been demonstrated through appropriate keyboard placement.[70] It is recommended that workstation ergonomic assessment and correction, use of proper seating, and use of assistive or supportive devices such as pillows or lumbar rolls be used in an attempt to reduce forward head posture.

Prolonged positioning contributes to the development of TrPs in as little as 1 hour of typing.[71] Individuals who have an occupation that involves prolonged sitting and typing are recommended to relieve muscle tension 1 to 2 times per hour by simply standing and walking a short distance. Stretching the pectoralis major and minor muscles (refer to Chapters 42 and 43) can also assist in correcting posture and may improve scapular mobility.

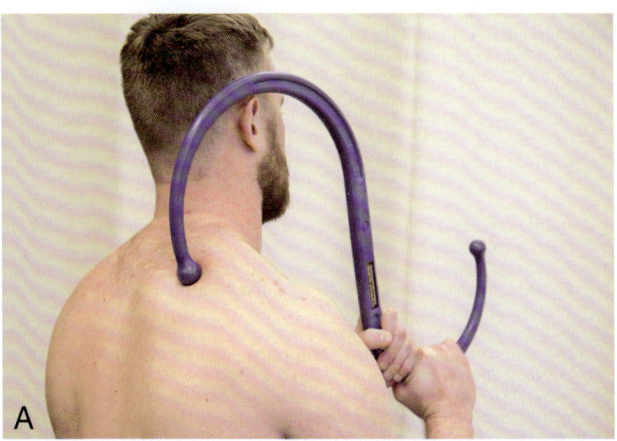
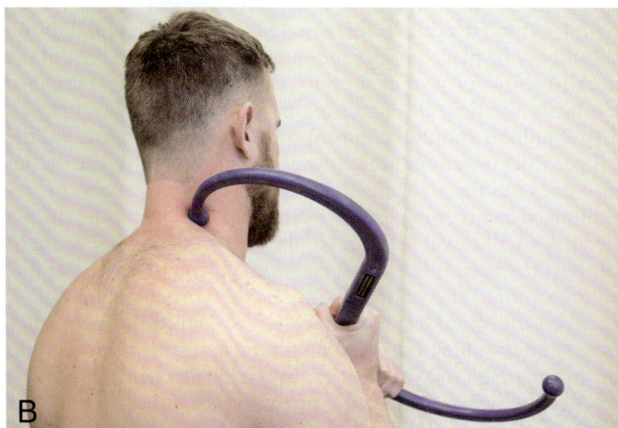

Figure 19-4. Trigger point self-pressure release. A, Attachment at scapula. B, Mid-muscle belly.

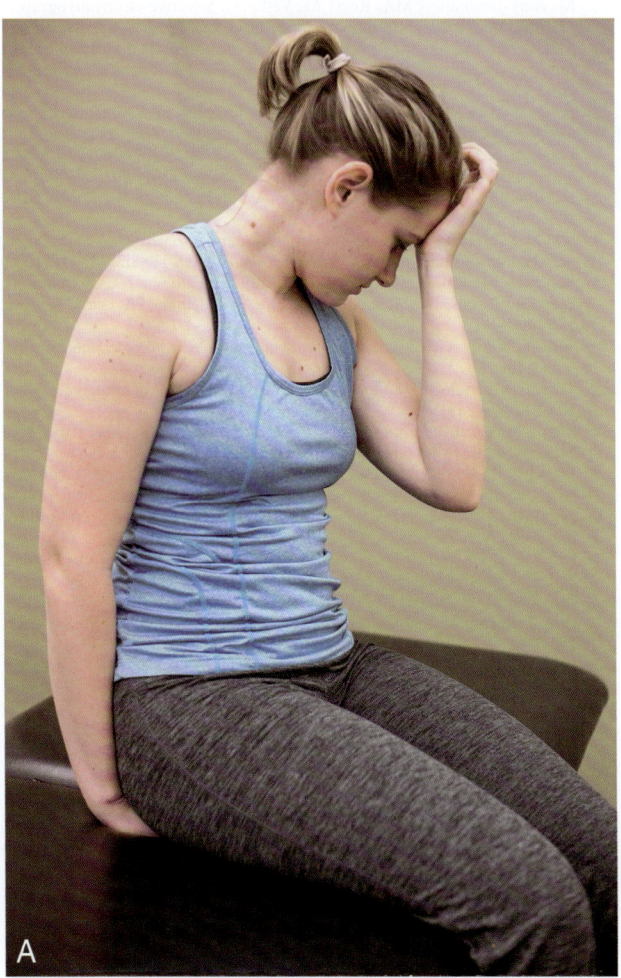
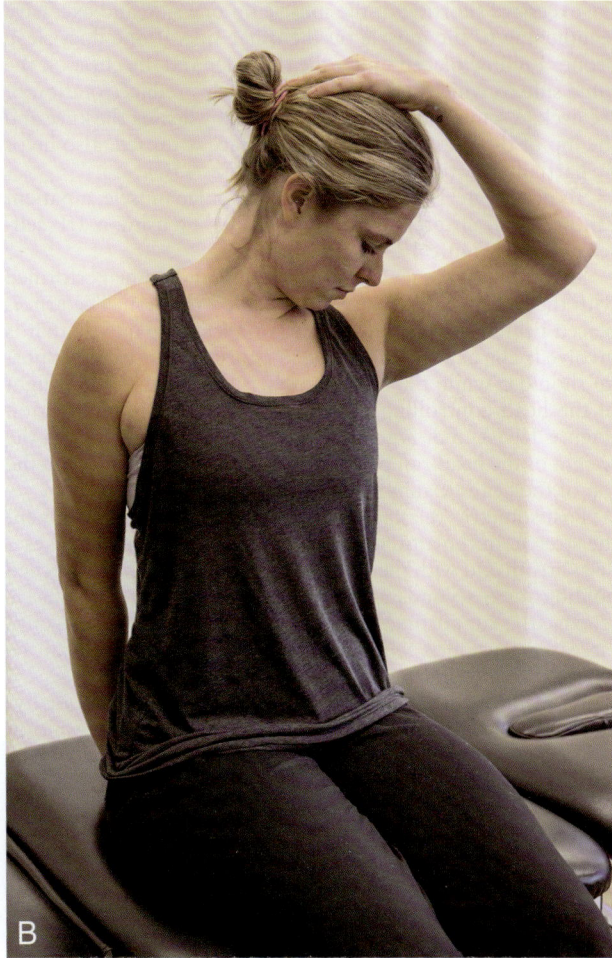

Figure 19-5. Self-stretch. A, Supporting the weight of the head. B, Augmenting the stretch with a gentle overpressure.

Individuals who talk on a phone frequently during the day should avoid holding the phone to the ear with the hand or shoulder. The most effective solution is a headset with a microphone or other hands-free technology that removes the need for prolonged levator scapulae activation.

When turning over in bed, the patient should roll the head on the pillow instead of lifting the head. When getting out of bed, the patient should roll onto one side and swing the legs off the bed to sit up, instead of pulling the trunk straight up because this action places additional strain on the levator scapulae muscles.

When using pillows at night to sleep, foam pillows tend to be more uncomfortable than softer pillows for patients with levator TrPs due to increased firmness and recoil. Pillows should not be placed under the shoulder but instead behind the neck to allow for proper support. Depending on the amount of kyphosis a patient has and the thickness of his or her pillows, 1 to 2 pillows should be appropriate. In a supine position, the proper thickness does not allow any extension of the head, but also does not place the head in excessive flexion, as this causes prolonged lengthening or shortening of the neck muscles during sleep. A small towel roll can be placed inside the pillowcase to support the neck in a neutral position, placing the face parallel to the ceiling. The patient can tuck the corner of the pillow between the shoulder and the chin (see Figure 7-5A) but not under the shoulder. For sleeping on the side, the pillow should be thick enough to keep the head and neck in a neutral position so that the head is not bent excessively to either side as this causes excessive lengthening of the muscle on the top side and excessive shortening of the muscle on the pillow side. The patient can tuck the corner of the pillow between the shoulder and the chin in the side-lying position as well (see Figure 7-5B) but not under the shoulder. Sleeping prone should be avoided due to the excessive shorting of the muscle on one side and excessive lengthening of the muscle on the other side. If one does sleep prone, a pillow placed under the shoulder and the chest on the same side to which the face is turned helps reduce rotation of the neck. A semiprone position, achieved by flexing the knee and the hip of the side toward which the face is turned, also helps by partially rotating the torso (see Figure 7-5C).

To deactivate TrPs in the levator scapulae muscle, a patient can perform self-pressure release of TrPs by using a TrP self-release tool (Figure 19-4A and B).

Stretching of the levator scapulae muscle can be performed with the patient in the seated or standing position. The arm is placed behind the back for the levator scapulae muscle that is involved. The head, is then rotated and side-bent to the opposite shoulder while the hand on that side supports the weight of the head controlling head motion in a forward direction (Figure 19-5A). For a greater stretch, the hand supporting the weight of the head can be taken away and placed lightly on the top of the head to augment the stretch (Figure 19-5B).

Postisometric relaxation may also be utilized to augment the stretch. In the aforementioned position the patient takes a deep breath and with their eyes looks to the side being stretched holding for 6 seconds and slowly exhaling. Once the muscle relaxes, the supporting hand can slowly lower the head until increased tension is felt in the muscle. This technique can be repeated 3 to 6 times.

As mentioned previously, UCS results in facilitated or hypertonic levator scapulae muscles. This condition also results in weakened or inhibited lower trapezius and deep cervical flexor muscles. Strengthening or activation of these muscles in addition to stretching of the levator scapulae muscles is essential.

References

1. Standring S. *Gray's Anatomy: The Anatomical Basis of Clinical Practice.* 41st ed. London, UK: Elsevier; 2015.
2. Kamibayashi LK, Richmond FJ. Morphometry of human neck muscles. *Spine.* 1998;23(12):1314-1323.
3. Macbeth RA, Martin CP. A note on the levator scapulae muscle in man. *Anat Rec.* 1953;115(4):691-696.
4. Menachem A, Kaplan O, Dekel S. Levator scapulae syndrome: an anatomic-clinical study. *Bull Hosp Jt Dis.* 1993;53(1):21-24.
5. Loukas M, Louis RG Jr, Merbs W. A case of atypical insertion of the levator scapulae. *Folia Morphol (Warsz).* 2006;65(3):232-235.
6. Chotai PN, Loukas M, Tubbs RS. Unusual origin of the levator scapulae muscle from mastoid process. *Surg Radiol Anat.* 2015;37(10):1277-1281.
7. Bergman RA. Anatomy atlases. An anatomy digital library. 2015. http://www.anatomyatlases.org/. Revised January 5, 2017.
8. Frank DK, Wenk E, Stern JC, Gottlieb RD, Moscatello AL. A cadaveric study of the motor nerves to the levator scapulae muscle. *Otolaryngol Head Neck Surg.* 1997;117(6):671-680.
9. Tubbs RS, Tyler-Kabara EC, Aikens AC, et al. Surgical anatomy of the dorsal scapular nerve. *J Neurosurg.* 2005;102(5):910-911.
10. Nguyen VH, Liu HH, Rosales A, Reeves R. A cadaveric investigation of the dorsal scapular nerve. *Anat Res Int.* 2016;2016:4106981.
11. Huelke DF. A study of the transverse cervical and dorsal scapular arteries. *Anat Rec.* 1958;132(3):233-245.
12. Smith R, Sanders WJ, Stewart KC. Blood supply to the levator scapulae muscle relative to carotid artery protection. *Trans Am Acad Ophthalmol Otolaryngol.* 1974;78(3):ORL128-ORL134.
13. De Freitas V, Vitti M, Furlani J. Electromyographic analysis of the levator scapulae and rhomboideus major muscle in movements of the shoulder. *Electromyogr Clin Neurophysiol.* 1979;19(4):335-342.
14. De Freitas V, Vitti M, Furlani J. Electromyographic study of levator scapulae and rhomboideus major muscles in movements of the shoulder and arm. *Electromyogr Clin Neurophysiol.* 1980;20(3):205-216.
15. Behrsin JF, Maguire K. Levator scapulae action during shoulder movement: a possible mechanism for shoulder pain of cervical origin. *Aust J Physiother.* 1986;32(2):101-106.
16. Ludewig PM, Cook TM, Nawoczenski DA. Three-dimensional scapular orientation and muscle activity at selected positions of humeral elevation. *J Orthop Sports Phys Ther.* 1996;24(2):57-65.
17. Escamilla RF, Andrews JR. Shoulder muscle recruitment patterns and related biomechanics during upper extremity sports. *Sports Med.* 2009;39(7):569-590.
18. Magnusson ML, Pope MH, Hasselquist L, et al. Cervical electromyographic activity during low-speed rear impact. *Eur Spine J.* 1999;8(2):118-125.
19. Olafsdottir JM, Brolin K, Blouin JS, Siegmund GP. Dynamic spatial tuning of cervical muscle reflexes to multidirectional seated perturbations. *Spine.* 2015;40(4):E211-E219.
20. Mayoux-Benhamou MA, Revel M, Vallee C. Selective electromyography of dorsal neck muscles in humans. *Exp Brain Res.* 1997;113(2):353-360.
21. McLean L. The effect of postural correction on muscle activation amplitudes recorded from the cervicobrachial region. *J Electromyogr Kinesiol.* 2005;15(6):527-535.
22. Janda V. Muscles and cervicogenic pain syndromes. In: Grant R, ed. *Physiotherapy of the Cervical and Thoracic Spine*. New York, NY: Churchill Livingstone; 1988.
23. Simons DG, Travell J, Simons L. *Travell & Simon's Myofascial Pain and Dysfunction: The Trigger Point Manual.* Vol 1. 2nd ed. Baltimore, MD: Williams & Wilkins; 1999:104.
24. Schuldt K, Harms-Ringdahl K. Activity levels during isometric test contractions of neck and shoulder muscles. *Scand J Rehabil Med.* 1988;20(3):117-127.
25. Bonica J. Neck pain, Chapter 47. In: Bonica JJ, Loeser JD, Chapman C, Fordyce WE, eds. *The Management of Pain*. Philadelphia, PA: Lea & Febiger; 1990:848-867.
26. Sola AE, Williams RL. Myofascial pain syndromes. *Neurology.* 1956;6(2):91-95 (p. 93, Fig. 1).
27. Travell J, Rinzler SH. The myofascial genesis of pain. *Postgrad Med.* 1952;11(5):425-434.
28. Kraus H. *Clinical Treatment of Back and Neck Pain*. New York, NY: McGraw-Hill; 1970: page 98.
29. Travell J. Rapid relief of acute stiff neck by ethyl chloride spray. *J Am Med Womens Assoc.* 1949;4(3):89-95 (pp. 92-93, Fig. 3, Case 1).
30. Zohn DA. *Musculoskeletal Pain: Diagnosis and Physical Treatment*. 2nd ed. Boston, MA: Little Brown; 1988 (Fig. 12-1).
31. Lewit K. *Manipulative Therapy in Rehabilitation of the Locomotor System*. 2nd ed. Oxford, England: Butterworth Heinemann; 1991:195, 196.
32. Grosshandler SL, Stratas NE, Toomey TC, Gray WF. Chronic neck and shoulder pain. Focusing on myofascial origins. *Postgrad Med.* 1985;77(3):149-151, 154-148.
33. Sola AE, Rodenberger ML, Gettys BB. Incidence of hypersensitive areas in posterior shoulder muscles; a survey of two hundred young adults. *Am J Phys Med.* 1955;34(6):585-590.
34. Sola AE, Kuitert JH. Myofascial trigger point pain in the neck and shoulder girdle; report of 100 cases treated by injection of normal saline. *Northwest Med.* 1955;54(9):980-984.
35. Fernández de las Peñas C, Grobli C, Ortega-Santiago R, et al. Referred pain from myofascial trigger points in head, neck, shoulder, and arm muscles reproduces pain symptoms in blue-collar (manual) and white-collar (office) workers. *Clin J Pain.* 2012;28(6):511-518.
36. Cerezo-Tellez E, Torres-Lacomba M, Mayoral-Del Moral O, Sanchez-Sanchez B, Dommerholt J, Gutierrez-Ortega C. Prevalence of myofascial pain syndrome in chronic non-specific neck pain: a population-based cross-sectional descriptive study. *Pain Med.* 2016;17(12):2369-2377.
37. Fernández de las Peñas C, Alonso-Blanco C, Miangolarra JC. Myofascial trigger points in subjects presenting with mechanical neck pain: a blinded, controlled study. *Man Ther.* 2007;12(1):29-33.
38. Campa-Moran I, Rey-Gudin E, Fernandez-Carnero J, et al. Comparison of dry needling versus orthopedic manual therapy in patients with myofascial

chronic neck pain: a single-blind, randomized pilot study. *Pain Res Treat.* 2015;2015:327307.
39. Neoh CA. Treating subjective shortness of breath by inactivating trigger points of levator scapulae muscles with acupuncture needles. *J Musculoskelet Pain.* 1996;4(3):81-85.
40. Goodman CC, Snyder TEK. *Differential Diagnosis for Physical Therapists: Screening for Referral.* 5th ed. St. Louis, MO: Saunders Elsevier; 2013.
41. Ludewig PM, Cook TM. The effect of head position on scapular orientation and muscle activity during shoulder elevation. *J Occup Rehabil.* 1996;6(3):147-158.
42. Cook C. *Orthopedic Manual Therapy: An Evidence Based Approach.* 2nd ed. Upper Saddle River, NJ: Pearson Education; 2012.
43. Lawrence RL, Braman JP, Laprade RF, Ludewig PM. Comparison of 3-dimensional shoulder complex kinematics in individuals with and without shoulder pain, part 1: sternoclavicular, acromioclavicular, and scapulothoracic joints. *J Orthop Sports Phys Ther.* 2014;44(9):636-645, A631-A638.
44. Ludewig PM, Cook TM. Alterations in shoulder kinematics and associated muscle activity in people with symptoms of shoulder impingement. *Phys Ther.* 2000;80(3):276-291.
45. Inman VT, Saunders M, Abbot LC. Observations on the function of the shoulder joint. *J Bone Joint Surg.* 1944;26(1):1-30.
46. Hidalgo-Lozano A, Fernández de las Peñas C, Alonso-Blanco C, Ge HY, Arendt-Nielsen L, Arroyo-Morales M. Muscle trigger points and pressure pain hyperalgesia in the shoulder muscles in patients with unilateral shoulder impingement: a blinded, controlled study. *Exp Brain Res.* 2010;202(4):915-925.
47. Ibarra JM, Ge HY, Wang C, Martinez Vizcaino V, Graven-Nielsen T, Arendt-Nielsen L. Latent myofascial trigger points are associated with an increased antagonistic muscle activity during agonist muscle contraction. *J Pain.* 2011;12(12):1282-1288.
48. Michele AA, Eisenberg J. Scapulocostal syndrome. *Arch Phys Med Rehabil.* 1968;49(7):383-387 (pp. 385, 386, Fig. 4).
49. Michele AA, Davies JJ, Krueger FJ, Lichtor JM. Scapulocostal syndrome (fatigue-postural paradox). *N Y State J Med.* 1950;50:1353-1356 (p. 1355, Fig. 4).
50. Pace JB. Commonly overlooked pain syndromes responsive to simple therapy. *Postgrad Med.* 1975;58(4):107-113 (p. 110).
51. Gerwin RD, Dommerholt J, Shah JP. An expansion of Simons' integrated hypothesis of trigger point formation. *Curr Pain Headache Rep.* 2004;8(6):468-475.
52. Ettlin T, Schuster C, Stoffel R, Bruderlin A, Kischka U. A distinct pattern of myofascial findings in patients after whiplash injury. *Arch Phys Med Rehabil.* 2008;89(7):1290-1293.
53. Castaldo M, Ge HY, Chiarotto A, Villafane JH, Arendt-Nielsen L. Myofascial trigger points in patients with whiplash-associated disorders and mechanical neck pain. *Pain Med.* 2014;15(5):842-849.
54. Fernandez-Perez AM, Villaverde-Gutierrez C, Mora-Sanchez A, Alonso-Blanco C, Sterling M, Fernández de las Peñas C. Muscle trigger points, pressure pain threshold, and cervical range of motion in patients with high level of disability related to acute whiplash injury. *J Orthop Sports Phys Ther.* 2012;42(7):634-641.
55. Cailliet R. *Neck and Arm Pain.* Philadelphia, PA: F.A. Davis; 1964: page 97.
56. Baker B. The muscle trigger: evidence of overload injury. *J Neurol Orthop Med Surg.* 1986;7(1):35-44.
57. Hong C-Z. Considerations and recommendations regarding myofascial trigger point injection. *J Musculoske Pain.* 1994;2(1):29-59.
58. Hsieh YL, Kao MJ, Kuan TS, Chen SM, Chen JT, Hong CZ. Dry needling to a key myofascial trigger point may reduce the irritability of satellite MTrPs. *Am J Phys Med Rehabil.* 2007;86(5):397-403.
59. Waldman SD. *Atlas of Uncommon Pain Syndromes.* 3rd ed. Philadelphia, PA: Elsevier Saunders; 2014.
60. Mills RR, Pagan FL. Patient considerations in the treatment of cervical dystonia: focus on botulinum toxin type A. *Patient Prefer Adherence.* 2015;9:725-731.
61. Albanese A, Bhatia K, Bressman SB, et al. Phenomenology and classification of dystonia: a consensus update. *Mov Dis.* 2013;28(7):863-873.
62. Jankovic J, Leder S, Warner D, Schwartz K. Cervical dystonia: clinical findings and associated movement disorders. *Neurology.* 1991;41(7):1088-1091.
63. Fernández de las Peñas C, Ge HY, Alonso-Blanco C, Gonzalez-Iglesias J, Arendt-Nielsen L. Referred pain areas of active myofascial trigger points in head, neck, and shoulder muscles, in chronic tension type headache. *J Bodyw Mov Ther.* 2010;14(4):391-396.
64. Fernández de las Peñas C, Cuadrado ML, Pareja JA. Myofascial trigger points, neck mobility and forward head posture in unilateral migraine. *Cephalalgia.* 2006;26(9):1061-1070.
65. Bogduk N. The anatomical basis for cervicogenic headache. *J Manipulative Physiol Ther.* 1992;15(1):67-70.
66. Moore MK. Upper crossed syndrome and its relationship to cervicogenic headache. *J Manipulative Physiol Ther.* 2004;27(6):414-420.
67. Fukui S, Ohseto K, Shiotani M, et al. Referred pain distribution of the cervical zygapophyseal joints and cervical dorsal rami. *Pain.* 1996;68(1):79-83.
68. Burkhart SS, Morgan CD, Kibler WB. The disabled throwing shoulder: spectrum of pathology Part III: the SICK scapula, scapular dyskinesis, the kinetic chain, and rehabilitation. *Arthroscopy.* 2003;19(6):641-661.
69. Timmons MK, Thigpen CA, Seitz AL, Karduna AR, Arnold BL, Michener LA. Scapular kinematics and subacromial-impingement syndrome: a meta-analysis. *J Sport Rehabil.* 2012;21(4):354-370.
70. Cook C, Burgess-Limerick R, Papalia S. The effect of upper extremity support on upper extremity posture and muscle activity during keyboard use. *Appl Ergon.* 2004;35(3):285-292.
71. Hoyle JA, Marras WS, Sheedy JE, Hart DE. Effects of postural and visual stressors on myofascial trigger point development and motor unit rotation during computer work. *J Electromyogr Kinesiol.* 2011;21(1):41-48.

Chapter 20

Scalene Muscles

"Pseudo-Radiculopathy"

Joseph M. Donnelly and Ingrid Allstrom Anderson

1. INTRODUCTION

The scalene muscles and the associated thoracic outlet entrapment syndrome (TOS) are often overlooked as a source of symptoms in patients with primary reports of pain, paresthesias, or dysesthesias in the upper extremity (UE). The scalene muscles have attachments throughout the cervical spine and to the first through the third ribs. All the scalene muscles are innervated by motor branches of the anterior primary divisions of spinal nerves C2 through C7 according to the segmental level of muscular attachment. Functionally, the scalene muscles stabilize the cervical spine against lateral movement and are well situated to elevate and stabilize the first and the second ribs during inhalation. The scalene muscles are one of 13 muscle groups that can refer pain to the medial border of the scapula. Referred pain from the scalene muscles can radiate anteriorly into the pectoral region; posteriorly to the medial border of the scapula; and laterally down the posterior arm, radial aspect of the forearm, and into the thumb and index finger. Patients may report pain as well as sensory and motor disturbances due to neurovascular entrapment. Distinctively, pain on the radial aspect of the hand is indicative of scalene involvement, whereas pain on the ulnar side of the hand with associated puffiness suggests brachial plexus and subclavian vein entrapment. Activation of scalene trigger points (TrPs) may result from excessive pulling and pushing, sporting activities, or chronic persistent coughing. Differential diagnosis includes C5-C6 radicular pain or radiculopathy, TOS, carpal tunnel syndrome, cervical spine dysfunction, and the first and/or second rib articular dysfunction. Entrapment of the lower trunk of the brachial plexus is a common result of TrPs in the scalenus anterior and medius muscles which can cause referred pain, paresthesia, and dysesthesia in an ulnar distribution in the UE and hand. Patients should be instructed on proper diaphragmatic breathing to decrease loading of the scalene muscles. Counsel regarding effective posture and positioning in sitting, standing, and lying positions is paramount to eliminate postural muscle strain. Ergonomic assessment of the work station is essential along with proper neck-stretching exercises and maintenance of adequate body warmth.

2. ANATOMIC CONSIDERATIONS

The scalene muscles consist of three muscle pairs located on the lateral aspect of the neck, posteromedial, and deep to the sternocleidomastoid (SCM) muscles. These muscles have a considerable variety in their fiber direction and attachments, but they also have varying lengths and functions. Because of these anatomic differences, each of the scalene muscles are addressed individually in the following.

Scalenus Anterior

The scalenus anterior muscle originates from the anterior tubercles on the transverse processes of vertebrae C3 through C6. The fibers blend and travel inferolaterally to insert into the scalene tubercle on the inner border of the first rib and on the upper surface anterior to the groove for the subclavian artery (Figure 20-1).[1] The scalenus anterior muscle serves as an important landmark in the anterior neck as there are several important anatomic structures in this region. The phrenic nerve passes anterior to the scalenus anterior muscle. Posteriorly, the suprapleural membrane and pleura, the cervical roots of the brachial plexus, and the subclavian artery all separate the scalenus anterior muscle from the scalenus medius muscle. The vertebral artery and vein pass to and from the transverse foramen of the sixth cervical vertebrae just below the muscle's attachment to C6 medially between the longus colli muscle and scalenus anterior muscle.[1]

Scalenus Medius

The scalenus medius muscle is the largest and the longest of the scalene muscles and originates from the posterior tubercles on the transverse processes of vertebrae C2 through C7 and occasionally to C1. The muscle slants diagonally and inserts onto the cranial surface of the first rib, posteriorly to, and partly deep to, the groove for the subclavian artery (Figure 20-1). A slip of the muscle sometimes extends to the second rib. As noted above, in the scalenus anterior muscle these two muscles are separated by the subclavian artery and the ventral rami of the cervical nerve roots. Anteriorly, the clavicle and the omohyoid muscle cross over this muscle. The SCM muscle crosses posterolateral and the levator scapula and scalenus posterior muscles lie posterior to the scalenus medius muscle.[1] The anterior rami of C4, C5 C6, and C7 pierce the scalenus medius muscle in route to form the dorsal scapular nerve and thoracodorsal nerve, respectively.[1]

Scalenus Posterior

The scalenus posterior muscle is the smallest and the deepest of the scalene muscles. This muscle originates from the posterior tubercles on the transverse processes of C4, C5, and C6, and inserts onto the lateral surface of the second rib just posterior to the attachment of the serratus anterior muscle and occasionally to the third rib. The scalenus posterior muscle crosses the first rib posterior to the scalenus medius muscle and deep to the anterior borders of the upper trapezius and levator scapulae muscles (Figure 20-1).

Scalenus Minimus

All the scalene muscles are variable in their attachments. The most variable is the scalenus minimus muscle that occurred on at least one side of the body in one third to three quarters of the

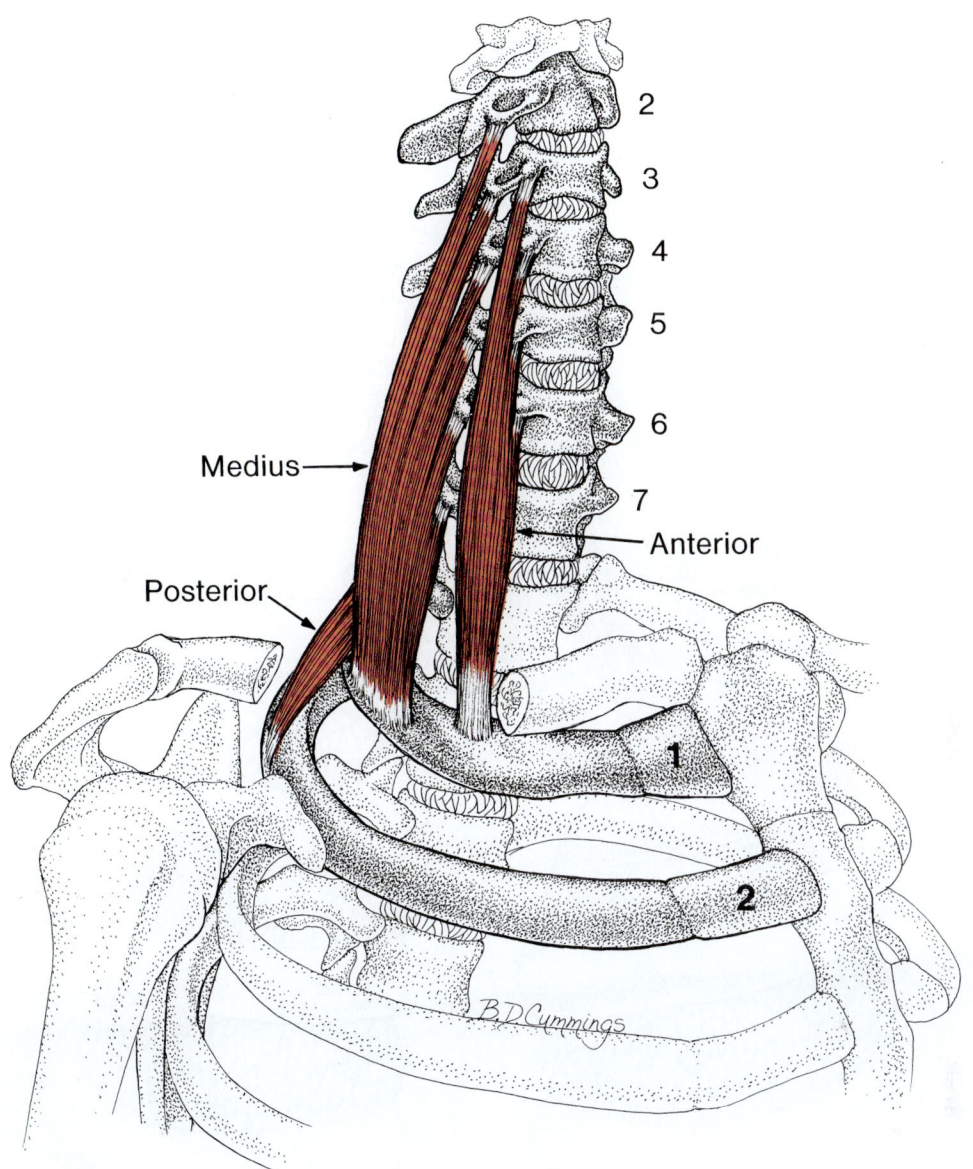

Figure 20-1. Oblique view of the attachments of the three major scalene muscles to the cervical vertebrae and to the first and the second ribs. The clavicle has been cut and the section that overlies the scalene muscles removed.

individuals studied.[2-4] This muscle usually originates from the anterior tubercle on the transverse process of vertebra C7, and sometimes also C6. It inserts onto the fascia supporting the pleural dome and beyond to the inner border of the first rib. The muscle lies deep to the scalenus anterior muscle and attaches posterior to the groove for the subclavian artery (Figure 20-2). The pleural dome, or cupola, is strengthened by the suprapleural membrane (Sibson's fascia) and anchored by this membrane to the anterior tubercle of C7 and the inner border of the first rib. The scalenus minimus muscle reinforces this fascia and can be up to 10 mm in diameter but is often much smaller.[1,2,4]

The scalenus minimus passes beneath and behind the subclavian artery to attach to the first rib, whereas the anterior scalene muscle passes over and in front of the artery (Figure 20-2).[4]

2.1. Innervation and Vascularization

All the scalene muscles are innervated by motor branches of the anterior primary divisions of spinal nerves C2 through C7 according to the segmental level of muscular attachment. The scalenus anterior muscle is specifically innervated by the anterior primary rami of C4-C6 nerves. The scalenus medius muscle is innervated by the anterior primary rami of C3-C8 nerves. The scalenus posterior and scalenus minimus muscles are innervated by the anterior primary rami of C6-C8 nerves.[1]

The vascular supply of all the scalene muscles comes from the ascending branch of the inferior thyroid artery. The scalenus posterior muscle also receives vascular supply from the superficial cervical artery.[1]

2.2. Function

The scalene muscles function to stabilize the cervical spine against lateral movement, and they serve a primary role in respiration. Their specific actions are dependent on whether they are fixed from below or from above.

Fixed From Below

Acting unilaterally, the scalene muscles laterally flex the cervical spine,[1,5] and when stimulated, they flex the head obliquely forward and sideways.[6] All four scalene muscles are poorly placed

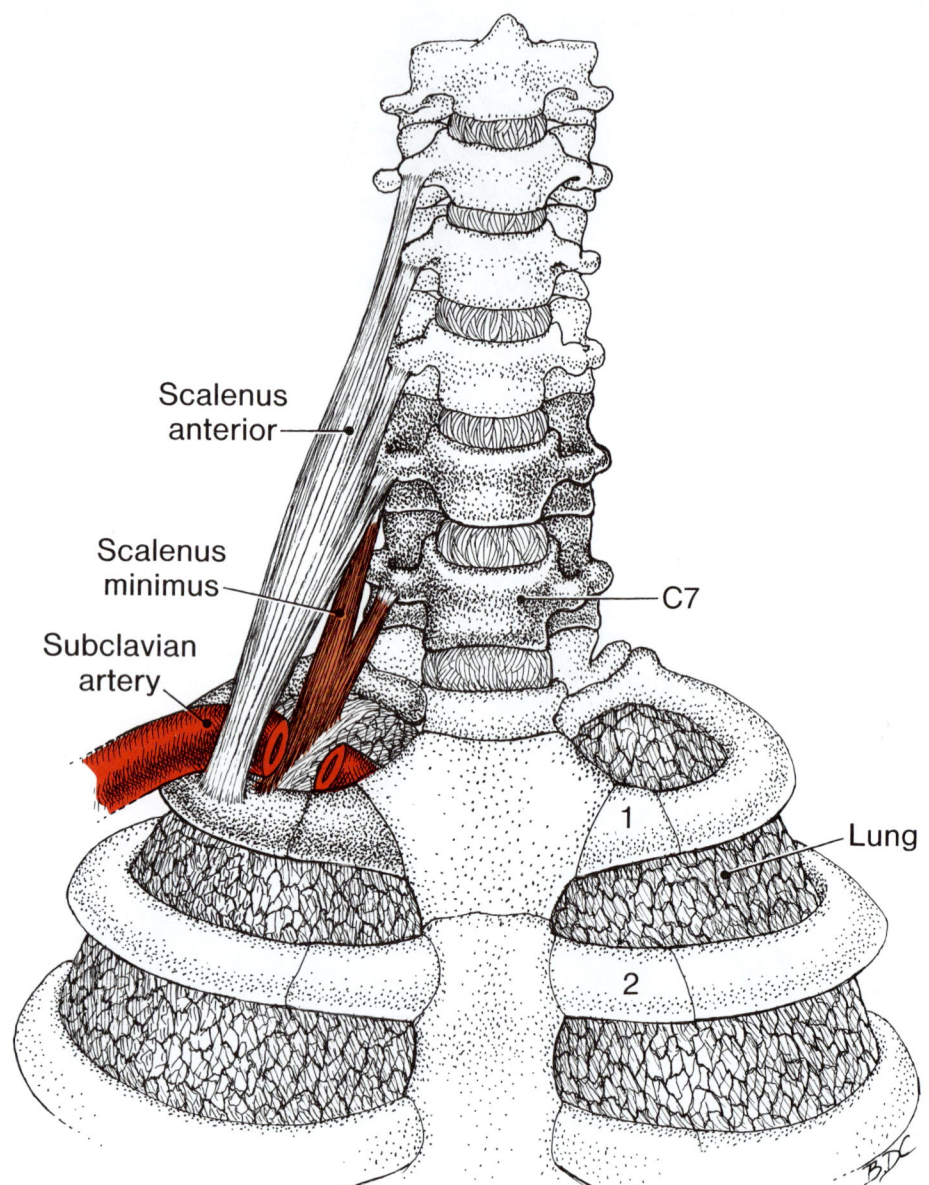

Figure 20-2. Anterior view of the attachments of the scalenus minimus muscle (medium red), which lies behind the dark red subclavian artery (cut), whereas the scalenus anterior muscle lies in front of the artery. The artery passes over the first rib between these two muscles. Note how high into this region the dome of the pleura extends, where it is vulnerable to needle penetration.

to influence rotation of the neck significantly. Acting bilaterally, the anterior scalene muscles assist in neck flexion.[1] In a study by Olinger and Homier,[7] seven cadaver specimens were examined using a mechanical approach to determine the function of the scalene muscles, specifically during cervical rotation. They concur with other authors that the primary function of the scalene muscles is to laterally flex the cervical spine ipsilaterally when contracting unilaterally and to assist with flexion of the cervical spine when acting bilaterally. Their model supports the notion that the anterior, middle, and posterior scalene muscles rotate the cervical spine ipsilaterally. Without stabilization of the cervical spine, the scalene muscles laterally flex the cervical spine ipsilaterally and elevate the first and the second ribs.[7] The much flatter angle of the scalenus posterior muscle makes it especially suited to stabilizing the base of the neck by controlling transverse forces in a manner similar to the lowest diagonal fibers of the quadratus lumborum muscle at the base of the lumbar spine.

Fixed From Above

The scalene muscles have long been recognized as important auxiliary muscles of respiration and are more commonly used for respiration than are the SCM muscles.[8,9] Electromyographic and muscle stimulation evidence supports elevation of the first and the second ribs during inspiration as a primary function, not just an accessory inspiratory function, especially the scalenus medius muscle.[1,6,10] The scalene muscles are active in normal quiet inhalation, though activation may be higher in those with a costal breathing pattern versus diaphragmatic breathing.[11,12] Scalenotomy causes an immediate decrease in the vital capacity, but considerable recovery occurs later.[8] When present, the scalenus minimus should also be effective for inhalation which may explain its hypertrophy in some persons. The scalene muscles often contract to stabilize the cervical spine when people carry, lift, or pull heavy objects.

> **Box 20-1** Functional unit of the scalene muscle
>
> | Action | Synergists | Antagonist |
> |---|---|---|
> | Cervical lateral flexion | Sternocleidomastoid
Longissimus capitis
Cervical multifidi | Scalenes (contralateral)
Sternocleidomastoid (contralateral) |
> | Inspiration | Diaphragm
External intercostal
Sternocleidomastoid | Rectus abdominis
External abdominal oblique
Internal abdominal oblique
Internal intercostal |

2.3. Functional Unit

The functional unit to which a muscle belongs includes the muscles that reinforce and counter its actions as well as the joints that the muscle crosses. The interdependence of these structures functionally is reflected in the organization and neural connections of the sensory motor cortex. The functional unit is emphasized because the presence of a TrP in one muscle of the unit increases the likelihood that the other muscles of the unit also develops TrPs. When inactivating TrPs in a muscle, one should be concerned about TrPs that may develop in muscles that are functionally interdependent. Box 20-1 grossly represents the functional unit of the scalene muscles.[13]

During labored breathing, the upper trapezius,[8] levator scapulae, and omohyoid muscles can assist inhalation by elevation of the shoulder that helps lift the weight of the shoulder girdle off the chest wall. The pectoralis minor muscle has a synergistic function with the scalene muscles for the elevation of the ribs when the scapula is stabilized.[8]

3. CLINICAL PRESENTATION

3.1. Referred Pain Pattern

Trigger points in the anterior, medial, or posterior scalene muscles may refer pain anteriorly to the chest, laterally to the upper limb, and posteriorly to the medial scapular border and adjacent interscapular region (Figure 20-3A).[9,14,15] It is important to remember that any one of the scalene muscles can produce any part of the referred pain pattern.

Posteriorly, pain is commonly referred from TrPs in the scalenus anterior muscle to the back, over the upper half of the vertebral border of the scapula, and to the adjacent interscapular region.[16] When the patient presents with posterior shoulder pain, particularly along the border of the scapula, one should be sure to check for scalene TrPs as they are one of the most common sources of this type of pain reported by patients.

Anteriorly, persistent aching pain is referred in two finger-like projections over the pectoral region down to about the nipple level.[17] This pattern commonly originates in the lower part of the scalenus medius or scalenus posterior muscle. Scalene pain referred to the anterior shoulder region is not characteristically described as deep in the joint, as is the pain referred from the infraspinatus muscle. It is often described as a tightness or a grabbing sensation, and on the left side of the thorax, this TrP referred pain may be mistaken for angina pectoris because it is likely to be associated with muscular activity.

Referred pain from the scalene muscles may extend down the front and back of the arm (over the biceps and triceps brachii muscles).[16] The referred pain often skips the elbow and reappears in the radial side of the forearm, the thumb, and the index finger. This upper limb pattern arises from TrPs in the scalenus anterior and scalenus medius muscles.

The less frequently seen pain referred from TrPs in the variable scalenus minimus muscle projects strongly to the thumb (Figure 20-3B). This pain covers the lateral aspect of the arm from the deltoid insertion to the elbow but skips the elbow to cover the dorsum of the forearm, wrist, hand, and all the five digits, accenting the thumb. Trigger points may refer a sensation that the patient describes as "numbness" of the thumb with or without demonstrable hypoesthesia to cold or touch.

Experimental injection of 0.2 to 0.5 mL of a 6% solution of sodium chloride into the scalenus anterior in seven subjects evoked referred pain primarily in the shoulder region in all subjects, pain down the arm in one subject, and a superficial hyperesthesia radiating upward over the neck in two subjects.[18]

3.2. Symptoms

Scalene TrPs should be considered as a source of symptoms in patients presenting with UE pain, paresthesias, or dysesthesias because TrPs in these muscles are a common source of neck, shoulder, and arm pain. Pain arising from TrPs in the scalene muscles is often under-diagnosed or misdiagnosed.[19,20] The most common diagnoses for symptoms associated with scalene myofascial pain is cervical disc pathology, cervical spondylosis, and TOS. Symptoms related to TOS are thoroughly addressed in Chapter 33. All these aforementioned conditions can cause neck and UE pain, paresthesias, and/or dysesthesias. Although scalene TrPs only occasionally refer pain to the head, they are commonly associated with TrPs in other muscles that do and therefore should be considered when a patient reports neck and head pain. In patients who report shoulder, medial border of scapula, and UE symptoms, TrPs in the scalene muscles should be considered. Patients may report pain and paresthesias that radiate into the lateral aspect of the hand. When the primary patient report is of UE pain that mimics C4-C7 radicular symptoms, the scalene muscles (especially the scalenus anterior and medius muscles) should be considered for specific examination.[20]

In a study by Jaeger et al, more than half of 11 patients with cervicogenic headache also had associated active scalene TrPs that contributed to their pain.[21] In an another recent study, increased mechanical sensitivity in the scalene muscles was noted in women with migraine headaches.[22] Of 72 patients with nontraumatic shoulder pain, active and latent TrPs were found in 12 and 17 individuals, respectively.[23] In a patient with a UE amputation, this referred pattern of the upper limb pain produced severe phantom limb pain that was relieved by one author[24] by the inactivation of scalene TrPs. Sherman[25] lists the elimination of TrPs as one treatment for relief of phantom limb pain.

When the patient reports pain in the upper back just medial to the superior angle of the scapula, the most likely myofascial source of these symptoms is a scalene TrP. Patients with TrPs in the scalene muscles sometimes speak of their "shoulder" pain while indicating the upper half of the arm. Sleep is often

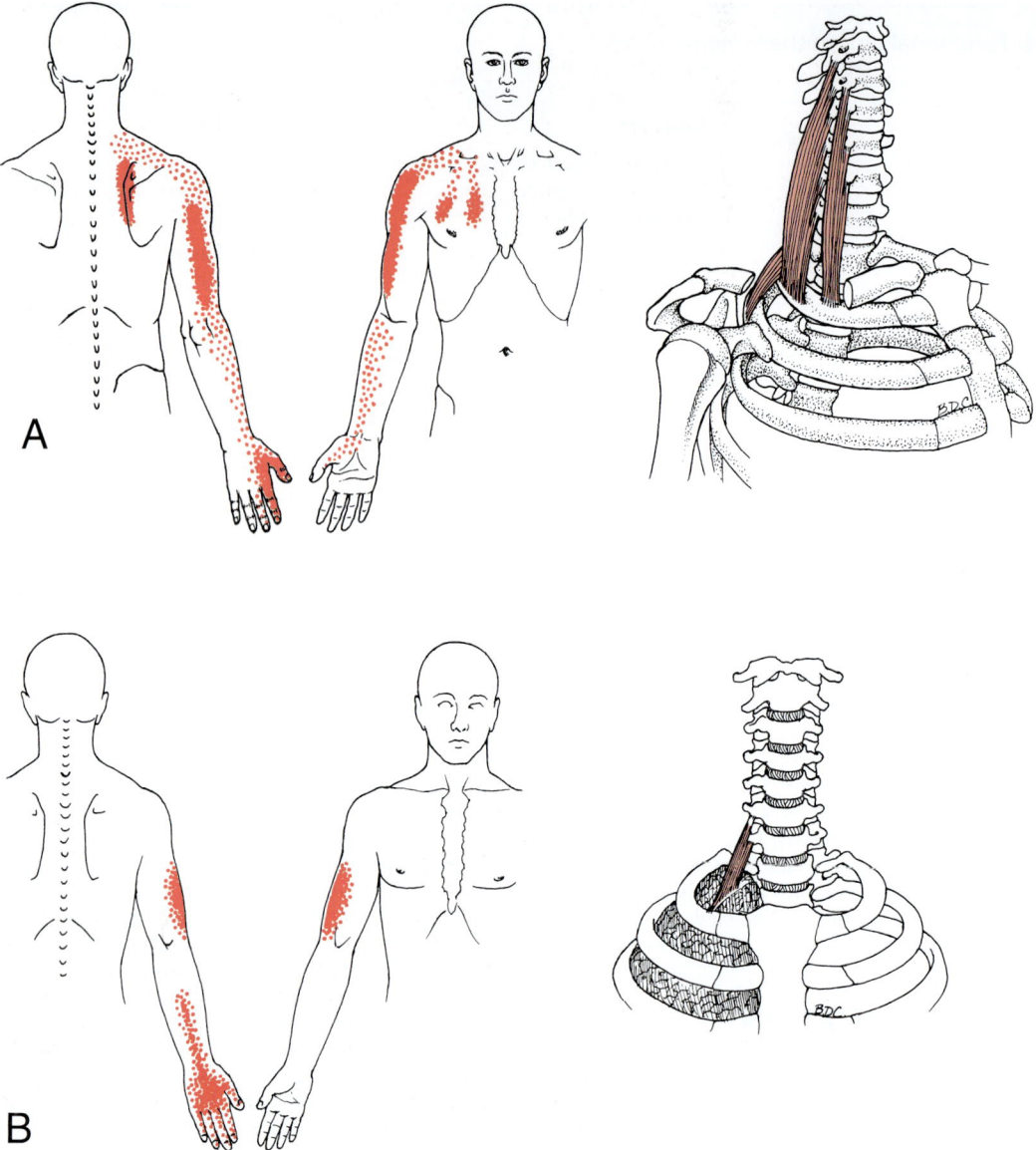

Figure 20-3. Composite pain patterns (solid red areas are the essential pain reference zones, and stippled red areas are the spillover reference zones) in the right scalene muscles (medium red). A, Scalenus anterior, medius, and posterior. Some TrPs may have only one essential reference zone. B, Scalenus minimus.

disturbed by pain. When the night pain is severe, the patient is likely to sleep sitting up on a sofa or propped up on pillows for relief. This position helps prevent the sustained shortening of the scalene muscles that tends to occur when the patient lies flat and the chest and the shoulders are elevated during sleep, particularly with an inappropriate pillow.

Neurologic symptoms of numbness and tingling in the hand (chiefly in the ulnar distribution) and the unexpected dropping of objects from the hand can result from the entrapment of the lower trunk of the brachial plexus. It exits the thorax by hooking over the first rib, indicating possible compression of the neurovascular bundle by the pectoralis minor muscle (refer to Chapter 33 for more clinical considerations).

Patients may also report swelling in the hand that, when present, appears diffusely distal to the wrist, particularly over the bases of the four fingers and the dorsum of the hand. Patients are likely to experience puffiness of the dorsum of the hand, stiffness of the fingers, and tightness of rings on fingers especially in the morning on waking. These symptoms are likely to be caused by entrapment of the subclavian vein and/or lymph duct as they pass across the first rib in front of the attachment of the scalenus anterior muscle. Scalene TrPs should be considered as a contributing factor to this entrapment. The swelling or reported puffiness may dissipate later in the day. The associated stiffness of the fingers is not solely due to the edema but also to myofascial tautness of the finger extensors that may have an autonomic reflex component.

3.3. Patient Examination

After a thorough subjective examination, the clinician should make a detailed drawing representing the pain pattern that the patient has described. This depiction will assist in planning the physical examination and can be useful in monitoring the progression of the patient as symptoms improve or change. In patients who report a history of falling or a motor vehicle accident, examination of the scalene and SCM muscles is a high priority. For proper examination of the scalene muscles, the clinician should observe head and neck postures, shoulder

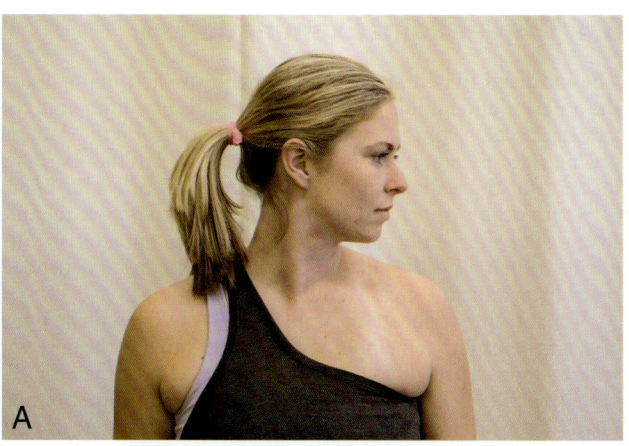 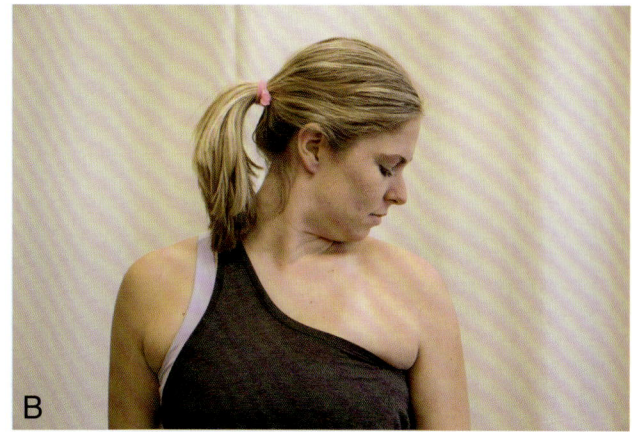

Figure 20-4. The Scalene Cramp Test elicits or increases pain from TrPs in the scalene muscles. A, The head rotates fully to the left side to test left scalene muscles. B, The chin dips down into the hollow behind the clavicle. This hard contraction in the shortened position of scalene muscles (with TrPs) causes a local ache at the TrP and pain that may be referred to a distance, as illustrated in Figure 20-3.

girdle posture, active and passive range of motion of the cervical spine, and the position and mobility of the first and the second ribs. It is extremely important to examine postures during functional activities because habitual postures or activities that require positioning the head off the center may overload the scalene muscles.

Cervical range of motion should be assessed using appropriate caution to avoid vertebral artery compromise. Neck rotation is painful only at the extreme range of motion to the same side, although it may not be painful because motion may be slightly restricted before the painful end range is reached. While the subject's neck is side-bent, the clinician should slowly and gently move the patient's head and neck into varying degrees of rotation. This maneuver often elicits increased pain or the report of a "tight feeling." If the patient is then instructed to point to the troublesome area, the clinician can use that as a starting point to palpate for TrPs. Side-bending of the neck to the opposite side is usually restricted if scalene TrPs are present. Scalene muscle involvement itself causes no restriction of motion at the glenohumeral joint, and pain is not significantly increased by tests of shoulder motion. However, the resultant first rib mobility deficits may cause a feeling of restricted shoulder elevation.

Scalene TrP activity alone causes a minimum restriction of neck rotation, whereas TrPs in the levator scapulae and splenius cervicis muscles markedly limit cervical rotation. Scalene TrPs are more closely associated with limited cervical side-bending and when moving the head in a combined cervical flexion, side-bending, and rotation pattern. Patients with a scalene myofascial pain syndrome tend to move the arm and neck restlessly, as if trying to relieve a "sore" muscle.

Diaphragmatic breathing should also be assessed because the scalene muscles function to elevate the first and the second ribs during inhalation. Inefficient respiration (chest breathing) is a contributing factor to scalene TrPs because this muscle activation pattern overly stresses the scalene muscles. In patients with chronic obstructive pulmonary disease, post bronchitis, or pneumonia, scalene TrPs are very common because the scalene muscles are overworked during inspiration.

Accessory joint motion should be tested in the cervical spine, the first and second ribs, acromioclavicular joint, sternoclavicular joint, and scapulothoracic joints. Seen clinically, joint hypomobility in the first and the second ribs can cause impairment in shoulder elevation contributing to alterations in normal muscle activation patterns. Articular dysfunctions in the cervical facet joints (C2-T1) and uncovertebral joints may also impair muscle activation patterns contributing to overload of the scalene muscles.

Travell and Simons described three tests they commonly utilized to identify scalene TrPs.[13] These tests include the scalene cramp test, scalene relief test, and the finger flexion test. The clinical utility of these tests have not been investigated; anecdotally, they appear to assist the clinician in the differential diagnosis of myofascial pain caused by scalene TrPs.

Scalene Cramp Test

To perform this test, the patient rotates the head fully to the side of the pain and actively pulls the chin down into the hollow above the clavicle by flexing the head and the neck (Figure 20-4), holding this position up to 60 seconds. During the last part of this movement, the anterior and the middle scalene muscles strongly contract while in the shortened position. This evokes a local cramp-like pain in the region of the TrP and may further activate the TrP causing continuing moderate or severe pain referred from it. If the patient was already in severe pain before attempting the test movement, the test result may not appear clearly positive because the patient does not perceive the additional pain caused by the test. In this situation of an existing severe pain, the Scalene Relief Test (Figure 20-5) should be tried first.

Scalene Relief Position

Referred pain from scalene TrPs may be relieved by the elevation of the arm and the clavicle[26] because this maneuver may remove pressure from structures traversing or attaching to the first rib (which can be elevated by TrP-shortened scalene muscles). The scalene relief position makes use of this principle. The patient places the painful forearm across the forehead while raising and pulling the shoulder *forward* to lift the clavicle off the underlying scalene muscles and brachial plexus (Figure 20-5). Pain relief, when it occurs, ensues immediately or within a few minutes. This position should not be confused with the shoulder abduction test as described by Wainner et al,[27] which is part of a test item cluster to rule in cervical radicular symptoms.

Finger Flexion Test

This test of finger flexion should be performed with the metacarpophalangeal (MCP) joints actively held straight in full extension. This position requires forceful contraction of the extensor digitorum muscle, but the tightly closed fist does not. The test is normal when the fingertips can firmly touch the volar pads of the MCP joints (Figure 20-6A). If one or more compartments of the extensor digitorum muscle have TrPs, each corresponding finger fails to flex completely. Figure 20-6B shows a positive test for TrPs in the extensor of the index finger. Voluntary hyperextension of the MCP joints strongly loads the finger extensors,

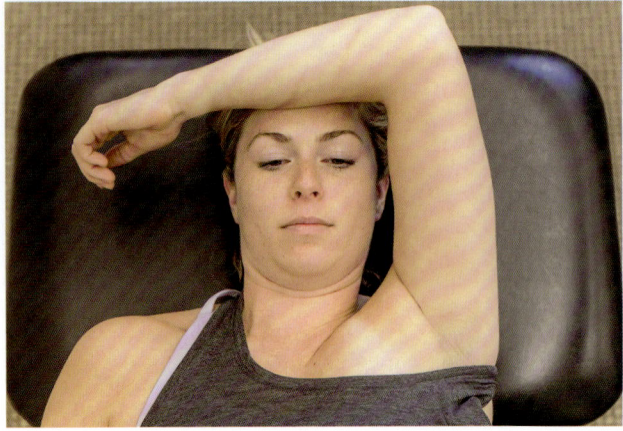

Figure 20-5. The scalene relief position helps identify the scalene TrPs source of referred pain that is caused or aggravated by clavicular pressure on the nerves passing over the elevated first rib or on an involved muscle. Clearance beneath the clavicle is maximized by swinging the shoulder forward, which protracts the scapula and pivots the clavicle forward and upward to fully relieve the clavicular pressure on neurovascular structures. Pain relief by this test should occur immediately or within a few minutes.

3.4. Trigger Point Examination

The localized twitch response is difficult to elicit manually in the anterior and middle scalene muscles and very difficult in the posterior scalene muscle. Based on the location and the data on the interrater reliability of TrP palpation, as well as the anatomic location of the scalene muscles, the detection of a taut band, a hyperirritable spot, and referred pain are the most reliable diagnostic criteria. Local twitch responses are characteristically elicited when a needle encounters the TrP. It can be depended on only as a diagnostically confirmatory finding.

When trying to locate the anterior and middle scalene muscles, it is helpful to remember that the digitations of the anterior scalene muscle attach to the anterior tubercles of the cervical vertebrae, the brachial plexus emerges between the anterior and posterior tubercles, and the fibers of the middle scalene muscle attach to the posterior tubercles. The brachial plexus descends in a palpable groove between the two muscles and becomes progressively more superficial to emerge from between the two muscles to exit the neck and thorax by crossing over the first rib. First, palpating the SCM muscle and finding the subclavian artery are the most reliable methods of locating the scalene muscles.

The TrPs in the scalenus anterior muscle are found by palpating the muscle behind the posterior border of the clavicular division of the SCM muscle. The posterior SCM border can be approximated by locating the external jugular vein with finger pressure just above the clavicle (Figure 20-8A). The omohyoid muscle is more superficial than the scalene muscles, emerges from behind the SCM muscle, and crosses diagonally over the anterior scalene. It can cross at about the same level as the scalene TrPs depending on which scalene digitation is involved and depending on the head and UE position. The omohyoid muscle tends to be thinner than the scalene muscles. To differentiate the scalene muscles from other structures, the patient should be asked to take a deep sniff through their nose. This action causes a significant contraction of the scalene muscles. If the inferior belly of the omohyoid muscle has a tender TrP and taut bands, it can easily be mistaken for the scalenus anterior muscle despite these muscles having different fiber directions (Figure 20-7). These TrPs frequently exist together as discussed earlier, and differentiation can be important in the treatment of whiplash-associated disorder (WAD) and TOS.

The patient should be positioned supine with the head slightly rotated in the contralateral direction with the cervical lordosis supported (Figure 20-8). The scalenus anterior muscle can be identified by positioning the patient's head to take up any slack in the muscle and then palpating its anterior and posterior

increasing the activity of these TrPs. This TrP activity apparently reflexively limits simultaneous distal interphalangeal flexion by inhibiting the corresponding finger flexor.

The test is also positive when TrPs are present in the scalene muscles. In this case, all four fingertips may fail to touch the MCP volar pads (Figure 20-6C). However, there is no difficulty in making a tight fist when the MCP joints are allowed to flex. Apparently, TrPs in the scalene muscles similarly inhibit finger flexors when the MCP joints are extended. Scalene TrPs are frequently the key to forearm extensor digitorum TrPs. The referred motor effects of TrPs are frequently independent of, and can affect different locations than, referred sensory effects.

A positive test is not simply due to edema, because this test of distal interphalangeal flexion is frequently restored to normal immediately after the treatment of the involved scalene muscles. Furthermore, edema is more likely to occur only with the involvement of the scalenus anterior, whereas active TrPs in any of the scalene muscles may be responsible for an abnormal finger flexion test.

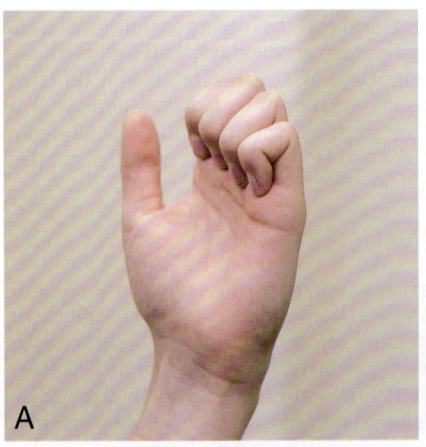 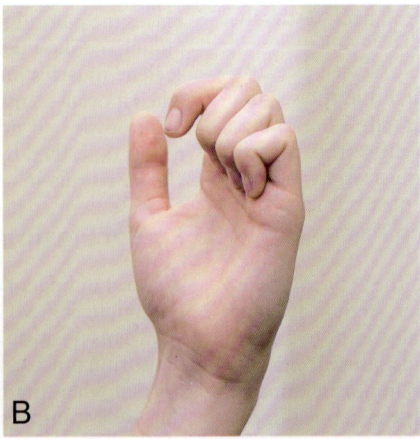 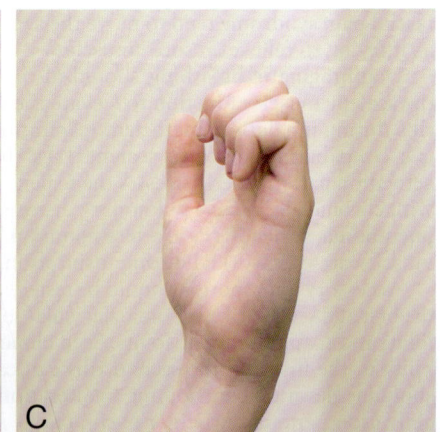

Figure 20-6. Finger flexion test. A, Normal finger closure with all fingers flexed tightly. B, Positive test for finger extensor muscle dysfunction. C, Positive scalene test, incomplete flexion of all fingers.

Chapter 20: Scalene Muscles 215

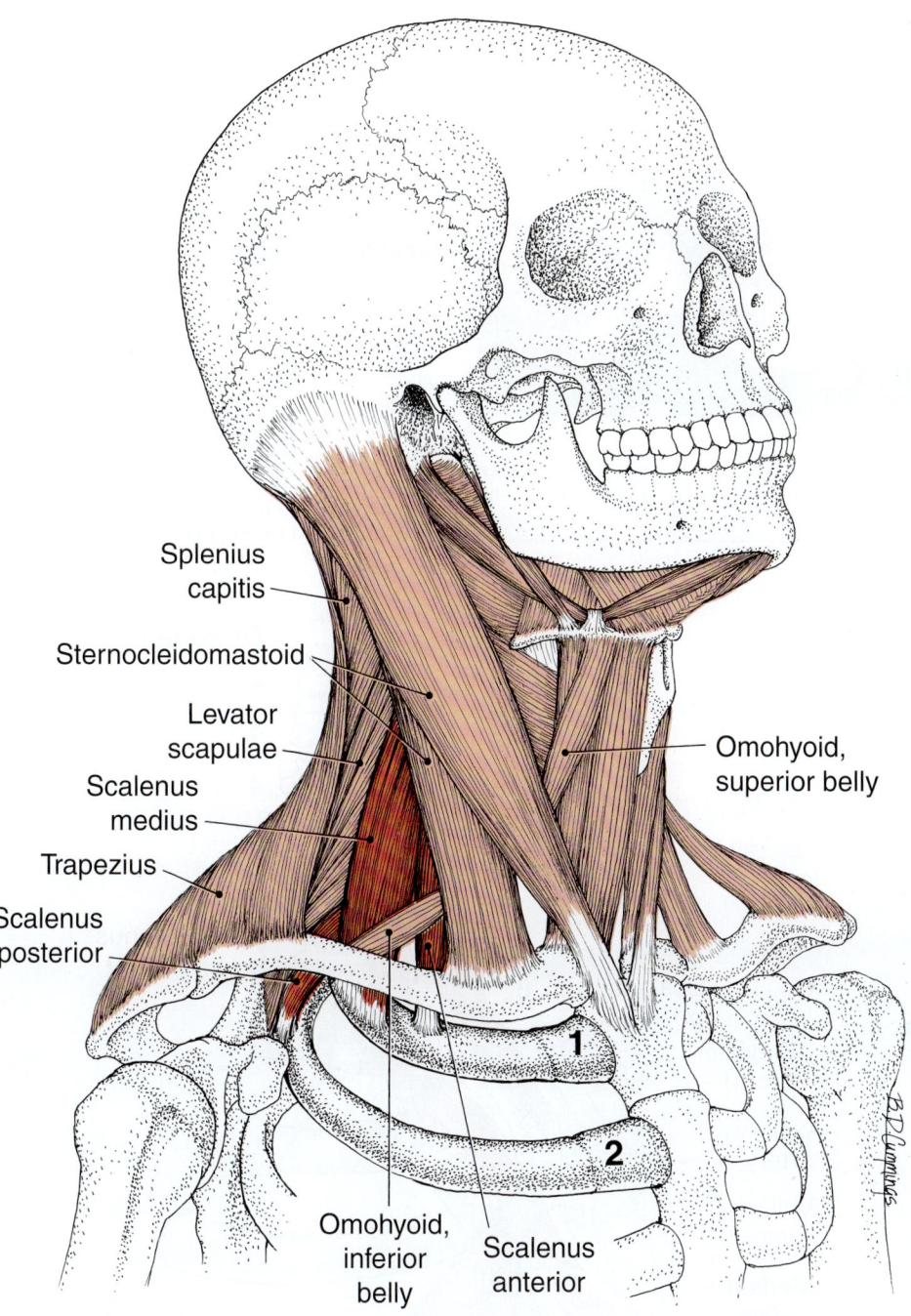

Figure 20-7. Neighboring muscles (medium red) that are useful landmarks in locating the scalene muscles (dark red). The inferior belly of the omohyoid muscle is easily mistaken for the anterior scalene muscle although they do not have the same fiber direction. It is superficial and is located where one could expect to find the scalene muscle.

borders. Its posterior border is confirmed by locating the groove between the anterior and middle scalene muscles that cradles the brachial plexus bundle of nerve fibers. In this groove, behind the clavicle, the subclavian artery is nearly always palpable where it passes between these two muscles to cross over the first rib (Figure 20-9). The fingers of one hand straddle the scalenus anterior muscle to establish its location, while the other hand utilizes cross-fiber flat palpation to precisely localize taut bands and TrPs (Figure 20-8).

The scalenus medius muscle is parallel to, and on the posterior side of, the groove described above that contains the bundle of brachial plexus nerve fibers. It is wider than the scalenus anterior muscle and lies anterior to the free border of the upper trapezius muscle (Figure 20-7). It can be palpated against the posterior tubercles of the transverse processes of the vertebrae utilizing cross-fiber flat palpation. Palpation should be carried out very carefully due to the neurovascular structures in the region. The sniff test can be utilized to identify the scalenus medius muscle.

The scalenus posterior muscle lies more horizontal than, and dorsal to, the scalenus medius muscle. It passes anterior to the levator scapula muscle, which should be pushed aside at the point where the levator scapula muscle emerges near the free anterior border of the upper trapezius muscle (Figure 20-7). Finding TrP tenderness requires cross-fiber flat palpation posterior to the scalenus medius muscle and to the depth of the first rib. This attachment is often tender in the absence of TrPs in the muscle belly.

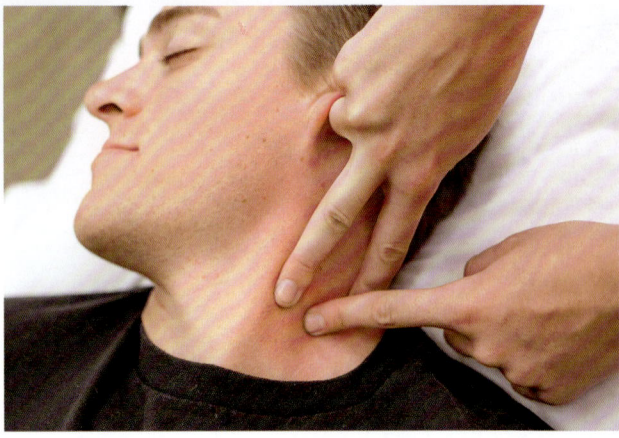

Figure 20-8. Palpation of anterior and middle scalene muscles between the sternocleidomastoid muscle anteriorly and the levator scapulae and upper trapezius muscles posteriorly.

Because of the location and variance of the scalenus minimus muscle in terms of existence, composition, and size, reliable TrP palpation is difficult. It may manifest into residual tenderness in the scalenus anterior muscle following treatment.

4. DIFFERENTIAL DIAGNOSIS

4.1. Activation and Perpetuation of Trigger Points

A posture or activity that activates a TrP, if not corrected, can also perpetuate it. In any part of the scalene muscles, TrPs may be activated by unaccustomed eccentric loading, eccentric exercise in an unconditioned muscle, or maximal or submaximal concentric loading.[28] Trigger points may also be activated or aggravated when the muscle is placed in a shortened or lengthened position for an extended period of time. Side-sleeping without proper pillow support or sleeping supine with too many pillows may place the scalene muscles in a shortened or lengthened position.

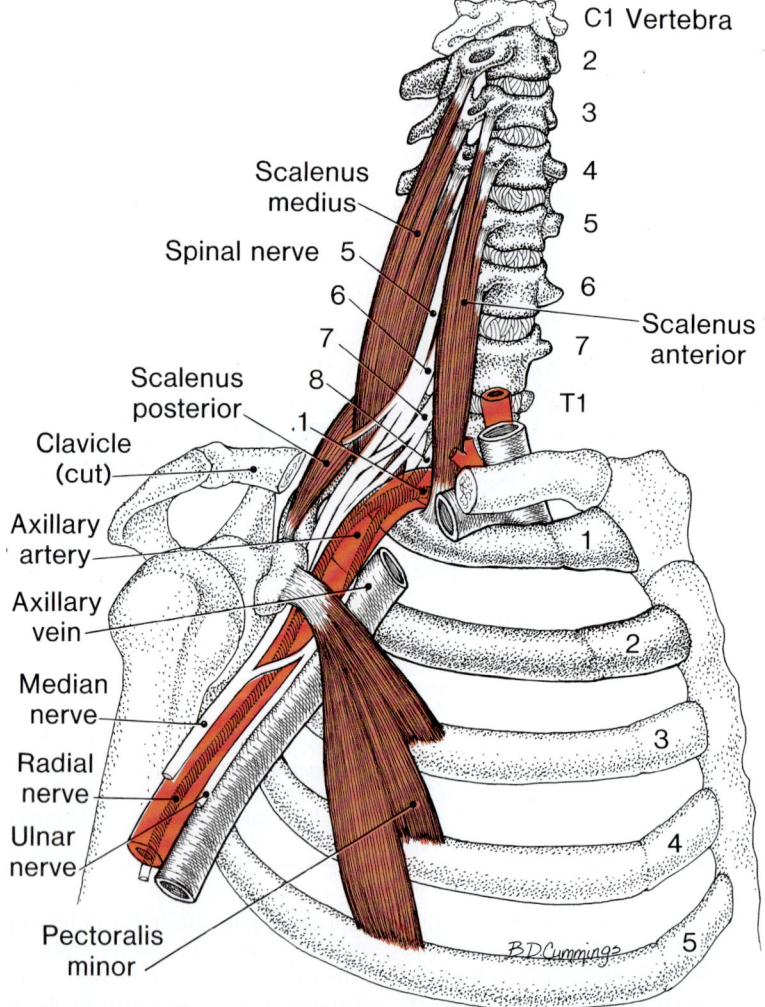

Figure 20-9. Thoracic outlet entrapment by the scalene muscles (medium red). The neurovascular bundle is spread out to show the relations of its component parts. A portion of the clavicle has been removed. The brachial plexus and subclavian artery (dark red) emerge above the first rib and behind the clavicle between the scalenus anterior and scalenus medius muscles. The spinal nerves are numbered on the left, the vertebrae on the right. The T1 nerve lies dorsal to and beneath the subclavian artery. These structures crossing over the first rib can be compressed when the rib becomes elevated. Trigger points in the scalenus anterior and/or the scalenus medius muscles are associated with taut bands that increase muscle tension and elevate the first rib, compressing the neurovascular structures.

Scalene TrPs are common following a cold with a bad cough, pneumonia, bronchitis, or allergies as all these conditions require the scalene muscles to be overloaded due to their respiratory functions. Scalene TrPs may also be activated by a fall or motor vehicle accident, prolonged pushing or pulling, or lifting and carrying awkwardly large objects with the UEs. Hiking with a heavy backpack for long hours is particularly demanding on the scalene muscles in addition to the upper trapezius, SCM, and pectoralis minor muscles. Playing handheld string instruments such as the violin or wind instruments such as the flute, which require a tilted head and neck position for proper use, may activate scalene TrPs. Swimming may also place the scalene muscles at risk for developing TrPs due to the cardiorespiratory demands, repetitive cervical spine rotation, and UE use.[29]

Biomechanical malalignment such as a tilted shoulder girdle axis due to a leg length discrepancy when standing, a small hemi-pelvis when seated, and a structural or functional scoliosis may also place the scalene muscles at a mechanical disadvantage and overload them. Changes in the rib cage that are common with a structural scoliosis may place increased demands on the scalene muscles during inspiration. Habitual chest breathing and poor diaphragmatic breathing patterns cause repetitive overload in the scalene muscles leading to TrP formation.

Prolonged computer work with improper or awkward workstation setup where an individual spends hours each day with the dominant arm in an elevated, abducted, and slightly internally rotated position while using a mouse can shorten and activate TrPs in all three or four scalene muscles. Visual stressors during computer work may also contribute to TrP formation as this causes an alteration in the head position from a centered neutral posture.[30] In addition, prolonged flexion and side-bending of the neck to hold a phone between the head and a slightly elevated shoulder contributes to the formation of scalene TrPs.

A whiplash-type injury from a motor vehicle accident is likely to activate TrPs in the scalene muscles in addition to several other muscles in the cervical spine and shoulder girdle. In a study by Hong et al, 81% of patients with WAD with a report of pain had at least one active scalene TrP.[31] In a more recent study, Fernandez-Perez et al investigated the prevalence of TrPs in patients with WAD and healthy controls. In individuals with acute WAD they found a high prevalence of active and latent TrPs compared with those in a healthy control group. They also found that subjects with acute WAD and higher levels of disability had more active TrPs resulting in higher reports of pain and widespread pressure hypersensitivity.[32]

The scalene muscles can be affected by movement impairments that produce a severe deviation from the normal pattern of gait. An antalgic gait pattern or limping on a weight-bearing lower extremity (with resultant torso and head adjustments) and lack of normal push-off at the end of the stance phase can activate TrPs in the scalene (and levator scapulae and SCM) muscles, because those muscles contract excessively in their reflexive attempt to compensate for, and/or maintain, equilibrium and efficiency of movement.

4.2. Associated Trigger Points

Associated TrPs can develop in the referred pain areas caused by primary TrPs.[33] Therefore, muscles in the referred pain areas of the scalene muscles should also be considered. The scalenus anterior and medius muscles are often involved together. When the scalenus minimus is involved or has TrPs, all the scalene muscles are usually affected. Scalene TrPs are often activated by TrPs in the SCM muscle, which form a functional unit with the scalene muscles. The SCM muscle is also an important part of the functional unit for vigorous or labored inhalation and is therefore likely to become involved if scalene TrPs have been active or present for a considerable period of time. Trigger points in the scalenus medius muscle are likely to be found in association with TrPs in the upper trapezius, SCM, and splenius capitis muscles.[34]

Associated TrPs may develop in several of the areas to which the scalene muscles refer pain. Both the pectoralis major and minor muscles commonly develop TrPs in regions that correspond to the scalene-referred pattern of anterior chest pain. Associated TrPs may also be found in the rhomboids, middle trapezius, and infraspinatus muscles due to the referral of pain from scalene muscles to the medial border of the scapula. Associated TrPs in the long head of the triceps brachii correspond to the scalene pattern of the posterior arm pain, and those in the deltoid muscle correspond to the anterior pattern.[23,31] Although the dorsal forearm is a less common site of scalene-referred pain, associated TrPs tend to develop in the extensor carpi radialis, extensor digitorum, extensor carpi ulnaris,[35] and brachioradialis muscles. When TrPs in the lateral part of the brachialis muscle are induced from scalene TrPs, both the brachialis and scalene muscles refer pain to the thumb, making this digit especially painful.

When the omohyoid muscle (see Chapter 12) develops TrPs and becomes tense, it can act as a constricting band across the brachial plexus.[36] Because the tense muscle stands out prominently when the head is side-bent to the contralateral side, it can be mistaken for the upper trapezius or a scalene muscle. When the omohyoid has TrPs, it can prevent full stretch of the trapezius and/or scalene muscles and therefore should also be released.

In individuals with a primary report of shoulder pain, scalene TrPs are likely to coexist with those in the rotator cuff, deltoid, biceps brachii, and triceps brachii muscles.[37] The pain from these muscles may correspond to the referred pain pattern of the scalene muscles.

4.3. Associated Pathology

Trigger points in the scalene muscles are associated with and can mimic a variety of different conditions that cause UE symptoms including TOS, scalenus anticus syndrome, C5 and C6 radicular pain and/or radiculopathy, poor posture, and carpal tunnel syndrome. It is essential to perform a thorough medical screening and examination to determine if referral to another healthcare practitioner is necessary. Appropriate medical management should be utilized to reduce the excessive demand on auxiliary muscles of respiration that is caused by coughing and sneezing (eg, in patients with allergic rhinitis, bronchitis, pneumonia, emphysema, asthma, and sinusitis).

The scalenus anticus (anterior scalene) syndrome, which in most literature has been subsumed under the broader TOS diagnosis, was identified as early as 1935 by pain in the anterior or posterior aspect of the arm and at the upper medial border of the scapula, as well as by the tenderness of the muscle to palpation.[9,26,38] In 1942, Travell et al[24] reported signs caused by scalene TrPs that included venous obstruction, vasomotor changes, and if the syndrome was severe, evidence of arterial insufficiency with compression of the motor and sensory nerves of the affected arm. The literature is clear that a scalene muscle problem is primarily responsible for neural or vascular entrapment in many patients who are commonly diagnosed as having TOS (refer to Chapter 33 for more clinical considerations).

Relief of pain by infiltrating the scalene muscles was used by Adson[39] as a diagnostic test to distinguish the scalenus anterior syndrome from structural causes of cephalobrachialgia. The TrP nature of the syndrome was not recognized. After an initial wave of enthusiasm for scalenotomy following Adson's report, interest waned because emphasis shifted to carpal tunnel syndrome and radiculopathy from nerve root compression by a protruded cervical disc. Research continues to use botulinum toxin injection and anesthetic block of the scalenus anterior muscle diagnostically, for treatment, and predicting successful scalenotomy.[40-43]

Braun et al investigated the effect of an anterior scalene muscle block (ASMB) on work production and time to fatigue in 34 individuals disabled with UE symptoms consistent with a diagnosis of TOS.[44] They studied work production and time to fatigue pre and post ASMB. They utilized three UE test positions: push pull at waist level and overhead and shoulder abduction to 90° with elbow flexion to 90° and repetitive hand gripping. All patients had improvement in power generation and time to fatigue post ASMB. The investigators conclude that the scalenus anterior muscle may hold the first rib in an elevated position and the ASMB allows a change in contour of the costoclavicular space and thoracic outlet. Therefore, if TrPs are present in the scalene muscles, they may have an effect on the first rib position and the contour of the costoclavicular space. While it has not been studied as such, this research indicates that injection of the scalenus anterior muscle provides relief for those with neurogenic TOS. This theory seems to suggest that scalenus anterior syndrome or neurogenic TOS may instead frequently be caused or perpetuated by scalene TrPs.

Many disciplines recognize the importance of diagnosing and treating TrPs in patients with symptoms of a TOS. An osteopathic physician[45] reported that in most cases of TOS, scalene or pectoral TrPs are responsible and treated them with myofascial release and self-stretching.[46] A physician practicing physical medicine and rehabilitation[47] noted that scalene TrPs commonly mimic the symptoms of a C6 radiculitis component of a TOS and that pectoralis minor TrPs create symptoms of medial cord compression. A physical therapist[48] identified TrPs in the scalene, supraspinatus, infraspinatus, and pectoral muscles as most commonly mimicking TOS. This topic is covered under the clinical considerations section in Chapter 33.

A C5-C6 radiculitis can produce pain very similar to that reported by patients with scalene TrPs. Cervical radiculitis in the C5 or C6 nerve roots often result in the formation of TrPs in those muscles innervated by the same nerve roots. Often patients with C5-C6 radicular symptoms report having deep anterior shoulder pain, anterolateral arm and forearm pain, and pain into the radial aspect of the hand and lateral two-and-a-half digits. Wainer et al[27] identified a test item cluster to determine the likelihood that a patient is presenting with cervical radicular symptoms. The following five predictor variables were identified: a positive Spurling sign, cervical rotation less than 60° to the same side, positive cervical compression test, relief of symptoms with axial distraction, and a positive neurodynamic upper limb test. Patients presenting with four of these positive variables have a 90% posttest probability of cervical radiculopathy. Patients with three positive variables have a 65% posttest probability of cervical radiculopathy.[27]

Carpal tunnel syndrome may occur as a concurrent entrapment with TOS, or the symptoms of carpal tunnel syndrome may be caused by scalene TrPs. Loss of normal mobility of the structures forming the carpal tunnel often contribute to the entrapment of the median nerve. Edema, reflexively originating from scalene TrPs, can be another important contributing factor.

Articular dysfunctions in C4, C5, and C6 are commonly associated with TrPs in the anterior and middle scalene muscles. Another articular dysfunction that is commonly observed with scalene muscle involvement is the elevation of the first and/or the second rib(s) (Figure 20-10). An apparent elevation of the first rib is typically concurrent with a T1 articular dysfunction.

A tilted shoulder girdle axis, sometimes caused by the functional scoliosis associated with a leg length discrepancy and/or a small hemi-pelvis, places chronic strain on the scalene muscles that should help straighten the tilted neck to level the eyes for good vision. An uncorrected leg length discrepancy or other

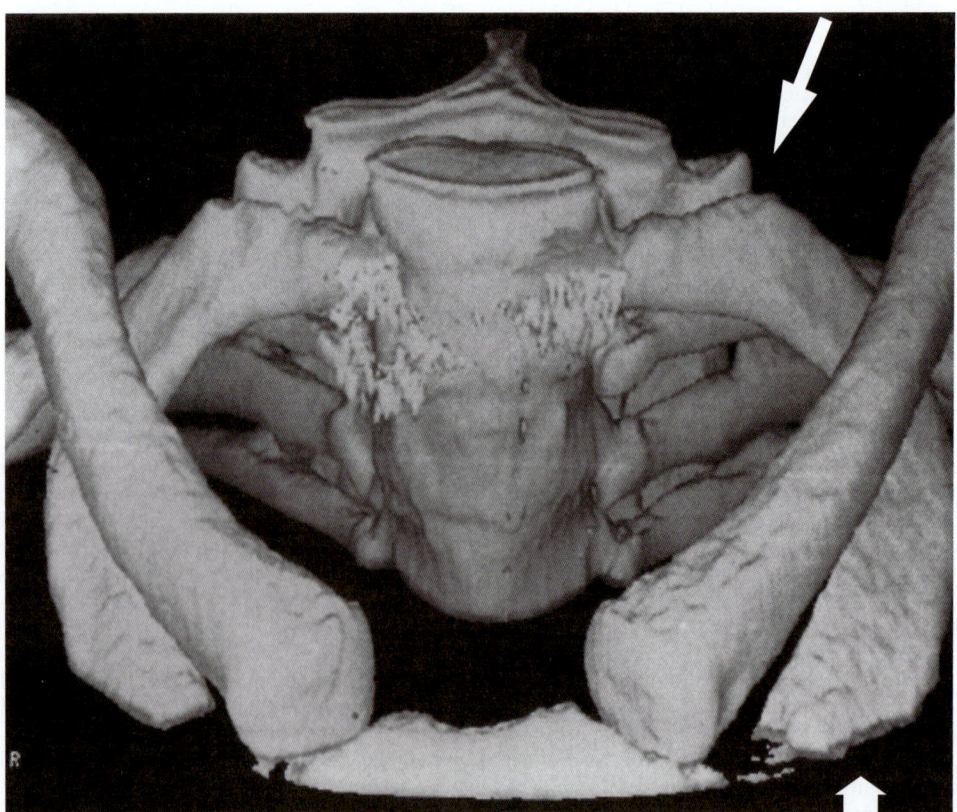

Figure 20-10. Computed tomographic view of the thoracic outlet viewed from front with three-dimensional shaded surface display. The first rib at the costotransverse joint on the left side (long arrow above) is displaced upward compared with the asymptomatic right side. This displacement is associated with an abnormal position of the whole first rib (short white arrow at the bottom right of figure). Reproduced with permission from Lindgren KA, Manninen H, Rytkönen H. Thoracic outlet syndrome—a functional disturbance of the thoracic upper aperture? *Muscle Nerve*. 1995;18:526-530.

Chapter 20: Scalene Muscles   219

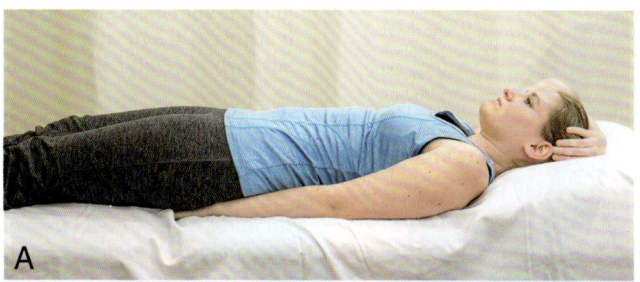
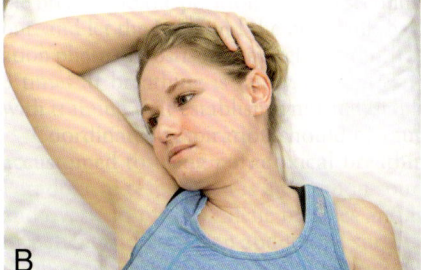
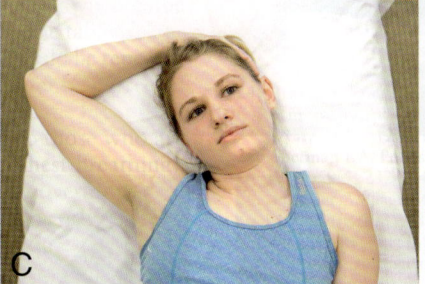
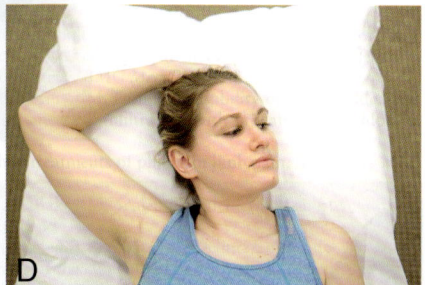

Figure 20-11. Self-stretch of the scalene muscles. A, Starting position. B, Posterior scalene. C, Middle scalene. D, Anterior scalene.

frontal plane asymmetry as little as 1 cm (3/8th in), sometimes less, can perpetuate scalene TrPs despite all other efforts in management.[13]

5. CORRECTIVE ACTIONS

The patient should avoid habitual sustained or repetitive motions that overload the scalene muscles such as carrying awkward packages that require lifting with the arms extended out in front of the body and hauling, pulling, or tugging strenuously. Increasing intra-abdominal pressure by performing Valsalva during lifting or defecating should be avoided. Carrying a heavy backpack for prolonged periods of time, as well as sporting activities such as swimming, may lead to the formation of scalene TrPs and modifications to these behaviors may be necessary for full relief of symptoms and prevention of reoccurrence.

Correction of poor posture (particularly "rounded shoulder" posture with an excessive forward head position) and maintenance of good posture in sitting, standing, and sleeping are primary in any treatment approach both for initial relief of pain and for lasting relief. Refer to Chapter 76 for discussions of posture and body mechanics.

Utilizing progressive lenses during work-related activity that requires typing, reading, and writing might place the scalene muscles in a prolonged shortened position by moving the head from a balanced neutral position to a flexed position to perform the work task effectively.

For sleeping, the patient should use only one soft comfortable pillow of the right thickness to maintain a normal cervical lordosis. In a supine position, the proper thickness does not allow any extension of the head but also does not place the head in excessive flexion, as this causes prolonged shortening of the scalene and anterior neck muscles during sleep. A small towel roll can be placed inside the pillowcase to support the neck in a neutral position, thus placing the face parallel to the ceiling. The patient can tuck the corner of the pillow between the shoulder and chin in the side-lying position but not under both the head and the shoulder. During side-sleeping, the pillow should be thick enough to keep the head and neck in a neutral position so that the head is not bent excessively to either side because this causes excessive lengthening of the muscle on the top side and excessive shortening of the muscle on the pillow side. It is recommended to avoid sleeping prone due to the excessive rotation and extension placing the scalene muscles in

a lengthened position. If one does sleep prone, a pillow placed under the shoulder and the chest on the same side to which the face is turned helps reduce rotation and extension of the neck. A semi-prone position can also be utilized, achieved by flexing the knee and the hip of the side toward which the face is turned, partly rotating the torso (Figure 7-5A to C).

If reading in bed, the light should be located directly overhead, on the headboard, on the wall, or suspended from the ceiling. It should not illuminate only one side of the bed because this placement can place excessive strain on the scalene muscles if the head is turned and tilted downward to maximize the light cast on the reading material.

When using a phone, it should not be held between the head and the shoulder. Instead, a headset, headphones, or hands-free speaker function should be utilized.

Correction of a posture is of paramount importance, as is the use of safe and efficient body mechanics for a long-term relief from muscle pain. Postural correction and body mechanics are discussed thoroughly in Chapter 76. Critical to recovery of patients with scalene TrPs is daily passive stretching of the scalene muscles at home. Stretching of the scalene muscles is illustrated in Figure 20-11A to D. With the patient lying supine, the shoulder of the side to be stretched (left side in this photo) is lowered and the hand anchored under the buttock (Figure 20-11A). The patient should learn to reach over the head to the ear with the hand of the contralateral side. They will assist the head and the neck to tilt it to the side away from the involved muscles while concentrating on relaxation of the neck muscles (Figure 20-11B). The head is drawn smoothly down toward the shoulder. The degree of head rotation determines which of the scalene muscles is specifically placed on stretch.

To stretch the scalenus posterior muscle (Figure 20-11B), the patient uses the assistive hand to gently pull the head and the neck into side-bending away from the side of the TrPs. They then turn the face away from the affected muscle. For the scalenus medius muscle, the patient looks straight up toward the ceiling (neutral position) or slightly toward the pulling arm (Figure 20-11C). To stretch the scalenus anterior muscle, the patient turns the face toward the affected muscle (Figure 20-11D). The patient concentrates the stretch on those directions in which the muscles feel tightest, holds each stretch for a slow count of 6 to 10 seconds while inhaling and slowly exhaling to give the stretched muscles time to release, and then gently taking up the slack. The head is then returned to the neutral mid-position. A pause, with deep diaphragmatic breathing between each passive stretch, helps reestablish complete muscular

Chapter 21

Supraspinatus Muscle

"Overhead Activity Archenemy"

Joseph M. Donnelly

1. INTRODUCTION

The supraspinatus muscle, a chief rotator cuff muscle, has three muscular heads and originates from the medial two-thirds of the supraspinous fossa of the scapula and the supraspinous fascia. It is thinner at the medial attachment, and becomes thicker as it travels laterally under the acromion to attach to the humerus. The three intertwined muscular heads give the muscle an increased ability to absorb tensile loads. The primary roles of this muscle are abduction and dynamic stability of the glenohumeral joint by compressive loading of the humeral head into the scapular glenoid fossa with the other rotator cuff musculature. It is considered to be the most active rotator cuff muscle and is involved with any functional activities that require the elevation of the upper extremity. Trigger points (TrPs) in the supraspinatus muscle produce a deep ache in the mid-deltoid region of the shoulder and can refer partway down the arm. It often refers pain to the lateral epicondyle of the humerus but rarely to the wrist. Symptoms may be exacerbated with sleeping on the affected side, carrying heavy objects with the arm hanging at the side, and reaching out to the side. Activation and perpetuation of TrPs in the supraspinatus muscle usually result from lifting objects to, or above, shoulder height with the arm outstretched or by performing tasks that demand repeated and/or moderately prolonged elevation of the arm. Differential diagnosis should include assessment for dysfunction of other rotator cuff and shoulder musculature, faulty scapulohumeral joint mobility, C5-C6 radicular symptoms, subdeltoid or subacromial bursitis, and scapular dyskinesia. Corrective actions include postural reeducation, effective sleep positioning, avoiding activities that overload the muscle, self-pressure release of TrPs, and self-stretch exercises.

2. ANATOMIC CONSIDERATIONS

The supraspinatus muscle originates from the medial two thirds of the supraspinous fossa of the scapula and the supraspinous fascia.[1] The muscle is thinner at its most medial attachment and becomes thicker as it travels laterally to attach to the humerus. As the muscle courses laterally, the obliquely oriented anterior fibers converge with the more parallel posterior fibers of the muscle to form a thick tendon under the acromion that passes over the humeral head to insert on the superior facet of the greater tubercle of the humerus (Figure 21-1). The tendon is thicker at its anterior attachment and is continuous with the transverse humeral and coracohumeral ligaments.[1] The tendon is flatter at the attachment of the superior facet, and the deeper portion of the tendon blends with the glenohumeral joint capsule.[1] The supraspinatus tendon lies between the coracoacromial ligament anteriorly and the infraspinatus muscle posteriorly.

The supraspinatus muscle has been described as having three different muscular heads that give it the appearance of a braided rope.[2] Arising from the spine of the scapula, the posterior head travels anteriorly, while the middle head travels laterally, and the anterior head courses posteriorly. The thin posterior tendon overlaps the anterior and middle heads, intertwining all three heads, thus increasing the muscle's ability to mitigate tensile loading.[2] An aponeurotic expansion was identified in approximately 50% of 150 shoulders studied with magnetic resonance imaging (MRI). This aponeurotic expansion continues inferiorly from the supraspinatus tendon parallel to the long head of the biceps tendon in the bicipital groove, outside the synovial sheath, and inserts into the humerus at the superior aspect of the pectoralis major tendon.[3]

Deeper vertical fibers from the infraspinatus muscle conjoin with the supraspinatus tendon superiorly and cross the rotator cuff interval, extending anteriorly to the biceps brachii muscle. This thick fibrous tendon is referred to as the rotator cable,[4] which links the posterior rotator cuff musculature to the anterior cuff muscle, and is commonly demonstrated in shoulder MRI scans.[5] The rotator crescent is the distal arrangement of the tendon that consists of the insertion of the supraspinatus and infraspinatus tendons lateral to the rotator cable that inserts onto the humerus. The rotator cable is thought to protect the rotator crescent[4] by transferring forces intrinsically from the posterosuperior rotator cuff to the anterior rotator cuff.[1] This complex insertion is thought to allow the rotator cuff to work in a coordinated fashion during all shoulder motions. Figure 21-1A identifies the attachments of the other three muscles that comprise the rotator cuff.

2.1. Innervation and Vascularization

The supraspinatus muscle is innervated by the suprascapular nerve through the upper trunk of the brachial plexus, primarily from the C5 to C6 spinal nerves,[1] and also from C4 in some individuals.[6] The suprascapular nerve travels parallel with the clavicle and courses posteriorly through the suprascapular notch onto the supraspinous fossa to innervate the supraspinatus muscle. It abruptly changes its course around the spinoglenoid notch of the scapula, giving rise to motor branches that innervate the infraspinatus.[6]

The vascular supply to the supraspinatus muscle arises from the suprascapular and dorsal scapular arteries.[1] The suprascapular artery courses above the transverse scapular ligament; whereas the suprascapular nerve travels below the transverse scapular ligament in most cases.[7]

2.2. Function

The supraspinatus muscle is an important dynamic stabilizer of the glenohumeral joint along with the infraspinatus, teres minor, and subscapularis muscles. The supraspinatus muscle plays a key role in dynamic stability during shoulder abduction. The supraspinatus, middle deltoid, and middle trapezius muscles are activated prior to arm movement during abduction in the coronal plan, and the supraspinatus muscle achieves its peak

Chapter 21: Supraspinatus Muscle   223

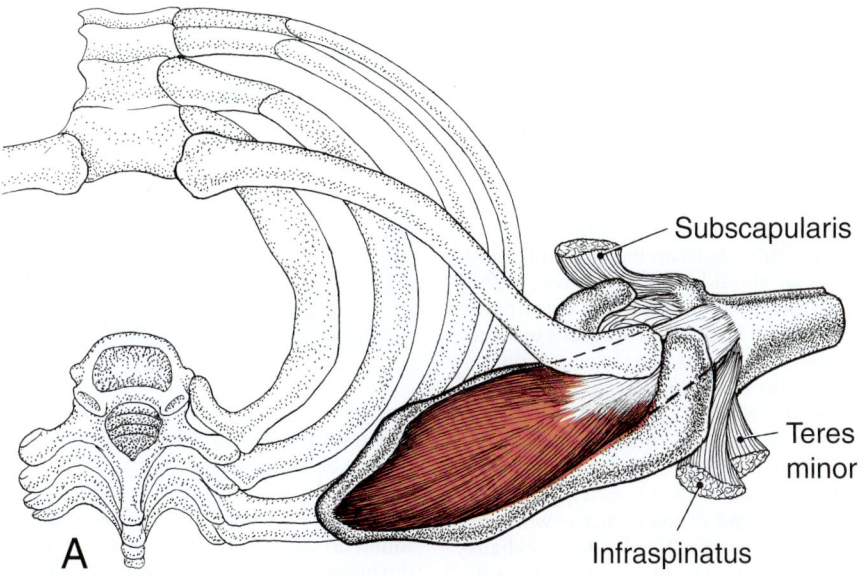

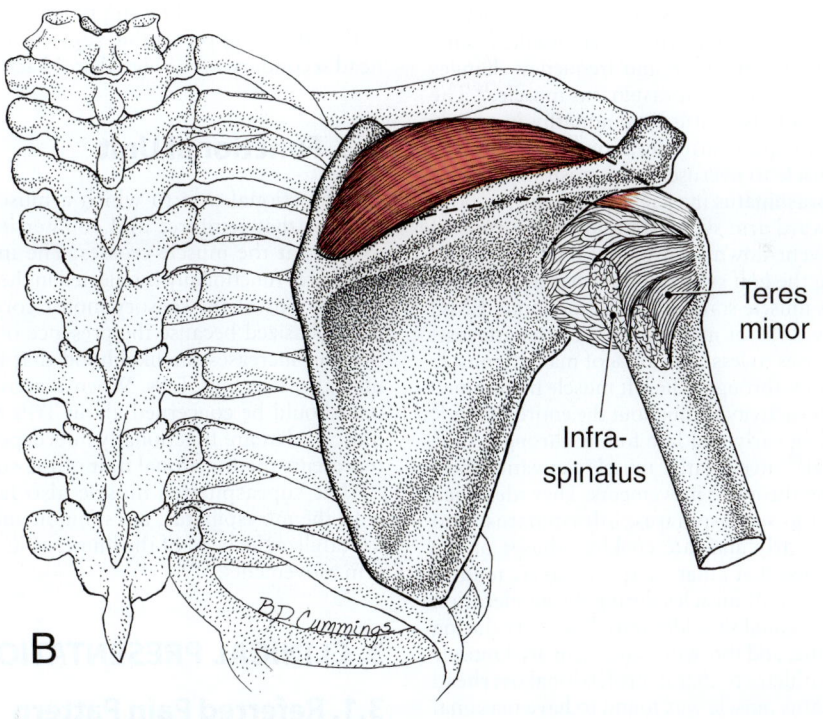

Figure 21-1. Attachments of the supraspinatus muscle (red). The other rotator cuff muscles are cut and reflected to show their attachments more clearly. A, Seen from above, including the relation of the humeral attachment of the supraspinatus muscle to the attachments of the other three rotator cuff muscles. B, Posterior view. If one envisions the trapezius attachments to the clavicle, the acromion, and the spine of the scapula, it becomes obvious how deep the muscle is due to the overlying trapezius muscle.

of maximal volitional contraction (MVC) at 88° of abduction. The infraspinatus muscle achieves its peak MVC at 165° and the subscapularis muscle at 108° of abduction. The supraspinatus muscle appears to have a larger contribution to abduction earlier in the range of motion. The rotator cuff muscles are recruited early and increase throughout the range of motion contributing to coaptation of the humeral head in the glenoid.[8] Kwon et al[9] studied the cross-sectional area of the supraspinatus muscle at various degrees of glenohumeral abduction and found the largest cross-sectional area of this muscle to be between 60° and 90° of shoulder abduction, signifying its greatest activation in this range. This description is consistent with the findings from that of other researchers.[8] Other authors have found that the pattern of activation in elevation in the coronal plane and plane of the scapula is similar in the supraspinatus, infraspinatus, and subscapularis muscles with all loads.[10-12] There is a strong correlation of the activation of the supraspinatus muscle with that of the deltoid muscle, whereas the infraspinatus and subscapularis muscles' activation patterns are strongly correlated with those of axioscapular musculature.[10,11] Witte et al[13] reported similar findings; however, they conclude that the supraspinatus and deltoid muscles may contribute to glenohumeral elevation moments in a complimentary manner. They also found that the response of the supraspinatus muscle to an increase in loading during multiple directions of shoulder elevation was highly variable as compared with the deltoid muscle which consistently increased activation with increased loading.[13] The results of recent research do not support historical notions that the supraspinatus muscle is more effective than the deltoid muscle at initiation of abduction when the arm is at the side.

In an electromyographic (EMG) study, Basmajian and Deluca[14] demonstrated that supraspinatus muscle activity alone, in the absence of other muscular activity at the shoulder, prevented downward displacement of the head of the humerus when the upper extremity, hanging at the side, was either loaded to exhaustion with a 7-kg weight or loaded with sudden downward jerks. This mechanism is effective because of the wedge action from the angulation of the glenoid fossa and the cartilaginous labrum.[14]

The EMG activity of the supraspinatus muscle during abduction of the arm increases almost linearly from resting to vigorous activity at 150° of abduction. During flexion, EMG activity increases rapidly at first, reaches a plateau, and increases again as flexion approaches 150°.[15] During sustained flexion or abduction to 90°, the supraspinatus muscle was the first to show evidence of fatigue compared with other shoulder muscles. After 5 minutes, both amplitude and frequency changes indicated advancing fatigue of the supraspinatus muscle.[16] The common occurrence of supraspinatus tendinopathy in people who carry out work that requires arm elevation[17] highlights the vulnerability of this muscle to overuse in this position.

During gait, the supraspinatus muscle is active during both the forward and backward arm swing (but not at the ends of the swing) to help prevent downward migration of the head of the humerus. During the golf swing in right-handed golfers, the right supraspinatus muscle starts out with moderate EMG activity (approximately 25% of manual muscle strength test) and progressively decreases to less than 10% of manual muscle strength test by late follow-through. The left muscle maintained relatively moderate EMG activity throughout the entire swing,[18] with more activity during early and late follow-through. Jobe et al[19] and Gowan et al[20] investigated muscle activation patterns and activity during throwing movements. They identified maximum activity of the supraspinatus, infraspinatus, and deltoid muscles during early and late cocking phases of the throw. They also identified that amateur sport players tend to utilize more of the rotator cuff muscles during the acceleration phase. Illyes et al[21] investigated shoulder muscle activity during pushing, pulling, elevating, and throwing, and compared muscle activity in recreational athletes to that in professional overhead athletes. The supraspinatus muscle was found to have maximal activity during pulling, elevation, and fast overhead throwing. The time to peak activity was much higher and the duration of activity lasted longer in recreational athletes as compared with professional throwers. Their findings are consistent with those of Gowan et al,[20] who identified the deltoid, supraspinatus, and infraspinatus muscles as stabilizers and the subscapularis, pectoralis major, latissimus dorsi, and triceps brachii muscles as accelerators of the glenohumeral joint during throwing activities.[21]

Activation of the shoulder musculature has also been studied during different driving conditions. The supraspinatus and deltoid muscles were both found to have moderate to high muscle activation during driving (30%-50% MVC).[22] If there is an injury or TrPs in one of these muscles, the other may not be able to compensate for the increased load as both muscles exhibit a high activation during normal driving conditions. Adjusting the driver's seat closer to the steering wheel so the shoulders can assume a resting position decreases average supraspinatus muscle activation by 45%.[22]

Reinold et al[23,24] investigated muscle activation in common rehabilitation exercises prescribed for the shoulder girdle. They found no statistical difference in supraspinatus muscle activation during any of the exercises tested. The "full can" exercise produced significantly less activity in the deltoid muscle; therefore, they conclude that this may be the best position to target the supraspinatus muscle for strength testing and exercises. High supraspinatus muscle activation was also demonstrated with standing external rotation with the arm abducted to 90°, prone external rotation with the arm at 90° abduction, and prone horizontal abduction at 100° with full external rotation. They also suggest using the "empty can" test to assess the rotator cuff's efficacy in preventing superior migration of the humeral head secondary to the high deltoid activation in this position.[24]

Box 21-1 Supraspinatus muscle

Action	Synergists	Antagonists
Shoulder elevation (abduction)	Deltoid	Teres major Pectoralis major Latissimus dorsi Coracobrachialis Long head triceps brachii

2.3. Functional Unit

The functional unit to which a muscle belongs includes the muscles that reinforce and counter its actions as well as the joints that the muscle crosses. The interdependence of these structures functionally is reflected in the organization and neural connections of the sensory motor cortex. The functional unit is emphasized because the presence of a TrP in one muscle of the unit increases the likelihood that the other muscles of the unit also develops TrPs. When inactivating TrPs in a muscle, one should be concerned about TrPs that may develop in the muscles that are functionally interdependent. Box 21-1 grossly represents the functional unit of the supraspinatus muscle.[25]

The supraspinatus muscle also functions synergistically with the infraspinatus, teres minor, and subscapularis muscles to stabilize the head of the humerus in the glenoid fossa during arm movements.[10,14]

3. CLINICAL PRESENTATION

3.1. Referred Pain Pattern

The referred pain pattern from TrPs in the supraspinatus muscle causes a deep ache of the shoulder, concentrating in the mid-deltoid region. The tenderness and pain that it projects to the mid-deltoid region can be easily mistaken for subdeltoid bursitis. This ache often refers down the arm and the forearm, and sometimes focuses strongly over the lateral epicondyle of the elbow (Figure 21-2).[26] This epicondylar component helps distinguish supraspinatus TrPs from infraspinatus TrPs, which do not typically refer concentrated pain to the elbow.[26,27] Occasionally, pain from supraspinatus TrPs is also referred to the wrist.

Other authors have described the pain referred from the supraspinatus muscle as traveling toward (or into) the shoulder,[28-30] to the outer side of the arm,[28,31] and from the scapula to the mid-humerus.[29]

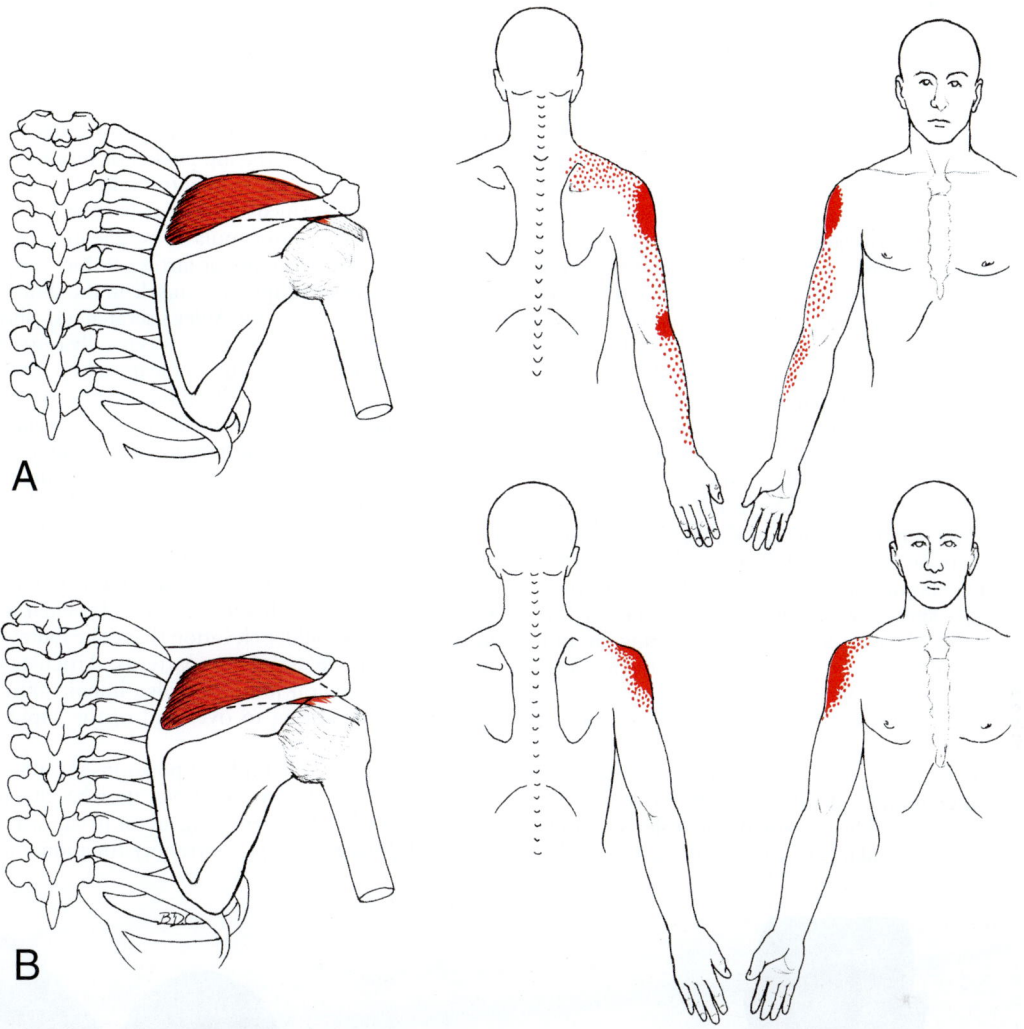

Figure 21-2. A and B, Referred pain patterns (essential reference zone solid red, spillover zone stippled red) of TrPs in the supraspinatus muscle. A, Trigger points may be located in any region of the muscle. B, In addition, a tender area located in the region of attachment of the supraspinatus tendon to the capsule of the glenohumeral joint may be indicative of an enthesopathy.

Experimental injection of 6% hypertonic saline into normal supraspinatus muscles caused referred pain to the shoulder (three subjects), to the upper back (two subjects), and to the elbow (one subject).[32]

3.2. Symptoms

The rotator cuff muscles are commonly implicated in patients who report shoulder pain with the supraspinatus muscle being one of the most frequently involved muscles.[33] Active TrPs in the supraspinatus muscle were found in 38% of individuals with nonspecific shoulder pain[34] and 65% of patients with a medical diagnosis of shoulder impingement.[35] Patients with supraspinatus TrPs often describe intense pain in the lateral aspect of the shoulder over the deltoid region with pain that may spread as far distally to the lateral epicondyle and forearm (Figure 21-2). The pain is usually felt intensely during the elevation of the arm at the glenohumeral joint, especially on initiation of the movement. Patients may experience a deep ache in the lateral aspect of the shoulder at rest that may mimic the pain of bursitis.[36] Pain usually prevents the patients from getting their arm above their head causing activity limitations. When the supraspinatus muscle on the dominant side is affected, the patients commonly report difficulty in reaching the head to comb their hair, brush teeth, or shave facial hair. Patients also report difficulty during sports activities that require arm elevation, such as serving in tennis. Patients with supraspinatus TrPs on the nondominant side may be unaware of even moderate restriction of these motions if the dominant arm usually performs these overhead activities. Ohmori et al[37] found that active TrPs in the supraspinatus and infraspinatus muscles were associated with shoulder pain during ipsilateral upper-extremity elevation in patients receiving a muscle-sparing thoracotomy; thus evaluation of shoulder muscles after surgical procedures that may require prolonged or unusual arm positioning is imperative for optimal postoperative recovery.

Supraspinatus TrPs alone rarely cause severe, sleep-disturbing nocturnal pain. Other authors have observed stiffness of the shoulder and nighttime ache secondary to the involvement of the supraspinatus muscle.[29] In patients older than 65 who report having nocturnal pain that disturbs sleep, examination for a rotator cuff tear should be performed. In some cases, if the supraspinatus TrP is highly irritable, the patient may report increased shoulder pain while walking due to supraspinatus activation during arm swing. In individuals who have recurrent lateral elbow pain or epicondylagia, the supraspinatus muscle should be examined. Some patients may report snapping or clicking sounds around the shoulder joint that is resolved when the supraspinatus TrPs are inactivated.

3.3. Patient Examination

After a thorough subjective examination, the clinician should make a detailed drawing representing the pain pattern that the patient has described. This depiction will assist in planning the physical examination and can be useful in monitoring the progression of the patient as symptoms improve or change. For a proper examination of the supraspinatus muscle, the clinician should observe the shoulder girdle posture, note the scapular position, and examine the active and passive ranges of motion of the shoulder girdle, paying special attention to muscle activation patterns and the scapulohumeral rhythm. The clinician should observe when and where the pain occurs. Supraspinatus TrPs can produce pain at rest or during movement particularly during arm elevation in any plane. The pain usually occurs throughout the abduction range of motion. If pain occurs only in one small arc of motion, evaluate for a rotator cuff injury. Clinically, this muscle is seldom involved in isolation. This muscle is commonly involved in association with the infraspinatus, deltoid, or the upper trapezius muscles that can also have TrPs.

To identify the range of motion deficits, and thus biomechanical dysfunction, that may be caused by TrPs in the supraspinatus muscle, the clinician should identify the limited range of motion by performing a specific range of motion testing for the supraspinatus muscle. Muscle-specific resisted testing should be carried out to identify impairments in muscle function and reproduction of painful symptoms. If active TrPs are present in the supraspinatus muscle, resisted elevation in the plane of the scapula is painfully inhibited.

The Apley's scratch test (shoulder extension, medial rotation, and adduction) can be used to identify restriction due to TrPs in the supraspinatus muscle. This version of the Apley's scratch test requires full adduction and medial rotation of the arm at the glenohumeral joint. It is performed by placing the hand of the affected side behind the back and reaching as far up toward the opposite scapula as possible. The fingertips should reach the inferior angle of the scapula (Figure 21-3A). This test also stretches the shoulder abductors and the infraspinatus muscle. When the range of these muscles is limited due to TrPs, the fingers may barely reach the hip pocket or thoracolumbar region. The limitation from supraspinatus TrPs is similar to when the movement is performed actively or passively. Conversely, TrPs in the antagonistic subscapularis muscle may allow the fingers to reach the spinal column, or farther, if done passively without contracting the subscapularis muscle in the shortened position.

The other version of the Apley's scratch test (shoulder flexion, lateral rotation, and abduction) is typically restricted by supraspinatus TrPs (Figure 21-3B). In the upright position, the patient is unable to hold the arm fully abducted due to pain because this contracts the supraspinatus muscle in the shortened position and compresses any present enthesopathy at its humeral attachment. When in a supine position, the patient with supraspinatus TrPs has less difficulty performing the overhead Apley's scratch test because the muscle does not lift the weight of the arm.

Accessory joint motion should be tested in the glenohumeral, acromioclavicular, sternoclavicular, and scapulothoracic joints. Often, joint hypomobility in the sternoclavicular joint can cause impairment in shoulder elevation that contributes to alterations in normal muscle activation patterns. Articular dysfunctions in the glenohumeral joint may also impair muscle activation patterns, contributing to overload of the supraspinatus and other rotator cuff muscles.

Scapular and humeral head positions should be assessed at rest and during upper extremity elevation because malalignment can be a significant contributing factor to supraspinatus muscle overload during all upper extremity functional activities. The

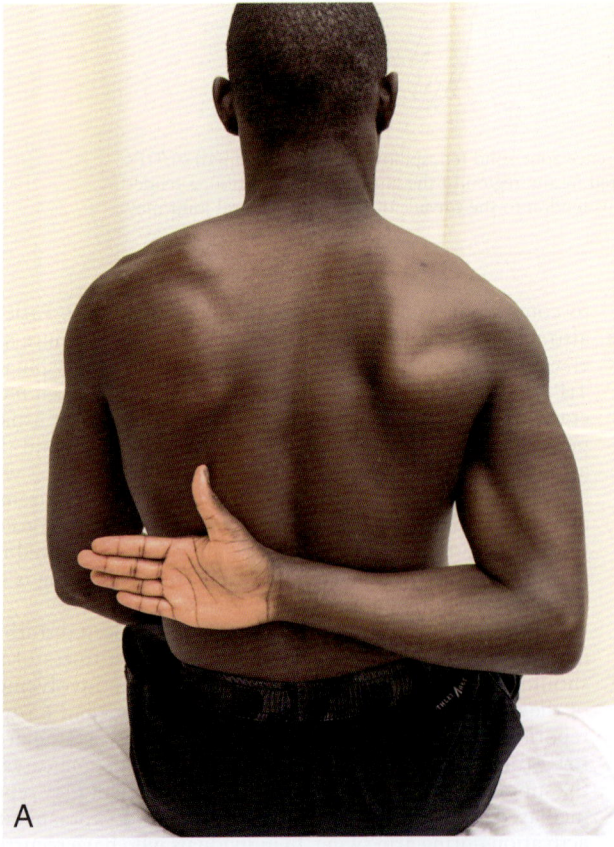
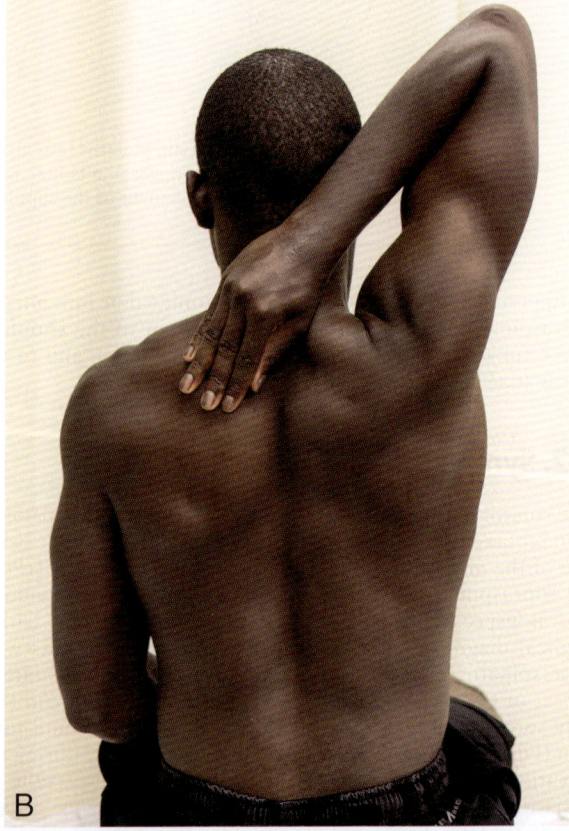

Figure 21-3. A, Apley's scratch test (extension, medial rotation, and adduction) to put the shoulder abductors and lateral rotators on stretch and to shorten the shoulder adductors and medial rotators. B, Apley's scratch test (flexion, lateral rotation, and abduction) to put the shoulder adductors and medial rotators on stretch and to shorten the shoulder abductors and lateral rotators.

elbow complex should be included in the examination because the supraspinatus muscle often refers pain to that region.

Patients with supraspinatus TrPs may be aware of, and be concerned about, clicking in the shoulder during movement. The clicking can be heard and palpated when the patient moves the arm at the glenohumeral joint in a way that incriminates the involved fibers of the supraspinatus muscle. Inactivating the supraspinatus TrPs eliminates the symptoms. The mechanism of this clicking is unknown but may relate to enthesopathy because the palpable source is also tender, or it may be associated with the inhibition of the supraspinatus muscle.

The humeral attachment of the supraspinatus tendon is most easily palpated if the hand of the upper limb being examined is placed behind the back at the waist level with the arm medially rotated. This position brings the tendon within the reach from beneath the acromion. Palpation often reveals a marked tenderness beneath the deltoid at the attachment of the supraspinatus tendon.

3.4. Trigger Point Examination

The patient sits comfortably, or lies on the uninvolved side, with the affected arm close to the body and is relaxed. In the case of less active TrPs, it may be desirable to place the arm behind the back, putting the supraspinatus muscle on stretch. The supraspinatus muscle should be palpated through the trapezius muscle utilizing cross-fiber flat palpation. The muscle should be palpated along its entire length within the supraspinous fossa to identify TrPs (Figure 21-4). Trigger points are typically located in the supraspinous fossa of the scapula underneath a relatively thick part of the trapezius muscle. Therefore, a local twitch response of the supraspinatus muscle is unreliably elicited by cross-fiber flat palpation and is not always perceived by needle penetration. Tenderness to palpation is often elicited in the mid-region of the supraspinous fossa (the midportion of some fibers pass here at about half the thickness of the muscle) but can be elicited anywhere in the supraspinous fossa because supraspinatus fibers attach throughout the medial two thirds of the fossa. The presence of spot tenderness in the lateral region, between the spine of the scapula and the clavicle, just medial to the acromion, most likely represents involvement of the musculotendinous junction secondary to increased muscle tension associated with the overuse of the supraspinatus muscle.

The severity and the extent of the referred pain evoked by needling TrPs in the muscular area are usually out of proportion to the slight degree of tenderness due to deep palpation reported by the patient, probably because of the depth of the muscle that should be penetrated diffuses the specificity of manual palpation pressure.

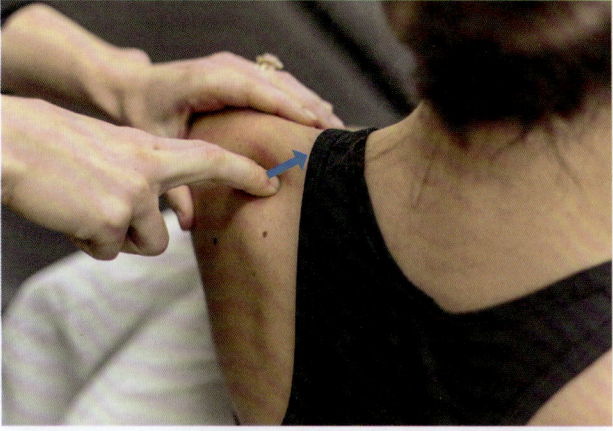

Figure 21-4. Cross-fiber flat palpation for TrPs in the supraspinatus muscle. The arrow depicts palpation direction.

The tendinous attachment into the head of the humerus, where the tendon of the muscle blends with the joint capsule to form part of the rotator cuff under the acromion, can be also be tender to palpation (Figure 21-2B). This tender region corresponds to the poorly vascularized area described by Hagberg[17] that is particularly vulnerable to sustained or repeated overload.

4. DIFFERENTIAL DIAGNOSIS

4.1. Activation and Perpetuation of Trigger Points

A posture or activity that activates a TrP, if not corrected, can also perpetuate it. In any part of the supraspinatus muscle, TrPs may be activated by unaccustomed eccentric loading, eccentric exercise in an unconditioned muscle, or maximal or submaximal concentric loading.[38] Trigger points may also be activated or aggravated when the muscle is placed in a shortened and/or lengthened position for an extended period of time.

Supraspinatus TrPs can be activated by carrying heavy objects such as a suitcase, briefcase, or package with the arm hanging down at the side, or by regularly walking a large dog that pulls on a leash. Trigger points in this muscle can also be activated by lifting an object to, or above, shoulder height with the arm outstretched or by performing tasks that demand repeated and/or moderately prolonged elevation of the arms.[17]

4.2. Associated Trigger Points

Associated TrPs can develop in the referred pain areas caused by other TrPs,[39] therefore, musculature in the referred pain areas for each muscle should also be considered. Release of the TrP in the muscle often allows for an immediate decrease in the pressure pain threshold of the associated TrPs.[39] This relationship is most commonly observed when TrPs in the supraspinatus muscle cause associated TrPs in the deltoid, lateral head of the triceps, and anconeus muscles.

Unlike the referred pain from the infraspinatus TrPs, which go deep into the shoulder and are easily mistaken for the arthritis of the glenohumeral joint,[40] the shoulder pain from supraspinatus TrPs lacks a deep, aching quality.

Clinical experience suggests that the supraspinatus, infraspinatus, deltoid, and biceps brachii muscles frequently develop TrPs at the same time and that the trapezius muscle may become involved as part of the functional unit. This notion is supported by recent research studies that investigated the prevalence and treatment of TrPs in patients presenting with shoulder pain.[41-43]

4.3. Associated Pathology

Cervical radiculitis in the C5 or C6 nerve roots often result in the formation of TrPs in those muscles innervated by the same nerve roots. Often patients with C5-C6 radicular symptoms report deep anterior shoulder pain, anterolateral shoulder pain, brachium and forearm pain, and pain into the radial aspect of the hand and the lateral two-and-a-half digits. Wainner et al[44] identified a test item cluster to determine the likelihood that a patient is presenting with a cervical radiculopathy. The following five predictor variables were identified: a positive spurling sign, cervical rotation less than 60° to the same side, positive cervical compression test, relief of symptoms with axial distraction, and a positive neurodynamic upper limb test. Patients presenting with four of these positive variables have a 90% posttest probability of cervical radiculopathy. Patients with three positive variables have a 65% posttest probability of cervical radiculopathy.[44]

Other diagnoses to consider include cervical arthritis or spurs with nerve root irritation and brachial plexus injuries. These neurogenic sources of pain are likely to exhibit EMG evidence of denervation (positive sharp waves and fibrillation potentials) in the muscles supplied by the compromised nerves. Muscles with TrPs show no EMG evidence of denervation because EMG evidence of muscle entrapment of a nerve would present in the muscles that are distal to the muscle causing the entrapment.

Shoulder pain accounts for approximately 12% of musculoskeletal conditions, and subacromial impingement syndrome (SIS) is the most prevalent diagnosis.[45] The direct cost for the treatment of shoulder pain in the United States was estimated to be $7 billion in the year 2000.[46] In a systematic review of the evidence related to the diagnosis of impingement syndrome of the shoulder by Papadonikolakis et al,[47] they concluded that the original diagnosis of impingement syndrome was developed to cover the breadth of rotator cuff disorders including tendinosis and complete and incomplete tears that were difficult to differentiate. These authors suggest that we drop the impingement syndrome diagnosis due to recent advancements in the diagnostics that allow differentiation of these diagnoses.[47] Diercks et al[48] suggested a guideline for the diagnosis and treatment of subacromial pain syndrome that includes the examination and treatment of TrPs. This syndrome is further discussed in Chapter 33 under Clinical Considerations.

Investigators have looked at the prevalence of TrPs, pressure pain threshold (PPT), and reproduction of shoulder pain in patients with nonspecific shoulder pain[49] or the diagnosis of impingement syndrome.[35,43] Hidalgo-Lozano et al[35] assessed 12 patients and 10 matched controls for the prevalence of TrPs and PPT. The inclusion criteria were: pain greater than 3-month duration, pain greater than 4/10 with shoulder elevation, and positive Neer and Hawkin's impingement tests. Patients with SIS had a greater number of active and latent TrPs. The highest prevalence of active TrPs was noted in the supraspinatus (62%), infraspinatus (42%), and subscapularis (42%) muscles. Patients with SIS demonstrated a decreased PPT that directly correlated with the number of TrPs. Each patient with SIS had up to three active TrPs. The greater the number of TrPs present, the lower the PPT. The results of their study lend credence to the idea that both peripheral and central pain mechanisms are present in patients with SIS. Manual treatment of these TrPs reduced shoulder pain and pressure sensitivity in individuals with SIS.[50] Similarly, the presence of TrPs in 10 muscles was investigated in 27 patients with a diagnosis of SIS and 20 matched controls.[43] The number of muscles with TrPs was significantly greater in the SIS group as compared with the control group, with the infraspinatus, subscapularis, and trapezius muscles having a significant number of active and latent TrPs. The infraspinatus muscle had the highest prevalence of active TrPs in the SIS group. The greater prevalence of TrPs in the SIS group signals the significance of myofascial pain in the presentation of SIS. Interestingly, TrPs in the supraspinatus muscle were found bilaterally in patients with SIS. Therefore, bilateral examination is important in patients with a diagnosis of SIS.[43]

In patients with unilateral shoulder pain and a diagnosis of SIS with associated positive impingement tests, it is essential to examine neck and shoulder muscles bilaterally for the presence of both active and latent TrPs. In addition to supraspinatus TrPs, subdeltoid bursitis, subacromial bursitis, adhesive capsulitis, and rotator cuff pathology may all cause tenderness at the tendinous attachment to the rotator cuff (capsule) beneath the acromion. Only TrPs, however, cause spot tenderness in the muscle belly of the supraspinatus muscle. Bursitis, adhesive capsulitis, and rotator cuff pathology are discussed in greater detail in Chapter 33 under Clinical Considerations.

Suprascapular nerve entrapment is a relatively rare entrapment seen in athletes performing repetitive cocking motions.[51] The cocking position requires shoulder abduction, extension, and external rotation, followed by rapid flexion and internal rotation.[19] Suprascapular nerve injury has also been identified in older individuals with degenerative changes in the glenohumeral joint and with capsular laxity associated with the aging process. This nerve entrapment is typically caused by repetitive overhead sports activity, ganglion cysts, or scapular fractures. Areas of entrapment include the suprascapular notch under the superior transverse ligament and the spinoglenoid notch in the presence of a space-occupying lesion.[52] Diagnosis by nerve conduction and EMG of both the infraspinatus and supraspinatus muscles is required to make this diagnosis. If the patient does not respond to rest and other conservative measures, surgery is indicated. A patient with suprascapular nerve entrapment reports vague shoulder girdle pain and demonstrates atrophy over the supraspinatus and infraspinatus muscles, limited shoulder range of motion, and fatigue in the shoulder girdle.[52] The patient's reports of pain may be similar to those caused by TrPs in shoulder girdle musculature especially the supraspinatus and infraspinatus muscles.

Scapulohumeral muscle imbalances, more commonly referred to as scapular dyskinesia, is defined as an alteration of normal motor recruitment pattern of muscle contraction of the shoulder girdle musculature during upper extremity movements. This alteration of normal muscle recruitment can lead to poor coordination, early fatigue, and overloading of the rotator cuff muscles. The role of scapular dyskinesia in myofascial pain and dysfunction is described in Chapter 33 under Clinical Considerations.

For patients with shoulder pain whose symptoms do not match their diagnosis or who have failed to improve with other conservative measures, supraspinatus TrP diagnosis and treatment can be invaluable.

5. CORRECTIVE ACTIONS

The patient with supraspinatus TrPs should avoid habitual, sustained, or repetitive motions that overload the supraspinatus muscle. This includes refraining from carrying heavy objects in the hand of the affected shoulder with the arm hanging down at the side, reaching backward or out to the side to retrieve objects, and lifting heavy items overhead. The patient should also avoid sustained contraction of the muscle, as when maintaining the arm in an elevated position (eg, holding the arms up continuously for several minutes to style hair or to work overhead). Occasionally, lowering the arms to relax the muscles can replenish their blood supply and prevent TrP formation.

When the patient lies on the uninvolved side, sleep is improved by supporting the uppermost elbow and forearm (painful limb) on a bed pillow, as described in Figure 22-4, to avoid the "watershed position" (Figure 22-4), which places undue tensile stress on the supraspinatus muscle. Another option is to place the pillow under the arm, perpendicular to the body so that the arm is out of the adducted position, thereby eliminating the

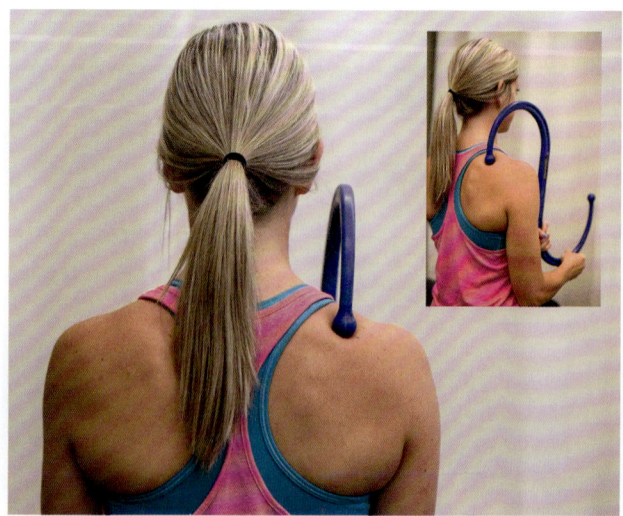

Figure 21-5. Trigger point self-pressure release of the supraspinatus muscle.

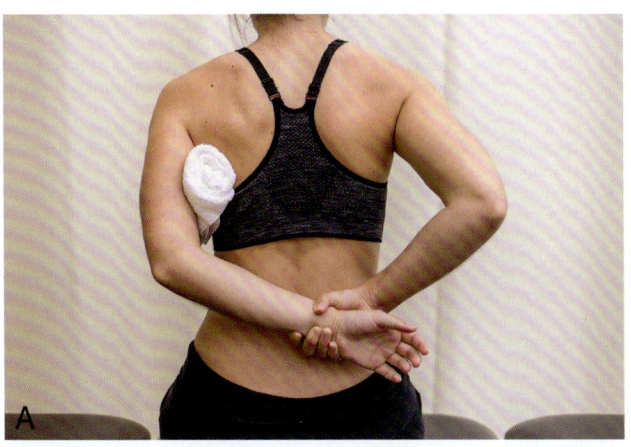 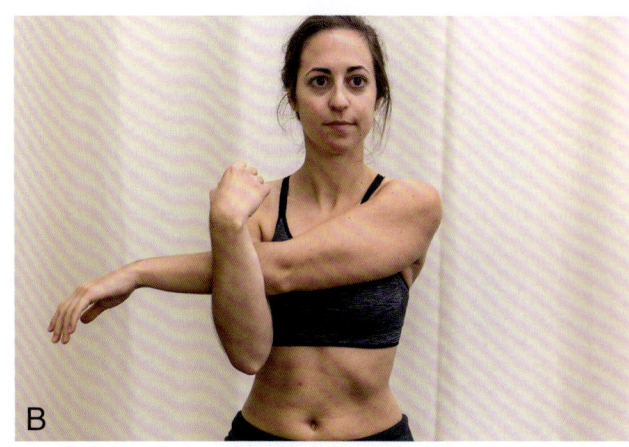

Figure 21-6. A, Self-stretch of the supraspinatus muscle. B, Self-stretch of supraspinatus and infraspinatus muscles if position A is unattainable due to pain.

supraspinatus muscle from being kept under tension. Patients should be cautioned regarding lying in bed with their arm(s) above their head in an abducted and externally rotated position because this position keeps the supraspinatus and infraspinatus muscles in a prolonged shortened position, causing increased tension.

The patient may inactivate supraspinatus TrPs using a TrP pressure release tool (Figure 21-5). This treatment is most comfortable if the pressure is applied while the involved arm is relaxed and supported in a comfortably adducted position. A more aggressive approach of this release involves taking up slack in the muscle (while TrP pressure release is continued) by sliding the hand behind the back, activating the antagonists to the supraspinatus muscle and thereby, allowing it to relax through reciprocal inhibition. A cold pack may be of therapeutic benefit post pressure release, especially in the case of acute shoulder pain.

The patient can stretch the supraspinatus muscle by slowly and firmly pulling the forearm behind the back in an upward direction with the other hand to position the involved arm as in Figure 21-6A. This passive stretch may be performed most effectively under a warm shower with the water beating on the muscle.

If both supraspinatus and infraspinatus TrPs are extremely sensitive and the patient has difficulty placing the hand behind the back, the arm may be brought across the front of the chest instead (Figure 21-6B). An effective self-stretch technique is the application of post-isometric relaxation (progressive contract-relax) with respiratory augmentation. The patient stretches the muscle by bringing the elbow of the involved side across the front of the chest with the other hand to take up slack in the muscle. As the patient takes slow deep breaths and during exhalation relaxes the muscle, the arm is brought further across the body passively with the unaffected arm. Lewit[53] illustrates this across-chest position and describes patient application of post-isometric relaxation that can be very helpful.

When prescribing neuromuscular reeducation or therapeutic exercises for the supraspinatus muscle, activation is greater with standing elevation in the plane of the scapula with thumbs up (full can), thumbs down (empty can), and in prone horizontal abduction 100° with full external rotation (full can).[24] Decker et al[54] found the greatest activity of the infraspinatus (115% MVC) and supraspinatus (125% MVC) muscles during the push-up plus activity. To minimize muscle activation of the supraspinatus and infraspinatus muscles, other authors suggest utilizing supported vertical and diagonal wall slides.[55,56]

Posterior glenohumeral joint tightness, when present, must be addressed to restore efficient shoulder girdle mechanics while concomitantly treating TrPs in the supraspinatus muscle. Treatment solely focused on TrPs in the supraspinatus muscle, which does not address the shoulder joint, results in treatment failure and only temporary relief of pain arising from TrPs in the supraspinatus muscle.

References

1. Standring S. *Gray's Anatomy: The Anatomical Basis of Clinical Practice.* 41st ed. London, UK: Elsevier; 2015.
2. Porterfield JA, DeRosa C. *Mechanical Shoulder Disorders: Perspectives in Functional Anatomy.* St. Louis, MO: Saunders; 2004:68-69.
3. Moser TP, Cardinal É, Bureau NJ, Guillin R, Lanneville P, Grabs D. The aponeurotic expansion of the supraspinatus tendon: anatomy and prevalence in a series of 150 shoulder MRIs. *Skeletal Radiol.* 2015;44(2):223-231.
4. Burkhart SS, Esch JC, Jolson RS. The rotator crescent and rotator cable: an anatomic description of the shoulder's "suspension bridge." *Arthroscopy.* 1993;9(6):611-616.
5. Sheah K, Bredella MA, Warner JJ, Halpern EF, Palmer WE. Transverse thickening along the articular surface of the rotator cuff consistent with the rotator cable: identification with MR arthrography and relevance in rotator cuff evaluation. *AJR Am J Roentgenol.* 2009;193(3):679-686.
6. Greiner A, Golser K, Wambacher M, Kralinger F, Sperner G. The course of the suprascapular nerve in the supraspinatus fossa and its vulnerability in muscle advancement. *J Shoulder Elbow Surg.* 2003;12(3):256-259.
7. Massimini DF, Singh A, Wells JH, Li G, Warner JJ. Suprascapular nerve anatomy during shoulder motion: a cadaveric proof of concept study with implications for neurogenic shoulder pain. *J Shoulder Elbow Surg.* 2013;22(4):463-470.
8. Wickham J, Pizzari T, Stansfeld K, Burnside A, Watson L. Quantifying "normal" shoulder muscle activity during abduction. *J Electromyogr Kinesiol.* 2010;20(2):212-222.
9. Kwon W, Jang H, Jun I. Comparison of supraspinatus cross-sectional areas according to shoulder abduction angles. *J Phys Ther Sci.* 2015;27(2):539-541.
10. Reed D, Cathers I, Halaki M, Ginn K. Does supraspinatus initiate shoulder abduction? *J Electromyogr Kinesiol.* 2013;23(2):425-429.
11. Reed D, Cathers I, Halaki M, Ginn KA. Does load influence shoulder muscle recruitment patterns during scapular plane abduction? *J Sci Med Sport.* 2015;15:207-208.
12. Wattanaprakornkul D, Halaki M, Boettcher C, Cathers I, Ginn KA. A comprehensive analysis of muscle recruitment patterns during shoulder flexion: an electromyographic study. *Clin Anat.* 2011;24(5):619-626.
13. de Witte PB, Werner S, ter Braak LM, Veeger HE, Nelissen RG, de Groot JH. The Supraspinatus and the Deltoid—not just two arm elevators. *Hum Mov Sci.* 2014;33:273-283.
14. Basmajian J, Deluca C. *Muscles Alive.* 5th ed. Baltimore, MD: Williams & Wilkins; 1985:185, 240-242, 263, 268, 274, 275, 385.
15. Ito N. Electromyographic study of shoulder joint. *Nihon Seikeigeka Gakkai Zasshi.* 1980;54(11):1529-1540.
16. Herberts P, Kadefors R. A study of painful shoulder in welders. *Acta Orthop Scand.* 1976;47(4):381-387.
17. Hagberg M. Local shoulder muscular strain—symptoms and disorders. *J Hum Ergol (Tokyo).* 1982;11(1):99-108.
18. Pink M, Jobe FW, Perry J. Electromyographic analysis of the shoulder during the golf swing. *Am J Sports Med.* 1990;18(2):137-140.
19. Jobe FW, Moynes DR, Tibone JE, Perry J. An EMG analysis of the shoulder in pitching. A second report. *Am J Sports Med.* 1984;12(3):218-220.
20. Gowan ID, Jobe FW, Tibone JE, Perry J, Moynes DR. A comparative electromyographic analysis of the shoulder during pitching. Professional versus amateur pitchers. *Am J Sports Med.* 1987;15(6):586-590.
21. Illyes A, Kiss RM. Shoulder muscle activity during pushing, pulling, elevation and overhead throw. *J Electromyogr Kinesiol.* 2005;15(3):282-289.

22. Pandis P, Prinold JA, Bull AM. Shoulder muscle forces during driving: Sudden steering can load the rotator cuff beyond its repair limit. *Clin Biomech (Bristol, Avon)*. 2015;30(8):839-846.
23. Reinold MM, Wilk KE, Fleisig GS, et al. Electromyographic analysis of the rotator cuff and deltoid musculature during common shoulder external rotation exercises. *J Orthop Sports Phys Ther*. 2004;34(7):385-394.
24. Reinold MM, Macrina LC, Wilk KE, et al. Electromyographic analysis of the supraspinatus and deltoid muscles during 3 common rehabilitation exercises. *J Athl Train*. 2007;42(4):464-469.
25. Simons DG, Travell J, Simons L. *Travell & Simon's Myofascial Pain and Dysfunction: The Trigger Point Manual*. Vol 1. 2nd ed. Baltimore, MD: Williams & Wilkins; 1999:104.
26. Travell J, Rinzler SH. The myofascial genesis of pain. *Postgrad Med*. 1952;11(5):425-434.
27. Zohn DA. *Musculoskeletal Pain: Diagnosis and Physical Treatment*. 2nd ed. Boston, MA: Little Brown; 1988:211.
28. Kelly M. The nature of fibrositis: III. Multiple lesions and the neural hypothesis. *Ann Rheum Dis*. 1946;5(5):161-167.
29. Kelly M. Some rules for the employment of local analgesic in the treatment of somatic pain. *Med J Aust*. 1947;1:235-239.
30. Kraus H. *Clinical Treatment of Back and Neck Pain*. New York, NY: McGraw-Hill; 1970:98.
31. Kellgren JH. A preliminary account of referred pains arising from muscle. *Br Med J*. 1938;1:325-327.
32. Steinbrocker O, Isenberg SA, Silver M, Neustadt D, Kuhn P, Schittone M. Observations on pain produced by injection of hypertonic saline into muscles and other supportive tissues. *J Clin Invest*. 1953;32(10):1045-1051.
33. Holtby R, Razmjou H. Validity of the supraspinatus test as a single clinical test in diagnosing patients with rotator cuff pathology. *J Orthop Sports Phys Ther*. 2004;34(4):194-200.
34. Bron C, Dommerholt J, Stegenga B, Wensing M, Oostendorp RA. High prevalence of shoulder girdle muscles with myofascial trigger points in patients with shoulder pain. *BMC Musculoskelet Disord*. 2011;12(1):139-151.
35. Hidalgo-Lozano A, Fernández de las Peñas C, Alonso-Blanco C, Ge HY, Arendt-Nielsen L, Arroyo-Morales M. Muscle trigger points and pressure pain hyperalgesia in the shoulder muscles in patients with unilateral shoulder impingement: a blinded, controlled study. *Exp Brain Res*. 2010;202(4):915-925.
36. Weed ND. When shoulder pain isn't bursitis. The myofascial pain syndrome. *Postgrad Med*. 1983;74(3):97-98, 101-102, 104.
37. Ohmori A, Iranami H, Fujii K, Yamazaki M, Doko Y. Myofascial involvement of supra- and infraspinatus muscles contributes to ipsilateral shoulder pain after muscle-sparing thoracotomy and video-assisted thoracic surgery. *J Cardiothorac Vasc Anesth*. 2013;27(6):1310-1314.
38. Gerwin RD, Dommerholt J, Shah JP. An expansion of Simons' integrated hypothesis of trigger point formation. *Curr Pain Headache Rep*. 2004;8(6):468-475.
39. Hsieh YL, Kao MJ, Kuan TS, Chen SM, Chen JT, Hong CZ. Dry needling to a key myofascial trigger point may reduce the irritability of satellite MTrPs. *Am J Phys Med Rehabil*. 2007;86(5):397-403.
40. Reynolds MD. Myofascial trigger point syndromes in the practice of rheumatology. *Arch Phys Med Rehabil*. 1981;62(3):111-114.
41. Hains G, Descarreaux M, Hains F. Chronic shoulder pain of myofascial origin: a randomized clinical trial using ischemic compression therapy. *J Manipulative Physiol Ther*. 2010;33(5):362-369.
42. Bron C, de Gast A, Dommerholt J, Stegenga B, Wensing M, Oostendorp RA. Treatment of myofascial trigger points in patients with chronic shoulder pain: a randomized, controlled trial. *BMC Med*. 2011;9:8.
43. Alburquerque-Sendin F, Camargo P, Viera A, Salvini TF. Bilateral myofascial trigger points and pressure pain thresholds in the shoulder muscles in patients with unilateral shoulder impingement syndrome. A blinded controlled study. *Clin J Pain*. 2013;29:478-486.
44. Wainner RS, Fritz JM, Irrgang JJ, Boninger ML, Delitto A, Allison S. Reliability and diagnostic accuracy of the clinical examination and patient self-report measures for cervical radiculopathy. *Spine*. 2003;28(1):52-62.
45. Pribicevic M, Pollard H, Bonello R. An epidemiologic survey of shoulder pain in chiropractic practice in australia. *J Manipulative Physiol Ther*. 2009;32(2):107-117.
46. Meislin RJ, Sperling JW, Stitik TP. Persistent shoulder pain: epidemiology, pathophysiology, and diagnosis. *Am J Orthop*. 2005;34(12 suppl):5-9.
47. Papadonikolakis A, McKenna M, Warme W, Martin BI, Matsen FA III. Published evidence relevant to the diagnosis of impingement syndrome of the shoulder. *J Bone Joint Surg Am*. 2011;93(19):1827-1832.
48. Diercks R, Bron C, Dorrestijn O, et al. Guideline for diagnosis and treatment of subacromial pain syndrome: a multidisciplinary review by the Dutch Orthopaedic Association. *Acta Orthop*. 2014;85(3):314-322.
49. Ge HY, Fernández de las Peñas C, Madeleine P, Arendt-Nielsen L. Topographical mapping and mechanical pain sensitivity of myofascial trigger points in the infraspinatus muscle. *Eur J Pain*. 2008;12(7):859-865.
50. Hidalgo-Lozano A, Fernández de las Peñas C, Diaz-Rodriguez L, Gonzalez-Iglesias J, Palacios-Cena D, Arroyo-Morales M. Changes in pain and pressure pain sensitivity after manual treatment of active trigger points in patients with unilateral shoulder impingement: a case series. *J Bodyw Mov Ther*. 2011;15(4):399-404.
51. Fritz RC, Helms CA, Steinbach LS, Genant HK. Suprascapular nerve entrapment: evaluation with MR imaging. *Radiology*. 1992;182(2):437-444.
52. Jacob PJ, Arun K, Binoj R. Suprascapular nerve entrapment syndrome. *Kerala J Orthop*. 2011;25:21-24.
53. Lewit K. *Manipulative Therapy in Rehabilitation of the Locomotor System*. 3rd ed. Oxford, England: Butterworth Heinemann; 1999:204-205.
54. Decker MJ, Tokish JM, Ellis HB, Torry MR, Hawkins RJ. Subscapularis muscle activity during selected rehabilitation exercises. *Am J Sports Med*. 2003;31(1):126-134.
55. Gaunt BW, McCluskey GM, Uhl TL. An electromyographic evaluation of subdividing active-assistive shoulder elevation exercises. *Sports Health*. 2010;2(5):424-432.
56. Wise MB, Uhl TL, Mattacola CG, Nitz AJ, Kibler WB. The effect of limb support on muscle activation during shoulder exercises. *J Shoulder Elbow Surg*. 2004;13(6):614-620.

Chapter 22

Infraspinatus Muscle

"Side-Sleeper's Nemesis"

Joseph M. Donnelly

1. INTRODUCTION

The infraspinatus muscle is a thick, irregularly shaped muscle, consisting of three muscle bellies: superior, middle, and inferior. The muscle originates from the medial two-thirds of the infraspinous fossa below the spine of the scapula and the adjacent fascia from the lower fibers of the trapezius, rhomboids, and serratus anterior muscles. The infraspinatus muscle inserts onto the middle facet on the posterior aspect of the greater tuberosity of the humerus. The infraspinatus muscle is innervated by the suprascapular nerve. The irregular shape and morphology of the infraspinatus muscle allow it to be a major contributor to glenohumeral joint stability, providing force to seat the humeral head in the glenoid of the scapula during upper extremity movement. Its chief action is external rotation of the shoulder along with the teres minor muscle. Trigger points (TrPs) in the infraspinatus muscle produce shoulder joint pain deep in the anterior deltoid region and are distally referred into the lateral forearm and radial aspect of the hand. Pain may be referred to the medial scapular border, to the suboccipital region, and occasionally to the posterior cervical region. Symptoms may be exacerbated with sleeping on the affected side, reaching behind the back, and performing activities of daily living that require combined movements of shoulder elevation and external rotation. Activation and perpetuation of TrPs in the infraspinatus muscle usually result from acute overload while reaching backward and upward or with overhead lifting with the upper extremity in external rotation. Differential diagnosis should include assessment for posterior glenohumeral joint capsule tightness, neurodynamic testing to rule out neural pathomechanics, C5-C6 radiculitis, bicipital tendonitis, and suprascapular nerve entrapment. Corrective actions should include postural reeducation (including proper sleep position), elimination of positions that cause recurrent overload on the muscle, self-pressure release of TrPs, and self-stretch exercises.

2. ANATOMIC CONSIDERATIONS

The infraspinatus muscle is contained within the infraspinatus fascia which is described as a tough sheet of connective tissue, that covers the infraspinous fossa and envelopes the infraspinatus muscle. Muscle fibers originate from both the fascia and the fossa.[1] The infraspinatus muscle originates from the medial two thirds of the infraspinous fossa below the spine of the scapula and the adjacent fascia from the lower fibers of the trapezius, rhomboids, and serratus anterior muscles. A fascial connection has also been identified between the posterior deltoid and infraspinatus muscles.[1] The infraspinatus inserts onto the middle facet on the posterior aspect of the greater tuberosity of the humerus[2] (Figure 22-1). The tendon may blend superiorly and posteriorly with the shoulder joint capsule[3] and can be separated by a small bursa.[2] The infraspinatus tendon fuses with the supraspinatus tendon just lateral to the spine of the scapula.[2] Investigators utilizing cadaver specimens demonstrated the gross anatomic structure of the infraspinatus muscle as being comprised of three distinct muscle partitions (heads).[4] These partitions were described as the superior, the middle, and the inferior partitions. The fibers of the superior partition are horizontally aligned, whereas the fibers of the middle and inferior partitions are oriented superolateral and terminate into the central thickened tendon. The middle partition of the muscle has a distinct fibrous band that inserts deep to the superior and inferior partitions and is thought to attach to the middle and superior facet with the supraspinatus muscle.[2] The deeper fibers pass at acute angles to conjoin with the supraspinatus muscle superiorly and cross the rotator cuff interval, attaching to the subscapularis tendon. This thick fibrous tendon is referred to as the rotator cable[5] that links the posterior rotator cuff muscles to the anterior cuff muscle. Lateral to the rotator cable, the distal arrangement of the tendon that inserts onto the humerus is called the rotator crescent. It consists of the distal insertions of the infraspinatus and supraspinatus tendons. The rotator cable is thought to protect the rotator crescent[5] by transferring forces intrinsically from the posterosuperior rotator cuff to the anterior rotator cuff.[2] This complex insertion allows the rotator cuff to work in a coordinated fashion during all the shoulder motions.

2.1. Innervation and Vascularization

The infraspinatus muscle is innervated by the suprascapular nerve that is derived from the upper trunk of the brachial plexus and the primary ventral rami of C5 and C6, with C5 contributing the majority of fibers.[6,7] The suprascapular nerve passes dorsolaterally through the posterior triangle of the neck and under the superior transverse scapular ligament into the supraspinous fossa. In the supraspinous fossa, the nerve provides innervation to the supraspinatus muscle before coursing laterally through the spinoglenoid notch to enter the infraspinous fossa. In the infraspinous fossa, primary, secondary, and tertiary branches provide innervation to the infraspinatus muscle. In more than 60% of specimens evaluated, the three partitions of the infraspinatus muscle were all innervated by a first-order branch of the suprascapular nerve.[4] The suprascapular nerve is subject to compression and potential entrapment as it passes under the transverse scapular ligament and in the spinoglenoid notch.[8,9]

The vascular supply to the infraspinatus muscle is provided by the suprascapular and circumflex scapular arteries.[2]

2.2. Function

The infraspinatus, teres minor, supraspinatus, and subscapularis muscles insert into the greater and lesser tuberosities of the humerus to form a musculotendinous rotator cuff. These rotator cuff muscles

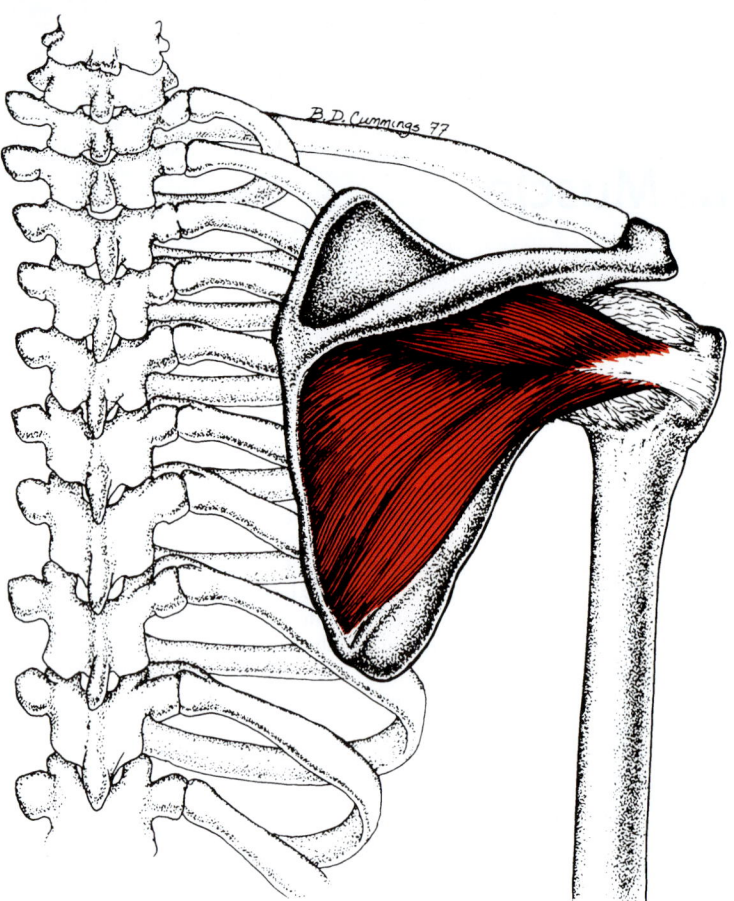

Figure 22-1. Infraspinatus muscle attachments from the medial two thirds of the infraspinous fossa to the middle facet on the posterior aspect of the greater tuberosity of the humerus. Deeper fibers attach to the superior facet conjoining with fibers of the supraspinatus to form the rotator cable.

provide dynamic stability to the glenohumeral joint. Motion at the shoulder is a complex coordinated activity, and the moment arms of the rotator cuff muscles exert inferiorly and medially directed forces that resist upward shear of the deltoid muscle during shoulder elevation while keeping the head of the humerus in close contact with the glenoid fossa.[10] The primary function of the infraspinatus muscle, along with the other three rotator cuff muscles, is to stabilize and center the head of the humerus in the glenoid fossa with any upper extremity movement. It also serves as a passive restraint to posterior subluxation and as a dynamic restraint against anterior subluxation of the head of the humerus.[11] The infraspinatus muscle has a primary action of external rotation at the glenohumeral joint, with the arm in any position.[12-14]

Some authors have reported the infraspinatus muscle as having a moderate maximum voluntary contraction (% MVC) in standing and side-lying external rotation movements; whereas peak activity was noted with prone horizontal abduction between 90° and 100° with full external rotation.[13,14] More recent research demonstrated that the infraspinatus muscle is active prior to humeral movement during shoulder flexion,[15] elevation in the plane of the scapula, and abduction in the coronal plane, and it reaches peak intensity at 165° of abduction.[10,14,16,17] Investigators theorize that the infraspinatus muscle has a role in counterbalancing the deltoid and pectoralis major muscles during shoulder elevation in addition to externally rotating the humerus to achieve full elevation. In abduction, multiple muscles contribute both to the abductive force and to the stabilization of the humeral head in the glenoid fossa.

Electromyographical studies have demonstrated that infraspinatus muscle activity increased linearly with increasing abduction, with additional peaks of activity during flexion.[17,18] The maximum isometric rotation moment capacity was greater at 0° abduction compared with 90° abduction.[14] Because of the superior belly's horizontal arrangement, it may be primarily responsible for the action of external rotation in neutral to 10°.[19]

The infraspinatus muscle serves as one of the primary decelerators of the throwing arm[18,20-22] and the follow-through arm in a golf swing.[23] The deceleration function, which requires an eccentric contraction, may be a contributing factor to the formation of TrPs[24,25] and breakdown on the undersurface of the infraspinatus tendon.[20] In throwers, near the moment of ball release, there is a large distraction force between the glenoid cavity and the humerus during this deceleration phase. The large distraction force is resisted by a strong eccentric contraction of the infraspinatus muscle, placing it at risk for tensile overload.[26] Other investigators found that the infraspinatus muscle is maximally activated during a fast overhead throw and moderately active during pushing and pulling activities.[27]

Basmajian and Deluca[28] described how the angulation of the glenoid fossa, together with the activity of horizontal fibers in several muscles, provides a coaptation force that prevents downward displacement of the head of the humerus. They showed that the activity of the supraspinatus muscle and the posterior fibers of the deltoid muscle prevented downward displacement of the humeral head, even with considerable downward loading of the adducted arm. In other positions, however, additional protection of the joint by rotator cuff muscular activity, which includes contraction of the infraspinatus muscle, becomes critical.[28]

Functionally, as the position of the arm changes, the function of the shoulder girdle muscles also change. The infraspinatus muscle is best aligned at 100° of scaption to exert an active compressive force between the humeral head and the glenoid along with combined motions of external rotation and horizontal abduction. This position may be optimal for resistance exercises of the infraspinatus muscle.[13,14]

Reed et al[16] found that as an external load increased during abduction in the plane of the scapula, the activity levels in the infraspinatus muscle increased systematically. The muscle activation pattern established with low loads is maintained as the load increases. They conclude that this activation pattern supports the law of proportional activation against the law of minimal activation based on activation of muscles with the least synergistic activity. Lucas et al[29] reported similar findings; however, they observed increased infraspinatus muscle activity level and early activation with an external load and presence of TrPs in the scapular upward rotators.[29]

The infraspinatus muscle's level of activity increases significantly with turning a car wheel, and to a much lesser extent, when the wheel is centered.[30] The highest level of activation noted in the infraspinatus muscle is following a steering maneuver when the wheel is being placed back to the center position. When the steering wheel is held in the center position, there is a cocontraction of shoulder muscles to stabilize the wheel.[30]

2.3. Functional Unit

The functional unit to which a muscle belongs includes the muscles that reinforce and counter its actions as well as the joints that the muscle crosses. The functional interdependence of these structures is reflected in the organization and neural connections of the sensory motor cortex. The functional unit is emphasized because the presence of a TrP in one muscle of the unit increases the likelihood that the other muscles of the unit also develops TrPs. When inactivating TrPs in a muscle, one should be concerned about TrPs that may develop in muscles that are functionally interdependent. Box 22-1 grossly represents the functional unit of the infraspinatus muscle.[24]

In addition, the infraspinatus muscle functions synergistically with the teres minor, the supraspinatus, and the subscapularis muscles to stabilize the head of the humerus in the glenoid fossa during arm movements.[10,28]

3. CLINICAL PRESENTATION

3.1. Referred Pain Pattern

Trigger points in the infraspinatus muscle refer pain deep in the anterior aspect of the shoulder.[31] Most reports of the referred pain pattern from the infraspinatus identify the anterior aspect of the shoulder as the major target area (Figure 22-2).[31-36] In 193 cases of referred pain from the infraspinatus muscle, all patients identified the anterior aspect of the shoulder as painful.[33] The pain was described as also projecting down the anterolateral aspect of the arm,[31,33-37] to the lateral forearm,[31,33-36] to the radial aspect of the hand,[31,33-37] and occasionally to the fingers[33,37] or to the upper posterior cervical region and medial border of the scapula (Figure 22-2). Patients usually identify the most painful area by covering the front of the shoulder with their hand.

Trigger points in the infraspinatus muscle have also been found to refer pain to the posterior aspect of the shoulder; however, this pain may result from TrPs simultaneously present in the adjacent teres minor muscle.[24] Bonica and Sola[38] described aching pain referring primarily to the region of the deltoid muscle. Rachlin[39] emphasized pain to the posterior aspect of the shoulder and also included referral along the medial border of the scapula as well as to the base of the neck in the region of the levator scapulae muscle.

Much of the variation among these reports is probably due to the appearance of referred pain in the variable spillover zones. Among 193 subjects with infraspinatus TrPs, 6% experienced pain in the deltoid and the biceps brachii regions, none reported elbow pain, 21% reported pain in the radial forearm, 13% in the radial side of the hand, and 14% in the suboccipital posterior cervical area.[33] No distinction was made in the pain patterns arising from these TrPs.

One patient with an aberrant pain pattern of infraspinatus TrPs was described. In that case, the pain was referred superficially to the front part of the chest. After the initial injection, the patient returned with the expected infraspinatus pain pattern that resolved with additional injections of infraspinatus TrPs.[40]

Experimentally, pressure stimulation of an active infraspinatus TrP increased alpha motor neuron excitability in the anterior fibers of the deltoid that in turn induced a referred pain pattern to the anterior aspect of the shoulder. Motor unit activity appeared at rest in the deltoid muscle during referred pain elicited by the application of digital pressure. The patient was unable to eliminate the motor unit activity by relaxation, although surrounding muscles not within the pain reference zone were electrically silent. This finding supports recent evidence that TrPs can refer increased alpha motor neuron excitability as well as pain. Fernández-Carnero et al[41] showed that an increased nociceptive activity in latent TrPs in the infraspinatus muscle might increase motor activity and sensitivity of a TrP in distant muscles, eg, the extensor carpi radialis brevis muscle, at the same segmental level.

Referred pain from the infraspinatus muscle was induced experimentally by injecting the normal muscle with 6% hypertonic saline. Deep pain was felt at the tip of the shoulder, in the posterior and lateral aspects of the shoulder, and in the anterolateral aspect of the arm.[42]

3.2. Symptoms

Trigger points in the infraspinatus muscle typically cause shoulder pain at rest, interfering with functional activities and sleep. Patients may report a deep ache in the anterior aspect of the shoulder and often describe the pain as being "deep in the joint." The pain can spread down the anterolateral aspect of the arm, the lateral forearm, the radial side of the hand, and occasionally into the fingers. The patient's symptoms may be similar to those of C5-C6 radicular pain or carpal tunnel syndrome. One study observed that approximately one third of patients referred with a clinical suspicion of carpal tunnel syndrome but with negative EMG findings had TrPs in the infraspinatus muscle.[43] In fact, Hains et al[44] observed that TrP therapy using ischemic compression was a useful approach to reduce symptoms associated with the carpal tunnel syndrome. Patients may also report pain along the medial border of the scapula over the insertion of the rhomboid muscles, significant activity limitations, and participation restrictions due to TrPs in the infraspinatus muscle.

When the patient's chief report is pain in the anterior aspect of the shoulder, infraspinatus, supraspinatus, deltoid (anterior and middle), biceps brachii, coracobrachialis, scaleni, pectoralis major and minor, and subclavius muscles are the most likely muscular sources of symptoms.[45] In fact, active TrPs in the infraspinatus muscle can contribute to symptoms in patients

---

Box 22-1 Functional unit in the infraspinatus muscle

Action	Synergists	Antagonists
Shoulder lateral rotation	Teres minor Posterior deltoid	Subscapularis Pectoralis major Latissimus dorsi Anterior deltoid

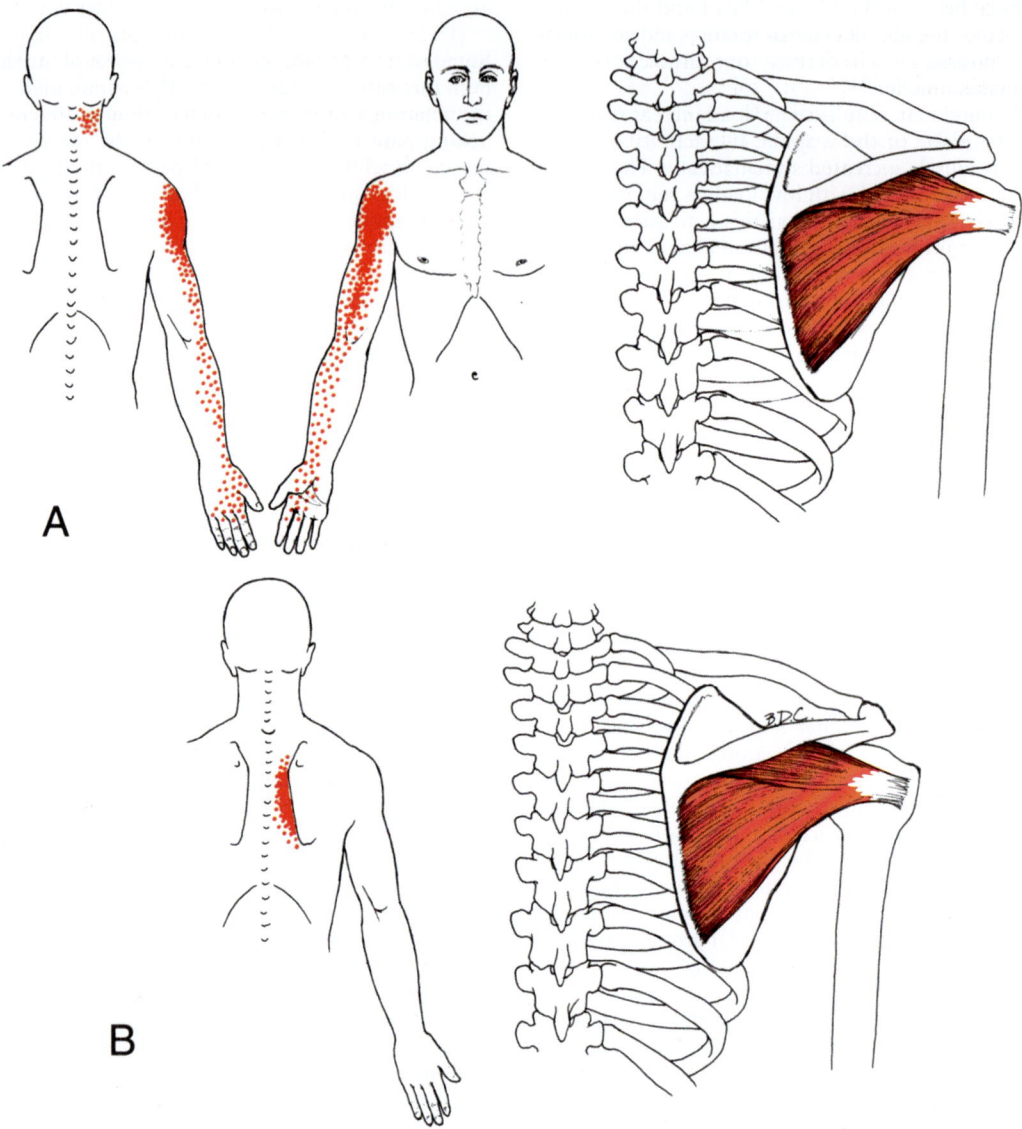

Figure 22-2. Referred pain patterns (red) in the right infraspinatus muscle. Solid red shows essential referred pain zones, stippled red areas show spillover zones.

with mechanical neck pain,[46] women with postmastectomy pain,[47] desk or industrial workers,[48] or individuals with medical diagnosis of subacromial impingement syndrome.[49] A thorough examination for the presence of TrPs in the shoulder girdle musculature is essential to improve patient functional outcomes for shoulder pain.[50,51]

Common reports of pain in patients with TrPs in the infraspinatus muscle are presented in Box 22-2. Sola and Williams[52] identified the symptoms of shoulder girdle fatigue, weakness of grip, loss of mobility at the shoulder, and hyperhidrosis in the referred pain area as due to TrP activity in the infraspinatus muscle.

The patient with TrPs in the infraspinatus muscle may also report increased local and/or referred pain at night due to sleeping postures and spontaneous activation of active TrPs (Figure 22-2). The weight of the thorax compresses and stimulates the infraspinatus TrPs while the patient is lying on the painful side (and sometimes on the back).[31] This hypothesis is supported by Ohmori et al[53] who reported that active TrPs in the supraspinatus and infraspinatus muscles are associated with shoulder pain in patients receiving muscle-sparing thoracotomy. The authors suggested that the position of the shoulder against the table was one of the main factors for activation of infraspinatus TrPs.[53] When the patient lies on the pain-free side for relief, the uppermost arm is likely to fall forward causing a painful stretch of the affected infraspinatus muscle, again disturbing sleep. Thus, patients with active infraspinatus TrPs may find that they can

> **Box 22-2 Common reports from patients with active TrPs in the infraspinatus**
>
> I can't reach into my back pants pocket.
> I can't fasten my brassiere behind my back.
> I have to put this arm into my coat sleeve first.
> I can't reach into the back seat of my car.
> I have difficulty combing or brushing my hair.
> Brushing my teeth is painful.
> I can't play overhead sports.

sleep only by propping themselves up while seated in a reclined position for the night.

A major part of the shoulder girdle pain associated with hemiplegia is commonly due to TrPs in the trapezius, levator scapulae, supraspinatus, infraspinatus, subscapularis, deltoid, and rhomboids muscles. In the absence of spasticity at rest, TrPs in these muscles usually respond well to local treatment.[54] These authors found that all patients after stroke who were randomly assigned to the dry needling group (n = 54) plus standard rehabilitation, exhibited infraspinatus TrPs in addition to TrPs in other shoulder girdle muscles. Following an intervention with dry needling, the patients reported restoration of sleep, significant decrease in frequency and intensity of pain during the day, and less pain and discomfort during rehabilitation as compared with those in the control group receiving standard rehabilitation only.[54]

3.3. Patient Examination

After a thorough subjective examination, the clinician should make a detailed drawing representing the pain pattern that the patient has described. This depiction will assist in planning the physical examination and can be useful in monitoring the progression of the patient as symptoms improve or change. For proper examination of the infraspinatus muscle, the examiner should observe the shoulder girdle posture, active and passive ranges of motion of the shoulder girdle, muscle activation patterns, and the scapulohumeral rhythm. Investigators have found that the presence of TrPs in the infraspinatus muscle can cause an inconsistent muscle activation pattern during shoulder elevation,[55] and that the infraspinatus muscle fires first and consistently in the presence of latent TrPs in the scapular upward rotators.[29] To identify TrPs in the infraspinatus muscle that may be limiting the range of motion and thus influencing dysfunction, the clinician should identify the limited range of motion by performing specific range of motion tests for all parts of the infraspinatus muscle. In addition to examination of passive medial rotation in neutral, the examiner should also include horizontal adduction as the superior belly of the infraspinatus muscle is lengthened with this motion, often reproducing the patient's pain. Muscle-specific resisted testing should be performed to identify impairments in muscle function and reproduction of painful symptoms. If active TrPs are present in the infraspinatus muscle, resisted lateral rotation in the neutral position is painfully inhibited.

The Apley's scratch test (extension, adduction, and medial rotation) can be used to identify restriction in the infraspinatus muscle due to TrPs. The hand-to-shoulder-blade test requires full adduction and medial rotation of the arm at the glenohumeral joint. This test is performed by placing the hand of the affected side behind the back and reaching as far up toward the opposite scapula as possible. The fingertips should reach the inferior angle of the scapula (Figure 21-3 in Chapter 21). This test stretches the shoulder abductors and the infraspinatus muscle. When the range of these muscles is limited due to TrPs, the fingers may barely reach to the hip pocket or thoracolumbar region. Range of motion limitation is similar when the movement is performed actively or passively. Conversely, TrPs in the antagonistic subscapularis muscle may allow the fingers to reach the spinal column, or farther, if done passively without contracting the subscapularis muscle in the shortened position, while an active limitation of this same motion is evident.

Accessory joint motion should be tested in the glenohumeral joint, acromioclavicular joint, sternoclavicular joint, and scapulothoracic joints. Many times, joint hypomobility in the sternoclavicular joint can cause impairment in shoulder elevation, contributing to alterations in the normal muscle activation patterns. Articular dysfunctions in the glenohumeral joint may also impair muscle activation patterns, contributing to overload of the infraspinatus and other rotator cuff muscles.

The glenohumeral joint should be carefully assessed for Glenohumeral Internal Rotation Deficit, which may be indicative of posterior capsule tightness. Scapular position and humeral head position should also be assessed at rest and during upper extremity elevation, as malalignment can be a significant contributing factor to infraspinatus muscle overload during all upper extremity functional activities.

3.4. Trigger Point Examination

Trigger points in the infraspinatus muscle are common in patients who report shoulder pain. The prevalence of active infraspinatus TrPs in patients with nontraumatic chronic shoulder pain is significant. In a study of 72 subjects with chronic shoulder pain, the most affected muscle was the infraspinatus muscle, which demonstrated active TrPs in 77% of subjects.[45] This study reinforces the findings from Ge et al[56] who commonly reported active TrPs patients with unilateral shoulder pain. Infraspinatus TrPs have also been associated with whiplash-associated disorders,[46] chronic work-related shoulder and neck complaints,[48] women with postmastectomy pain,[47] or shoulder impingement syndrome.[49] It is not uncommon to find multiple TrPs, both active and latent, in the infraspinatus muscles of patients with shoulder pain.[56]

In a study of 126 patients, investigators found referred pain to the shoulder region arose from the infraspinatus muscle in 31% of the cases, a frequency second only to that of the levator scapulae muscle (55%).[34] In an unpublished research project, Donnelly found that the prevalence of latent TrPs in 92 healthy pain-free adults was 70% in the infraspinatus muscle, as compared with 13% in the biceps brachii and 27% in the triceps brachii muscles.

The infraspinatus muscle may be examined for TrPs with the patient seated, side-lying on the pain-free side, or in prone. When the patient is seated, the arm may be supported by the side of the body (Figure 22-3). Cross-fiber flat palpation frequently reveal multiple taut bands containing TrPs in this muscle.[45,56] Trigger points are typically found in the midportion (endplate zone) of the infraspinatus muscle; however, the entire muscle needs to be palpated for an accurate diagnosis. Ge et al[56] investigated topographical mapping and pain pressure threshold (PPT) of TrPs in the infraspinatus muscles in 21 female patients with primary reports of unilateral shoulder pain. They found multiple active TrPs on the painful side but not on the uninvolved side. They also found multiple latent TrPs both on the painful side and unpainful side. A majority of the active and latent TrPs were found to be located in the mid-fiber region of the infraspinatus muscle.[56] Occasionally, a TrP may cause pain referral to the medial border of the scapula and adjacent rhomboid muscles (Figure 22-2).

Each of the three distinct muscle partitions (superior, middle, and inferior) should be examined carefully. Knowledge of fiber direction is critical, as cross-fiber flat palpation should be performed along the length of the entire infraspinatus muscle to locate the taut bands and identify spot tenderness within the taut band.

Firm bands in this superficial muscle may be more difficult to identify than one might expect. Local twitch responses (LTRs) are moderately difficult to elicit by cross-fiber flat snapping palpation. The overlying skin is often thick and indurated by associated panniculosis. Referred pain can usually be evoked or aggravated by sustained pressure on an infraspinatus TrP. Trigger points in the infraspinatus muscle typically have a referred pain latency when pressure is applied to the TrP, which can take up to 30 seconds for distal referral of symptoms.

In a study by Bron et al,[57] the interrater reliability of palpation of TrPs in three shoulder muscles (infraspinatus, biceps brachii, and deltoid) was investigated in asymptomatic subjects, patients with unilateral shoulder pain, and patients with bilateral shoulder pain.[57] They found that experienced clinicians

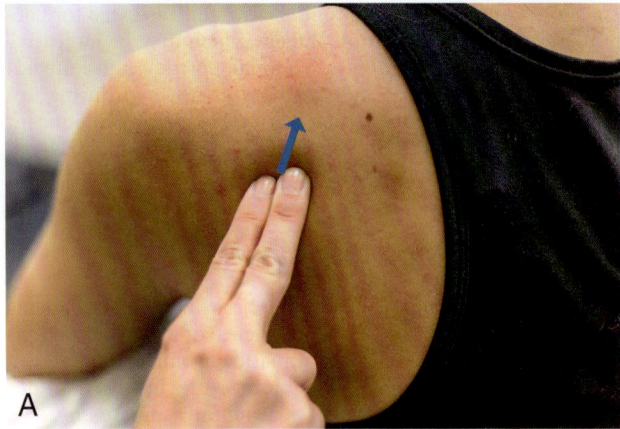
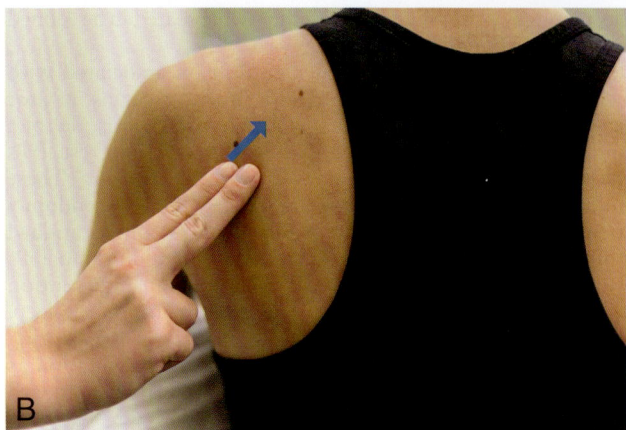
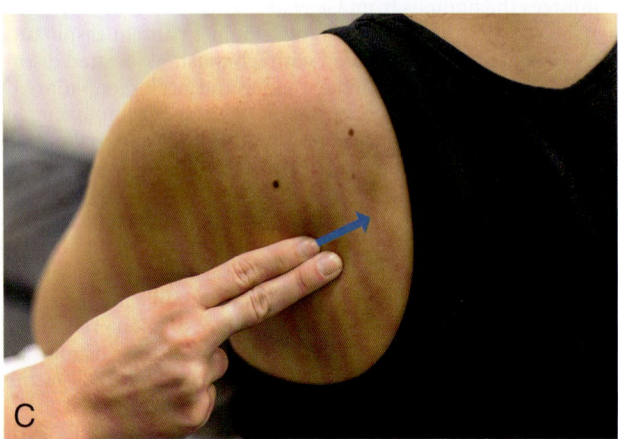

Figure 22-3. Cross-fiber flat palpation for TrPs in the infraspinatus muscle. A, Superior fibers. B, Middle fibers. C, Inferior fibers.

had a greater than 70% agreement in identifying TrPs in the infraspinatus muscle. They also found that referred pain was the most reliable feature in all muscles, whereas identification of the taut band, LTR, and jump sign were the most reliable criteria for identifying TrPs in the infraspinatus muscle. Their findings were also consistent with those of Ge et al[56] who identified latent TrPs bilaterally in those patients presenting with unilateral shoulder pain and a more frequent location of TrPs in the mid-fiber region of the muscle.

4. DIFFERENTIAL DIAGNOSIS

4.1. Activation and Perpetuation of Trigger Points

A posture or activity that activates a TrP, if not corrected, can also perpetuate it. In any part of the infraspinatus muscle, TrPs may be activated by unaccustomed eccentric loading, eccentric exercise in an unconditioned muscle, or maximal or submaximal concentric loading.[25] Trigger points may also be activated or aggravated when the muscle is placed in a shortened or lengthened position for an extended period of time. Infraspinatus TrPs are usually activated by an acute overload or by repeated overload, such as the stress of frequently reaching to the back seat of a car, reaching back from an office chair, grabbing behind for support to regain balance (eg, grasping the railing when slipping on stairs), twisting the arm that holds a ski pole during a fall, delivering an especially hard tennis serve when off balance, or with dragging a novice ice skater around by the arm for a long period of time. Vigorous weight training with heavy overhead loads or eccentric loading can also precipitate the formation of

TrPs in the infraspinatus muscle. The onset of shoulder pain is usually within a few hours of the initiating trauma. The patient can generally identify when the muscle was overloaded.

Baker[58] found that between 20% and 30% of the infraspinatus muscles of patients experiencing their first motor vehicle accident had active TrPs following the accident, regardless of the direction of impact. This was slightly lesser than the number of TrPs that developed in the supraspinatus muscles of these patients.

Bron et al[51] investigated the role of TrPs in chronic shoulder pain and dysfunction. Patients were randomly assigned to either a treatment group or a control group. The control group was placed on a waiting list (wait and see) for 12 weeks. The number of active TrPs present was less in the intervention group at 12 weeks as compared with the control group; however, there was no difference in the number of latent TrPs. Active TrPs in the infraspinatus and other rotator cuff musculature were responsible for reproduction of the patients pain. There was a positive correlation in the number of active TrPs and the score on the Disability of Arm, Shoulder, and Hand (DASH) that demonstrated a change of 24% as active TrPs were inactivated. They reported a 55% improvement in pain and function in the intervention group with a significant reduction in the number of active TrPs at 12 weeks.[51]

Hidalgo-Lozano et al[59] investigated the prevalence and mechanical sensitivity of several shoulder and neck muscles in elite swimmers with and without shoulder pain. They demonstrated that elite swimmers with shoulder pain had significantly decreased PPT as compared with that in controls. However, swimmers without shoulder pain showed no significant difference in PPT as compared with those with shoulder pain. Swimmers with shoulder pain had a significant number of active TrPs present in the infraspinatus and subscapularis muscles, which on palpation reproduced the swimmers pain. Surprisingly, they found active TrPs in swimmers without shoulder pain as well. When the swimmers were questioned about this finding, they reported that it was a historically familiar pain. Both elite swimmers with and without shoulder pain had a significant number of latent TrPs; however, the latter had a higher prevalence.[59]

Repetitive overuse is also seen in competitive overhead athletes. The overhead volleyball or tennis serve can cause repetitive strain and TrP formation in the rotator cuff muscles especially the infraspinatus muscle. Osborne et al[60] identified TrPs in volleyball players that developed after several long days of training and tournament play. Release of the TrPs restored an active range of motion and allowed the athletes to quickly return to competitive play.

4.2. Associated Trigger Points

Associated TrPs can develop in the referred pain areas caused by TrPs.[61] Therefore, musculature in the referred pain areas for each muscle should also be considered. Three groups of muscles develop TrPs in association with the infraspinatus muscle. Any given patient typically exhibits involvement of one of the three groups. The first group consists of the anterior deltoid muscle, which lies in the essential pain reference zone of the infraspinatus muscle, and the biceps brachii muscle, which may also become involved with prolonged activation of the infraspinatus muscle. The second group includes the teres major and latissimus dorsi muscles. The third group includes the subscapularis and pectoralis major muscles, which are antagonistic to the infraspinatus muscle in lateral rotation of the humerus.

Other muscles that can refer pain to the same region as the infraspinatus muscle are the upper, middle, and lower trapezius; supraspinatus; scalene; teres minor; middle deltoid; triceps brachii; and pectoralis minor muscles. All these muscles should be examined for the presence of TrPs, especially when resolution of the patient's shoulder pain is not being achieved with the treatment of TrPs in the infraspinatus muscle.

4.3. Associated Pathology

Cervical radiculitis in the C5 or C6 nerve roots often result in the formation of TrPs in those muscles innervated by the same nerve roots. Often patients with a C5 or C6 radiculopathy report having deep anterior shoulder pain, anterolateral arm and forearm pain, and pain into the radial aspect of the hand and lateral two-and-a-half digits. Wainner et al[62] identified a test item cluster to determine the likelihood that a patient is presenting with a cervical radiculopathy. The following predictor variables were identified: a positive Spurling sign, cervical rotation less than 60° to the same side, positive cervical compression test, relief of symptoms with axial distraction, and a positive neurodynamic upper limb test. Patients presenting with four of these positive variables have a 90% posttest probability of cervical radiculopathy. Patients with three positive variables have a 65% posttest probability of cervical radiculopathy.[62]

Often times, it is clinically seen that patients who are administered postoral steroid or epidural spinal injection for cervical radicular symptoms have residual pain in the upper extremity that is often related to TrP activity in the infraspinatus muscle. Treatment of infraspinatus TrPs can alleviate the remaining upper extremity pain in this type of patient.

Shoulder pain accounts for approximately 12% of musculoskeletal conditions, with subacromial impingement syndrome being the most prevalent diagnosis.[63] The direct cost for the treatment of shoulder pain to the United States was estimated to be $7 billion in the year 2000.[64] In a systematic review of the evidence related to the diagnosis of impingement syndrome of the shoulder, Papadonikolakis et al[65] concluded that the original diagnosis of shoulder impingement syndrome was developed to cover the breadth of rotator cuff disorders including tendinosis, as well as complete and incomplete tears that were difficult to differentiate. They suggest that the impingement syndrome diagnosis no longer be utilized due to recent advancements in diagnostics that allow these diagnoses to be differentiated.[65] Diercks et al[66] suggested a guideline for the diagnosis and treatment of subacromial pain syndrome, that includes clinical examination and treatment of TrPs.

As discussed in Chapter 21, authors have investigated the prevalence of TrPs, PPT, and reproduction of shoulder pain in patients with a diagnosis of impingement syndrome.[49,67] The greatest prevalence of active TrPs was noted in the supraspinatus (62%), the infraspinatus (42%), and the subscapularis (42%) muscles. This study clearly supports that the number of active TrPs in the shoulder musculature was related to increased pressure pain sensitivity in individuals with "shoulder impingement syndrome."[49] This association suggests that active TrPs in the infraspinatus muscle could be associated with sensitization mechanisms in patients with shoulder pain. This hypothesis is also confirmed by the association of both active and latent TrPs in the infraspinatus muscle with lower PPT[56] and the presence of bilateral TrPs in the infraspinatus muscle in patients with unilateral shoulder symptoms.[67]

Because the infraspinatus muscle is one of the rotator cuff muscles, differential diagnosis should rule out rotator cuff dysfunction. With rotator cuff dysfunction, the pain is severe and is usually exhibited through a limited arc of motion. It has been identified as a test item cluster of signs and symptoms indicative of rotator cuff pathology. The variables identified were age, supraspinatus weakness, weakness in external rotation, and impingement. Any two positive variables in combination with age more than 60 was associated with a posttest probability of 98% and at any age with three positive variables was associated with a 98% posttest probability. Any two positive variables with age less than 60 was associated with a 64% posttest probability of rotator cuff pathology.[68]

Suprascapular nerve entrapment is a relatively rare entrapment seen in athletes performing repetitive cocking motions. The cocking position requires abduction, extension, and external rotation followed by rapid flexion and internal rotation.[21] Suprascapular nerve injury has also been identified in individuals with degenerative changes in the glenohumeral joint and with capsular laxity in an aging population. Entrapment is typically caused by repetitive overhead activity in overhead athletes, by ganglion cysts, or by scapular fractures. Areas of entrapment include the suprascapular notch under the superior transverse ligament or at the spinoglenoid notch secondary to a space-occupying lesion.[69] Diagnosis by nerve conduction and electromyography of both the infraspinatus and supraspinatus muscles is required to make this diagnosis. If the patient does not respond to rest and other conservative measures, surgery is indicated. Typical signs and symptoms include a vague report of shoulder girdle pain, atrophy over the supraspinatus and infraspinatus muscles, limited shoulder range of motion, and fatigue in the shoulder girdle.[69] The patient's pain may be similar to that caused by TrPs in the shoulder girdle musculature, especially the supraspinatus and infraspinatus muscles.

5. CORRECTIVE ACTIONS

The patient with infraspinatus TrPs should avoid habitual sustained or repetitive motions that overload the muscle, such as repetitive overhead lifting with the upper extremity in abduction and external rotation and reaching backward into the back seat of the car.

When the patient lies on the uninvolved side, sleep is improved by supporting the uppermost elbow and forearm (painful limb) on a bed pillow (Figure 22-4A) to avoid overstretching the affected infraspinatus muscle that can cause referred pain. For back sleepers, a pillow may be placed between the arm and the trunk, so that the pillow rests under the arm to keep the shoulder in a

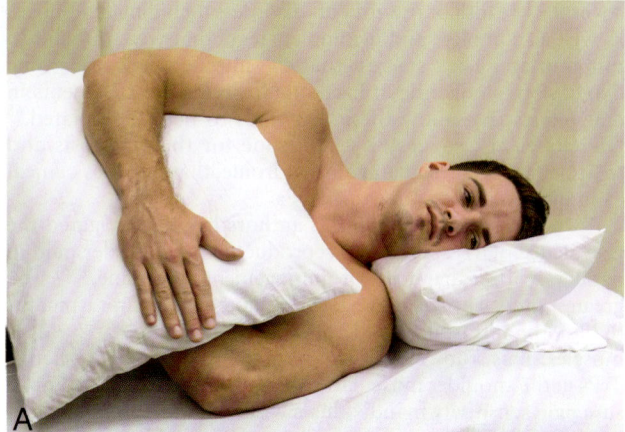
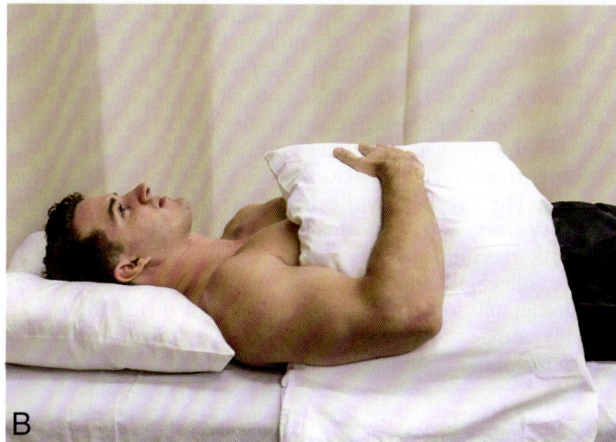
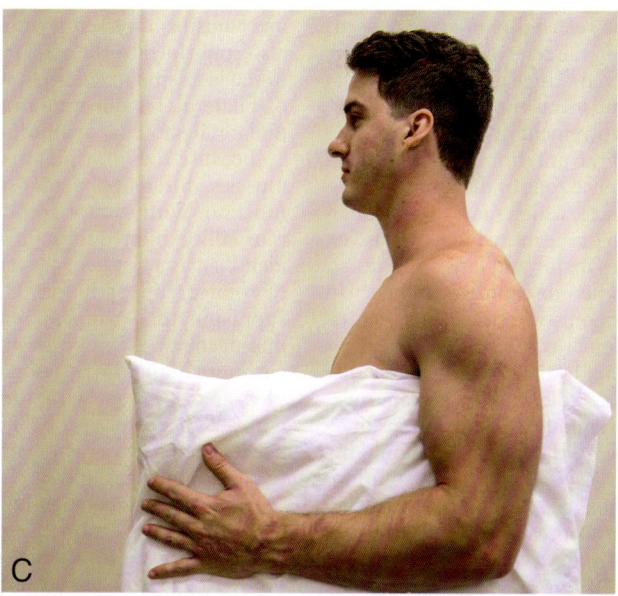

Figure 22-4. Pain-relieving positions for active right infraspinatus TrPs. A, Side-lying position of relief is with the affected side up with arm in slight abduction, passively placing the infraspinatus muscle in a resting position. B, Supine position of relief is with the arm supported in slight abduction. Note the right arm is not allowed to fall behind the body due to the support of the pillow. C, Seated position of relief is with the affected arm supported in slight abduction, neutral rotation by a pillow.

relaxed position (Figure 22-4B). A neutral sleeping posture is best. Patients should be cautioned regarding lying in bed with their arm(s) above their head in an abducted and externally rotated position, as this will keep the infraspinatus muscle in a prolonged shortened position causing increased tension in the TrP region. When seated, a pillow may be used in the same manner to place the shoulder in a resting position (Figure 22-4C).

When prescribing neuromuscular reeducation or therapeutic exercises for the infraspinatus muscle, activation is greater with standing external rotation with the arm at the side (44% MVC), and in side-lying (42% MVC). Utilizing a towel roll in the axilla during external rotation activates the posterior deltoid muscle to assist the infraspinatus muscle with external rotation.[12] Decker et al[70] found the greatest activity of the infraspinatus (115% MVC) and supraspinatus (125% MVC) muscles during the push-up plus activity.

The patient may inactivate an infraspinatus TrP with self-pressure release of TrPs by lying on a tennis ball placed directly under a tender spot in the muscle or standing with their back against the wall utilizing the aforementioned technique. Body weight is used to maintain increasing pressure for 1 to 2 minutes, as described in the interventions section. The self-pressure release of TrPs may be repeated several times daily until the TrP is inactivated. A cold pack may be of therapeutic benefit post pressure release, especially in the case of acute shoulder pain.

There are a variety of commercialized products that can be used for pressure release techniques.

The patient may stretch the muscle daily while seated or while taking a warm shower. To stretch all three heads of the muscle, the arm first be stretched across the chest in front, then up the back from behind (Figure 22-5A and B).

Another effective self-stretch technique is the application of post-isometric relaxation (progressive contract–relax) with respiratory augmentation. The patient lies supine with the affected upper limb placed such that the elbow extends over the edge of the bed or sofa with the elbow flexed 90° (Figure 22-6A).[71-73] The patient inhales slowly and deeply and then relaxes during exhalation, while gravity assists the arm in slowly falling downward to stretch the infraspinatus muscle (Figure 22-6B). Additional release of infraspinatus muscle tightness may be achieved by a voluntary effort to lower the hand (medially rotate the arm), providing additional stretch within a comfortable range.

In cases of glenohumeral posterior capsule tightness, it is imperative that the connective tissue dysfunction be addressed in addition to restoration of scapulohumeral mechanics while concomitantly treating TrPs in the infraspinatus muscle. Treatment isolated to TrPs in the infraspinatus muscle that does not address the arthrokinematics of the scapulohumeral joints results in a treatment failure and only a temporary relief of pain.

Chapter 22: Infraspinatus Muscle 239

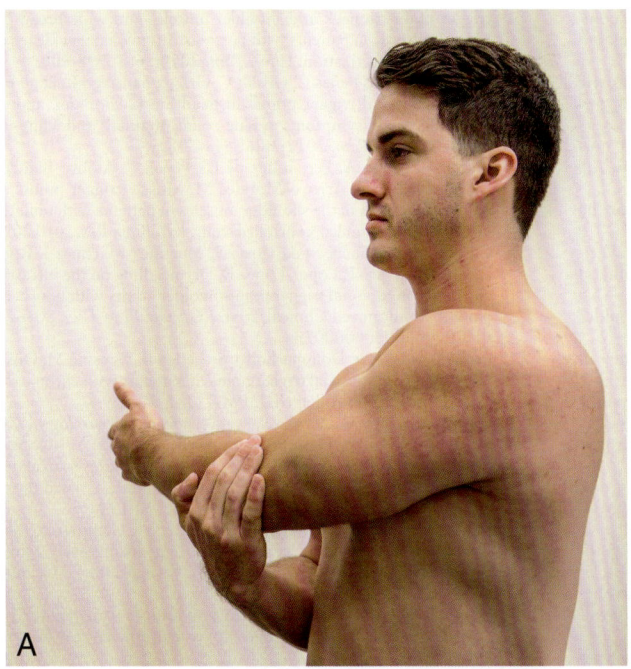
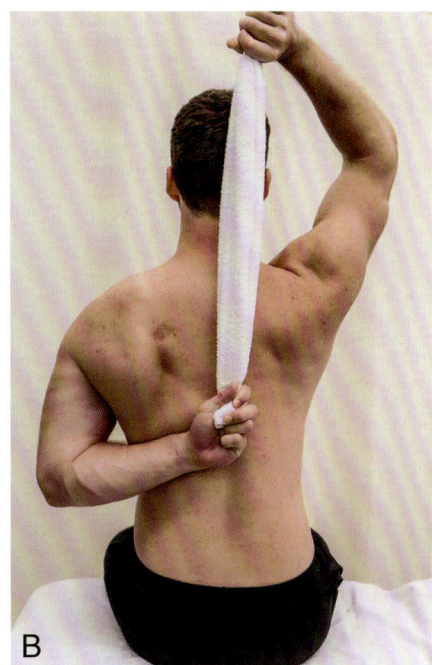

Figure 22-5. Stretch positions for the infraspinatus muscle. A, To stretch the superior belly, the affected shoulder is placed in maximum horizontal adduction at 90° of shoulder elevation with overpressure supplied by the unaffected extremity. B, To stretch the middle and inferior bellies, the affected arm is placed behind the patient's back in extension, medial rotation, and adduction. A towel is used to allow the unaffected arm to passively pull the affected arm into more medial rotation stretching the infraspinatus muscle. The stretch can be augmented with a contract–relax or postisometric relaxation technique.

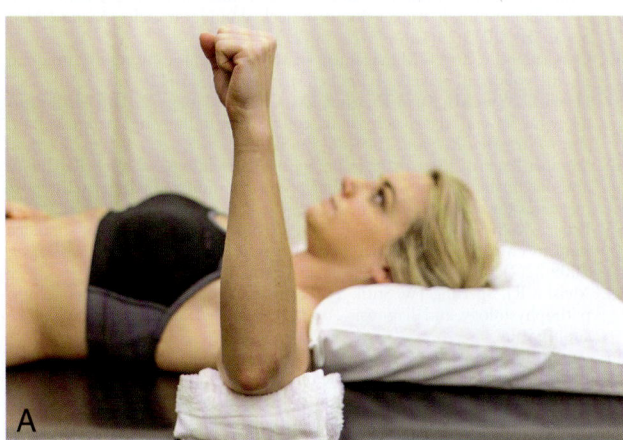
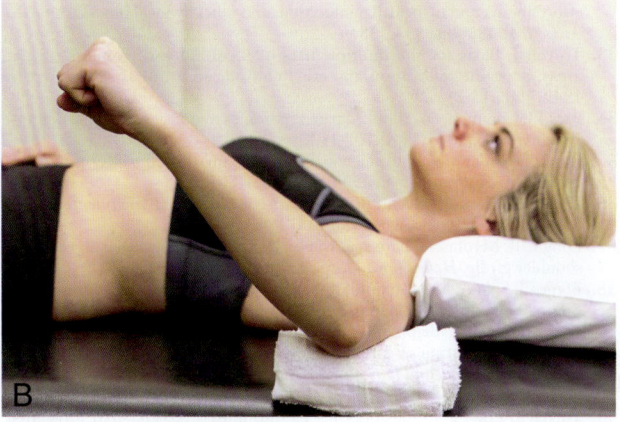

Figure 22-6. Postisometric relaxation for the infraspinatus muscle. A, Starting position. B, Stretch position.

References

1. Moccia D, Nackashi AA, Schilling R, Ward PJ. Fascial bundles of the infraspinatus fascia: anatomy, function, and clinical considerations. *J Anat.* 2016;228(1):176-183.
2. Standring S. *Gray's Anatomy: The Anatomical Basis of Clinical Practice.* 41st ed. London, UK: Elsevier; 2015.
3. Moore KL, Agur AMR, Dalley AF. *Clinically Oriented Anatomy.* Baltimore, MD: Lippincott Williams & Wilkins; 2014:700-707.
4. Fabrizio PA, Clemente FR. Anatomical structure and nerve branching pattern of the human infraspinatus muscle. *J Bodyw Mov Ther.* 2014;18(2):228-232.
5. Burkhart SS, Esch JC, Jolson RS. The rotator crescent and rotator cable: an anatomic description of the shoulder's "suspension bridge". *Arthroscopy.* 1993;9(6):611-616.
6. Shin C, Lee SE, Yu KH, Chae HK, Lee KS. Spinal root origins and innervations of the suprascapular nerve. *Surg Radiol Anat.* 2010;32(3):235-238.
7. Ozer Y, Grossman JA, Gilbert A. Anatomic observations on the suprascapular nerve. *Hand Clin.* 1995;11(4):539-544.
8. Clemente C. *Gray's Anatomy of the Human Body.* 30th ed. Philadelphia, PA: Lea & Febiger; 1985:523-524.
9. Aktekin M, Demiryurek D, Bayramoglu A, Tuccar E. The significance of the neurovascular structures passing through the spinoglenoid notch. *Saudi Med J.* 2003;24(9):933-935.
10. Reed D, Cathers I, Halaki M, Ginn K. Does supraspinatus initiate shoulder abduction? *J Electromyogr Kinesiol.* 2013;23(2):425-429.
11. Porterfield JA, DeRosa C. *Mechanical Shoulder Disorders: Perspectives in Functional Anatomy.* St. Louis, MO: Saunders; 2004:65-66.
12. Sakita K, Seeley MK, Myrer JW, Hopkins JT. Shoulder-muscle electromyography during shoulder external-rotation exercises with and without slight abduction. *J Sport Rehabil.* 2015;24(2):109-115.
13. Marta S, Pezarat-Correla P, Fernandes O, et al. Electromyographic analysis of posterior deltoid, posterior rotator cuff and trapezius musculature in different shoulder exercises. *In J Sports Med.* 2013;14:1-15.
14. Reinold MM, Wilk KE, Fleisig GS, et al. Electromyographic analysis of the rotator cuff and deltoid musculature during common shoulder external rotation exercises. *J Orthop Sports Phys Ther.* 2004;34(7):385-394.

15. Wattanaprakornkul D, Halaki M, Boettcher C, Cathers I, Ginn KA. A comprehensive analysis of muscle recruitment patterns during shoulder flexion: an electromyographic study. *Clin Anat.* 2011;24(5):619-626.
16. Reed D, Cathers I, Halaki M, Ginn KA. Does load influence shoulder muscle recruitment patterns during scapular plane abduction? *J Sci Med Sport.* 2015;15:207-208.
17. Wickham J, Pizzari T, Stansfeld K, Burnside A, Watson L. Quantifying 'normal' shoulder muscle activity during abduction. *J Electromyogr Kinesiol.* 2010;20(2):212-222.
18. Inman VT, Saunders M, Abbot LC. Observations on the function of the shoulder joint. *J Bone Joint Surg.* 1944;26(1):1-30.
19. Langenderfer JE, Patthanacharoenphon C, Carpenter JE, Hughes RE. Variability in isometric force and moment generating capacity of glenohumeral external rotator muscles. *Clin Biomech.* 2006;21(7):701-709.
20. Jobe FW, Moynes DR, Tibone JE, Perry J. An EMG analysis of the shoulder in pitching. A second report. *Am J Sports Med.* 1984;12(3):218-220.
21. Jobe FW, Tibone JE, Perry J, Moynes D. An EMG analysis of the shoulder in throwing and pitching. A preliminary report. *Am J Sports Med.* 1983;11(1):3-5.
22. Digiovine NM, Jobe FW, Pink M, Perry J. An electromyographic analysis of the upper extremity in pitching. *J Shoulder Elbow Surg.* 1992;1(1):15-25.
23. Jobe FW, Moynes DR, Antonelli DJ. Rotator cuff function during a golf swing. *Am J Sports Med.* 1986;14(5):388-392.
24. Simons DG, Travell J, Simons L. *Travell & Simon's Myofascial Pain and Dysfunction: The Trigger Point Manual.* Vol 1. 2nd ed. Baltimore, MD: Williams & Wilkins; 1999.
25. Gerwin RD, Dommerholt J, Shah JP. An expansion of Simons' integrated hypothesis of trigger point formation. *Curr Pain Headache Rep.* 2004;8(6):468-475.
26. Werner SL, Gill TJ, Murray TA, Cook TD, Hawkins RJ. Relationships between throwing mechanics and shoulder distraction in professional baseball pitchers. *Am J Sports Med.* 2001;29(3):354-358.
27. Illyes A, Kiss RM. Shoulder muscle activity during pushing, pulling, elevation and overhead throw. *J Electromyogr Kinesiol.* 2005;15(3):282-289.
28. Basmajian J, Deluca C. *Muscles Alive.* 5th ed. Baltimore, MD: Williams & Wilkins; 1985:270, 273-276.
29. Lucas KR, Rich PA, Polus BI. Muscle activation patterns in the scapular positioning muscles during loaded scapular plane elevation: the effects of Latent Myofascial Trigger Points. *Clin Biomech.* 2010;25(8):765-770.
30. Gao ZH, Fan D, Wang D, Zhao H, Zhao K, Chen C. Muscle activity and co-contraction of musculoskeletal model during steering maneuver. *Biomed Mater Eng.* 2014;24(6):2697-2706.
31. Travell J, Rinzler SH. The myofascial genesis of pain. *Postgrad Med.* 1952;11(5):425-434.
32. Travell J, Rinzler SH. Pain syndromes of the chest muscles; resemblance to effort angina and myocardial infarction, and relief by local block. *Can Med Assoc J.* 1948;59(4):333-338.
33. Travell J. Basis for the multiple uses of local block of somatic trigger areas; procaine infiltration and ethyl chloride spray. *Miss Valley Med J.* 1949;71(1):13-21.
34. Pace JB. Commonly overlooked pain syndromes responsive to simple therapy. *Postgrad Med.* 1975;58(4):107-113.
35. Rubin D. An approach to the management of myofascial trigger point syndromes. *Arch Phys Med Rehabil.* 1981;62:107-110.
36. Zohn DA. *Musculoskeletal Pain: Diagnosis and Physical Treatment.* 2nd ed. Boston, MA: Little Brown; 1988:211.
37. Long C II. Myofascial pain syndromes. II. Syndromes of the head, neck and shoulder girdle. *Henry Ford Hosp Med Bull.* 1956;4(1):22-28.
38. Bonica J, Sola A. Other painful disorders of the upper limb, Chapter 52. In: Bonica JJ, Loeser JD, Chapman A, Fordyce WE, eds. *The Management of Pain.* 2nd ed. Philadelphia, PA: Lea & Febiger; 1990:947-958 (page 949).
39. Rachlin ES. Injection of specific trigger points, Chapter 10. In: Rachlin ES, ed. *Myofascial Pain and Fibromyalgia.* St. Louis, MO: Mosby; 1994:197-360 (pages 322-325).
40. Travell J. Ethyl chloride spray for painful muscle spasm. *Arch Phys Med Rehabil.* 1952;33(5):291-298.
41. Fernández-Carnero J, Ge HY, Kimura Y, Fernández de las Peñas C, Arendt-Nielsen L. Increased spontaneous electrical activity at a latent myofascial trigger point after nociceptive stimulation of another latent trigger point. *Clin J Pain.* 2010;26(2):138-143.
42. Kellgren JH. Observations on referred pain arising from muscle. *Clin Sci.* 1938;3:175-190.
43. Qerama E, Kasch H, Fuglsang-Frederiksen A. Occurrence of myofascial pain in patients with possible carpal tunnel syndrome—a single-blinded study. *Eur J Pain.* 2009;13(6):588-591.
44. Hains G, Descarreaux M, Lamy AM, Hains F. A randomized controlled (intervention) trial of ischemic compression therapy for chronic carpal tunnel syndrome. *J Can Chiropr Assoc.* 2010;54(3):155-163.
45. Bron C, Dommerholt J, Stegenga B, Wensing M, Oostendorp RA. High prevalence of shoulder girdle muscles with myofascial trigger points in patients with shoulder pain. *BMC Musculoskelet Disord.* 2011;12(1):139-151.
46. Castaldo M, Ge HY, Chiarotto A, Villafane JH, Arendt-Nielsen L. Myofascial trigger points in patients with whiplash-associated disorders and mechanical neck pain. *Pain Med.* 2014;15(5):842-849.
47. Fernández-Lao C, Cantarero-Villanueva I, Fernández de las Peñas C, Del-Moral-Avila R, Arendt-Nielsen L, Arroyo-Morales M. Myofascial trigger points in neck and shoulder muscles and widespread pressure pain hypersensitivity in patients with postmastectomy pain: evidence of peripheral and central sensitization. *Clin J Pain.* 2010;26(9):798-806.
48. Fernández de las Peñas C, Grobli C, Ortega-Santiago R, et al. Referred pain from myofascial trigger points in head, neck, shoulder, and arm muscles reproduces pain symptoms in blue-collar (manual) and white-collar (office) workers. *Clin J Pain.* 2012;28(6):511-518.
49. Hidalgo-Lozano A, Fernández de las Peñas C, Alonso-Blanco C, Ge HY, Arendt-Nielsen L, Arroyo-Morales M. Muscle trigger points and pressure pain hyperalgesia in the shoulder muscles in patients with unilateral shoulder impingement: a blinded, controlled study. *Exp Brain Res.* 2010;202(4):915-925.
50. Calvo-Lobo C, Pacheco-da-Costa S, Martinez-Martinez J, Rodriguez-Sanz D, Cuesta-Alvaro P, Lopez-Lopez D. Dry needling on the infraspinatus latent and active myofascial trigger points in older adults with nonspecific shoulder pain: A Randomized Clinical Trial. *J Geriatr Phys Ther.* 2016. doi:10.1519/JPT.0000000000000079.
51. Bron C, de Gast A, Dommerholt J, Stegenga B, Wensing M, Oostendorp RA. Treatment of myofascial trigger points in patients with chronic shoulder pain: a randomized, controlled trial. *BMC Med.* 2011;9:8.
52. Sola AE, Williams RL. Myofascial pain syndromes. *Neurology.* 1956;6(2):91-95.
53. Ohmori A, Iranami H, Fujii K, Yamazaki A, Doko Y. Myofascial involvement of supra- and infraspinatus muscles contributes to ipsilateral shoulder pain after muscle-sparing thoracotomy and video-assisted thoracic surgery. *J Cardiothorac Vasc Anesth.* 2013;27(6):1310-1314.
54. DiLorenzo L, Traballesi M, Morelli D, et al. Hemiparetic shoulder pain syndrome treated with deep dry needling during early rehabilitation: a prospective, open-lavel, randomized investigation. *J Musculoskelet Pain.* 2004;12(2):25-34.
55. Lucas KR, Polus PA, Rich J. Latent myofascial trigger points: their effect on muscle activation and movement efficiency. *J Bodyw Mov Ther.* 2004;8:160-166.
56. Ge HY, Fernández de las Peñas C, Madeleine P, Arendt-Nielsen L. Topographical mapping and mechanical pain sensitivity of myofascial trigger points in the infraspinatus muscle. *Eur J Pain.* 2008;12(7):859-865.
57. Bron C, Franssen J, Wensing M, Oostendorp RA. Interrater reliability of palpation of myofascial trigger points in three shoulder muscles. *J Man Manip Ther.* 2007;15(4):203-215.
58. Baker B. The muscle trigger: evidence of overload injury. *J Neurol Orthop Med Surg.* 1986;7(1):35-44.
59. Hidalgo-Lozano A, Fernández de las Peñas C, Calderon-Soto C, Domingo-Camara A, Madeleine P, Arroyo-Morales M. Elite swimmers with and without unilateral shoulder pain: mechanical hyperalgesia and active/latent muscle trigger points in neck-shoulder muscles. *Scand J Med Sci Sports.* 2013;23(1):66-73.
60. Osborne NJ, Gatt IT. Management of shoulder injuries using dry needling in elite volleyball players. *Acupunct Med.* 2010;28(1):42-45.
61. Hsieh YL, Kao MJ, Kuan TS, Chen SM, Chen JT, Hong CZ. Dry needling to a key myofascial trigger point may reduce the irritability of satellite MTrPs. *Am J Phys Med Rehabil.* 2007;86(5):397-403.
62. Wainner RS, Fritz JM, Irrgang JJ, Boninger ML, Delitto A, Allison S. Reliability and diagnostic accuracy of the clinical examination and patient self-report measures for cervical radiculopathy. *Spine.* 2003;28(1):52-62.
63. Pribicevic M, Pollard H, Bonello R. An epidemiologic survey of shoulder pain in chiropractic practice in australia. *J Manipulative Physiol Ther.* 2009;32(2):107-117.
64. Meislin RJ, Sperling JW, Stitik TP. Persistent shoulder pain: epidemiology, pathophysiology, and diagnosis. *Am J Orthop (Belle Mead NJ).* 2005;34(12 suppl):5-9.
65. Papadonikolakis A, McKenna M, Warme W, Martin BI, Matsen FA III. Published evidence relevant to the diagnosis of impingement syndrome of the shoulder. *J Bone Joint Surg Am.* 2011;93(19):1827-1832.
66. Diercks R, Bron C, Dorrestijn O, et al. Guideline for diagnosis and treatment of subacromial pain syndrome: a multidisciplinary review by the Dutch Orthopaedic Association. *Acta Orthop.* 2014;85(3):314-322.
67. Alburquerque-Sendin F, Camargo P, Viera A, Salvini TF. Bilateral myofascial trigger points and pressure pain thresholds in the shoulder muscles in patients with unilateral shoulder impingement syndrome. A blinded controlled study. *Clin J Pain.* 2013;29:478-486.
68. Murrell GA, Walton JR. Diagnosis of rotator cuff tears. *Lancet.* 2001;357(9258):769-770.
69. Jacob PJ, Arun K, Binoj R. Suprascapular nerve entrapment syndrome. *Kerala J Orthop.* 2011;25:21-24.
70. Decker MJ, Tokish JM, Ellis HB, Torry MR, Hawkins RJ. Subscapularis muscle activity during selected rehabilitation exercises. *Am J Sports Med.* 2003;31(1):126-134.
71. Lewit K. Role of manipulation in spinal rehabilitation, Chapter 11. In: Liebenson C, ed. *Rehabilitation of the Spine: A Practitioner's Guide.* Baltimore, MD: Williams & Wilkins; 1996:195-224 (page 208).
72. Liebenson C. Manual resistance techniques and self-stretches for improving flexibility/mobility, Chapter 13. In: Liebenson C, ed. *Rehabilitation of the Spine: A Practitioner's Guide.* Baltimore, MD: Williams & Wilkins; 1996:253-292 (pages 282-283).
73. Lewit K. *Manipulative Therapy in Rehabilitation of the Locomotor System.* 3rd ed. Oxford, England: Butterworth Heinemann; 1999:204-205.

Chapter 23

Teres Minor Muscle

"Throwers Trial"

Joseph M. Donnelly

1. INTRODUCTION

The small, slightly fusiform teres minor muscle is one of the four rotator cuff muscles of the shoulder. It attaches from the posterior aspect of the scapula to the inferior facet of the greater tubercle of the humerus, and it acts to dynamically stabilize the humeral head in the glenoid fossa of the scapula and to laterally rotate the arm at the glenohumeral joint. Trigger points (TrPs) in the teres minor muscle produce pain deep in the posterior deltoid region of the shoulder, near its insertion on the humerus. Symptoms may be exacerbated by sleeping on the affected side, reaching behind the back, and performing activities of daily living that require combined movements of shoulder elevation and external rotation (ER). Activation and perpetuation of TrPs in the teres minor muscle usually result from acute overload while reaching backward and upward, or with repetitive overhead activities. Differential diagnosis should include assessment for posterior glenohumeral joint capsule tightness, rotator cuff tears, quadrilateral space syndrome, and C8-T1 radicular symptoms. Corrective actions include postural training (including effective sleep positioning), behavior change to eliminate positions that cause recurrent overload on the muscle, self-pressure release, and self-stretch exercises.

2. ANATOMIC CONSIDERATIONS

The teres minor muscle originates medially from the upper two thirds of the flattened area of the dorsal surface of the scapula that roughly extends from the medial aspect of the inferior angle to the posterior and the inferior aspects of the glenoid fossa of the scapula and from the aponeurosis that separates this muscle from the infraspinatus and teres major muscles that border it superiorly and inferiorly, respectively. It inserts lateral to the inferior facet of the greater tubercle of the humerus and onto the humerus, proximal to the origin of the lateral head of the triceps brachii muscle (Figure 23-1). The tendon blends with the lower posterior aspect of the glenohumeral joint capsule. In some cases, the teres minor muscle may fuse with the infraspinatus muscle.[1] Two distinct fascial variations have been reported: the teres minor muscle may be contained in its own inflexible facial compartment or it may share the facial compartment of the infraspinatus muscle.[2]

2.1. Innervation and Vascularization

The teres minor muscle is innervated by the axillary nerve through the posterior cord from the C5 and C6 spinal segments. This innervation differs from that of the infraspinatus muscle above, which is supplied by the suprascapular nerve, and from that of the teres major muscle below, supplied by the lower subscapular nerve. All three muscles are supplied at least in part from the cervical spinal segments C5 and C6.[1]

Loukas et al[3] investigated the course of the axillary nerve in 100 nerve specimens. In 65% of the cases, the axillary nerve split within the quadrangular space into an anterior and a posterior branch. The remaining 35% split within the deltoid muscle. Irrespective of the origin, the posterior deltoid branch gave off a branch to the teres minor muscle in 100% of the cases.[3,4]

The teres minor muscle receives its vascular supply through the posterior humeral circumflex and circumflex scapular arteries.[1]

2.2. Function

The teres minor, infraspinatus, supraspinatus, and subscapularis muscles insert into the greater and lesser tuberosities of the humerus and form a musculotendinous rotator cuff. These rotator cuff muscles provide dynamic stability to the glenohumeral joint. Motion at the shoulder is a complex, coordinated activity performed by the rotator cuff muscles, which exert inferior and medially directed forces that resist upward shear forces of the deltoid muscle during shoulder elevation while keeping the head of the humerus in a close contact with the glenoid fossa.[5] The teres minor muscle functions with the other rotator cuff muscles to stabilize and center the head of the humerus in the glenoid with upper extremity movement.

Apart from its stabilizing role, the teres minor (along with the infraspinatus) muscle is a prime mover at the glenohumeral joint for ER with the arm in any position.[6,7] The teres minor muscle has a moderate maximal volitional contraction (%MVC) in standing and side-lying ER movements.[7] Peak activity for the teres minor muscle is with prone horizontal abduction at 90° of abduction and full ER with the elbow extended. The teres minor muscle demonstrates the least activity during ER in the plane of the scapula and with a towel roll in the axilla.[6] The teres minor muscle activation patterns mirror those of the infraspinatus muscle with both muscles having greater than a 40% MVC during six of seven motions studied.[6]

Investigators have utilized positron emission tomography to look at the function of the teres minor muscle in shoulder adduction (0°) and abduction positions (90° in the frontal plane) on healthy volunteers. Their results showed that the teres minor muscle had a more definitive role in ER in the abducted position.[8]

Although weak adduction has been identified as an action of the teres minor muscle on the basis of anatomic orientation,[1] there is no electromyographic evidence to date to support adduction as a function of this muscle.[5-7,9,10] However, a weak adduction function may be extrapolated from the teres minor muscle's role in dynamic stabilization of the glenohumeral joint by providing a medial and inferiorly directed force during shoulder elevation.

2.3. Functional Unit

The functional unit to which a muscle belongs includes the muscles that reinforce and counter its actions as well as the

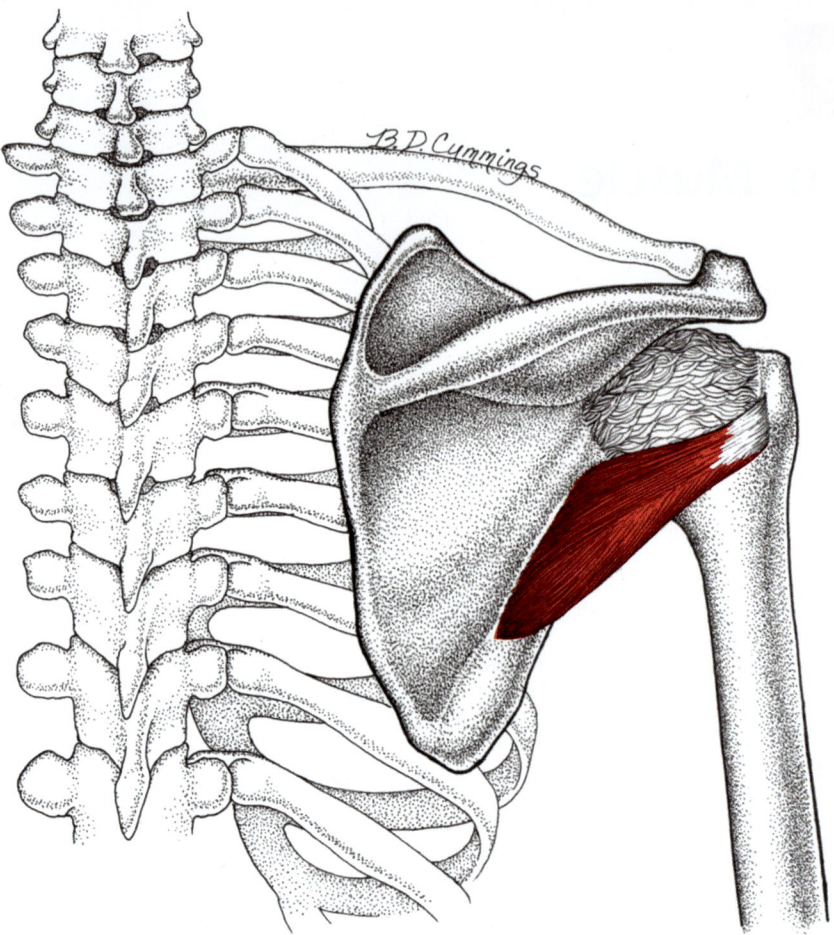

Figure 23-1. Attachments of the teres minor muscle showing location and direction of muscle fibers.

joints that the muscle crosses. The interdependence of these structures is functionally reflected in the organization and neural connections of the sensory motor cortex. The functional unit is emphasized because the presence of a TrP in one muscle of the unit increases the likelihood that the other muscles of the unit also develops TrPs. When inactivating TrPs in a muscle, one should be concerned about TrPs that may develop in muscles that are functionally interdependent. The teres minor muscle functions in parallel with the infraspinatus muscle, to which it is a "little brother," having similar attachments but a different nerve supply. Box 23-1 grossly represents the functional unit of the teres minor muscle.[11] The teres minor muscle also functions synergistically with the infraspinatus, supraspinatus, and subscapularis muscles to stabilize the head of the humerus in the glenoid fossa during arm movements.[5,9]

Box 23-1 Functional unit of the teres minor muscle

Action	Synergists	Antagonists
Shoulder external rotation	Infraspinatus Posterior deltoid	Subscapularis Pectoralis major Latissimus dorsi Anterior deltoid

3. CLINICAL PRESENTATION

3.1. Referred Pain Pattern

Trigger points in the teres minor muscle primarily refer deep pain in the region of the posterior deltoid muscle toward the insertion of the teres minor muscle (Figure 23-2). This area of pain lies proximal to the deltoid muscle's attachment at the deltoid tubercle of the humerus. It can be concentrated in a small area (about the size of a prune) well below the subacromial bursa but could feel like "bursitis" because of its sharp localization and deep quality. A broadly distributed aching pain in the arm and the shoulder posteriorly is rarely due to TrPs in the teres minor muscle alone. Bonica and Sola[12] illustrate a broader distribution of pain in the region of the posterior deltoid muscle.

One report of four patients[13] indicates that referred dysesthesia of tingling and numbness to the fourth and fifth fingers may be as common as pain referred to the shoulder by active TrPs in the teres minor muscle.

3.2. Symptoms

Compared with other rotator cuff muscles, the teres minor muscle is less commonly involved in primary shoulder pain despite active TrPs being found in 45% of individuals with nonspecific shoulder pain.[14] A patient with teres minor TrPs may earn a diagnosis of "painful bursa" due to the report of pain deep in the posterior deltoid muscle close to the attachment of the teres minor muscle on the humerus. The patient's primary concern

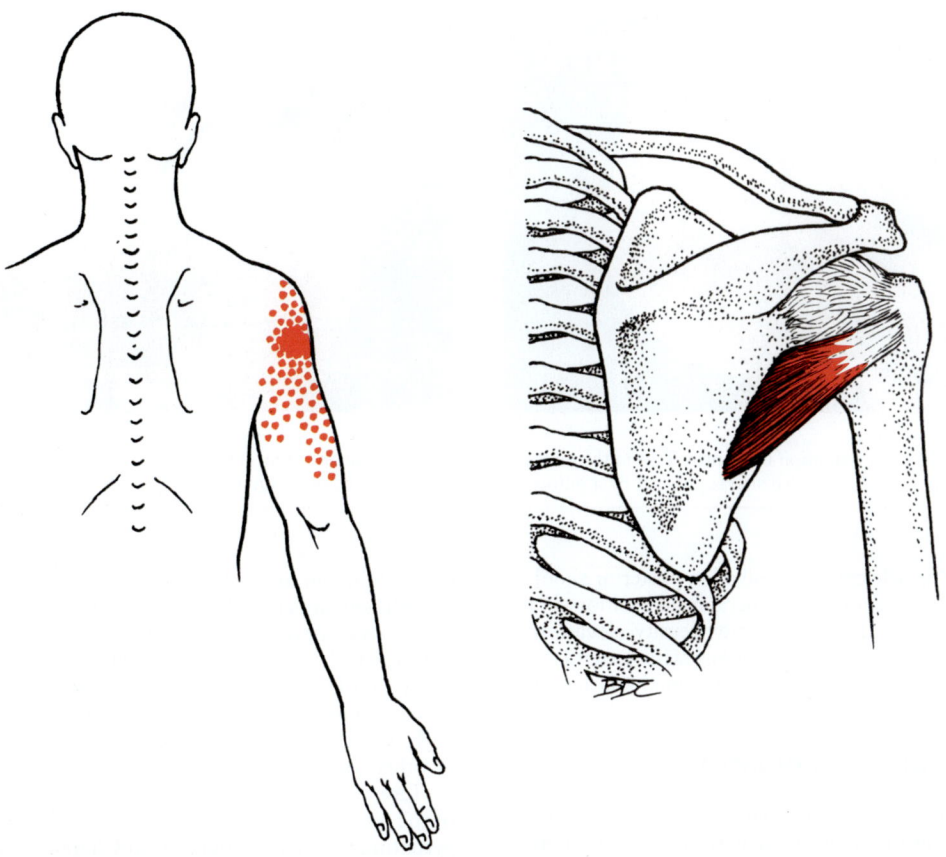

Figure 23-2. Referred pain pattern (essential zone solid red, spillover zone stippled red) of TrPs in the right teres minor muscle.

is typically posterior shoulder pain rather (Figure 23-2) than restricted shoulder range of motion (ROM). Clinically, teres minor TrPs occur concomitantly with infraspinatus TrPs. When the patient presents with pain deep in the anterior shoulder, the symptom is likely due to active TrPs in the infraspinatus muscle rather than the teres minor muscle. When pain from infraspinatus TrPs is relieved and normal infraspinatus muscle length is restored, the patient may become aware of the pain in the back of the shoulder referred by the teres minor muscle.

Escobar and Ballesteros[13] reported four patients with isolated active teres minor TrPs. All four described symptoms of numbness and/or tingling of the fourth and fifth fingers aggravated by shoulder activity that required reaching above the shoulder height or behind them. These movements also caused pain in three of the patients. In a more recent case report, a patient with posterior shoulder tightness was successfully treated after application of dry needling to the teres minor and infraspinatus muscles.[14] Pain and restricted ROM of the shoulder improved after dry needling of these muscles restored more normative sensory and motor function.[15]

3.3. Patient Examination

After a thorough subjective examination, the clinician should make a detailed drawing representing the pain pattern that the patient has described. This depiction will assist in planning the physical examination and can be useful in monitoring the progression of the patient as symptoms improve or change. For proper examination of the teres minor muscle, the clinician should observe the shoulder girdle posture, examine active and passive ranges of the motion of the shoulder girdle, and observe muscle activation patterns as well as the scapulohumeral rhythm.

The teres minor muscle has been considered one of the less commonly involved shoulder muscles. About 7% of patients with myofascial pain in the shoulder region were found to have TrPs in the teres minor muscle in earlier studies.[16,17] Only 3% of healthy young adults had latent TrPs in the teres minor or teres major muscles.[16] Bron et al[14] investigated the prevalence of TrPs in nontraumatic unilateral chronic shoulder pain and found a high prevalence of active TrPs in the teres minor (45%) muscle. They also found a high prevalence of latent TrPs (20%) in the teres minor muscle. The authors recommend examination for the presence of TrPs in patients who present with shoulder pain.[14]

Usually, the patient presents with primary TrPs in the infraspinatus muscle. Active TrPs in the teres minor muscle may show some restricted ROM in the Apley's scratch test (see Figure 22-3) even after TrPs in the infraspinatus muscle have been inactivated by treatment. When the pain report shifts from the front of the shoulder (in the case of infraspinatus TrPs) to the back of the shoulder (pain distribution of teres minor TrPs), assessment of TrPs in the teres minor muscle is indicated.

Accessory joint motion should be tested in the glenohumeral, acromioclavicular, sternoclavicular, and scapulothoracic joints. Often, joint hypomobility in the sternoclavicular joint can cause impairment in shoulder elevation, which contributes to alterations in the normal muscle activation patterns. Articular dysfunctions in the glenohumeral joint may also impair muscle activation patterns contributing to overload of the teres minor and other rotator cuff muscles.

The glenohumeral joint should be carefully assessed for Glenohumeral Internal Rotation Deficit, which may be indicative of posterior capsule tightness. A recent case report suggests that TrPs

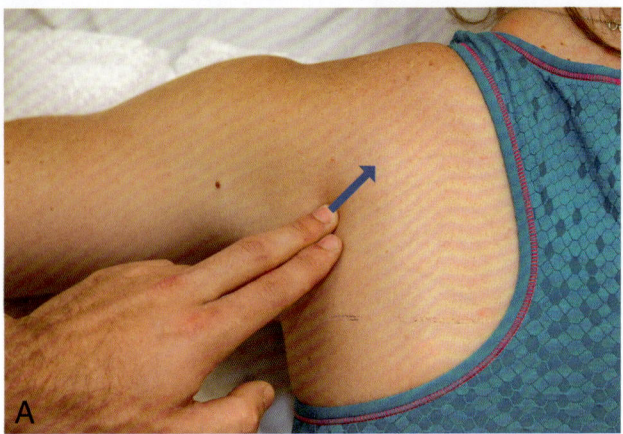 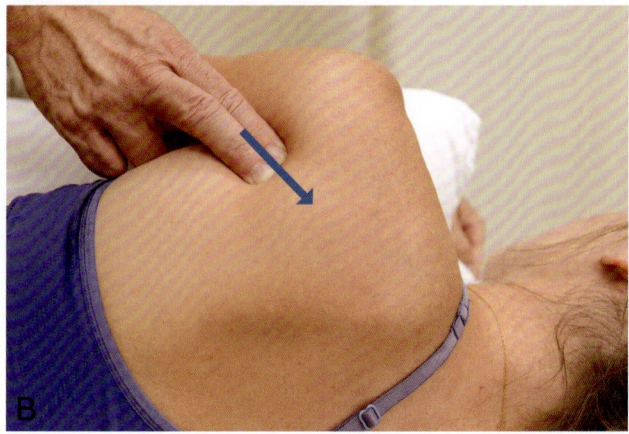

Figure 23-3. Cross-fiber flat palpation to identify TrPs in the teres minor muscle. A, Patient in prone with arm in 90° of abduction. B, Patient lies on the unaffected side with the affected side supported by a pillow in approximately 30° of abduction.

in the teres minor muscle can be involved in posterior shoulder tightness.[15] Scapular position and humeral head position should be assessed at rest and during upper extremity elevation as malalignment can be a significant contributing factor to teres minor muscle overload during all upper extremity functional activities.

3.4. Trigger Point Examination

Several positions may be useful when examining a patient for teres minor TrPs. One option is for the patient to assume a prone position with the arm in 90° of abduction supported on the table and the elbow bent to 90° with the forearm hanging from the table's edge (Figure 23-3A). This position may be useful to allow for ease of glenohumeral internal and ER ROM testing to help differentiate between the teres major and the teres minor muscles. The teres minor muscle can be identified by palpating the muscle while the patient alternately attempts internal and external rotation of the arm against minimal resistance. It contracts during ER and relaxes during internal rotation. Cross-fiber flat or pincer palpation may be utilized at the lateral edge of the scapula to identify TrPs (Figure 23-3B).

In an another option for examination, the patient lies on the unaffected side with the uppermost (involved) arm resting on a pillow placed against the chest. The clinician faces the patient and utilizes cross-fiber flat palpation along the lateral edge of the scapula, between the infraspinatus above and the teres major muscle below, to locate TrPs in the teres minor muscle (Figure 23-3). Figure 23-4 illustrates these anatomic relationships with the surrounding muscles. The long head of the triceps brachii muscle passes between the teres minor and teres major muscles, and these muscles form three sides of the quadrangular space (Figure 23-4).

4. DIFFERENTIAL DIAGNOSIS

4.1. Activation and Perpetuation of Trigger Points

A posture or activity that activates a TrP, if not corrected, can also perpetuate it. In any part of the teres minor muscle, TrPs may be activated by unaccustomed eccentric loading, eccentric exercise in an unconditioned muscle, or maximal or submaximal concentric loading.[18] Trigger points may also be activated or aggravated when the muscle is placed in a shortened and/or lengthened position for an extended period of time.

The teres minor muscle is not usually involved in isolation. Its TrPs are activated by the same overload stresses—reaching up or reaching out and behind the shoulder—that activate TrPs in the infraspinatus muscle (see Chapter 22). Patients may activate acute teres minor TrPs in the following ways: as a result of a motor vehicle accident (particularly when holding on to something such as the steering wheel), by loss of balance while lifting a heavy object overhead, while working in cramped quarters with the arm reaching overhead, and while playing volleyball or other overhead sports.[13]

Teres minor TrPs are perpetuated by continued overloading of the muscle when reaching up and back and by systemic perpetuating factors, as discussed in Chapters 1 to 4.

4.2. Associated Trigger Points

Associated TrPs can develop in the referred pain areas caused by TrPs in other muscles[19] therefore muscles in the referred pain areas for each muscle should also be considered. The infraspinatus muscle is the primary synergist of the teres minor muscle and clinically, almost always becomes involved when there are TrPs in the teres minor muscle.

Other muscles that should be considered for TrP examination include the supraspinatus muscle, posterior fibers of the deltoid muscle, the teres major muscle, the latissimus dorsi muscle, the scalene muscles, and the levator scapula muscles. In addition, the subscapularis and pectoralis major muscles that are antagonistic to the teres minor muscle in ER of the humerus should be examined as part of the functional unit.

4.3. Associated Pathology

Patients usually do not describe a small arc of severely painful motion with teres minor TrPs; rather, the entire movement or just end of the range of movement is painful. Because the teres minor muscle is one of the rotator cuff muscles, rotator cuff tears should be ruled out. The teres minor muscle is very rarely involved in rotator cuff tears, unless the infraspinatus muscle is also involved.[20] To test the integrity of the teres minor muscle, the external rotation lag test, the drop sign, and Patte test can be utilized. A positive external rotation lag test greater than 40° has been shown to have 100% sensitivity in detecting teres minor tears.[21] In a retrospective study of 279 subjects, investigators found hypertrophic changes in the teres minor muscle in cases where rotator cuff tears included the infraspinatus muscle. The integrity of the teres minor muscle is a prognostic factor for positive outcomes with total shoulder arthroplasty.[22]

The teres minor muscle itself does not seem to contribute to axillary nerve entrapment; however, two anatomic variations

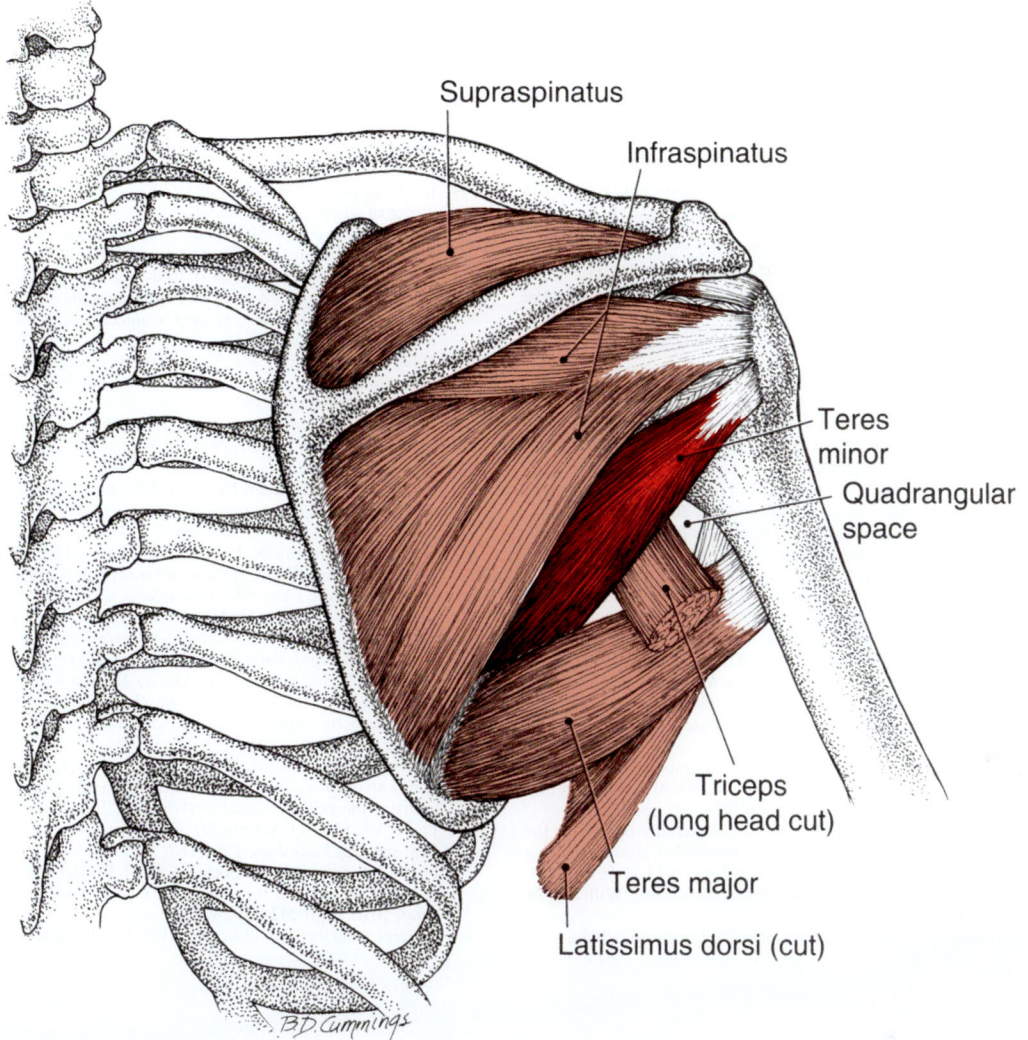

Figure 23-4. Anatomic relations of the teres minor muscle (dark red) to other dorsal scapular muscles (light red). The lateral border of the scapula is usually palpable as an orienting landmark and can be located in the space between the teres minor and the teres major muscles while using pincer palpation. The long head of the triceps muscle also passes through that space and, with the teres minor and teres major muscles and the humerus, helps define the quadrangular (quadrilateral) space.

have been identified in the posterior fascia of the shoulder. One half of the shoulders studied demonstrated a stout fascial sling that the authors believe could be a site for compression and possible tethering of the posterior branch of the axillary nerve to the teres minor muscle. Further understanding of this anatomic abnormality may be helpful when evaluating patients with primary teres minor atrophy and associated reports of pain.[2]

Quadrilateral space syndrome is characterized by intermittent and poorly localized shoulder pain, paresthesias in the upper extremity in a nondermatomal pattern, point tenderness over the quadrilateral space,[23] and selective atrophy of the teres minor and deltoid muscles.[24] This syndrome results from the compression of the axillary nerve by fibrous bands of tissue as the nerve passes through the quadrilateral space. This etiology was demonstrated in three patients by MRI.[24] More recently, authors have proposed that quadrilateral space syndrome and isolated teres minor atrophy are distinct clinical entities. The former is typically seen in younger patients and the latter in older adults.[23,25,26]

As the four case reports of Escobar and Ballesteros[13] demonstrate, dysesthesia in the fourth and fifth fingers that is caused by active teres minor TrPs can easily be mistaken for an ulnar neuropathy or C8 radiculopathy. The neuropathy and radiculopathy can be ruled out by appropriate electrodiagnostic evaluation.

5. CORRECTIVE ACTIONS

The patient should avoid habitual, sustained, or repetitive motions that overload the teres minor and infraspinatus muscles, such as repetitive overhead lifting with the upper extremity in abduction and ER, and reaching backward into the back seat of the car.

When prescribing or performing neuromuscular reeducation or therapeutic exercises for the teres minor muscle, it is effective to remember that teres minor muscle activation is greater with side-lying ER with the arm at the side and in standing with the shoulder in the plane of the scapula.[7] The teres minor muscle demonstrates minimal to moderate activity in standing with the arm at the side.[6,7]

Corrective actions for the teres minor muscle are essentially the same as those described in detail for the infraspinatus muscle (see Chapter 22, Section 5). They include avoidance of excessive or repetitive load on the muscle, correct position of the arm to avoid full shortening during sleep (see Figure 22-4A to C), home application of heat or cold packs, TrP pressure release, and self-stretch exercises.

The patient may inactivate teres minor TrP with the application of TrP compression by lying on a tennis ball placed directly on a tender spot in the muscle or by standing with their back against the wall utilizing the aforementioned technique. In either position, body weight is used to maintain increasing pressure for 1 or 2 minutes, as described in the interventions section. This self-release technique may be repeated several times daily until TrP tenderness disappears. A cold pack may be of therapeutic benefit immediately following pressure release, especially in the case of acute shoulder pain. There are a variety of TrP self-release tools on the market.

References

1. Standring S. *Gray's Anatomy: The Anatomical Basis of Clinical Practice.* 41st ed. London, UK: Elsevier; 2015.
2. Chafik D, Galatz LM, Keener JD, Kim HM, Yamaguchi K. Teres minor muscle and related anatomy. *J Shoulder Elbow Surg.* 2013;22(1):108-114.
3. Loukas M, Grabska J, Tubbs RS, Apaydin N, Jordan R. Mapping the axillary nerve within the deltoid muscle. *Surg Radiol Anat.* 2009;31(1):43-47.
4. Zhao X, Hung LK, Zhang GM, Lao J. Applied anatomy of the axillary nerve for selective neurotization of the deltoid muscle. *Clin Orthop Relat Res.* 2001(390):244-251.
5. Reed D, Cathers I, Halaki M, Ginn K. Does supraspinatus initiate shoulder abduction? *J Electromyogr Kinesiol.* 2013;23(2):425-429.
6. Marta S, Pezarat-Correla P, Fernandes O, Carita A, Cabri J, de Moraes A. Electromyographic analysis of posterior deltoid, posterior rotator cuff and trapezius musculature in different shoulder exercises. *Int J Sports Med.* 2013;14:1-15.
7. Reinold MM, Wilk KE, Fleisig GS, et al. Electromyographic analysis of the rotator cuff and deltoid musculature during common shoulder external rotation exercises. *J Orthop Sports Phys Ther.* 2004;34(7):385-394.
8. Kurokawa D, Sano H, Nagamoto H, et al. Muscle activity pattern of the shoulder external rotators differs in adduction and abduction: an analysis using positron emission tomography. *J Shoulder Elbow Surg.* 2014;23(5):658-664.
9. Basmajian J, Deluca C. *Muscles Alive.* 5th ed. Baltimore: Williams & Wilkins; 1985:270.
10. Duchenne G. *Physiology of Motion.* Philadelphia, PA: Lippincott; 1949:64, 66.
11. Simons DG, Travell JG, Simons LS. *Myofascial Pain and Dysfunction: The Trigger Point Manual. Volume 1: Upper Half of Body.* 2nd ed. Philadelphia, PA: Lippincott Williams & Wilkins; 1999.
12. Bonica J, Sola A. Other painful disorders of the upper limb, Chapter 52. In: Bonica JJ, Loeser JD, Chapman C, Fordyce WE, eds. *The Management of Pain.* 2nd ed. Philadelphia, PA: Lea & Febiger; 1990:947-958.
13. Escobar PL, Ballesteros J. Teres minor. Source of symptoms resembling ulnar neuropathy or C8 radiculopathy. *Am J Phys Med Rehabil.* 1988;67(3):120-122.
14. Bron C, Dommerholt J, Stegenga B, Wensing M, Oostendorp RA. High prevalence of shoulder girdle muscles with myofascial trigger points in patients with shoulder pain. *BMC Musculoskelet Disord.* 2011;12:139.
15. Passigli S, Plebani G, Poser A. Acute effects of dry needling on posterior shoulder tightness. A case report. *Int J Sports Phys Ther.* 2016;11(2):254-263.
16. Sola AE, Kuitert JH. Myofascial trigger point pain in the neck and shoulder girdle; report of 100 cases treated by injection of normal saline. *Northwest Med.* 1955;54(9):980-984.
17. Sola AE, Rodenberger ML, Gettys BB. Incidence of hypersensitive areas in posterior shoulder muscles; a survey of two hundred young adults. *Am J Phys Med.* 1955;34(6):585-590.
18. Gerwin RD, Dommerholt J, Shah JP. An expansion of Simons' integrated hypothesis of trigger point formation. *Curr Pain Headache Rep.* 2004;8(6):468-475.
19. Hsieh YL, Kao MJ, Kuan TS, Chen SM, Chen JT, Hong CZ. Dry needling to a key myofascial trigger point may reduce the irritability of satellite MTrPs. *Am J Phys Med Rehabil.* 2007;86(5):397-403.
20. Collin P, Matsumura N, Ladermann A, Denard PJ, Walch G. Relationship between massive chronic rotator cuff tear pattern and loss of active shoulder range of motion. *J Shoulder Elbow Surg.* 2014;23(8):1195-1202.
21. Collin P, Treseder T, Denard PJ, Neyton L, Walch G, Ladermann A. What is the best clinical test for assessment of the teres minor in massive rotator cuff tears? *Clin Orthop Relat Res.* 2015;473(9):2959-2966.
22. Kikukawa K, Ide J, Kikuchi K, Morita M, Mizuta H, Ogata H. Hypertrophic changes of the teres minor muscle in rotator cuff tears: quantitative evaluation by magnetic resonance imaging. *J Shoulder Elbow Surg.* 2014;23(12):1800-1805.
23. Wilson L, Sundaram M, Piraino DW, Ilaslan H, Recht MP. Isolated teres minor atrophy: manifestation of quadrilateral space syndrome or traction injury to the axillary nerve? *Orthopedics.* 2006;29(5):447-450.
24. Linker CS, Helms CA, Fritz RC. Quadrilateral space syndrome: findings at MR imaging. *Radiology.* 1993;188(3):675-676.
25. Friend J, Francis S, McCulloch J, Ecker J, Breidahl W, McMenamin P. Teres minor innervation in the context of isolated muscle atrophy. *Surg Radiol Anat.* 2010;32(3):243-249.
26. Masters S, Burley S. Shoulder pain. *Aust Fam Physician.* 2007;36(6):385-480.

Chapter 24

Latissimus Dorsi Muscle
"Mid-back Manipulator"

Sophia Maines

1. INTRODUCTION

The latissimus dorsi muscle is an expansive muscle that links the upper and the lower halves of the body through its attachments to the thoracic and lumbar spine via the thoracolumbar fascia and to the proximal humerus. The muscle originates from the spinous processes of T6-L2, the posterior layer of the thoracolumbar fascia, and the posterior aspect of iliac crest lateral to the erector spinae muscles. It inserts onto the humerus at the floor of the intertubercular sulcus. The muscle is innervated by the thoracodorsal nerve from the posterior cord of the brachial plexus. With direct, as well as fascial, connections to the spine, ribs, pelvis, scapula, and humerus, the latissimus dorsi muscle has a myriad of functions for both movement and stability. The muscle functions to extend, adduct, and internally rotate the humerus, and it can influence depression of the shoulder. Its development is key for athletes such as swimmers and baseball players who utilize it for propulsion through the water or throwing. It is one of the most commonly used muscle flaps for a variety of surgical procedures including breast reconstruction. Pain arising due to latissimus dorsi trigger points (TrPs) may be referred to the anterior shoulder, the inferior angle of the scapula, the axillary region, or down the medial aspect of the arm to the fourth and fifth digits. Activities that require straining to reach overhead or out in front of the body, such as hanging, climbing, swimming, or repetitive throwing, may activate and/or perpetuate TrPs in the latissimus dorsi muscle. Differential diagnosis should include cervical radicular pain or radiculopathy, suprascapular nerve entrapment, and bicipital tendinopathy. Altering sleeping posture to prevent prolonged shoulder extension while in a supine position or adduction with internal rotation while lying on the side is essential for managing the patient's pain. Self-stretching and TrP self-pressure release can be very effective in managing symptoms caused by TrPs in the latissimus dorsi muscle.

2. ANATOMIC CONSIDERATIONS

The latissimus dorsi muscle originates from the spinous processes of T6-L2,[1,2] the posterior layer of the thoracolumbar fascia, and the posterior aspect of iliac crest lateral to the erector spinae muscles[1] (Figure 24-1). The muscle fibers fan from their origins at the trunk toward each shoulder. The upper fibers are nearly horizontal, the middle fibers have a more oblique path, and the lower fibers course almost vertically.[1] The upper fibers pass over, and sometimes attach to, the inferior angle of the scapula.[1] In a study of 100 cadavers, Pouliart and Gagey[3] found muscular attachments to the scapula 43% of the time. On others, they observed a small fibrous attachment or an intervening bursa with no connecting tissue. The lower fibers of the latissimus dorsi muscle, which run nearly vertically, have anterior attachments to the lower three or four ribs.[1,2] In the scapular region, the muscle curves around the inferior border of the teres major muscle, forming the posterior axillary fold.[1] The muscle fibers in this region twist around one another with the lowest originating fibers inserting at the highest point on the humerus and those originating highest at the midline of the body inserting at the lowest point on the humerus.[1] The muscle then inserts onto the humerus at the floor of the intertubercular sulcus, posterior to pectoralis major muscle and anterior to teres major muscle. A bursa separates the latissimus dorsi and teres major tendons near their insertions.[1]

Rarely, a variant axillary arch muscle has been identified as a slip of muscle extending from the latissimus dorsi muscle's upper border to the humerus, where it inserts deep to the pectoralis major tendon.[4]

2.1. Innervation and Vascularization

The latissimus dorsi muscle is supplied by the thoracodorsal nerve from the posterior cord of the brachial plexus. It arises from the ventral rami of the cervical nerves C6, C7, and C8. The thoracodorsal nerve branches from the posterior cord between the upper and lower subscapular nerves. It accompanies the subscapular artery along the posterior axillary wall, where it supplies the latissimus dorsi muscle.[1]

The muscle receives vascular supply primarily from the thoracodorsal artery; the terminal branch of the subscapular artery; from branches of the ninth, tenth, and eleventh posterior intercostal arteries; and the first through third lumbar arteries, which supply the inferior and medial muscle fibers. The thoracodorsal artery enters the muscle near the lateral border and bifurcates into two branches, one that travels parallel to the upper border of the muscle and the other travels medially at a 45° angle. In a rare variation, the thoracodorsal artery can trifurcate with a third branch that may supply the muscle proximally or distally.[1]

2.2. Function

With direct, as well as fascial, connections to the spine, ribs, pelvis, scapula, and humerus, the latissimus dorsi muscle has a myriad of functions for both movement and stability. It primarily functions in the movement and positioning of the upper limb and trunk; it also plays a role in lumbar extension, trunk and pelvic stability, and respiration.

The latissimus dorsi muscle functions to extend, adduct, and internally rotate the humerus and[1] it can also influence shoulder depression.[5,6] Following a dissection and analysis of the muscle's fascicles, Bogduk and Johnson et al[2] concluded that the latissimus dorsi muscle's primary actions are movement of the upper extremity and lifting the trunk, such as in a wheelchair transfer.

Using electromyographic (EMG) analysis of the shoulder girdle muscles during various internal rotation exercises, Alizadehkhaiyat and colleagues[7] found the greatest activity of the

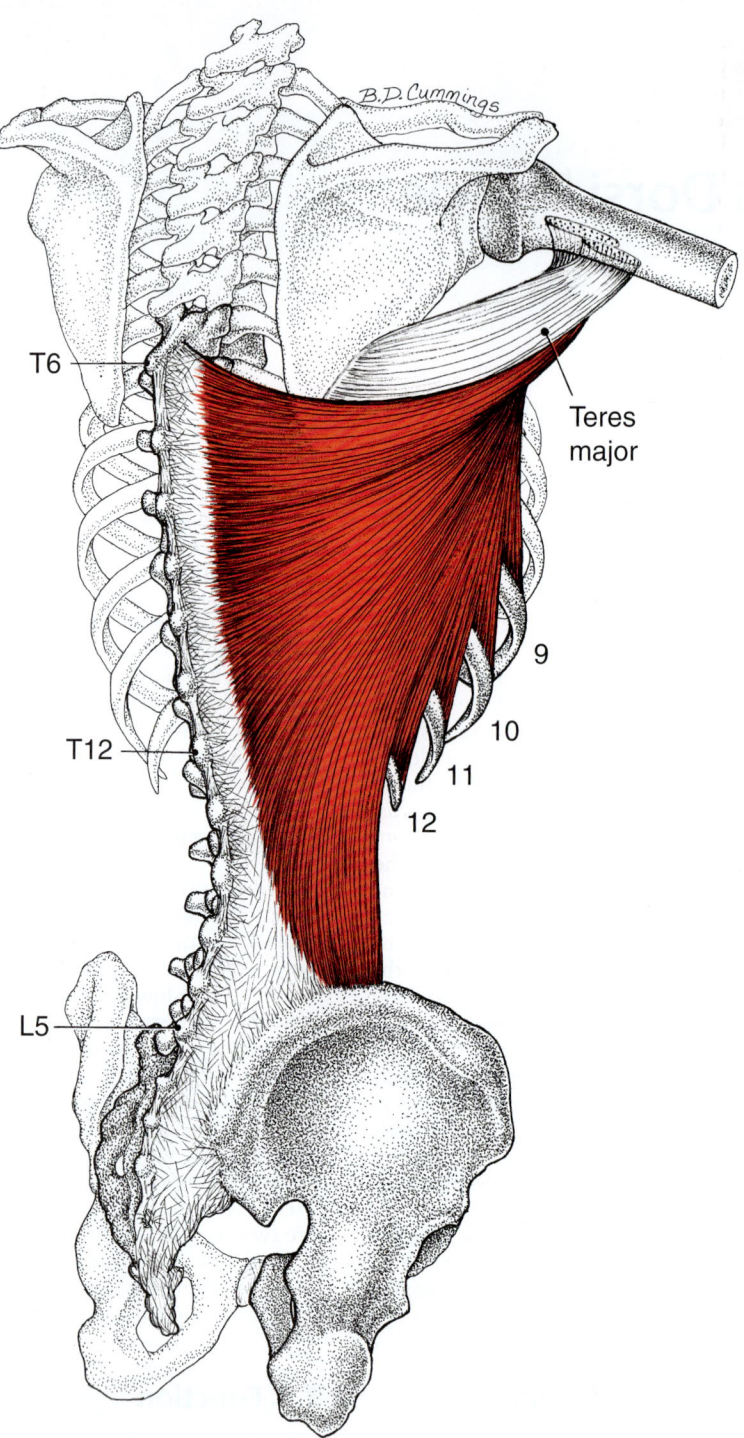

Figure 24-1. Attachments of the latissimus dorsi muscle (red), and its relation to the teres major muscle, which arises from the edge of the scapula. The superior (horizontal) fibers of the latissimus dorsi muscle swing around the teres major muscle, and the tendons attach near each other (the teres major muscle to the medial lip of the intertubercular groove of the humerus, and the latissimus dorsi muscle to the floor of the groove). Both muscles are elongated by flexion and external rotation of the humerus.

latissimus dorsi muscle with an internal rotation of shoulder elevation at 155° in the scapular plane.

The latissimus dorsi muscle often contributes to power and acceleration movements of the upper limb during various sporting activities such as swimming, throwing, and golfing.[8] When swimming the butterfly stroke, the latissimus dorsi muscle assists with propulsion through the water.[9] During the golf swing, it is highly active during the acceleration phase, from a horizontal club position to ball impact.[10,11] The latissimus dorsi muscle is considered a power muscle, along with the subscapularis, pectoralis major, and serratus anterior muscles for the trail arm to accelerate during the golf downswing.[12]

During the overhead baseball pitch, the latissimus dorsi muscle is most active during the acceleration phase, from maximum shoulder external rotation to ball release,[12-15] when it works with the subscapularis and pectoralis major muscles for rapid internal rotation of the shoulder.[12] In a study using intramuscular EMG analysis of the throwing shoulder, Jobe et al[16] found that the activity of pectoralis major and latissimus dorsi muscles occurred at the end of the cocking phase and continued through the acceleration phase. They concluded that these two muscles provided the "power and driving force" of forward shoulder movement. Comparing the muscle activity of professional against amateur pitchers, Gowan et al[17] found that professional pitchers demonstrated a stronger activity of latissimus dorsi and subscapularis muscles than amateurs.

Surgical transfer of the latissimus dorsi muscle most often leads to deficits of endurance in shoulder extension and adduction, observed on an earlier onset of fatigue with activities such as swimming or ladder climbing.[18] In a study involving 26 men and women, Fraulin et al[19] found deficits in power as well as endurance of shoulder adduction and extension post transfer.

Studies have sought to functionally differentiate the parts of the muscle.[20] In one such study involving a surface EMG analysis of 17 subjects, Park and Yoo[5] separated the muscle into medial and lateral compartments. They examined the medial compartment with a surface electrode placed over the muscle belly lateral to T9. Activity in the lateral compartment was observed with an electrode placement 4 cm below the inferior angle of the scapular midway between the spine and the lateral edge of the torso. They found more activity in the medial compartment with shoulder adduction, extension, and internal rotation, whereas more activity was present in the lateral compartment with shoulder depression. Paton and Brown[20] found functional differentiation within the latissimus dorsi muscle when they used surface EMG to record isometric muscle contractions. They concluded that adduction from an abducted position preferentially involved the muscle's most caudal fibers, whereas isometric adduction in the anatomic position involved muscle activity across the entire muscle.

The latissimus dorsi muscle also functions as an accessory muscle for respiration, with both deep inspiration and forced expiration as with coughing.[1]

Whereas the latissimus dorsi muscle is generally recognized for its role in the movement of the upper limb, its fascial connections have been investigated for their contribution to lumbar movement and trunk and pelvic stability. The latissimus dorsi aponeurosis is continuous with the superficial lamina of the posterior layer of the thoracolumbar fascia. This fascial layer also has fibrous connections with the trapezius, gluteus maximus, and external oblique muscles.[21] In a study involving embalmed cadavers, Vleeming et al[22] found that traction on the latissimus dorsi muscle displaced the superficial lamina both ipsilaterally and, in some areas, contralaterally. Similarly, a study involving unembalmed cadavers found that tensioning the latissimus dorsi muscle displaced the posterior layer of the lumbar fascia.[23] When studied in vivo, researchers observed that tensioning of the latissimus dorsi muscle produced myofascial force transmission, likely through the thoracolumbar fascia, which moved the contralateral hip into external rotation.[24] Mooney et al[25] used surface EMG to confirm a reciprocal relationship between the latissimus dorsi and the contralateral gluteus maximus muscles during a torso rotation exercise and gait in healthy participants.

In a study of force closure of the sacroiliac joint (SIJ) involving six subjects, muscle activation was found to effect SIJ stiffness, although activation of the latissimus dorsi muscle was found to have only a small effect, less than that with activation of the erector spinae, biceps femoris, and gluteus maximus muscles. One subject was able to nearly isolate the latissimus dorsi muscle with no change in joint stiffness. The authors reported that SIJ stiffness found in other subjects with latissimus dorsi muscle activation could be due to activity of other muscles.[26]

The latissimus dorsi muscle's contribution to lumbar extension has also been studied. Mathematical models used to study how tension from the latissimus dorsi muscle on the lumbodorsal fascia could affect the extension moment on the spine during a dynamic squat lift found negligible contributions on extension during the lifts studied.[27] De Ridder et al[28] used functional MRI to study muscle activation during prone trunk and leg extension exercises and found the latissimus dorsi muscle was the least activated muscle compared with the paraspinal and multifidi muscles.

Box 24-1 Functional unit of the Latissimus Dorsi muscle[18]

Action	Synergists	Antagonists
Shoulder internal rotation	Subscapularis Pectoralis major Teres major Anterior deltoid	Infraspinatus Teres minor Posterior deltoid
Shoulder extension	Teres major Triceps brachii Posterior deltoid	Anterior deltoid Long head biceps brachii Coracobrachialis
Shoulder adduction	Pectoralis major Teres major Coracobrachialis	Middle deltoid Supraspinatus
Shoulder girdle depression	Teres major Pectoralis major External abdominal oblique	Scalene muscles Upper trapezius

2.3. Functional Unit

The functional unit to which a muscle belongs includes the muscles that reinforce and counter its actions as well as the joints that the muscle crosses. The interdependence of these structures functionally is reflected in the organization and neural connections of the sensory motor cortex. The functional unit is emphasized because the presence of a TrP in one muscle of the unit increases the likelihood that the other muscles of the unit also develops TrPs. When inactivating TrPs in a muscle, one should be concerned about TrPs that may develop in muscles that are functionally interdependent. Box 24-1 grossly represents the functional unit of the latissimus dorsi muscle.[29]

When the arm is abducted, the latissimus dorsi muscle works with the triceps brachii muscle to stabilize the glenohumeral joint. When the arm is by the side of the body, the latissimus dorsi muscle and the long head of the triceps brachii muscle act as antagonists of glenohumeral joint stabilization. The latissimus dorsi muscle also works with the external abdominal oblique muscle to stabilize the lower ribs.

3. CLINICAL PRESENTATION

3.1. Referred Pain Pattern

The latissimus dorsi muscle is a frequently overlooked cause of mid-thoracic back pain of myofascial origin. Trigger points are commonly found in the posterior axillary fold (Figure 24-2A). Pain may refer to the inferior angle of the scapula and ipsilateral mid-thoracic region. It also may extend to the posterior aspect of the shoulder, down the medial aspect of the arm, forearm, and hand to the fourth and the fifth fingers (Figure 24-2B).

Trigger points may also be present at the lateral aspect of the muscle in the region of the lower ribs (Figure 24-2C, D). Trigger points in this area commonly refer pain to the front of

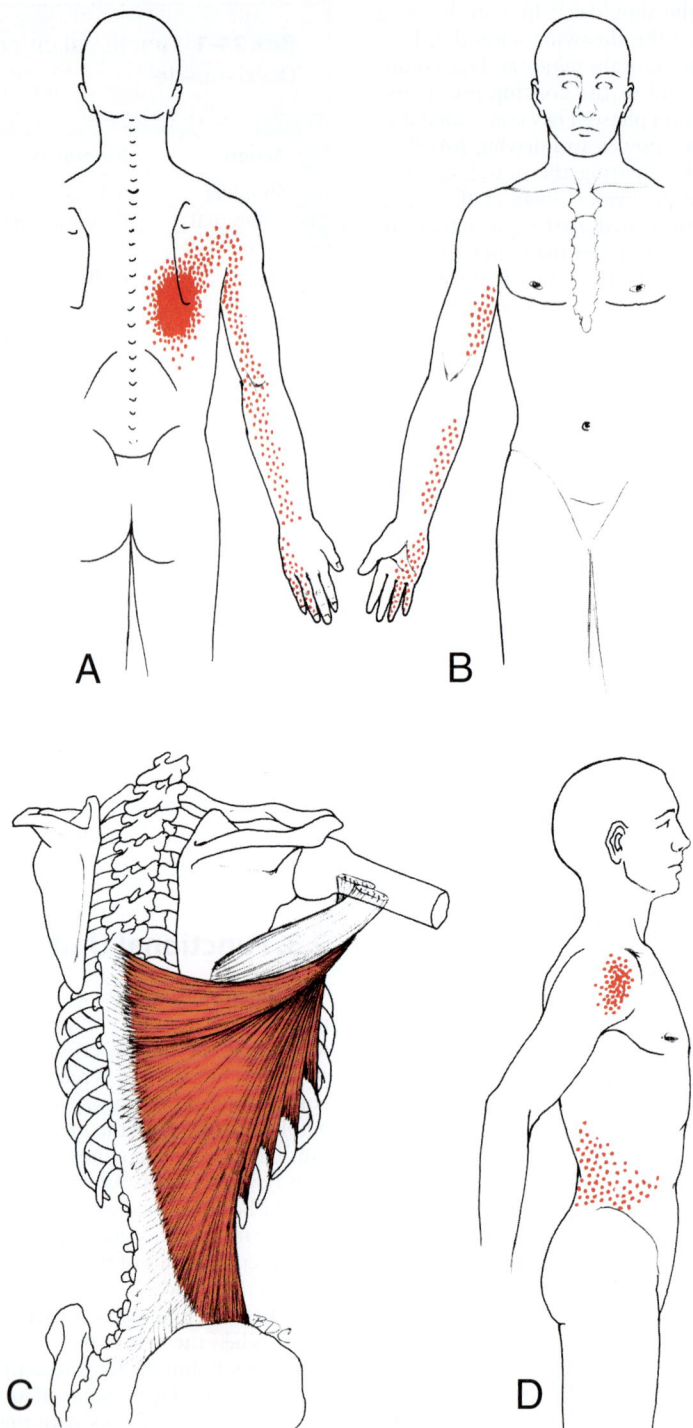

Figure 24-2. Referred pain patterns (essential portion is solid red, spillover portion is stippled red) referred from TrPs in the right latissimus dorsi muscle. A, Back view of the pain pattern from TrPs in their most common location within the axillary portion of the muscle. B, Front view of the same. C, Right latissimus dorsi muscle and attachments. D, Pain pattern of TrPs in the inferior portion of the muscle which may also refer pain down the arm.

the shoulder and to the side of the torso above the iliac crest. A TrP in the thoracolumbar region may refer pain locally to the inferior aspect of the posterior axillary fold.[30]

In a study using 7.5% saline injections to determine referred pain patterns, injection to the vertically oriented fibers in the axillary region next to teres major muscle most commonly referred pain to the dorsum at the scapular region. Injection to the superficial, horizontal fibers most commonly referred pain to the upper limb.[31]

Pain patterns have not been identified for the latissimus dorsi muscle's anterior fibers that attach to the ribs. Some cases of low back pain have historically been attributed to latissimus dorsi dysfunction in the lumbosacral area, but this pain may have been caused by enthesopathy.[32]

3.2. Symptoms

Patients with TrPs in the latissimus dorsi muscle usually do not report pain until the TrPs are active and cause pain at rest. Furthermore, patients are often unable to identify a particular activity that aggravates their pain. They may give a long history of negative diagnostic procedures, such as bronchoscopy or computerized tomography, as well as a history of unsuccessful therapy aimed at the area of referred pain in the back rather than at its source.

The patient with latissimus dorsi TrPs may report a constant aching pain referring to the inferior scapular angle and surrounding mid-thoracic region. When asked to draw the pain, a patient is apt to mark a circle centered on the inferior scapular angle. Alternatively, pain from TrPs in the latissimus dorsi muscle can also mimic cervical radicular pain with symptoms down the posterior and/or medial aspects of the arm into the fingers. Numbness and tingling along this area are frequently reported.

Pain from TrPs in the latissimus dorsi muscle may be recreated by shoulder girdle depression movements that load the muscle or weighted overhead stretching in front of the body, such as to retrieve an object from a high shelf.

3.3. Patient Examination

After a thorough subjective examination, the clinician should make a detailed drawing representing the pain pattern that the patient has described. This depiction will assist in planning the physical examination and can be useful in monitoring the progression of the patient as symptoms improve or change. For a proper examination of the latissimus dorsi muscle, the clinician should observe shoulder girdle and trunk posture and scapular position, examining active and passive ranges of motion of the shoulder girdle and taking note of muscle activation patterns and the scapulohumeral rhythm.

To identify TrPs in the latissimus dorsi muscle that may be limiting the range of motion and thus influencing dysfunction, the clinician should identify the limited range of motion by performing specific range of motion tests for all parts of the latissimus dorsi muscle. Because a patient with latissimus dorsi TrPs often presents with a shoulder range of motion limitations, a thorough examination of all contributing factors to the lost range of motion should be completed.

There are several variations of testing procedures for latissimus dorsi muscle length. In the Vladimir Janda approach, the patient lies supine with knees bent and feet on the table. The clinician moves one of the patient's arms through shoulder elevation. According to this assessment, with sufficient latissimus dorsi muscle length, the lumbar spine should remain flat on the table and not extended when the arm is horizontal and resting on the table. Extension of the spine or lack of full shoulder elevation motion may indicate muscle shortness.[33]

Accessory joint motions of the glenohumeral, acromioclavicular, sternoclavicular, and scapulothoracic joints should be tested. The thoracic spine, rib cage, and lumbar intervertebral accessory joint motion should also be assessed manually. Often, joint hypomobility in the sternoclavicular joint, thoracic spine, and rib cage can cause impairment in shoulder elevation, contributing to alterations in the normal muscle activation patterns. Articular dysfunctions in the glenohumeral joint may also impair muscle activation patterns contributing to the overload of the latissimus dorsi and other shoulder girdle muscles.

3.4. Trigger Point Examination

Clinical examination may be performed in supine, prone, or a side-lying position (Figure 24-3A to C). The side-lying position is preferred as the entirety of the muscle is accessible, and the clinician is able to see the patient's face during the examination. When examining the left latissimus dorsi muscle, the patient should be positioned on the right side with left arm elevated and placed on a pillow. The clinician can cue the patient to adjust trunk flexion and extension as needed. Trigger points in the dorsal and caudal fibers can be palpated with a cross-fiber flat palpation (Figure 24-3A). The clinician should be cognizant of fiber direction to ensure accuracy with palpation. The most lateral fibers, which attach to the iliac crest, are the most vertical and run about 15° to the sagittal plane.[2] Fiber direction, which is always oblique, becomes more horizontal superiorly with fibers from the thoracic region running about 50° to 60° to the sagittal plane.[2] Cross-fiber pincer palpation may also be used in the axillary region or at the lateral trunk to identify TrPs (Figure 24-3B, C).

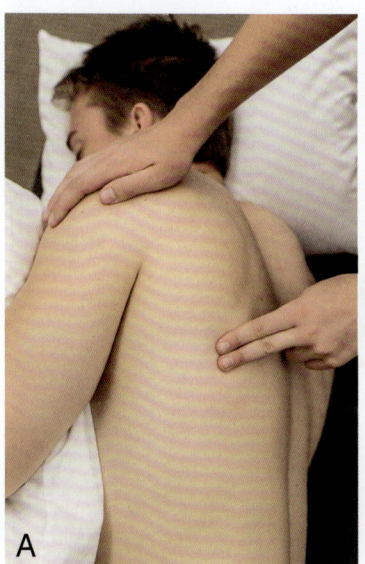
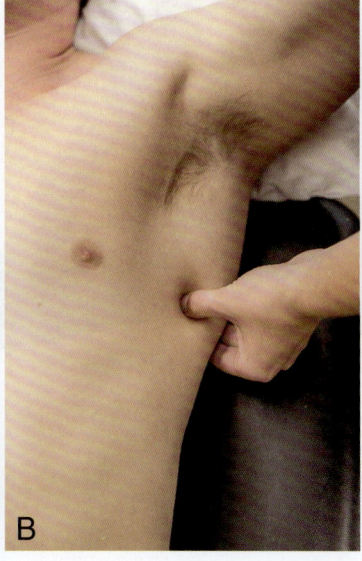
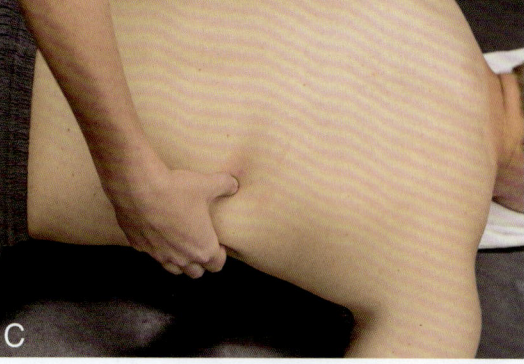

Figure 24-3. Palpation of the latissimus dorsi muscle. A, Side-lying cross-fiber flat palpation. B, Supine cross-fiber pincer palpation in the axillary region. C, Prone cross-fiber pincer palpation at the lateral trunk.

4. DIFFERENTIAL DIAGNOSIS

4.1. Activation and Perpetuation of Trigger Points

A posture or activity that activates a TrP, if not corrected, can also perpetuate it. In any part of the latissimus dorsi muscle, TrPs may be activated by unaccustomed eccentric loading, eccentric exercise in an unconditioned muscle, or maximal or submaximal concentric loading.[34] Trigger points may also be activated or aggravated when the muscle is placed in a shortened and/or lengthened position, such as side sleeping or sitting with increased internal rotation of the shoulders. Compression from a restrictive undergarment or bra can also activate and perpetuate TrPs and may be implicated if there is visible indentation from the band on the skin.

Finding the source of TrPs in the latissimus dorsi muscle requires a careful analysis of activities that require repetitive shoulder girdle depression, shoulder extension or adduction, or trunk movement. Activities that utilize the latissimus dorsi muscle and may activate TrPs include walking with axillary crutches, wheelchair use or wheelchair transfers, throwing, and climbing or hanging from the upper limbs.[2] Activities that require straining to reach overhead or out in front of the body may also activate and/or perpetuate TrPs in the latissimus dorsi muscle.

4.2. Associated Trigger Points

Muscles in the referred pain areas of the latissimus dorsi muscle should be considered because associated TrPs can develop within them.[35] These include the biceps brachii, deltoid, coracobrachialis, flexor carpi ulnaris, triceps brachii, infraspinatus, teres major, trapezius, rhomboids, and abdominal oblique muscles.

The teres major muscle frequently develops TrPs with the latissimus dorsi muscle due to its anatomic proximity. Similarly, the long head of the triceps brachii muscle is also prone to associated TrPs, particularly in chronic cases.

Because the latissimus dorsi muscle is one of 13 muscles that refer pain to the medial border of the scapula, the other referring muscles should also be considered when pain here is reported. These include the scalenes, cervical and thoracic multifidi, levator scapula, rhomboid major and minor, serratus anterior, serratus posterior superior, iliocostalis thoracis, infraspinatus, and the middle and lower trapezius muscles.

4.3. Associated Pathology

The latissimus dorsi muscle (along with the pectoralis major, teres major, and subscapularis muscles) is implicated in myofascial presentation of thoracic outlet syndrome. Referred pain from any one of these four muscles can mimic thoracic outlet syndrome. Trigger points in at least three of these muscles are strongly suggestive of the syndrome and often misdiagnosed as such, though these muscles do not cause compression of structures in the thoracic outlet. The thoracic outlet syndrome is further discussed in Chapter 33.

Other conditions that should be considered include cervical radicular pain or radiculopathy, bicipital tendinopathy, and entrapment of the suprascapular nerve at the spine of the scapula.

Both latissimus dorsi and quadratus lumborum TrPs have been associated with innominate dysfunction. However, the muscles have distinctly different pain referral patterns. Quadratus lumborum TrPs are associated with sacroiliac dysfunction, whereas isolated latissimus dorsi TrPs are associated with innominate upslips. Therefore, a positive SIJ testing may implicate quadratus lumborum muscle involvement, but not the latissimus dorsi muscle.[29]

5. CORRECTIVE ACTIONS

A patient with latissimus dorsi TrPs should avoid habitual, sustained, or repetitive motions that overload the latissimus dorsi muscle. These motions may include retrieving heavy objects from a shelf that requires straining or overreaching or activities that require excessive pulling such as gymnastics, tennis, swimming, rowing, chopping wood, or throwing.

Sleeping positions can be particularly troublesome for assuming prolonged aggravating postures. The individual with latissimus dorsi TrPs may be most comfortable sleeping on the back or on the pain-free side. When lying on the uninvolved side, sleep may be improved by supporting the uppermost elbow and forearm of the painful limb on a pillow (Figure 22-4A) in a neutral position to avoid prolonged shortening of the affected latissimus dorsi muscle that can cause referred pain. This pillow positioning technique can also help keep the arm in a neutral position while lying on the back (Figure 22-4C). Another option is to place the pillow under the arm perpendicular to the body to keep the arm out of adduction and internal rotation and in a resting length-tension position for the latissimus dorsi muscle. Patients should be cautioned regarding lying in bed with their

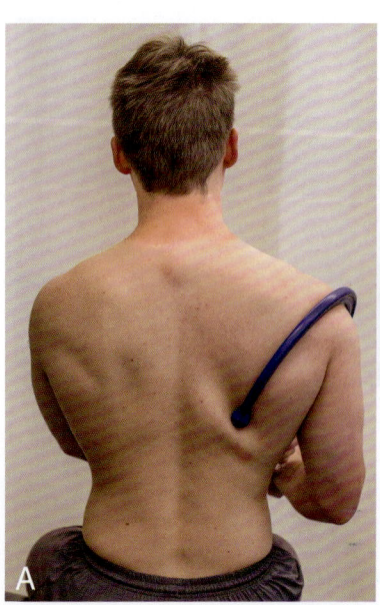
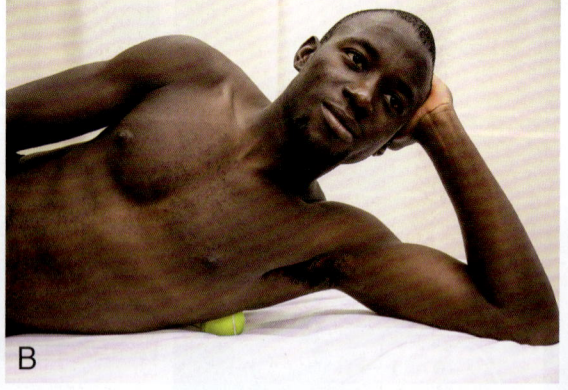
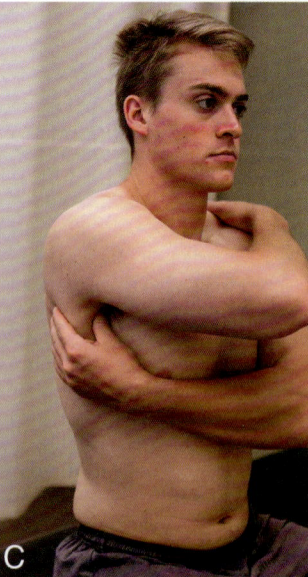

Figure 24-4. TrP self-release. A, Self-pressure release of TrPs with tool. B, Lying on tennis ball. C, Manual self-pressure release of TrPs.

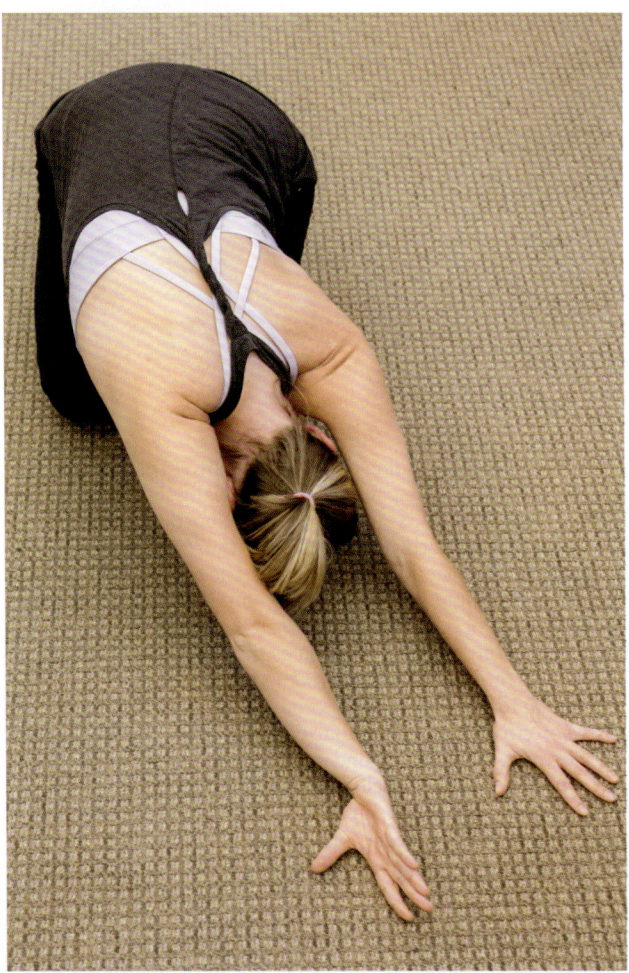

Figure 24-5. Latissimus dorsi muscle self-stretch. The patient can begin in child's pose, then walk the hands away from the side being stretched. The exercise can be modified by internally or externally rotating the arm.

arm(s) above their head in an abducted and an externally rotated position, as this position keeps the latissimus dorsi muscle in a prolonged lengthened position and may cause increased tensile stress in the muscle.

A patient can also learn self-treatment for latissimus dorsi TrPs using a round TrP self-release tool (Figure 24-4A, B). The patient lies on the affected side with the shoulder abducted to stretch the latissimus dorsi muscle. The body position is adjusted over the tennis ball at the TrP site. A gentle pressure is applied while the patient performs gentle isometric contractions followed by muscle relaxation. The patient can perform manual self-pressure release of TrPs by grasping the muscle belly where it is most tender (Figure 24-4C). The patient should be instructed to exhale during the relaxation phase to encourage muscle relaxation.

The patient can be instructed in a self-stretch for the muscle as well. The patient begins in a quadruped position and then move backward into a "child's pose," achieved by bringing the buttocks to rest on the feet and chest atop the knees with arms forward on the floor. To stretch the left side of the muscle, the patient can walk the hands along the floor to the right. The patient can modify the stretch by turning the palm up on the side that is being stretched (Figure 24-5).

References

1. Standring S. *Gray's Anatomy: The Anatomical Basis of Clinical Practice.* 41st ed. London, UK: Elsevier; 2015.
2. Bogduk N, Johnson G, Spalding D. The morphology and biomechanics of latissimus dorsi. *Clin Biomech (Bristol, Avon).* 1998;13(6):377-385.
3. Pouliart N, Gagey O. Significance of the latissimus dorsi for shoulder instability. I. Variations in its anatomy around the humerus and scapula. *Clin Anat.* 2005;18(7):493-499.
4. Bakirci S, Kafa IM, Uysal M, Sendemir E. Langer's axillary arch (axillopectoral muscle): a variation of latissimus dorsi muscle. *Int J Anat Variations.* 2010;3:91-92.
5. Park SY, Yoo WG. Differential activation of parts of the latissimus dorsi with various isometric shoulder exercises. *J Electromyogr Kinesiol.* 2014;24(2):253-257.
6. Townsend H, Jobe FW, Pink M, Perry J. Electromyographic analysis of the glenohumeral muscles during a baseball rehabilitation program. *Am J Sports Med.* 1991;19(3):264-272.
7. Alizadehkhaiyat O, Hawkes DH, Kemp GJ, Frostick SP. Electromyographic analysis of shoulder girdle muscles during common internal rotation exercises. *Int J Sports Phys Ther.* 2015;10(5):645-654.
8. Pink M, Jobe FW, Perry J. Electromyographic analysis of the shoulder during the golf swing. *Am J Sports Med.* 1990;18(2):137-140.
9. Pink M, Jobe FW, Perry J, Kerrigan J, Browne A, Scovazzo ML. The normal shoulder during the butterfly swim stroke. An electromyographic and cinematographic analysis of twelve muscles. *Clin Orthop Relat Res.* 1993;(288):48-59.
10. Marta S, Silva L, Castro MA, Pezarat-Correia P, Cabri J. Electromyography variables during the golf swing: a literature review. *J Electromyogr Kinesiol.* 2012;22(6):803-813.
11. Jobe FW, Moynes DR, Antonelli DJ. Rotator cuff function during a golf swing. *Am J Sports Med.* 1986;14(5):388-392.
12. Escamilla RF, Andrews JR. Shoulder muscle recruitment patterns and related biomechanics during upper extremity sports. *Sports Med.* 2009;39(7):569-590.
13. Escamilla RF, Fleisig GS, Barrentine SW, Zheng N, Andrews JR. Kinematic comparisons of throwing different types of baseball pitches. *J Appl Biomech.* 1998;14(1):1-23.
14. Escamilla R, Fleisig G, Barrentine S, Andrews J, Moorman C III. Kinematic and kinetic comparisons between American and Korean professional baseball pitchers. *Sports Biomech.* 2002;1(2):213-228.
15. Fleisig GS, Andrews JR, Dillman CJ, Escamilla RF. Kinetics of baseball pitching with implications about injury mechanisms. *Am J Sports Med.* 1995;23(2):233-239.
16. Jobe FW, Moynes DR, Tibone JE, Perry J. An EMG analysis of the shoulder in pitching. A second report. *Am J Sports Med.* 1984;12(3):218-220.
17. Gowan ID, Jobe FW, Tibone JE, Perry J, Moynes DR. A comparative electromyographic analysis of the shoulder during pitching. Professional versus amateur pitchers. *Am J Sports Med.* 1987;15(6):586-590.
18. Spear SL, Hess CL. A review of the biomechanical and functional changes in the shoulder following transfer of the latissimus dorsi muscles. *Plast Reconstr Surg.* 2005;115(7):2070-2073.
19. Fraulin FO, Louie G, Zorrilla L, Tilley W. Functional evaluation of the shoulder following latissimus dorsi muscle transfer. *Ann Plast Surg.* 1995;35(4):349-355.
20. Paton ME, Brown JM. Functional differentiation within latissimus dorsi. *Electromyogr Clin Neurophysiol.* 1995;35(5):301-309.
21. Vleeming A, Stoeckart R. The role of the pelvic girdle in coupling the spine and the legs: a clinical-anatomical perspective on pelvic stability. In: Vleeming A, Mooney V, Stoeckart R, eds. *Movement, Stability and Lumbopelvic Pain.* Edinburgh: Churchill Livingstone; 2007:113-137.
22. Vleeming A, Pool-Goudzwaard AL, Stoeckart R, van Wingerden JP, Snijders CJ. The posterior layer of the thoracolumbar fascia. Its function in load transfer from spine to legs. *Spine (Phila Pa 1976).* 1995;20(7):753-758.
23. Barker PJ, Briggs CA, Bogeski G. Tensile transmission across the lumbar fasciae in unembalmed cadavers: effects of tension to various muscular attachments. *Spine (Phila Pa 1976).* 2004;29(2):129-138.
24. Carvalhais VO, Ocarino Jde M, Araujo VL, Souza TR, Silva PL, Fonseca ST. Myofascial force transmission between the latissimus dorsi and gluteus maximus muscles: an in vivo experiment. *J Biomech.* 2013;46(5):1003-1007.
25. Mooney V, Pozos R, Vleeming A, Gulick J, Swenski D. Exercise treatment for sacroiliac pain. *Orthopedics.* 2001;24(1):29-32.
26. van Wingerden JP, Vleeming A, Buyruk HM, Raissadat K. Stabilization of the sacroiliac joint in vivo: verification of muscular contribution to force closure of the pelvis. *Eur Spine J.* 2004;13(3):199-205.
27. McGill SM, Norman RW. Potential of lumbodorsal fascia forces to generate back extension moments during squat lifts. *J Biomed Eng.* 1988;10(4):312-318.
28. De Ridder EM, Van Oosterwijck JO, Vleeming A, Vanderstraeten GG, Danneels LA. Muscle functional MRI analysis of trunk muscle recruitment during extension exercises in asymptomatic individuals. *Scand J Med Sci Sports.* 2015;25(2):196-204.
29. Simons DG, Travell J, Simons L. *Travell & Simon's Myofascial Pain and Dysfunction: The Trigger Point Manual.* Vol 1. 2nd ed. Baltimore: Williams & Wilkins; 1999:104.
30. Travell J, Rinzler SH. Pain syndromes of the chest muscles; resemblance to effort angina and myocardial infarction, and relief by local block. *Can Med Assoc J.* 1948;59(4):333-338.
31. Simons DG, Travell J. The latissimus dorsi syndrome: a source of mid-back pain. *Arch Phys Med Rehabil.* 1976;57:561.
32. Winter Z. Referred pain in fibrositis. *Med Rec.* 1944;157:34-37.
33. Page P, Frank C, Lardner R. *Assessment and Treatment of Muscle Imbalance. The Janda Approach.* Champaign, IL: Human Kinetics; 2010.
34. Gerwin RD, Dommerholt J, Shah JP. An expansion of Simons' integrated hypothesis of trigger point formation. *Curr Pain Headache Rep.* 2004;8(6):468-475.
35. Hsieh YL, Kao MJ, Kuan TS, Chen SM, Chen JT, Hong CZ. Dry needling to a key myofascial trigger point may reduce the irritability of satellite MTrPs. *Am J Phys Med Rehabil.* 2007;86(5):397-403.

Chapter 25

Teres Major Muscle

"Forgotten Shoulder Aggravator"

Sophia Maines

1. INTRODUCTION

The teres major muscle is a thick, round muscle that is significantly shorter than its neighbor, the latissimus dorsi muscle. The teres major muscle originates from the inferior angle of the scapula and travels laterally to insert on the medial lip of the bicipital groove. The teres major attachment on the lowest part of the scapula becomes the superior attachment on the humerus, twisting like its counterpart, the latissimus dorsi muscle. This unique arrangement of fiber orientation allows it to generate exceptional tensile forces. The teres major muscle is entwined with the larger latissimus dorsi muscle in the posterior axillary fold. It is innervated by the lower subscapular nerves, C5, C6, and C7, and it assists the latissimus dorsi muscle with shoulder internal rotation as well as shoulder adduction and extension. The teres major muscle refers pain to the region of the posterior deltoid muscle, posterior glenohumeral joint, over the long head of the triceps brachii muscle, and occasionally into the posterior aspect of the forearm. Patients often report minimal pain at rest but sharp pain in the posterior shoulder with overhead movements, especially with retrieving items from a high shelf. Trigger points (TrPs) are easily activated and perpetuated by activities that require excessive amounts of pulling such as rowing, playing tennis, or throwing. The teres major muscle is a common site for TrPs in patients with unilateral, nontraumatic shoulder pain, and it should be examined when patients report pain, weakness, tenderness, or paresthesias in the upper quarter. Altering the sleeping posture to prevent prolonged shoulder extension while supine, or adduction with internal rotation while lying on the side, is essential for managing pain. Self-stretching and TrP self-pressure release can be very effective in managing symptoms caused by TrPs in the teres major muscle.

2. ANATOMIC CONSIDERATIONS

The teres major muscle originates from the middle third of the lateral posterior aspect of the scapula;[1] from the inferior angle of the scapula, and from a fibrous septa between the teres minor muscle and the infraspinatus muscle (Figure 25-1). Its fibers spiral laterally toward the humerus, passing anteriorly to the long head of triceps brachii muscle, where they insert onto the medial aspect of the intertubercular sulcus of the humerus.[2] Roughly 4 cm in width, the teres major tendon inserts posterior to the latissimus dorsi tendon.[3] In a study of cadavers, Pearle et al[3] found variable merging of the teres major and latissimus dorsi tendons near their insertion site. Due to its spiraling structure, similar to that of the latissimus dorsi muscle, the lowest portion of the origin of the muscle on the scapula is attached to the highest point of its insertion on the humerus. Therefore, the fibers of the teres major muscle that originally faced posterior at its origin, face anterior at its insertion.[1]

The teres major muscle marks a border for several clinically important regions including the upper and lower triangular spaces and the quadrangular space. The upper triangular space, which houses the circumflex scapular vessels, is bordered by the teres major muscle inferiorly. The other borders are the subscapularis, teres minor, and the long head of the triceps brachii muscles. The lower triangular space, which contains the radial nerve and profunda brachii vessels, is bordered by the subscapularis muscle, the long head of the triceps muscle, and the humerus. The teres major muscle forms its posterior border.[2]

The quadrangular space contains the axillary nerve and posterior circumflex humeral artery and veins. The teres major muscle forms its inferior boundary. It is bordered by the long head of the triceps brachii muscle medially and the humerus laterally. At its anterior aspect, the superior borders are the subscapularis muscle, the glenohumeral joint capsule, and the teres minor muscle. Posteriorly, its superior border is the teres minor muscle.[2]

2.1. Innervation and Vascularization

The teres major muscle is innervated by the lower subscapular nerves, C5, C6, and C7.[2] A variant nerve supply from the thoracodorsal nerve has also been identified.[4]

The teres major muscle receives its vascular supply from either the thoracodorsal artery or the circumflex scapular artery, both of which are branches of the subscapular artery.[4]

2.2. Function

The teres major muscle is a thick fusiform muscle able to produce great tensile forces due to its shape and structure. The teres major muscle and the latissimus dorsi muscle have very similar actions at the glenohumeral joint.[1] The teres major muscle assists with shoulder extension, adduction, and internal rotation.[2,5] Perhaps more interesting is its role in static posture and arm swing during gait.[2] The muscle is active during the backward arm swing.[6] Studies also have found that the muscle is active during typing, handwriting, and turning a car steering wheel.[5,7,8] In a small study, the teres major muscle was found to be active during shoulder depression, adduction behind the line of the body, and extension.[5]

2.3. Functional Unit

The functional unit to which a muscle belongs includes the muscles that reinforce and counter its actions as well as the joints that the muscle crosses. The functional interdependence of these structures is reflected in the organization and neural connections of the sensory motor cortex. The functional unit is emphasized because the presence of a TrP in one muscle of the

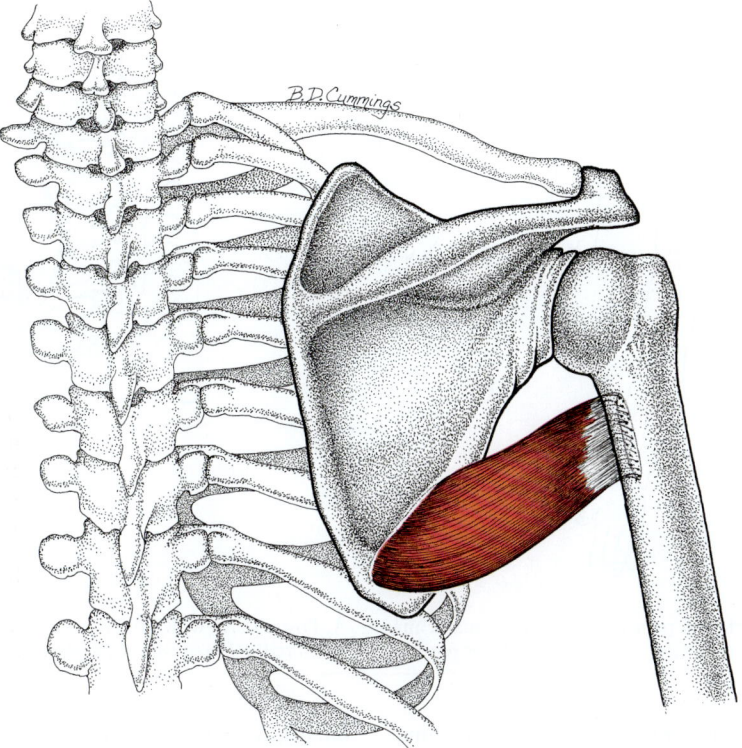

Figure 25-1. Attachments of the teres major muscle. See Figure 24-2 for its anatomic relation to the latissimus dorsi muscle, and Figure 26-3 for its relation to other shoulder girdle muscles.

Box 25-1 Functional Unit of the Teres Major Muscle

Action	Synergists	Antagonist
Shoulder internal rotation	Latissimus dorsi Pectoralis major Subscapularis	Infraspinatus Teres minor
Shoulder extension	Latissimus dorsi Posterior deltoid Triceps brachii long head	Anterior deltoid Pectoralis major Biceps brachii long head Coracobrachialis
Shoulder adduction	Pectoralis major Latissimus dorsi Subscapularis Coracobrachialis	Deltoid Supraspinatus

unit increases the likelihood that the other muscles of the unit also develops TrPs. When inactivating TrPs in a muscle, one should be concerned about TrPs that may develop in muscles that are functionally interdependent. Box 25-1 grossly represents the functional unit of the teres major muscle.[9]

3. CLINICAL PRESENTATION

3.1. Referred Pain Pattern

The prevalence of teres major TrPs in patients with shoulder pain may be higher than thought earlier. In an observational study of 72 patients with nontraumatic unilateral shoulder pain, Bron et al[10] observed latent TrPs in the teres major muscle in 49% of subjects. These were the most frequently observed latent TrPs, followed by anterior deltoid TrPs found in 38% of the patients.[10]

Trigger points in the teres major muscle are most commonly found in three areas. Medially, TrPs may be found in the region of the inferior angle of the scapula. They may also be found in the middle of the muscle in the posterior axillary fold, where the teres major muscle is overlapped by the latissimus dorsi muscle. Last, TrPs are often located laterally in the region of the musculotendinous junction.

Trigger points in this muscle commonly refer pain to the posterior deltoid region and to the region of the long head of the triceps brachii muscle (Figure 25-2A to C). Trigger points may refer pain into the posterior aspect of the glenohumeral joint and occasionally, to the posterior aspect of the forearm.

3.2. Symptoms

Patients with TrPs in the teres major muscle may complain of mild pain at rest; however the primary complaint often is pain with motion. Patients often report sharp pain in the posterior aspect of the shoulder, especially when reaching up to retrieve an object from a shelf or cabinet. Pain in the teres major muscle is often elicited by a stretching movement such as passive shoulder flexion, abduction, or external rotation.[11] Similarly, pain may occur with loading during resisted shoulder extension or internal rotation of the humerus.[11]

Teres major muscle involvement does not significantly restrict shoulder movement as observed with adhesive capsulitis, but patients may experience significant pain, which limits full overhead range of motion.

3.3. Patient Examination

After a thorough subjective examination, the clinician should make a detailed drawing representing the pain pattern that the

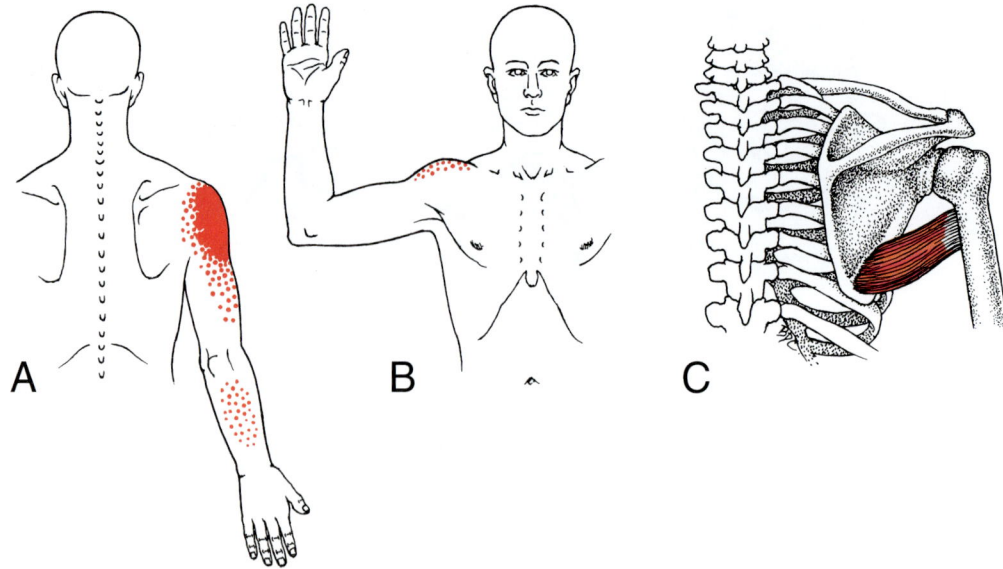

Figure 25-2. Referred pain pattern of teres major muscle. A, Posterior view. B, Anterior view of referred pain patterns (essential portion is solid red, spillover portion is stippled red) referred from C, Right teres major muscle.

patient has described. This depiction will assist in planning the physical examination and can be useful in monitoring the progression of the patient as symptoms improve or change.

Proper assessment of the teres major muscle should include examination of shoulder range of motion and strength. Patients with TrPs in the teres major muscle may exhibit weakness or pain with resisted testing. Increased upward scapular rotation can be observed with shoulder flexion secondary to restrictions in the teres major muscle length. Limited shoulder abduction with an inability to bring the involved arm in contact with the ear can suggest TrPs in the teres major muscle. Frequently, involvement of this muscle causes pain at the end of the range of motion. Restrictions of 3 to 5 cm (1-2 in) and/or pain with the Apley's scratch test (abduction, flexion, and external rotation) may also suggest teres major muscle involvement (Figure 21-3).

3.4. Trigger Point Examination

Once the teres major muscle is identified properly, the reliability of identifying TrPs should be comparable with that of the latissimus dorsi muscle. In a study of reliability of TrP examination, Gerwin et al[12] included the latissimus dorsi muscle among four muscles examined. They reported a high degree of agreement for the detection of a taut band, the presence of spot tenderness, referred pain, and reproduction of the symptomatic pain.

Clinical examination may be performed in a supine (Figure 25-3A), prone (Figure 25-3B), seated, or side-lying position. For all these positions, a cross-fiber flat palpation may be utilized to detect taut bands and TrPs. Cross-fiber pincer palpation may also be utilized to identify TrPs in the mid-muscle belly; however, the clinician should be able to differentiate between the latissimus dorsi and teres major muscles.

To examine the muscle in the supine position, the shoulder should be positioned in 90° of shoulder abduction and external rotation (Figure 25-3B). Landmarks to locate the teres major muscle include the axillary border of the scapula cranially, the latissimus dorsi muscle, and the inferior border of the scapula caudally. To locate the axillary border of the scapula, the clinician can use deep pincer palpation of the axillary fold approximately 1 in below the humerus. This location is cranial to the teres major muscle's attachment site on the scapula. Just caudal to this site

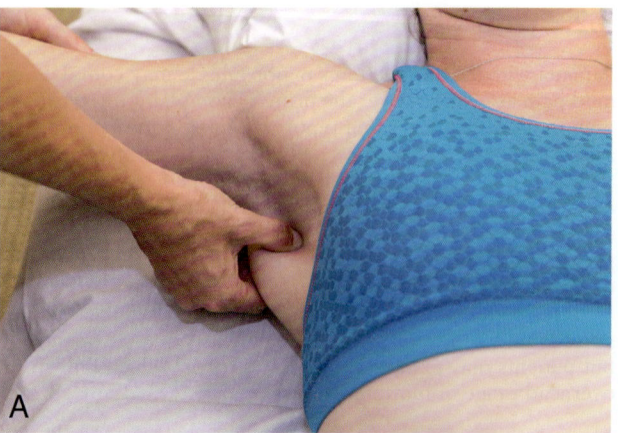
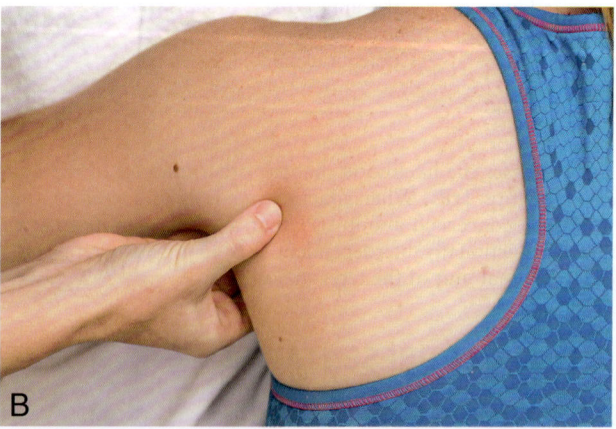

Figure 25-3. Examination of TrPs in the teres major muscle. In the axilla, the examiner's digits should fully encompass the latissimus dorsi muscle to reach the teres major muscle. The groove between the teres major and the latissimus dorsi muscles is confirmed when the examiner's finger tips can identify the lateral border of the scapula between the two muscles. A, Patient supine; B, Patient prone.

lies a palpable groove between the scapular border and the teres major muscle. Sliding the pincer grasp slightly caudally allows palpation of the axillary portion of teres major muscle. Below this location, at the level of the inferior angle of the scapula, lies the latissimus dorsi muscle. The latissimus dorsi muscle forms the free border of the posterior axillary fold as it wraps around the teres major muscle. The clinician may instruct the patient to perform shoulder internal rotation to confirm the location of the muscle.

The muscle is easily palpated in the prone position with the arm abducted 70-90° and the forearm off the table. Resisted shoulder internal rotation helps distinguish the muscle from the teres minor and latissimus dorsi muscles.

To access the muscle in a side-lying position, the patient lies on the uninvolved side with the involved arm resting on a pillow. The teres major muscle can be located in the axillary fold by following its fibers from the dorsal surface of the scapula. Cross-fiber flat palpation across the fibers can be used to locate TrPs in the region of the lateral border of the lower third of the scapula.

4. DIFFERENTIAL DIAGNOSIS

4.1. Activation and Perpetuation of Trigger Points

A posture or activity that activates a TrP, if not corrected, can also perpetuate it. In any part of the teres major muscle, TrPs may be activated by unaccustomed eccentric loading, eccentric exercise in an unconditioned muscle, or maximal or submaximal concentric loading.[13] Trigger points may also be activated or aggravated when the muscle is placed in a shortened and/or lengthened position for an extended period of time. Inquiry into possible aggravating activities such as sitting or standing with the shoulder in a position of increased internal rotation, prolonged driving with exertional movement of the steering wheel, or repetitive shoulder movement is necessary to modify behaviors that might result in continued pain. Activities that require excessive pulling actions such as playing tennis or golf, rowing, and throwing a ball may also activate TrPs in the teres major muscle. Finding the driving cause of these TrPs requires careful analysis of activities that require repetitive shoulder extension, internal rotation, or adduction.

4.2. Associated Trigger Points

Trigger points may develop in muscles in the referred pain area from other muscles that have TrPs.[14] Muscles that can develop TrPs due to pain referral from teres major muscle include the posterior deltoid, middle deltoid, the long head of the triceps, and the wrist extensor muscles. Trigger points in the teres major muscle can also develop due to TrPs of other muscles including the deltoid, the subscapularis, and the latissimus dorsi muscles.

Clinically, associated TrPs have also been located in the latissimus dorsi muscle. Involvement of the teres minor and subscapularis muscles may lead to pain and significant functional impairment in a condition that can mimic "frozen shoulder."

4.3. Associated Pathology

The teres major muscle (along with latissimus dorsi, pectoralis major, and subscapularis muscles) is one of the four muscles implicated in myofascial pseudothoracic outlet syndrome. Active TrPs in at least three of these muscles is strongly suggestive of thoracic outlet syndrome and often misdiagnosed as such. However, these muscles do not cause compression of the neurovascular structures of the thoracic outlet. Implications of myofascial dysfunction in thoracic outlet syndrome are further discussed in Chapter 33.

Other conditions that can mimic teres major TrPs include subacromial or subdeltoid bursitis, supraspinatus tendinopathy, and C6-C7 radicular pain and/or radiculopathy. The associated pathology also includes triangular interval syndrome and quadrilateral space syndrome.

Sebastian[15] described a case study of triangular interval syndrome. The patient presented with right scapular pain with radiating symptoms into the posterior arm to the radius. Onset of symptoms, described as sharp and shooting pain, followed punching during a kickboxing class. Testing did not meet the standards for the clinical prediction rule established by Wainer et al[16] for cervical radiculopathy. The patient demonstrated a negative Spurling's test, relief of symptoms with cervical distraction, and ipsilateral neck rotation greater than 60°. The patient had a positive radial nerve-biased upper limb tension test. On palpation, the patient exhibited tenderness at the long and lateral heads of the triceps brachii muscle superiorly and at the lateral portion of the teres major muscle along with reduced pain pressure threshold with reproduction of the patient's symptoms. After the patient was treated for soft-tissue dysfunction at the triangular interval and adverse radial nerve tension, resolution of symptoms was reported.[15]

Patients with quadrilateral space syndrome, a rare condition of compression of the axillary nerve and posterior circumflex artery, may report symptoms of shoulder pain, tenderness, and paresthesias aggravated by shoulder abduction and rotation.[17-19]

5. CORRECTIVE ACTIONS

The patient with teres major TrPs should modify any activity that repeatedly stresses the muscle, such as prolonged driving and lifting weights overhead. To prevent full shortening of this muscle while sleeping on the affected side, a small pillow can be placed between the elbow and the lateral aspect of the trunk to maintain a neutral position of the muscle (Figure 22-4C). A pillow support can also be used for this purpose while sleeping on the uninvolved side (Figure 22-4A).

The patient can self-treat the muscle with TrP self-pressure release utilizing a tennis ball or TrP self-pressure release tool in a technique similar to that used for the latissimus dorsi muscle (Figure 25-4). The patient lies on the affected side with the shoulder flexed to stretch the muscle. Body position can be adjusted over the tennis ball at the TrP site. This treatment could also be

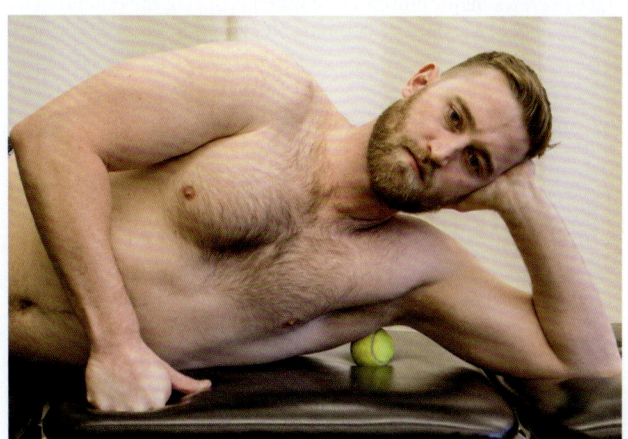

Figure 25-4. To self-treat the teres major muscle. The patient lies on the involved side with the shoulder flexed and the tennis ball situated in the axillary region, slightly posterior to the latissimus dorsi muscle. A gentle pressure is applied. The patient may perform gentle isometric contractions by pushing the elbow gently into the floor and holding for 6 to 10 seconds followed by relaxation.

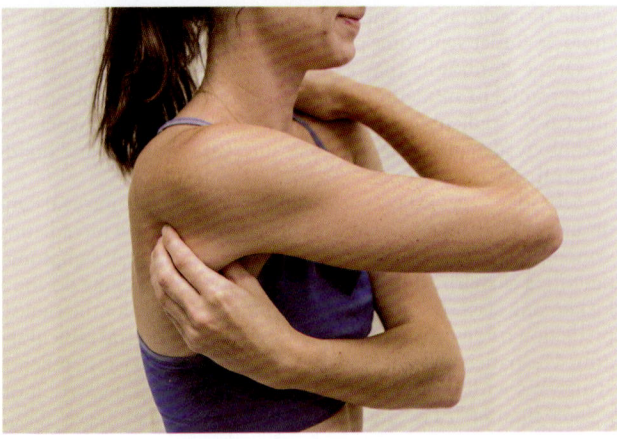

Figure 25-5. The patient can perform manual TrP self-pressure release by grasping the teres major muscle between the thumb and fingers holding compression for 15 to 30 seconds, repeating as necessary.

performed in a sitting position with pressure applied using the opposite hand with or without a tennis ball. The patient can also perform pressure release by grasping the muscle belly between the thumb and fingers and holding compression for 15 to 30 seconds, repeating as necessary (Figure 25-5).

Stretching techniques for this muscle are similar to those for the latissimus dorsi muscle (Figure 24-5); however, it is important to stabilize the scapula from abducting for maximal efficacy.

References

1. Porterfield JA, DeRosa C. *Mechanical Shoulder Disorders: Perspectives in Functional Anatomy*. St. Louis, MO: Saunders; 2004:53-54.
2. Standring S. *Gray's Anatomy: The Anatomical Basis of Clinical Practice*. 41st ed. London, UK: Elsevier; 2015.
3. Pearle AD, Kelly BT, Voos JE, Chehab EL, Warren RF. Surgical technique and anatomic study of latissimus dorsi and teres major transfers. *J Bone Joint Surg Am*. 2006;88(7):1524-1531.
4. Dancker M, Lambert S, Brenner E. The neurovascular anatomy of the teres major muscle. *J Shoulder Elbow Surg*. 2015;24(3):e57-e67.
5. Jonsson B, Olofsson BM, Steffner LC. Function of the teres major, latissimus dorsi and pectoralis major muscles. A preliminary study. *Acta Morphol Neerl Scand*. 1972;9(4):275-280.
6. Basmajian J, Deluca C. *Muscles Alive*. 5th ed. Baltimore: Williams & Wilkins; 1985:270, 271, 385.
7. Lundervold AJ. Electromyographic investigations of position and manner of working in typewriting. *Acta Physiol Scand Suppl*. 1951;24(84):1-171:66-68, 80-81, 94-95, 101, 157.
8. Jonsson S, Jonsson B. Function of the muscles of the upper limb in car driving. V: The supraspinatus, infraspinatus, teres minor and teres major muscles. *Ergonomics*. 1976;19(6):711-717.
9. Simons DG, Travell JG, Simons LS. *Myofascial Pain and Dysfunction: The Trigger Point Manual. Volume 1: Upper Half of Body*. 2nd ed. Philadelphia, PA: Lippincott Williams & Wilkins;1999.
10. Bron C, Dommerholt J, Stegenga B, Wensing M, Oostendorp RA. High prevalence of shoulder girdle muscles with myofascial trigger points in patients with shoulder pain. *BMC Musculoskelet Disord*. 2011;12:139.
11. Macdonald AJ. Abnormally tender muscle regions and associated painful movements. *Pain*. 1980;8(2):197-205.
12. Gerwin RD, Shannon S, Hong C-Z, Hubbard DR, Gevirtz R. Interrater reliability in myofascial trigger point examination. *Pain*. 1997;69:65-73.
13. Gerwin RD, Dommerholt J, Shah JP. An expansion of Simons' integrated hypothesis of trigger point formation. *Curr Pain Headache Rep*. 2004;8(6):468-475.
14. Hsieh YL, Kao MJ, Kuan TS, Chen SM, Chen JT, Hong CZ. Dry needling to a key myofascial trigger point may reduce the irritability of satellite MTrPs. *Am J Phys Med Rehabil*. 2007;86(5):397-403.
15. Sebastian D. Triangular interval syndrome: a differential diagnosis for upper extremity radicular pain. *Physiother Theory Pract*. 2010;26(2):113-119.
16. Wainner RS, Fritz JM, Irrgang JJ, Boninger ML, Delitto A, Allison S. Reliability and diagnostic accuracy of the clinical examination and patient self-report measures for cervical radiculopathy. *Spine (Phila Pa 1976)*. 2003;28(1):52-62.
17. McClelland D, Paxinos A. The anatomy of the quadrilateral space with reference to quadrilateral space syndrome. *J Shoulder Elbow Surg*. 2008;17(1):162-164.
18. Cahill BR, Palmer RE. Quadrilateral space syndrome. *J Hand Surg Am*. 1983;8(1):65-69.
19. Chautems RC, Glauser T, Waeber-Fey MC, Rostan O, Barraud GE. Quadrilateral space syndrome: case report and review of the literature. *Ann Vasc Surg*. 2000;14(6):673-676.

Chapter 26

Subscapularis Muscle

"Pseudo Frozen Shoulder"

Joseph M. Donnelly and Laura Gold

1. INTRODUCTION

The subscapularis muscle is the largest of the four rotator cuff muscles. It attaches to the periosteum of the costal surface of the scapula beneath the serratus anterior muscle from its vertebral border to the axillary border. Other fibers attach at the intramuscular septa and aponeurosis separating the subscapularis muscle from the lateral scapular musculature. The tendon attaches anteriorly at the lesser tubercle of the humerus and anterior articular capsule. The subscapularis muscle is innervated by the upper and lower subscapular nerves, branches of the posterior cord of the brachial plexus that arise from spinal levels C5 and C6. It is responsible for internal rotation and adduction of the humerus, as well as dynamic stabilization of the glenohumeral joint along with the other rotator cuff muscles. One of the most important functions of the subscapularis muscle is to provide dynamic restraint to the posterior aspect of the glenohumeral joint. Trigger points (TrPs) in the subscapularis muscle will produce severe pain in the posterior shoulder that can refer down the back of the arm and to the dorsal and volar aspect of the wrist. Subscapularis TrPs often play a role in frozen shoulder syndrome (FSS). Trigger points in this muscle are frequently the foundation in a tower of shoulder dysfunction. Symptoms may be aggravated by sleeping on the affected side, reaching the arm out to the side, or performing functional activities that require flexion and adduction. Activation and perpetuation of TrPs in the subscapularis muscle usually result from acute overload, repeated forceful overhead lifting while exerting strong adduction forces, and catching oneself from a fall with an outstretched arm. Differential diagnosis should include assessment for posterior glenohumeral joint capsule tightness; C5, C6, or C7 radicular pain; subacromial pain (impingement) syndrome (SIS); FSS (adhesive capsulitis); rotator cuff pathology; thoracic outlet syndrome; and scapulothoracic or subacromial bursitis. Corrective actions should include postural reeducation (including proper sleep position), elimination of positions that cause recurrent overload on the muscle, self-pressure release of TrPs, and self-stretch exercises. Clinically, this muscle produces an easily recognizable, distinct pain pattern that may be key in unraveling a number of shoulder conditions, both acute and chronic in nature.

2. ANATOMIC CONSIDERATIONS

The subscapularis muscle is the largest and most anterior of the four rotator cuff muscles. The subscapularis muscle has two heads, and its triangular mass fills the subscapular fossa.[1] The subscapularis muscle is quite thick and has a similar arrangement to that of the infraspinatus muscle in that the muscle fibers converge from a broad medial portion toward a central tendon that covers the anterior aspect of the glenohumeral joint.[2] Medially, the subscapularis muscle attaches to the periosteum of the costal surface of the scapula beneath the serratus anterior muscle from its vertebral border to the axillary border. Other fibers attach at the intramuscular septa and aponeurosis, separating the subscapularis muscle from the lateral scapular musculature. Multipennate in appearance, the horizontally oriented superior fibers converge with the more vertically oriented inferior fibers to form a tendon that runs laterally and attaches anteriorly at the lesser tubercle of the humerus and anterior articular capsule (Figure 26-1). The thick inferior head of the subscapularis muscle provides a majority of the structure of the subscapular tendon. Cleeman et al[3] performed a detailed cadaveric dissection of the tendon insertion of the subscapularis muscle. They describe the subscapularis tendon as consisting of three distinct sections: "a thick superior tubular tendon, a flat middle tendon, and an inferior portion where the muscle fibers insert directly into the humerus." The cross-sectional area of the subscapularis tendon is the largest of all tendons in the shoulder, and it dynamically reinforces the glenohumeral ligaments and the anterior glenoid labrum.[2] The large subscapular bursa, which usually communicates with the cavity of the shoulder joint, separates the tendon from the scapular neck and joint capsule medially.[1]

2.1. Innervation and Vascularization

The subscapularis muscle is innervated by the upper and lower subscapular nerves, branches of the posterior cord of the brachial plexus that arise from spinal levels C5 and C6.[1] Two upper subscapular nerves typically supply the upper portion of the subscapularis muscle, whereas the lower subscapular nerve, which terminates in the teres major muscle, supplies the lower, more distal, portion of the muscle. The separate innervation of these upper and lower fibers is consistent with the findings of Electromyography (EMG) studies that show these "compartments" as functioning independently.[4-6]

The vascular supply of subscapularis muscle comes from branches off the suprascapular, axillary, and subscapular arteries.[1] Detailed cadaveric dissection described by Serita et al,[6] however, revealed variable distribution that also included supply from the circumflex scapular, brachial, thoracodorsal, and lateral thoracic arteries. These authors also noted correspondence between areas of relatively poor vascular supply (ie, possible areas of local ischemia) and common possible locations for TrPs in the rotator cuff muscles.[6]

2.2. Function

The subscapularis, infraspinatus, teres minor, and supraspinatus muscles are inserted, respectively, into the lesser and greater tuberosities of the humerus and form a musculotendinous rotator cuff. These rotator cuff muscles provide dynamic stability to the glenohumeral joint. Motion at the shoulder joint is a complex coordinated activity and the moment arms of the rotator cuff

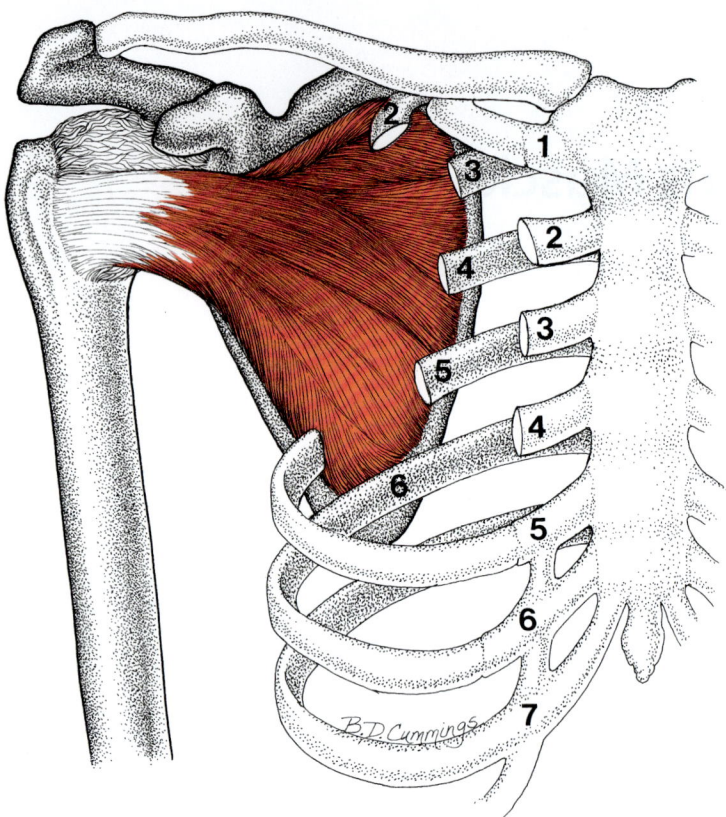

Figure 26-1. Attachments of the right subscapularis muscle, as seen from the front with the arm externally rotated. Parts of ribs two through five have been removed for clarity.

muscles exert inferior and medially directed forces, resisting upward shear of the deltoid muscle during shoulder elevation while keeping the head of the humerus in close contact with the glenoid fossa.[7] The subscapularis muscle functions alone as a powerful internal rotator of the humerus, but equally important is its role as a dynamic stabilizer of the glenohumeral joint.[1,8] The subscapularis muscle prevents anterior displacement of the humeral head, especially in lower ranges of abduction.[9,10] It is also established as acting in concert with the infraspinatus muscle to depress the humeral head in opposition to the upward displacement caused by the deltoid muscle during arm elevation.[11,12] Heuberer et al[12] published data from an EMG study supporting that the subscapularis muscle has a major role during glenohumeral flexion and abduction. The authors speculate at the possibility of the subscapularis muscle acting as an abductor given the superior portion of the tendon's high insertion point on the lesser tubercle of the humerus (rather than solely stabilizing during the motion). In contrast, it has been previously reported that the subscapularis muscle functions as a humeral adductor.[13] This dual functionality may be possible given the likely separate roles of the upper and lower muscular compartments. A number of EMG studies reinforce the idea that the subscapularis muscle is composed of two (upper and lower) functional units[5,14]; however, consensus has not been reached regarding the specific role each functional unit plays except to note that varying degrees of abduction result in differing levels of activation in the upper and lower units.

Reed et al[15] studied the influence of loads on the recruitment patterns of the rotator cuff muscles during abduction. They found that the activation patterns that were established with low loads continued as the load increases and they concluded that the role of the subscapularis and infraspinatus muscles is to counterbalance the upward migration of the humerus caused by the strong torque produced by the middle deltoid. The patterns of activation of the subscapularis and infraspinatus muscles were strongly correlated to the axioscapular muscle activation pattern.[15] In another study looking at shoulder abduction in the plane of the scapula and coronal plane, it was found that all rotator cuff muscles activated before movement of the humerus during all abduction movements.[7] The subscapularis muscle was recruited later than the other three rotator cuff muscles but still before humerus motion. They conclude that shoulder abduction in the coronal plane and elevation in the plane of the scapula is a complex coordinated activity initiated and controlled by several muscles.[7] Wickham et al[16] found the upper and lower subscapularis peak muscle activation to be 18% and 25% maximum volitional contraction (MVC) between 80° and 120° of abduction, respectively.

EMG analysis of the rotator cuff muscles was performed during forward flexion with no load, 20%, and 60% of the subject's maximum load. These studies found that the supraspinatus and infraspinatus muscles were activated at significantly higher levels than the subscapularis muscle at all load levels. The authors conclude that the posterior rotator cuff muscles are recruited at higher levels to prevent translation of the humeral head during flexion similarly to the inferior cuff muscles during abduction.[7,17]

EMG analysis of subscapularis muscle activity during functional movements is well documented, especially in sporting activities. Jobe et al[18] and Gowan et al[19] investigated muscle activation patterns and activity during throwing movements. They identified maximum activity of the supraspinatus, infraspinatus, and deltoid muscles during early and late cocking phases of the throw, whereas the subscapularis and latissimus dorsi muscles were more active during the acceleration phase of the throw. They also identified that amateurs tend to utilize more of the rotator cuff muscles during the acceleration phase. This notion is further supported by a study of healthy, skilled throwers in which the EMG activity of the subscapularis muscle was lower during wind up, increased dramatically by late cocking, increased further during acceleration to 185% of test value, and tapered to 97% during follow-through.[20] Athletes with painful shoulders in the same study reached only one-third to one-half the normal values during the throwing motion.

Subscapularis muscle function has also been studied with other overhead sporting movements. During a tennis serve, the subscapularis muscle is most heavily recruited during late cocking and early acceleration.[21] During the golf swing, subscapularis muscle activity tends to increase through acceleration in the dominant shoulder and tends to maintain a moderate level of activation throughout the swing in the nondominant shoulder.[22,23] In EMG analysis of healthy freestyle swimmers, the subscapularis muscle remains at a constant level of significant activation throughout the stroke.[24] However, this pattern does not hold true for swimmers with a painful shoulder who exhibit an approximate 50% drop in subscapularis muscle activity during the recovery phase (the last phase of a freestyle stroke when the airborne arm is about to return to the water at the front of the body).[23] This drop in activity may be due to muscle inhibition from TrPs, or it could represent an attempt to avoid aggravation of painful TrPs during the extreme internal rotation and extension of this phase of the freestyle stroke.[13]

2.3. Functional Unit

The functional unit to which a muscle belongs includes the muscles that reinforce and counter its actions as well as the joints that the muscle crosses. The interdependence of these structures is functionally reflected in the organization and neural connections of the sensory motor cortex. The functional unit is emphasized because the presence of a TrP in one muscle of the unit increases the likelihood that the other muscles of the unit will also develop TrPs. When inactivating TrPs in a muscle, one must be concerned about TrPs that may develop in muscles that are functionally interdependent. Box 26-1 grossly represents the functional unit of the subscapularis muscle.[13]

The subscapularis muscle also functions synergistically with the infraspinatus, teres minor, and supraspinatus muscles to stabilize the head of the humerus in the glenoid fossa during arm movements.[7,25]

3. CLINICAL PRESENTATION
3.1. Referred Pain Pattern

Subscapularis TrPs result in severe pain of the upper limb at rest and during motion.[13] Pain is primarily referred to the posterior aspect of the shoulder (Figure 26-2). Spillover reference zones may extend over the scapula and down the posterior aspect of the arm to the elbow. A distal reference zone is sometimes present as a strap-like band of pain around the wrist with the dorsum of the wrist more painful than the volar aspect.[26] Although not reported in the classic Travell study, Jalil et al[27] provided a case study including two individuals who presented with atypical chest pain that responded to treatment (TrP injection) of subscapularis TrPs.

3.2. Symptoms

The rotator cuff muscles are commonly involved in patients who report having shoulder pain. The subscapularis muscle is one of the most prevalent muscles found to have TrPs. Hidalgo-Lozano et al[28] found active TrPs in 42% of individuals diagnosed with shoulder impingement syndrome. During early stages of subscapularis myofascial dysfunction, patients demonstrate decreased function when reaching into abduction and external rotation (as if reaching back to throw a ball)[13] or with reaching toward the rear of a vehicle from the front seat (as when soothing a crying child in her car seat). As the dysfunction progresses, lifting the arm becomes increasingly painful and difficult with abduction limited to 45° or less. The patient will likely describe pain at rest, pain with movement, and the inability to reach the opposite armpit (as when applying deodorant). Because of the severe pain and range of motion (ROM) limitations, the patient may be diagnosed with adhesive capsulitis or "frozen shoulder." If presenting with referred pain at the wrist, the patient

Box 26-1 Functional unit of the subscapularis muscle

Action	Synergists	Antagonist
Shoulder internal rotation	Teres major Latissimus dorsi Pectoralis major	Infraspinatus Teres minor
Shoulder adduction	Teres major Latissimus dorsi Pectoralis major	Deltoid Supraspinatus

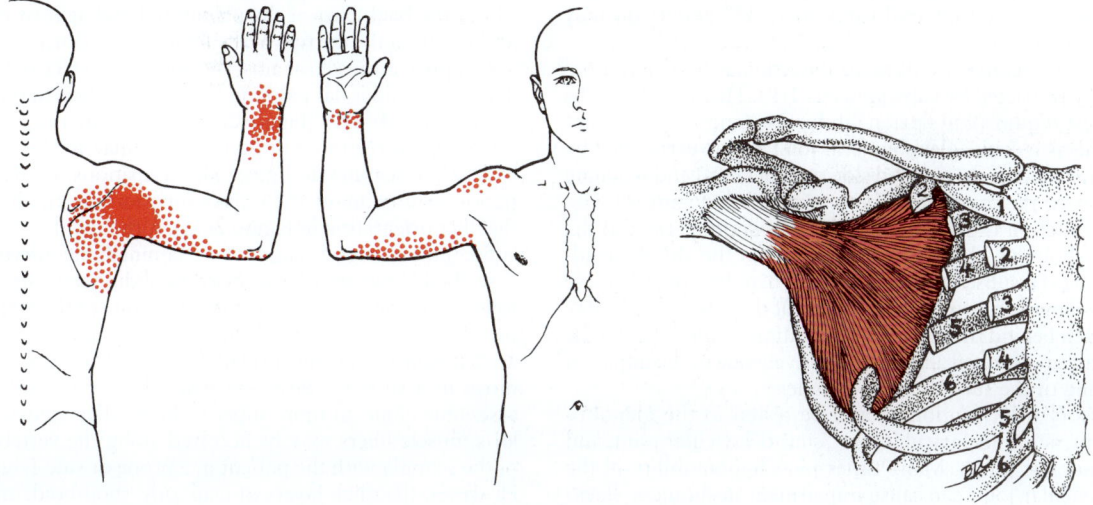

Figure 26-2. Referred pain pattern from TrPs in the right subscapularis muscle. The essential referred pain zone is solid red; the spillover zone is stippled red. Portions of the second through the fifth ribs have been removed for clarity.

may complain of soreness in a strap-like area and may move a wristwatch or bracelet to the opposite hand. In mild cases of subscapularis TrP involvement, these authors have observed reports of "tightness" at the wrist upon maximal overhead reaching. Subscapularis muscle shortening due to the presence of TrPs may also contribute to subluxation of the head of the humerus. This concept is consistent with the observations of anatomic architecture of rotator cuff musculature by Ward et al[8] who pointed out that the stabilizing function of these muscles is sensitive to length changes. Some patients will also describe snapping or clicking sounds around the shoulder joint with arm movements, which is usually associated with subscapularis and/or supraspinatus TrPs.

3.3. Patient Examination

After a thorough subjective examination the clinician should make a detailed drawing representing the pain pattern that the patient has described. This depiction assists in planning the physical examination and can be useful in monitoring the progression of the patient as symptoms improve or change. For proper examination of the subscapularis muscle, the clinician should observe shoulder girdle posture, scapular position, and active and passive ROM of the shoulder girdle, paying close attention to muscle activation patterns and the scapulohumeral rhythm. The clinician should note when and where pain occurs. Subscapularis TrPs can produce pain at rest or during movement, particularly during arm elevation in the coronal plane and especially when combined with external rotation. The pain usually occurs throughout abduction ROM. Clinically, this muscle is seldom involved by itself but rather in association with the infraspinatus, supraspinatus, or the levator scapulae muscles, which also commonly have TrPs.

In order to identify TrPs in the subscapularis muscle that may be limiting ROM and thus influencing dysfunction, the clinician should identify limited ROM by performing specific ROM testing for all parts of the muscle. Because the patient with subscapularis TrPs often presents with major ROM limitations, a thorough examination of all contributing factors to the lost ROM should be completed. The clinician can expect external rotation to be restricted due to subscapularis TrPs, but must also consider that full elevation may be limited due to the prerequisite external rotation required to achieve full elevation (abduction or flexion).[13] One helpful sign in determining subscapularis muscle restriction is greater loss of external rotation at 45° versus 90° of abduction.[29]

Muscle-specific resisted testing should be carried out to identify impairments in muscle function and reproduction of painful symptoms. If active TrPs are present in the subscapularis muscle, resisted internal rotation at 45° abduction may be painfully limited.

The Apley's Scratch test (flexion, abduction, external rotation) is typically restricted by subscapularis TrPs. This version of the Apley's test requires full flexion, abduction, and external rotation of the arm at the glenohumeral joint and is performed by placing the hand of the affected side over the head and reaching as far toward the opposite scapula as possible (Figure 21-3B). If no dysfunction is present, the fingertips should reach to the opposite shoulder blade. This test stretches the shoulder adductors and the subscapularis muscle. When the range of these muscles is limited due to TrPs, the hand of the affected side may barely reach behind the head. This limitation is similar when the movement is performed actively or passively due to the impaired lengthening of the subscapularis muscle.

Accessory joint motion should be tested in the glenohumeral joint, acromioclavicular joint, sternoclavicular joint, and scapulothoracic joints. Many times joint hypomobility in the sternoclavicular joint can cause impairment in shoulder elevation contributing to alterations in the normal muscle activation patterns. Articular dysfunctions in the glenohumeral joint may also impair muscle activation patterns contributing to overload of the subscapularis and other rotator cuff muscles.

Scapular and humeral head positions should be assessed at rest and during upper extremity elevation because malalignment can be a significant contributing factor to subscapularis muscle overload during upper extremity functional activities that require combined internal rotation and adduction.

A general cervical screen, testing for neurologic signs, and neural mobility testing of the upper extremity should also be investigated to eliminate radicular symptoms as causative. If referred wrist pain is present, a clinical examination of local tissues at the wrist should also be conducted.

3.4. Trigger Point Examination

The patient should be positioned in supine with the arm abducted to 90° (if tissue tension allows) to expose the chest wall and axilla. Many patients with significant TrP activity such as those presenting with a diagnosis of adhesive capsulitis may be limited to only 20° to 30° of abduction. If sufficient abduction for examination is not available, the contract–relax technique may be used to achieve additional ROM.[13,29,30] Before palpation, the relation to other structures should be considered: the subscapularis muscle constitutes much of the posterior axillary wall. Anterior to the subscapularis muscle is the serratus anterior (inferomedially) and the coracobrachialis muscles, the biceps brachii muscle, the axillary and subscapular vessels, and the brachial plexus (superolaterally). Posterior to the subscapularis muscle lies its attachment sites at the scapula and glenohumeral capsule. Inferiorly, the subscapularis muscle meets its synergists, the teres major and latissimus dorsi muscles (Figure 26-3).[1] The subscapularis muscle can exhibit TrPs in any portion of its muscle belly; however, secondary to its deep anatomic location, proper access to the different muscle fibers is difficult. The most easily accessed lateral site lies along axillary border of the scapula on its costal surface within the vertical fibers of the muscle; the second lateral site lies just superior to this among the more horizontally oriented fibers (Figure 26-2). Harrison et al[31] identified common motor points within the horizontal fibers of the subscapularis muscle that aimed at developing a technique for botulinum toxin injection for neuromuscular blockade. The plotted motor points of 20 subscapularis muscle dissections are consistent with the common TrP sites described in the previous edition of this book.[13]

Adequate abduction of the scapula is also required to access the subscapularis muscle for manual palpation and may be achieved by maintaining traction on the humerus or when possible, by hooking the fingers of the nonpalpating hand along the vertebral border of the scapula and pulling it laterally (as shown by the arrow in Figure 26-4A).

While maintaining scapular abduction, the clinician then places the back part of the palpating hand against the rib cage and slowly sinks the tips of the fingers posteriorly to palpate the subscapularis muscle against the anterior surface of the scapula. Then, cross-fiber flat palpation over the surface of the scapula is used to identify TrPs (Figure 26-4B). In the inferior, more vertical fibers, this direction will be perpendicular to the longitudinal axis of the scapula and gradually transitions to an inferior-superior strumming as the moves superiorly in the muscle (note the fiber orientation in Figure 26-1). Although the entirety of the subscapularis muscle cannot be examined, the inferolateral site described above may be accessed by sliding the palpating finger toward the chest wall, such that the dorsum of the finger contacts the serratus anterior muscle and the subscapularis muscle fibers are felt beneath the finger (Figure 26-4B). The clinician may then move in a superior direction toward the coracoid process to assess the clinician more superior fibers. The medial subscapularis muscle fibers may be accessed along the vertebral border of the scapula with the patient in a prone or side-lying position. However, the thick layers of trapezius, rhomboid, and serratus anterior musculature through which the clinician must palpate make this a nonspecific assessment of the subscapularis muscle.

In the presence of a TrP, sustained light to moderate pressure will reproduce the patient's posterior shoulder and

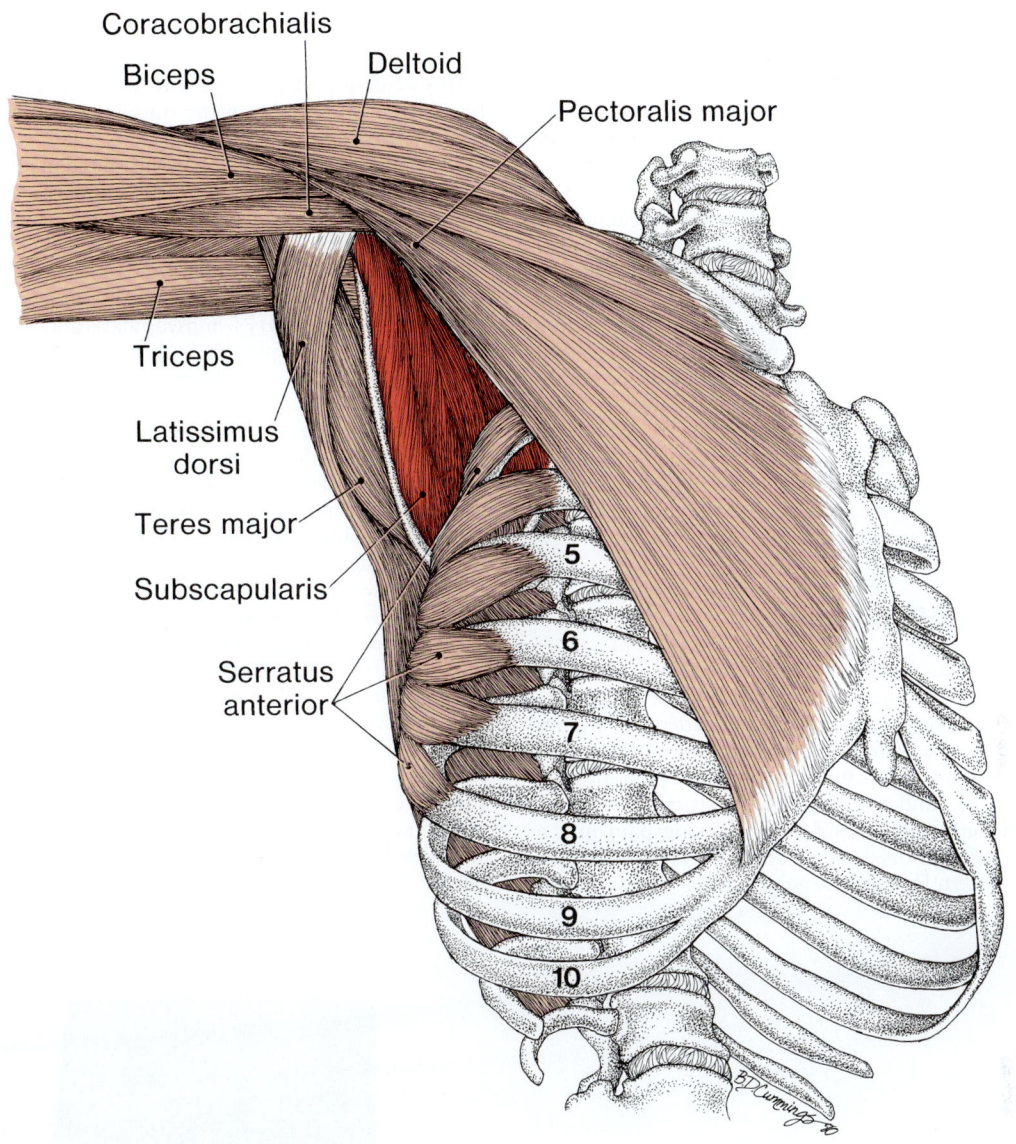

Figure 26-3. Relation of the subscapularis muscle (dark red) to the surrounding muscles (lighter red) when the scapula (shown as a vertical white line) has been pulled away from the chest wall by the clinician.

scapular pain, as well as, an occasional "twinge in the wrist."[13] Local twitch responses may be visually observed but are more likely to be felt given the muscle's location. Although not essential to diagnosis, the local twitch response is strongly confirmatory. The axillary region and subscapularis muscle are sensitive areas for many patients and may be exquisitely tender or ticklish with even light pressure in the presence of TrPs. Care should be taken (and fingernails kept short) to avoid confusion of skin pain.

Al-Shenqiti et al[32] found good test–retest reliability of TrP detection in patients with rotator cuff tendonitis when the criteria of presence or absence of the taut band, spot tenderness, jump sign, and pain recognition were used.

4. DIFFERENTIAL DIAGNOSIS

4.1. Activation and Perpetuation of Trigger Points

A posture or activity that activates a TrP, if not corrected, can also perpetuate it. In any part of the subscapularis muscle, TrPs may be activated by unaccustomed eccentric loading, eccentric exercise in an unconditioned muscle, or maximal or submaximal concentric loading.[33] Trigger points may also be activated or aggravated when the muscle is placed in a shortened and/or lengthened position for an extended period of time.[13]

Subscapularis TrPs can be activated by activities involving repetitive exertion with forceful internal rotation such as free-style swimming,[24,34,35] throwing a baseball,[20,36] or serving in tennis.[21,37] Other movements that may activate subscapularis TrPs include repeated forceful overhead lifting while exerting strong adduction (as in swinging a child back and forth from between the legs to overhead or as in poorly performed kettle bell swings); sudden stress overload as in reaching back abruptly at the shoulder level to catch oneself when falling[13]; local traumatic injury such as glenohumeral dislocation, tear of the shoulder joint capsule, or proximal humeral fracture; prolonged immobilization of the shoulder in an adducted, internally rotated position; or surgical or medical procedures such as mastectomy, lumpectomy, or radiation treatment.[38-40] Once established, these TrPs may be perpetuated by repetitive movements requiring internal rotation or typical poor "slumped" posture fostering prolonged positioning in internal rotation of the humerus.

4.2. Associated Trigger Points

Associated TrPs can develop in the muscles within the referred pain areas resultant from an active TrP.[41] Therefore, muscles in the referred pain areas for each muscle should also be considered for examination. Pain referral from subscapularis TrPs could activate TrPs in the deltoid, infraspinatus, supraspinatus, triceps brachii, teres major and minor, and latissimus dorsi muscles. When TrPs are present in the subscapularis muscle, arm movement may be significantly restricted without associated TrP activity in other shoulder girdle muscles. Once the TrPs become active, further pain-induced movement restriction becomes severe such that functionally related muscles develop TrPs. Ultimately, motion at the shoulder may be "frozen" and mimic adhesive capsulitis (see Chapter 33 for more on this diagnosis). Often the pectoralis major muscle first develops associated TrPs, followed by teres major, latissimus dorsi, and the long head of the triceps brachii muscles. Finally the anterior deltoid muscle becomes involved. Once TrPs occur in all these muscles, their combined shortened lengths may severely limit all movement of the shoulder, mimicking the medical diagnosis of adhesive capsulitis.[42]

4.3. Associated Pathology

Cervical radicular pain or radiculopathy in the C5 or C6 nerve roots often results in the formation of TrPs in those muscles innervated by the same nerve roots. Oftentimes patients with C5-6 radiculitis describe deep anterior shoulder pain, anterolateral shoulder pain, brachium and forearm pain, and pain into the radial aspect of the hand and lateral digits. Patients with C7 radicular symptoms will often describe having pain in the shoulder, arm, and the dorsal aspect of the wrist which is part of the referral pattern from subscapularis TrPs.

Other diagnoses to consider include cervical arthritis or spurs with nerve root irritation and brachial plexus injuries. All of these neurogenic sources of pain are likely to exhibit EMG evidence of denervation (positive sharp waves and fibrillation potentials) in the muscles supplied by the compromised nerves.

Although further research is warranted in all cases to better understand their relationships, subscapularis TrPs are closely associated with subacromial pain syndrome; primary and secondary FSS[43]; rotator cuff pathology; C5, C6, or C7 radicular pain/radiculopathy; thoracic outlet syndrome; and scapulothoracic or subacromial bursitis, which can cause similar pain that is not due to subscapularis TrPs. Subscapularis and other rotator cuff muscle TrPs may be present with any of these conditions and can also mimic these conditions, which are further discussed in Chapter 33.

FSS or adhesive capsulitis has been defined by the American Elbow and Shoulder Surgeons as "a condition of uncertain etiology characterized by significant restriction of both active and passive shoulder motion that occurs in the absence of a known intrinsic shoulder disorder."[43] The diagnosis, FSS or adhesive capsulitis, may be the result of other shoulder pathology or systemic disease or may be idiopathic in the case of primary FSS or adhesive capsulitis. Secondary FSS is typically related to an event that can be described by the patient.[43] The symptoms of subscapularis TrPs, including pain and significant limitations in external rotation and abduction, are similar to those associated with FSS. Myofascial dysfunction resulting from subscapularis TrPs should certainly be considered as a potential cause of pain and impairment in any patient presenting with a diagnosis of FSS. Given the ambiguous etiology of primary FSS, clinicians may question the potential for subscapularis TrP involvement in its development. Interestingly, thyroid disease, which is considered a systemic cause of secondary FSS, is also a systemic

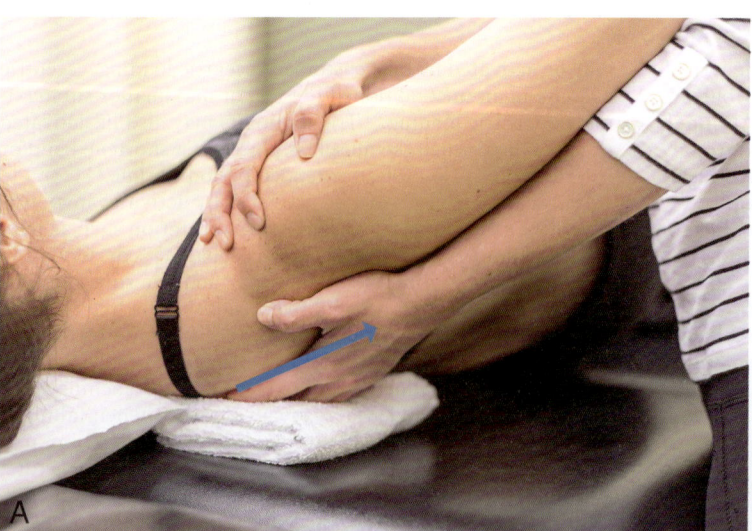
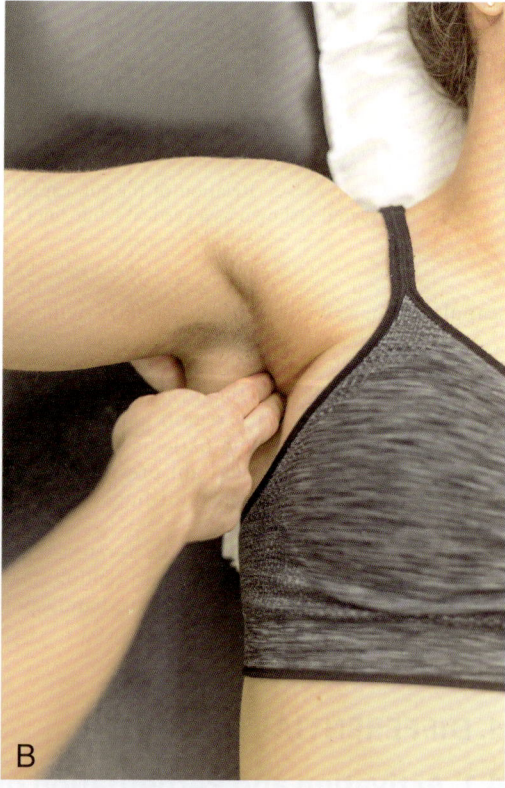

Figure 26-4. Examination of the subscapularis muscle. A, The clinician grasps the vertebral border of the scapula and passively pulls it as far laterally as possible to expose the subscapularis muscle. B, Palpation of the subscapularis muscle.

perpetuating factor of TrPs.[13] In fact, there is only one case report describing the clinical reasoning behind the use of TrP dry needling in the treatment of an individual with adhesive capsulitis.[44] This case report describes a rapid improvement in pain and ROM following the initiation of dry needling applied to upper trapezius, levator scapulae, deltoid, and infraspinatus muscles. Surprisingly, there is no mention of subscapularis TrPs in this case report. Trigger point contribution to FSS is further discussed in Chapter 33.

Investigators have looked at the prevalence of TrPs, pain pressure threshold (PPT), and reproduction of shoulder pain in patients with a diagnosis of SIS.[28,45,46] Investigators[28] assessed 12 patients and 10 matched controls for the prevalence of TrPs and PPT. The inclusion criteria was pain of greater than 3 month duration, pain greater than 4/10 with shoulder elevation, and a positive Neer and Hawkin's impingement test. Patients with SIS had a greater number of active and latent TrPs. The greatest prevalence of active TrPs was found in the subscapularis (42%), infraspinatus (42%), and supraspinatus muscles (62%). Decreased PPT in patients with SIS was directly correlated with the number of TrPs present. Patients who experienced reproduction of their pain with TrP palpation had significantly decreased PPT. Each patient with SIS had up to three active TrPs. The greater number of TrPs present, the lower the PPT. The results of this study lend credence to the theory that both peripheral and central pain mechanisms contribute to the pain experience of patients with SIS.[28]

The presence of TrPs in 10 muscles was investigated in 27 patients with a diagnosis of SIS and 20 matched controls.[46] The number of muscles with TrPs was significantly greater in the SIS group as compared with the control group with the subscapularis, infraspinatus, and trapezius muscles having a significant number of active and latent TrPs. The infraspinatus muscle had the highest prevalence of active TrPs in the SIS group. The greater prevalence of TrPs in the SIS group adds relevance to the contribution of myofascial pain in the signs and symptoms of SIS.[46]

In patients presenting with unilateral shoulder pain and a diagnosis of SIS with associated positive impingement tests, it is essential to examine neck and shoulder muscles bilaterally for the presence of both active and latent TrPs.

A number of studies implicate subscapularis TrPs in individuals with hemiplegia-related shoulder pain. Dysfunction often attributed to spasticity may actually be a result of subscapularis TrPs.[47] Dilorenzo et al[47] published the results of a trial in which TrP dry needling was used in conjunction with standard rehabilitative therapy to improve pain and functional outcomes in individuals with hemiparetic shoulder pain syndrome (hemiplegia-related shoulder pain). More recently, Mendigutía-Gómez et al[48] observed that dry needling applied to shoulder muscles, including the subscapularis muscle, was effective for reducing pressure pain sensitivity and spasticity in patients who have had a stroke.

Scapulohumeral muscle imbalances, more commonly referred to as scapular dyskinesia, are defined as an alteration of normal motor recruitment patterns of muscle contractions of the shoulder girdle musculature during upper extremity movements. This alteration of muscle recruitment can lead to incoordination, early fatigue, and overloading of the rotator cuff muscles and must be assessed and treated for the effective resolution of shoulder pain due to shoulder girdle TrPs.

5. CORRECTIVE ACTIONS

The patient should avoid habitual, sustained, or repetitive motions that overload the subscapularis muscle, such as retrieving heavy objects from a high shelf and lifting heavy objects from the floor. Reaching up to fasten the seatbelt when it is on the same side as the affected arm can be quite painful and challenging. During the acute phase, the unaffected arm should be utilized to fasten the seatbelt.

Attaining restful sleep may be difficult due to the inability to assume comfortable sleeping positions for prolonged periods. The individual with subscapularis TrPs may be most comfortable sleeping on the back or pain-free side. When the patient lies on the uninvolved side, sleep is improved by supporting the uppermost elbow and forearm (painful limb) on a bed pillow (Figure 22-4A) avoiding prolonged shortening of the affected subscapularis muscle that can cause referred pain. This technique can also be used to keep the arm in a neutral position when lying supine (Figure 22-4B) or when seated (Figure 22-4C). Another option is to place the pillow under the arm perpendicular to the body keeping the arm out of adduction and internal rotation and in a resting length-tension position for the subscapularis muscle. Patients should be cautioned regarding the lying in bed with their arm(s) above their head in an abducted and externally rotated position because this posture will keep the subscapularis muscle in a prolonged lengthened position.

During waking hours, the individual with subscapularis TrPs should be careful to avoid forward head and rounded shoulder postures, which are typically adopted during seated desk and computer work, texting, and driving. Setting an alarm every half hour to cue frequent standing, stretching, and arm movement can be beneficial in preventing the arm from remaining too close to the side for prolonged periods. When driving long distances, using the armrest or placing a small towel roll in the axilla may allow the arm to rest in some abduction (preventing full shortening). Stretches of the arm up and behind the head, or across to behind the opposite seat or headrest, can be helpful.

When prescribing neuromuscular reeducation or therapeutic exercises early in a supervised rehabilitation program, research supports utilization of supported vertical and diagonal wall slides, which decrease loading of the rotator cuff muscles.[49,50] As pain decreases and ROM increases, the addition of exercises that target the subscapularis muscle should be added. These exercises include internal rotation at 0° and 90° abduction, scapular punch, a diagonal movement pattern simulating throwing acceleration, high row, low row, dynamic hug, and push up plus. These exercises produce a muscle activation ranging from 20% to 136% MVC.[5,36,49]

The patient may inactivate subscapularis TrPs with the application of self-pressure release of TrPs in seated, standing, and/or lying positions. In the seated position, hanging the affected arm down between the legs is desired when motion in abduction is extremely painful and ROM is limited (Figure 26-5A). Most of the subscapularis muscle is accessible from this position. In the seated position, the affected arm is raised to allow improved access to the subscapularis muscle (Figure 26-5B). The fingertips or thumb of the opposite hand are placed inside the edge of the shoulder blade and pressed back into the subscapularis muscle. Placing the affected arm's hand on the opposite shoulder, if possible, brings the shoulder blade around the side of the body and can improve access (Figure 26-5C). This technique can also be employed supine if the seated position is too painful or not tolerated well (Figure 26-5D). If the shoulder is too acute, a towel roll can be placed under the arm instead of reaching the affected arm across the body (Figure 26-5E). The tenderest spot should be identified and pressure held for 30 seconds until pain subsides. This technique can be repeated up to 5 times. Massage across the taut bands in the same position may also be effective for symptom relief.[51]

A patient can learn to release tightness in the subscapularis muscle by slowly and firmly stretching it using the middle hand positions in the doorway, stretching into external rotation (Figure 26-6). A firm, gentle, pain-free stretch can be held for 30 seconds and repeated up to 3 to 5 times. To augment the stretch, a PNF hold relax technique can be used. The patient gently pushes into the door frame (internal rotation) to minimally contract the subscapularis muscle for 5 to 10 seconds followed by relaxation and gentle stretching of the muscle into further external rotation by rotating the body away from the doorframe. Alternatively, the stretch can be augmented through respiration

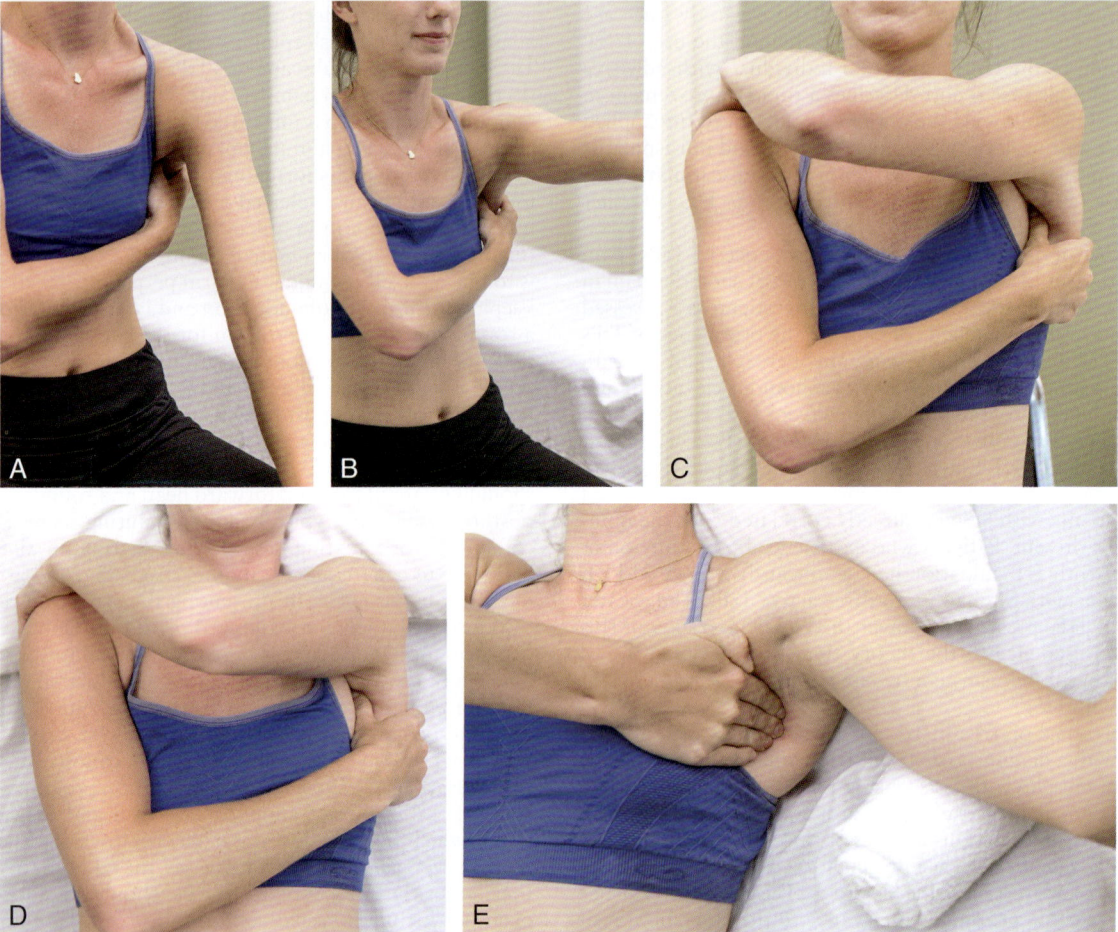

Figure 26-5. Self-pressure release of TrPs in the subscapularis muscle. A, Seated position for an acutely painful shoulder. B, Starting position for self-pressure release of TrPs in the subscapularis muscle. C, Placing hand on opposite shoulder improves accessibility to the muscle. D, Supine option. E, Supine option for acutely painful shoulder.

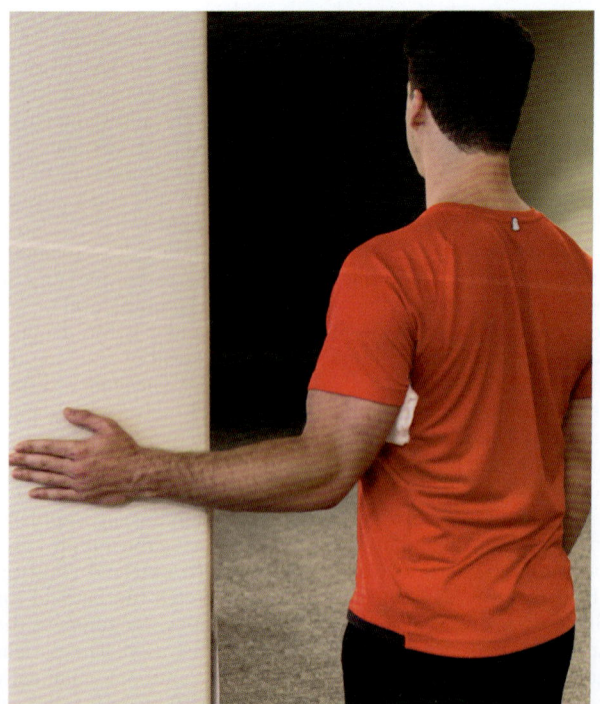

Figure 26-6. Self-stretch of the subscapularis muscle in a doorway with a towel placed in the axilla for optimal alignment.

by timing the inhale with a gentle push into the doorframe and the exhale with a gentle stretch further into external rotation by rotating the body away from the door frame. This sequence can be repeated 3 to 5 times, up to 3 to 4 times per day. A cold pack may be of therapeutic benefit immediately following pressure release or stretching, especially in the case of acute shoulder pain.

It is imperative that any glenohumeral posterior joint tightness be addressed, in addition to restoration of efficient shoulder girdle mechanics, while concomitantly treating TrPs in the supraspinatus muscle. Treatment isolated to TrPs in the supraspinatus muscle that does not address the shoulder joint will result only in temporary relief of pain arising from TrPs in the supraspinatus muscle and may warrant further assessment.

References

1. Standring S. *Gray's Anatomy: The Anatomical Basis of Clinical Practice.* 41st ed. London, UK: Elsevier; 2015.
2. Porterfield JA, DeRosa C. *Mechanical Shoulder Disorders: Perspectives in Functional Anatomy.* St. Louis, MO: Saunders; 2004:78-79.
3. Cleeman E, Brunelli M, Gothelf T, Hayes P, Flatow EL. Releases of subscapularis contracture: an anatomic and clinical study. *J Shoulder Elbow Surg.* 2003;12(3):231-236.
4. McCann PD, Cordasco FA, Ticker JB, et al. An anatomic study of the subscapular nerves: A guide for electromyographic analysis of the subscapularis muscle. *J Shoulder Elbow Surg.* 1994;3(2):94-99.
5. Decker MJ, Tokish JM, Ellis HB, Torry MR, Hawkins RJ. Subscapularis muscle activity during selected rehabilitation exercises. *Am J Sports Med.* 2003;31(1):126-134.
6. Serita T, Kudoh H, Sakai T. Variability of the arterial distribution to the rotator cuff muscles and its correlation with the diversity of arterial origin. *Juntendo Med J.* 2014;60(2):137-146.

7. Reed D, Cathers I, Halaki M, Ginn K. Does supraspinatus initiate shoulder abduction? *J Electromyogr Kinesiol.* 2013;23(2):425-429.
8. Ward SR, Hentzen ER, Smallwood LH, et al. Rotator cuff muscle architecture: implications for glenohumeral stability. *Clin Orthop Relat Res.* 2006;448:157-163.
9. Turkel SJ, Panio MW, Marshall JL, Girgis FG. Stabilizing mechanisms preventing anterior dislocation of the glenohumeral joint. *J Bone Joint Surg Am.* 1981;63(8):1208-1217.
10. Ovesen J, Nielsen S. Stability of the shoulder joint. Cadaver study of stabilizing structures. *Acta Orthop Scand.* 1985;56(2):149-151.
11. Halder AM, Zhao KD, Odriscoll SW, Morrey BF, An KN. Dynamic contributions to superior shoulder stability. *J Orthop Res.* 2001;19(2):206-212.
12. Heuberer P, Kranzl A, Laky B, Anderl W, Wurnig C. Electromyographic analysis: shoulder muscle activity revisited. *Arch Orthop Trauma Surg.* 2015;135(4):549-563.
13. Simons DG, Travell J, Simons L. *Travell & Simon's Myofascial Pain and Dysfunction: The Trigger Point Manual.* Vol 1. 2nd ed. Baltimore: Williams & Wilkins; 1999:104.
14. Kadaba MP, Cole A, Wootten ME, et al. Intramuscular wire electromyography of the subscapularis. *J Orthop Res.* 1992;10(3):394-397.
15. Reed D, Cathers I, Halaki M, Ginn KA. Does load influence shoulder muscle recruitment patterns during scapular plane abduction? *J Sci Med Sport.* 2015;15:207-208.
16. Wickham J, Pizzari T, Stansfeld K, Burnside A, Watson L. Quantifying 'normal' shoulder muscle activity during abduction. *J Electromyogr Kinesiol.* 2010;20(2):212-222.
17. Wattanaprakornkul D, Halaki M, Boettcher C, Cathers I, Ginn KA. A comprehensive analysis of muscle recruitment patterns during shoulder flexion: an electromyographic study. *Clin Anat.* 2011;24(5):619-626.
18. Jobe FW, Moynes DR, Tibone JE, Perry J. An EMG analysis of the shoulder in pitching. A second report. *Am J Sports Med.* 1984;12(3):218-220.
19. Gowan ID, Jobe FW, Tibone JE, Perry J, Moynes DR. A comparative electromyographic analysis of the shoulder during pitching. Professional versus amateur pitchers. *Am J Sports Med.* 1987;15(6):586-590.
20. Glousman R, Jobe F, Tibone J, Moynes D, Antonelli D, Perry J. Dynamic electromyographic analysis of the throwing shoulder with glenohumeral instability. *J Bone Joint Surg Am.* 1988;70(2):220-226.
21. Ryu RK, McCormick J, Jobe FW, Moynes DR, Antonelli DJ. An electromyographic analysis of shoulder function in tennis players. *Am J Sports Med.* 1988;16(5):481-485.
22. Jobe FW, Perry J, Pink M. Electromyographic shoulder activity in men and women professional golfers. *Am J Sports Med.* 1989;17(6):782-787.
23. Pink M, Jobe FW, Perry J. Electromyographic analysis of the shoulder during the golf swing. *Am J Sports Med.* 1990;18(2):137-140.
24. Pink M, Perry J, Browne A, Scovazzo ML, Kerrigan J. The normal shoulder during freestyle swimming. An electromyographic and cinematographic analysis of twelve muscles. *Am J Sports Med.* 1991;19(6):569-576.
25. Basmajian J, Deluca C. *Muscles Alive.* 5th ed. Baltimore: Williams & Wilkins; 1985:385.
26. Travell J, Rinzler SH. The myofascial genesis of pain. *Postgrad Med.* 1952;11(5):425-434.
27. Jalil NA, Prateepavanich P, Chaudakshetrin P. Atypical chest pain from myofascial pain syndrome of subscapularis muscle. *J Musculoske Pain.* 2010;18(2):173-179.
28. Hidalgo-Lozano A, Fernández de las Peñas C, Alonso-Blanco C, Ge HY, Arendt-Nielsen L, Arroyo-Morales M. Muscle trigger points and pressure pain hyperalgesia in the shoulder muscles in patients with unilateral shoulder impingement: a blinded, controlled study. *Exp Brain Res.* 2010;202(4):915-925.
29. Godges JJ, Mattson-Bell M, Thorpe D, Shah D. The immediate effects of soft tissue mobilization with proprioceptive neuromuscular facilitation on glenohumeral external rotation and overhead reach. *J Orthop Sports Phys Ther.* 2003;33(12):713-718.
30. Al Dajah SB, Unnikrishnan R. Subscapularis trigger release and contract relax technique in patients with shoulder impingement syndrome. *Eur Scientific J.* 2014;10:408-416.
31. Harrison TP, Sadnicka A, Eastwood DM. Motor points for the neuromuscular blockade of the subscapularis muscle. *Arch Phys Med Rehabil.* 2007;88(3):295-297.
32. Al-Shenqiti AM, Oldham JA. Test-retest reliability of myofascial trigger point detection in patients with rotator cuff tendonitis. *Clin Rehabil.* 2005;19(5):482-487.
33. Gerwin RD, Dommerholt J, Shah JP. An expansion of Simons' integrated hypothesis of trigger point formation. *Curr Pain Headache Rep.* 2004;8(6):468-475.
34. Hidalgo-Lozano A, Fernández de las Peñas C, Calderon-Soto C, Domingo-Camara A, Madeleine P, Arroyo-Morales M. Elite swimmers with and without unilateral shoulder pain: mechanical hyperalgesia and active/latent muscle trigger points in neck-shoulder muscles. *Scand J Med Sci Sports.* 2013;23(1):66-73.
35. Blanch P. Conservative management of shoulder pain in swimming. *Phys Ther in Sport.* 2004;5:109-124.
36. Myers JB, Pasquale MR, Laudner KG, Sell TC, Bradley JP, Lephart SM. On-the-field resistance-tubing exercises for throwers: an electromyographic analysis. *J Athl Train.* 2005;40(1):15-22.
37. Ingber RS. Shoulder impingement in tennis/racquetball players treated with subscapularis myofascial treatments. *Arch Phys Med Rehabil.* 2000;81(5):679-682.
38. Katz J, Poleshuck EL, Andrus CH, et al. Risk factors for acute pain and its persistence following breast cancer surgery. *Pain.* 2005;119(1-3):16-25.
39. Fernandez-Lao C, Cantarero-Villanueva I, Fernández de las Peñas C, Del-Moral-Avila R, Arendt-Nielsen L, Arroyo-Morales M. Myofascial trigger points in neck and shoulder muscles and widespread pressure pain hypersensitivty in patients with postmastectomy pain: evidence of peripheral and central sensitization. *Clin J Pain.* 2010;26(9):798-806.
40. Shin HJ, Shin JC, Kim WS, Chang WH, Lee SC. Application of ultrasound-guided trigger point injection for myofascial trigger points in the subscapularis and pectoralis muscles to post-mastectomy patients: a pilot study. *Yonsei Med J.* 2014;55(3):792-799.
41. Hsieh YL, Kao MJ, Kuan TS, Chen SM, Chen JT, Hong CZ. Dry needling to a key myofascial trigger point may reduce the irritability of satellite MTrPs. *Am J Phys Med Rehabil.* 2007;86(5):397-403.
42. Ferguson L, Gerwin R. *Shoulder Dysfunction and Frozen Shoulder. Clinical Mastery in the Treatment of Myofascial Pain.* Baltimore: Lippincott Williams & Wilkins; 2005:91-121.
43. Zuckerman JD, Rokito A. Frozen shoulder: a consensus definition. *J Shoulder Elbow Surg.* 2011;20(2):322-325.
44. Clewley D, Flynn TW, Koppenhaver S. Trigger point dry needling as an adjunct treatment for a patient with adhesive capsulitis of the shoulder. *J Orthop Sports Phys Ther.* 2014;44(2):92-101.
45. Ge HY, Fernández de las Peñas C, Madeleine P, Arendt-Nielsen L. Topographical mapping and mechanical pain sensitivity of myofascial trigger points in the infraspinatus muscle. *Eur J Pain.* 2008;12(7):859-865.
46. Alburquerque-Sendin F, Camargo P, Viera A, Salvini TF. Bilateral myofascial trigger points and pressure pain thresholds in the shoulder muscles in patients with unilateral shoulder impingement syndrome. A blinded controlled study. *Clin J Pain.* 2013;29:478-486.
47. DiLorenzo L, Traballesi M, Morelli D, Pompa A, Brunelli S, Buzzi MG. Hemiparetic shoulder pain syndrome treated with deep dry needling during early rehabilitation: a prospective, open-lavel, randomized investigation. *J Musculoske Pain.* 2004;12(2):25-34.
48. Mendigutia-Gomez A, Martin-Hernandez C, Salom-Moreno J, Fernández de las Peñas C. Effect of dry needling on spasticity, shoulder range of motion, and pressure pain sensitivity in patients with stroke: a crossover study. *J Manipulative Physiol Ther.* 2016;39(5):348-356.
49. Wise MB, Uhl TL, Mattacola CG, Nitz AJ, Kibler WB. The effect of limb support on muscle activation during shoulder exercises. *J Shoulder Elbow Surg.* 2004;13(6):614-620.
50. Gaunt BW, McCluskey GM, Uhl TL. An electromyographic evaluation of subdividing active-assistive shoulder elevation exercises. *Sports Health.* 2010;2(5):424-432.
51. Davies C. *The Trigger Point Therapy Workbook.* Oakland CA: New Harbinger Publications; 2001:90-91.

Chapter 27

Rhomboid Minor and Major Muscles

"Shoulder Blade Sorcerers"

Matthew Vraa

1. INTRODUCTION

The rhomboid minor and major muscles are important stabilizers of the scapula. The rhomboid minor muscle originates from the distal ligamentum nuchae and the spinous processes of C7 and T1 and descends inferolaterally to the base of the triangular medial surface of the spine of the scapula. The rhomboid major muscle originates from the spinous processes and supraspinous ligaments of T2-T5 and descends inferolaterally to the medial border of the scapula between the root of the scapular spine and the inferior angle. The muscles are innervated by a branch of the dorsal scapular nerve. Functionally, the muscles are involved in scapular retraction, downward (internal) rotation, and components of scapular elevation. They also provide dynamic stabilization during lifting, pushing, and pulling as well as activities of daily living tasks such as styling hair, tucking in a shirt, putting on a seat belt, and picking up a workbag. The referred pain from rhomboid trigger points (TrPs) expands over the medial border of the scapula and spreads superolaterally over the supraspinatus muscle and spine of the scapula. Trigger points in the rhomboid muscles have been associated with upper quarter myofascial pain syndrome and reduced upper extremity strength. Trigger points in these muscles can be activated or perpetuated by prolonged poor posture, holding the arms overhead for extended periods of time, or structural causes such as scoliosis or leg length discrepancies. The rhomboid muscles are involved in pain syndromes of the cervical spine, particularly cervical radicular pain. Individuals with space-occupying lesions at C4-C5, C5-C6, or C6-C7 commonly present with TrPs in the rhomboid muscles. Additionally, dorsal scapular nerve entrapment, thoracic facet syndrome, and costovertebral joint dysfunction can present with a pain pattern (interscapular pain) similar to rhomboid muscle TrPs and must be considered in the differential diagnosis. Corrective actions include TrP self-pressure release and correcting abnormal postures during sitting (especially driving and deskwork) to decrease excessive loading of the rhomboid muscles in a prolonged lengthened position.

2. ANATOMIC CONSIDERATIONS

Rhomboid Minor

The rhomboid minor muscle originates from the distal ligamentum nuchae and the spinous processes of C7 and T1.[1] The muscle descends inferolaterally to the base of the triangular medial surface of the spine of the scapula. The rhomboid minor muscle sits just inferior to the levator scapula muscle attachment on the scapula.[1] The rhomboid minor muscle can have attachments of the ligamentum nuchae of C4-C6.[2]

Rhomboid Major

The rhomboid major muscle originates from the spinous processes and supraspinous ligaments of T2-T5.[1] The quadrilateral sheet of the muscle descends inferolaterally to the medial border of the scapula between the foot of the spine and the inferior angle (Figure 27-1). A case study of a 49-year-old Korean male demonstrated a trapezoid-shaped rhomboid major muscle with different attachments on the right and left sides.[2] The muscle attached superiorly to the ligamentum nuchae at C6, extending to the spinous process of T2 on the right and to T4 on the left.[2]

Rhomboid Tertius

Although there is little anatomic variation of the rhomboid major and minor muscles, there are documented cases of a third rhomboid muscle (tertius). In one case, the muscle originated from the spinous processes of T6-T8 on the left side and from T6 to T7 on the right with muscle fibers running nearly horizontally as it inserted into the most inferior part of the medial border of the scapula.[3] The maximal width was noted at 40 mm on the left side and 27 mm on the right.[3]

Another documented case of the rhomboid tertius muscle noted the inferior origin as the spinous process of T5 bilaterally. However, the superior border was T4 spinous process on the left and T2 spinous process on the right.[2] The insertion was similar bilaterally to the other rhomboid tertius muscle variation with an attachment to the inferior medial border of the scapula.[2,3]

Rhomboid Interdigitating

Other variations exist with slips of the surrounding muscles (teres major, latissimus dorsi, and serratus anterior) interdigitating into rhomboid muscles.[3] This variation is unlikely to alter the function of the rhomboid major or minor muscles.

2.1. Innervation and Vascularization

The rhomboid minor and major muscles are innervated by a branch of the dorsal scapular nerve.[1] This nerve originates from the C4-C5 nerve root and becomes the dorsal scapular nerve via the upper trunk of the brachial plexus.[4-6] The nerve can also originate from the C6 root and pierce the middle scalene muscle as it passes the vertebral border of the scapula between the serratus posterior superior, posterior scalene, and levator scapulae muscles to innervate the rhomboid muscles.[7] The dorsal scapular nerve also innervates the levator scapulae muscle.

Vascular supply of the rhomboid minor and major muscles is variable. The dorsal scapular artery or a deep branch of the transverse cervical artery typically supplies the muscles.[1]

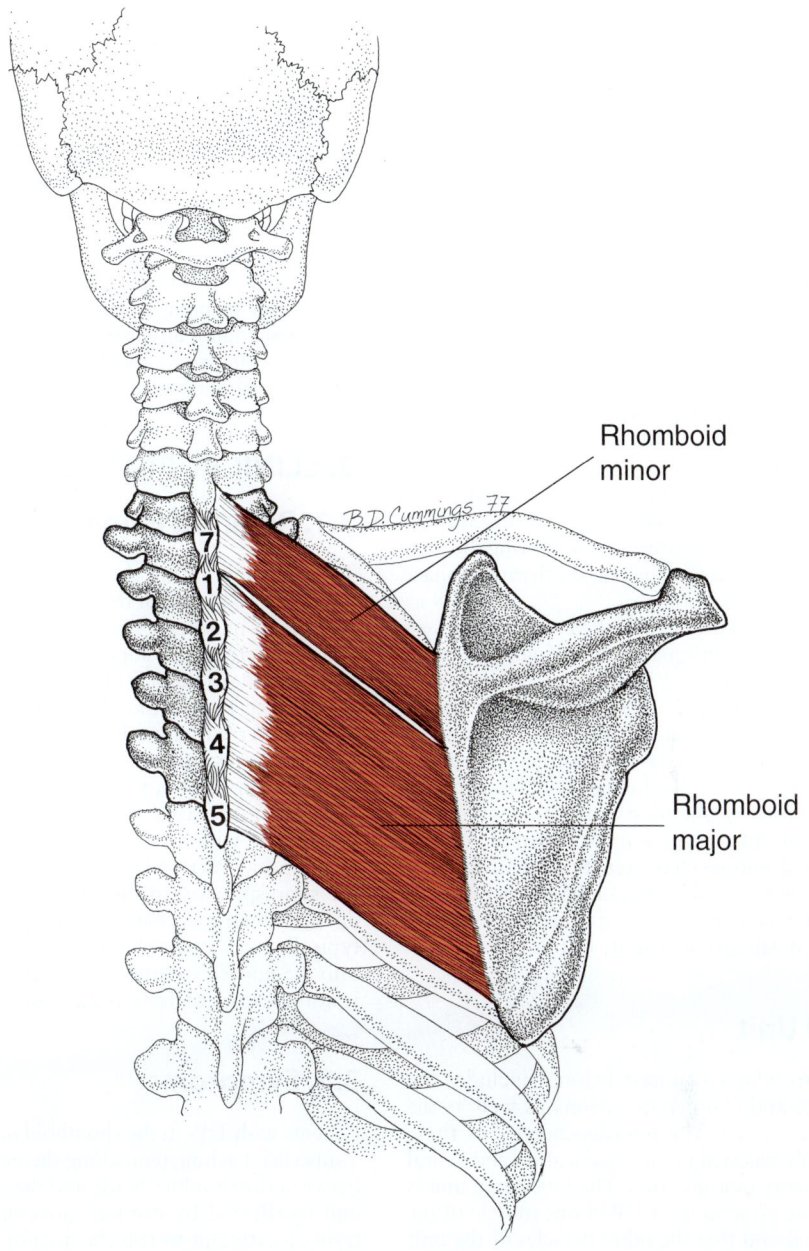

Figure 27-1. Attachments of the rhomboid minor and major muscles to the vertebral spinous processes and the medial border of the scapula, showing the direction and extent of the muscle fibers.

The dorsal branches from the posterior intercostal arteries can also supply the rhomboid muscles.[1]

2.2. Function

The rhomboid muscles adduct and elevate the scapula.[1,4,5,8] The attachment of the rhomboid major muscle fibers to the lower vertebral border of the scapula tends to downwardly rotate the scapula causing the glenoid fossa to tilt inferiorly.[1,4,5,8] Both rhomboid muscles assist in shoulder abduction, adduction, flexion, extension, and scaption motions of the arm by stabilizing the scapula in the retracted position.[1,4,5,8-13]

No distinction in function has been noted between the rhomboid minor and major muscles. Because of the differences in attachments of both muscles to the scapula, the rotation effect of the rhomboid major muscle may be much greater than that of the minor. However, because the majority of electromyography (EMG) studies conducted on the rhomboid muscles only studied the rhomboid major muscle, it is difficult to make a definitive statement regarding individual functions of each muscle.

EMG data demonstrate that the rhomboid major muscle is active to varying degrees in just about all upper extremity activities. The rhomboid muscles are more active during shoulder abduction, circumduction, and scapular elevation than during glenohumeral flexion or extension.[14,15] Ito[16] noted that the rhomboid muscles exhibited steadily increasing activity throughout abduction and similarly during flexion, but in the latter case, the EMG activity reached only about two-thirds of the amplitude seen with abduction. In another study, the electrical activity of the rhomboid muscles rapidly increased in intensity between 160° and 180° of abduction and flexion.[17] This activity was not predicted by any of the aforementioned anatomic-based actions. The increase may be due to the stabilization actions that the rhomboid muscles provide during upper extremity activities. Wickham et al[18] found maximal voluntary isometric contraction (MVIC) in shoulder abduction between 90° and 135° but less activity upon lowering the arm from the maximal abducted position. Castelein et al[10] showed MVIC activity at 135° of flexion against a downward force applied at the elbow. The results of the MVIC testing were not statistically different in a prone horizontal abduction test position versus a prone position against resistance with the arm in an overhead position (similar to the position to test lower trapezius muscle strength).[10]

The rhomboid muscles are active in both forward and backward swings of the arm during walking, probably to stabilize the scapula.[15] Although the strength of adduction and extension of the humerus is diminished by loss of rhomboid muscle fixation of the scapula, ordinary function of the arm is affected less by loss of rhomboid muscle fixation of the scapula than by loss of either the trapezius or the serratus anterior muscles.[4]

EMG activity has been examined in some sport activities. During overhead baseball pitching, MVIC activity of the rhomboid muscles was highest during the acceleration and deceleration phases of throwing mechanics.[19] Similar high MVIC activity is recorded during the acceleration phase of the windmill softball pitch.[20] The rhomboid muscles were most active during the start of the forward golf swing followed by the acceleration phase (hitting the golf ball).[19]

Scovazzo et al[21] compared fine wire EMG recordings of rhomboid muscle activity during aquatic swimming between 14 subjects with a painful shoulder and 12 subjects with pain-free shoulders. EMG activity in painful shoulders was only one-fourth that in normal subjects. But during middle pull-through, it was 4 times that of normal, falling back to less than normal throughout early recovery.[21] The initial pattern of inhibition could be expected because this muscle is prone to inhibition and weakness.[22] However, the subsequent abnormally high level of rhomboid muscle activity is surprising and is more characteristic of a muscle that is strongly compensating for the dysfunction of another muscle. Identification of which muscles had TrPs and which muscles were free of TrPs would be invaluable in a study of this type.

2.3. Functional Unit

The functional unit to which a muscle belongs includes the muscles that reinforce and counter its actions as well as the joints that the muscle crosses. The interdependence of these structures is functionally reflected in the organization and neural connections of the sensory motor cortex. The functional unit is emphasized because the presence of a TrP in one muscle of the unit increases the likelihood that the other muscles of the unit will also develop TrPs. When inactivating TrPs in a muscle, one must be concerned about TrPs that may develop in muscles that are functionally interdependent. Box 27-1 grossly represents the functional unit of the rhomboid minor and major muscles.[23]

Box 27-1 Functional unit of the rhomboid minor and major muscles

Action	Synergists	Antagonists
Scapular elevation	Levator scapulae Upper trapezius	Latissimus dorsi Lower trapezius Pectoralis minor
Scapular retraction	Middle trapezius Latissimus dorsi	Serratus anterior Pectoralis major Pectoralis minor
Scapular downward rotation	Levator scapulae Latissimus dorsi	Upper trapezius Lower trapezius Serratus anterior

It should be noted that the fasciae of the rhomboid minor muscle and the serratus anterior muscle are interdigitated.[1] This relationship is the main reason these muscles are clinically correlated in dysfunction.

During the initiation of upper extremity glenohumeral flexion, the action of downward rotation by the levator scapulae and the rhomboid muscles is dominant over the action of upward rotation by the upper trapezius and the serratus anterior muscles.[24] This stabilization of the scapula then allows for scapular upward rotation during later stages of glenohumeral flexion and abduction.[8,25,26] A length deficit in the rhomboid muscles and/or the levator scapulae muscle can cause movement impairments during scapular upward rotation. If the glenohumeral joint does not compensate for the deficient scapular motion, shoulder flexion or abduction range of motion will be limited.

3. CLINICAL PRESENTATION

3.1. Referred Pain Pattern

Trigger points in the rhomboid muscles usually refer pain to the vertebral border of the scapula between the scapula and the paraspinal muscles (Figure 27-2). This interscapular pain can project laterally and superiorly over the supraspinatus muscle and the spine of the scapula on the affected side.[23] Experimental injection of hypertonic saline into normal rhomboid muscles caused referred pain felt over the medial part of the scapula, extending upward and laterally over to the acromion.[27]

The pain pattern somewhat resembles that of the levator scapulae or the scalene muscles but without the cervical component and without loss of motion in rotation or side bending in the neck. Part of the pain pattern can also mimic that of the supraspinatus, infraspinatus, middle trapezius, latissimus dorsi, and serratus posterior superior muscles, but these muscles typically have a pain that refers beyond the acromion or down into the upper extremity.[23] Referred pain extending to the arm is not a feature of TrPs in the rhomboid muscles.

3.2. Symptoms

Patients with TrPs in the rhomboid muscles will typically report a superficial aching pain along the medial border of the scapula between the shoulder blade and the spine that is present at rest and unaffected by normal movements. Patients may report trying to attempt to rub the area of pain for relief. Often, the patient reports soliciting a loved one to "rub it out" or that they have leaned against the corner of a wall to apply pressure to the area. Patients may also report snapping and crunching feelings during movement of the scapula, which may be due to TrPs in the rhomboid muscles. The skin overlying the area of reported pain may even be bruised or discolored if the patient has repeatedly been applying firm pressure in attempts to relieve the pain.

A retracted position of the shoulder girdle is commonly associated with muscle facilitation dysfunctions of the scapular retractors (trapezius muscle, levator scapula muscle, and latissimus dorsi muscles). A protracted position with rounded shoulder posture can be associated with facilitated/adaptive shortening of the serratus anterior and/or pectoralis muscles (major and minor).[24,28] In this protracted position, facilitated upper trapezius and levator scapulae muscles are common.[24,28] This pattern is often clinically correlated with muscle inhibition of the rhomboid and middle and lower trapezius muscles.[28] This overstretch/inhibition pain from a protracted scapular position will gradually subside if the muscle remains in a neutral length tension position that places it neither under tension nor in a shortened position.[4]

The lack of literature related to TrPs in the rhomboid muscles may be due to the fact that the rhomboid TrPs are less common than other shoulder girdle muscles.[29-32] Trigger points in the rhomboid muscle are often associated with other impairments

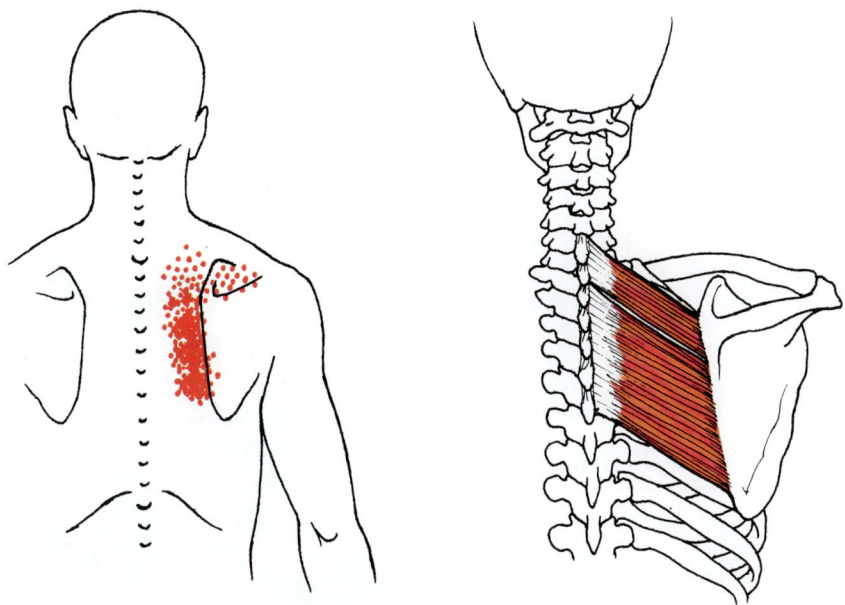

Figure 27-2. Composite referred pain pattern (essential zone solid red, spillover zone stippled red) caused by TrPs of the right rhomboid muscles.

and upper quarter conditions.[30-33] Pain is rarely identified as originating in these muscles until TrPs in neighboring affected muscles (such as the levator scapulae, supraspinatus, infraspinatus, middle trapezius, and the serratus posterior superior muscles) have been deactivated.

In a case study by Kellgren in 1938, an individual presented with TrPs as he described in the rhomboid muscles. The TrPs presented ipsilateral interscapular pain with referred pain that was reported from the base of the head, along the upper trapezius muscle down to the acromion on the affected side.[27] Upon injections of the TrPs with 16 mL of novocaine, the left-sided neck and interscapular pain of 6 months' duration was fully resolved within 1 week.[27]

3.3. Patient Examination

After a thorough subjective examination, the clinician should make a detailed drawing representing the pain pattern that the patient has described. This depiction will assist in planning the physical examination and can be useful in monitoring the progression of the patient as symptoms improve or change. A static posture analysis provides a wealth of information regarding the length-tension relationships of scapular muscles and their relationship to the resting position of the scapula. A rounded shoulder posture may indicate shortening and tightness of the pectoralis major and minor muscles and can put sustained stretch on the rhomboid and middle trapezius muscle fibers. Tightness of the latissimus dorsi muscle can lead to increased internal rotation of the humerus, causing an appearance of a forward shoulder position. Postural scapular elevation can be caused by facilitation of the levator scapula and upper trapezius muscles and inhibition of the lower trapezius muscle. Scapular winging is often associated with inhibition or weakness of the serratus anterior muscle.[24] Refer to Chapter 76 for more on posture.

After a comprehensive postural screen of the upper and lower quadrants, a movement screen of the shoulder girdle and upper extremity should be performed to identify movement impairments that need to be examined more closely.[4,34] Active and passive range of motion of the shoulder girdle complex should be thoroughly examined with specific observation of scapular motion. Clinicians should also screen the cervical, thoracic, and lumbar spine for mobility impairments as well as the scapulothoracic, glenohumeral, acromioclavicular, sternoclavicular, and elbow joints.[34] Impairments in any of the aforementioned joints can directly or indirectly affect rhomboid muscles' activation patterns or those of its functional unit. Examination of these joints may help to identify soft tissue, muscular, or accessory motion limitations.[4,5,24,34]

Additionally, clinical screening for proper resting and contracted muscle length may reveal muscle facilitation/inhibition patterns (including the rhomboid muscles) that need to be addressed.[4,5,24,34,35]

Although no research currently exists to describe the relationship of upper quarter movement impairments and rhomboid TrPs, it is expected that biomechanical faults may occur with rhomboid muscle dysfunction. Inefficient strength and length of the rhomboid muscles do alter movement patterns of the scapula and the upper extremity.[35-38] Furthermore, TrPs in other shoulder girdle muscles affect movement patterns and shoulder pain.[38-43] Assessing the scapulothoracic rhythm during upper extremity flexion and abduction may provide useful information on muscle function and performance.

Passive range of motion of the joints of the upper quarter can aid in the differentiation of soft tissue dysfunction versus faulty joint mechanics.[24,34] Assessing the mobility of the scapula in elevation, depression, protraction, retraction, and rotation can be achieved by manual assessment. This assessment of the scapula for mobility over the thoracic cage can reveal the source of movement restrictions. Restrictions in upward rotation or protraction implicate the rhomboid or levator scapulae muscles. Difficulty with retraction could be caused by a length deficit in anterior structures (pectoralis major/minor muscles), whereas the inability to depress the scapula would implicate the levator scapulae and upper trapezius muscles. Length deficits of the latissimus dorsi and lower fibers of the trapezius muscles could cause restriction of scapular elevation. Some patients may report, or the clinician may palpate, snapping and crepitus during mobility assessment of the scapula, and these phenomena may be due to TrPs in the rhomboid muscles.

Additional testing should include muscle length examination in abduction and adduction.[4,5,24,34] Classic muscle testing of the rhomboid muscles involves prone position of the patient with horizontal adduction scapula being tested.[4,5] Typically, differentiation for middle trapezius muscle versus rhomboid muscle is determined by the testing position: the arm in a externally rotated position for the trapezius muscle and the arm internally rotated for the rhomboid muscles.[4,5]

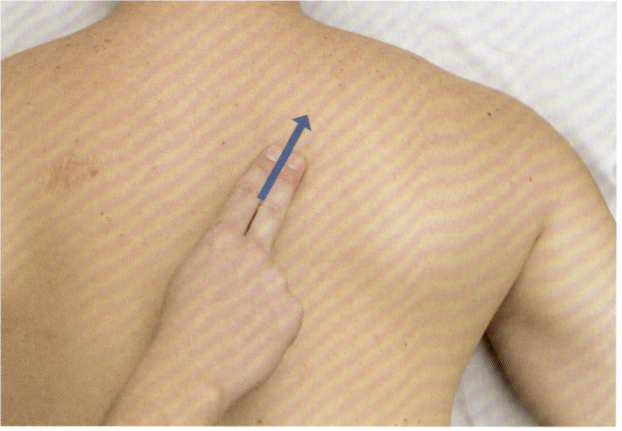

Figure 27-3. Palpation of the rhomboid muscles in prone.

The most reliable clinical indication of rhomboid major weakness is obtained by palpation of the rhomboid major muscle during adduction and elevation of the scapula with downward rotation of the scapula. Muscle fiber orientation along with depth will aid in differentiation between muscle activation of the middle trapezius muscle and the rhomboid muscles.

3.4. Trigger Point Examination

Cross-fiber flat palpation is preferred to identify taut bands and TrPs in the rhomboid minor and major muscles with the patient in the prone position (Figure 27-3). The muscle can also be palpated with the patient in the seated position, with the arm supported in 90° elevation in the sagittal plane or with the arm in the hammerlock position. A TrP within a taut band of the rhomboid muscle can be distinguished from the overlying trapezius muscle by fiber orientation. The rhomboid muscle fibers are directed obliquely, in an inferolateral direction away from the vertebrae; the lower trapezius muscle fibers are angled superolaterally, and the middle trapezius muscle fibers run relatively horizontally.

To define the precise borders of these muscles, the patient should lie prone or sit with his or her hand resting on the lumbar spine (hammerlock position). This position will raise the vertebral boarder of the scapula off the thoracic cage. The clinician can then place a finger (reinforced with the opposite hand, if necessary) deep to the medial border of the scapula. When the patient lifts the hand up off the back, the rhomboid muscles contract vigorously, pushing the clinician's finger out from under the scapula. Once the rhomboid muscles have been outlined, deep cross-fiber flat palpation along the rhomboid muscle fibers can be used to identify any taut bands that contain TrPs (Figure 27-4).

The rhomboid muscles are examined for taut bands along the entire muscle with a cross-fiber flat palpation. Trigger points can be anywhere along the length of the taut band and anywhere within the muscle. All but the caudal ends of the lowermost fibers of the rhomboid major muscle will be palpable through the trapezius muscle.

4. DIFFERENTIAL DIAGNOSIS

4.1. Activation and Perpetuation of Trigger Points

A posture or activity that activates a TrP, if not corrected, can also perpetuate it. In any part of the rhomboid muscles, TrPs may be activated by unaccustomed eccentric loading, eccentric exercise in an unconditioned muscle, or maximal or submaximal concentric loading.[44] Trigger points may also be activated or aggravated when the muscle is placed in a shortened and/or lengthened position for an extended period of time. Therefore, it is essential to examine workloads, strength, and length of other upper extremity and scapular stabilizing muscles.

Trigger points in the rhomboid muscles may be activated by holding the arm in abduction or flexion above 90° for a prolonged period, such as when painting overhead, installing drywall, or with certain sport/recreational activities (rock climbing, volleyball, tennis, throwing sports, etc.). Trigger points can also be activated and perpetuated by working at a desk with a rounded shoulder posture and prolonged forward leaning. These positions are common with poor office workstation ergonomics and using handheld electronic devices, respectively.

Even when postural and behavioral corrections are made, some individuals may present with TrPs due to structural causes. A prolonged stretch due to prominence of the scapula on the convex side in upper thoracic scoliosis can create a structural dilemma. Adaptation in length can occur after certain disease process or injuries to the patient (congenital elevation of the scapula, cerebrovascular accident, accessory nerve disorder, brachial plexus injury). Other events and circumstances, like chest surgery or a limb-length discrepancy in the upper or lower extremity, can cause changes in how the upper extremity is held or used and can perpetuate TrPs in the rhomboid muscles.

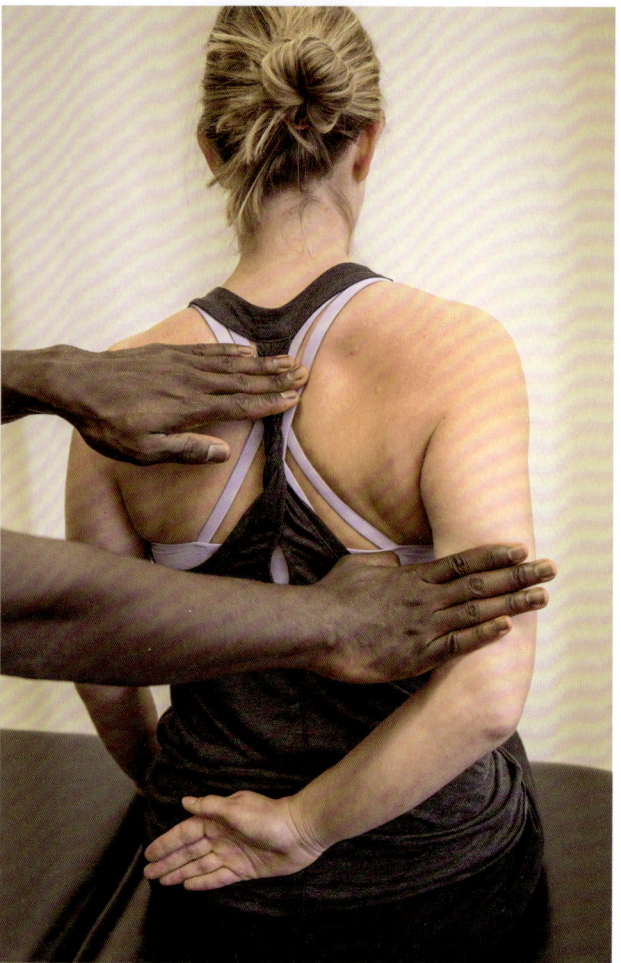

Figure 27-4. Differentiation of rhomboid muscles in the seated posture with the arm in the hammerlock position.

4.2. Associated Trigger Points

Associated TrPs can develop in the referred pain areas caused by other TrPs[45]; therefore, muscles in the referred pain areas for each muscle should also be considered. Several muscles refer pain in a similar pattern to that of the rhomboid muscles, including the scalene, levator scapulae, middle trapezius, infraspinatus, supraspinatus, serratus posterior superior, and latissimus dorsi muscles. These muscles should also be examined for the presence of TrPs, especially if the therapeutic response to rhomboid muscle treatment does not resolve pain. The anatomic proximity of the splenius capitis, splenius cervicis, spinalis muscle, longissimus, and iliocostalis muscles should also be evaluated for muscle dysfunction in the midthoracic region. Occasionally, rhomboid TrPs become obvious only after inactivation of TrPs in the scalene, levator scapulae, middle trapezius, infraspinatus, or supraspinatus muscles.

Patients with rhomboid TrPs frequently present with a rounded shoulder posture and are unable to achieve effective postural alignment due to tightness and TrPs in the pectoralis major and/or minor muscles. The rhomboid and middle trapezius muscles are then placed on prolonged stretch or experience overload as a consequence of the shortened pectoral muscles. This maladaptive position can perpetuate TrPs and muscle inhibition in both muscle groups, exacerbating the rounded shoulder position. Trigger points in the serratus anterior muscle can also contribute to rhomboid muscle overload.

4.3. Associated Pathology

Trigger points in the rhomboid muscles may be associated with, and can mimic, many different conditions. A thorough medical screening and physical examination are essential, and referral to another healthcare practitioner may be necessary. Systemic conditions from cardiopulmonary, gastrointestinal (upper portions), renal, hepatic, and biliary systems all have the potential to refer pain to the same anatomic location and pain referral areas as the rhomboid muscles.[46-48] A systems review and review of systems (heart rate, blood pressure, respiratory rate, oxygen saturation, etc.) can aid in clinical reasoning.[34,46-48]

Due to the attachment sites and the innervation of the rhomboids muscles, articular or neural involvement may be associated with impairments in the rhomboid muscle function. Trigger points in the rhomboid muscles are often associated with other impairments or upper quarter conditions.[30-33] Hsueh et al[33] observed that individuals with neural involvement at C4-C5, C5-C6, or C6-C7 can present with TrPs in the rhomboid muscles. There is additional evidence to support the role of scapular mobility in subjects with neck pain.[10,49-52] These studies recommend evaluating and treating using a regional impairment-based approach.[53,54] Refer to other texts for descriptions of manual therapy and exercises to address thoracic spine or rib cage dysfunctions that can perpetuate TrPs in the rhomboid muscles.[55-59]

Articular dysfunction of spinal segments from C7 to T5 is associated with rhomboid TrPs. Usually two or more segments are involved. Occasionally, a T3 spinal segmental dysfunction of extension as well as ipsilateral lateral flexion and rotation is noted. This single-segment fault usually presents as reduced upper thoracic kyphosis with limited flexion mobility and concurrent scapular adduction with rhomboid muscle involvement. This segmental dysfunction must be recognized and appropriately treated. Concurrent rhomboid TrP deactivation often occurs with correction of this articular dysfunction.

5. CORRECTIVE ACTIONS

A patient with rhomboid TrPs should modify or limit any activity that involves holding the arm above shoulder height for a prolonged period, such as when painting or working overhead, and certain sport/recreational activities such as rock climbing. The use of a lumbar pillow or a thoracolumbar support may help to correct a rounded shoulder posture and place the muscles in a neutral length-tension position, especially while working at a desk or driving a car.

Patients should avoid any chair that pushes the upper torso, shoulders, and head/neck forward. Some backward slope of the backrest with lumbar support is needed for a comfortable and effective seated posture. When evaluating sitting posture at a desk, consideration of table height, keyboards, and computer screen distance/height to optimize ergonomic support (see Chapter 76).

For a patient who becomes preoccupied at a desk and forgets to take frequent breaks to change position and thus relieve the strain on the muscles, an interval timer can be placed across the room and set to ring every 20 to 30 minutes. This aid will promote intermittent movement, encouraging the patient to get up at regular intervals to reset the timer.

Scapular protraction, or any other observed faulty scapular position, due to functional scoliosis caused by a leg length discrepancy or an asymmetric pelvis, can be corrected by leveling the pelvis and straightening the spine with appropriate lifts in standing or sitting. Several options are available to address these structural asymmetries to normalize posture.

The patient should be cognizant of posture at work and during sleep for successful management of TrPs in the rhomboid muscles. Once local strength of the muscle is improved, addressing controlled and functional dynamic stability of the scapula will be important for successful return to sport.

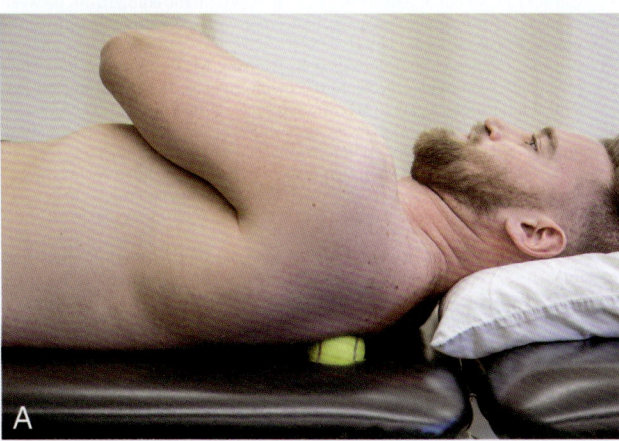 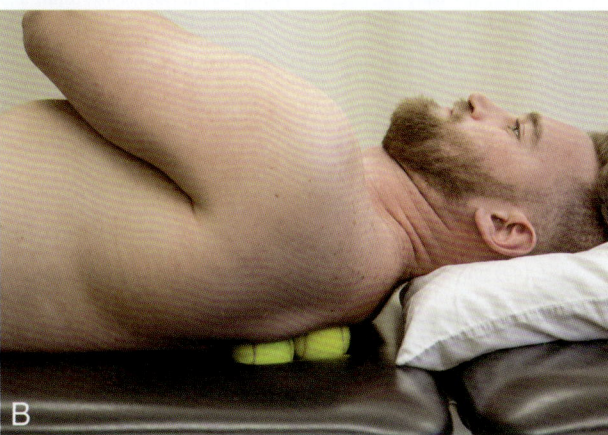

Figure 27-5. Rhomboid muscle self-pressure release of TrPs utilizing A, one tennis ball; B, two tennis balls.

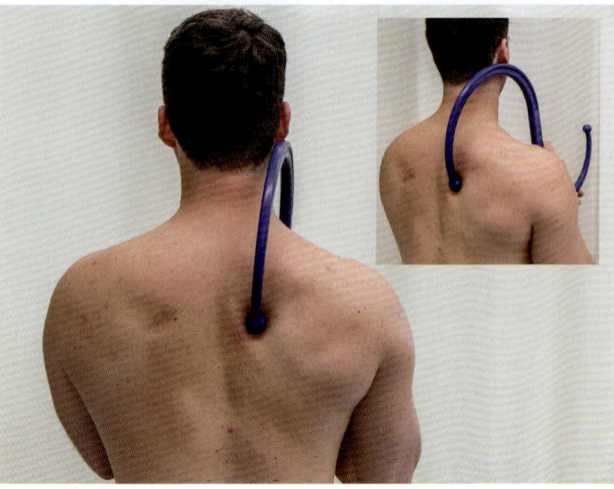

Figure 27-6. Rhomboid TrP self-release with TrP self-release tool.

Rarely do the rhomboid muscles need active stretching exercises. However, their antagonists, the pectoralis major and minor muscles, are often tight or shortened. Stretching the pectoral muscles, if shortened or tight, will assist in the maintenance of proper posture by placing the scapula in a better resting position, thus decreasing stretch tension on the rhomboid muscles (see Figs. 42-10, 11 and Fig. 44-6).

Additionally, the patient can treat the rhomboid muscles with pressure release by utilizing instrument-assisted techniques. Inexpensive options like laying on tennis balls (Figure 27-5A) or a rolled up towel are often effective. The patient can lie on the tennis ball and position the body and shoulder blade so the ball is over the TrP. The patient can locate each rhomboid TrP by rolling a single tennis ball along the medial border of the scapula. If there is involvement of both rhomboid muscles on one side, a pair of tennis balls can be used (Figure 27-5B). The pressure is centered on the most tender spot until the tenderness fades, usually holding firm pressure for 15 to 30 seconds and repeated as necessary. Other options include commercially available TrP self-release tools (Figure 27-6).

References

1. Standring S. *Gray's Anatomy: The Anatomical Basis of Clinical Practice*. 41st ed. London, UK: Elsevier; 2015.
2. Lee J, Jung W. A pair of atypical rhomboid muscles. *Korean J Phys Anthropol*. 2015;28(4):247-251.
3. Jelev L, Landzhov B. A rare muscular variation: the third of the rhomboids. *Anatomy*. 2013;6-7:63-64.
4. Kendall FP, McCreary EK. *Muscles: Testing and Function, with Posture and Pain*. Baltimore: Lippincott Williams & Wilkins; 2005.
5. Hislop H, Avers D, Brown M. *Daniels and Worthingham's Muscle Testing: Techniques of Manual Examination and Performance Testing*. 9th ed. Philadelphia, PA: WB Saunders Co; 2014.
6. Sultan HE, Younis El-Tantawi GA. Role of dorsal scapular nerve entrapment in unilateral interscapular pain. *Arch Phys Med Rehabil*. 2013;94(6):1118-1125.
7. Tubbs RS, Tyler-Kabara EC, Aikens AC, et al. Surgical anatomy of the dorsal scapular nerve. *J Neurosurg*. 2005;102(5):910-911.
8. Neumann DA. *Kinesiology of the Musculoskeletal System: Foundations for Rehabilitaion*. 2nd ed. St. Louis, MO: Mosby; 2010.
9. Moseley JB Jr, Jobe FW, Pink M, Perry J, Tibone J. EMG analysis of the scapular muscles during a shoulder rehabilitation program. *Am J Sports Med*. 1992;20(2):128-134.
10. Castelein B, Cagnie B, Parlevliet T, Danneels L, Cools A. Optimal normalization tests for muscle activation of the levator scapulae, pectoralis minor, and rhomboid major: an electromyography study using maximum voluntary isometric contractions. *Arch Phys Med Rehabil*. 2015;96(10):1820-1827.
11. Ginn KA, Halaki M, Cathers I. Revision of the Shoulder Normalization Tests is required to include rhomboid major and teres major. *J Orthop Res*. 2011;29(12):1846-1849.
12. Smith J, Padgett DJ, Kaufman KR, Harrington SP, An KN, Irby SE. Rhomboid muscle electromyography activity during 3 different manual muscle tests. *Arch Phys Med Rehabil*. 2004;85(6):987-992.
13. Castelein B, Cools A, Parlevliet T, Cagnie B. Modifying the shoulder joint position during shrugging and retraction exercises alters the activation of the medial scapular muscles. *Man Ther*. 2016;21:250-255.
14. De Freitas V, Vitti M, Furlani J. Electromyographic study of levator scapulae and rhomboideus major muscles in movements of the shoulder and arm. *Electromyogr Clin Neurophysiol*. 1980;20(3):205-216.
15. Basmajian J, Deluca C. *Muscles Alive*. 5th ed. Baltimore: Williams & Wilkins; 1985.
16. Ito N. Electromyographic study of shoulder joint. *Nihon Seikeigeka Gakkai Zasshi*. 1980;54(11):1529-1540.
17. Inman VT, Saunders JB, Abbott LC. Observations of the function of the shoulder joint. 1944. *Clin Orthop Relat Res*. 1996(330):3-12.
18. Wickham J, Pizzari T, Stansfeld K, Burnside A, Watson L. Quantifying 'normal' shoulder muscle activity during abduction. *J Electromyogr Kinesiol*. 2010;20(2):212-222.
19. Escamilla RF, Andrews JR. Shoulder muscle recruitment patterns and related biomechanics during upper extremity sports. *Sports Med*. 2009;39(7):569-590.
20. Oliver GD, Plummer HA, Keeley DW. Muscle activation patterns of the upper and lower extremity during the windmill softball pitch. *J Strength Cond Res*. 2011;25(6):1653-1658.
21. Scovazzo ML, Browne A, Pink M, Jobe FW, Kerrigan J. The painful shoulder during freestyle swimming. An electromyographic cinematographic analysis of twelve muscles. *Am J Sports Med*. 1991;19(6):577-582.
22. Lewit K. *Manipulative Therapy in Rehabilitation of the Locomotor System*. 2nd ed. Oxford: Butterworth Heinemann; 1991.
23. Simons DG, Travell J, Simons L. *Travell & Simon's Myofascial Pain and Dysfunction: The Trigger Point Manual*. Vol 1. 2nd ed. Baltimore: Williams & Wilkins; 1999:104.
24. Sahrmann S. *Diagnosis and Treatment of Movement Impairment Syndromes*. St. Louis, MO: Mosby; 2002.
25. Mottram SL. Dynamic stability of the scapula. *Man Ther*. 1997;2(3):123-131.
26. Struyf F, Nijs J, Mottram S, Roussel NA, Cools AM, Meeusen R. Clinical assessment of the scapula: a review of the literature. *Br J Sports Med*. 2014;48(11):883-890.
27. Kellgren JH. Observations on referred pain arising from muscle. *Clin Sci*. 1938;3:175-190.
28. Page P, Frank C, Lardner R. *Assessment and Treatment of Muscle Imbalance. The Janda Approach*. Champaign, IL: Human Kinetics; 2010.
29. Sola AE, Kuitert JH. Myofascial trigger point pain in the neck and shoulder girdle; report of 100 cases treated by injection of normal saline. *Northwest Med*. 1955;54(9):980-984.
30. Oh S, Kim HK, Kwak J, et al. Causes of hand tingling in visual display terminal workers. *Ann Rehabil Med*. 2013;37(2):221-228.
31. Sari H, Akarirmak U, Uludag M. Active myofascial trigger points might be more frequent in patients with cervical radiculopathy. *Eur J Phys Rehabil Med*. 2012;48(2):237-244.
32. Chiarotto A, Clijsen R, Fernández de Las Peñas C, Barbero M. Prevalence of myofascial trigger points in spinal disorders: a systematic review and meta-analysis. *Arch Phys Med Rehabil*. 2016;97(2):316-337.
33. Hsueh TC, Yu S, Kuan TS, Hong CZ. Association of active myofascial trigger points and cervical disc lesions. *J Formos Med Assoc*. 1998;97(3):174-180.
34. Magee DJ. *Orthopedic Physical Assessment*. 6th ed. St Louis, Missouri: Saunders Elsevier; 2014.
35. Page P. Shoulder muscle imbalance and subacromial impingement syndrome in overhead athletes. *Int J Sports Phys Ther*. 2011;6(1):51-58.
36. Paine R, Voight ML. The role of the scapula. *Int J Sports Phys Ther*. 2013;8(5):617-629.
37. Ludewig PM, Reynolds JF. The association of scapular kinematics and glenohumeral joint pathologies. *J Orthop Sports Phys Ther*. 2009;39(2):90-104.
38. Lucas KR, Rich PA, Polus BI. How common are latent myofascial trigger points in the scapular positioning muscles? *J Musculoske Pain*. 2008;16(4):279-286.
39. Celik D, Yeldan I. The relationship between latent trigger point and muscle strength in healthy subjects: a double-blind study. *J Back Musculoskelet Rehabil*. 2011;24(4):251-256.
40. Gerber LH, Sikdar S, Armstrong K, et al. A systematic comparison between subjects with no pain and pain associated with active myofascial trigger points. *PM R*. 2013;5(11):931-938.
41. Bron C, Dommerholt J, Stegenga B, Wensing M, Oostendorp RA. High prevalence of shoulder girdle muscles with myofascial trigger points in patients with shoulder pain. *BMC Musculoskelet Disord*. 2011;12(1):139-151.
42. Osborne NJ, Gatt IT. Management of shoulder injuries using dry needling in elite volleyball players. *Acupunct Med*. 2010;28(1):42-45.
43. Alburquerque-Sendin F, Camargo P, Viera A, Salvini TF. Bilateral myofascial trigger points and pressure pain thresholds in the shoulder muscles in patients with unilateral shoulder impingement syndrome. A blinded controlled study. *Clin J Pain*. 2013;29:478-486.
44. Gerwin RD, Dommerholt J, Shah JP. An expansion of Simons' integrated hypothesis of trigger point formation. *Curr Pain Headache Rep*. 2004;8(6):468-475.
45. Hsieh YL, Kao MJ, Kuan TS, Chen SM, Chen JT, Hong CZ. Dry needling to a key myofascial trigger point may reduce the irritability of satellite MTrPs. *Am J Phys Med Rehabil*. 2007;86(5):397-403.
46. Goodman CC, Fuller KS. *Pathology: Implications for the Physical Therapist*. 5th ed. St. Louis, MO: Saunders Elsevier; 2009.
47. Boissonnault WG. *Primary Care for the Physical Therapist*. 2nd ed. Philadelphia, PA: Elsevier/Saunders; 2010.
48. Goodman CC, Snyder TEK. *Differential Diagnosis for Physical Therapists: Screening for Referral*. 5th ed. St. Louis, MO: Saunders Elsevier; 2013.

49. Szeto GP, Straker L, Raine S. A field comparison of neck and shoulder postures in symptomatic and asymptomatic office workers. *Appl Ergon.* 2002;33(1):75-84.
50. Helgadottir H, Kristjansson E, Mottram S, Karduna AR, Jonsson H Jr. Altered scapular orientation during arm elevation in patients with insidious onset neck pain and whiplash-associated disorder. *J Orthop Sports Phys Ther.* 2010;40(12):784-791.
51. Cools AM, Struyf F, De Mey K, Maenhout A, Castelein B, Cagnie B. Rehabilitation of scapular dyskinesis: from the office worker to the elite overhead athlete. *Br J Sports Med.* 2014;48(8):692-697.
52. Cagnie B, Struyf F, Cools A, Castelein B, Danneels L, O'Leary S. The relevance of scapular dysfunction in neck pain: a brief commentary. *J Orthop Sports Phys Ther.* 2014;44(6):435-439.
53. Wainner RS, Whitman JM, Cleland JA, Flynn TW. Regional interdependence: a musculoskeletal examination model whose time has come. *J Orthop Sports Phys Ther.* 2007;37(11):658-660.
54. Sueki DG, Cleland JA, Wainner RS. A regional interdependence model of musculoskeletal dysfunction: research, mechanisms, and clinical implications. *J Man Manip Ther.* 2013;21(2):90-102.
55. Warmerdam A. *Manual Therapy: Improving Muscle and Joint Functioning.* Wantagh, NY: Pine Publications; 1999.
56. Isaacs ER, Bookhout MR. *Bourdillon's Spinal Manipulation.* 6th ed. Wodurn, MA: Butterworth-Heinemann; 2002.
57. DiGiovanna EL, Schiowitz S, Dowling DJ. *An Osteopathic Approach to Diagnosis and Treatment.* 3rd ed. Philadelphia, PA: Wolters Kluwer; 2005.
58. Gibbons P, Tehan P. *Manipulation of the Spine, Thorax and Pelvis: An Osteopathic Perspective.* 3rd ed. St. Louis, MO: Elsevier 2010.
59. DeStefano L. *Greenman's Principles of Manual Medicine.* 5th ed. Philadelphia, PA: Wolters Kluwer; 2016.

Chapter 28

Deltoid Muscle

"Overt Botherer"

Joseph M. Donnelly and Leigh E. Palubinskas

1. INTRODUCTION

The deltoid muscle consists of three parts that together form the rounded shape of the shoulder area. The anterior deltoid portion originates from the anterior border and superior surface of the lateral one-third of the clavicle. The middle deltoid portion originates from the lateral margin and superior surface of the acromion. The posterior deltoid portion originates from the lower edge of the crest of the spine of the scapula. All three portions insert onto the deltoid tubercle of the humerus. The deltoid muscle is innervated by the axillary nerve. The anterior, middle, and posterior deltoid portions can function individually or in conjunction with one another to perform motion at the glenohumeral joint. Simultaneous contraction of the anterior, middle, and posterior parts of the deltoid muscle abduct the arm, with the middle deltoid generating the most abduction force. The anterior fibers are active during forward elevation and adduction of the glenohumeral joint, whereas the posterior fibers function to extend the shoulder and externally rotate the humerus. Trigger points (TrPs) in the deltoid muscle do not refer pain to distant areas; the pain is localized and rarely refers past the elbow. A patient with deltoid TrPs typically reports having shoulder pain, particularly with an active movement of the glenohumeral joint. Pain may be felt deeply when moving the humerus into horizontal adduction across the front of the chest and rotating the humerus internally and externally during functional activities. Activating and perpetuating factors for TrPs in this muscle include impact trauma from contact sports or getting hit by a ball, sudden overload to the muscles in an effort to break a fall, poor workstation setup, and repetitive activities. Deltoid TrPs are commonly misdiagnosed as rotator cuff (RTC) tears, bicipital tendinitis, subdeltoid bursitis, glenohumeral joint arthritis, subacromial pain (impingement) syndrome, or C5 radicular pain. Corrective actions for this muscle include addressing ergonomic setup, wearing protective padding during contact sports, ensuring proper arm support during exercise, and performing self-pressure release of TrPs.

2. ANATOMIC CONSIDERATIONS

The deltoid muscle is a large muscle that forms the rounded shape of the shoulder.[1] It is divided into three parts: the anterior, the middle, and the posterior fibers. The directions of the anterior and the posterior fibers are essentially parallel to each other, covering the anterior and the posterior aspects of the shoulder. The anterior and the posterior fibers exhibit a fusiform arrangement of long fiber bundles that extend directly from the origin to the insertion. The middle deltoid fibers are multipennate in their structure. The muscle fibers of the entire muscle converge distally near the midpoint of the lateral aspect of the shaft of the humerus and attach to the deltoid tubercle near the brachialis origin.[2] The muscle also gives off an expansion into the deep brachial fascia that may reach the forearm and allows for reciprocal feedback between the muscles and fascia of the upper arm and the forearm during functional activities.[3]

Anterior Deltoid Fibers

The anterior fibers of the deltoid muscle originate from the anterior border and the superior surface of the lateral one-third of the clavicle and travel posterolaterally to insert midshaft on the lateral aspect of the humerus at the deltoid tubercle (Figure 28-1). The distal tendon is thick and fibrous and joins the middle and posterior deltoid fibers to form a central tendon at the insertion on the lateral tubercle.[2]

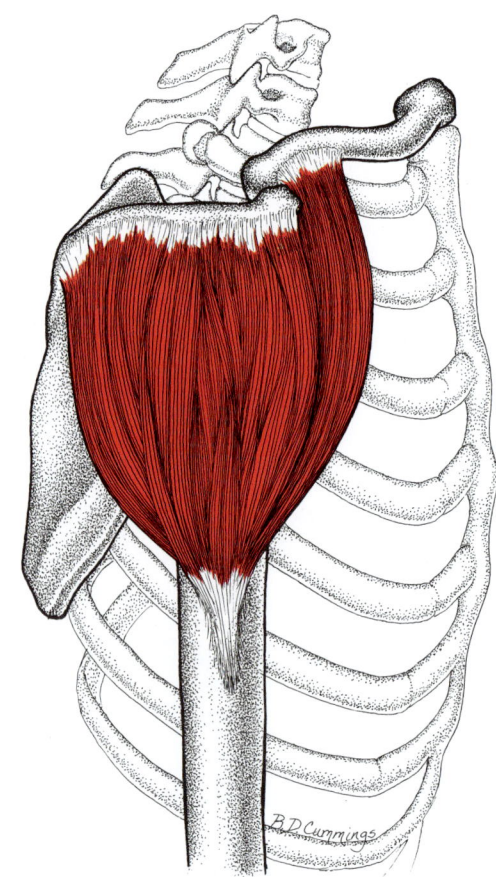

Figure 28-1. Attachments of the right deltoid muscle (dark red). Compare the diagonal and complexly interwoven fibers of the middle fibers with the simple fusiform arrangement in the anterior and posterior fibers. The schematic of Figure 28-3 shows how, in principle, these fiber arrangements affect endplate distribution.

Middle Deltoid Fibers

The middle fibers originate from the lateral margin and the superior surface of the acromion and travel inferiorly to join the anterior and posterior deltoid muscle bellies to insert midshaft on the lateral tubercle of the humerus. The middle deltoid fibers are multipennate and slant obliquely between proximal tendons (usually four) that extend downward from the acromion into the substance of the muscle. Three interdigitating tendons extend upward from the lateral tubercle and are connected by short muscle fibers that generate powerful traction.[2]

Posterior Deltoid Fibers

The posterior fibers originate on the lower edge of the crest of the spine of the scapula and travel anterolaterally and join the middle and anterior fibers to insert midshaft on the lateral tubercle of the humerus. Its fiber direction is essentially parallel to the anterior fibers.[2]

2.1. Innervation and Vascularization

The deltoid muscle is innervated by the anterior rami of the C5 and C6 spinal roots via a branch of the posterior cord known as the axillary nerve. The axillary nerve divides into anterior and posterior branches just distal to the subscapularis muscle. The anterior branch innervates the anterior and middle deltoid muscles and the posterior branch innervates the posterior deltoid and teres minor muscles.[4] Loukas et al[5] analyzed 100 nerve specimens from 50 cadavers and in 18% of the cases, the anterior branch of the axillary nerve provided a branch to the posterior part of the deltoid muscle, and in 38% of specimens the middle part of the deltoid muscle received dual innervation from both the anterior and posterior parts of the axillary nerve.

The deltoid muscle receives its vascularization via the deltoid branches of the thoracoacromial, and acromial arteries, and the anterior and posterior circumflex humeral arteries. The deltoid branches of the thoracoacromial and acromial arteries supply the anterior deltoid muscle and the posterior circumflex humeral artery supplies the middle and posterior fibers of the muscle. The anterior circumflex humeral artery also supplies the anterior fibers of the deltoid muscle.[2]

2.2. Function

The anterior, middle, and posterior deltoid muscles can act separately or in conjunction with one another to generate motion at the glenohumeral joint. The efficiency of the deltoid muscle is dependent on the health of the RTC muscles because movements of the shoulder girdle are complex and require coordinated muscle activation patterns.[6] A simultaneous contraction of the anterior, middle, and posterior fibers of the deltoid muscle contribute to shoulder elevation.[2]

Earlier it was thought that the deltoid and the supraspinatus muscles had different activation patterns during shoulder abduction. However, the electrical activity of both the deltoid and supraspinatus muscles increases progressively throughout abduction. With elevation in the plane of the scapula, the supraspinatus muscle activity is higher in the first arc of motion and the anterior and middle deltoid muscle bellies have higher activity in the second and third arcs of motion. This is primarily due to the differing lengths of the lever arms of each muscle as they move through the shoulder elevation motion. Electromyography (EMG) activity was found to be greatest in the middle deltoid and supraspinatus muscles in the 30° to 60° range of scapular elevation.[7] Witte et al[8] found a significant increase in deltoid muscle activation (all three portions) in response to glenohumeral elevation moments. The supraspinatus muscle response to increasing glenohumeral moments was highly variable without a consistent increase in activity. They conclude that the deltoid and supraspinatus muscles may contribute to glenohumeral moments in a complimentary manner.

Other authors have also found utilizing surface and fine wire EMG that the deltoid (all portions), supraspinatus, infraspinatus, upper trapezius, lower trapezius, and serratus anterior muscles all activate prior to the onset of the humerus motion during coronal plane abduction, elevation in the plane of the scapula, and elevation in the sagittal plane.[6,9] This activation pattern was observed regardless of the external load of the arm.[6] Peak activity of the middle deltoid fibers was observed at 100° abduction, anterior deltoid fibers at 125°, and posterior deltoid fibers at 140°.[9]

Anterior Deltoid Fibers

During shoulder flexion, the anterior deltoid fibers, supraspinatus, infraspinatus, pectoralis major, serratus anterior, upper and lower trapezius muscles activate moderately prior to limb movement and increase proportionally with a 20% and 60% load of the subject's repetition maximum.[10] In an older study, the anterior deltoid fibers were recruited most strongly when flexion and adduction movements were combined to move the arm obliquely upward inclining toward midline.[11] The attachments of the anterior deltoid fibers appear as though they should internally rotate the arm, but the use of this action is questioned by electromyographers and the deltoid muscle appears to contribute little to internal or external rotation.[12] However, when the humerus is rotated internally to 45° during an elevation task, the anterior deltoid muscle is maximally activated. In fact, during pushing the anterior deltoid muscle is maximally active.[13]

Middle Deltoid Fibers

The middle fibers of the deltoid muscle are designed structurally for abduction, during which they show strong EMG response. The linear increase in EMG activity during abduction of the arm indicates a primary abduction function of the middle part of these fibers with a peak activity at 110° abduction.[9] With increasing loads, the middle deltoid muscle activation pattern increased similarly to the supraspinatus muscle pattern, systematically supporting the "law of proportional activation."[14] The activation pattern of abduction in the plane of the scapula is established with low loads and is maintained as the load is increased in subjects with no history of neck or shoulder dysfunction.[14] However, during flexion, a nonlinear increase in the activity of the middle fibers between 60° and 90° of arm elevation indicates that its flexor action is enhanced as arm elevation increases,[15] and an overall increase in maximal voluntary contraction was noted with an external load in the upper extremity.[10] Gregory et al[16] investigated the role of the middle deltoid fibers in the elevation and coaptation of the glenohumeral joint in five healthy subjects and 10 with full-thickness RTC tears. They found that the anterior fibers of the middle deltoid muscle have an increased coaptation role in elevation and may improve shoulder function in the presence of an RTC tear. They conclude that a stronger efficient anterior portion of the middle deltoid muscle may assist a weakened RTC during elevation due to its coaptation forces.[16] During pushing, the middle deltoid fibers were found to be moderately active along with the pectoralis major, infraspinatus, biceps brachii, and triceps brachii muscles.[13]

Posterior Deltoid Fibers

The posterior fibers of the deltoid muscle extend the arm with the latissimus dorsi and teres major muscles. This function is essential to reach behind the body for dressing and toileting activities. Anatomically, the posterior fibers should assist the external rotation of the shoulder,[2] but that function has not been substantiated electromyographically. It is now thought that these fibers do not lend a significant clinical contribution to the rotational movement of the shoulder.[17] The moment arms of the middle and posterior deltoid muscles also increased with rotation, but the changes were not considered clinically relevant.[17] In addition to shoulder extension, the posterior deltoid fibers act during abduction in the coronal plane and elevation in the plane of scapula and in the forward elevation of the shoulder. However, Wickham et al[9] found that the peak activity of the posterior deltoid fibers was at 140° of abduction in the coronal plane and this activity was thought to counterbalance the abduction moment. The posterior deltoid muscle was found to be maximally active during pulling activity and during quick throwing activities.[13]

Driving a car with the hands on top of the steering wheel chiefly activated the anterior, and to a lesser extent the middle, part(s) of the muscle.[18] When the steering wheel is held in the center position, there is a co-contraction of shoulder muscles to stabilize the wheel. During steering maneuvers, the posterior deltoid fibers provide the greatest contribution as steering torque increases.[18]

During freestyle swimming, of which the crawl stroke has been studied the most,[19-21] an EMG analysis of 12 muscles found the anterior and middle deltoid fibers had an 80% maximal voluntary contraction during early to late recovery phases. In a study that looked at EMG activity in swimmers with painful shoulders, the normally marked increase in the middle deltoid fiber activity during the beginning and the end recovery phases was significantly inhibited. In the anterior deltoid muscle, the marked activity of the early recovery and the late recovery phases was significantly inhibited. Unfortunately, the structures responsible for the pain were not identified in this study.[19] Trigger points can cause this kind of a muscle inhibition when a person performs a well-learned and repetitive activity.

2.3. Functional Unit

The functional unit to which a muscle belongs includes the muscles that reinforce and counter its actions as well as the joints that the muscle crosses. The functional interdependence of these structures is reflected in the organization and neural connections of the sensory motor cortex. The functional unit is emphasized because the presence of a TrP in one muscle of the unit increases the likelihood that the other muscles of the unit will also develop TrPs. When inactivating TrPs in a muscle, one should be concerned about TrPs that may develop in muscles that are functionally interdependent. Box 28-1 grossly represents the functional unit of the deltoid muscle.[22]

The supraspinatus, infraspinatus, subscapularis, upper trapezius, lower trapezius, and serratus anterior muscles act synergistically during abduction in the coronal plane (shoulder abduction), elevation in the plane of the scapula, and elevation in the sagittal plane (shoulder flexion).

3. CLINICAL PRESENTATION

3.1. Referred Pain Pattern

Trigger points in the anterior deltoid fibers (Figure 28-2A) refer pain to the anterior and middle areas of the shoulder[23,24] and the anterolateral aspect of the upper arm. Trigger points in the posterior deltoid muscle (Figure 28-2B) refer pain that concentrates over the posterior shoulder area, sometimes referring into the adjacent posterior aspect of the upper extremity. Trigger points in the middle deltoid muscle produce pain centered in that region of the shoulder with some referred pain to adjacent areas (Figure 28-2C). Typically, pain is deeply localized to the shoulder and rarely refers past the elbow. The deltoid muscle lacks any distant projection of referred pain. Referred pain from this muscle was demonstrated experimentally by the injection of hypertonic saline.[25]

3.2. Symptoms

Trigger points in the anterior deltoid muscle cause pain in the front of the shoulder and may refer into the front of the upper arm. In contrast, TrPs in the posterior deltoid muscle cause pain in the back of the shoulder with referral occasionally into the back and side of the upper arm and less frequently in the front of the shoulder joint. Trigger points in the middle deltoid muscle most often cause pain only in the lateral aspect of the shoulder over the muscle belly, without referral into the upper arm. Clinical experience suggests that TrPs in the deltoid muscle are usually related to inhibition of the supraspinatus muscle caused by TrPs in that muscle.

Often, a patient with deltoid TrPs presents with symptoms that began after a traumatic impact to the shoulder during contact sports or other activities. Trigger points in the deltoid muscle can also be activated during repetitive strain injuries on work activities. In fact, Fernández de las Peñas et al[26] observed that manual and office workers had a similar number of TrPs in the shoulder muscles. Patients with TrPs in the deltoid muscle complain of pain that is deep in the shoulder area with active shoulder motion and, less frequently, of pain at rest (Figure 28-2). The patient with anterior deltoid TrPs has difficulty raising the upper extremity to the shoulder level and reaching behind the body at the shoulder level. A patient with multiple deltoid TrPs may present with impairment of strength or a total inability to raise the upper extremity to the shoulder level due to painful weakness. Hains et al[27] found that the application of ischemic compression on TrPs in the shoulder muscles, including the deltoid muscle, was effective for reducing the symptoms of patients experiencing chronic shoulder pain.

3.3. Patient Examination

After a thorough subjective examination, the clinician should make a detailed drawing representing the pain pattern that the patient has described. This depiction will assist in planning the physical examination and can be useful in monitoring the progression of the patient as symptoms improve or change. For effective examination of the deltoid muscle, the clinician should assess the shoulder girdle posture, active and passive ranges of motion of the shoulder, and scapulohumeral rhythm, paying close attention to muscle activation patterns. To identify TrPs in the deltoid muscle that may be limiting the range of motion and thus influencing dysfunction, the clinician should identify the limited range of motion by performing specific excitability testing for all parts of the deltoid muscle.

Box 28-1 Functional unit of the deltoid muscle

Action	Synergists	Antagonist
Shoulder abduction	Supraspinatus	Teres major Latissimus dorsi Pectoralis major
Shoulder flexion	Coracobrachialis Pectoralis major Biceps brachii long head	Triceps brachii long head Teres major Latissimus dorsi
Shoulder extension	Triceps brachii long head Teres major Latissimus dorsi	Coracobrachialis Pectoralis major Biceps brachii long head

Chapter 28: Deltoid Muscle 279

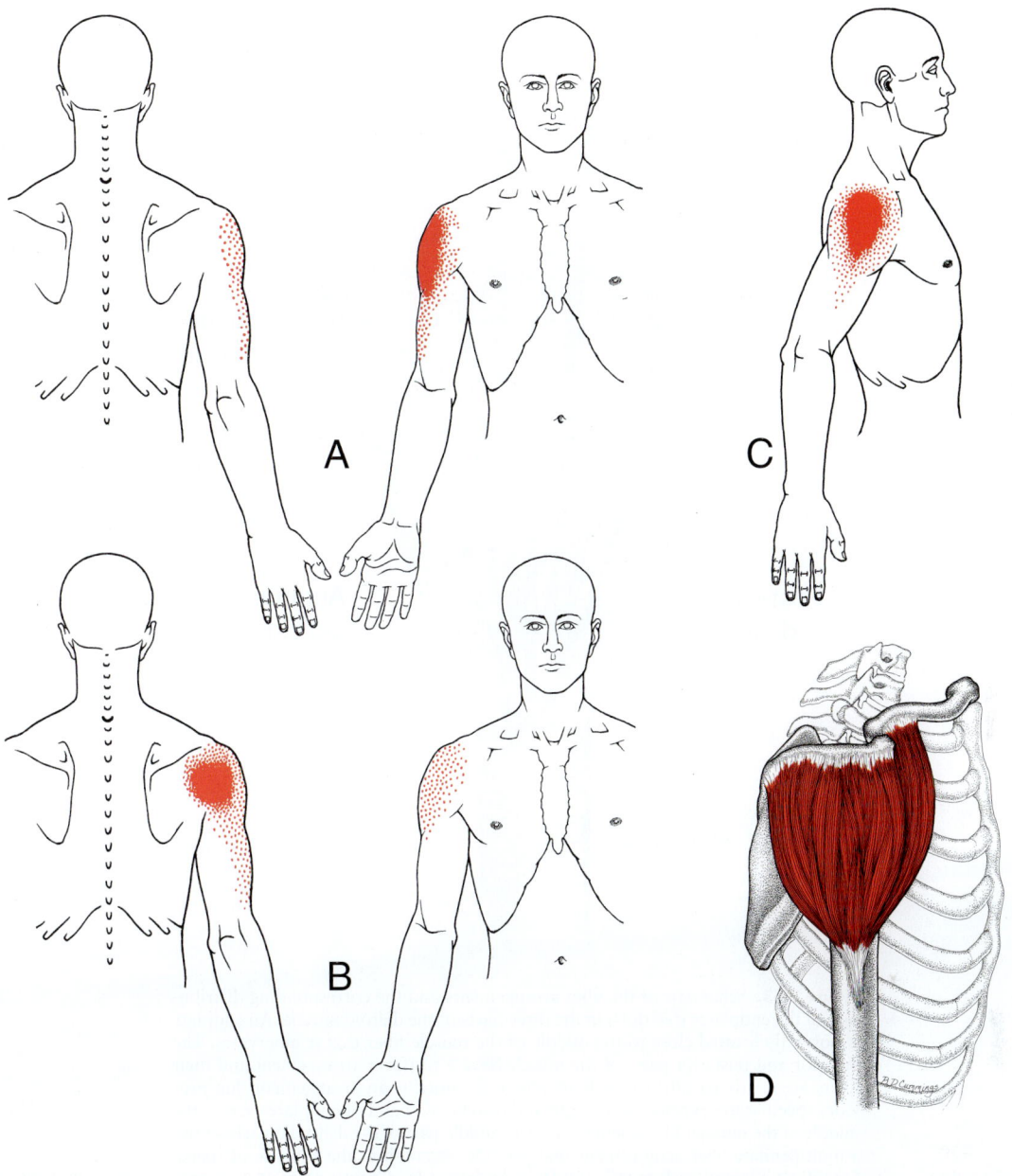

Figure 28-2. Referred pain patterns (dark red) from TrPs in the right deltoid muscle (light red). A, Pain pattern from TrPs in the anterior fibers of the muscle. B, Pain pattern from the posterior fibers. C, Pain pattern from TrPs in the middle fibers of the muscle. The distribution of TrPs in the anterior and posterior parts of the deltoid muscle has a different pattern from the distribution of TrPs in the middle deltoid muscle. Figure 28-3 provides a possible explanation for this clinical phenomenon. D, Right deltoid muscle.

Examination of muscle activation patterns is particularly important for individuals with TrPs of shoulder muscles because TrPs have been found to induce delayed and inconsistent activation of the upper trapezius and serratus anterior muscles during arm elevation.[28,29] Also, TrPs in the posterior deltoid fibers are able to reduce the efficiency of reciprocal inhibition of the anterior deltoid fibers during arm elevation.[30] In the light of the above findings and those of Bron et al,[31] 38% of patients with non-specific shoulder pain exhibited TrPs in the anterior fibers of the deltoid muscle, and a thorough examination of the deltoid muscle in any patient presenting with shoulder pain is very important.

Accessory joint motion of the glenohumeral, acromioclavicular, sternoclavicular, and scapulothoracic joints should be manually tested. Often, restrictions in the sternoclavicular joint can cause impairment in shoulder elevation, contributing to alterations in muscle activation patterns. Articular dysfunctions in the glenohumeral joint may also impair muscle activation patterns contributing to the overload of the deltoid muscle by inhibiting supraspinatus muscle function. Muscle-specific resisted testing should be carried out to identify impairments in muscle function and reproduction of painful symptoms.

Involvement of the anterior deltoid fibers impairs the performance of the Apley's extension, internal rotation, and adduction test (Figure 21-3A); whereas TrPs in the posterior deltoid fibers bar the execution of the Apley scratch test (flexion, abduction and external rotation) (Figure 21-3B): the arm can reach over the head but not behind it, secondary to pain induced by a forceful contraction of the affected posterior deltoid fibers in the shortened position.

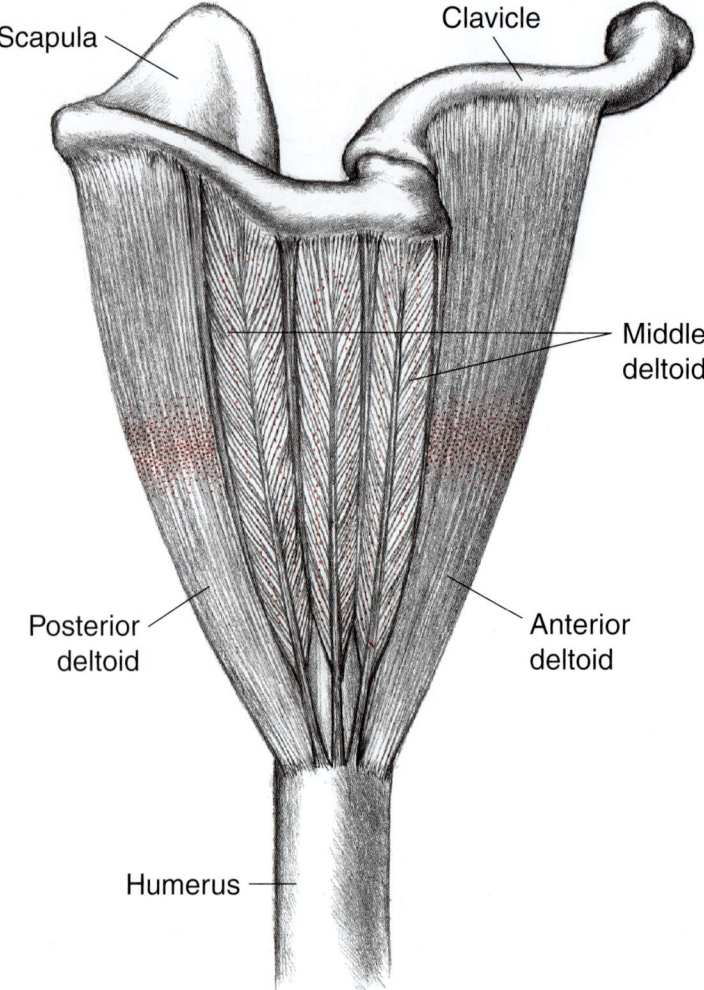

Figure 28-3. Schematic of the fiber arrangements and the corresponding distribution of the endplates (red dots) in the three parts of the deltoid muscle. An endplate is normally located close to the middle of the muscle fiber that it innervates. The anterior and posterior parts of the muscle have a fusiform arrangement and their fibers are nearly parallel to the long axis of the muscle, an arrangement that provides speed at the expense of strength and results in a band of endplates across the middle of the muscle. The schematic for the middle part of the deltoid muscle shows a multipennate fiber arrangement that provides strength at the expense of speed. Schematic adapted with permission from Anderson JE. *Grant's Atlas of Anatomy*. 7th ed. Baltimore, MD: Williams & Wilkins; 1978.

3.4. Trigger Point Examination

The deltoid muscle's superficial location makes it easy to palpate the muscle bellies utilizing cross-fiber flat palpation to identify a taut band and TrP. Examination is best performed with the arm slightly abducted (to ~30°) to relax the muscle. Bron et al[31] reported moderate reliability for palpation of TrPs in the anterior and middle fibers of the deltoid muscle. The most reliable characteristics identified by the study of Bron et al[32] were a palpable taut band, a jump sign, and the presence of referred pain.

The location of endplates in the deltoid muscle is illustrated schematically in Figure 28-3 and reflects the difference in endplate distribution within each part of the muscle. An endplate is normally located close to the mid-portion of the muscle fiber that it supplies. The endplate zone in a fusiform muscle, like the anterior and posterior deltoid fibers, is a single, sometimes irregular, band of motor endplates extending across the mid-portion of the muscle. However, the endplates in the angulated fibers of the middle deltoid are widely distributed throughout the muscle.[33] Therefore, TrPs in the deltoid muscle can be located in any fibers of the muscle. Clinicians should carefully explore all the fibers to determine the most affected portion.

Trigger points are common in patients complaining of shoulder pain. In a study of 72 subjects with chronic shoulder pain, 50% of patients had active TrPs in the middle deltoid fibers, 47% in the anterior deltoid muscle and 44% in the posterior deltoid fibers. The anterior fibers of the deltoid muscle also had a significant number of latent TrPs with 27% of the subjects affected.[31] Deltoid TrPs have also been associated with whiplash-associated disorders[34] and work-related shoulder and neck complaints.[26] Trigger point involvement exclusive to the deltoid muscle is rare. During the examination, muscles that typically have associated TrPs should be evaluated and treated for full resolution of shoulder pain complaints.

Anterior Deltoid Fibers

Cross-fiber flat palpation of the muscle fibers is utilized to identify the taut bands associated with anterior deltoid TrPs (Figure 28-4A). Trigger points in this portion of the muscle are readily identifiable.

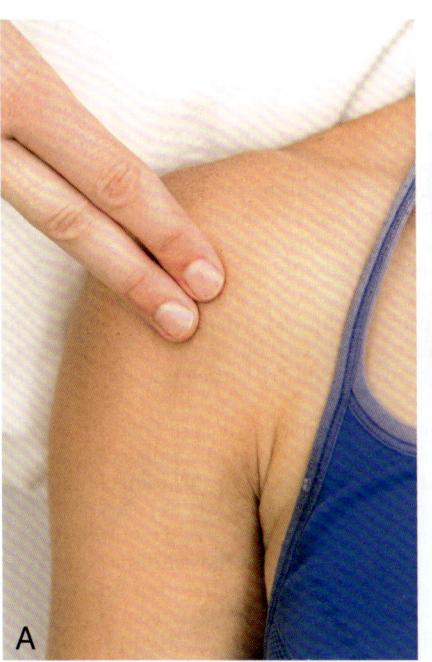
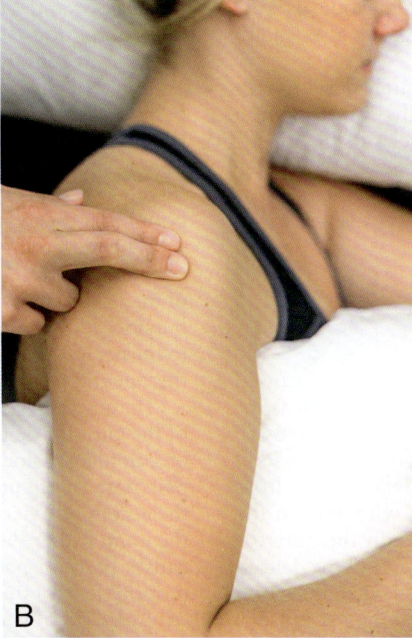
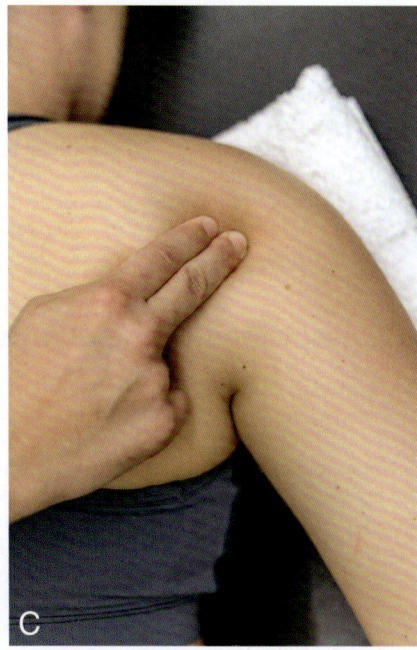

Figure 28-4. Cross-fiber flat palpation to identify trigger points in the (A) anterior, (B) middle, and (C) posterior fibers of the deltoid muscle.

Middle Deltoid Fibers

Trigger points in the middle fibers of the deltoid muscle may develop almost anywhere along the length of the muscle belly because this middle part of the muscle is multipennate and its motor endplates are widely distributed. Tenderness from enthesopathy of the supraspinatus attachment at the superior facet of the greater tuberosity of the humerus can be confused with tenderness associated with deltoid muscle TrPs. To differentiate tenderness from supraspinatus enthesopathy and that of a deltoid TrP, the arm is passively abducted to 90°, which protects the supraspinatus muscle attachment from digital pressure beneath the acromion while the deltoid TrPs remain tender to palpation (Figure 28-4B).

Posterior Deltoid Fibers

Posterior deltoid TrPs are typically located along the posterior margin of the muscle, slightly more distal than those of the anterior fibers. Cross-fiber flat palpation along the muscle belly should be utilized to identify TrPs in this portion of the muscle (Figure 28-4C).

4. DIFFERENTIAL DIAGNOSIS

4.1. Activation and Perpetuation of Trigger Points

A posture or activity that activates a TrP, if not corrected, can also perpetuate it. In any part of the deltoid muscle, TrPs may be activated by unaccustomed eccentric loading, eccentric exercise in an unconditioned muscle, or maximal or submaximal concentric loading.[35] Trigger points may also be activated or aggravated when the muscle is placed in a shortened and/or lengthened position for an extended period of time. Trauma is a common cause of TrP formation in the deltoid muscle. The deltoid muscle is often overloaded in athletic activities such as swimming, overhead throwing, tennis, weight lifting, and skiing. Many of these activities require forceful flexion that can overload the deltoid muscle. Impact trauma may occur from a hit by a tennis or golf ball, from falling directly on the muscle, or from collisions during contact sports. The repeated recoil of a gun when shooting can also cause traumatization of the anterior deltoid muscle. Trauma by sudden overload can occur during a loss of balance when going down steps and reaching out to a bannister or railing to "catch a fall" causing a sudden overexertion and overstretch trauma to the deltoid muscle. Whiplash-associated disorders can be exacerbated by TrPs that form in the shoulder and cervical muscles as a result of trauma from a motor vehicle accident and are often the cause of the intractable neck and shoulder pain or headaches suffered by these patients.[34] Carrying heavy objects or lifting and holding children may also overload the deltoid and RTC muscles.

Trigger point formation in the anterior deltoid muscle can be caused by overload activation of the muscle, such as holding a power tool at the shoulder height or working at an improperly adjusted workspace. Improper ergonomics of an office workstation can cause increased and sustained activity in the deltoid muscle. Conte et al[36] investigated muscle co-contractions in the trunk and upper arm muscles utilizing superficial EMG during controlled use of a computer touch pad and a traditional mouse control. These authors found that even though the use of the mouse required shoulder abduction, the use of the touchpad required a greater degree of movement accuracy and therefore more stabilization of the shoulder. They conclude that the use of a mouse with a laptop may reduce biomechanical risks for injury of shoulder and upper arm injuries.[36]

Repetitive activities that require work with the arms elevated to shoulder or eye height for hours at a time may activate TrPs and can perpetuate them if the task is continued without alteration. Workers with chronic arm, neck, and shoulder pain often have TrPs in the shoulder and the cervical musculature including the deltoid muscle.[26] As expected, sustained computer work and poor posture may predispose subjects to increased TrP prevalence. Also, the prevalence of TrPs is similar between desk and manual workers, suggesting that they overuse the same muscles even though their work activities may be very different.[26]

Repetitive overuse is also seen in competitive overhead athletes. The overhead volleyball or tennis serve can cause repetitive strain and TrP formation in the deltoid muscle. Osborne and Gatt[37] identified TrPs in volleyball players that developed after several long days of training and tournament play. Release of the TrPs restored an active range of motion and allowed the athletes to quickly return to competitive play. Episodic overexertion, such as unaccustomed deep-sea fishing, can also lead to TrP formation in the anterior deltoid fibers.

The posterior fibers of the deltoid muscle rarely develop TrPs as the result of activity in isolation. Typically, TrP formation occurs in association with TrPs in other muscles of the kinetic chain. However, specific overexercise may activate TrPs in the posterior deltoid muscle and may occur from activities such as excessive poling when skiing, or other repetitive exercises that require a pulling action.[13]

4.2. Associated Trigger Points

Associated TrPs can develop in the referred pain areas caused by TrPs.[37] Therefore, musculature in the referred pain areas for each muscle should also be considered. Often, release of the TrP in the associated muscle allows for an immediate decrease in the pressure pain threshold of the associated TrPs in the deltoid muscle.[38] This relationship is most common with TrPs in the infraspinatus muscle causing associated TrPs in the anterior deltoid muscle. Trigger points in the anterior part of the deltoid muscle are often associated with TrPs in the clavicular section of the pectoralis major muscle, the pectoralis minor muscle, the biceps brachii muscle, and in the posterior fibers of the deltoid muscle.

When a TrP is identified in posterior deltoid fibers, one should also examine the proximal third of the long head of the triceps brachii, the latissimus dorsi, and the teres major muscles for associated TrPs. The teres minor fibers are only aligned with the posterior deltoid muscle when the arm is held in full abduction; therefore, it is less likely to develop associated TrPs. Isolated TrPs in the posterior deltoid fibers rarely occur unless TrPs become activated by local injection of an irritant solution into the muscle. In these instances, the TrP activity tends to be self-sustaining.

Because the deltoid muscle lies in the referred pain areas of both the infraspinatus and supraspinatus muscles, it rarely escapes the development of associated TrPs when these muscles have TrPs. Hong[39] reported that TrPs in the scalene or supraspinatus muscles can induce associated TrPs in the deltoid muscle. Pressure was applied to a TrP in the infraspinatus muscle, which caused referred pain over the front area of the shoulder. The pressure caused increased motor unit activity, or referred spasm, in the anterior deltoid muscle while recording needles in the biceps and triceps brachii muscles showed electrical silence.[38] Release of the TrP in the infraspinatus muscle caused a decrease in the pain pressure threshold of the TrP in the anterior deltoid muscle, despite the fact that no treatment was performed on the deltoid muscle.

If inactivation of deltoid TrPs restores only about 90° of abduction, then any active supraspinatus TrPs should be located and eliminated. This intervention usually restores the full range of arm motion in the overhead position, unless antagonists to shoulder abduction are also involved. Trigger points in the antagonists can negatively affect shoulder elevation. When TrPs are present in the posterior deltoid muscle, there is decreased reciprocal inhibition of the muscle during shoulder elevation.[30] This relationship can cause reduced efficiency of movement, which may lead to decreased muscle relaxation, disordered muscle activation patterns, and a sustained muscle overload to the anterior deltoid muscle. These are all precursors to TrP formation in the muscle agonist.

4.3. Associated Pathology

Deltoid TrPs are commonly misdiagnosed as RTC tears, bicipital tendinitis, subdeltoid bursitis, glenohumeral joint arthritis, impingement syndrome, or C5 radiculopathy. These conditions need to be considered in the differential diagnosis of shoulder pain symptoms. They may cause deep shoulder pain and tenderness and referred pain similar to that from deltoid TrPs, but they lack the specific physical signs of palpable bands, spot tenderness, and local twitch responses in the muscle. One of these conditions often coexist with deltoid TrPs, and in these cases, both conditions should be treated.

Referred pain from any part of the deltoid muscle can mimic pain arising from the glenohumeral joint[40] and thus, can easily be misdiagnosed as arthritis of that joint. Any TrP in the deltoid muscle should be inactivated and the therapeutic response observed before deciding to inject the shoulder joint. Sometimes both the muscle and the joint have to be treated.

When attention is directed only to the subacromial area of referred pain and tenderness, and TrPs in any or all three parts of the deltoid muscle are overlooked, a diagnosis of "subdeltoid bursitis" is often rendered. A normal bursa may then be injected, to the neglect of the active deltoid TrPs, often resulting in a poor therapeutic result.

The acromioclavicular joint underlies the proximal attachment of the anterior deltoid muscle. Pain due to sprain, subluxation, or complete dislocation or separation of this joint mimics the pain pattern of anterior deltoid TrPs, or vice versa. A sprain of the acromioclavicular joint produces localized tenderness over the joint, rather than TrP tenderness in the deltoid muscle, and causes pain on passive mobilization of the joint and by arm motion that rotates or elevates the scapula. Acromioclavicular subluxation and dislocation are more likely during sports activities and following an automobile accident in which the patient was holding on to the steering wheel or stretched the arm out for protection. Passive horizontal abduction is painful at the acromioclavicular joint if it is involved.

Adhesive capsulitis, or frozen shoulder, is a condition of unknown etiology that will limit the available range of motion at the glenohumeral joint and is associated with considerable pain during active and passive movements of the shoulder. Often, these patients have TrPs present in the scapulothoracic and glenohumeral muscles, particularly the subscapularis muscle, which can contribute to the patient's pain and cause limited motion. Clewley et al[41] treated a patient with adhesive capsulitis using TrP release. When an initial bout of cervicothoracic and thoracic thrust manipulation of the spine was ineffective, the surrounding shoulder musculature was evaluated for TrPs. They found TrPs present in the upper trapezius, levator scapula, deltoid, and infraspinatus muscles. Often the subscapularis muscle is also involved. Trigger point release by dry needling reduced the patient's pain significantly after two visits, which allowed for improved shoulder motion during functional activities and the introduction of higher grades of manual intervention for further progression of motion.[41] This case demonstrates that releasing the TrPs decreases the pain and may allow for improved motion so that further manual treatment options may be tolerable for the patient.

5. CORRECTIVE ACTIONS

Chronic shoulder pain in desk workers has been associated with both active and latent TrPs in the shoulder muscles including the deltoid muscle.[26,31] As stated earlier, a poor ergonomic setup can cause prolonged strain through the deltoid muscle, and this may be a main generator of neck and shoulder pain for employees who work long hours at a desk. Therefore, a thorough ergonomic assessment of the workspace and proper adjustment of the keyboard so that the elbow is supported at approximately 90° of flexion helps decrease the overload to the muscle and potentially eliminate pain. Several checklists can be found on the Internet regarding proper workstation arrangement and many companies have employees on staff who can provide an ergonomic assessment of a workspace. Physical or occupational therapists may be consulted to provide proper recommendations for adjustments to improve comfort.

In addition to postural adjustments, other mechanical stress factors also need to be corrected. Heavy lifting should be performed with the arm rotated such that the thumb is turned in the direction that unloads the affected part of the deltoid muscle. To effectively unload the anterior deltoid fibers, the arm should be rotated externally. Internal rotation thus unloads the posterior fibers.

The patient should take precautions on stairs and prevent potential deltoid muscle overload that can result from being forced to quickly grab a hand railing. Traversing stairs slowly while holding onto railings, in addition to visually watching foot placement, may prevent a near fall and recurrence of muscle overload.

Athletes participating in contact sports should use protective padding over the anterior portion of the shoulder. Shooting enthusiasts should place a pad in front of the shoulder or use a garment specifically designed to minimize the direct trauma of gun recoil. This helps prevent further pain and irritation and helps prevent TrP formation.

Supporting the arm with a towel roll in the axilla during targeted exercises and placing the shoulder in 30° of abduction do not alter middle deltoid muscle activation but significantly increases posterior deltoid activation. In a side-lying position, using a towel roll in the axilla increases the maximal voluntary contraction of the posterior deltoid muscle, while significantly decreasing it in the middle deltoid muscle. Utilization of a towel roll in standing and side-lying should be considered for focused training of the posterior deltoid muscle or relaxation of the middle deltoid muscle.[42,43] Investigators have demonstrated that prone horizontal abduction at 90° abduction with full external rotation[44] or 100° abduction with full external rotation[43] produces 80% to 88% maximal voluntary contraction of the middle and posterior deltoid portions, respectively. Although the deltoid muscle does not have a specific role in the rotation of the humerus, internal and external rotation exercises in standing can be used as a starting point for neuromuscular reeducation of this muscle.[42-44]

Trigger point pressure release applied with the deltoid muscle relaxed in a position of ease (supported at about 45° of abduction is optimal) can be particularly effective (Figure 28-5). Pressure should be uncomfortable but tolerable, and it can be effectively applied for bouts as short as 15 seconds in duration.[26] If the TrP is not readily accessible for digital compression, a tennis ball can be used against a wall to apply pressure over the TrP. Patients can also use commercially available tools to assist with pressure application.

Clinicians can teach the patient self-pressure release of TrPs in the deltoid muscle. Daily gentle passive stretching of the affected part of the muscle may also be performed for pain relief and to maintain gains achieved after TrP release (Figure 28-6A and B). These stretches can be performed under a warm shower with water directed over the muscle for increased comfort during stretching.

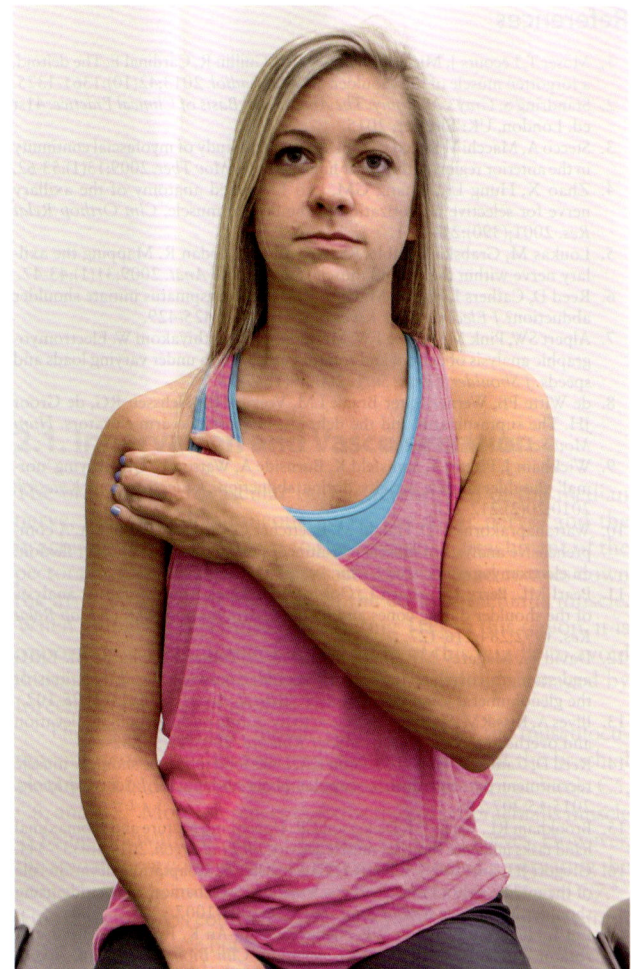

Figure 28-5. Self-pressure release of TrPs of anterior fibers of the deltoid.

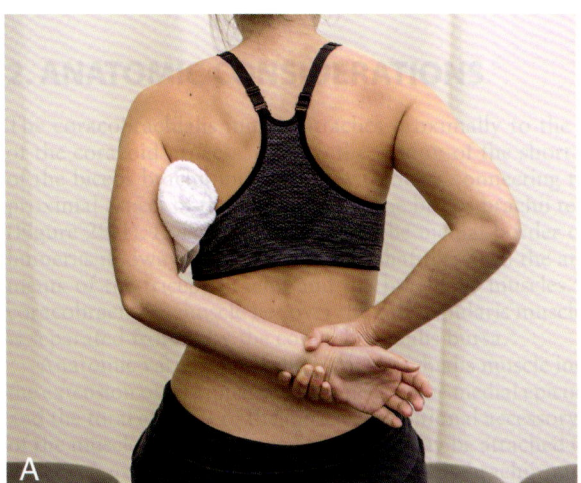
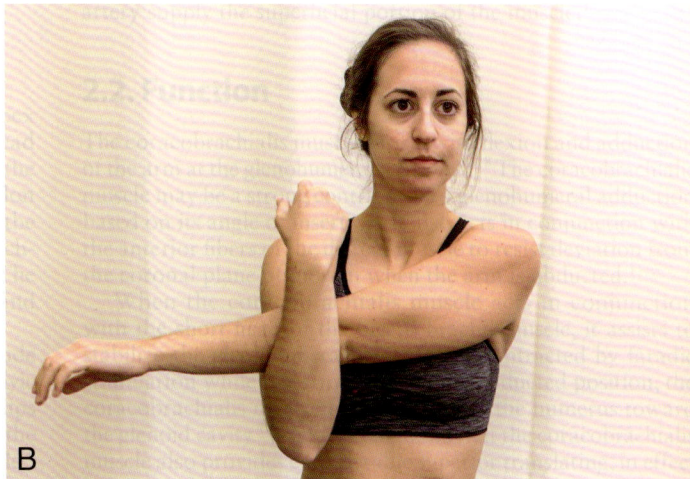

Figure 28-6. Self-stretch of deltoid muscle. A, Middle fibers. B, Posterior fibers.

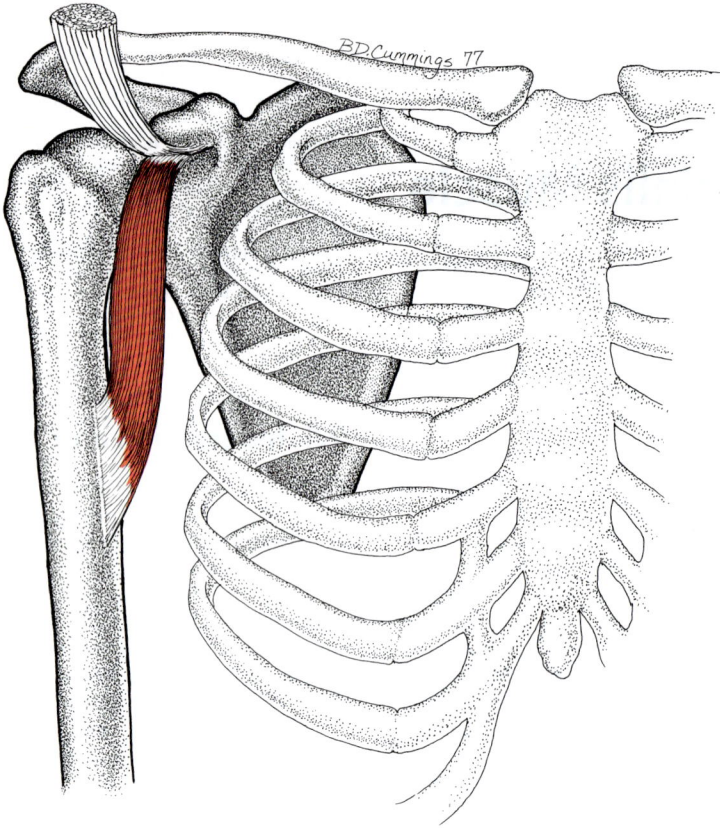

Figure 29-1. Usual attachments of the coracobrachialis muscle (red): proximally to the tip of the coracoid process, and distally to a line along the humerus extending almost to midshaft. The short head of the biceps brachii muscle (which has been cut and turned up) has a shared origin with the coracobrachialis muscle at the coracoid process.

Box 29-1 Functional unit of the coracobrachialis muscle

Action	Synergists	Antagonist
Shoulder flexion	Deltoid (anterior fibers) Biceps brachii short head Pectoralis major	Teres major Latissimus dorsi Triceps brachii long head Deltoid (posterior fibers)
Shoulder adduction	Teres major Latissimus dorsi Pectoralis major	Deltoid Supraspinatus

when the arm is moved into abduction.[20] When the shoulder is moved into extension, the coracobrachialis muscle provides an anterior stabilizing force to the humeral head. This function is most prevalent when confirmed anterior shoulder instability is present, and therefore, the coracobrachialis muscle provides positional dynamic stability as it wraps across the anterior humeral head just over the subscapularis muscle.

The muscle's insertion on the medial shaft of the humerus allows it to be elongated by both internal and external rotation of the shoulder. It has been reported that the muscle assists in returning the arm to neutral from these positions.[3,18]

2.3. Functional Unit

The functional unit to which a muscle belongs includes the muscles that reinforce and counter its actions as well as the joints that the muscle crosses. The functional interdependence of these structures is reflected in the organization and neural connections of the sensory motor cortex. The functional unit is emphasized because the presence of a TrP in one muscle of the unit increases the likelihood that the other muscles of the unit also develops TrPs. When inactivating TrPs in a muscle, one should be concerned about TrPs that may develop in muscles that are functionally interdependent. Box 29-1 grossly represents the functional unit of the coracobrachialis muscle.[21]

3. CLINICAL PRESENTATION

3.1. Referred Pain Pattern

Referred pain from TrPs in the coracobrachialis muscle is primarily located in the anterior aspect of the shoulder in the region of the anterior fibers of the deltoid muscle (Figure 29-2). Pain may also spread down the posterior aspect of the arm, concentrating over the triceps brachii muscle, the dorsum of the forearm, and the dorsum of the hand extending to the tip of the middle finger. Often, the elbow and wrist joints are not involved in the patient's report of symptoms.

The more active the TrPs, the greater the extent of the referred pain, the more intense the pain, and the more likely the pain is to persist at rest. Also, the TrPs are tenderer, the taut bands are tenser, and the local twitch responses are more vigorous.

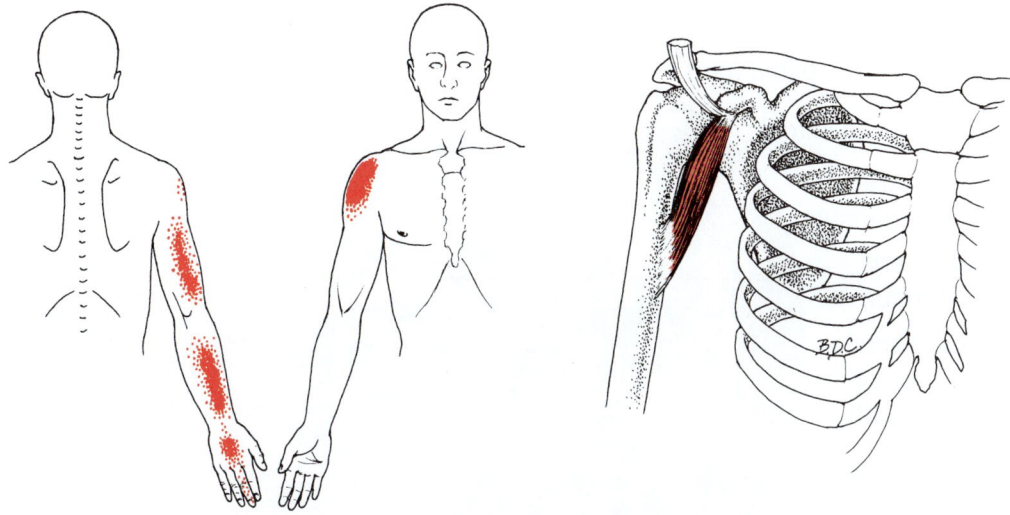

Figure 29-2. Pain pattern (red) referred from a TrP in the right coracobrachialis muscle. Trigger points are likely to be found as far distally as the middle of the muscle belly. In patients with milder involvement, the pain may extend only to the elbow.

3.2. Symptoms

Trigger points in the coracobrachialis muscle should be considered when the patient reports having upper limb pain, particularly in the front of the shoulder or the back of the arm. Patients with TrPs in the coracobrachialis muscle may experience pain and difficulty when reaching behind the body and across the lower back. The patient may report pain when reaching into a back pocket or tucking in a shirt. When only the coracobrachialis muscle is involved, neither reaching the arm up nor reaching out to the side with the elbow bent (as in touching the top of the head) is painful. However, reaching up into full forward elevation and then moving the arm behind the ear toward the middle of the body causes pain because of the contraction of the coracobrachialis muscle in the shortened position.

3.3. Patient Examination

After a thorough subjective examination, the clinician should make a detailed drawing representing the pain pattern that the patient has described. This depiction will assist in planning the physical examination and can be useful in monitoring the progression of the patient as symptoms improve or change. A comprehensive examination of the coracobrachialis muscle should include observation of shoulder girdle posture and scapular position as well as active and passive ranges of motion of the shoulder girdle, with special attention paid to muscle activation patterns and scapulohumeral rhythm. The clinician should note when and where pain occurs.

With coracobrachialis TrPs, the arm can be flexed as far as the ear but not behind it as this adds an aggravating adduction moment. Contracting the muscle in the shortened position causes pain.

Muscle-specific resisted testing should be performed to identify impairments in muscle function and reproduction of painful symptoms. To test the strength of the coracobrachialis muscle, the patient first elevates the arm to about 45° of flexion with external rotation. The patient's elbow should be flexed and the forearm fully supinated to minimize biceps brachii muscle's assistance.[17] Inability to adequately resist pressure applied by the clinician can indicate inhibition caused by TrPs in the coracobrachialis muscle. If the coracobrachialis muscle has TrPs, resistance effort by the patient is likely to elicit pain.

The Apley's scratch test (extension, internal rotation, and adduction) (Figure 20-3A) reveals restriction in shoulder range of motion when there are TrPs in the involved coracobrachialis muscle. Reaching behind the body and across the lower back puts the muscle in a painful position due to the stretch of the coracobrachialis muscle that is caused by extreme internal rotation and extension. Typically, the patient has difficulty reaching past the midline of the back secondary to pain. Stretching the involved coracobrachialis muscle by passively extending the arm at the shoulder joint also causes pain particularly with the addition of an abduction component.[22]

Accessory joint motion should be tested in the glenohumeral, acromioclavicular, sternoclavicular, and scapulothoracic joints. Often, joint hypomobility in the sternoclavicular joint can cause impairment in shoulder elevation, which contributes to alterations in normal muscle activation patterns. Articular dysfunctions in the glenohumeral joint may also impair muscle activation patterns, contributing to the overload of the coracobrachialis muscle.

Scapular position and humeral head position should be assessed at rest and during upper extremity elevation, as malalignment can be a significant contributing factor to coracobrachialis muscle overload during upper extremity functional activities that require combined flexion and adduction.

3.4. Trigger Point Examination

The patient should be positioned in a supine position with the arm abducted to 60° to allow access to the coracobrachialis muscle. Prior to palpation, the relation to other structures should be considered. The coracobrachialis muscle crosses superficially to the attachments of the subscapularis, latissimus dorsi, and teres major muscles but lies deep to the pectoralis major and anterior deltoid muscles (Figure 29-3). Coracobrachialis TrPs are found by palpating the muscle against the humerus, sliding the finger into the axilla deep to the deltoid and pectoralis major muscles (Figure 29-4). The tip of the digit encounters the adjacent bellies of the short head of the biceps brachii muscle and, more posteriorly, the coracobrachialis muscle at a level where about half of the biceps brachii muscle fibers become attached to their common tendon. The axillary neurovascular bundle passes along the coracobrachialis muscle[23] and should be displaced posteriorly to permit the digit to explore the fibers of the coracobrachialis muscle for taut bands by strumming the muscle against the humerus. Trigger points are typically found approximately mid-muscle. The attachment area may also feel indurated and respond to digital pressure with referred pain.

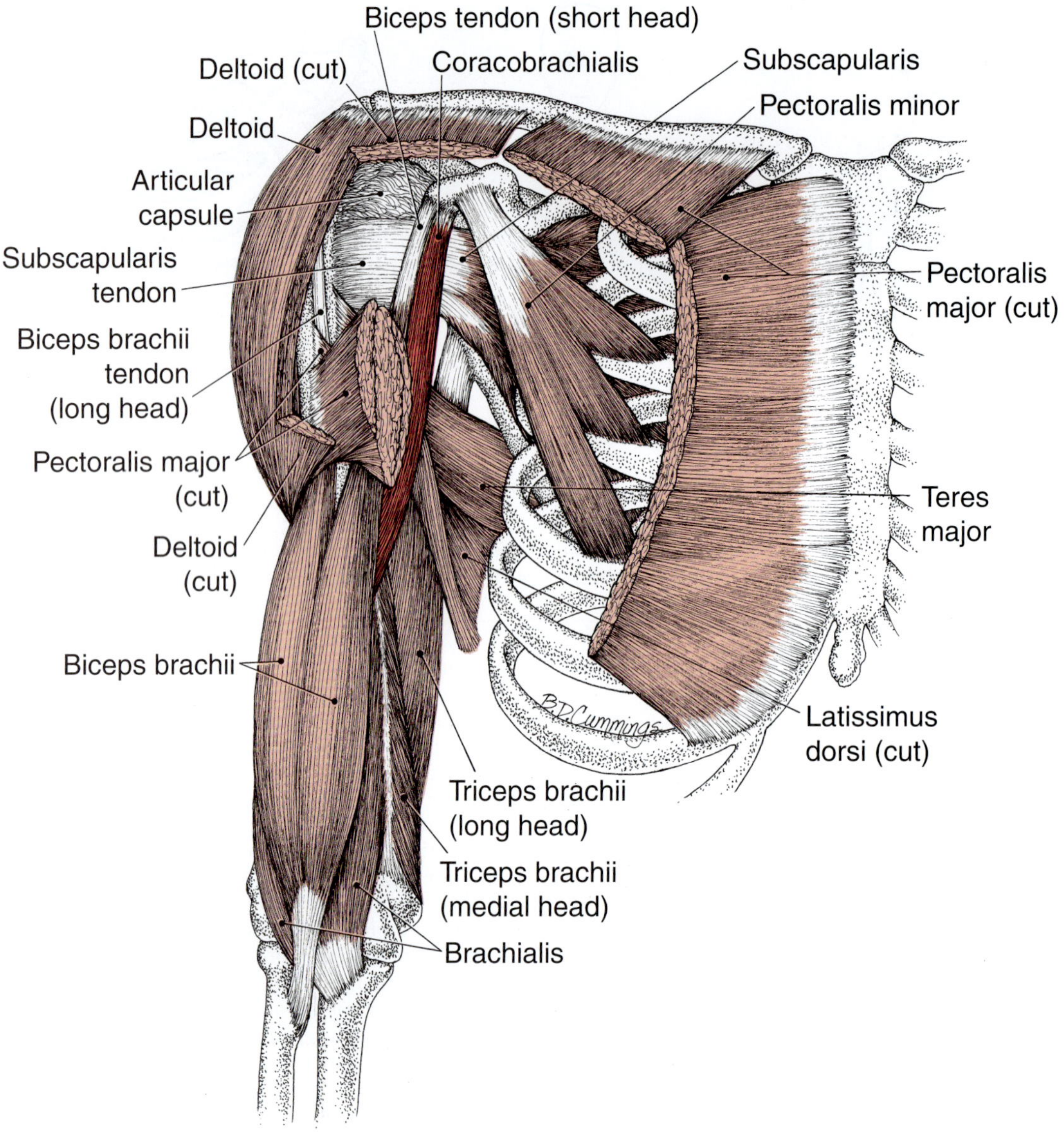

Figure 29-3. Muscular regional anatomy of the right shoulder, seen from the front. The coracobrachialis muscle (dark red) crosses superficial to the attachments of the subscapularis, latissimus dorsi, and teres major muscles but lies deep to the pectoralis major and anterior deltoid muscles. For clarity, the serratus anterior muscle is not shown. The coracobrachialis muscle lies medial to the short head of the biceps brachii muscle and is palpated for TrPs against the humerus in the anterior axillary fossa, deep to the pectoralis major muscle.

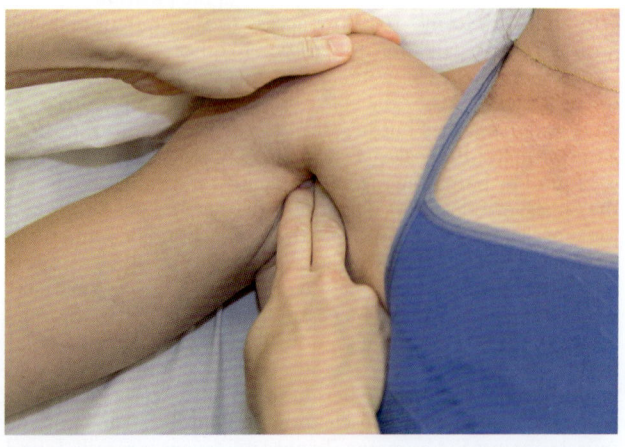

Figure 29-4. Palpation of coracobrachialis muscle for TrPs.

Evaluation for Trigger Points

Evaluation for TrPs should include cross-fiber flat palpation of the whole muscle. Two areas of tenderness are common in this muscle, more proximally and more distally. Trigger point tenderness is typically located approximately mid-muscle but could be present anywhere throughout the muscle belly. Attachment tenderness may also be located in the region of the proximal musculotendinous junction, although it also can be distal and most likely represents enthesopathy secondary to sustained tension caused by taut bands of the TrPs.[24]

Trigger points may be identified by passively moving the arm through a range that lengthens or stretches the coracobrachialis muscle. However, involvement of the coracobrachialis muscle is usually discovered when the patient returns following a successful inactivation of multiple TrPs in other shoulder muscles, especially the anterior deltoid and biceps brachii muscles. Although there is no recurrence of tenderness or taut bands in the muscles treated earlier, the patient reports posterior arm pain and deep tenderness that remains in the region of the anterior deltoid muscle. Careful examination reveals tenderness that lies deeper than that in the deltoid muscle.

4. DIFFERENTIAL DIAGNOSIS

4.1. Activation and Perpetuation of Trigger Points

A posture or an activity that activates a TrP, if not corrected, can also perpetuate it. In any part of the coracobrachialis muscle, TrPs may be activated by unaccustomed eccentric loading, eccentric exercise in an unconditioned muscle, or maximal or submaximal concentric loading.[25] Trigger points may also be activated or aggravated when the muscle is placed in a shortened and/or lengthened position for an extended period of time.

Because it is a strong shoulder adductor, coracobrachialis TrPs can be activated by activities involving repetitive upper limb exertion such as push-ups, rock climbing, swimming, throwing a ball, and playing tennis or golf. Occupations that require pulling objects downward, lowering objects from the shoulder height or above down to the floor, or lifting heavy objects with the arms extended may put a patient at risk to develop coracobrachialis TrPs. Prolonged immobilization of the shoulder joint in an adducted, internally rotated position from a surgical procedure, or self-immobilization due to pain, may also activate TrPs in the coracobrachialis muscle.

4.2. Associated Trigger Points

Associated TrPs can develop in muscles within the referred pain areas resultant from an active TrP. Therefore, muscles in the referred pain areas for each involved muscle should also be considered for examination.[26] Patients rarely present with symptoms of TrPs in this muscle alone. Coracobrachialis TrPs may generally develop in association with TrPs in functionally related muscles, such as the anterior or posterior deltoid portions, the biceps brachii (short head), the supraspinatus, and the triceps brachii (long head) muscles. Therefore, when evaluating a patient with pain in the anterior shoulder or posterior arm, it is necessary to evaluate muscles of the functional unit and treat TrPs in these muscles first. Often, coracobrachialis TrPs are identified after these associated TrPs have been treated and pain continues to persist.

4.3. Associated Pathology

Diagnoses that can present similarly to coracobrachialis TrPs includes C7 radicular pain (due to the area of pain reported by the patient), carpal tunnel syndrome, subacromial bursitis, subacromial pain syndrome (impingement), supraspinatus tendinopathy, and acromioclavicular joint dysfunction. Tenderness elicited slightly inferior to the acromioclavicular joint could implicate an enthesopathy of the coracobrachialis muscle. If tenderness to palpation is more distal, coracobrachialis TrPs in the muscle belly are more likely.

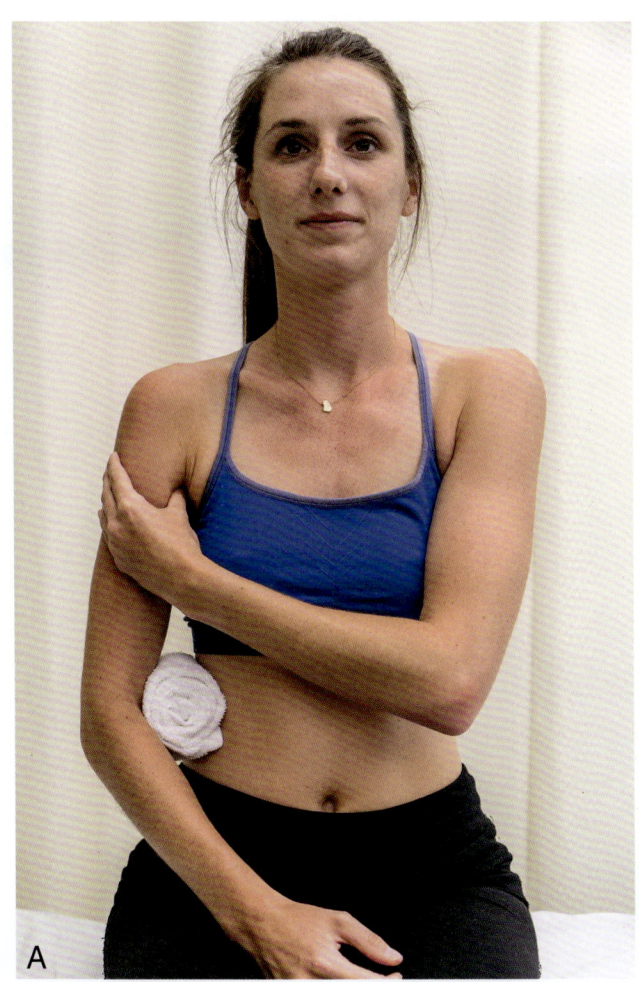
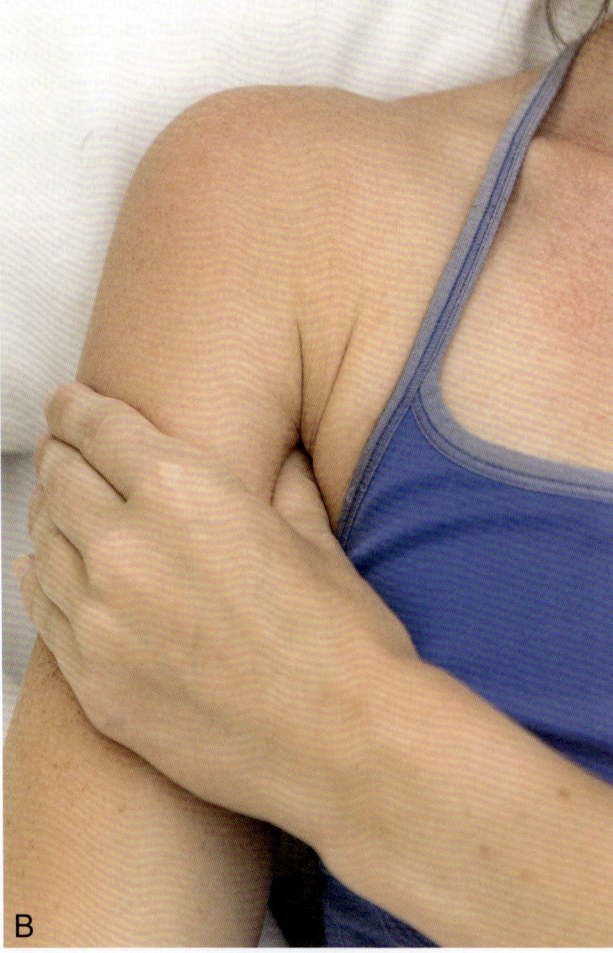

Figure 29-5. Self-pressure release of TrPs in the coracobrachialis muscle. A, Seated with towel roll to provide better access to the muscle. B, Lying down.

An important differential diagnostic procedure to distinguish acromioclavicular joint dysfunction from coracobrachialis TrPs is performed by passively placing the affected arm in full horizontal adduction to stress the acromioclavicular joint. Additional application of resistance to horizontal abduction in this fully adducted position increases the sensitivity of the test.[27] Either or both of these maneuvers elicit pain if there is an acromioclavicular joint dysfunction and should not elicit pain with coracobrachialis TrPs in isolation.

Tears of this muscle are rare and typically occur in combination with other shoulder muscles,[28] though three cases of isolated tears of the coracobrachialis muscle have been reported.[29] All resulted from forceful extension of the arm with the humerus in external rotation and abduction.

Entrapment of the musculocutaneous nerve by the coracobrachialis muscle can lead to weakness and wasting of the brachialis and biceps brachii muscles. Entrapment of the musculocutaneous nerve can be distinguished from a C5 or C6 radiculopathy or from a lateral cord lesion of the brachial plexus by the sparing of the coracobrachialis muscle. Pećina and Bojanić[30] reported the case of an oarsman who practiced 500 push-ups daily and who presented with reduced size and strength of the biceps brachii muscle, absent biceps brachii tendon reflex, reduced biceps brachii muscle tone, and diminished sensation of the lateral surface of the forearm. Electrodiagnostic testing showed prolonged distal latencies and decreased amplitude of evoked responses in the biceps brachii and brachialis muscles, indicating musculocutaneous nerve compression. Three months after stopping the daily push-ups, muscle mass, strength, and sensation in the forearm had returned. Electrodiagnostic studies showed improvement as well. Because the coracobrachialis muscle function was unimpaired, entrapment of the musculocutaneous nerve must have been distal to the motor branch to the coracobrachialis muscle.

Additional case reports[31-33] describe similar painless loss of musculocutaneous nerve function distal to the coracobrachialis muscle following heavy exercise (weight lifting and building a rock wall) with functional recovery within a few months after cessation of the strenuous activity. Exercise-induced hypertrophy of the coracobrachialis muscle that caused pressure compromise of the nerve as it penetrated the muscle was assumed to be responsible in these cases. No mention was made of examining the coracobrachialis muscle for TrPs. Latent TrPs that cause no clinical report of pain can be associated with well-developed taut bands that produce serious dysfunction and muscle inhibition.[34-36]

There have also been several cases of proximal musculocutaneous nerve injury in baseball and softball pitchers.[37-40] In these cases, the patients presented with acute pain in the anterior shoulder and weakness in the forearm supinators and elbow flexors. Sensory changes were present in the volar forearm, but onset was variable and in one case it was absent.[38] EMG testing showed isolated musculocutaneous nerve injury with sparing of the coracobrachialis muscle. Treatment for these players involved rest, anti-inflammatory medication, and physical therapy. In all cases, each of the throwers were able to return to their previous level of play without any surgical intervention. It is unclear why these throwers developed this condition, but it is hypothesized that a combination of anatomic variance and exercise-specific training contributed to the cause.[37] In both softball and baseball pitching, the arm is placed in a position that applies significant traction along the course of the nerve that could cause damage.[39]

5. CORRECTIVE ACTIONS

If coracobrachialis TrPs are suspected to be the cause of pain, repetitive or habitual movements that overuse the shoulder flexors such as repetitive or heavy lifting overhead, push-ups, bench press or inclined bench press, and repetitive throwing should be avoided. Lifting should be modified to keep elbows close to the body.

Sleeping positions can be particularly troublesome due to prolonged aggravating postures. The individual with coracobrachialis TrPs may be most comfortable sleeping on the back or on the pain-free side. When the patient lies on the uninvolved side, sleep comfort is improved by supporting the uppermost arm in a neutral position with the elbow and forearm placed on a pillow (Figure 22-4A) to avoid prolonged shortening of the affected coracobrachialis muscle. A pillow placed between the arm and the body can also be used to keep the arm in a neutral position when lying face up (Figure 22-4B). Another option is to place the pillow under the arm, perpendicular to the body, to keep the arm out of adduction and internal rotation and in a resting length–tension position for the coracobrachialis muscle. Patients should be cautioned regarding lying in bed with their arm(s) above their head in an abducted and externally rotated position, as this position keeps the coracobrachialis muscle in a shortened position and could cause increased pain from TrPs.

The patient may inactivate coracobrachialis TrPs with the application of self-release in the seated (Figure 29-5A), standing, or lying position (Figure 29-5B). Taking the hand of the unaffected side, the patient places the pad of the thumb along the humerus in the underarm beneath the pectoralis major muscle (Figure 29-5B). The thumb is pressed on the inner side of the bone in the underarm. The elbow is pressed into the side of the body to feel the coracobrachialis muscle contract. After finding the tender spot, a gentle pressure is applied for 30 seconds or until the pain decreases. This release may be repeated three to five times. Forceful pressure should be avoided as many nerves travel through this region. If any numbness or tingling occurs, the position of the thumb should be modified.

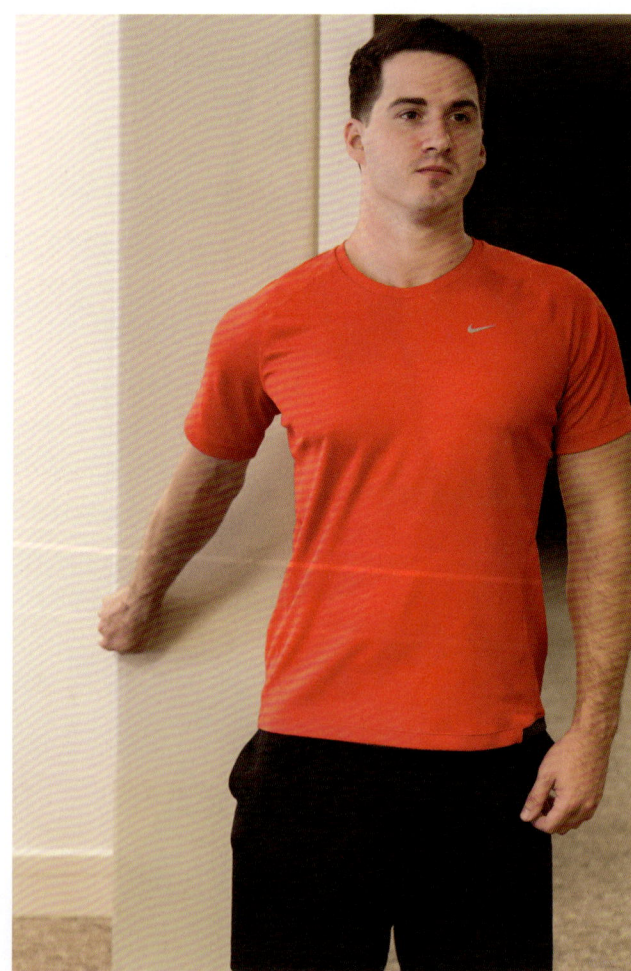

Figure 29-6. Self-stretch in doorway with arm in mid-position.

The patient should learn to release the TrP tightness by slowly and firmly stretching the coracobrachialis muscle by using the mid-arm position in a doorway to stretch into horizontal abduction with the humerus in internal rotation and the forearm in pronation (thumb and arm turned down) (Figure 29-6). The gentle stretch should be held for 30 seconds and repeated three to five times as needed, taking care not to overstretch. This sequence should be performed daily for optimal benefit.

Local application of moist heat to the muscle before or after the passive stretch exercise can reduce soreness. If soreness is a problem, an alternate-day program may be best and a post-stretching cold pack may help. Stretching too vigorously by using excessive body weight in the stretch should be avoided, and form may need to be checked by a professional to assist in modification for efficacy. Trigger points in this muscle rarely exist in isolation and all other associated TrPs in the shoulder girdle should therefore be addressed to achieve full resolution of pain.

References

1. Standring S. *Gray's Anatomy: The Anatomical Basis of Clinical Practice.* 41st ed. London, UK: Elsevier; 2015.
2. Porterfield JA, DeRosa C. *Mechanical Shoulder Disorders: Perspectives in Functional Anatomy.* St. Louis, MO: Saunders; 2004.
3. Morris H, Jackson CM. *Morris' Human Anatomy: A Complete Systematic Trastise by English and American Authors.* Vol 6. Philadelphia, PA: P. Blakiston; 1921.
4. El-Naggar MM, Al-Saggaf S. Variant of the coracobrachialis muscle with a tunnel for the median nerve and brachial artery. *Clin Anat.* 2004;17(2):139-143.
5. Kopuz C, Icten N, Yildirim M. A rare accessory coracobrachialis muscle: a review of the literature. *Surg Radiol Anat.* 2003;24(6):406-410.
6. El-Naggar MM, Zahir FI. Two bellies of the coracobrachialis muscle associated with a third head of the biceps brachii muscle. *Clin Anat.* 2001;14(5):379-382.
7. Ray B, Rai AL, Roy TS. Unusual insertion of the coracobrachialis muscle to the brachial fascia associated with high division of brachial artery. *Clin Anat.* 2004;17(8):672-676.
8. Lindner H. *Clinical Anatomy.* Norwalk, CT: Appleton & Lange; 1989.
9. Woo JS, Shin C, Hur MS, Kang BS, Park SY, Lee KS. Spinal origins of the nerve branches innervating the coracobrachialis muscle: clinical implications. *Surg Radiol Anat.* 2010;32(7):659-662.
10. el-Naggar MM. A study on the morphology of the coracobrachialis muscle and its relationship with the musculocutaneous nerve. *Folia Morphol (Warsz).* 2001;60(3):217-224.
11. Remerand F, Laulan J, Couvret C, et al. Is the musculocutaneous nerve really in the coracobrachialis muscle when performing an axillary block? An ultrasound study. *Anesth Analg.* 2010;110(6):1729-1734.
12. Apaydin N, Bozkurt M, Sen T, et al. Effects of the adducted or abducted position of the arm on the course of the musculocutaneous nerve during anterior approaches to the shoulder. *Surg Radiol Anat.* 2008;30(4):355-360.
13. Nakatani T, Mizukami S, Tanaka S. Three cases of the musculocutaneous nerve not perforating the coracobrachialis muscle. *Kaibogaku Zasshi.* 1997;72(3):191-194.
14. Guerri-Guttenberg RA, Ingolotti M. Classifying musculocutaneous nerve variations. *Clin Anat.* 2009;22(6):671-683.
15. Loukas M, Aqueelah H. Musculocutaneous and median nerve connections within, proximal and distal to the coracobrachialis muscle. *Folia Morphol (Warsz).* 2005;64(2):101-108.
16. Jenkins DB. *Hollinshead's Functional Anatomy of the Limbs and Back.* 6th ed. Philadelphia, PA: W.B. Saunders; 1991.
17. Kendall FP, McCreary EK. *Muscles: Testing and Function, with Posture and Pain.* Baltimore, MD: Lippincott Williams & Wilkins; 2005.
18. Rasch PJ, Burke RK. *Kinesiology and Applied Anatomy: The Science of Human Movement.* 6th ed. Philadelphia, PA: Lea & Febiger; 1978.
19. Duchenne G. *Physiology of Motion.* Philadelphia, PA: Lippincott; 1949.
20. Halder AM, Halder CG, Zhao KD, O'Driscoll SW, Morrey BF, An KN. Dynamic inferior stabilizers of the shoulder joint. *Clin Biomech (Bristol, Avon).* 2001;16(2):138-143.
21. Simons DG, Travell J, Simons L. *Travell & Simon's Myofascial Pain and Dysfunction: The Trigger Point Manual.* Vol 1. 2nd ed. Baltimore, MD: Williams & Wilkins; 1999:104.
22. Macdonald AJ. Abnormally tender muscle regions and associated painful movements. *Pain.* 1980;8(2):197-205.
23. Agur AM. *Grant's Atlas of Anatomy.* 9th ed. Baltimore, MD: Williams & Wilkins; 1991.
24. Karim MR, Fann AV, Gray RP, Neale DF, Escarda JD. Enthesitis of biceps brachii short head and coracobrachialis at the coracoid process: a generator of shoulder and neck pain. *Am J Phys Med Rehabil.* 2005;84(5):376-380.
25. Gerwin RD, Dommerholt J, Shah JP. An expansion of Simons' integrated hypothesis of trigger point formation. *Curr Pain Headache Rep.* 2004;8(6):468-475.
26. Hsieh YL, Kao MJ, Kuan TS, Chen SM, Chen JT, Hong CZ. Dry needling to a key myofascial trigger point may reduce the irritability of satellite MTrPs. *Am J Phys Med Rehabil.* 2007;86(5):397-403.
27. Dutton M. *Dutton's Orthopaedic Examination, Evaluation and Intervention.* 3rd ed. New York, NY: McGraw Hill; 2012:537.
28. Saltzman BM, Harris JD, Forsythe B. Proximal coracobrachialis tendon rupture, subscapularis tendon rupture, and medial dislocation of the long head of the biceps tendon in an adult after traumatic anterior shoulder dislocation. *Int J Shoulder Surg.* 2015;9(2):52-55.
29. Wardner JM, Geiringer SR, Leonard JA. Coracobrachialis muscle injury [abstract]. *Arch Phys Med Rehabil.* 1988;69:783.
30. Pecina M, Bojanic I. Musculocutaneous nerve entrapment in the upper arm. *Int Orthop.* 1993;17(4):232-234.
31. Mastaglia FL. Musculocutaneous neuropathy after strenuous physical activity. *Med J Aust.* 1986;145(3-4):153-154.
32. Braddom RL, Wolfe C. Musculocutaneous nerve injury after heavy exercise. *Arch Phys Med Rehabil.* 1978;59(6):290-293.
33. Swain R. Musculocutaneous nerve entrapment: a case report. *Clin J Sport Med.* 1995;5(3):196-198.
34. Lucas KR. The impact of latent trigger points on regional muscle function. *Curr Pain Headache Rep.* 2008;12(5):344-349.
35. Lucas KR, Rich PA, Polus BI. Muscle activation patterns in the scapular positioning muscles during loaded scapular plane elevation: the effects of Latent Myofascial Trigger Points. *Clin Biomech (Bristol, Avon).* 2010;25(8):765-770.
36. Ibarra JM, Ge HY, Wang C, Martinez Vizcaino V, Graven-Nielsen T, Arendt-Nielsen L. Latent myofascial trigger points are associated with an increased antagonistic muscle activity during agonist muscle contraction. *J Pain.* 2011;12(12):1282-1288.
37. Stephens L, Kinderknecht JJ, Wen DY. Musculocutaneous nerve injury in a high school pitcher. *Clin J Sport Med.* 2014;24(1):e68-e69.
38. Hsu JC, Paletta GA Jr, Gambardella RA, Jobe FW. Musculocutaneous nerve injury in major league baseball pitchers: a report of 2 cases. *Am J Sports Med.* 2007;35(6):1003-1006.
39. DeFranco MJ, Schickendantz MS. Isolated musculocutaneous nerve injury in a professional fast-pitch softball player: a case report. *Am J Sports Med.* 2008;36(9):1821-1823.
40. Henry D, Bonthius DJ. Isolated musculocutaneous neuropathy in an adolescent baseball pitcher. *J Child Neurol.* 2011;26(12):1567-1570.

Chapter 30

Biceps Brachii Muscle
"Upper Arm Agitator"

Joseph M. Donnelly and Leigh E. Palubinskas

1. INTRODUCTION

The powerful biceps brachii muscle spans the shoulder, elbow, and proximal radioulnar joints. It is a fusiform muscle with two distinct heads. Proximally, the long head of the biceps brachii muscle attaches to the superior margin of the glenoid cavity and glenoid labrum (biceps–labral complex), whereas the short head attaches with the coracobrachialis muscle to the coracoid process of the scapula. The two muscle heads fuse into a common tendon that attaches to the posterior aspect of the tuberosity of the radius. The muscle is innervated by the musculocutaneous nerve, which is comprised of spinal nerve root levels C5 and C6. The function of the biceps brachii muscle is complex because it spans three joints. Both heads of the muscle act synergistically to perform elbow flexion and supination of the forearm, and they both assist with flexion of the shoulder. The long head also assists with shoulder abduction when the arm is externally rotated and helps provide passive stability for the head of the humerus in the glenoid fossa. The short head assists with horizontal adduction of the shoulder. Pain referred from biceps brachii TrPs is typically located over the muscle and over the anterior region of the shoulder. Occasionally, pain is also referred to the suprascapular region and the antecubital space. Symptoms are most often exaggerated by repetitive flexion of the elbow or supination of the forearm. Patients may have difficulty reaching behind them with the elbow extended and the forearm supinated such as when pulling a rolling suitcase or when lifting items overhead with the arm outstretched and supinated. Examination of the patient should include testing to rule out bicipital tendinitis or biceps–labral complex dysfunction, subdeltoid bursitis, C5-C6 radicular pain, bicipital bursitis, and glenohumeral arthritis. The patient with TrPs in the biceps brachii muscle should avoid carrying or lifting items with the arm outstretched or supinated. Altering the sleeping posture to prevent prolonged flexion of the elbow can be helpful and self-stretch techniques can minimize pain associated with dysfunction of this muscle.

2. ANATOMIC CONSIDERATIONS

Long Head of Biceps Brachii

The biceps brachii muscle spans the shoulder, elbow, and proximal radioulnar joints (Figure 30-1). It is a fusiform muscle with two distinct proximal parts or "heads."[1] The long head of the biceps brachii muscle originates from the supraglenoid tubercle at the superior margin of the glenoid cavity, the posterior–superior aspect of the glenoid labrum, and the glenoid rim of the scapula (Figure 30-1).[1,2] This proximal region is commonly referred to as the biceps–labral complex.[3] The tendon is enclosed in a synovial sheath within an opening of the glenohumeral joint capsule. This anatomic arrangement allows the long head tendon to be

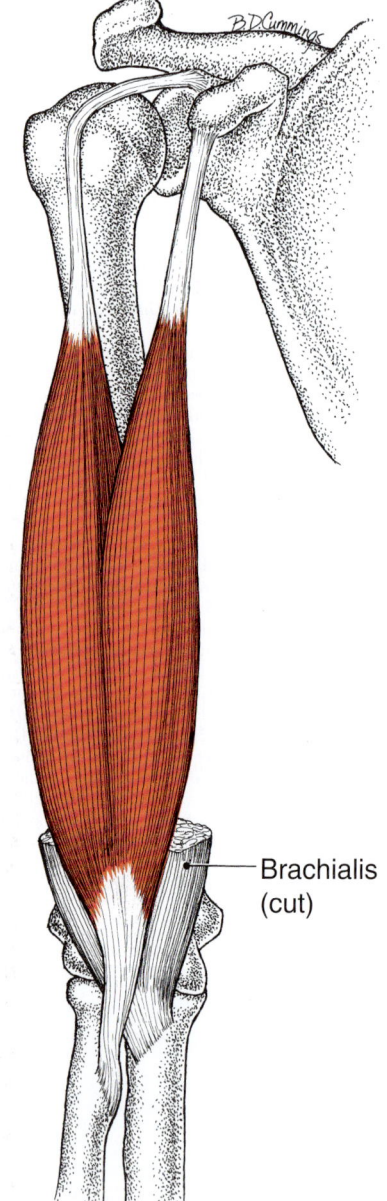

Figure 30-1. Separate proximal attachments of the two heads of the biceps brachii muscle (red), which covers most of the brachialis muscle. The two heads of the biceps brachii muscle join distally to attach to the tuberosity of the radius. The forearm is fully supinated in this figure. The biceps brachii tendon wraps more than halfway around the radius in pronation. The brachialis muscle has been cut for clarity.

intracapsular but extrasynovial. The tendon travels distally over the humeral head and exits the joint capsule to reside within the bicipital (intertubercular) groove. The tendon of the long head is stabilized proximally within the glenohumeral joint capsule by the coracohumeral and superior glenohumeral ligaments, the supraspinatus tendon, and the superior portion of the subscapularis tendon. These structures are commonly referred to as the "biceps pulley" and are clearly visualized arthroscopically.[4] On exiting the joint capsule into the bicipital groove, the tendon is supported by the transverse humeral ligament. The part of the tendon that resides in the main part of the bicipital groove is stabilized by a fascial expansion of the pectoralis major muscle (falciform ligament).[2] The falciform ligament attaches to both the medial and lateral lips of the bicipital grove and the glenohumeral joint capsule, adding stability to the tendon within the groove. The tendon is therefore stabilized by a variety of soft-tissue structures proximally. This orientation keeps the tendon stationary within the bicipital groove under a moving humerus during functional activities. The two heads of the biceps brachii muscle can be identified as individual heads from the glenohumeral joint distally approximately 7 to 10 cm proximal to the elbow joint.[1]

Short Head of Biceps Brachii

The short head originates from the coracoid process of the scapula by a thick, flat tendon with the coracobrachialis muscle. The tendon of the short head is lateral to the coracobrachialis muscle and anterior to the glenohumeral joint capsule. The short head travels inferolaterally, where it conjoins the long head of the biceps brachii muscle.

The common tendon of the two heads of the biceps brachii muscle attaches laterally to the posterior area of the tuberosity of the radius. The attachment faces the ulna when the forearm is supinated,[1] but in pronation the tendon wraps more than halfway around the radius.[5] The distal tendon also fuses medially with the bicipital aponeurosis, which attaches to the deep fascia of the forearm flexors. The muscle also has fibrous attachments to the brachial and antebrachial fascia of the anterior arm and forearm, respectively.[6,7]

The median and radial nerves lie along the medial and lateral borders of the distal portion of the biceps brachii and brachialis muscles. The endplates of a mature muscle form a somewhat ragged V-shaped band through the middle of the two heads.[8] Postmortem examination of six biceps brachii muscles for innervation and corresponding distribution of motor endplates indicated that each head was divided into three distinct longitudinal compartments.[9] The endplate zone of the long head is located slightly more proximal than that of the short head because of the difference in tendon arrangement and the innervation zone.[10]

Studies exploring the fiber composition of the biceps brachii muscle demonstrate an almost equal number of type-I (slow twitch) and type-II (fast twitch) fibers.[11,12] This finding of two older studies suggests that the biceps brachii muscle acts both as a power muscle for quicker vigorous activities such as sport play as well as an active contributor to lower-level sustained activities of daily living, though more research is needed.

This muscle rarely has anatomic anomalies. A third head may attach at the origin of the coracobrachialis muscle on the coracoid process[13] or may arise from the superomedial part of the brachialis muscle beneath the brachial artery, attaching to the bicipital aponeurosis and the medial side of the tendon of insertion.[1]

2.1. Innervation and Vascularization

The musculocutaneous nerve, arising from the lateral cord of the brachial plexus and spinal nerve roots C5 and C6, innervates the biceps brachii muscle after it passes through or over the coracobrachialis muscle. A separate branch of the musculocutaneous nerve innervates each head of the muscle.[1]

The biceps brachii muscle receives its vascular supply primarily via multiple vessels originating from the brachial artery. It also receives some vascularization from the anterior humeral circumflex artery and the deltoid branch of the thoracoacromial artery; however, a great variation in vascularization has been identified.[1]

2.2. Function

Due to its attachment sites, the biceps brachii muscle acts at the glenohumeral, humeroulnar, and humeroradial joints, as well as the proximal radioulnar articulation that lies within the elbow joint capsule. The fact that this muscle has two heads and spans three joints helps explain the complexity of its functions. The biceps brachii muscle functions to flex the elbow[1,5,14-17] and to supinate the forearm when the elbow is partially flexed.[15,18] The biceps brachii muscle functions at the shoulder to assist in flexion,[1,15,17] to assist in abduction of the shoulder when the arm is externally rotated (long head),[17] to assist in horizontal adduction of the arm (short head),[1] to pull the humerus down to the side of the body from an elevated position, and to seat the head of the humerus in the glenoid fossa to counteract superior translation from the deltoid (long head).[1,5,17]

During elbow flexion, the two heads of the biceps brachii, the brachialis, and the brachioradialis muscles distribute a sustained forearm flexion load that is irregular and variable.[14] Earlier research suggested that electrical activity is most vigorous in the biceps brachii muscle during flexion at the elbow when the forearm is supinated but is markedly inhibited when the forearm is pronated.[14,19] Recent research of muscle activity during elbow flexion demonstrates no significant changes with any hand position for the biceps brachii muscle. In contrast, significant differences in the contribution of the brachioradialis muscle were found during elbow flexion in the pronated, supinated, and neutral hand positions.[20] Elbow flexion can still be achieved by the brachialis and brachioradialis muscles if atrophy of the biceps brachii muscle is present.

Support from the biceps brachii muscle is needed at the shoulder to keep the head of the humerus seated in the glenoid cavity and to resist the upward translation of the humerus by the deltoid muscle. When the distal attachment (forearm) is fixed, the biceps brachii muscle flexes the elbow by moving the humerus toward the forearm, as in a pull-up.[21,22]

The biceps brachii muscle also functions as a synergist to the supinator muscle to reinforce fast supination or forceful supination of the forearm against resistance.[18] When electrically stimulated, the supination force supplied by the biceps brachii muscle is strongest when the elbow is held in a flexed position.[16,19] With the elbow flexed, motor unit activity in the biceps brachii muscle appears during resistance to supination but disappears when the elbow is fully extended.[14]

Each head of the biceps brachii muscle can also function independently of one another when abducting and adducting the shoulder. The long head of the biceps brachii muscle is active during both flexion and abduction of the shoulder.[5] However, it assists with abduction only when the glenohumeral joint is externally rotated with the forearm in a supinated position.[14] During shoulder flexion, both heads of the muscle contribute to the movement but the long head is more active than the short head.[14] The short head assists with horizontal adduction of the shoulder due to its attachment at the coracoid.[1]

The long head also affords increased stability of the glenohumeral joint by providing static restraint to superior migration of the humeral head. This role is primarily passive as active contraction only slightly depresses the humeral head.[23] The static contribution is dependent on the positioning of the tendon within the bicipital groove, which is supported by the biceps brachii pulley mechanism. Tears in the rotator cuff muscles can affect the long head tendon position in the groove due to their role in the biceps brachii pulley mechanism. The biceps brachii tendon is not able to provide a contribution to glenohumeral stability when rotator cuff tears are present. The long head tendon is vulnerable to compression under the acromion and at its attachment to the labrum where it can be avulsed.[2]

The biceps brachii muscle often performs lengthening eccentric contractions during activities of daily living (eg, when one is required to lower a load from torso level down to the floor) as well as during sports play.[1] During eccentric contractions, the muscle fibers contract while the muscle lengthens. This kind of contraction can cause an acute overload to the muscle that may lead to TrP formation, particularly during sports activities or strengthening exercises. Biceps–labral complex injuries occur more commonly in young athletes and within older manual laborers.

Overload and injury commonly occur in sports activities such as baseball pitching, softball, tennis, swimming, volleyball, and other overhead activities.[24] Unusually vigorous motor unit responses of the biceps brachii muscle appear near the end of the tennis serve[25] and during the deceleration phase of a baseball pitch. When playing basketball, the muscle is active when blocking a shot or performing a layup. Interestingly, minimal motor unit activity develops during the tennis forehand drive, batting a baseball, or during the golf drive.[25] Ilyes et al conducted an EMG analysis of shoulder and upper extremity muscles in five conditions comparing professional javelin throwers with a control group and found the biceps brachii muscle to be moderately active during pulling with the shoulder in 45° flexion and elbow fully extended, and during pushing with the shoulder in a neutral position and the elbow flexed to 90° (45%-55% of maximum volitional contraction [MVC]). During shoulder elevation to 140° in the plane of the scapula, they found the biceps brachii muscle to be moderately active in the control group (58% MVC) and maximally active in the professional athletes (71% MVC).[26] During a goal-oriented slow throw, the biceps brachii muscle was minimally active in both the groups, and during a fast throw the biceps brachii muscle was maximally active in both the groups (87% MVC).

Conte et al investigated the EMG activity of the upper extremity, shoulder, and trunk muscles during the use of both a touch pad and an external mouse while utilizing a laptop computer. They found a greater activity in the biceps brachii and triceps brachii muscles while utilizing the touch pad against the external mouse. They found that the touch pad required a greater degree of movement accuracy and stabilization than the external mouse. They concluded that frequent laptop computer users should utilize an external mouse instead of a touch pad to decrease muscle overload.[27]

2.3. Functional Unit

The functional unit to which a muscle belongs includes the muscles that reinforce and counter its actions as well as the joints that the muscle crosses. The functional interdependence of these structures is reflected in the organization and neural connections of the sensory motor cortex. The functional unit is emphasized because the presence of a TrP in one muscle of the unit increases the likelihood that the other muscles of the unit also develops TrPs. When inactivating TrPs in a muscle, one should be concerned about TrPs that may develop in muscles that are functionally interdependent. Box 30-1 grossly represents the functional unit of the biceps brachii muscle.[28]

In addition, the biceps brachii muscle is synergistic with the anterior deltoid muscle during shoulder flexion, and the middle deltoid and the supraspinatus muscles when abducting the arm at the shoulder. The coracobrachialis, the clavicular head of the pectoralis major, and the latissimus dorsi muscles act with the short head of the biceps brachii muscle to adduct the arm at the shoulder.

The shoulder adductors, subscapularis, latissimus dorsi, teres major, coracobrachialis, and pectoralis major muscles, act as antagonists to glenohumeral abduction. The supraspinatus, middle deltoid, and shoulder abductor muscles counteract adduction of the shoulder performed by the short head of the biceps brachii muscle.

Box 30-1 Functional unit of the biceps brachii muscle

Action	Synergists	Antagonist
Elbow flexion	Brachialis Brachioradialis	Triceps brachii Anconeus
Forearm supination	Supinator	Pronator teres Pronator quadratus

3. CLINICAL PRESENTATION

3.1. Referred Pain Pattern

Trigger points in the biceps brachii muscle are usually found in the midportion of the muscle but can be located anywhere throughout the length of the muscle. They refer pain upward over the biceps brachii muscle and over the anterior deltoid region of the shoulder.[29] Occasionally, pain is also located in the suprascapular region (Figure 30-2). Biceps brachii TrPs may also refer less-intense pain downward in the antecubital space.

Experimental injection of 6% sodium chloride solution into the biceps brachii tendon at the antecubital space in 10 healthy subjects caused pain that was referred locally and also proximally over the biceps brachii muscle, including the acromion in one case. Other phenomena that referred distally to some part of the volar forearm and hand included deep tenderness, erythema, paresthesia, pallor, and a feeling of weakness.[30]

3.2. Symptoms

Biceps brachii TrPs cause pain that is superficial in the front of the shoulder and may travel down the front of the upper arm over the length of the muscle. Pain may also be present in front of the elbow at the crease. Unlike the infraspinatus muscle, biceps brachii TrP pain is not described as "deep" in the shoulder joint and spares the side of the shoulder. Pain often increases during the elevation of the arm above the shoulder level either to the side or in front of the body.[31]

Tenderness may be present over the upper portion of the front of the shoulder in the area of the biceps brachii tendon. Diffuse aching over the front of the upper arm that rarely includes the elbow and weakness with pain on raising the arm above the head are also symptoms of biceps brachii TrPs. The patient may feel snapping or grating sounds in the upper portion of the shoulder when reaching the arm out to the side. Aching and soreness may be present in the upper shoulder and neck in the region of the upper trapezius muscle.

In contrast to patients with TrPs of the infraspinatus muscle, the patient with biceps brachii TrPs can lie comfortably on the affected side and can reach behind the waistline without pain.

3.3. Patient Examination

After a thorough subjective examination the clinician should make a detailed drawing representing the pain pattern that the patient has described. This depiction will assist in planning the physical examination and can be useful in monitoring the progression of the patient as symptoms improve or change. For proper examination of the biceps brachii muscle, the clinician

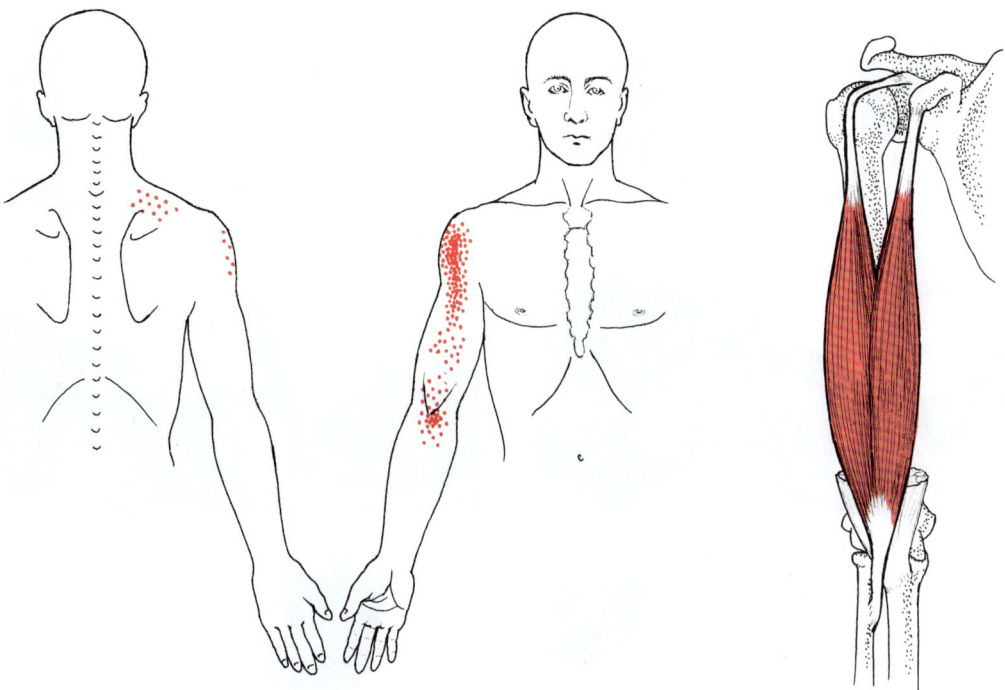

Figure 30-2. Referred pain pattern (essential zone is solid red, spillover zone stippled red) of TrPs in the right biceps brachii muscle.

should assess upper extremity posture in standing with arms at the side (elbow carrying position should be noted), shoulder girdle posture, active and passive ranges of motion of the elbow and the forearm, muscle activation patterns, and scapulohumeral rhythm. To identify TrPs in the biceps brachii muscle that may be limiting the range of motion and thus influencing dysfunction, the clinician should identify the limited range of motion by performing a specific range of motion testing for all parts of the biceps brachii muscle. The bicep brachii muscle crosses three joints and it is therefore difficult to identify length deficits in the muscle or restricted elbow or shoulder motion due to the presence of TrPs. The muscle should be lengthened across all three joints simultaneously to accurately test for abnormal tension of the muscle fibers. The biceps-extension test (Figure 30-3) can be used to evaluate the length of the long head of the biceps brachii muscle. With the patient seated in a low-backed chair and leaning back to stabilize the scapula against the backrest, the patient's arm is abducted to about 45° (Figure 30-3A). With the clinician's hand stabilizing the shoulder, the elbow is then fully extended and the forearm pronated to stretch the muscle across the elbow (Figure 30-3B). Finally, without letting the arm internally rotate at the shoulder, the arm is moved posteriorly into extension. Normally, the arm achieves a fully extended position (Figure 30-3B). If the muscle has been shortened by TrPs, the elbow flexes to relieve tension caused by the increased stretch across the shoulder joint (Figure 30-3C). This compensatory flexion of the elbow indicates a shortened biceps brachii muscle. Stretching the involved biceps brachii muscle by passively extending the forearm causes pain.

The patient may report a sudden painful "catch" in the shoulder when abducting the arm in slight extension to 15° or 20°, and careful examination may reveal tenderness or enthesopathy near the attachment of the long head of the biceps brachii tendon to the glenoid labrum. When the tender area of enthesopathy presses against the acromion during the elevation of the arm, the patient experiences pain that is commonly referred to as an "impingement syndrome." The tendon of the long head can be palpated against the head of the humerus only with the arm in external rotation. Otherwise, it is covered by the acromion.

Hidalgo-Lozano et al[32] identified that patients diagnosed with shoulder impingement had a higher prevalence of active and latent TrPs in the biceps brachii muscle than asymptomatic control subjects. Patients with TrPs in the biceps brachii and subscapularis muscles (active or latent) had higher levels of pain with an active elevation of the shoulder when compared with patients without TrPs in those muscles. When TrPs in the long head of the biceps brachii muscle were inactivated, patients experienced a spontaneous resolution of their pain and restoration of a full range of motion at the shoulder.

Muscle-specific resisted testing should be performed to identify impairments in muscle function and reproduction of painful symptoms. Inhibition of the biceps brachii and brachialis muscles can be identified by strength testing of elbow flexion in forearm supination and then pronation, while the elbow is extended. The biceps brachii muscle activation pattern remains the same with the forearm supinated, pronated, or in the neutral position, whereas the brachioradialis muscle activation varies depending on the hand position. Brachialis muscle function increases with forearm pronation.[20]

Accessory joint motion of the shoulder, elbow, and radioulnar joints should be manually tested when biceps brachii TrPs are suspected. Specifically, treatment of the acromioclavicular and sternoclavicular joints may be necessary to establish a free movement of the entire shoulder complex, if pathologic arthrokinematics are a contributing factor to biceps brachii TrPs.

3.4. Trigger Point Examination

To examine the biceps brachii muscle, the patient is positioned supine with the scapula flat on the examining table or seated with the elbow supported on a well-padded surface and with the trunk stabilized against the back of the chair. Palpation for TrPs in the biceps brachii muscle should include the evaluation of the whole muscle including both the short and long heads. To slacken the biceps brachii muscle slightly, the elbow is flexed to about 15° and the forearm is supinated and supported. Cross-fiber flat or

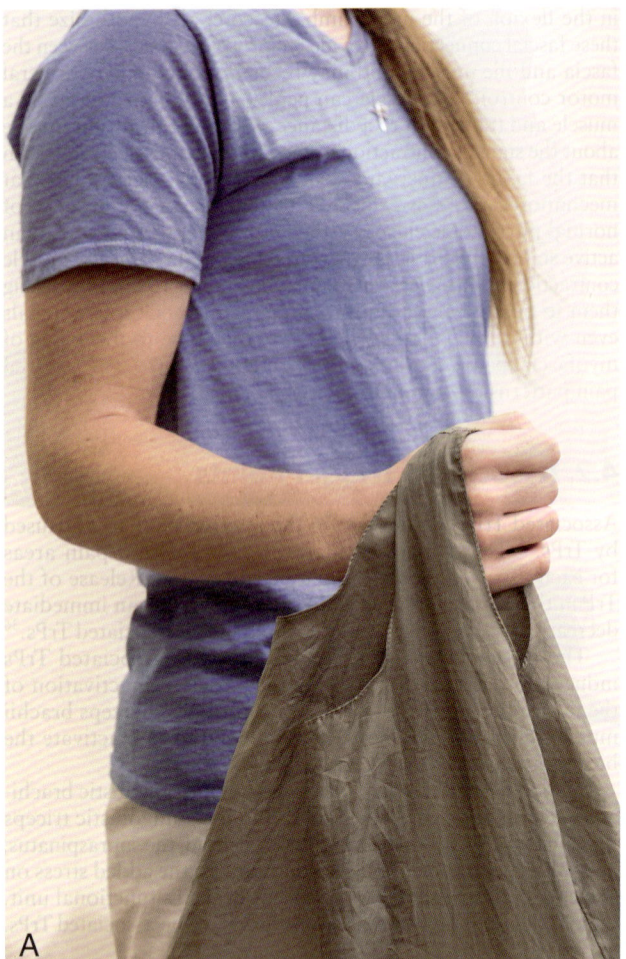 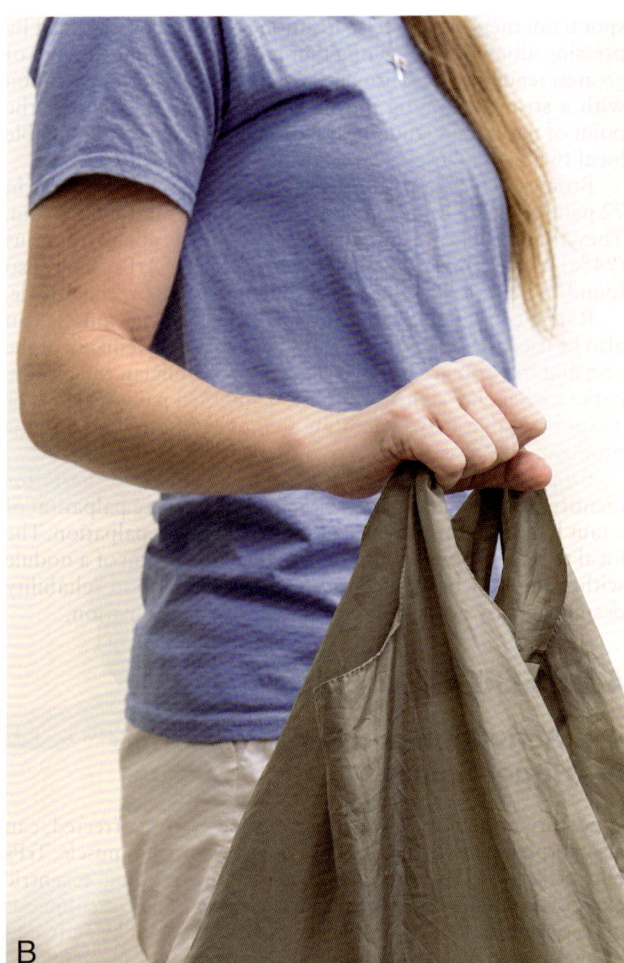

Figure 30-5. Carrying an object with different forearm positions. A, Forearm in neutral. B, Forearm pronated.

back into external rotation.[15] Biceps brachii tendon instability is unlikely to be related to biceps brachii TrPs. If dysfunction of the biceps–labral complex is suspected, specific diagnostic testing should be carried out to determine the structures at fault. Similarly, tenderness elicited by deep palpation over the deltoid muscle but referred from biceps brachii TrPs may be misidentified as subdeltoid bursitis. Refer to orthopedic examination textbooks and journal articles for more on these conditions.

Proximal forearm pain experienced when the forearm is flexed at the elbow with supination but not felt during flexion with pronation, may be attributed to bursitis of the bicipital bursa located at the radial attachment of the biceps brachii muscle or to active TrPs in the biceps brachii or supinator muscles. Trigger points and bursitis can also occur simultaneously and both should be considered when evaluating a patient who reports this type of pain.

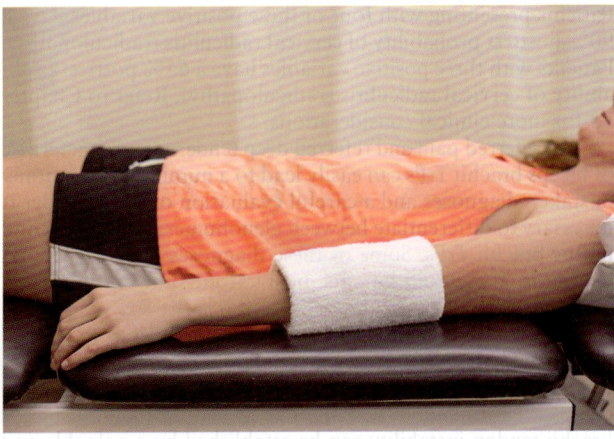

Figure 30-6. The correct sleeping position for a patient with TrPs in the left biceps brachii muscle.

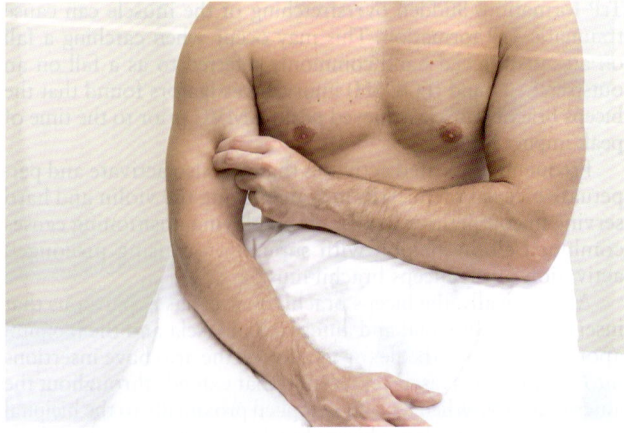

Figure 30-7. Self-pressure release of TrPs using a pincer palpation technique.

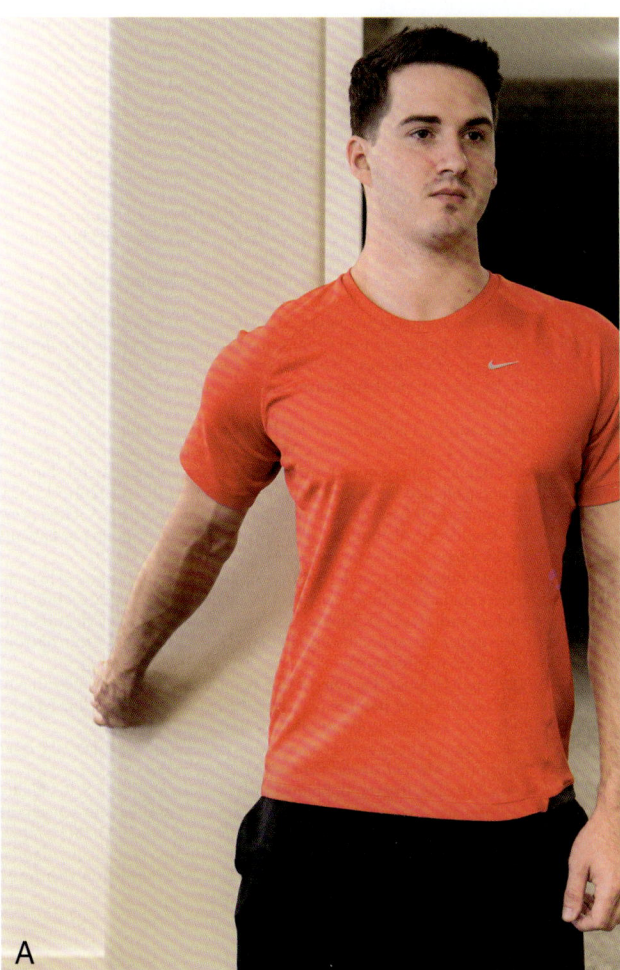 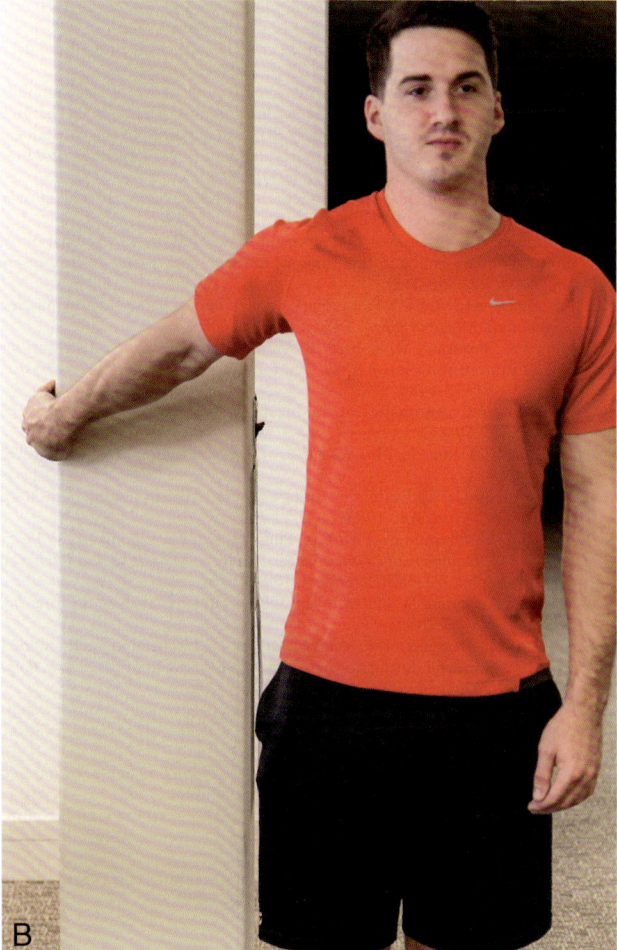

Figure 30-8. Self-stretch of the biceps brachii, anterior deltoid, and coracobrachialis muscles. A, The patient starts by placing their hand on the door frame in the lower position. B, If no stretch is felt, the hand can be placed higher on the door frame just below shoulder height. This stretch should not be performed with the hand above the shoulder height. Slow exhalation during the stretch phase enhances the effectiveness of this exercise.

5. CORRECTIVE ACTIONS

Trigger points in the biceps brachii muscle can be treated through activity modification to avoid excessive muscle strain, self-pressure release, and self-stretch techniques. The patient with biceps brachii TrPs should avoid habitual, sustained, or repetitive motions that overload the biceps brachii muscle by not carrying heavy objects such as grocery bags or a briefcase with the elbow fully straightened or slightly bent. The patient should also avoid lifting and carrying objects with the forearms supinated. Placing the forearm in a neutral position with the thumb up (Figure 30-5A) or pronating the forearm by turning the palm down (Figure 30-5B) when lifting will transfer some of the load from the biceps brachii muscle to the brachioradialis, brachialis, and supinator muscles. The muscle activation of the biceps brachii muscle does not change, but the muscles that assist with this function are activated more strongly.[20]

The patient should avoid sleeping with the elbow tightly flexed by placing a small pillow in the crook of the elbow or by wrapping a small towel loosely around the elbow to avoid bending the elbow past 90° (Figure 30-6). This simple technique prevents the prolonged shortening of the muscle while sleeping.

The patient may inactivate a biceps brachii TrPs by applying self-pressure release using a pincer palpation technique (Figure 30-7). Trigger point compression alone has been found to be effective in treating chronic shoulder pain. Pressure should be painful but bearable, and it can be applied for bouts as short as 15 seconds in duration to be effective.[39] The patient can perform the examination for TrPs in the biceps brachii muscle as mentioned earlier, and then apply pressure over the TrP while the arm is allowed to relax. The elbow can be gently flexed and extended in turn to help facilitate release.

Following treatment for inactivation of TrPs in the biceps brachii muscle, the patient should gently stretch both heads of the muscle daily by doing a self-stretch in a doorway (Figure 30-8A and B). The patient externally rotates the arm at the shoulder joint and pronates the forearm to hook the fingers, thumb down, against the doorjamb. With the hand slightly below the shoulder level, the patient rotates the torso away from that arm, applying a gentle traction to the straightened elbow (Figure 30-8A and B). Bouncing and jerking should be avoided to achieve a steady passive stretch of the muscle. Slow exhalation during the stretch enhances relaxation and improves tension release in the muscle.

References

1. Standring S. *Gray's Anatomy: The Anatomical Basis of Clinical Practice*. 41st ed. London, UK: Elsevier; 2015.
2. Porterfield JA, DeRosa C. *Mechanical Shoulder Disorders: Perspectives in Functional Anatomy*. St. Louis, MO: Saunders; 2004:65-66.
3. Taylor SA, O'Brien SJ. Clinically relevant anatomy and biomechanics of the proximal biceps. *Clin Sports Med*. 2016;35(1):1-18.
4. Habermeyer P, Magosch P, Pritsch M, Scheibel MT, Lichtenberg S. Anterosuperior impingement of the shoulder as a result of pulley lesions: a prospective arthroscopic study. *J Shoulder Elbow Surg*. 2004;13(1):5-12.

5. Rasch PJ, Burke RK. *Kinesiology and Applied Anatomy: The Science of Human Movement*. 6th ed. Philadelphia, PA: Lea & Febiger; 1978.
6. Stecco C, Porzionato A, Lancerotto L, et al. Histological study of the deep fasciae of the limbs. *J Bodyw Mov Ther*. 2008;12(3):225-230.
7. Stecco A, Macchi V, Stecco C, et al. Anatomical study of myofascial continuity in the anterior region of the upper limb. *J Bodyw Mov Ther*. 2009;13(1):53-62.
8. Aquilonius SM, Askmark H, Gillberg PG, Nandedkar S, Olsson Y, Stalberg E. Topographical localization of motor endplates in cryosections of whole human muscles. *Muscle Nerve*. 1984;7(4):287-293.
9. Segal RL. Neuromuscular compartments in the human biceps brachii muscle. *Neurosci Lett*. 1992;140(1):98-102.
10. Amirali A, Mu L, Gracies JM, Simpson DM. Anatomical localization of motor endplate bands in the human biceps brachii. *J Clin Neuromuscul Dis*. 2007;9(2):306-312.
11. Jozsa L, Demel S, Reffy A. Fibre composition of human hand and arm muscles. *Gegenbaurs Morphol Jahrb*. 1981;127(1):34-38.
12. Elder GC, Bradbury K, Roberts R. Variability of fiber type distributions within human muscles. *J Appl Physiol Respir Environ Exerc Physiol*. 1982;53(6):1473-1480.
13. Khaledpour C. Anomalies of the biceps muscle of the arm. *Anat Anz*. 1985;158(1):79-85.
14. Basmajian J, Deluca C. *Muscles Alive*. 5th ed. Baltimore, MD: Williams & Wilkins; 1985.
15. Curtis AS, Snyder SJ. Evaluation and treatment of biceps tendon pathology. *Orthop Clin North Am*. 1993;24(1):33-43.
16. Duchenne G. *Physiology of Motion*. Philadelphia, PA: Lippincott; 1949.
17. Jenkins DB. *Hollinshead's Functional Anatomy of the Limbs and Back*. 6th ed. Philadelphia, PA: W.B. Saunders; 1991.
18. Travill A, Basmajian JV. Electromyography of the supinators of the forearm. *Anat Rec*. 1961;139:557-560.
19. Sullivan WE, Mortensen OA, Miles M, Greene LS. Electromyographic studies of m. biceps brachii during normal voluntary movement at the elbow. *Anat Rec*. 1950;107(3):243-251.
20. Kleiber T, Kunz L, Disselhorst-Klug C. Muscular coordination of biceps brachii and brachioradialis in elbow flexion with respect to hand position. *Front Physiol*. 2015;6:215.
21. Kendall FP, McCreary EK. *Muscles: Testing and Function, with Posture and Pain*. Baltimore, MD: Lippincott Williams & Wilkins; 2005.
22. Doma K, Deakin GB, Ness KF. Kinematic and electromyographic comparisons between chin-ups and lat-pull down exercises. *Sports Biomech*. 2013;12(3):302-313.
23. Sharkey NA, Marder RA, Hanson PB. The entire rotator cuff contributes to elevation of the arm. *J Orthop Res*. 1994;12(5):699-708.
24. Abrams GD, Safran MR. Diagnosis and management of superior labrum anterior posterior lesions in overhead athletes. *Br J Sports Med*. 2010;44(5):311-318.
25. Broer M, Houtz S. *Patterns of Muscular Activity in Selected Sports Skills, an Electromyographic Study*. Springfield, IL: Charles C. Thomas; 1967.
26. Illyes A, Kiss RM. Shoulder muscle activity during pushing, pulling, elevation and overhead throw. *J Electromyogr Kinesiol*. 2005;15(3):282-289.
27. Conte C, Ranavolo A, Serrao M, et al. Kinematic and electromyographic differences between mouse and touchpad use on laptop computers. *Int J Ind Ergon*. 2014;44:413-420.
28. Simons DG, Travell JG, Simons LS. *Myofascial Pain and Dysfunction: The Trigger Point Manual. Volume 1: Upper Half of Body*. 2nd ed. Philadelphia, PA: Lippincott Williams & Wilkins;1999.
29. Gutstein M. Diagnosis and treatment of muscular rheumatism. *Br J Phys Med*. 1938;1:302-321.
30. Steinbrocker O, Isenberg SA, Silver M, Neustadt D, Kuhn P, Schittone M. Observations on pain produced by injection of hypertonic saline into muscles and other supportive tissues. *J Clin Invest*. 1953;32(10):1045-1051.
31. Gutstein M. Common rheumatism and physiotherapy. *Br J Phys Med*. 1940;3:46-50.
32. Hidalgo-Lozano A, Fernandez-de-las-Penas C, Alonso-Blanco C, Ge HY, Arendt-Nielsen L, Arroyo-Morales M. Muscle trigger points and pressure pain hyperalgesia in the shoulder muscles in patients with unilateral shoulder impingement: a blinded, controlled study. *Exp Brain Res*. 2010;202(4):915-925.
33. Bron C, Dommerholt J, Stegenga B, Wensing M, Oostendorp RA. High prevalence of shoulder girdle muscles with myofascial trigger points in patients with shoulder pain. *BMC Musculoskelet Disord*. 2011;12:139.
34. Gerwin RD, Dommerholt J, Shah JP. An expansion of Simons' integrated hypothesis of trigger point formation. *Curr Pain Headache Rep*. 2004;8(6):468-475.
35. Burkhart TA, Andrews DM. Kinematics, kinetics and muscle activation patterns of the upper extremity during simulated forward falls. *J Electromyogr Kinesiol*. 2013;23(3):688-695.
36. Hsieh YL, Kao MJ, Kuan TS, Chen SM, Chen JT, Hong CZ. Dry needling to a key myofascial trigger point may reduce the irritability of satellite MTrPs. *Am J Phys Med Rehabil*. 2007;86(5):397-403.
37. Hong C-Z. Considerations and recommendations regarding myofascial trigger point injection. *J Musculoskelet Pain*. 1994;2(1):29-59.
38. Wainner RS, Fritz JM, Irrgang JJ, Boninger ML, Delitto A, Allison S. Reliability and diagnostic accuracy of the clinical examination and patient self-report measures for cervical radiculopathy. *Spine (Phila Pa 1976)*. 2003;28(1):52-62.
39. Hains G, Descarreaux M, Hains F. Chronic shoulder pain of myofascial origin: a randomized clinical trial using ischemic compression therapy. *J Manipulative Physiol Ther*. 2010;33(5):362-369.

Chapter 31

Brachialis Muscle

"Snuffbox Scourge"

Joseph M. Donnelly and Leigh E. Palubinskas

1. INTRODUCTION

The brachialis muscle is a powerful one-joint elbow flexor that originates proximally from the shaft of the humerus and attaches distally to the ulna. This orientation allows the brachialis muscle to function independently from forearm rotation unlike the biceps brachii muscle. The brachialis muscle is innervated by the musculocutaneous nerve. Trigger points (TrPs) in the brachialis muscle chiefly refer pain to the dorsum of the carpometacarpal joint at the base of the thumb and often elicit pain reports in the region of the anterior upper arm and the antecubital space. Trigger points in the brachialis muscle can be aggravated by holding the elbow in positions of flexion for prolonged periods or by repetitive overload of the muscle during activities such as lifting with the elbows flexed. Brachialis TrPs most often occur in conjunction with those found in the biceps brachii muscle. Evaluation of the patient should include testing to rule out C5-C6 radicular pain, lateral epicondylalgia, De Quervain's tenosynovitis, carpal tunnel syndrome, and radial nerve entrapment. The patient with TrPs in the brachialis muscle should be instructed to avoid repetitive elbow flexion and lifting techniques that foster overload stress to the brachialis muscle. Sleeping postures should be altered to avoid prolonged positioning of the muscle in a shortened flexed posture. To independently manage pain related to the brachialis muscle, the patient may perform TrP self-pressure release and self-stretch techniques.

2. ANATOMIC CONSIDERATIONS

The brachialis muscle originates from the distal half of the anterior surface of the shaft of the humerus and from the medial and lateral intermuscular septa (medial more than lateral). The proximal attachment reaches the distal attachment of the deltoid muscle (Figure 31-1). The muscle fibers converge into a thick broad tendon that attaches to the ulnar tuberosity and the anterior surface of the coronoid process on the proximal end of the ulna.[1]

Anatomical variations of the brachialis muscle have been identified but are quite rare. The brachialis muscle may be divided into two or more parts. It may be fused with the brachioradialis, pronator teres, or biceps brachii muscles. In some cases, it may send tendinous slips to the radius or bicipital aponeurosis.[1] Anatomical variations can also include accessory brachialis muscles arising from the distal portion of the muscle.[2-4] In two of these reported cases,[2,4] the accessory muscle crossed over the median nerve creating a point of possible entrapment. In a third case,[3] the brachialis muscle split into two distally, encompassing the radial nerve. Capsular fibers from the deepest part of the brachialis muscle may insert into the anterior joint capsule of the elbow.[4,5] Originally, it was thought that these fibers may cause retraction of the elbow joint capsule to prevent impingement when the elbow flexes.[4] This notion has since been refuted and these capsular attachments are believed to serve as an additional attachment site for the muscle with no functional significance.[5] Proximally, variation of the muscle origin is less frequent; however, one study found the brachialis muscle attached by a strong tendon to the lateral lip of the intertubercular sulcus close to the

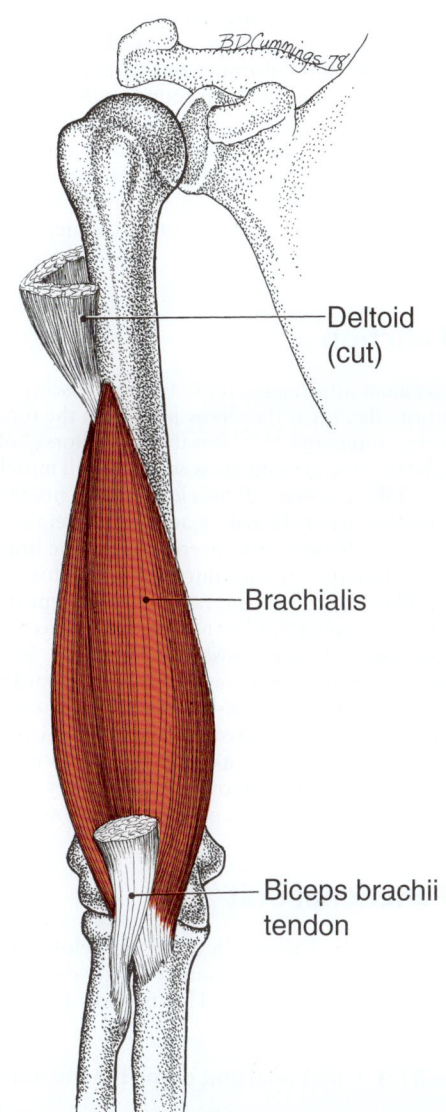

Figure 31-1. Attachments of the right brachialis muscle to the humerus above, and ulna below. The cut end of the overlying biceps brachii tendon appears below. The deltoid muscle, above, also has been cut for clarity.

deltoid tuberosity.[6] This tendinous insertion did not appear to play a functional role, and it has been speculated that it could be used for reconstructive surgeries.

2.1. Innervation and Vascularization

The brachialis muscle is innervated by the musculocutaneous nerve via the lateral cord of the brachial plexus arising from the C5 and C6 nerve roots. The musculocutaneous nerve supplies a branch to the shoulder joint and then passes through the coracobrachialis muscle and between the biceps brachii and brachialis muscles, sending branches to both before descending through the cubital fossa.[1]

A small inferolateral part of the brachialis muscle is typically innervated by the radial nerve via the posterior cord from the C7 nerve root.[1,7] Radial nerve innervation is present in approximately 67% to 100% of the population.[8-13] This variation in findings is thought to be due to race, sample size, and research techniques.[12] Originally, it was believed that the radial nerve served only a sensory function, but more recent research has confirmed the radial nerve provides motor innervation as well.[10,12,14]

In some instances, the median nerve may also innervate the brachialis muscle. This variation is typically observed when there is damage to the musculocutaneous nerve, but in some cases, the brachialis muscle has been found with triple innervation from the musculocutaneous, radial, and median nerves.[12,15,16]

Vascular supply to the brachialis muscle is primarily provided by the brachial artery (superiorly) and the superior ulnar collateral artery (inferiorly). The brachialis muscle may also receive vascularization from the inferior ulnar collateral artery or the profunda brachii artery.[1]

2.2. Function

Due to its ulnar attachment, the brachialis muscle performs only one motion: flexion at the elbow joint with the forearm either pronated or supinated.[1,17-21] It is the "workhorse" of the elbow flexors, having the greatest cross section of all muscles near the elbow.[1,22] Like the deltoid muscle, it shows no activity when the dependent arm is heavily loaded with weights.[17] There is a fine interplay between the biceps brachii, the brachialis, and the brachioradialis muscles during resisted forearm flexion. The interplay shows striking variability on repeated trials.[17]

When the proximal attachment (humerus) is fixed, the brachialis muscle moves the forearm toward the humerus. With the distal attachment (ulna) fixed, it moves the humerus toward the forearm, as in pull-up exercises.[20] The brachialis muscle often contracts eccentrically to decelerate and control the lowering of heavy objects.

During the act of driving a car, the brachialis muscle demonstrates a relatively constant low level of activity and only occasionally showed short bursts of more intense activity.[23]

2.3. Functional Unit

The functional unit to which a muscle belongs includes the muscles that reinforce and counter its actions as well as the joints that the muscle crosses. The functional interdependence of these structures is reflected in the organization and neural connections of the sensory motor cortex. The functional unit is emphasized because the presence of a TrP in one muscle of the unit increases the likelihood that the other muscles of the unit also develops TrPs. When inactivating TrPs in a muscle, one should be concerned about TrPs that may develop in muscles that are functionally interdependent. Box 31-1 grossly represents the functional unit of the Brachialis muscle.[24]

3. CLINICAL PRESENTATION

3.1. Referred Pain Pattern

Pain from brachialis TrPs chiefly refers to the dorsum of the carpometacarpal joint at the base of the thumb and to the dorsal web of the thumb (Figure 31-2).[25] The referred pain pattern may also include the anterior aspect of the upper arm and the antecubital space.

Pain referral from mid-fiber TrPs may cover the antecubital space. The pain that occasionally extends upward over the deltoid muscle is more likely to arise from the most proximal TrPs in the brachialis muscle (Figure 31-2).[26]

3.2. Symptoms

Trigger points in the brachialis muscle are often associated with diffuse soreness of the thumb. The patient's main report of pain is typically present when the joint is at rest and may be aggravated with an active thumb motion. The patient may also report pain in the crease of the elbow and in the anterior aspect of the shoulder and upper arm.

Pain in the anterior shoulder that is caused solely by brachialis TrPs are not associated with impairment of the shoulder motion. Because the brachialis muscle is a one-joint muscle that crosses the elbow, decreased flexibility or pain with muscle activation does not have an effect on the glenohumeral joint function.

Pain symptoms in the carpometacarpal thumb joint may arise from radial nerve entrapment due to TrPs in the brachialis muscle. Symptoms caused by the entrapment of the superficial sensory (cutaneous) branch of the radial nerve include dysesthesia, tingling, and numbness at the dorsum of the thumb. The aching pain of referred TrPs and the symptoms of radial nerve entrapment are both experienced in the thumb and may be relieved by inactivating brachialis TrPs.

3.3. Patient Examination

After a thorough subjective examination, the clinician should make a detailed drawing representing the pain pattern that the patient has described. This depiction will assist in planning the physical examination and can be useful in monitoring the patient's progression as symptoms improve or change. Pain referred from brachialis TrPs is increased by full passive extension of the elbow, although limitation of motion is not often a report. The range of elbow extension may be restricted by only a few degrees and may be detectable only by comparison with the other side or by improvement after treatment. Active motion of the thumb in the pain referral zone is typically painful, but active movement of the elbow is not.

Weakness or inhibition of the biceps brachii and brachialis muscles can be distinguished by testing the strength of the elbow flexion in supination and then in pronation of the forearm while the elbow is extended. This change in position has no effect on brachialis muscle strength because it attaches to the ulna, but historical theory states that the biceps brachii muscle may demonstrate functional weakness with forearm pronation by placing it in a lengthened position. A recent research utilizing

Box 31-1 Functional unit of the brachialis muscle

Action	Synergists	Antagonist
Elbow flexion	Biceps brachii Brachioradialis Pronator teres	Triceps brachii Anconeus

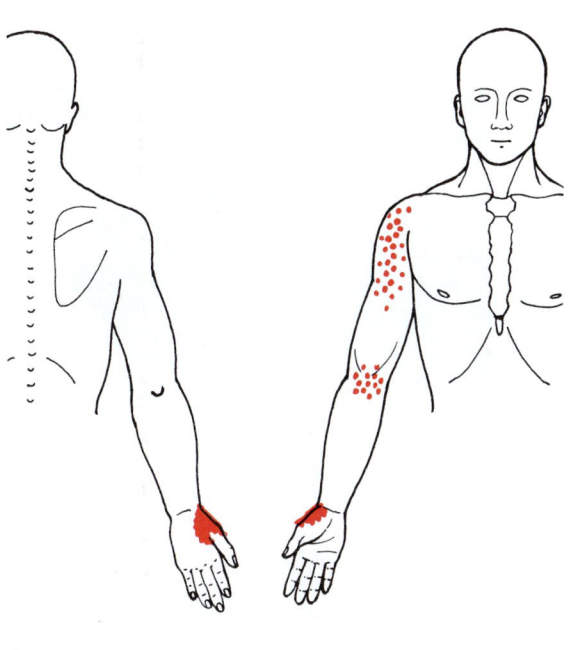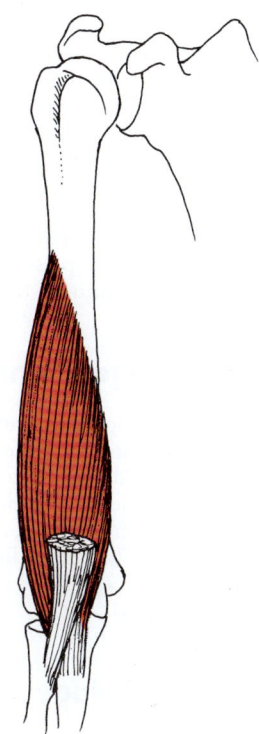

Figure 31-2. The pain pattern (essential portion, solid red; spillover portion, stippled red) that is referred from TrPs in the right brachialis muscle. Taut bands associated with mid-muscle TrPs may cause entrapment of the radial nerve.

EMG analysis of the biceps brachii and brachioradialis muscles during elbow flexion with altering the hand positions demonstrates no change in biceps brachii muscle activation with a change in the hand position.[27] Therefore, it may be more beneficial to test resisted forearm supination to differentiate the biceps brachii muscle from the brachialis muscle.

Radial nerve compression is indicated when a tingling in the thumb results from the pressure exerted on the region where the nerve exits the musculospiral groove and pierces the lateral intermuscular septum (Figure 32-2). Pressure should be applied about mid-arm, just below the dimple that marks the apex, or the distal end, of the triangular bulge produced by the deltoid muscle. In this area the radial nerve passes between the brachialis and the brachioradialis muscles, creating a possible site of compression.[28]

If a limited elbow range of motion is present, the humeroulnar, humeroradial, and proximal radioulnar joints should be examined for accessory joint motion and should be treated, if restricted.[29]

3.4. Trigger Point Examination

When evaluating for TrPs in the brachialis muscle, the patient should be positioned with the elbow flexed between 30° and 45° and the forearm in a comfortable resting position. If there is increased tension in the biceps brachii muscle the patient's forearm can be placed in a supinated position to slacken the biceps brachii muscle. The bulk of the biceps brachii muscle should be pushed aside, medially, to palpate the underlying brachialis TrPs (Figure 31-3). The biceps brachii muscle has more slack if the forearm is placed in supination and is relaxed. Brachialis TrPs are typically located in the distal half of the muscle (Figure 31-2) and are likely to refer pain to the thumb and sometimes to the front of the elbow. Trigger points may be located deep to the lateral edge of the undisplaced biceps brachii muscle, but others are found toward the middle of the brachialis muscle, sometimes under the biceps brachii muscle. The more proximal TrPs, which refer pain to the upper arm and anterior aspect of the shoulder, are covered by the biceps brachii muscle, making identification and palpation more difficult.

4. DIFFERENTIAL DIAGNOSIS

4.1. Activation and Perpetuation of Trigger Points

Trigger points may be activated by unaccustomed eccentric loading, eccentric exercise in an unconditioned muscle, or maximal or submaximal concentric loading.[30] Trigger points may also be activated or aggravated when the muscle is placed in a shortened or lengthened position for an extended period of time. Brachialis TrPs can be activated and can be perpetuated by repeated and prolonged overload of elbow flexion during heavy lifting. Examples of stress overloads are holding a power tool, carrying groceries, holding a baby, picking up children, and playing a violin or guitar with the forearm supinated such that the biceps brachii muscle is shortened and inhibited. Computer work where the arms are held out for long periods of time requires a static low-level contraction of the brachialis muscle in both arms and can lead to activation and perpetuation of TrPs in the brachialis muscle.

Elbow pain associated with TrPs in the brachialis muscle may be misdiagnosed as lateral epicondylalgia or "tennis elbow." With this condition, brachialis muscle involvement tends to develop together with that of the biceps brachii muscle after initial activation of TrPs in the supinator muscle (Chapter 36). The repetitive nature of the tennis swing during a match play or practice is another example of repetitive overload to the elbow flexors and supinators. This phenomenon is especially observed with forehand ground strokes in tennis.

Recent research indicates that brachialis TrPs may also form as a result of rotator cuff pathology. Suh et al[31] found brachialis TrPs to cause anterior shoulder pain in a sample of patients with rotator cuff pathology, whose anterior shoulder pain did not respond to subacromial injections of local anesthetics or steroid. Palpation of the brachialis muscle revealed TrPs in 23 of the 24 patients who did not respond to injection. It is hypothesized that the biceps brachii muscle may perform a greater role as a shoulder stabilizer in this population, causing increased overload pressure on the brachialis muscle during elbow flexion. The one-joint nature of the brachialis muscle also causes it to be more involved in posture, which may be distorted due to shoulder pain and a change in scapula position. Each of these would lead to increased overload pressure through the muscle, which may promote TrP formation.[31]

4.2. Associated Trigger Points

Associated TrPs can develop in the referred pain areas of TrPs.[32] Therefore, musculature in the referred pain areas for each involved muscle should also be considered. Associated TrPs of the brachialis muscle can develop in the deltoid, biceps brachii, supinator, brachioradialis, and the adductor and opponens pollicis muscles. The brachialis muscle is also likely to be involved when the biceps brachii, brachioradialis, or supinator muscles have TrPs.

4.3. Associated Pathology

Anterior shoulder pain in the region of referred pain from brachialis TrPs may also be caused by bicipital or supraspinatus tendinitis, or by TrPs of the infraspinatus, anterior deltoid, posterior deltoid, and/or latissimus dorsi muscles. These conditions should be ruled out with a thorough examination of the shoulder region. Active movement of the shoulder should not be painful if brachialis TrPs are the sole source of pain and dysfunction.

Cervical radicular symptoms from the C5 or C6 nerve roots may cause pain in the anterior shoulder, anterolateral upper arm, forearm, and the radial portion of the wrist and hand encompassing the thumb and index finger. These symptoms could easily be confused with the referral pattern associated with brachialis TrPs (Figure 31-2). A test item cluster has been identified to rule out cervical radicular pain and/or radiculopathy (refer to Chapter 33).[33]

As mentioned earlier, lateral epicondylalgia (tennis elbow) is often the result of TrPs in the biceps brachii, supinator, and potentially, the brachialis muscles. Trigger points should be considered in the absence of tenderness over the lateral epicondyle of the humerus.

Other hand pathologies should be considered when evaluating the patient with thumb pain. Carpal tunnel syndrome may cause pain perceived as isolated over the thenar eminence. De Quervain's tenosynovitis can also cause pain in the region of the carpometacarpal joint. If TrPs are responsible for the pain, Finkelstein's test yields different results if performed with the elbow extended or flexed. Because the abductor pollicis longus and extensor pollicis brevis tendons do not cross the elbow, the position of the elbow joint should not change the patient's pain if De Quervain's tenosynovitis is the cause.

Entrapment of the radial nerve should also be considered as part of the differential diagnosis. Symptoms of nerve entrapment include numbness, hypoesthesia or hyperesthesia, and dysesthesia. These symptoms, like the referred pain from brachialis TrPs, appear over the dorsum of the thumb and its adjacent web space. An entrapment of the sensory branch of the radial nerve can be caused by a TrP, usually in the lateral border of the brachialis muscle, which produces a taut band of muscle fibers extending to the level where the radial nerve exits the musculospiral groove and pierces the lateral intermuscular septum (Figure 32-2). These symptoms of entrapment caused by brachialis TrPs are relieved by the release of the TrP, which feels like a palpable knot in the lateral border of the muscle, just

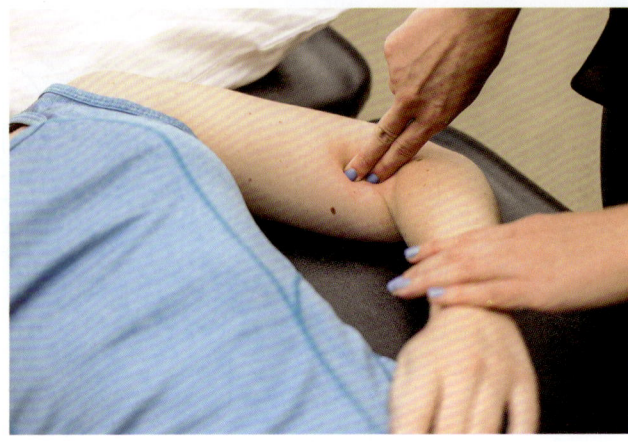

Figure 31-3. Examination of the brachialis muscle for TrPs by pushing the biceps brachii muscle aside in a medial direction to perform cross-fiber flat palpation to identify the TrPs. The biceps brachii muscle has additional slack if the forearm is supinated rather than pronated as shown here.

proximal to the nerve. A resultant resolution of the taut band and the relief of nerve entrapment symptoms strongly suggest that muscle shortening associated with the TrPs produced the nerve compression.

5. CORRECTIVE ACTIONS

To prevent stress overload of elbow flexion, the patient should lift only light or moderate loads with the forearms pronated. This position more readily activates the brachioradialis muscle, avoiding additional load on the brachialis muscle.[27] Avoiding repetitive lifting with the elbows flexed also decreases the overload on the muscle.

To avoid immobilizing the brachialis muscle in a shortened position, a towel can be wrapped around the elbow to prevent a prolonged flexed or extended position while sleeping (Figure 30-6). This prevents tension through the muscle. Likewise, the elbow should not be held sharply flexed while talking on a phone. The phone should be switched between hands occasionally, or a speaker function may be utilized. A purse should be held in the fingers with the elbow straight or hung over the opposite shoulder, not hung from the affected forearm with the elbow bent, to avoid prolonged strain through the elbow flexors. When playing a musical instrument that requires bent elbow positioning, like the violin or guitar, the elbow should be allowed to hang down straight at every opportunity.

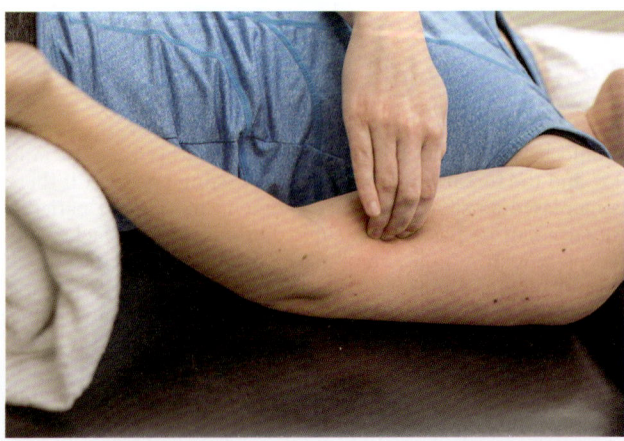

Figure 31-4. Self-pressure release of TrPs in the brachialis muscle.

Patients can perform self-pressure release of TrPs in either the supine or seated position. The patient should support the forearm in a flexed position to slacken the biceps brachii muscle and to allow access to the deep brachialis muscle (Figure 31-4). After finding a tender spot, a gentle pressure is applied with either the thumb or a tier of digits for 30 seconds or until the pain decreases. This release may be repeated three to five times as needed. Forceful pressure should be avoided as many nerves travel through this region. If any numbness or tingling occurs, the position of the thumb or digits should be modified.

Initially, the arm should be allowed to rest in this position using only the force of gravity to assist post-isometric relaxation without any assistance from the other hand. The patient should then perform a series of contracting and relaxing maneuvers synchronized with respiration to obtain maximum efficacy. During these maneuvers, the patient may also apply firm pressure with the opposite fingers over an identified active TrP. This action may help facilitate the TrP release. After several cycles of post-isometric relaxation, additional release and lengthening may be achieved by gently assisting a stretch into elbow extension (straightening) with the other hand. This process should not be painful, but a sense of stretch tension may be perceived. The patient should do several of these augmented stretches two to three times daily.

References

1. Standring S. *Gray's Anatomy: The Anatomical Basis of Clinical Practice*. 41st ed. London, UK: Elsevier; 2015.
2. Loukas M, Louis RG Jr, South G, Alsheik E, Christopherson C. A case of an accessory brachialis muscle. *Clin Anat*. 2006;19(6):550-553.
3. Pai MM, Nayak SR, Vadgaonkar R, et al. Accessory brachialis muscle: a case report. *Morphologie*. 2008;92(296):47-49.
4. Vadgaonkar R, Rai R, Nayak SR, D'Costa S, Saralaya V, Dhanya. An anatomical and clinical insight on brachialis with emphasis on portal's muscle. *Rom J Morphol Embryol*. 2010;51(3):551-553.
5. Tubbs RS, Yablick MW, Loukas M, Shoja MM, Ardalan M, Oakes WJ. Capsular attachment of the brachialis muscle (Portal's muscle): an anatomical and functional study. *Surg Radiol Anat*. 2008;30(3):229-232.
6. Mehta V, Suri RK, Arora J, Rath G, Das S. Peculiar tendinous origin of the brachialis muscle: anatomic and clinical insight. *Rom J Morphol Embryol*. 2009;50(1):141-143.
7. Oh CS, Won HS, Lee KS, Chung IH. Origin of the radial nerve branch innervating the brachialis muscle. *Clin Anat*. 2009;22(4):495-499.
8. Prakash, Kumari J, Singh N, Rahul Deep G, Akhtar T, Sridevi NS. A cadaveric study in the Indian population of the brachialis muscle innervation by the radial nerve. *Rom J Morphol Embryol*. 2009;50(1):111-114.
9. Blackburn SC, Wood CP, Evans DJ, Watt DJ. Radial nerve contribution to brachialis in the UK Caucasian population: position is predictable based on surface landmarks. *Clin Anat*. 2007;20(1):64-67.
10. Bendersky M, Bianchi HF. Double innervation of the brachialis muscle: anatomic-physiological study. *Surg Radiol Anat*. 2012;34(9):865-870.
11. Mahakkanukrauh P, Somsarp V. Dual innervation of the brachialis muscle. *Clin Anat*. 2002;15(3):206-209.
12. Won SY, Cho YH, Choi YJ, et al. Intramuscular innervation patterns of the brachialis muscle. *Clin Anat*. 2015;28(1):123-127.
13. Frazer EA, Hobson M, McDonald SW. The distribution of the radial and musculocutaneous nerves in the brachialis muscle. *Clin Anat*. 2007;20(7):785-789.
14. Spinner RJ, Pichelmann MA, Birch R. Radial nerve innervation to the inferolateral segment of the brachialis muscle: from anatomy to clinical reality. *Clin Anat*. 2003;16(4):368-369.
15. Nasr AY. Morphology and clinical significance of the distribution of the median nerve within the arm of human cadavers. *Neurosciences (Riyadh)*. 2012;17(4):336-344.
16. Parchand MP, Patil ST. Absence of musculocutaneous nerve with variations in course and distribution of the median nerve. *Anat Sci Int*. 2013;88(1):58-60.
17. Basmajian J, Deluca C. *Muscles Alive*. 5th ed. Baltimore, MD: Williams & Wilkins; 1985.
18. Duchenne G. *Physiology of Motion*. Philadelphia, PA: Lippincott; 1949.
19. Jenkins DB. *Hollinshead's Functional Anatomy of the Limbs and Back*. 6th ed. Philadelphia, PA: W.B. Saunders; 1991.
20. Kendall FP, McCreary EK. *Muscles: Testing and Function, with Posture and Pain*. Baltimore, MD: Lippincott Williams & Wilkins; 2005.
21. Rasch PJ, Burke RK. *Kinesiology and Applied Anatomy: The Science of Human Movement*. 6th ed. Philadelphia, PA: Lea & Febiger; 1978.
22. Hu SN, Zhou WJ, Wang H, et al. Origination of the brachialis branch of the musculocutaneous nerve: an electrophysiological study. *Neurosurgery*. 2008;62(4):908-911; discussion 911-912.
23. Jonsson S, Jonsson B. Function of the muscles of the upper limb in car driving. *Ergonomics*. 1975;18(4):375-388.
24. Simons DG, Travell JG, Simons LS. *Myofascial Pain and Dysfunction: The Trigger Point Manual. Volume 1: Upper Half of Body*. 2nd ed. Philadelphia, PA: Lippincott Williams & Wilkins;1999.
25. Kelly M. The nature of fibrositis: I. The myalgic lesion and its secondary effects: a reflex theory. *Ann Rheum Dis*. 1945;5(1):1-7.
26. Kellgren JH. Observations on referred pain arising from muscle. *Clin Sci*. 1938;3:175-190.
27. Kleiber T, Kunz L, Disselhorst-Klug C. Muscular coordination of biceps brachii and brachioradialis in elbow flexion with respect to hand position. *Front Physiol*. 2015;6:215.
28. Lee YK, Kim YI, Choy WS. Radial nerve compression between the brachialis and brachioradialis muscles in a manual worker: a case report. *J Hand Surg Am*. 2006;31(5):744-746.
29. Mennell JM. *Joint Pain: Diagnosis and Treatment using Manipulative Techniques*. 1st ed. Boston, MA: Little Brown; 1964.
30. Gerwin RD, Dommerholt J, Shah JP. An expansion of Simons' integrated hypothesis of trigger point formation. *Curr Pain Headache Rep*. 2004;8(6):468-475.
31. Suh MR, Chang WH, Choi HS, Lee SC. Ultrasound-guided myofascial trigger point injection into brachialis muscle for rotator cuff disease patients with upper arm pain: a pilot study. *Ann Rehabil Med*. 2014;38(5):673-681.
32. Hsieh YL, Kao MJ, Kuan TS, Chen SM, Chen JT, Hong CZ. Dry needling to a key myofascial trigger point may reduce the irritability of satellite MTrPs. *Am J Phys Med Rehabil*. 2007;86(5):397-403.
33. Wainner RS, Fritz JM, Irrgang JJ, Boninger ML, Delitto A, Allison S. Reliability and diagnostic accuracy of the clinical examination and patient self-report measures for cervical radiculopathy. *Spine (Phila Pa 1976)*. 2003;28(1):52-62.

Chapter 32

Triceps Brachii and Anconeus Muscles
"Elbow Excruciators"

Leigh E. Palubinskas and Joseph M. Donnelly

1. INTRODUCTION

The triceps brachii muscle is commonly overlooked as a source of symptoms for lateral or medial epicondylalgia. It is a three-headed fusiform muscle that occupies the posterior extensor compartment of the upper arm along with the anconeus muscle. The long head of the triceps brachii muscle is biarticular, crossing both the shoulder and the elbow, allowing it to act at both joints. The other heads (medial and lateral) are uniarticular and act only at the elbow. The long and lateral heads of the triceps brachii muscle and the anconeus muscle are innervated by branches of the radial nerve. The innervation of the medial head of the triceps brachii muscle is controversial. It is generally accepted that the muscle is also innervated by the radial nerve, but others have shown that the ulnar nerve innervates the medial head of the triceps brachii muscle. The primary function of the triceps brachii muscle is extension of the elbow. The medial head of the triceps brachii muscle is most active in elbow extension and is considered the "workhorse" of the three heads. The long head of the triceps brachii muscle stabilizes the glenohumeral joint from below by providing a superior force, which counteracts the tendency of the latissimus dorsi and pectoralis major muscles to pull the head of the humerus downward out of the glenoid fossa. It also adducts and extends the arm at the shoulder. The anconeus muscle assists the triceps brachii muscle in elbow extension and acts as an active lateral stabilizer of the humeroulnar joint. Trigger points (TrPs) in the triceps brachii muscle primarily refer pain to the posterior upper arm with referral into the posterior shoulder and upper trapezius muscles proximally. Distally, the referral pattern can encompass the posterior forearm and fourth and fifth digits of the hand. Pain is often localized over the lateral epicondyle and/or medial epicondyle, mimicking the symptoms of tennis and golfer's elbow, respectively. Trigger points in the anconeus muscle refer to the lateral epicondyle. Triceps brachii and anconeus TrPs are activated by repetitive overuse of elbow extension such as when using forearm crutches, playing tennis, or repeatedly pressing down on a surface. Differential diagnoses include lateral or medial epicondylitis, olecranon bursitis, and thoracic outlet syndrome. Postural adjustments to support the elbow when performing activities with the arms in front of the body can help prevent TrP formation. Corrective actions include modification of sports activities with a gradual return to sport following treatment; TrP self-pressure release and self-stretch are also effective in releasing TrPs in the triceps brachii muscle.

2. ANATOMIC CONSIDERATIONS

Triceps Brachii

Long Head
The triceps brachii muscle is a three-headed fusiform muscle that fills the majority of the extensor compartment of the upper arm (Figure 32-1A and B). The long head of the triceps brachii muscle crosses both the shoulder and elbow joints. Proximally, it originates from a flat tendon attached to the infraglenoid tubercle of the scapula and blends superiorly with the glenohumeral joint capsule.[1] The muscle travels inferomedially, passing between the teres major and teres minor muscles to form the quadrangular and triangular spaces.[1,2] The quadrangular space contains the posterior humeral circumflex artery and the axillary nerve. The subscapularis muscle, teres minor muscle, and glenohumeral joint capsule make up the superior border. The inferior border is defined by the teres major muscle. The medial border is defined by the long head of the triceps brachii muscle, and the lateral border is defined by the humerus. The triangular space contains the scapular circumflex vessels and is defined superiorly by the teres minor muscle, inferiorly by the teres major muscle, and laterally by the long head of the triceps brachii muscle.[1] These spaces and boundaries are important to identify when performing a TrP injection or dry needling.

Medial Head
The medial head of the triceps brachii muscle, sometimes referred to as the deep head, originates from the entire posterior surface of the proximal humerus, at the insertion of the teres major muscle and below the radial groove, extending inferiorly just proximal to the trochlea of the humerus.[1] It also originates from the medial humerus and from the lower portion of the lateral intermuscular septum. It covers the posterior humerus both medially and laterally. The medial head of the triceps brachii muscle lies deep against the bone and attaches just above the elbow (Figure 32-2). The lateral and long heads of the muscle overlap it posteriorly. The distal portion of the medial head converges with the common triceps brachii tendon with some muscle fibers inserting directly into the olecranon.[1]

Lateral Head
Proximally, the lateral head of the triceps brachii muscle originates from a flat tendon on the posterior surface of the shaft of the humerus, the lateral intermuscular septum just superior to the radial groove, and posterior to the deltoid tuberosity, extending to the surgical neck of the humerus near the insertion of the teres minor muscle. It bridges the radial nerve and covers much of the medial head of the triceps brachii muscle (Figure 32-1B). The fibers of the lateral head of the triceps brachii muscle converge with the common tendon medially. The medial and lateral heads of the triceps brachii muscle are uniarticular, crossing only the elbow joint.[1]

The three heads of the triceps brachii muscle insert distally to the upper surface of the olecranon process of the ulna via a common tendon (Figure 32-1), which begins in the middle of the muscle and consists of a superficial lamina and a deep lamina that join near their insertion. On the lateral side of the olecranon, a band of fibers continue down over the anconeus muscle to blend with the antebrachial fascia.[1]

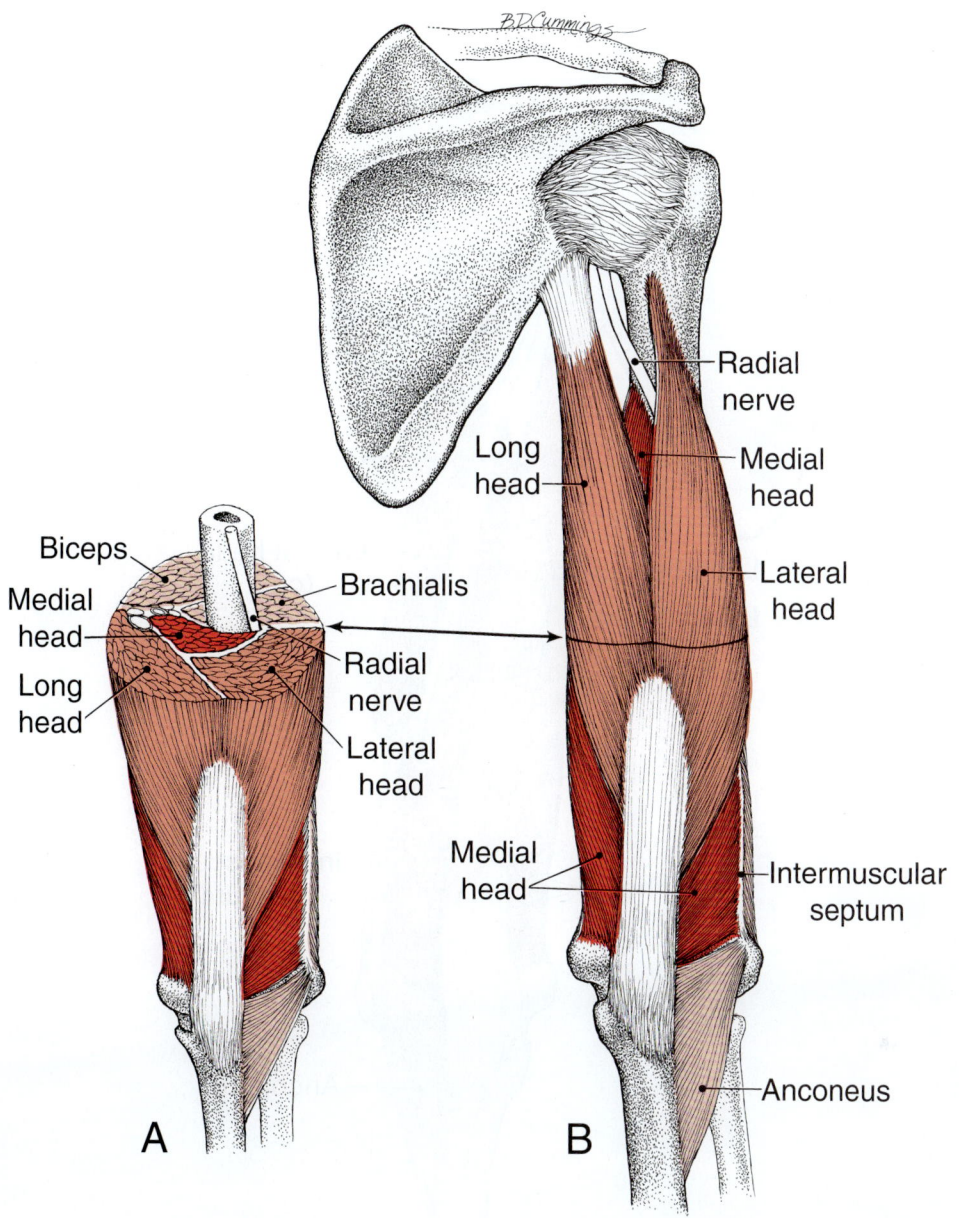

Figure 32-1. A, Cross section of the right arm just proximal to the level where the radial nerve penetrates the lateral intermuscular septum (the horizontal double arrow and black line in [B] across the muscle indicate the level of cross section). The biceps brachii, brachialis, and anconeus muscles are light red. B, Attachments of the right triceps brachii muscle (two darker reds) seen from behind. The medial (deep) head is dark red and the lateral and long heads are medium red and the anconeus is in light red.

The distribution of fiber types in the triceps brachii muscle has been studied by taking samples of the triceps brachii muscles post mortem.[3-5] Both the lateral head and long head of the triceps brachii muscle had ~60% to 65% fast twitch (type II) fibers and ~40% slow twitch (type I) fibers. However, the medial head was comprised of 60% slow twitch fibers and only 40% fast twitch fibers.[3] Samples taken near the surface of the muscle and from deep in the triceps brachii muscles showed no significant difference in this composition.

Anconeus

The anconeus muscle is a small triangular muscle that is partially blended with the triceps brachii muscle posterior to the elbow joint. It originates from the posterior surface of the lateral epicondyle, covers the posterior aspect of the annular ligament, and attaches distally to the lateral side of the olecranon process and to the dorsal surface of the ulna.[1] Fibers of the muscle are also adhered to the lateral aspect of the humeroulnar joint, adding stability to the joint.[6] An anomalous anconeus epitrochlearis muscle may attach between the medial aspect of the olecranon and the medial epicondyle overlying the ulnar nerve.[7]

The anconeus muscle is composed of ~60% to 67% type I fibers and ~35% type II fibers.[5] This fiber composition supports the function of the anconeus muscle as an elbow stabilizer rather than a force producing muscle.

2.1. Innervation and Vascularization

The long and lateral heads of the triceps brachii muscle and the anconeus muscle are innervated by branches of the radial

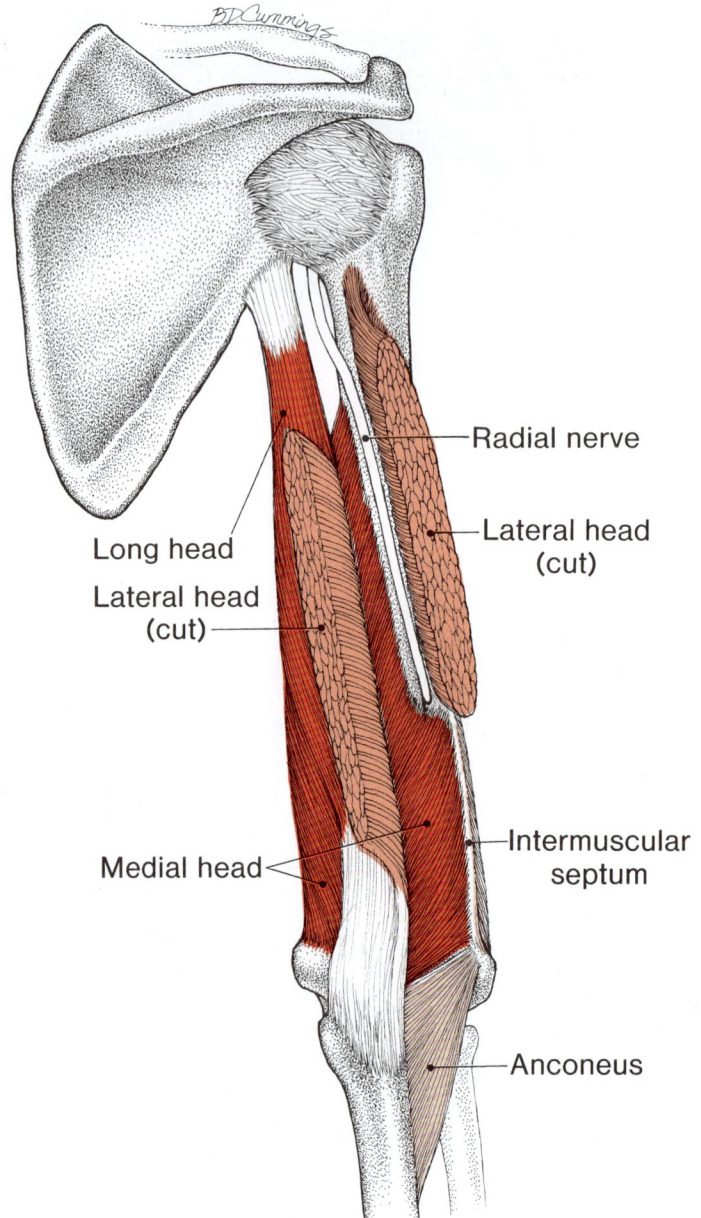

Figure 32-2. Posterior view of the triceps brachii muscle with the lateral head cut and reflected, showing the course of the radial nerve, which separates the humeral attachments of the medial and lateral heads of the triceps brachii muscle.

nerve via the posterior cord of the brachial plexus from spinal roots C6, C7, and C8.[1]

The innervation of the medial head of the triceps brachii muscle is controversial. Several recent cadaveric studies have identified ulnar nerve innervation in 28% to 61% of samples.[8-10] This finding is contrary to the generally accepted belief that the muscle is innervated by the radial nerve. It is hypothesized that the high incidence of ulnar nerve innervation may be due to the fact that in these studies the nerve was not traced far enough proximally to make an accurate identification of the nerve.[11,12] In addition, the radial and ulnar nerves travel for a distance within the same nerve sheath making conclusive identification of the fibers difficult. Innervation of this shoulder remains debatable and no conclusive data from large-scale research studies have confirmed innervation of the medial head of the muscle by either the radial or the ulnar nerve.

The long head of the triceps brachii muscle receives its vascular supply from the axillary artery and the brachial or ulnar collateral arteries. The medial and lateral heads of the triceps brachii muscle receive vascularization primarily from the profunda brachii artery, superior ulnar collateral artery, and a branch of the posterior circumflex artery.[1]

The anconeus muscle receives its vascularization via branches of the posterior interosseous recurrent artery.[1]

2.2. Function

All parts of the triceps brachii muscle extend the forearm at the elbow joint.[13-19] The medial (deep) head, however, is the "workhorse" among elbow extensors and is active in all forms of extension.[1] It exhibits the earliest and the greatest electromyographic (EMG) activity.[13,20] The position of the elbow changes the effectiveness of the triceps brachii muscle. The triceps brachii muscle produces maximum torque with the elbow flexed to 90°.[21] But the position of the forearm does not change triceps brachii muscle activation, due to its attachment on the ulna and not on the radius. The triceps brachii muscle acts concentrically to perform elbow extension during a push-up and works eccentrically in a reverse action, controlling elbow flexion during the lowering phase of the push-up. Two studies investigated the muscle activation patterns of the three heads of the triceps brachii muscle to determine load sharing of the muscles during elbow movement.[18,22] Considerable differences were present between subjects in both studies indicating that there is not a consistent load-sharing pattern for activation of the triceps brachii muscle during elbow movement.

Only the activity of the long head of the triceps brachii muscle is altered by shoulder position because it crosses both the shoulder and the elbow joints. With the shoulder joint in extension and the muscle in a shortened position, the long head of the triceps brachii muscle cannot produce as much torque at the elbow. The long head also extends the arm at the shoulder and acts to adduct the arm, pulling the humerus back to the anatomic position from an elevated shoulder position.[2,13,15-17,23] During stimulation of the long head, adduction appeared to be the dominant action.[14] The long head of the triceps brachii muscle is most active during shoulder extension in ranges from 80° to 120° of shoulder flexion, and elbow flexion has little effect on muscle activation of the long head at the shoulder joint.[23]

The long head of the triceps brachii muscle also produces arthrokinematic forces at the glenohumeral joint. It mitigates inferior translation of the humeral head when downward forces are transmitted through the joint. It also pulls the head of the humerus superiorly. The scapular attachment of the long head of the triceps brachii muscle influences actions at the glenohumeral joint. Older electrical stimulation studies[14] demonstrated that the activation of the long head of the triceps brachii muscle alone, with the arm hanging down at the side of the body, elevated the head of the humerus toward the acromion. Stimulation with the arm abducted to 90° forced the head of the humerus into the glenoid cavity. The long head of the triceps brachii, the pectoralis major, and latissimus dorsi muscles all strongly adduct the arm, but the long head of the triceps brachii muscle counteracts the strong tendency of the other two muscles to pull the head of the humerus downward out of the glenoid fossa.[14] Stimulation of the long head of the triceps brachii muscle suggests that adduction of the arm at the glenohumeral joint is achieved by drawing the humerus to the scapula without rotating the scapula, whereas stimulating the teres major muscle tended to draw the inferior angle of the scapula toward the humerus without moving the arm.[14] These differences in function are not surprising because these two muscles have reverse long and short lever arms resulting in different moments of force at the glenohumeral joint.

Myers et al[24] investigated EMG activity using maximal volitional contraction (MVC) in the shoulder and the upper extremity muscles during 12 rubber-tubing exercises commonly used for shoulder rehabilitation. They found maximum activation of the triceps brachii muscle (67% MVC) during shoulder extension from 90° of shoulder flexion to a neutral position. They also found moderate activation during acceleration and deceleration while throwing, external and internal rotation at 0° shoulder abduction, scapular punches, middle and low scapular rows, and during shoulder flexion.[24]

Bilateral triceps brachii muscles were monitored electromyographically with surface electrodes during 13 sports activities including overhand and underhand throws, tennis, golf, baseball batting, and one-foot jumps. Most of the records showed briefer, more intense contraction of the dominant triceps brachii muscle than the nondominant muscle. The more prolonged activity of the nondominant triceps brachii muscle appeared to function in counterbalance. Two outstanding exceptions were batting a baseball and golf swings, in which the nondominant triceps brachii muscle acted as a prime mover.[25] There is also a relationship between triceps brachii muscle activation and the velocity of the forehand drive in tennis. Increasing the velocity of a tennis swing causes earlier activation of the muscle. The muscle may activate earlier to provide stabilization to the elbow at impact and to prepare for the increased deceleration force needed during a follow through.[26-28]

EMG analysis of muscle activation patterns during the crawl swimming stroke have been studied extensively over the past 50 years.[29] Rouard et al[30] concluded that the triceps brachii and biceps brachii muscles served antagonistic roles during the crawl stroke to stabilize the elbow joint to improve the performance of the prime movers. Lauer et al[31] found the greatest coactivation to be during early pull through to stabilize the elbow joint. Both investigators[30,31] found the triceps brachii muscle to have approximately 40% MVC during mid-to-late pull through, having a large function in propulsion, and the least activity (15% MVC) during early recovery.

In an EMG analysis of the shoulder and the upper extremity muscles in five conditions comparing professional javelin throwers with a control group found that the triceps brachii muscle is moderately active during pulling, starting with the shoulder in 45° flexion and elbow fully extended, and with pushing, starting with the shoulder in neutral and the elbow flexed to 90° (40–51% MVC). With shoulder elevation, they found the triceps brachii muscle to be moderately active in the control group (47% MVC) and minimally active in the professional athletes (29% MVC) in the plane of the scapula to 140° elevation. During a goal-oriented slow throw, the triceps brachii muscle was moderately active in both the groups (53% MVC) and during a quick throw the biceps brachii muscle was maximally active in both the groups (98% MVC). The professional throwers achieved peak activation much sooner in the motion, but it was not statistically significant.[32]

Conte et al[33] investigated EMG activity of the upper extremity, shoulder, and trunk muscles in two different conditions while utilizing a laptop, a touch pad, and an external mouse. They found greater activity in the triceps brachii and biceps brachii muscles while utilizing the touch pad against the external mouse. They believe the touch pad requires a greater degree of movement accuracy and, therefore, stabilization than the external mouse. They conclude that using an external mouse should be preferred to a touch pad by frequent users of a laptop to decrease muscle overload.

EMG analysis of the upper extremity muscles during driving[34,35] demonstrates that the triceps brachii muscle is moderately active during turning to the same side the wheel was turning. Also, driving positions with the arm outstretched produced greater muscular activity than a driving position with the arms closer to the body in a more vertical position.

Anconeus

The anconeus muscle assists the triceps brachii muscle in extension at the elbow joint.[13] The muscle contributes approximately 15% of the extension movement at low torque levels.[19] As elbow flexion increases, the activity of the anconeus decreases, and at greater than 45° of elbow flexion, the anconeus muscle becomes a lateral stabilizer of the humeroulnar joint.[36] Its adherence to the lateral humeroulnar capsule allows it to actively stabilize the elbow, preventing posterolateral dislocation and providing an active constraint to protect the passive lateral collateral ligament and joint capsule.[6] This role as a stabilizer has also been confirmed electromyographically. The medial head of the triceps brachii, anconeus, and supinator muscles work together to stabilize the elbow joint during pronation and supination of the forearm by abducting the ulna.[13,37] The anconeus muscle is also active during all index finger movements and during maximal gripping.[38,39] During gripping, the anconeus muscle may be activated to stabilize the elbow and counteract the elbow flexion moment caused by forceful activation of the wrist flexor muscles.[40]

> **Box 32-1** Functional unit of the triceps brachii/anconeus muscles
>
> | Action | Synergists | Antagonist |
> |---|---|---|
> | Elbow extension | Triceps brachii
Anconeus | Biceps brachii
Brachioradialis
Brachialis
Pronator teres |

2.3. Functional Unit

The functional unit to which a muscle belongs includes the muscles that reinforce and counter its actions as well as the joints that it crosses. The functional interdependence of these structures is reflected in the organization and neural connections of the sensory motor cortex. The functional unit is emphasized because the presence of a TrP in one muscle of the unit increases the likelihood that the other muscles of the unit also develop TrPs. When inactivating TrPs in a muscle, one should be concerned about TrPs that may develop in muscles that are functionally interdependent. Box 32-1 grossly represents the functional unit of the triceps brachii muscle.[41]

The long head of the triceps brachii muscle is synergistic with the latissimus dorsi, teres major, and teres minor muscles, which can all act as adductors and extensors of the arm at the shoulder joint. The long head of the triceps brachii muscle works synergistically with the coracobrachialis, the short head of the biceps brachii, the clavicular head of the pectoralis major, and the deltoid muscles to pull the humerus superiorly and also to eccentrically control inferior translation of the humerus. The subscapularis and costal portion of the pectoralis major muscle provide a stabilizing antagonistic pull.[2]

The deltoid and supraspinatus muscles are antagonistic to shoulder adduction and the pectoralis major, anterior deltoid, and coracobrachialis muscles are antagonistic to shoulder extension.

3. CLINICAL PRESENTATION
3.1. Referred Pain Pattern

Triceps Brachii

Trigger points in the triceps brachii muscle occur frequently and can be found in any of the three heads of the muscle. They are most commonly found in the long head and the lateral portion of the medial head of the muscle. The referral patterns for each portion of the muscle vary and can refer pain to the posterior or anterior portions of the upper arm and elbow. In this muscle, it is important to distinguish TrPs in the distal portion of the muscle from attachment enthesopathy of the common triceps brachii tendon.

Long Head

Trigger points in the long head of the triceps brachii muscle (Figure 32-3A, left) refer pain and tenderness upward over the posterior arm to the back of the shoulder, occasionally to the base of the neck in the region of the upper trapezius muscle, and sometimes down the dorsum of the forearm, skipping the elbow. Trigger points are often located in the central portion of the long head muscle belly.

Medial Head

The medial head of the triceps brachii muscle may have TrPs that lie mid-fiber in the lateral portion (Figure 32-3A, right) or in the deeper segment of the medial portion of the muscle (Figure 32-3C). Trigger points in the lateral portion of the medial head presents with referred pain to the lateral epicondyle and are often a common component of the epicondylalgia more commonly known as "tennis elbow" (Figure 32-3B, right). Pain may also extend to the radial aspect of the forearm (Figure 32-3A, right). If the deep portion of the medial head is involved, pain and tenderness is present over the medial epicondyle and may extend to the volar surface of the fourth and fifth digits and occasionally into the adjacent palm and the middle finger (Figure 32-3C). Pain may also occur along the inner side of the forearm from these TrPs at this location.[42]

Lateral Head

Pain and tenderness from TrPs in the lateral head of the triceps brachii muscle (Figure 32-3B, left) refer over the arm posteriorly, sometimes to the dorsum of the forearm, and occasionally to the fourth and fifth digits. Taut bands in the lateral head may cause entrapment of the radial nerve.

Distal Triceps Brachii

Trigger points in the distal portion (Figure 32-3B, right) of the triceps brachii muscle cause local tenderness over the olecranon process. Trigger points in this region typically occur secondarily to TrPs in the long head, lateral head, and deep portion of the medial head of the triceps brachii muscle.

Anconeus

A TrP in the anconeus muscle refers pain and tenderness locally to the lateral epicondyle (Figure 32-4) and is often involved in cases of lateral epicondylalgia and chronic "tennis elbow" that persist after TrPs in the wrist extensor and triceps brachii muscles have been inactivated.

3.2. Symptoms

Patients who have TrPs in the triceps brachii muscle often report pain that is vague and hard to localize in the back of the shoulder and the upper arm. In highly irritable cases, the patient may report pain in the dorsal and volar aspect of the forearm and into the fourth and fifth digits of the hand. They may also report pain localized at the medial or lateral aspect of the elbow joint and often present with symptoms similar to "tennis elbow" or "golfer's elbow." Patients do not typically report restricted motion though they may be unaware of any elbow or forearm joint restriction because of the automatic tendency to keep the elbow slightly flexed and out of the painful range. They may compensate for the slightly reduced reach by additional shoulder blade or trunk movements. Because of tenderness referred to the inner elbow, the elbow may be held away from the side to avoid body contact and the patient may be unable to place their elbow on a supporting surface. Patients may report that they cannot place the elbow on the center console or arm rest while driving or performing computer work secondary to pain.

The patient may also report pain during activities that require forceful extension of the elbow such as playing tennis (dominant arm), playing golf (nondominant arm), or while swimming (crawl stroke). Pain from TrPs in the lateral head of the triceps brachii muscle can play an important role in the pain experience and loss of function of patients diagnosed with lateral epicondylalgia or "tennis elbow" (see Chapter 41).

3.3. Patient Examination

After a thorough subjective examination the clinician should make a detailed drawing representing the pain pattern that the patient has described. This depiction will assist in planning the physical examination and can be useful in monitoring the

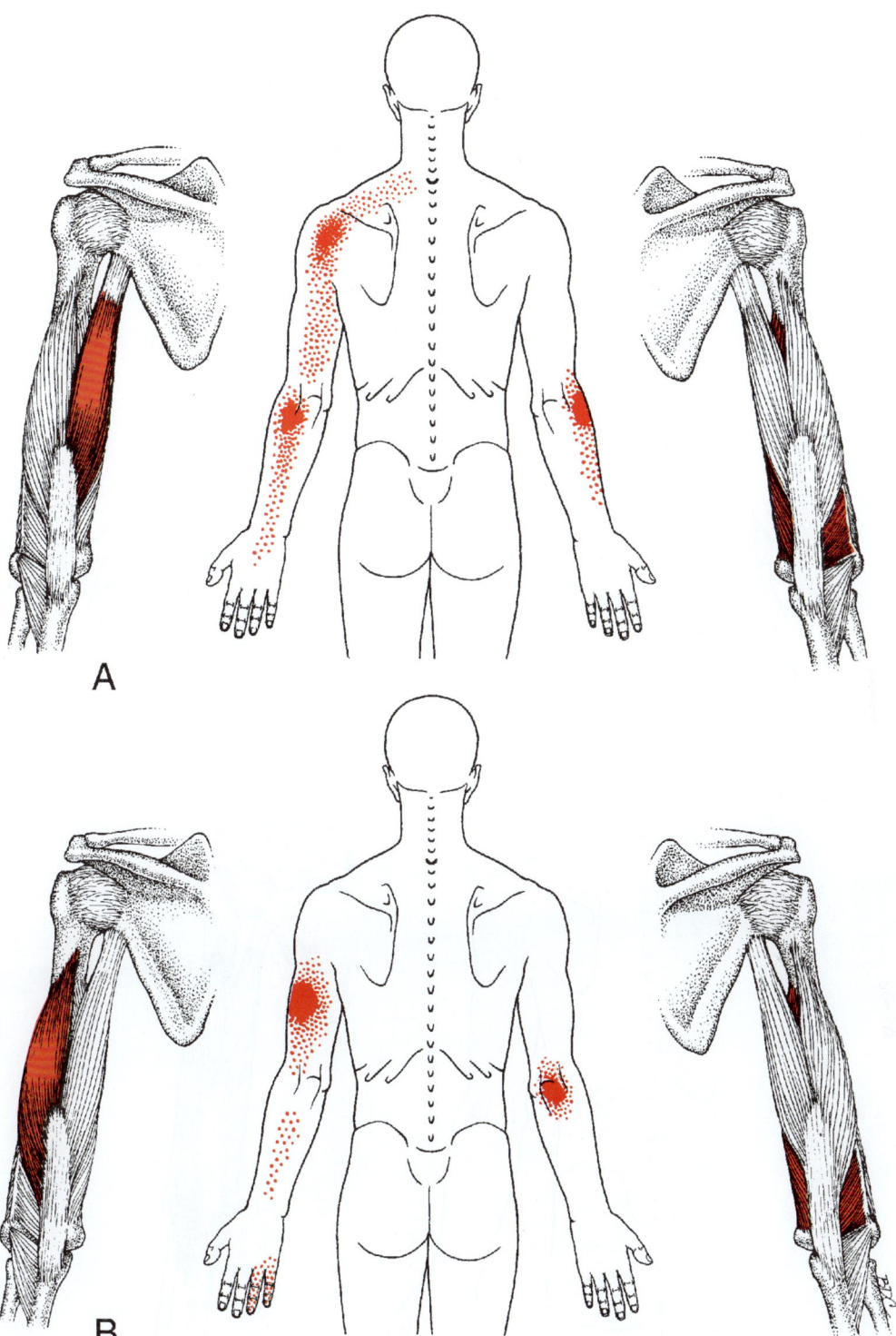

Figure 32-3. Referred pain patterns (dark red) from TrPs in the triceps brachii muscle (medium red). A, Trigger points in the left long head and in the lateral portion of the right medial (deep) head. B, Trigger points in the left lateral head and deep in the right medial head under the tendon in the musculotendinous attachment region. C, Additional pain referral pattern for TrPs in the right medial (deep) head of the triceps brachii muscle.

patient's progress as symptoms improve or change. For proper examination of the triceps brachii and anconeus muscles, the clinician should assess the patient's upper extremity and shoulder girdle posture while standing with arms at the side, elbow carrying position, active and passive ranges of motion of the upper extremity joints, muscle activation patterns in the shoulder girdle, and scapulohumeral rhythm. To identify TrPs in the triceps brachii muscle that may be limiting the range of motion and thus influencing dysfunction, the clinician should identify the limited range of motion by performing a specific range of motion testing for all parts of the triceps brachii muscle. The long head of the triceps brachii muscle crosses both the elbow and shoulder joints and therefore shoulder position should be considered while evaluating this portion of the triceps brachii muscle. By increasing muscle tension, TrPs can produce biomechanical dysfunction.

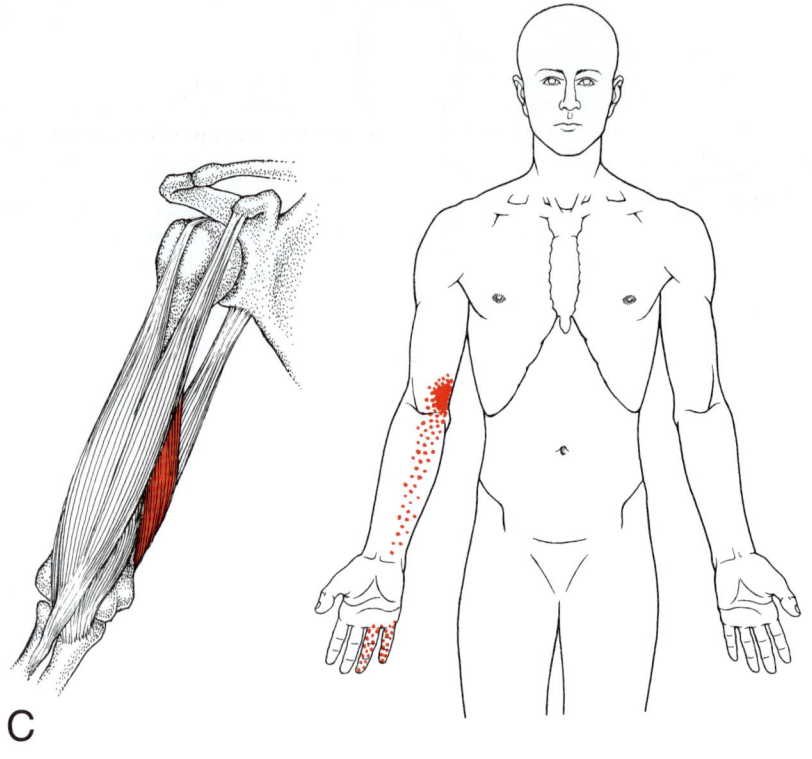

Figure 32-3. (continued)

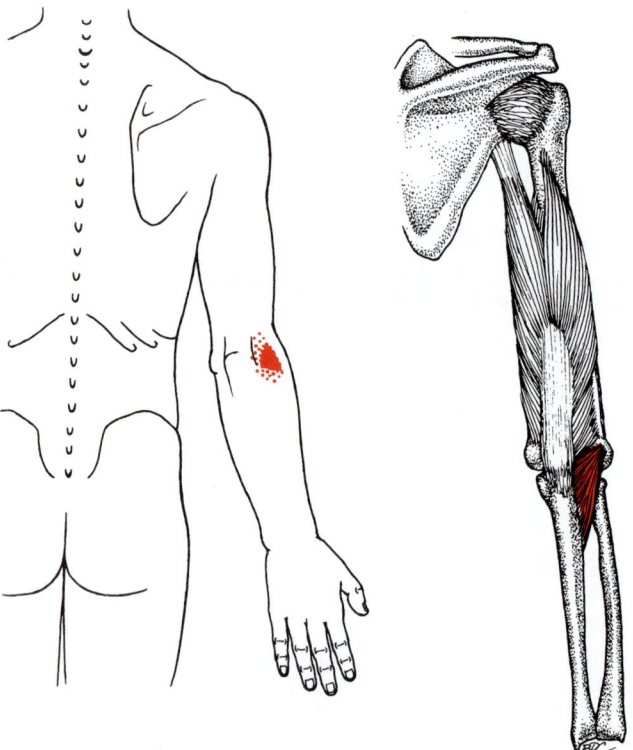

Figure 32-4. Anconeus muscle pain referral pattern (dark red) for TrPs located within the muscle (light red).

Bron et al[43] assessed the prevalence of muscles with TrPs in 72 patients with chronic nontraumatic unilateral shoulder pain. They found the highest prevalence of muscles with TrPs in the infraspinatus (93%) and upper trapezius (94%) muscles. They also found that 56% of the patients had TrPs in the triceps brachii muscle, though they did not report the specific prevalence of TrPs in the three different heads of the triceps brachii muscle.

Muscle-specific resisted testing should be carried out to identify impairments in muscle function and reproduction of painful symptoms with loading. Weakness or inhibition of the triceps brachii muscle can be identified by resisting elbow extension in 90° of elbow flexion. Resisting shoulder extension (between 80° and 120° of shoulder flexion) with the elbow straight maximally activates the long head of the muscle and helps differentiate it from the medial and lateral heads. The forearm position does not affect triceps brachii muscle activation patterns due to its attachment on the ulna.[23] To differentiate the activation of the anconeus muscle, resistance to elbow extension should be applied with the elbow in less than 45° of flexion or resistance can be applied at the end range of forearm pronation.

Accessory joint motion of the elbow and shoulder joints (including the acromioclavicular and sternoclavicular joints) should be manually tested to determine if faulty arthrokinematics are a contributing factor to triceps brachii TrPs. If the shoulder girdle is found to be a contributing factor to activation and perpetuation of TrPs in the triceps brachii muscle, effective joint movement should be restored.

If a humeral epicondyle is painful due to TrPs, it may also be sensitive to tapping or vibration because of referred tenderness. Pain in the lateral epicondyle due to triceps brachii TrPs often persists in patients diagnosed with "tennis elbow" after the supinator, biceps brachii, and brachioradialis TrPs have been inactivated. Residual percussion tenderness of the posterior aspect of the epicondyle indicates that triceps brachii TrPs are likely referring pain to this area.

3.4. Trigger Point Examination

The patient is positioned supine or prone to gain access to the triceps brachii and anconeus muscles. Cross-fiber pincer palpation can be utilized to identify TrPs in the long head of the triceps brachii muscle and cross-fiber flat palpation technique can be used to identify TrPs in the medial and lateral heads of the triceps brachii muscle and in the anconeus muscle.

Triceps Brachii

Long Head

Trigger points in the long head of the triceps brachii muscle are typically found deep in the midportion of the muscle, a few centimeters distal to where the long head of the triceps brachii muscle crosses the teres major muscle. Cross-fiber pincer palpation is usually necessary to locate TrPs in this muscle. The fingers should encircle the triceps brachii muscle (Figure 32-5A), reaching in until they encounter the humerus. The long head of the triceps brachii muscle can be separated slightly from the humerus and its fibers can be rolled between the digits. Clusters of TrPs are often present and are identified by their multiple taut bands, by reproduction of the patient's pain, and often by local twitch responses. The taut bands associated with TrPs in the long head of the triceps brachii muscle are likely to contribute to the tenderness of TrPs near the musculotendinous junction.

Medial Head

Trigger points in the lateral portion of the medial head are found with cross-fiber flat palpation (Figure 32-5B). Trigger points can also be found deep in the medial border of the mid-fiber region of the medial head, just above the medial epicondyle. Trigger points here are found by cross-fiber flat palpation with the patient lying supine and the arm externally rotated at the shoulder joint to expose the muscle belly (Figure 32-5C).

Lateral Head

Trigger points in the lateral head of the triceps brachii muscle can be identified by a cross-fiber flat palpation at the mid-belly in the lateral border of the lateral head, just above the point where the radial nerve exits from the radial groove (Figure 32-5D). The taut bands of TrPs in this part of the muscle may entrap the sensory fibers of the radial nerve as it passes through this area. In this case, firm palpation along the lateral intermuscular septum, in

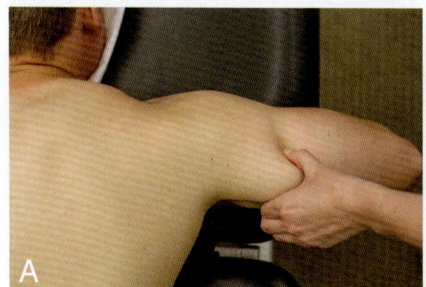
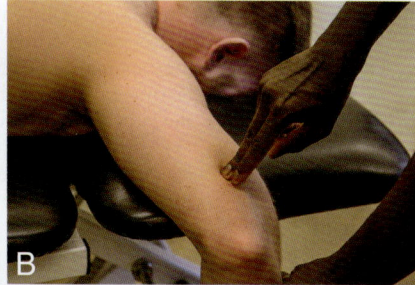
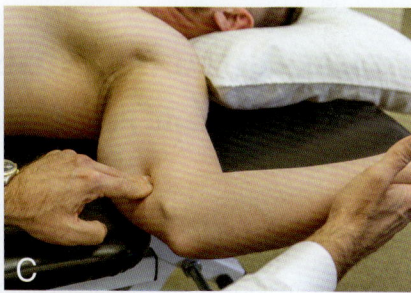
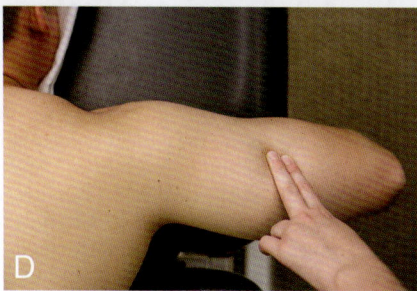
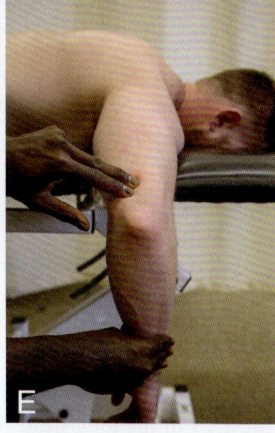

Figure 32-5. Trigger point examination of the triceps brachii muscle. A, Cross-fiber pincer palpation to identify TrPs in the long head of the right triceps brachii muscle. B, Cross-fiber flat palpation to identify TrPs in the lateral portion of the medial head. C, Cross-fiber flat palpation to identify TrPs in the medial portion of the medial head. D, Cross-fiber flat palpation to identify TrPs in the lateral head. E, Cross-fiber flat palpation to identify TrPs in the distal portion of the muscle, where all three heads conjoin.

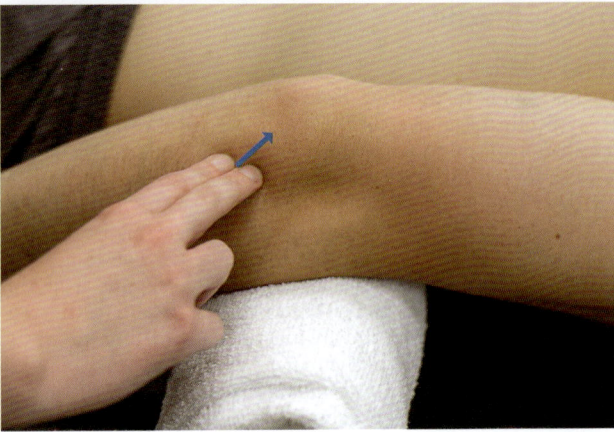

Figure 32-6. Trigger Point examination of the anconeus muscle using cross-fiber palpation.

the region where the radial nerve penetrates the septum, is likely to cause a tingling sensation in the hand.

Distal Triceps Brachii

Trigger points that are present near the tendon insertion of the triceps brachii muscle are found deep in the distal medial head with a cross-fiber flat palpation near the area of fusion of the three heads, just above the olecranon, to which it refers pain (Figure 32-5E).

Anconeus

Although the muscle is thin, TrPs in the anconeus muscle are deep and can be palpated using cross-fiber flat palpation lateral and inferior to the olecranon with the elbow slightly flexed and supported (Figure 32-6).

4. DIFFERENTIAL DIAGNOSIS

4.1. Activation and Perpetuation of Trigger Points

A posture or activity that activates a TrP, if not corrected, can also perpetuate it. In any part of the triceps brachii muscle, TrPs may be activated by unaccustomed eccentric loading, eccentric exercise in an unconditioned muscle, or maximal or submaximal concentric loading.[44] Trigger points may also be activated or aggravated when the muscle is placed in a shortened and/or lengthened position(s) for an extended period of time.

Activation of TrPs in the triceps brachii muscle may occur due to repetitive overload from overuse of forearm or axillary crutches, the stress of using a cane that is too long, short upper arms, excessive city driving in a car with manual transmission requiring extensive and repetitive manual gear shifting, or from any strong repetitive pushing action. Formation of TrPs may also occur due to traumatic overuse such as a catching the weight of the body during a fall on an outstretched hand. Investigators found that the triceps brachii muscle achieved peak %MVC prior to the time of peak impact force during three different fall scenarios from two different heights.[45] Activities such as tennis or overenthusiastic conditioning exercises (golf practice or push-ups) may also perpetuate TrPs in the triceps brachii muscle. Interestingly, the TrPs in the long head of the triceps brachii muscle are also likely to be activated by sitting for long periods with the elbow held forward in front of the plane of the chest or abdomen without proper elbow support (eg, driving a car on a long trip, or other handwork without elbow support).

Triceps brachii TrPs were activated by jackknife positioning of a patient during nephrolithotomy in a way that held the muscle in the stretched position for a prolonged period of time.[46] The TrPs were inactivated by deep massage of the TrPs and passive stretch, and the patient was relieved of the previously enigmatic pain.

Pain alters muscle activation patterns and this can also cause TrP formation. Investigators have induced pain in the triceps brachii and biceps brachii muscles with repetitive dynamic reaching, and the muscle activation patterns of the muscles in the upper arm changed.[47] When pain was induced, the activity of the biceps brachii and brachioradialis muscles decreased, but the activity in the triceps brachii muscle increased. A decreased activity in the biceps brachii muscle was compensated for by an increased activity in the other flexor muscles. In extension, compensation for decreased triceps brachii muscle activity is not possible, therefore the muscle should continue to act to complete the task at the same speed. The lack of redundancy of muscles in the posterior arm to perform extension motion may predispose the triceps brachii muscle to injury and TrP formation, especially from repetitive overuse because the muscle should continue to function to complete dynamic tasks despite pain and injury.

4.2. Associated Trigger Points

Associated TrPs can develop in the referred pain areas caused by primary TrPs.[48] Therefore, musculature in the referred pain areas for each muscle should also be evaluated. Release of the TrP in the associated muscle often allows for an immediate decrease in the pressure pain threshold of the associated TrPs.[47]

When a TrP is identified in the long head of the triceps brachii muscle, one should also examine the posterior deltoid, latissimus dorsi, teres major, and teres minor muscles for associated TrPs.

When elbow pain persists in the lateral epicondylar area after eliminating TrPs in the medial head of the triceps brachii muscle, the anconeus, supinator, brachioradialis, and extensor carpi radialis longus muscles should be examined for associated TrPs.

Trigger points in the ipsilateral latissimus dorsi, serratus posterior superior,[49] coracobrachialis, or subscapularis muscles may cause associated TrPs in the triceps brachii muscle. For lasting release of the triceps brachii TrPs, TrPs in these other muscles should be inactivated.

As antagonists to the triceps brachii muscle are part of the functional unit, the biceps brachii and brachialis muscles are prone to develop TrPs (often latent) during chronic TrP involvement of the triceps brachii muscle.

4.3. Associated Pathology

Because pain from the triceps brachii muscle may concentrate on the back of the arm and extend into the hand, it is sometimes erroneously thought to result from C7 radicular pain.[50]

Whenever the patient reports lateral or medial elbow pain, and diagnoses of "tennis elbow," "golfers elbow," lateral or medial epicondylitis, olecranon bursitis, or thoracic outlet syndrome are being considered; evaluation for TrPs in the triceps brachii muscle should also be performed. Tennis elbow (lateral epicondylitis) is discussed in detail in Chapter 41 and thoracic outlet syndrome in Chapter 33. Special tests for lateral epicondylitis in most cases are negative, but the patient reports pain in the area of the lateral epicondyle. Careful palpation of the triceps brachii and anconeus muscles may reveal that TrPs in this area have been causing referred pain to the epicondyle. The same is true of special tests for thoracic outlet syndrome, except for the Roos' test, which may reproduce the patient's pain due to prolonged use of the triceps brachii muscle to stabilize the arm in the testing position.

Pain referred from the triceps brachii muscle to the vicinity of the elbow joint may be mistakenly attributed to arthritis.[50]

Osteoarthritic changes in the joint may also be associated with locking or grinding and the range of motion limitations may be evident in both flexion and extension. With triceps brachii TrPs, a passive range of motion is limited to flexion only, if at all.

Cubital tunnel syndrome is more likely to cause hypoesthesia of the skin in the ulnar distribution of the hand and weakness and clumsiness of the hand, rather than pain.[51] This syndrome is associated with slowing of ulnar nerve conduction through the cubital tunnel, whereas the pain from triceps brachii TrPs is not.

Lateral elbow pain that may mimic referred pain from TrPs in the lateral portion of the medial head of the triceps brachii muscle may also be caused by entrapment of the motor branch of the radial nerve, the posterior interosseous nerve, by the arcade of Frohse, or other soft tissues overlying the head of the radius. This nerve pathology is primarily characterized by functional deficits at the wrist, atypical of triceps brachii TrPs.[52]

Entrapment of the radial and ulnar nerves may occur from TrPs in the lateral head of the triceps brachii muscle or from the presence of an anomalous anconeus epitrochlearis muscle, respectively. Nerve compression by these muscles can cause neurologic symptoms such as dysesthesias and loss of motor control in the forearm and hand.

Trigger points in the lateral border of the lateral head of the triceps brachii muscle (Figure 32-3B, left), just proximal to the exit of the radial nerve from the musculospiral (radial) groove (Figure 32-2), are often associated with sensory signs and symptoms of compression of the radial nerve. The patient commonly reports tingling and numbness (dysesthesias) over the dorsum of the lower forearm, wrist, and hand to the base of the middle finger, which lies in the sensory distribution of the radial nerve. By comparison, the pain from TrPs in the lateral head of the triceps brachii muscle appears in the two "ulnar" digits (fourth and fifth) and typically aches in nature. Symptoms of nerve compression may be relieved within minutes to days after the release of the TrP that eliminates the responsible taut band of the muscle. An injection of a local anesthetic solution into the TrP may also temporarily block the radial nerve.

Radial nerve entrapment can also occur beneath the triceps brachii muscle. Careful postmortem dissection revealed an accessory band of the lateral head of the triceps brachii muscle originating below the spiral groove in almost every cadaver studied. The attachment of this slip of muscle to the humerus forms a fibrotic arch of variable tightness over the radial nerve. This arch is distinct from the opening of the lateral intermuscular septum.[53] A patient with a 3-year history of an atraumatic radial paresis progressing to a paralysis was relieved by surgical release of the fibers of the lateral head of the triceps brachii muscle that attached near the radial nerve.[54] The taut fibers caused by TrPs in this portion of the muscle may tense this arch, contributing to a nerve entrapment.

The anconeus epitrochlearis muscle is an anomalous muscle that attaches from the inferior surface of the medial epicondyle to the medial olecranon.[6] It overlies the ulnar nerve and becomes taut in flexion, potentially causing compression at the cubital tunnel. The presence of the muscle has been confirmed by multiple cadaveric studies, and its incidence in the general population has been estimated between 4% and 34%.[7,55,56] Compression of the ulnar nerve by an edematous or hypertrophied anconeus epitrochlearis muscle can cause compression of the nerve, and it has been identified as such in several studies.[7,55,57-63] Pain from compression by the anconeus epitrochlearis muscle often presents as medial elbow pain that does not respond well to conservative treatment.

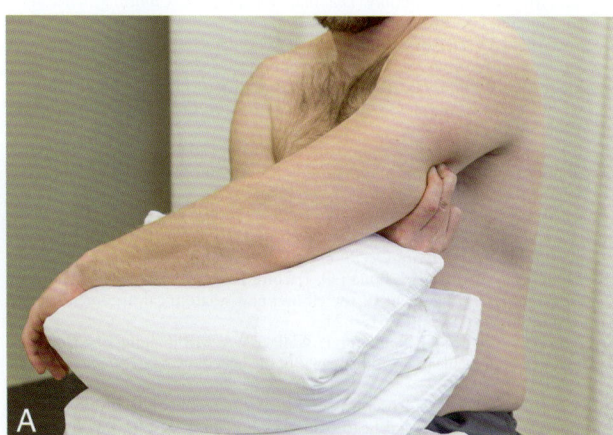
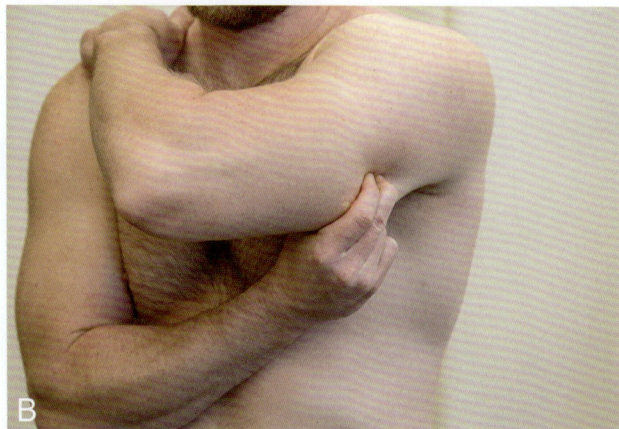
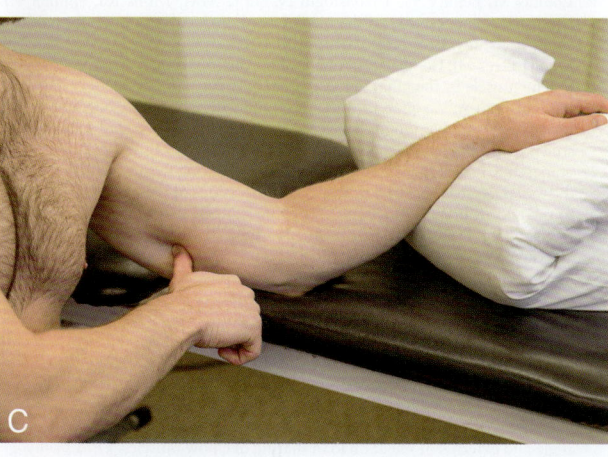
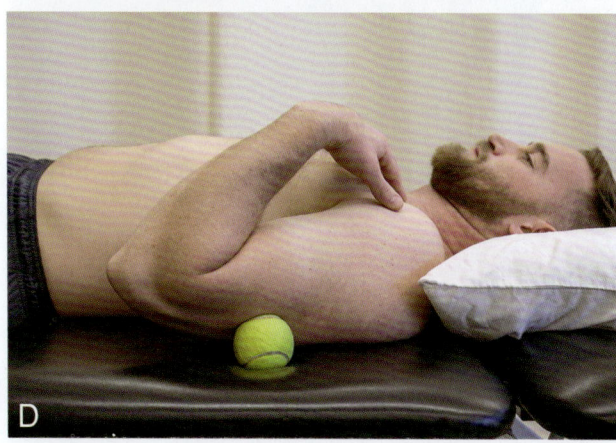

Figure 32-7. Self-pressure release of TrPs. A, Long head of triceps brachii muscle with arm supported. B, Long head of triceps brachii muscle. C, Medial head. D, Lateral head with tennis ball.

Surgical release of the muscle is often recommended for relief of symptoms. It has been postulated that the anconeus epitrochlearis muscle may be a cause of unrelenting medial elbow pain in overhead athletes.[64] Compression of the ulnar nerve by the anconeus epitrochlearis muscle was identified as the cause of medial elbow pain in three baseball pitchers.[54] Surgical release of the muscle was performed for all and each was able to return to their prior level of play.

5. CORRECTIVE ACTIONS

The patient should avoid habitual, sustained, or repetitive motions that overload the triceps brachii muscle, including activities that require excessive pushing or sustained positions with the elbows straight and the arms held away from the body. Postural adjustments when typing, writing, and reading should be made to keep the arm vertical with the elbow behind the plane of the chest and not projected forward. Whenever possible, an armrest of suitable height should support the elbow. To correct for short upper arms in relation to the torso height, a chair with adjustable armrests is recommended. The height of the armrests should always be adjusted properly to support the arms when seated (see Figure 6-9).

The patient should avoid sleeping postures that tightly flex the elbow or extend the shoulder (elbow falling behind the body). To assist in avoiding these positions, the patient can wrap a small towel loosely around the elbow to avoid bending it past 90° (see Figure 30-6) and place a pillow under the arm while lying supine so that the shoulder is maintained in a neutral position.

Sporting activities and exercises should also be addressed. In tennis, the patient may change to a lighter-weight racquet. Also, it may be helpful to shorten the grip on the racquet handle or "choke up," which reduces the leverage on the triceps brachii muscle. When training to increase the velocity of a swing, the progression should be done in a gradual manner to decrease traumatic overload of the triceps brachii muscle.[28] Pull-ups, push-ups, bench press, and military press, which easily overload the arm muscles, should be avoided until after recovery and then resumed gradually.

Trigger point self-pressure release techniques can also be helpful in resolving pain from triceps brachii TrPs. The patient may inactivate TrPs in the long head of the triceps brachii muscle by firmly grasping and holding the muscle belly with the elbow in slight flexion and the upper extremity supported (Figure 32-7A) or by resting the affected hand on the opposite shoulder (Figure 32-7B). Massage to the tender area may be more tolerable if pain with the above technique is too intense. Pressure applied with the flat aspect of the thumb can be utilized to release TrPs in the medial head (Figure 32-7C), and finger pressure or a tennis ball can be utilized to release TrPs in the lateral head (Figure 32-7D).

Trigger point compression alone has been found to be effective in treating chronic shoulder complaints. Pressure should be mildly painful but tolerable and can be applied for bouts as short as 15 seconds in duration to be effective.[65] Following treatment for inactivation of TrPs in the triceps brachii muscle, the patient should passively and gently stretch the entire muscle daily (Figure 32-8).

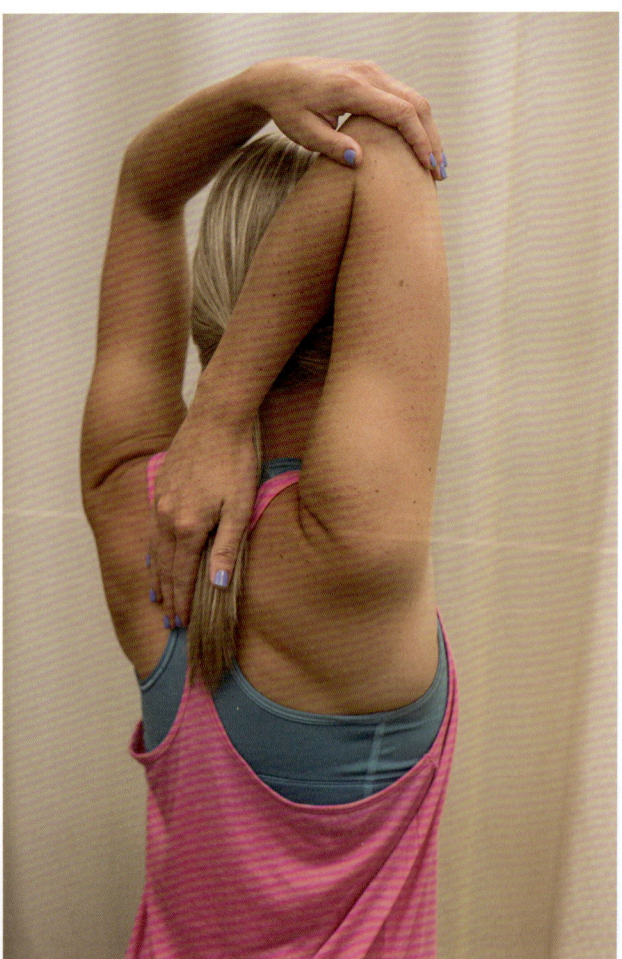

Figure 32-8. Self-stretch of the triceps brachii muscle.

References

1. Standring S. *Gray's Anatomy: The Anatomical Basis of Clinical Practice*. 41st ed. London, UK: Elsevier; 2015.
2. Porterfield JA, DeRosa C. *Mechanical Shoulder Disorders: Perspectives in Functional Anatomy*. St. Louis, MO: Saunders; 2004:73-74.
3. Elder GC, Bradbury K, Roberts R. Variability of fiber type distributions within human muscles. *J Appl Physiol Respir Environ Exerc Physiol*. 1982;53(6):1473-1480.
4. Johnson MA, Polgar J, Weightman D, Appleton D. Data on the distribution of fibre types in thirty-six human muscles. An autopsy study. *J Neurol Sci*. 1973;18(1):111-129.
5. Le Bozec S, Maton B. Differences between motor unit firing rate, twitch characteristics and fibre type composition in an agonistic muscle group in man. *Eur J Appl Physiol Occup Physiol*. 1987;56(3):350-355.
6. Molinier F, Laffosse JM, Bouali O, Tricoire JL, Moscovici J. The anconeus, an active lateral ligament of the elbow: new anatomical arguments. *Surg Radiol Anat*. 2011;33(7):617-621.
7. Jeon IH, Fairbairn KJ, Neumann L, Wallace WA. MR imaging of edematous anconeus epitrochlearis: another cause of medial elbow pain? *Skeletal Radiol*. 2005;34(2):103-107.
8. Bekler H, Wolfe VM, Rosenwasser MP. A cadaveric study of ulnar nerve innervation of the medial head of triceps brachii. *Clin Orthop Relat Res*. 2009;467(1):235-238.
9. Loukas M, Bellary SS, Yuzbasioglu N, Shoja MM, Tubbs RS, Spinner RJ. Ulnar nerve innervation of the medial head of the triceps brachii muscle: a cadaveric study. *Clin Anat*. 2013;26(8):1028-1030.
10. Miguel-Perez MI, Combalia A, Arandes JM. Abnormal innervation of the triceps brachii muscle by the ulnar nerve. *J Hand Surg Eur Vol*. 2010;35(5):430-431.
11. Pascual-Font A, Vazquez T, Marco F, Sanudo JR, Rodriguez-Niedenfuhr M. Ulnar nerve innervation of the triceps muscle: real or apparent? An anatomic study. *Clin Orthop Relat Res*. 2013;471(6):1887-1893.
12. Stanescu S, Post J, Ebraheim NA, Bailey AS, Yeasting R. Surgical anatomy of the radial nerve in the arm: practical considerations of the branching patterns to the triceps brachii. *Orthopedics*. 1996;19(4):311-315.
13. Basmajian J, Deluca C. *Muscles Alive*. 5th ed. Baltimore, MD: Williams & Wilkins; 1985.
14. Duchenne G. *Physiology of Motion*. Philadelphia, PA: Lippincott; 1949.
15. Jenkins DB. *Hollinshead's Functional Anatomy of the Limbs and Back*. 6th ed. Philadelphia, PA: W.B. Saunders; 1991.
16. Kendall FP, McCreary EK. *Muscles: Testing and Function, with Posture and Pain*. Baltimore, MD: Lippincott Williams & Wilkins; 2005.
17. Rasch PJ, Burke RK. *Kinesiology and Applied Anatomy: The Science of Human Movement*. 6th ed. Philadelphia, PA: Lea & Febiger; 1978.
18. Praagman M, Chadwick EK, van der Helm FC, Veeger HE. The effect of elbow angle and external moment on load sharing of elbow muscles. *J Electromyogr Kinesiol*. 2010;20(5):912-922.
19. Davidson AW, Rice CL. Effect of shoulder angle on the activation pattern of the elbow extensors during a submaximal isometric fatiguing contraction. *Muscle Nerve*. 2010;42(4):514-521.

20. Travill AA. Electromyographic study of the extensor apparatus of the forearm. *Anat Rec.* 1962;144:373-376.
21. Bohannon RW. Shoulder position influences elbow extension force in healthy individuals. *J Orthop Sports Phys Ther.* 1990;12(3):111-114.
22. Grabiner MD, Jaque V. Activation patterns of the triceps brachii muscle during sub-maximal elbow extension. *Med Sci Sports Exerc.* 1987;19(6):616-620.
23. Landin D, Thompson M. The shoulder extension function of the triceps brachii. *J Electromyogr Kinesiol.* 2011;21(1):161-165.
24. Myers JB, Pasquale MR, Laudner KG, Sell TC, Bradley JP, Lephart SM. On-the-field resistance-tubing exercises for throwers: an electromyographic analysis. *J Athl Train.* 2005;40(1):15-22.
25. Broer M, Houtz S. *Patterns of Muscular Activity in Selected Sports Skills, an Electromyographic Study.* Springfield, IL: Charles C. Thomas; 1967.
26. Bazzucchi I, Riccio ME, Felici F. Tennis players show a lower coactivation of the elbow antagonist muscles during isokinetic exercises. *J Electromyogr Kinesiol.* 2008;18(5):752-759.
27. Rogowski I, Creveaux T, Faucon A, et al. Relationship between muscle coordination and racket mass during forehand drive in tennis. *Eur J Appl Physiol.* 2009;107(3):289-298.
28. Rota S, Hautier C, Creveaux T, Champely S, Guillot A, Rogowski I. Relationship between muscle coordination and forehand drive velocity in tennis. *J Electromyogr Kinesiol.* 2012;22(2):294-300.
29. Martens J, Figueiredo P, Daly D. Electromyography in the four competitive swimming strokes: a systematic review. *J Electromyogr Kinesiol.* 2015;25(2):273-291.
30. Rouard AH, Clarys JP. Cocontraction in the elbow and shoulder muscles during rapid cyclic movements in an aquatic environment. *J Electromyogr Kinesiol.* 1995;5(3):177-183.
31. Lauer J, Figueiredo P, Vilas-Boas JP, Fernandes RJ, Rouard AH. Phase-dependence of elbow muscle coactivation in front crawl swimming. *J Electromyogr Kinesiol.* 2013;23(4):820-825.
32. Illyes A, Kiss RM. Shoulder muscle activity during pushing, pulling, elevation and overhead throw. *J Electromyogr Kinesiol.* 2005;15(3):282-289.
33. Conte C, Ranavolo A, Serrao M, et al. Kinematic and electromyographic differences between mouse and touchpad use on laptop computers. *Int J Ind Ergon.* 2014;44:413-420.
34. Gao ZH, Fan D, Wang D, Zhao H, Zhao K, Chen C. Muscle activity and co-contraction of musculoskeletal model during steering maneuver. *Biomed Mater Eng.* 2014;24(6):2697-2706.
35. Pandis P, Prinold JA, Bull AM. Shoulder muscle forces during driving: sudden steering can load the rotator cuff beyond its repair limit. *Clin Biomech (Bristol, Avon).* 2015;30(8):839-846.
36. Pereira BP. Revisiting the anatomy and biomechanics of the anconeus muscle and its role in elbow stability. *Ann Anat.* 2013;195(4):365-370.
37. Spalteholz W. *Handatlas der Anatomie des Menschen.* Vol 2. 11th ed. Leipzig, Germany: S. Hirzel; 1922.
38. Sano S, Ando K, Katori I, et al. Electromyographic studies on the forearm muscle activities during finger movements. *J Jpn Orthop Assoc.* 1977;51:331-337.
39. Ali A, Sundaraj K, Badlishah Ahmad R, Ahamed NU, Islam A, Sundaraj S. Muscle fatigue in the three heads of the triceps brachii during a controlled forceful hand grip task with full elbow extension using surface electromyography. *J Hum Kinet.* 2015;46:69-76.
40. Bergin MJ, Vicenzino B, Hodges PW. Functional differences between anatomical regions of the anconeus muscle in humans. *J Electromyogr Kinesiol.* 2013;23(6):1391-1397.
41. Simons DG, Travell JG, Simons LS. *Myofascial Pain and Dysfunction: The Trigger Point Manual. Volume 1: Upper Half of Body.* 2nd ed. Philadelphia, PA: Lippincott Williams & Wilkins;1999.
42. Winter Z. Referred pain in fibrositis. *Med Rec.* 1944;157:34-37.
43. Bron C, Dommerholt J, Stegenga B, Wensing M, Oostendorp RA. High prevalence of shoulder girdle muscles with myofascial trigger points in patients with shoulder pain. *BMC Musculoskelet Disord.* 2011;12(1):139-151.
44. Gerwin RD, Dommerholt J, Shah JP. An expansion of Simons' integrated hypothesis of trigger point formation. *Curr Pain Headache Rep.* 2004;8(6):468-475.
45. Burkhart TA, Andrews DM. Kinematics, kinetics and muscle activation patterns of the upper extremity during simulated forward falls. *J Electromyogr Kinesiol.* 2013;23(3):688-695.
46. Prasanna A. Myofascial pain as postoperative complication. *J Pain Symptom Manage.* 1993;8(7):450-451.
47. Ervilha UF, Farina D, Arendt-Nielsen L, Graven-Nielsen T. Experimental muscle pain changes motor control strategies in dynamic contractions. *Exp Brain Res.* 2005;164(2):215-224.
48. Hsieh YL, Kao MJ, Kuan TS, Chen SM, Chen JT, Hong CZ. Dry needling to a key myofascial trigger point may reduce the irritability of satellite MTrPs. *Am J Phys Med Rehabil.* 2007;86(5):397-403.
49. Hong C-Z. Considerations and recommendations regarding myofascial trigger point injection. *J Musculoskelet Pain.* 1994;2(1):29-59.
50. Reynolds MD. Myofascial trigger point syndromes in the practice of rheumatology. *Arch Phys Med Rehabil.* 1981;62(3):111-114.
51. Craven PR Jr, Green DP. Cubital tunnel syndrome. Treatment by medial epicondylectomy. *J Bone Joint Surg Am.* 1980;62(6):986-989.
52. Minami M, Yamazaki J, Kato S. Lateral elbow pain syndrome and entrapment of the radial nerve. *Nihon Seikeigeka Gakkai Zasshi.* 1992;66(4):222-227.
53. Lotem M, Fried A, Levy M, Solzi P, Najenson T, Nathan H. Radial palsy following muscular effort. A nerve compression syndrome possibly related to a fibrous arch of the lateral head of the triceps. *J Bone Joint Surg Br.* 1971;53(3):500-506.
54. Manske PR. Compression of the radial nerve by the triceps muscle: a case report. *J Bone Joint Surg Am.* 1977;59(6):835-836.
55. Li X, Dines JS, Gorman M, Limpisvasti O, Gambardella R, Yocum L. Anconeus epitrochlearis as a source of medial elbow pain in baseball pitchers. *Orthopedics.* 2012;35(7):e1129-e1132.
56. Chalmers J. Unusual causes of peripheral nerve compression. *Hand.* 1978;10(2):168-175.
57. Nellans K, Galdi B, Kim HM, Levine WN. Ulnar neuropathy as a result of anconeus epitrochlearis. *Orthopedics.* 2014;37(8):e743-e745.
58. Byun SD, Kim CH, Jeon IH. Ulnar neuropathy caused by an anconeus epitrochlearis: clinical and electrophysiological findings. *J Hand Surg Eur Vol.* 2011;36(7):607-608.
59. Yalcin E, Demir SO, Dizdar D, Buyukvural S, Akyuz M. Hypertrophic anconeus epitrochlearis muscle as a cause of ulnar neuropathy at elbow. *J Back Musculoskelet Rehabil.* 2013;26(2):155-157.
60. Morgenstein A, Lourie G, Miller B. Anconeus epitrochlearis muscle causing dynamic cubital tunnel syndrome: a case series. *J Hand Surg Eur Vol.* 2016;41(2):227-229.
61. Dekelver I, Van Glabbeek F, Dijs H, Stassijns G. Bilateral ulnar nerve entrapment by the M. anconeus epitrochlearis. A case report and literature review. *Clin Rheumatol.* 2012;31(7):1139-1142.
62. Tiong WH, Kelly J. Ulnar nerve entrapment by anconeus epitrochlearis ligament. *Hand Surg.* 2012;17(1):83-84.
63. Masear VR, Hill JJ Jr, Cohen SM. Ulnar compression neuropathy secondary to the anconeus epitrochlearis muscle. *J Hand Surg Am.* 1988;13(5):720-724.
64. Chen FS, Rokito AS, Jobe FW. Medial elbow problems in the overhead-throwing athlete. *J Am Acad Orthop Surg.* 2001;9(2):99-113.
65. Hains G, Descarreaux M, Hains F. Chronic shoulder pain of myofascial origin: a randomized clinical trial using ischemic compression therapy. *J Manipulative Physiol Ther.* 2010;33(5):362-369.

Chapter 33

Clinical Considerations of Upper Back Shoulder and Arm Pain

César Fernández de las Peñas and José L. Arias-Buría

1. CERVICAL RADICULAR PAIN

1.1. Overview

The presence of symptoms in the upper extremity is usually associated with the presence of nerve entrapment or radicular pain. However, once any nerve involvement is excluded, clinicians should consider the presence of TrPs in the musculature for which referred pain could mimic this condition, for example, the infraspinatus or scalene muscles.

Cervical radiculopathy is defined as an abnormality of a nerve root with an origin in the cervical spine.[1] Cervical radiculopathy has a prevalence ranging[1] from 83.2 per 100 000 people to 3.3 cases per, 1 000,[2] affecting men more frequently than women. It has a peak annual incidence of 2.1 cases per 1 000 and it occurs most commonly in the fourth and fifth decades of life.[3] The seventh (60%) and the sixth (25%) cervical nerve roots are the most commonly affected.[4] Cervical radiculopathy is caused by a cascade of events that lead to nerve root distortion, intraneural edema, impaired circulation and focal nerve ischemia, localized inflammatory response, and altered nerve conduction. The localized inflammatory response of the nerve is stimulated by chemical mediators in the disk that may incite the production of inflammatory cytokines, substance P, bradykinin, tumor necrosis factor α, and prostaglandins.[5]

The most common compressive causes of cervical radiculopathy include disk herniation and degenerative spine components such as osteophytes, facet joint hypertrophy, and ligament hypertrophy. Disk herniation causes occur when nuclear material from the acute soft disk herniation impinges on a nerve root; whereas the degenerative causes are associated with a loss of disk height and a "hard disk" bulging with resultant compressive elements such as the ligaments and osteophytes.[5]

1.2. Initial Evaluation of a Patient with Cervical Radicular Pain

In patients with cervical radicular pain, the neurologic symptoms may lead to pain, motor weakness, and/or sensory deficits along the affected nerve root.[5] Depending on the nerve root affected, symptoms may exist concurrently in the neck, shoulder, upper arm, or forearm.[1] Often, pain and sensory changes are not consistent and may result in a dull ache to a severe burning pain in the neck and upper extremity. Pain is typically noted in the medial border of the scapula and shoulder that can progress down the ipsilateral arm and hand along the sensory distribution of the involved nerve root.[6] Clinicians should disregard the muscle involvement because the referred pain elicited by TrPs in some muscles can be similar to the dermatomal patterns of spinal nerve roots.[7]

Motor weakness associated with radiculopathy may provide a variety of clinical scenarios and is associated with specific nerve root levels.[1] Specific nerve root weakness typically presents in the following patterns: scapular weakness with C4; shoulder abduction or elbow flexion weakness with C5; wrist extension/supination with C6; triceps brachii, wrist flexion/pronation with C7; and finger flexor/interossei with C8.[8] Muscle weakness should be complemented with examination of deep tendon reflexes because TrPs can also be responsible for muscle weakness. In fact, cervical radicular pain typically presents with diminished deep tendon reflexes (muscle stretch reflex). Loss of deep tendon reflexes is usually said to be the most reliable clinical finding and has been noted in 70% of the cases.[8] Generally, the decline in reflexes follows a predictable radicular pattern.

Sensibility changes (sensation variations) of the affected nerve roots may help localize the level of the lesion. C4 nerve root distribution tends to affect the shoulder and upper arm; C5 nerve root distribution the lateral aspect of the arm; C6 nerve root affects the lateral aspect of the forearm, hand, and thumb; the C7 nerve root the dorsal lateral forearm and third digit; and the C8 nerve root the medial forearm, hand, and fourth and fifth digits.[9] It is important to consider that referred pain areas from TrPs may also exhibit sensory changes, so it is important to complement neurologic examination with musculoskeletal assessment.

Patients with cervical radicular pain often hold their head away from the injurious side, avoiding rotation to the affected side.[6] Cervical range of motion is typically decreased, specifically rotation to the affected side[2] and also extension. Clinicians should take into account that cervical spine movement should reproduce radicular pain symptoms in these patients. The Spurling's test is one of the most common clinical tests used for assessment of cervical radicular pain. This test combines cervical lateral flexion and compression and is considered positive if symptoms of radicular pain are reproduced or worsen during the compression.[8] Other authors have proposed the Upper Limb Tension Test (ULTT) as a good screening test for ruling out cervical radicular pain. Wainner et al[2] developed a clinical prediction rule for diagnosis of cervical radicular pain: positive Spurling's test, cervical rotation range of motion <60°, positive cervical distraction test, and positive ULTT. When all four tests are positive, the specificity was 99% with an LR+ of 30.0.[2]

1.3. Trigger Points and Cervical Radiculopathy

The presence of cervical radicular pain and symptoms does not exclude a potential relevance of TrPs. In fact, some patients with symptoms in the upper extremity are mistakenly diagnosed as having cervical radicular pain when the problem is entirely TrPs. In patients with real cervical radiculopathy, TrPs can be a worsening musculoskeletal factor for their symptoms. In addition, patients with cervical radicular pain reported a higher number of tender spots on the side of the radiculopathy, with predilection toward muscles innervated by the involved nerve root.[10] Hsueh et al[11] observed that C3-C4 lesions were associated with levator scapulae and latissimus dorsi TrPs; C4-C5 lesions with splenius capitis, levator scapulae, and rhomboid minor TrPs; C5-C6 lesions with splenius capitis, deltoid, levator scapulae, infraspinatus, upper paraspinal, and latissimus dorsi TrPs; and C6-C7 lesions with latissimus dorsi and rhomboid minor TrPs. Sari et al[12] described the presence of active TrPs in the upper trapezius, multifidus, splenius capitis, levator scapulae, rhomboids, and deep paraspinal muscles in individuals with cervical radiculopathy. These authors hypothesized that in patients with nerve involvement, the cervical root compression can be considered a precipitating factor for the development of active TrPs in the associated muscles.[12] This finding has been also observed in individuals with lumbosacral radicular symptoms who reported the presence of TrPs in the gluteal muscles.[13] Proper identification of TrPs in patients with radicular pain can be crucial because lack of treatment of TrPs could lead to further aggravation of the symptoms in these patients. In fact, a recent study found that injection of TrPs in the affected muscles in patients with radicular pain was effective for decreasing pain.[14]

However, these studies examined muscles showing a segmental relationship with the affected radicular segment but did not include examination of other muscles that referred pain may mimic cervical radicular pain. For instance, active TrPs in the scalene, infraspinatus, supraspinatus, teres minor, latissimus dorsi, or pectoralis minor muscles can refer to the upper extremity, mimicking symptoms consistent with radicular pain diagnosis. In an older report, Escobar and Ballesteros[15] described four case reports where active TrPs in the teres minor muscle mimic ulnar neuropathy or C8 radiculopathy symptoms. More recently, Qerama et al[16] found the presence of active TrPs in the infraspinatus muscle in individuals with symptoms compatible with carpal tunnel syndrome but normal nerve conduction study. In this study, approximately two-thirds of patients referred with a clinical suspicion of carpal tunnel syndrome, but normal nerve conduction studies, exhibited active TrPs in the infraspinatus muscle.[16]

2. THORACIC OUTLET SYNDROME

2.1. Overview

Thoracic outlet syndrome (TOS) is a broad term used to describe upper extremity symptoms, and it is usually defined as "compression of the brachial plexus and subclavian artery by attached muscles in the region of the first rib and clavicle," which highlights the structures usually considered involved. The anatomic relation of these structures is illustrated in Figure 20-9 (from which a portion of the clavicle has been removed). Both the brachial plexus and the subclavian artery emerge through the interscalene triangle bounded by the anterior and middle scalene muscles and the first rib, where nerves of the brachial plexus and the subclavian artery pass over the first (or, rarely, the cervical) rib. The subclavian vein, accompanied by a lymphatic duct, passes over the first rib anteriorly (medially) to the attachment of the anterior scalene muscle. Entrapment symptoms may be of neural, vascular, and/or lymphatic origin. The lower trunk of the brachial plexus is formed from spinal nerves C8 and T1. The T1 nerve exits the spinal foramen between the first and second thoracic vertebrae, and courses cephalad to hook over the first rib where its fibers, and those of the C8 spinal nerve, are wedged between the subclavian artery and the rib attachment of the middle scalene muscle.

Symptoms experienced by these patients are related to compression or tension of the brachial plexus and the subclavian artery and vein in an area located above the first rib and behind the clavicle. The scalenus anterior muscle, the scalenus medius muscle, and the first rib define borders of the thoracic outlet. Pathology or dysfunction of these structures as well as that of the clavicle, a cervical rib or transverse process of C7, pectoralis minor, omohyoid, subclavius, and scalene minimus muscles are associated with TOS. In their course from the interscalene triangle to the axilla, these neurovasculature structures are covered with a fascial sheath (part of the deep cervical fascia), which can become problematic.[17] Fibrous bands, both congenital and acquired, also restrict movements of the clavicle and first rib. The term TOS does not specify the compressing agent and does not identify the structure being compressed.

The thoracic outlet region includes three major areas in which the compression can occur: interscalene triangle, costoclavicular space, and subpectoralis minor space. Other causes include congenital bony structures (eg, cervical rib), fibromuscular anomalies, postural deviations, and muscle imbalance.

Entrapment at the Interscalene Triangle

Because the brachial plexus runs between the scalenus anterior and medius muscles, increased tension from either muscle can be responsible for the entrapment of neurovascular structures in the interscalene triangle causing potential symptoms. The reason for this increased muscle tension remains enigmatic in the literature. One reason for an increased muscle tone in the scalene muscles may be the presence of TrPs. In addition, the scalene muscles can hypertrophy with trauma or repetitive motion. Sanders[18] found 25% increase in connective tissue in the scalene muscles following injury.

Thomas et al[19] emphasized the middle scalene muscle as being just as important as the anterior scalene muscle in producing TOS. Because the middle scalene muscle is usually a larger, more powerful muscle and has leverage as good as, if not better than, the anterior muscle for elevating the first rib, the middle scalene muscle likely is more important. Of 108 patients who received operative care for TOS, 23% had an anterior insertion of the middle scalene muscle that placed the lower trunk of the brachial plexus and the subclavian artery in direct contact with the muscle's anterior margin. This relationship would make the nerves and artery more vulnerable to abnormal sustained tension of the middle scalene muscle caused by TrPs. In a study of 56 cadavers, the lower trunk of the brachial plexus rested on the inferior portion of the margin of the middle scalene muscle in practically all cases.[19]

Entrapment at the Costoclavicular Space/First Rib

The compression of the neurovascular bundle of the upper extremity between the clavicle and the first rib is denominated costoclavicular syndrome. Any muscle tightness that tends to elevate the first rib (ie, scalene muscle tightness) could aggravate this syndrome. In addition to the scalene muscles, increased tension of the pectoralis minor muscle can contribute indirectly to first rib elevation when the third through fifth ribs (sometimes also the first and second ribs) are upward.

Makhoul and Machleder[20] reviewed the surgical findings in patients who received operative care for costoclavicular syndrome and found numerous references to compression of the subclavian vein against the first rib because of enlargement of the subclavius muscle. An abnormality of the subclavius muscle was found in 19.5% of their 200 surgical cases, and an exostosis at the subclavius tubercle was observed in 15.5%, suggesting abnormally increased tension of that muscle. The subclavius muscle attaches laterally to the middle third of the clavicle and medially to the first rib and its cartilage at their junction.[21] Prolonged shortening of this muscle, for instance, because of a rounded shoulder posture, could produce a force that would tend to elevate the rib.

Some authors emphasized the important relationship between the TOS and dislocation or subluxation of the first rib.[22-24] The treatment, which the authors found to successfully restore normal relations of the first rib and relieve the patient's symptom, was essentially an isometric contract–relax technique specifically for the scalene muscles. This finding raises the question of whether the release of the first rib elevation is not primarily a matter of effectively inactivating scalene TrPs and releasing the abnormal tension in these muscles. Clinicians would expect that downward pressure, applied to the posterior portion of the first rib after the scalene tension is released, facilitates restoration of the normal anatomic relations at the costotransverse joint.

Entrapment at the Subpectoralis Minor Space

The subpectoralis minor space is located below the coracoid process and under the pectoralis minor muscle insertion. Kendall et al[25] defined coracoid pressure syndrome as "a condition of arm pain in which there is compression of the brachial plexus ... [that] is associated with muscle imbalance and faulty postural alignment." Shortening of the pectoralis minor muscle can lead to a narrowing of the subpectoralis minor space by increasing pressure on the blood vessels and brachial plexus. Forward depression of the coracoid process tends to narrow the space available for the three cords of the brachial plexus, the axillary artery, and the axillary vein to pass between the attachment of the pectoralis minor muscle to the coracoid process and the rib cage. Some muscles demonstrate weakness because of the forward and downward tilting of the coracoid process (lower portion of the trapezius muscle), whereas others tend to be tight (pectoralis minor muscle). In fact, TrPs and their taut bands commonly shorten the pectoralis minor muscle and most likely contribute to this syndrome. The pull of tight pectorals can overstretch and weaken the lower trapezius muscle and this weakness can allow the scapula to ride upward and tilt forward, favoring adaptive shortening of the pectoralis minor muscle, creating a perpetuating cycle. Clinicians should consider that TrPs can also inhibit muscular activity, for example, in the lower portion of the trapezius muscle. Finally, a tight pectoralis minor muscle may also compress the neurovascular structures during hyperabduction of the shoulder. Wright termed this syndrome as hyperabduction syndrome.[26]

Entrapment due to Congenital Abnormalities

The incidence of a cervical rib is less than 1% and may be bilateral. Among 40 000 consecutive chest x-ray examinations of army recruits, completely articulated cervical ribs were found in 0.17% and anomalous or deformed first ribs in 0.25%.[20] The cervical rib size varies from a bony exostosis to a full-grown cervical rib with ligamentous cartilaginous or bony attachment to the first rib. The female:male ratio is 2:1.[17] When present, a cervical rib can intensify the symptoms that result from elevation of the rib by the scalene muscles because all structures crossing over a cervical rib are more sharply angulated than usual. In fact, a cervical rib causes the brachial plexus to be pulled against the scalene fascial bands and C8-T1 symptoms can develop. A cervical rib, in a patient exhibiting rounded shoulder and forward head posture, can cause pressure on both the plexus and the vessels.

A higher number of congenital anomalies can also increase the likelihood of entrapment at the thoracic outlet. A congenital abnormally narrow space between the attachments of the two scalene muscles at the first rib will restrict the opening and make the neurovascular structures more vulnerable to compression. An additional space-occupying structure, such as an accessory muscle or fibrous band that passes through the interscalene triangle, will have the same effect. Sharp fibrous edges of the scalene muscles or fibrous bands bordering or within the interscalene triangle can make components of the brachial plexus more vulnerable to compression as well. Makhoul and Machleder[20] analyzed 200 consecutive surgically treated cases of TOS for developmental anomalies and reviewed the literature. A congenital abnormality was found in 66% of cases, higher than that in unselected populations. A cervical rib or first rib abnormality appeared in 8.5% of cases. Supernumerary scalene muscles were found in 10%, developmental variations of scalene muscles in 43%, and variations of the subclavius muscle in 19.5%. However, the only correlation between the clinical and the morphologic characteristics was thrombosis of the subclavian vein due to enlargement of the subclavius muscle system.

2.2. Initial Evaluation of a Patient with Thoracic Outlet Syndrome

The history and physical examination have proved to be the most useful for making the diagnosis of TOS. Further testing may help confirm that there is entrapment and may indicate where it is, but usually tells the clinician little about what is causing the entrapment, which is what a surgeon needs to know. The exception to this is venous entrapment, implicating the subclavius muscle. Physical signs may reflect entrapment of the brachial plexus, subclavian artery, subclavian vein, or the lymph duct from the arm. Electrodiagnostic procedures test for compromise of nerve function, and provocative maneuvers are commonly used to detect both arterial and nerve involvement. Neural involvement is reported to be much more common than arterial involvement,[20] and the literature rarely mentions venous/lymphatic compromise except in connection with the costoclavicular syndrome.

Patients typically report pain in the subscapular, scapular, cervical, and cervicothoracic areas as well as occipital headaches. Paraesthesia and numbness may be present in the entire hand region or parts of it. Often, using the arms in an elevated position exacerbates the symptoms, and reports are of a heavy, tired, aching sensation along with numbness or paraesthesia. Common clinical presentation of TOS includes (1) numbness/tingling in ring and small finger but can encompass entire hand; (2) paraesthesias at night and/or during daily activities; (3) vague pain in the uninvolved extremity can occur in the hand, elbow, shoulder, and/or cervical spine; (4) subjective reports of hand/arm weakness, especially with arms raised overhead; and, (5) subjective reports of swelling in the absence of true swelling.

Electrodiagnostic tests have been disappointingly unreliable for diagnosing TOS, except in more severe cases.[27] On the other hand, electrodiagnostic test results should be negative in the case of myofascial involvement. Needle electromyography (EMG) was the most sensitive to a neuropathy caused by TOS, but was positive only in more chronic and severe cases.[28]

Diagnosis is based on a total clinical picture, comprised of a careful meticulous history, review of medical records, and clinical examination. Clinical examination also includes tenderness over the scalene muscles, anterior chest wall, a positive Tinel sign over the brachial plexus in the cervical spine, reduced sensation to light touch in the fingers, and a positive response to several provocative maneuvers that put stress on the brachial plexus to elicit symptoms. The most common provocative maneuvers used include Adson test, costoclavicular maneuver, Wright test (hyperabduction test), and Roos test.[29] Roos[30] reported that the only maneuver, which he found helpful, was a test that required the patient to hold the hands up with both arms abducted to 90° and the elbows bent at 90° as if told to "stick 'em up." A study of 200 healthy volunteers observed that vascular responses were too common to be a reliable indicator of TOS. The Adson maneuver produced 13.5% positive responses, the costoclavicular maneuver produced positive responses in 47%, and the hyperabduction maneuver in 57% of normal extremities.[31] On the other hand, evaluation of neurologic responses produced positive results to the Adson maneuver in only 2% of normal extremities, to the costoclavicular maneuver in 10%, and to the hyperabduction maneuver in 16.5% of normal extremities. Nevertheless, identification of the structure suffering compression does not by itself identify the cause of compression.

2.3. Trigger Points and Thoracic Outlet Syndrome

Abnormal tension of the scalene muscles is frequently identified as being responsible for the symptoms of TOS, but why the scalene muscles become abnormally tense remains enigmatic in most of the literature. Trigger points are not considered as a potential source of this syndrome. In addition, the scalene muscles cannot exhibit high tension but only TrPs. In fact, the referred pain elicited by the scalene muscles themselves can mimic TOS pain symptoms. In addition to the scalene muscles, other muscles can have TrPs that refer pain in locations mimicking TOS symptoms. The four primary muscles that can mimic TOS symptoms and that are particularly confusing if several of them develop TrPs at the same time are the pectoralis major, latissimus dorsi, teres major, and the subscapularis muscles.[32] Because all of these muscles commonly develop TrPs and are infrequently, if ever, examined by surgeons as a likely source of TOS symptoms, it is not surprising that some patients who undergo surgery for TOS, in whom no anatomic abnormality is clearly found, experience limited clinical benefit from surgery. Also, overlooking active TrPs in conservative treatment helps account for many of those patients who do not respond to conservative treatment. In addition, because pectoralis minor TrPs are likely to be associated with scalene TrPs, the arterial flow may suffer a double entrapment where the subclavian artery emerges from the thorax wedged between the first rib and the tendon of the anterior scalene muscle and where the axillary artery hooks behind the pectoralis minor muscle. Nevertheless, entrapment of the axillary artery is more often due to TrP activity and taut bands of the pectoralis minor muscle than to TrP activity of the scalene muscles.

The presence of TrPs does not exclude a real TOS. For instance, the increased angulation of the neurovascular bundle over a cervical rib instead of the first rib increases its vulnerability to entrapment. An increased tension caused by TrPs will likely cause more severe symptoms when a cervical rib is present. Release of the TrPs may also relieve the symptoms they precipitated, if the TrPs have not been allowed to persist for too long a time and if the tension has not produced permanent nerve damage.

Conservative treatment for TOS almost always includes a treatment procedure that would be likely to release scalene muscle tightness, usually a stretching exercise or a myofascial release procedure. Both can be effective ways of inactivating TrPs if applied in a suitable manner to release TrPs in the involved muscles. Effective management may also need to include correction of ineffective posture (particularly rounded shoulder posture), elimination of unnecessary stress on the muscles during daily activities, counsel on proper care of the muscles, mobilization of articular dysfunctions, and attention to life stresses and coping strategies. A few patients with symptoms of TOS will have anatomic abnormalities that require surgical correction for complete relief. Tardif[33] noted that scalene TrPs commonly mimicked the symptoms of a C6 radiculopathy component of TOS and that pectoralis minor TrPs can create symptoms of medial cord compression. Walsh[34] identified TrPs in the scalene, supraspinatus, infraspinatus, and pectoral muscles as the most common muscles that mimic TOS. Unfortunately, no studies have critically tested a TrP-based approach as a nonoperative intervention for TOS.

3. SUBACROMIAL PAIN SYNDROME

3.1. Overview

Shoulder pain is a significant health problem with a prevalence of 25% in the general population.[35] Neither rotator cuff disease nor impingement syndrome, as each term is commonly used, is a specific or satisfactory diagnosis. Tekavec et al[36] found that the most prevalent diagnosis in individuals with shoulder pain is subacromial pain syndrome. The societal burden of shoulder pain is substantial. The annual cost of a patient with shoulder pain is €4 139 in primary health care in Sweden,[37] and the direct costs for the treatment of shoulder disorders in the United States are $7 billion.[38] Reports of shoulder pain are also a common reason for patients to seek therapy. In a survey of US outpatient physical therapy services, 11% of 1 258 patients indicated the shoulder as their chief area of pain.[39] Below is a review and analysis of problems of the rotator cuff in relation to muscle imbalance, particularly applicable to the supraspinatus, infraspinatus, teres minor, and subscapularis muscles as it relates to shoulder impingement.

Rotator Cuff Syndrome and Shoulder Impingement

The rotator cuff consists of the supraspinatus, infraspinatus, teres minor, and subscapularis muscles and it is considered the main stabilizing complex of the glenohumeral joint. Traditionally, the rotator cuff muscles were thought of as humeral head depressors maintaining a physiologic subacromial space against mainly the deltoid muscle imparting superior translation. However, the rotator cuff muscles are poorly positioned to produce effective depression of the humeral head.[40] More likely, the main role consists of producing proper compressive forces required for concavity compression of the humeral head into the concave glenoid fossa. This is clinically important for avoiding superior translation of the humeral head induced by the deltoid muscle that may easily cause narrowing of the subacromial space and subsequent impingement.[41]

Shoulder impingement as a clinical entity is currently under debate because no clear evidence of real impingement has been found. The coracoacromial arch defines the subacromial space consisting of the acromion and coracoid processes with the coracoacromial ligament spanned between them. The subacromial bursa, the rotator cuff tendons, and the tendon of the long head of the biceps brachii muscle are located between the head of the humerus and the coracoacromial arch, in a space measuring 1 to 1.5 cm on radiographs taken in the anatomic position.[41] Variations in the shape of the acromion have been suggested as playing a role in shoulder impingement, although classification of acromion morphology has been questioned.[42] A study conducted on 216 patients found that the presence of an acromial spur was associated with the presence of a full-thickness rotator cuff tear in both symptomatic and asymptomatic patients.[42]

In primary impingement, the combination of repetitive overhead activity and external narrowing of the subacromial space is thought to be responsible for tendon injury. Mechanical compression occurs between the rotator cuff tendons and the coracoacromial arch. Secondary impingement is mostly associated with glenohumeral instability. Congenital laxity, labral and rotator cuff tears, and posterior glenohumeral capsular tightness have all been implicated in secondary impingement.[43] The most common type of shoulder impingement is the posterosuperior internal impingement, whereby the articular side of the supraspinatus tendon is impinged between the posterosuperior labrum, the glenoid and the greater tuberosity.[44] With coracoid impingement, the tendon of the subscapularis muscle and, occasionally, the long head of the biceps brachii tendon are impinged between the lesser tuberosity and the coracoid process. This impingement occurs during flexion, internal rotation, and cross-body adduction of the shoulder.[45]

Another diagnosis that is commonly seen is bursitis, sometimes identified specifically as subdeltoid or subacromial bursitis. The subdeltoid bursa is large and lies beneath the deltoid muscle against the joint capsule. The subacromial bursa is more superficial and lies between the deep surface of the acromion and the tendon of the supraspinatus muscle overlying the capsule.[21] Bursitis is diagnosed by palpation of tenderness directly under the acromial process with the arm in the neutral resting position at the patient's side and duplicating the patient's pain at the point of pressure. However, by palpation, bursitis alone is indistinguishable from supraspinatus enthesopathy. In fact, the tendinous attachment region of the supraspinatus muscle is in contact with the bursa. Enthesopathy (nociceptive sensitization) of that muscle attachment may become inflammatory enthesitis that, by its direct contact, causes inflammatory changes in the subacromial bursa.

Finally, some patients with subacromial pain syndrome develop calcific tendinopathy. In the shoulder, the supraspinatus tendon is most commonly affected with deposits located around 1 to 1.5 cm proximal to its humeral insertion. Symptoms are due to exudation of cells, rupture of the calcific deposit into the bursa, and vascular proliferation. An acute episode can last up to 2 weeks, but the subsequent subacute episode with pain and restricted movement lasts 3 to 8 weeks.[46]

3.2. Initial Evaluation of a Patient with Subacromial Pain Syndrome

Subacromial pain syndrome often presents with a poorly localized pain in the anterior to lateral part of the shoulder. In some patients, particularly those developing sensitization mechanisms, symptoms can spread toward the upper extremity, particularly during overhead movements.[47] The pain may be present spontaneously at rest or at night when the patient sleeps on the affected shoulder, but it is usually most pronounced with motion, especially overhead. Generally, the intensity of the pain is moderate, but in some patients, severe pain may indicate pathology requiring referral for further medical screening.

Clinical diagnosis of subacromial pain syndrome has mostly focused on rotator cuff or shoulder impingement symptoms. In fact, there is consensus that a cluster of tests should be used for diagnosis of this syndrome. The painful arc sign is the test most commonly used in clinical practice for diagnosis of subacromial pain syndrome. A painful arc sign is defined as pain on active frontal or scapular plane elevation that is most pronounced during midrange (60°-120°). Sensitivity and specificity of the painful arc sign was 0.45 to 0.98 and 0.10 to 0.79, respectively, for rotator cuff tear diagnosis and 0.33 to 0.71 and 0.47 to 0.81 for shoulder impingement.[48] A recent meta-analysis found that a positive painful arc test during abduction had a +LR of 3.7 (95% CI 1.9-7.0).[49] In another review, Alqunaee et al[50] reported the psychometric data for the following clinical tests: Hawkins–Kennedy test (+LR 1.70, 1.29-2.26), Neer's sign (+LR 1.86, 1.49-2.31), empty can test (pooled specificity 0.62), drop arm test (pooled specificity 0.92), and lift-off test (pooled specificity 0.97).

In individuals with suspicion of rotator cuff tear, the Dutch Orthopedic Association Clinical Practice Guideline for subacromial pain syndrome recommends the use of ultrasound for the diagnosis.[51] A literature review by Dinnes et al[52] found that for full-thickness tears, sensitivity and specificity ranges from 0.58 to 1.00 and from 0.78 to 1.00 respectively, suggesting that ultrasound can be used as a confirmatory diagnostic test for subacromial pain syndrome. Magnetic resonance imaging can be also used for proper diagnosis of rotator cuff tear, but it is more expensive than ultrasound and can produce false-positives.

After proper diagnosis of the condition, the clinician should examine the glenohumeral joint, shoulder girdle and scapula, cervical spine, thoracic spine, and the ribs for the presence of joint hypomobility and scapular dyskinesia. In addition, TrPs should be considered to be among the most common causes of shoulder pain. In fact, the Dutch Orthopedic Association Clinical Practice Guideline for subacromial pain syndrome specifically recommends examination and management of TrPs.[51] It is important to determine whether a diagnosis has been properly conducted, or the symptoms experienced by the patient can be exclusively related to TrPs. For instance, TrPs in the biceps brachii muscle refer pain to the long bicipital tendon area. Therefore, tenderness to palpation of the bicipital tendon in the referred pain area from TrPs in the biceps brachii muscle may be mistaken for bicipital tendinitis or subdeltoid bursitis. Although a positive Yergason's sign (pain in the proximal aspect of the bicipital groove when the patient supinates the forearm against resistance) is usually interpreted as a sign of bicipital tendinitis, it can be also referred pain elicited by biceps brachii TrPs. Similarly, tenderness elicited by deep palpation over the deltoid muscle, but referred from biceps brachii muscle TrPs, may be misidentified as subdeltoid bursitis.

3.3. Trigger Points and Subacromial Pain Syndrome

It seems clear that the presence of TrPs in the shoulder musculature can play a relevant role in the sensory and motor symptoms in individuals with subacromial pain syndrome.[53] For instance, active TrPs in the infraspinatus, supraspinatus, teres minor, or subscapularis muscles may cause referred pain, which can be felt deep in the shoulder and can mimic symptoms like subacromial bursitis or rotator cuff tendinopathy.[54] Development of TrPs in the shoulder muscles may be caused by different circumstances, for example, sudden contractions,[54] overload during sports,[55] shoulder surgery,[56] or even thorax surgery.[57]

In a reliability study on palpation of the shoulder muscles, Bron et al[58] reported that the most reliable features of TrPs were the referred pain sensation and jump sign with a percentage of pair-wise agreement of 70% (range 63-93%) and 70% (range 67-77%), respectively. This data suggests that identification of TrPs in the shoulder girdle muscles is reliable. Trigger point prevalence in the shoulder muscles has been explored in different studies. Bron et al[59] included individuals with nontraumatic unilateral shoulder pain, without specifying particular diagnosis, and found that all patients exhibited a median number of six active TrPs. Trigger points were found to be present in the infraspinatus, upper trapezius, deltoid, teres minor, and middle trapezius muscles. In this study, the number of active TrPs was associated with pain-related disability, pain intensity, and the duration of the shoulder pain supporting a potential role of active TrPs in this condition. In another study, the same authors observed that manual therapy targeting active TrPs in the shoulder musculature was more effective than a wait-and-see strategy for improving pain and function in individuals with nonspecific shoulder pain in the short term.[60] Other studies have also demonstrated that proper management of TrPs in the shoulder muscles is effective for shoulder pain and disability.[61,62] Another study observed the presence of bilateral TrPs in the infraspinatus muscles in people with chronic unilateral myofascial shoulder pain supporting the role of sensitization mechanisms in TrP pain.[63] Active TrPs were only found in the symptomatic side, but the most interesting finding was the presence of latent TrPs in the non-symptomatic side. Another important finding from this study was the presence of multiple, rather than single, active TrPs in the infraspinatus muscle, underscoring the importance of searching for multiple active TrPs within one muscle in patients with myofascial pain.[63]

Other studies including people with specific diagnosis of shoulder impingement have observed similar data. Hidalgo Lozano et al[64] found that patients with shoulder impingement had a larger number of both active and latent TrPs than did healthy subjects and that the presence of active TrPs was associated with greater shoulder pain intensity. Active TrPs within

Table 33-1	Active Myofascial Trigger Points Found in Subacromial Pain Syndrome.

Nonspecific Shoulder Pain

Infraspinatus 77% active TrPs
Upper trapezius 58% active TrPs
Deltoid 40% active TrPs
Teres minor 35% active TrPs
Middle trapezius 30% active TrPs

Shoulder Impingement

Supraspinatus 67% active TrPs
Infraspinatus 42-48% active TrPs
Upper trapezius 44% active TrPs
Subscapularis 40-42% active TrPs
Scalene 40% active TrPs

The table summarizes the percentage of active TrPs found in patients with nonspecific shoulder pain[59] and those with medical diagnosis of shoulder impingement.[64,65]

the supraspinatus, infraspinatus, and subscapularis muscles were the most prevalent. A relevant finding for clinical practice was that the presence of active TrPs in some muscles was related to pain during specific movements of the shoulder. For instance, the presence of active TrPs in the infraspinatus muscle was related to more pain at rest, whereas the presence of active TrPs in the biceps brachii muscle was related to more pain during arm elevation.[64] Another study found that people with unilateral shoulder impingement exhibited latent TrPs in the unaffected shoulder.[65] Patients with shoulder impingement showed at least four active TrPs in the shoulder musculature, and the number of TrPs was related to shoulder pain. In this study, the supraspinatus, infraspinatus, subscapularis, and deltoid muscles were the most affected by active TrPs. Table 33-1 summarizes which muscles exhibit active TrPs in patients with subacromial pain syndrome.

There is clear evidence supporting a potential role of active TrPs in shoulder pain. In addition, the fact that exercise and manual therapies are the most common therapeutic strategies used for the management of this condition[66] supports this assumption. Exercise programs are supported in systematic reviews for producing improvements in both pain and function in individuals with shoulder pain.[67]

4. SCAPULAR DYSKINESIA

4.1. Overview

Scapular dyskinesia can be defined as a motor alteration of the normal recruitment pattern of muscle contraction of the shoulder girdle musculature. It seems that a consistent recruitment pattern of the shoulder muscles during abduction in the scapular plane is found in asymptomatic shoulders.[68,69] The upper trapezius muscle is activated first, followed by serratus anterior, middle trapezius, and finally, the lower trapezius muscles. The temporal characteristics are delayed but not changed by fatigue in asymptomatic subjects.[68]

Reflecting the role of the glenohumeral joint as part of the multijoint shoulder girdle, scapular dyskinesia has been suggested as a potential cause for shoulder pain. In fact, a reasonably consistent pattern of decreased activity has been demonstrated in both the lower trapezius and serratus anterior muscles and increased activity in upper trapezius muscles in individuals with shoulder pain.[69-72] In a more recent study, Kibler et al[73] observed that inhibition of lower trapezius and serratus anterior muscles was a nonspecific response to shoulder pain, irrespective of the underlying pathology. Decreased activity in the lower trapezius and serratus anterior muscles associated with arm elevation[70,74] in patients with shoulder dysfunction supports the observation of delayed or reduced upward rotation in the clinical setting. Increased upper trapezius muscle activity under heavier load[70] and in the upper ranges of elevation[74] possibly reflects a compensation for decreased activity in lower trapezius and serratus anterior muscles and/or an attempt to overcome the increased tone in the antagonists.

External rotator fatigue significantly reduced scapular upward rotation, posterior tilt, and external rotation during shoulder arm elevation, thereby decreasing the amount of subacromial space.[75] Cools et al[71] showed significant delays in activation of the middle and lower trapezius muscles in individuals with shoulder impingement. Further, indicating the possible role of pain-related inhibition in scapular dyskinesia, Falla et al[76] demonstrated that the injection of hypertonic saline injection in the upper trapezius muscle was sufficient to result in altered motor control of this muscle, not only locally at the site of pain but also in non-painful regions within the same muscle and on the contralateral side. A modification of motor strategy resulting in compensatory muscle activity is likely to lead to muscle overload and perpetuate pain and dyskinesia.

Nevertheless, clinicians should consider that not all responses to shoulder pain are consistent,[71,74] possibly reflecting the different patterns demonstrated in subgroups within sample populations with the same medical diagnosis.[69] The observation of variations in patterns of muscle activity supports the need to address each patient's impairment individually during assessment.

4.2. Initial Evaluation of a Patient with Scapular Dyskinesia

Several exploratory tests can be used for proper evaluation of scapula kinematics. The Apley's test (flexion, abduction, external rotation) may be used to grossly evaluate for TrP involvement in the shoulder girdle musculature. The test is performed by placing the forearm and hand of the affected side behind the head and reaching as far toward the opposite scapula as possible (Figure 21-3B). This test requires full active abduction and external rotation of the arm at the glenohumeral joint. It also requires normal scapular mobility. If the clinician looks closely at how the subject raises the arm, scapulohumeral rhythm can also be assessed. If no dysfunction is present, the fingertips should reach to the opposite shoulder blade.

Moving the hand to the end position or holding this position may be painful because of strong contraction of the abductors and external rotators of the shoulder that are in the shortened position. However, movement also may be limited by a tight adductors or internal rotators. Although any of these muscles might cause pain-limited restriction during this test, the muscles most likely to limit the movement in this way are the strongly contracted infraspinatus and middle deltoid muscles. In this case, the pain is most likely to be in the immediate vicinity of the TrPs. The test movement also passively stretches the subscapularis muscle and if that muscle has TrPs, it is likely to refer pain behind the shoulder and to the wrist. Trigger points of the latissimus dorsi muscle can also cause pain at the end of its extensive range of motion only if no other muscle were restricting the movement. Clinicians are encouraged to consider the presence of TrPs in all clinical tests used for assessing motor impairments in scapular kinematics.

4.3. Trigger Points and Scapular Dyskinesia

Examination of all components of the neuromuscular system including dysfunction of synergistic control, timing of muscle activation, patterns of co-contraction, and proprioceptive control in a patient with shoulder pain is clinically recommended, especially pain of long duration and/or high intensity. Although there is no study investigating the presence of TrPs in patients with scapular dyskinesia, there is clear evidence showing that TrPs can cause altered motor control patterns, accelerated muscle fatigability, and increased motor activation in the affected and related musculature.[77] This relationship is particularly and clinically important in the case of latent TrPs, because latent TrPs do not produce sensory pain symptoms but they clearly induce motor disorders. For instance, Ibarra et al[78] observed that intramuscular, but not superficial, EMG activity of antagonist muscles (ie, posterior portion of the deltoid muscle) was significantly higher at rest and during agonist contraction (ie, anterior portion of the deltoid muscle) with the presence of latent TrPs in the related muscle, signifying reduced antagonist reciprocal inhibition. Ge et al[79] found that latent TrPs were associated with an accelerated development of muscle fatigue, as depicted by early decrease in intramuscular EMG mean power frequency, and also by simultaneously overloading active motor units close to the TrP expressed as early and significant increase in surface EMG root mean square amplitude. In another study, the same authors observed that latent TrPs were also associated with an increased intramuscular, but not surface muscle, activity during synergistic muscle contraction.[80] This study explains that active motor units from latent TrPs have to work more than the active motor units from non-TrP fibers to maintain the similar level of force output, leading to an incoherent muscle activation pattern of synergist muscle fibers. Therefore, a chaotic muscle recruitment pattern may lead to muscle overuse and premature fatigue of musculature harboring TrPs. In such a scenario, TrPs provide a potent source for disturbance of muscular imbalances observed in people with scapular dyskinesia. This is also related to the fact that TrPs in some muscles, for example, the lower portion of the trapezius muscle, induce muscle inhibition.

Different studies have demonstrated that the presence of latent TrPs in the neck/shoulder muscles induces change in motor recruitment patterns and decreases efficiency of movement during scapular plane elevation of the shoulder girdle musculature during unloaded and low-load tasks.[77,81,82] These studies found that people with latent TrPs exhibited different temporal sequences of activation in the scapular and rotator cuff muscles during upper extremity low-load tasks. However, there were inconsistencies in the order of muscle activation. The only common feature observed was early activation of the infraspinatus muscle.[77,81,82] Current findings suggest that in individuals with latent TrPs, the timing of muscle activation is altered and more variable not only in the muscles containing the TrPs (upward scapular rotators) but also in functionally related muscles (infraspinatus muscle as a glenohumeral stabilizer and middle deltoid muscle as abductor of upper extremity) during scapular plane elevation. A recent study confirmed that the presence of latent TrPs in the upper trapezius muscle produces a delayed timing activation of the upper trapezius and serratus anterior muscles during rapid arm elevation in all planes of movement.[83]

These changes in timing recruitment may predispose individuals to increased risk of subacromial impingement. It would be reasonable to expect that treatment of TrPs may lead to normalization of motor activation patterns and facilitate spontaneous recovery of shoulder pain, either without exercising or by making therapeutic exercise more effective. This thinking was partially confirmed in a follow-up experiment when half of the subjects presenting with latent TrPs were treated, deactivating their TrPs using dry needling and passive muscle stretching.[81] The individuals in whom latent TrPs were treated demonstrated a normalized motor recruitment pattern, resulting in no significant differences in the timing of muscle activation compared with the control group.

5. FROZEN SHOULDER

5.1. Overview

The descriptive terms "frozen shoulder" and "adhesive capsulitis" are not specific diagnoses and frequently are based only on the presence of a painful shoulder that exhibits severely restricted range of motion in all directions. The label "frozen shoulder," when presented as the diagnosis that accounts for the patient's symptoms, serves as a warning that the patient is in need of a more specific diagnosis. The etiology of this condition is unknown, and it is commonly differentiated between primary and secondary frozen shoulder. Primary frozen shoulder is idiopathic and not related to other diseases; whereas secondary frozen shoulder is related to known systemic pathology, such as diabetes mellitus, thyroid disease, Parkinson's disease, post-surgery, post-trauma, or after long periods of immobilization. It can be difficult to differentiate, but post-surgical shoulder stiffness is not the same as secondary post-surgical frozen shoulder.

Although the pathologic process in primary frozen shoulder is unclear, it is generally accepted as the presence of an underlying inflammatory process of the synovial membrane followed by a fibrotic reaction of the fibrous layer of the glenohumeral capsule. Especially in the area of the coracohumeral ligament and the rotator cuff interval, scar and contracture formation is initiated by the expression of vimentin (a cytocontractile protein, usually seen in fibromyocytes), whereas in the entire joint capsule there is fibroplasia (thickening of the joint capsule) without contraction.[84,85] Nevertheless, despite all the scientific research done on primary frozen shoulder, the trigger for the cascade of inflammatory and fibrogenetic processes is still unclear.

5.2. Initial Evaluation of a Patient with Frozen Shoulder

Primary frozen shoulder is mainly characterized by restriction of shoulder motion without major shoulder injury; global stiffness of the shoulder joint in all directions without the loss of strength, joint stability, or joint surface integrity; and plain shoulder radiographs showing a normal glenohumeral joint space and no peri-articular abnormalities. The pain is usually experienced in the shoulder region, the deltoid muscle insertion, and upper arm, but it often refers to the neck and more distal regions of the upper extremity. In the freezing phase, the pain is felt during rest and intensified during movement and during sleep. The amount of pain depends on the clinical phase of the disease. In fact, clinical diagnosis of a primary frozen shoulder includes proper recognition of each phase of the condition (freezing, frozen, and thawing) and the practitioner's clinical challenge is formed by the discrimination of the exact phase and appropriate duration of symptoms or signs. Frozen shoulder is generally considered a self-limiting disease with a mean average duration of 1 to 3 years, but a part of the population presents with substantial limitations in shoulder passive range of motion for up to 10 years after the onset of the condition.[86]

Physical examination of a patient with frozen shoulder includes palpation of the cervical spine and the shoulder girdle for tendon and ligament tenderness. The shoulder should be examined for signs of muscle atrophy, former trauma, and swelling. During assessment of shoulder mobility, attention should be paid to the contribution of the glenohumeral joint isolated to active and passive range of motion. Clinicians should consider that in the freezing phase, pain is the most limiting factor and joint restriction of glenohumeral motion may be less clear. In the frozen phase, the characteristic global limitation of passive range of motion of the glenohumeral joint is present. In the thawing phase, the global limitation fades out and usually the contracture of the rotator interval causes a marked limitation of external rotation. It is interesting to note that all these clinical signs can be also a manifestation of TrPs in the shoulder girdle musculature, particularly the subscapularis, supraspinatus, and infraspinatus muscles.

5.3. Trigger Points and Frozen Shoulder

Clinicians should consider that the primary symptoms of frozen shoulder, namely shoulder pain referred to the upper extremity and restricted range of motion, are also primary symptoms of active TrPs in the shoulder girdle musculature. For instance, the shoulder becomes more restricted in external rotation (up to 45° or more) when the subscapularis muscle exhibits active TrPs. Trigger points in the infraspinatus muscle seem to be responsible for shoulder pain during internal rotation; whereas TrPs in the teres major muscle may be responsible for a restriction in abduction. Probably, the subscapularis muscle is the most important muscle to consider in frozen shoulder. Lewit[87] voiced the observation of clinicians skilled at identifying TrPs that "painful spasm of the subscapularis, with TrPs, accompanies frozen shoulder from the onset." Because the humeral tendinous attachment region of the subscapularis is not accessible to direct palpation, its tendency to develop enthesitis is not well recognized. The humeral attachment of the subscapularis tendon lies in close approximation to the subscapular bursa. Because adhesions in the subscapular bursa are identified as a major component of adhesive capsulitis or frozen shoulder, it is possible that a chronic enthesitis of the subscapularis muscle adjacent to its bursa could induce an inflammatory reaction that could lead to fibrosis of the bursa, which requires either forceful manipulation, inflation of the bursa, or arthroscopic surgery to release it. In this case, the stage of fibrosis could be prevented by prompt recognition and treatment of the subscapularis TrPs.

In addition, one potential reason for the shoulder becoming so painful and motion so limited when a patient develops subscapularis TrPs is that other shoulder girdle muscles, for example, supraspinatus, infraspinatus, or deltoid muscles, can be also involved, adding their pain patterns and movement restrictions. For instance, the supraspinatus muscle is prone to develop enthesopathy or enthesitis. Similar considerations apply to supraspinatus TrPs and enthesitis of the supraspinatus tendon in the region where it blends with the joint capsule. Both the subacromial bursa and the coracohumeral ligament lie in close approximation to this region of supraspinatus attachment. Therefore, proper treatment of TrPs could potentially prevent subsequent pain, disability, and expense in individuals with frozen shoulder.

The frozen shoulder literature often refers to the importance of trying conservative interventions first and frequently identifies physical therapy as an essential part of a conservative care plan. When a patient presents with a diagnosis of adhesive capsulitis or frozen shoulder, clinicians need to consider TrP as a potential source of symptoms. Nevertheless, specific identification of subscapularis TrPs as a focus of therapeutic attention in frozen shoulder has been rarely mentioned in the literature, and no controlled trials that specifically addressed the TrP component of frozen shoulder have been found. There is only one case report describing the clinical reasoning behind the use of TrP dry needling in the treatment of an individual with adhesive capsulitis.[88] This case report observed a rapid improvement in pain and range of motion following the initiation of dry needling applied to upper trapezius, levator scapula, deltoid, and infraspinatus muscles. Surprisingly, there is no mention of the subscapularis muscle TrPs in this case report.

6. NECK PAIN (STIFF NECK)

Clinically, patients can present with cervical spine dysfunction with a predominant symptom of stiffness in the neck (see Chapter 18). Patients with a "stiff neck" syndrome exhibit extremely reduced cervical range of motion (some patients cannot move their neck) and they perceive their neck as feeling "like a stick." One cause of this syndrome may be increased tone in the cervical muscles that cross the craniocervical and cervicothoracic junctions vertically. The levator scapulae muscle is the main example. Active trigger points (TrPs) in both levator scapulae muscles combined with an increased muscle tone by their respective taut bands can precipitate a "stiff neck" syndrome. In addition, the splenius cervicis, scalenus medius, and iliocostalis cervicis muscles can also be involved. Contrary to what might be expected, rhomboid TrP activity is rarely associated with levator scapulae muscle involvement. If the patient's head is strongly tilted to one side (wry neck), TrPs in the sternocleidomastoid muscle are more likely to be responsible than are levator scapulae TrPs.

The common physical finding of crepitation and the relatively frequent presence of bursae near the upper (superior) angle of the scapula indicate that the tenderness and referred pain elicited may be caused by a bursitis instead of, or in addition to, enthesopathy caused by unrelieved tension of taut bands associated with TrPs in the levator scapulae muscle. Nevertheless, tightness of the levator scapulae muscle or taut bands associated with TrPs can be also responsible for crepitation in the superior angle of the scapula. In such cases, release of TrPs in the muscle belly of the levator scapula muscle is critical for relief of these reported or observed symptoms.

It is known that referred pain from zygapophysial joints can appear confusingly similar to that of TrPs in muscles at approximately the same segment.[89] The referred pain of levator scapulae TrPs overlaps the lower two-thirds of referred pain from the C4-C5 zygapophysial joints but also extends more inferiorly.[90] In fact, articular dysfunctions commonly associated with levator scapulae TrPs can be at C3, C4, C5, or C6 levels. However, there are important differences. Even though joints and muscles are innervated by the same or overlapping neural segments, myofascial pain referral patterns can be distinctively different for different muscles innervated by the same neural segments. The patterns are not always limited to the sclerotomes or myotomes of the segments that innervate the muscle. Trigger points are confirmed by physical examination of the muscle, whereas zygapophysial joint dysfunction is assessed by passive manual tests including evaluation of end-feel, tissue resistance, and reproduction of the patient's symptoms.

The etiology of scapulocostal syndrome has been considered enigmatic by many authors in the past, but a number of authors have empirically attributed the symptoms to TrPs.[91,92] Ormandy[93] presented a review of this diagnosis including anatomic outlines of the muscles this author considered responsible: the levator scapulae, rhomboid minor, subscapularis, and trapezius muscles. It seems that the levator scapulae muscle is the major, if not the primary, cause of this condition.

References

1. Polston DW. Cervical radiculopathy. *Neurol Clin*. 2007;25(2):373-385.
2. Wainner RS, Fritz JM, Irrgang JJ, Boninger ML, Delitto A, Allison S. Reliability and diagnostic accuracy of the clinical examination and patient self-report measures for cervical radiculopathy. *Spine (Phila Pa 1976)*. 2003;28(1):52-62.
3. Wainner RS, Gill H. Diagnosis and nonoperative management of cervical radiculopathy. *J Orthop Sports Phys Ther*. 2000;30(12):728-744.
4. Malanga GA. The diagnosis and treatment of cervical radiculopathy. *Med Sci Sports Exerc*. 1997;29(7 suppl):S236-S245.
5. Rhee JM, Yoon T, Riew KD. Cervical radiculopathy. *J Am Acad Orthop Surg*. 2007;15(8):486-494.
6. Wolff MW, Levine LA. Cervical radiculopathies: conservative approaches to management. *Phys Med Rehabil Clin N Am*. 2002;13(3):589-608, vii.
7. Lauder TD. Musculoskeletal disorders that frequently mimic radiculopathy. *Phys Med Rehabil Clin N Am*. 2002;13(3):469-485.
8. Tsao BE, Levin KH, Bodner RA. Comparison of surgical and electrodiagnostic findings in single root lumbosacral radiculopathies. *Muscle Nerve*. 2003;27(1):60-64.
9. Chien A, Eliav E, Sterling M. Whiplash (grade II) and cervical radiculopathy share a similar sensory presentation: an investigation using quantitative sensory testing. *Clin J Pain*. 2008;24(7):595-603.
10. Letchuman R, Gay RE, Shelerud RA, VanOstrand LA. Are tender points associated with cervical radiculopathy? *Arch Phys Med Rehabil*. 2005;86(7):1333-1337.
11. Hsueh TC, Yu S, Kuan TS, Hong CZ. Association of active myofascial trigger points and cervical disc lesions. *J Formos Med Assoc*. 1998;97(3):174-180.
12. Sari H, Akarirmak U, Uludag M. Active myofascial trigger points might be more frequent in patients with cervical radiculopathy. *Eur J Phys Rehabil Med*. 2012;48(2):237-244.
13. Adelmanesh F, Jalali A, Jazayeri Shooshtari SM, Raissi GR, Ketabchi SM, Shir Y. Is there an association between lumbosacral radiculopathy and painful gluteal trigger points?: a cross-sectional study. *Am J Phys Med Rehabil*. 2015;94(10):784-791.
14. Saeidian SR, Pipelzadeh MR, Rasras S, Zeinali M. Effect of trigger point injection on lumbosacral radiculopathy source. *Anesth Pain Med*. 2014;4(4):e15500.

15. Escobar PL, Ballesteros J. Teres minor. Source of symptoms resembling ulnar neuropathy or C8 radiculopathy. *Am J Phys Med Rehabil*. 1988;67(3):120-122.
16. Qerama E, Kasch H, Fuglsang-Frederiksen A. Occurrence of myofascial pain in patients with possible carpal tunnel syndrome—a single-blinded study. *Eur J Pain*. 2009;13(6):588-591.
17. Atasoy E. Thoracic outlet syndrome: anatomy. *Hand Clin*. 2004;20(1):7-14, v.
18. Sanders RJ, Jackson CG, Banchero N, Pearce WH. Scalene muscle abnormalities in traumatic thoracic outlet syndrome. *Am J Surg*. 1990;159(2):231-236.
19. Thomas GI, Jones TW, Stavney LS, Manhas DR. The middle scalene muscle and its contribution to the thoracic outlet syndrome. *Am J Surg*. 1983;145(5):589-592.
20. Makhoul RG, Machleder HI. Developmental anomalies at the thoracic outlet: an analysis of 200 consecutive cases. *J Vasc Surg*. 1992;16(4):534-542; discussion 542-545.
21. Standring S. *Gray's Anatomy: The Anatomical Basis of Clinical Practice*. 41st ed. London, UK: Elsevier; 2015.
22. Lindgren KA, Leino E. Subluxation of the first rib: a possible thoracic outlet syndrome mechanism. *Arch Phys Med Rehabil*. 1988;69(9):692-695.
23. Lindgren KA. Thoracic outlet syndrome with special reference to the first rib. *Ann Chir Gynaecol*. 1993;82(4):218-230.
24. Lindgren KA. Reasons for failures in the surgical treatment of thoracic outlet syndrome. *Muscle Nerve*. 1995;18(12):1484-1486.
25. Kendall FP, McCreary EK, Provance PG. *Muscles, Testing and Function*. 4th ed. Baltimore, MD: Williams & Wilkins; 1993:317-343.
26. Beyer JA. The hyperabduction syndrome, with special reference to its relationship to Raynaud's syndrome. *Circulation*. 1951;4(2):161-172.
27. Schnyder H, Rosler KM, Hess CW. The diagnostic significance of additional electrophysiological studies in suspected neurogenic thoracic outlet syndrome. *Schweiz Med Wochenschr*. 1994;124(9):349-356.
28. Passero S, Paradiso C, Giannini F, et al. Diagnosis of thoracic outlet syndrome. Relative value of electrophysiological studies. *Acta Neurol Scand*. 1994;90(3):179-185.
29. Gillard J, Perez-Cousin M, Hachulla E, et al. Diagnosing thoracic outlet syndrome: contribution of provocative tests, ultrasonography, electrophysiology, and helical computed tomography in 48 patients. *Joint Bone Spine*. 2001;68(5):416-424.
30. Roos DB. Pathophysiology of congenital anomalies in thoracic outlet syndrome. *Acta Chir Belg*. 1980;79(5):353-361.
31. Rayan GM, Jensen C. Thoracic outlet syndrome: provocative examination maneuvers in a typical population. *J Shoulder Elbow Surg*. 1995;4(2):113-117.
32. Sucher BM. Thoracic outlet syndrome—a myofascial variant: Part 1. Pathology and diagnosis. *J Am Osteopath Assoc*. 1990;90(8):686-696, 703-684.
33. Tardif GS. Myofascial pain syndromes in the diagnosis of thoracic outlet syndromes. *Muscle Nerve*. 1990;13(4):362-363.
34. Walsh MT. Therapist management of thoracic outlet syndrome. *J Hand Ther*. 1994;7(2):131-144.
35. Luime JJ, Koes BW, Hendriksen IJ, et al. Prevalence and incidence of shoulder pain in the general population; a systematic review. *Scand J Rheumatol*. 2004;33(2):73-81.
36. Tekavec E, Joud A, Rittner R, et al. Population-based consultation patterns in patients with shoulder pain diagnoses. *BMC Musculoskelet Disord*. 2012;13:238.
37. Virta L, Joranger P, Brox JI, Eriksson R. Costs of shoulder pain and resource use in primary health care: a cost-of-illness study in Sweden. *BMC Musculoskelet Disord*. 2012;13:17.
38. Meislin RJ, Sperling JW, Stitik TP. Persistent shoulder pain: epidemiology, pathophysiology, and diagnosis. *Am J Orthop (Belle Mead NJ)*. 2005;34(12 suppl):5-9.
39. Boissonnault WG. Prevalence of comorbid conditions, surgeries, and medication use in a physical therapy outpatient population: a multicentered study. *J Orthop Sports Phys Ther*. 1999;29(9):506-519; discussion 520-525.
40. Halder AM, Zhao KD, Odriscoll SW, Morrey BF, An KN. Dynamic contributions to superior shoulder stability. *J Orthop Res*. 2001;19(2):206-212.
41. Limb D, Collier A. Impingement syndrome. *Curr Orthop*. 2000;14:161-166.
42. Hamid N, Omid R, Yamaguchi K, Steger-May K, Stobbs G, Keener JD. Relationship of radiographic acromial characteristics and rotator cuff disease: a prospective investigation of clinical, radiographic, and sonographic findings. *J Shoulder Elbow Surg*. 2012;21(10):1289-1298.
43. Pyne SW. Diagnosis and current treatment options of shoulder impingement. *Curr Sports Med Rep*. 2004;3(5):251-255.
44. Belling Sorensen AK, Jorgensen U. Secondary impingement in the shoulder. An improved terminology in impingement. *Scand J Med Sci Sports*. 2000;10(5):266-278.
45. Radas CB, Pieper HG. The coracoid impingement of the subscapularis tendon: a cadaver study. *J Shoulder Elbow Surg*. 2004;13(2):154-159.
46. Hughes PJ, Bolton-Maggs P. Calcifying tendonitis. *Curr Orthop*. 2002;16:389-394.
47. Sanchis MN, Lluch E, Nijs J, Struyf F, Kangasperko M. The role of central sensitization in shoulder pain: a systematic literature review. *Semin Arthritis Rheum*. 2015;44(6):710-716.
48. Park HB, Yokota A, Gill HS, El Rassi G, McFarland EG. Diagnostic accuracy of clinical tests for the different degrees of subacromial impingement syndrome. *J Bone Joint Surg Am*. 2005;87(7):1446-1455.
49. Hermans J, Luime JJ, Meuffels DE, Reijman M, Simel DL, Bierma-Zeinstra SM. Does this patient with shoulder pain have rotator cuff disease?: the Rational Clinical Examination systematic review. *JAMA*. 2013;310(8):837-847.
50. Alqunaee M, Galvin R, Fahey T. Diagnostic accuracy of clinical tests for subacromial impingement syndrome: a systematic review and meta-analysis. *Arch Phys Med Rehabil*. 2012;93(2):229-236.
51. Diercks R, Bron C, Dorrestijn O, et al. Guideline for diagnosis and treatment of subacromial pain syndrome: a multidisciplinary review by the Dutch Orthopaedic Association. *Acta Orthop*. 2014;85(3):314-322.
52. Dinnes J, Loveman E, McIntyre L, Waugh N. The effectiveness of diagnostic tests for the assessment of shoulder pain due to soft tissue disorders: a systematic review. *Health Technol Assess*. 2003;7(29):iii, 1-166.
53. Sergienko S, Kalichman L. Myofascial origin of shoulder pain: a literature review. *J Bodyw Mov Ther*. 2015;19(1):91-101.
54. Simons DG, Travell J, Simons L. *Travell & Simon's Myofascial Pain and Dysfunction: The Trigger Point Manual*. Vol 1. 2nd ed. Baltimore, MD: Williams & Wilkins; 1999.
55. Hidalgo-Lozano A, Fernández de las Peñas C, Calderon-Soto C, Domingo-Camara A, Madeleine P, Arroyo-Morales M. Elite swimmers with and without unilateral shoulder pain: mechanical hyperalgesia and active/latent muscle trigger points in neck-shoulder muscles. *Scand J Med Sci Sports*. 2013;23(1):66-73.
56. Arias-Buria JL, Valero-Alcaide R, Cleland JA, et al. Inclusion of trigger point dry needling in a multimodal physical therapy program for postoperative shoulder pain: a randomized clinical trial. *J Manipulative Physiol Ther*. 2015;38(3):179-187.
57. Ohmori A, Iranami H, Fujii K, Yamazaki A, Doko Y. Myofascial involvement of supra- and infraspinatus muscles contributes to ipsilateral shoulder pain after muscle-sparing thoracotomy and video-assisted thoracic surgery. *J Cardiothorac Vasc Anesth*. 2013;27(6):1310-1314.
58. Bron C, Franssen J, Wensing M, Oostendorp RA. Interrater reliability of palpation of myofascial trigger points in three shoulder muscles. *J Man Manip Ther*. 2007;15(4):203-215.
59. Bron C, Dommerholt J, Stegenga B, Wensing M, Oostendorp RA. High prevalence of shoulder girdle muscles with myofascial trigger points in patients with shoulder pain. *BMC Musculoskelet Disord*. 2011;12(1):139-151.
60. Bron C, de Gast A, Dommerholt J, Stegenga B, Wensing M, Oostendorp RA. Treatment of myofascial trigger points in patients with chronic shoulder pain: a randomized, controlled trial. *BMC Med*. 2011;9:8.
61. Hsieh YL, Kao MJ, Kuan TS, Chen SM, Chen JT, Hong CZ. Dry needling to a key myofascial trigger point may reduce the irritability of satellite MTrPs. *Am J Phys Med Rehabil*. 2007;86(5):397-403.
62. Hains G, Descarreaux M, Hains F. Chronic shoulder pain of myofascial origin: a randomized clinical trial using ischemic compression therapy. *J Manipulative Physiol Ther*. 2010;33(5):362-369.
63. Ge HY, Fernández de las Peñas C, Madeleine P, Arendt-Nielsen L. Topographical mapping and mechanical pain sensitivity of myofascial trigger points in the infraspinatus muscle. *Eur J Pain*. 2008;12(7):859-865.
64. Hidalgo-Lozano A, Fernández de las Peñas C, Alonso-Blanco C, Ge HY, Arendt-Nielsen L, Arroyo-Morales M. Muscle trigger points and pressure pain hyperalgesia in the shoulder muscles in patients with unilateral shoulder impingement: a blinded, controlled study. *Exp Brain Res*. 2010;202(4):915-925.
65. Alburquerque-Sendin F, Camargo P, Viera A, Salvini TF. Bilateral myofascial trigger points and pressure pain thresholds in the shoulder muscles in patients with unilateral shoulder impingement syndrome. A blinded controlled study. *Clin J Pain*. 2013;29:478-486.
66. Gebremariam L, Hay EM, van der Sande R, Rinkel WD, Koes BW, Huisstede BM. Subacromial impingement syndrome—effectiveness of physiotherapy and manual therapy. *Br J Sports Med*. 2014;48(16):1202-1208.
67. Saltychev M, Aarimaa V, Virolainen P, Laimi K. Conservative treatment or surgery for shoulder impingement: systematic review and meta-analysis. *Disabil Rehabil*. 2015;37(1):1-8.
68. Moraes GF, Faria CD, Teixeira-Salmela LF. Scapular muscle recruitment patterns and isokinetic strength ratios of the shoulder rotator muscles in individuals with and without impingement syndrome. *J Shoulder Elbow Surg*. 2008;17(1 suppl):48S-53S.
69. Roy JS, Moffet H, McFadyen BJ. Upper limb motor strategies in persons with and without shoulder impingement syndrome across different speeds of movement. *Clin Biomech (Bristol, Avon)*. 2008;23(10):1227-1236.
70. Ludewig PM, Cook TM. Alterations in shoulder kinematics and associated muscle activity in people with symptoms of shoulder impingement. *Phys Ther*. 2000;80(3):276-291.
71. Cools AM, Witvrouw EE, Declercq GA, Danneels LA, Cambier DC. Scapular muscle recruitment patterns: trapezius muscle latency with and without impingement symptoms. *Am J Sports Med*. 2003;31(4):542-549.
72. Ludewig PM, Reynolds JF. The association of scapular kinematics and glenohumeral joint pathologies. *J Orthop Sports Phys Ther*. 2009;39(2):90-104.
73. Kibler WB, Ludewig PM, McClure PW, Michener LA, Bak K, Sciascia AD. Clinical implications of scapular dyskinesis in shoulder injury: the 2013 consensus statement from the 'Scapular Summit'. *Br J Sports Med*. 2013;47(14):877-885.
74. Cools AM, Declercq GA, Cambier DC, Mahieu NN, Witvrouw EE. Trapezius activity and intramuscular balance during isokinetic exercise in overhead athletes with impingement symptoms. *Scand J Med Sci Sports*. 2007;17(1):25-33.
75. Tsai NT, McClure PW, Karduna AR. Effects of muscle fatigue on 3-dimensional scapular kinematics. *Arch Phys Med Rehabil*. 2003;84(7):1000-1005.
76. Falla D, Farina D, Graven-Nielsen T. Experimental muscle pain results in reorganization of coordination among trapezius muscle subdivisions during repetitive shoulder flexion. *Exp Brain Res*. 2007;178(3):385-393.
77. Lucas KR. The impact of latent trigger points on regional muscle function. *Curr Pain Headache Rep*. 2008;12(5):344-349.
78. Ibarra JM, Ge HY, Wang C, Martinez Vizcaino V, Graven-Nielsen T, Arendt-Nielsen L. Latent myofascial trigger points are associated with an increased antagonistic muscle activity during agonist muscle contraction. *J Pain*. 2011;12(12):1282-1288.

79. Ge HY, Arendt-Nielsen L, Madeleine P. Accelerated muscle fatigability of latent myofascial trigger points in humans. *Pain Med*. 2012;13(7):957-964.
80. Ge HY, Monterde S, Graven-Nielsen T, Arendt-Nielsen L. Latent myofascial trigger points are associated with an increased intramuscular electromyographic activity during synergistic muscle activation. *J Pain*. 2014;15(2):181-187.
81. Lucas KR, Polus PA, Rich J. Latent myofascial trigger points: their effect on muscle activation and movement efficiency. *J Bodyw Mov Ther*. 2004;8:160-166.
82. Lucas KR, Rich PA, Polus BI. Muscle activation patterns in the scapular positioning muscles during loaded scapular plane elevation: the effects of latent myofascial trigger points. *Clin Biomech (Bristol, Avon)*. 2010;25(8):765-770.
83. Bohlooli N, Ahmadi A, Maroufi N, Sarrafzadeh J, Jaberzadeh S. Differential activation of scapular muscles, during arm elevation, with and without trigger points. *J Bodyw Mov Ther*. 2016;20(1):26-34.
84. Uhthoff HK, Boileau P. Primary frozen shoulder: global capsular stiffness versus localized contracture. *Clin Orthop Relat Res*. 2007;456:79-84.
85. Schultheis A, Reichwein F, Nebelung W. Frozen shoulder. Diagnosis and therapy. *Orthopade*. 2008;37(11):1065-1066, 1068-1072.
86. Miller MD, Wirth MA, Rockwood CA Jr. Thawing the frozen shoulder: the "patient" patient. *Orthopedics*. 1996;19(10):849-853.
87. Lewit K. *Manipulative Therapy in Rehabilitation of the Locomotor System*. 3rd ed. Oxford, UK: Butterworth Heinemann; 1999.
88. Clewley D, Flynn TW, Koppenhaver S. Trigger point dry needling as an adjunct treatment for a patient with adhesive capsulitis of the shoulder. *J Orthop Sports Phys Ther*. 2014;44(2):92-101.
89. Fernández de las Peñas C, Fernandez-Carnero J, Miangolarra-Page J. Musculoskeletal disorders in mechanical neck pain: myofascial trigger points versus cervical joint dysfunction—a clinical study. *J Musculoskelet Pain*. 2005;13(1):27-35.
90. Bogduk N, Simons D. Chapter 20, Neck pain: joint pain or trigger points? In: Vaeroy H, Merskey H, eds. *Progress in Fibromyalgia and Myofascial Pain*. Vol 6, *Pain Research and Clinical Management*. Amsterdam, Netherlands: Elsevier; 1993:267-273.
91. Michele AA, Davies JJ, Krueger FJ, et al. Scapulocosal syndrome (fatigue-postural paradox). *N Y State J Med*. 1950;50:1353-1356.
92. Michele AA, Eisenberg J. Scapulocostal syndrome. *Arch Phys Med Rehabil*. 1968;49(7):383-387.
93. Ormandy L. Scapulocostal syndrome. *Va Med Q*. 1994;121(2):105-108.

Section 4: Forearm, Wrist, and Hand Pain

Chapter 34

Wrist Extensor and Brachioradialis Muscles

"Pseudo Tennis Elbow"

Orlando Mayoral del Moral and Enrique Lluch Girbés

1. INTRODUCTION

The wrist extensor muscles are anatomically located in the dorsal forearm and include the extensor carpi radialis longus (ECRL), extensor carpi radialis brevis (ECRB), and the extensor carpi ulnaris (ECU) muscles. The main function of these muscles is wrist extension with a component of either radial or ulnar deviation. Despite also being located in the dorsal forearm, the brachioradialis muscle does not exert its main function at the wrist; its primary role is to flex the elbow, regardless of forearm position. The referred pain elicited by trigger points (TrPs) from the wrist extensor and brachioradialis muscles spreads upward to the lateral epicondyle and downward toward the dorsum of the forearm, wrist, and base of the thumb, in the space between the thumb and the index finger. Symptoms may be exacerbated by repetitive lifting and grasping activities, as well as sleeping postures that promote elbow and wrist flexion. Activation and perpetuation of TrPs in the wrist extensor and brachioradialis muscles are caused by repetitive forceful grasping and sporting activities. The larger the object being grasped, and the greater the amount of ulnar deviation required of the hand, the more likely the muscles are to develop TrPs. Compelling evidence supports a role of myofascial pain derived from the wrist extensor and brachioradialis muscles as part of the etiology of lateral elbow pain or lateral epicondylalgia. Differential diagnosis includes true tennis elbow, ECRB tendinopathy, local arthritis, radiocapitellar pathology, radial tunnel syndrome, posterior interosseous nerve syndrome, cervical radicular pain or radiculopathy (C7), and de Quervain syndrome. Corrective actions include eliminating strain of the involved muscles, correcting grasp, establishing a home program of TrP self-pressure release and self-stretch exercises, and the gradual resumption of normal activities after inactivating the TrPs.

2. ANATOMIC CONSIDERATIONS

The muscles of the forearm can be divided into two major compartments: the flexors and extensors. The extensor muscles can be further divided into five dorsal compartments: (1) a radial compartment enclosing the brachioradialis muscle; (2) a radial compartment enclosing the ECRB and ECRL muscles; (3) an abductor compartment with the abductor pollicis longus and extensor pollicis brevis muscles; (4) a central compartment with the extensor digitorum, extensor digiti minimi, extensor pollicis longus, and extensor indicis muscles; and (5) an ulnar compartment housing the ECU muscle.[1]

The wrist extensor musculature is located over the radial and ulnar aspects of the forearm. The ECRL and ECRB muscles are located radially and the ECU muscle is located ulnarly. Together with the brachioradialis, supinator, extensor digitorum, and extensor digiti minimi muscles, they constitute the extensor-supinator muscle group.[2] Each muscle belonging to this group originates near or directly onto the lateral epicondyle of the humerus. Anatomic variations of radial wrist extensor muscles are common, and several varieties from the norm are documented in the literature.[3-7] The tendons of the ECRB, ECRL, and brachioradialis muscles are quite useful in tendon transfer operations, such as in correction of finger clawing and restoration of thumb opposition.[7-9] The extensor retinaculum prevents the extensor tendons from "bowstringing" away from the radiocarpal joint during functional activities. Under the extensor retinaculum are six fibro-osseous tunnels that contain the extensor tendons and their synovial sheaths. The tendons of the ECRL and ECRB muscles are within the same tunnel but have independent synovial sheaths.[10]

Extensor Carpi Radialis Longus

The ECRL muscle originates from the distal third of the lateral supracondylar ridge of the humerus, between the lateral epicondyle and the attachment of the brachioradialis muscle (Figure 34-1A).[2,9,11,12] Distally, the ECRL muscle inserts onto the base of the 2nd metacarpal bone on its dorsoradial aspect and may also send slips to the 1st and 3rd metacarpal bones. The muscle fibers extend one-third of the length of the forearm, and its tendon extends the remaining two-thirds.[13]

Extensor Carpi Radialis Brevis

The ECRB muscle arises mainly from the lateral epicondyle of the humerus, radial collateral ligament, intermuscular septa and is covered by a strong aponeurosis.[13] The ECRB muscle lies deep to the belly of the ECRL muscle.[2,11] The belly of the ECRB muscle expands to full thickness near the junction of the upper and middle thirds of the forearm where the more lateral ECRL muscle belly fades to a tendon.[14] The ECRB muscle passes behind and deep to the ECRL muscle, and under the extensor retinaculum distally, inserting onto the base of the 3rd metacarpal bone and sometimes with a slip to the 2nd metacarpal on its dorsoradial aspect (Figure 34-3A).[2,13]

The ECRB muscle origin comprises a superficial, narrow tendinous attachment to the lateral epicondyle and a broad attachment to an intermuscular septum.[15,16] The deeper aspect of the ECRB origin merges directly with the lateral collateral ligament that in turn also fuses with the annular ligament of the proximal radioulnar joint.[16] This relationship may explain the progressive involvement of the lateral collateral ligament in some clinical presentations of lateral epicondylalgia.[17] In addition, the interdigitation between the origins of the ECRB muscle and the portion of extensor digitorum muscle that extends to the 3rd digit explains Maudsley's test, that is, pain with resisted extension of the 3rd finger.[18]

The ECRB muscle is the only wrist extensor that has a proximal attachment with a long tendinous portion without any muscle fascicles, whereas the other wrist extensors originate as a mixture of tendon and muscle.[12] The tendinous portion of the ECRB muscle is most substantial at its origin and gradually transitions into muscle as it descends in the forearm.[12] The tendinous origin of the ECRB muscle has less vascularity in comparison with the other extensor origins, which have muscular portions, explaining why an injury to the origin of the ECRB muscle may take longer or be less likely to heal.[12] In addition, the attachment of the articular capsule to the anterior part of the ECRB muscle origin has been hypothesized to be a causative factor of lateral epicondylalgia.[12]

Proximally, the strong aponeurosis of the ECRB muscle forms a bridge of fascia, which stretches between the lateral epicondyle of the humerus and the deep fascia of the dorsal forearm. It may become thickened[19,20] where the deep (motor) branch of the radial nerve passes beneath it to enter the supinator muscle (Figure 34-1C). Usually, the superficial radial nerve has branched off before the deep radial nerve dips beneath the ECRB muscle (Figure 34-1B). In some cases, however, the nerve divides more distally (Figure 34-1C), so that the superficial branch must penetrate the belly of the ECRB muscle to return to its own course beneath the brachioradialis muscle.[19] Therefore, the radial nerve may get entrapped in the superolateral part of the ECRB muscle.[21]

Extensor Carpi Ulnaris

The ECU muscle originates proximally from the lateral epicondyle (where it forms the most medial part of the common extensor origin), the upper two-thirds of the posterior border of the ulna (by an aponeurosis shared with the flexor carpi ulnaris and flexor digitorum profundus muscles), and the overlying fascia.[13] Distally, it attaches to a tubercle on the ulnar side of the base of the 5th

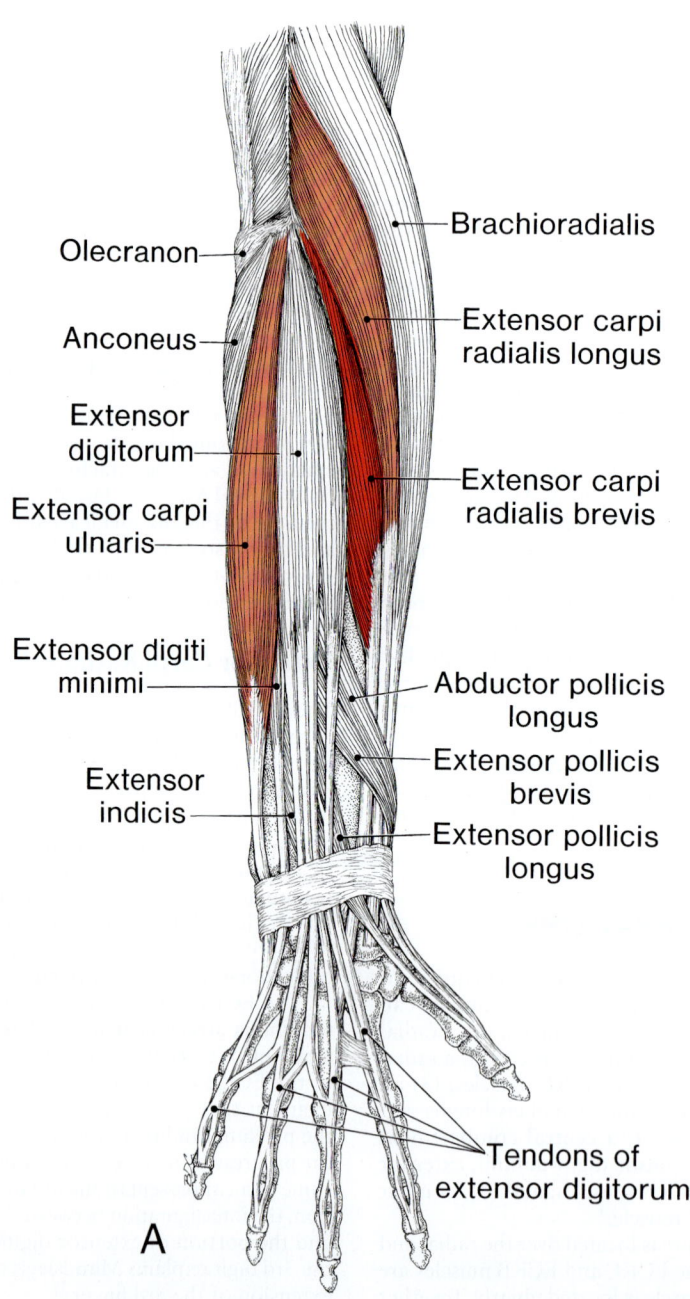

Figure 34-1. The relations of the hand extensor muscles and part of the radial nerve in the right forearm. A, Dorsal view showing the attachments of the extensor carpi radialis longus and brevis, and extensor carpi ulnaris muscles.

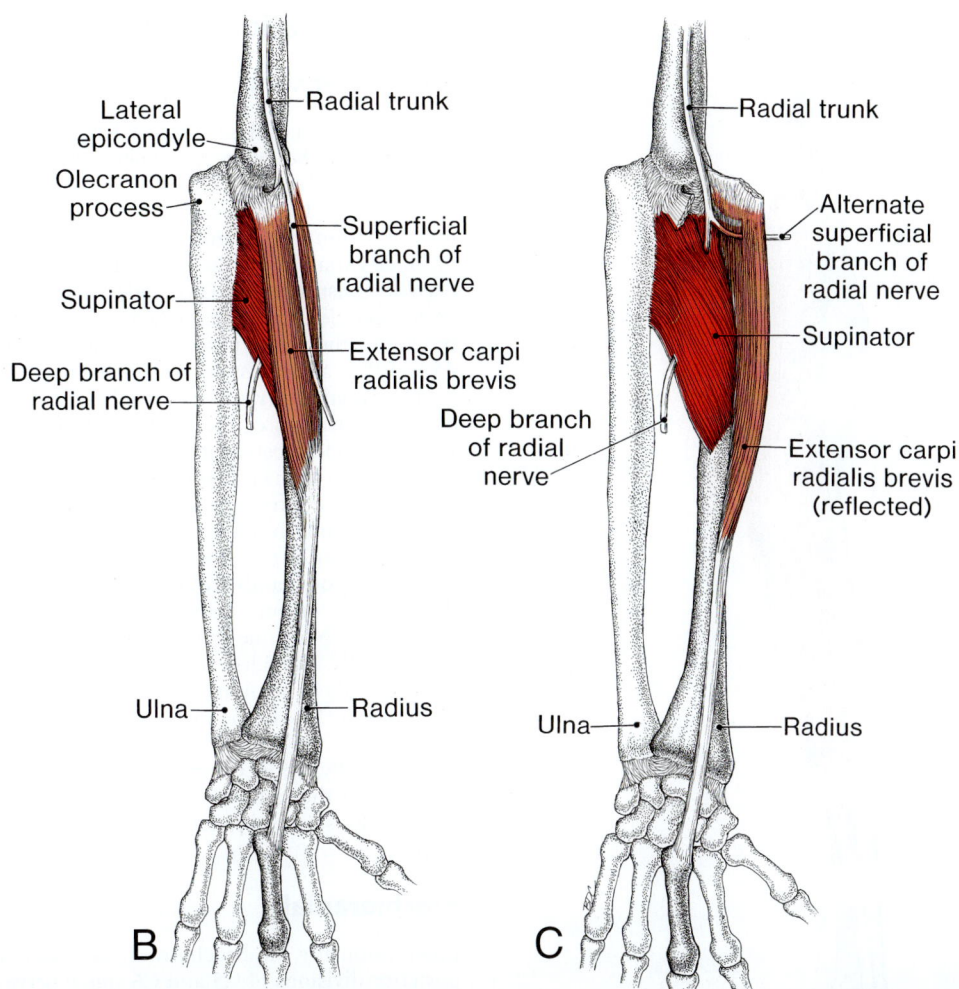

Figure 34-1. (*continued*) B, Lateral view showing the deep branch of the radial nerve before it passes beneath the fibrous arch formed by the proximal attachments of the extensor carpi radialis brevis (light red), and showing the normal course of the superficial (sensory) branch. C, Variant course of the superficial branch of the radial nerve *through* the (reflected) extensor carpi radialis brevis muscle. Adapted from Kopell HP, Thompson WA. *Peripheral Entrapment Neuropathies.* 2nd ed. Baltimore, MD: Williams & Wilkins; 1963.

metacarpal bone (Figure 34-1A).[2,11,13] The ECU muscle is composed of a muscular portion and a thin membranous tendon.[12]

Brachioradialis

The brachioradialis muscle originates from the proximal two-thirds of the lateral supracondylar ridge of the humerus and along the anterior surface of the lateral intermuscular septum,[13] distal to the spiral groove, where the radial nerve penetrates the septum at mid-arm level (Figure 34-2).[2,18] It forms the lateral border of the cubital fossa.[13] The muscle fibers end above mid-forearm level and transition to a flat tendon that runs distally over the anterolateral aspect of the radioulnar joint and inserts onto the lateral side of the distal end of the radius, just proximal to the styloid process.[2,13,18] It is composed of a muscular portion and only a thin, short tendon.[12] The brachioradialis muscle has a series-fibered architecture that consists of multiple, overlapping bands of muscle fibers in most individuals.[22] In some individuals, however, a simple parallel-fibered architecture is observed.[22]

Anatomic Variations

Several anatomic variations have been reported for the wrist extensor and brachioradialis muscles.[3-7] In particular, different varieties of additional radial wrist extensor muscle bellies with independent tendons have been reported by Nayak et al.[7] These additional muscles originated either from the ECRL or the ECRB muscles and were inserted at the base of the 2nd or 3rd metacarpal bones. The two classic variants described for the radial wrist extensors are named the extensor carpi radialis intermedius and extensor carpi radialis accessorius muscles.[5,7] The extensor carpi radialis intermedius muscle originates from the ECRB muscle, becomes tendinous, and travels between the two radial extensor tendons. It inserts independently into the 2nd metacarpal bone.[5,7] The extensor carpi radialis accessorius muscle arises from below the ECRL muscle and inserts into the 1st metacarpal bone.[5,7]

A rare extensor carpi radialis accessorius muscle was reported originating from the ECRL muscle, passing superficially over the parent tendon, and inserting into the abductor pollicis brevis muscle.[5] Another additional extensor carpi radialis muscle originating from the common extensor origin, between the ECRL and extensor digitorum muscles, has been noted and dubbed the extensor carpi radialis tertius muscle.[6] The tendon of this muscle divides below the abductor pollicis longus muscle and attaches to the base of the 2nd and 3rd metacarpal bones.[6] Mitsuyasu et al[4] reported the origin of the ECRB muscle from the fascia/tendon of the extensor digitorum muscle, without any of its origin at the usual location on the lateral epicondyle.

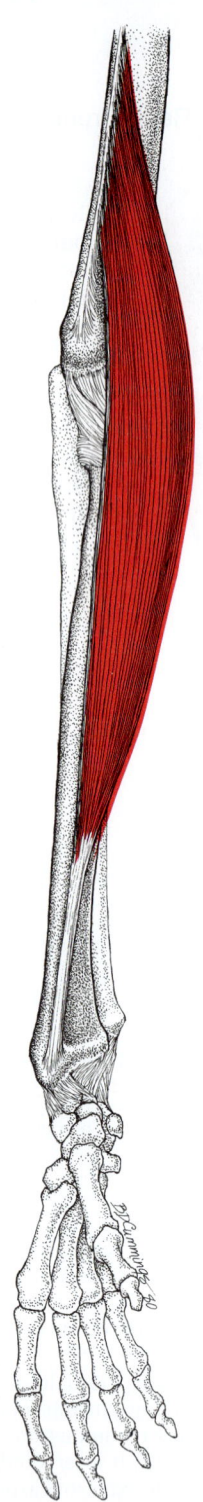

Figure 34-2. The attachments of the right brachioradialis muscle, from the radial view.

2.1. Innervation and Vascularization

Wrist Extensors

The innervation of the ECRL, ECRB, and ECU muscles is provided by branches of the radial nerve, particularly the posterior interosseous nerve.[24] The ECRL muscle innervation is from C6 and C7,[13] the ECRB muscle from C7 and C8,[13] and the ECU muscle[13] from the C7 and C8 nerve roots.[13,25]

Wide variability of the innervation of the ECRB muscle has been demonstrated, with no single consistent pattern.[9,26,27] The ECRB muscle can be innervated by the radial nerve, the deep branch of the radial nerve (the posterior interosseous nerve; 45%-50%), and the superficial radial nerve (25%-35%).[9,26,27]

The radial artery and its branches are the principal sources of vascularization of the ECRL and ECRB muscles.[28,29] The ECRL muscle receives its principal vascular supply from a single branch of the radial recurrent artery.[13] Additional vascularization comes from branches of the radial collateral branch of the profunda brachii artery and from the radial artery in the distal part of the muscle.[13] The ECRB muscle receives its vascularization mainly from two pedicles: a single branch from the radial recurrent artery and a branch of the radial artery that arises about one-third of the way down the forearm.[13] Additionally, branches from the radial collateral branch of the profunda brachii artery supply the muscle proximally.[13] The undersurface of the ECRB tendon was found to be almost avascular.[29]

Proximally, the ECU muscle receives its vascularization from branches of the radial recurrent artery, whereas distally, it is supplied by several branches from the posterior interosseous artery.[13]

Brachioradialis

Innervation for the brachioradialis muscle comes from the posterior divisions of C5 and C6 spinal nerve roots.[2,13]

Latev and Dalley in 2005 investigated the innervation of the brachioradialis muscle in 43 embalmed cadaveric specimens.[30] A wide anatomic variation was observed in the innervation pattern. A single primary nerve branch arising from the radial nerve, 30 mm proximal to the lateral epicondyle, was found in the majority of cases (46.5%). In 16 of these cases, the primary branch split into two to four secondary branches, and in four cases, there was only one branch entering the muscle.[30]

Vascularization of the brachioradialis muscle is supplied by branches of the radial recurrent artery that pierce the posteromedial surface of the muscle.[13] It is also supplied by branches from the radial collateral branch of the profunda brachii artery and from the radial artery in the distal part of the muscle.[13]

2.2. Function

The wrist extensors ensure effective length-tension ratios of the opposite finger flexors during their contraction for grasping. The wrist extensor muscles activate strongly in this stabilizing role to prevent wrist flexion produced by contraction of the finger flexor muscles with gripping or pinching functional activities.[31-33] Most textbooks of anatomy briefly describe that the ECRL and ECRB muscles act as extensors and radial deviators of the wrist, and the ECU muscle acts as an extensor and ulnar deviator of the wrist.[13,34-36] However, cadaver studies and some studies that measure topographic relationships among the tendons of the wrist extensor muscles and the axes of the joint have shown that strict actions of the ECRL muscle differ from those of the ECRB muscle.[37-39] Furthermore, actions of the extensor muscles, including direction of the motion and force of each muscle, change depending on forearm position.[38]

A number of variations in the attachments of the brachioradialis muscle have been reported. The distal attachment of the brachioradialis muscle may be more proximal than usual.[13] It may fuse proximally with the brachialis muscle, and the tendon may, occasionally, divide into two or three separately attached slips.[13] In rare instances, it is double or absent.[13] A variable slip of the muscle may attach distally to several carpal bones and to the 3rd metacarpal.[23]

Wrist Extensors

Sagae et al[40] analyzed strict actions of the human wrist extensors using electrical neuromuscular stimulation, a method that has the ability to activate each muscle individually. This method is thought to be superior to electromyography (EMG) recording of wrist extensor muscle activity during voluntary movements because EMG shows activities of two or more wrist extensor muscles during wrist-bending motion, making it difficult to determine the activation of each individual muscle.[40] The ECRL muscle was found to act as a wrist extensor rather than a radial deviator with the forearm in a pronated position and as a wrist radial deviator rather than an extensor with the forearm in neutral and in supinated positions.[40] The ECRB muscle behaved as a wrist extensor rather than a radial deviator with the pronated, neutral, and supinated forearm positions, and the ECU muscle acts as a wrist ulnar deviator rather than an extensor with the neutral and supinated forearm positions and as a wrist ulnar deviator with the pronated forearm position.[40] Therefore, the ECRL muscle is a wrist radial deviator and extensor, and the ECRB muscle is a wrist extensor rather than a radial deviator. Supporting this argument, a previous study by Fujii et al[41] found that electrical neuromuscular stimulation to the ECRL muscle induced motions of wrist extension and radial deviation regardless of the positions of the forearm.

In addition to performing extension and radial deviation of the wrist, the ECRL muscle has a good moment arm to act as an elbow flexor with the forearm pronated.[42] The ECRL muscle may also provide some valgus force at the elbow joint.[42] Interestingly, co-contraction of the pronator teres and ECRL muscles occurs during wrist extension movements to prevent supination of the forearm. Contraction of the ECRL muscle induced 30° to 80° supination of the forearm from the pronated position.[41] Therefore, forearm supination from the pronated position should be considered one of the actions of the ECRL muscle.[10,41]

In addition to extension and ulnar deviation of the wrist, the ECU muscle may also provide some valgus force at the elbow joint.[42] It is a better wrist extensor with the forearm supinated than pronated because the tendon slips anteriorly during forearm pronation.[43,44] It also stabilizes the wrist during thumb abduction.[45]

Brachioradialis

Initially, this muscle was named the "supinator longus" on the assumption that its primary action was supination of the forearm. The brachioradialis muscle has the largest mechanical advantage of any of the elbow flexors because it inserts a long distance from the joint axis.[46] Duchenne clearly demonstrated, through stimulation studies, that it functioned chiefly as a flexor of the elbow,[34] which led to its current name, the brachioradialis muscle. The primary role of the brachioradialis muscle appears to be that of an elbow flexor together with the biceps brachii and brachialis muscles.[13] Information regarding this muscle's role as a forearm supinator or pronator remains controversial in the literature.[47] A study using fine-wire EMG electrodes in the brachioradialis muscle, along with kinematic data, showed that the greatest EMG activity recorded from the brachioradialis muscle occurs during elbow flexion, regardless of the forearm position.[47] In this same study, during tasks that required pronation and supination, the brachioradialis muscle was more active during pronation tasks compared with supination tasks, indicating a secondary function of the brachioradialis muscle as a forearm pronator.[47]

Electromyographically,[35] brachioradialis muscle activity is usually reserved for speedy movement and lifting weight by flexing the elbow, especially if the forearm is in the neutral position. It is minimally active in slow flexion or with the forearm supinated but generates a powerful burst of activity in both flexion and extension when movement is rapid.[13] However, none of the elbow flexors is used to counteract gravity when a weight is held in the dependent hand with the elbow straight.[35] The brachioradialis muscle attaches in such a manner as to prevent separation of the elbow joint with centrifugal force by contracting during rapid elbow movement. This pronounced transarticular component of its force helps stabilize the elbow joint.[13] In contrast, the biceps brachii and brachialis muscles accelerate movement at the elbow without counteracting distraction of the elbow joint.

Historically, a specific tennis racquet grip size (following Nirschl's recommended measurement) was linked to less risk of lateral epicondylalgia. However, Hatch et al,[48] using fine-wire EMG in different forearm musculature, including the ECRB and ECRL muscles, demonstrated that alterations in tennis racquet grip size do not have a significant effect on forearm muscle activity, and therefore racquet grip does not represent a significant risk factor for lateral epicondylalgia. Another accessory, string dampers, is often used by tennis players to supposedly reduce the amount of racket frame vibration received at the forearm and thus ameliorate the stress on the wrist extensor muscles, but no mechanical advantage has been demonstrated for string dampers.[49]

Tennis players with TrPs in the wrist extensor muscles should avoid a "leading elbow" or an open racquet face near the time of ball impact. In addition, ball contact in the lower half of the strings should be minimized. Poor racquet mechanics can make the wrist extensor muscles more vulnerable to potential injury.[50] Performance of the backhand stroke should be done with the wrist extended (ie, neutral alignment of the forearm and hand dorsum). In expert players, collision of the ball and racket during the backhand stroke normally occurs with the wrist extended, and the wrists move further into extension at impact.[51] Expert players demonstrate greater wrist extensor activity than novice players after ball contact, consistent with the accompanying wrist extension.[51] An eccentric contraction of the wrist extensor muscles throughout the stroke is observed in novice players. Because muscle overload as a result of eccentric muscle contractions is one recognized factor that leads to the development of TrPs,[52,53] novice tennis players should be instructed to quickly release their grip tightness during backhand strokes after ball impact in order to reduce shock impact transmission to the wrist and elbow.[54]

2.3. Functional Unit

The functional unit to which a muscle belongs includes the muscles that reinforce and counter its actions as well as the joints that the muscle crosses. The interdependence of these structures is functionally reflected in the organization and neural connections of the sensory motor cortex. The functional unit is emphasized because the presence of a TrP in one muscle of the unit increases the likelihood that the other muscles of the unit will also develop TrPs. When inactivating TrPs in a muscle, one must be concerned about TrPs that may develop in muscles that are functionally interdependent. Box 34-1 grossly represents the functional unit of the wrist extensor muscles, and Box 34-2 grossly represents the functional unit of the brachioradialis muscle.[55]

The ECRL muscle co-contracts with the pronator teres muscle during wrist extension movements to prevent supination of the forearm.[41] During the grasping of an object, the wrist extensors act synergistically to prevent flexion of the wrist that the extrinsic finger flexors would otherwise produce.[31-33]

3. CLINICAL PRESENTATION

Travell and Simons[55] described the referred pain patterns from TrPs in most forearm muscles that produce similar pain features of lateral epicondylalgia. Similar pain referral patterns as those described for the TrPs of the wrist extensors, with some

Box 34-1 Functional unit of the ECRL, ECRB, and ECU muscles

Action	Synergists	Antagonists
Wrist extension	Extensor digitorum longus Extensor indicis Extensor pollicis longus	Flexor carpi radialis Flexor carpi ulnaris Flexor digitorum superficialis Flexor digitorum profundus
Radial deviation (ECRL)	Flexor carpi radialis	ECU Flexor carpi ulnaris
Ulnar deviation (ECU)	Flexor carpi ulnaris	ECRL ECRB Flexor carpi radialis

Box 34-2 Functional unit of the brachioradialis muscle

Action	Synergists	Antagonists
Elbow flexion	Biceps brachii Brachialis	Triceps brachii Anconeus

differences, have been described in experimental pain models of lateral epicondylalgia.[56,57] In these studies, injection of hypertonic saline[56,58] or nerve growth factor[57] into the wrist extensor muscles (ECRB, supinator, common wrist extensor origin)[57] or into the ECRB muscle[56,58] reproduced pain over the lateral epicondyle and spread distally into the forearm. Furthermore, infusion of hypertonic saline into latent TrPs in the brachioradialis muscle produced referred pain to the dorsum of the wrist in 35% of infusions.[59] Three clinical studies[60-62] demonstrated that referred pain elicited by manual palpation of TrPs in the forearm musculature share similar patterns of sustained lateral elbow and forearm pain that is characteristic of people with lateral epicondylalgia.

3.1. Referred Pain Pattern

Wrist Extensors

Pain elicited by TrPs in the ECRL muscle is referred to the lateral epicondyle and to the dorsum of the hand next to the region of the anatomic snuff box (Figure 34-3C), which is often described by the patient as "the thumb."[63,64] In a study of patients with lateral epicondylalgia, ECRL active TrPs reproduced lateral epicondylar pain in 72.2% of the cases.[62]

ECRB TrPs project pain to the back of the hand and wrist (Figure 34-3B).[63] This referred pain is one of the most common myofascial sources of pain in the back of the wrist. Some studies have also found that pain referral to the lateral aspect of the elbow or the forearm, elicited by active TrPs in the ECRB muscle, reproduced the symptoms of 85% to 100% of patients with lateral epicondylalgia.[61,62,65] These studies, as well as the results of the injection studies mentioned earlier,[56-58] suggest that pain referred to the lateral epicondyle (Figure 34-3B) should also be considered as an important pattern of the ECRB muscle.[56-58]

Pain elicited by TrPs in the ECU muscle primarily refers to the ulnar side of the dorsal aspect of the wrist (Figure 34-3A). It has also been reported that ECU TrPs sometimes refer pain to the posterior aspect of the lateral epicondyle (Figure 34-3A).[65]

Brachioradialis

In patients with lateral epicondylalgia, the brachioradialis muscle exhibits TrPs less often than the ECRL and ECRB muscles (50%-66%).[60-62] The essential pain pattern of the brachioradialis muscle is into the lateral epicondyle, the radial aspect of the forearm, the wrist, and the base of the thumb (in the web space between the thumb and the index finger) (Figure 34-4). Bonica and Sola[66] illustrated the referred pain of the brachioradialis muscle to the lateral epicondyle, and Kelly[67] identified a pattern of pain and tenderness close to the elbow and a diffuse referred pain and tenderness across the dorsum of the hand.

3.2. Symptoms

Patients will typically report pain and dysfunction in the form of limited elbow, wrist, and/or hand movements. However, pain will be their primary report. The patients often describe an onset of pain that appears first in the lateral epicondyle and then spreads progressively to the wrist and hand. When the patient primarily reports lateral elbow pain, TrPs of the wrist extensors and brachioradialis muscles can be responsible for these symptoms. If TrPs go unidentified or are not addressed, persistent chronic pain could result, leading to functional disability and high costs because of loss of productivity and increased utilization of healthcare.[68]

If the ECU muscle has TrPs, the patient will typically report pain and limitations in ulnar deviation of the wrist; however, TrPs in this muscle may be responsible for atypical posterior lateral epicondyle pain. Although patients with TrPs in the forearm muscles will classically report pain as the main feature of their condition, they may also present with limited movement and/or inhibition weakness.

Pain caused by TrPs in the forearm muscles is usually manifested during loading activities of the wrist extensor muscles, such as those involving gripping or manipulating an object (eg, lifting a coffee cup, shaking hands, dressing, typing, and house work). However, some patients do not refer to a previous history of overload of the forearm extensor muscles, and the pain may have an insidious onset with no specific causal activity. Patients may also report grip weakness that can lead to objects slipping out of the hand, particularly with wrist ulnar deviation (eg, letting the head of the tennis racquet drop and lacking control when pouring milk from a carton or just before the mug reaches the lip when drinking coffee). Pain can also be felt when forceful supination or pronation is added to the grasp, as when turning a doorknob or using a screwdriver, especially when the ECU muscle is involved. When the brachioradialis muscle is involved, resisted movements of elbow flexion or thumb extension may also reproduce symptoms.

3.3. Patient Examination

After a thorough subjective examination, the clinician should make a detailed drawing representing the pain pattern that the patient has described. This depiction will assist in planning the physical examination and can be useful in monitoring the progression of the patient as symptoms improve or change. Evaluation of the cervical and thoracic spine,[69,70] as well as neurodynamic testing of the radial nerve,[71] can help to identify spinal contribution to symptoms felt in the forearm region. These tests are important even if patients do not report symptoms in the cervical or thoracic spine.[70] Subjects with lateral epicondylalgia exhibit impairments at C4 and C5 spinal levels more frequently than healthy subjects.[70]

Chapter 34: Wrist Extensor and Brachioradialis Muscles

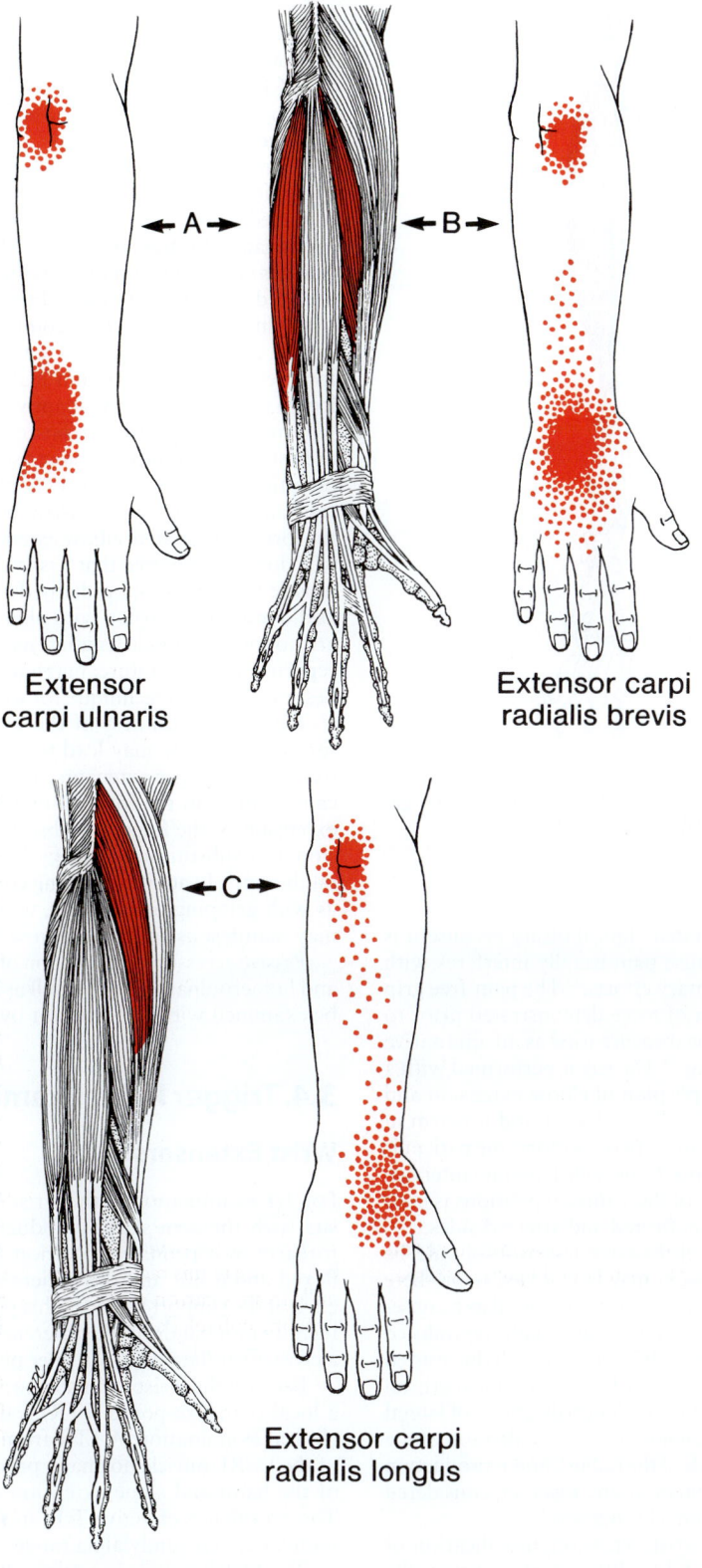

Figure 34-3. Referred pain patterns (dark red) from TrPs in the three primary hand extensor muscles (medium red) in the right forearm. A, Extensor carpi ulnaris muscle. B, Extensor carpi radialis brevis muscle. C, Extensor carpi radialis longus muscle.[65]

Observation of posture should focus on the elbow, wrist, and hand. Resting static posture of wrist radial deviation with extension can indicate stiffness, shortness, or overuse of the ECRL and ECRB muscles relative to the ECU muscle.[72] Overuse of the ECU muscle may result in wrist ulnar deviation and extension at rest.[72]

Functional assessment should include gripping tasks, along with maximal grip strength and pain-free grip strength tests using a hand-held dynamometer. This assessment allows the therapist to quantify strength deficits, inhibition weakness, and/or pain with gripping in order to evaluate treatment effects and monitor progress. In patients with lateral epicondylalgia,

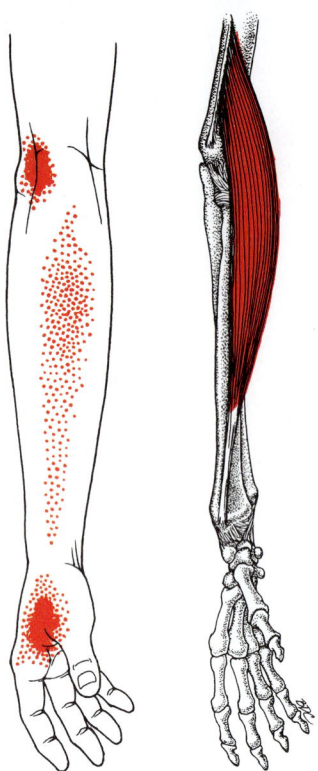

Figure 34-4. Referred pain pattern (dark red) from a TrP in the right brachioradialis muscle (medium red).

maximal grip strength is of limited clinical utility because it is not always impaired and because pain usually interferes with maximal or submaximal voluntary efforts.[73] The pain-free grip test, which reflects the amount of force demonstrated prior to the onset of pain, is an outcome measure used as an alternative to maximal grip strength testing.[74] The test is performed with a dynamometer starting from a position of elbow extension and forearm pronation or from 90° elbow flexion and forearm in neutral rotation. From either of these two positions, the patient is asked to perform three gripping actions with 1-minute intervals between trials, and the average of these three repetitions is used for comparison between the unaffected and affected sides.[74]

Resisted movement testing of the wrist extensors should be performed to identify which muscles may be involved and if there are associated neurologic deficits. Symptoms reported as a consequence of TrPs in the wrist extensor muscles are usually reproduced with the resisted wrist extension test (Cozen test), with the resisted middle finger test (Maudsley's test), or by having the patient grip an object. These tests are also used for the clinical diagnosis of lateral epicondylalgia. Maudsley's test, tenderness with palpation of the radial tunnel (anterior to the neck of the radius), and reproduction of symptoms with resisted supination are, together, considered clinical signs indicating radial tunnel syndrome.[75]

When performing resisted wrist extension, modification of the elbow position can be helpful to differentiate between the ECRL and ECRB muscles as the source of symptoms. Symptoms reproduced with resisted wrist extension with the elbow flexed bias the ECRB muscle, whereas painful wrist extension with the elbow extended biases the ECRL muscle.[76] It is important to note that reproduction of familiar pain by resisted extension of the wrist, index, or middle finger; pain upon gripping; and pain with palpation of the lateral epicondyle are considered the cardinal physical signs for diagnosing lateral epicondylalgia.[77,78]

Passive physiologic range of motion should be tested at the wrist, both with the elbow extended and flexed. Length deficit of the ECRL muscle may be a contributing factor to limited elbow extension range of motion when the wrist is flexed. Therefore, elbow extension range of motion should be tested with and without a stretch on the ECRL muscle.[74] Maximum stretch on the ECRL and ECRB muscles occurs with combined passive wrist flexion, forearm pronation, and elbow extension, with the humerus stabilized in neutral rotation.[79] Length deficits of the ECRL and ECRB muscles result in wrist extension and radial deviation range of motion limitations when the arm is pronated with the elbow extended and the humerus stabilized in neutral.[75] Takasaki et al[80] investigated effective positions for elongating the ECRB and ECRL muscles and found that the maximal strain on those muscles was obtained with elbow extension, forearm pronation, and wrist flexion with ulnar deviation. These combined positions should not only be utilized to assess muscle length but also be subsequently used for stretching the ECRL and ECRB muscles,[80] if found to have length deficits because of adaptive shortening or TrPs.

Symptoms reported as a consequence of TrPs in the ECU muscle are usually reproduced with resisted wrist extension with ulnar deviation.[76] Shortness of the ECU muscle is identified by increased resistance to stretch during wrist flexion and radial deviation with the forearm pronated, elbow extended, and humerus stabilized.[72] Macdonald[81] reported that passively stretching an involved ECU muscle by flexing and radially deviating the wrist caused pain, as did resisted extension with ulnar deviation of the wrist. There are no specific muscle length tests for the brachioradialis muscle reported in the literature; manual palpation of this muscle is the best examination technique for identifying a dysfunction.

Inhibition weakness of the wrist extensor muscles, which results from TrPs, may lead to a compensatory increase in activity of the finger extensors. This neuromuscular dysfunction can manifest in the form of movement impairments in which extension of the fingers is observed during active wrist extension as a substitution strategy for wrist extensor weakness or inhibition.[72] In addition, during contraction of the finger flexors, as with gripping or pinching, weakness in the wrist extensors may manifest as an increase in wrist flexion during the action.

Passive accessory joint motion of the radioulnar, radiohumeral, and humeroulnar joints, as well as the radiocarpal joints should be examined with and without overpressure.[82,83]

3.4. Trigger Point Examination

Wrist Extensors

For TrP examination of the wrist extensor muscles, the patient sits with the arm slightly abducted and supported with the forearm in a pronated position (Figure 34-5). The elbow is flexed about 30° and the patient's hand hangs down over the edge of the support surface. This position allows the clinician to identify taut bands of the different forearm muscles using either a cross-fiber flat or a cross-fiber pincer palpation (Figure 34-5).

Because the wrist extensors are superficial muscles, eliciting a local twitch response (LTR) is usually easy to obtain during clinical examination. A LTR from cross-fiber pincer palpation of the ECRL muscle normally produces strong radial deviation of the hand and some extension at the wrist (Figure 34-5A). The prevalence of active TrPs in the ECRL muscle in patients with lateral epicondylalgia ranges between 70% and 95%.[60-62]

The ECRB muscle is a relatively thin muscle that lies almost parallel to the axis of the forearm, together with the finger extensors. Trigger points in the ECRB muscle are usually located in the muscle mass on the ulnar side of the brachioradialis muscle, distal to those in the ECRL muscle. The muscle may be examined by cross-fiber flat palpation against the radius to elicit its LTR, which produces hand extension with slight radial deviation at the wrist (Figure 34-5B). Active TrPs in the ECRB muscle range between 65% and almost 100% in patients with lateral epicondylalgia.[60-62]

The ECU muscle can be located in the dorsal ulnar side of the forearm. The patient is asked to perform wrist extension with ulnar deviation or thumb abduction[45] to make the muscle more

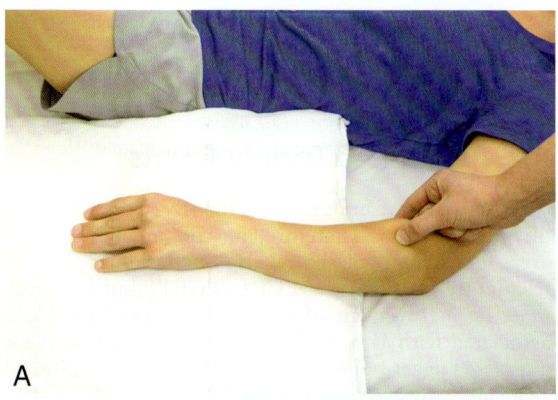
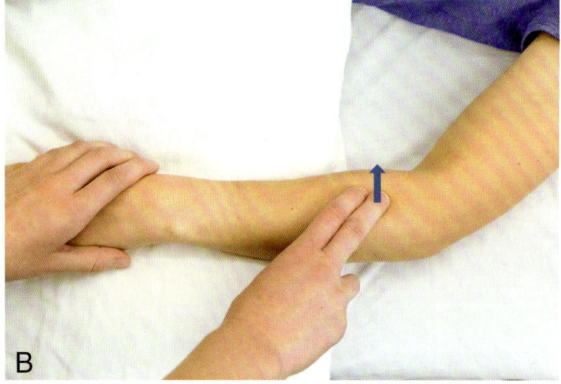
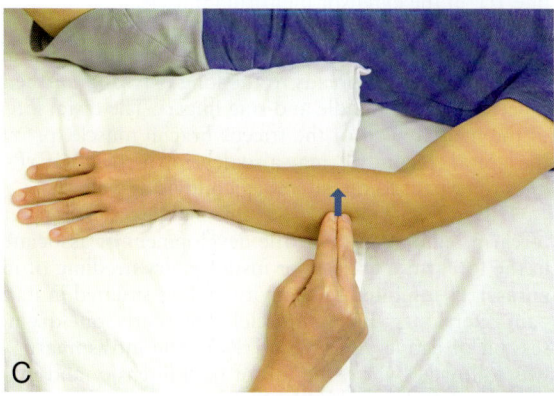

Figure 34-5. Palpation for TrPs in the wrist extensor muscles. A, Cross-fiber pincer palpation of extensor carpi radialis longus muscle. B, Cross-fiber flat palpation of extensor carpi radialis brevis muscle. Arrow showing direction of palpation. C, Cross-fiber flat palpation of extensor carpi ulnaris muscle. Arrow shows direction of palpation.

prominent. Cross-fiber flat palpation is applied just distal to the lateral epicondyle and medially from the sharp edge of the ulna toward the dorsal surface of the forearm (Figure 34-3A). If the clinician is able to elicit a LTR with cross-fiber flat palpation, it produces extension and ulnar deviation of the wrist (Figure 34-5C), although a LTR in this muscle is difficult to elicit.

Brachioradialis

The brachioradialis muscle is the most superficial muscle at the lateral elbow. It is a relatively thin muscle that is located immediately overlying and parallel to the ECRL muscle. Cross-fiber pincer palpation is preferred for examining the brachioradialis muscle because the clinician can encircle the muscle between the thumb and fingers and separate it from the underlying ECRL and ECRB muscles. For palpation of TrPs in the brachioradialis muscle, the patient sits comfortably with the forearm resting on a padded armrest, forearm pronated or in neutral and the elbow slightly flexed (Figure 34-6). The patient is asked to flex the elbow against resistance with the forearm in a neutral position. In this position, and especially when the elbow flexion is resisted at 90° of flexion, the brachioradialis muscle becomes more pronounced and it is easy for the clinician to palpate it using a pincer grasp.

Mora-Relucio et al[84] evaluated the interexaminer reliability of three clinicians (two experienced and one novice) on TrP location (at a distance <1.5 cm) and classification (relevant, nonrelevant, absent) in the wrist extensor musculature. Data showed 81.73% of agreement on TrP classification and 85.58% on TrP location between the two experienced clinicians for the ECRB muscle. The agreement on TrP classification between experienced and inexperienced clinicians was 54.81% and 51.92%, respectively, for the ECRB muscle, and the agreement between experienced and inexperienced clinicians on TrP location was 54.81% and 60.58%, respectively, for the ECRB muscle. Findings from this study also demonstrate that experienced clinicians were able to reliably identify and palpate TrPs in the extensor digitorum muscle. The level of interexaminer agreement was significantly better with experienced clinicians as compared to inexperienced clinicians.[84]

4. DIFFERENTIAL DIAGNOSIS

4.1. Activation and Perpetuation of Trigger Points

A posture or activity that activates a TrP, if not corrected, can also perpetuate it. In any part of the extensor muscle group or brachioradialis muscle, TrPs may be activated by unaccustomed eccentric loading, eccentric exercise in an unconditioned muscle, or maximal or submaximal concentric loading.[85] Trigger points may also be activated or aggravated when the muscle is placed in a shortened and/or lengthened position for an extended period of time.

Trigger points are activated in the ECRL, ECRB, and brachioradialis muscles by repetitive forceful grasping. The larger the object being grasped, and the greater the amount of ulnar deviation required of the hand, the more likely the muscles are to develop TrPs. This theory means that TrPs in the wrist extensor and brachioradialis muscles are common in tennis players and in individuals working in professions requiring handling of heavy loads or tools, forceful gripping or pronation/supination manual tasks with a combination of force, repetition, and awkward postures. Adopting awkward postures such as a non-neutral wrist position during work activity (eg, gripping with a more flexed wrist position)[73] can produce high eccentric loads and overelongation of the wrist extensor muscles, thus activating and/or perpetuating TrPs in these muscles. The optimal wrist posture for maximal grip force in healthy adults is reported in slight wrist extension.[86]

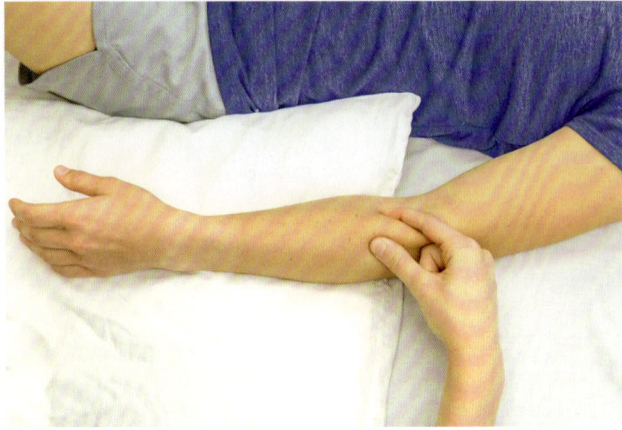

Figure 34-6. Cross-fiber pincer palpation for TrPs in the brachioradialis muscle.

Other examples of activities that can activate or perpetuate TrPs in these muscles are: dressing, house work, racquet sports, weeding with a trowel, extensive handshaking, scraping ice off a windshield, ironing of clothes, and repetitive frisbee-throwing. Carrying heavy objects, poor posture while at the computer keyboard, or playing musical instruments can also act as activating or perpetuating activities. Chen et al[87] found significant decrease in pain pressure thresholds over latent TrPs in the forearm muscles of piano students after only 20 minutes of playing.

The ECU muscle, which is seldom required to support a load against gravity, develops TrPs to a lesser extent than the other wrist extensors. Its involvement is usually secondary to gross trauma, such as fracture of the ulna, or as a sequela of frozen shoulder syndrome, in which most of the shoulder muscles and many of the elbow muscles develop TrPs.

Motor control dysfunctions may also activate or perpetuate TrPs in the forearm muscles. For instance, abnormal activation patterns of forearm extensor muscles and poor posture of the upper limb have been reported in people with lateral epicondylalgia.[50] In particular, during the performance of a backhand tennis stroke, tennis players with pain developed higher levels of electrical activity of the wrist extensors at ball impact when compared to asymptomatic subjects. In addition, the ECRB muscle of tennis players with lateral epicondylalgia was less active in the early preparatory phase prior to ball impact, reflecting impaired stability at the wrist, whereas activity was greater at ball impact. Individuals with lateral epicondylalgia showed a "leading elbow" posture during the backhand at ball impact in which the wrist was extended more in individuals with lateral epicondylalgia than the tennis players without lateral epicondylalgia.[50] Reduced activity of the ECRL and ECRB muscles was demonstrated in subjects with lateral epicondylalgia during isometric wrist extension[88] and gripping tasks.[89] The relationship between these neuromuscular imbalances and development of TrPs in the forearm muscles needs to be investigated further.

Joint dysfunctions in the elbow or wrist may also perpetuate TrPs of the forearm muscles. For instance, restriction of scaphoid mobility at the wrist in a volar direction may limit wrist extension and thus impart muscle overload in the forearm muscles. In this regard, a scaphoid thrust manipulation technique has been successfully used in the treatment of lateral epicondylalgia.[90]

Different counterforce braces[91-94] and taping techniques[95] applied to the forearm region can be helpful to reduce the lateral elbow pain provoked by TrPs of the wrist extensors and brachioradialis muscles. Because results may be similar with different types of braces, the choice will depend on factors such as patient preference, comfort, and cost.[94] If a forearm support band is used, it may be most effective for reducing strain in the ECRB muscle when applied at a force of 40 to 50 mm Hg and used during light-duty activities.[96] Moreover, the strain on the ECRB muscle origin is less when the forearm support band is applied at four-fifths the distance from the wrist to the elbow.[97]

4.2. Associated Trigger Points

Associated TrPs can develop in the referred pain areas caused by primary TrPs.[98] Therefore, musculature in the referred pain areas for each muscle should also be considered. Trigger points frequently occur in the ECRL, ECRB, and brachioradialis muscles; involvement of one of these muscles is likely to be associated with TrPs in the extensor digitorum and supinator muscles. Trigger points are rarely observed in the ECU muscle as a single muscle syndrome and typically occur with at least one TrP in the extensor digitorum muscle.

Trigger points in the brachioradialis muscle often develop in association with TrPs in the supinator and ECRL muscles. Involvement then spreads to the long extensors of the fingers, especially to the middle and ring fingers. The distal lateral end of the medial head of the triceps brachii muscle, proximal to the lateral epicondyle, may also develop associated TrPs. These TrPs refer pain to the lateral epicondyle as well.

Trigger points located in remote muscles referring pain to the forearm region can favor the development of associated TrPs in the forearm muscles. For instance, dry needling of infraspinatus TrPs inhibited the activity of TrPs situated in its zone of pain referral (eg, ECRL muscle).[98] Similarly, one dry needling session of active and latent TrPs of the infraspinatus muscle was followed by a reduction of pain intensity and irritability of latent TrPs located in the ECRB muscle in older adults with nonspecific shoulder pain.[99] This remote influence seems to occur in a reciprocal direction as well. Tsai et al[100] showed that dry needling of the ECRL muscle could reduce the irritability of proximal TrPs located in the upper trapezius muscle. Trigger points in the scalene or supraspinatus muscles may induce associated TrPs in the ECRL, ECRB, and ECU muscles. Trigger points in the serratus posterior superior muscle can also induce TrPs in the ECU muscle.[101]

Similarly, patients can develop TrPs bilaterally in the same musculature, that is, a "mirror" affectation. This phenomenon has been explored in individuals with lateral epicondylalgia because latent TrPs in the ECRB and ECRL muscles were found in a similar percentage in the unaffected forearm in patients with strictly unilateral elbow symptoms.[61]

4.3. Associated Pathology

Clinical entities producing lateral elbow pain include ECRB tendinopathy, true tennis elbow, local arthritis at the elbow,[102] radiocapitellar pathology (ie, synovial plica at the humeroradial joint),[103-105] radial tunnel syndrome,[75,106] posterior interosseous nerve entrapment,[107] cervical radicular pain or radiculopathy,[108] posterolateral rotatory instability,[109] and nonspecific arm pain,[110] which is defined as diffuse forearm pain not associated with any particular structure.

When pain or paresthesia is felt distally in the upper extremity and/or the brachium, along with diffuse arm pain or concomitant neck pain, the clinician should suspect the presence of cervical radicular pain, radiculopathy, or radial nerve entrapment.[78,111,112]

Local tendon pathology at the tendinous insertion of the ECRB muscle is one of the underlying pathophysiologic mechanisms in lateral epicondylalgia.[111,112] The most common site of focal degeneration in lateral epicondylalgia has been reported in the deep and anterior fibers of the proximal insertion of the ECRB tendon.[113-115] These pathologic changes were considered by several authors as the primary candidate for the pathologic basis of lateral epicondylalgia.[113,114]

Pain mechanism changes (eg, central sensitization)[58,61,116-121] and motor system impairments[111,112] also contribute to the clinical picture of lateral epicondylalgia and elbow pain. Several neuromuscular impairments have been demonstrated in people with lateral epicondylalgia including reductions in pain-free grip force,[74] weakness in the wrist extensors with compensatory increased activity in the finger extensors,[89,122] morphologic changes in the ECRB muscle,[123] widespread muscle weakness in the affected limb,[89,122] and motor control deficits.[73]

In addition, triangular fibrocartilage complex tear, distal radioulnar joint injury or instability, and ECU tendinopathy should be considered as potential sources of symptoms in the dorsum of the ulnar distal wrist.

The pain referral elicited by TrPs to the dorsum of the hand and wrist, especially in the region of the base of the thumb, may easily be mistaken for tenosynovitis (de Quervain's disease), which presents with similar symptoms.[124] In both conditions, the pain is aggravated by either loading or stretching the involved tendons and muscles.

When symptoms are located at the base of the thumb, other causes of pain besides TrPs and de Quervain's disease should be taken into consideration such as carpometacarpal entrapment of the superficial radial nerve (Wartenberg syndrome).

Dorsal wrist pain may be caused by pathologies including intersection syndrome, Kienbock's disease, or wrist instability (eg, scapholunate dissociation). Details about key features and clinical examination procedures for identifying all these clinical syndromes can be found elsewhere.[112,125]

Unfortunately, many of the above-mentioned diagnostic labels lack accepted definitions and diagnostic criteria. For instance, nonspecific arm pain is a diagnosis often reached by exclusion of other specific conditions. However, there are some clues from the clinical history and physical examination that can orient clinicians for effective diagnosis. Clicking at the elbow, loss of control, or difficulty with pushing up with the forearm supinated may indicate posterolateral instability of the radial head.[112] Reproduction of lateral elbow pain during manual palpation and/or active, passive, or combined movements of the cervical spine, concomitant neck pain, or diffuse arm pain or paresthesias should raise suspicion of radicular or referred pain.[112] Patients with posterior interosseous nerve entrapment usually report pain over the dorsal aspect of the forearm and exhibit muscle weakness of the finger and thumb extensors without sensory loss.[126]

5. CORRECTIVE ACTIONS

The patient with TrPs in the radial wrist extensors should avoid forceful and repeated activity with the wrist flexed and ulnarly deviated. It may be helpful to adapt certain activities and provide adequate rest and recovery periods during prolonged and repetitive tasks as follows: liquid should be poured from a container by rotating the arm at the shoulder joint, instead of by ulnarly deviating or twisting at the wrist, or by providing support to the bottom of the container with the unaffected hand. The patient should learn to avoid activities that can aggravate brachioradialis TrPs, such as digging with a trowel, prolonged shaking of hands, and playing tennis with a racquet that is too heavy. If the patient is an avid tennis or golf player, he/she should seek professional consultation for a movement analysis of their swing and for any equipment modifications.

Some workplace and ergonomic modifications can be made to minimize work tasks requiring awkward wrist postures, forceful exertions, and highly repetitive movements. For instance, a computer keyboard with a downward slope may reduce the wrist extension angle and the activity of the forearm muscles, in particular the wrist extensors.[127] A similar effect on the wrist extension angle has been observed when the keyboard was higher than elbow height.[128]

The patient with TrPs in the ECRL muscle or pain at the lateral aspect of the elbow should bend the elbow with the palms facing up in order to increase the use of the biceps brachii muscle and avoid overuse of the ECRL muscle when lifting objects, especially if repetitive lifting is required.[72] Repeated lifting and grasping activities with the elbows fully straightened can be associated with relatively overused wrist extensors because of the excessive force placed on the outside of the elbow.

Self-pressure release for TrPs in the ECRL (Figure 34-7A), ECRB (Figure 34-7B), or ECU (Figure 34-7C) muscles can be performed in sitting by placing the forearm on the armrest of a chair or on a table with the palm down, using manual pressure or with a TrP self-release tool. Trigger point self-pressure release

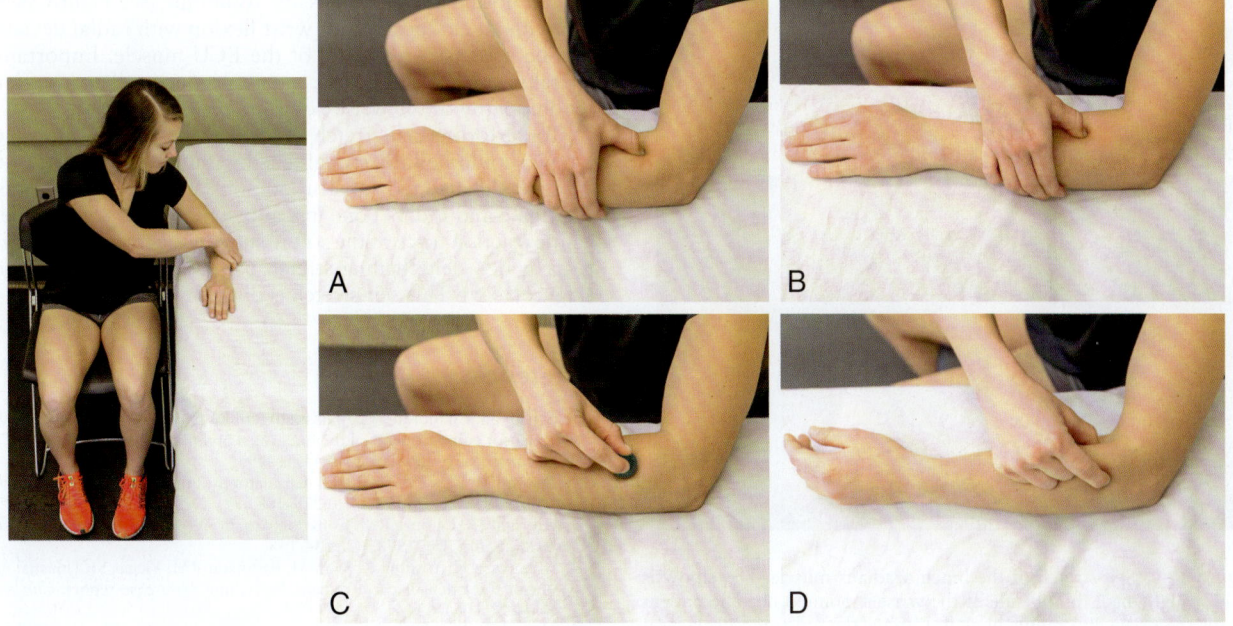

Figure 34-7. Self-pressure release of TrPs. A, Extensor carpi radialis longus muscle. B, Extensor carpi radialis brevis muscle. C, Extensor carpi ulnaris muscle. D, Brachioradialis muscle.

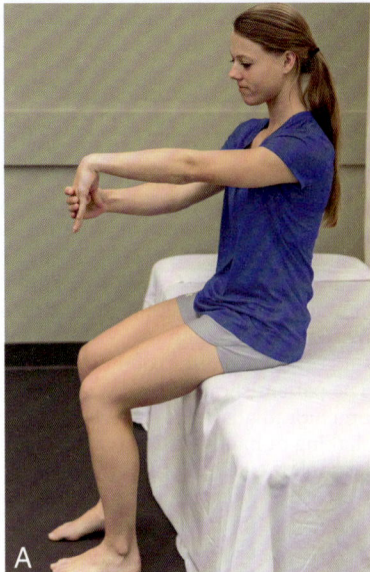
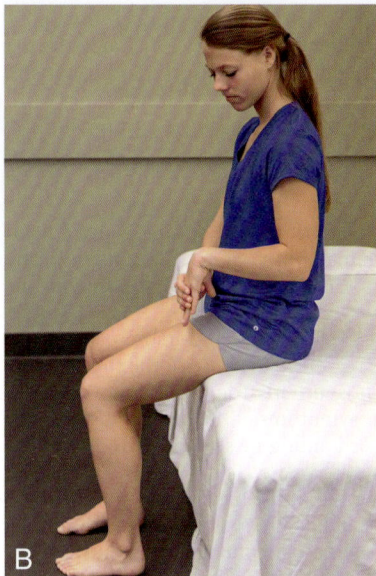

Figure 34-8. Self-stretch of wrist extensors. A, Elbow straight, wrist gently pulled down and slightly out to focus stretch of the extensor carpi radialis longus muscle. B, Elbow is bent, wrist gently pulled down and slightly out to focus stretch on the extensor carpi radialis brevis muscle. Not pictured: to stretch the extensor carpi ulnaris muscle the same position as in B is utilized but the wrist is pulled slightly in.

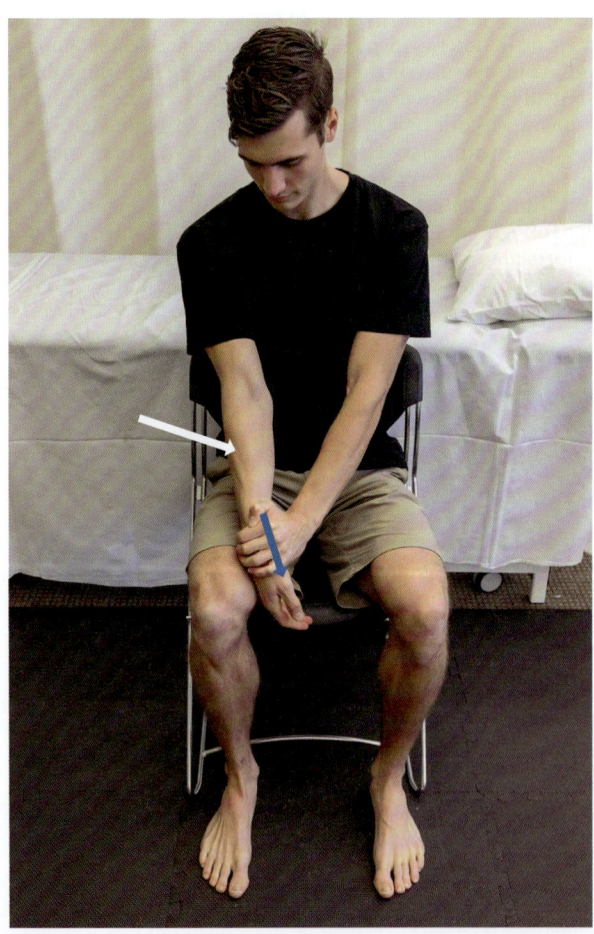

Figure 34-9. Self-stretch of the brachioradialis muscle. The elbow is fully straightened, thumb side of the wrist is pointed up. The patient grasps the tissue and radius bone just above the wrist and provides a gentle traction force (blue arrow) of the soft tissues on the top of the forearm to provide a lengthening stretch of the myofascial structures. White arrow is the area of the forearm where the stretch should be felt.

of the brachioradialis muscle is performed in the same position with manual pincer grasp (Figure 34-7D). For any of these self-pressure release techniques, the sensitive spot is located with the fingers or a tool, and light pressure (no more than 4/10 pain) is applied and held for 15 to 30 seconds or until pain reduces. This can be repeated five times, several times per day.

The patient can easily perform self-stretching techniques as part of self-management for TrPs located in the forearm muscles. Stretching of the ECRL and ECRB muscles should be performed with the elbow fully straightened, palm facing down, and wrist flexion with ulnar deviation (Figure 34-8A). The same procedure can be followed with the elbow bent (Figure 34-8B).[80] These self-stretches should be carried out gently, and attention to the reproduction of pain versus stretch is paramount. These stretches should not be painful. The same technique (see Figure 34-8B) but with an end position of wrist flexion with radial deviation can be used for stretching of the ECU muscle. Importantly, stretching techniques may be counterproductive if an insertional tendinopathy of the wrist extensors is present.[129]

To perform a self-stretch of the brachioradialis muscle, the elbow should be fully straightened with the thumb side of the wrist of the affected forearm pointing up. The patient grasps the tissue and radius bone just above the wrist and provides a gentle traction force of the soft tissues on the top of the forearm to provide a lengthening stretch of the myofascial structures (Figure 34-9). This self-stretch is difficult to perform.

References

1. Selvan SS, Chandran TC, Alalasundaram KV, Muthukumaran R, Suresh S. Extensor compartments of the forearm: a preliminary cadaveric study. *Plast Reconstr Surg*. 2005;115(5):1447-1449.
2. Stroyan M, Wilk KE. The functional anatomy of the elbow complex. *J Orthop Sports Phys Ther*. 1993;17(6):279-288.
3. Albright JA, Linburg RM. Common variations of the radial wrist extensors. *J Hand Surg Am*. 1978;3(2):134-138.
4. Mitsuyasu H, Yoshida R, Shah M, Patterson RM, Viegas SF. Unusual variant of the extensor carpi radialis brevis muscle: a case report. *Clin Anat*. 2004;17(1):61-63.
5. Hong MK, Hong MK. An uncommon form of the rare extensor carpi radialis accessorius. *Ann Anat*. 2005;187(1):89-92.
6. Nayak SR, Madhan Kumar SJ, Krishnamurthy A, et al. An additional radial wrist extensor and its clinical significance. *Ann Anat*. 2007;189(3):283-286.

7. Nayak SR, Krishnamurthy A, Prabhu LV, Rai R, Ranade AV, Madhyastha S. Anatomical variation of radial wrist extensor muscles: a study in cadavers. *Clinics (Sao Paulo)*. 2008;63(1):85-90.
8. Friden J, Albrecht D, Lieber RL. Biomechanical analysis of the brachioradialis as a donor in tendon transfer. *Clin Orthop Relat Res*. 2001(383):152-161.
9. Kerver AL, Carati L, Eilers PH, Langezaal AC, Kleinrensink GJ, Walbeehm ET. An anatomical study of the ECRL and ECRB: feasibility of developing a preoperative test for evaluating the strength of the individual wrist extensors. *J Plast Reconstr Aesthet Surg*. 2013;66(4):543-550.
10. Neumann DA. *Kinesiology of the Musculoskeletal System: Foundations for Rehabilitation*. 2nd ed. St. Louis, MO: Mosby; 2010.
11. Cohen MS, Romeo AA, Hennigan SP, Gordon M. Lateral epicondylitis: anatomic relationships of the extensor tendon origins and implications for arthroscopic treatment. *J Shoulder Elbow Surg*. 2008;17(6):954-960.
12. Nimura A, Fujishiro H, Wakabayashi Y, Imatani J, Sugaya H, Akita K. Joint capsule attachment to the extensor carpi radialis brevis origin: an anatomical study with possible implications regarding the etiology of lateral epicondylitis. *J Hand Surg Am*. 2014;39(2):219-225.
13. Standring S. *Gray's Anatomy: The Anatomical Basis of Clinical Practice*. 41st ed. London, UK: Elsevier; 2015.
14. McMinn RMH, Hutchings RT, Pegington J, Abrahams PH. *Color Atlas of Human Anatomy*. 3rd ed. St. Louis, MO: Mosby Year Book; 1993.
15. Stoeckart R, Vleeming A, Snijders CJ. Anatomy of the extensor carpi radialis brevis muscle related to tennis elbow. *Clin Biomech*. 1989;4(4):210-212.
16. Milz S, Tischer T, Buettner A, et al. Molecular composition and pathology of entheses on the medial and lateral epicondyles of the humerus: a structural basis for epicondylitis. *Ann Rheum Dis*. 2004;63(9):1015-1021.
17. Bredella MA, Tirman PF, Fritz RC, Feller JF, Wischer TK, Genant HK. MR imaging findings of lateral ulnar collateral ligament abnormalities in patients with lateral epicondylitis. *AJR Am J Roentgenol*. 1999;173(5):1379-1382.
18. Villasenor-Ovies P, Vargas A, Chiapas-Gasca K, et al. Clinical anatomy of the elbow and shoulder. *Reumatol Clin*. 2012;8 suppl 2:13-24.
19. Kopell HP, Thompson WA. *Peripheral Entrapment Neuropathies*. Baltimore, MD: William & Wilkins; 1963.
20. Goldman S, Honet JC, Sobel R, Goldstein AS. Posterior interosseous nerve palsy in the absence of trauma. *Arch Neurol*. 1969;21(4):435-441.
21. Clavert P, Lutz JC, Adam P, Wolfram-Gabel R, Liverneaux P, Kahn JL. Frohse's arcade is not the exclusive compression site of the radial nerve in its tunnel. *Orthop Traumatol Surg Res*. 2009;95(2):114-118.
22. Lateva ZC, McGill KC, Johanson ME. The innervation and organization of motor units in a series-fibered human muscle: the brachioradialis. *J Appl Physiol (1985)*. 2010;108(6):1530-1541.
23. Clemente C. *Gray's Anatomy of the Human Body*. 30th ed. Philadelphia, PA: Lea & Febiger; 1985.
24. Cricenti SV, Deangelis MA, Didio LJ, Ebraheim NA, Rupp RE, Didio AS. Innervation of the extensor carpi radialis brevis and supinator muscles: levels of origin and penetration of these muscular branches from the posterior interosseous nerve. *J Shoulder Elbow Surg*. 1994;3(6):390-394.
25. Zhang L, Zhang CG, Dong Z, Gu YD. Spinal nerve origins of the muscular branches of the radial nerve: an electrophysiological study. *Neurosurgery*. 2012;70(6):1438-1441; discussion 1441.
26. Abrams RA, Ziets RJ, Lieber RL, Botte MJ. Anatomy of the radial nerve motor branches in the forearm. *J Hand Surg Am*. 1997;22(2):232-237.
27. Ravichandiran M, Ravichandiran N, Ravichandiran K, et al. Neuromuscular partitioning in the extensor carpi radialis longus and brevis based on intramuscular nerve distribution patterns: a three-dimensional modeling study. *Clin Anat*. 2012;25(3):366-372.
28. Zbrodowski A, Gajisin S, Grodecki J. Vascularization of the tendons of the extensor pollicis longus, extensor carpi radialis longus and extensor carpi radialis brevis muscles. *J Anat*. 1982;135(pt 2):235-244.
29. Schneeberger AG, Masquelet AC. Arterial vascularisation of the proximal extensor carpi radialis brevis tendon. *Clin Orthop Relat Res*. 2002(398):239-244.
30. Latev MD, Dalley AF II. Nerve supply of the brachioradialis muscle: surgically relevant variations of the extramuscular branches of the radial nerve. *Clin Anat*. 2005;18(7):488-492.
31. Hazelton FT, Smidt GL, Flatt AE, Stephens RI. The influence of wrist position on the force produced by the finger flexors. *J Biomech*. 1975;8(5):301-306.
32. Snijders CJ, Volkers AC, Mechelse K, Vleeming A. Provocation of epicondylagia lateralis (tennis elbow) by power grip or pinching. *Med Sci Sports Exerc*. 1987;19(5):518-523.
33. al-Qattan MM. The nerve supply to extensor carpi radialis brevis. *J Anat*. 1996;188(pt 1):249-250.
34. Duchenne G. *Physiology of Motion*. Philadelphia, PA: Lippincott; 1949.
35. Basmajian J, Deluca C. *Muscles Alive*. 5th ed. Baltimore, MD: Williams & Wilkins; 1985.
36. Livingston BP, Segal RL, Song A, Hopkins K, English AW, Manning CC. Functional activation of the extensor carpi radialis muscles in humans. *Arch Phys Med Rehabil*. 2001;82(9):1164-1170.
37. Lieber RL, Jacobson MD, Fazeli BM, Abrams RA, Botte MJ. Architecture of selected muscles of the arm and forearm: anatomy and implications for tendon transfer. *J Hand Surg Am*. 1992;17(5):787-798.
38. Horii E, An KN, Linscheid RL. Excursion of prime wrist tendons. *J Hand Surg Am*. 1993;18(1):83-90.
39. Loren GJ, Shoemaker SD, Burkholder TJ, Jacobson MD, Friden J, Lieber RL. Human wrist motors: biomechanical design and application to tendon transfers. *J Biomech*. 1996;29(3):331-342.
40. Sagae M, Suzuki K, Fujita T, et al. Strict actions of the human wrist extensors: a study with an electrical neuromuscular stimulation method. *J Electromyogr Kinesiol*. 2010;20(6):1178-1185.
41. Fujii H, Kobayashi S, Sato T, Shinozaki S, Naito A. Co-contraction of the pronator teres and extensor carpi radialis during wrist extension movements in humans. *J Electromyogr Kinesiol*. 2007;17(1):80-89.
42. An KN, Hui FC, Morrey BF, Linscheid RL, Chao EY. Muscles across the elbow joint: a biomechanical analysis. *J Biomech*. 1981;14(10):659-669.
43. Brand PW, Hollister AM. *Clinical Mechanics of the Hand*. St. Louis, MO: Mosby; 1999.
44. Levangie PK, Norkin CC. *Joint Structure and Function: A Comprehensive Analysis*. 5th ed. Philadelphia, PA: FA Davis; 2011.
45. Tubiana R, Thomine J, Mackin E. *Examination of the Hand and Wrist*. London, England: Informa Healthcare; 1996.
46. Murray WM, Delp SL, Buchanan TS. Variation of muscle moment arms with elbow and forearm position. *J Biomech*. 1995;28(5):513-525.
47. Boland MR, Spigelman T, Uhl TL. The function of brachioradialis. *J Hand Surg Am*. 2008;33(10):1853-1859.
48. Hatch GF III, Pink MM, Mohr KJ, Sethi PM, Jobe FW. The effect of tennis racket grip size on forearm muscle firing patterns. *Am J Sports Med*. 2006;34(12):1977-1983.
49. Li FX, Fewtrell D, Jenkins M. String vibration dampers do not reduce racket frame vibration transfer to the forearm. *J Sports Sci*. 2004;22(11-12):1041-1052.
50. Kelley JD, Lombardo SJ, Pink M, Perry J, Giangarra CE. Electromyographic and cinematographic analysis of elbow function in tennis players with lateral epicondylitis. *Am J Sports Med*. 1994;22(3):359-363.
51. Blackwell JR, Cole KJ. Wrist kinematics differ in expert and novice tennis players performing the backhand stroke: implications for tennis elbow. *J Biomech*. 1994;27(5):509-516.
52. Itoh K, Okada K, Kawakita K. A proposed experimental model of myofascial trigger points in human muscle after slow eccentric exercise. *Acupunct Med*. 2004;22(1):2-12; discussion 12-13.
53. Bron C, Dommerholt JD. Etiology of myofascial trigger points. *Curr Pain Headache Rep*. 2012;16(5):439-444.
54. Wei SH, Chiang JY, Shiang TY, Chang HY. Comparison of shock transmission and forearm electromyography between experienced and recreational tennis players during backhand strokes. *Clin J Sport Med*. 2006;16(2):129-135.
55. Simons DG, Travell J, Simons L. *Travell & Simon's Myofascial Pain and Dysfunction: The Trigger Point Manual*. Vol 1. 2nd ed. Baltimore, MD: Williams & Wilkins; 1999:104.
56. Slater H, Arendt-Nielsen L, Wright A, Graven-Nielsen T. Experimental deep tissue pain in wrist extensors—a model of lateral epicondylalgia. *Eur J Pain*. 2003;7(3):277-288.
57. Bergin MJ, Hirata R, Mista C, et al. Movement evoked pain and mechanical hyperalgesia after intramuscular injection of nerve growth factor: a model of sustained elbow pain. *Pain Med*. 2015;16(11):2180-2191.
58. Slater H, Arendt-Nielsen L, Wright A, Graven-Nielsen T. Sensory and motor effects of experimental muscle pain in patients with lateral epicondylalgia and controls with delayed onset muscle soreness. *Pain*. 2005;114(1-2):118-130.
59. Graven-Nielsen T, Arendt-Nielsen L, Svensson P, Jensen TS. Experimental muscle pain: a quantitative study of local and referred pain in humans following injection of hypertonic saline. *J Musculoske Pain*. 1997;5(1):49-69.
60. Fernandez-Carnero J, Fernández-de-las-Peñas C, de la Llave-Rincon AI, Ge HY, Arendt-Nielsen L. Prevalence of and referred pain from myofascial trigger points in the forearm muscles in patients with lateral epicondylalgia. *Clin J Pain*. 2007;23(4):353-360.
61. Fernandez-Carnero J, Fernández-de-las-Peñas C, de la Llave-Rincon AI, Ge HY, Arendt-Nielsen L. Bilateral myofascial trigger points in the forearm muscles in patients with chronic unilateral lateral epicondylalgia: a blinded, controlled study. *Clin J Pain*. 2008;24(9):802-807.
62. Mayoral O, de Felipe JA, Velasco S, Jimenez F, Miota J, Lopez P. Prevalence of Myofascial Pain Syndrome in Lateral Epicondyle Enthesopathy. Paper presented at: MYOPAIN 2010. VIII World Congress on Myofascial Pain and Fibromyalgia 2010; Todedo, Spain.
63. Travell J. Pain mechanisms in connective tissue. Paper presented at: Connective Tissues, Transactions of the Second Conference 1951; New York, NY.
64. Travell J, Rinzler SH. The myofascial genesis of pain. *Postgrad Med*. 1952;11(5):425-434.
65. Mayoral del Moral O, Gimenez Donoso C, Salvat Salvat I, Fernandez Carnero J. Puncion seca de los musculos del brazo, el antebrazo y la mano. In: Mayoral del Moral O, Salvat Salvat I, eds. *Fisioterapia Invasiva del Sindrome de Dolor Miofascial Manual de puncion seca de punto gatillo*. Madrid, Spain: Editorial Medica Panamericana; 2017:265-309.
66. Bonica J, Sola A. Chapter 52, Other painful disorders of the upper limb. In: Bonica JJ, Loeser JD, Chapman C, Fordyce WE, eds. *The Management of Pain*. 2nd ed. Philadelphia, PA: Lea & Febiger; 1990:947-958.
67. Kelly M. Pain in the forearm and hand due to muscular lesions. *Med J Aust*. 1944;2:185-188.
68. Shiri R, Viikari-Juntura E, Varonen H, Heliovaara M. Prevalence and determinants of lateral and medial epicondylitis: a population study. *Am J Epidemiol*. 2006;164(11):1065-1074.
69. Berglund KM, Persson BH, Denison E. Prevalence of pain and dysfunction in the cervical and thoracic spine in persons with and without lateral elbow pain. *Man Ther*. 2008;13(4):295-299.
70. Coombes BK, Bisset L, Vincenzino B. Bilateral cervical dysfunction in patients with unilateral lateral epicondylalgia without concomitant cervical or upper limb symptoms: a cross-sectional case-control study. *J Manipulative Physiol Ther*. 2014;37(2):79-86.
71. Manvell JJ, Manvell N, Snodgrass SJ, Reid SA. Improving the radial nerve neurodynamic test: an observation of tension of the radial, median and ulnar nerves during upper limb positioning. *Man Ther*. 2015;20(6):790-796.

72. Sahrmann S. *Movement System Impairment Syndromes of the Extremities, Cervical and Thoracic Spines*. St Louis, MO: Elsevier; 2010.
73. Bisset LM, Russell T, Bradley S, Ha B, Vicenzino BT. Bilateral sensorimotor abnormalities in unilateral lateral epicondylalgia. *Arch Phys Med Rehabil*. 2006;87(4):490-495.
74. Lim EC. Pain free grip strength test. *J Physiother*. 2013;59(1):59.
75. Lutz FR. Radial tunnel syndrome: an etiology of chronic lateral elbow pain. *J Orthop Sports Phys Ther*. 1991;14(1):14-17.
76. Kendall FP, McCreary EK. *Muscles: Testing and Function, with Posture and Pain*. 5th ed. Baltimore, MD: Lippincott Williams & Wilkins; 2005.
77. Haker E. Lateral epicondylalgia: diagnosis, treatment, and evaluation. *Crit Rev Phys Rehabil Med*. 1993;5:129-154.
78. Vicenzino B. Lateral epicondylalgia: a musculoskeletal physiotherapy perspective. *Man Ther*. 2003;8(2):66-79.
79. Dutton M. *Dutton's Orthopaedic Examination, Evaluation and Intervention*. 3rd ed. New York, NY: McGraw Hill; 2012.
80. Takasaki H, Aoki M, Muraki T, Uchiyama E, Murakami G, Yamashita T. Muscle strain on the radial wrist extensors during motion-simulating stretching exercises for lateral epicondylitis: a cadaveric study. *J Shoulder Elbow Surg*. 2007;16(6):854-858.
81. Macdonald AJ. Abnormally tender muscle regions and associated painful movements. *Pain*. 1980;8(2):197-205.
82. Hengeveld E, Banks K. *Maitland's Peripheral Manipulation: Management of Neuromusculoskeletal Disorders*. London, UK: Churchill Livingstone; 2013.
83. Kaltenborn FM. *Manual Mobilization of the Joints: The Extremities*. Vol 1. 8th ed. Minneapolis, MN Orthopedic Physical Therapy Products; 2014.
84. Mora-Relucio R, Nunez-Nagy S, Gallego-Izquierdo T, et al. Experienced versus inexperienced interexaminer reliability on location and classification of myofascial trigger point palpation to diagnose lateral epicondylalgia: an observational cross-sectional study. *Evid Based Complement Alternat Med*. 2016;2016:6059719.
85. Gerwin RD, Dommerholt J, Shah JP. An expansion of Simons' integrated hypothesis of trigger point formation. *Curr Pain Headache Rep*. 2004;8(6):468-475.
86. Pryce JC. The wrist position between neutral and ulnar deviation that facilitates the maximum power grip strength. *J Biomech*. 1980;13(6):505-511.
87. Chen S-M, Chen JT, Kuan T-S, Hong J, Hong C-Z. Decrease in pressure pain thresholds of latent myofascial trigger points in the middle finger extensors immediately after continuous piano practice. *J Musculoske Pain*. 2000;8(3):83-92.
88. Rojas M, Mananas MA, Muller B, Chaler J. Activation of forearm muscles for wrist extension in patients affected by lateral epicondylitis. *Conf Proc IEEE Eng Med Biol Soc*. 2007;2007:4858-4861.
89. Alizadehkhaiyat O, Fisher AC, Kemp GJ, Vishwanathan K, Frostick SP. Upper limb muscle imbalance in tennis elbow: a functional and electromyographic assessment. *J Orthop Res*. 2007;25(12):1651-1657.
90. Struijs PA, Damen PJ, Bakker EW, Blankevoort L, Assendelft WJ, van Dijk CN. Manipulation of the wrist for management of lateral epicondylitis: a randomized pilot study. *Phys Ther*. 2003;83(7):608-616.
91. Faes M, van Elk N, de Lint JA, Degens H, Kooloos JG, Hopman MT. A dynamic extensor brace reduces electromyographic activity of wrist extensor muscles in patients with lateral epicondylalgia. *J Orthop Sports Phys Ther*. 2006;36(3):170-178.
92. Jafarian FS, Demneh ES, Tyson SF. The immediate effect of orthotic management on grip strength of patients with lateral epicondylosis. *J Orthop Sports Phys Ther*. 2009;39(6):484-489.
93. Sadeghi-Demneh E, Jafarian F. The immediate effects of orthoses on pain in people with lateral epicondylalgia. *Pain Res Treat*. 2013;2013:353597.
94. Bisset LM, Collins NJ, Offord SS. Immediate effects of 2 types of braces on pain and grip strength in people with lateral epicondylalgia: a randomized controlled trial. *J Orthop Sports Phys Ther*. 2014;44(2):120-128.
95. Vicenzino B, Brooksbank J, Minto J, Offord S, Paungmali A. Initial effects of elbow taping on pain-free grip strength and pressure pain threshold. *J Orthop Sports Phys Ther*. 2003;33(7):400-407.
96. Meyer NJ, Pennington W, Haines B, Daley R. The effect of the forearm support band on forces at the origin of the extensor carpi radialis brevis: a cadaveric study and review of literature. *J Hand Ther*. 2002;15(2):179-184.
97. Takasaki H, Aoki M, Oshiro S, et al. Strain reduction of the extensor carpi radialis brevis tendon proximal origin following the application of a forearm support band. *J Orthop Sports Phys Ther*. 2008;38(5):257-261.
98. Hsieh YL, Kao MJ, Kuan TS, Chen SM, Chen JT, Hong CZ. Dry needling to a key myofascial trigger point may reduce the irritability of satellite MTrPs. *Am J Phys Med Rehabil*. 2007;86(5):397-403.
99. Calvo-Lobo C, Pacheco-da-Costa S, Martinez-Martinez J, Rodriguez-Sanz D, Cuesta-Alvaro P, Lopez-Lopez D. Dry needling on the infraspinatus latent and active myofascial trigger points in older adults with nonspecific shoulder pain: a randomized clinical trial. *J Geriatr Phys Ther*. 2018;41:1-13.
100. Tsai CT, Hsieh LF, Kuan TS, Kao MJ, Chou LW, Hong CZ. Remote effects of dry needling on the irritability of the myofascial trigger point in the upper trapezius muscle. *Am J Phys Med Rehabil*. 2009;89(2):133-140.
101. Hong C-Z. Considerations and recommendations regarding myofascial trigger point injection. *J Musculoske Pain*. 1994;2(1):29-59.
102. Papatheodorou LK, Baratz ME, Sotereanos DG. Elbow arthritis: current concepts. *J Hand Surg Am*. 2013;38(3):605-613.
103. Duparc F, Putz R, Michot C, Muller JM, Freger P. The synovial fold of the humeroradial joint: anatomical and histological features, and clinical relevance in lateral epicondylalgia of the elbow. *Surg Radiol Anat*. 2002;24(5):302-307.
104. Ruch DS, Papadonikolakis A, Campolattaro RM. The posterolateral plica: a cause of refractory lateral elbow pain. *J Shoulder Elbow Surg*. 2006;15(3):367-370.
105. Steinert AF, Goebel S, Rucker A, Barthel T. Snapping elbow caused by hypertrophic synovial plica in the radiohumeral joint: a report of three cases and review of literature. *Arch Orthop Trauma Surg*. 2010;130(3):347-351.
106. Stanley J. Radial tunnel syndrome: a surgeon's perspective. *J Hand Ther*. 2006;19(2):180-184.
107. Carter GT, Weiss MD. Diagnosis and treatment of work-related proximal median and radial nerve entrapment. *Phys Med Rehabil Clin N Am*. 2015;26(3):539-549.
108. Wainner RS, Fritz JM, Irrgang JJ, Boninger ML, Delitto A, Allison S. Reliability and diagnostic accuracy of the clinical examination and patient self-report measures for cervical radiculopathy. *Spine (Phila Pa 1976)*. 2003;28(1):52-62.
109. Anakwenze OA, Kancherla VK, Iyengar J, Ahmad CS, Levine WN. Posterolateral rotatory instability of the elbow. *Am J Sports Med*. 2014;42(2):485-491.
110. Huisstede BM, Miedema HS, Verhagen AP, Koes BW, Verhaar JA. Multidisciplinary consensus on the terminology and classification of complaints of the arm, neck and/or shoulder. *Occup Environ Med*. 2007;64(5):313-319.
111. Coombes BK, Bisset L, Vicenzino B. A new integrative model of lateral epicondylalgia. *Br J Sports Med*. 2009;43(4):252-258.
112. Coombes BK, Bisset L, Vicenzino B. Management of lateral elbow tendinopathy: one size does not fit all. *J Orthop Sports Phys Ther*. 2015;45(11):938-949.
113. Nirschl RP, Pettrone FA. Tennis elbow. The surgical treatment of lateral epicondylitis. *J Bone Joint Surg Am*. 1979;61(6A):832-839.
114. Regan W, Wold LE, Coonrad R, Morrey BF. Microscopic histopathology of chronic refractory lateral epicondylitis. *Am J Sports Med*. 1992;20(6):746-749.
115. Benjamin M, Toumi H, Ralphs JR, Bydder G, Best TM, Milz S. Where tendons and ligaments meet bone: attachment sites ('entheses') in relation to exercise and/or mechanical load. *J Anat*. 2006;208(4):471-490.
116. Fernandez-Carnero J, Fernández-de-las-Peñas C, de la Llave-Rincon AI, Ge HY, Arendt-Nielsen L. Widespread mechanical pain hypersensitivity as sign of central sensitization in unilateral epicondylalgia: a blinded, controlled study. *Clin J Pain*. 2009;25(7):555-561.
117. Fernandez-Carnero J, Fernández-de-las-Peñas C, Sterling M, Souvlis T, Arendt-Nielsen L, Vicenzino B. Exploration of the extent of somato-sensory impairment in patients with unilateral lateral epicondylalgia. *J Pain*. 2009;10(11):1179-1185.
118. Ruiz-Ruiz B, Fernández-de-las-Peñas C, Ortega-Santiago R, Arendt-Nielsen L, Madeleine P. Topographical pressure and thermal pain sensitivity mapping in patients with unilateral lateral epicondylalgia. *J Pain*. 2011;12(10):1040-1048.
119. Coombes BK, Bisset L, Vicenzino B. Thermal hyperalgesia distinguishes those with severe pain and disability in unilateral lateral epicondylalgia. *Clin J Pain*. 2012;28(7):595-601.
120. Lim EC, Sterling M, Pedler A, Coombes BK, Vicenzino B. Evidence of spinal cord hyperexcitability as measured with nociceptive flexion reflex (NFR) threshold in chronic lateral epicondylalgia with or without a positive neurodynamic test. *J Pain*. 2012;13(7):676-684.
121. Jespersen A, Amris K, Graven-Nielsen T, et al. Assessment of pressure-pain thresholds and central sensitization of pain in lateral epicondylalgia. *Pain Med*. 2013;14(2):297-304.
122. Alizadehkhaiyat O, Fisher AC, Kemp GJ, Vishwanathan K, Frostick SP. Assessment of functional recovery in tennis elbow. *J Electromyogr Kinesiol*. 2009;19(4):631-638.
123. Ljung BO, Lieber RL, Friden J. Wrist extensor muscle pathology in lateral epicondylitis. *J Hand Surg Br*. 1999;24(2):177-183.
124. Huisstede BM, Coert JH, Friden J, Hoogvliet P, European HG. Consensus on a multidisciplinary treatment guideline for de Quervain disease: results from the European HANDGUIDE study. *Phys Ther*. 2014;94(8):1095-1110.
125. Magee DJ. *Orthopedic Physical Assessment*. 6th ed. St Louis, MO: Saunders Elsevier; 2014.
126. Bisset LM, Vicenzino B. Physiotherapy management of lateral epicondylalgia. *J Physiother*. 2015;61(4):174-181.
127. Simoneau GG, Marklin RW, Berman JE. Effect of computer keyboard slope on wrist position and forearm electromyography of typists without musculoskeletal disorders. *Phys Ther*. 2003;83(9):816-830.
128. Simoneau GG, Marklin RW. Effect of computer keyboard slope and height on wrist extension angle. *Hum Factors*. 2001;43(2):287-298.
129. Cook JL, Purdam C. Is compressive load a factor in the development of tendinopathy? *Br J Sports Med*. 2012;46(3):163-168.

Chapter 35

Extensor Digitorum and Extensor Indicis Muscles
"Painful Pointers"

Orlando Mayoral del Moral and Robert D. Gerwin

1. INTRODUCTION

The extensor digitorum (ED) muscle arises from the lateral epicondyle of the humerus via the common extensor tendon. The muscle belly divides in the distal third of the forearm into four tendons, one to each finger. The tendons to the index and small fingers are accompanied by the extensor indicis (EI) and extensor digiti minimi tendons. The tendinous expansions and their complicated connections to intrinsic hand muscles provide for intricate interplay, producing fine finger movements. The juncturae tendinae and the intertendinous bands that stabilize each tendon to the finger it crosses limit the specificity with which the extensor muscles can control individual finger movements, which also depend on the lumbricals, interossei, and individual finger flexor muscles for precise movement. The referred pain and tenderness from trigger points (TrPs) in the ED muscle are projected distally in the forearm to the back of the hand, often to the fingers it moves, and proximally to the lateral epicondyle region. Pain from the EI is felt most strongly at the junction of the wrist and the dorsum of the hand. Symptoms may also include weakness, stiffness, and tenderness of the proximal interphalangeal joints. Differential diagnosis includes true tennis elbow, C7 radicular pain or radiculopathy (occasionally C6), and De Quervain's stenosing tenosynovitis. Consideration of TrPs as the cause of symptoms identified as lateral epicondylalgia or TrPs in functionally related muscles including the supinator, brachioradialis, and extensor carpi radialis longus and brevis muscles should be differentiated. Corrective actions include avoidance of unnecessary muscular strain, postural education for grasping, proper sleeping and work postures, and establishing a home exercise program of TrP self-pressure release and self-stretching exercises to achieve and maintain full range of motion and functional muscle strength.

2. ANATOMIC CONSIDERATIONS

Extensor Digitorum

The ED muscle arises proximally from the lateral epicondyle of the humerus, from intermuscular septa, and from the antebrachial fascia (Figure 35-1A).[1] The ED muscle occupies the space on the dorsal surface of the forearm between the extensor carpi radialis brevis and extensor carpi ulnaris muscles. The three muscles form a common tendon at the lateral epicondyle. The muscle belly of the ED muscle divides into three muscle bundles, two of which have one tendon each, and the lateral muscle bundle which gives rise to two tendons, one to the long finger and one to the index finger.[2] The four tendons pass through the 4th compartment or tunnel under the extensor retinaculum[2,3] in a common synovial sheath with the tendon of the EI muscle.[1] The tendons diverge on the dorsum of the hand, one to each finger.[1] The tendon to the index finger is accompanied by the EI muscle, which lies medial to it.[1] The tendon to the ring finger is connected by intertendinous junctions (juncturae tendinae)[1] to the tendons of the extensor digiti minimi muscle and the tendon to the long finger, so that the medial three fingers move together. Independent movement of these digits is most difficult with the wrist flexed. Distally, each tendinous slip of the ED muscle is bound by fibrous bands to the collateral ligaments of its metacarpophalangeal joint, as the tendon crosses the joint. The tendon spreads into an aponeurotic expansion (also called the extensor hood) to cover the dorsal surface of the proximal phalanx of each finger. Here, it is joined by tendons of the lumbrical and interosseous muscles.[1,4] This aponeurosis then divides into a central and two collateral slips; the central slip inserts on the base of the 2nd phalanx, and the collateral slips continue on to unite and insert onto the dorsal surface of the distal phalanx of each finger as the terminal tendon.[2,5] The ED muscle has tendons to the three middle digits (index, long, and ring) in 77% of dissections in one study but only 34% of the time to the extensor digiti minimi muscle.[6]

Extensor Digiti Minimi

The extensor digiti minimi muscle (Figure 35-1A) is not considered separately in this chapter because its muscle belly is often connected to, indistinct from,[1] and sometimes fused[7] to the adjacent ED muscle and is usually covered by it.[1] The extensor digiti minimi muscle forms a long tendon that constitutes the 5th dorsal compartment as it proceeds beneath the extensor retinaculum.[1] Distal to it, the tendon typically splits into two, and the lateral slip is joined by a tendon from the ED muscle.

Extensor Indicis

The EI muscle (Figure 35-1B) is a pennate muscle[8] that originates from the dorsal and lateral surface of the body of the ulna distal to the extensor pollicis longus muscle, from the interosseous membrane,[1] and in part, from the extensor pollicis longus septum.[9] The muscle at the interosseous membrane arises directly from its dense connective tissue.[10] The muscle belly of the EI muscle is the only muscle belly to enter the 4th tendon compartment, where its tendon runs under the extensor retinaculum deep to the tendons of the ED muscle.[9] The musculotendinous junction of the EI muscle is under the extensor retinaculum in 95% of cases and is at its proximal edge in 5% of cases.[8] Distally, at the level of the head of the 2nd metacarpal, it joins the ulnar side of the slip of the ED muscle going to the index finger and attaches into the extensor expansion.[1,11]

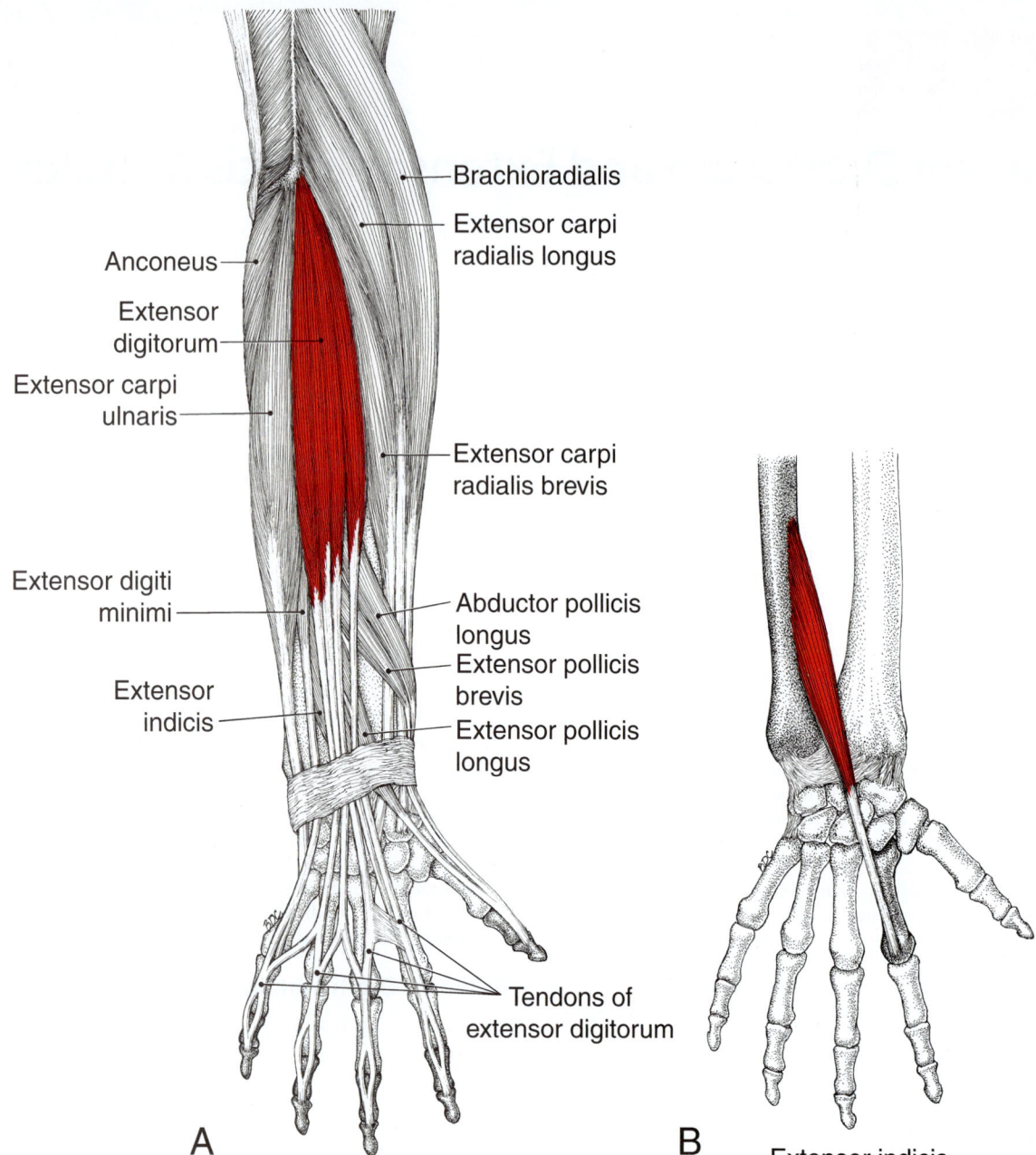

Figure 35-1. Attachments of the right finger extensor muscles and dorsal forearm muscles. A, ED muscle (red), showing oblique bands that interconnect the distal tendons, and the junction of the EI tendon with the index finger tendon of the ED muscle. Note that the tendon to the ring finger is connected by junctional tendons to the tendons of the long and small fingers, so that extension of the ring finger is usually accompanied by extension of all three fingers. Also note that there are no junctional tendons to the index finger which can move independently. B, EI (red), which passes beneath the ED tendons.

Anatomic Variations

Anatomic variations of the extensor muscles of the hand are common[12,13] and may be important causes of wrist pain and sources of misdiagnosis. The tendons of the ED muscle may be variably deficient,[1] although more commonly, they are doubled, or even tripled, in one or more digits: most frequently, the index finger or the middle finger. Rarely, a slip of tendon passes to the thumb. The arrangement of the intertendinous connections on the dorsum of the hand is highly variable. The medial connection is rather strong and pulls the tendon of the little finger toward that of the ring finger, whereas the connection between the middle two tendons is weak and may be absent.[1]

The ED brevis manus muscle is a relatively rare anatomic variation occurring in 38 (1.1%) of 3,304 hands examined. When present, it is commonly symptomatic (50% of the 38 cases).[11,14] It is clinically important because it may become painful when overexercised[15] and may be misdiagnosed as a ganglion cyst or tumor, resulting in unnecessary surgery.[15] It originates on the distal margin of the radius or from the dorsal capsule of the wrist joint and inserts on the dorsal aponeurosis of the index finger.[16] This muscle frequently appears as a variation of the EI muscle because when the ED brevis manus muscle is present, the EI muscle is usually absent.[14]

There are many variations of the EI muscle belly and tendon anatomy. The EI tendon is important because it is considered the best substitute for reconstruction of the hand after trauma or disease,[11] especially for the abductor pollicis longus and extensor pollicis longus tendons. Furthermore, variants of the EI muscle may result in a predisposition toward isolated neuropathy of the posterior interosseous nerve.[12,17]

Yoshida[9] lists a number of variants encountered in his anatomic study of 832 upper limbs. An EI ulnaris muscle (2.9%) lies medial to the EI muscle and is attached to the index finger more medial to the tendon of the EI muscle. The EI et medii accessorius muscle (1.4%) originates more medially on the dorsal surface of the ulna. Its tendon bifurcates: one part attaches to the index finger and the other one attaches to the middle finger. An extensor pollicis et indicis communis muscle arises from the interosseous membrane and the intermuscular septum. The tendon passes through the 4th compartment and bifurcates, the medial slip attaching to the medial aspect of the thumb and the ulnar slip to the radial dorsum of the index finger.[11] When this rare variant is present, it is always in addition to both the extensor pollicis longus and the EI muscles, and never replaces either. A variant of this is the supernumerary muscle that arises from an independent belly of muscle that is part of the muscle mass of the extensor pollicis longus muscle. The tendon from this supernumerary muscle follows an oblique course radial to the 2nd metatarsal bone, attaches to a thickening of the fascia between the accessory tendon and the ulnar portion of the extensor pollicis longus tendon. This accessory muscle corresponds to the EI radialis muscle, but the fascial connection results in its functioning as an extensor pollicis and extensor digitorum muscle.[18] The importance of this description is emphasis on the relationship of the intertendinous fascia to the course of the tendons.

Variations of the origin of the EI muscle are also reported. The origin of the EI muscle can be the articular upper surface of the lunate bone and the dorsal radiocarpal ligament rather than the ulna. In this variant, the tendon of the EI muscle passes along with and joins the tendons from the ED muscle to the EI muscle, inserting on the base of the distal phalanx.[19] There are variations of other extensor forearm muscles that affect the EI muscle. For example, a duplication of the extensor pollicis longus muscle gives rise to a tendon that courses with the tendon of the EI muscle and inserts with it. Likewise, a duplicated tendon and partial muscle belly of the EI muscle was found to arise from the normal muscle mass of the EI muscle and the ulna, its tendon inserting with the tendon of the extensor pollicis longus muscle.[20]

2.1. Innervation and Vascularization

Both the ED and EI muscles are innervated by the deep branch of the radial (posterior interosseous) nerve, from spinal nerves[1] C7 and C8 through the posterior cord of the lower trunk of the brachial plexus.[12,21]

Regarding vascular supply, the ED and EI muscles are supplied by branches of the brachial artery. The proximal third of the ED muscle is supplied by branches from the radial recurrent artery, and the distal two-thirds are supplied by branches from the posterior interosseous artery.[1] The very distal portion is supplied by a perforating branch from the anterior interosseous artery that passes through the interosseous membrane.[1,22] The EI muscle is supplied on its superficial surface by branches from the posterior interosseous artery and on its deep surface by perforating branches from the anterior interosseous artery.[1]

2.2. Function

The muscles controlling wrist and finger movements are important because of their constant use during functional activities and for their contribution to fine motor control. Consequently, musculoskeletal disorders involving muscle and tendon are very common in the hand and forearm. The ED muscle extends all phalanges of the fingers (2nd through 5th digits),[1,23,24] especially the proximal phalanges,[25] and assists in extension of the wrist.[1,23] It assists in abducting (spreading) the index, ring, and little fingers away from the middle finger.[1,24] All of the extrinsic hand muscles become involved in a power grip, in proportion to the strength of the grip.[23,26] The ED muscle acts in conjunction with the lumbrical and interosseous muscles to extend the middle and distal phalanges of the 2nd through 5th digits. When the proximal phalanges are held in flexion, the ED muscle extends the more distal phalanges, but when the proximal phalanges and the hand are held in extension, then, its contraction has little additional effect on the last two phalanges.[24,27] These intrinsic and extrinsic digit extensors provide an essential synergistic function to permit selective control of individual fingers; recent research shows that the independent control of the output of the ED muscle is limited, which may reflect "spillover" of motor commands to other digital extensor compartments.[28] The movements are coordinated, so that extension of one finger coactivates the extension of additional fingers.[28,29] Only extension of the index and small fingers occurs[28] more independently of extension of the other fingers because of both neurologic control[29] and anatomic reasons related to the tendons, reviewed earlier, and the presence of the EI and extensor digiti minimi muscles.

The EI muscle, in addition to acting on the index finger in the same way that the ED muscle acts, thus extending it, may assist in adducting the index finger toward the middle finger[24,25] because of the angulation of its tendon across the dorsum of the hand. The EI muscle allows the index finger to function independently of the 3rd and 4th digits. Alone, or with the ED muscle, it extends the index finger[1] at the metacarpophalangeal joint and proximal interphalangeal joint and assists in wrist extension.[1,12]

Hand grip is enhanced by wrist extension. Hand grip requires stabilization of the wrist through coactivation of forearm extensor and flexor muscles to counteract the force of the finger flexors that unopposed would cause wrist flexion. Therefore, the ED muscle and EI muscles improve hand grip by assisting in wrist extension.[12,30]

2.3. Functional Unit

The functional unit to which a muscle belongs includes the muscles that reinforce and counter its actions as well as the joints that the muscle crosses. The interdependence of these structures is functionally reflected in the organization and neural connections of the sensory motor cortex. The functional unit is emphasized because the presence of a TrP in one muscle of the unit increases the likelihood that the other muscles of the unit will also develop TrPs. When inactivating TrPs in a muscle, one must be concerned about TrPs that may develop in muscles that are functionally interdependent. Box 35-1 grossly represents the functional unit of the ED and EI muscles.[31]

Strong agonist–antagonist interactions are needed between the flexors and extensors of the hand and fingers to produce finger dexterity as well as to produce forceful hand grip. The flexor digitorum are antagonist muscles, but the synergic coactivation of both flexor digitorum muscles and the ED muscle increases grip strength and wrist stability.[32] In fact, it has been shown

Box 35-1 Functional unit of the ED and EI muscles

Action	Synergists	Antagonists
Finger extension	Lumbricals Interossei	Flexor digitorum superficialis Flexor digitorum profundus

that coactivation of the flexor digitorum muscles and the ED muscle requires cutaneous sensory feedback because elimination of cutaneous sensation in the digit reduces the maximum voluntary force of the ED muscle affecting that digit, thereby reducing the agonist–antagonist coactivation.[32]

Powerful flexion of the distal phalanges requires strong activity also of the finger extensors. On the other hand, for the ED muscle to extend the interphalangeal joints, the lumbrical and interosseous muscles need to function.

The ring and little finger extensors form a functional unit with the supinator muscle for twisting motions, such as closing jar tops and door knobs.

The EI muscle is activated independently and is coactivated with the ED muscle and is thereby an agonist of the ED muscle. It is an agonist of all muscles that extend the wrist, including both extensor carpi radialis, extensor carpi ulnaris, and the short and long extensor muscles of the thumb. It is both an antagonist to the finger flexors in finger extension, and an agonist with these same muscles in stiffening the index finger and in stabilizing the wrist.[29] It shares the action of wrist stabilization with the ED muscle and the forearm flexor muscles.

3. CLINICAL PRESENTATION
3.1. Referred Pain Pattern

Extensor Digitorum

According to Simons et al[31] involvement of the fibers of the ED muscle associated with the middle finger is extremely common. The pain, which is felt most intensely in the hand, forms a line that extends onto the dorsum of the forearm, wrist, and hand, including the metacarpophalangeal and proximal interphalangeal joints of the middle finger. There may also occasionally be an area of pain on the volar side of the wrist (Figure 35-2A). Patients report pain in the hand and finger and of stiffness and soreness in the painful finger joints.[33-35] The original report of this pain referral was based on 38 patients.[34]

Fibers of the ED muscle associated with the ring finger refer pain similarly to the same finger.[35] However, unlike the middle finger extensor, TrPs in the ring and little finger extensors are likely also to project pain and tenderness proximally into the region of the lateral epicondyle (Figure 35-2B).

Other authors described the ED muscle as referring pain to the elbow or lateral epicondyle[36,37] even from the middle finger[38] in patients with lateral epicondylalgia,[39,40] to the forearm,[33,36,37] and to the hand.[36]

Kellgren[41] injected 0.2 mL of 6% sodium chloride solution into the belly of a normal ED muscle. Pain was developed in the dorsal forearm and more severely over the back of the hand. During the sensation of pain, there was slight tenderness to deep pressure, definite tenderness to tapping, but no hypersensitivity of the skin in the painful area. Dejung et al[42] described the referred pain pattern from the ED muscle derived from examination of 10 patients. The referred pain in these patients extended from the elbow to the fingers, over the dorsum of the forearm, but most commonly over the wrist. Specifically, pain referred to the long axis of the wrist and forearm as opposed to encircling the wrist and into the finger of the affected slip of extensor muscle.

Extensor Indicis

Trigger points in the EI muscle refer pain toward the radial side of the dorsum of the wrist and hand but not into the fingers (Figure 35-2C).

3.2. Symptoms

Patients with TrPs in the finger extensor muscles report pain in the dorsal aspect of the forearm, wrist, and fingers. When asked whether the pain is felt more on the top or the underside of the fingers, the patient may not be able to isolate the pain but is likely to show the location by rubbing the dorsal surface of the fingers. Pain from TrPs in the ED muscle may also be associated with symptoms of lateral epicondylalgia[39,40,43] or with arthritis of the fingers. When the fibers of the middle finger alone are involved, the patient may report weakness in their grip, without pain.[44] The finger extensors are essential to a powerful grip, and this weakness in grip reported by the patient presents another example of inhibition weakness caused by the TrPs.

Symptoms of impaired finger flexion may be due to TrPs in the finger extensor muscles. Patients may complain of stiffness and tenderness of the proximal interphalangeal joints. Stiffness and painful cramping of the fingers prevented one patient from milking his cows until TrPs in his ED muscle had been inactivated.[33] A patient seen by Dr. Travell could not type because the ring and little fingers would "not work separately" until the TrPs were injected in the extensor fibers of those fingers.

The presence of an anomalous ED profundus muscle may cause pain and swelling over the dorsal aspect of the 2nd and 3rd metacarpals of the left hand in a guitar player.[45]

3.3. Patient Examination

After a thorough subjective examination, the clinician should make a detailed drawing representing the pain pattern that the patient has described. This depiction will assist in planning the physical examination and can be useful in monitoring the progression of the patient as the symptoms improve or change. Because the ED muscle crosses the elbow, the wrist, and all joints of the fingers, the clinician needs to assess passive range of motion to identify limitations caused by TrPs or joint dysfunctions. It is best to extend the elbow and fully flex the fingers first, then slowly and gently flex the wrist, and finally, move the wrist into ulnar deviation to reveal increased muscle tension caused by either adaptive shortening of the muscle or TrPs. To examine the length of the EI muscle, the clinician passively flexes the wrist and the index finger joints together with some radial deviation.

Limitation of active range of motion can be tested with the finger flexion test by having the patient flex the interphalangeal joints to bring the tips of the fingers against the palmar pads, while extending the metacarpophalangeal joints (Figure 35-3A). Increased tension of an affected finger extensor muscle due to a TrP results in that finger standing out from the others, away from the palm, such as the index finger in Figure 35-3B. Passive flexion of the finger beyond this point is painful and differentiated from lumbrical muscle tightness. Should the 2nd digit be affected, possible contribution by EI muscle should be considered.

Inhibition weakness due to finger extensor TrPs is detected in the grip during a handshake by testing and comparing both hands simultaneously. This bilateral handgrip test is more painful when the patient holds the hands in ulnar deviation and flexed at the wrist. This test may reveal weakness without pain with latent TrPs.

Resisted extension of the middle finger produces pain over the lateral epicondyle (Maudsley's test) in persons with potential lateral epicondylalgia.[46] The muscle fascicle of the ED muscle to the long finger arises from the lateral epicondyle. Tenderness at the origin of the ED muscle directly correlates with pain on Maudsley's test.[46] These observations have led to the hypothesis that the pain of lateral epicondylalgia comes from the ED muscle.[46,47] Trigger points in ED muscle are very prevalent in patients with lateral epicondylalgia, ranging between 25%[39] and 83.3%.[38,40]

Weakness of the ED muscle can also be tested by resisting extension of the metacarpophalangeal joints of the 2nd through 5th digits with the arm resting on a table, as illustrated by Kendall et al.[48] Weakness in this muscle causes weakness in wrist extension. Weakness of the 2nd digit could also result from TrPs in the EI muscle.

Chapter 35: Extensor Digitorum and Extensor Indicis Muscles

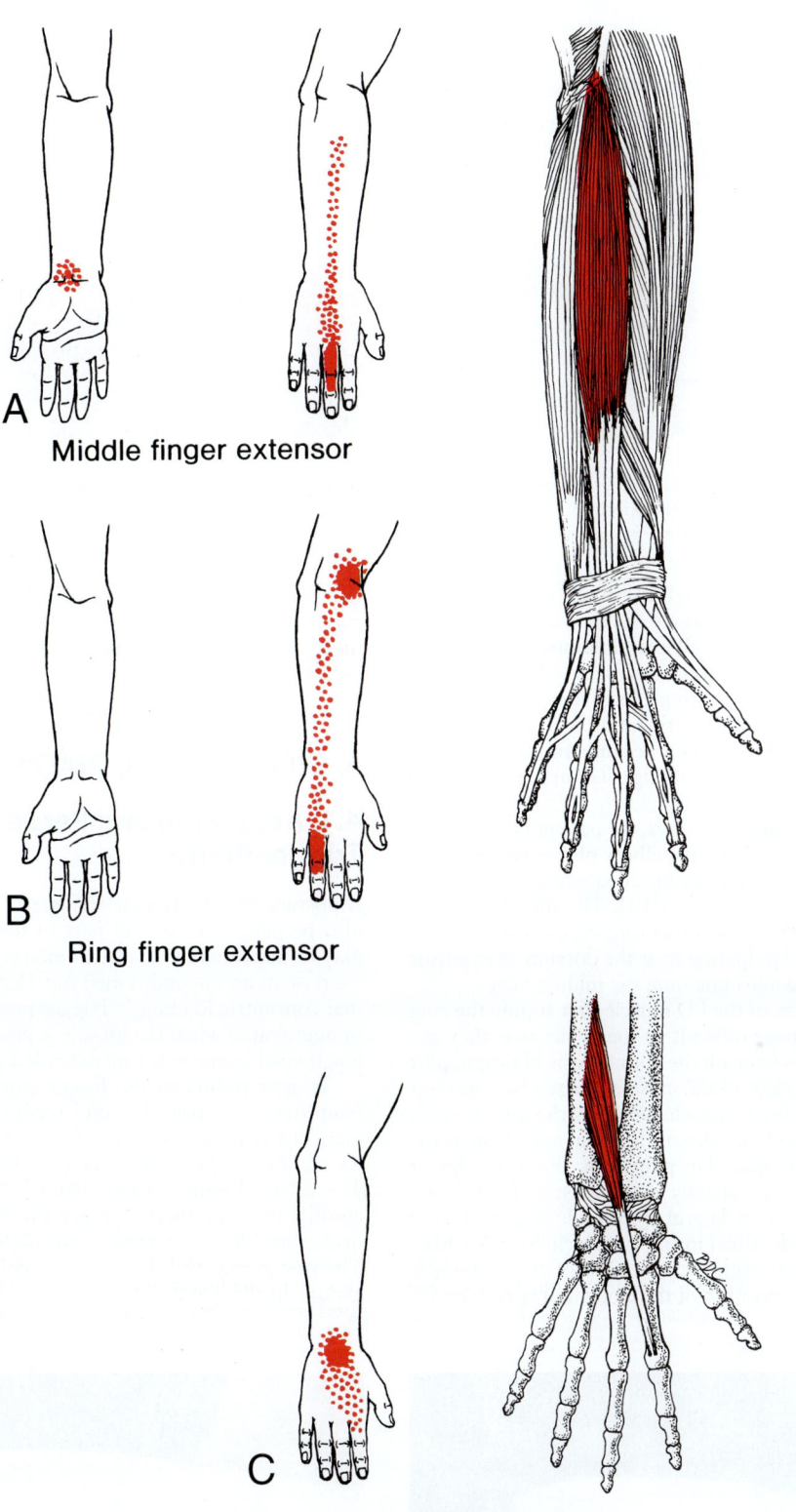

Figure 35-2. Pain patterns (dark red) from TrPs in right ED and EI muscles (medium red). A, Pain pattern from TrPs in fibers of the middle finger. B, Pain pattern from TrPs in fibers of the ring finger. C, Pain pattern from TrPs in the EI muscle, dorsal view.

Tenderness of the proximal interphalangeal joint is commonly associated with the finger stiffness and "soreness" because of finger extensor TrPs, sometimes without referred pain in the joint.[44] Accessory joint motion should be examined in the elbow, wrist, and hand. Decreased accessory joint motion may be a contributing factor to ED and EI muscle overload.[49]

3.4. Trigger Point Examination

Gerwin et al[50] established that among experienced and trained clinicians, reliable criteria for diagnosing TrPs were the detection of a taut band, the presence of spot tenderness, the presence of referred pain, and reproduction of the patient's symptomatic pain.

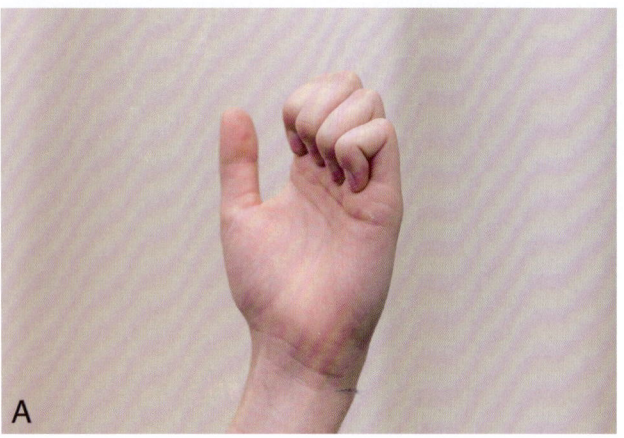
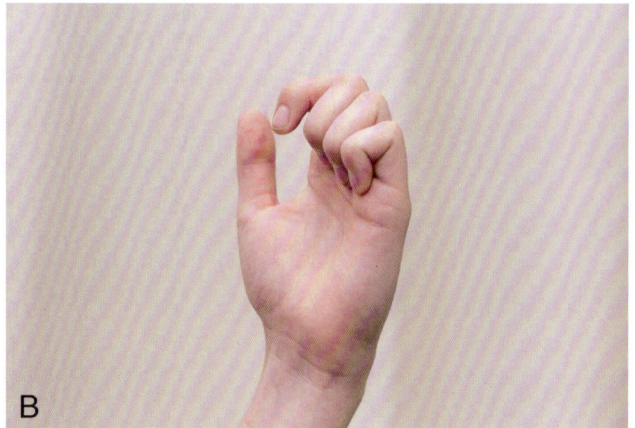

Figure 35-3. Finger flexion test. A, Normal finger closure with all fingers flexed. B, Positive test for finger extensor muscle dysfunction. Note that the index finger is unable to achieve full flexion.

Although for some muscles tested, local twitch responses were not identified reliably, the ED muscle in this study scored very high on interrater reliability for all examinations including the local twitch response. It is one of the easiest muscles to examine reliably for TrPs and also for eliciting a local twitch response. In fact, a recent study found that identification of TrPs within the forearm muscles is a skilled activity because an inexperienced clinician had more difficulty identifying a TrP in the ED muscle than an experienced clinician.[51]

To examine the ED muscle for TrPs, the patient is positioned with the forearm supported and the elbow placed between 90° and 135° of flexion, which allows for adequate cross-fiber flat palpation of the muscle (Figure 35-4A). The muscle may be identified and distinguished from other forearm extensor muscles by flexing the wrist and palpating over the dorsum or extensor surface of the muscle while extending the middle finger.

The TrPs in the fibers of the ED muscle that supply the ring and little fingers are more difficult to locate because they are deep in the muscle mass beneath the aponeurosis of origin, part of which covers the surface of the muscle. These fibers lie next to the extensor carpi ulnaris muscle, which is the muscle mass just lateral to the palpable border of the ulna, and close to the underlying supinator muscle. On palpation, these two finger extensors tend to refer pain distally to the wrist and hand, and sometimes proximally to the lateral epicondyle (Figure 35-2).

Trigger points are identified in the EI muscle by cross-fiber flat palpation (Figure 35-4B). Examination of the EI muscle does not depend on the position of the elbow but is easier with the wrist slightly extended to put the muscle in mid-length. The patient is asked to move the index finger into extension at the metacarpophalangeal joint, allowing the contracting muscle to be identified.

4. DIFFERENTIAL DIAGNOSIS

4.1. Activation and Perpetuation of Trigger Points

A posture or activity that activates a TrP, if not corrected, can also perpetuate it. In any part of the ED or EI muscles, TrPs may be activated by unaccustomed eccentric loading, eccentric exercise in an unconditioned muscle, or maximal or submaximal concentric loading.[52] Trigger points may also be activated or aggravated when the muscle is placed in a shortened and/or lengthened position for an extended period of time.

Trigger points in the finger extensors commonly result from overuse during forceful repetitive finger movements or vigorous grip by professional musicians, carpenters, butchers, ice cream scoopers, plumbers, tennis players, mechanics, etc. The referred pain patterns from TrPs in the upper body, including the arm muscles, reproduced the pain patterns in the neck, shoulders, and arms of both laborers and office workers. The prevalence and distribution of TrPs were similar in both groups in this study.[53]

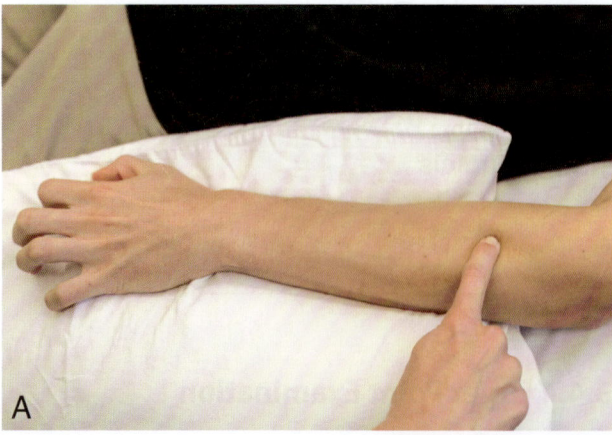
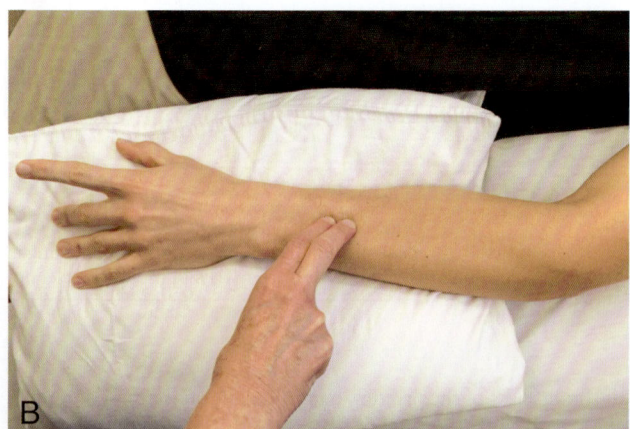

Figure 35-4. Cross-fiber flat palpation for TrPs in finger extensor muscles. A, Extensor digitorum muscle. B, Extensor indicis muscle.

Overuse of muscles arising in the forearm that control the thumb, wrist, and finger extension produces pain in the thumb and forearm as well as pain in the hand and digits. The widespread use of handheld devices like mobile phones and gaming controllers requires repeated movements of the thumb and digits. A retrospective study of individuals with musculoskeletal disorders who participated in a tertiary level rehabilitation center showed an important association between usage of these handheld devices and tendinosis of the extensor pollicis longus muscle and myofascial pain syndrome of the ED, the 1st interosseous, and the thenar musculature.[54]

Trigger points in the ED and EI muscles occur with eccentric contraction when elongated.[52,55] Office workers using computers are particularly susceptible. This phenomenon occurs with keyboard activity when the wrist is extended and the fingers flexed. Prolonged or repeated wrist extension, whether computer keyboard related factory work, or playing a musical instrument, can produce this condition. Forearm pain can be seen in guitarists and other string instrument players. Muscle- and tendon-related pain is reported in 64% to 76% of all instrumentalists surveyed.[56,57] In sports activities, the backhand stroke in tennis overloads the wrist extensors, and the forceful grip overloads the finger extensors.[58]

People with Ehlers-Danlos syndrome, who have hypermobility, often show signs of muscle pain and TrP formation.[59] Hyperextension of the finger joints commonly produces joint pain and can also produce forearm myofascial pain. Use of "silver rings" designed to prevent overextension of the small joints can prevent forearm and hand pain.

4.2. Associated Trigger Points

Associated TrPs can develop in the referred pain areas caused by primary TrPs.[60] Therefore, musculature in the referred pain areas for each muscle should also be considered. Trigger points can occur concomitantly in any of the muscles of the functional unit. The most commonly involved muscles are the extensor carpi radialis brevis and longus muscles, as they share action at the elbow and the wrist. However, the association with other muscles such as the supinator, brachioradialis, extensor carpi ulnaris, triceps brachii, and brachialis muscles or with the forearm antagonists in the flexor–pronator group is very common.

Moreover, pain in the dorsum of the forearm when using the hand, specifically when grasping and lifting, may alter the use of shoulder muscles and induce the formation of TrPs and pain in the shoulder muscles, particularly the infraspinatus, upper trapezius, and levator scapulae muscles, as the shoulder braces or stabilizes during the activity. In addition to these related TrPs, Hong[61] found that TrPs in either the scalene muscles or the serratus posterior superior muscle could induce associated TrPs in the ED muscle.

4.3. Associated Pathology

Differential diagnoses for TrPs in the finger extensors include lateral epicondylalgia, C7 (and occasionally C6) radicular pain or radiculopathy, and De Quervain's stenosing tenosynovitis. The common diagnosis of lateral epicondylalgia is frequently caused by TrPs in at least one muscle that attaches to the lateral epicondyle. Often several of them are involved,[38-40,43] and the prevalence of myofascial pain syndrome in patients with lateral epicondylalgia ranges between 90%[40] and 100%.[43] ED muscle activity may be altered in patients with lateral epicondylalgia where it contributes more to wrist extension than in normal controls, whereas the contribution of the extensor carpi radialis brevis muscle to wrist extension is reduced.[30]

Common causes of dorsal hand pain are ganglion cyst, tenosynovitis, direct trauma, and soft-tissue tumors.[12] Reports of pain from muscle pathology itself are rare.[11] However, reports of pain from TrPs in these muscles are generally not found in the literature.

Acute spontaneous compartment syndrome following repetitive exertional stress produces severe pain and swelling. Pain can occur over the dorsum of the forearm one to several days prior to the onset of swelling. Pain may worsen with finger extension when the ED muscle is involved.[62,63] Decreased range of motion at the wrist may be seen in both compartment syndrome and in pain caused by TrPs. Pain can worsen with wrist or finger extension in both conditions. Neurologic impairment is more likely with compartment syndrome, except that it is also possible that patients may report paresthesias as a result of TrPs in the wrist and finger extensor muscles.

The sagittal bands are the primary stabilizers of the ED tendons over the metacarpal phalangeal joints in the hand. If disrupted due to a disease process such as rheumatoid arthritis or due to trauma, the ED muscle may sublux or become dislocated and lodged on the ulnar side of the joint. This condition is a serious source of muscular strain because of the resultant ulnar deviation of the finger, and the tendon displacement must be surgically repaired for restoration of function.

Closed wrist trauma can rupture muscle tendons, with or without distal radial fracture, but this condition occurs most commonly with the extensor pollicis longus muscle and only infrequently with the EI muscle. Spontaneous tendon rupture can also occur after corticosteroid injection.[8] Wrist pain may also be caused by aberrant extensor tendon variants and their complications. One such variant from the extensor pollicis longus muscle passed over the extensor retinaculum and was associated with radial wrist pain and limited thumb extension, related to stenosing tenosynovitis. The symptoms improved after decompressive surgery.[64]

5. CORRECTIVE ACTIONS

One of the most important corrective actions is to avoid extreme, prolonged, or repetitive wrist extension. These actions are not only considered a risk factor for carpal tunnel syndrome but also increase the activity of wrist extensors, including the ED muscle.[65] Nevertheless, when it comes to ED muscle overload, wrist extension past 45° should be avoided,[65] especially when performing repetitive flexion/extension activity of the fingers on a keyboard, a computer or a musical instrument, or a computer mouse.

If TrPs in the ED or EI muscles are highly irritable, the patient should be instructed in sleeping positions that keep the wrist and fingers from adapting a prolonged flexed posture that can perpetuate pain and symptoms from TrPs in the finger and wrist extensors. The patient can be instructed in the use of a support to prevent maximum finger flexion while maintaining the wrist in a neutral position. A small towel or pad can be placed on the front of the wrist and hand and then secured with a wrap to keep the wrist in a neutral position and the fingers in a relaxed position while sleeping (Figure 35-5A). If the patient's pain is acute or has spread to the elbow, a small towel can be wrapped around the elbow to prevent it from adapting a flexed posture during sleep (Figure 35-5B).

Interrupting prolonged typing or data entry every 30 minutes or so to do the finger-flutter exercise by dropping the hands to the sides of the body, completely relaxed, and moving the arms and elbows to cause passive relaxed shaking of the hands and fingers helps the extensor forearm muscles recover from prolonged activity. Regarding the use of virtual keyboards in tablets or in other devices, the split keyboard design proved better for the use of the tablet in bed,[66] while the wide keyboard gave better results in the traditional desk setting.[66]

The patient must learn to avoid overload of the finger extensors. During grasping or repetitive gripping activities, it is best to keep the wrist in a neutral position, with the wrist stabilized to decrease the demand on the finger extensor muscles. When gripping or twisting with the hand, as in playing tennis, the patient should maintain the hand slightly extended and radially

350 Section 4: Forearm, Wrist, and Hand Pain

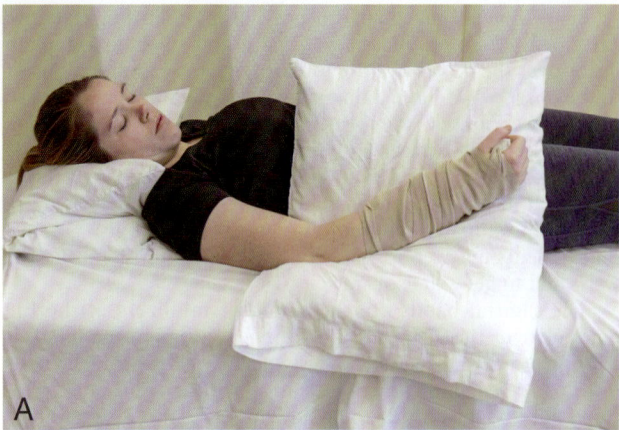 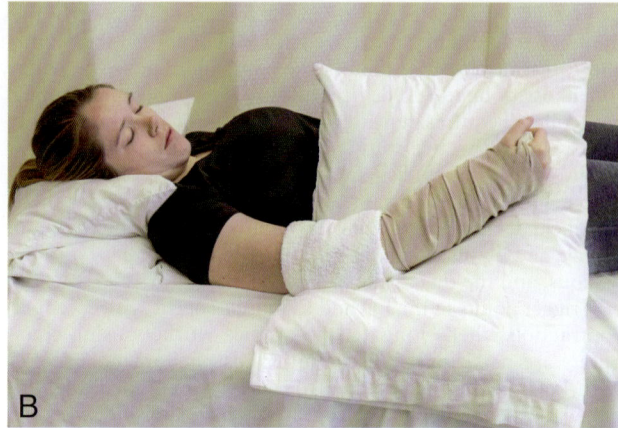

Figure 35-5. Sleeping position for supporting finger extensors. A, Wrist supported in neutral with fingers in a relaxed position and blocked from making a full fist. B, Towel wrapped around the elbow to prevent elbow flexion with wrist supported as in A for acute lateral epicondylalgia or irritable wrist extensor and finger extensor TrPs.

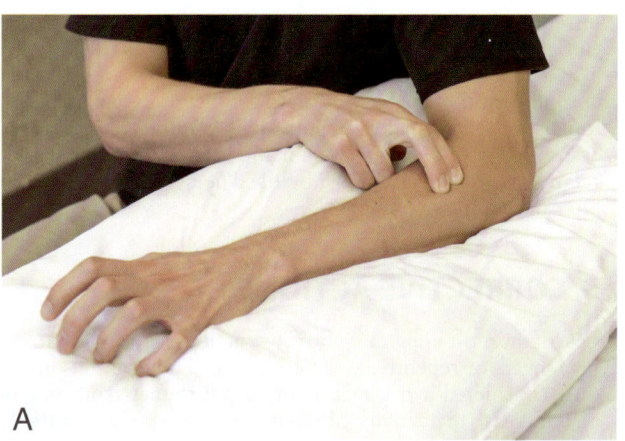 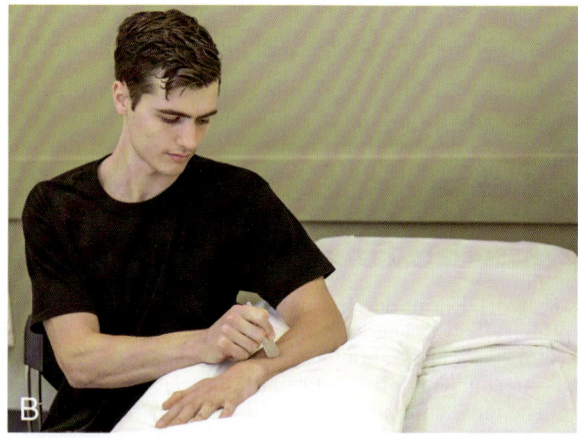

Figure 35-6. Self-pressure release of TrPs. A, Extensor digitorum muscle. B, Extensor indicis muscle.

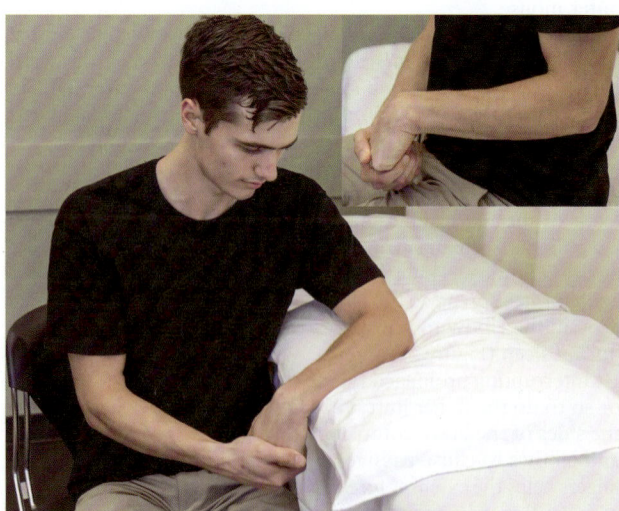

Figure 35-7. Self-stretch of finger extensor muscles. Note in small picture the fingers being passively taken into full finger flexion with wrist flexion.

Self-pressure release for TrPs in the ED (Figure 35-6A) and EI (Figure 35-6B) muscles can be performed in sitting position by placing the forearm on the arm rest of a chair or on a table with the palm down with manual pressure or a TrP release tool. For any self-pressure release techniques, the TrP should be identified with the fingers or a TrP self-release tool. Light pressure (no more than 4/10 pain) is held for 15 to 30 seconds or until pain reduces. This technique can be repeated five times, several times per day.

The patient can easily perform self-stretch techniques as part of a self-management program for TrPs in the finger extensor muscles.[67] Stretching of the ED and EI muscles should be performed with the elbow bent, palm facing down, and wrist and fingers in full flexion (Figure 35-7). The same procedure can be followed with the elbow straight to thoroughly stretch the ED muscle (see Figure 34-9). These self-stretches should be carried out gently, and attention to the reproduction of pain versus stretch is paramount. These stretches should not be painful. The self-stretch enables the patient to relieve the tension of the taut finger extensors. It is essential for the wrist and finger joints to be fully flexed. Addition of postisometric relaxation with a gentle contraction can be helpful.

deviated (in a cock-up position of the wrist), rather than flexed and ulnarly deviated. Avid tennis and golf players should seek professional advice regarding appropriate grip positions and biomechanics.

References

1. Standring S. *Gray's Anatomy: The Anatomical Basis of Clinical Practice.* 41st ed. London, UK: Elsevier; 2015.
2. Precerutti M, Garioni E, Ferrozzi G. Dorsal forearm muscles: US anatomy Pictorial Essay. *J Ultrasound.* 2010;13(2):66-69.

3. Rousset P, Vuillemin-Bodaghi V, Laredo JD, Parlier-Cuau C. Anatomic variations in the first extensor compartment of the wrist: accuracy of US. *Radiology.* 2010;257(2):427-433.
4. McMinn RMH, Hutchings RT, Pegington J, Abrahams PH. *Color Atlas of Human Anatomy.* 3rd ed. St. Louis, MO: Mosby Year Book; 1993.
5. Saladin KS. *Human Anatomy.* New York, NY: McGraw Hill; 2016.
6. Dass P, Prabhu LV, Pai MM, Nayak V, Kumar G, Janardhanan JP. A comprehensive study of the extensor tendons to the medial four digits of the hand. *Chang Gung Med J.* 2011;34(6):612-619.
7. Bettencourt Pires MA, Casal D, Mascarenhas de Lemos L, Godinho CE, Pais D, Goyri-O'Neill J. An unusual variety of the extensor digiti muscles: report with notes on repetition strain injuries. *Acta Med Port.* 2013;26(3):278-283.
8. Lepage D, Tatu L, Loisel F, Vuillier F, Parratte B. Cadaver study of the topography of the musculotendinous junction of the finger extensor muscles: applicability to tendon rupture following closed wrist trauma. *Surg Radiol Anat.* 2015;37(7):853-858.
9. Yoshida Y. Anatomical study on the extensor digitorum profundus muscle in the Japanese. *Okajimas Folia Anat Jpn.* 1990;66(6):339-353.
10. Schwarzkopf R, DeFrate LE, Li G, Herndon JH. The quantification of the origin area of the deep forearm musculature on the interosseous ligament. *Bull NYU Hosp Jt Dis.* 2008;66(1):9-13.
11. Yammine K. The prevalence of the extensor indicis tendon and its variants: a systematic review and meta-analysis. *Surg Radiol Anat.* 2015;37(3):247-254.
12. Kumka M. A variant extensor indicis muscle and the branching pattern of the deep radial nerve could explain hand functionality and clinical symptoms in the living patient. *J Can Chiropr Assoc.* 2015;59(1):64-71.
13. Shereen R, Loukas M, Tubbs RS. Extensor digitorum brevis manus: a comprehensive review of this variant muscle of the dorsal hand. *Cureus.* 2017;9(8):e1568.
14. Gama C. Extensor digitorum brevis manus: a report on 38 cases and a review of the literature. *J Hand Surg Am.* 1983;8(5, pt 1):578-582.
15. Kuschner SH, Gellman H, Bindiger A. Extensor digitorum brevis manus. An unusual cause of exercise-induced wrist pain. *Am J Sports Med.* 1989;17(3):440-441.
16. Shaw JA, Manders EK. Extensor digitorum brevis manus muscle. A clinical reminder. *Orthop Rev.* 1988;17(9):867-869.
17. Feneis H, Dauber W. *Pocket Atlas of Human Anatomy. Based on the International Nomenclature.* New York, NY: Thieme Stuttgart; 2000.
18. Casanova Martinez D, Valdivia Gandur I, Golano P. Extensor pollicis et indicis communis or extensor indicis radialis muscle. *Anat Sci Int.* 2013;88(3):153-155.
19. Arathala R, Sankaran PK, Ragunath G, Harsha SS, Sugumar TS. The extensor indicis brevis—a rare variation and its significance. *J Clin Diagn Res.* 2016;10(2):AD03-AD04.
20. Talbot CE, Mollman KA, Perez NM, et al. Anomalies of the extensor pollicis longus and extensor indicis muscles in two cadaveric cases. *Hand (N Y).* 2013;8(4):469-472.
21. Li WJ, Wang SF, Li PC, et al. Electrophysiological study of the dominant motor innervation to the extensor digitorum communis muscle and long head of triceps brachii at posterior divisions of brachial plexus. *Microsurgery.* 2011;31(7):535-538.
22. Revol MP, Lantieri L, Loy S, Guerin-Surville H. Vascular anatomy of the forearm muscles: a study of 50 dissections. *Plast Reconstr Surg.* 1991;88(6):1026-1033.
23. Basmajian J, Deluca C. *Muscles Alive.* 5th ed. Baltimore, MD: Williams & Wilkins; 1985.
24. Kendall FP, McCreary EK, Provance PG. *Muscles, Testing and Function.* 4th ed. Baltimore, MD: Williams & Wilkins; 1993.
25. Duchenne G. *Physiology of Motion.* Philadelphia, PA: Lippincott; 1949.
26. Long C II, Conrad PW, Hall EA, Furler SL. Intrinsic-extrinsic muscle control of the hand in power grip and precision handling. An electromyographic study. *J Bone Joint Surg Am.* 1970;52(5):853-867.
27. Rasch PJ, Burke RK. *Kinesiology and Applied Anatomy: The Science of Human Movement.* 6th ed. Philadelphia, PA: Lea & Febiger; 1978.
28. van Duinen H, Yu WS, Gandevia SC. Limited ability to extend the digits of the human hand independently with extensor digitorum. *J Physiol.* 2009;587(pt 20):4799-4810.
29. Birdwell JA, Hargrove LJ, Kuiken TA, Weir RF. Activation of individual extrinsic thumb muscles and compartments of extrinsic finger muscles. *J Neurophysiol.* 2013;110(6):1385-1392.
30. Heales LJ, Vicenzino B, MacDonald DA, Hodges PW. Forearm muscle activity is modified bilaterally in unilateral lateral epicondylalgia: a case-control study. *Scand J Med Sci Sports.* 2016;26(12):1382-1390.
31. Simons DG, Travell J, Simons L. *Travell & Simon's Myofascial Pain and Dysfunction: The Trigger Point Manual.* Vol 1. 2nd ed. Baltimore, MD: Williams & Wilkins; 1999:104.
32. Kim Y, Shim JK, Hong YK, Lee SH, Yoon BC. Cutaneous sensory feedback plays a critical role in agonist-antagonist co-activation. *Exp Brain Res.* 2013;229(2):149-156.
33. Kelly M. Pain in the forearm and hand due to muscular lesions. *Med J Aust.* 1944;2:185-188.
34. Travell J. Pain mechanisms in connective tissue. Paper presented at: Connective Tissues, Transactions of the Second Conference; 1951; New York, NY.
35. Travell J, Rinzler SH. The myofascial genesis of pain. *Postgrad Med.* 1952;11(5):425-434.
36. Kelly M. New light on the painful shoulder. *Med J Aust.* 1942;1:488-493.
37. Good MG. The role of skeletal muscles in the pathogenesis of diseases. *Acta Med Scand.* 1950;138(4):284-292.
38. Mayoral del Moral O, Gimenez Donoso C, Salvat Salvat I, Fernandez Carnero J. Puncion seca de los musculos del brazo, el antebrazo y la mano. In: Mayoral del Moral O, Salvat Salvat I, eds. *Fisioterapia Invasiva del Sindrome de Dolor Miofascial Manual de puncion seca de punto gatillo.* Madrid, Spain: Editorial Medica Panamericana; 2017:265-309.
39. Fernandez-Carnero J, Fernández-de-las-Peñas C, de la Llave-Rincon AI, Ge HY, Arendt-Nielsen L. Prevalence of and referred pain from myofascial trigger points in the forearm muscles in patients with lateral epicondylalgia. *Clin J Pain.* 2007;23(4):353-360.
40. Mayoral O, de Felipe JA, Velasco S, Jimenez F, Miota J, Lopez P. Prevalence of Myofascial Pain Syndrome in Lateral Epicondyle Enthesopathy. Paper presented at: MYOPAIN 2010. VIII World Congress on Myofascial Pain and Fibromyalgia; 2010; Todedo, Spain.
41. Kellgren JH. Observations on referred pain arising from muscle. *Clin Sci.* 1938;3:175-190.
42. Dejung B, Grobli C, Colla F, Weissman R. *Triggerpunkt-Therapie (Trigger Point Therapy).* Bern, Switzerland: Verlag Hans Huber; 2003.
43. Fernandez-Carnero J, Fernández-de-las-Peñas C, de la Llave-Rincon AI, Ge HY, Arendt-Nielsen L. Bilateral myofascial trigger points in the forearm muscles in patients with chronic unilateral lateral epicondylalgia: a blinded, controlled study. *Clin J Pain.* 2008;24(9):802-807.
44. Travell J, Bigelow NH. Role of somatic trigger areas in the patterns of hysteria. *Psychosom Med.* 1947;9(6):353-363.
45. Reeder CA, Pandeya NK. Extensor indicis proprius syndrome secondary to an anomalous extensor indicis proprius muscle belly. *J Am Osteopath Assoc.* 1991;91(3):251-253.
46. Fairbank SM, Corlett RJ. The role of the extensor digitorum communis muscle in lateral epicondylitis. *J Hand Surg Br.* 2002;27(5):405-409.
47. Shmushkevich Y, Kalichman L. Myofascial pain in lateral epicondylalgia: a review. *J Bodyw Mov Ther.* 2013;17(4):434-439.
48. Kendall FP, McCreary EK. *Muscles: Testing and Function, with Posture and Pain.* 5th ed. Baltimore, MD: Lippincott Williams & Wilkins; 2005.
49. Lewit K. *Manipulative Therapy. Musculoskeletal Medicine.* London, England: Churchill Livingstone; 2010.
50. Gerwin RD, Shannon S, Hong C-Z, Hubbard DR, Gevirtz R. Interrater reliability in myofascial trigger point examination. *Pain.* 1997;69:65-73.
51. Mora-Relucio R, Nunez-Nagy S, Gallego-Izquierdo T, et al. Experienced versus inexperienced interexaminer reliability to location and classification of myofascial trigger point palpation to diagnose lateral epicondylalgia: an observational cross-sectional study. *Evid Based Complement Alternat Med.* 2016;2016:6059719.
52. Gerwin RD, Dommerholt J, Shah JP. Expansion of Simons' integrated hypothesis. *J Musculoske Pain.* 2004;12(suppl 9):23.
53. Fernández-de-las-Peñas C, Grobli C, Ortega-Santiago R, et al. Referred pain from myofascial trigger points in head, neck, shoulder, and arm muscles reproduces pain symptoms in blue-collar (manual) and white-collar (office) workers. *Clin J Pain.* 2012;28(6):511-518.
54. Sharan D, Mohandoss M, Ranganathan R, Jose J. Musculoskeletal disorders of the upper extremities due to extensive usage of hand held devices. *Ann Occup Environ Med.* 2014;26:22.
55. Itoh K, Okada K, Kawakita K. A proposed experimental model of myofascial trigger points in human muscle after slow eccentric exercise. *Acupunct Med.* 2004;22(1):2-12; discussion 12-13.
56. Brandfonbrener AG. Musculoskeletal problems of instrumental musicians. *Hand Clin.* 2003;19(2):231-239, v-vi.
57. Lederman RJ. Neuromuscular and musculoskeletal problems in instrumental musicians. *Muscle Nerve.* 2003;27(5):549-561.
58. Kim PS. Role of injection therapy: review of indications for trigger point injections, regional blocks, facet joint injections, and intra-articular injections. *Curr Opin Rheumatol.* 2002;14(1):52-57.
59. Tewari S, Madabushi R, Agarwal A, Gautam SK, Khuba S. Chronic pain in a patient with Ehlers-Danlos syndrome (hypermobility type): the role of myofascial trigger point injections. *J Bodyw Mov Ther.* 2017;21(1):194-196.
60. Hsieh YL, Kao MJ, Kuan TS, Chen SM, Chen JT, Hong CZ. Dry needling to a key myofascial trigger point may reduce the irritability of satellite MTrPs. *Am J Phys Med Rehabil.* 2007;86(5):397-403.
61. Hong C-Z. Considerations and recommendations regarding myofascial trigger point injection. *J Musculoske Pain.* 1994;2(1):29-59.
62. Johnson AL, Maish D, Darowish M. Isolated compartment syndrome of the extensor digitorum communis: a case report. *Hand (N Y).* 2011;6(4):442-444.
63. Dalton DM, Munigangaiah S, Subramaniam T, McCabe JP. Acute bilateral spontaneous forearm compartment syndrome. *Hand Surg.* 2014;19(1):99-102.
64. Turker T, Robertson GA, Thirkannad SM. A classification system for anomalies of the extensor pollicis longus. *Hand (N Y).* 2010;5(4):403-407.
65. Chen HM, Leung CT. The effect on forearm and shoulder muscle activity in using different slanted computer mice. *Clin Biomech (Bristol, Avon).* 2007;22(5):518-523.
66. Lin MI, Hong RH, Chang JH, Ke XM. Usage position and virtual keyboard design affect upper-body kinematics, discomfort, and usability during prolonged tablet typing. *PLoS One.* 2015;10(12):e0143585.
67. Van Eerd D, Munhall C, Irvin E, et al. Effectiveness of workplace interventions in the prevention of upper extremity musculoskeletal disorders and symptoms: an update of the evidence. *Occup Environ Med.* 2016;73(1):62-70.

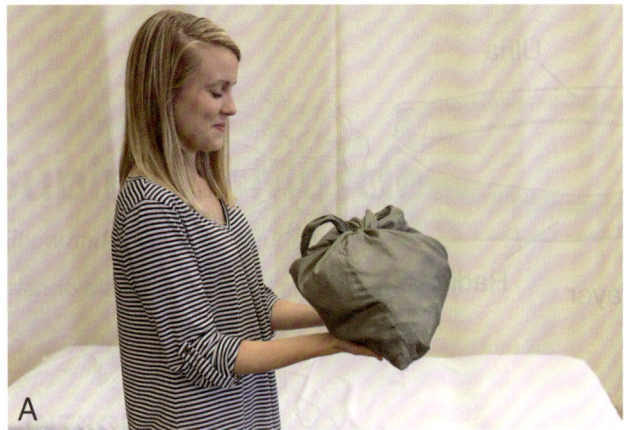

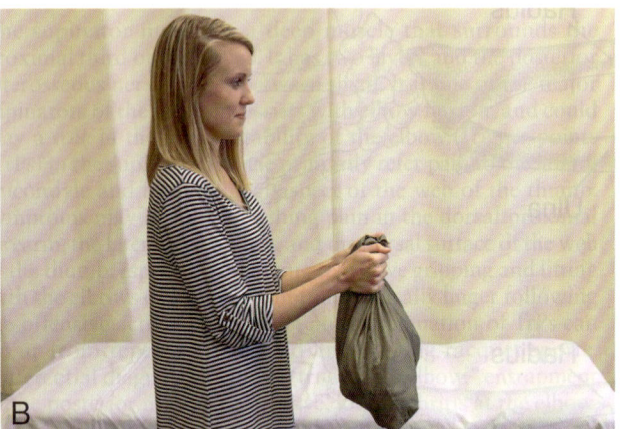

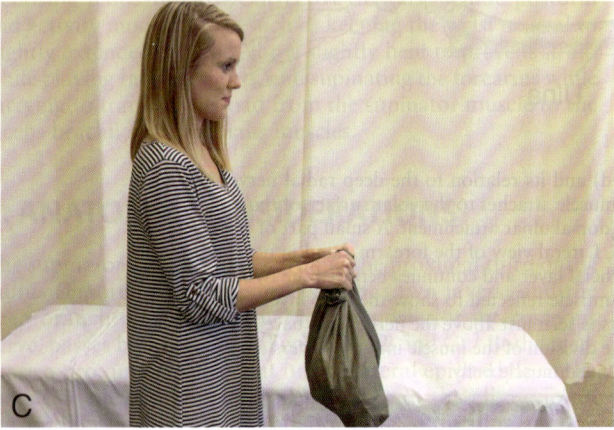

Figure 36-2. Three hand positions for carrying a heavy object with the elbow flexed. A, Forearms supinated, which loads the biceps brachii muscle and unloads the supinator muscle. B, Hands in the neutral position, which loads both the muscles. C, Forearms pronated, which tends to unload the biceps brachii muscle and to load the brachialis, brachioradialis, and the few fibers of the supinator muscles that contribute to elbow flexion.

Box 36-1	Functional unit of the supinator muscle	
Action	Synergists	Antagonists
Supination	Biceps brachii Extensor carpi radialis longus	Pronator teres Pronator quadratus
Elbow flexion	Biceps brachii Brachialis Brachioradialis Extensor carpi radialis longus	Triceps brachii Anconeus

and pronator teres muscles.[11] This result may have implications regarding the application of the principle of superposition for muscle forces in the estimation of distal radioulnar joint loading.

3. CLINICAL PRESENTATION

3.1. Referred Pain Pattern

Trigger points in the supinator muscle refer pain primarily to the lateral epicondyle and the anterior and posterior surrounding areas. They also project pain to the dorsal aspect of the web of the thumb[m], and if sufficiently intense, the pain may include some of the dorsal forearm[12] (Figure 36-3).

Dejung et al[13] described a pain referral pattern observed in 27 patients. The essential pattern was very similar to the one described in Figure 36-3, but it also included some spread of pain to the anterior and the posterior aspects of the shoulder and to the parietal part of the head, close to its vertex.

Slater et al[14] injected hypertonic saline in several parts of the forearm, including the supinator muscle. The injection of this muscle produced a very diffuse pain pattern, and the pain spread both proximally to the deltoid region and distally to the metacarpal and intercarpal joints.[14] The referred pain evoked by the injection of the supinator muscle varied in subjects participating in the study, with reports of pain felt in the dorsolateral forearm, extending to the distal radioulnar joint and to the hand, and immediately proximal to the common extensor origin.[14] A more recent study found that the referred pain elicited by active supinator TrPs contributed to the overall pain of patients with unspecific arm pain but without describing a specific pattern of pain for TrPs in this muscle.[15]

3.2. Symptoms

Patients with active TrPs in the supinator muscle primarily report aching pain in the dorsal proximal forearm, the lateral epicondyle, and the dorsal surface of the web space of the thumb. The patient's pain is aggravated by activities such as carrying a heavy briefcase with the elbow fully extended, playing tennis, and other functional activities that require excessively forceful, repetitive, or sustained supination of the forearm, especially with the elbow straight. Patients may also report pain that persists even after these activities have ceased.

According to Simons et al,[3] nearly every patient with lateral epicondylar pain has a supinator TrP, and they state that the supinator muscle is the muscle most frequently contributing to the pain of "tennis elbow." Nevertheless, the only TrP prevalence study in lateral epicondylalgia that included the supinator muscle among the muscles studied reported just a 50% involvement rate of this muscle in patients diagnosed clinically and with ultrasound imaging as having an enthesopathy of the extensor–supinator muscle complex.[16] Despite this discrepancy, the relevance of supinator TrPs in this condition is considered very important when it is involved, in which case its treatment can be decisive in the outcome.[17]

3.3. Patient Examination

After a thorough subjective examination, the clinician should make a detailed drawing representing the pain pattern that the patient has described. This depiction will assist in planning

Chapter 36: Supinator Muscle 355

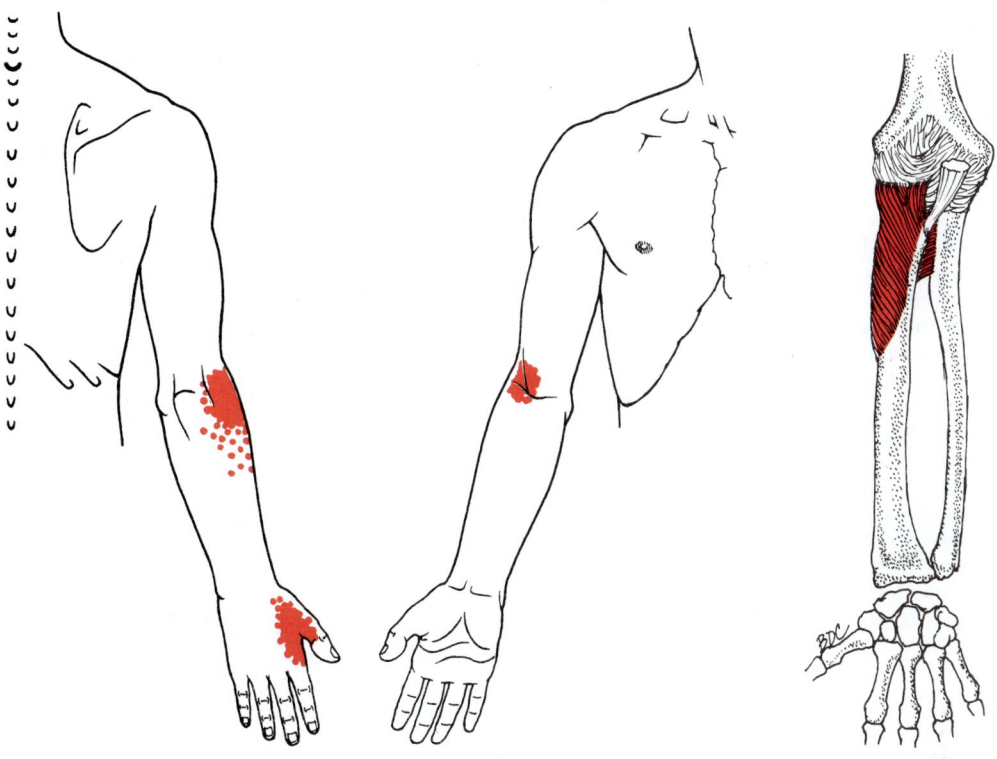

Figure 36-3. Referred pain pattern (dark red) of TrPs in the right supinator muscle.

the physical examination and can be useful in monitoring the progression of the patient as symptoms improve or change. Screening of the cervical spine and shoulder girdle should be conducted to identify any possible sources of symptoms or contributing factors to the patient's presentation of lateral elbow or thumb pain.

Active and passive range of motion including elbow flexion and extension, forearm pronation and supination, and a combination of elbow extension with forearm pronation should be examined. The clinician should test specifically for supinator muscle length by simultaneously passively pronating the forearm and extending the elbow. This test may show range of motion restriction if the supinator muscle is adaptively shortened or has TrPs. If the subjective reports include pain in the region of the web space of the thumb, the range of motion of the thumb and carpometacarpal joints should be assessed. Thumb motion is usually not restricted and often is not painful; however, the patient may be sensitive to palpation in this region, especially if the supinator muscle has active TrPs.

To test the supinator muscle for strength with minimum interfering assistance from the biceps brachii muscle, have the patient in a supine position with the elbow extended along the side of the body and the hand and forearm in a neutral position and resist a supination effort by the patient.

The Apley's Scratch Test (see Figure 21-3A) shows slight restriction, and causes pain in the distribution described in Figure 36-3. A handshake with a firm grip becomes painful when extensor muscles of the wrist and fingers have developed associated TrPs.

There has been some speculation that the eccentric function of the supinator muscle is compromised in individuals with lateral epicondylalgia.[14] Hypothetically, this dysfunction might lead to excessive medial and inferior displacement of the radius, with increased load on the common extensor origin[14] and on radial joints. Accessory joint motion of the radioulnar (proximal and distal), radiohumeral, and humeroulnar joints should be assessed because hypomobility in any of these joints may overload the supinator muscle. The radioulnar (proximal and distal) and radiohumeral joints are most critical for normal supinator muscle function,[3,18] and hypomobility in these joints can not only be a consequence of supinator TrPs but also act as an activating and perpetuating factor of TrPs in this and in other muscles in the area.[17]

Neurodynamic testing of the radial nerve should be conducted to identify potential neuropathic contributions to the patient's reported symptoms. A thorough sensory and motor examination of the radial nerve and C7 nerve root should be conducted because of the structural interface of the arcade of Frohse and the supinator muscle.

Two studies related the development of lateral epicondylalgia with inadequate grip strength.[19,20] With slight extension and no ulnar deviation of the hand at the wrist, the increase in strength protects the supinator muscle from overload and is easily demonstrated on a grip-strength meter. A slight extension places the forearm flexors at some mechanical advantage. Ulnar deviation places the ring and little finger flexors at a mechanical disadvantage. The bent elbow provides biceps brachii muscle assistance in supination and helps prevent supinator muscle overload. The two-handed backhand stroke protects the supinator muscle by preventing complete elbow extension during the stroke. Tennis players who use a two-handed backhand have much less trouble with tennis elbow.[21,22]

If the player still has difficulty with the racket slipping from the hand because the grip is weak, the size of the racquet handle should be reduced[19,20] so that the fingers wrap fully around it. Otherwise the extensors, especially those of the ring and little fingers that are essential for a strong grip, function at a disadvantage. The additional effort required to keep a tight grip on a large handle further strains the finger extensors. Sometimes, it is also recommended to change the grip position.[23]

3.4. Trigger Point Examination

Gerwin et al[24] established that, among experienced and trained clinicians, three reliable criteria for diagnosing TrPs were the detection of a taut band, the presence of spot tenderness, and patient's recognition of pain elicited from the tender spot in the taut band. In several muscles, local twitch responses were not identified as reliable. The supinator muscle was not one of the muscles tested in this study, but based on comparable muscles that were tested, the supinator muscle would likely be one of the more difficult and skill-demanding muscles to reliably examine for a local twitch response. A recent study by Mora-Relucio et al[25] evaluated the interexaminer reliability of two experienced and one inexperienced clinicians on TrP location in extensor carpi radialis brevis and extensor digitorum muscles, and it proved that diagnosis of TrPs in both muscles through palpation is reliable when the evaluators are expert practitioners. The authors warn that the validity of their findings is limited to superficial forearm muscles and may not be generalized to deeper muscles such as the supinator muscle.[25] Nevertheless, clinical experience and some studies show that TrPs in supinator muscle can be readily identified[15,16] and its pain referral evoked by palpation,[13,15] dry needling,[13] or injection.[14]

The supinator muscle can develop TrPs in any part of the muscle belly, but it is common to identify them on the ventral aspect of the radius, just lateral and somewhat distal to the biceps brachii tendon (Figure 36-4A). The forearm must be fully supinated, otherwise the TrPs may be hidden by the ulna. In this position, the supinator TrPs lie directly over the radius and immediately beneath the skin between the biceps brachii tendon and the brachioradialis muscle. Both muscular landmarks are readily identified by asking the patient to flex the forearm against resistance. Cross-fiber flat palpation of irritable TrPs may occasionally produce a confirmatory supination twitch response of the hand in spite of the shortened position of the muscle. The muscular nature of the deep layer and of the deep aspect of the superficial layer[2] makes it more likely that the TrPs are deeply located. A monofilament or injection needle may be necessary to accurately identify TrPs in the supinator muscle because palpation of the deeper portion can be highly unreliable.

Sometimes, TrPs in the supinator muscle may be found by pressing downward against the ulna on the posterolateral side of the forearm, close to the radius as the muscle approaches its attachment where the lateral joint capsule meets the ulna (Figure 36-4B). This TrP area is evidenced by deep palpation through the mass of the extensors, especially through the extensor carpi ulnaris[3] or the extensor digitorum[17] muscles. Trigger points in the supinator muscle can be associated with posterior interosseous nerve entrapment.

4. DIFFERENTIAL DIAGNOSIS

4.1. Activation and Perpetuation of Trigger Points

A posture or activity that activates a TrP, if not corrected, can also perpetuate it. In any part of the supinator muscle, TrPs may be activated by unaccustomed eccentric loading, eccentric exercise in an unconditioned muscle, or maximal or submaximal concentric loading.[26] Trigger points may also be activated or aggravated when the muscle is placed in a shortened and/or lengthened position for an extended period of time.

Supinator muscle strain may occur when resisting unexpected pronation, as when the tennis player hits the ball "off-center," twisting the racquet with the elbow completely extended as in a one-hand backhand stroke. During full elbow extension, the biceps brachii muscle cannot assist the supinator muscle to resist the added force. This sudden overload could activate TrPs in the supinator muscle, which could give rise to "tennis elbow" symptoms (lateral epicondylalgia).

Elbow pain often begins when a person gets a new racquet that is too heavy, has a larger handle, or is unbalanced and too heavy at the head end. The position of the grip on the racquet may be shortened to reduce the length of the lever arm against which the forearm muscles must operate.

Tennis players with this elbow dysfunction should not play on consecutive days, but should rest the supinator muscle until the postexercise soreness from overuse has worn off, usually in a day or two. There is some evidence that the frequency of playing and/or the volume of play is important in the prevention of the condition.[21,23] The use of bracing systems is controversial and there is not much evidence of its usefulness in the prevention or in the treatment of lateral epicondylalgia.[19,27]

Any excessively forceful, repetitive, or sustained supination of the forearm, especially with the elbow straight, may initiate activation of TrPs in the supinator muscle. A forceful elbow flexion motion when the forearm is held in pronation may also activate or perpetuate TrPs (Figure 36-2C). Carrying a heavy briefcase, suitcase, or heavy bag with the elbow straight when it must be stabilized by the supinator muscle with each step is also traumatic, especially if the leg bumps the back end of the object during ambulation.

Additional activating and perpetuating stresses include turning stiff doorknobs, wringing out wet clothing or a washcloth, using a screwdriver, unscrewing a tight jar lid by movement only at the wrist, walking an undisciplined dog excessively pulling on a leash, washing floors by hand, and raking leaves.

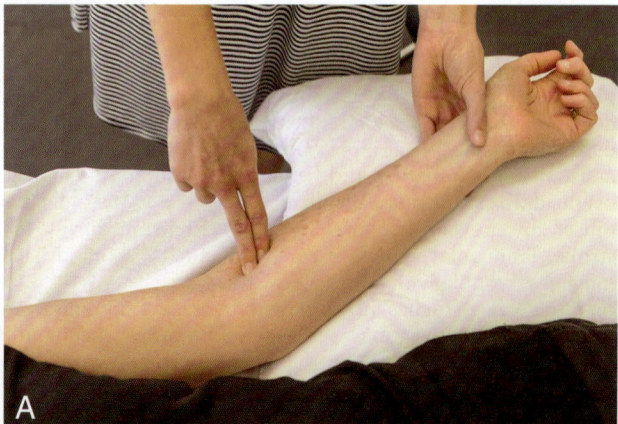 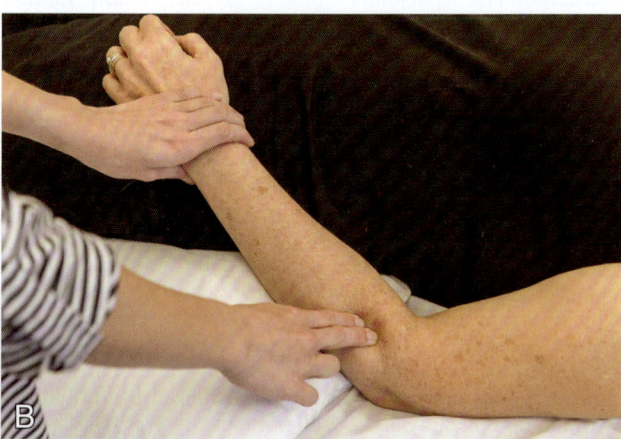

Figure 36-4. Cross-fiber flat palpation for TrPs in the supinator muscle. A, Ventral approach. B, Dorsal approach.

4.2. Associated Trigger Points

Associated TrPs can develop in the referred pain areas caused by primary TrPs.[28] Therefore, musculature in the referred pain areas for each muscle should also be considered. With the symptoms of pain and tenderness in the region of the lateral epicondyle, TrPs are often also found in the triceps brachii muscle (in the lower end of the lateral margin of its medial head) in the long extensors of the fingers, in the extensor carpi radialis longus and brevis muscles, and in the anconeus and brachioradialis muscles. Other TrPs involved in this pain are the scalene muscles, the infraspinatus muscle, the supraspinatus muscle, and less commonly, the subclavius muscle. Additional muscles that may become involved as part of the supinator muscle's functional unit but which do not refer pain to the lateral epicondyle are the brachialis, the biceps brachii, and sometimes the palmaris longus muscles.

4.3. Associated Pathology

Differential diagnosis of the symptoms caused by supinator TrPs include lateral elbow pain or epicondylalgia, entrapment of the deep branch of the radial nerve (radial tunnel syndrome or posterior interosseous nerve entrapment), local arthritis at the elbow,[29] radiocapitellar pathology (ie, synovial plica at the humeroradial joint),[30-32] C5-C6 radicular pain or radiculopathy,[33] posterolateral rotatory instability,[34,35] and nonspecific arm pain[36] (defined as diffuse forearm pain not associated with any particular structure), De Quervain's stenosing tenosynovitis, trapeziometacarpal joint arthritis, recurring articular dysfunction at the distal radioulnar joint, and entrapment of the superficial radial nerve (cheiralgia paresthetica or Wartenberg syndrome).

Lateral epicondylalgia (tennis elbow, radial epicondylalgia, or lateral elbow tendinosis) is a fairly commonly diagnosed upper limb musculoskeletal disorder, and the most common cause of lateral elbow pain in adults. Its incidence is lower than 10% in the general population.[37]

Some studies have investigated the degree of involvement of TrPs in individuals with lateral epicondylalgia reaching as high as 90%[16] or even 100%.[38] As described earlier, the only TrP prevalence study on lateral epicondylalgia, which included the supinator muscle, reported an involvement rate of 50% in patients diagnosed clinically with ultrasound imaging confirmation as having an enthesopathy of the common wrist extensor tendon.[16] Other muscles involved in lateral epicondylalgia are the extensor carpi radialis brevis muscle: 65%,[39] 83.3%,[16] or 100%[38]; the brachioradialis muscle: 50%[38,39] or 66.6%[16]; the extensor carpi radialis longus muscle: 70%,[39] 96%,[38] or 72.2%[16]; and the extensor digitorum muscle: 35%[38,39] or 83.3%.[16] In a cadaveric study,[40] the authors tensile-loaded different muscles arising in the lateral epicondyle and measured their contribution to the tensile force generated in the common extensor tendon. They concluded that there is a biomechanical basis for the superficial head of supinator muscle in the etiology of lateral epicondylalgia.

Several controlled trials have demonstrated significant improvement in pain and dysfunction after the application of soft tissue techniques, focusing on the myofascial component of patients with lateral epicondylalgia.[41] Although the isolated contribution of TrPs in the supinator muscle is not accurately known, TrPs could be a major contributor to pain and dysfunction in lateral epicondylalgia.

As discussed earlier in the wrist extensors and brachioradialis muscles chapter (see Chapter 34), it is currently unknown as to what degree myofascial pain coexists, causes, or predisposes sensory and motor impairments reported in individuals with lateral epicondylalgia. Nevertheless, given the high prevalence of TrPs found in people with lateral epicondylalgia,[16,38,39] their contribution to pain symptoms,[16,38,39] and the effectiveness of treatments focusing on myofascial components in this population,[41,42] clinicians are encouraged to evaluate and treat TrPs as an essential component for the routine management of lateral epicondylalgia (see Chapters 34 and 35 for further information on this issue).

Entrapment of the deep branch of the radial nerve[43] (posterior interosseous nerve[1]) as it enters the supinator muscle has been commonly accepted in the literature as a cause of neuropathic epicondylalgia,[40,44] and it is sometimes referred to as "radial tunnel syndrome."[44] It may or may not produce symptoms often identified in patients presenting with lateral epicondylalgia. The clinician should note that: (1) the painless weakness of muscles supplied by the radial nerve is frequently caused by a tumor[45]; (2) a painful lateral epicondyle without muscular weakness or signs of nerve entrapment (usually diagnosed as lateral epicondylalgia) is often caused by TrPs without radial nerve compromise; and (3) the mixture of lateral epicondylalgia and evidence of radial nerve entrapment in the region of the supinator muscle suggests the possibility of both nerve entrapment and supinator TrPs. A study in cadavers demonstrated a biomechanical basis for the superficial head of the supinator muscle in the etiology of both lateral epicondylalgia and radial tunnel syndrome.[40]

True posterior interosseous neuropathy causes neurogenic weakness in the muscles innervated by the nerve,[46] distal to the point of entrapment. The typical pattern of weakness does not involve the extensor carpi radialis muscle, so wrist drop is absent, but because of weakness of the extensor carpi ulnaris muscle, the patient may radially deviate the wrist during wrist extension.[46] Finger extension at the metacarpophalangeal joints is impaired, as is the action of the abductor pollicis longus and extensor pollicis longus and brevis muscles.[46] Pain and focal tenderness are not necessarily present in patients with this presentation and no sensory deficits are reported.[46]

Surgical reports of radial nerve entrapment make it clear that the problem frequently occurs as the posterior interosseous nerve enters the supinator muscle (Figure 36-1B and C).[47] An anatomic study showed that the proximal edge of the superficial layer of muscle fibers formed a tendinous thickened border in 30% of 50 "normal" adult arms.[48] As stated earlier, different studies have shown that it is muscular in newborn full-term fetuses, and it has been suggested that repetitive pronation and supination movements probably form this semicircular fibrous arcade in adults.[2] Actually, the thickened arch was much more common in patients who received surgical intervention for a supinator syndrome than in "normal" arms.

Moreover, supinator TrPs can also cause entrapment of the deep radial nerve if those supinator fibers that are attached to an arcade with a thick tendinous edge are shortened by activity of these TrPs and create tension on the arcade of Frohse.

Clinically, it is often found that inactivation of all TrPs relieves the pain, and usually relieves the deep radial nerve entrapment, without surgical intervention. Patients with a hypertrophied arcade[40] may be more vulnerable to entrapment of the radial nerve by supinator TrPs. There is a paucity in the literature, and not one paper could be located that reported systematic examination of patients for TrPs with this entrapment or for the results of treating TrPs. Competent research studies of this type are sorely needed.

5. CORRECTIVE ACTIONS

According to the literature, the prevalence of lateral epicondylalgia in tennis players ranges between 14.1%[19] and 35%,[21] or even up to 50% throughout their tennis career.[49] To decrease these rates, tennis players should keep the wrist slightly extended[50] and the elbow slightly bent during play (Figure 36-5A). Allowing the head of the racquet to drop (Figure 36-5B) reduces grip strength. Consultation with a professional for appropriate racquet size, weight, and grip is highly recommended.

A patient with supinator TrPs or lateral epicondylalgia is encouraged to use rolling luggage, or carry his or her briefcase or

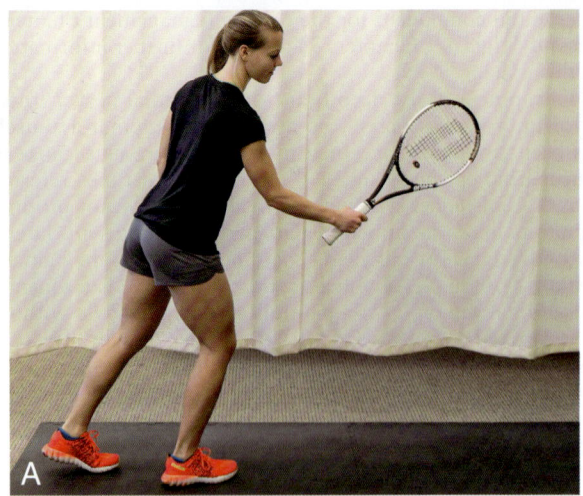 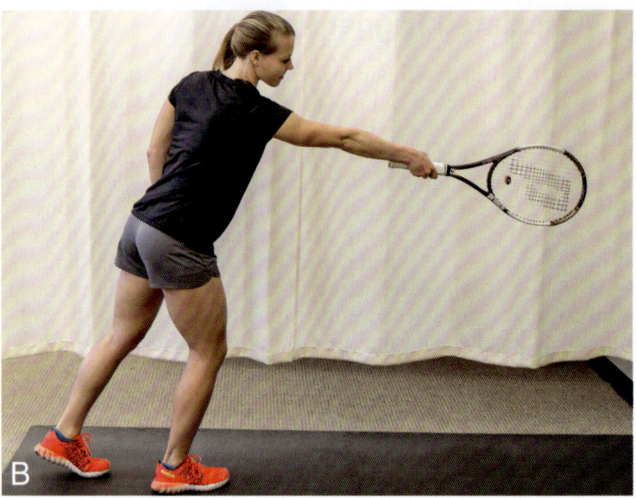

Figure 36-5. Use and misuse of the tennis racquet (backhand stroke). A, Effective position. The elbow is slightly bent and the wrist cocked in radial extension to raise the head of the racquet. B, Ineffective position. The elbow is straight and the wrist dropped, which overloads the supinator muscle during supination at the end of the stroke and weakens the grip.

purse tucked under the arm with the elbow bent. While pulling the luggage, the patient should be sure to keep the elbow in slight flexion and the wrist in slight extension with radial deviation to decrease the external load on the supinator muscle.

For some activities, wrist-rotation stress may be avoided temporarily by using the other hand or by using the affected hand differently. Instead of wringing washed clothes or a cleaning rag, they may be pressed against the bottom of the sink to drain the water from them. Raking leaves and walking a large dog that pulls on a leash should be discontinued. If shaking hands in a receiving line is unavoidable, the patient is encouraged to do a fist bump.

The patient with supinator TrPs should learn to carry packages with the forearms supinated (Figure 36-2A) rather than pronated (Figure 36-2C). This position substitutes the biceps brachii muscle for the supinator muscle as an assistant to the brachialis muscle in flexing the elbow while lifting loads. The biceps brachii muscle is much stronger than the supinator muscle for this purpose. Patients may also need to assume a sleeping posture as described in Figure 35-5B.

It is very difficult to perform self-pressure release or self-stretching exercises for self-management of supinator TrPs. Patients with lateral elbow pain are encouraged to seek care from a clinician who has knowledge and expertise in myofascial pain and dysfunction.

References

1. Standring S. *Gray's Anatomy: The Anatomical Basis of Clinical Practice*. 41st ed. London, UK: Elsevier; 2015.
2. Berton C, Wavreille G, Lecomte F, Miletic B, Kim HJ, Fontaine C. The supinator muscle: anatomical bases for deep branch of the radial nerve entrapment. *Surg Radiol Anat*. 2013;35(3):217-224.
3. Simons DG, Travell J, Simons L. *Travell & Simon's Myofascial Pain and Dysfunction: The Trigger Point Manual*. Vol 1. 2nd ed. Baltimore, MD: Williams & Wilkins; 1999:104.
4. Paraskevas GK, Ioannidis O. Accessory muscles around the superior radioulnar joint: a morphological study. *Ital J Anat Embryol*. 2011;116(1):45-51.
5. Hast MH, Perkins RE. Secondary tensor and supinator muscles of the human proximal radio-ulnar joint. *J Anat*. 1986;146:45-51.
6. Travill A, Basmajian JV. Electromyography of the supinators of the forearm. *Anat Rec*. 1961;139:557-560.
7. Basmajian J, Deluca C. *Muscles Alive*. 5th ed. Baltimore, MD: Williams & Wilkins; 1985.
8. Gordon KD, Pardo RD, Johnson JA, King GJ, Miller TA. Electromyographic activity and strength during maximum isometric pronation and supination efforts in healthy adults. *J Orthop Res*. 2004;22(1):208-213.
9. Stroyan M, Wilk KE. The functional anatomy of the elbow complex. *J Orthop Sports Phys Ther*. 1993;17(6):279-288.
10. Stuart PR. Pronator quadratus revisited. *J Hand Surg Br*. 1996;21(6):714-722.
11. Gordon KD, Kedgley AE, Ferreira LM, King GJ, Johnson JA. Effect of simulated muscle activity on distal radioulnar joint loading in vitro. *J Orthop Res*. 2006;24(7):1395-1404.
12. Travell J, Rinzler SH. The myofascial genesis of pain. *Postgrad Med*. 1952;11(5):425-434.
13. DeJung B, Grobli C, Colla F, Weissman R. *Triggerpunkt-Therapie (Trigger Point Therapy)*. Bern, Switzerland: Verlag Hans Huber; 2003.
14. Slater H, Arendt-Nielsen L, Wright A, Graven-Nielsen T. Experimental deep tissue pain in wrist extensors—a model of lateral epicondylalgia. *Eur J Pain*. 2003;7(3):277-288.
15. Fernández-de-las-Peñas C, Grobli C, Ortega-Santiago R, et al. Referred pain from myofascial trigger points in head, neck, shoulder, and arm muscles reproduces pain symptoms in blue-collar (manual) and white-collar (office) workers. *Clin J Pain*. 2012;28(6):511-518.
16. Mayoral O, de Felipe JA, Velasco S, Jimenez F, Miota J, Lopez P. Prevalence of Myofascial Pain Syndrome in Lateral Epicondyle Enthesopathy. Paper presented at: MYOPAIN 2010. VIII World Congress on Myofascial Pain and Fibromalgia 2010; Todedo, Spain.
17. Mayoral del Moral O, Gimenez Donoso C, Salvat Salvat I, Fernandez Carnero J. Puncion seca de los musculos del brazo, el antebrazo y la mano. In: Mayoral del Moral O, Salvat Salvat I, eds. *Fisioterapia Invasiva del Sindrome de Dolor Miofascial Manual de puncion seca de punto gatillo*. Madrid, Spain: Editorial Medica Panamericana; 2017:265-309.
18. Baeyens JP, Van Glabbeek F, Goossens M, Gielen J, Van Roy P, Clarys JP. In vivo 3D arthrokinematics of the proximal and distal radioulnar joints during active pronation and supination. *Clin Biomech (Bristol, Avon)*. 2006;21 suppl 1:S9-S12.
19. Gruchow HW, Pelletier D. An epidemiologic study of tennis elbow. Incidence, recurrence, and effectiveness of prevention strategies. *Am J Sports Med*. 1979;7(4):234-238.
20. Rossi J, Vigouroux L, Barla C, Berton E. Potential effects of racket grip size on lateral epicondilalgy risks. *Scand J Med Sci Sports*. 2014;24(6):e462-e470.
21. Carroll R. Tennis elbow: incidence in local league players. *Br J Sports Med*. 1981;15(4):250-256.
22. Roetert EP, Brody H, Dillman CJ, Groppel JL, Schultheis JM. The biomechanics of tennis elbow. An integrated approach. *Clin Sports Med*. 1995;14(1):47-57.
23. Abrams GD, Renstrom PA, Safran MR. Epidemiology of musculoskeletal injury in the tennis player. *Br J Sports Med*. 2012;46(7):492-498.
24. Gerwin RD, Shannon S, Hong C-Z, Hubbard DR, Gevirtz R. Interrater reliability in myofascial trigger point examination. *Pain*. 1997;69:65-73.
25. Mora-Relucio R, Nunez-Nagy S, Gallego-Izquierdo T, et al. Experienced versus inexperienced interexaminer reliability on location and classification of myofascial trigger point palpation to diagnose lateral epicondylalgia: an observational cross-sectional study. *Evid Based Complement Alternat Med*. 2016;2016:6059719.
26. Gerwin RD, Dommerholt J, Shah JP. An expansion of Simons' integrated hypothesis of trigger point formation. *Curr Pain Headache Rep*. 2004;8(6):468-475.
27. Groppel JL, Nirschl RP. A mechanical and electromyographical analysis of the effects of various joint counterforce braces on the tennis player. *Am J Sports Med*. 1986;14(3):195-200.
28. Hsieh YL, Kao MJ, Kuan TS, Chen SM, Chen JT, Hong CZ. Dry needling to a key myofascial trigger point may reduce the irritability of satellite MTrPs. *Am J Phys Med Rehabil*. 2007;86(5):397-403.
29. Papatheodorou LK, Baratz ME, Sotereanos DG. Elbow arthritis: current concepts. *J Hand Surg Am*. 2013;38(3):605-613.

30. Duparc F, Putz R, Michot C, Muller JM, Freger P. The synovial fold of the humeroradial joint: anatomical and histological features, and clinical relevance in lateral epicondylalgia of the elbow. *Surg Radiol Anat.* 2002;24(5):302-307.
31. Ruch DS, Papadonikolakis A, Campolattaro RM. The posterolateral plica: a cause of refractory lateral elbow pain. *J Shoulder Elbow Surg.* 2006;15(3):367-370.
32. Steinert AF, Goebel S, Rucker A, Barthel T. Snapping elbow caused by hypertrophic synovial plica in the radiohumeral joint: a report of three cases and review of literature. *Arch Orthop Trauma Surg.* 2010;130(3):347-351.
33. Wainner RS, Fritz JM, Irrgang JJ, Boninger ML, Delitto A, Allison S. Reliability and diagnostic accuracy of the clinical examination and patient self-report measures for cervical radiculopathy. *Spine (Phila Pa 1976).* 2003;28(1):52-62.
34. Anakwenze OA, Kancherla VK, Iyengar J, Ahmad CS, Levine WN. Posterolateral rotatory instability of the elbow. *Am J Sports Med.* 2014;42(2):485-491.
35. Coombes BK, Bisset L, Vicenzino B. Management of lateral elbow tendinopathy: one size does not fit all. *J Orthop Sports Phys Ther.* 2015;45(11):938-949.
36. Huisstede BM, Miedema HS, Verhagen AP, Koes BW, Verhaar JA. Multidisciplinary consensus on the terminology and classification of complaints of the arm, neck and/or shoulder. *Occup Environ Med.* 2007;64(5):313-319.
37. Descatha A, Albo F, Leclerc A, et al. Lateral epicondylitis and physical exposure at work? A review of prospective studies and meta-analysis. *Arthritis Care Res (Hoboken).* 2016;68(11):1681-1687.
38. Fernandez-Carnero J, Fernández-de-las-Peñas C, de la Llave-Rincon AI, Ge HY, Arendt-Nielsen L. Bilateral myofascial trigger points in the forearm muscles in patients with chronic unilateral lateral epicondylalgia: a blinded, controlled study. *Clin J Pain.* 2008;24(9):802-807.
39. Fernandez-Carnero J, Fernández-de-las-Peñas C, de la Llave-Rincon AI, Ge HY, Arendt-Nielsen L. Prevalence of and referred pain from myofascial trigger points in the forearm muscles in patients with lateral epicondylalgia. *Clin J Pain.* 2007;23(4):353-360.
40. Erak S, Day R, Wang A. The role of supinator in the pathogenesis of chronic lateral elbow pain: a biomechanical study. *J Hand Surg Br.* 2004;29(5):461-464.
41. Shmushkevich Y, Kalichman L. Myofascial pain in lateral epicondylalgia: a review. *J Bodyw Mov Ther.* 2013;17(4):434-439.
42. Gonzalez-Iglesias J, Cleland JA, del Rosario Gutierrez-Vega M, Fernández-de-las-Peñas C. Multimodal management of lateral epicondylalgia in rock climbers: a prospective case series. *J Manipulative Physiol Ther.* 2011;34(9):635-642.
43. Feneis H, Dauber W. *Pocket Atlas of Human Anatomy. Based on the International Nomenclature.* New York, NY: Thieme Stuttgart; 2000.
44. Naam NH, Nemani S. Radial tunnel syndrome. *Orthop Clin North Am.* 2012;43(4):529-536.
45. Goldman S, Honet JC, Sobel R, Goldstein AS. Posterior interosseous nervepalsy in the absence of trauma. *Arch Neurol.* 1969;21(4):435-441.
46. Rosenbaum R. Disputed radial tunnel syndrome. *Muscle Nerve.* 1999;22(7):960-967.
47. Cravens G, Kline DG. Posterior interosseous nerve palsies. *Neurosurgery.* 1990;27(3):397-402.
48. Spinner M. *Injuries to the Major Branches of peripheral Nerves of the Forearm.* 2nd ed. Philadelphia, PA: W.B. Saunders; 1978.
49. Chung KC, Lark ME. Upper extremity injuries in tennis players: diagnosis, treatment, and management. *Hand Clin.* 2017;33(1):175-186.
50. Dines JS, Bedi A, Williams PN, et al. Tennis injuries: epidemiology, pathophysiology, and treatment. *J Am Acad Orthop Surg.* 2015;23(3):181-189.

Chapter 37

Palmaris Longus Muscle

"Variant Vandal"

Wesley J. Wedewer

1. INTRODUCTION

The palmaris longus muscle is a highly variable muscle of the anterior forearm that, when present, is commonly observed in clinical practice to have trigger points (TrPs). It mainly functions to flex the wrist and tense the palmar fascia and may contribute to abduction of the thumb. Trigger points in this muscle refer a superficial, needle-like prickling pain that centers in the palm and extends to the base of the thumb and to the distal crease of the palm. Occasionally, the referred pain may include the distal volar forearm. Palmaris longus TrPs frequently develop in manual laborers, carpenters, and novice athletes who improperly grip their equipment. Patients often report pain in the palm and difficulty in handling tools or equipment. This muscle may be involved in several different conditions including carpal tunnel syndrome and Guyon canal syndrome. Modification of tools or correction of improper gripping techniques can help decrease stress and pressure onto the palm and is a critical component of management of TrPs in this muscle for laborers and athletes. Self-stretches to the palmar fascia and the palmaris longus muscles are effective for resolution of TrPs.

2. ANATOMIC CONSIDERATIONS

In its most frequent form, the palmaris longus muscle arises from the medial epicondyle of the humerus via the common flexor origin and from adjacent intermuscular septa and deep fascia. It is a long slender fusiform muscle with its belly located in the proximal half of the forearm between the flexor carpi radialis and flexor carpi ulnaris muscles. It becomes tendinous in the mid-forearm, and the long tendon overlies the flexor digitorum superficialis muscle. At the wrist, its tendon passes superficial to the flexor retinaculum. A few fibers leave the tendon and interweave with the transverse fibers of the retinaculum, but most of the tendon passes distally. As the tendon crosses the retinaculum, it broadens out to become a flat sheet that becomes incorporated into the triangular palmar aponeurosis (Figure 37-1).[1] The tendon stands out clearly when the hand is actively flexed and the palm cupped, because the tendon is superficial to the carpal tunnel and ends in the hand as the palmar aponeurosis (Figure 37-1).[2]

The palmar aponeurosis comprises two layers. A superficial layer of longitudinal fibers extends directly from the palmaris longus tendon at the wrist to the fingers. There, the fibers fan out in bundles to cover the flexor tendons of each finger and often of the thumb. Some of the superficial fibers attach to the skin of the flexor crease at the base of the fingers. Others continue into the digits to merge with the digital sheaths. The rest of the distal superficial fibers arch as bands transversely across the underlying tendons and muscles. The deep layer, which consists mainly of transverse fibers, blends with the transverse metacarpal and transverse palmar ligaments. The fibers of the two layers of aponeurosis intertwine.[3] A lateral slip from the palmaris longus tendon attaches to the superficial surface of the abductor pollicis brevis muscle, and this connection may account for a role of thumb abduction.[4-6] The palmaris longus muscle is occasionally absent on one or both sides and is anatomically highly variable.[7]

Variations of the palmaris longus muscle include congenital absence, unilateral,[8,9] or more commonly, bilateral[10,11]; reversal of the muscle belly-tendon relationship (tendinous at its proximal end and muscular at its distal end); a distally placed muscle belly[12]; a double-bellied muscle[6]; and a distally placed anomalous muscle that may demonstrate a variety of attachments.[1,6] The incidence of total absence or so-called agenesis is estimated at 15% of the global population.[6] There have been numerous studies that have objectively assessed palmaris longus muscle presence, and the results showed that its absence ranges between 1.5% and 63.9% among different populations.[2,13-19] Current evidence is conflicting, but there appears to be a trend that palmaris longus muscle absence is more common in women[6,15-18,20] and on the left side.[14,16,18] Bilateral agenesis presents to be more common as compared with the absence of just one muscle,[14,15,18,20] but evidence is contradictory.[2,13,19] One study showed a high correlation in individuals with palmaris longus agenesis to be left hand dominant.[21] Palmaris longus agenesis is postulated to be inherited as a sex-linked dominant trait.[6] Anomalies other than absence occur in approximately 9% of individuals.[12,22,23]

Palmaris longus muscle variations can contribute to painful syndromes of the forearm and wrist, including carpal tunnel syndrome and Guyon canal syndrome. Cases are infrequently reported, but when anomalies are discovered intraoperatively, they typically require surgical removal of the muscle to relieve patient's symptoms.

Several reports of patients having signs and symptoms consistent with Guyon canal syndrome were discovered during surgery to be due to having a hypertrophied accessory palmaris longus muscle.[24-26] An anomalous reversed palmaris longus muscle that entered the Guyon canal has been observed in several patients,[27,28] but it did not always cause symptoms related to overcrowding.[29]

Multiple cases of what appeared to be carpal tunnel syndrome were found to have a variation of the palmaris longus muscle in which the tendon passed beneath, rather than above, the volar carpal ligament.[30,31] A dual palmaris longus tendon, central muscle belly variant, was observed to cause median nerve compression in the mid-forearm.[32] Three other cases proved to have anomalous distal bellies of the palmaris longus muscle that compressed the median nerve against the underlying tendons.[33] The surgical decompressions described all produced successful outcomes.[30-33] A cross-sectional study examined the influence on the presence or absence of the palmaris longus tendon on median sensory nerve latencies across the wrist. Werner and Spiegelberg found the presence of a palmaris longus tendon did not influence the median nerve function across the wrist in 462 healthy subjects.[34]

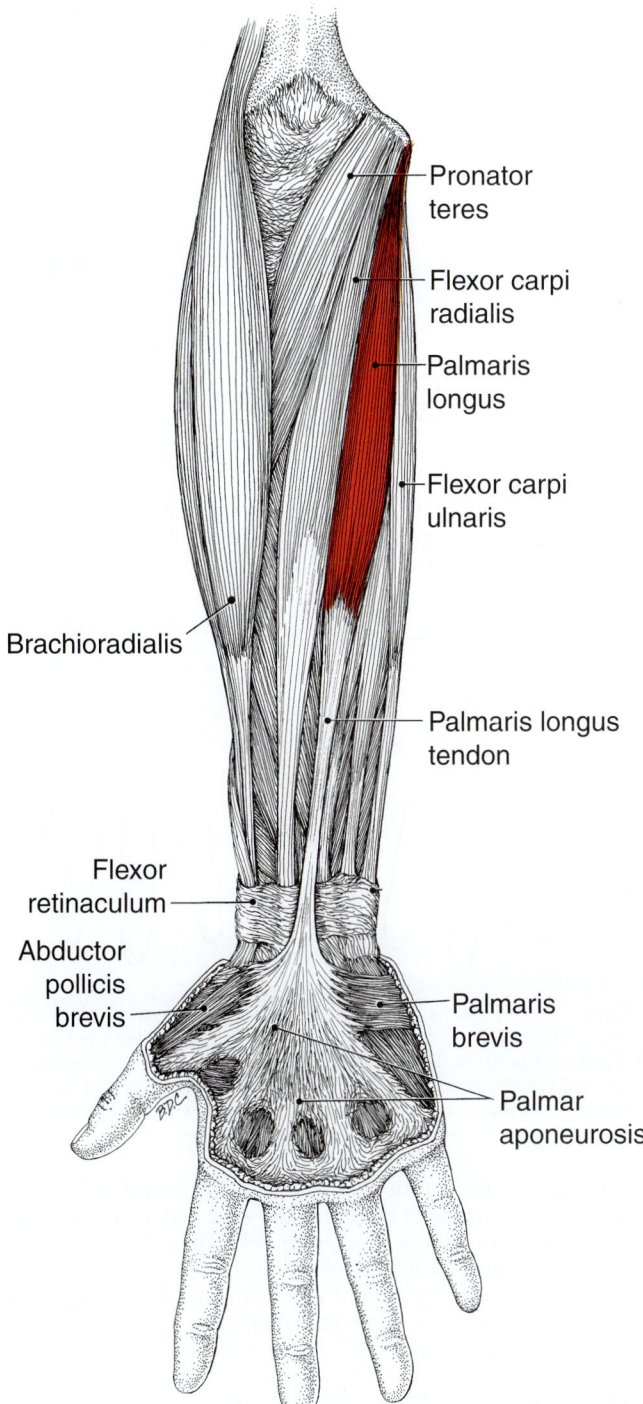

Figure 37-1. Ventral forearm muscles including the usual attachments of the palmaris longus muscle (red). It originates at the medial epicondyle, and attaches distally to the palmar aponeurosis. The superficial layer of the palmar aponeurosis has fibrous bands that extend into the fingers and often to the thumb.

The palmaris longus muscle is considered an accessory muscle and is not essential for normal muscle function. Therefore, the palmaris longus tendon is commonly used for various reconstruction surgeries because of its lack of importance in function, low donor site morbidity, and easy accessibility for harvesting.[35,36] Wehbé concluded that the palmaris longus tendon should be the prime choice for tendon grafts when a strong tendon is required.[36] Examples of its use vary to include ulnar collateral ligament reconstructive surgery in overhead athletes,[37] acromioclavicular joint reconstruction,[38] sternoclavicular joint reconstruction,[39] triangular fibrocartilage complex reconstruction,[40] interposition arthroplasty of the carpometacarpal joint,[41] and facial palsy,[42] among others.[7,43]

2.1. Innervation and Vascularization

The median nerve supplies the palmaris longus muscle through a branch from spinal roots C6-C7,[44,45] C7-C8 (the usual arrangement),[1,46,47] or C7-T1.[48] The median nerve forms from the union of the lateral root (C6-C7) from the lateral cord, and the medial root (C8-T1) from the medial cord that meet anterior to the third part of the axillary artery. The median nerve branch to the palmaris longus muscle is variable; it may penetrate the flexor carpi radialis muscle[46] or the superficial fibers of the flexor digitorum superficialis muscle.[49]

A small vascular branch from the anterior ulnar recurrent artery supplies the vascularization of the palmaris longus muscle.[1,50] A contribution is sometimes made by the median artery (a branch of the anterior interosseous artery)[1] or brachial[50] artery. The arterial branches penetrate the muscle through the posterior aspect, either through the proximal third or middle third of the belly.[50]

2.2. Function

The distinctive primary function of the palmaris longus muscle is to tense the palmar fascia and weakly flex the wrist.[1,47,51] It also acts as an anchor for the skin and fascia of the hand, stabilizing the structures against shearing forces.[1,7,16] This muscle may also contribute to abduction of the thumb.[4,20]

Functions of the palmaris longus muscle have been substantiated in the literature. Duchenne,[52] upon neuromuscular stimulation of the palmaris longus muscle, observed only wrist flexion without pronation or deviation of the hand to either side. Authors have consistently noted this flexor function.[44,47,49,51,53] Historically, Beevor[53] observed that the palmaris longus muscle contracted with the flexor carpi radialis muscle as the hand was pronated against resistance; others have agreed with this pronator function.[49,54] Pai and colleagues examined cadavers and concluded that the distal tendinous segments of the palmaris longus muscle appear to contribute to stabilizing the mobile end of the long axis, around which supination and pronation of the forearm occur.[22] Because of the muscle's attachment to the medial epicondyle of the humerus, some authors propose a possible weak flexor action at the elbow.[47,49] Although several secondary functions of the palmaris longus muscle have been proposed, the literature is inconclusive and is based off weak evidence at best.

Generally, the palmaris longus muscle's role is negligible, which is why it is used in many reconstruction operations without any cost to the function of the forearm or the wrist.[7] Absence of the palmaris longus muscle is not associated with a decrease in grip or pinch strength.[55] It has also been demonstrated that utilizing the ipsilateral palmaris longus tendon for ulnar collateral ligament reconstruction does not appear to compromise pitching mechanics in baseball players.[56,57]

2.3. Functional Unit

The functional unit to which a muscle belongs includes the muscles that reinforce and counter its actions as well as the joints that the muscle crosses. The interdependence of these structures is functionally reflected in the organization and neural connections of the sensory motor cortex. The functional unit is emphasized because the presence of a TrP in one muscle of the unit increases the likelihood that the other muscles of the unit will also develop TrPs. When inactivating TrPs in a muscle, one must be concerned about TrPs that may develop in muscles that

Box 37-1 Functional unit of the palmaris longus muscle

Action	Synergists	Antagonists
Wrist flexion	Flexor carpi radialis Flexor digitorum superficialis Flexor carpi ulnaris	Extensor carpi radialis longus Extensor carpi radialis brevis Extensor digitorum Extensor carpi ulnaris
Thumb abduction	Abductor pollicis longus and brevis Flexor pollicis brevis Opponens pollicis	Adductor pollicis Extensors of the thumb

are functionally interdependent. Box 37-1 grossly represents the functional unit of the palmaris longus muscle.[58]

3. CLINICAL PRESENTATION

3.1. Referred Pain Pattern

The palmaris longus muscle can exhibit TrPs in any part of the muscle. Trigger points in the palmaris longus muscle refer a superficial, needle-like prickling pain rather than the deep-tissue aching pain of most other muscles. This is similar to the platysma, which also acts primarily on the cutaneous tissue. The referred pain pattern typically centers in the palm (Figure 37-2). It can extend to the base of the thumb and to the distal crease of the palm but not into the digits. The prickling sensation feels as if many fine needles are producing it. The pain may also spread to the distal volar forearm.

3.2. Symptoms

In addition to pain, patients with TrPs in the palmaris longus muscle may report difficulty in handling tools because of soreness and tenderness in the palm, and the soreness may call attention to tender nodules there. The pressure of working with the handle of a screwdriver or trowel in the palm can become intolerably painful. For instance, a construction worker may be unable to firmly grip tools to secure a bolt or screw.

Most manipulative activities involve thumb abduction. Patients may report overuse symptoms from TrPs in the palmaris longus muscle after performing repetitive activities (eg, when playing a musical instrument that requires a wide span of the hand, such as when repeatedly striking a key on a piano with the thumb, or when performing a recurring manual task in a factory or on a computer requires a similar movement).[4] Overuse may be more pronounced when the activities are resisted.

3.3. Patient Examination

After a thorough subjective examination, the clinician should make a detailed drawing representing the pain pattern that the patient has described. This depiction will assist in planning the physical examination and can be useful in monitoring the progression of the patient as symptoms improve or change. For proper assessment and examination of the palmaris longus muscle, the clinician should first assess the general and resting hand posture, range of motion of the wrist and fingers, and the presence of the palmaris longus muscle. The palm and fingers should be palpated for nodules that may be associated with Dupuytren contracture (most commonly at the ring and little fingers) as a potential differential diagnosis.

To assess for the presence of the palmaris longus muscle, the patient should have his or her arm supported with the forearm supinated and elbow flexed before the patient cups the hand forcefully (Figure 37-3) abducting and opposing the thumb toward the little finger with the wrist partially flexed to make the tendon stand out at the wrist superficial to the transverse carpal ligament. The prominence of the tendon depends on the degree of wrist flexion or extension. This becomes evident when the strongly cupped hand is moved slowly from extension to flexion. Palpation of the muscle during contraction helps to identify variations of the usual structure. There are more than 10 different clinical tests that have been established and referred to in the literature to identify presence, absence, and variations in the palmaris longus muscle.[2,13,20,59-61]

3.4. Trigger Point Examination

Currently, there are no reliability studies specific to the examination of the palmaris longus muscle for TrPs. However, in other muscles, Gerwin et al[62] found that the most reliable

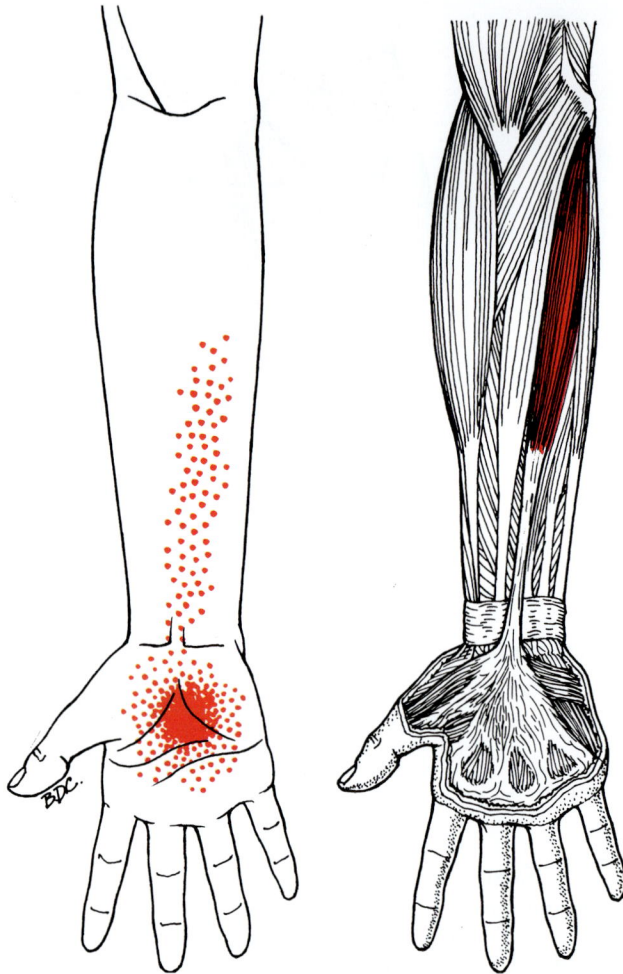

Figure 37-2. Patterns of the referred prickling sensation (dark red) arising from TrPs in a right palmaris longus muscle (light red) in its usual configuration. The referred sensation is described as a superficial painful prickle, rather than an aching pain. The belly of this variable muscle, and therefore its TrPs, may lie high or low in the forearm.

Chapter 37: Palmaris Longus Muscle

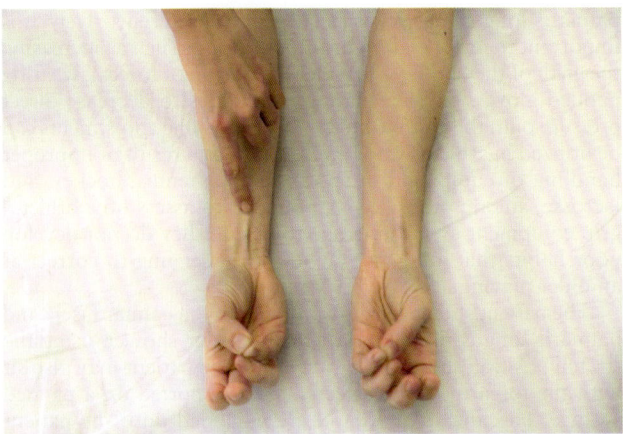

Figure 37-3. Identification that the individual has a palmaris longus muscle. Finger points to palmaris longus tendon in the right arm. Note its absence in the left forearm.

examination criteria for making the diagnosis of TrPs were the identification of a taut band by palpation, the presence of spot tenderness in the band, the presence of referred pain, and reproduction of the patient's symptomatic pain. Although identification of a local twitch response by palpation was unreliable, it is a valuable objective confirmatory finding when present.

For examination of the palmaris longus muscle, the patient can be seated in a chair with his or her forearm relaxed and in contact with the armrest. Alternatively, a supine position with the shoulder slightly abducted and externally rotated and the forearm relaxed on a pillow (Figure 37-4) may be assumed. Cross-fiber flat palpation is utilized to locate a TrP in the palmaris longus muscle. The TrP usually responds with a local twitch response seen as wrist flexion. Stimulation of this TrP by pressure often elicits the projection of referred prickling pain into the volar forearm and up to the base of the thumb and distal crease of the palm (Figure 37-4).

No nerve entrapments have been observed because of TrPs in this muscle. However, anatomic variations may cause median nerve entrapment at the wrist[30,32] or ulnar nerve entrapment in the region of the ulnar tunnel at the wrist.[25-28,63] In addition, increased tension and nodular enlargement characteristic of TrPs in one of these variant muscle configurations could aggravate entrapment symptoms.

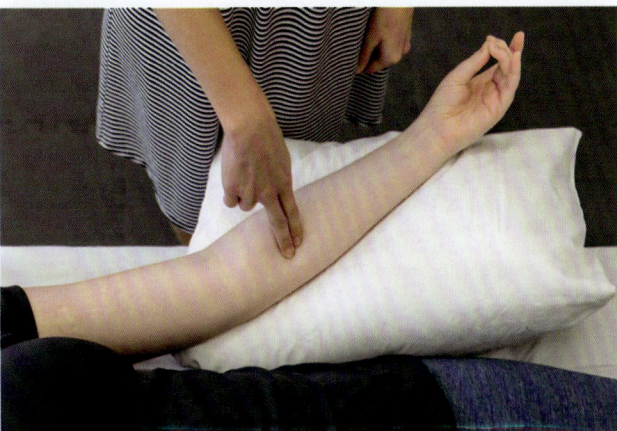

Figure 37-4. Cross-fiber flat palpation for TrPs in the palmaris longus muscle.

4. DIFFERENTIAL DIAGNOSIS

4.1. Activation and Perpetuation of Trigger Points

A posture or activity that activates a TrP, if not corrected, can also perpetuate it. Unaccustomed eccentric loading, eccentric exercise in an unconditioned muscle, or maximal or submaximal repetitive concentric loading can activate TrPs in any part of the palmaris longus muscle.[64] Trigger points may also be activated or aggravated when the muscle is placed in a shortened and/or lengthened position for an extended period of time.

In addition, TrPs in the palmaris longus muscle may also be activated by direct trauma, such as a fall on the outstretched hand. The use of a tool forcibly pressed or held firmly in the cupped palm can aggravate and possibly initiate TrP activity in the palmaris longus muscle. Examples include gardening and using a screwdriver or other carpenter's tools. Holding a tennis racquet with the end of the handle against the palm, and leaning on a cane with an angular, rather than a round handle pressing into the palm may also activate or perpetuate TrPs in this muscle. The novice worker or athlete is apt to maintain the palm in a more tightly cupped position for longer periods when holding equipment, whereas the skilled more experienced individual does not.

4.2. Associated Trigger Points

Associated TrPs can develop in the referred pain areas caused by primary TrPs. Therefore, musculature in the referred pain areas for each muscle should also be considered.[65] Muscles in the referred pain regions of the palmaris longus muscle are frequently associated with TrPs in the wrist and finger flexors. However, palmaris longus TrPs are rarely associated with TrPs in the muscles that refer pain to the elbow, as in "tennis elbow" or "golfer's elbow." Associated TrPs in the palmaris longus muscle may develop secondary to TrPs in the distal medial head of the triceps brachii muscle,[66] which can also refer pain to the region of the palmaris longus muscle.

4.3. Associated Pathology

Trigger points in this muscle are associated with or can mimic several different conditions; therefore, a thorough medical screening and examination are essential and a possible referral to another healthcare practitioner may be necessary.

The volar wrist and hand pain and tenderness may tempt some clinicians to diagnose the symptoms caused by palmaris longus TrPs as carpal tunnel syndrome. When the palmaris longus muscle anomalously extends under the carpal ligament, TrPs in it can cause a genuine carpal tunnel syndrome. Active TrPs in such a muscle would increase tendon tension and tend to aggravate the carpal tunnel symptoms.

In 2005, Wainner et al published a clinical prediction rule to aid clinicians in diagnosing carpal tunnel syndrome. The components include: (1) shaking hands for symptom relief; (2) wrist ratio index >0.67; (3) Symptom Severity Scale score >1.9; (4) reduced median sensory field of the first digit; and (5) age >45 years. The likelihood ratio was 18.3 when all five tests were positive and was 4.6 when at least four of the tests were positive.[67]

Electrodiagnostic examination of the median nerve is commonly used as the reference standard, with separate guidelines established by the American Association of Electrodiagnosis, the American Academy of Neurology, and the American Physical Medicine and Rehabilitation Academy to classify patients as having minimal, moderate, or severe carpal tunnel syndrome.[68] Interestingly, positive electrodiagnostic findings do not necessarily correlate to symptom development,[69] severity, or clinical presentation.[70,71] Therefore, diagnosis of carpal tunnel syndrome presents a clinical challenge that must incorporate clinical pain presentation and full clinical examination, and integrate imaging/electrodiagnostic studies as necessary. Because of its distinctive prickling pain, TrPs in the palmaris longus muscle are usually easily distinguished from carpal tunnel syndrome, but nonetheless, should still be examined in the event of a positive electrodiagnostic finding. Other painful conditions of the volar wrist and hand such as referred pain from TrPs in the flexor carpi radialis, pronator teres, and the brachialis muscles should also be assessed.

Patients with Dupuytren contracture may present with symptoms that could be confused with active TrPs in the palmaris longus muscle. In the case of Dupuytren contracture, dimpling over the palmar crease on the ulnar side of the hand is evident along with digital flexion contractures, most typically involving the metacarpophalangeal and proximal interphalangeal joints of the ring or little finger. Palpation of the palm during the early development of Dupuytren contracture reveals discretely tender nodules and patient reports of diffuse referred palmar tenderness, typically responding as "soreness" to the applied pressure. In contrast, the TrP-referred sensation has a prickling quality. The presence of digital flexion contractures, discrete nodules, and diffuse tenderness rather than a cutaneous prickling sensation enables the practitioner to differentiate TrPs from Dupuytren contracture. Conservative rehab for Dupuytren contracture is not warranted.

5. CORRECTIVE ACTIONS

Correction of aggravating activities is an essential first step for anyone who experiences pain during manual labor. Using ill-fitted tools such as a screwdriver or jackhammer with the end of the handle held directly against the palm can activate TrPs in the palmaris longus muscle, especially when used repetitively. It is important to make ergonomic modifications such as increasing the girth of the handle (for wider dispersion of forces), wearing padded gloves, and alternating techniques to decrease direct pressure onto the palm from the tool. The same adjustments can be utilized in athletes who develop TrPs as a result of improper handling of equipment in sports such as tennis, hockey, and lacrosse, among others. It is important to assess how athletes grip equipment at a young age to ensure they do not develop poor habits that are generally more challenging to correct at an older playing age.

The patient should learn to self-stretch the palmar fascia and palmaris longus muscle in a warm bath or shower, using the stretch position shown in Figure 37-5. The patient may also sit with the forearm of the affected side supported on a padded surface. The fingers and hand are extended until the patient feels a moderate stretch. Extending the forearm at the elbow normally does not add to the passive stretch. Simultaneously extending the thumb may increase further gains. As always, it is important to avoid stretching muscles to full range of motion in hypermobile joints. Patients with osteoarthritis in any of the joints in the thumb likely will not be able to tolerate the addition of thumb extension.

After stretching, the entire group of forearm flexor muscles, particularly the wrist and finger flexors, may then be stretched to eliminate any associated TrP involvement of parallel muscles (see Chapter 38). After inactivation of the palmaris longus TrPs, firmly extending the fingers and splaying the palm under warm water may stretch mild to moderate contractures of the palmar fascia.

References

1. Standring S. *Gray's Anatomy: The Anatomical Basis of Clinical Practice*. 41st ed. London, UK: Elsevier; 2015.
2. Eric M, Krivokuca D, Savovic S, Leksan I, Vucinic N. Prevalence of the palmaris longus through clinical evaluation. *Surg Radiol Anat*. 2010;32(4):357-361.
3. Agur AM. *Grant's Atlas of Anatomy*. 9th ed. Baltimore, MD: Williams & Wilkins; 1991:412-441.
4. Gangata H, Ndou R, Louw G. The contribution of the palmaris longus muscle to the strength of thumb abduction. *Clin Anat*. 2010;23(4):431-436.
5. Oudit D, Crawford L, Juma A, Howcroft A. The "four-finger" sign: to demonstrate the palmaris longus tendon. *Plast Reconstr Surg*. 2005;116(2):691-692.
6. Reimann AF, Daseler EH, Anson BJ, Beaton LE. The palmaris longus muscle and tendon. A study of 1600 extremities. *Anat Rec*. 1944;89:495-505.
7. Ioannis D, Anastasios K, Konstantinos N, Lazaros K, Georgios N. Palmaris longus muscle's prevalence in different nations and interesting anatomical variations: review of the literature. *J Clin Med Res*. 2015;7(11):825-830.
8. Murabit A, Gnarra M, Mohamed A. Reversed palmaris longus muscle: anatomical variant—case report and literature review. *Can J Plast Surg*. 2013;21(1):55-56.
9. Cope JM, Looney EM, Craig CA, Gawron R, Lampros R, Mahoney R. Median nerve compression and reverse palmaris longus. *Int J Anat Var*. 2009;2:102-104.
10. Heck L, Campos D. Embryological considerations on the bilateral reversed palmaris longus muscle: a case report in human. *J Morphol Sci*. 2014;31(1):58-61.
11. Salgado G, Cantin M, Inzunza O, Munoz A, Saez J, Macuer M. Bilateral reversed palmaris longus muscle: a rare anatomical variation. *Folia Morphol (Warsz)*. 2012;71(1):52-55.
12. Natsis K, Didagelos M, Manoli S, et al. Fleshy palmaris longus muscle—a cadaveric finding and its clinical significance: a case report. *Hippokratia*. 2012;16(4):378-380.
13. Gangata H. The clinical surface anatomy anomalies of the palmaris longus muscle in the Black African population of Zimbabwe and a proposed new testing technique. *Clin Anat*. 2009;22(2):230-235.
14. Ceyhan O, Mavt A. Distribution of agenesis of palmaris longus muscle in 12 to 18 years old age groups. *Indian J Med Sci*. 1997;51(5):156-160.
15. Raouf HA, Kader GA, Jaradat A, Dharap A, Fadel R, Salem AH. Frequency of palmaris longus absence and its association with other anatomical variations in the Egyptian population. *Clin Anat*. 2013;26(5):572-577.
16. Osonuga A, Mahama HM, Brown AA, et al. The Prevalence of Palmaris Longus Agenesis Among the Ganaian Population. *Asian Pac J Trop Dis*. 2012;2 (suppl 2):S887-S889.
17. Sater MS, Dharap AS, Abu-Hijleh MF. The prevalence of absence of the palmaris longus muscle in the Bahraini population. *Clin Anat*. 2010;23(8):956-961.
18. Thompson NW, Mockford BJ, Cran GW. Absence of the palmaris longus muscle: a population study. *Ulster Med J*. 2001;70(1):22-24.
19. Venter G, Van Schoor AN, Bosman MC. Degenerative trends of the palmaris longus muscle in a South African population. *Clin Anat*. 2014;27(2):222-226.

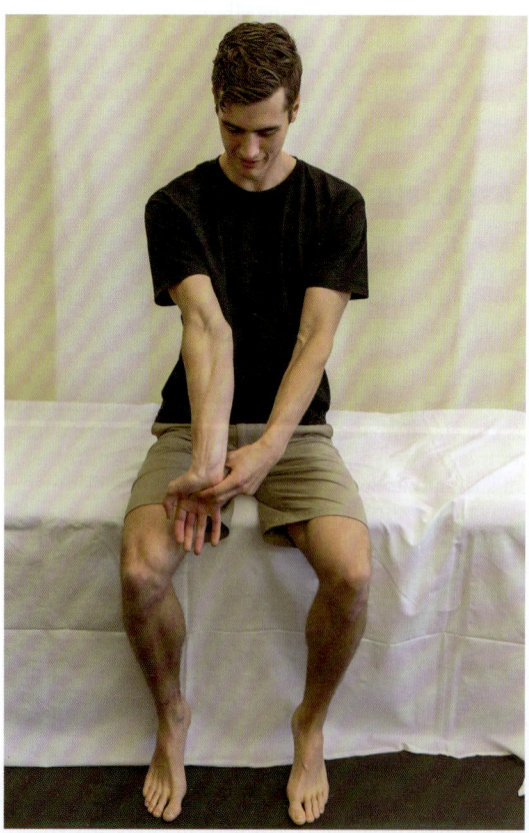

Figure 37-5. Self-stretch position for the palmaris longus muscle. To fully stretch the muscle, the patient simultaneously extends his or her fingers and hand at the wrist. Adducting the thumb with his or her contralateral index finger can enhance the stretch of the muscle.

20. Kose O, Adanir O, Cirpar M, Kurklu M, Komurcu M. The prevalence of absence of the palmaris longus: a study in Turkish population. *Arch Orthop Trauma Surg.* 2009;129(5):609-611.
21. Abdolahzadeh Lahiji F, Ashoori K, Dahmardehei M. Prevalence of palmaris longus agenesis in a hospital in Iran. *Arch Iran Med.* 2013;16(3):187-188.
22. Pai MM, Prabhu LV, Nayak SR, et al. The palmaris longus muscle: its anatomic variations and functional morphology. *Rom J Morphol Embryol.* 2008;49(2):215-217.
23. Tiengo C, Macchi V, Stecco C, Bassetto F, De Caro R. Epifascial accessory palmaris longus muscle. *Clin Anat.* 2006;19(6):554-557.
24. Barkats N. Hypertrophy of palmaris longus muscle, a rare anatomic aberration. *Folia Morphol (Warsz).* 2015;74(2):262-264.
25. Lal RA, Raj S. Guyon's canal syndrome due to accessory palmaris longus muscle: aetiological classification: a case report. *Cases J.* 2009;2:9146.
26. Santoro TD, Matloub HS, Gosain AK. Ulnar nerve compression by an anomalous muscle following carpal tunnel release: a case report. *J Hand Surg Am.* 2000;25(4):740-744.
27. Bhashyam AR, Harper CM, Iorio ML. Reversed palmaris longus muscle causing volar forearm pain and ulnar nerve paresthesia. *J Hand Surg Am.* 2017;42(4):298.e291-298.e295.
28. Lisanti M, Rosati M, Maltinti M. Ulnar nerve entrapment in Guyon's tunnel by an anomalous palmaris longus muscle with a persisting median artery. *Acta Orthop Belg.* 2001;67(4):399-402.
29. Ogun TC, Karalezli N, Ogun CO. The concomitant presence of two anomalous muscles in the forearm. *Hand (N Y).* 2007;2(3):120-122.
30. Christos L, Konstantinos N, Evagelos P. Revision of carpal tunnel release due to palmaris longus profundus. *Case Rep Orthop.* 2015;2015:616051.
31. Brones MF, Wilgis EF. Anatomical variations of the palmaris longus, causing carpal tunnel syndrome: case reports. *Plast Reconstr Surg.* 1978;62(5):798-800.
32. Markeson D, Basu I, Kulkarni MK. The dual tendon palmaris longus variant causing dynamic median nerve compression in the forearm. *J Plast Reconstr Aesthet Surg.* 2012;65(8):e220-e222.
33. Backhouse KM, Churchill-Davidson D. Anomalous palmaris longus muscle producing carpal tunnel-like compression. *Hand.* 1975;7(1):22-24.
34. Werner RA, Spiegelberg T. Does the presence of the palmaris longus tendon influence median nerve function? *Muscle Nerve.* 2012;45(6):895-896.
35. Jakubietz MG, Jakubietz DF, Gruenert JG, Zahn R, Meffert RH, Jakubietz RG. Adequacy of palmaris longus and plantaris tendons for tendon grafting. *J Hand Surg Am.* 2011;36(4):695-698.
36. Wehbe MA. Tendon graft donor sites. *J Hand Surg Am.* 1992;17(6):1130-1132.
37. Langer P, Fadale P, Hulstyn M. Evolution of the treatment options of ulnar collateral ligament injuries of the elbow. *Br J Sports Med.* 2006;40(6):499-506.
38. Gogna P, Mukhopadhyay R, Singh A, et al. Mini incision acromio-clavicular joint reconstruction using palmaris longus tendon graft. *Musculoskelet Surg.* 2015;99(1):33-37.
39. Bak K, Fogh K. Reconstruction of the chronic anterior unstable sternoclavicular joint using a tendon autograft: medium-term to long-term follow-up results. *J Shoulder Elbow Surg.* 2014;23(2):245-250.
40. Bain GI, Eng K, Lee YC, McGuire D, Zumstein M. Reconstruction of chronic foveal TFCC tears with an autologous tendon graft. *J Wrist Surg.* 2015;4(1):9-14.
41. Pegoli L, Parolo C, Ogawa T, Toh S, Pajardi G. Arthroscopic evaluation and treatment by tendon interpositional arthroplasty of first carpometacarpal joint arthritis. *Hand Surg.* 2007;12(1):35-39.
42. Toyserkani NM, Bakholdt V, Sorensen JA. Using a double-layered palmaris longus tendon for suspension of facial paralysis. *Dan Med J.* 2015;62(3).
43. Angelini Junior LC, Angelini FB, de Oliveira BC, Soares SA, Angelini LC, Cabral RH. Use of the tendon of the palmaris longus muscle in surgical procedures: study on cadavers. *Acta Ortop Bras.* 2012;20(4):226-229.
44. Clemente C. *Gray's Anatomy of the Human Body.* 30th ed. Philadelphia, PA: Lea & Febiger; 1985.
45. Rasch PJ, Burke RK. *Kinesiology and Applied Anatomy: The Science of Human Movement.* 6th ed. Philadelphia, PA: Lea & Febiger; 1978.
46. Hollinshead WH. *Functional Anatomy of the Limbs and Back.* 4th ed. Philadelphia, PA: Saunders; 1976.
47. Kendall FP, McCreary EK. *Muscles: Testing and Function, with Posture and Pain.* 5th ed. Baltimore, MD: Lippincott Williams & Wilkins; 2005.
48. Spalteholz W. *Handatlas der Anatomie des Menschen.* Vol 2. 11th ed. Leipzig, Germany: S. Hirzel; 1922.
49. Bardeen C. The musculature, Sect. 5. In: Jackson CM, ed. *Morris's Human Anatomy.* 6th ed. Philadelphia, PA: Blakiston's Son & Co; 1921:432.
50. Wafae N, Itezerote AM, Laurini Neto H. Arterial branches to the Palmaris Longus muscle. *Morphologie.* 1997;81(253):25-28.
51. Rasch PJ, Burke RK. *Kinesiology and Applied Anatomy.* 3rd ed. Philadelphia, PA: Lea & Febiger; 1967.
52. Duchenne G. *Physiology of Motion.* Philadelphia, PA: Lippincott; 1949:120.
53. Beevor CE. Muscular movements and their representation in the central nervous system. *Lancet.* 1903;1:1715-1724, 1718-1719.
54. Jenkins DB. *Hollinshead's Functional Anatomy of the Limbs and Back.* 6th ed. Philadelphia, PA: W.B. Saunders; 1991:125-127.
55. Sebastin SJ, Lim AY, Bee WH, Wong TC, Methil BV. Does the absence of the palmaris longus affect grip and pinch strength? *J Hand Surg Br.* 2005;30(4):406-408.
56. Fleisig GS, Leddon CE, Laughlin WA, et al. Biomechanical performance of baseball pitchers with a history of ulnar collateral ligament reconstruction. *Am J Sports Med.* 2015;43(5):1045-1050.
57. Azar FM, Andrews JR, Wilk KE, Groh D. Operative treatment of ulnar collateral ligament injuries of the elbow in athletes. *Am J Sports Med.* 2000;28(1):16-23.
58. Simons DG, Travell J, Simons L. *Travell & Simon's Myofascial Pain and Dysfunction: The Trigger Point Manual.* Vol 1. 2nd ed. Baltimore, MD: Williams & Wilkins; 1999:104.
59. Sankar KD, Bhanu PS, John SP. Incidence of agenesis of palmaris longus in the Andhra population of India. *Indian J Plast Surg.* 2011;44(1):134-138.
60. Kyung DS, Lee JH, Choi IJ, Kim DK. Different frequency of the absence of the palmaris longus according to assessment methods in a Korean population. *Anat Cell Biol.* 2012;45(1):53-56.
61. Kigera JW, Mukwaya S. Frequency of agenesis Palmaris longus through clinical examination—an East African study. *PLoS One.* 2011;6(12):e28997.
62. Gerwin RD, Shannon S, Hong C-Z, Hubbard DR, Gevirtz R. Interrater reliability in myofascial trigger point examination. *Pain.* 1997;69:65-73.
63. Regan PJ, Feldberg L, Bailey BN. Accessory palmaris longus muscle causing ulnar nerve compression at the wrist. *J Hand Surg Am.* 1991;16(4):736-738.
64. Gerwin RD, Dommerholt J, Shah JP. An expansion of Simons' integrated hypothesis of trigger point formation. *Curr Pain Headache Rep.* 2004;8(6):468-475.
65. Hsieh YL, Kao MJ, Kuan TS, Chen SM, Chen JT, Hong CZ. Dry needling to a key myofascial trigger point may reduce the irritability of satellite MTrPs. *Am J Phys Med Rehabil.* 2007;86(5):397-403.
66. Hong C-Z. Considerations and recommendations regarding myofascial trigger point injection. *J Musculoske Pain.* 1994;2(1):29-59.
67. Wainner RS, Fritz JM, Irrgang JJ, Delitto A, Allison S, Boninger ML. Development of a clinical prediction rule for the diagnosis of carpal tunnel syndrome. *Arch Phys Med Rehabil.* 2005;86(4):609-618.
68. American Association of Electrodiagnostic Medicine, American Academy of Neurology, American Academy of Physical Medicine and Rehabilitation. Practice parameter for electrodiagnostic studies in carpal tunnel syndrome: summary statement. *Muscle Nerve.* 2002;25(6):918-922.
69. Nathan PA, Keniston RC, Myers LD, Meadows KD, Lockwood RS. Natural history of median nerve sensory conduction in industry: relationship to symptoms and carpal tunnel syndrome in 558 hands over 11 years. *Muscle Nerve.* 1998;21(6):711-721.
70. Duckworth AD, Jenkins PJ, Roddam P, Watts AC, Ring D, McEachan JE. Pain and carpal tunnel syndrome. *J Hand Surg Am.* 2013;38(8):1540-1546.
71. Nunez F, Vranceanu AM, Ring D. Determinants of pain in patients with carpal tunnel syndrome. *Clin Orthop Relat Res.* 2010;468(12):3328-3332.

Chapter 38

Wrist and Finger Flexors in the Forearm
Flexor Carpi Radialis and Ulnaris Muscles; Flexor Digitorum Superficialis and Profundus Muscles; Flexor Pollicis Longus, Pronator Teres, and Pronator Quadratus Muscles

"Pseudo Golfer's Elbow and Gripping Gripers"

Johnson McEvoy and Joseph M. Donnelly

1. INTRODUCTION

The wrist and finger flexor muscles and the pronator muscles of the forearm are important muscles in power gripping and in fine dexterous movements of the forearm, wrist, and hand. The synergy between the forearm extensor muscles and flexor muscles optimizes the wrist position and hand grip for efficient movement and function. These muscles are involved in pain syndromes of the elbow, forearm, wrist, hand, and fingers. Trigger points (TrPs) in these muscles may be primary pain generators or coexist with other diagnoses. Activation and perpetuation of TrPs in these muscles can occur with gripping and repetitive hand actions. Symptoms may include pain, paresthesias, and dysesthesias in the elbow, forearm, wrist, and hand. Differential diagnosis includes medial epicondylitis; ulnar neuropathy; carpal tunnel syndrome; osteoarthritis of the wrist; C5, C6, C7, C8, and T1 radicular pain or radiculopathy; and median and ulnar nerve entrapment syndromes. Corrective actions include modification of activities (especially those that require gripping), self-pressure TrP release, self-stretching, and strengthening.

2. ANATOMIC CONSIDERATIONS

Wrist Flexor Muscles

The flexor carpi radialis (FCR) muscle[1] is subcutaneous and nearly centered on the volar side of the forearm between the pronator teres muscle, which crosses the forearm above it on the radial side, and the palmaris longus muscle, which tends to overlap it on the ulnar side (Figure 38-1A). This radial wrist flexor muscle originates from the medial epicondyle via the common flexor tendon and to the intermuscular septa. The muscle belly extends only to the mid-forearm. Its tendon inserts mainly onto the base of the 2nd metacarpal bone, with a slip extending to the base of the 3rd metacarpal bone.

The flexor carpi ulnaris (FCU) muscle[1] lies superficially along the volar side of the sharp edge of the ulna. It originates proximally by two heads: the humeral head attaches to the medial epicondyle of the humerus via the common flexor tendon, and the ulnar head attaches to the medial margin of the olecranon and to the proximal two-thirds of the dorsal border of the ulna through an aponeurosis shared in common with the extensor carpi ulnaris and flexor digitorum profundus (FDP) muscles, and to intermuscular septa. Distally, its tendon inserts onto the pisiform bone.

Finger Flexor Muscles

Proximally, the flexor digitorum superficialis (FDS) muscle[1] has three heads: humeral, ulnar, and radial (Figure 38-1B). The humeral head originates from the medial epicondyle of the humerus via the common flexor tendon and to the intermuscular septa. The ulnar head attaches to the medial side of the coronoid process of the ulna, proximal to the attachment of the pronator teres muscle, beneath the humeral head. The radial head attaches to the oblique line of the radius between the attachments of the biceps brachii and pronator teres muscles. The median nerve passes beneath the fibrous archway between the attachments of the ulnar and radial heads. This muscle covers most of the volar forearm, beneath the palmaris longus muscle and flexor carpi muscles (Figure 38-1B).

The tendons at the wrist, and to some extent the fibers of the FDS muscle, lie in a deep and superficial plane. The superficial plane carries tendons to the middle and ring fingers, and the deep plane carries tendons to the index and little fingers.[1]

Distally, at the first phalanx, each tendon of the FDS muscle divides to pass around the deep tendon of the FDP muscle, as each superficialis tendon attaches to the sides of a middle phalanx.[1]

The fibers of the FDP muscle[1] (Figure 38-1C) extend through the proximal half on the ulnar side of the forearm. The muscle originates from the proximal three-fourths of the volar, medial, and dorsal surfaces of the ulna to an aponeurosis shared by the flexor and extensor carpi ulnaris muscles, to the medial side of the coronoid process of the ulna, and to the ulnar half of the interosseous membrane. Each tendon inserts onto the base of the terminal phalanx of the respective finger.

The flexor pollicis longus (FPL) muscle[1] (Figure 38-1C) extends throughout the forearm under more superficial muscles, chiefly on the radial side. It originates proximally from the radius, the adjacent interosseous membrane, and by a slip to the humerus, and it inserts onto the base of the distal phalanx of the thumb. The belly of the FDS muscle covers both the deep finger flexor and the long thumb flexor muscles.[1]

Pronator Muscles

The pronator teres muscle[1] originates above and medially by two heads. The humeral head attaches proximally to the medial epicondyle and to the adjacent fascia. The ulnar head attaches to the medial side of the coronoid process of the ulna, and the median nerve enters the forearm between these two heads. The muscle travels distally and laterally and inserts onto the lateral surface of the radius at its midpoint in the forearm.

366

The pronator quadratus muscle is a deep flat muscle that covers the distal ends of the ulna and radius anteriorly. It originates from the anterior surface of the shaft of the distal ulna and by a strong aponeurosis that covers the medial one-third of the muscle. The muscle travels obliquely and downward to insert onto the distal aspect of the anterior surface of the radius.[1] Cadaveric studies have shown that the pronator quadratus muscle has a superficial head and a deep head.[2-4] The superficial head has a transverse orientation from the distal anterior ulna to the distal anterior radius. The deep head has an oblique orientation arising from the anterior surface of the ulna and traveling downward and laterally to insert onto the anterior surface of the radius and onto the distal radioulnar joint.[2-4] Sakamoto et al[2] describe two or more muscle fascicles with multiple arrangements both in the superficial and deep head in 80% of the forearms investigated. They also found a slip of muscle in 26 of 40 forearms that inserted onto the head of the ulna extending to the styloid process. They suspect that this slip of muscle would provide additional stabilization to the distal radioulnar joint.

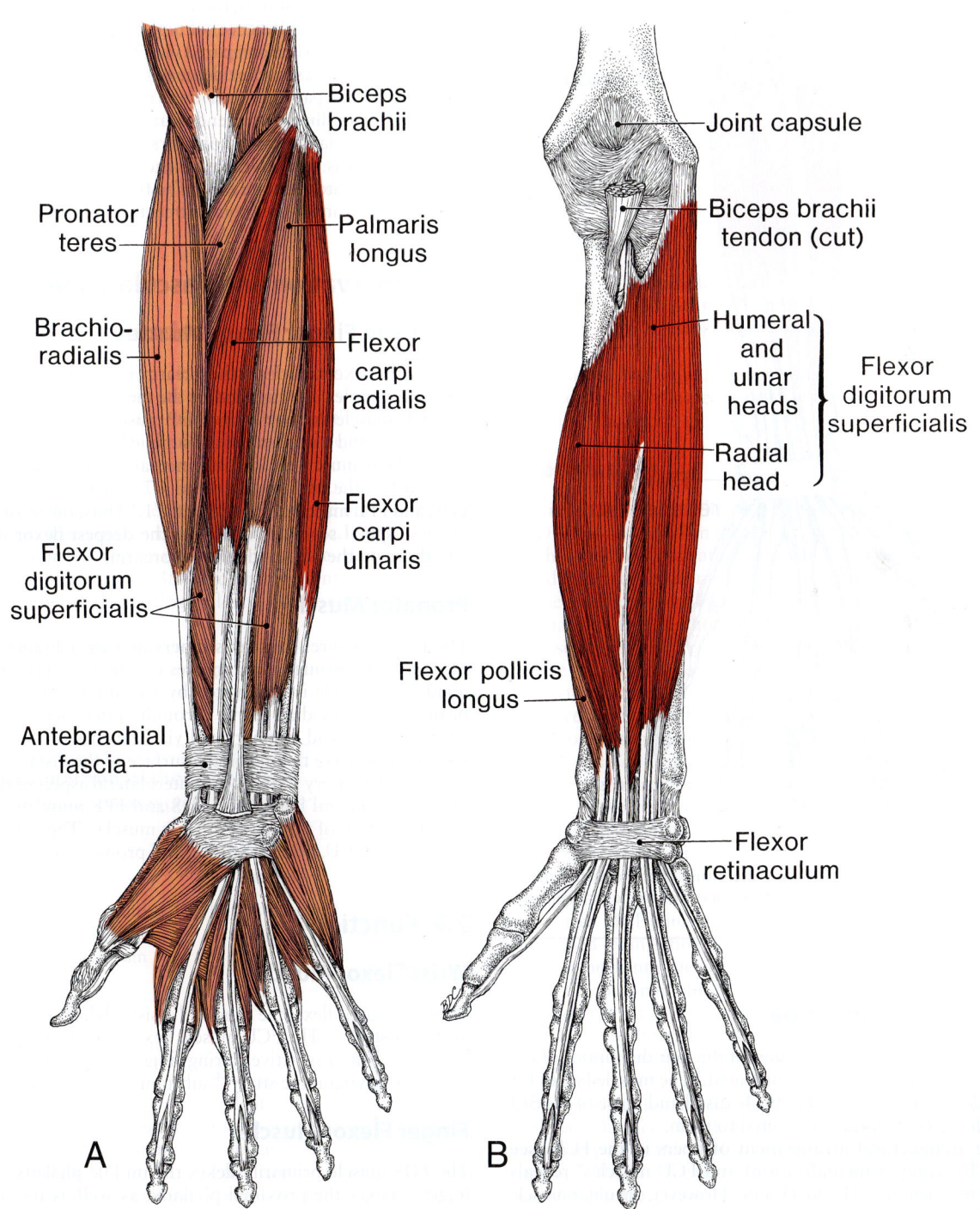

Figure 38-1. Volar view of the right upper extremity showing the attachments of the wrist and finger flexor muscles in the forearm. A, Flexor carpi radialis and flexor carpi ulnaris muscles are dark red, other muscles including the pronator teres muscle are medium red. B, Flexor digitorum superficialis muscle (dark red). The ulnar head lies unseen beneath the humeral head.

370 Section 4: Forearm, Wrist, and Hand Pain

Trigger points in the FPL muscle project pain throughout the volar aspect of the thumb to its tip (and possibly "beyond") (Figure 38-2C).

Pronator Muscles

Pronator teres TrPs refer pain deep in the volar radial region of the wrist and the forearm (Figure 38-2D).

Trigger point referral pattern for the pronator quadratus muscle has not been previously described by Simons et al.

Hwang and Kang[24] investigated the pain referral pattern of the pronator quadratus muscle in the nondominant arm of 35 healthy individuals using 0.3 mL of 6% hypertonic saline injection. They used electromyographic guidance for accurate placement of the injection solution into the pronator quadratus muscle. In 57% of the individuals, a pain referral pattern was reported from the injection site both proximally and distally along the medial aspect of the forearm. Fifty percent of these individuals reported that the pain spread as far proximally to

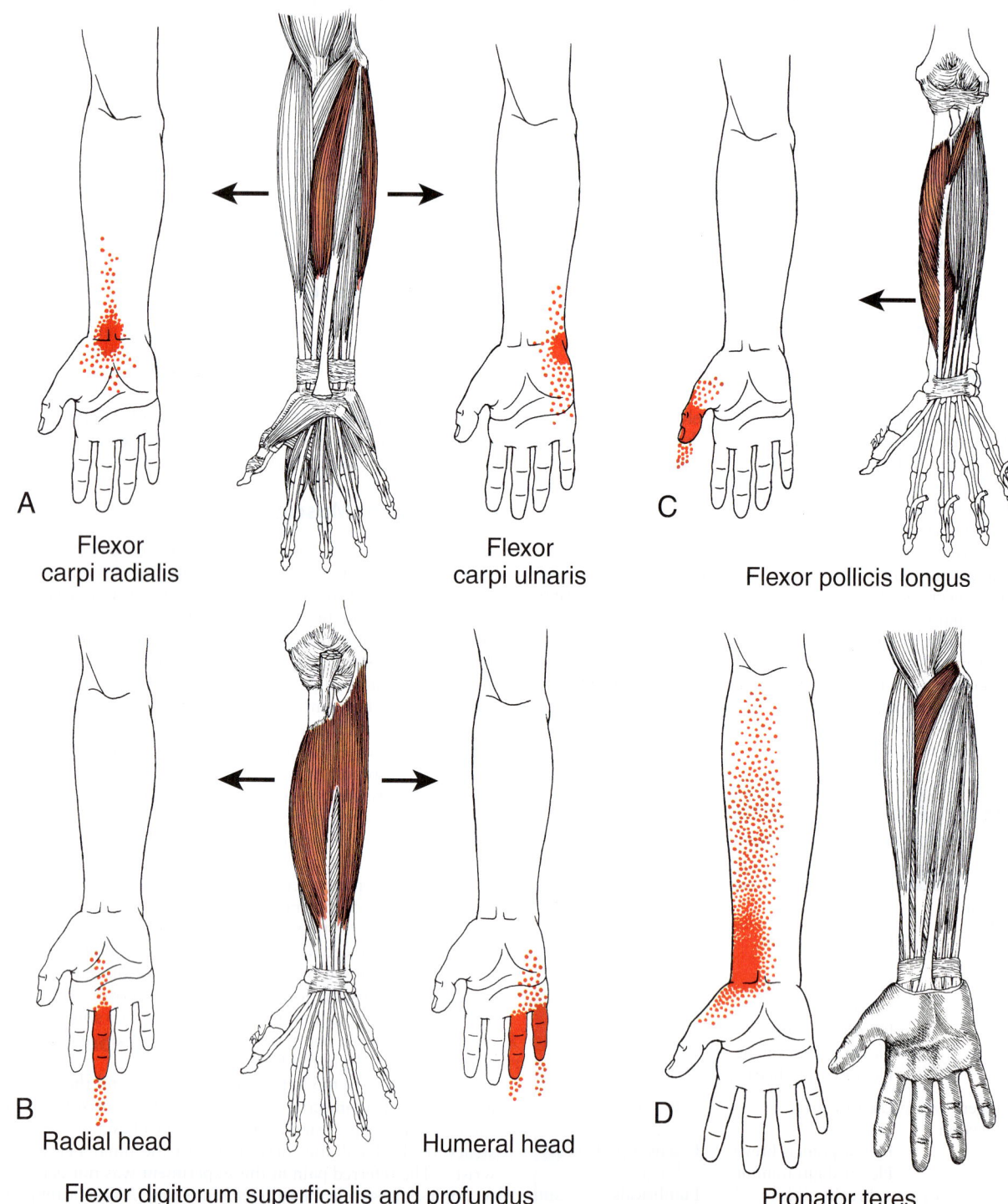

Figure 38-2. Composite referred pain patterns (dark red) in the right wrist and finger flexor muscles (medium red) for all muscles. A, Flexor carpi radialis and flexor carpi ulnaris muscles. B, Flexor digitorum superficialis and profundus muscles: left—superficialis middle finger pattern; right—superficialis 4th and 5th digit pattern and profundus pattern. The index finger pattern, not shown, is comparable. C, Flexor pollicis longus muscle. D, Pronator teres muscle.

Chapter 38: Wrist and Finger Flexors in the Forearm   371

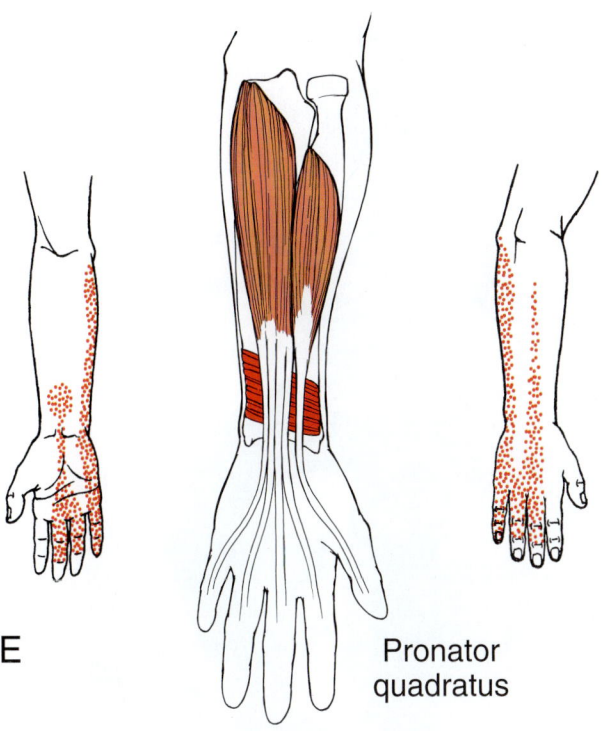

Figure 38-2. (*continued*) E, Pronator quadratus muscle.[24]

the medial epicondyle of the humerus and distally to the 5th digit. Twenty-nine percent of the individuals described a pain referral pattern from the volar and dorsal aspect of the mid-distal forearm spreading to the 3rd and 4th digits, both volarly and dorsally to the distal interphalangeal joints. The referred pain patterns from the pronator quadratus muscle resemble the C8-T1 dermatomal pattern as well as the ulnar and medial nerve sensory distribution (Figure 38-2E).[24]

In their illustrations of the referred pain patterns for all of these flexor muscles located in the forearm, Bonica and Sola strongly emphasized local pain in the region of the TrP and minimized pain referred to the wrist and beyond.[25] Rachlin, however, emphasized the more distal pain pattern of the FDS muscle but did not include the other wrist and finger flexor muscles.[26]

3.2. Symptoms

Patients with TrPs in the flexor muscles of the forearm report difficulty in using scissors for cutting heavy cloth, handling tools while gardening, or using tools that require stability and a forceful grasp. These symptoms are typically reported in the volar aspect of the forearm and/or fingers and may or may not be associated with lateral epicondylalgia because of the reciprocal role the extensor muscles play in grasp.

Patients with TrPs in the finger flexor muscles typically report increasing difficulty with fine motor skills such as writing, picking up coins from a flat surface, or other functional activities that require fine coordinated finger movements and grasping. When patients with TrPs in the finger flexor muscles are asked whether the pain is more on the top or underside of the finger, they may rub the volar aspect and reply, "I don't know." Where the patient rubs his or her fingers will lead the clinician to investigate either the finger flexor or extensor muscles.

Patients with TrPs in the pronator teres muscle are likely to be unable to supinate the cupped hand, as when coins are placed into it or when trying to use a screwdriver to loosen a screw or a jar in a right-hand dominant person. The combined motion of full supination, slight extension, and cupping of the hand becomes prohibitively painful because of the stretch and overload on the pronator teres muscle. These patients usually compensate by rotating the arm at the shoulder, thus overloading the shoulder muscles.

If a patient presents with signs and symptoms of a trigger finger, TrPs may be associated with but not be the primary cause of the presenting dysfunction. Pain produced by TrPs may be in the region of the trigger finger on the volar aspect of the thumb or first two digits.

3.3. Patient Examination

After a thorough subjective examination, the clinician should make a detailed drawing, representing the pain pattern that the patient has described. This depiction will assist in planning the physical examination and can be useful in monitoring the progression of the patient as symptoms improve or change.

Evaluation of the cervical and thoracic spine as well as neurodynamic testing of the median and ulnar nerves is also helpful in identifying any spinal contribution to symptoms felt in the forearm region. This assessment is important even if patients do not report symptoms that are directly related to the cervical or thoracic spine. Wainner et al[27] identified a test item cluster to determine the likelihood that a patient presents with a cervical radiculopathy. The following four predictor variables were identified: a positive Spurling sign, cervical rotation less than 60° to the same side, positive cervical compression test, relief of symptoms with axial distraction, and a positive neurodynamic upper limb test. Patients presenting with four of these positive variables have a 90% posttest probability of cervical radiculopathy. Patients with three positive variables have a 65% posttest probability of cervical radiculopathy.

Active and passive range of motion of the elbow, wrist, forearm, and hand should be carefully examined. When testing for TrP dysfunction, painful restriction of the range of motion is a better indicator of TrPs than is weakness. All of the wrist and finger flexor muscles can be screened for restriction at one time by fully supinating the forearm with the fingers (including the distal phalanges) and wrist fully extended. The long thumb flexor can be tested by extending the wrist and thumb. Hand-held dynamometer can be employed to objectify wrist and hand power grip.[28,29]

The finger extension test can screen both hands at once by first placing the fingertips of the right and left hands together (Figure 38-3A), and then pushing the palms tightly against each other while bringing the forearms into as straight a line as possible (Figure 38-3B). If there are TrPs present in the flexor muscles, they are revealed by a feeling of tightness in the muscle and pain in the pain reference areas specific to the involved muscles as described in Section 3 (Figure 38-2A to E).

Involvement of individual finger flexor muscles can be tested by passive extension of each digit first by extending the wrist and just the middle phalanx, and then both the middle and distal phalanges are tested for painful limitation of extension.

If weakness is an issue, individual muscles can be tested as clearly described and illustrated by Kendall et al.[12]

Accessory joint motion should be examined in the proximal and distal radioulnar, radiocarpal, and intercarpal joints, and also the MCP and interphalangeal joints of all five digits. Loss in accessory motion in any of these joints may lead to wrist, finger, and pronator quadratus muscle overload.[30,31]

3.4. Trigger Point Examination

Trigger points in the wrist flexor, finger flexor, and pronator muscles are easily examined with the patient side-lying on the affected side with the shoulder elevated, forearm fully supinated,

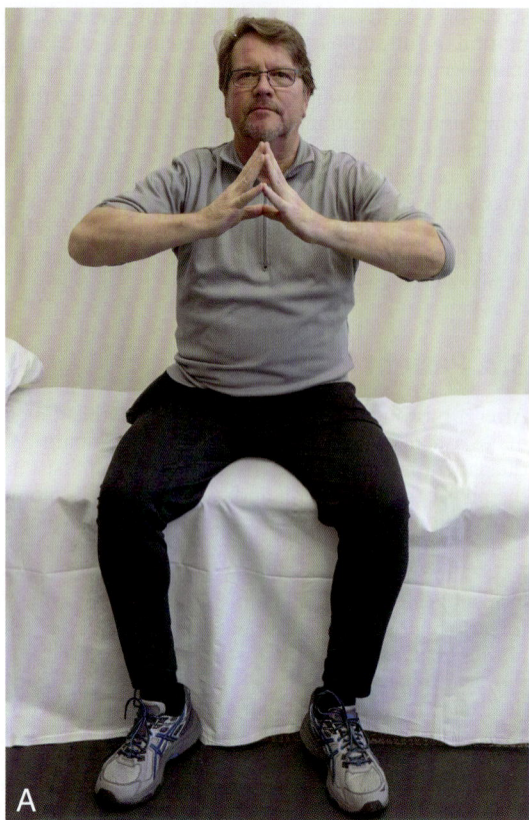
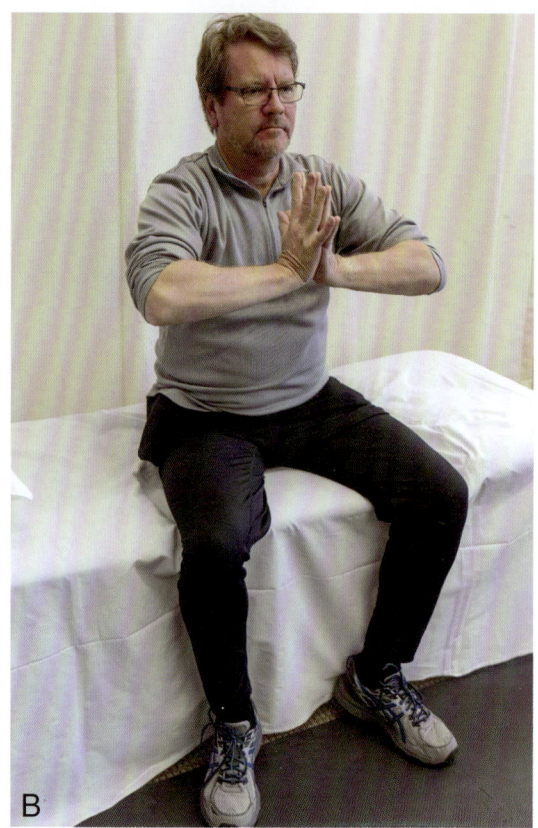

Figure 38-3. The finger extension test showing some tightness of the wrist and finger flexor muscles. A, Starting position. B, Nearly normal extension. The final position must have the palms together and both forearms in a horizontal line for a completely negative, normal test.

and the wrist and hand in neutral position (Figure 38-4A). If full forearm supination is not tolerated, a towel roll can be used to place the forearm in a comfortable position. Trigger points in the flexor muscles are typically located in the mid-fiber portions of the muscle bellies; however, the entire muscle should be examined. Both the FCR and FCU muscles are sufficiently superficial, and their TrPs can be identified by cross-fiber flat palpation (Figure 38-4C and E). FDS and FDP TrPs are identified using a cross-fiber flat palpation (Figure 38-4D) and are typically palpated together. Depth and location of the referred pain pattern assist the clinician in identifying the affected muscle. A monofilament needle or injection needle may be utilized to differentiate and identify the FDP TrPs from FDS TrPs. FPL TrPs are identified by cross-fiber flat palpation against the proximal volar surface of the radius (Figure 38-4F).

Pronator teres TrPs are identified with cross-fiber flat palpation near its origin at the medial epicondyle of the humerus (Figure 38-4B) or near its insertion on the radius at the midpoint of the forearm. The pronator quadratus muscle cannot be reliably palpated. A trained clinician can use a monofilament needle or injection needle to identify TrPs in the pronator quadratus muscle. A dorsal approach is encouraged to avoid the anterior interosseous nerve on the volar aspect of the muscle.

4. DIFFERENTIAL DIAGNOSIS

4.1. Activation and Perpetuation of Trigger Points

A posture or activity that activates a TrP, if not corrected, can also perpetuate it. In any part of the wrist or finger flexors or pronator muscles, TrPs may be activated by unaccustomed eccentric loading, eccentric exercise in an unconditioned muscle, or maximal or submaximal concentric loading.[32] Trigger points may also be activated or perpetuated when the muscle is placed in a shortened and/or lengthened position for an extended period of time.

Trigger points in the wrist and finger flexor muscles are not aggravated by the fine pincer movements that tend to activate TrPs in the intrinsic hand muscles but rather are aggravated by repetitive overload from gross gripping movements. The TrPs in the wrist and finger flexor muscles are activated and perpetuated by any functional or work-related activities that require excessive use through gripping, twisting, and pulling. The skier who grips ski poles hard for long periods and the carpenter who tightly grips small-handled tools are likely to activate TrPs in these muscles. Playing a musical instrument that requires grasp and fine finger movements such as the guitar, saxophone, or other wind instruments may also activate and perpetuate TrPs in these muscles.

The finger flexor muscles may develop TrPs as a result of driving a car with the fingers tightly gripping the steering wheel, especially when the hand grasps the top of the wheel so that the finger flexion is combined with wrist flexion. Symptoms are especially likely to occur after long, focused driving as is required in a rain or snowstorm. FDS and FDP TrPs may be specifically activated with sporting activities that require intense grasping such as tennis, golf, or rowing.

Activation of FPL TrPs causes symptoms that have been termed "weeder's thumb." These TrPs are activated by forceful rocking, twisting, and then pulling motions, all of which can strain the FPL and other thumb muscles.

The pronator teres TrP can be activated as a result of a fracture at the wrist or elbow. In addition, along with the pronator quadratus muscle, these TrPs can also be caused by rapid forceful pronation movements, for example, a "top spin" forehand technique used by high-level recreational or professional tennis

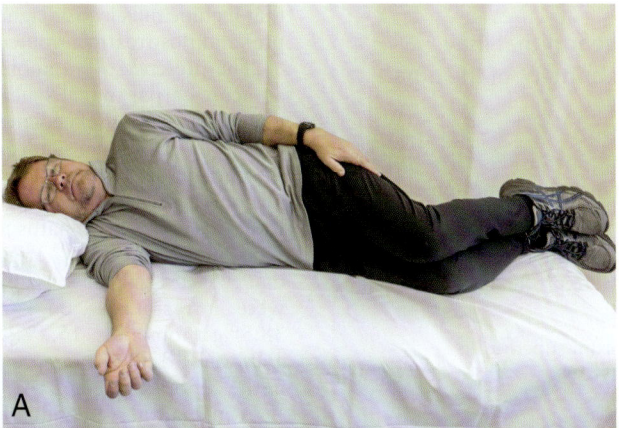
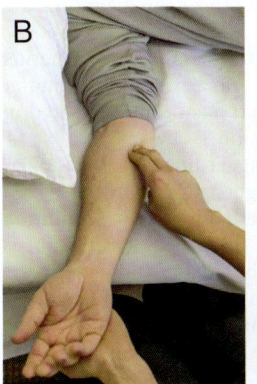 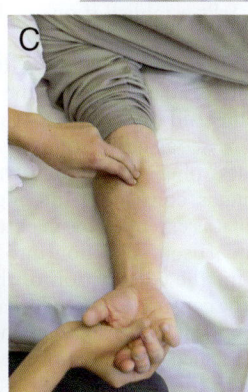 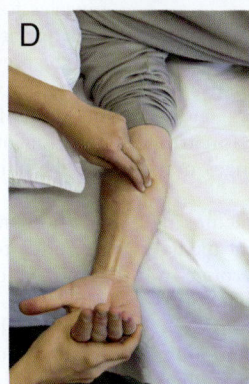 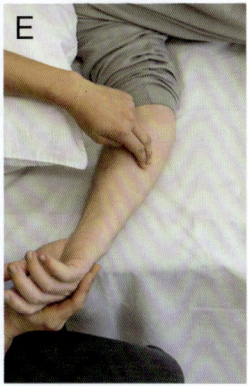 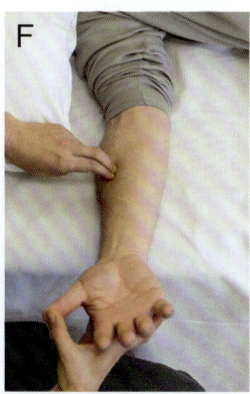

Figure 38-4. Cross-fiber flat palpation for TrPs in the wrist and finger flexor muscles. A, Side-lying with the volar aspect of the forearm exposed. B, Pronator teres muscle. C, Flexor carpi radialis muscle. D, Flexor digitorum superficialis/profundus muscle. E, Flexor carpi ulnaris muscle. F, Flexor pollicis longus muscle.

players. They can also be activated or perpetuated by loosening screws with a manual screwdriver for right-handed individuals, and tightening screws for left-handed individuals.

4.2. Associated Trigger Points

Associated TrPs can develop in the referred pain areas caused by primary TrPs.[33] Therefore, musculature in the referred pain areas for each muscle should also be considered. Trigger points tend to develop in the parallel FDS and FDP muscles together and in the FCR and FCU muscles together. However, TrPs may appear in the FCR muscle alone following an elbow fracture or comparable trauma. Associated TrPs may develop in the FCR muscle from active TrPs in the pectoralis minor muscle.[34] Associated TrPs may develop in the FCU muscle from TrPs in the pectoralis minor, latissimus dorsi, or serratus posterior superior muscles.[33,34]

Trigger points in the finger flexor muscles may develop as a result of TrPs in muscles of the shoulder and neck that refer pain into the volar forearm, most commonly the infraspinatus, scalene, and pectoralis minor muscles.

Trigger points in the FPL muscle tend to develop independently of TrPs in the other forearm flexor muscles.

4.3. Associated Pathology

Differential diagnoses that are commonly identified when TrPs in flexor muscles of the forearm are responsible for or contribute to the symptoms include medial epicondylitis, ulnar neuropathy, carpal tunnel syndrome, osteoarthritis of the wrist, C5 radicular pain or radiculopathy (when there are TrPs in the FPL muscle), C7 radicular pain or radiculopathy (with TrPs in the radial head of the FDS muscle), and C8 or T1 radicular pain or radiculopathy (with TrPs in the humeral head of the FDS muscle and/or the pronator quadratus muscle).[24] Erroneous diagnosis of thoracic outlet syndrome with active TrPs in the proximal part of the FDS or pronator quadratus muscles is possible, as some practitioners are prone to apply the term thoracic outlet syndrome to any disturbance of the 4th and 5th digits in the presence of a normal or nonfocal neurologic examination.

Medial common flexor tendinopathy (golfer's elbow) is basically similar to lateral common extensor tendinopathy (tennis elbow), as discussed in Chapter 36 under Associated Pathology.

Adaptive shortening and/or TrPs in the muscles of this chapter can contribute to entrapment syndromes in both the ulnar and median nerves. The forearm muscles serve as a structural interface for the course of the nerves as it travels distally to innervate target tissues. Trigger points may cause localized tension and fascial restrictions where the nerve travels over, through, or under these muscles and fascial components. Box 38-2 lists, for each nerve, the muscles that may be a source of or contributing factor for the patient's symptoms.

Entrapments or compressions correlated with the ulnar nerve are typically associated with muscles in the forearm and are likely to begin immediately distal to the condylar groove (cubital tunnel) that the nerve fills going around the elbow. Any entrapment within the cubital tunnel is often called a cubital tunnel syndrome and is classified as neuropathic pain. Symptoms of entrapment or compression commonly begin with a disturbed sensation in the 4th and 5th digits, including dysesthesia, burning pain, and a feeling of numbness. Hypoesthesia may also be present. Motor involvement leads to clumsiness and weakness of the grip because of neuropraxia in half of the lumbrical and the interossei muscles. The diagnosis is confirmed by delayed

> **Box 38-2** Muscles of the forearm that may develop TrPs that cause entrapment of the ulnar or median nerve
>
> | Nerve | Muscles that may cause entrapment |
> |---|---|
> | Ulnar nerve | Flexor carpi ulnaris
Flexor digitorum superficialis
Flexor digitorum profundus |
> | Median nerve | Pronator teres
Flexor digitorum superficialis |

nerve conduction velocity across, and to a lesser extent beyond, the point of entrapment.[35] The region of entrapment can usually be identified in this way as somewhere beyond the distal end of the condylar groove and within the first third of the forearm. Electromyographic data that show neuropathic changes may further localize the lesion.

The ulnar nerve exits the upper arm through the medial intermuscular septum, to pass through a groove behind the medial epicondyle (Figure 38-5A). The nerve is held in this groove by a fibrous expansion of the common flexor tendon that forms the roof of the cubital tunnel. From there, it enters the forearm beneath an aponeurotic arch formed by the humeral and ulnar heads of the FCU muscle,[36] commonly called the humeroulnar arcade. In 130 cadaver elbows, the arcade was identified 3 to 20 mm distal to the medial epicondyle, and the nerve then coursed through the FCU muscle for 18 to 70 mm.[37] The ulnar nerve then occupies the triangular space bounded by three flexor muscles: the FCU muscle covers the space superficially toward the ulnar side of the forearm, the FDS muscle is located superficially and radially, and the FDP muscles lies beneath, deep to the nerve.[38] The ulnar nerve continues through the proximal half of the forearm between the FCU muscle above it and the FDP muscle beneath it (Figure 38-5B).

Trigger points in the FCU muscle are most likely to be associated with entrapment or compression of the ulnar nerve. This entrapment may be caused by adaptive muscle shortening, myofascial tension pulling the humeroulnar arcade tight against the nerve, or by compressing the nerve where the nerve penetrates the muscle.

Clinically, TrPs in the FDP muscle also seem to contribute to ulnar nerve entrapment symptoms; however, the specifics of this mechanism are not clear. Symptoms related to TrP and localized tension leading to entrapment or compression causing symptoms of neuropathic pain are relieved by inactivating all contributing TrPs.

Median nerve entrapment or compression below the elbow will typically cause paresthesias, dysesthesia, and hyperesthesia of the 3rd and 4th digits, and occasionally the adjacent digits, and it is commonly called pronator teres syndrome.[39,40] The median nerve generally passes between the humeral and ulnar heads of the pronator teres muscle beneath the fibrous arch between the two heads but sometimes pierces the humeral head.[40] The nerve then passes beneath the aponeurotic arch of the FDS muscle that bridges between its radial and humeroulnar heads and clings to the underside of that muscle.[41] Adaptive shortening of fascial structures and/or local tension caused by TrPs might promote entrapment or compression of the median nerve in the pronator teres or FDS muscles through increased tension of the aponeurotic arch against the nerve or by direct compression of the nerve, where the nerve penetrates the humeral head of the pronator teres muscle.

Although clinical experience indicates TrPs can cause some of these entrapments, well-planned case studies of these conditions that include full electrodiagnostic documentation and adequate pre- and posttreatment outcome measures are sorely needed.

The presence of an anomalous FDS indicis muscle caused an acute carpal tunnel syndrome that was relieved by freeing the muscle from the median nerve.[42]

The carpal tunnel syndrome is likely to be diagnosed when the patient has TrPs in the pronator teres, FCR, and/or brachialis muscles. The referred pain from even more distant TrPs in trapezius and infraspinatus muscles can mimic a carpal tunnel syndrome diagnosis.[43,44] Trigger points in the respective muscles that evoked a tingling sensation in the hand in order of frequency were: infraspinatus, 65.4%; upper trapezius, 57.7%; FCR, 38.5%; rhomboids, 15.4%; and FPL, 11.5%.[44] Infraspinatus TrPs were 13 times more prevalent than carpal tunnel syndrome in the cohort studied.[44]

A median nerve conduction study and examination of the muscles for TrPs establish if one or both of the diagnoses are appropriate.

The presence of an anomalous FCR brevis muscle originating in the proximal radial aspect of the forearm and inserting at the base of the 2nd or 3rd metacarpal has been implicated in anterior interosseous nerve compression.[45]

The painless phenomenon of a trigger finger,[19] a "trick" or "locking" finger, consists of the finger sticking in the flexed position until it is extended by an external force. This condition responds to cortisone injection into the fascial sheath that is responsible for the constriction of the flexor tendon near the MCP joint. The constriction may ensnare a knot-like enlargement of the tendon itself. Such a fascial band that might anchor the tendon is described just short of the end of the distal palmar synovial sheath for digits 2, 3, and 4.[36]

Several techniques are available for noninvasive treatment of the trigger finger. Blocking or splinting the MCP joint of the affected finger in extension will typically eliminate or reduce the triggering. With the finger in the MCP extended position, the patient should flex and extend the interphalangeal joints while maintaining the MCP joint extended position. This maneuver mechanically limits the nodule from exiting the finger pulley system and often will eliminate "locking" of the finger.

Amirfeyz et al[46] report in a systematic review that there is moderate evidence to support the use of a cortisone injection early on in treatment; however, there is strong evidence that cortisone injection is associated with recurrence and ongoing symptoms at 6 months following injection. There is weak evidence to support conservative interventions or splinting for management of adult trigger finger. There is also strong evidence to support the management of trigger finger through percutaneous surgical intervention. They conclude that a cortisone injection may be the first line of intervention, but if symptoms recur, surgical intervention is the best option.[46]

5. CORRECTIVE ACTIONS

When prolonged gripping is required, as in tightly holding a ski pole or a steering wheel, lifting weights, or climbing, the patient should learn to relax the grip frequently. They should also be taught alternative strategies such as gripping with the palm down versus the palm up and stretching the flexor muscles at frequent intervals. Taking micro breaks or rotating activities can also be a useful strategy. Relaxation is aided by occasionally performing the finger-flutter exercise with a gentle shaking motion of the hands with the arms hanging down at the side to release tension. Grasping the sides of the steering wheel at the 9 and 3 position of a clock places the wrist in a more neutral position and is the recommended position for holding the steering wheel while driving by the National Highway Traffic Administration.

If the patient rows on a crew or paddles a canoe, he or she should fully open the fingers on the return stroke while holding the oar or paddle between the thumb and palm to relieve tension and to stretch the flexor muscles. For those playing racquet

Chapter 38: Wrist and Finger Flexors in the Forearm   375

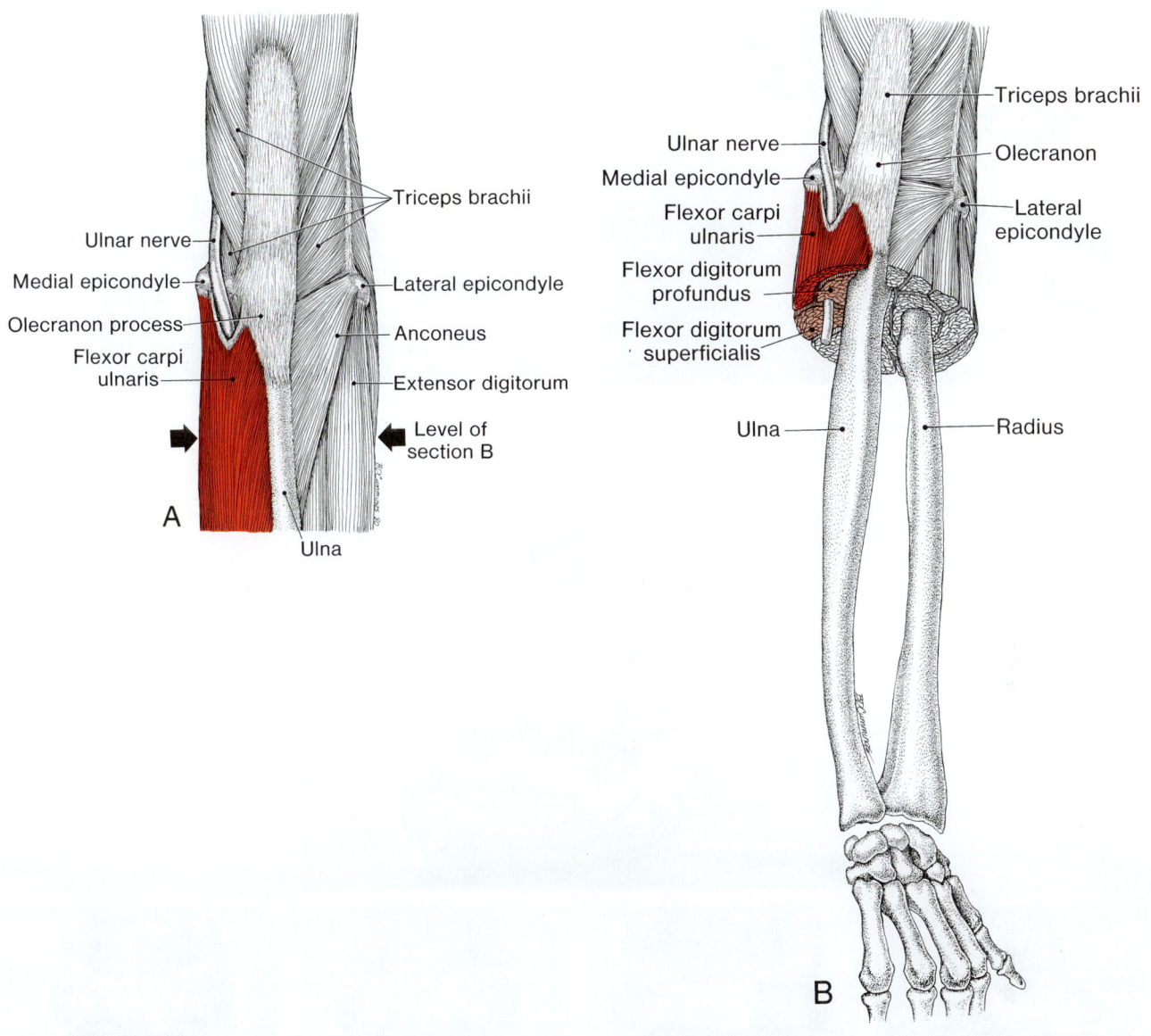

Figure 38-5. Dorsal view of the normal relation between the right ulnar nerve and the FCU muscle (dark red). A, The tendinous arch between the muscle's humeral and ulnar heads, through which the ulnar nerve passes, is called the cubital tunnel. B, Cross-section showing the relation of the ulnar nerve to the FCU muscle (dark red), and the flexor digitorum superficialis and profundus muscles (light red). The section is several centimeters below the elbow in the region of TrPs that may cause the nerve entrapment.

games, the wrist should be held in a neutral or slightly "cock-up" position and should not allow the head of the racquet to tilt downward (see Figure 36-5A). A patient with TrPs in the flexor muscles should learn to keep the wrist, as well as the forearm, supported on the armrest while sitting and not to let the wrist dangle over the end, thus avoiding leaving the wrist and finger flexor muscles in a shortened position.

Individuals who are required to work at the computer should take frequent breaks, especially with prolonged mouse or touch screen work as these activities keep the finger flexor muscles in a shortened position. Frequent breaks will prevent overload of the muscles that may activate and perpetuate TrPs.

Self-pressure release for TrPs in the wrist flexor, finger flexor, and pronator muscles can be performed in a sitting position by placing the forearm on the armrest of a chair or on a table with the palm up, using manual pressure (Figure 38-6A) or a TrP release tool (Figure 38-6B). For any self-pressure release techniques, the sensitive spot in your forearm is identified with the fingers, light pressure (no more than 4/10 pain) is applied and held for

15 to 30 seconds, or until pain reduces. This technique can be repeated five times, several times per day.

The patient can easily perform self-stretch techniques as part of self-management for TrPs located in the wrist flexor, finger flexor, or pronator muscles. Stretching of the pronator teres and pronator quadratus muscles should be performed with the elbow straightened and bent, respectively, with the palm facing up. The patient grasps the forearm above the wrist and gently turns the forearm into more supination (palm up) (Figure 38-7B). To stretch the wrist flexor muscles, the elbow is supported on the armrest and the opposite hand pushes the wrist down into extension with pressure on the palm of the hand (Figure 38-7C). To stretch the finger flexor muscles, the same procedure is used as in the wrist flexor muscles, but the pressure is applied into extension across the four fingers of the hand (Figure 38-7D). This technique can also be performed one finger at a time. The same procedure may be followed with the elbow straight to thoroughly stretch the wrist flexor and finger flexor muscles that have a humeral attachment. To stretch the long flexor muscle

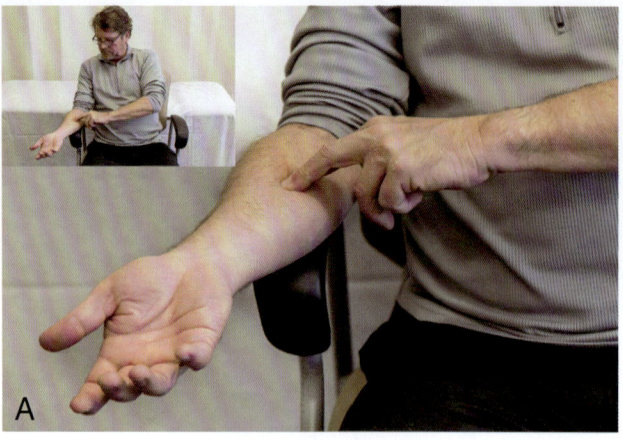
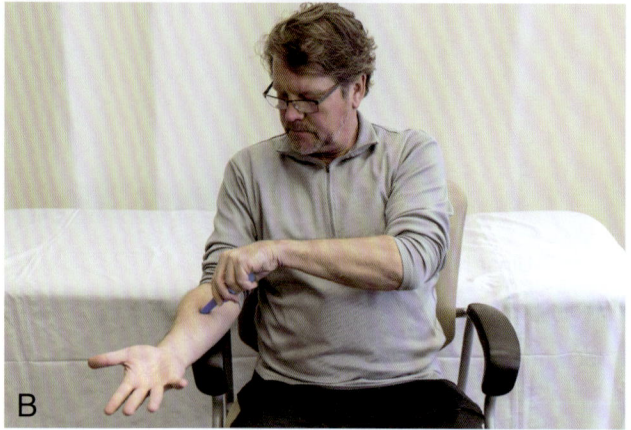

Figure 38-6. Self-pressure release technique for pronator teres, wrist and finger flexor muscles. A, Manual. B, Trigger point release tool.

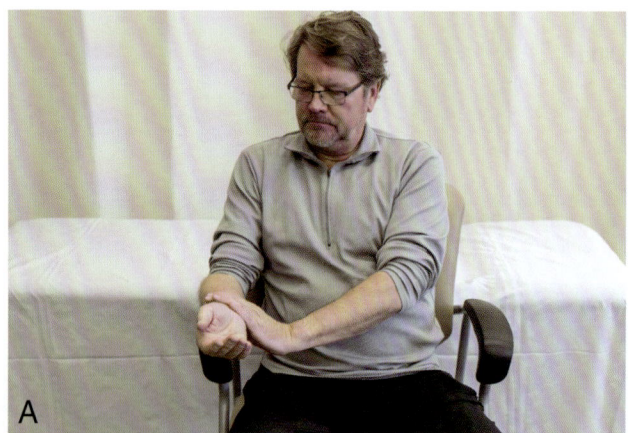

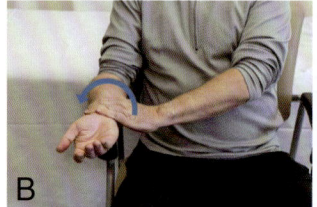
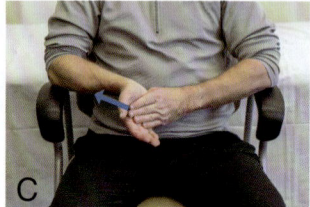
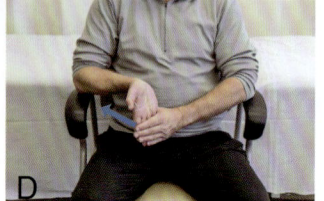
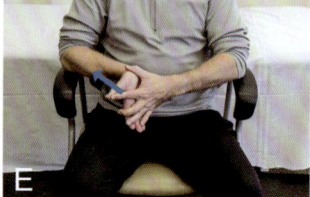

Figure 38-7. Self-stretch of pronator teres, wrist and finger flexor muscles. A, Starting position with elbow supported. B, Pronator teres muscles stretch into supination. C, Wrist flexor muscle stretch. D, Finger flexor muscle stretch. E, Thumb flexor muscle stretch.

of the thumb, the same procedure is used as in stretching of the finger flexor muscles with the addition of the thumb being pushed out and down with the index finger of the unaffected hand (Figure 38-7E). These self-stretches should be carried out gently, and attention to the reproduction of pain versus stretch is paramount. These stretches should not be painful, nor should they cause tingling or numbness in the hand or forearm.

References

1. Standring S. *Gray's Anatomy: The Anatomical Basis of Clinical Practice*. 41st ed. London, UK: Elsevier; 2015.
2. Sakamoto K, Nasu H, Nimura A, Hamada J, Akita K. An anatomic study of the structure and innervation of the pronator quadratus muscle. *Anat Sci Int*. 2015;90(2):82-88.
3. Stuart PR. Pronator quadratus revisited. *J Hand Surg Br*. 1996;21(6):714-722.
4. Koebke J, Werner J, Piening H. The quadrate pronator muscle—a morphological and functional analysis [in German]. *Anat Anz*. 1984;157(4):311-318.
5. Bickerton LE, Agur AM, Ashby P. Flexor digitorum superficialis: locations of individual muscle bellies for botulinum toxin injections. *Muscle Nerve*. 1997;20(8):1041-1043.
6. Lieber RL, Fazeli BM, Botte MJ. Architecture of selected wrist flexor and extensor muscles. *J Hand Surg*. 1990;15(2):244-250.
7. Lieber RL, Jacobson MD, Fazeli BM, Abrams RA, Botte MJ. Architecture of selected muscles of the arm and forearm: anatomy and implications for tendon transfer. *J Hand Surg*. 1992;17(5):787-798.
8. Segal RL, Wolf SL, DeCamp MJ, Chopp MT, English AW. Anatomical partitioning of three multiarticular human muscles. *Acta Anat (Basel)*. 1991;142(3):261-266.
9. Jozsa L, Demel S, Reffy A. Fibre composition of human hand and arm muscles. *Gegenbaurs Morphol Jahrb*. 1981;127(1):34-38.
10. Bonica J, Sola A. Chapter 52, Other painful disorders of the upper limb. In: Bonica JJ, Loeser JD, Chapman C, Fordyce WE, eds. *The Management of Pain*. 2nd ed. Philadelphia, PA: Lea & Febiger; 1990:947-958.
11. Rasch PJ, Burke RK. *Kinesiology and Applied Anatomy: The Science of Human Movement*. 6th ed. Philadelphia, PA: Lea & Febiger; 1978: 185-206.
12. Kendall FP, McCreary EK. *Muscles: Testing and Function, with Posture and Pain*. 5th ed. Baltimore, MD: Lippincott Williams & Wilkins; 2005:264, 280-283, 286.
13. Sano S, Ando K, Katori I, et al. Electromyographic studies on the forearm muscle activities during finger movements. *J Jpn Orthop Assoc*. 1977;51:331-337.
14. McFarland GBJ, Kursen UL, Weathersby HT. Kinesiology of selected muscles acting on the wrist: electromyographic study. *Arch Phys Med Rehabil*. 1962;43:165-171.

15. Basmajian J, Deluca C. *Muscles Alive*. 5th ed. Baltimore, MD: Williams & Wilkins; 1985:280, 281, 290, 294.
16. Weathersby HT, Sutton LR, Krusen UL. The kinesiology of muscles of the thumb: an electromyographic study. *Arch Phys Med Rehabil*. 1963;44:321-326.
17. Ok N, Agladioglu K, Gungor HR, et al. Relationship of side dominance and ultrasonographic measurements of pronator quadratus muscle along with handgrip and pinch strength. *Med Ultrason*. 2016;18(2):170-176.
18. Simons DG, Travell J, Simons L. *Travell & Simon's Myofascial Pain and Dysfunction: The Trigger Point Manual*. Vol 1. 2nd ed. Baltimore, MD: Williams & Wilkins; 1999:104.
19. Cooper C. *Fundamentals of Hand Therapy: Clinical Reasoning and Treatment Guidelines for Common Diagnoses of the Upper Extremity*. St. Louis, MO: Mosby, Elsevier; 2007:chap 15.
20. Winter Z. Referred pain in fibrositis. *Med Rec*. 1944;157:34-37.
21. Good MG. What is fibrositis? *Rheumatism*. 1949;5(4):117-123.
22. Good MG. The role of skeletal muscles in the pathogenesis of diseases. *Acta Med Scand*. 1950;138(4):284-292.
23. Kellgren JH. Observations on referred pain arising from muscle. *Clin Sci*. 1938;3:175-190.
24. Hwang M, Kang YK, Kim DH. Referred pain pattern of the pronator quadratus muscle. *Pain*. 2005;116(3):238-242.
25. Bonica JJ. *The Management of Pain*. Philadelphia, PA: Lea & Febiger; 1953.
26. Rachlin ES. Chapter 10, Injection of specific trigger points. In: Rachlin ES, ed. *Myofascial Pain and Fibromyalgia*. St. Louis, MO: Mosby; 1994:197-360, 342.
27. Wainner RS, Fritz JM, Irrgang JJ, Boninger ML, Delitto A, Allison S. Reliability and diagnostic accuracy of the clinical examination and patient self-report measures for cervical radiculopathy. *Spine (Phila Pa 1976)*. 2003;28(1):52-62.
28. Steiber N. Strong or weak handgrip? Normative reference values for the German population across the life course stratified by sex, age, and body height. *PLoS One*. 2016;11(10):e0163917.
29. Wong SL. Grip strength reference values for Canadians aged 6 to 79: Canadian Health Measures Survey, 2007 to 2013. *Health Rep*. 2016;27(10):3-10.
30. Mennell JM. *Joint Pain: Diagnosis and Treatment Using Manipulative Techniques*. 1st ed. Boston, MA: Little Brown; 1964.
31. Lewit K. *Manipulative Therapy in Rehabilitation of the Locomotor System*. 3rd ed. Oxford, England: Butterworth Heinemann; 1999.
32. Gerwin RD, Dommerholt J, Shah JP. An expansion of Simons' integrated hypothesis of trigger point formation. *Curr Pain Headache Rep*. 2004;8(6):468-475.
33. Hsieh YL, Kao MJ, Kuan TS, Chen SM, Chen JT, Hong CZ. Dry needling to a key myofascial trigger point may reduce the irritability of satellite MTrPs. *Am J Phys Med Rehabil*. 2007;86(5):397-403.
34. Hong C-Z. Considerations and recommendations regarding myofascial trigger point injection. *J Musculoske Pain*. 1994;2(1):29-59.
35. Kanakamedala RV, Simons DG, Porter RW, Zucker RS. Ulnar nerve entrapment at the elbow localized by short segment stimulation. *Arch Phys Med Rehabil*. 1988;69(11):959-963.
36. Clemente C. *Gray's Anatomy of the Human Body*. 30th ed. Philadelphia, PA: Lea & Febiger; 1985:532-535.
37. Campbell WW, Pridgeon RM, Riaz G, Astruc J, Sahni KS. Variations in anatomy of the ulnar nerve at the cubital tunnel: pitfalls in the diagnosis of ulnar neuropathy at the elbow. *Muscle Nerve*. 1991;14(8):733-738.
38. Carter B, Morehead J, Wolpert S, al e. *Cross-Sectional Anatomy*. New York, NY: Appleton-Century-Crofts; 1977:sections 53-58.
39. Bayerl W, Fischer K. The pronator teres syndrome. Clinical aspects, pathogenesis and therapy of a non-traumatic median nerve compression syndrome in the space of the elbow joint [in German]. *Handchirurgie*. 1979;11(2):91-98.
40. Fuss FK, Wurzl GH. Median nerve entrapment. Pronator teres syndrome. Surgical anatomy and correlation with symptom patterns. *Surg Radiol Anat*. 1990;12(4):267-271.
41. Agur AM. *Grant's Atlas of Anatomy*, 9th ed. Baltimore, MD: Williams & Wilkins; 1991.
42. al-Qattan MM, Duerksen F. A variant of flexor carpi ulnaris causing ulnar nerve compression. *J Anat*. 1992;180 (pt 1):189-190.
43. Qerama E, Kasch H, Fuglsang-Frederiksen A. Occurrence of myofascial pain in patients with possible carpal tunnel syndrome—a single-blinded study. *Eur J Pain*. 2009;13(6):588-591.
44. Oh S, Kim HK, Kwak J, et al. Causes of hand tingling in visual display terminal workers. *Ann Rehabil Med*. 2013;37(2):221-228.
45. Lahey MD, Aulicino PL. Anomalous muscles associated with compression neuropathies. *Orthop Rev*. 1986;15(4):199-208.
46. Amirfeyz R, McNinch R, Watts A, et al. Evidence-based management of adult trigger digits. *J Hand Surg Eur Vol*. 2017;42(5):473-480.

Chapter 39

Adductor and Opponens Pollicis Muscles

"Clumsy Thumb"

Johnson McEvoy and Joseph M. Donnelly

1. INTRODUCTION

The adductor pollicis and opponens pollicis muscles are intrinsic muscles of the hand and along with the flexor pollicis brevis and abductor pollicis brevis muscles make up the thenar muscle group. The adductor pollicis and opponens pollicis muscles are important for gripping and fine dexterous movements between the thumb and fingers. The synergy between the thumb and fingers is important in human hand function, fine motor skills, power and pincer gripping. It is also a vital component of activities of daily living and of occupational, recreational, and sporting activities. Pain from trigger points (TrPs) is referred over the distal radial wrist and hand. In addition to pain, patients will report a feeling of clumsiness and difficulty with fine motor movements of the thumb and hand. Activation and perpetuation of TrPs in these muscles can result from repetitive or forceful gripping actions and fine motor activities such as typing, moussing, or phone usage. Differential diagnosis includes cervical radicular pain or radiculopathy, local wrist and thumb joint dysfunction, and osteoarthritis. Corrective actions include modification of activities, ergonomics assessment and training, TrP self-pressure release, self-stretch, and strengthening of the upper extremity and hand muscles.

2. ANATOMIC CONSIDERATIONS

Adductor Pollicis

The adductor pollicis muscle is the largest and most powerful of the intrinsic hand muscles.[1] The adductor pollicis muscle spans the web space between the thumb and index finger. Both the oblique and transverse heads lie beneath (dorsal to) the tendon of the flexor pollicis longus muscle and originate laterally to the ulnar side of the base of the proximal phalanx of the thumb (Figure 39-1A) along with the flexor pollicis brevis and abductor pollicis brevis muscles (Figure 39-2B). Medially, the oblique head of the adductor pollicis muscle inserts into the bases of the 2nd and 3rd metacarpals and to the capitate bone. The transverse head inserts medially onto the distal two-thirds of the palmar surface of the 3rd metacarpal bone (Figure 39-2A).[1]

Opponens Pollicis

The opponens pollicis muscle originates medially to a tubercle of the trapezium bone of the wrist and to the flexor retinaculum, and it inserts laterally and distally along the whole length of the radial side and the adjoining lateral half of the palmar surface of the 1st metacarpal bone (Figure 39-1A).[1]

This muscle lies partly under the abductor pollicis brevis muscle and between the superficial and deep heads of the flexor pollicis brevis muscle (Figure 39-1B).[1] It is not easy to distinguish from the other two muscles that may contain TrPs that are attributed to the opponens pollicis muscle.

A bulbous enlargement of the flexor pollicis longus tendon may become ensnared by a restricted flexor sheath at the head of the 1st metacarpal bone, where the tendon becomes firmly attached to the thumb after it has passed over the adductor pollicis muscle and between the two heads of the flexor pollicis brevis muscle (Figure 39-1B).[1] This "triggering" phenomenon is similar to that described for the tendons of the finger flexors (see Chapter 38).

2.1. Innervation and Vascularization

Adductor Pollicis

The adductor pollicis muscle is innervated by the deep palmar branch of the ulnar nerve via the medial cord and lower trunk of the brachial plexus from spinal nerves C8 and T1.[1]

Opponens Pollicis

The opponens pollicis muscle is innervated by a branch of the median nerve via the lateral cord and upper and middle trunks from spinal nerves C6 and C7.[1]

The adductor and opponens pollicis muscles receive their vascularization by the superficial palmar branches of the radial artery.[1]

2.2. Function

The meaning of terms used to describe the direction of movement of the thumb is specific and requires definition. Flexion and extension movement at the metacarpophalangeal (MCP) and interphalangeal (IP) joints is perpendicular to the thumb nail and in the plane of the palm. Flexion is in the ulnar direction and extension in the radial direction. Abduction and adduction are movements perpendicular to the plane of the palm, away from and toward the palm, respectively. Opposition brings the palmar surfaces of the thumb and fifth finger in direct contact (not just fingertip contact).[1-5]

Adductor Pollicis

This muscle adducts the thumb. It also assists in flexion at the MCP joint of the thumb.

The adductor pollicis muscle has been shown to be electromyographically active during any adduction, opposition, and MCP flexion movements[6] and especially during forceful opposition of the thumb, which rotates the thumb to face the other fingers.[2,4]

Opponens Pollicis

The opponens pollicis muscle of the thumb abducts,[2] flexes,[2,3] and rotates the metacarpal bone of the thumb into a position of opposition.[1-5,7]

Electromyographically, the opponens pollicis muscle is consistently active during opposition of the thumb and, surprisingly, is moderately active during extension, and markedly active during abduction of the thumb.[2]

2.3. Functional Unit

The functional unit to which a muscle belongs includes the muscles that reinforce and counter its actions as well as the joints that the muscle crosses. The interdependence of these structures is functionally reflected in the organization and neural connections of the sensory motor cortex. The functional unit is emphasized because the presence of a TrP in one muscle of the unit increases the likelihood that the other muscles of the unit will also develop TrPs. When inactivating TrPs in a muscle, one must be concerned about TrPs that may develop in muscles that are functionally interdependent. Box 39-1

Box 39-1 Functional unit of the adductor pollicis and opponens pollicis muscles

Action	Synergists	Antagonists
Thumb adduction	First dorsal interosseous	Abductor pollicis longus Abductor pollicis brevis
Thumb opposition	Abductor pollicis brevis Flexor pollicis brevis	Adductor pollicis Extensor pollicis longus Extensor pollicis brevis

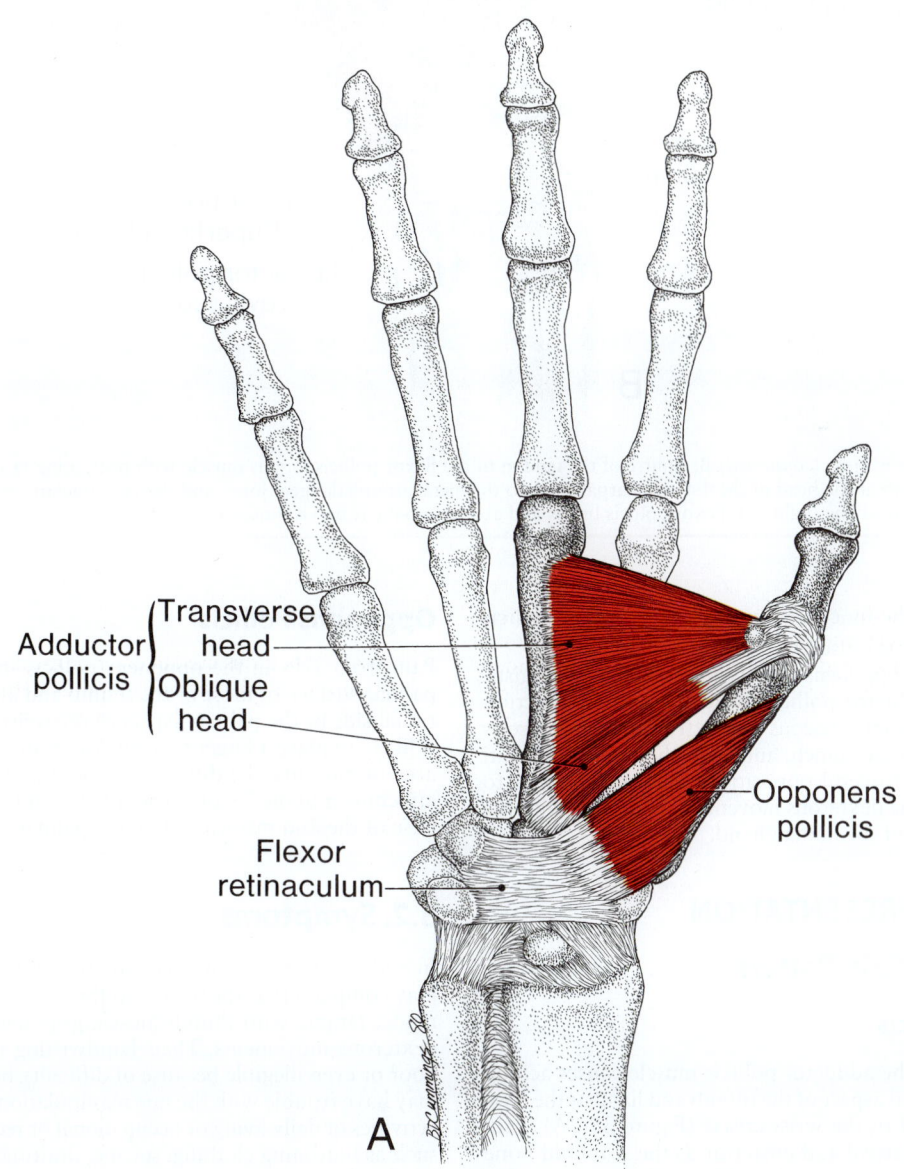

Figure 39-1. Attachments of thumb muscles. A, The adductor pollicis and opponens pollicis (dark red) muscles after removal of the flexor pollicis brevis and abductor pollicis brevis muscles.

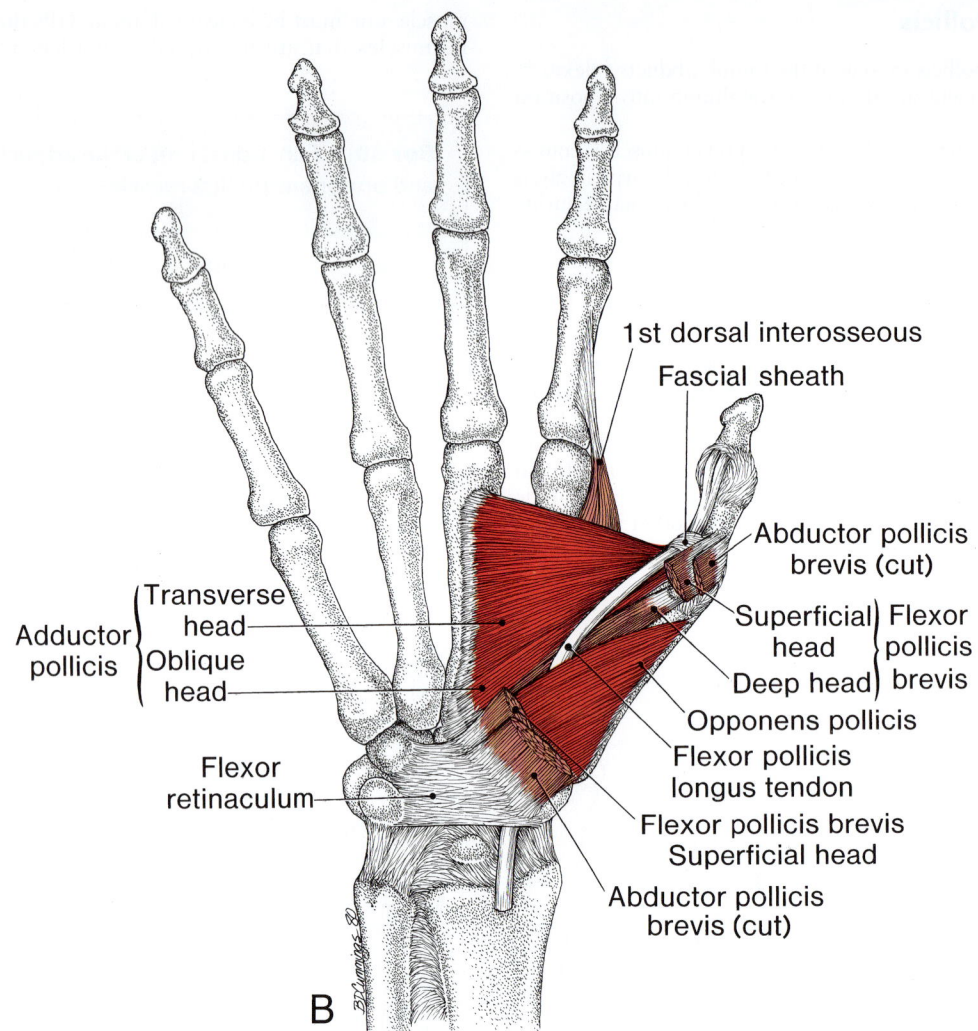

Figure 39-1. *(continued)* B, Course of the tendon of the flexor pollicis longus muscle with restraining fascial sheath at the head of the 1st metacarpal close to the metacarpophalangeal joint, and the cut attachments of the overlying (light red) flexor pollicis brevis and abductor pollicis brevis muscles.

grossly represents the functional unit of the adductor pollicis and opponens pollicis muscles.[8]

Functionally, the opponens pollicis muscle and its synergists, along with the adductor pollicis muscle, act in conjunction with the first dorsal interosseous and extrinsic finger muscles for forceful index-finger pinch, and with the opponens digiti minimi muscle for forceful opposition. This synergy acts to allow power and fine dexterous movement associated with the functional nuances of the human hand.

3. CLINICAL PRESENTATION
3.1. Referred Pain Pattern

Adductor Pollicis

Pain from TrPs in the adductor pollicis muscle causes aching pain along the lateral aspect of the thumb and hand at the base of the thumb distal to the wrist crease (Figure 39-2A). Pain may spread as far lateral and posterior as the scaphoid bone in the vicinity of the anatomical snuffbox. The pain may also spread over the palmar surface of the 1st MCP joint, and it may include most of the thumb, thenar eminence, and dorsal web space.[9,10]

Opponens Pollicis

Pain from TrPs in the opponens pollicis muscle refers to the palmar surface of most of the thumb and also to a spot on the radial side of the palmar aspect of the wrist, where the patient is likely to place a finger to locate the pain (Figure 39-2B). This area of pain may be diffuse and located in the vicinity of the attachment of the flexor carpi radialis tendon insertion into the base of the 2nd metacarpal on the palmar aspect of the wrist.

3.2. Symptoms

In addition to pain, patients with TrPs in these thumb muscles may complain that the hand and thumb is "clumsy." They may report fatigue with thumb muscle gripping or continued fine dexterous movements. Their handwriting may often become poor or even illegible because of difficulty holding a pen. They may have trouble with the fine manipulations necessary for the activities of daily living or occupational or recreational activities such as buttoning clothing, sewing, drafting, and painting that require the prehensile pincer grip provided by the thumb. In athletes, gripping and squeezing a water bottle may be painful or difficult. Smartphone and tablets create new challenges for the hand and thumb in terms of fine repeated dexterous movements,

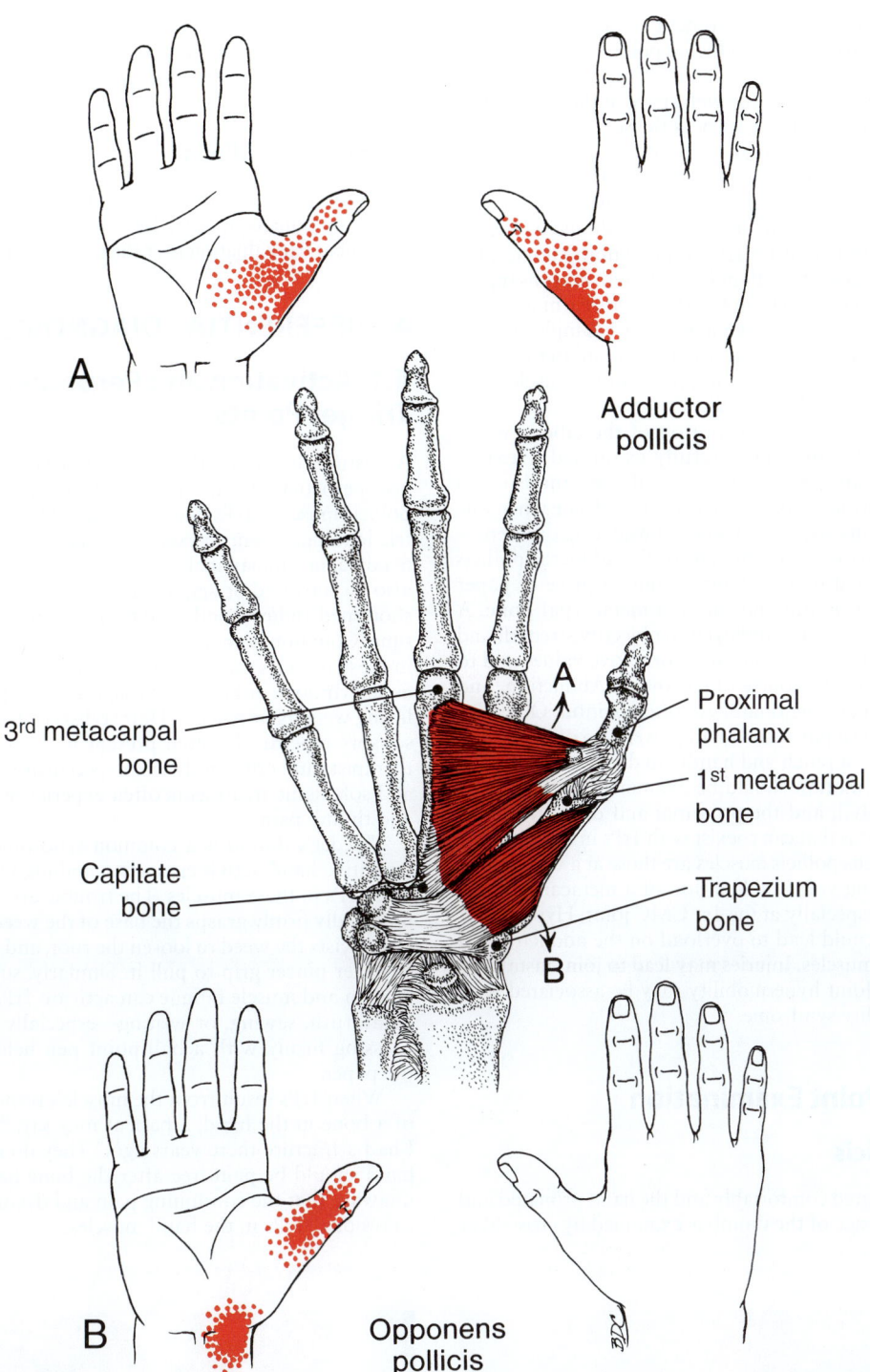

Figure 39-2. Referred pain patterns (dark red) for two thumb muscles (medium red), right hand. A, Adductor pollicis muscle. B, Opponens pollicis muscle.

often over extended periods of time. Adductor pollicis myofascial pain is commonly seen in patients who frequently use handheld devices.[11] See Chapter 41 for further discussion.

3.3. Patient Examination

After a thorough subjective examination, the clinician should make a detailed drawing representing the pain pattern that the patient has described. This depiction will assist in planning the physical examination and can be useful in monitoring the progression of the patient as symptoms improve or change.

Evaluation of the cervical and thoracic spine (as well as neurodynamic testing of the median, radial, and ulnar nerves) is also helpful in identifying any spinal or peripheral nerve contribution to symptoms felt in the wrist and hand region. This assessment is important even if patients don't report symptoms that are directly related to the cervical or thoracic spine. When ulnar nerve compression or entrapment is suspected, special tests for motor integrity of the adductor pollicis muscle should be conducted.

Because deep tenderness in the web space of the thumb may be referred from other muscles such as the scalene, brachialis, supinator, extensor carpi radialis longus, or brachioradialis muscles, these muscles should be examined for TrPs as well. The infraspinatus is another muscle that can refer sensory phenomena to the hand. If these muscles are involved, they should be treated before attempting to inactivate TrPs in the thumb muscles; the tenderness in the region of the thumb, if referred, may disappear following inactivation of TrPs in the distant forearm and arm muscles. In "weeder's thumb" syndrome, for example, TrPs in the first dorsal interosseous muscle usually respond to treatment immediately, leaving the more complex thumb muscles still causing symptoms (see Chapter 40).

Active and passive range of motion of the elbow, wrist, forearm, and hand should be carefully examined. Flexion, adduction, and abduction movements of the thumb often demonstrate inhibition weakness on the affected side when one of these muscles is involved, even when considering differences due to hand dominance. The strength of the adductor pollicis muscle is easily tested by the ability to hold a piece of paper tightly between the thumb and the 2nd metacarpal bone. A pinch strength gauge can be employed to objectify strength and compare to the contralateral side and normative values and to measure change over the course of treatment. Abduction, and especially extension, of the thumb are often painful. Objective strength assessment of pinch and hand power grip of the thumb can be measured by a pinch and handheld dynamometer.

Accessory joint motion should be examined in the 1st carpometacarpal (CMC), and the proximal and distal IP joints. Articular dysfunctions that can coexist with TrPs in the adductor pollicis and opponens pollicis muscles are those at a CMC joint, the most likely being volar subluxation of a metacarpal bone on a carpal bone, especially at the 1st CMC joint. Hypomobility in these joints could lead to overload on the adductor and opponens pollicis muscles. Injuries may lead to joint instability or hypermobility. Joint hypermobility may be associated with benign hypermobility syndrome.[12,13]

3.4. Trigger Point Examination

Adductor Pollicis

With the patient seated comfortably and the hand pronated and relaxed, the web space of the thumb is examined by cross-fiber pincer palpation (Figure 39-3A). The first dorsal interosseous muscle, which lies superficial to the transversely oriented adductor fibers, is pushed aside to improve access to the adductor pollicis muscle.

Opponens Pollicis

With the patient seated as noted for the examination of the adductor pollicis muscle, TrPs in this muscle are identified by cross-fiber flat palpation over the thenar eminence (Figure 39-3B).

4. DIFFERENTIAL DIAGNOSIS

4.1. Activation and Perpetuation of Trigger Points

A posture or activity that activates a TrP, if not corrected, can also perpetuate it. In any part of the adductor and opponens pollicis muscles, TrPs may be activated by unaccustomed eccentric loading, eccentric exercise in an unconditioned muscle, or maximal or submaximal concentric loading.[14] Trigger points may also be activated or aggravated when the muscle is placed in a shortened and/or lengthened position for an extended period of time. Common activities associated with the activation of TrPs in these muscles include repetitive fine motor movements such as smartphone or keyboard usage and gripping actions such as lifting weights or rowing. Hair stylists or barbers manipulating scissors repetitively often present with thumb pain. Physical therapists and other body work specialists who perform manual and soft tissue treatments often experience occupational hand and thumb pain.

Weeder's thumb is a common syndrome that results from repetitive hand activities, such as pulling weeds, that can activate TrPs in these muscles. The trouble arises when the patient repeatedly firmly grasps the base of the weed in a strong pincer grip, twists the weed to loosen the root, and then exerts an even stronger pincer grip to pull it. Similarly, sustained, unrelieved tension and muscle fatigue can activate TrPs when using a fine paintbrush, sewing, or writing—especially if writing requires pressing firmly with a ball-point pen held perpendicular to the paper.

When TrPs result from the muscle's response to the fracture of a bone in the hand, a patient may say, "Of course it hurts, I had a fracture there years ago." They do not realize that the hand should be pain-free after the bone has healed. They are unaware that the continuing pain and dysfunction may be due to residual TrPs in the hand muscles.

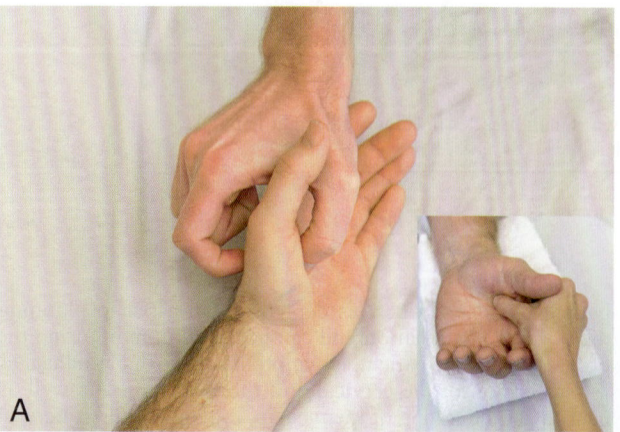
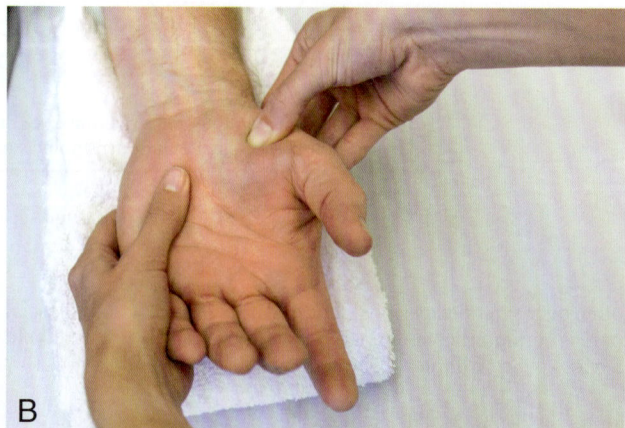

Figure 39-3. Palpation for TrPs in thumb muscles. A, Cross-fiber pincer palpation of the adductor pollicis muscle. B, Cross-fiber flat palpation of the opponens pollicis muscle.

Psychophysiologic patterns during text messaging revealed that subjects showed significant increases in respiration rate, heart rate, skin conductance, and shoulder and thumb surface electromyography (EMG) when compared with baseline measures.[15] Eighty-three percent of subjects reported hand and neck pain during texting and held their breath and experienced increased arousal when receiving text messages. Most participants were unaware of these changes. The study suggests that frequent triggering of these physiologic patterns may increase muscle discomfort symptoms. This study may have implications with patients presenting with hand and thumb pain and who regularly use handheld devices.[15]

4.2. Associated Trigger Points

Associated TrPs can develop in the referred pain areas caused by primary TrPs.[16] Therefore, musculature in the referred pain areas for each muscle should also be considered. Trigger points are nearly always found in the first dorsal interosseous muscle when they are present in the adductor and opponens pollicis muscles. Clinically, it appears that the thumb muscles are involved primarily, and the first dorsal interosseous muscle is affected secondarily because of its synergistic function. The flexor pollicis brevis and abductor pollicis brevis muscles eventually are also likely to become involved.

These muscles may also develop associated TrPs from the scalene, brachialis, supinator, infraspinatus, extensor carpi radialis longus, or brachioradialis muscles as they are located within the pain referral pattern of these muscles.

4.3. Associated Pathology

The symptoms produced by TrPs in the adductor and opponens pollicis muscles are most commonly mistakenly for carpal tunnel syndrome, DeQuervain's stenosing tenosynovitis, and CMC osteoarthritis. These conditions can exist in isolation but more commonly they coexist with TrPs in the thumb muscles and must be differentially diagnosed for effective treatment. An accessory flexor pollicis longus muscle, when present, can cause compression neuropathy of the anterior interosseous nerve.[17]

Osteoarthrosis of the CMC or MCP of the thumb is common in patients over age 55 and especially in individuals with thumb trauma. It is estimated that greater than 90% of people will have CMC osteoarthritis after 80 years of age.[18] Trigger points are often present in this condition, and treatment can assist with pain management and movement impairment.

Hand pain and weakness can be associated with neuropathic mechanisms such as nerve root compression, radiculopathy, and other neurologic disorders. Assessment with EMG, nerve conduction studies, and imaging may be required to assist in differential diagnosis. Guyon's canal syndrome may lead to weakness of the adductor pollicis muscle, resulting in diminished grip strength (refer to Chapter 40).[19]

Pain and tenderness referred to the 1st MCP joint from TrPs in the adductor pollicis muscle are easily mistaken for evidence of joint disease if the myofascial origin of the symptoms is not recognized.[20] On the other hand, pain and dysfunction of the MCP and IP joints may be due to loss of accessory joint motion, which should be identified and corrected.[21]

Heberden's nodes have been observed on the ulnar side of the thumb. When a node is present there, an associated TrP can sometimes be found in the adductor pollicis muscle.

The phenomenon of "trigger thumb" is identified by the patient's inability to extend the thumb without external assistance after flexing it; the thumb "locks" in flexion. The corresponding phenomenon, trigger finger, is considered in detail in Chapter 38.

Trigger thumb may be associated with a TrP located lateral to the tendon of the flexor pollicis longus muscle, possibly in

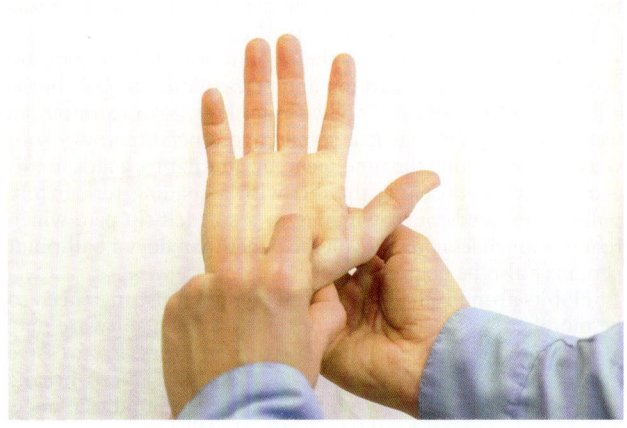

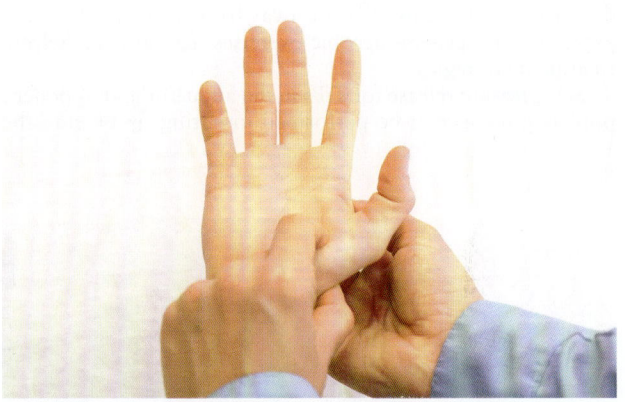

Figure 39-4. Technique for palpating the TrP of a "trigger thumb." The distal phalanx is wiggled back and forth to help identify the flexor pollicis longus tendon. Pressure against the head of the metacarpal bone, radial (lateral) to the tendon, elicits spot tenderness.

the flexor pollicis brevis muscle. To locate this TrP, the patient supinates the forearm, fully extends the MCP joint of the thumb (Figure 39-4A), and then alternately flexes and extends the distal phalanx, while the clinician identifies the tendon and corresponding TrP (Figure 39-4B). To identify the tendon of the flexor pollicis longus muscle, the clinician places a finger against the bulge of the MCP joint, pressing on the space between the flexor pollicis brevis and adductor pollicis muscles where the tendon of the flexor pollicis longus muscle enters the fascial sheath of the thumb (Figure 39-1B). As the patient moves the distal phalanx back and forth, the cord of the subcutaneous tendon is located proximal to where it enters the securing arch of fibers at the head of the 1st metacarpal bone in the region of the "trigger" phenomenon. The TrP is usually located several millimeters lateral (radial) to the tendon, just proximal to the bony bulge of the MCP joint.

Locking of the IP joint of the thumb may be caused by a sesamoid bone of that joint.[22] Of 30 patients presenting with trigger thumb, 25 were followed to spontaneous resolution without treatment. Five demanded treatment. The average duration of symptoms to spontaneous recovery was 6.8 months (range 2-15 months).[23]

5. CORRECTIVE ACTIONS

An attempt should be made to identify and correct the causative and/or contributing factors of the patient's symptoms. Ergonomic aids for activities of daily living and occupational activities may be required. Ergonomic assessment may play an important role in the adaptation of habitual tasks.[19]

Modification of activities that require forceful gripping are necessary to reduce activation and perpetuation of TrPs in the adductor and opponens pollicis muscles. As an example, in weeder's thumb, the patient should avoid persistent, vigorous weeding by limiting the time spent, by alternating hands in this activity, or by loosening the dirt with a spading fork before pulling the weeds out. Switching to a soft felt-tip pen, which requires much less pressure on the paper than does a ball-point pen, may also be helpful.

Habits around smartphone and computer use may need to be modified. Voice activation or text to speech software may assist in reducing load in keyboard operators. Progressive graded exposure to activities, coupled with micro-breaks and rotation of activities, may be required to build tolerance. Patient education should include mindfulness of patterns of increased psychophysiologic arousal and muscle tension during smartphone use.[15] Time away from devices, relaxation exercises, and general aerobic exercises may also be helpful treatment strategies.

Self-pressure release for TrPs in the adductor and opponens pollicis muscles can be performed in sitting by placing the forearm on the arm rest of a chair or on a table with the palm up. Manual pressure is the best method for performing self-pressure release of the adductor pollicis (Figure 39-5A) and opponens pollicis muscles (Figure 39-5B). As with any self-pressure release technique, the sensitive spot in the web space of the hand or the front of the thumb is identified with the fingers; light pressure (no more than 4/10 pain) is applied and held for 15 to 30 seconds, or until pain reduces. This technique can be repeated five times, several times per day.

The patient can easily perform self-stretch techniques as part of self-management for TrPs located in the adductor or opponens pollicis muscles. Stretching of the adductor and opponens pollicis muscles is performed with the patient seated, forearm supported with the palm up (Figure 39-6). To stretch the adductor pollicis muscle, the patient spreads the thumb away from the first finger using the unaffected thumb and index finger. Pressure is applied on the bone just below the finger and the base of the thumb (Figure 39-6A). To stretch the opponens pollicis muscle, the patient pushes the thumb down so the stretch is felt in the pad of the thumb (Figure 39-6B). These self-stretches should be carried out gently, and attention to the reproduction of pain versus stretch is paramount. These stretches should not be painful.

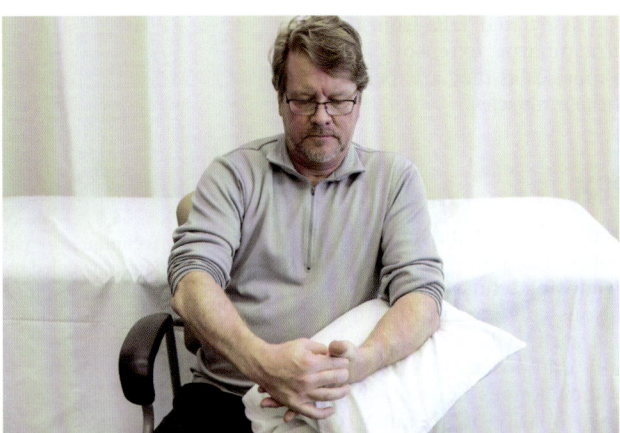

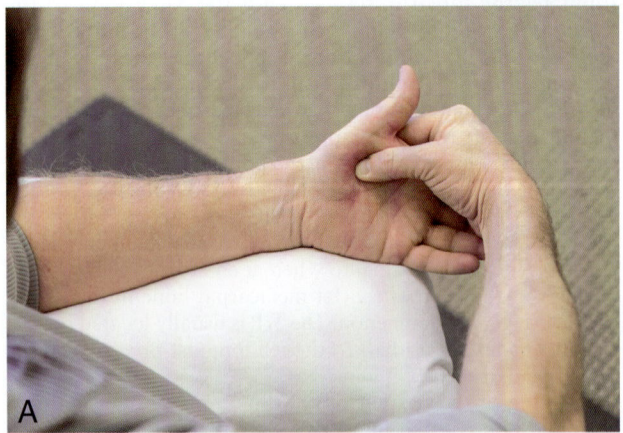
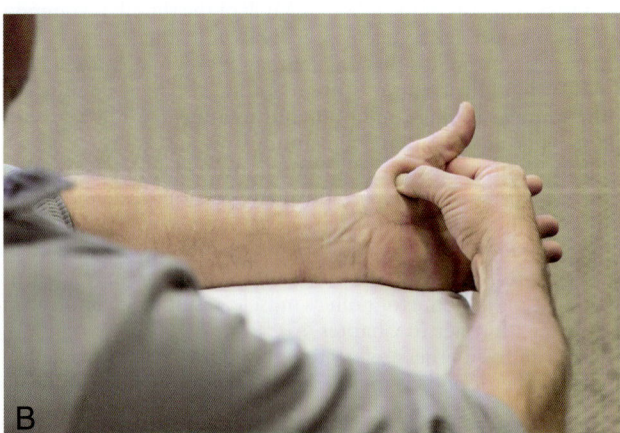

Figure 39-5. Self-pressure release seated with forearm supported. A, Manual pincer grasp for the adductor pollicis muscle. B, Manual release for the opponens pollicis muscle.

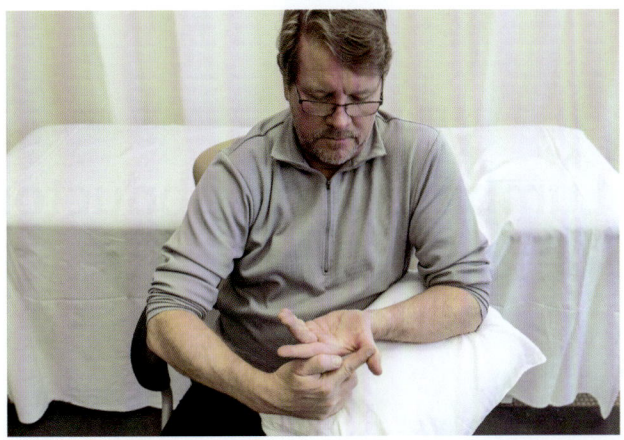
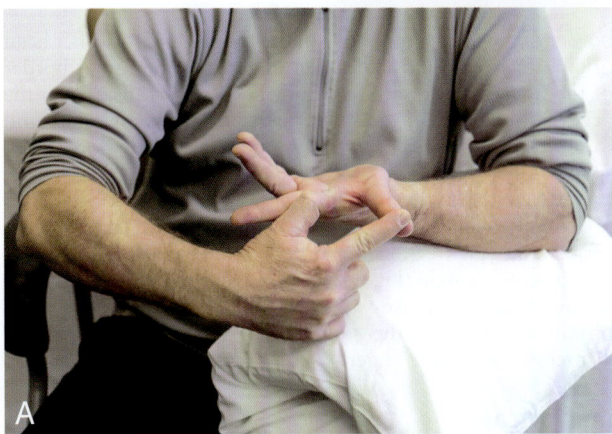
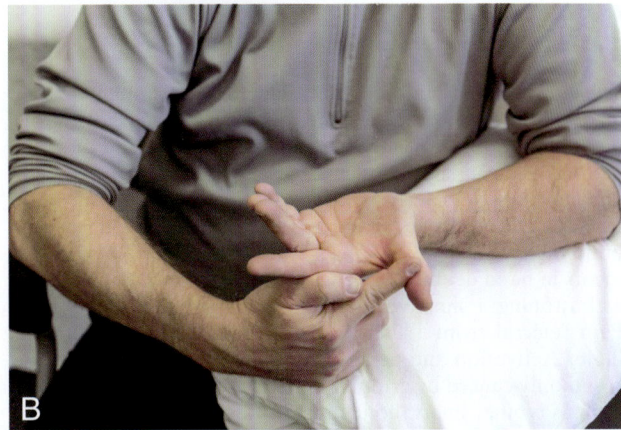

Figure 39-6. Self-stretch. A, Adductor pollicis muscle. B, Opponens pollicis muscle.

References

1. Standring S. *Gray's Anatomy: The Anatomical Basis of Clinical Practice.* 41st ed. London, UK: Elsevier; 2015.
2. Basmajian J, Deluca C. *Muscles Alive.* 5th ed. Baltimore, MD: Williams & Wilkins; 1985 (pp. 297, 306, 307).
3. Jenkins DB. *Hollinshead's Functional Anatomy of the Limbs and Back.* 6th ed. Philadelphia, PA: W.B. Saunders; 1991 (pp. 16-166).
4. Oatis C. *Kinesiology: The Mechanics and Pathomechanics of Human Movement.* Philadelphia, PA: Lippincott Williams & Wilkins; 2004:chap 19.
5. Kendall FP, McCreary EK. *Muscles: Testing and Function, with Posture and Pain.* 5th ed. Baltimore, MD: Lippincott Williams & Wilkins; 2005 (pp. 261, 263).
6. Weathersby HT, Sutton LR, Krusen UL. The kinesiology of muscles of the thumb: an electromyographic study. *Arch Phys Med Rehabil.* 1963;44:321-326.
7. Forrest WJ, Basmajian JV. Functions of human thenar and hypothenar muscles; an electromyographic study of twenty-five hands. *J Bone Joint Surg Am Vol.* 1965;47(8):1585-1594.
8. Simons DG, Travell J, Simons L. *Travell & Simon's Myofascial Pain and Dysfunction: The Trigger Point Manual.* Vol 1. 2nd ed. Baltimore, MD: Williams & Wilkins; 1999 (p. 104).
9. Travell J, Rinzler SH. The myofascial genesis of pain. *Postgrad Med.* 1952;11(5):425-434.
10. Zohn DA. *Musculoskeletal Pain: Diagnosis and Physical Treatment.* 2nd ed. Boston, MA: Little Brown; 1988 (p. 211, Fig. 12-2).
11. Sharan D, Ajeesh PS. Risk factors and clinical features of text message injuries. *Work.* 2012;41 suppl 1:1145-1148.
12. Beighton P, Solomon L, Soskolne CL. Articular mobility in an African population. *Ann Rheum Dis.* 1973;32(5):413-418.
13. Remvig L, Jensen DV, Ward RC. Epidemiology of general joint hypermobility and basis for the proposed criteria for benign joint hypermobility syndrome: review of the literature. *J Rheumatol.* 2007;34(4):804-809.
14. Gerwin RD, Dommerholt J, Shah JP. An expansion of Simons' integrated hypothesis of trigger point formation. *Curr Pain Headache Rep.* 2004;8(6):468-475.
15. Lin IM, Peper E. Psychophysiological patterns during cell phone text messaging: a preliminary study. *Appl Psychophysiol Biofeedback.* 2009;34(1):53-57.
16. Hsieh YL, Kao MJ, Kuan TS, Chen SM, Chen JT, Hong CZ. Dry needling to a key myofascial trigger point may reduce the irritability of satellite MTrPs. *Am J Phys Med Rehabil.* 2007;86(5):397-403.
17. Lahey MD, Aulicino PL. Anomalous muscles associated with compression neuropathies. *Orthop Rev.* 1986;15(4):199-208.
18. Gelberman RH, Boone S, Osei DA, Cherney S, Calfee RP. Trapeziometacarpal arthritis: a prospective clinical evaluation of the thumb adduction and extension provocative tests. *J Hand Surg Am.* 2015;40(7):1285-1291.
19. Cooper C. *Fundamentals of Hand Therapy: Clinical Reasoning and Treatment Guidelines for Common Diagnoses of the Upper Extremity.* St. Louis, MO: Mosby, Elsevier; 2007 (pp. 236-239).
20. Reynolds MD. Myofascial trigger point syndromes in the practice of rheumatology. *Arch Phys Med Rehabil.* 1981;62(3):111-114.
21. Mennell JM. *Joint Pain: Diagnosis and Treatment Using Manipulative Techniques.* 1st ed. Boston, MA: Little Brown; 1964.
22. Brown M, Manktelow RT. A new cause of trigger thumb. *J Hand Surg Am.* 1992;17(4):688-690.
23. Schofield CB, Citron ND. The natural history of adult trigger thumb. *J Hand Surg Br.* 1993;18(2):247-248.

Chapter 40

Interosseous, Lumbrical, and Abductor Digiti Minimi Muscles

"Hand Crampers"

Johnson McEvoy and Joseph M. Donnelly

1. INTRODUCTION

The interosseous, lumbrical, and abductor digiti minimi muscles are intrinsic muscles of the hand involved in specific dexterous fine-hand motor movements, including gripping and pinching motions. Pain and dysfunctions, such as contracture and strength deficits, can significantly impact hand function. Symptoms from trigger points (TrPs) in the intrinsic hand muscles include a deep boney ache in the fingers, finger stiffness that produces impairments in hand dexterity, strength, and function. Activities such as buttoning a shirt, writing, and grasping may be impaired. Pain referral from TrPs in these muscles is primarily to the digits. Activation and perpetuation of TrPs in these muscles is commonly caused by gripping actions and fine motor activities such as typing, smartphone usage, and sporting activities such as boxing. Differential diagnosis includes cervical radicular pain or radiculopathy, local wrist and hand joint dysfunction, and osteoarthritis. Corrective actions include modification of activities, ergonomic assessment and training, TrP self-pressure release, self-stretch, and strengthening exercises.

2. ANATOMIC CONSIDERATIONS

Interossei

As the name denotes, the interosseous muscles lie between adjacent metacarpal bones. The interosseous muscles are divided into two groups: palmar and dorsal interossei muscles.[1] The dorsal interosseous muscles are larger and more expansive. Each dorsal interosseous muscle originates proximally by two heads (Figure 40-1A) with significantly different structures that may be important to know when examining for injection of TrPs. The attachment of the head on the side nearest the middle finger covers nearly three-fourths of that metacarpal bone,[2] giving it a pennate structure, as clearly illustrated for the first dorsal interosseous muscle.[3] The other head has a much shorter attachment to its metacarpal bone[2] and more parallel arrangement of fibers.[3] This structure indicates that the head on the side nearest the middle finger (designed for strength) has a long endplate zone running nearly the length of the muscle belly, whereas the other head (designed for speed and large range of motion) has a nearly transverse endplate zone near the middle of the muscle belly. Each bipennate muscle inserts distally at the base of the proximal phalanx of the related finger and to that finger's extensor aponeurosis. Each muscle attaches on the side of the phalanx away from the midline of the hand.[1]

The first dorsal interosseous muscle is larger than the other interosseous muscles, but it follows the same attachment pattern (Figure 40-1A). One head originates proximally from the ulnar border of the metacarpal bone of the thumb, and the other head originates from almost the entire length of the radial border of the 2nd metacarpal bone. Both heads insert distally to the proximal phalanx of the index finger on the radial side (and to the extensor aponeurosis). This muscle fills the dorsal web space of the thumb.

Each of the three palmar interosseous muscles originates proximally from the palmar interosseous surface of one metacarpal bone (Figure 40-1B) and lies palmar to the related dorsal interosseous muscle (Figure 40-1C). Each then inserts distally to that finger's extensor aponeurosis and to the base of the proximal phalanx on the side closest to the midline of the hand (center of the middle finger).

Lumbricals

The four lumbrical muscles are worm-shaped muscles that originate proximally from the four tendons of the flexor digitorum profundus muscle in mid-palm and insert distally to the radial side of the extensor aponeurosis on each of the four fingers.[1] The first and second lumbrical muscles lie palmar to the first and second dorsal interosseous muscles, but the transverse head of the adductor pollicis muscle is interposed between these two lumbrical muscles and the dorsal interosseous muscles. The third and fourth lumbrical muscles lie palmar and adjacent to the second and third palmar interosseous muscles (Figure 40-1C).

Abductor Digiti Minimi

The abductor digiti minimi muscle provides half of what would be the next dorsal interosseous muscle and exhibits a parallel fiber arrangement[3] that has a transverse endplate zone in mid-muscle (light red, Figure 40-1A and B). The muscle originates proximally from the pisiform bone, and it inserts distally onto the ulnar side of the base of the first phalanx of the fifth finger and to its associated extensor aponeurosis.[1]

2.1. Innervation and Vascularization

All of the interosseous muscles and the abductor digiti minimi muscle are innervated by branches of the ulnar nerve, through the medial cord and lower trunk of the brachial plexus from spinal nerves C8 and T1.[1] The first and second lumbrical muscles are innervated by the median nerve, and the 3rd and 4th are innervated by the ulnar nerve.[1]

The dorsal interosseous muscles receive vascularization through the dorsal and palmar metacarpal arteries. The dorsal metacarpal arteries arise from the dorsal carpal arch of the anastomosis of the dorsal carpal branch of the radial and ulnar

Chapter 40: Interosseous, Lumbrical, and Abductor Digiti Minimi Muscles 387

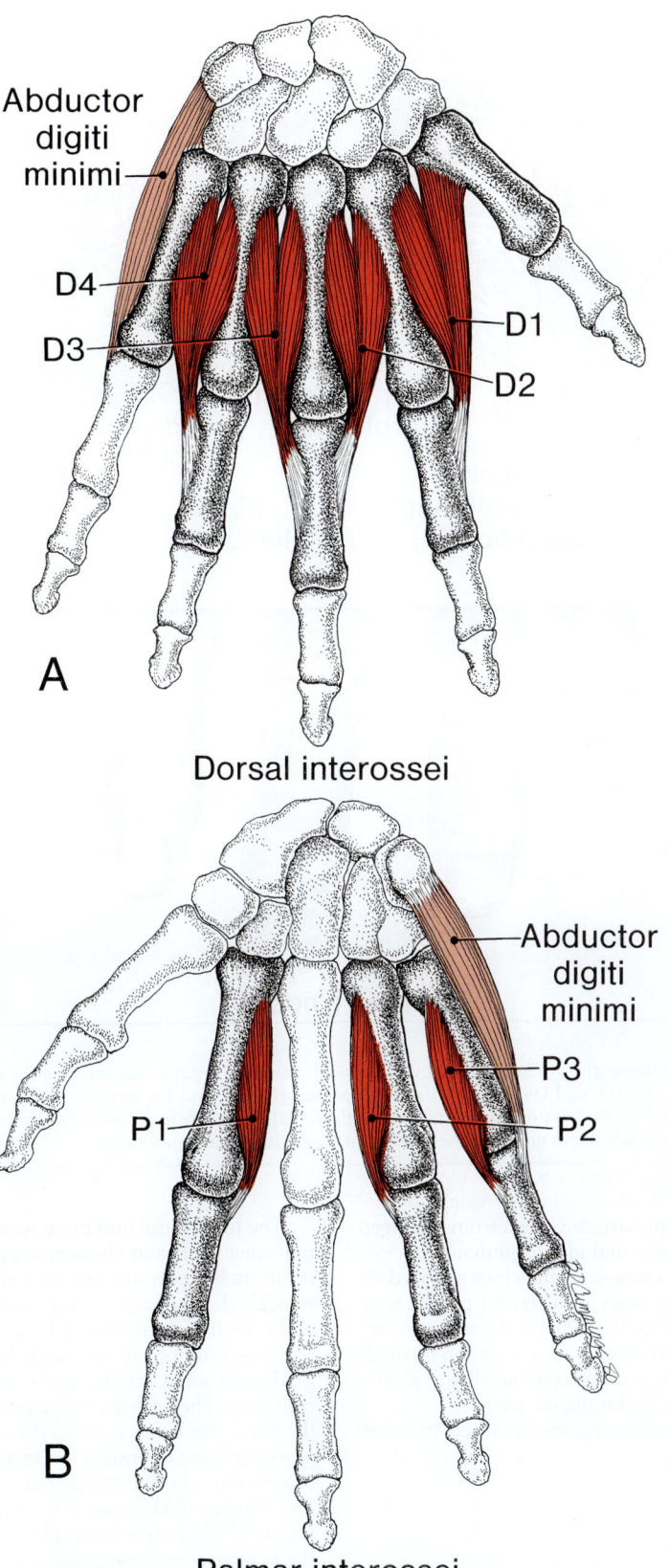

Figure 40-1. Attachments of the right interossei muscle. A, Dorsal view of the dorsal interosseous muscles (dark red), which move the fingers away from the midline of the middle finger, and of the abductor digiti minimi muscle (light red). B, Palmar view of all (the first, second, and third) palmar interossei (dark red) muscles.

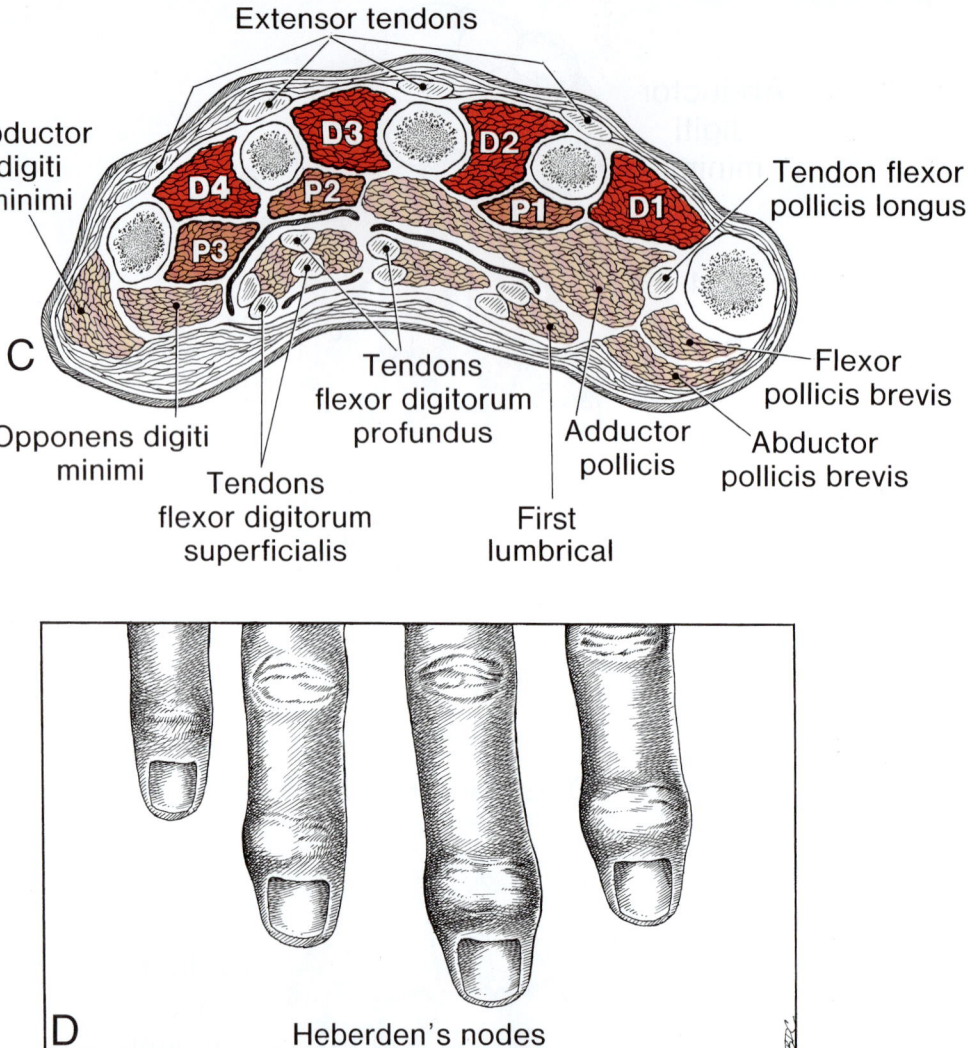

Figure 40-1. *(continued)* C, Cross-sectional view through the metacarpal bones showing the relationship between the dorsal (D1, D2, D3, and D4, dark red) and the palmar (P1, P2, and P3, medium red) interossei muscles. The lumbrical muscles are the light red muscle masses on the radial side of the four flexor digitorum profundus tendons. D, Appearance of Heberden's nodes on the sides of the distal interphalangeal joints.

arteries. The palmar metacarpal arteries arise from the deep palmar arch formed by the radial and ulnar arteries.[1]

Vascularization of the palmar interosseous muscles is provided via the palmar metacarpal artery that arises from the deep palmar arch. The deep palmar arch is formed by the radial and ulnar arteries.[1]

The lumbrical muscles receive their vascularization through the superficial palmar arch, the common palmar digital artery, the deep palmar arch, and the dorsal digital artery.[1]

The abductor digiti minimi muscle receives its vascularization through the ulnar artery.[1]

2.2. Function

The interosseous and lumbrical muscles are important intrinsic muscles of the hand that assist in fine dexterous movement, stability, and function. To understand the actions of these intrinsic hand muscles, it is important to remember that the extensor digitorum muscle strongly extends the proximal phalanx of each finger but only weakly extends the middle and distal phalanges. The flexor digitorum superficialis muscle attaches to the center of the middle phalanx, thus acting to flex the proximal and middle phalanges. The flexor digitorum profundus muscle attaches to the distal phalanx, flexing it and the more proximal phalanges.

The four dorsal and three palmar interosseous muscles have opposing actions in abduction and adduction, respectively, and rotation. Both groups of interosseous, along with the lumbrical muscles, flex the fingers at the metacarpophalangeal (MCP) joints and extend the middle and distal phalanges.[1,4-7] It is the interosseous and lumbrical muscles that extend the middle and distal phalanges when any degree of flexion of the proximal phalanx is present. The flexion or extension of the latter is controlled by the flexor digitorum superficialis and extensor digitorum muscles, working as antagonists. The **D**orsal interosseous muscles *ab*duct (mnemonic—DAB), and the *p*almar interosseous muscles *ad*duct (mnemonic—PAD) with reference to the midline of the middle finger.[1,4,5,7,8] Electromyographic (EMG) studies have shown that the interosseous hand muscles act as flexors of the MCP joints only when this function does *not* conflict with their extensor function at the interphalangeal joints (IP) joints.[4]

The flexion–extension function of the interosseous muscles requires considerably less force than the lateral motions of abduction and adduction. Therefore, in disease, the lateral motions are lost earlier and recover more slowly than flexion–extension. The abduction–adduction functions of the interosseous muscles must be tested with the fingers extended at the MCP joints. Spreading the fingers apart is normally significantly limited when the fingers are flexed at the MCP joint.[8]

Chapter 40: Interosseous, Lumbrical, and Abductor Digiti Minimi Muscles 389

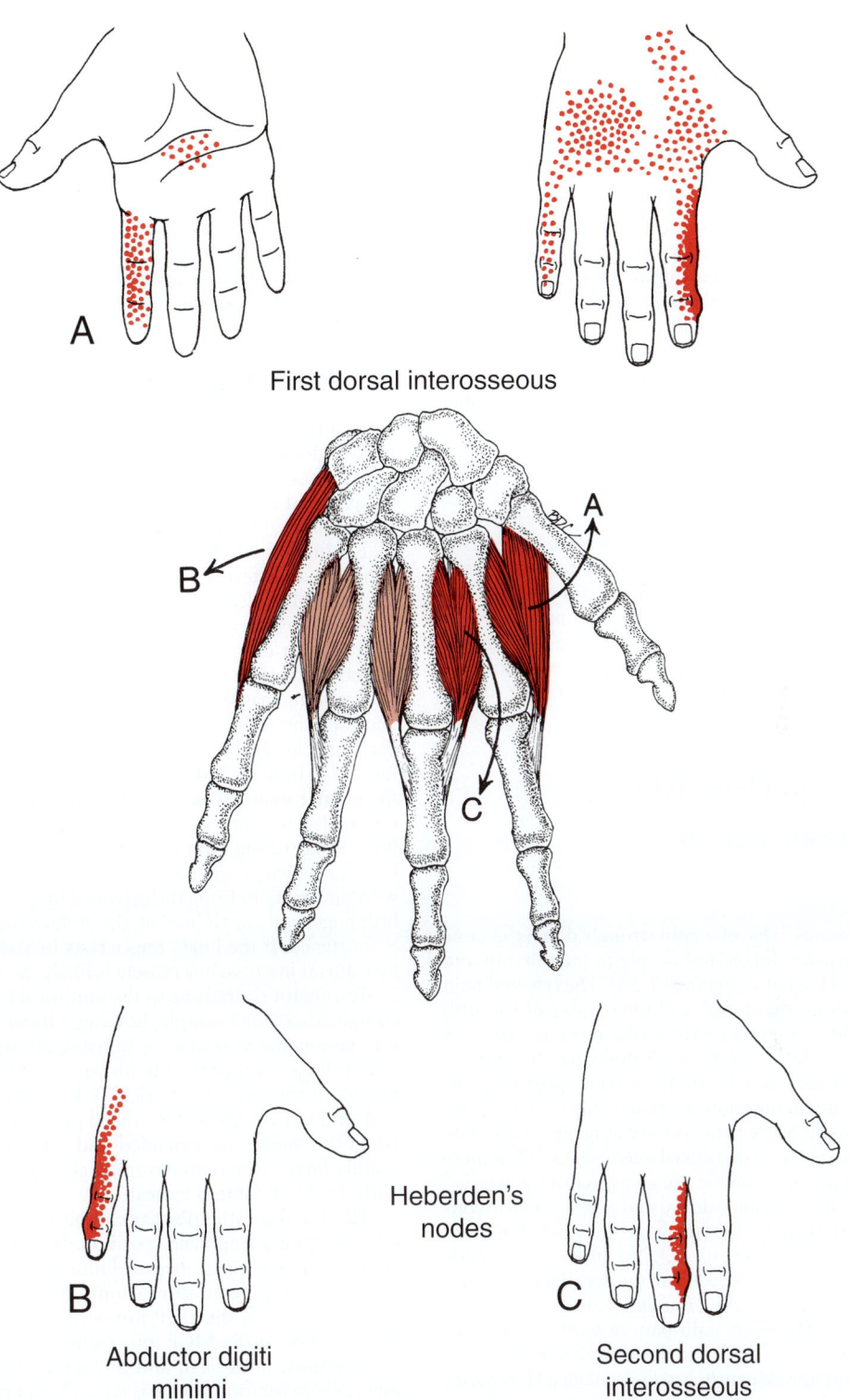

Figure 40-2. Referred pain patterns (dark red) for selected intrinsic muscles of the right hand. Essential zones are solid red, spillover zones are stippled red. A, The first dorsal interosseous muscle (medium red). B, The abductor digiti minimi muscle (medium red). C, The second dorsal interosseous muscle (medium red) and the third and fourth dorsal interosseous muscles (light red). Trigger points may be found anywhere in the interossei muscles, proximally or distally. This is to be expected because the two heads converge in a bipenniform manner and have endplate zones running in the shape of a horse-shoe the length of the muscles. Note the small Heberden's nodes in the essential pain reference zones.

The first dorsal interosseous muscle rotates the proximal phalanx to make the index finger pad face the ulnar side of the hand, whereas the first palmar interosseous muscle rotates it in the opposite direction. The first dorsal and first palmar interosseous muscles counter-balance their rotational movements while combining their flexion–extension actions. In precision handling of objects, the interosseous muscles function mainly as abductors and adductors of the fingers. In spherical grip, their rotational forces were found to position the proximal phalanges for best finger pad contact.[9]

Weakness of the interosseous muscles may lead to loss of pinch and grasp grip strength and muscle balance associated with claw hand dysfunction.[6]

The lumbrical muscles are unusual in that they don't attach to bone but to the tendons of other muscles.[1] Thus, the lumbrical muscles function as the equivalent of an adjustable physiologic tendon transplant. Contraction of these muscles converts the distal phalanx flexion action of the flexor digitorum profundus muscle to extension of the distal phalanges. The lumbrical muscles specifically permit the flexor digitorum superficialis muscle to strongly grip with the proximal and middle phalanges, yet release the distal phalanx grip in the presence of flexor digitorum profundus muscle activity. The usual test of the intrinsic muscles' flexion–extension function, by resisting IP joint extension with the MCP joint flexed, tests both the interosseous and lumbrical muscles.[7] The lumbrical muscles' function is most important when a strong grip is required in the absence of finger-tip pressure.

Isolated weakness of the lumbrical muscles is unusual and hard to identify. It may, with combined weakness of the interosseous muscles, contribute to claw hand deformity.[6]

2.3. Functional Unit

The dorsal and palmar interosseous muscles are synergistic for flexion at the metacarpophalangeal joint and extension of the two most distal phalanges. They are antagonistic for adduction–abduction and for rotation of the proximal phalanges.

The interosseous and lumbrical muscles are synergistic. Full effectiveness of these intrinsic muscles for grip, holding, and grasping objects also requires the assistance of the thumb muscles in the thenar eminence.

3. CLINICAL PRESENTATION

3.1. Referred Pain Pattern

Interossei

First dorsal interosseous TrPs refer pain strongly down the same (radial) side of the index finger and deeply in the dorsum and through the palm of the hand (Figure 40-2A). The referred pain may also extend along the dorsal and ulnar sides of the fifth finger.[10,11] Generally, patients experience the most intense pain at the distal IP joint where a Heberden's node may be noted.

First dorsal interosseous TrPs are the second most frequent source of referred pain in the palm, exceeded only by TrPs in the palmaris longus muscle. Some patients have difficulty in deciding whether the pain referred from first dorsal interosseous TrPs is more prominent on the palmar or on the dorsal aspect of the hand.[12]

Trigger points in the remaining dorsal and palmar interosseous muscles refer pain along the side of the finger to which that interosseous muscle attaches (Figure 40-2C). No distinction is made between the patterns of pain referred from the dorsal interosseous, palmar interosseous, and lumbrical muscles. Pain extends as far as the distal IP joint. The exact pain pattern varies somewhat, depending on the location of the TrP in the interosseous muscle. A TrP in an interosseous muscle may be associated with a Heberden's node located within the TrP zone of referred pain and tenderness.

Experimental injection of hypertonic saline solution into the third dorsal interosseous of one subject referred pain to the ulnar aspect of both the dorsal and palmar surfaces of the hand[13] but not to the fingers.[14]

Abductor Digiti Minimi

The abductor digiti minimi muscle refers pain similarly along the outer aspect of the fifth finger to which it attaches (Figure 40-2B).

3.2. Symptoms

Patients with TrPs in an interosseous muscle characteristically report an achy "arthritis pain in my finger." The pain is often described as a deep boney ache. They may also report finger stiffness that produces impairments in hand dexterity and strength and in functions such as buttoning a shirt, writing, and grasping. Numbness and paresthesia is not expected to accompany these TrPs unless there was involvement of the sensory digital nerves. Some patients will identify and describe the Heberden's node as a "sore inflamed joint." Careful examination indicates a tender Heberden's node but, as a rule, no true synovial or bony swelling. In time, the Heberden's node becomes less tender. Clinically, it appears that TrPs in muscles can be associated with joint disease,[15] but there is little quality research on this association.

3.3. Patient Examination

After a thorough subjective examination, the clinician should make a detailed drawing representing the pain pattern that the patient has described. This depiction will assist in planning the physical examination and can be useful in monitoring the progression of the patient as symptoms improve or change.

Evaluation of the cervical and thoracic spine, as well as neurodynamic testing of the median, radial, and ulnar nerves is also helpful in identifying any spinal or neurogenic contribution to symptoms felt in the wrist and hand region. This assessment is important even if patients don't report symptoms that are directly related to the cervical or thoracic spine.

Active and passive range of motion of the elbow, wrist, forearm, and hand should be carefully examined. Kendall et al[7] describe and illustrate clearly the effect of shortening of the interosseous and lumbrical muscles. Adaptive shortening or local TrP tension of the palmar interosseous muscles that produce adduction of the fingers (PAD) compromises the ability to fully spread the extended fingers. Shortening, pain, or dysfunction of the dorsal interosseous muscles, which produce abduction of the fingers (DAB), interferes with the ability to bring the extended fingers close together. If the fifth finger rests in abduction, the abductor digiti minimi muscle is shortened. If the index finger rests in abduction, a shortened first dorsal interosseous muscle is likely the cause.

Testing for shortening of the lumbrical muscles is a bit more complicated. For example, holding a hand of cards or holding up a newspaper to read it[7] by pressing the middle phalanx of the middle finger against the thumb but avoiding finger-tip pressure overloads the second lumbrical. When it becomes shortened, it will tend to hyperextend the distal phalanx of the middle finger when the fingers are extended and prevent full closure of the middle finger when attempting a claw position (fingers flexed with the MCP joint extended).

The muscles with TrPs may exhibit some weakness, especially when tested in a lengthened position. Tests of interosseous muscle strength are well described and illustrated by Kendall et al.[7]

Accessory joint motion should be examined in the MCP, proximal IP, and distal IP joints of all five fingers. Articular dysfunctions of the MCP joints often coexist with TrPs in the interosseous, lumbrical, and abductor digiti minimi muscles, especially in rotation, which is typically not examined. Hypomobility in these joints could lead to overload on the interosseous, lumbrical, and abductor digiti minimi muscles, especially during forceful grasping.

3.4. Trigger Point Examination

Trigger points in the interosseous or lumbrical muscles are difficult to palpate. The first dorsal interosseous muscle can be palpated with the forearm supported and in a neutral position. Cross-fiber flat palpation is used to identify TrPs in this muscle (Figure 40-3A). Separating the fingers widely moves the metacarpal bones apart and permits pincer palpation of the other interosseous and lumbrical muscles between the metacarpal bones. A counter-pressure is produced with

Chapter 40: Interosseous, Lumbrical, and Abductor Digiti Minimi Muscles

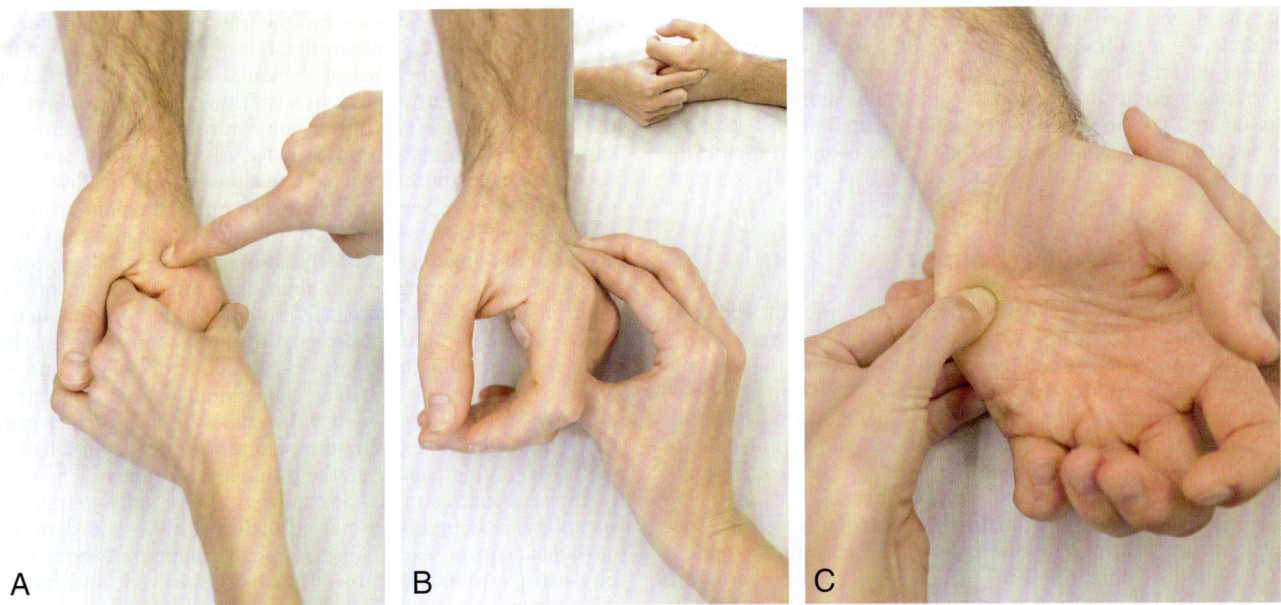

Figure 40-3. Palpation for TrPs in intrinsic hand muscles. A, Cross-fiber flat palpation of the first dorsal interosseous muscle. B, Cross-fiber pincer palpation of interossei and lumbrical muscles. C, Cross-fiber pincer palpation of the abductor digiti minimi muscle.

a finger against the palm, beneath the muscle to be palpated (Figure 40-3B). Deep tenderness can be localized in the interosseous and lumbrical muscles but, except for the first dorsal interosseous muscle, referred pain and local twitch responses are rarely induced unless a monofilament or injection needle penetrates the TrPs.

To examine the abductor digiti minimi muscle, the patient's forearm and hand is supported with the palm facing up, and the TrPs are identified using cross-fiber pincer palpation (Figure 40-3C).

Cutaneous hypoesthesia may be noted along one side of a finger where the patient reports a sensation of numbness when an active TrP lies in the corresponding interosseous muscle. This apparent neurologic phenomenon may disappear following inactivation of the TrP, suggesting that the median or ulnar digital nerve had been affected by the increased tension of the involved interosseous muscle. However, this symptom could be sensory referred phenomena related to the presence of TrPs. It should be noted that no evidence exists to support this hypothesis, and more research is warranted.

On their way through the palm to the digits, the median and ulnar nerves lie next to the lumbrical and palmar interosseous muscles. The deep (motor) branch of the ulnar nerve pierces the opponens digiti minimi muscle before supplying all the interosseous muscles, the third and fourth lumbrical muscles, the adductor pollicis muscle, and the deep head of the flexor pollicis brevis muscle.[1] Trigger points in the opponens digiti minimi muscle can be responsible for weakness of these ulnarly innervated muscles, and if weakness is present, the opponens digiti minimi muscle should be examined for TrPs.

4. DIFFERENTIAL DIAGNOSIS

4.1. Activation and Perpetuation of Trigger Points

A posture or activity that activates a TrP, if not corrected, can also perpetuate it. In any part of the interosseous, lumbrical, and abductor digiti minimi muscles, TrPs may be activated by unaccustomed eccentric loading, eccentric exercise in an unconditioned muscle, or maximal or submaximal concentric loading.[16] Trigger points may also be activated or aggravated when the muscle is placed in a shortened and/or lengthened position for an extended period of time.

Trigger points in the interosseous muscles are activated by sustained or repetitive pincer grasp, as performed by a tailor, hair stylist, painter, sculptor, mechanic, or wind instrument player. Balancing and sustaining a smartphone between the index finger and thumb may fatigue intrinsic muscles of the hand. Text message–related injuries are a relatively new phenomenon, with myofascial pain syndrome of the adductor pollicis muscle, first interosseous muscle, and extensor digitorum muscle being common (70%).[17] Activities requiring sustained forceful finger movements, such as pulling weeds, manipulation of hand muscles by a physical or massage therapist, or the actions of an aesthetician, can initiate interosseous TrPs. "Golf hands" have been associated with constant tight grip on the handle of the golf club, especially when the handle has a very small diameter.

Clinically, "boxer's fractures" of the 2nd and 5th metacarpal have been seen to activate TrPs in patient's first interosseous (2nd metacarpal) muscle or abductor digiti minimi (5th metacarpal) muscle, causing persistent pain and impairment. Trigger point dry needling into the muscle with several local twitch responses rapidly reduced pain and improved function. In several cases, recognized pain to the related digit was elicited. One patient, who presented with suspected complex regional pain syndrome of 5 months' duration after surgical pinning of a 2nd metacarpal fracture, rapidly achieved long-term relief of pain after two sessions of TrP dry needling. Strength gains were significant and seen within several days of relief of pain. Subsequent graded return to sport was achieved within 2 weeks of the amelioration of the pain in the first interosseous muscle and a return of grip strength. The boxer continued to box for years without return of pain or recurrence.

4.2. Associated Trigger Points

Associated TrPs can develop in the referred pain areas caused by primary TrPs.[18] Therefore, musculature in the referred pain areas for each muscle should also be considered. When the interosseous muscles are involved, the intrinsic thumb muscles should be examined for associated TrPs. Other TrPs that may refer pain into the fingers include the long flexors and extensors of the fingers, the infraspinatus muscle, the latissimus dorsi muscle, the pectoralis major muscle, the scalene muscles, and either the lateral or medial head of the triceps brachii muscle.

Trigger points in the pronator quadratus muscle may cause associated TrPs in the abductor digiti minimi muscle because it is located in the pain referral zone of the pronator quadratus muscle.

4.3. Associated Pathology

The distal IP joints of the fingers preferentially develop Heberden's nodes. This phenomenon can be evidence of an osteoarthritic process[19] and is most common in the finger joint that has the highest load per unit area of joint surface and in those individuals who commonly load that joint.[20] The increased strain on the interosseous muscles caused by abnormal hand mechanics associated with the distorted joint function of arthritis may activate and perpetuate these TrPs. Vice versa, TrPs may also contribute to the pain of arthritis,[15] potentially through peripheral and central pain mechanisms. Inactivating the related TrPs and the elimination or management of their perpetuating factors may be important in rehabilitation and management of patients with osteoarthritis of the fingers and hand.

Heberden's nodes are often identified with osteoarthritis,[19,21] particularly with the primary idiopathic form, rather than the traumatic secondary form.[22] The node is an enlargement of soft tissue, sometimes partly bony, on the dorsal surface on either side of the terminal phalanx at the distal IP joint (Figure 40-2D). A positive association between Heberden's and radiographic evidence of osteoarthritis has been demonstrated ($n = 1939$; mean age 68 years, 54% women).[19] The patient may eventually develop a flexion deformity with lateral or medial deviation of the distal phalanx.[23] Similar nodes located at the proximal IP joints are called Bouchard's nodes, but they are seen in only 25% of individuals with Heberden's nodes.[24]

Not all swollen painful distal IP joints of the hands should be assumed to be Heberden's nodes as, for example, the prevalence of distal IP joint rheumatoid arthritic involvement is estimated at 10%.[25,26]

The presence of Heberden's nodes is a common finding in patients with TrPs in the interosseous muscles. A node is palpable as an excrescence on the dorsal margin of the distal phalanx or the distal end of the middle phalanx on either side, always near the distal IP joint (Figure 40-2D). A Heberden's node may also appear on the thumb, usually on its ulnar side, in conjunction with TrPs in the adductor pollicis muscle. Idiopathic Heberden's nodes are most commonly seen on the index and middle fingers.[5] They may appear on the side of the interosseous muscle attachment to the finger. A well-designed research study is needed to study the relationship between TrPs and Heberden's nodes and the efficacy of TrP treatment.

The diagnoses most likely to be confused with interosseous TrPs include C6 radicular pain or radiculopathy, ulnar neuropathy, C8 or T1 radicular pain or radiculopathy, and when the TrPs are primarily in the abductor digiti minimi muscle, thoracic outlet syndrome. Rarely, one may see the pain misdiagnosed as an isolated digital nerve entrapment when, in fact, it is associated with TrPs in one of the dorsal interosseous muscles. When the TrP is inactivated, this finger pain resolves completely. Finger pain and numbness may also result from neuropathy of the brachial plexus including compression from the scalene muscles (scalene syndrome) or compression as the plexus passes beneath the scapular attachment of the pectoralis minor muscle (see Figure 44-2B). The infraspinatus muscle has been associated with hand symptoms similar to those of carpal tunnel syndrome[27] and in one study was 12 times more likely than true carpal tunnel syndrome.[28]

Guyon's canal is a passageway on the medial palmar aspect of the wrist that allows the ulnar nerve and artery to enter the hand.[29,30] The canal is created between the hook of the hamate bone and the pisiform bone and the transverse carpal ligament proximally and the aponeurotic arch of the hypothenar muscles distally with the roof of the canal covered by the flexor retinaculum.[1,30] Entrapment or irritation of the ulnar nerve in the canal is termed Guyon's canal syndrome after the French surgeon who first described it in 1861.[29,30] Entrapment can lead to sensory and motor deficits as well as significant disability of hand function. Sensory deficits can affect the palmar ulnar aspect of the hand, both sides of the fifth finger, and the ulnar aspect of the ring finger.[30] Motor effects include loss of strength and potential wasting of the ulnar innervated muscles of the hand including the hypothenar muscles (abductor, opponens, and flexor digiti minimi muscles), the interosseous muscles, the third and fourth lumbrical muscles, the adductor pollicis muscle, and the flexor pollicis muscle.[1,30] Functional loss of normal grip is demonstrated by claw hand and weakness or loss of pinch grip strength.[30] Clinical examination, along with nerve conduction and EMG studies, assists in the differential diagnosis.[30,31]

Intrinsic contracture of the hand may also result from trauma, spasticity, ischemia, rheumatoid arthritis (RA) disorders, or iatrogenic causes. A diagnosis is usually made by history and physical examination; however, imaging, EMG, and blood testing may be required.[32]

Articular dysfunctions, including the loss of joint play, that are associated with interosseous TrPs can occur at either the level of the carpometacarpal joint or at the level of the MCP joint, and any of these joint dysfunctions need to be treated concurrently with the associated interosseous TrPs.

Diseases such as RA and disorders of the skin, vascular, and musculoskeletal systems may influence the hand, making differential diagnosis even more important.[33] Imaging of the hand may prove useful for differential diagnosis in hand trauma or persistent hand pain. The occurrence of hand stress fractures in athletes is not uncommon, and imaging plays an integral role in timely diagnosis and management.[34] The complex nature of the hand may require consultation with specialists in the diagnosis and treatment of orthopedic hand disorders for optimal medical and/or surgical management to maximize functional and occupational outcomes.

5. CORRECTIVE ACTIONS

The patient should learn to reduce the force and duration of pincer grip activities in order to lessen strain on the interosseous muscles. Patients who use ballpoint pens should, if their work permits, write with a more freely flowing felt-tip pen that needs a much lighter touch. Reducing texting through habit modification, alternate modes of communication, or speech-to-text applications can lessen intrinsic hand muscle fatigue and overload. Patient education should also include mindfulness of patterns of increased psychophysiologic arousal and muscle tension during smartphone use.[35] Time away from devices, relaxation exercises, and general aerobic exercises may be helpful treatment strategies.

The patient should interrupt prolonged fine manual activity with the finger-flutter exercise to lessen tension of the intrinsic muscles of the hand. With the arms and hands by the side, the patient gently shakes the hands and arms to release tension. Ergonomic aids for activities of daily living and occupational activities may be required. Ergonomic assessment may play an important role in the adaptation of habitual tasks. Splinting may be helpful in managing specific hand dysfunctions.[30]

Self-pressure release for TrPs in the interosseous, lumbrical, and abductor digiti minimi muscles can be performed in sitting by placing the forearm on the arm rest of a chair or on a table with the thumb pointed up toward the ceiling for the first dorsal interosseous muscle (Figure 40-4A) as well as the other interosseous and lumbrical muscles (Figure 40-4B). Manual pressure is the best method for performing self-pressure release of these muscles. With the palm facing up, a pincer grasp can be

Chapter 40: Interosseous, Lumbrical, and Abductor Digiti Minimi Muscles   393

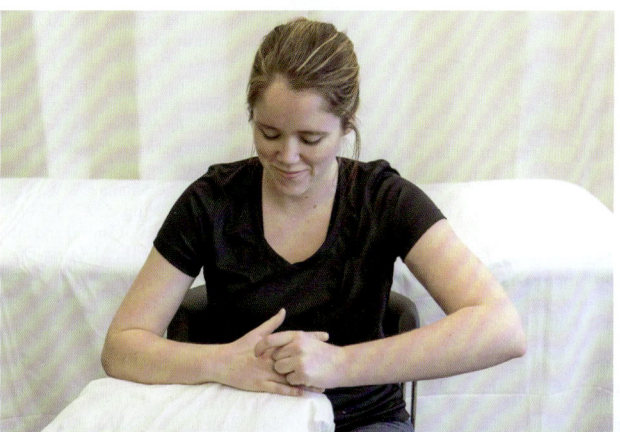

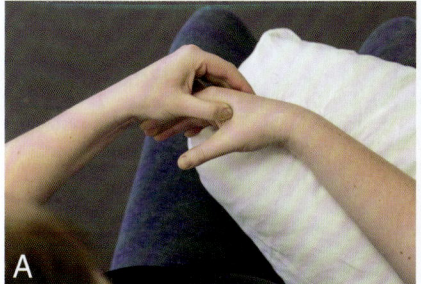 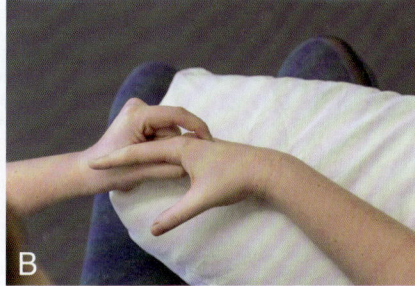 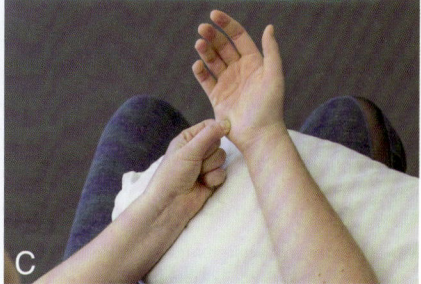

Figure 40-4. Self-pressure release of hand muscle TrPs. A, First dorsal interosseous muscle. B, Interossei and lumbrical muscles. C, Abductor digiti minimi muscle.

used for manual release of TrPs in the abductor digiti minimi muscle (Figure 40-4C). As with any self-pressure release technique, the sensitive spot on the pinky finger side of the hand or in the palm is identified with the fingers, light pressure (no more than 4/10 pain) is applied and held for 15 to 30 seconds or until pain reduces. This technique can be repeated five times several times per day.

When indicated, the patient should perform the interosseous self-stretch exercise, illustrated in Figure 40-5. In doing this exercise, it is important that the forearms form a straight line. When active TrPs are present in the first dorsal interosseous muscle, regular use of the adductor pollicis self-stretch exercise (see Figure 39-6A) may also help ensure continued recovery. These self-stretches should be carried out gently, and attention to the reproduction of pain versus stretch is paramount. These stretches should not be painful.

Strengthening of the upper limb, wrist, thumb, and hand is an important component of upper extremity rehabilitation. Strength deficits identified from a professional assessment can be addressed with the use of hand putty, hand grippers, and weights. The restoration of strength and grip function is an important component of rehabilitation.

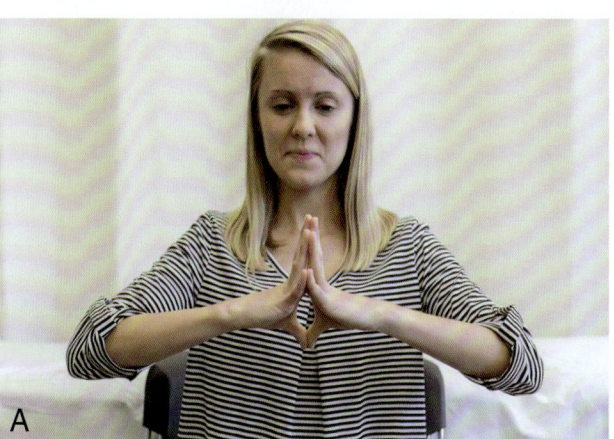 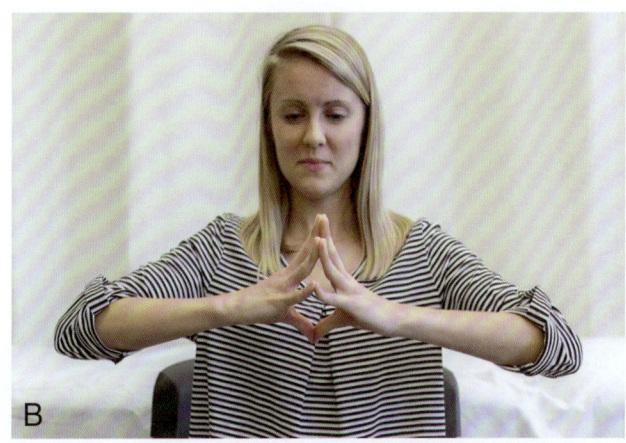

Figure 40-5. Two views of the interosseous-stretch exercise. Both hand positions are effective. The forearms are held in a straight line with the arms abducted. A, An effort is made to firmly oppose the palmar aspects of the metacarpal heads and the fingers, whereas the fingers and thumbs are spread apart. B, Only the finger pads contact each other while the fingers and thumbs are spread apart, with the uninvolved fingers assisting the stretch of the involved interossei muscle.

References

1. Standring S. *Gray's Anatomy: The Anatomical Basis of Clinical Practice.* 41st ed. London, UK: Elsevier; 2015.
2. Bardeen C. The musculature, Section 5. In: Jackson CM, ed. *Morris's Human Anatomy.* 6th ed. Philadelphia, PA: Blakiston's Son & Co; 1921 (p. 444).
3. McMinn RMH, Hutchings RT, Pegington J, Abrahams PH. *Color Atlas of Human Anatomy.* 3rd ed. St. Louis, MO: Mosby Year Book; 1993 (pp. 35D, 147D).
4. Basmajian J, Deluca C. *Muscles Alive.* 5th ed. Baltimore, MD: Williams & Wilkins; 1985 (pp. 291, 292).
5. Jenkins DB. *Hollinshead's Functional Anatomy of the Limbs and Back.* 6th ed. Philadelphia, PA: W.B. Saunders; 1991 (pp. 167-168).
6. Oatis C. *Kinesiology: The Mechanics and Pathomechanics of Human Movement.* Philadelphia, PA: Lippincott Williams & Wilkins; 2004 (pp. 337, 338, 340-344).
7. Kendall FP, McCreary EK. *Muscles: Testing and Function, with Posture and Pain.* 5th ed. Baltimore, MD: Lippincott Williams & Wilkins; 2005 (pp. 270, 272-276).
8. Duchenne G. *Physiology of Motion.* Philadelphia, PA: Lippincott; 1949 (p. 612).
9. Long C II, Conrad PW, Hall EA, Furler SL. Intrinsic-extrinsic muscle control of the hand in power grip and precision handling. An electromyographic study. *J Bone Joint Surg Am Vol.* 1970;52(5):853-867.
10. Travell J, Rinzler SH. The myofascial genesis of pain. *Postgrad Med.* 1952;11(5):425-434.
11. Zohn DA. *Musculoskeletal Pain: Diagnosis and Physical Treatment.* 2nd ed. Boston, MA: Little Brown; 1988 (p. 211, Fig. 12-2).
12. Simons DG, Travell J, Simons L. *Travell & Simon's Myofascial Pain and Dysfunction: The Trigger Point Manual.* Vol 1. 2nd ed. Baltimore, MD: Williams & Wilkins; 1999.
13. Kellgren JH. Observations on referred pain arising from muscle. *Clin Sci.* 1938;3:175-190.
14. Heberden W. *Commentaries on the History and Cure of Diseases.* New York, NY: Hafner Pub. Co.; 1962 (pp 148-149).
15. Reynolds MD. Myofascial trigger point syndromes in the practice of rheumatology. *Arch Phys Med Rehabil.* 1981;62(3):111-114.
16. Gerwin RD, Dommerholt J, Shah JP. An expansion of Simons' integrated hypothesis of trigger point formation. *Curr Pain Headache Rep.* 2004;8(6):468-475.
17. Sharan D, Ajeesh PS. Risk factors and clinical features of text message injuries. *Work.* 2012;41 suppl 1:1145-1148.
18. Hsieh YL, Kao MJ, Kuan TS, Chen SM, Chen JT, Hong CZ. Dry needling to a key myofascial trigger point may reduce the irritability of satellite MTrPs. *Am J Phys Med Rehabil.* 2007;86(5):397-403.
19. Rees F, Doherty S, Hui M, et al. Distribution of finger nodes and their association with underlying radiographic features of osteoarthritis. *Arthritis Care Res (Hoboken).* 2012;64(4):533-538.
20. Radin EL, Parker HG, Paul IL. Pattern of degenerative arthritis. Preferential involvement of distal finger-joints. *Lancet.* 1971;1(7695):377-379.
21. Altman R, Alarcon G, Appelrouth D, et al. The American College of Rheumatology criteria for the classification and reporting of osteoarthritis of the hand. *Arthritis Rheum.* 1990;33(11):1601-1610.
22. Boyle JA, Buchanan WW. *Clinical Rheumatology.* Philadelphia, PA: F.A. Davis; 1971 (pp. 5, 27, 32-34).
23. Moskowitz RW. Clinical and laboratory findings in osteoarthritis, Chapter 56. In: Hollander JL, McCarty DJ, eds. *Arthritis and Allied Conditions.* 8th ed. Philadelphia, PA: Lea & Febiger; 1972 (pp. 1034, 1037, 1045).
24. Mannik M, Gilliland BC. Degenerative joint disease, Chapter 361. In: Wintrobe MM, eds. *Harrison's Principles of Internal Medicine.* 7th ed. New York, NY: McGraw-Hill Book Co.; 1974:2006.
25. Ichikawa N, Taniguchi A, Kobayashi S, Yamanaka H. Performance of hands and feet radiographs in differentiation of psoriatic arthritis from rheumatoid arthritis. *Int J Rheum Dis.* 2012;15(5):462-467.
26. Menegola M, Daikeler T. Painful swollen distal interphalangeal joints are not always Heberden's nodes! *Arthritis Rheumatol.* 2014;66(8):2312.
27. Qerama E, Kasch H, Fuglsang-Frederiksen A. Occurrence of myofascial pain in patients with possible carpal tunnel syndrome—a single-blinded study. *Eur J Pain.* 2009;13(6):588-591.
28. Oh S, Kim HK, Kwak J, et al. Causes of hand tingling in visual display terminal workers. *Ann Rehabil Med.* 2013;37(2):221-228.
29. Maroukis BL, Ogawa T, Rehim SA, Chung KC. Guyon canal: the evolution of clinical anatomy. *J Hand Surg Am.* 2015;40(3):560-565.
30. Cooper C. *Fundamentals of Hand Therapy: Clinical Reasoning and Treatment Guidelines for Common Diagnoses of the Upper Extremity.* St. Louis, MO: Mosby Elsevier; 2007 (pp. 236-239).
31. O'Brien C. *Peripheral Nerve Injuries.* Dublin, Ireland: Eireann Healthcare Publications; 2004.
32. Tosti R, Thoder JJ, Ilyas AM. Intrinsic contracture of the hand: diagnosis and management. *J Am Acad Orthop Surg.* 2013;21(10):581-591.
33. Fontaine C, Staumont-Salle D, Hatron PY, Cotten A, Couturier C. The hand in systemic diseases other than rheumatoid arthritis. *Chir Main.* 2014;33(3):155-173.
34. Anderson MW. Imaging of upper extremity stress fractures in the athlete. *Clin Sports Med.* 2006;25(3):489-504, vii.
35. Lin IM, Peper E. Psychophysiological patterns during cell phone text messaging: a preliminary study. *Appl Psychophysiol Biofeedback.* 2009;34(1):53-57.

Chapter 41

Clinical Considerations of Elbow, Wrist, and Hand Pain

Ann M. Lucado, Gustavo Plaza-Manzano, and César Fernández de las Peñas

1. INTRODUCTION

Potential competing diagnoses are abundant in nontraumatic distal upper extremity pain–producing conditions. A thorough medical history, an upper quarter regional examination, and a detailed assessment of local anatomic structures are required in the clinical diagnosis of conditions causing elbow, wrist, and/or hand pain symptoms. The tight confines in which multiple anatomic structures function in the distal upper extremity make it particularly challenging to isolate pathologic disorders; in fact, symptoms are often attributable to multiple sources. Moreover, movement strategies that an individual may use to avoid or compensate for pain from a primary diagnosis may result in altered motor patterns and overload of muscles. These compensatory movement strategies may result in trigger point (TrP) development in the distal upper extremity musculature, further complicating the isolation of a clinical diagnosis. Nonetheless, it is important to address faulty or compensatory movement patterns along with the primary condition(s). Recent or past trauma to the region can directly or indirectly impact current symptoms. Soft-tissue tumors, other space-occupying lesions, vascular compromise or occlusion, and proximal pathology are all known to mimic painful local musculoskeletal conditions in this region. Systemic disorders such as endocrine dysfunction including diabetes, autoimmune diseases, rheumatologic and neurologic conditions directly impact clinical presentation and must be ruled out or taken into account, if present, as potential contributors to symptoms in the upper extremity. Appropriate medical management is essential for successful outcomes; yet, its comprehensive discussion is beyond the scope of this text. This chapter provides an overview of the most common nontraumatic musculoskeletal clinical considerations of elbow, wrist, and hand pain.

2. LATERAL EPICONDYLALGIA

2.1. Overview

The presence of symptoms in the lateral aspect of the elbow may be primarily associated with local tendinopathy, joint pathology (arthritis, radiocapitellar pathology, posterolateral rotatory instability), or nerve compression (radial tunnel syndrome, posterior interosseous nerve entrapment). Any of these diagnoses may occur in isolation or in combination and do not preclude the presence of referred pain from TrPs in the associated muscles.

Lateral epicondylalgia is commonly considered a tendinopathy of the common wrist extensor tendon at the lateral epicondyle. Although a diagnosis of lateral epicondylalgia may be an accurate term for the patient presenting with pain over the lateral epicondyle, it provides little information about the underlying pathology. In fact, multiple, essentially synonymous, names are associated with this disorder, including, tennis elbow, lateral elbow pain, and lateral epicondylitis. Additionally, several derivations of the term related to tendinopathy have been used to describe the pathophysiology thought to accompany the condition, including tendinitis and tendinosis. Symptoms typically arise in middle-aged active adults.[1] Although it has been commonly associated with tennis players, lateral epicondylalgia also develops in individuals who repetitively use their arms at work or in other sporting activities. The annual incidence of lateral epicondylalgia is less than 10% in the general population,[2] but it continues to be highly prevalent in tennis players, particularly those who are less skilled and play recreationally.[3]

Loading of the wrist extensor muscles in a forceful or repetitive manner, especially in extreme positions of the wrist or elbow, is associated with an onset of lateral epicondylalgia[4]; although symptoms develop gradually. Extrinsic reaction forces from using tools, such as a hammer or tennis racquet, or internal forces generated to manipulate a mouse or type on a keyboard can contribute to the overload of the wrist extensor muscle-tendon unit. Over time, the excessive loading results in a cascade of pathophysiologic events within the tendon, leading to pain. Nirschl[5] and Kraushaar[6] first described tendinopathy in stages that ranged in severity symptoms and tendon pathology. The earliest stage consists of a peritendinous inflammation, whereas later and more severe stages are characterized by angiofibroblastic degeneration and ultimately fibrosis of the tendon.[5] Nevertheless, most histologic studies on lateral epicondylalgia have not found clear evidence of an inflammatory process,[7] and it is likely that individuals may experience acute on chronic aggravation of symptoms after loading an inferior quality tendon. The presence of neuropeptides, substance P, and calcitonin gene-related peptide in local sensory nerve fibers implicates neurogenic inflammation as a possible mediator of pain in patients with lateral epicondylalgia.[8-10] Neurochemical and tissue changes associated with chronic tendinopathy can also result in central sensitization, compounding the potential complexity of this diagnosis.[11] In an effort to adequately explain different clinical presentations, Cook and Purdam[12] proposed a clinical model of histopathologic changes across a continuum from (a) reactive tendinopathy, (b) tendon disrepair to (c) degenerative tendinopathy.

Ultrasonography has been extensively used for the identification of grey-scale hypoechoic lesions that imply dysfunction in the connective tissues; however, hypoechoic lesions identified in the wrist extensor common tendon in patients with lateral epicondylalgia are not linked to pain in the tendon.[12-14] This discrepancy between imaging and clinical pain symptoms has led to some authors claiming that there is a relevant role of nociceptive pain mechanisms in lateral epicondylalgia and other tendinopathies.[15] Today, there is strong evidence implicating the central nervous system in the symptoms experienced in patients with lateral epicondylalgia, which could explain why several patients with unilateral symptoms, if they are not properly treated, develop bilateral symptoms.

Several conservative treatments, such as medication, exercise, and manual therapy, are advocated for the management of lateral epicondylalgia. Therapeutic exercise is probably the physical therapy strategy with the highest evidence for lateral epicondylalgia,[16,17] but eccentric exercise is not necessarily better than concentric exercise.[18] The exercise program should be graduated and progressive from isometric to isotonic contractions of the wrist and forearm muscles, culminating in pragmatic exercises that replicate the patient's required function. This functional management supports a role of the wrist extensor muscles, and hence the presence of TrPs, in lateral epicondylalgia.

2.2. Initial Evaluation of a Patient With Lateral Epicondylalgia

Lateral epicondylalgia is by definition a clinical entity; therefore, imaging studies for confirmatory diagnosis are not usually required. The diagnosis of lateral epicondylalgia can be achieved most easily in the early stages of its onset. Focal pain is located directly over, or immediately distal to, the lateral epicondyle. With time, most patients report pain spreading to the forearm and the wrist. The pain is aggravated with palpation, contractile unit testing of the wrist, and occasionally the finger extensors, and any activity that loads the wrist extensor muscles, including lifting in a pronated position or gripping made worse when the elbow is in an extended position. Stretching of the wrist extensor muscles may also reproduce symptoms. Although muscular tightness may be detected, passive and active elbow, forearm, wrist, and hand range of motion are generally unaffected.[19-21] Patients presenting with lateral epicondylalgia will have pain and weakness with tests that challenge the wrist extensor muscles. Pain-free grip strength is a commonly used outcome measure and has been shown to be more sensitive to change than maximal grip strength in patients with lateral epicondylalgia.[22] Grip strength deficits are generally greater when tested in an elbow extended position than when tested with the elbow at 90° of flexion.[23] Cozen test (resisted wrist radial deviation), Mill stretch maneuver (long extensor stretch), and pain with palpation to the lateral epicondyle are all special tests associated with making this clinical diagnosis; however, the diagnostic utility of these tests has not been established. Because each of these tests stresses other soft tissue located in the region, it is important to interpret the results of the special tests in the context of the entire clinical examination considering the role of muscle tissue instead of just the tendon. The assessment should include examination for TrPs in the wrist extensor muscles including the brachioradialis[24] that may be the source or a contributing factor to the symptoms. In fact, a recent study has reported that the identification of TrPs in the wrist extensor muscles is reliable.[25] Similarly, TrPs in the antagonist muscles, ie wrist flexor muscles, should also be explored.

A detailed clinical examination that systematically rules out other potential causes of lateral elbow pain is essential to improving the confidence in making this differential diagnosis.

3. RADIOCAPITELLAR JOINT PATHOLOGY

3.1. Overview

Patients with arthritic changes at the radiocapitellar joint are typically middle-aged to older adults who present with gradual increasing stiffness and pain in the lateral elbow.[26] Stiffness due to osteoarthritis will be most noticeable in the morning or after periods of rest. If arthritis is due to an inflammatory condition, like rheumatoid arthritis, visible generalized joint effusion may be present. Noninflammatory arthritic conditions can be degenerative in nature or post-traumatic; eg, post-traumatic arthritis may present years following a radial head fracture because of structural changes to the joint causing pain and loss of motion. Articular cartilage tears, loose bodies, and bone spurs can develop and potentially cause mechanical blocks to motion, particularly loss of full elbow extension.

In younger, more athletic, individuals, richly innervated synovial plica at the humeroradial joint may become inflamed, hypertrophied, and symptomatic.[27-29] Although plica, also known as synovial folds, in the elbow are normal, pathologic changes in the lateral synovial fold associated with repetitive elbow motion will cause a vague posterolateral elbow pain and often a palpable "snapping" when the elbow is moved passively or actively.[28]

Posterolateral rotatory instability is most commonly seen in subjects who sustained a traumatic injury to the elbow, particularly a fall on an outstretched arm.[30] The traumatic event tears the lateral collateral ligamentous complex. This will result in gross instability or subluxation of the radial head and ulna from the humerus in a posterolateral direction. In other cases, individuals may present with a slower onset of symptoms because of a gradual attenuation of the lateral collateral ligament complex. The subluxation may be subtle in cases of gradual onset. Assuming that obvious signs of gross instability are not present, a painful click or clunk with motion may be noted, particularly when a person is using the arm to push up to standing from a seated position. Patients will typically report vague, lateral-sided elbow pain. Camp et al[30] hypothesize that repeated cortisone injections commonly used for lateral epicondylalgia may contribute to posterolateral rotatory instability in certain patients because of the steroid's damaging effects on the ligamentous tissue. As in other joint instabilities, it is possible that overactivity of muscles in the region that provide dynamic stability to the joint may lead to TrP formation.

3.2. Initial Evaluation of a Patient With Radiocapitellar Joint Pathology

If radial joint pathology is suspected, clinicians must differentiate between radiocapitellar arthritis, hypertrophied and inflamed synovial plica, and posterolateral rotatory instability. All may produce mechanical limits in passive as well as active range of motion of the elbow and forearm rotation. They may be associated with audible crepitus, clicking, or clunks with motion and will likely present with vague lateral elbow pain.[26] Contractile unit testing is typically normal and not painful in these joint conditions. If associated muscular symptoms are present, the examination should include examination for TrPs in regional muscles that could be contributing to symptoms concurrently, particularly the supinator and pronator teres muscles, among others.[31]

It may be difficult to differentiate between radiocapitellar joint pathologies using clinical evaluation alone. Plain radiographs are useful in confirming the presence of arthritis in the radiocapitellar joint, whereas magnetic resonance imaging is better at identifying hypertrophied and inflamed synovial plica. Provocation of posterolateral rotary instability is difficult without anesthesia because of muscle guarding and pain. The chair push-up or prone push-up tests with the forearm in a supinated position are the most convenient clinical special tests to attempt to provoke subluxation in the elbow. Lateral elbow pain, posterior subluxation of the radial head (as evidenced by dimpling of the skin between the radial head and the capitellum), and a clunk as the subluxed joint reduces are signs of a positive test. The chair and push-up tests are specific for detecting posterolateral rotatory instability but may produce a high percentage of false-negative results. Special tests such as the lateral pivot-shift test or posterolateral rotatory drawer test provide more accurate results, especially when the individual can be fully relaxed under anesthesia.[30]

4. RADIAL (CERVICAL) NERVE ENTRAPMENT

4.1. Overview

The incidence of cervical pathology ranges from 10% to 20% in the general population; it is more common in women than in men, and its onset increases in middle age.[32] In fact, patients with elbow pain and concomitant neck pain typically experience a poorer outcome.[33] Further, several studies show the benefits of adding treatment of the cervical spine to elbow local treatment.[34,35] Cervical radiculopathy is characterized by pain that radiates into the arm that can be associated with loss of sensation and/or weakness. Irritation of the C7 (or occasionally of the C6) nerve root refers symptoms into the lateral elbow region, may mimic symptoms of lateral epicondylalgia, and should be ruled out as a potential proximal cause of elbow pain.[36] Refer to Chapter 33 for further information on cervical radicular pain.

Compression of the posterior interosseous branch of the radial nerve at the dorsal forearm is called radial tunnel syndrome when lateral elbow pain is the primary symptom.[37] The condition referred to as posterior interosseous nerve compression occurs when a pain-free weakness or paresis is present in the finger and thumb extensors, while the wrist extensor muscle strength essentially appears intact. Compression of the posterior interosseous nerve has an estimated annual incidence of 0.03% and is less common than other upper extremity compression syndromes.[38] The nerve can be entrapped within thickened fascial layers close to the radiocapitellar joint, along fibrous bands associated with the extensor carpi radialis brevis muscle, the proximal (arcade of Frohse) or distal borders of the supinator muscle, or can be compressed by abnormalities within the radial recurrent blood vessels in the region referred to as the leash of Henry. Fibro-fatty tumors in the region may also compress the nerve. Characterized by the absence of motor deficits, radial tunnel syndrome is often differentiated from lateral epicondylalgia by the location of pain which is typically located over the supinator muscle belly approximately 5 cm distal to the lateral epicondyle. Although individuals with pathology in the musculotendinous unit of contractile structures tend to have pain associated with activity, individuals with radial tunnel syndrome often report pain at night and may have trouble sleeping.[38]

4.2. Initial Evaluation of a Patient With Cervical or Radial Nerve Entrapment

When radial nerve entrapment is suspected, clinicians must differentiate between more proximal sources of nerve compression in the cervical spine versus compression of the posterior interosseous branch of the radial nerve in the forearm. All individuals with lateral elbow pain should undergo a cervical spine screening. Any reproduction of lateral elbow pain with neck movement, palpation, or during assessment of accessory mobility of the cervical vertebrae will implicate the cervical spine as a potential contributor to lateral elbow pain.[17] Individuals with cervical radiculopathy will likely have associated neck pain and may report paresthesias and/or weakness in the upper extremity. A positive neurodynamic test of the median nerve may also implicate cervical radiculopathy.[32]

Local examination of the elbow is necessary and should include a history and physical examination. Individuals with either posterior interosseous nerve compression or radial tunnel syndrome will report no sensory deficits because of the lack of cutaneous sensory fibers in this deep branch of the radial nerve. Sensation testing may reveal deficits along the C7 or C6 dermatomes in cervical radiculopathy, including the dorsal arm and hand or thumb. In true posterior interosseous nerve compression, the absence of pain and the presence of defined weakness or complete paralysis in the extensor digitorum, extensor indicis, extensor digiti minimi, extensor pollicis longus and brevis, and abductor pollicis longus muscles as well as possibly the extensor carpi ulnaris muscle is evident. Testing procedures will confirm the diagnosis. It is likely that individuals with posterior interosseous nerve compression will demonstrate incomplete or no active digit and thumb extension range of motion, and wrist extension may deviate toward the radial side because of weakness of the extensor carpi ulnaris muscle, while the strength of the radial wrist extensor muscles is spared.

Range-of-motion deficits in the upper extremity are not common in either cervical radiculopathy or radial tunnel syndrome. Strength deficits associated with cervical radiculopathy, if present, are not as clearly defined as in posterior interosseous nerve compression. Palpation over the course of the posterior interosseous nerve in the forearm is generally not painful in individuals with cervical radiculopathy or with posterior interosseous nerve compression; however, the nerve will typically be exquisitely tender in those with radial tunnel syndrome. A positive neurodynamic test of the radial nerve is typical in radial tunnel syndrome but not necessarily in cervical radiculopathy.[32]

Special tests for radial tunnel syndrome may be positive for pain in the region of the supinator muscle, approximately 5 cm distal to the lateral epicondyle. Resisted supination, resisted wrist extension, and resisted middle-finger extension can all load the musculature that forms the roof of the radial tunnel; theoretically, these tests will all potentially cause irritation of the posterior interosseous nerve and replicate symptoms of pain by loading the roof of the tunnel.[38] However, the diagnostic utility of these tests in accurately identifying radial tunnel syndrome have not been clearly established. Peripheral nerve conduction velocity and electromyographic (EMG) testing can also produce false-negative results and are therefore not considered to be useful in many cases of radial tunnel syndrome.[38]

4.3. Trigger Points and Lateral Elbow Pain

Several studies have reported a high prevalence of active TrPs in the wrist extensor muscles, particularly the extensor carpi radialis brevis and longus muscles, in subjects with lateral epicondylalgia[24,39] and blue-collar and white-collar workers.[40] Obviously, any wrist extensor muscle, and potentially the brachioradialis, can be affected (Chapters 34 and 35). It is still unclear as to whether TrPs predispose individuals to lateral epicondylalgia or if they coexist.[41]

The role of TrPs in lateral epicondylalgia is also supported by preliminary evidence showing that myofascial release and dry needling have been found to be effective for reducing symptoms related to lateral epicondylalgia.[42] However, soft-tissue mobilization and manual myofascial release techniques plus ultrasound were no more effective than no treatment or laser for elbow pain.[43] Shmushkevich and Kalichman[41] have called for more research examining the effectiveness of myofascial techniques on reducing symptoms of lateral elbow pain and advocate the use of manual myofascial techniques in the treatment of lateral epicondylalgia. Krey et al[44] conducted a systematic review examining the effectiveness of dry needling alone in the treatment of tendinopathy and concluded that dry needling seems to have a positive effect on self-reported function in the midterm in these patients. Because dry needling is still an emerging intervention for the treatment of TrPs in the treatment of lateral elbow pain, more clinical trials are clearly needed.

Trigger points in other neck and shoulder muscles, such as the scalenes or infraspinatus muscles, and elbow muscles, such as the triceps brachii or anconeus muscles, can also refer pain to the lateral area of the elbow and contribute to symptoms compatible with lateral epicondylalgia; however, limited evidence is available. Clinically, TrPs within the triceps brachii, supinator, and anconeus muscles are more related to individuals with localized elbow pain, whereas TrPs in the wrist extensor muscles are more related to individuals with symptoms spreading throughout the forearm.

Pain in peripheral nerve compression syndromes can be replicated/provoked by maneuvers that either stretch the irritated nerve or exacerbate compressive forces. Because neural tissues are pain-sensitive and are relatively mobile within the musculoskeletal system under normal conditions, nerves have the potential to be responsible for painful movement and dysfunction. However, compression neuropathy often results from a nerve that is chronically compressed by some adjacent anatomic structure. In many cases this structure may be a muscle with taut bands from TrPs or overactivity. Therefore, examination of muscles adjacent to the nerve for TrPs should be conducted in patients with suspected nerve compression syndromes. A clear example of the close association of myofascial pain syndrome and radial tunnel syndrome is seen in patients with symptoms of radial tunnel syndrome who exhibit TrPs in the supinator muscle (Chapter 36).

5. MEDIAL EPICONDYLALGIA

5.1. Overview

Medial epicondylalgia is a condition that causes medial elbow pain that may result from tendinopathy of the common flexor tendon at the medial epicondyle.[45] It is considered analogous to lateral epicondylalgia in terms of its pathophysiology[8]; however, medial epicondylalgia is less prevalent and less often studied than lateral epicondylalgia. Medial epicondylalgia is said to occur more often in golfers than in tennis players, but any activity that cyclically loads the wrist flexor muscles and forearm pronators in a forceful or repetitive manner can cause symptoms.[46]

Management of medial epicondylalgia is more limited than that for lateral epicondylalgia and generally includes a combination of activity modification, ice, oral analgesics, anti-inflammatory medications, physical therapy, iontophoresis, and dry needling. Similar to lateral epicondylalgia, therapeutic exercise would probably lead to positive outcomes in medial epicondylalgia; however, no clinical trials exist on this topic.[47]

5.2. Initial Evaluation of a Patient With Medial Epicondylalgia

Similar to lateral epicondylalgia, a definitive diagnosis is easier to establish early in the onset of its development. Pain is generally localized to the medial epicondyle or just distal to it. The focal pain is aggravated with palpation, contractile unit testing of wrist flexion, and possibly pronation, and with any activity that loads the wrist flexor muscles or pronators. Strength of the wrist flexor muscles and pronators may be inhibited by pain. Stretching of the wrist flexor muscles may also replicate symptoms; although muscular tightness may be detected, passive and active elbow, forearm, wrist, and hand range of motion are generally unaffected.[45] Similarly, as with lateral epicondylalgia, most clinical tests stress other soft tissue located in the region; therefore, it is important to interpret their results in the context of the entire clinical examination and to consider the role of muscle tissue and of the tendon. The assessment should include examination for TrPs in the wrist flexor muscles and forearm pronators that may be the source or a contributing factor to the symptoms. A thorough differential examination should be conducted to rule out other sources of medial elbow pain.

6. HUMEROULNAR JOINT PATHOLOGY

6.1. Overview

Patients with arthritic changes at the humeroulnar joint are typically middle-aged or older adults who present with gradually increasing stiffness and pain in the medial elbow region. Stiffness due to osteoarthritis will be most noticeable in the morning or after periods of rest.[26] If arthritis is due to an inflammatory condition, such as rheumatoid arthritis, visible joint effusion and olecranon bursitis may be present, and oftentimes, the swollen bursa is apparent to visual inspection. Noninflammatory arthritic conditions can be degenerative in nature or post-traumatic, following elbow dislocation and/or fracture. Articular cartilage tears, loose bodies, and bone spurs can develop and potentially cause mechanical blocks to motion, particularly loss of full elbow extension.

In overhead throwing athletes, such as baseball pitchers, javelin throwers, and other athletes who repeatedly use a throwing motion, ulnar collateral ligament (UCL) injuries are common.[48] The ligament originates from the medial epicondyle and runs distally to insert on the ulna. It is the main restraint of the elbow joint to valgus stresses. The valgus stresses on the medial elbow can overload the UCL in time, causing a gradual over-lengthening resulting in ligamentous insufficiency or a tear that could cause joint instability. Both UCL insufficiency and instability are typically associated with medial elbow pain with activity that subsides with rest. Additionally, the athlete may report loss of throwing speed or accuracy.[48] Late stages of UCL insufficiency as a result of repetitive throwing activities is called valgus extension overload syndrome and can be associated with posteromedial osteophyte formation, loose bodies, and flexor-pronator muscle injury.[45]

6.2. Initial Evaluation of a Patient With Humeroulnar Joint Pathology

When medial elbow joint pathology is suspected, it is fairly easy to differentiate between humeroulnar arthritis and UCL/medial joint instability. To start with, the history and the behavior of symptoms are quite different, as outlined above; although both conditions present with vague medial elbow pain. Humeroulnar arthritis may produce mechanical limits in passive as well as active flexion/extension of the elbow because of bone spurs or loose bodies in the joint associated with the arthritic condition. Movement may be associated with audible crepitus or clicking. In contrast, elbow motion is typically full and smooth in individuals with UCL insufficiency or instability.[48]

Pain and stiffness with motion is typically worse in the morning for individuals with arthritic changes at the medial elbow, whereas with UCL injury, motion without resistance is typically pain free. Contractile unit testing is typically normal and not painful in either of these joint conditions. Also, plain radiographs are useful in confirming the presence of arthritis in the humeroulnar joint. Special tests to assess medial elbow joint stability have demonstrated acceptable diagnostic utility in detecting UCL injuries. The moving valgus stress test has demonstrated a superior estimated positive likelihood ratio of 4.0 (95% CI 0.73, 21.8) and a negative likelihood ratio of 0.04 (95% CI 0.00, 0.72) over valgus stress tests to the elbow at varying degrees of elbow flexion. It is important to compare the results of these tests with the contralateral extremity and assess for both pain and instability.[49]

7. POTENTIAL NERVE ENTRAPMENTS CAUSING MEDIAL ELBOW PAIN

7.1. Overview

Thoracic outlet syndrome, as discussed in detail in Chapter 33, is a potential cause of medial elbow pain when the lower trunk of the brachial plexus is affected. Symptoms aside from medial elbow pain may also include neurologic and/or vascular components. Neurologic symptoms are evidenced by sensory disturbance, or even strength deficits in severe cases, in the ulnar nerve distribution. Vascular symptoms may present as arterial compromise associated with a coldness and whitish hue to the hand, venous congestion associated with a purplish hue to the hand, or vasospasm resulting in Raynaud phenomenon characterized by cold insensitivity.

Cubital tunnel syndrome is a condition that results from ulnar nerve compression, stretching or friction irritation anywhere along the medial elbow region. Irritation of the ulnar nerve in the region of the elbow is a potential source of medial elbow pain. Cubital tunnel syndrome is the second most common upper extremity nerve entrapment after carpal tunnel syndrome (CTS).[50] Its prevalence ranges from 0.6% to 0.8% in the general population but may be even more prevalent in individuals with certain occupations. Individuals with high occupational force requirements have a worse prognosis for complete symptom resolution.[50]

Along the course of the ulnar nerve, multiple potential compression sites exist. In the upper extremity, the ulnar nerve pierces the medial intermuscular septum, travels along the posterior aspect of the humerus, and passes through a deep fascial band in the distal arm, called the arcade of Struthers, before it crosses the elbow in the cubital tunnel, posterior to the medial epicondyle, leading into the forearm.[51] The medial intermuscular septum and the arcade of Struthers are potential sites of compression of the ulnar nerve if these fascial bands become thickened, if the muscular attachments become hypertrophied, or through a friction irritation of the nerve associated with repetitive flexion and extension of the elbow.[52] The cubital tunnel itself can be a source of compression as the tunnel floor is formed by the rigid ulna and roof is formed by an unyielding retinaculum that keeps the nerve in place. An attenuation of the cubital tunnel retinaculum can allow the ulnar nerve to sublux anteriorly. Repetitive elbow flexion and extension movements can cause a friction irritation of the ulnar nerve that is compounded if the ulnar nerve is not firmly situated in the ulnar groove. In many subjects, the subluxation may be asymptomatic, but if the ulnar nerve should become symptomatic, the repeated friction irritation from the nerve subluxing anteriorly out of the cubital tunnel perpetuates symptoms and may require surgical intervention in advanced cases.[53] The ulnar nerve can also be compressed as it travels distal to the cubital tunnel into the forearm. An aponeurosis between the humeral and ulnar heads of the flexor carpi ulnaris (FCU) muscle can be a source of ulnar nerve irritation.[51] Forearm flexor muscle hypertrophy can exacerbate irritating forces along the ulnar nerve.[54]

Because there is little subcutaneous tissue protecting the nerve at the elbow, the ulnar nerve is also susceptible to direct pressure from leaning the elbow region on a table or arm rest. Because the nerve courses posterior to the axis of rotation of the elbow, when the joint is flexed, the nerve is stretched. If the elbow is held in a flexed position and tension is placed on the ulnar nerve for prolonged periods of time, symptoms of cubital tunnel syndrome are evoked. Holding a phone up to the ear for a prolonged period of time can cause ulnar nerve irritation at the elbow, as can a sleeping posture of acute elbow flexion. Cubital tunnel syndrome is typically associated with paresthesias and sensory disturbance, and in the long term can result in weakness in muscles innervated by the ulnar nerve including the FCU muscle, the flexor digitorum profundus muscle to the fourth and fifth digits, and most of the intrinsic muscles of the hand. Muscle strength deficits are often associated with reports of clumsiness and the inability to grip tightly.[45]

The median nerve also travels in the medial arm and forearm and can be a potential source of medial elbow pain, although in a lesser extent than the ulnar nerve. Entrapment of the median nerve in the elbow region is referred to as pronator syndrome. It has been reported to be more common in women and occurs primarily in middle-aged adults.[55] Pronator syndrome is associated with variations in local muscular architecture and is characterized by vague medial elbow pain and sensory disturbance in the median nerve distribution at the hand.[56] The sensory symptoms may be similar to those of CTS; however, sensation in the palm is impaired in pronator syndrome and spared in CTS because the anterior cutaneous branch splits from the median nerve proximal to the carpal canal. Symptoms are aggravated with repetitive forearm rotational tasks in occupations requiring assembly-line work.[55] Anecdotally, it is also seen in active individuals who are avid rock climbers. Finally, compression of the anterior interosseous nerve is referred to as anterior interosseous nerve compression syndrome, and it is mainly differentiated from pronator syndrome by its characteristic nonpainful weakness or paresis of the muscles it innervates. No sensory disturbance is noted in anterior interosseous nerve compression.[56]

7.2. Initial Evaluation of a Patient With Potential Nerve Entrapments Causing Medial Elbow Pain

The examination for identifying thoracic outlet syndrome has been described in detail in Chapter 33. When examining individuals suspected of having either ulnar or median nerve entrapment associated with medial elbow pain, common symptoms denoting a nerve compression issue will include sensory disturbance and possible weakness in the peripheral nerve distribution of the involved nerve. Therefore, in addition to the history, visual inspection, and general orthopedic examination assessing range of motion and contractile unit testing, a full sensory examination and manual muscle test may be required to fully differentiate the source and location of nerve compression. Results of the examination will vary greatly depending on the extent and severity of nerve entrapment. Severe cases of entrapment can be easy to identify, but the subtle signs of either cubital tunnel or pronator syndrome may be more difficult to discern early in the stages of compression. Provocative maneuvers include Tinel test over the involved nerve, neurodynamic testing of the ulnar or median nerve, and muscle length tests (which may irritate the nerve if taut). All muscles related to each particular nerve should be examined for the presence of TrPs, including, the flexor digitorum profundus and FCU muscles in patients with a potential involvement of the ulnar nerve. Electrodiagnostic tests for compromise of ulnar nerve function have demonstrated excellent diagnostic utility in cubital tunnel syndrome but not for pronator syndrome. This difference may be related to the depth at which the median nerve travels compared with the more superficial ulnar nerve.

Multiple nerve entrapments may occur simultaneously and are commonly referred to as a "double crush" phenomenon. One compression site on a nerve will lower its threshold for occurrence of a second neuropathy along the same nerve, by blocking the axonal transport mechanism by which the nerve cell body provides nutrition and removes breakdown products. This block makes a nerve that has a more proximal (or distal) entrapment more susceptible to a second location of entrapment. It is therefore important to examine the structures along the entire path of the nerve. It is common to see multiple neuropathy situations occur along the median nerve at the level of the cervical spine, the pronator teres, and the carpal canal and along the ulnar nerve at the thoracic outlet, the elbow, and the wrist.

7.3. Trigger Points and Medial Elbow Pain

Trigger points in the wrist flexor muscles or forearm pronator muscles could lead to symptoms associated to medial epicondylalgia; however, there is no epidemiologic study in the literature investigating this topic. In all nerve entrapment syndromes that are associated with medial elbow pain, muscle hypertrophy and/or overactivity due to taut bands resulting from TrPs are potential contributors to the irritation of the involved peripheral nerve. For instance, in thoracic outlet syndrome, overactivity of the scalene muscles related to excessive use of these muscles for breathing, or of the pectoralis musculature in weight lifters due to excessive training of the anterior chest muscles, can cause compression of the lower portion of the brachial plexus; hypertrophy of the FCU muscle can cause entrapment of the ulnar nerve; pronator teres hypertrophy, such as in rock climbers, can result in the compression of the median nerve of the elbow. Although there is a scarcity of studies examining the relationship, it stands to reason that abnormal tone related to taut bands resulting from TrP in musculature adjacent to these nerves may also be related to nerve compression syndromes. Therefore, all muscles related to a particular peripheral nerve should be evaluated for TrPs and managed appropriately. Trigger points in the proximal upper quarter musculature that also contribute to medial elbow pain may include the scalene, pectoralis major, latissimus dorsi, teres major, and subscapularis muscles.

8. RADIAL WRIST/THUMB PAIN

8.1. Overview

The presence of symptoms in the radial area of the wrist and thumb may be primarily associated with local tendinopathy (DeQuervain tenosynovitis, intersection syndrome, extensor pollicis longus muscle irritation), joint pathology (carpometacarpal joint [CMCJ] arthritis, ganglion cyst), or local nerve compression (Wartenburg syndrome, CTS). Any of these diagnoses may occur in isolation or in combination.

DeQuervain tenosynovitis, intersection syndrome, and irritation of the extensor pollicis longus tendon are all tendinopathies that can contribute to radial wrist pain. DeQuervain tenosynovitis refers to a painful tendonitis of the first dorsal compartment tendons including the abductor pollicis longus and extensor pollicis brevis muscles. Repetitive movements of the thumb and loading of the involved tendons are thought to be causative factors. The meta-analysis conducted by Stahl et al[57] found 2.89 (95% CI 1.4-5.97) increased odds of developing DeQuervain tenosynovitis with repetitive, forceful, or ergonomically stressful manual work. It is also a common condition in new mothers that seems to be related to lifting a newborn or toddler child and in people who do needle work, use a computer mouse, and in phlebotomists. Pain along the thumb that increases with activity or lifting with the forearms in a neutral position is typical in people with DeQuervain tenosynovitis.

Intersection syndrome refers to tendonitis at the intersection site where the abductor pollicis longus and extensor pollicis brevis muscles cross over the extensor carpi radialis longus and brevis tendons in the distal radial forearm.[58] Hypertrophy of the abductor pollicis longus and extensor pollicis brevis muscles at the dorsal distal forearm can be often visually appreciated. Extensor pollicis longus tendon irritation can occur where the tendon is redirected at Lister tubercle on the distal radius. Attenuation and eventually rupture of the extensor pollicis longus tendon is known to occur in subjects with rheumatoid arthritis. The onset of each of these tendinopathies at the radial wrist is associated with repetitive thumb and/or wrist movements.

The most common nontraumatic joint pathologies causing radial wrist pain include CMCJ or metacarpal phalangeal (MCP) joint osteoarthritis of the thumb and development of a dorsal wrist ganglion. As in other osteoarthritic conditions, the onset typically occurs in middle-aged adults and may have a genetic component, or it may be associated with previous trauma to the joint. Osteoarthritis in any joint of the hand is characterized by pain, stiffness, and deformity. In the thumb CMCJ, a visible bump represents the dorsal subluxation of the 1st metacarpal on the trapezium. Nodules can also develop in the finger joints causing generalized hand pain: the proximal interphalangeal (PIP) joint nodules are referred to as Bouchard nodes and those at the distal interphalangeal (IP) joint are called Heberden nodes. Activities including opening jars, turning keys, and writing are often reported to be painful in patients with CMCJ or hand arthritis.

Ganglion cysts are fluid-filled lumps that occur commonly at the dorsal wrist and sometimes the fingers.[59] The cause of ganglion cysts is unknown, although they seem to occur in subjects who use the wrist in repetitively or in extreme positions and may be associated with tendon or joint irritation or mechanical changes. They occur in patients of all ages, genders, and ethnic backgrounds. Ganglion cysts vary in size, location, and may or not cause pain. They may cause sensory disturbance if located in the region of a nerve. A common site for ganglion cyst formation is at the scapholunate joint and therefore can be the cause of radial wrist/thumb pain. Ganglions can also form at other joints and can therefore be the cause of pain anywhere in the hand depending on its location. Because ganglion cysts are known to resolve naturally in time with no intervention, many times no treatment is offered. If the ganglion cyst is causing symptoms of pain, loss of motion, or causing nerve compression, the cyst can be aspirated or surgically removed.

Irritation of the radial nerve can also cause radial wrist/thumb pain. Wartenburg syndrome is a radial nerve irritation at wrist level where the superficial branch of the radial nerve emerges between the brachioradialis and extensor carpi radialis longus tendons. Pronation of the forearm causes these two tendons to come together and compress the radial nerve. Repetitive pronation and supination may cause irritation at this site secondary to the creation of a scissoring effect between the brachioradialis and extensor carpi radialis longus muscles. Blunt local trauma, a wrist watch applied too tightly, or a surgical incision in the region can also cause the nerve irritation. The annual incidence rate for Wartenburg syndrome is 0.003%.[38] This condition may affect cutaneous sensation to the radial thenar area and the dorsal hand and wrist and can cause extreme hypersensitivity in the cutaneous nerve distribution including the dorsum of the 1st and 2nd metacarpals. In some cases, pain may extend proximally and radially into the forearm and is typically described as sharp and shooting.

8.2. Initial Evaluation of Patients With Radial Wrist/Thumb Pain

A detailed history is imperative to allow the clinician to obtain as much information as possible regarding the causes of the patient's symptoms. Information must be gathered regarding the physical demands and postural requirements of the patient at work, at home, and at play. In addition, what activities exacerbate and relieve the symptoms must be noted. This knowledge will be critical for the recommendation and implementation of activity modifications.

Patients with Dequervain tenosynovitis and intersection syndrome will report no sensory deficits, and Tinel test will be negative in both conditions. Pain reports are local to the anatomic snuffbox and thumb in DeQuervain tenosynovitis and are located in the distal third of the dorsal forearm (approximately 4-6 cm proximal to the first dorsal compartment) in intersection syndrome. Application of resistance to the affected tendons will aggravate the pain; abductor pollicis longus and extensor pollicis brevis–resisted testing may produce pain in both conditions, but resisted wrist extension is typically painful in intersection syndrome as well. Crepitus is often palpated at the intersection site with wrist range of motion, and swelling in the area may be visible; these findings are absent in DeQuervain tenosynovitis. Finkelstein test is a highly sensitive test that results in many positive, including false-positive, results. It can be positive in patients with intersection syndrome, but pain is usually located over the intersection site. If Finkelstein test is negative, it is likely that the patient does not have DeQuervain tenosynovitis.[60]

The evaluation of patients with CMCJ arthritis should include a close visual inspection of the region. The appearance of the thumb is distinct because of the arthritic changes, but may not be fully appreciated in early stages. Dorsal subluxation of the 1st metacarpal on the trapezium is evident as a dorsal bump at the base of the thumb. In advanced cases, a thumb CMCJ adduction contracture and MCP joint extension contracture can develop. Sensory deficits are not typical, but pain can be elicited with palpation directly of the CMCJ and with resisted or sustained pinch activities that compound the dorsally directed forces of the 1st metacarpal on the trapezium. Other resisted tests may be variably uncomfortable but not associated with specific tendon loading. Tinel tests over regional nerves are typically negative. Approximation and rotation of the 1st metacarpal on the trapezium through the grind test may elicit pain, especially earlier in the disease process, and joint surface changes may be appreciated as crepitus type sensation by the clinician.

Visual inspection is also an important component when a ganglion cyst is suspected. A visible discrete bump located at the dorsal wrist is the most typical presentation. Although palpation may reveal a soft fluid or gel filled nodule that becomes more noticeable with wrist flexion, the presentation of ganglion cysts is quite variable in the hand. Referral to a hand specialist is recommended for definitive medical treatment if it is highly symptomatic.

As it has been previously mentioned, a screen of the cervical spine is necessary for all patients who are thought to have a peripheral nerve compression, because of the potential of a multiple neuropathy syndrome along the nerve segment or referred pain from a cervical radiculopathy. A proximal origin of symptoms should be suspected if pain is radiating into the chest wall or posteriorly along the medial border of the scapula. A cervical radiculopathy or radicular pain may present if symptoms increase with a Valsalva maneuver, coughing, or sneezing. The examination may include the assessment of motor weakness in the C6 distribution (elbow flexion or wrist extension) or C7 distribution (elbow extension, finger extension, and flexion).

The examination of patients with Wartenburg syndrome will demonstrate symptoms consistent with an isolated neuritis of the superficial radial nerve including loss of cutaneous sensation to the radial thenar area and the dorsal hand and wrist, and it is often associated with extreme hypersensitivity including the dorsum of the 1st and 2nd metacarpals. Range of motion and strength are typically intact, although movements of the forearm or wrist may aggravate pain. Provocative tests for Wartenberg syndrome will produce tingling or an "electric" type pain along the course of the superficial radial nerve when positive including the Tinel test over the superficial radial nerve. Placing the proximal portions of the superficial radial nerve in a stretched position (extended elbow, pronated forearm, and ulnarly deviated wrist) will likely increase symptoms as will the Finklestein position, because the simultaneous thumb flexion and wrist ulnar deviation places the distal portion of the superficial radial nerve on stretch.

8.3. Trigger Points and Radial Wrist and Thumb Pain

The role of forearm musculature in radial wrist and thumb pain may be lower than in other pain syndromes of the forearm. Obviously, tension induced by taut bands resulting from TrPs in these muscles could lead to an increased load in the respective tendon and therefore be a contributing or perpetuating factor for the pain symptoms. There is no study investing this topic.[61]

9. ULNAR WRIST PAIN

9.1. Overview

The presence of symptoms in the ulnar area of the wrist may be primarily associated with local tendinopathy (FCU or extensor carpi ulnaris tendinopathy), joint pathology (triangular fibrocartilage complex [TFCC] degeneration, distal radial ulnar joint instability, or ulnar impaction syndrome), or local nerve compression (Guyon tunnel syndrome).

Pain at the ulnar aspect of the wrist can be challenging to diagnose because of the multiple interrelated anatomic structures on the ulnar side that contribute to wrist joint stability as well as to its mobility and are required to place the hand in numerous positions for function.[62] There are multiple causes of ulnar wrist pain that all have similar symptoms.[63] Activities that require repeated forearm rotation, radial/ulnar deviation of the wrist, and/or sudden impact involving the forearm, wrist, or hand can result in overload of the ulnar wrist structures and may result in ulnar wrist injury and pain. It is common in athletes such as golfers, baseball players, lacrosse players, and many others who use equipment to aggressively impact or throw a ball or puck.[64] Gymnasts and weight lifters who bear high loads of weight on the wrist are also susceptible to ulnar-sided wrist injuries. Occupations that have similar force requirements can also result in workers who sustain ulnar-sided wrist injury and subsequent pain.

It is the intricate connections between the tendons, ligaments, and joints at the ulnar wrist that make it difficult to differentiate involved tissues in patients with ulnar-sided wrist pain. The TFCC is an arrangement of ligamentous and cartilaginous tissue at the ulnar wrist joint that acts as a cushion in the space between the ulna and ulnar carpal bones preventing ulnocarpal abutment. This complex acts as a major stabilizing structure for the distal radioulnar joint. It distributes loads at the ulnar wrist and contributes to the complex, fine movements of the wrist and forearm. The TFCC consists of the articular disc structures, UCL, dorsal and palmar radioulnar ligaments, floor of extensor carpi ulnaris sub-sheath, and the ulnolunate and ulnotriquetral ligaments.[51] These structures provide anatomic links connecting the joint structures to the stabilizing ligaments and to the movers of the joint through the tendons. Injury to one of these structures can impact the function of the other structures.

In patients with suspected tendon pathology, extensor carpi ulnaris irritation or subluxation is more common and potentially problematic than irritation to the FCU muscle.[62] Injury to the extensor carpi ulnaris complex is common in elite male (76%) over female tennis players (45%) as well as other elite athletes.[65] The location of the extensor carpi ulnaris tendon within the sixth dorsal compartment of the wrist is recognized as the second most common location of stenosing tenosynovitis. The spectrum of extensor carpi ulnaris injury ranges from a painful tenosynovitis, subluxation of the extensor carpi ulnaris with corresponding irritation to the tendon, to complete rupture of the extensor carpi ulnaris tendon.[65] Dynamic instability of the extensor carpi ulnaris tendon is associated with a shallow ulna groove, a weakened sheath due to repetitive impact, or an acute injury. Subluxation will not present in static situations; therefore, it is important to palpate the tendon for shifting during forearm rotation.[65]

If joint or ligamentous pathology is suspected, a TFCC tear should be ruled out as a potential source of pathology. In the absence of a traumatic incident, this ulnar stabilizing complex may have been exposed to stresses over time causing degenerative changes to the TFCC complex. Compressive loading of the TFCC or repetitive forearm rotation stresses can result in TFCC injury and is a cause of ulnar wrist pain, and in severe cases, instability of the distal radial ulnar joint.[64]

Normally, the TFCC absorbs approximately 20% of compressive loads of the wrist, with the radiocarpal joint taking the rest of the load.[64] However, alterations in ulnar variance, referring to the relative position of the articular surfaces of the radius and ulna at the wrist, will change this load distribution. A positive ulnar variance refers to a situation where the ulna projects more distally than normal. Ulnar impaction syndrome may result in positive ulnar variance leading to excessive loads on the ulnar aspect of the wrist and the TFCC. Over time, the excessive ulnar forces can lead to TFCC degeneration and tears. Ulnar impaction syndrome most commonly presents in middle-aged patients and may be associated with a previous wrist or forearm fracture or simply repetitive use in a person whose normal wrist architecture presents with positive ulnar variance. Conversely, Keinbock disease is associated with negative ulnar variance and excessive loading of the radius on the carpus, and results in avascular necrosis of the lunate and in mid-dorsal wrist pain. Local pain with palpation directly over the lunate and wrist radiographs can confirm the diagnosis. The etiology of Keinbock disease is unknown.

Guyon tunnel syndrome is a neuropathy of the ulnar nerve at the wrist level that causes ulnar-sided symptoms at the wrist and hand. It is associated with either external compression (handlebar palsy in cyclists, using the hand as a hammer) or a space-occupying lesion (ulnar artery thrombosis, ganglion). It can be easily confused with cubital tunnel syndrome and should also be differentiated from thoracic outlet syndrome and cervical radiculopathy affecting the C8/T1 segments.

9.2. Initial Evaluation of Patients With Ulnar Wrist Pain

When evaluating a patient with tendinopathy, resisted or muscle length testing will reproduce pain in the involved tendon in either the extensor carpi ulnaris or FCU muscles. Palpation along the distal portion of the tendon will also elicit pain. Range of motion will typically demonstrate no restrictions; however, the dorsal ulnar wrist should be palpated and visualized during forearm rotation to identify subluxation of the extensor carpi ulnaris tendon. A painful snapping or clicking sensation over the dorsoulnar side of the wrist is a typical finding in a patient who has an unstable extensor carpi ulnaris tendon. The extensor carpi ulnaris synergy test is positive if bowstringing is visible and/or pain is replicated when the patient radially abducts the thumb against resistance with the forearm in supination and wrist in neutral (causing a synergistic co-contraction of the extensor carpi ulnaris muscle).[66]

The FCU muscle has no tendon sheath and is not physically attached to the TFCC and is therefore more straightforward to evaluate its contribution to ulnar wrist pain.[62] Range of motion and sensation are typically without restriction in FCU tendinopathy. Contractile unit testing in wrist flexion and ulnar deviation and sometimes palpation will result in volar ulnar wrist pain approximately 3 cm proximal to the pisiform along the FCU tendon.[62]

A click or pop may also be noticeable with forearm rotation in patients with TFCC injury, although joint motion is typically full. Visual inspection will often reveal a more prominent ulnar styloid compared with the uninvolved extremity. Pain or distal radioulnar joint instability may be detected with special tests. The ulnomeniscotriquetral dorsal glide test (piano key test) may reveal distal radioulnar joint instability because of a TFCC tear. Testing in various degrees of pronation and supination may elicit pain, tenderness, and increased mobility compared with the contralateral side, and all may suggest distal radioulnar joint injury/instability.[67] Tenderness with palpation immediately distal to the distal radioulnar joint and between the head of the ulna and triquetrum may indicate a TFCC problem or an ulnocarpal abutment. The TFCC can also be loaded axially while ulnarly deviating the wrist and moving the wrist into flexion and extension. Any crepitus and/or reproduction of symptoms may indicate a TFCC tear or ulnocarpal abutment or impaction.[28] Forearm pronation or ulnar deviation of the wrist effectively increases positive ulnar variance; therefore, grip testing in a pronated position compared with a supinated position will accentuate symptoms when ulnar impaction and/or TFCC injury is present.

Sensory examination helps differentiate neural compression that may be contributing to ulnar-sided wrist pain. In local ulnar nerve compression, referred to as "Guyon tunnel syndrome," sensation on the volar ulnar aspect of the hand is affected, but the dorsoulnar hand sensation is spared. If the compression is more proximal, as in cubital tunnel syndrome, dorsoulnar hand sensation deficits will be apparent. Symptoms of Guyon syndrome include pain along the ulnar side of palm as well as the fourth and fifth digits, sensation deficits in the same distribution, and weakness of the ulnar innervated intrinsic muscles. Muscle testing will reveal compression of superficial branch leading to possible weakness/atrophy of the hypothenar muscle group, most notably the first dorsal interosseous muscles and the third/fourth lumbrical muscles. In advanced cases, complete paralysis will present as a clawed hand in the fourth and fifth digits. Compression of the deep branch of the ulnar nerve is more common in chronic compression and may also lead to weakness of the flexor pollicis brevis and adductor pollicis muscles. Motor involvement will grossly impact grip and pinch strength of the hand; therefore, weakness in both may be detected. Froment sign may be positive. With attempts to perform lateral pinch against resistance, the IP joint of the thumb flexes, indicating weakness of the abductor pollicis muscle and the deep head of the flexor pollicis brevis muscle. Wartenberg sign may be seen where the fifth digit is held in an abducted position from the fourth digit secondary to weakness of the volar interosseous muscle. These tests may also be positive in cubital tunnel syndrome; therefore, location of pain, Tinel test, and sensory examination may be helpful in differentiating the location of ulnar nerve compression. In cubital tunnel syndrome, motor weakness to the FCU muscle and the flexor digitorum profundus muscle to the fourth and fifth digit may be present and can result in less of a clawed position of the ulnar digits secondary to lack of strength in the flexor digitorum profundus muscle which is no longer pulling unopposed to the lumbrical muscles.[68] The examination should also include differential tests to rule out the cervical spine (C8, T1) or thoracic outlet as being the cause of ulnar nerve symptoms. Tinel and Phalen tests at the wrist will often times be positive over the ulnar nerve at the wrist in Guyon tunnel syndrome, but is negative in the more proximal nerve compressions.

9.3. Trigger Points and Ulnar Wrist Pain

The role of forearm musculature in ulnar wrist pain may be lower than in other pain syndromes of the forearm. Again, tension induced by TrP taut bands in these muscles could lead to an increased load in the respective tendon and therefore becomes a contributing or perpetuating factor for the pain symptoms. Experimentally induced pain through saline injections in the extensor carpi ulnaris muscle results in pain spreading distally on the ulnar side of the forearm toward the hand, although no changes in motor activity are found when mechanical circumstances remain the same.[69] Because of the complexity of the anatomy and differential diagnosis at the ulnar wrist, examining TrPs in the extensor carpi ulnaris or FCU muscles should not be neglected.

10. CARPAL TUNNEL SYNDROME

10.1. Overview

CTS is a compression of the median nerve at the wrist under the transverse carpal ligament, which extends from the tuberosity of the scaphoid and part of trapezium to the pisiform and hook of the hamate. It is the most common nerve compression syndrome in the upper extremity and is characterized by pain and paresthesia in the median nerve distribution of the hand usually including the thumb, index finger, middle finger, and radial aspect of the ring finger. Dale et al[70] pooled the epidemiologic data of CTS and reported an overall prevalence rate of 7.8% and an incidence rate of 2.3/100 persons/year. Symptoms increase with repetitive hand or wrist movements. Patients report clumsiness and weakness in the hand. Paresthesia and pain tend to be worse at night. Some studies have observed that patients with CTS also exhibit symptoms throughout the upper extremity.[71]

The underlying causes of CTS are highly variable, but are associated with several conditions that cause increased pressure within the carpal tunnel, including pregnancy or thyroid disorders that may cause fluid retention. Repetitive movements of the wrist and/or fingers or use of the wrist in extreme positions can cause swelling around the wrist flexor muscle tendons, referred to as tenosynovitis, which imparts increased pressure in the carpal tunnel. Trauma resulting in carpal joint dislocations, fractures in the region, or arthritic conditions can increase pressure in the canal resulting in symptoms of CTS.[72,73]

Potential compression sites of the median nerve include those at the ligament of Struthers (a ligament that links the supracondylar ridge and medial epicondyle of the humerus) in the distal arm, under the lacertus fibrosus of the biceps brachii tendon (if present), where the median nerve passes between the aponeurotic arch linking the humeral and ulnar heads of the pronator teres, and where it travels under the arch of the flexor digitorum superficialis muscle between the radial and humeral heads of that muscle.[51]

Management of CTS is still controversial because some authors propose a conservative approach, whereas others suggest surgery. It is interesting to note that conservative treatments applied just locally to the carpal tunnel have shown limited results.[74,75] Similarly, outcomes are not clearly different between conservative and surgical treatments. Current theories propose that treatment of patients with CTS should include soft-tissue treatment of those areas anatomically related to the median nerve, ie, muscles, and neural mobilization interventions, suggesting a role for TrPs.

10.2. Initial Evaluation of a Patient With Carpal Tunnel Syndrome

Reports of transient symptoms as well as nocturnal pain and paresthesia within the hand are extremely common in patients with CTS; therefore, an assessment of the behavior of symptoms should be obtained. The gold standard for a diagnosis of CTS is the following clinical presentation: paresthesia, pain, swelling, weakness, or clumsiness of the hand provoked or worsened by sleep, sustained hand or arm positions, repetitive action of the hand or wrist that is mitigated by changing postures or by shaking of the hand, sensory deficits in the median-innervated region of the hand, and motor deficit or hypotrophy of the median-innervated thenar muscles. Provocative tests may replicate patient's symptoms or cause a tingling or "electric" type pain along the course of the median nerve when positive. Phalen test, reverse Phalen test, Tinel test, carpal compression test, and neurodynamic testing have been studied for their diagnostic utility and have shown variable results; however, the majority of tests demonstrate positive and negative likelihood ratios close to one and/or nonsignificant results, indicating that none of these tests alone are particularly consistently useful in confirming the diagnosis of CTS. The presence of clusters of factors improves the diagnostic accuracy of CTS. The presence of four of the following factors increases the probability of having CTS by over four times (+LR = 4.6): shaking hands for symptom relief, wrist-ratio index greater than 0.67, symptom severity scale score >1.9 points, reduced median sensory field of the first digit, and age greater than 45 years.[36]

Another gold standard for the confirmation of CTS diagnosis is the EMG. In fact, some studies have identified the relationship between the distribution of sensory pain symptoms and the severity of CTS, according to the neurophysiologic classification. Patients with lower severity of pathology report sensory symptoms with a glove distribution, whereas patients with a higher severity of pathology report sensory symptoms with the "classical" median distribution, suggesting that affectation of the median nerve depends on its compression. Sensitivity testing reveals reduced light touch, pain, and temperature detection in the distal median nerve distribution. The palmar cutaneous branch of the median nerve distribution at the palm of the hand will demonstrate intact sensation in CTS but may be impaired in more proximal nerve compressions. Two-point discrimination tests (sensor receptor density) may be normal in CTS; therefore, the more sensitive Semmes Weinstein Monofilament test (threshold sensory examination) is preferred when attempting to detect sensory changes in CTS. Stress testing along with, before, and after volumetric and sensory measurements can objectify increases in hand volume and sensory changes after provoking activities.

Motor dysfunction may be noted in severe or more chronic cases; weakness and atrophy may be present in the median-innervated musculature including the abductor pollicis brevis, opponens pollicis, and first and second lumbrical muscles. Grip and pinch strength may be reduced secondary to weakness of these intrinsic muscles.

Cervical radicular pain or radiculopathy involving the C6 and C7 nerve roots may mimic CTS symptoms including mild to moderate aching in the forearm, and if symptoms are associated with neck or shoulder pain, one should suspect more proximal compression at the level of the pronator teres, cervical spine, or a multiple neuropathy syndrome at either of those locations. Therefore, examination of the cervical spine should be included in CTS.

Finally, clinicians should examine all muscles anatomically related to the median nerve for TrPs, particularly the scalene, pectoralis minor, biceps brachii, pronator teres, flexor digitorum, and lumbrical muscles.

10.3. Trigger Points and Carpal Tunnel Syndrome

Chapter 38 outlines the association of TrPs in the pronator teres muscle with symptoms of CTS. Cervical radicular pain or radiculopathy involving the C6 or C7 nerve roots is known to appear symptomatically similar to CTS, but symptoms may be aggravated by TrPs in muscles innervated by the affected nerve root. Active TrPs in infraspinatus or upper trapezius muscles proximally and in the pronator teres, flexor carpi radialis, palmaris longus, and/or biceps brachii muscles are potential sources of referred pain that cause symptoms that can be confused with CTS or other conditions causing radial hand pain. Qerama et al[76] found that one-third of patients referred with clinical symptoms compatible with CTS, but EMG negative, exhibited active TrPs in the infraspinatus muscle reproducing their symptoms. Nevertheless, local neuropathy of the median nerve could also activate TrPs. In such scenarios, Azadeh et al[77] observed that 70% of patients with clinical and electrophysiologic evidence of CTS showed TrPs in the upper trapezius muscle, probably related to nerve irritation. Therefore, an assessment of upper extremity muscles for the presence of TrPs is imperative in the differential diagnosis of CTS.

11. OTHER CAUSES OF HAND PAIN

11.1. Overview

Other causes of symptoms in the hand may be associated with Dupuytren contracture or trigger finger (stenosing tenosynovitis of the flexor tendons). Dupuytren contracture is an abnormal thickening of the tissue just beneath the skin. This thickening occurs in the palm and can extend into the fingers. Firm pits, bumps, and firm cords can develop in the palm, and occasionally at the dorsal PIP joints, resulting in flexion contractures of the fingers, primarily at the MCP and PIP joints. The cause of Dupuytren contracture is unknown. This condition is more common in men, people over age 40, and people of Caucasian/European descent.[78] There is no evidence that hand injuries or specific jobs lead to a higher risk of developing Dupuytren contracture. In the case of Dupuytrens, dimpling over the palmar crease on the ulnar side of the hand is evident along with digital flexion contractures, most typically involving the MCP and PIP joints of the ring or little finger. Palpation of the palm in early development of Dupuytren contracture reveals discretely tender nodules and patient reports of diffuse palmar tenderness.[79] The presence of digital flexion contractures, discrete nodules, and diffuse tenderness are typical findings of Dupuytren contracture. Estimations of the prevalence of the disease vary considerably, depending on where monitoring occurs, as it is more common in Europe.[78]

Although uncomfortable in some people, Dupuytren contracture is not typically painful. As the fingers contract into the palm, it may be more difficult to wash hands, wear gloves, shake hands, and get hands into pockets. It is difficult to predict how the disease will progress. Some people have only small lumps or cords, whereas others will develop severe contractures.

Trigger finger is a stenosing tenosynovitis of the flexor tendons at the fingers or thumb. Changes, including thickening or a nodule formation, around the digital pulley system or to the flexor tendons cause snapping or locking of the finger in a flexed position, both of which can cause pain in some patients. The prevalence of trigger digit is 2% to 3% in the general population. Its etiology is unknown, but individuals with diabetes or rheumatoid arthritis have a much higher prevalence of the condition compared with the general population.[80] Repeated use of the hand seems to be associated with symptoms. Patients typically present with a painful nodule at the volar MCP corresponding with the level of the A1 pulley and a noticeable catching or locking of the finger with active flexion or extension. In severe cases, the finger can become locked in a flexed position and may resemble and ultimately result in a PIP joint flexion contracture. It can interfere with most activities that require grasping.[80] A concern is that repeated triggering of the tendon can result in tendon fraying and ultimately tendon rupture over time; therefore, proper and early management is important.

11.2. Initial Evaluation of a Patient With Hand Pain

Visual observations for deformity such as nodules, cords, or joint contractures at the hand can help differentiate some local causes of hand pain. Enlargement of joints or node formation at the joints, as described for radial hand pain previously, can implicate an arthritic condition; in osteoarthritis, these changes often occur at the IP joints of the fingers or at the CMC joint of the thumb. Nodules at the dorsal PIP joints, thick cord formations in the palm, dimpling of the skin in the palm, and flexion contractures of the MCPs and proximal phalangeal joints are consistent with Dupuytren contracture. Range-of-motion assessment will often reveal specific deficits. End-range motion deficits may be noted in osteoarthritic hands, and if it affects the CMC joint of the thumb, passive adduction and flexion contracture may be noted in advanced cases. Patients with Dupuytren contracture demonstrate incomplete digit extension, both passively and actively. Attempts to passively extend the affected fingers will be met with unyielding resistance, and the tight cords in the palm may be more visible. Patients with Dupuytren contracture may present with symptoms that could be confused with active TrPs in the palmaris longus muscle.

Active motion assessment in patients with trigger finger will reveal the characteristic triggering with flexion and extension. In advanced cases, the finger may get stuck in flexion, unable to extend without an external passive force applied by the patient or clinician. Passive motion is generally full with trigger finger. Strength will be variably affected in each of these conditions, depending on symptom severity.

11.3. Trigger Points and Hand Pain

Intrinsic muscles of the hand can develop TrPs that cause pain and replicate symptoms of common hand diagnoses. Chapter 39 overviews TrPs in the adductor and opponens pollicis muscles mimicking pain conditions, such as trigger thumb, CMCJ arthritis, CTS, and DeQuervain tenosynovitis. The symptoms may be aggravated with gross grasping activities or using the thumbs for smart phone use and texting. As adduction contractures form in advanced stages of CMCJ arthritis, self-release techniques and stretching will help alleviate associated TrPs and may slow or halt the progression of contracture development at the thumb index web space. The interosseous, lumbrical, and hypothenar muscles may emulate arthritic conditions in the hand. Following trauma or after conditions that result in considerable swelling in the hand, it is important to assess the intrinsic musculature. Tightness and local TrPs may cause difficulty in making a full fist and may lead to generalized or local hand pain, depending on the extent the intrinsic muscles are involved. Being such small muscles, they are often disregarded once swelling has subsided. Yet, intrinsic muscles can become adaptively shortened and result in an inability to make a complete fist.

Trigger points in the flexor pollicis longus, flexor digitorum superficialis, or flexor digitorum profundus muscles may result in pain reports similar to trigger finger or an arthritic condition in the corresponding digit. Trigger points in the palmaris longus muscle can result in volar hand pain that may associated with the fascial changes corresponding with Dupuytren contracture, as outlined in Chapter 37.

References

1. Sanders TL Jr, Maradit Kremers H, Bryan AJ, Ransom JE, Smith J, Morrey BF. The epidemiology and health care burden of tennis elbow: a population-based study. *Am J Sports Med*. 2015;43(5):1066-1071.
2. Descatha A, Albo F, Leclerc A, et al. Lateral epicondylitis and physical exposure at work? A review of prospective studies and meta-analysis. *Arthritis Care Res (Hoboken)*. 2016;68(11):1681-1687.
3. Chung KC, Lark ME. Upper extremity injuries in tennis players: diagnosis, treatment, and management. *Hand Clin*. 2017;33(1):175-186.
4. Ellenbecker TS, Nirschl R, Renstrom P. Current concepts in examination and treatment of elbow tendon injury. *Sports Health*. 2013;5(2):186-194.
5. Nirschl RP. Elbow tendinosis/tennis elbow. *Clin Sports Med*. 1992;11(4):851-870.
6. Kraushaar BS, Nirschl RP. Tendinosis of the elbow (tennis elbow). Clinical features and findings of histological, immunohistochemical, and electron microscopy studies. *J Bone Joint Surg Am*. 1999;81(2):259-278.
7. Alfredson H, Ljung BO, Thorsen K, Lorentzon R. In vivo investigation of ECRB tendons with microdialysis technique—no signs of inflammation but high amounts of glutamate in tennis elbow. *Acta Orthop Scand*. 2000;71(5):475-479.
8. Ljung BO, Alfredson H, Forsgren S. Neurokinin 1-receptors and sensory neuropeptides in tendon insertions at the medial and lateral epicondyles of the humerus. Studies on tennis elbow and medial epicondylalgia. *J Orthop Res*. 2004;22(2):321-327.
9. Wood WA, Stewart A, Bell-Jenje T. Lateral epicondylalgia: an overview. *Phys Ther Rev*. 2006;11(3):155-160.
10. Rees JD, Stride M, Scott A. Tendons—time to revisit inflammation. *Br J Sports Med*. 2014;48(21):1553-1557.
11. Plinsinga ML, Brink MS, Vicenzino B, van Wilgen CP. Evidence of nervous system sensitization in commonly presenting and persistent painful tendinopathies: a systematic review. *J Orthop Sports Phys Ther*. 2015;45(11):864-875.
12. Cook JL, Purdam CR. Is tendon pathology a continuum? A pathology model to explain the clinical presentation of load-induced tendinopathy. *Br J Sports Med*. 2009;43(6):409-416.
13. Cook JL, Khan KM, Kiss ZS, Coleman BD, Griffiths L. Asymptomatic hypoechoic regions on patellar tendon ultrasound: a 4-year clinical and ultrasound followup of 46 tendons. *Scand J Med Sci Sports*. 2001;11(6):321-327.
14. du Toit C, Stieler M, Saunders R, Bisset L, Vicenzino B. Diagnostic accuracy of power Doppler ultrasound in patients with chronic tennis elbow. *Br J Sports Med*. 2008;42(11):872-876.
15. Rio E, Moseley L, Purdam C, et al. The pain of tendinopathy: physiological or pathophysiological? *Sports Med*. 2014;44(1):9-23.
16. Bisset LM, Vicenzino B. Physiotherapy management of lateral epicondylalgia. *J Physiother*. 2015;61(4):174-181.
17. Coombes BK, Bisset L, Vicenzino B. Management of lateral elbow tendinopathy: one size does not fit all. *J Orthop Sports Phys Ther*. 2015;45(11):938-949.

18. Woodley BL, Newsham-West RJ, Baxter GD. Chronic tendinopathy: effectiveness of eccentric exercise. *Br J Sports Med.* 2007;41(4):188-198; discussion 199.
19. Plancher KD, Halbrecht J, Lourie GM. Medial and lateral epicondylitis in the athlete. *Clin Sports Med.* 1996;15(2):283-305.
20. Urban MO, Gebhart GF. Central mechanisms in pain. *Med Clin North Am.* 1999;83(3):585-596.
21. Gellman H. Tennis elbow (lateral epicondylitis). *Orthop Clin North Am.* 1992;23(1):75-82.
22. Stratford PW, Norman GR, McIntosh JM. Generalizability of grip strength measurements in patients with tennis elbow. *Phys Ther.* 1989;69(4):276-281.
23. De Smet L, Fabry G. Grip strength in patients with tennis elbow. Influence of elbow position. *Acta Orthop Belg.* 1996;62(1):26-29.
24. Fernandez-Carnero J, Fernández de las Peñas C, de la Llave-Rincon AI, Ge HY, Arendt-Nielsen L. Prevalence of and referred pain from myofascial trigger points in the forearm muscles in patients with lateral epicondylalgia. *Clin J Pain.* 2007;23(4):353-360.
25. Mora-Relucio R, Nunez-Nagy S, Gallego-Izquierdo T, et al. Experienced versus inexperienced interexaminer reliability on location and classification of myofascial trigger point palpation to diagnose lateral epicondylalgia: an observational cross-sectional study. *Evid Based Complement Alternat Med.* 2016;2016:6059719.
26. Papatheodorou LK, Baratz ME, Sotereanos DG. Elbow arthritis: current concepts. *J Hand Surg Am.* 2013;38(3):605-613.
27. Duparc F, Putz R, Michot C, Muller JM, Freger P. The synovial fold of the humeroradial joint: anatomical and histological features, and clinical relevance in lateral epicondylalgia of the elbow. *Surg Radiol Anat.* 2002;24(5):302-307.
28. Ruch DS, Papadonikolakis A, Campolattaro RM. The posterolateral plica: a cause of refractory lateral elbow pain. *J Shoulder Elbow Surg.* 2006;15(3):367-370.
29. Steinert AF, Goebel S, Rucker A, Barthel T. Snapping elbow caused by hypertrophic synovial plica in the radiohumeral joint: a report of three cases and review of literature. *Arch Orthop Trauma Surg.* 2010;130(3):347-351.
30. Camp CL, Smith J, O'Driscoll SW. Posterolateral rotatory instability of the elbow: part I. Mechanism of injury and the posterolateral rotatory Drawer test. *Arthrosc Tech.* 2017;6(2):e401-e405.
31. Simons DG, Travell J, Simons L. *Travell & Simon's Myofascial Pain and Dysfunction: The Trigger Point Manual.* Vol 1. 2nd ed. Baltimore, MD: Williams & Wilkins; 1999.
32. Blanpied PR, Gross AR, Elliott JM, et al. Neck pain: revision 2017. *J Orthop Sports Phys Ther.* 2017;47(7):A1-A83.
33. Smidt N, Lewis M, Van Der Windt DA, Hay EM, Bouter LM, Croft P. Lateral epicondylitis in general practice: course and prognostic indicators of outcome. *J Rheumatol.* 2006;33(10):2053-2059.
34. Cleland J, Flynn TW, Palmer JA. Incorporation of manual therapy directed at the cervicothoracic spine in patients with lateral epicondylalgia: a pilot clinical trial. *J Man Manip Ther.* 2005;13:143-151.
35. Cleland JA, Whitman JM, Fritz JM. Effectiveness of manual physical therapy to the cervical spine in the management of lateral epicondylalgia: a retrospective analysis. *J Orthop Sports Phys Ther.* 2004;34(11):713-722; discussion 722-714.
36. Wainner RS, Fritz JM, Irrgang JJ, Boninger ML, Delitto A, Allison S. Reliability and diagnostic accuracy of the clinical examination and patient self-report measures for cervical radiculopathy. *Spine (Phila Pa 1976).* 2003;28(1):52-62.
37. Naam NH, Nemani S. Radial tunnel syndrome. *Orthop Clin North Am.* 2012;43(4):529-536.
38. Moradi A, Ebrahimzadeh MH, Jupiter JB. Radial tunnel syndrome, diagnostic and treatment dilemma. *Arch Bone Joint Surg.* 2015;3(3):156-162.
39. Fernandez-Carnero J, Fernández de las Peñas C, de la Llave-Rincon AI, Ge HY, Arendt-Nielsen L. Bilateral myofascial trigger points in the forearm muscles in patients with chronic unilateral lateral epicondylalgia: a blinded, controlled study. *Clin J Pain.* 2008;24(9):802-807.
40. Fernández de las Peñas C, Grobli C, Ortega-Santiago R, et al. Referred pain from myofascial trigger points in head, neck, shoulder, and arm muscles reproduces pain symptoms in blue-collar (manual) and white-collar (office) workers. *Clin J Pain.* 2012;28(6):511-518.
41. Shmushkevich Y, Kalichman L. Myofascial pain in lateral epicondylalgia: a review. *J Bodyw Mov Ther.* 2013;17(4):434-439.
42. Ajimsha MS, Chithra S, Thulasyammal RP. Effectiveness of myofascial release in the management of lateral epicondylitis in computer professionals. *Arch Phys Med Rehabil.* 2012;93(4):604-609.
43. Blanchette MA, Normand MC. Augmented soft tissue mobilization vs natural history in the treatment of lateral epicondylitis: a pilot study. *J Manipulative Physiol Ther.* 2011;34(2):123-130.
44. Krey D, Borchers J, McCamey K. Tendon needling for treatment of tendinopathy: a systematic review. *Phys Sportsmed.* 2015;43(1):80-86.
45. Barco R, Antuna SA. Medial elbow pain. *EFORT Open Rev.* 2017;2(8):362-371.
46. Shiri R, Viikari-Juntura E. Lateral and medial epicondylitis: role of occupational factors. *Best Pract Res Clin Rheumatol.* 2011;25(1):43-57.
47. Hoogvliet P, Randsdorp MS, Dingemanse R, Koes BW, Huisstede BM. Does effectiveness of exercise therapy and mobilisation techniques offer guidance for the treatment of lateral and medial epicondylitis? A systematic review. *Br J Sports Med.* 2013;47(17):1112-1119.
48. Savoie FH, O'Brien M. Chronic medial instability of the elbow. *EFORT Open Rev.* 2017;2(1):1-6.
49. O'Driscoll SW, Lawton RL, Smith AM. The "moving valgus stress test" for medial collateral ligament tears of the elbow. *Am J Sports Med.* 2005;33(2):231-239.
50. Fadel M, Lancigu R, Raimbeau G, Roqueleure Y, Descatha A. Occupational prognosis factors for ulnar nerve entrapment at the elbow: a systematic review. *Hand Surg Rehabil.* 2017;36(4):244-249.
51. Standring S. *Gray's Anatomy: The Anatomical Basis of Clinical Practice.* 41st ed. London, UK: Elsevier; 2015.
52. Assmus H, Antoniadis G, Bischoff C, et al. Cubital tunnel syndrome—a review and management guidelines. *Cent Eur Neurosurg.* 2011;72(2):90-98.
53. Richard MJ, Messmer C, Wray WH, Garrigues GE, Goldner RD, Ruch DS. Management of subluxating ulnar nerve at the elbow. *Orthopedics.* 2010;33(9):672.
54. Harrelson JM, Newman M. Hypertrophy of the flexor carpi ulnaris as a cause of ulnar-nerve compression in the distal part of the forearm. Case report. *J Bone Joint Surg Am Vol.* 1975;57(4):554-555.
55. Lee MJ, LaStayo PC. Pronator syndrome and other nerve compressions that mimic carpal tunnel syndrome. *J Orthop Sports Phys Ther.* 2004;34(10):601-609.
56. Strohl AB, Zelouf DS. Ulnar tunnel syndrome, radial tunnel syndrome, anterior interosseous nerve syndrome, and pronator syndrome. *J Am Acad Orthop Surg.* 2017;25(1):e1-e10.
57. Stahl S, Vida D, Meisner C, et al. Systematic review and meta-analysis on the work-related cause of de Quervain tenosynovitis: a critical appraisal of its recognition as an occupational disease. *Plast Reconstr Surg.* 2013;132(6):1479-1491.
58. Skinner TM. Intersection syndrome: the subtle squeak of an overused wrist. *J Am Board Fam Med.* 2017;30(4):547-551.
59. Kumka M. A variant extensor indicis muscle and the branching pattern of the deep radial nerve could explain hand functionality and clinical symptoms in the living patient. *J Can Chiropr Assoc.* 2015;59(1):64-71.
60. Ahuja NK, Chung KC. Fritz de Quervain, MD (1868-1940): stenosing tendovaginitis at the radial styloid process. *J Hand Surg Am.* 2004;29(6):1164-1170.
61. Villafane JH, Herrero P. Conservative treatment of Myofascial Trigger Points and joint mobilization for management in patients with thumb carpometacarpal osteoarthritis. *J Hand Ther.* 2016;29(1):89-92; quiz 92.
62. Watanabe A, Souza F, Vezeridis PS, Blazar P, Yoshioka H. Ulnar-sided wrist pain. II. Clinical imaging and treatment. *Skeletal Radiol.* 2010;39(9):837-857.
63. Buterbaugh GA, Brown TR, Horn PC. Ulnar-sided wrist pain in athletes. *Clin Sports Med.* 1998;17(3):567-583.
64. Pang EQ, Yao J. Ulnar-sided wrist pain in the athlete (TFCC/DRUJ/ECU). *Curr Rev Musculoskelet Med.* 2017;10(1):53-61.
65. Singh R, Patel A, Roulohamin N, Turner R. A classification for extensor carpi ulnaris groove morphology as an aid for ulnar sided wrist pain. *J Hand Surg Asian Pac Vol.* 2016;21(2):246-252.
66. Crosby NE, Greenberg JA. Ulnar-sided wrist pain in the athlete. *Clin Sports Med.* 2015;34(1):127-141.
67. LaStayo P, Howell J. Clinical provocative tests used in evaluating wrist pain: a descriptive study. *J Hand Ther.* 1995;8(1):10-17.
68. Nakazumi Y, Hamasaki M. Electrophysiological studies and physical examinations in entrapment neuropathy: sensory and motor functions compensation for the central nervous system in cases with peripheral nerve damage. *Electromyogr Clin Neurophysiol.* 2001;41(6):345-348.
69. Birch L, Christensen H, Arendt-Nielsen L, Graven-Nielsen T, Sogaard K. The influence of experimental muscle pain on motor unit activity during low-level contraction. *Eur J Appl Physiol.* 2000;83(2-3):200-206.
70. Dale AM, Harris-Adamson C, Rempel D, et al. Prevalence and incidence of carpal tunnel syndrome in US working populations: pooled analysis of six prospective studies. *Scand J Work Environ Health.* 2013;39(5):495-505.
71. Zanette G, Marani S, Tamburin S. Proximal pain in patients with carpal tunnel syndrome: a clinical-neurophysiological study. *J Peripher Nerv Syst.* 2007;12(2):91-97.
72. Zyluk A, Waskow B. Symptoms of the compression of median nerve in patients after fractures of the distal radius treated operatively [in Polish]. *Chir Narzadow Ruchu Ortop Pol.* 2011;76(4):189-192.
73. Karadag O, Kalyoncu U, Akdogan A, et al. Sonographic assessment of carpal tunnel syndrome in rheumatoid arthritis: prevalence and correlation with disease activity. *Rheumatol Int.* 2012;32(8):2313-2319.
74. Shi Q, MacDermid JC. Is surgical intervention more effective than non-surgical treatment for carpal tunnel syndrome? A systematic review. *J Orthop Surg Res.* 2011;6:17.
75. Page MJ, O'Connor D, Pitt V, Massy-Westropp N. Exercise and mobilisation interventions for carpal tunnel syndrome. *Cochrane Database Syst Rev.* 2012;(6):CD009899.
76. Qerama E, Kasch H, Fuglsang-Frederiksen A. Occurrence of myofascial pain in patients with possible carpal tunnel syndrome—a single-blinded study. *Eur J Pain.* 2009;13(6):588-591.
77. Azadeh H, Dehghani M, Zarezadeh A. Incidence of trapezius myofascial trigger points in patients with the possible carpal tunnel syndrome. *J Res Med Sci.* 2010;15(5):250-255.
78. Eaton C. Evidence-based medicine: dupuytren contracture. *Plast Reconstr Surg.* 2014;133(5):1241-1251.
79. von Campe A, Mende K, Omaren H, Meuli-Simmen C. Painful nodules and cords in Dupuytren disease. *J Hand Surg Am.* 2012;37(7):1313-1318.
80. Adams JE, Habbu R. Tendinopathies of the hand and wrist. *J Am Acad Orthop Surg.* 2015;23(12):741-750.

Section 5: Trunk and Pelvis Pain

Chapter 42

Pectoralis Major and Subclavius Muscles

"Chest and Shoulder Nuisance"

Joseph M. Donnelly and Deanna Hortman Camilo

1. INTRODUCTION

The pectoralis major muscle is a broad, multipennate muscle comprising of two distinct divisions. Its unique shape and large size allow the pectoralis major muscle to have an influence on three different joints in the upper quarter (sternoclavicular, acromioclavicular, and glenohumeral joints) in addition to participating in the gliding movement of the scapula over the ribs. Both divisions may act separately to achieve different glenohumeral joint motions, but the primary role of the pectoralis major muscle as a whole is to adduct and internally rotate the humerus. Trigger points (TrPs) within the pectoralis major muscle will generate referred pain over the anterior deltoid muscle, the chest region, and the medial aspect of the arm. Pain from pectoralis major TrPs may also extend toward the volar aspect of the forearm and ulnar side of the hand, including the last two or two-and-a-half digits. Symptoms may be exacerbated by rounded shoulder posture, heavy lifting, overhead sporting activities, weight training, and sustained lifting in a fixed position. Differential diagnosis should include pectoralis major muscle tear, angina pectoris, medial and lateral epicondylalgia, C5-C6 and C7-C8 radicular symptoms, and thoracic outlet syndrome (TOS). Corrective actions to prevent perpetuation and/or recurrence of pectoralis major TrPs should include techniques to address postural imbalances, work place ergonomics, and sleeping positions, as well as self-pressure release and self-stretching.

The subclavius is a small muscle that lies between the clavicle and first rib and indirectly assists in protraction of the shoulder. TrPs within the subclavius muscle commonly refer pain ipsilaterally into the anterior aspect of the shoulder area and arm, extending to the radial side of the forearm and hand. Differential diagnosis for subclavius TrPs should include vascular TOS. Access to this muscle is limited; therefore, indirect treatments can be used for management of TrPs in this muscle.

2. ANATOMIC CONSIDERATIONS

Pectoralis Major

The pectoralis major muscle is a multipennate fan-shaped muscle commonly described as having clavicular, sternal, costal, and abdominal heads with a complex morphologic arrangement. The most superior division of the pectoralis major muscle, the clavicular head, originates from the sternal half of the clavicle.[1,2] The sternal head has been described as consisting of six to seven muscle segments[3]; other researchers have found as few as two segments.[4] Regardless of the number of segments, muscle fibers that comprise the sternal head originate from the manubrium, the sternum, the costal cartilage of the upper six ribs, and the external oblique aponeurosis (abdominal head) (Figure 42-1). The clavicular and sternal heads come to form a bilaminar flat tendon, approximately 5 cm wide, and travel laterally to insert into the lateral lip of the intertubercular groove of the humerus and the glenohumeral joint capsule.[1-3,5] The tendon comprises a thicker anterior tendon lamina and a posterior tendon lamina.[1-4]

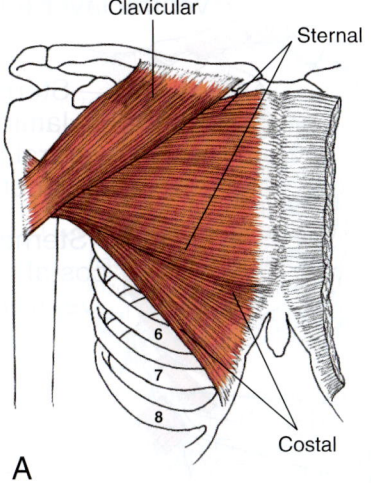
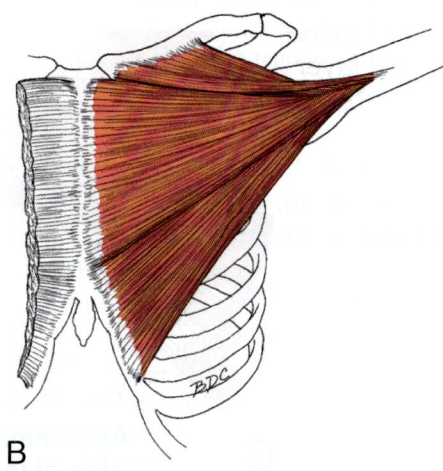

Figure 42-1. Attachments of the pectoralis major muscle (red), anterior (ventral) view. A, Fibers of the uppermost clavicular section overlap fibers of the sternal section to form part of the ventral layer at the humeral attachment. B, Costal fibers curl around the lateral border (anterior axillary fold) to form most of the dorsal layer at the humerus.

The forward punch and internal rotation at 90° of elevation produced the lowest average and peak amplitudes (18%–25% MVC).[11]

Among 13 professional right-handed golfers, the greatest pectoralis major muscle activity occurred during the acceleration and early follow-through phases of the swing.[12] The left side showed more activity than the right, and men showed higher activity than did women. The power in the shoulder for the drive came first from the latissimus dorsi muscle and then the pectoralis major muscle, which showed more activity than any of the other seven tested muscles.[12] This activity provided the powerful arm adduction and internal rotation required.[13]

Electromyographic analysis of shoulder girdle muscle activity during functional movements is well documented. Jobe et al[12] and Gowan et al[14] investigated muscle activation patterns and activity during throwing movements. They identified maximum activity of the supraspinatus, infraspinatus, and deltoid muscles during early and late cocking phases of the throw; whereas the pectoralis major, subscapularis, and latissimus dorsi muscles were more active during the arm cocking and acceleration phase of the throw. They also identified that amateurs tend to utilize more of the rotator cuff muscles during the acceleration phase.[12,14] This notion is further supported in a study of healthy, skilled throwers where EMG activity of the pectoralis major muscle increased dramatically with arm cocking and remained high during arm acceleration (56% of MVC) tapering to 30% during follow-through.[15,16] During a tennis serve, the pectoralis major muscle is the most heavily recruited during acceleration.[17]

Bankoff et al[18] performed an EMG study of the pectoralis major (sternocostal portion) and the middle deltoid muscles in volleyball sequential actions. They found the pectoralis major muscle to have its peak activity during the spike and serve between 180° and 90° flexion. Peak activity was achieved during interaction with the ball versus movement without the ball.[18] This conclusion is consistent with the findings reported by Rokito et al.[19]

During freestyle swimming, the clavicular section of the pectoralis major muscle in normal subjects was active during the pull-through phase, with peaks of activity during early and late pull-through as internal rotation of the arm progressed.[20] During the butterfly stroke, the pectoralis major muscle is the first muscle recruited, and it reaches peak activity rapidly during the pulling phase of the stroke during which it is considered to be a primary propulsive muscle.[21]

During simulated driving, the clavicular section showed more activity bilaterally during left turns than during right turns, and the clavicular section showed more activity than the sternocostal section.[22] Other investigators found that the pectoralis major muscle reached the peak MVC during a pushing activity.[23]

Subclavius

The subclavius muscle assists with protraction of the shoulder indirectly by approximating the clavicle and the first rib.[7,8] It is also thought that the subclavius muscle resists elevation and rotation of the clavicle during activities that require rapid elevation of the shoulder girdle.[2]

2.3. Functional Unit

The functional unit to which a muscle belongs includes the muscles that reinforce and counter its actions as well as the joints that the muscle crosses. The interdependence of these structures is functionally reflected in the organization and neural connections of the sensory motor cortex. The functional unit is emphasized because the presence of a TrP in one muscle of the unit increases the likelihood that the other muscles of the unit will also develop TrPs. When inactivating TrPs in a muscle, one must be concerned about TrPs that may develop in muscles that are functionally interdependent. Box 42-1 grossly represents the functional unit of the pectoralis major muscle.[24]

Box 42-1 Functional unit of the pectoralis major muscle

Action	Synergists	Antagonist
Shoulder internal rotation	Latissimus dorsi Teres major Subscapularis	Infraspinatus Teres minor
Shoulder flexion	Anterior deltoid Biceps brachii long head Coracobrachialis	Latissimus dorsi Posterior deltoid Triceps brachii long head
Shoulder adduction	Teres major Latissimus dorsi Subscapularis Coracobrachialis	Deltoid Supraspinatus
Shoulder protraction (sternal head)	Serratus anterior Pectoralis minor Subclavius	Rhomboid major Rhomboid minor Middle trapezius

Agonist muscles in parallel and in series, which may assist the clavicular section of the pectoralis major muscle, include the anterior deltoid, coracobrachialis, subclavius, scalenus anterior, and sternocleidomastoid muscles on the same side. The clavicular head and the anterior deltoid muscle work very closely together because they lie side by side, with adjacent attachments, and are separated only by the groove of the cephalic vein.

The more vertically oriented, lower fibers of the sternal sections of the pectoralis major muscle depress the shoulder with the help of corresponding fibers of the latissimus dorsi, lower trapezius, and lower serratus anterior muscles. The subclavius and the pectoralis minor muscles also assist these lower pectoralis major fibers.

3. CLINICAL PRESENTATION
3.1. Referred Pain Pattern

Pectoralis Major

Although the pectoralis major muscle may develop TrPs in any portion of the muscle, with pain and tenderness referred unilaterally without crossing midline, five areas are classically described, each with a distinctive pain reference pattern.[24]

The TrPs located in the clavicular section (Figure 42-3A) often refer pain over the anterior deltoid muscle and locally to the clavicular section of the pectoralis major muscle itself.

Trigger points within the sternal section of the pectoralis major muscle (Figure 42-3B) are likely to refer pain to the anterior chest,[25–27] down the medial aspect of the arm toward the medial epicondyle. Pain may also be referred to the volar aspect of the forearm and ulnar side of the hand to include the last two or two-and-a-half digits.[28] The uppermost of these sternal TrP areas (Figure 42-3B) lies at the three-way overlap of the clavicular and manubrial sections of the pectoralis major and the underlying pectoralis minor muscles.

In the costal and abdominal portions of the pectoralis major muscle, TrPs develop in two pectoral regions. One of these regions lies along the lateral border of the muscle; however, the full length of the fibers should be examined for the presence of TrPs. Trigger points closest to the border (Figure 42-3C) can cause breast tenderness with hypersensitivity of the nipple, intolerance to clothing, and often breast pain.[29]

More medially, a TrP associated with somatovisceral cardiac arrhythmias[30] may be located on the right side between the fifth

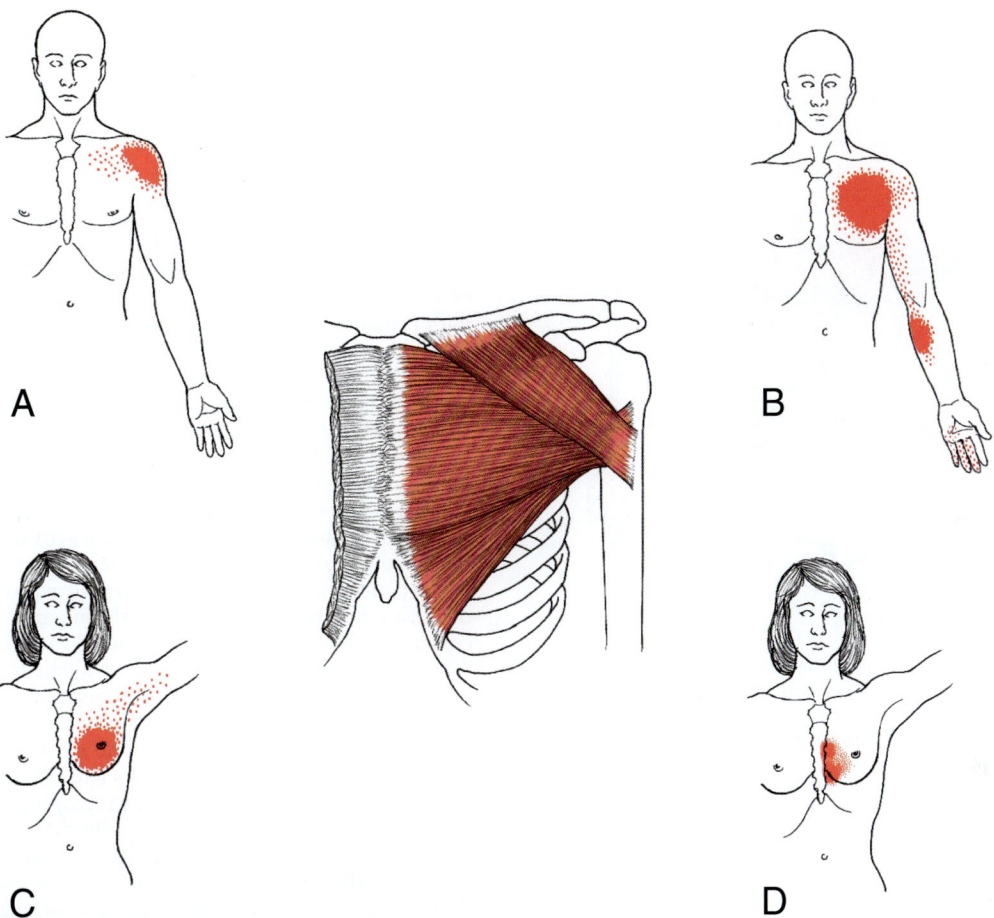

Figure 42-3. Referred pain patterns (red) and TrP areas in the left pectoralis major muscle. Solid red shows essential areas of referred pain, and stippled red shows the spillover pain areas. A, The clavicular section. B, Intermediate sternal section. C, The lateral free margin of the pectoralis major muscle, which includes fibers of the costal and abdominal sections that form the anterior axillary fold. D, Parasternal pectoralis major TrPs.

and sixth ribs, just below the point where the lower border of the fifth rib crosses a vertical line that lies midway between the margin of the sternum and the nipple (Figure 42-4). This TrP area has been observed only on the right side, except in situs inversus. The spot tenderness of this TrP is associated with ectopic cardiac rhythms but not with any pain complaint. There may be nearby tender points over or between adjacent ribs that are not pertinent to cardiac arrhythmia.

It is important for the clinician to note that TrPs within the left pectoralis major muscle may mimic pain symptoms of cardiac ischemia. In addition, patients may develop TrPs within this muscle after a myocardial infarction (viscerosomatic activation).

Subclavius

The subclavius muscle can develop TrPs that refer pain ipsilaterally into the upper extremity (Figure 42-5B). The pain may travel across the front of the shoulder, down the front of the arm, and along the radial side of the forearm bypassing the elbow and wrist to reappear on the radial half of the hand. In addition, the patient may experience pain in the dorsal and volar aspects of the thumb, the index finger, and the middle finger.

3.2. Symptoms

When patients report pain in the chest, anterior shoulder, medial aspect of the arm, medial elbow, medial aspect of the hand, and the fourth and fifth digits, TrPs in the pectoralis major muscle should be considered as a possible source of symptoms. Patients may report pain and symptoms that appear to be cardiac in nature and, in fact, can be caused by TrPs in the pectoralis major muscle. Conversely, TrPs in the pectoralis major muscle can be activated by cardiac disease or events resulting in complaints of persistent chest pain even though the heart may have recovered (viscerosomatic reflex).

When the patient reports primary pain in the anterior aspect of the shoulder, the pectoralis major and minor, subclavius, infraspinatus, supraspinatus, deltoid (anterior, middle), biceps brachii, coracobrachialis, and scalene muscles are the most likely muscular sources of symptoms.[31] Other investigators found a high prevalence (66%) of TrPs in the pectoralis major muscle in patients with unilateral shoulder impingement syndrome as compared to a matched control group,[32] and still others found expansive pain referral patterns in both blue collar and white collar workers.[33] In addition, Alonso-Blanco et al[34] observed that active TrPs in the pectoralis major muscle were also highly prevalent in women with fibromyalgia syndrome.

When patients present with autonomic symptoms and pain in the subclavicular region (Figure 42-3A), it is important to consider TrPs within the clavicular head of the pectoralis major muscle. This phenomenon occurs when shortening of the clavicular portion produces a downward and forward pull on the medial part of the clavicle, placing tension on the clavicular portion of the sternocleidomastoid muscle, thus perpetuating or activating TrPs in this muscle.

Patients with pectoralis major TrPs are likely to be as aware of their interscapular back pain as they are of the pain referred

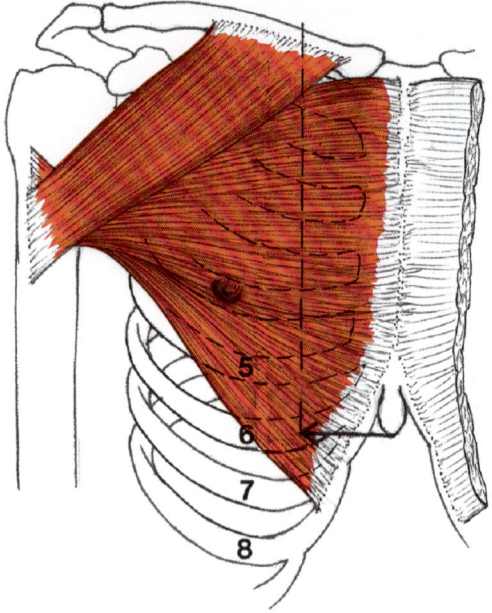

Figure 42-4. Right pectoralis major muscle TrP phenomena. Location of the "cardiac arrhythmia" TrP below the lower border of the fifth rib in the vertical line that lies midway between the sternal margin and the nipple line. On this line, the sixth rib is found at the level of the tip of the xiphoid process (arrow).

by their pectoralis major TrPs. In fact, the pectoral muscle TrPs may be painlessly latent but potent as the cause of pain-producing overload of scapular adductors including the middle trapezius and rhomboid muscles. Trigger points in the pectoralis major muscle should be considered as a potential source of symptoms when the patient experiences pain in the interscapular region when performing scapular adduction or when attempting to lie supine. Patients may also experience difficulty or pain when performing glenohumeral abduction (particularly horizontal abduction).

Patients may report breast tenderness or pain with hypersensitivity of the nipple and intolerance to clothing (allodynia). Trigger points in the sternal head of the pectoralis major muscle are likely to be the source of these symptoms.[29] This pain referral is most common in women, but may also be seen in men. Trigger points in the central part of the pectoralis major muscle refer pain widely over the precordium (if on the left side) and may cause a sense of chest constriction that is readily confused with angina pectoris. A patient with TrPs in the intermediate fibers of the left sternal section is likely to complain of intermittent, intense chest pain (Figure 42-5A) that appears in the precordial region with upper limb activity and also at rest if the TrPs are severe.

Different studies reported that examination of TrPs reproduced pain symptoms in the neck, shoulder, and axillary regions in women following breast cancer surgery.[35,36] In fact, development of active TrPs in the pectoralis major muscle was similar in woman who underwent mastectomy or lumpectomy.[37] Therefore, examination and treatment of TrPs should be part of the postoperative care for women experiencing pain in the neck, shoulder, arm, or axilla after mastectomy or lumpectomy surgery.

When patients report symptoms consistent with TOS (see Chapter 33), the subclavius muscle should be considered as a possible source of symptoms because the pain referral pattern from the subclavius muscle is in the same distribution of symptoms from TOS.

3.3. Patient Examination

After a thorough subjective examination, the clinician should make a detailed drawing representing the pain pattern described by the patient. This activity will assist in planning the physical examination and can be useful in monitoring the progression of the patient as symptoms improve or change. Any patient with primary reports of chest pain should alert the clinician to perform a thorough review of the cardiovascular and pulmonary systems. Any concerns regarding the involvement of the cardiovascular or respiratory systems as a source of symptoms should result in an immediate referral to the emergency room or a physician. For proper examination of the pectoralis major muscle, the clinician should observe shoulder girdle posture and scapula position, examine active and passive range of motion of the shoulder girdle, and observe muscle activation patterns and the scapulohumeral rhythm. The clinician should note when and where pain occurs. Pectoralis major TrPs can produce pain at rest or during movement, particularly during arm elevation in the coronal plane especially when combined with external rotation. The pain may or may not be present throughout abduction range of motion. Clinicians find that this muscle may be involved by itself, or be associated with other TrPs in the subclavius, scalene, anterior deltoid, pectoralis minor, and rotator cuff muscles.

A patient with significant TrP-associated shortening of the pectoralis major muscle will present with a stooped, rounded shoulder, and forward head posture. When observing the patient from the rear, the clinician may note faulty scapular position and asymmetries. Scapular and humeral head positions should be assessed at rest and during upper extremity elevation because malalignment can be a significant contributing factor to pectoralis major muscle overload during upper extremity functional activities requiring combined internal rotation and adduction especially from an overhead position. Trigger points in the pectoral muscles may restrict scapular adduction, which can be tested by having the patient place the back of the ipsilateral hand on the hip and move the elbow posteriorly for range of backward movement. Bilateral comparison is the most sensitive indicator of restriction if muscle involvement is unilateral. Reproduction of interscapular pain is another indicator of restriction. With these postural imbalances, manual muscle testing will reveal weak or inhibited interscapular muscles.

To identify TrPs in the pectoralis major muscle that may or may not be limiting range of motion and thus influencing dysfunction, the clinician should identify limited range of motion by performing specific range of motion testing for all parts of the muscle. Because the patient with pectoralis major TrPs in isolation often presents with minimal to no range of motion limitations, a thorough examination of all factors contributing to the patient's pain report should be completed. The clinician can expect external rotation to be restricted because of pectoralis major TrPs, but must also consider that full shoulder elevation may be limited due to the prerequisite external rotation required to achieve full elevation (abduction or flexion).[24] One helpful sign in differentiating pectoralis major muscle restriction from subscapularis muscle restriction is greater loss of external rotation at 90° versus 45° of abduction.[38]

TrPs in the pectoralis major muscle, when it is involved alone, cause minimal restriction of motion at the shoulder. The Apley's Scratch Test (shoulder extension, internal rotation, and adduction, Figure 21-3A) may be helpful in identifying muscle length deficits due to TrPs especially in the clavicular portion of the muscle. During this test, the shoulder girdle should not anteriorly tip forward while the patient attempts to reach the hand of the affected side behind the back and reaching as far

Chapter 42: Pectoralis Major and Subclavius Muscles   413

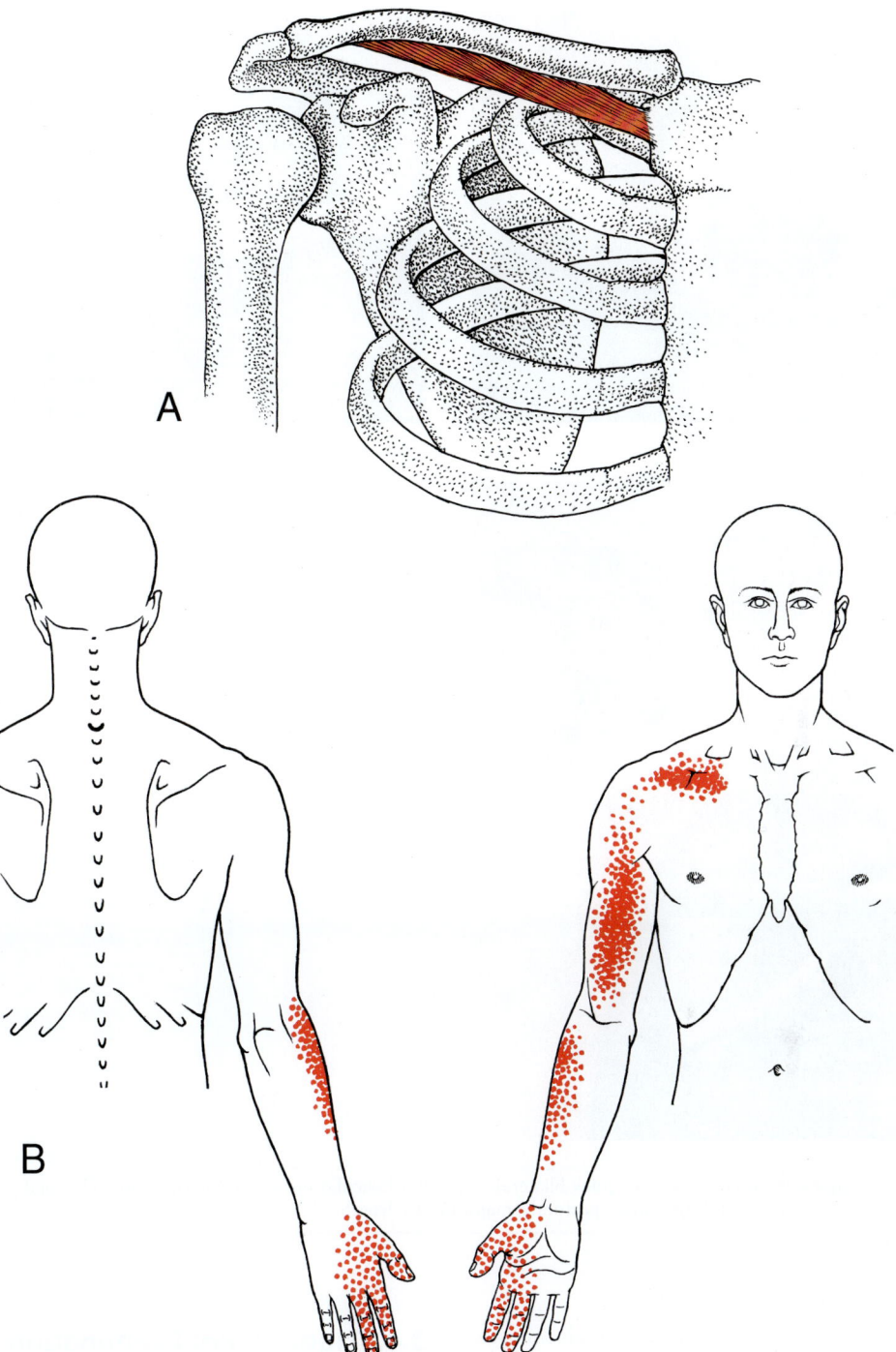

Figure 42-5. Subclavius muscle. A, Attachments of the muscle (medium red). B, Referred pain pattern (dark red) of a subclavius TrP. Stippled red is possible spillover in the lateral aspect of the hand.

up toward the opposite scapula as possible. Additional pectoralis major muscle length tests can be carried out in the supine position (Figure 42-6A to C).

Accessory joint motion should be tested in the glenohumeral joint, acromioclavicular joint, sternoclavicular joint, scapulothoracic joints, and thoracic rib cage. Oftentimes, joint hypomobility in the sternoclavicular joint or rib cage can cause impairment in shoulder elevation, contributing to alterations in the normal muscle activation patterns. Articular dysfunctions in the glenohumeral joint may also impair muscle activation patterns that can contribute to overload of the pectoralis major and rotator cuff muscles.

A cervical screen, neurologic examination including mobility testing of the neural tissues of the shoulder girdle should be done to eliminate radicular symptoms as causative. If referred hand and/or finger pain is present, a clinical examination of local tissues at the wrist and hand should be also conducted.

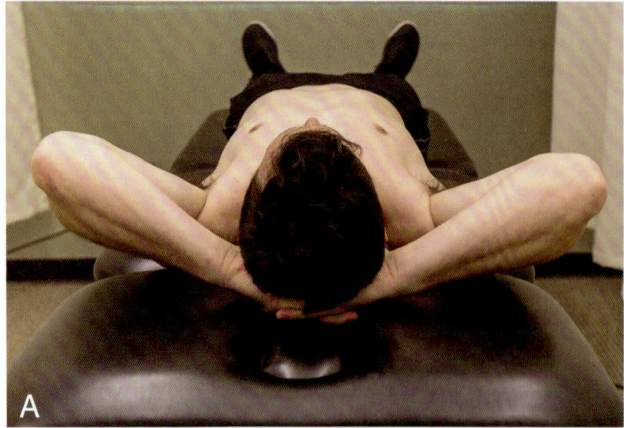
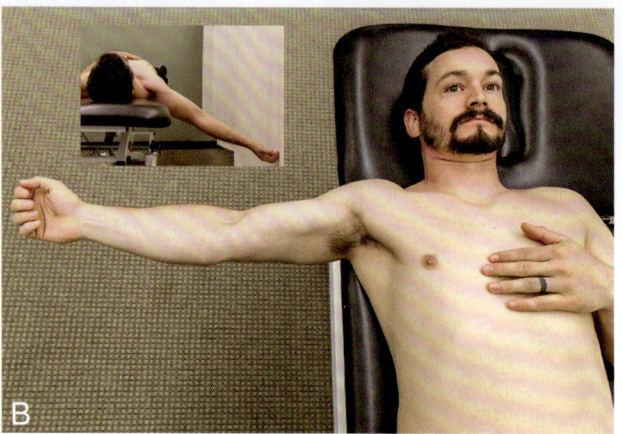
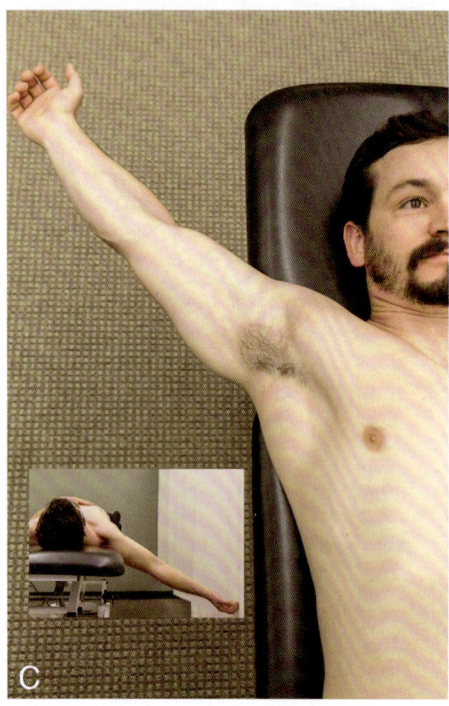

Figure 42-6. Pectoralis major muscle length test. A, Quick bilateral screen. B, Clavicular portion. C, Sternal and abdominal portion. The humerus should be able to fall below the horizontal for normal pectoralis major muscle length.

Symptoms from TrPs within the pectoralis major muscle should be differentiated from symptoms being driven by the subclavius and scalene muscles. The subclavius muscle is more closely associated with lateral forearm and lateral hand pain, whereas the pectoralis major muscle is associated with medial elbow, forearm, and hand pain. The scalene muscle referred pain is similar to the subclavius muscle referred pain pattern. The Finger-flexion Test (see Figure 20-6) may be utilized to differentiate scalene from subclavius or pectoralis major muscle involvement. If this test is positive, the scalene muscles may be implicated because TrPs or restrictions in the pectoralis major or subclavius muscles will not presumably affect this test.

The patient with chest pain due to pectoralis major TrPs is likely to report additional referred pain and restriction of movement at the shoulder because of associated TrPs in functionally related shoulder girdle muscles, which also need to be considered.

3.4. Trigger Point Examination

Pectoralis Major

Most of the TrPs found in the clavicular section, and TrPs in the parasternal section of the muscle, are identified by cross-fiber flat palpation (Figure 42-7A and B). Trigger points in the intermediate and lateral parts of the sternal and costal sections are best located by cross-fiber flat palpation (Figure 42-7B). The muscle may be placed on minimal to moderate tension by abducting the shoulder between 60° and 90° to maximize the spot tenderness found in a taut band. Local twitch responses may or may not be elicited, although they are easily obtained because this is a superficial muscle. The lateral part of the pectoralis major muscle is one of the easier muscles in which to identify taut bands by cross-fiber pincer palpation (Figure 42-7C). In women who have large breasts, the side-lying position can be utilized because gravity will aid in moving the breast

Chapter 42: Pectoralis Major and Subclavius Muscles

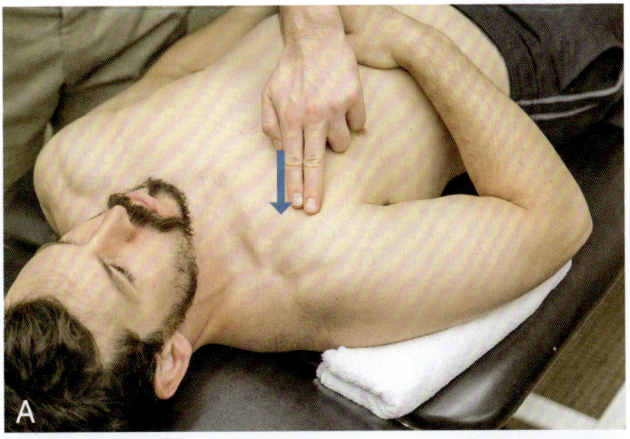
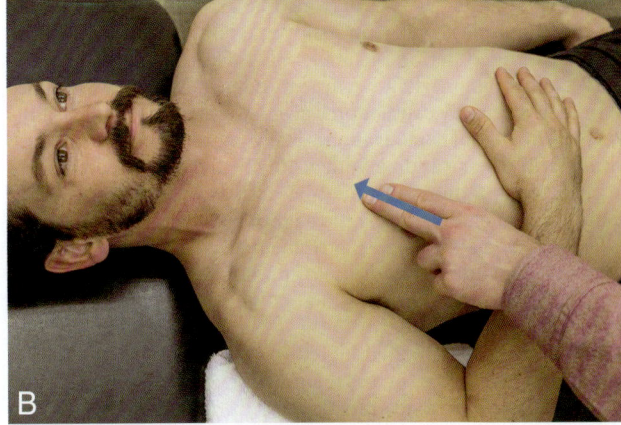
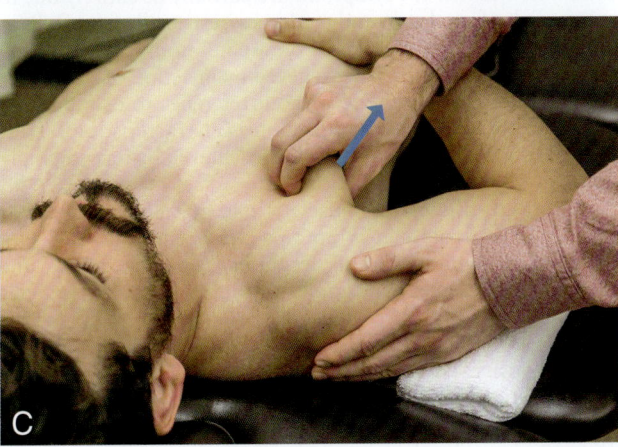
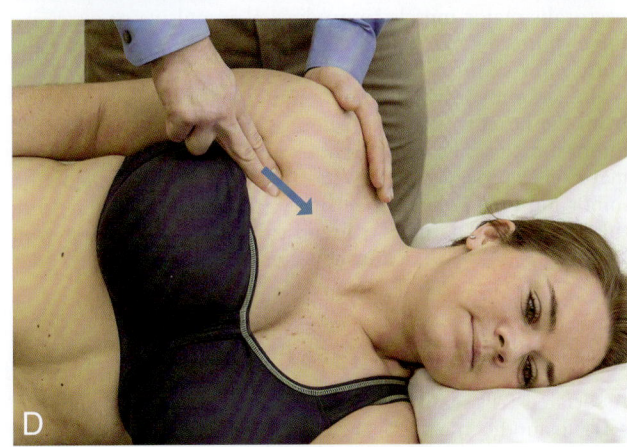

Figure 42-7. Palpation for TrPs in the pectoralis major muscle. A, Clavicular head cross-fiber flat palpation. B, Sternal head cross-fiber flat palpation. C, Lateral portion with cross-fiber pincer palpation. D, Side-lying cross-fiber flat palpation for a female patient.

tissue medially to allow better access to the pectoralis major muscle fibers (Figure 42-7D).

To find the "cardiac arrhythmia" TrP (Figure 42-5B), the tip of the xiphoid process is located. Then, at this level on the right side, in a vertical line midway between the sternal border and the nipple line, the region of the hollow between the fifth and sixth ribs is examined for a tender spot. This TrP is found by pressing upward against the inferior edge of the fifth rib and exploring for spot tenderness. Tenderness here may be also be caused by a TrP in an intercostal muscle rather than the sought pectoralis major muscle TrP.

Subclavius

The subclavius muscle must be palpated through the clavicular division of the pectoralis major muscle, and localization of its TrPs is best achieved with the pectoralis major muscle placed on slack. To do this, the relaxed patient's shoulder is placed in adduction and internal rotation. The clinician can palpate subclavius TrPs at the lateral portion of the medial third of the clavicle by rolling the palpating finger underneath the clavicle, deep into the recess and across the tense fibers (Figure 42-8). Palpation of the taut band of a TrP is not reliable through the pectoralis major muscle. Trigger points may also be found at the attachment of the muscle, just lateral to and below the costoclavicular joint from the central subclavius TrPs that are found closer to the mid-clavicle.

4. DIFFERENTIAL DIAGNOSIS

4.1. Activation and Perpetuation of Trigger Points

In any part of the pectoralis major muscle, TrPs may be activated by unaccustomed eccentric loading, eccentric exercise in unconditioned pectoralis major muscle, or maximal or submaximal

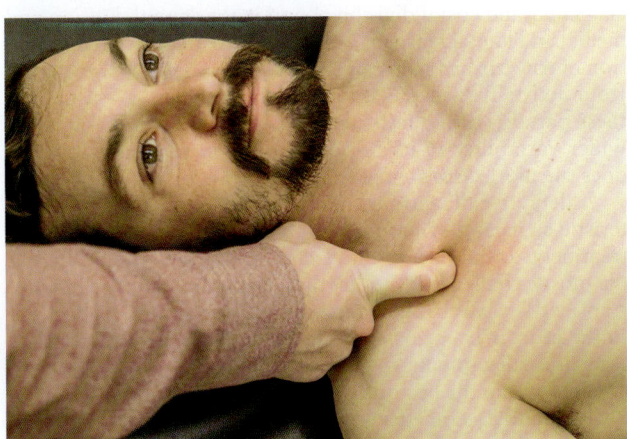

Figure 42-8. Palpation of the subclavius muscle.

concentric loading.[39] TrPs may also be activated or aggravated when the muscle is placed in a shortened or lengthened position for an extended period of time.

Pectoralis major TrPs are activated and perpetuated by a rounded shoulder posture because it produces sustained shortening of the pectoral muscles. This activation is likely to occur during prolonged sitting and when standing with a slouched, flat-chested posture.

Pectoralis major TrPs may be activated or reactivated in many ways including heavy lifting or weight training (especially when reaching out in front), carrying a heavy backpack, overuse of arm adduction (as with use of manual hedge clippers), sustained lifting in a fixed position (as with use of a power saw), immobilization of the arm in the adducted position (arm in a sling or cast), or sustained high levels of anxiety.

Sporting activities such as tennis, volleyball, swimming, baseball, and golf may place repetitive or excessive forces through the pectoralis major muscle. These activities, which require the pectoralis major muscle to produce a propulsive or excessive force (butterfly stroke, spiking a ball, bench press), place the muscle at risk for development of TrPs.

In acute myocardial infarction, pain is commonly referred from the heart to the mid-region of the pectoralis major and minor muscles. The injury to heart muscle initiates a viscerosomatic reflex process that activates TrPs in the pectoral major and minor muscles. Following recovery from the acute infarction, these self-perpetuating TrPs tend to persist in the chest wall unless wiped away like dust collected on a shelf.

4.2. Associated Trigger Points

Associated TrPs can develop in the referred pain areas caused by a TrP in another muscle.[58] Therefore, musculature in the referred pain areas for each muscle should also be considered. The sternalis (see Chapter 43) and pectoralis minor muscles (see Chapter 44) have a similar pain referral pattern and a close anatomic relationship to the pectoralis major muscle. Trigger points in the scalene muscles (see Chapter 20) also refer pain to the pectoral region and should be considered when pectoralis major TrPs are suspected.[28]

Many muscles of the shoulder and upper extremity should be examined for associated TrPs when treating dysfunction of the pectoralis major muscle. Trigger points in the iliocostalis thoracis muscle between the second and the sixth thoracic vertebrae on the left[59] and the region of the left upper rectus abdominis muscle induce chest pain that strongly mimics pain of cardiac origin and can coexist with pectoralis major TrPs.[60] The anterior deltoid, coracobrachialis, biceps brachii, brachialis, flexor carpi ulnaris, flexor digitorum superficialis, and profundus and abductor digiti minimi muscles are all within the pain referral pattern of the pectoralis major muscle and could harbor associated TrPs. The subclavius muscle shares the proximal pain referral pattern in the chest, anterior shoulder, and upper arm; however, its pain referral pattern spreads to the radial aspect of the forearm and hand instead of the ulnar aspect. The pronator teres, supinator, extensor digitorum, brachioradialis, and extensor carpi radialis longus muscles should be also examined for the presence of associated TrPs.

In addition, muscles that comprise the functional unit may also have associated TrPs. The anterior deltoid and coracobrachialis muscles are synergists that substitute for impaired function of the pectoralis major muscle. The subscapularis, teres major, and latissimus dorsi muscles, which are also part of the synergistic functional unit, may develop associated TrPs. Involvement of the serratus anterior, rhomboids, and middle trapezius muscles, which are antagonists, often follows, especially in a patient with a rounded shoulder posture. The antagonistic infraspinatus, teres minor, and posterior deltoid muscles may also develop TrPs, resulting in significant shoulder stiffness. In addition, tense pectoral muscles can overload posterior muscles, causing painful stretch weakness. In either case, the interscapular muscles should be addressed.

4.3. Associated Pathology

Pectoralis Major

Differential diagnosis of symptoms caused by TrPs in the pectoralis major muscle should include angina pectoris; tear of the muscle belly[40]; bicipital tendinitis; supraspinatus tendinitis; subacromial bursitis; medial epicondylalgia; lateral epicondylalgia; C5-C6 radicular pain; C7-C8 radicular pain; TOS; intercostal neuritis; irritation of the bronchi, pleura, and/or esophagus; mediastinal emphysema[41]; breast cancer; and lung cancer. Some of the less common noncardiac skeletal syndromes that cause pain and tenderness in the chest include the chest wall syndrome,[42] Tietze's syndrome,[43,44] costochondritis, hypersensitive xiphoid syndrome, precordial catch syndrome,[45,46] slipping rib syndrome,[47] and rib-tip syndrome.[48] Each patient should be carefully examined to determine whether the symptoms are partially or entirely due to myofascial referred pain and tenderness, especially from TrPs in the pectoralis major muscle. Of these conditions, each has been reported as sometimes being relieved by injection of the tender area with a local anesthetic without reference to examination for TrPs. Because relief by injection is characteristic of TrPs, the resolution of pain may have been achieved by unknowingly treating the muscle dysfunction.

The pectoralis major muscle is one of four muscles that can produce myofascial symptoms consistent with TOS (see Chapter 33 for more on this condition). This muscle and the latissimus dorsi, teres major, and subscapularis muscles individually, and especially in combination, produce referred pain that mimics a TOS. The patient may, however, have a true entrapment or compressive TOS with similar symptoms and referred pain from scalene TrPs may also be present.

When a patient reports having breast soreness (referred tenderness), she or he also may describe a feeling of congestion in that breast. When compared with the other side, the breast may be slightly enlarged and feel doughy. These signs of impaired lymph drainage, possibly due to entrapment or reflex inhibition of peristalsis, soon disappear after inactivation of the responsible TrPs in the lateral border of the tense pectoralis major muscle (Figure 42-3C). The patient who presents with a painful or tender breast, often with hypersensitivity of the nipple to light contact, may have TrPs in the lateral margin of the pectoralis major muscle[28,29] (Figure 42-3C). The thought of having cancer may be a serious, but unexpressed fear in patients, who later express enormous relief when they realize that the pain has a benign treatable myofascial cause.

Other authors have noted that pectoralis major TrPs can simulate the symptoms of angina pectoris[49] and have illustrated similar referred pain patterns for pectoralis major TrPs in the clavicular and costal divisions[50] and in the sternal division and medial and lateral margins.[51] The intensity, quality, and distribution of true cardiac pain can be reproduced by the pain referred from active TrPs in the anterior chest muscles.[52–54] Although these patterns can mimic cardiac pain, TrP pain shows a much wider variability in its response to day-to-day activity than does the more consistent exercise response of angina pectoris.

A definitive diagnosis of active TrPs based on their characteristic signs and symptoms and a dramatic response to local treatment does NOT exclude cardiac disease. Adding to this diagnostic challenge is the fact that noncardiac pain may induce transient T-wave changes in the electrocardiogram.[55] A disorder of the heart may coexist and must be ruled out by appropriate tests of cardiac function.[56]

TrPs within the pectoralis major muscle have been shown to have somatovisceral effects on the heart. A common example of this somatovisceral response is found in patients who experience episodes of supraventricular tachycardia, supraventricular premature contractions, or ventricular premature contractions without other evidence of heart disease. The patient with such an ectopic rhythm should be checked for TrP in the right pectoral region between the fifth and sixth ribs at the specific site described earlier[30] (Figure 42-5B). Although this TrP is tender to palpation, it is not usually a source of referred pain. Inactivation of the TrP promptly restores normal sinus rhythm when the TrP is contributing to an ectopic supraventricular rhythm and also can eliminate recurrences of the paroxysmal arrhythmia or frequent premature contractions for a long period of time.

In addition to somatovisceral effects, studies have demonstrated that there is a viscerosomatic effect between the visceral structures within the chest cavity and the musculature on the anterior chest wall. An example of this myofascial viscerosomatic interaction begins with coronary artery insufficiency, or other intrathoracic disease, that refers pain to the anterior chest. As a result of this pain referral, TrPs develop in the somatic pectoral muscles. Kennard and Haugen[57] related the presence of palpable TrPs in the chest muscles to chest and arm pain and to the disease process responsible for the pain. They found that 61% of 72 patients with cardiac disease, 48% of 35 patients with other visceral chest disease, and 20% of 46 patients with pelvic and lower extremity disease had tender TrPs in the chest muscles. In the patients with chest and arm pain due to cardiac and other unilateral intrathoracic disease, tender TrPs were strongly lateralized to the affected side.[57]

Subclavius

Subclavius muscle shortening by TrPs can contribute to symptoms of a vascular TOS. Shortening of the subclavius muscle because of TrPs will draw the clavicle down toward the subclavian artery and vein as they pass over the first rib. In some patients, this pressure can contribute to, if not cause, entrapment and the symptoms of a vascular TOS. See Chapter 33 for further information on TOS and myofascial considerations.

5. CORRECTIVE ACTIONS

The patient with pectoralis major TrPs should modify activities that repeatedly stress this muscle such as carrying a heavy backpack and weight training (especially bench press). Correction of rounded shoulder posture and maintenance of good dynamic posture are essential for lasting relief of pectoral TrPs. In standing, patients should not be encouraged to actively hold their shoulders back or stand in a "military posture" because this stance will aggravate pectoral muscle and interscapular TrPs. Focusing on the head position and standing tall will allow the shoulders to find their proper resting position.

Supportive sleeping posture is key to a lasting resolution of pectoralis major TrPs. When sleeping, the patient must avoid shortening of the pectoralis major muscle, as occurs when the arms are folded across the chest. A pillow can be used to support the arms to avoid this arm position. When lying on the pain-free side, the patient should support the uppermost forearm on a pillow to prevent the arm from dropping forward to the

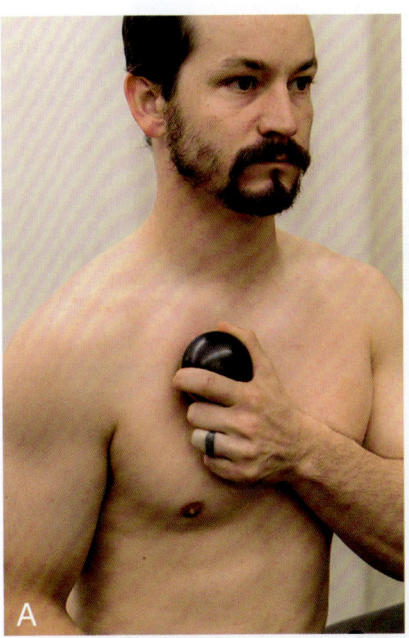
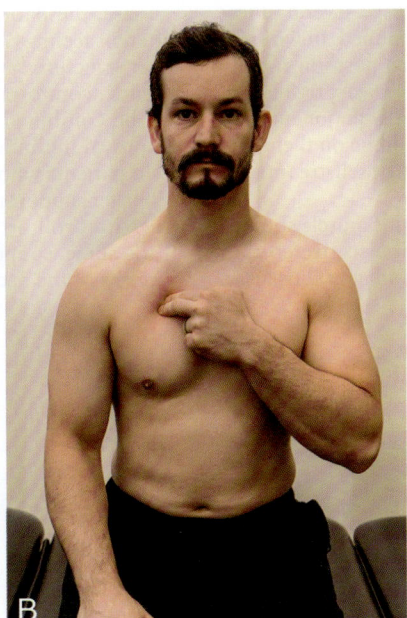
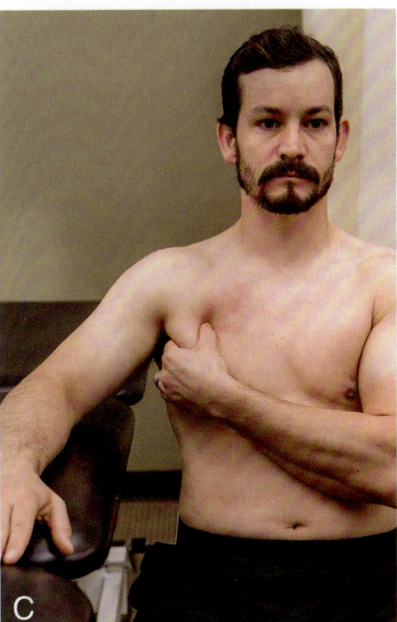
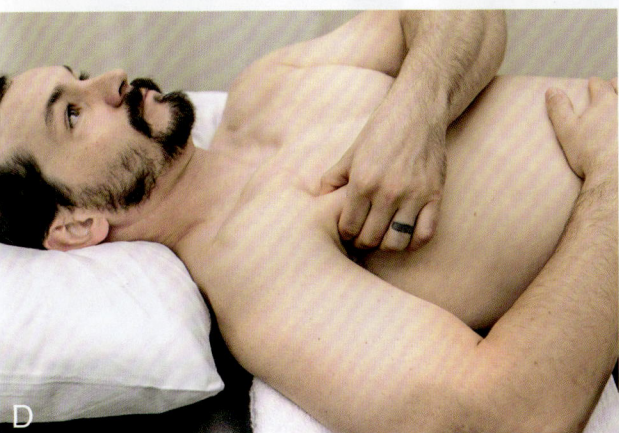
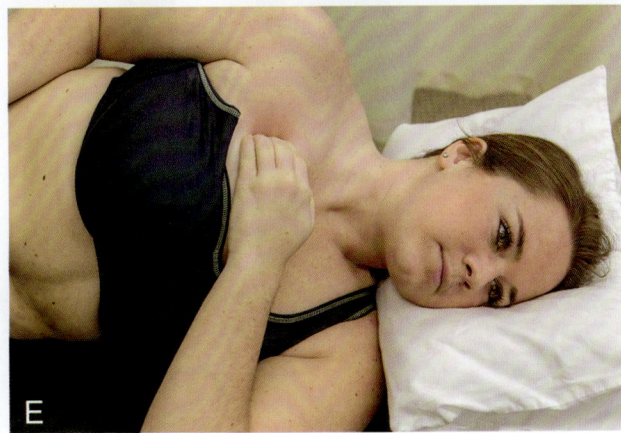

Figure 42-9. Self-pressure release of TrPs in the pectoralis major muscle. A, TrP pressure release tool. B, Self-pressure release. C, Self-pressure release using pincer grasp sitting. D, Supine. E, Side-lying position for a female patient.

bed and thus shortening the affected pectoralis major muscle (see Figure 22-4A). When the patient lies on the affected side, the pillow fits in the axilla between the arm and the chest to prevent undue shortening of the pectoralis major muscle (see Figure 7-5B). In addition, the corner of the pillow should be tucked between the head and shoulder to drop the shoulder backward, not tucked under the shoulder (see Figure 7-5A).

When sitting for a prolonged period or when working at a computer, the chair should be adjusted so as to support the natural lumbar lordosis and the keyboard and monitor should be adjusted appropriately to prevent a slouched rounded shoulder and forward head posture. Patients should be discouraged from forcing their shoulders back with muscle action because this will aggravate symptoms. For further information on posture, refer to Chapter 76.

Pectoralis major TrPs can be self-treated with pressure release utilizing a tennis ball or other TrP release tools. In men, the entire pectoralis major muscle can be easily accessed through the skin; in women, the upper portion of the pectoralis major muscle can be treated through the skin, and the sternal portion must be accessed by moving the breast tissue aside as much as possible. A tennis ball, TrP release tool, or self-pressure release may be utilized in a seated position using the unaffected side to perform the technique (Figure 42-9A and B). For the lateral aspect of the pectoralis major muscle, a pincer grasp can be used for self-pressure release treatment (Figure 42-9C and D). Pressure should be applied to the TrPs, held for 15 to 30 seconds, and repeated 6 to 10 times. This technique can be used several times a day as long as favorable results are being obtained. In women who have large breasts, the supine or side-lying position can be utilized because gravity will aid in moving the breast tissue out of the way. For example, if the right pectoralis major muscle has TrPs that need treatment, the patient would lie on their left side giving access to the right axillary border for self-treatment with the opposite hand (Figure 42-9E).

Stretching techniques for the pectoralis major muscle should be gentle because stretching this muscle will also stretch the other internal rotators of the shoulder joint and neural tissues.

The doorway stretch is useful to stretch all of the adductors and internal rotators of the shoulders. The patient stands in a narrow doorway with the forearms flat against the door facings to anchor the forearms and steps forward through the doorway to stretch the muscles (Figure 42-10). The patient should not grasp the doorjamb and hang on because that action interferes with the muscular relaxation needed for the stretch to be effective. One foot is placed in front of the other, and the forward knee is bent to accept the forward shift of bodyweight. The patient holds the head erect, looking straight ahead, neither craning the neck forward nor looking down at the floor. As the forward knee bends and the patient shifts the body through the doorway, a slow, gentle, passive stretch is exerted bilaterally on the pectoralis major muscle and on its synergistic muscles. The gentle stretch is held for 30 seconds and can be repeated up to five or six times. The patient pauses, relaxes, and takes a few slow abdominal breaths between each cycle to enhance relaxation.

The hand position against the doorjamb is adjusted to apply the stretch to different taut bands in the muscle. Fibers of the clavicular section are stretched best in the lower hand position (Figure 42-10A). By raising the hands to the middle hand position with the upper arms horizontal (Figure 42-10B), the sternal section is stretched. Moving the hands as high as possible, keeping the forearms against the doorjambs (Figure 42-10C), stretches the costal and more vertical abdominal fibers that form the lateral margin of the muscle. When doing this stretching exercise, the patient should be encouraged to distinguish the different feelings of stretch for each section of muscle. Because other structures are also placed on stretch with this technique, a gentle, comfortable stretch should be the goal. This exercise can be combined with the principles of contract–relax and reciprocal inhibition to good advantage.

In patients who require a less aggressive stretch, a towel roll or bolster support may be used in the supine hook-lying position. The towel roll or bolster is positioned vertically in the center of the spine, supporting both the head and thoracic spine. All portions of the pectoralis major muscle can be gently stretched

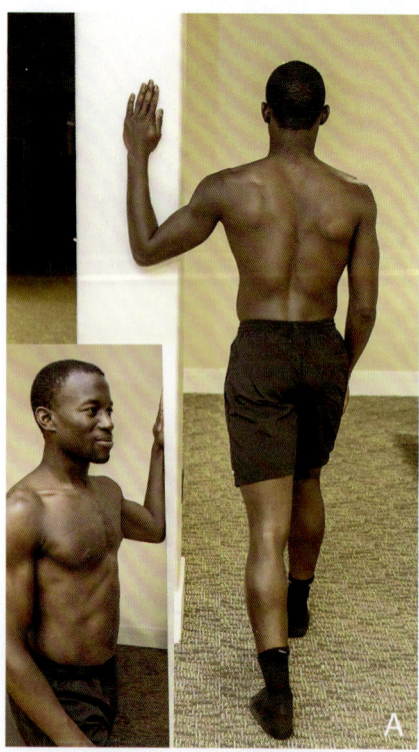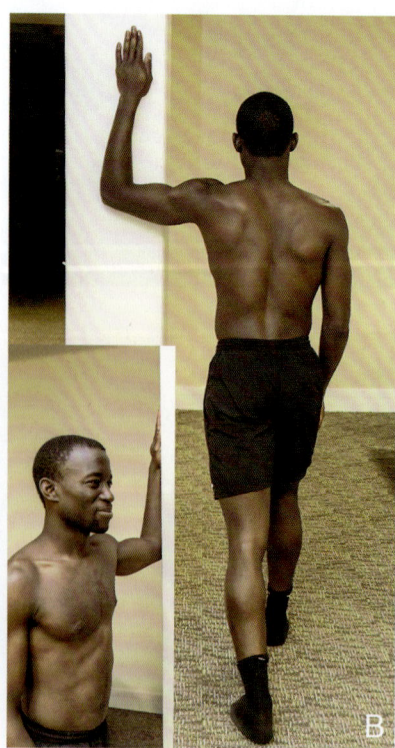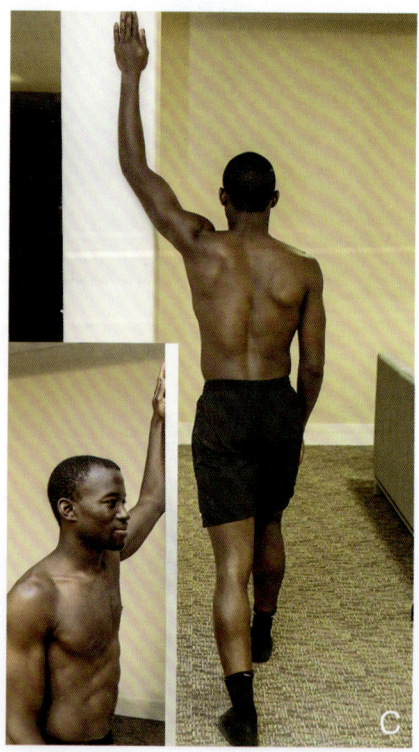

Figure 42-10. Self-stretch of pectoralis major muscle. A, Lower arm position. B, Mid position. C, High position.

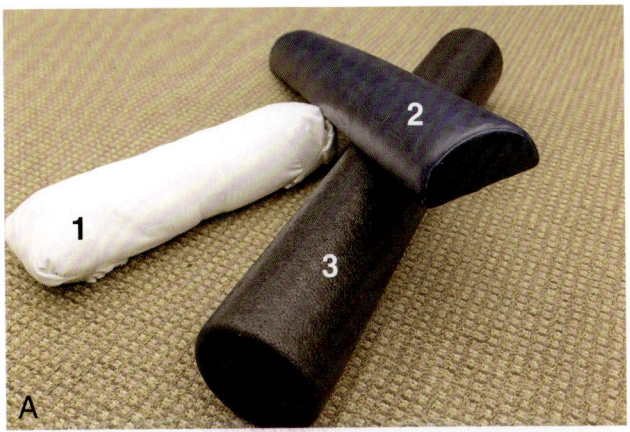
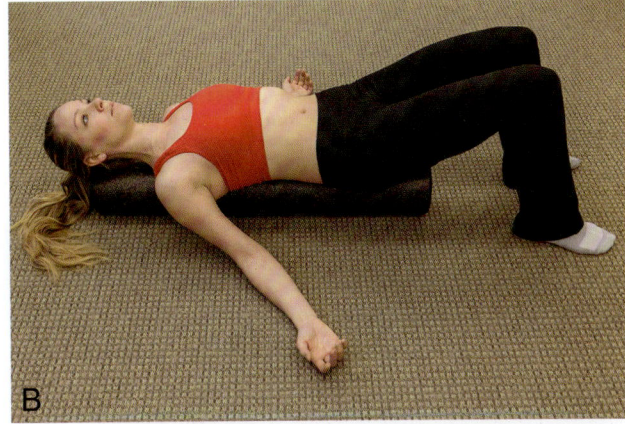
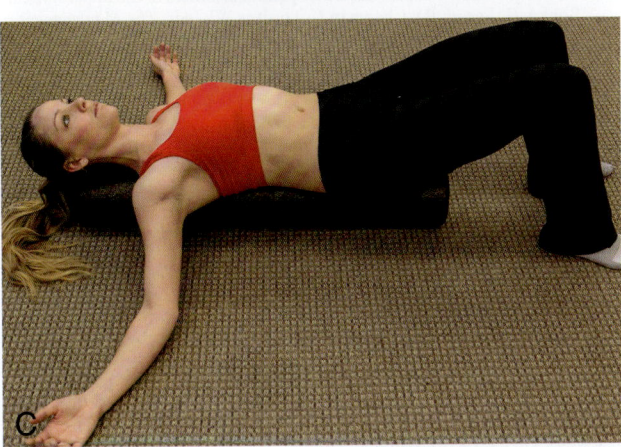
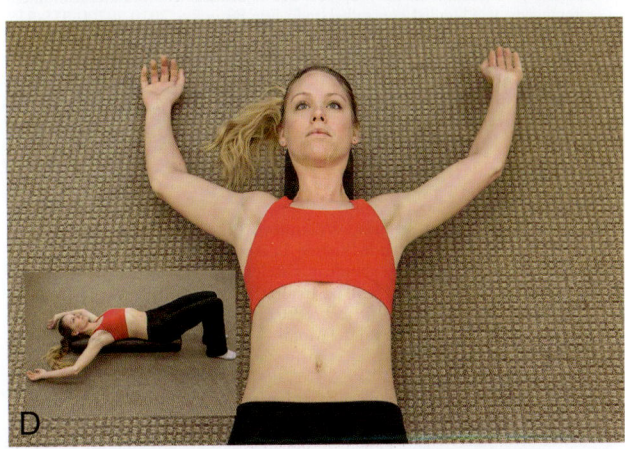

Figure 42-11. Supine bolster stretch. A, Examples of bolsters: *1*, Towel rolled in sheet; *2*, half foam roll; *3*, full foam roll. B, Low position. C, Mid position. D, High position.

---

in this position. Each stretch may be held for 30 seconds and repeated up to five times (Figure 42-11A to D).

Full effectiveness of both of these stretch techniques requires the patient to be mindful of the intensity of stretch. The patient should be instructed to stretch the muscle to the point of comfortable tension (without pain) paying attention to any unfamiliar shoulder symptoms or arm/hand numbness and tingling. If pain, numbness, and/or tingling is felt in the arm, forearm, or hands, this exercise should be stopped immediately, and the patient should seek guidance from an appropriate health care practitioner.

References

1. Petilon J, Ellingson CI, Sekiya JK. Pectoralis major muscle ruptures. *Oper Tech Sports Med.* 2005;13(3):162-168.
2. Standring S. *Gray's Anatomy: The Anatomical Basis of Clinical Practice.* 41st ed. London, UK: Elsevier; 2015.
3. ElMaraghy AW, Devereaux MW. A systematic review and comprehensive classification of pectoralis major tears. *J Shoulder Elbow Surg.* 2012;21(3):412-422.
4. Haley CA, Zacchilli MA. Pectoralis major injuries: evaluation and treatment. *Clin Sports Med.* 2014;33(4):739-756.
5. Porterfield JA, DeRosa C. *Mechanical Shoulder Disorders: Perspectives in Functional Anatomy.* St. Louis, MO: Saunders; 2004:81-82.
6. Ashley GT. The manner of insertion of the pectoralis major muscle in man. *Anat Rec.* 1952;113(3):301-307.
7. Kendall FP, McCreary EK. *Muscles: Testing and Function, with Posture and Pain.* 5th ed. Baltimore, MD: Lippincott Williams & Wilkins; 2005.
8. Neumann DA. *Kinesiology of the Musculoskeletal System: Foundations for Rehabilitaion.* 2nd ed. St. Louis, MO: Mosby; 2010.
9. Wattanaprakornkul D, Halaki M, Boettcher C, Cathers I, Ginn KA. A comprehensive analysis of muscle recruitment patterns during shoulder flexion: an electromyographic study. *Clin Anat.* 2011;24(5):619-626.
10. Wickham J, Pizzari T, Stansfeld K, Burnside A, Watson L. Quantifying 'normal' shoulder muscle activity during abduction. *J Electromyogr Kinesiol.* 2010;20(2):212-222.
11. Decker MJ, Tokish JM, Ellis HB, Torry MR, Hawkins RJ. Subscapularis muscle activity during selected rehabilitation exercises. *Am J Sports Med.* 2003;31(1):126-134.
12. Jobe FW, Perry J, Pink M. Electromyographic shoulder activity in men and women professional golfers. *Am J Sports Med.* 1989;17(6):782-787.
13. Pink M, Jobe FW, Perry J. Electromyographic analysis of the shoulder during the golf swing. *Am J Sports Med.* 1990;18(2):137-140.
14. Gowan ID, Jobe FW, Tibone JE, Perry J, Moynes DR. A comparative electromyographic analysis of the shoulder during pitching. Professional versus amateur pitchers. *Am J Sports Med.* 1987;15(6):586-590.
15. Glousman R, Jobe F, Tibone J, Moynes D, Antonelli D, Perry J. Dynamic electromyographic analysis of the throwing shoulder with glenohumeral instability. *J Bone Joint Surg Am.* 1988;70(2):220-226.
16. Digiovine NM, Jobe FW, Pink M, Perry J. An electromyographic analysis of the upper extremity in pitching. *J Shoulder Elbow Surg.* 1992;1(1):15-25.
17. Ryu RK, McCormick J, Jobe FW, Moynes DR, Antonelli DJ. An electromyographic analysis of shoulder function in tennis players. *Am J Sports Med.* 1988;16(5):481-485.
18. Bankoff AD, Fonseca Neto DR, Zago LC, Moraes AC. Electromyographical study of the pectoralis major (sternocostal part) and deltoid muscles (middle fibers) in volleyball sequential actions. *Electromyogr Clin Neurophysiol.* 2006;46(1):27-33.
19. Rokito AS, Jobe FW, Pink MM, Perry J, Brault J. Electromyographic analysis of shoulder function during the volleyball serve and spike. *J Shoulder Elbow Surg.* 1998;7(3):256-263.
20. Nuber GW, Jobe FW, Perry J, Moynes DR, Antonelli D. Fine wire electromyography analysis of muscles of the shoulder during swimming. *Am J Sports Med.* 1986;14(1):7-11.
21. Pink M, Jobe FW, Perry J, Kerrigan J, Browne A, Scovazzo ML. The normal shoulder during the butterfly swim stroke. An electromyographic and cinematographic analysis of twelve muscles. *Clin Orthop Relat Res.* 1993;(288):48-59.
22. Jonsson S, Jonsson B. Function of the muscles of the upper limb in car driving. IV: the pectoralis major, serratus anterior and latissimus dorsi muscles. *Ergonomics.* 1975;18(6):643-649.
23. Illyes A, Kiss RM. Shoulder muscle activity during pushing, pulling, elevation and overhead throw. *J Electromyogr Kinesiol.* 2005;15(3):282-289.

24. Simons DG, Travell J, Simons L. *Travell & Simon's Myofascial Pain and Dysfunction: The Trigger Point Manual.* Vol 1. 2nd ed. Baltimore, MD: Williams & Wilkins; 1999.
25. Kelly M. Pain in the chest: observations on the use of local anaesthesia in its investigation and treatment. *Med J Aust.* 1944;1:4-7.
26. Winter Z. Referred pain in fibrositis. *Med Rec.* 1944;157:34-37.
27. Long C 2nd. Myofascial pain syndromes. III. Some syndromes of the trunk and thigh. *Henry Ford Hosp Med Bull.* 1956;4(2):102-106.
28. Travell J, Rinzler SH. The myofascial genesis of pain. *Postgrad Med.* 1952;11(5):425-434.
29. Travell J. Referred pain from skeletal muscle; the pectoralis major syndrome of breast pain and soreness and the sternomastoid syndrome of headache and dizziness. *N Y State J Med.* 1955;55(3):331-340.
30. Travell J. *Office Hours: Day and Night.* New York, NY: The World Publishing Company; 1968:261, 263, 264.
31. Bron C, Dommerholt J, Stegenga B, Wensing M, Oostendorp RA. High prevalence of shoulder girdle muscles with myofascial trigger points in patients with shoulder pain. *BMC Musculoskelet Disord.* 2011;12(1):139-151.
32. Hidalgo-Lozano A, Fernández de las Peñas C, Alonso-Blanco C, Ge HY, Arendt-Nielsen L, Arroyo-Morales M. Muscle trigger points and pressure pain hyperalgesia in the shoulder muscles in patients with unilateral shoulder impingement: a blinded, controlled study. *Exp Brain Res.* 2010;202(4):915-925.
33. Fernández de las Peñas C, Grobli C, Ortega-Santiago R, et al. Referred pain from myofascial trigger points in head, neck, shoulder, and arm muscles reproduces pain symptoms in blue-collar (manual) and white-collar (office) workers. *Clin J Pain.* 2012;28(6):511-518.
34. Alonso-Blanco C, Fernández de las Peñas C, Morales-Cabezas M, Zarco-Moreno P, Ge HY, Florez-Garcia M. Multiple active myofascial trigger points reproduce the overall spontaneous pain pattern in women with fibromyalgia and are related to widespread mechanical hypersensitivity. *Clin J Pain.* 2011;27(5):405-413.
35. Fernandez-Lao C, Cantarero-Villanueva I, Fernández de las Peñas C, Del-Moral-Avila R, Arendt-Nielsen L, Arroyo-Morales M. Myofascial trigger points in neck and shoulder muscles and widespread pressure pain hypersensitivtiy in patients with postmastectomy pain: evidence of peripheral and central sensitization. *Clin J Pain.* 2010;26(9):798-806.
36. Torres Lacomba M, Mayoral del Moral O, Coperias Zazo JL, Gerwin RD, Goni AZ. Incidence of myofascial pain syndrome in breast cancer surgery: a prospective study. *Clin J Pain.* 2010;26(4):320-325.
37. Fernandez-Lao C, Cantarero-Villanueva I, Fernández de las Peñas C, Del-Moral-Avila R, Menjon-Beltran S, Arroyo-Morales M. Development of active myofascial trigger points in neck and shoulder musculature is similar after lumpectomy or mastectomy surgery for breast cancer. *J Bodyw Mov Ther.* 2012;16(2):183-190.
38. Godges JJ, Mattson-Bell M, Thorpe D, Shah D. The immediate effects of soft tissue mobilization with proprioceptive neuromuscular facilitation on glenohumeral external rotation and overhead reach. *J Orthop Sports Phys Ther.* 2003;33(12):713-718.
39. Gerwin RD, Dommerholt J, Shah JP. An expansion of Simons' integrated hypothesis of trigger point formation. *Curr Pain Headache Rep.* 2004;8(6):468-475.
40. Zeman SC, Rosenfeld RT, Lipscomb PR. Tears of the pectoralis major muscle. *Am J Sports Med.* 1979;7(6):343-347.
41. Smith JR. Thoracic pain. *Clinics.* 1944;2:1427-1459.
42. Epstein SE, Gerber LH, Borer JS. Chest wall syndrome, a common cause of unexplained cardiac pain. *JAMA.* 1979;241:2793-2797.
43. Levey GS, Calabro JJ. Tietze's syndrome: report of two cases and review of the literature. *Arthritis Rheum.* 1962;5:261-269.
44. Jelenko C 3rd. Tietze's syndrome at the xiphisternal joint. *South Med J.* 1974;67(7):818-820.
45. Stegman D, Mead BT. The chest wall twinge syndrome. *Nebr State Med J.* 1970;55(9):528-533.
46. Calabro JJ, Jeghers H, Miller KA, Gordon RD. Classification of anterior chest wall syndromes. *JAMA.* 1980;243(14):1420-1421.
47. Heinz GJ, Zavala DC. Slipping rib syndrome. *JAMA.* 1977;237(8):794-795.
48. McBeath AA, Keene JS. The rib-tip syndrome. *J Bone Joint Surg Am.* 1975;57A(6):795-797.
49. Harman JB, Young RH. Muscle lesions simulating visceral disease. *Lancet.* 1940;238:1111-1113.
50. Bonica J, Sola A. Chapter 52, Other painful disorders of the upper limb. In: Bonica JJ, Loeser JD, Chapman C, Fordyce WE, eds. *The Management of Pain.* 2nd ed. Philadelphia, PA: Lea & Febiger; 1990:947-958.
51. Bonica J, Sola A. Chapter 58, Chest pain caused by other disorders. In: Bonica JJ, Loeser JD, Chapman C, Fordyce WE, eds. *The Management of Pain.* 2nd ed. Philadelphia, PA: Lea & Febiger; 1990:1114-1145.
52. Landmann HR. Trigger areas as cause of persistent chest and shoulder pain in myocardial infarction or angina pectoris. *J Kans Med Soc.* 1949;50(2):69-71.
53. Reeves TJ, Harrison TR. Diagnostic and therapeutic value of the reproduction of chest pain. *AMA Arch Intern Med.* 1953;91(1):8-25, 15.
54. Travell J, Rinzler SH. Pain syndromes of the chest muscles; resemblance to effort angina and myocardial infarction, and relief by local block. *Can Med Assoc J.* 1948;59(4):333-338.
55. Gold H, Kwit NT, Modell W. The effect of extra-cardiac pain on the heart. *Proc Assoc Res Nerv Ment Dis.* 1943;23:345-357.
56. Travell J. Early relief of chest pain by ethyl chloride spray in acute coronary thrombosis; case report. *Circulation.* 1951;3(1):120-124.
57. Kennard MA, Haugen FP. The relation of subcutaneous focal sensitivity to referred pain of cardiac origin. *Anesthesiology.* 1955;16(3):297-311.
58. Hsieh YL, Kao MJ, Kuan TS, Chen SM, Chen JT, Hong CZ. Dry needling to a key myofascial trigger point may reduce the irritability of satellite MTrPs. *Am J Phys Med Rehabil.* 2007;86(5):397-403.
59. Young D. The effects of novocaine injections on simulated visceral pain. *Ann Intern Med.* 1943;19:749-756.
60. Kelly M. The treatment of fibrositis and allied disorders by local anesthesia. *Med J Aust.* 1941;1:294-298.

Chapter 43

Sternalis Muscle

"Alarming Agonizer"

Joseph M. Donnelly and Brian Yee

1. INTRODUCTION

The sternalis muscle is often forgotten, not only in human function, but just as notably as a contributor to myofascial pain. The sternalis muscle is highly variable and its fibers are superficial to the pectoralis major muscle, generally running parallel to the sternum. The muscle may be present on one or both sides. When trigger points (TrPs) exist in this muscle, the referred pain pattern is a deep substernal ache that is independent of movement. Patients will complain of a deep ache or soreness over the sternum, which cannot be reproduced with movements or posture alterations. Differential diagnosis should include costochondritis, Tietze's syndrome, gastroesophageal reflux, esophagitis, and an anginal presentation of C7 radicular symptoms. Corrective actions include addressing pectoral and sternocleidomastoid TrPs, postural imbalances, sleeping position alteration, and most importantly TrP self-pressure release.

2. ANATOMIC CONSIDERATIONS

The anomalous sternalis muscle is highly variable in presence, symmetry, length, bulk, attachments, and innervation. It may occur bilaterally (Figure 43-1) or more often unilaterally, on either side of the sternum, or rarely, the two muscles may fuse across the sternum. Its reported origins or superior attachments include a combination of the sternum, the inferior border of the clavicle, the sternocleidomastoid fascia, the pectoralis major muscle, and the upper ribs and their costal cartilages. The insertion or inferior attachments include structures such as the lower ribs and their costal cartilages, the pectoralis major muscle, rectus abdominis sheath, and the external oblique aponeurosis.[1,2] The muscle may be as thick as 2 cm (3/4 in) over the sternum, a depth through which it is difficult to palpate pectoralis major TrPs (Figure 43-1). Its maximum reported length ranges from a relatively short muscle of only 2.4 cm to very long specimens of 26.0 cm; the maximum width ranges from 0.48 to 7.0 cm.[1]

The sternalis muscle presents as a parasternal mass deep to the superficial fascia of the anterior thoracic wall and superficial to the pectoral fascia overlying the pectoralis major muscle.[1] It has been reported to be a cord-like structure, a flat band[3] or an irregular and flame-like shape.[4] A unilateral sternalis muscle is more common (67%) than bilateral (33%) with preferential occurrence on the right side (64% right, 36% left).

The sternalis muscle was found in 1.7% to 14.3% (median 4.4%) of cases in 13 studies of at least 10 200 cadaver specimens[5]; at most, in 48% of anencephalic specimens[5]; in 4.3% of 2 062 cadavers as summarized by Christian[6]; and in 6% of 535 cadavers according to Barlow.[7] Eisler,[5] Hollinshead,[8] Grant,[9] and Toldt[10] have each illustrated the sternalis muscle. Cadaveric investigations reveal that the sternalis muscle has an overall prevalence of around 7.8% in the general population.[1] Christian[6] illustrated two bilateral muscles while Shen et al reported one pair.[11] Barlow[7] reported no significant difference in the incidence of the sternalis muscle in white and black Americans. Some of the highest rates have been reported in Asian populations (11.5%) compared with 8.4% in populations of African descent, and 4.4% in those of European descent. Women may have a slightly higher rate of occurrence than men (8.6% and 7.5% respectively), although some studies report no gender difference.[7,12,13] Results from operating rooms seem to support the notion that the sternalis muscle is clinically underreported.[1] Harish and Gopinath[14] report 0.7% cases of a present sternalis muscle in their study.

Jelev et al[15] outlined four basic morphologic characteristics that must be satisfied for a muscle to be accepted as the sternalis muscle: (1) location between the superficial fascia of the anterior thoracic region and the pectoral fascia; (2) origin from the sternum or infraclavicular region; (3) insertion onto the lower ribs, costal cartilages, aponeurosis of the external abdominal oblique muscle, or the sheath of the rectus abdominis muscle; (4) innervation by the anterior thoracic (pectoral) and/or intercostal nerves.

2.1. Innervation and Vascularization

Based on the innervation patterns of 26 sternalis muscles in 20 cadavers,[6] the sternalis muscle was considered a variant of either the pectoralis major or rectus abdominis muscles. Sixteen of 26 sternalis muscles (62%) received their innervation from intercostal nerves (anterior primary divisions of thoracic spinal nerves) and were considered homologous to the rectus abdominis muscle. The remaining 38% received their innervation from the cervical plexus, usually via the medial pectoral nerve, which is derived from spinal nerves C8 and T1, so that these muscles were considered homologous with the sternal portion of the pectoralis major muscle. Two muscles received a dual innervation.[6] Whether the sternalis muscle has an exact analogue in other species has been the subject of unresolved controversy. Its diverse innervation suggests that it may represent variable remnants of several muscles.

The blood supply is primarily derived from the perforating branches of the internal thoracic artery[1,15-20] with additional supply from intermuscular connections from the pectoral branch of the thoracoacromial artery.[19]

2.2. Function

No skeletal movement is attributed to this muscle. No electromyographic data or clinical reports of muscular contraction of the sternalis muscle were located; thus, if, when, or why it contracts is unresolved. The sternalis muscle has no apparent physiologic function.[3] Owing to its parasternal location, the sternalis muscle has been reported to confuse radiologists by presenting as an irregular mass in the medial breast on routine mammograms, leading to the misdiagnosis of breast tumors[4,21,22] or hematomas.[23]

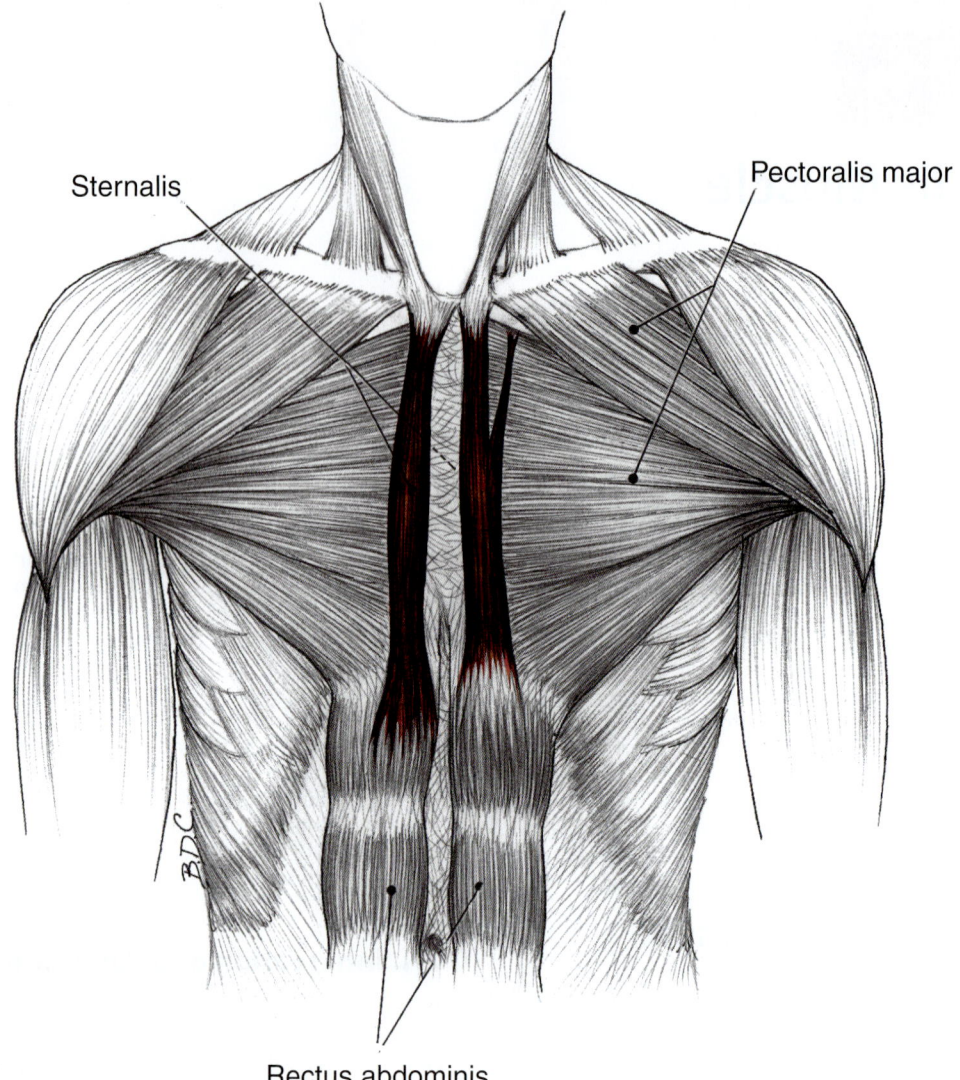

Figure 43-1. Commonly seen attachments of the anatomically variable sternalis muscle (*red*).

2.3. Functional Unit

The functional unit to which a muscle belongs includes the muscles that reinforce and counter its actions as well as the joints that the muscle crosses. The interdependence of these structures functionally is reflected in the organization and neural connections of the sensory motor cortex. The functional unit is emphasized because the presence of a TrP in one muscle of the unit increases the likelihood that the other muscles of the unit will also develop TrPs. When inactivating TrPs in a muscle, one must be concerned about TrPs that may develop in muscles that are functionally interdependent.[24] The functional relation of the sternalis muscle to other muscles must await determination of its specific function.

3. CLINICAL PRESENTATION

3.1. Referred Pain Pattern

The referred pain pattern of the sternalis muscle usually includes the entire sternal and substernal region and may extend on the ipsilateral side across the upper pectoral area and front of the shoulder to the underarm and to the ulnar aspect of the elbow (Figure 43-2).[25-27] This pattern closely mimics the substernal ache of myocardial infarction or angina pectoris. The chest pain referred from this muscle has a terrifying quality that is remarkably independent of body movement. The left-sided pattern of the sternalis muscle differs from the referred pain of the left pectoralis major muscle in that the latter is more likely to extend beyond the elbow into the ulnar aspect of the left forearm and hand. Both muscles may contribute simultaneously to the pain reported by the patient.[26,28,29]

Trigger points may be located anywhere within the sternalis muscle: as high as the manubrium, as low as the xiphoid process, and on either or both sides, including the midline of the sternum when the muscle fuses across the sternum. Sternalis TrPs usually occur over the upper two-thirds of the sternum and are most likely to be found in the central part of the muscle, slightly to the left of the midline at the midsternal level. Anatomically, a unilateral muscle is more common on the right than on the left, but active TrPs appear to be more common on the left side, probably because of their activation from the heart from a viscerosomatic reflex.

Though the sternalis muscle may be only a small remnant of muscle, the intensity of pain arising from TrPs in it (or any other muscle) is not related to the size of the muscle, but to the degree of irritability and size of the TrPs.

Chapter 43: Sternalis Muscle 423

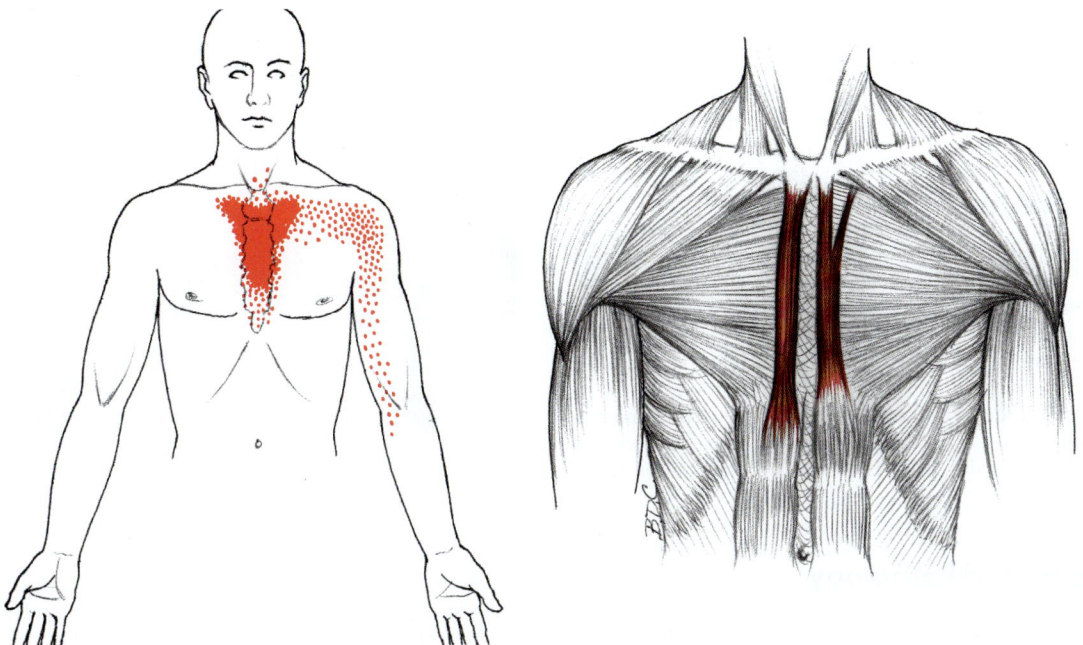

Figure 43-2. A TrP in the left sternalis muscle gives rise to the referred pain pattern shown in *red*.

At times, a TrP located at the confluence of the sternalis, pectoralis major, and sternal division of the sternocleidomastoid muscles can be the source of a dry, hacking cough. Palpation and treatment for the TrP may temporarily produce the cough but it slowly dissipates.

3.2. Symptoms

The symptoms associated with TrPs in this muscle are intense deep substernal pain and occasionally, soreness over the sternum. Since the pain arising from this muscle is not aggravated by movement, its musculoskeletal origin is easily overlooked.

3.3. Patient Examination

After a thorough subjective examination the clinician should make a detailed drawing representing the pain pattern that the patient has described. This depiction will assist in planning the physical examination and can be useful in monitoring the progression of the patient as symptoms improve or change. Any patient with primary reports of chest pain should alert the clinician to perform a thorough review of the cardiovascular and pulmonary systems. Any concerns regarding the involvement of the cardiovascular or respiratory systems as a source of symptoms should result in an immediate referral to the emergency room or a physician. Range-of-motion tests are typically negative in a patient with sternalis TrPs, since the pain is neither relieved nor aggravated by any musculoskeletal activity, such as movement of the shoulder girdle, deep breathing, or stooping. Trigger point palpation is the only confirming sign that TrPs in the sternalis muscle are the source of the patient's symptoms.

3.4. Trigger Point Examination

Sternalis TrPs are found by systematic cross-fiber flat palpation against the underlying sternum and costal cartilages (Figure 43-3). Firm pressure elicits focal deep tenderness at the TrP and projection of referred pain but rarely elicits a local twitch response. On examination, the patient has difficulty in distinguishing between

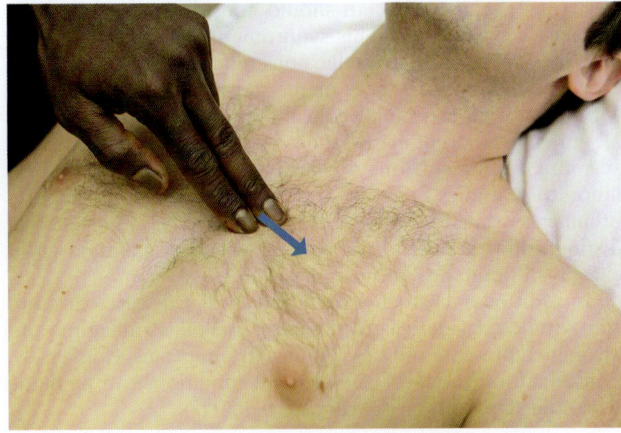

Figure 43-3. Palpation of left sternalis muscle.

the local and the referred pain that is elicited from this muscle, unless the pain radiates not only to the sternum but also to the shoulder or arm. Referred pain responses due to needle penetration of the TrP are more clearly distinguishable. Trigger points in the central part of the muscle are most commonly found to the left or right of the midline at the midsternal level.[26,30]

4. DIFFERENTIAL DIAGNOSIS

4.1. Activation and Perpetuation of Trigger Points

Since the sternalis muscle has no confirmed movement function, TrPs are thought to be activated, not by muscle loading or exercise, as is typical, but instead by its location within or proximity to the referral pain areas of other tissues. It is important to realize that patients with either acute myocardial infarction or angina pectoris are likely to develop active TrPs in both the sternalis and left pectoralis major and minor muscles. A sternalis TrP activated by an episode of myocardial ischemia, as in acute infarction, is likely to persist long after this initiating event.

4.2. Associated Trigger Points

Associated TrPs can develop in the referred pain areas caused by a TrP.[31] Therefore, musculature in the referred pain areas for each muscle should also be considered. One rarely observes sternalis TrPs alone without the presence of TrPs in the pectoralis major and/or minor muscles. The possibility that a sternalis TrP is associated with other TrPs makes it important to examine the lower portion of the sternal division of the sternocleidomastoid muscle, which may refer pain downward over the sternum. Activation of TrPs also may result from direct trauma to the costosternal area.

4.3. Associated Pathology

The sternalis muscle has major implications in breast and thoracic surgery. When undetected before surgery it can interfere with procedures, leading to longer operative times. Yet when detected preoperatively it can be used as a muscular flap in reconstructive surgery and improve aesthetic results in breast augmentation by providing extra cover for the prosthesis.[1]

When multiple areas of spot tenderness are found over the costochondral junctions without the referred pain feature of sternalis TrPs, the clinician should consider costochondritis or Tietze's syndrome.[32] This syndrome is identified by upper anterior chest pain with tender, nonsuppurative swelling in the area of the costal cartilages or the sternoclavicular junctions. Multiple lesions are more frequent than single lesions and usually involve adjacent articulations. Also, in Tietze's syndrome, systemic manifestations are absent and radiographic and laboratory studies are normal, except for occasional reports of increased calcification at affected sites.[32] The importance of distinguishing between chest pain of cardiac origin and that of chest wall origin has been emphasized.[33]

In addition to costochondritis and cardiac disease, the clinician should consider gastroesophageal reflux, esophagitis, and an anginal presentation of C7 radicular symptoms. Conversely, a mistaken diagnosis of one of these conditions can be made when the symptoms arise from sternalis TrPs.

5. CORRECTIVE ACTIONS

For acute pain situations, due to sternalis TrP pain, the patient should be instructed to lie on their back with a quarter turn toward the side of discomfort (in slight flexion and rotation/side bending to the side of pain, if unilateral) with slight neck flexion due to its connection to sternocleidomastoid muscle and its interaction with the pectoralis major muscle.

As pain becomes less severe, it is important to educate patients in appropriate postures that promote neutral spine positions and rib positioning. Instruction in proper breathing patterns, emphasizing diaphragmatic breathing patterns more than upper chest respiratory patterns, as well as core and scapular stability is also important.

The patient should learn to perform self-pressure release on his or her own sternalis TrPs, followed by application of moist heat. The patient selects a tender spot and presses on it steadily against the underlying bone with one finger to the point of discomfort and holds it until it fully releases (Figure 43-4). This release is assisted by slow relaxed exhalation. It may remain quiescent indefinitely, unless the TrP is reactivated, as by recurring angina pectoris.[34]

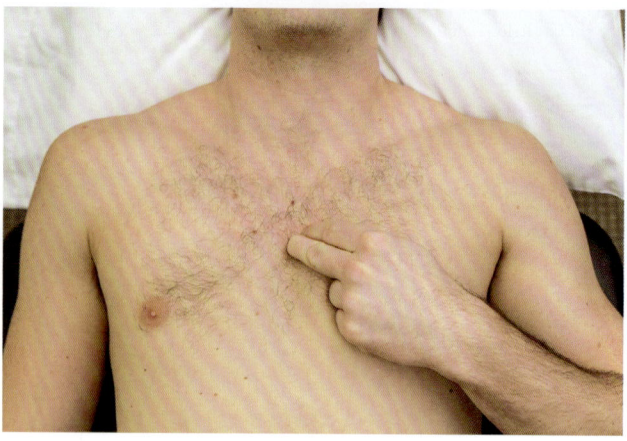

Figure 43-4. Trigger point self-pressure release.

Stretch of the sternalis muscle is not practical except for clinician applied myofascial release techniques, TrP injection, or dry needling techniques. Deep friction massage applied to the muscle fibers in the region of the TrP may also be beneficial.

Local treatment of sternalis TrPs is not complete until TrPs in the pectoralis major and/or minor muscles and the inferior end of the sternal division of the sternocleidomastoid muscle have been treated. The patient is less likely to experience recurrence of pain due to TrPs in the sternalis muscle if these other two muscles are also released.

References

1. Snosek M, Tubbs RS, Loukas M. Sternalis muscle, what every anatomist and clinician should know. *Clin Anat.* 2014;27(6):866-884, 867-870.
2. Standring S. *Gray's Anatomy: The Anatomical Basis of Clinical Practice.* 41st ed. London, UK: Elsevier; 2015.
3. Turner W. On the musculus sternalis. *J Anat Physiol.* 1867;1(2):246.25-378.25.
4. Bradley FM, Hoover HC Jr, Hulka CA, et al. The sternalis muscle: an unusual normal finding seen on mammography. *AJR Am J Roentgenol.* 1996;166(1):33-36.
5. Eisler P. *Die Muskeln des Stammes.* Jena, Germany: Gustav Fischer; 1912:470-475, Figs. 70 and 72.
6. Christian HA. Two instances in which the musculus sternalis existed-one associated with other anomalies. *Bull Johns Hopkins Hosp.* 1898;9:235-240.
7. Barlow RN. The sternalis muscle in American whites and Negroes. *Anat Rec.* 1935;61:413-426.
8. Hollinshead WH. *Anatomy for Surgeons.* Vol 1. 3rd ed. Hagerstown, MD: Harper & Row; 1982:281, Fig. 4-19.
9. Grant JCB. *An Atlas of Human Anatomy.* 7th ed (see Anderson for 1983 edition). Baltimore, MD: Williams & Wilkins; 1978, Fig. 6-120B.
10. Toldt C. *An Atlas of Human Anatomy.* Vol 1. 2nd ed. New York, NY: Macmillan; 1919:282.
11. Shen CL, Chien CH, Lee SH. A Taiwanese with a pair of sternalis muscles. *Kaibogaku Zasshi.* 1992;67(5):652-654.
12. Cunningham DJ. The musculus sternalis. *J Anat Physiol.* 1888;22(Pt 3):390.1-407.1.
13. Yap SE. Musculus sternalis in Filipinos. *Anat Rec.* 1921;21:353-371.
14. Harish K, Gopinath KS. Sternalis muscle: importance in surgery of the breast. *Surg Radiol Anat.* 2003;25(3-4):311-314.
15. Jelev L, Georgiev G, Surchev L. The sternalis muscle in the Bulgarian population: classification of sternales. *J Anat.* 2001;199(Pt 3):359-363.
16. Flint JM. On the use of clay models to record variations found in the dissecting room, with a note of two cases of M. sternalis and its influence on the growth of M. pectoralis major. *J Med Res.* 1902;8(3):496-501.
17. Jeng H, Su SJ. The sternalis muscle: an uncommon anatomical variant among Taiwanese. *J Anat.* 1998;193(Pt 2):287-288.
18. Motabagani MA, Sonalla A, Abdel-Meguid E, Bakheit MA. Morphological study of the uncommon rectus sterni muscle in German cadavers. *East Afr Med J.* 2004;81(3):130-133.
19. Schulman MR, Chun JK. The conjoined sternalis-pectoralis muscle flap in immediate tissue expander reconstruction after mastectomy. *Ann Plast Surg.* 2005;55(6):672-675.
20. Georgiev GP, Jelev L, Ovtscharoff VA. On the clinical significance of the sternalis muscle. *Folia Med (Plovdiv).* 2009;51(3):53-56.
21. Goktan C, Orguc S, Serter S, Ovali GY. Musculus sternalis: a normal but rare mammographic finding and magnetic resonance imaging demonstration. *Breast J.* 2006;12(5):488-489.

22. Pojchamarnwiputh S, Muttarak M, Na-Chiangmai W, Chaiwun B. Benign breast lesions mimicking carcinoma at mammography. *Singapore Med J.* 2007;48(10):958-968.
23. Raikos A, Paraskevas GK, Yusuf F, Kordali P, Ioannidis O, Brand-Saberi B. Sternalis muscle: a new crossed subtype, classification, and surgical applications. *Ann Plast Surg.* 2011;67(6):646-648.
24. Simons DG, Travell J, Simons L. *Travell & Simon's Myofascial Pain and Dysfunction: The Trigger Point Manual.* Vol 1. 2nd ed. Baltimore, MD: Williams & Wilkins; 1999.
25. Bonica J, Sola A. Chapter 58, Chest pain caused by other disorders. In: Bonica JJ, Loeser JD, Chapman C, Fordyce WE, eds. *The Management of Pain.* 2nd ed. Philadelphia, PA: Lea & Febiger; 1990:1114-1145.
26. Travell J, Rinzler SH. The myofascial genesis of pain. *Postgrad Med.* 1952;11(5):425-434, 429.
27. Zohn DA. *Musculoskeletal Pain: Diagnosis and Physical Treatment.* 2nd ed. Boston, MA: Little Brown; 1988:212, Fig. 12-4.
28. Travell J. Pain mechanisms in connective tissue. In: Ragan C, ed. Paper presented at: Connective Tissues, Transactions of the Second Conference 1951. New York, NY: Josiah Macy Jr. Foundation. 1952 (pp. 86-125).
29. Travell J, Rinzler SH. Pain syndromes of the chest muscles; resemblance to effort angina and myocardial infarction, and relief by local block. *Can Med Assoc J.* 1948;59(4):333-338, Cases 2 and 3.
30. Webber TD. Diagnosis and modification of headache and shoulder-arm-hand syndrome. *J Am Osteopath Assoc.* 1973;72(7):697-710, 10, 12; Fig. 32.
31. Hsieh YL, Kao MJ, Kuan TS, Chen SM, Chen JT, Hong CZ. Dry needling to a key myofascial trigger point may reduce the irritability of satellite MTrPs. *Am J Phys Med Rehabil.* 2007;86(5):397-403.
32. Levey GS, Calabro JJ. Tietze's syndrome: report of two cases and review of the literature. *Arthritis Rheum.* 1962;5:261-269.
33. Epstein SE, Gerber LH, Borer JS. Chest wall syndrome, a common cause of unexplained cardiac pain. *JAMA.* 1979;241:2793-2797.
34. Travell J, Rinzler SH. Therapy directed at the somatic component of cardiac pain. *Am Heart J.* 1958;35:248-268.

Chapter 44

Pectoralis Minor Muscle

"Thoracic Outlet Imposter"

Joseph M. Donnelly and Deanna Hortman Camilo

1. INTRODUCTION

The pectoralis minor muscle is a thin, flat muscle that lies under the pectoralis major muscle along the anterior portion of the third, fourth, and fifth ribs. It moves the scapula forward (anterior tilt), downward, and inward (internal rotation) to depress the glenohumeral joint and stabilize the scapula when the upper extremity is moving downward against resistance. Pectoralis minor muscle length deficit is thought to be an important contributing factor to subacromial pain syndrome. Trigger points (TrPs) in the pectoralis minor muscle refer pain over the anterior deltoid region, often extending along the ulnar side of the arm, elbow, forearm, and palmar aspect of the hand to include the last three fingers. Symptoms may be exacerbated by slumped or rounded shoulder posture as well as with repetitive activities including throwing, gardening, crutch walking, and paradoxical breathing. Differential diagnosis should include thoracic outlet syndrome, C7 and C8 radicular pain or radiculopathy, supraspinatus or bicipital tendinopathy, and medial epicondylalgia. Corrective actions involve techniques to improve posture, effective workplace ergonomics, neutral sleeping positions, TrP self-pressure release, and self-stretching techniques.

2. ANATOMIC CONSIDERATIONS

The pectoralis minor muscle is a thin triangular shaped muscle that is seated immediately posteriorly to the pectoralis major muscle and lies over the rib cage. Notably, the anatomic relationship between the costal origin of the pectoralis major and minor muscles is highly variable in relation to the intermuscular space.[1] It originates from the outer surface of ribs three, four, and five and occasionally as high as the first rib and as low as the sixth rib near their costal cartilage and from the fascia of the external intercostal muscles.[2] The fibers ascend laterally and insert onto the medial border and superior surface of the coracoid process of the scapula (Figure 44-1).[2,3] A slip of the pectoralis minor muscle may extend beyond the coracoid process in about 15% of bodies to attach to tendons of adjacent muscles or to the greater tuberosity of the humerus.[4] In fact, Lee et al[5] reported a prevalence of 13.4% of ectopic insertion of the pectoralis minor muscle. Weinstabl et al[6] also found that the pectoralis minor muscle had a continuous connection with the coracohumeral ligament in their study of 126 shoulder specimens, which is consistent with more recent sources.[2,6,7]

The tip of the coracoid process of the scapula also provides a site of attachment for the tendons of the coracobrachialis and short head of the biceps brachii muscles. These tendinous insertions are encased by the clavipectoral fascia.[2]

Although rare, other anatomic variations of the pectoralis minor muscle include the pectoralis minimus and pectoralis intermedius muscles. The pectoralis minimus muscle connects the first rib cartilage to the coracoid process, whereas the pectoralis intermedius muscle may attach more medially than the pectoralis minor muscle onto the third, fourth, and fifth rib cartilages and above the clavipectoral fascia covering the coracobrachialis and biceps brachii muscles. This arrangement sandwiches the pectoralis intermedius muscle between the pectoralis major and minor muscles.

Approximately 40% of pectoralis minor muscle fibers are type II, decreasing slightly after age 60. The volume of type II fibers is significantly decreased after that age.[8]

2.1. Innervation and Vascularization

The pectoralis minor muscle is innervated by branches of the medial and lateral pectoral nerves.[2] The lateral pectoral nerve is derived from spinal nerves C5, C6, and C7 and lies anterior to the muscle along with branches of the thoracoacromial artery. The medial pectoral nerve is a branch from the medial cord and is comprised of fibers from roots C8 and T1. It innervates and pierces the pectoralis minor muscle en route to innervate the sternal head of the pectoralis major muscle.[2,9,10] Mehta et al[11] described a case report of an unusual innervation presentation of the pectoralis minor muscle in which the pectoralis minor muscle was pierced extensively by multiple branches from the medial pectoral nerve, but none from the lateral pectoral nerve.

Porzionato et al[12] demonstrated that the medial pectoral nerve originates from the medial cord in 49.3% of specimens, the anterior division of the lower trunk in 43.8% of specimens, and the lower trunk in 4.7% of specimens. The distal portion of the brachial plexus passes deep to the pectoralis minor muscle where the muscle attaches to the coracoid process,[2] which may explain the potential role of this muscle in thoracic outlet syndrome symptoms.

The primary vascular supply of the pectoralis minor muscle is through the deltoid and pectoral branches of the thoracoacromial artery and by branches of the lateral and superior thoracic arteries.[2] Although the lateral thoracic artery shows morphologic variability, it usually descends on the lateral border of the pectoralis minor muscle.[13]

The pectoralis minor muscle is the landmark for anatomically dividing the axillary artery into three parts: the first part superior to its medial border, the second part of the artery deep to the muscle, and the third part inferior to its lateral border. The upper border of the pectoralis minor muscle is separated from the clavicle by a triangular gap created by the clavipectoral fascia and the axillary vessels, nerves, and lymphatics lie posterior to this structure, just before they pass under the pectoralis minor muscle into the brachium.[2] When the arm is abducted and externally rotated at the shoulder (Figure 44-2A), the artery, vein, and nerves are bent and stretched around the pectoralis minor muscle near its attachment (Figure 44-2B). The neurovascular structures are likely to be compressed if the pectoralis minor muscle is tightened by TrPs or from increased pectoralis minor

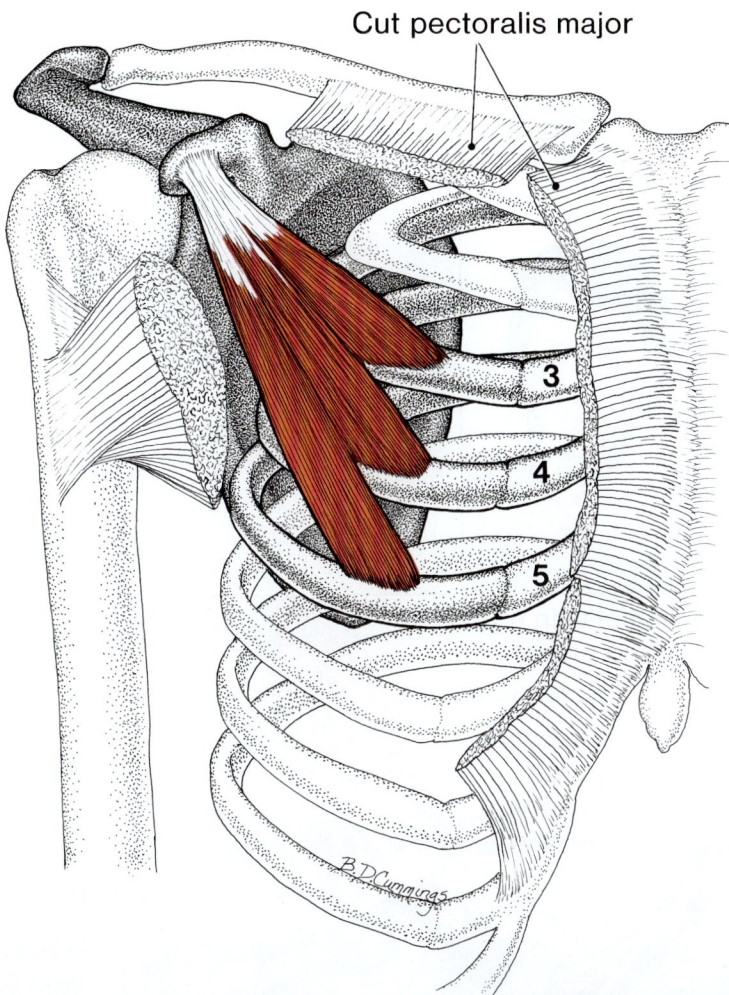

Figure 44-1. Attachments of the pectoralis minor muscle (*red*) to the coracoid process of the scapula and to the third, fourth, and fifth ribs.

muscle tension, which also increases the entrapment potential of the C7 and C8 roots that pass over the first rib, contributing to thoracic outlet syndrome symptoms.[14]

2.2. Function

The pectoralis minor muscle is one of five muscles that can both initiate and control scapular movement. The pectoralis minor muscle acts synergistically with the serratus anterior muscle to perform scapular protraction. If contracted independently, it performs a combination of movements including anterior tilting, protraction, and downward rotation of the scapula.[15] Since the inward force component is blocked by the clavicle when the pectoralis minor muscle contracts, there is an associated elevation of the scapula and a resultant force that draws the glenoid fossa of the scapula obliquely down and forward (anterior tilt). At the same time, this force tends to lift the scapula's medial border and inferior angle away from the rib cage (winging of the scapula).[16]

The shoulder depression function of the pectoralis major and latissimus dorsi muscles is assisted by the pectoralis minor muscle that directly depresses the scapula through its attachment on the coracoid process. Depression of the shoulder by the pectoralis minor muscle stabilizes the scapula when the arm exerts a downward pressure against resistance.[17] This coracoid depression is used to elevate and pull the shoulder forward. The pectoralis minor muscle stabilizes the scapula against any elevation force, as needed during activities such as crutch walking, driving a stake into the ground, and digging holes.[16]

Wickham et al[18] investigated muscle activity using electromyography (EMG) on 15 shoulder muscles during shoulder elevation. These authors found that the supraspinatus, middle deltoid, and middle trapezius muscles activated prior to limb movement and the pectoralis minor muscle was the second to last muscle to activate (at 16° of shoulder elevation) with a peak maximum volitional isometric contraction (MVIC) of 30% between 135° and 165° of shoulder elevation.[18] Castelein et al,[15] in an attempt to identify MVIC of the deep scapulothoracic muscles utilizing fine wire EMG, found six positions that maximally activated the pectoralis minor muscle. The test position that activated the pectoralis minor muscle to the highest MVIC was the combination of internal rotation and glenohumeral elevation to 90° in the coronal plane. The investigators surmised that this position requires the pectoralis minor muscle to pull the scapula anteriorly and inferiorly toward the ribs to stabilize the scapula during resisted glenohumeral internal rotation.[15] They also found that pure protraction from the supine position, as described by Kendall et al[19] for a manual muscle test of this muscle, produced 11% less MVIC than the other test positions. They conclude that clinical tests utilized to look at pectoralis minor muscle strength may not automatically lead to highest EMG activation, especially when utilizing fine wire EMG.[15]

Castelein et al[20] also investigated the role of the pectoralis minor muscle as a synergist to the serratus anterior muscle during

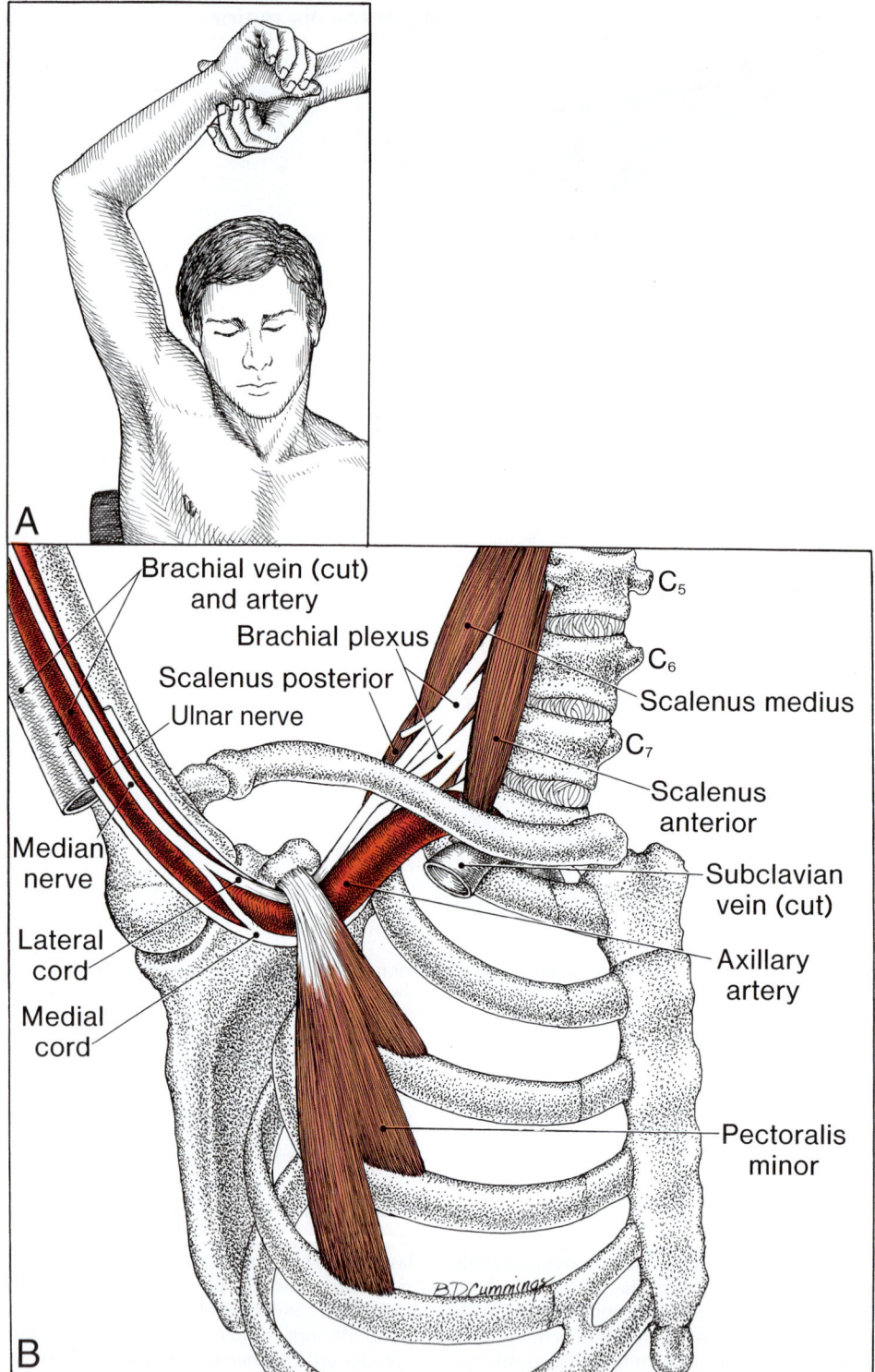

Figure 44-2. Entrapment of the lower brachial plexus and axillary artery by the right pectoralis minor muscle during the Wright full-abduction test. A, Abduction test position. B, Stretch and torsion of the brachial plexus and axillary artery can occur as they hook beneath the pectoralis minor muscle where it attaches to the coracoid process. The clavicle may also compress these neurovascular structures directly against the first rib as the scapula is forcefully pulled into adduction.

three common exercises (modified push up plus on the wall, modified knee push up on the floor, and serratus punch standing) utilizing surface and fine wire EMG. The wall pushup plus and the modified knee push up on the floor activated the pectoralis minor and serratus anterior muscles very similarly; however, the serratus anterior punch standing maximally activated the serratus anterior muscle with minimal synergistic activation of the pectoralis minor muscle.[20]

The main function of the pectoralis minor muscle is to provide scapular stabilization, especially during functional activities. Therefore, it has a propensity to lose its extensibility, which places the scapula in an abnormal position and leads to rounded shoulder posture, subacromial pain syndrome, and scapular dyskinesia.[3,21,22] The role of the pectoralis minor muscle in subacromial impingement syndrome during elevation activities was investigated using surface and fine wire EMG on the superficial and deep scapulothoracic muscle respectively.[23] This study compared scapulothoracic muscle activation during shoulder elevation between individuals with subacromial impingement syndrome and asymptomatic controls. They found that the pectoralis minor muscle was significantly more active in the patient group during all elevation activities as compared to the control group, a result that supports the theory that the pectoralis minor muscle has a role in subacromial impingement syndrome.

2.3. Functional Unit

The functional unit to which a muscle belongs includes the muscles that reinforce and counter its actions as well as the joints that the muscle crosses. The interdependence of these structures functionally is reflected in the organization and neural connections of the sensory motor cortex. The functional unit is emphasized because the presence of a TrP in one muscle of the unit increases the likelihood that the other muscles of the unit will also develop TrPs. When inactivating TrPs in a muscle, one must be concerned about TrPs that may develop in muscles that are functionally interdependent. Box 44-1 grossly represents the functional unit of the pectoralis minor muscle.[24]

The pectoralis minor muscle forms a synergistic functional unit that creates additional support for vigorous inhalation with the levator scapulae, upper trapezius, and sternocleidomastoid muscles in addition to the parasternal internal intercostals, lateral external intercostals, diaphragm, and scalene muscles. Additionally, electromyographically, the pectoralis minor muscle is active in forced inspiration but not in quiet breathing.[16]

3. CLINICAL PRESENTATION

3.1. Referred Pain Pattern

Trigger points in the pectoralis minor muscle refer pain most strongly over the anterior deltoid area. The pain may extend upward over the subclavicular area and sometimes covers the entire pectoral region on the ipsilateral side. Pain can also be referred along the ulnar side of the arm, elbow, forearm, and palmar aspect of the hand to include the medial three fingers (Figure 44-3). A similar referral pattern can be found with TrPs in the clavicular division of the pectoralis major muscle (see Figure 42-3B).[25] Pain from either pectoral muscle, and specifically the pectoralis minor muscle, can closely mimic the pain of cardiac ischemia.[26,27] In fact, Lawson et al[28] described a case report when the pectoralis minor muscle was the pain source in a patient with anterior chest pain. Proper treatment of the pectoralis muscle was effective for reducing symptoms.

3.2. Symptoms

Trigger points in the pectoralis minor muscle should be considered as a potential source of symptoms when a patient reports pain or difficulty with reaching forward and up or reaching backward with the arm at shoulder level. When the patient's primary report of pain

Box 44-1 Functional unit of the pectoralis minor muscle

Action	Synergists	Antagonist
Shoulder depression	Pectoralis major Subclavius Latissimus dorsi Teres major Trapezius (lower) Serratus anterior	Trapezius (upper) Levator scapulae Rhomboids
Shoulder protraction	Serratus anterior Pectoralis major Subclavius	Rhomboid major Rhomboid minor Trapezius (middle, lower)

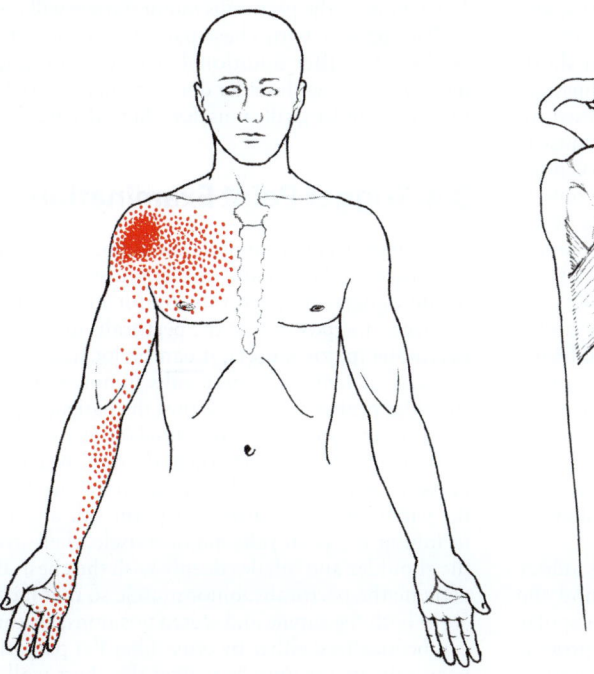
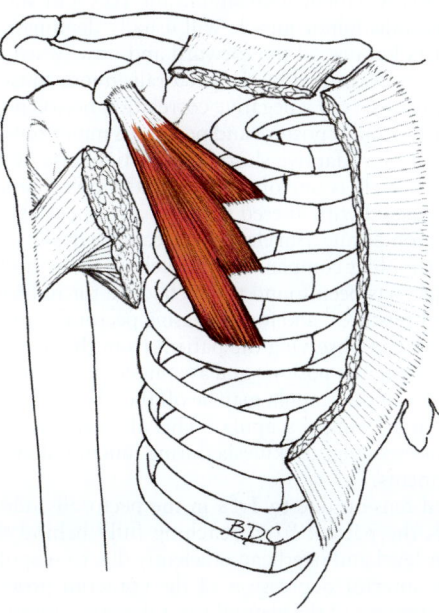

Figure 44-3. Referred pain pattern (solid red is the essential portion, stippled red shows the spillover portion) in the right pectoralis minor muscle.

is in the anterior aspect of the shoulder, the pectoralis major and minor, subclavius, infraspinatus, supraspinatus, deltoid (anterior, middle), biceps brachii, coracobrachialis, and scalene muscles are the most likely muscular sources of symptoms.[29] The intensity and quality, as well as the distribution, of cardiac pain may be reproduced by this pectoral muscle's referred pain pattern.[27,28]

The shortened pectoralis minor muscle may cause distinctive neurovascular symptoms through entrapment of the axillary neurovascular bundle below the clavicle.[30,31] This condition is known as pectoralis minor syndrome and may result in "pain, weakness, paresthesias, and arterial/venous insufficiency" of the affected upper extremity.[30] Pectoralis minor muscle shortening or tightness must also be considered in cases of brachial plexus compression.[31] The outcomes of patients with thoracic outlet syndrome and pectoralis minor syndrome vary and depend on duration of symptoms before initiation of physical therapy or surgical intervention.[30,31] In fact, in some patients with neurogenic thoracic outlet syndrome, the isolated treatment of pectoralis minor muscle can be very effective, thus supporting the role of this muscle in this symptomatology.[32]

When the patient reports swelling in the hand and fingers these symptoms are more closely associated with TrPs in the scalene muscles as the axillary vein is located under the scalene muscle but not under the pectoralis minor muscle. Thoracic outlet syndrome and TrP considerations are presented in Chapter 33.

3.3. Patient Examination

After a thorough subjective examination the clinician should make a detailed drawing representing the pain pattern that the patient has described. This depiction will assist in planning the physical examination and can be useful in monitoring the progression of the patient as symptoms improve or change. Any patient with primary reports of chest pain should alert the clinician to perform a thorough review of the cardiovascular and pulmonary systems. Any concerns regarding the involvement of the cardiovascular or pulmonary systems as a source of symptoms should result in an immediate referral to the emergency room or a physician. For proper examination of the pectoralis minor muscle, the clinician should observe shoulder girdle posture, scapular position, active and passive range of motion of the shoulder girdle, muscle activation patterns, and the scapulohumeral rhythm. The clinician should note when and where pain occurs. A patient with significant TrPs and shortening of the pectoralis minor muscle will usually demonstrate rounded shoulders because of the forward and downward tilt of the coracoid process caused by the pectoralis minor muscle. Lee et al[33] recently observed a negative correlation between the degree of forward scapular posture and pectoralis minor muscle shortening. In fact, the adaptive shortening or tightness of the pectoralis minor muscle is one of the potential biomechanical mechanisms associated with altered scapular alignment at rest and scapular motion during arm elevation (scapular dyskinesis) in patients with shoulder complaints.[34] Stretching of the pectoralis minor muscle has been found to be effective for reducing rounded shoulder posture[21] and for increasing pectoralis minor muscle length.[35] When observing the patient from the rear, the clinician may note scapular position and asymmetries. The medial and inferior border of the scapula may be off the rib cage giving the appearance of a "winged scapula." This abnormal resting position will cause scapular dyskinesia during functional upper extremity movements.

The increased tension due to TrPs in the pectoralis minor muscle prevents the patient from reaching fully behind the back at shoulder level and overhead efficiently due to scapular dyskinesia. The anterior depression of the coracoid process and downward rotation of the glenoid fossa that are caused by pectoralis minor muscle tension limits full elevation of the arm at the shoulder girdle. Examination of pectoralis minor muscle length is essential when the patient presents with subacromial impingement syndrome. Borstad[3] established excellent interrater reliability for examining pectoralis minor muscle length using the Pectoralis Minor Index (PMI) which accounts for the patient's anthropometrics. Other investigators have found excellent interrater reliability to determine pectoralis muscle length in patients with subacromial impingement syndrome and healthy controls.[36,37]

When the pectoralis minor and subscapularis muscles are shortened by TrPs, they restrict the combined movement of abduction and external rotation at the shoulder. However, subscapularis TrPs primarily restrict glenohumeral motion, whereas pectoralis minor TrPs restrict scapular mobility on the chest wall. With the arm abducted to 90°, external rotation is restricted markedly by both muscles; however, with the shoulder at 45° elevation,[38] the subscapularis muscle primarily restricts external rotation. Also, when elevation of the shoulder is restricted by pectoralis minor muscle tautness, the patient may be aware of pulling on the ribs or tightness in the anterior chest wall at the limit of elevation.

Accessory joint motion should be tested in the glenohumeral joint, acromioclavicular joint, sternoclavicular joint, scapulothoracic joints, and thoracic rib cage. Oftentimes, joint hypomobility in the sternoclavicular joint or rib cage can cause impairment in shoulder elevation contributing to alterations in the normal muscle activation patterns. Articular dysfunctions in the glenohumeral joint may also impair muscle activation patterns contributing to overload of the pectoralis minor and rotator cuff muscles.

A cervical screen, neurologic signs, and mobility of the neural tissues of the shoulder girdle and upper extremity should be investigated to eliminate neural symptoms as source of the patient's symptoms. If referred hand and/or finger pain is present, a clinical examination of local tissues at the wrist and hand should be also conducted. The Wright's test for hyper-abduction syndrome should also be performed to rule out vascular compromise from a shortened pectoralis minor muscle.[39]

Symptoms from TrPs in the pectoralis minor muscle must be differentiated from scalene TrPs as the pain referral pattern in the anterior chest and upper extremity is very similar. The Finger-flexion test (see Figure 20-6) may be utilized to differentiate scalene from pectoralis minor muscle involvement. If this test is positive, the scalene muscles may be implicated, as TrPs or restrictions in the pectoralis minor muscle will not affect this test.

The patient with chest pain due to pectoralis minor TrPs is likely to suffer additional referred pain and restriction of movement at the shoulder due to associated TrPs in functionally related shoulder girdle muscles which also need to be considered.

3.4. Trigger Point Examination

The pectoralis major muscle should be examined first for active TrPs that might obscure and confuse the localization of TrPs in the underlying pectoralis minor muscle. If the clinician is unsure of the position of the pectoralis minor muscle under the pectoralis major muscle, it can be located by palpation when the patient tenses the pectoralis minor muscle by performing shoulder protraction. To do this, the patient is positioned supine and is instructed to raise the shoulder away from the examining table, while relaxing the arm and carefully avoiding downward pressure against the table with the hand. In the seated position, the patient holds the arm close to the side and a little to the rear to inhibit the pectoralis major muscle, then strongly protracts the shoulder and inhales deeply with the chest. Both maneuvers activate the pectoralis minor muscle so that it can be identified.

In both the supine and seated positions, pectoralis minor TrPs can be localized either by cross-fiber flat palpation through the pectoralis major muscle against the chest wall (Figure 44-4A) or by cross-fiber pincer palpation (Figure 44-4B). With either approach, the pectoralis major muscle is slackened by keeping the patient's arm toward the front of the body and the forearm

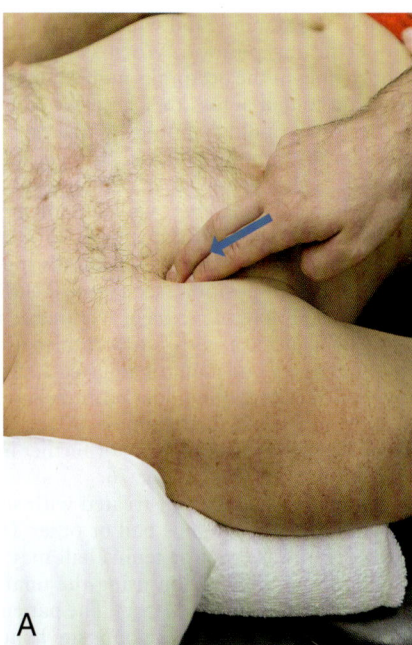
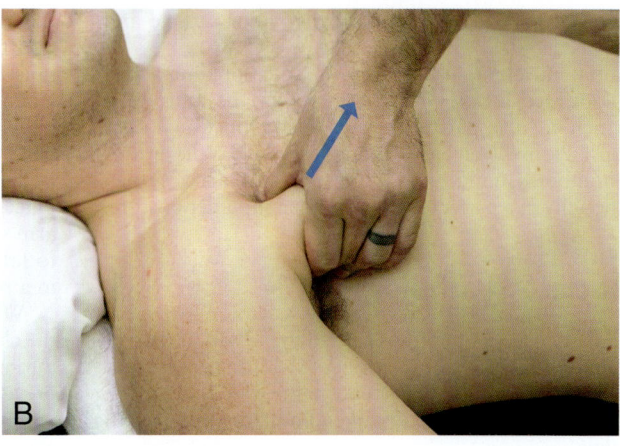

Figure 44-4. Palpation of TrPs in the pectoralis minor muscle. The overlying pectoralis major muscle is slackened by supporting the arm as shown, or by placing the forearm on the abdomen. A, Cross-fiber flat palpation of the pectoralis minor muscle through the pectoralis major muscle. B, Cross-fiber pincer palpation around the pectoralis major muscle. The thumb contacts the pectoralis minor muscle anteriorly and the fingers grasp it through the pectoralis major muscle. Together they can partially separate it from the chest wall. The pectoralis minor muscle may be tautened for better identification of its TrPs by elevating the shoulder.

on the abdomen, and the pectoralis minor muscle may be placed on the desired degree of stretch by adducting the scapula toward the military-brace position. The two pectoral muscles may be distinguished by noting the muscle fiber direction of palpable bands and of local twitch responses.

In the supine position, the pectoralis minor muscle can usually be palpated directly by cross-fiber pincer palpation (Figure 44-4B). The pectoralis major muscle may be further slackened by placing the arm in the position described above, and if additional relief is necessary, the shoulder is protracted by placing a towel roll under it. The clinician places the thumb in the apex of the axilla and slides it against the chest wall beneath the pectoralis major muscle toward the midline, until it encounters the muscle mass of the pectoralis minor muscle. That muscle (and the pectoralis major muscle above it) are then encompassed by a pincer grasp between the thumb and fingers (Figure 44-4B) partially separating it from the chest wall. The fibers of the pectoralis minor muscle can then be palpated directly through the skin for a taut band and hyperirritable spot tenderness. Identification of TrPs in the pectoralis minor muscle may be enhanced by elevating the shoulder cephalad to tauten the pectoralis minor muscle, which increases the sensitivity of its TrPs without tightening the pectoralis major muscle.

4. DIFFERENTIAL DIAGNOSIS

4.1. Activation and Perpetuation of Trigger Points

In any part of the pectoralis minor muscle, TrPs may be activated by unaccustomed eccentric loading, eccentric exercise in unconditioned pectoralis minor muscle, or maximal or submaximal concentric loading.[40] Trigger points may also be activated or aggravated when the muscle is placed in a shortened or lengthened position for an extended period of time.

Pectoralis minor TrPs may be activated due to their presence within the zone of pain induced by myocardial ischemia, by trauma (a gunshot wound through the upper chest, or fracture of upper ribs), by a whiplash type motor vehicle accident,[41] by strain through overuse as a shoulder depressor, by overload as an accessory muscle of inspiration (severe coughing or to assist paradoxical breathing), by poor seated posture, or by prolonged compression of the muscle with a backpack with a tight strap over the front of the shoulder. Habitually slumped posture, rounded shoulder posture, and forward head posture can also activate and perpetuate TrP formation in the pectoralis minor muscle. Repetitive forceful downward motions of the arms (crutch walking), working with arms out in front for a long period of time, heavy lifting, overhead throwing, volleyball, or tennis can overload the pectoralis minor muscle due to its association with scapular stabilization during shoulder internal rotation with the upper extremity in an elevated position. Weakness of the lower trapezius muscle can allow the scapula to anteriorly tilt and lead to adaptive shortening of the pectoralis minor muscle, activating or perpetuating TrPs in the muscle.

4.2. Associated Trigger Points

Associated TrPs can develop in the referred pain areas of TrPs in another muscle.[42] Therefore, musculature in the referred pain areas for each muscle should also be considered.

Trigger points within the pectoralis minor muscle rarely occur without TrPs in the pectoralis major muscle. Therefore, the same muscles that are commonly associated with pectoralis major muscle involvement are likely to have associated TrPs when the pectoralis minor muscle is involved. The anterior deltoid, scalene, and sternocleidomastoid muscles should be examined for the presence of TrPs. The coracobrachialis, biceps brachii, flexor carpi ulnaris, flexor digitorum superficialis and profundus, and abductor digiti minimi muscles are all within the pain referral pattern of the pectoralis minor muscle and should be considered.

In addition, muscles that comprise the functional unit may also have associated TrPs. The teres major and latissimus dorsi muscles, which are also part of the synergistic functional unit, may develop TrPs. Involvement of antagonists such as the levator scapulae, rhomboids, middle and lower trapezius muscles often follows, especially in a patient with a rounded shoulder posture.

4.3. Associated Pathology

Differential diagnosis of symptoms caused by TrPs in the pectoralis minor muscle includes thoracic outlet syndrome, pectoralis minor syndrome, C7 and C8 radicular pain or radiculopathy, supraspinatus tendinopathy, bicipital tendinopathy, and medial epicondylalgia.

Pectoralis minor syndrome is differentiated from thoracic outlet syndrome by the area in which the neurovascular bundle is compressed.[31] Thoracic outlet syndrome often involves compression of the neurovascular bundle above the clavicle in the scalene triangle.[31] Pectoralis minor syndrome involves compression of the subclavian artery, subclavian vein, and brachial plexus below the clavicle within the sub–pectoralis minor muscle space.[30,31] Typical clinical presentation of pectoralis minor syndrome includes tenderness over the pectoralis minor tendon in addition to weakness, pain, paresthesias, and/or temperature changes in the affected upper extremity.[30] Special tests used to diagnose pectoralis minor syndrome and thoracic outlet syndrome include Roos, Adson's, Halsted's, and Wright's hyper-abduction tests (see Chapter 33). These tests should be used in combination with neurodynamic testing, myotomal testing, and dermatomal testing in order to differentiate pectoralis minor syndrome from pectoralis minor TrPs.

Articular dysfunctions likely to be associated with pectoralis minor TrPs includes elevation of the third, fourth, and fifth ribs.

5. CORRECTIVE ACTIONS

The patient with pectoralis minor TrPs should modify activities that repeatedly stress this muscle such as carrying a heavy backpack, weight training (especially bench press), and any other activity that overwork the pectoral muscles. Correction of rounded shoulder posture[21] and maintenance of good dynamic posture are essential for lasting relief of pectoralis minor TrPs. In standing, patients should not be encouraged to actively hold their shoulders back or stand in a "military type posture" as this will aggravate the pectoral and interscapular TrPs. Focusing on the head position and standing tall will allow the shoulders to find their proper resting position. When sleeping, the patient must avoid shortening of the pectoralis minor muscle, as occurs when the arms are folded across the chest. When lying on the back, the corner of the pillow should be tucked between the head and shoulder to drop the shoulder backward, not tucked under the shoulder (see Figure 7-5A). A pillow should also be placed between the axilla and chest wall supporting the upper arm so that the arm is in a neutral position. Allowing the arm to fall behind the body will place the pectoralis minor muscle in a prolonged shortened position (see Figure 22-4B).

When sitting for a prolonged period or working at a computer, the chair should be adjusted so as to support the natural lumbar lordosis and the keyboard and monitor adjusted appropriately to prevent a slouched or rounded shoulder posture. Patients should be discouraged from forcing their shoulders back with muscle action as this will aggravate symptoms. For further information on posture retraining refer to Chapter 76.

Pectoralis minor TrPs can be self-treated with self-pressure release techniques utilizing a tennis ball or other TrP pressure release tools. A TrP release tool or tennis ball may be used in standing, seated, or supine position using the unaffected side to perform the technique (Figure 44-5A). The patient may also perform self-pressure release with the opposite hand as shown in Figure 44-5B. Pressure should be applied to the TrPs, held for 15 to 30 seconds, and repeated six times. This technique can be used several times a day as long as favorable results are being obtained. In women who have large breasts, the supine or side-lying position may be utilized as gravity will aid in moving the breast tissue out of the way. For example, if the right pectoralis minor muscle has TrPs that need treatment, the patient would lie on their left side giving access to the right axillary border for self-treatment with the opposite hand.

Stretching techniques for this muscle should be gentle and started with the upper extremity in the mid or lower position as stretching this muscle will also stretch the other internal rotators of the shoulder joint and neural tissues. Additionally, the in-doorway stretch is useful to stretch all of the adductors and internal rotators at the shoulders. The patient should learn to maintain full pectoral muscle length by using a corner/doorway stretch (see Figure 42-10) or lying on the back on a foam roller with the arms at the side (Figure 44-6A and B). A gentle stretch is held for 30 seconds and can be repeated up to five or six times. Post isometric relaxation can also be used by asking the patient to take a deep abdominal breath, hold for 6 seconds, and slowly breathe out to their toes and relax. In the relaxation phase, the patient is instructed to reach their hands toward their toes gently stretching the pectoralis minor muscle.

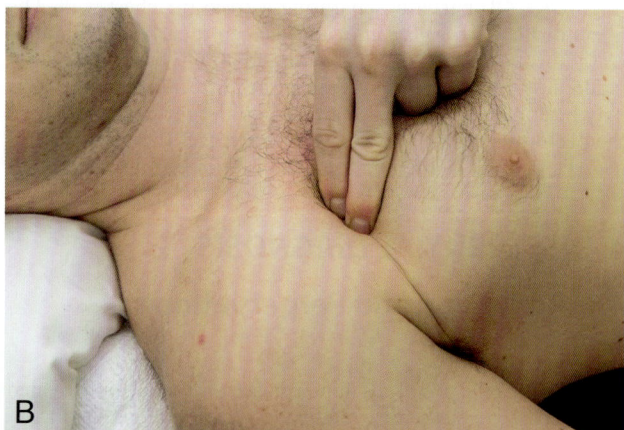

Figure 44-5. Pectoralis minor muscle self-pressure release techniques. A, Using a trigger point release tool in supine. B, Patient self-release using opposite hand.

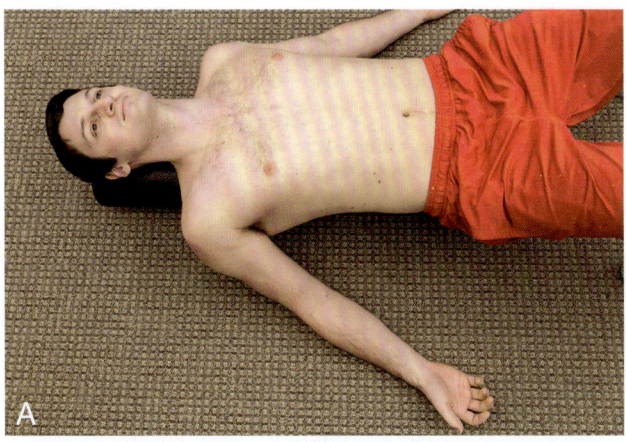 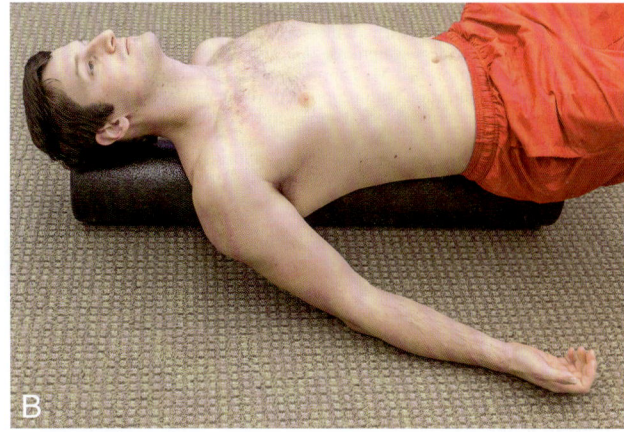

Figure 44-6. Pectoralis minor muscle stretch on bolster. A, Bird's-eye view. B, View from the side.

For full effectiveness with both of these stretch techniques, the patient needs to learn the concept of barrier release. The clinician should instruct the patient to properly stretch the muscle to the point of comfortable tension (without pain), paying attention to any unfamiliar shoulder, chest or interscapular pain, or arm/hand numbness and tingling. If numbness and tingling are felt in the upper arm, forearm, or hands, this exercise should be stopped immediately and the patient should seek guidance from an appropriate health care practitioner.

It is imperative that the clinician and/or patient identifies and limits activities that are leading to overuse of the pectoralis minor muscle. These offending activities may include gardening, working at a desk, ambulation with crutches, and apical breathing patterns.

References

1. Sanchez ER, Sanchez R, Moliver C. Anatomic relationship of the pectoralis major and minor muscles: a cadaveric study. *Aesthet Surg J*. 2014;34(2):258-263.
2. Standring S. *Gray's Anatomy: The Anatomical Basis of Clinical Practice*. 41st ed. London, UK: Elsevier; 2015.
3. Borstad JD. Measurement of pectoralis minor muscle length: validation and clinical application. *J Orthop Sports Phys Ther*. 2008;38(4):169-174.
4. Bardeen C. Section 5. The musculature. In: Jackson CM, ed. *Morris's Human Anatomy*. 6th ed. Philadelphia, PA: Blakiston's Son & Co; 1921:406-407.
5. Lee CB, Choi SJ, Ahn JH, et al. Ectopic insertion of the pectoralis minor tendon: inter-reader agreement and findings in the rotator interval on MRI. *Korean J Radiol*. 2014;15(6):764-770.
6. Weinstabl R, Hertz H, Firbas W. Connection of the ligamentum coracoglenoidale with the muscular pectoralis minor. *Acta Anat (Basel)*. 1986;125(2):126-131.
7. Moineau G, Cikes A, Trojani C, Boileau P. Ectopic insertion of the pectoralis minor: implication in the arthroscopic treatment of shoulder stiffness. *Knee Surg Sports Traumatol Arthrosc*. 2008;16(9):869-871.
8. Sato T, Akatsuka H, Kito K, Tokoro Y, Tauchi H, Kato K. Age changes in size and number of muscle fibers in human minor pectoral muscle. *Mech Ageing Dev*. 1984;28(1):99-109.
9. Petilon J, Ellingson CI, Sekiya JK. Pectoralis major muscle ruptures. *Oper Tech Sports Med*. 2005;13(3):162-168.
10. Haley CA, Zacchilli MA. Pectoralis major injuries: evaluation and treatment. *Clin Sports Med*. 2014;33(4):739-756.
11. Mehta V, Baliyan R, Arora J, Suri RK, Rath G, Kumar A. Unusual innervation pattern of pectoralis minor muscle-anatomical description and clinical implications. *Clin Ter*. 2012;163(6):499-502.
12. Porzionato A, Macchi V, Stecco C, Loukas M, Tubbs RS, De Caro R. Surgical anatomy of the pectoral nerves and the pectoral musculature. *Clin Anat*. 2012;25(5):559-575.
13. Loukas M, du Plessis M, Owens DG, et al. The lateral thoracic artery revisited. *Surg Radiol Anat*. 2014;36(6):543-549.
14. Sucher BM. Thoracic outlet syndrome-postural type: ultrasound imaging of pectoralis minor and brachial plexus abnormalities. *PM R*. 2012;4(1):65-72.
15. Castelein B, Cagnie B, Parlevliet T, Danneels L, Cools A. Optimal normalization tests for muscle activation of the levator scapulae, pectoralis minor, and rhomboid major: an electromyography study using maximum voluntary isometric contractions. *Arch Phys Med Rehabil*. 2015;96(10):1820-1827.
16. Oatis C. *Kinesiology: The Mechanics and Pathomechanics of Human Movement*. 2nd ed. Baltimore, MD: Lippinott, Williams & Wilkins; 2009:164.
17. Porterfield JA, DeRosa C. *Mechanical Shoulder Disorders: Perspectives in Functional Anatomy*. St. Louis, MO: Saunders; 2004:83.
18. Wickham J, Pizzari T, Stansfeld K, Burnside A, Watson L. Quantifying 'normal' shoulder muscle activity during abduction. *J Electromyogr Kinesiol*. 2010;20(2):212-222.
19. Kendall FP, McCreary EK. *Muscles: Testing and Function, with Posture and Pain*. 5th ed. Baltimore, MD: Lippincott Williams & Wilkins; 2005:68.
20. Castelein B, Cagnie B, Parlevliet T, Cools A. Serratus anterior or pectoralis minor: which muscle has the upper hand during protraction exercises? *Man Ther*. 2016;22:158-164.
21. Wong CK, Coleman D, diPersia V, Song J, Wright D. The effects of manual treatment on rounded-shoulder posture, and associated muscle strength. *J Bodyw Mov Ther*. 2010;14(4):326-333.
22. Tate A, Turner GN, Knab SE, Jorgensen C, Strittmatter A, Michener LA. Risk factors associated with shoulder pain and disability across the lifespan of competitive swimmers. *J Athl Train*. 2012;47(2):149-158.
23. Castelein B, Cagnie B, Parlevliet T, Cools A. Scapulothoracic muscle activity during elevation exercises measured with surface and fine wire EMG: a comparative study between patients with subacromial impingement syndrome and healthy controls. *Man Ther*. 2016;23:33-39.
24. Simons DG, Travell J, Simons L. *Travell & Simon's Myofascial Pain and Dysfunction: The Trigger Point Manual*. Vol 1. 2nd ed. Baltimore, MD: Williams & Wilkins; 1999.
25. Travell J, Rinzler SH. The myofascial genesis of pain. *Postgrad Med*. 1952;11(5):425-434.
26. Mendlowitz M. Strain of the pectoralis minor, an important cause of precordial pain in soldiers. *Am Heart J*. 1945;30:123-125.
27. Rinzler SH, Travell J. Therapy directed at the somatic component of cardiac pain. *Am Heart J*. 1948;35(2):248-268.
28. Lawson GE, Hung LY, Ko GD, Laframboise MA. A case of pseudo-angina pectoris from a pectoralis minor trigger point caused by cross-country skiing. *J Chiropr Med*. 2011;10(3):173-178.
29. Bron C, Dommerholt J, Stegenga B, Wensing M, Oostendorp RA. High prevalence of shoulder girdle muscles with myofascial trigger points in patients with shoulder pain. *BMC Musculoskelet Disord*. 2011;12(1):139-151.
30. Sanders RJ, Rao NM. The forgotten pectoralis minor syndrome: 100 operations for pectoralis minor syndrome alone or accompanied by neurogenic thoracic outlet syndrome. *Ann Vasc Surg*. 2010;24(6):701-708.
31. Sanders RJ, Annest SJ. Thoracic outlet and pectoralis minor syndromes. *Semin Vasc Surg*. 2014;27(2):86-117.
32. Vemuri C, Wittenberg AM, Caputo FJ, et al. Early effectiveness of isolated pectoralis minor tenotomy in selected patients with neurogenic thoracic outlet syndrome. *J Vasc Surg*. 2013;57(5):1345-1352.
33. Lee JH, Cynn HS, Yi CH, Kwon OY, Yoon TL. Predictor variables for forward scapular posture including posterior shoulder tightness. *J Bodyw Mov Ther*. 2015;19(2):253-260.
34. Morais N, Cruz J. The pectoralis minor muscle and shoulder movement-related impairments and pain: rationale, assessment and management. *Phys Ther Sport*. 2016;17:1-13.
35. Lee JH, Cynn HS, Yoon TL, et al. The effect of scapular posterior tilt exercise, pectoralis minor stretching, and shoulder brace on scapular alignment and muscles activity in subjects with round-shoulder posture. *J Electromyogr Kinesiol*. 2015;25(1):107-114.
36. Lewis JS, Valentine RE. The pectoralis minor length test: a study of the intra-rater reliability and diagnostic accuracy in subjects with and without shoulder symptoms. *BMC Musculoskelet Disord*. 2007;8:64.

37. Struyf F, Meeus M, Fransen E, et al. Interrater and intrarater reliability of the pectoralis minor muscle length measurement in subjects with and without shoulder impingement symptoms. *Man Ther*. 2014;19(4):294-298.
38. Godges JJ, Mattson-Bell M, Thorpe D, Shah D. The immediate effects of soft tissue mobilization with proprioceptive neuromuscular facilitation on glenohumeral external rotation and overhead reach. *J Orthop Sports Phys Ther*. 2003;33(12):713-718.
39. Beyer JA. The hyperabduction syndrome, with special reference to its relationship to Raynaud's syndrome. *Circulation*. 1951;4(2):161-172.
40. Gerwin RD, Dommerholt J, Shah JP. An expansion of Simons' integrated hypothesis of trigger point formation. *Curr Pain Headache Rep*. 2004;8(6):468-475.
41. Hong C-Z, Simons DG. Response to treatment for pectoralis minor myofascial pain syndrome after whiplash. *J Musculoskelet Pain*. 1993;1(1):89-131.
42. Hsieh YL, Kao MJ, Kuan TS, Chen SM, Chen JT, Hong CZ. Dry needling to a key myofascial trigger point may reduce the irritability of satellite MTrPs. *Am J Phys Med Rehabil*. 2007;86(5):397-403.

Chapter 45

Intercostal and Diaphragm Muscles
"Stich in the Side"

Joseph M. Donnelly

1. INTRODUCTION

The external and internal intercostal muscles are located between the ribs in a crisscross pattern. The dome-shaped diaphragm muscle has a unique central tendon and separates the thoracic and abdominal cavities. Its central tendon is surrounded by muscle fibers that attach to the inferior thoracic outlet peripherally. The intercostal muscles function in both postural and respiratory roles. The intercostal muscles are mechanically suited for active rotation and side-bending of the thoracic spine and rib cage. The function of the diaphragm muscle is inhalation. During quiet inhalation, the diaphragm, scalene, and parasternal intercostal muscles are active. Exhalation mainly occurs passively by the recoil of the lungs. The abdominal muscles are active during forced expiration. Pain from trigger points (TrPs) in the intercostal muscles primarily refers locally in the region of the TrP. Pain from TrPs in the diaphragm muscle refers to the upper border of the ipsilateral shoulder at the angle of the neck and to the anterolateral costal margin. Symptoms associated with TrPs in the intercostal muscles are pain and limited range of motion (ROM) when rotating to look behind and chest pain that increases with deep respiration, especially when coughing or sneezing. Shortness of breath may be associated with diaphragm TrPs. Patient examination should include a thorough assessment of posture, cervical, and thoracic spine ROM, and respiratory mechanics. Accessory motion testing of the cervical spine, especially C3-C5, thoracic spine and rib cage, and shoulder girdle joints, should be carried out. Trigger point examination for intercostal muscles should start with the painful segment looking for narrowed rib space and continue along the full segment looking for spot tenderness. Diaphragm TrPs are not palpable and can be difficult to differentiate from transverse abdominis muscle tenderness along the costal margin. Differential diagnosis should include rib articular dysfunctions, costochondritis, myocardial infarction, and pleural effusion. Corrective actions to prevent perpetuation and/or recurrence of intercostal or diaphragm TrPs should include postural education, instruction in diaphragmatic breathing, self-pressure release, and self-stretching.

2. ANATOMIC CONSIDERATIONS

Intercostals

The external and internal intercostal muscles have a crisscross arrangement, crossing each other at nearly a right angle, similar to the external and internal abdominal oblique muscles (see Chapter 49), and in the same directions. Each muscle spans the distance between two ribs (or costal cartilages). The external intercostal muscles are considerably thicker than the internal intercostal muscles. The vessels and nerves supplying these muscles run deep to the internal intercostal muscles and are protected by a slight overhang of the inferior margin of the more cephalad rib. The innermost intercostal muscles, which used to be considered variant subcostal muscles, are located deep to the vessels and nerve and have a fiber direction nearly the same as the corresponding internal intercostal muscles.[1]

External Intercostals

The 11 external intercostal muscles on each side do not extend quite the full length of each intercostal space, reaching only to the costal cartilage anteriorly, except between the lowest ribs (Figure 45-1). They do reach the end of the rib posteriorly at the tubercle (Figure 45-2) where they blend with the fibers of the superior costotransverse ligament. Anteriorly, the external intercostal muscles have only a fascial extension, the external intercostal membrane, that reaches to the sternum.[2] The external fibers are angled obliquely inferomedially as seen from in front (Figure 45-1) and obliquely inferolaterally as seen from behind (Figure 45-2). Each muscle attaches from the lower border of the rib above and to the upper border of the rib below.[2] Fibers from the lower ribs may blend with the external abdominal oblique muscle.[3] Figure 49-2 provides a convenient way of remembering the direction of each muscle.

Levatores Costarum

The 12 posterior, extrathoracic levatores costarum muscles can be considered an extrathoracic nonintercostal version of the external intercostal muscles (Figure 45-2 left side). They attach above to the tips of the transverse processes from C7 through T11 and attach below and more laterally to the adjacent rib (levator costae brevis muscle) between the rib's tubercle and its angle, or in the lower four ribs the muscle has two slips that span to the adjacent lower rib or to the second rib below its origin (levator costae longus muscle).[2]

Each muscle attaches above from the costal groove of the cephalad rib and inserts to the superior border of the rib below.[2] The internal intercostal fiber direction is the reverse of the direction of the external intercostal fibers; the internal intercostal fibers are angled obliquely inferolaterally in the front of the chest (Figures 45-1, 45-3 and 45-8). Since the muscle has the same fiber direction as it continues around the chest, the fibers appear to be angled obliquely inferomedially when viewed in the back of the chest (Figure 45-3).

Innermost Intercostals

The innermost intercostal muscles lie between the intercostal nerves and vessels and the endothoracic fascia and parietal pleura. When present, they run tandem with the inner intercostal muscles. They are often unsubstantiated in the highest levels of the thoracic spine and generally thicken into existence inferiorly. They may interdigitate with the neighboring subcostales muscles posteriorly.[1]

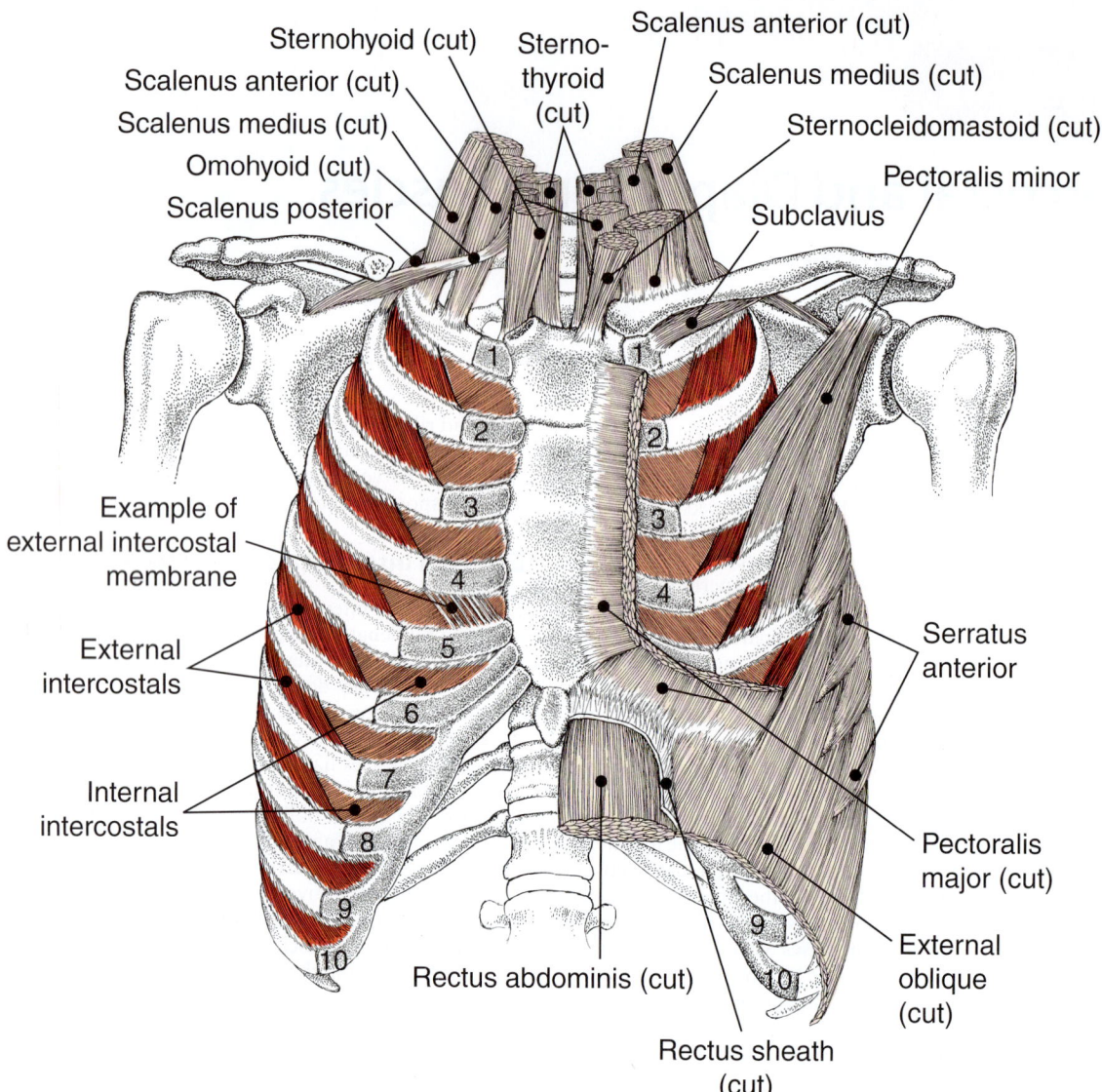

Figure 45-1. Exterior of anterior thoracic wall, showing the anatomic relations and attachments of intercostal and related respiratory muscles. The external intercostal muscles are darkest red, the internal intercostal muscles are intermediate red. The external intercostal muscles do not extend beyond the costochondral junctions medially, except between the lowest ribs. Other muscles are light red. All but the omohyoid muscle attach to the thoracic cage and could directly influence respiration.

Subcostales

The subcostales muscle can be considered a variation of the internal intercostal muscles. The subcostales muscle spans from the upper ribs internal surface near the rib angle and descends to attach to the second or third rib below. It has the same fiber direction as the internal intercostals and is most fully developed in the lower part of the thorax.[2] The subcostales muscle very likely functions in concert with the internal intercostal muscles of the lower thorax.

Transverse Thoracis

The transversus thoracis muscle is an interior, anterior chest muscle that covers the internal surface of the anterior thoracic wall and is not intercostal (Figure 45-4).[2] It lies deep to the sternum and the parasternal intercostal muscles and is composed of tendinous and muscular fibers that attach in a fan-like arrangement. The upper digitations of the muscle reach from the inner surface of the lower sternum and xiphoid process upward (craniad) to the costal cartilages of the second to sixth ribs in a vertical arrangement. The intermediate fibers have an oblique arrangement, and the lowest fibers are essentially horizontal and blend with the fibers of the transversus abdominis muscle. The transverse thoracis muscle varies in its attachments side to side in the same individual and is variable between individuals.[2]

Diaphragm

The diaphragm muscle is a dome-shaped musculofibrous structure that separates the thoracic and abdominal cavities (Figures 45-4 and 45-5).[4] The dome of the diaphragm muscle has a central tendon which is a strong aponeurosis situated near the center of the muscle. Centrally, it lies immediately inferior to and is blended with fibers of the pericardium.[2] It is surrounded by muscle fibers that form an extended "skirt" that attaches peripherally to the circumference of the inferior thoracic outlet. The muscle is divided into a sternal portion that attaches anteriorly to the sternum, a costal portion that attaches laterally to the costal margin, and a lumbar portion that attaches posteriorly by the paired medial and lateral arcuate ligaments. The sternal portion arises from the posterior aspect of the xiphoid process. The costal portion arises from the internal

Chapter 45: Intercostal and Diaphragm Muscles

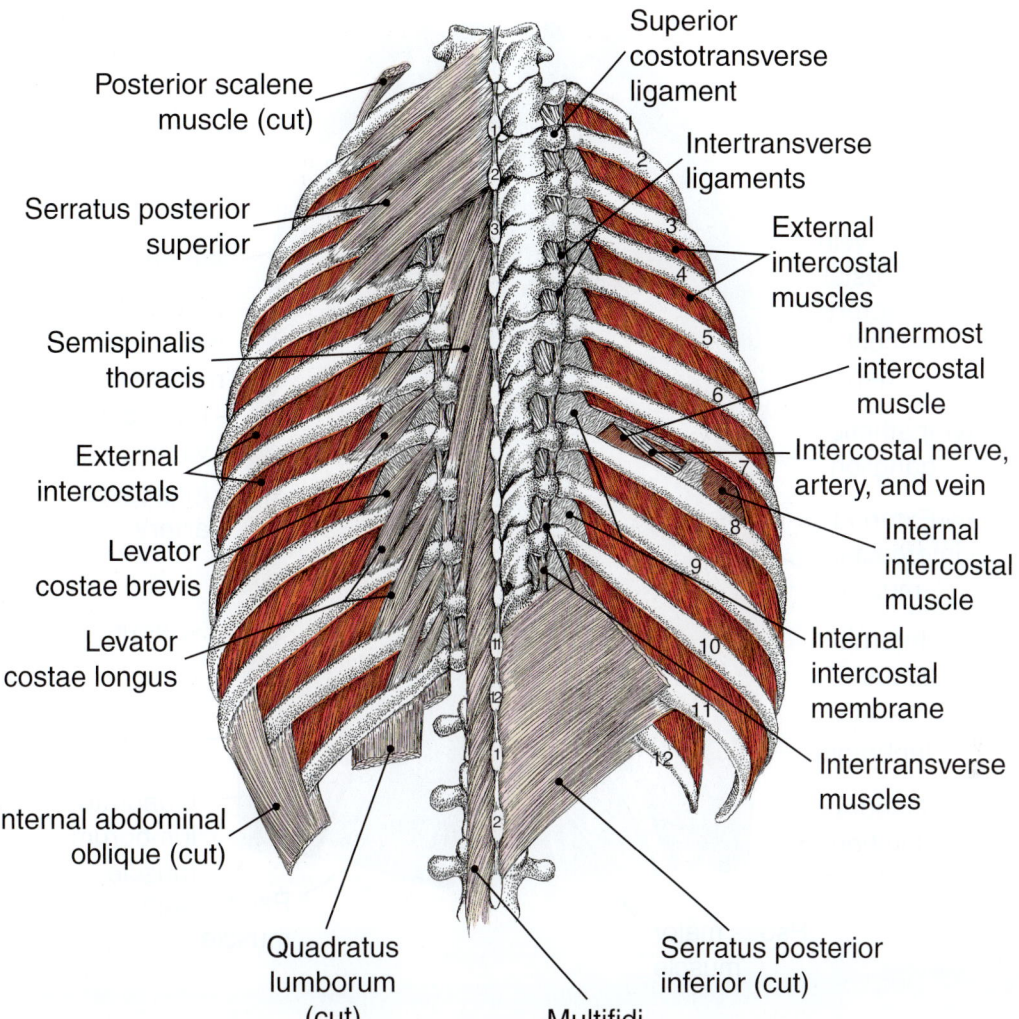

Figure 45-2. Exterior of posterior thoracic wall, showing anatomic relations and attachments of intercostal and related respiratory muscles. The external intercostal muscles are dark red, the internal intercostal muscles are intermediate red. Other muscles are light red. The posterior scalene (cut), external intercostal, and the levatores costarum muscles (levator costae longus and brevis) are primary muscles for inhalation that appear in this figure. The serratus posterior superior muscles help to elevate the ribs during forced inhalation. The serratus posterior inferior (cut), quadratus lumborum (cut), and internal abdominal oblique (cut) muscles shown here may assist exhalation. The detailed drawing between ribs 7 and 8 on the right side shows that the internal intercostal muscles are absent medial to the region of the angle of the ribs but are represented medially as the internal intercostal membrane. The neurovascular bundle runs between the internal intercostal muscle or membrane, which lies superficial to it, and the innermost intercostal muscle or membrane which lies deep to it. The internal intercostal and innermost intercostal muscles have an almost identical fiber direction and are usually referred to collectively as the internal intercostal muscles. The intercostal neurovascular bundle actually lies deep to the lower border of the cephalad rib and might not be visible from this view.

surfaces of the costal cartilages and internal surfaces of the lower six ribs which also interdigitates with the transverse abdominis muscle. The lumbar portion arises from two aponeurotic arches, the medial and lateral arcuate ligaments.[2] The medial arcuate ligament extends over the upper portion of the psoas major muscles as fibrous attachments between the L1 or L2 vertebral body and the transverse process of L1. The lateral arcuate ligaments are thickened fascial bands covering the quadratus lumborum muscle and extend from the transverse processes of the first lumbar vertebrae laterally to the midportion of the 12th ribs and by two muscular crura to the bodies of the upper lumbar vertebrae. The lumbar portion also attaches to two bilateral arcuate ligaments which span from the vertebrae to the transverse processes and from those processes to the 12th rib (Figure 45-5).[2]

The diaphragm muscle is penetrated by the aorta, vena cava, and esophagus. The arcuate ligaments provide passage posteriorly for the psoas major and quadratus lumborum muscles (Figures 45-3 and 45-5).

2.1. Innervation and Vascularization

Intercostals

Each intercostal muscle is supplied by adjacent branches of the corresponding intercostal nerve.[2]

The muscles of the thoracic wall receive their vascularization from the internal thoracic artery via the musculophrenic artery, the superior intercostal artery, posterior intercostal artery, subcostal and superior thoracic arteries, and the descending aorta. Additional vascular supply is provided by the vessels that supply the upper limb.[2]

Diaphragm

The diaphragm muscle receives motor innervation from the right and left phrenic nerves, which originate from cervical nerves C3-C5 and facilitate both sensory and motor function. The paired phrenic nerves are located posteriorly in the lateral

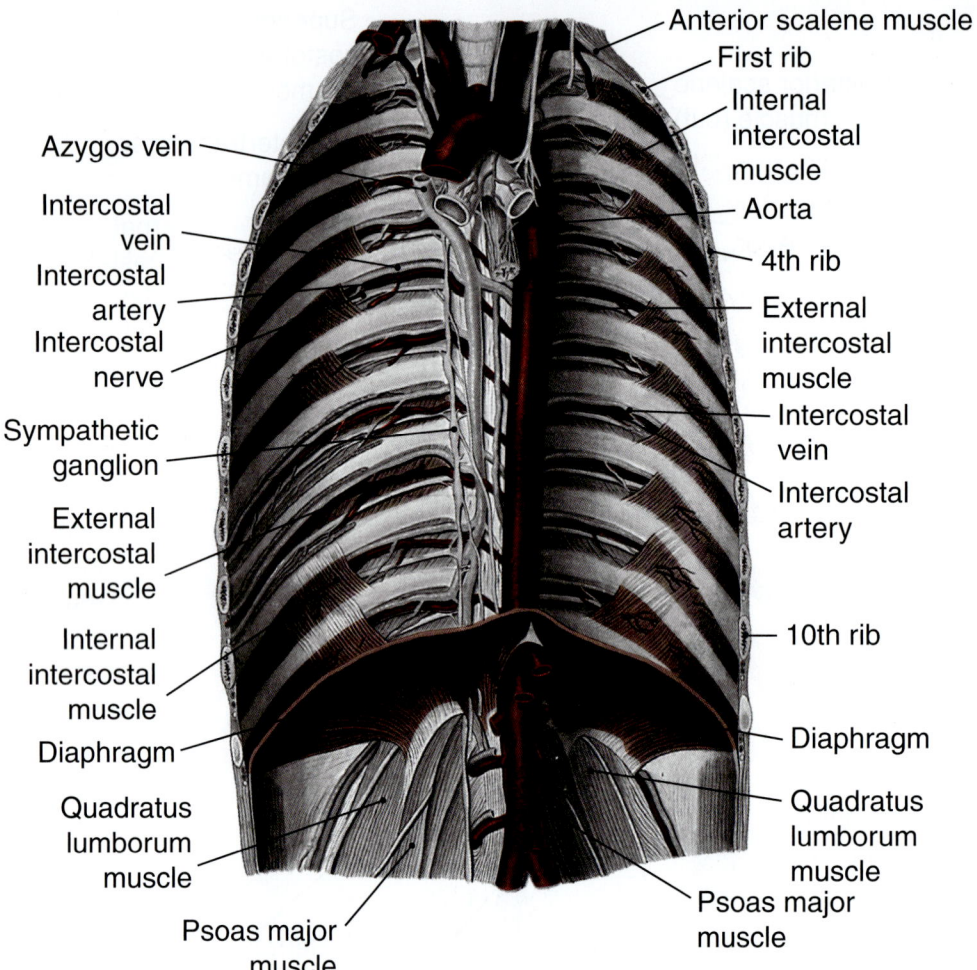

Figure 45-3. Interior of the posterior chest wall showing anatomic relations and attachments of the intercostal muscles and also major blood vessels. The internal intercostal muscles are intermediate red. The diaphragm and external intercostal muscles are dark red, and the arteries are darkest red. Other muscles are light red. Reproduced and adapted with permission from Ferner H, Staubesand J. *Sobotta Atlas of Human Anatomy.* Vol. 2. Munich: Urban & Schwarzenberg; 1983.

compartment of the neck and travel anteriorly as they course through the thorax. The phrenic nerves run along the anterior surface of the pericardium before they reach the diaphragm muscle, where they arborize on the superior and inferior surfaces. Sensory innervation to the peripheral part of the muscle is through the lower six to seven intercostal nerves.[2,4]

The diaphragm muscle receives its vascularization from the subcostal and lower five intercostal arteries, the superior and inferior phrenic arteries, the musculophrenic and pericardiacophrenic arteries. The major vascular supply to the diaphragm muscle is provided by the right and left inferior phrenic arteries.[2]

2.2. Function

Recent studies have helped clarify much of the controversy associated with the activity and role of several respiratory muscles, including the intercostal and diaphragm muscles. To understand their function, it is helpful to understand basic respiratory mechanics. Inhalation is an active process requiring muscular effort. Exhalation during quiet breathing is largely a passive process performed by the elastic recoil of the lungs.[5] In that sense, all expiratory muscles are to some degree accessory muscles of respiration recruited with increased respiratory demand.

Intercostals

The function of the intercostal muscles depends on their internal–external position, on their anteroposterior position, and on their transverse location on the rib cage. In addition, the muscle's superior–inferior position on the rib cage affects the relative order and magnitude of recruitment. The only portion of the intercostal muscles associated with primary inspiration are the parasternal portion of the internal intercostal muscles. It is believed that both the internal and external intercostal muscles are active during both phases of ventilation.[6]

It is of fundamental importance that the lateral portion of intercostal muscles are tailor-made for rotating the thoracic spine and rib cage, a function that is frequently overlooked. During right trunk rotation, the left external intercostal muscles and the right internal intercostal muscles are activated to perform this motion.[6]

Diaphragm

The diaphragm muscle is the primary muscle of ventilation during quiet breathing and responsible for producing up to 80% of the inspirational force.[7] It also aids in emesis, urination, and defecation by increasing intra-abdominal pressure and helps prevent gastroesophageal reflux by exerting external pressure at the esophageal hiatus.

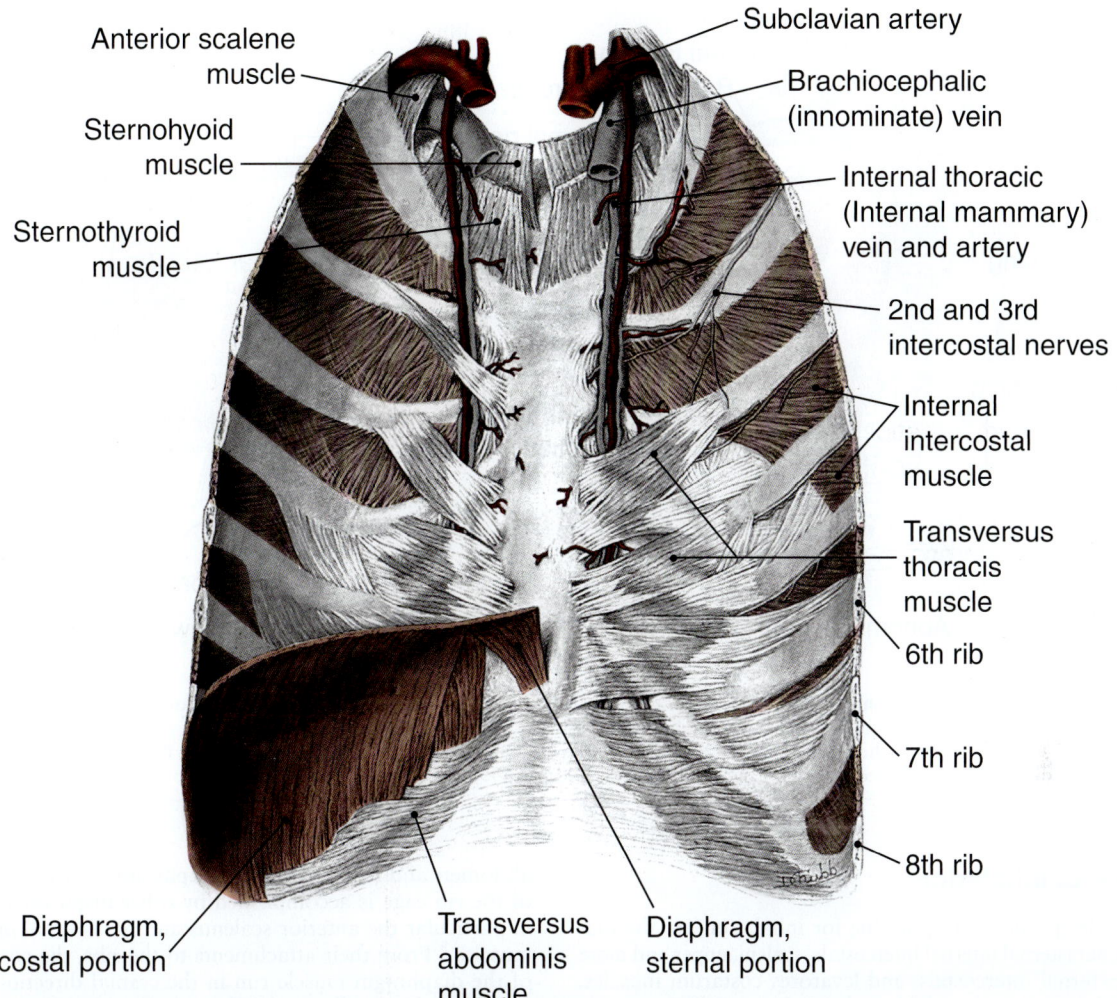

Figure 45-4. Interior of the anterior thoracic wall. The subclavian and internal thoracic arteries are darkest red, the diaphragm muscle (shown in part and only on the left side) is dark red, the internal intercostal muscles are intermediate red, and the remaining muscles are light red. Note that, generally, only the internal intercostal muscles continue anteriorly and as far medially as the sternum (completing coverage of the anterior costal interspaces). The external intercostal muscles (not seen in this view) stop short at the costochondral junctions. The diaphragm muscle is a primary muscle for inhalation. Note how it extends downward to lie against the lowest rib. Reproduced and adapted with permission from Agur AM. *Grant's Atlas of Anatomy*. 9th ed. Baltimore, MD: Williams & Wilkins; 1991.

Respiratory Mechanics

Movement of the chest wall during inhalation is a complex integrated process that requires sophisticated coordination of numerous muscles. Lung volume is controlled by three basic movements. Figure 45-6 illustrates two of the movements: (1) elevation of the sternum (Figure 45-6A) that increases the anteroposterior diameter by rotating the ribs around the spinal attachments, and (2) spreading of the lower ribs (Figure 45-6B) that increases the lateral diameter of the thorax by rotating the ribs around their sternal attachments.[8] The downward piston-like motion of the diaphragm muscle provides the third movement (Figure 45-7). The sternal elevation movement is often compared to that of an old-fashioned pump handle, and the lateral rib movement to that of a bucket handle (one on each side).

The axis of rotation of a rib is defined by its articulations with the vertebral body and the transverse process. Since most ribs are inclined obliquely approximately 45° to the horizontal, when the rib rotates upward it increases the volume within the rib cage, which is associated with inhalation. The upper ribs that attach to the sternum with short costal cartilages tend to move in unison, whereas the lower ribs that are attached with longer costal cartilages have more freedom to move independent of sternal motion.[9]

The pump-handle movement of inhalation that elevates the sternum (and produces predominantly anteroposterior expansion) depends primarily on the intercostal muscles located at the sides of the thorax for which these muscles are mechanically well-situated.[8] The intercostal muscles suited to raising the bucket handles on each side of the chest (expanding the transverse diameter of the rib cage) are located nearly midline close to the sternum and the spine, especially the parasternally located internal intercostal muscles and the paraspinally located levatores costarum muscles. These relationships were identified by calculations using three dimensional finite element analysis of the human rib cage[8] and were confirmed experimentally in dogs.[10]

The depression of the diaphragm muscle, by its activity during inhalation and its passive elevation during exhalation, is illustrated in the sagittal sections in Figure 45-7. The corresponding effect on lung volume is shown in the frontal sections in Figure 45-7. Contraction of the diaphragm muscle tends to elevate and spread the lower costal margin and lower ribs when support and resistance are supplied to the central tendon by the abdominal contents.[11] The muscles largely responsible for these movements are illustrated in Figure 45-8 in greatly simplified form with arrows that indicate the force vector produced by contraction of the muscle.

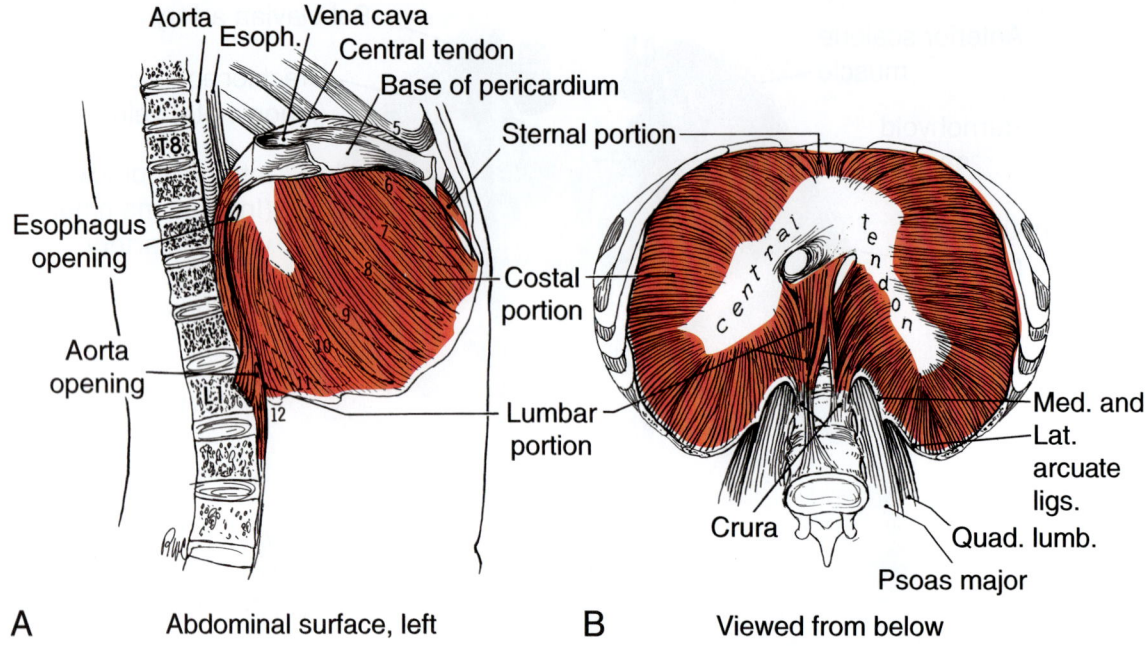

Figure 45-5. Caudal (abdominal) surface of diaphragm muscle (red), which is the most important muscle for inhalation. A, Internal aspect of left hemidiaphragm as seen from the right side of body. B, Diaphragm muscle viewed from below, showing its attachment to the caudal margins of the thoracic cage. Reproduced with permission from Kendall FP, McCreary EK, Provance PG. *Muscles: Testing and Function.* 4th ed. Baltimore, MD: Williams & Wilkins; 1993.

Muscles of Inhalation

The muscles primarily responsible for inhalation are the diaphragm, parasternal internal intercostals, scaleni, upper and more lateral external intercostals, and levatores costarum muscles. The diaphragm muscle, which is the main respiratory muscle in humans, does not expand the entire chest wall but just the abdomen and lower rib cage. Expansion of the cranial half of the rib cage is accomplished by other inspiratory muscles, in particular the anterior scalenus and parasternal intercostal muscles.[9] From their attachments to the ribs, the costal fibers of the diaphragm muscle run in the cranial direction next to the ribs for some distance.[9] This relationship is important because contraction of these fibers elevates the lower ribs when

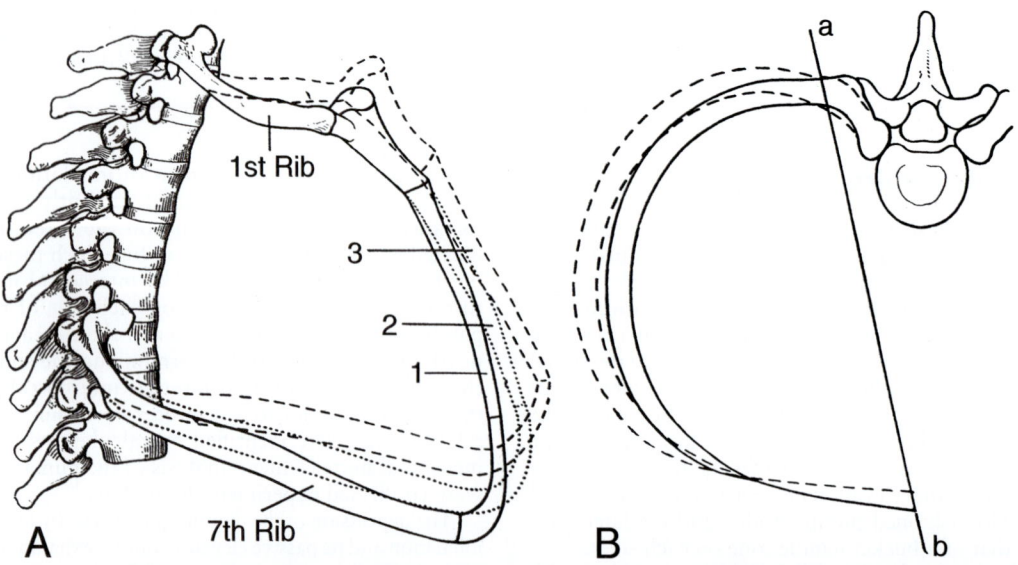

Figure 45-6. Change of sternum and rib positions with inhalation. A, Lateral view of the chest showing the upward and outward (forward) movement of the anterior rib cage during inhalation, which increases intrathoracic volume. This can be compared to a "pump-handle" movement. Position 1, ordinary exhalation; position 2 (dotted lines), quiet inhalation; position 3 (dashed lines) deep inhalation. B, View from above showing how, for ribs attaching to the costal cartilages below the sternum (vertebrochondral ribs), the movement is upward and lateral, which increases intrathoracic volume. The dashed lines represent the position of the rib during inhalation. The line labeled a-b represents the axis of movement. This upward and lateral rib movement can be compared on each side to the movement of a bucket handle. Reprinted with permission from Clemente CD. *Gray's Anatomy.* 30th ed. Philadelphia, PA: Lea & Febiger; 1985.

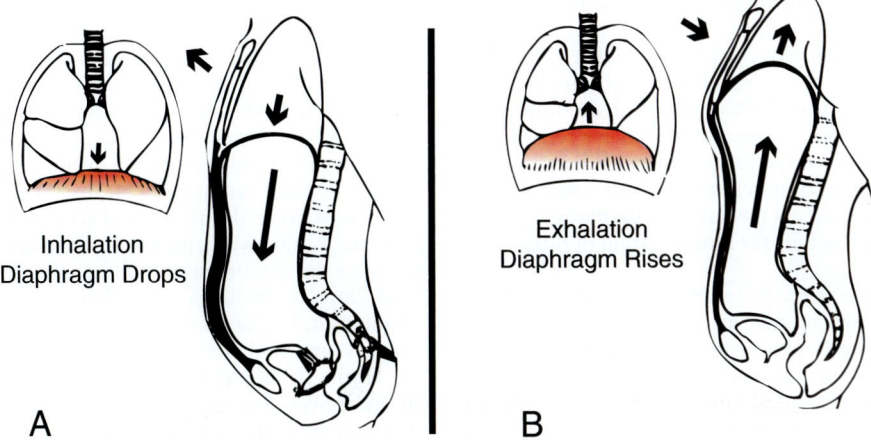

Figure 45-7. Schematic of respiration dynamics. A, Inhalation. The sagittal section (right figure of A) shows how the combination of depression (contraction) of the diaphragm muscle (long down arrow) that is displacing the abdominal contents downward and simultaneous expansion of the thoracic cage (diagonal up arrow) reduce intrathoracic pressure. This sucks air into the lungs (short down arrow), inflating them. The frontal section (left figure in A) shows the depressed diaphragm muscle and inflated lungs. B, Exhalation. The sagittal section (right figure in B) shows how depression of the thoracic cage (diagonal down arrow) and elevation (relaxation) of the diaphragm muscle (long up arrow) tend to increase intrathoracic pressure. During quiet respiration the elastic recoil of the lungs and chest forces air out of the lungs (short up arrow), deflating them. The frontal section (left figure) shows the elevated diaphragm muscle and deflated lungs. In forced exhalation, the abdominal muscles displace the abdominal contents inward and upward and pull the thoracic cage downward and inward, accelerating airflow out of the lungs.

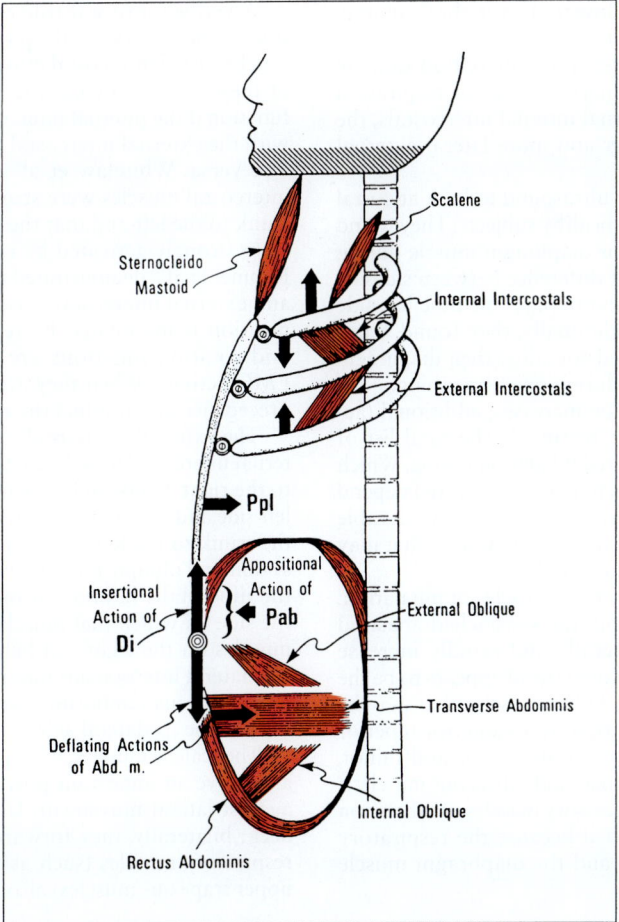

Figure 45-8. Schematic of respiratory mechanics illustrating some of the most important respiratory muscles and their actions (thick black arrows). Abd. m., abdominal muscles; Di, diaphragm muscle; Pab, abdominal pressure; Ppl, pleural pressure. Reprinted with permission from Roussos C. Function and fatigue of the respiratory muscle. *Chest*. 1985;88(suppl):124s-132s.

depression of the dome of the diaphragm muscle is resisted by the abdominal contents.[9,12]

During quiet inhalation, electrical activity of the diaphragm muscle precedes that of the external intercostal muscles[13]; the diaphragm muscle produces 70% to 80% of the inhalation force.[5] This is why paradoxical breathing is such a serious dysfunction. Hyperinflation of the lungs due to obstructive lung disease puts the diaphragm muscle at a serious disadvantage, and under some circumstances the flattened diaphragm muscle can reverse its effect by pulling the costal margin in rather than lifting it up and out.[10]

During quiet breathing, the first external intercostal muscles (between the first and second ribs) are always active, the second pair of muscles are usually active, and the third, only occasionally. With increasingly more forced respiration, successively more caudal external intercostal muscles are recruited during inhalation.[13]

The anterior scalene muscles are always active in quiet inhalation (Figure 45-8) and are likely to activate shortly before the parasternal internal intercostal muscles.[13] The activity of the scalene muscles is needed during inhalation to prevent the downward suction produced by the piston action of the diaphragm muscle from pulling the sternum down and in. A downward motion of the sternum tends to reduce intrathoracic volume rather than increase it. The scalene muscles respond increasingly vigorously to increasing respiratory effort.[13]

The posteriorly located levatores costarum muscles (Figure 45-2), which also show some activity in quiet respiration,[13] become increasingly active with increasing ventilatory demand.[10] They are anchored proximally to the vertebral column, not to another rib. They elevate the rib cage with effective leverage. A small upward movement of the ribs, so close to the vertebral column, is greatly magnified at the sternum.

The diaphragm muscle initiates quiet inhalation quickly followed by activity of other primary muscles of respiration including the scalene, the parasternal internal intercostals, the levatores costarum, and the upper and more lateral external intercostal muscles.

Harper et al,[14] utilized B-mode ultrasound to look at costal diaphragm muscle function in 150 healthy subjects. They found that most of the subjects used their diaphragm muscle during quiet breathing with no significant difference between sides or across age ranges. They did find that in older men the left side thickens more than the right. Additionally, they found a fair number of individuals who either did not utilize their diaphragm muscle at all or did so minimally during quiet breathing.

As the vigor of forced respiration increases, additional (accessory) muscles of inhalation are recruited. The total list of muscles that can contribute to labored inhalation is long. Which muscles are activated and how much they are activated depend strongly on the circumstances. Therefore, there is considerable diversity of opinion as to the relative roles of muscles that may serve as accessory muscles of respiration.[15]

The scalene muscles serve as primary muscles of inhalation. With increased ventilatory demand, the sternocleidomastoid muscles also become active bilaterally and rapidly increase their level of activity. The sternocleidomastoid appears to be the most important accessory muscle. Other muscles that may be recruited include the upper trapezius, serratus anterior superior and serratus posterior superior, pectoralis major and minor, latissimus dorsi, thoracic erector spinae, and subclavius muscles.[7]

With paradoxical respiration, accessory muscles of inhalation must carry a major part of the load because the respiratory effects of the intercostal muscles and the diaphragm muscle largely cancel each other's efforts.

Muscles of Exhalation

During quiet respiration, exhalation is largely a passive process dependent on the elasticity of the lungs. The muscles primarily responsible for exhalation during periods of increased demand are the abdominal, interosseous internal intercostal, transversus thoracis, and subcostal muscles. The lowest (11th) intercostal pair is most important for exhalation, and an electromyogram (EMG) study showed that as intercostal activity developed during forced exhalation, recruitment progressed upward from the 11th pair of muscles. Electrical activity of the transversus thoracis muscle appeared only during exhalation.[13]

When functioning as expiratory muscles, the abdominal muscles squeeze the abdominal contents upward and pull the chest cage downward, increasing intra-abdominal pressure that elevates the diaphragm muscle, accelerates expiratory airflow, and empties the lungs more than would occur with passive expiration. In this way, these muscles regulate end-expiratory lung volume and breathing efficiency.[16]

During forced exhalation, the abdominal muscles are the prime movers assisted by the internal intercostal muscles (with the exception of the parasternal internal intercostal muscles, which support inhalation). With increased ventilatory demand, the latissimus dorsi, quadratus lumborum, and erector spinae muscles may also be recruited.[3]

Postural Functions

Experimental evidence[17] supports the view that intercostal muscles, particularly the laterally located external intercostal muscles in the more cephalic spaces, are mainly involved in postural functions. The opposite appears to be the case for the intercartilaginous muscles (located anteriorly) and the levatores costarum muscles (located posteriorly), which in all circumstances, exhibit phasic inspiratory activity quite similar to the diaphragm muscle.[17]

A verified postural role of the intercostal muscles is rotation of the thorax.[6,18] Respiration is executed with bilaterally synchronized intercostal muscle activity. The crisscross pattern of these muscles makes them admirably suited to a rotation function if the internal intercostal muscles on one side contract with the external intercostal muscles on the opposite side and vice versa. Whitelaw et al[6] reported that the right external intercostal muscles were strongly activated by rotation of the trunk to the left and that the right internal intercostal muscles were strongly activated by rotation of the trunk to the right. Rimmer et al[18] demonstrated that the tonic discharge of internal and external intercostal muscles induced by holding a rotated position is modulated by respiration. When the respiration and rotation functions are compatible, they reinforce the EMG activity. When they are incompatible, respiration takes precedence and inhibits the rotation function.[18]

The external intercostal muscles on the left side and the internal intercostal muscles on the right side both rotate the trunk to the right. Conversely, the internal intercostal muscles on the left side and external intercostal muscles on the right side rotate the trunk to the left. The corresponding internal and external abdominal oblique muscles would augment these rotations and the iliocostalis lumborum muscle augments rotation toward the side on which that muscle lies. The multifidi and rotatores muscles on the right can help to rotate the trunk to the left. The lateral interosseous intercostal, the lateral abdominal, and the quadratus lumborum muscles help to side bend the trunk toward the ipsilateral side.

The scalene muscles, which are primary players in respiration, also serve an important postural role. They stabilize the neck against lateral movement. Unilaterally, they laterally flex the neck; bilaterally, they forward flex the neck. Other accessory respiratory muscles (such as the sternocleidomastoid and the upper trapezius muscles) also flex the neck and rotate the head.

Special Functions

Many complex special functions including coughing, sneezing, vomiting, gasping, running, and speech depend on the muscles of the trunk.

Both coughing and sneezing are protective reflexes that defend the airways against inhaled particles and noxious substances and remove mucus by inducing high airflow velocities during forced exhalation. A cough has three phases: inhalation, compression, and expulsion. Following reflex inhalation, the brief compressive phase involves continued activity of the diaphragm muscle and activation of ribcage and abdominal expiratory muscles against a closed glottis. The expulsive phase begins with opening of the glottis as relaxation of the diaphragm muscle and vigorous reflex expiratory muscle activity produce high airflow velocities.[19] Repeated coughing can induce enthesopathy in the attachments of, and activate and perpetuate TrPs in, the expiratory muscles (especially the abdominal muscles). A coughing spell can become excruciatingly painful for this reason.

The neurogenesis for sneezing is somewhat different than for coughing. During this reflex, there are often intermittent pauses during the inspiratory effort, and expired air is diverted through the nose in addition to the mouth.[19] Since a prolonged series of sneezes is much less likely to occur than a protracted period of coughing, sneezing is less likely to produce muscular distress.

The inhalations and exhalations of gasping, which are induced by severe hypoxia (or during panic attacks), are more sudden in beginning and ending compared to the rhythmic respirations of eupnea (normal breathing). This unique pattern of autonomic ventilatory activity differs fundamentally from eupnea because the neurogenesis of gasping depends on a specific region of the medulla.[20]

Another reflex respiratory activity, vomiting, involves violent contraction of expiratory muscles. Vomiting can be induced by reverse peristalsis of the duodenum, by motion sickness, pregnancy, or other systemic causes. It is such a primitive reflex that it is preserved in decerebrate animal preparations and is produced by the thoracoabdominal respiratory muscles. Expulsion of the gastric bolus by vomiting is usually preceded by retching, which involves successive waves of reflex cocontraction of the diaphragm and abdominal muscles that override the respiratory cycle. Recurrent attacks of retching are feared by clinicians and patients because of the severe fatigue they can induce in respiratory muscles, and attacks have occasionally led to rib fractures.[21] Again, this muscle overload can produce severely painful enthesopathy and can activate TrPs that persist after an attack.

Most conditioned runners show a tight locomotor-respiratory coupling which is established during the first four or five strides of the run. The ratio is usually two strides to one respiratory cycle. Inexperienced runners show little or no tendency for such coupling.[22] During prolonged maximal exercise, the blood flow requirements of respiratory muscles are comparable to those of propulsive limb muscles.[23]

Mantilla and Sieck 2013 found changes in diaphragm muscle structure and function in various disease and clinical conditions, which affected more fatigable, but less frequently activated, motor units that are not required for vital ventilator function. They suggest that improving muscle strength may be advantageous in diseases that affect diaphragm muscle fatigability. They conclude that future studies should investigate how atrophy and reduced fatigability of fast twitch motor units containing Type IIx and/or IIb fibers can be improved.[24]

2.3. Functional Unit

The functional unit to which a muscle belongs includes the muscles that reinforce and counter its actions as well as the joints that the muscle crosses. The interdependence of these structures functionally is reflected in the organization and neural connections of the sensory motor cortex. The functional unit is emphasized because the presence of a TrP in one muscle of the unit increases the likelihood that the other muscles of the unit will also develop TrPs. When inactivating TrPs in a muscle, one must be concerned about TrPs that may develop in muscles that are functionally interdependent. Box 45-1 grossly represents the functional unit of the intercostal and diaphragm muscles.[25]

The role of the internal and external intercostal muscles during ventilation remains controversial with the exception of the parasternal internal intercostal muscles (active during inspiration); however, their role in trunk rotation is well established.[6,18] Muscles that attached the thorax to the shoulder girdle, vertebral column, head, or pelvis may assist with ventilation depending on the ventilatory demand.

Muscles around the lumbo-pelvic region contribute to its stability by an internal positive pressure that creates functional strength and stability. This pressure is regulated mostly by an intra-abdominal pressure mechanism provided by such key muscles

Box 45-1 Functional unit of the intercostal and diaphragm muscles

Action	Synergists	Antagonist
Inspiration	Diaphragm Parastenal intercostals Scalenes Sternocleidomastoid Levatoris costarum Upper and lateral external intercostals	External oblique abdominis Internal oblique abdominis Rectus abdominis Transversus abdominis Qudratus lumborum Erector spinae
Expiration	External oblique abdominis Internal oblique abdominis Rectus abdominis Transversus abdominis Transversus thoracis Qudratus lumborum Erector spinae	Diaphragm Parastenal intercostals Scalenes Sternocleidomastoid Levatoris costarum Upper and lateral external intercostals
Trunk rotation	Ipsilateral internal intercostals Contralateral external intercostals Ipsilateral internal oblique abdominis Contralateral oblique external abdominis	Contralateral internal intercostals Ipsilateral external intercostals Contralateral internal oblique abdominis Ipsilateral external oblique abdominis

as transversus abdominis, pelvic floor, and diaphragm muscles. Other muscles such as lumbar multifidus, internal and external oblique abdominales, psoas major, quadratus lumborum, rectus abdominis, and gluteal muscles also all provide lumbo-pelvic stability. The concept of intra-abdominal pressure may be compared to a sealed can of soda as the coordination of the key muscles (ie, diaphragm, pelvic floor, transversus abdominis) provides a stable chamber for the pressurized abdominal contents. In the absence of muscle dysfunction, which would be comparable to damage of the soda can, the contents are securely contained despite inevitable changes in pressure. The lumbo-pelvic girdle then allows larger, more superficial muscles around the trunk to provide further stability as well as gross movement and torque needed for daily and athletic activities.

3. CLINICAL PRESENTATION

3.1. Referred Pain Pattern

Intercostal Muscles

Trigger points in intercostal muscles refer pain locally in the region of the TrP and tend to refer pain anteriorly along that interspace toward the front of the thorax, rather than toward the back (Figure 45-9). The more posteriorly the TrP is located, the stronger is its tendency to refer pain toward the front. Active TrPs may refer pain to the intercostal spaces above and below the TrP. Bonica and Sola[26] illustrated a similar local intercostal muscle pain pattern around the TrP.

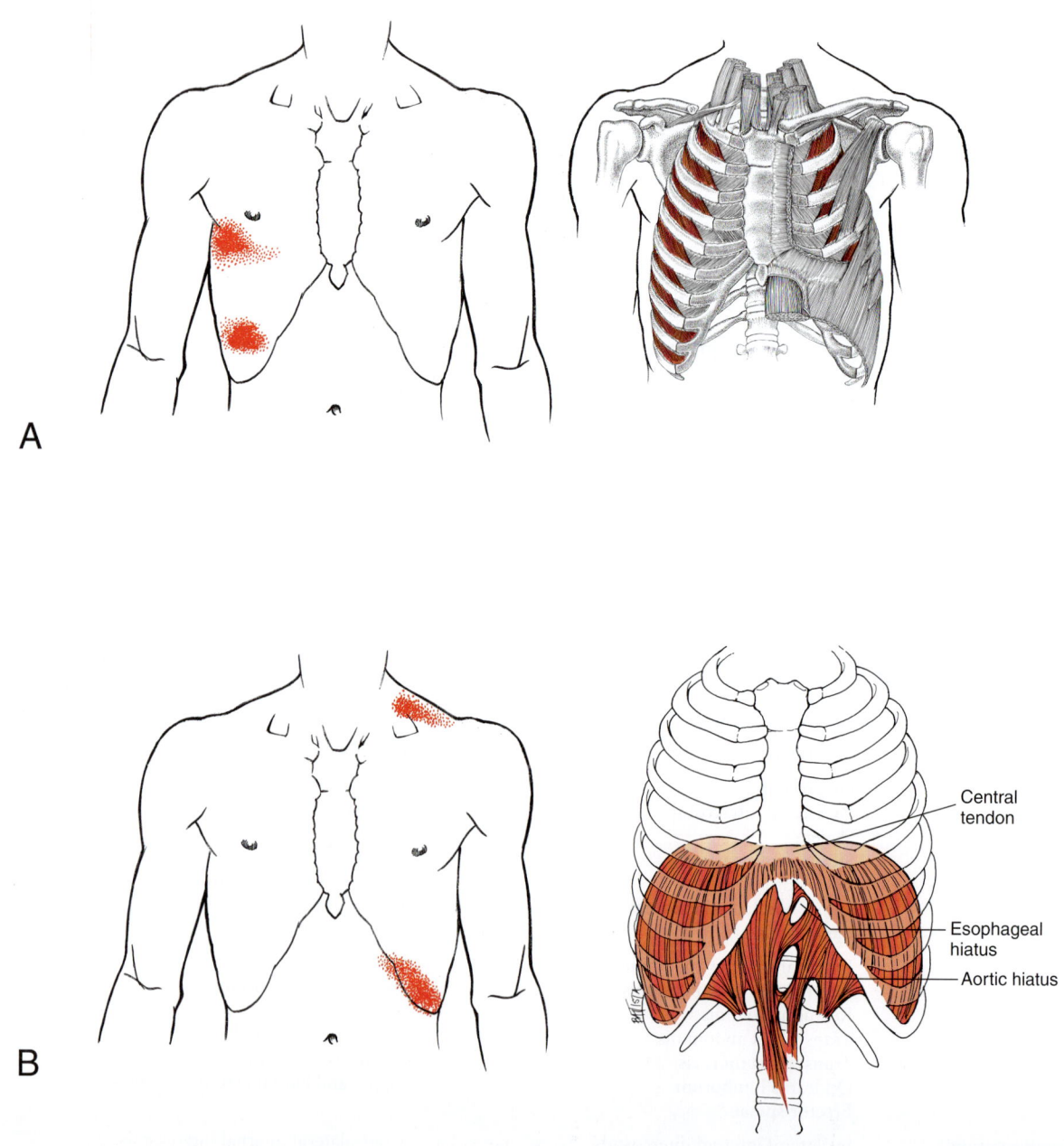

Figure 45-9. A, Examples of referred pain patterns (dark red) of TrPs in intercostal muscles (light red). A TrP can occur in any intercostal muscle. The more dorsally the TrP is located, the farther the pain pattern tends to extend toward the sternum. Patterns tend to follow the curvature of the ribs. B, TrPs in the central diaphragm muscle can refer pain to the upper border of the ipsilateral shoulder at the angle of the neck, and other TrPs refer to the anterolateral aspect of the lower border of the rib cage as in a "stitch in the side."

Diaphragm

During vigorous exercise, diaphragm TrPs can produce the pain commonly described as a "stitch in the side" that is felt deep anterolaterally in the region of the lower border of the rib cage. The pain tends to be aggravated by continued exercise and relieved by rest (Figure 45-9B).

Pain arising from stimulation of the central dome portion of the diaphragm muscle can be referred to the upper border of the ipsilateral shoulder. Stimulation of the peripheral part is referred as an aching pain to the region of the adjacent costal margin. The difference in pain distribution depends on the innervation of the stimulated site.[27] Among a series of 17 patients complaining of chest pain and dyspnea attributed to spasm of the diaphragm muscle,[28] nine complained of pain in the substernal region and eight located their pain in or near the right hypochondrial region, which suggests that the location of the pain identified the nerve supply and identified from which part of the diaphragm muscle the pain originated. This principle may also apply to pain referred from diaphragm TrPs.

Fields[27] called attention to experiments of Capps[29] that involved direct stimulation of the peritoneal (caudal) surface of the diaphragm muscle with a smooth bead or the rough end of a wire. In three subjects, stimulation of the central portion of the diaphragm muscle with the bead caused a sharp, localized pain that was illustrated as referring to the middle region of the anterior border of the upper trapezius muscle about half way between the acromion and the base of the neck. Stimulation with the rough end of the wire produced pain of great intensity at the same location. One subject described the sensation as, "the wire sticking into my neck," and could point to the precise spot with a fingertip. When pressed, that spot was abnormally tender. On the other hand, in one subject tested, stimulation of the peripheral margin of the diaphragm muscle produced a diffuse pain referred to the costal border. The patient indicated the area with his hand placed transversely over the lower ribs and over the right hypochondrium. The difference in the quality and location of the pain referred from the central compared to the peripheral parts of the diaphragm muscle may reflect the marked differences in their sources of innervation and a difference in spatial resolution of receptors in these tendon and muscle.

3.2. Symptoms

When the patient reports an aching pain along the rib interface and is unable to lie in the position that places body weight on the affected side, the intercostal muscles should be considered as a possible source of the patient's symptoms. Patients may also report increased pain and symptoms during cardiorespiratory exercises that increase the ventilatory demand, especially inspiration. The patient may also report significant exacerbation of painful symptoms with either coughing or sneezing.

Cardiac arrhythmia, including auricular fibrillation, can depend on the arrhythmia TrP considered in detail in Chapter 42. It may be located in intercostal muscles on the right side between the fifth and sixth ribs midway between the sternal border and nipple line. When a TrP of this nature occurs, cardiac arrhythmia may be one symptom of intercostal TrPs.

When a patient's primary report of pain is that of a "stitch in the side," especially when performing cardiorespiratory exercise that requires rapid deep breaths, the diaphragm muscle should be considered as a source of symptoms. The pain is likely to be most intense at the end of a full exhalation when the diaphragm fibers are stretched. Coughing can also be excruciatingly painful.

Seventeen patients diagnosed with episodic spasms of the diaphragm muscle[28] complained of chest pain, dyspnea, and inability to get a full breath. Sometimes attacks were precipitated by anxiety-producing situations. Patients sometimes had so much difficulty breathing that they feared they might die. This demonstrates the importance of the diaphragm muscle. The author[28] did not consider TrPs as a source of these patient's symptoms.

A hiccup represents a reflex contraction of the diaphragm muscle. The anatomy, physiology, and clinical aspects of hiccups were thoroughly reviewed by Travell.[30] Often hiccups can be relieved by mechanical (and cold) stimulation of the uvula, suggesting that an area in the mucosa or musculature of the uvula can be a major factor in causing hiccups.[30] Also, TrPs of the diaphragm muscle are suggested by the observation that exhalation tends to relieve the hiccups, and deep inhalation (shortening the muscle fibers) tends to aggravate them. However, this respiratory effect may also be an example of respiratory synkinesis.[31]

3.3. Patient Examination

After a thorough subjective examination the clinician should make a detailed drawing representing the pain pattern that the patient has described. This depiction will assist in planning the physical examination and can be useful in monitoring the progression of the patient as symptoms improve or change. Any patient with primary reports of chest pain should alert the clinician to perform a thorough review of the cardiovascular and pulmonary systems. Any concerns regarding the involvement of the cardiovascular or respiratory systems as a source of symptoms should result in an immediate referral to the emergency room or a physician.

In myofascial pain disorders, patients will very commonly (if not exclusively) present with an asynchrony between respiratory mechanics and posture that not only affects the function of the lumbo-pelvic area but also affects the function of the upper and lower quarter regions and extremities as a whole. Especially in patients with chronic myofascial pain, physical observation of the patient's static posture can indicate much about their respiratory state as well as trunk stability that ultimately provides information about the patient's pain state.

For proper examination of the intercostal and diaphragm muscles, the clinician should observe standing posture, especially shoulder girdle posture, scapula position, and spinal curves. The clinician should also monitor the ventilation cycle and breathing patterns. The clinician should examine diaphragmatic breathing, and if the patient presents with a paradoxical breathing pattern, high priority should be given to effectively correct this ineffective breathing pattern, both during initial therapy and at follow-up visits. This treatment is discussed further in Section 5 of this chapter.

Respiratory mechanics should be assessed during resting respiration and with forced inhalation and exhalation from an anterior, lateral, and posterior perspective. The clinician should note upward and outward motion (pump handle) in the anterior rig cage, upward and lateral motion (bucket handle) in the vertebrochondral rib cage, and caliper motion in ribs 11 and 12.

The vital capacity of the patients with intercostal and/or diaphragm TrPs is likely to be reduced because the TrPs often painfully restrict deep inhalation or full exhalation even with normal coordinated diaphragmatic breathing pattern. In normal respiratory mechanics, the diaphragm muscle would expand primarily with a secondary upper chest rib expansion. However, when the diaphragm muscle no longer provides the volumetric exchange of oxygen that it is intended to provide, excessive upper chest respiration develops to compensate for the lack of diaphragmatic contributions. As time goes on, a feed forward loop develops and the patient develops a learned pattern of a predominate upper chest breathing pattern (paradoxical breathing). This respiratory pattern results in static resting postures with an elevated lower rib cage, increased thoracolumbar extension and increased myofascial tension of the upper rib and neck muscles such as the scalenes, sternocleidomastoid, and upper trapezius muscles—as if the patient were holding an inspired breath. The paradoxical respiratory pattern results in an 'inspired rib cage position' such that the patient not only presents with flared out lower ribs and increased upper chest muscle tone, but also reduced abdominal expansion. This posture indicates that the diaphragm muscle may not be contracting appropriately and a lack of lateral rib cage expansion may result in an overall loss of pulmonary function.

This alteration in breathing mechanics and resting postures adds more stress to the thoracolumbar spine and can be a major contributing factor not only to low back pain (LBP), but as well as upper and lower quarter injuries since these regions rely heavily on the foundation of the thoracolumbar and pelvic region stability. As in any other muscle that develops TrPs due to excessive use and poor mechanics, the diaphragm and intercostal muscles can also easily develop myofascial dysfunction.

Active and passive movement testing of the trunk may reveal a loss of rotation in one or both directions, and/or limited lateral flexion due to TrPs in the intercostal muscles. The clinician should also examine for TrPs in the abdominal oblique, serratus posterior inferior, and iliocostalis lumborum muscles, which may also restrict trunk rotation and lateral flexion.

The patient may present with limited shoulder elevation on the affected side because of painfully restricted rib mobility due to TrPs in the intercostal muscles. Intercostal TrPs are usually aggravated by contralateral trunk lateral flexion, and may be somewhat relieved by ipsilateral trunk lateral flexion.

Patients with TrPs in the diaphragm muscle are likely to experience pain at the end of a maximal exhalation due to stretching of the muscle. To increase the sensitivity of testing, the patient can increase stretch tension on the diaphragm muscle near the end of full exhalation by a vigorous contraction of the abdominal muscles. If the abdominal musculature is weak, the patient can apply external pressure to the abdomen to increase intra-abdominal pressure forcing the diaphragm muscle upward and stretching it. Performing this abdominal maneuver during continued exhalation ensures an open glottis. The effectiveness of this effort is blocked if the patient closes the glottis, which is what patients normally do when contracting the abdominal muscles to increase intra-abdominal pressure. Vigorous coughing at nearly complete exhalation can also elicit pain from TrPs in the diaphragm muscle. If the TrPs have caused appreciable enthesopathy, any vigorous cough is likely to be painful.

Among 17 patients with episodes that were diagnosed as diaphragmatic spasm, the author[28] was able to induce an attack in 12 of them during fluoroscopic examination. As the patient had increasing difficulty taking in a full breath, the diaphragm muscle became progressively contracted until it was essentially flat across the abdomen and the patient was in serious respiratory distress because of inability to inhale adequately. Episodes were usually precipitated by engaging the patients in discussion of topics known to be very emotionally stressful to them. The diaphragmatic spasm (or contracture) eliminated diaphragmatic function and was blocking both the pump-handle and bucket-handle movements of the thorax.[28] Increased diaphragmatic muscle tension caused by TrPs would produce a similar effect to a significantly lesser degree and would also be aggravated by emotional distress.

Accessory joint motion should be tested in the cervical spine (especially C3-C5 due to the relationship of the phrenic nerve roots), thoracic intervertebral and facet joints, costovertebral joints, rib cage, sternoclavicular joint, manubriosternal joint, xiphisternal joint, and scapulo-thoracic joints. Oftentimes, joint hypomobility in the thoracic spine or rib cage can cause impairment in respiratory mechanics leading to overload and TrP formation in the intercostal and diaphragm muscles.

Additional testing of all muscles which attach from the shoulder girdle, head and neck, and pelvis to the thorax should be carried out as all these muscles can act as accessory respiratory muscles depending on the position of the trunk and upper extremities.

3.4. Trigger Point Examination

Intercostal Muscles

Intercostal TrPs are usually located anterolaterally or posterolaterally and less commonly in the extreme anterior and posterior portions of the muscle (Figure 45-10A). The parasternal internal

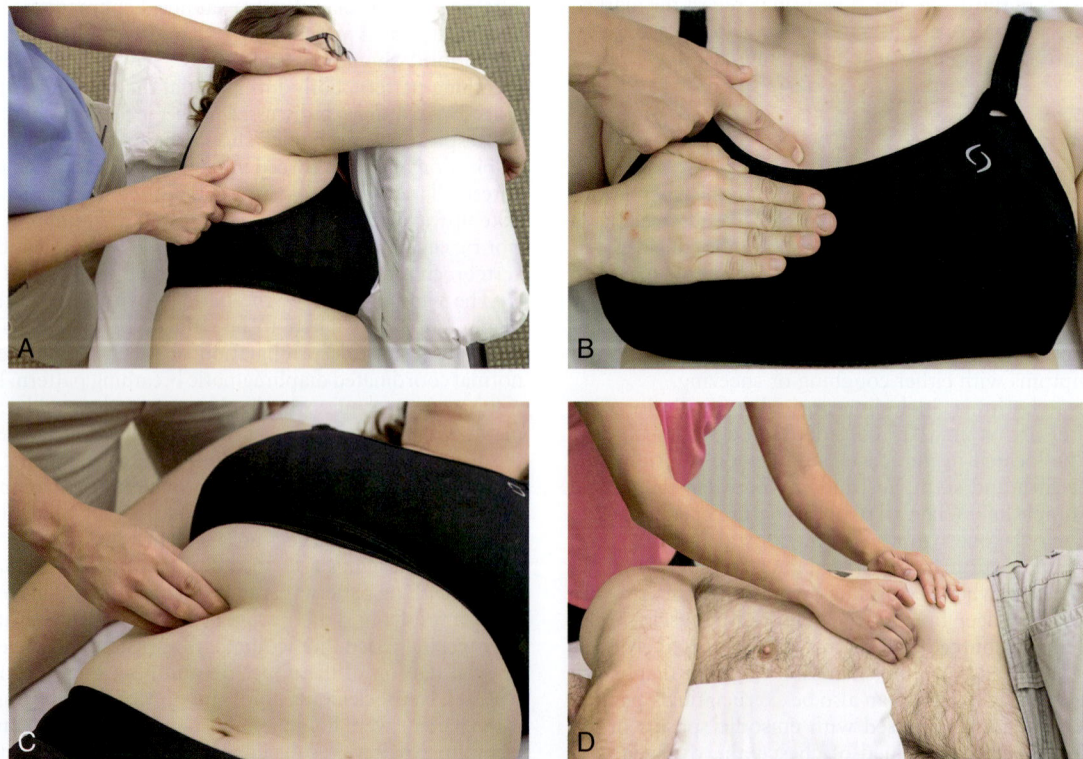

Figure 45-10. Cross-fiber flat palpation for identification of intercostal TrPs. A, Posterolateral trunk. B, Cross-fiber flat palpation of parasternal internal intercostal TrPs. For female patients modesty may be maintained by the patient using their own hand to move and cover their breast tissue. C, Cross-fiber flat palpation near the costal fibers of diaphragm muscle. D, Palpation of the diaphragm muscle side-lying.

intercostal muscles are an exception to this finding and should be carefully investigated utilizing cross-fiber flat palpation in the supine position (Figure 45-10B). Careful examination of the parasternal internal intercostal muscles should be performed in cases of suspected costochondritis and Tietze syndrome. These syndromes may be caused by, or associated with, TrPs in these workhorse respiratory muscles.

To locate intercostal TrPs, the clinician should examine the rib cage for abnormally narrow rib interspaces that could indicate tense intercostal muscles or a rib dysfunction. This can be performed in supine, side-lying, and prone positions depending on the patients report of pain. The patient usually describes pain along a narrowed interspace if active intercostal TrPs are the source of the patient's symptoms. The region of increased muscle tension and of TrP tenderness can be found by running the palpating finger between the ribs for the full length of the suspected segment and can be identified with cross-fiber flat palpation (Figure 45-10A and B).

Dr Travell observed that a TrP in the intercostal muscle located posteriorly between ribs 4 and 5, close to the rhomboid minor muscle, initiated a hiccup when pressed before TrP injection but not following the TrP injection.[25]

Diaphragm

Palpation for TrPs in the diaphragm muscle can be performed in side-lying, supine, or seated position. The midfiber central TrPs of the diaphragm muscle are not accessible to palpation. However, TrPs in the costal portion of the diaphragm muscle are detectable just inside the anterior lower border of the thoracic rib cage (Figure 45-10C and D). Tenderness detected in this region could originate in the diaphragm, the external oblique abdominis, internal oblique abdominis, or transversus abdominis muscles. The external and internal oblique abdominis muscles attach to the ribs externally above the costal margin (Figure 49-4), whereas the transversus abdominis muscle attaches to the costal margin and interdigitates with angulated diaphragm fibers (see Figures 45-4 and 49-3). Palpation of the abdominal muscle during an active contraction will assist in the identification of the specific muscle based on fiber direction and can help the clinician to differentiate taut bands and TrP tenderness in the more superficial abdominal muscles from tenderness in the deeper muscles.

The ambiguity of distinguishing between the attachment tenderness of the transversus abdominis and diaphragm muscles at the costal margin can be resolved by testing sensitivity to stretch. To differentiate between the transversus abdominis and the diaphragm muscles the clinician can assess whether pain and tenderness are increased by stretching the abdominal muscles (protruding the abdomen) or by stretching the diaphragm muscle (compressing the abdomen near the end of exhalation).

4. DIFFERENTIAL DIAGNOSIS

4.1. Activation and Perpetuation of Trigger Points

In any part of the intercostal or diaphragm muscles, TrPs may be activated by unaccustomed eccentric loading, eccentric exercise in unconditioned muscle, or maximal or sub-maximal concentric loading.[32] Trigger points may also be activated or aggravated when the muscle is placed in a shortened or lengthened position for an extended period of time. A slumped or forward head posture may activate TrPs in the intercostal or diaphragm muscles. Chronic coughing as many individuals with chronic obstructive pulmonary disease (COPD) or individuals who smoke experience will activate and perpetuate TrPs in the respiratory muscles.

Intercostal Muscles

A posture or activity that activates a TrP, if not corrected, can also perpetuate it. For the intercostal muscles, postural considerations are very important.

Intercostal TrPs may be activated by gross or local impact trauma, excessive coughing, and chest surgery.[26,33] Chest retractors used during surgery were found likely to leave painful clusters of intercostal TrPs.[34] Open heart surgery that employed incision of the sternum rather than ribs was more likely to result in TrPs in the pectoralis major and minor muscles than in the anterior intercostal muscles.[34] Other causes for activation include an attack of herpes zoster,[35] fracture of a rib to which the muscle attaches, and possibly a breast implant.

Intercostal TrPs also may become active in association with intrathoracic lesions, such as pneumothorax, pyothorax, and pleural effusion (secondary to a tumor). These associated TrPs are likely to involve the last three intercostal muscles and a complaint of posterolateral low chest pain.

Significant perpetuating factors can be anxiety, repetitive trunk rotation, overexertion in sports, or a chronic cough. Trigger points in the overlying pectoralis major muscle, and paradoxical breathing may also activate and perpetuate intercostal TrPs. It is not always clear which comes first as the abnormal respiratory pattern and the TrPs seem to reinforce each other.

Diaphragm

Anxiety, chest breathing, and overexertion in exercise, such as rapid walking or running or a persistent cough, can activate and perpetuate TrPs in the diaphragm muscle. Any condition that causes labor intensive respiration can also cause TrPs to develop in the diaphragm muscle. Keeping the stomach flat at all times to demonstrate a slim physique will alter normal respiratory mechanics and cause the diaphragm muscle to develop TrPs. A slumped posture with forward head position can also activate TrPs in the diaphragm muscle. It is likely they could appear following gastrectomy or any chest surgery.

4.2. Associated Trigger Points

Associated TrPs can develop in the referred pain areas caused by TrPs.[36] Therefore, musculature in the referred pain areas for each muscle should also be considered.

Spot tenderness of the chest wall in locations where the serratus anterior muscle attaches to ribs may appear to be intercostal TrPs. A palpable taut band in the serratus anterior muscle over the rib rather than in the intercostal space helps to identify the TrP in the serratus anterior muscle versus intercostal muscles. The pectoralis major and minor, scalenii, sternocleidomastoid, upper trapezius and latissimus dorsi muscles should also be assessed for the presence of TrPs. In addition, muscles that comprise the functional unit may also have or produce associated TrPs.

Full elevation of an upper limb opens up the intercostal spaces on the same side and stretches fascial tissues over the chest wall. This movement is painful to patients who have intercostal TrPs, who are recovering from thoracotomy, or who have herpes zoster with or without intercostal TrPs. Patients with these conditions are vulnerable to developing a painful myofascial "frozen" shoulder because of the pain-induced restricted ROM at the shoulder that encourages the development and perpetuation of subscapularis TrPs as described in Chapter 26.

At times, the cardiac arrhythmia TrP associated with the pectoralis major muscle (see Chapter 42) appears just as likely to be located in an intercostal muscle between rib 5 and 6 on the right.

Diaphragmatic TrPs may form as a result of referred pain in the upper portion of the rectus abdominis muscle on the same side. On examination, the tenderness of rectus abdominis TrPs is increased by stretching that muscle or by asking the supine patient to raise the feet off of the examining table. If these movements do not increase the TrP sensitivity, then tenderness to pressure applied inside the lower border of this region of the rib cage most likely indicates diaphragm TrP involvement.

Articular dysfunction associated with intercostal TrPs is usually isolated to one or two rib levels and presents as an exhalation restriction or a depressed rib. This dysfunction is best treated by inactivating the TrPs, by using respiration to augment relaxation, or by functional (indirect) techniques. Diaphragm TrPs have no recognized articular dysfunctions related to them other than generalized loss of accessory motion in the thoracic spine and rib cage.

4.3. Associated Pathology

Intercostal Muscles

Differential diagnoses of symptoms caused by intercostal TrPs should include herpes zoster, rib articular dysfunctions, fibromyalgia, cardiac diseases (in cases of left unilateral intercostal TrPs), painful rib syndrome,[37] Tietze syndrome or costochondritis (which was clearly differentiated by Calabro et al[38]), thoracic radiculopathy, and intercostal muscle spasm (considered one of the most common and generally unrecognized, benign causes of chest pain).[39]

Serious intrathoracic disease that can mimic the symptoms of intercostal TrPs include myocardial infarction, tumor, pleural effusion, and pyothorax. These conditions must be ruled out and when present, they also can induce and perpetuate TrP activity in the respiratory muscles. Thus, if intercostal TrPs respond poorly to treatment, imaging of the chest and a search for other conditions is indicated.

Intercostal TrPs commonly develop in conjunction with an attack of herpes zoster.[35] In a study by Chen, the neurogenic pain of herpes was often described as a shooting pain that was generally responsive to Tegretol therapy. Pain from TrPs was described as a localized ache that, in these cases, persisted despite Tegretol therapy but responded to TrP treatment.[35] The TrP pain is most likely to be prominent in the chronic stage of a herpes attack and may be the only remaining source of chest pain. The intercostal TrP pain tends to be well localized, most commonly in the posterolateral part of the chest.

Diaphragm

With regard to diaphragm TrPs, differential diagnoses include diaphragmatic spasm,[28] peptic ulcer, gastroesophageal reflux, and gallbladder diseases (in cases of right-side unilateral diaphragmatic TrPs).

Atypical chest pain (which, when in the lower sternal area, has also been called "slipping rib syndrome," xiphoidalgia, or precordial catch syndrome) was shown in one characteristic example to be due to a TrP in the diaphragm muscle.[40] Clinical research studies are still needed to clarify the relation between these syndromes and TrPs.

When chest pain is closely associated with increased tension of the diaphragm muscle it must not be assumed that the tension is caused by spasm. Increased muscle tension and pain in the absence of spasm are cardinal features of TrPs.

Kolar et al[41] investigated the function of the diaphragm muscle during postural limb isometric activities in patients with chronic LBP and healthy controls. Both groups had normal pulmonary function test results prior to the study. Dynamic resonance imaging and specialized spirometer readings were used in all subjects to measure diaphragm muscle function. They found patients with chronic LBP had a higher diaphragm muscle resting position with smaller diaphragm muscle excursions during tidal breathing measurements. They conclude that the abnormal postural function of the diaphragm muscle may serve as one underlying factor in patients with chronic LBP.

Janssens et al[42] investigated diaphragm muscle fatigability in 10 individuals with LBP as compared to 10 healthy normal controls. They utilized transdiaphragmatic twitch pressure measurements prior to, 20, and 45 minutes after inspiratory muscle loading. They found a failure in the diaphragm muscle to potentiate is much more common in individuals with LBP as compared to the healthy normal controls. They conclude that individuals with LBP exhibit significant diaphragm muscle fatigue at 20 and 45 minutes following inspiratory muscle loading. They suggest that fatigability of the diaphragm muscle may be an underlying mechanism of persistent LBP, and this may contribute to impaired spinal motor control anteriorly. Inspiratory muscle training may be indicated to decrease diaphragm muscle fatigability however further studies are warranted.

Vostatek et al[43] investigated changes in the diaphragm muscle in regards to shape and motion when postural demands on the body were increased utilizing magnetic resonance imaging (MRI). They included 17 subjects with chronic LBP and 16 healthy normal controls. The ROM of the diaphragm muscle was two to three times greater in the control group with a diaphragm muscle excursion of 40 mm in the control group as compared to 22 mm in the LBP group. The control group also demonstrated a lower breathing frequency during postural demands. They conclude that the postural and breathing components are better balanced and more harmonious within its movement in the control group, and their findings confirmed worse diaphragm muscle cooperation in the subjects with LBP.

Although there is no specific evidence that hiccups are directly related to diaphragm TrPs, it is interesting that breathing while in the position of as full exhalation as possible (which stretches the diaphragm muscle) tends to reduce hiccup activity and discourage its return, while taking a deep inhalation (which shortens diaphragm muscle fibers) can reactivate hiccups.[30] The fact that severance of both phrenic nerves may not terminate hiccups suggests that hiccups can be produced by reflex activity of the inspiratory chest muscles without diaphragmatic contraction. Dr Travell spent many years exploring ways to end persistent hiccups in challenging cases, and in 1977[30] summarized some of the techniques she had found to be most effective.

5. CORRECTIVE ACTIONS

Forward head, slumped posture needs to be corrected to facilitate erect posture which improves respiratory efficiency. Proper posture and respiratory mechanics are interdependent of each other, and both must be addressed when patient's present with TrPs in the intercostal or diaphragm muscles. When posture and respiratory mechanics are not optimized, evidence suggests that not only is there a decrease in oxygen exchange, but also a decrease in lumbo-pelvic stability as well as an overall loss in movement efficiency.[41,43] The initial resting posture of the thorax and rib cage are crucial for the ideal synergy of the structure of the rib cage, spine, and pelvis and the muscles surrounding these areas that allow for proper respiration and lumbo-pelvic stability.

Therefore, it is vital that education and correction of the patient's posture and respiratory mechanics are provided by the clinician. Good posture is also essential for maintenance of muscle length and effective respiratory patterns. The clinician should educate the patient about what the inspired rib cage position indicates and how it relates to their pain and dysfunction. The patient should be trained in how to self-correct their posture to attain a more optimal position and should employ proper breathing technique with an emphasis on a diaphragmatic breathing pattern (Figure 45-11).

When lower thoracic intercostal and/or diaphragm TrPs are identified on one side, the release technique illustrated and described in Figure 45-12 can be used as a self-pressure release technique. This procedure is done in the supine position with the hips and knees flexed to relax the abdominal musculature. The patient hooks his or her fingers under the lower ribs of the affected side and then inhales deeply in a slow, relaxed manner. During slow exhalation, the patient's fingers follow the diaphragm muscle in and under the ribs and then apply upward traction on the ribs for the actual release. This procedure also helps to release lower intercostal TrPs as well.

Chapter 45: Intercostal and Diaphragm Muscles   **449**

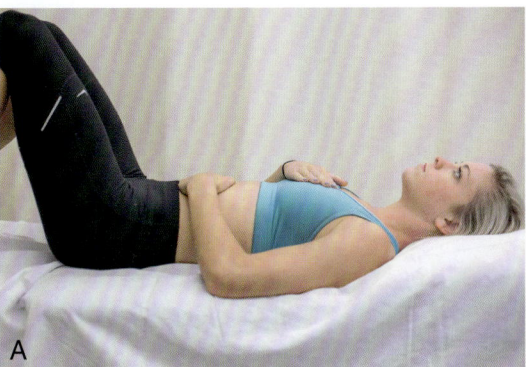
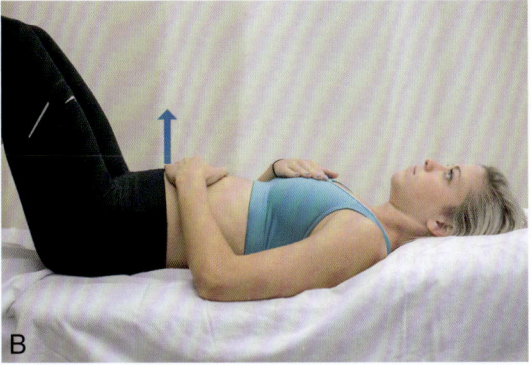
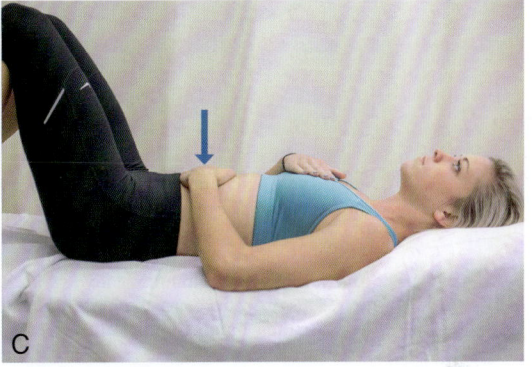

Figure 45-11. Diaphragmatic breathing. A, The patient places one hand on the stomach and the other on the chest. B, The patient takes a deep breath through their nose. The patient should feel their stomach rise and minimal to no motion in the chest. C, At the end of the inspiration the patient should hold for 3 to 5 seconds and slowly exhale through their mouth with pursed lips.

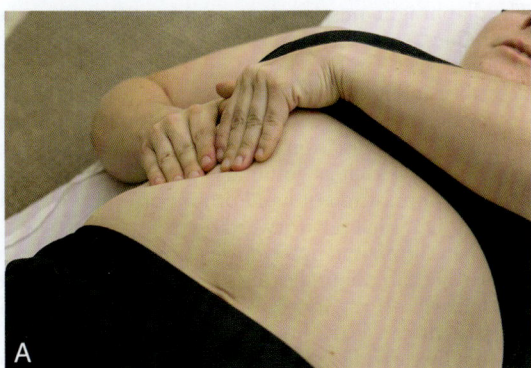
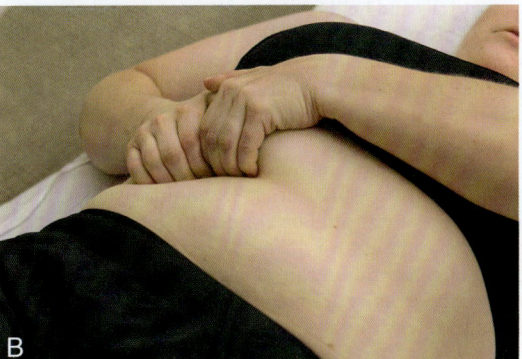
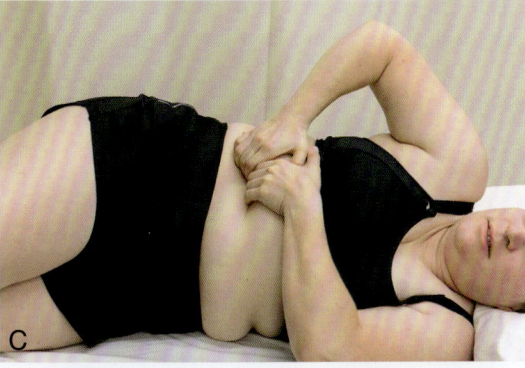

Figure 45-12. Self-release of the diaphragm muscle. This self-stretch procedure is done in the supine position with the hips and knees flexed to relax the abdominal musculature. A, The patient hooks his or her fingers under the lower ribs of the affected side and then inhales deeply in a slow, relaxed manner. B, During slow exhalation, the patient's fingers follow the diaphragm muscle in and under the ribs and then apply upward traction on the ribs for the actual release. This self-stretch procedure also helps to release lower intercostal TrPs. C, This technique may also be performed in side-lying.

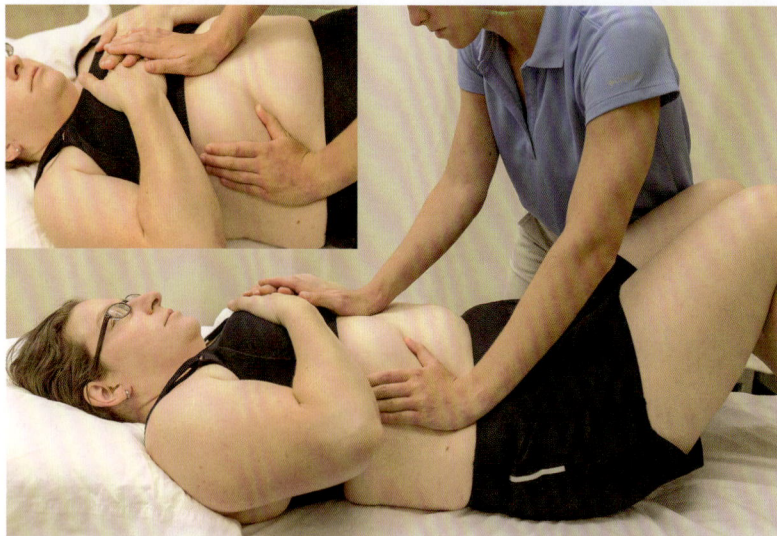

Figure 45-13. Diaphragm muscle release with the patient supine. The clinician stands at the patient's side opposite to the side to be released and places both hands anteriorly at the lower border of the patient's rib cage. The patient is instructed to breathe in normally in a relaxed manner and then breathe out slowly. During exhalation, the clinician's thumbs follow the diaphragm muscle inward under the rib cage and then lift the rib cage anteriorly. This procedure is also helpful for releasing lower intercostal TrPs. Female patients may use their hands to block the breast tissue.

Maximum elevation of the diaphragm muscle is achieved in the supine position by letting the breath out completely and then contracting the abdominal muscles. This places the diaphragm muscle on maximum passive stretch with some additional help from reciprocal inhibition supplied by the voluntary contraction of the abdominal muscles.[44] Pressure should be applied to the area of sensitive TrPs and held for 15 to 30 seconds and repeated 6 to 10 times. This technique can be used several times a day as long as favorable results are being obtained. In some cases the clinician may need to perform a manual technique to assist in release of TrPs in the diaphragm and intercostal muscles (Figure 45-13).

Inactivation of TrPs in the intercostal muscles can be achieved by application of self-pressure release technique using a finger (Figure 45-14). Pressure should be applied to the sensitive TrPs between two ribs and held for 15 to 30 seconds and repeated 6 to 10 times. This technique can be used several times a day as long as favorable results are being obtained.

In addition to releasing the specific pain-producing TrPs, it is helpful to release all tense myofascial tissues in that region. In the lower thorax, an effective approach to release TrPs in these lower intercostal muscles is illustrated and described in Figure 45-15.[45,46]

The muscle fibers of the diaphragm muscle are placed on stretch by maximum exhalation, which moves the dome of the diaphragm muscle up into the chest cavity. The fibers are also stretched by any compression of the abdomen at full exhalation. The diaphragm muscle is inaccessible to direct manual therapy techniques, such as TrP release. However, it and the lower intercostal TrPs can be released by the technique illustrated and described in Figure 45-15.

An increase in intra-abdominal pressure for added stretch to the diaphragm muscle on full exhalation can be accomplished in various ways, such as voluntary contraction of the abdominal muscles, application of hand or arm pressure to the abdomen, and bending the body forward on exhalation.

When the patient has a chronic cough, it must be controlled before one can obtain lasting relief from TrPs in these respiratory muscles. If the source of the cough cannot be eliminated, the patient can learn how to suppress a cough and raise the sputum by clearing the throat, assisted by a cough suppressant, if necessary.

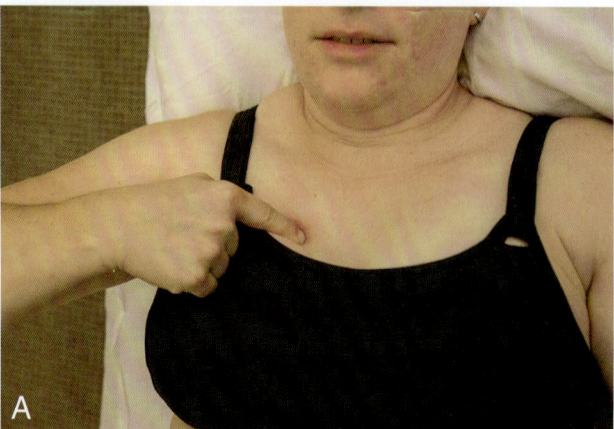 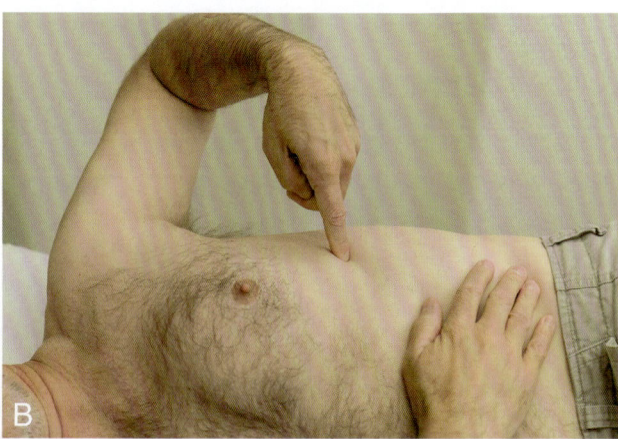

Figure 45-14. Self-pressure release of trigger points in the intercostal muscles. A, Anterior release technique. B, Lateral release technique.

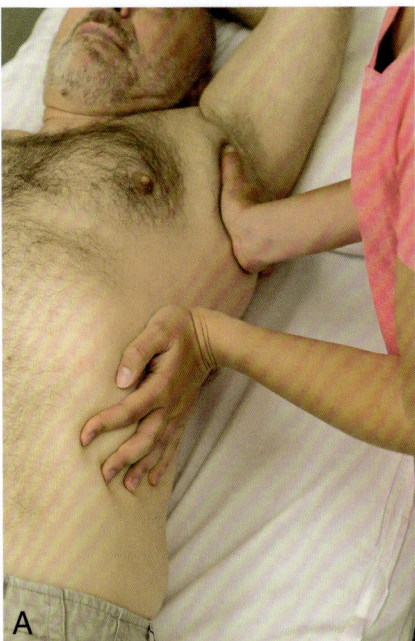
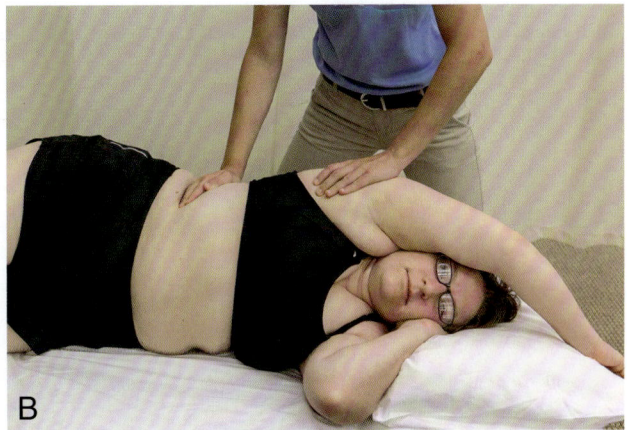

Figure 45-15. Release of lower intercostal muscle tension caused by TrPs. This technique is sometimes called "lower rib release" and can also be used to release TrP tension of the latissimus dorsi muscle. Patient is A, supine or B, side-lying with the arm on the affected side positioned upward and reaching over the head. One hand of the clinician (the right hand in this figure) is placed so as to span the lateral aspect of the patient's lower ribs; the other hand is placed in the patient's axillary region for stabilization. The patient is then instructed to take a deep breath. During the exhalation phase, the clinician's right hand applies gentle downward pressure (caudally directed) on the patient's lower ribs. As the patient inhales, the clinician resists elevation of the lower ribs, and as the patient exhales, the clinician's downward pressure facilitates depression and release of the lower ribs. The patient is instructed to reach overhead toward the opposite shoulder during exhalation, which accentuates the stretch of the intercostal and latissimus dorsi muscles. The stretch cycle is repeated until release is satisfactory.

References

1. Clemente C. *Gray's Anatomy of the Human Body*. 30th American ed. Philadelphia, PA: Lea & Febiger; 1985:476-477.
2. Standring S. *Gray's Anatomy: The Anatomical Basis of Clinical Practice*. 41st ed. London, UK: Elsevier; 2015:940-942.
3. Oatis C. *Kinesiology: The mechanics and Pathomechanics of Human Movement*. 2nd ed. Baltimore, MD: Lippinott, Williams & Wilkins; 2009:546-553.
4. Nason LK, Walker CM, McNeeley MF, Burivong W, Fligner CL, Godwin JD. Imaging of the diaphragm: anatomy and function. *Radiographics*. 2012;32(2):E51-E70.
5. Reid WD, Dechman G. Considerations when testing and training the respiratory muscles. *Phys Ther*. 1995;75(11):971-982.
6. Whitelaw WA, Ford GT, Rimmer KP, De Troyer A. Intercostal muscles are used during rotation of the thorax in humans. *J Appl Physiol (1985)*. 1992;72(5):1940-1944.
7. Levangie PK, Norkin CC. *Joint Structure and Function: A Comprehensive Analysis*. 5th ed. Philadelphia, PA: FA Davis; 2011:201-212.
8. Loring SH. Action of human respiratory muscles inferred from finite element analysis of rib cage. *J Appl Physiol (1985)*. 1992;72(4):1461-1465.
9. De Troyer A. Chapter 6, Mechanics of the chest wall muscles. In: Miller AD, Bianchi AL, Bishop BP, eds. *Neural Control of the Respiratory Muscles*. New York, NY: CRC Press; 1997:59-73.
10. Han JN, Gayan-Ramirez G, Dekhuijzen R, Decramer M. Respiratory function of the rib cage muscles. *Eur Respir J*. 1993;6(5):722-728.
11. Roussos C. Function and fatigue of respiratory muscles. *Chest*. 1985;88(2 Suppl):124S-132S.
12. De Troyer A. Actions of the respiratory muscles or how the chest wall moves in upright man. *Bull Eur Physiopathol Respir*. 1984;20(5):409-413.
13. Basmajian J, Deluca C. *Muscles Alive*. 5th ed. Baltimore, MD: Williams & Wilkins; 1985:409-426.
14. Harper CJ, Shahgholi L, Cieslak K, Hellyer NJ, Strommen JA, Boon AJ. Variability in diaphragm motion during normal breathing, assessed with B-mode ultrasound. *J Orthop Sports Phys Ther*. 2013;43(12):927-931.
15. Walker DJ, Walterspacher S, Schlager D, et al. Characteristics of diaphragmatic fatigue during exhaustive exercise until task failure. *Respir Physiol Neurobiol*. 2011;176(1-2):14-20.
16. Bishop BP. Chapter 4, The abdominal muscles. In: Miller AD, Bianchi AL, Bishop BP, eds. *Neural Control of the Respiratory Muscles*. New York, NY: CRC Press; 1997:35-46.
17. Duron B, Rose D. Chapter 3, The intercostal muscles. In: Miller AD, Bianchi AL, Bishop BP, eds. *Neural Control of the Respiratory Muscles*. New York, NY: CRC Press; 1997:21-33.
18. Rimmer KP, Ford GT, Whitelaw WA. Interaction between postural and respiratory control of human intercostal muscles. *J Appl Physiol (1985)*. 1995;79(5):1556-1561.
19. Shannon R, Bolser DC, Lindsey BG. Chapter 18, Neural control of coughing and sneezing. In: Miller AD, Bianchi AL, Bishop BP, eds. *Neural Control of the Respiratory Muscles*. New York, NY: CRC Press; 1997:213-222.
20. St John WM. Chapter 16, Gasping. In: Miller AD, Bianchi AL, Bishop BP, eds. *Neural Control of the Respiratory Muscles*. New York, NY: CRC Press; 1997:195-202.
21. Grelot L, Miller AD. Chapter 20, Neural control of respiratory muscle activation during vomiting. In: Miller AD, Bianchi AL, Bishop BP, eds. *Neural Control of the Respiratory Muscles*. New York, NY: CRC Press; 1997:239-248.
22. Viala D. Chapter 24, Coordination of locomotion and respiration. In: Miller AD, Bianchi AL, Bishop BP, eds. *Neural Control of the Respiratory Muscles*. New York, NY: CRC Press; 1997:285-296.
23. Ainsworth DM. Chapter 14, Respiratory muscle recruitment during exercise. In: Miller AD, Bianchi AL, Bishop BP, eds. *Neural Control of the Respiratory Muscles*. New York, NY: CRC Press; 1997:171-180.
24. Mantilla CB, Sieck GC. Impact of diaphragm muscle fiber atrophy on neuromotor control. *Respir Physiol Neurobiol*. 2013;189(2):411-418.
25. Simons DG, Travell J, Simons L. *Travell & Simon's Myofascial Pain and Dysfunction: The Trigger Point Manual*. Vol 1. 2nd ed. Baltimore, MD: Williams & Wilkins; 1999.
26. Bonica J, Sola A. Chapter 58, Chest pain caused by other disorders. In: Bonica JJ, Loeser JD, Chapman C, Fordyce WE, eds. *The Management of Pain*. 2nd ed. Philadelphia, PA: Lea & Febiger; 1990:1114-1145.
27. Fields H. *Pain*. New York, NY: McGraw-Hill Book Co.; 1987.
28. Wolf SG. Diaphragmatic spasm: a neglected cause of dyspnoea and chest pain. *Integr Physiol Behav Sci*. 1994;29(1):74-76.
29. Capps JA. *An Experimental and Clinical Study of Pain in the Pleura, Pericardium and Peritoneum*. New York, NY: The MacMillan Company; 1932:69-99.
30. Travell JG. A trigger point for hiccup. *J Am Osteopath Assoc*. 1977;77(4):308-312.
31. Lewit K, Berger M, Holzmuller G, Lechner-Steinleitner S. Breathing movements: the synkinesis of respiration with looking up and down. *J Musculoskelet Pain*. 1997;5(4):57-69.
32. Gerwin RD, Dommerholt J, Shah JP. An expansion of Simons' integrated hypothesis of trigger point formation. *Curr Pain Headache Rep*. 2004;8(6):468-475.
33. Nguyen JT, Buchanan IA, Patel PP, Aljinovic N, Lee BT. Intercostal neuroma as a source of pain after aesthetic and reconstructive breast implant surgery. *J Plast Reconstr Aesthet Surg*. 2012;65(9):1199-1203.
34. Sola A. Personal communication. In: David G. Simons MD, ed. 1986.
35. Chen S-M, Chen JT, Wu V-C, Kuan T-S, Hong C-Z. Myofascial trigger points in intercostal muscles secondary to herpes zoster infection to the intercostal nerve [abstract]. *Arch Phys Med Rehabil*. 1996;77:961.

36. Hsieh YL, Kao MJ, Kuan TS, Chen SM, Chen JT, Hong CZ. Dry needling to a key myofascial trigger point may reduce the irritability of satellite MTrPs. *Am J Phys Med Rehabil*. 2007;86(5):397-403.
37. Dyer NH. Painful rib syndrome. *Gut*. 1994;35(3):429.
38. Calabro JJ, Jeghers H, Miller KA, Gordon RD. Classification of anterior chest wall syndromes. *JAMA*. 1980;243(14):1420-1421.
39. Blumer I. Chest pain and intercostal spasm. *Hosp Pract (Off Ed)*. 1989;24(5A):13.
40. Ingber RS. Atypical chest pain due to myofascial dysfunction of the diaphragm muscle: a case report. *Arch Phys Med Rehabil*. 1988;69:729.
41. Kolar P, Sulc J, Kyncl M, et al. Postural function of the diaphragm in persons with and without chronic low back pain. *J Orthop Sports Phys Ther*. 2012;42(4):352-362.
42. Janssens L, Brumagne S, McConnell AK, Hermans G, Troosters T, Gayan-Ramirez G. Greater diaphragm fatigability in individuals with recurrent low back pain. *Respir Physiol Neurobiol*. 2013;188(2):119-123.
43. Vostatek P, Novak D, Rychnovsky T, Rychnovska S. Diaphragm postural function analysis using magnetic resonance imaging. *PLoS One*. 2013;8(3):e56724.
44. Wanke T, Lahrmann H, Formanek D, Zwick H. Effect of posture on inspiratory muscle electromyogram response to hypercapnia. *Eur J Appl Physiol Occup Physiol*. 1992;64(3):266-271.
45. Goodridge JP, Kuchera WA. Chapter 54, Muscle energy treatment techniques for specific areas. In: Ward RC, ed. *Foundations for Osteopathic Medicine*. Baltimore, MD: Williams & Wilkins; 1997:697-761.
46. DeStefano L. *Greenman's Principles of Manual Medicine*. 5th ed. Philadelphia, PA: Wolters Kluwer; 2016:274.

Chapter 46

Serratus Anterior Muscle
"Flank Foe"

Deanna Hortman Camilo and César Fernández de las Peñas

1. INTRODUCTION

The serratus anterior muscle is a broad, flat muscle that is structurally divided into three groups of muscle fibers. These three groups of muscle fibers work together as scapular stabilizers to keep the scapula seated against the thoracic wall. Trigger points (TrPs) in the serratus anterior muscle can refer pain in the anterolateral chest, the inferior angle of the scapula, the medial aspect of the arm, and into the palm and ring finger. Rarely, serratus anterior TrPs may cause chest pain and pain with deep inhalation. Activation and perpetuation of TrPs can result from prolonged running, heavy overhead lifting, push-ups, and strenuous coughing. Damage during surgical procedures, such as a mastectomy for the treatment of breast cancer, can also activate TrPs in the serratus anterior muscle. Differential diagnosis should include assessment of the diaphragm and pectoralis major muscles, thoracic spine, rib cage, and long thoracic nerve. Corrective actions should include proper training of diaphragmatic breathing, correction of sleeping position, improving mechanics with sporting activities, and self-pressure release and/or self-stretching.

2. ANATOMIC CONSIDERATIONS

The serratus anterior muscle is composed of three groups of fibers. The most superior group of fibers lies parallel with the underlying ribs. These fibers originate from the first and second ribs and insert onto the superior angle of the scapula.[1] The middle portion runs at a 45° angle to the underlying ribs. This group of fibers originates from the second, third, and fourth ribs and inserts onto the anterior aspect of the medial scapular border.[1] The most inferior portion of the muscle is the strongest part of the muscle and originates from ribs five through nine and inserts onto the inferior angle of the scapula (Figure 46-1).[1] This anatomic division has been recently confirmed by Webb et al.[2] The lower fibers of the serratus anterior muscle attaches to the lower ribs and interdigitates anteriorly with the external oblique muscle that becomes continuous with the contralateral internal oblique and femoral adductor muscles.[1] This anatomic connection among the serratus anterior, external oblique, internal oblique, and the femoral adductor muscles has been termed the "serape effect," and it demonstrates the impact that upper extremity function has on the trunk and lower extremity since simultaneous recruitment of the lower extremity and trunk muscles increases the activation of the serratus anterior muscle during the forward punch plus exercise.[3]

2.1. Innervation and Vascularization

The serratus anterior muscle is innervated by the long thoracic nerve which is derived from the anterior rami of spinal nerves C5-C7 and sometimes C8 nerve root.[4] The fibers of the upper portion of the muscle receive innervation mainly from C5; the middle portion is innervated by C5 and C6, and the lower portion from C6 and C7.[1] The long thoracic nerve lies superficial to the serratus anterior muscle in the line of the anterior axillary fold. Smith et al[5] demonstrated that a separate superior branch of the long thoracic nerve innervates the upper fibers of the serratus anterior muscle. The remaining parts of the muscle are innervated by the descending portion of the long thoracic nerve following its passage over the upper portion of the serratus anterior muscle. The long thoracic nerve is not vulnerable to entrapment within the serratus anterior muscle; however, branches from C5 and C6 (two of the nerve roots that form the long thoracic nerve) pass between the anterior and middle scalene muscle,[6] and the branches are therefore vulnerable to entrapment by TrP activity in the middle scalene muscle. Trauma to the long thoracic nerve may cause paralysis of the serratus anterior muscle that results in winging of the scapula (ie, the scapula does not remain stabilized snugly against the thoracic wall).

The serratus anterior muscle receives its vascular supply from the superior thoracic artery, lateral thoracic artery, and thoracodorsal artery.[1]

2.2. Function

The serratus anterior muscle is active during all upper extremity motions; however, it is most active during shoulder flexion and abduction due to its stabilizing effect on the scapula, and its contribution to upward rotation. This is particularly relevant for the upper part of the muscle since the middle part provides the scapular abduction, and the lower part contributes to upward rotation, abduction, and posterior tilting of the scapula.[7] When elevating the upper extremity, as with flexion and abduction, the scapula undergoes upward rotation, external rotation, and posterior tilting. As the serratus anterior muscle contracts to move the scapula laterally around the chest wall, the displacement is resisted by the lower fibers of the trapezius muscle. In order to achieve 180° of humeral elevation, the scapula must depress, adduct, and tilt posteriorly at end-range upward rotation.[8] These motions are coordinated by the serratus anterior muscle.

The superior portion of the serratus anterior muscle forms the main axis of rotation for the scapula, and the middle fibers draw the scapula forward.[4] The inferior fibers of the muscle upwardly rotate the scapula while maintaining scapular position against the thorax during upper extremity elevation.[4,9]

By abducting the scapula, the serratus anterior muscle protracts the shoulder girdle, as when the individual exerts effort to push an object forward. Thus, this muscle helps to stabilize the scapula against the posterior thorax during forward-pushing efforts.[9] With the upper extremity fixed against a surface, it displaces the thorax posteriorly during a push-up from the floor or during a push back from the wall.

Because of its contribution to scapular mechanics and stabilization, the serratus anterior muscle plays a large role

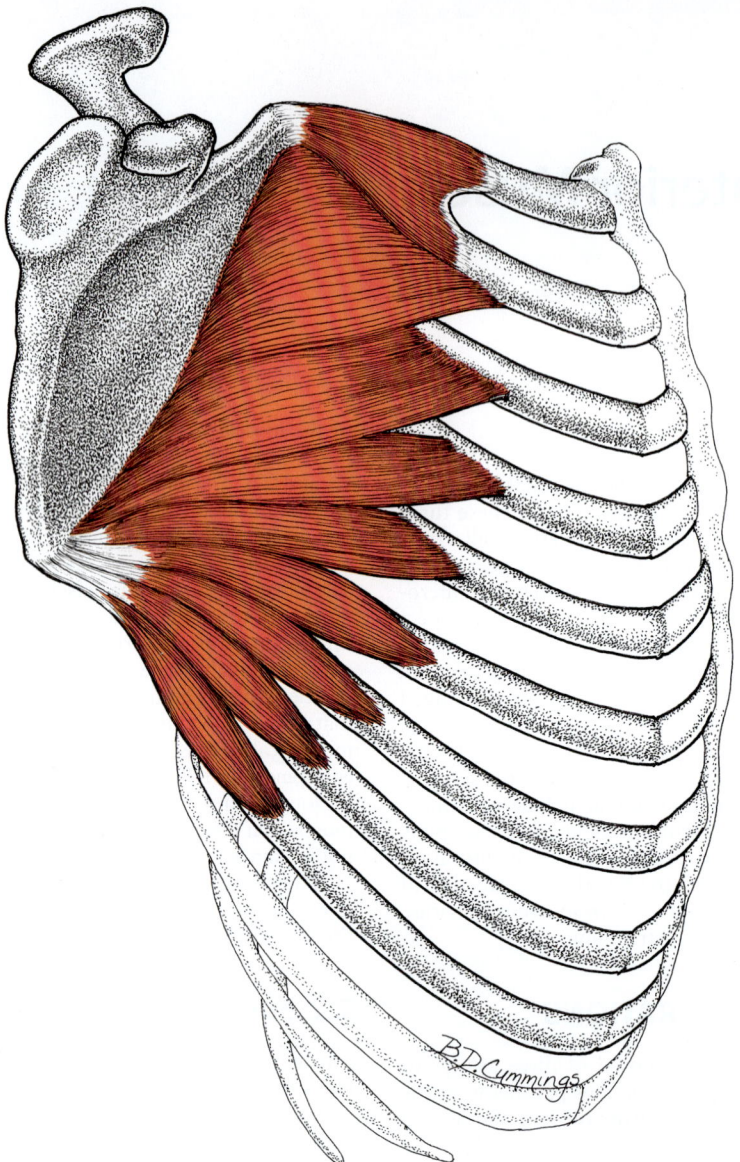

Figure 46-1. Attachments of the right serratus anterior muscle (*red*). The clavicle has been removed and the scapula rotated backward. The fibers of the muscle are divided into three groups and are identified by their fiber direction and the rib to which each digitation or segment attaches.

in overhead sporting activities. The serratus anterior muscle, in combination with the upper trapezius and anterior deltoid muscles, is active during the wind-up phase of the baseball pitch.[10] These muscles work together to upwardly rotate and elevate the scapula when the arm is brought overhead. As the pitching arm is lowered to the chest level, the serratus anterior muscle eccentrically contracts to control downward rotation of the scapula.[10] Additionally, electromyography (EMG) evidence demonstrates that maximum serratus anterior muscle contraction occurs during the cocking phase of the baseball pitch. Baseball pitchers with decreased activity from the serratus anterior muscle may be at an increased risk of subacromial pain syndrome and rotator cuff pathology due to a lack of scapular upward rotation, which may lead to misalignment of the scapula while the humerus is externally rotating and horizontally adducting.[10] Electrocardiogam analysis of the golf swing has also demonstrated moderate activity of the serratus anterior muscle in the lead arm during the take-away phase of the swing and of the trail arm in the acceleration and deceleration phases.[10]

The serratus anterior muscle illustrates a paradoxical situation that sometimes arises with regard to the effect of TrPs and their functional implications. Because of the increased tension caused by the taut bands, one would not expect winging of the scapula to be a symptom of TrPs in the serratus anterior muscle. However, TrPs can have some effects that are largely uninvestigated and poorly understood. Clinically, scapular winging can sometimes be relieved by inactivating serratus anterior TrPs. Weakness in this case could reflect a combination of reflex facilitation of antagonist muscles and inhibition of the serratus anterior muscle. Janda[11] identified this muscle as one prone to weakness and inhibition leading to biomechanical imbalance in the shoulder girdle. This muscle inhibition, if left untreated, may lead to poor scapular positioning with upper extremity movements and secondary impingement as well as rotator cuff tears.[3] In fact, athletes with shoulder and scapular dyskinesia exhibit weakness within the serratus anterior muscle that is associated with decreased upward rotation of the scapula.[12] Decreased muscle activation of the serratus anterior muscle is also found in non-athlete subjects with shoulder and scapular dyskinesia.[13]

2.3. Functional Unit

The functional unit to which a muscle belongs includes the muscles that reinforce and counter its actions as well as the joints that the muscle crosses. The interdependence of these structures is functionally reflected in the organization and neural connections of the sensory motor cortex. The functional unit is emphasized because the presence of a TrP in one muscle of the unit increases the likelihood that the other muscles of the unit will also develop TrPs. When inactivating TrPs in a muscle, one must be concerned about TrPs that may develop in muscles that are functionally interdependent. Box 46-1 grossly represents the functional unit of the serratus anterior muscle.[14]

3. CLINICAL PRESENTATION

3.1. Referred Pain Pattern

Trigger points in the serratus anterior muscle can refer pain to the anterolateral part of the chest, the inferior angle of the scapula, medial aspect of the arm, and into the palm and ring finger (Figure 46-2). Kelly[15] suggested that TrPs in the serratus anterior muscle should be considered as a source of symptoms when a patient reports pain anterolaterally at mid-chest level. Others suggested that serratus anterior TrPs are a common source of pain referral to the medial aspect of the arm, extending to the palm and ring finger.[16,17]

In some patients, TrPs in the serratus anterior muscle contribute to abnormal breast sensitivity, in combination with TrPs in the pectoralis major muscle,[18] which are usually responsible for this patient reported symptom. Trigger points in the serratus anterior muscle can be found in any fiber of the muscle; however, the posterior attachment of the muscle located along the underside of the medial border of the scapula is difficult, if not impossible to localize and treat.

3.2. Symptoms

Chest pain from serratus anterior TrPs may be present at rest, during respiration, or during functional activities. When the TrPs are latent, pain may be precipitated by deep breathing (ie, a "stitch in the side") while running. Similar pain may also arise from TrPs in the external abdominal oblique muscle, which interdigitates with the lowest group of serratus anterior fibers; or if the "stitch" is a little lower, it may result from diaphragm TrPs. A runner may press against, or squeeze, the painful area for relief in order to keep going; taking a few slow full breaths may also help. Patients report having difficulty finding a comfortable position at night and often are unable to lie on the affected side. In fact, chronic chest pain is a challenge for clinicians, and serratus anterior muscle pain is often overlooked. Vargas-Schaffer et al[19] described a case series where patients experienced a significant reduction in pain after injection of serratus anterior TrPs.

Patients with TrPs in the serratus anterior muscle may report that they are "short of breath" or that they "can't take a deep breath because it hurts." Although patients are likely to receive a cardiopulmonary work-up for dyspnea, at least part of the cause is reduced tidal volume due to restriction of chest expansion by pain or by increased tension caused by TrPs in the serratus anterior muscle. Serratus anterior TrPs can enhance the pain associated with myocardial infarction when the left serratus anterior muscle is affected. The enahnced referred pain from these TrPs has been relieved by inactivating the pectoral and serratus anterior TrPs on the left side.[20] Pain is rarely aggravated by the usual tests for range of motion at the shoulder but may result from a strong effort to protract the shoulder girdle, for example during a serratus anterior punch. Trigger points may alter muscle activation patterns altering scapulo-humeral rhythm in the shoulder girdle.

Additionally, following breast cancer surgery, women may experience symptoms that mimick neuropathic post-mastectomy pain, which can also be caused or exacerbated by TrPs in the serratus anterior muscle. Torres-Lacomba et al[21] found that 24% of 106 women who had undergone breast cancer surgery exhibited active TrPs in the serratus anterior muscle 1-year after surgery.

3.3. Patient Examination

After a thorough subjective examination, the clinician should make a detailed drawing representing the pain pattern that the patient has described. This depiction will assist in planning the physical examination and can be useful in monitoring the progression of the patient as symptoms improve or change. A patient's reports of chest pain should alert the clinician to perform a thorough review of the cardiovascular and pulmonary systems. Any concerns regarding the involvement of the cardiovascular or pulmonary systems as a source of symptoms should result in an immediate referral to the emergency room or a physician. For proper examination of the serratus anterior muscle, the clinician should observe shoulder girdle posture and scapula position, examine active and passive range of motion of the shoulder girdle, and observe muscle activation patterns and the scapulo-humeral rhythm. The clinician should note when and where pain occurs during testing motions.

Rounded shoulder posture and prominence of the superior border and spine of the scapula on the affected side can result from abduction and rotation of the scapula by restrictions in serratus anterior muscle fibers. Lee et al[22] observed that slouched sitting posture affects scapular movement, inducing a scapular dyskinesia during arm elevation leading to overactive scapular stabilizers, including the serratus anterior muscle. The patient with a unilateral rounded shoulder posture is similar to that seen when the pectoralis major or minor muscles develop unilateral TrPs, but the pectoralis major muscle is often nearly equally affected on both sides of the body. Some patients may show winging of the scapula due to TrP inhibition of the serratus anterior muscle and facilitation of its antagonists.

The clinician should observe the patient's rib cage movement during respiration. Active TrPs in the serratus anterior muscle inhibit expansion of the lower chest due to pain. Upon inspiration, the patient can expand the upper thoracic rib cage, but measurement of chest expansion around the lower margin of the rib cage is likely to show marked restriction. After inactivation of TrPs in the serratus anterior muscle, a smaller minimum and a larger maximum lower chest circumference should be observed. The resultant marked increase in volume of tidal air is associated with relief of respiratory pain and dyspnea. Also, in the patients who experience a feeling of "air hunger" associated with rapid shallow respirations, the respiratory cycles usually

---

Box 46-1 Functional unit of the serratus anterior muscle

Action	Synergists	Antagonist
Shoulder protraction	Pectoralis major Subclavius Pectoralis minor	Rhomboid major Rhomboid minor Middle trapezius
Scapular upward rotation	Trapezius (upper, lower fibers)	Rhomboid major Rhomboid minor Levator scapulae Latissimus dorsi

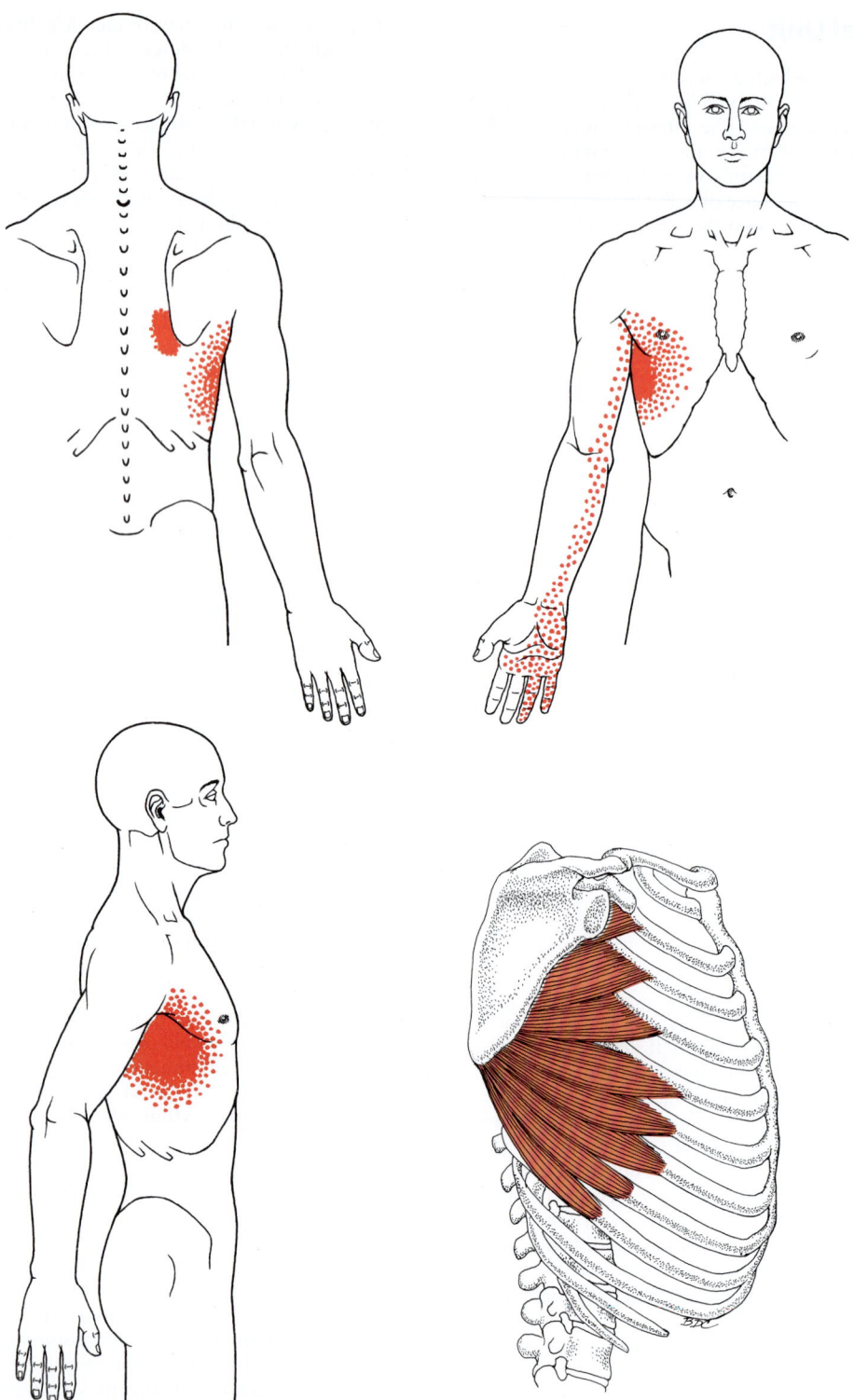

Figure 46-2. Referred pain pattern (essential areas *solid dark red*, spillover areas *stippled dark red*) from TrPs in the right serratus anterior muscle (*medium red*), as seen from the back, front, and side view. Trigger points in fibers covering the first two ribs can be difficult or nearly impossible to reach for examination.

revert to normal depth when all active serratus anterior TrPs have been inactivated.

Before treatment for serratus anterior TrPs, the patient is likely to underuse the diaphragm muscle and overuse the muscles of respiration in the neck, eg, scalene muscles. The diaphragmatic dysfunction and the reduced lower chest expansion appear to represent reflex inhibitory influences on respiration since the serratus anterior muscle is normally an accessory respiratory muscle for increased demand rather than a primary muscle of respiration along with the diaphragm and scalene muscles.

The clinician should stand behind the patient and observe scapular motion and scapulo-humeral rhythm while the patient performs shoulder flexion and elevation movements. Although the range of arm elevation may be within normal limits, scapulo-humeral rhythm and muscle activation can be disrupted by serratus anterior TrPs. Differences in scapular position, specifically tilt, between affected and unaffected shoulders in patients with shoulder pain are significantly associated with pain and disability and changes in serratus anterior muscle activity.[23] The presence of either active or latent TrPs in the shoulder girdle musculature, including the serratus anterior muscle, may provoke an inconsistent pattern of motor activation and control during shoulder motion.[24] Therefore, the presence of TrPs in upward scapular rotators can alter the muscle activation pattern during scapular plane elevation, potentially predisposing the patient to overuse conditions including impingement syndrome, rotator cuff pathology, and myofascial pain.[24]

The serratus anterior muscle should be tested directly for weakness or inhibition. Trigger points in the serratus anterior muscle may limit scapular range of adduction and the patient is likely to experience pain at the end of available movement, in contrast to the greater and pain-free range of motion on the uninvolved side. Subacromial pain syndrome can involve over-activation of the upper fibers of the trapezius muscle and a decrease in maximal activation of the serratus anterior muscle.[25]

The serratus anterior muscle can also exhibit over-activity, which is dysfunctional in patients who have undergone neck dissection surgery for cancer and whose surgical side demonstrated clinical signs of accessory nerve injury.[26] Therefore, it is important that clinicians conduct a complete clinical examination of the shoulder girdle in patients with suspicion of serratus anterior TrPs.

3.4. Trigger Point Examination

Due to its superficial position, parts of the serratus anterior muscle are easy to palpate. Trigger points can be located in the any of the muscle fibers of the muscle. Cross-fiber flat palpation is used to identify a taut band and TrPs. Since the serratus anterior muscle lies over the ribs, clinicians should differentiate between rib jumps and taut bands. Snapping palpation of the serratus anterior muscle can induce a local twitch response in the palpable taut band. For examination, the patient is side-lying, with the ipsilateral arm partly extended and the elbow bent (Figure 46-3). With the arm extended, the clinician locates the mid-axillary line, which is the optimal anatomic reference for palpation of TrPs in the serratus anterior muscle.

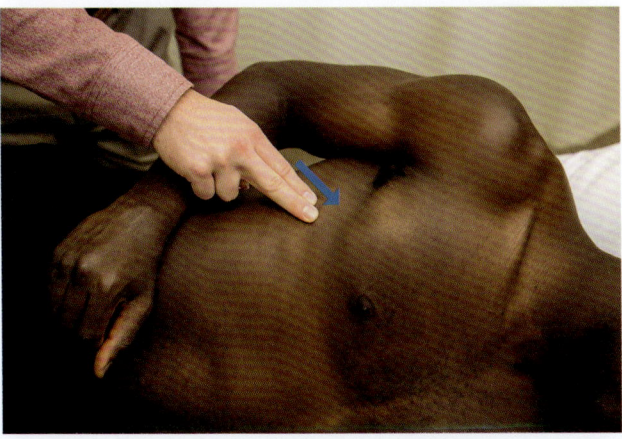

Figure 46-3. Cross-fiber flat palpation for TrPs in serratus anterior muscle.

4. DIFFERENTIAL DIAGNOSIS

4.1. Activation and Perpetuation of Trigger Points

In any part of the serratus anterior muscle, TrPs may be activated by unaccustomed eccentric loading, eccentric exercise in an unconditioned serratus anterior muscle, or maximal or sub-maximal concentric loading.[27] Trigger points may be also activated or aggravated when the muscle is placed in a shortened or lengthened position for an extended period of time.

Serratus anterior TrPs may be activated by muscle overload during excessively fast or prolonged running, push-ups, lifting heavy weights overhead, or strenuous coughing due to respiratory disease. Serratus anterior TrPs appear to be particularly vulnerable to torsional stresses, for example, when an automobile driver makes an abrupt forceful turn of a steering wheel in an attempt to avoid an accident or when the thorax rotates vigorously while the upper limb is in a fixed position.

Another cause of TrP activation in the serratus anterior muscle is surgery, particularly mastectomy for breast cancer[21] or any surgery involving the nine uppermost ribs.

4.2. Associated Trigger Points

Associated TrPs can develop in the referred pain areas of TrPs in another muscle.[28] Therefore, muscles in the referred pain areas for each involved muscle should also be considered for examination. The latissiumus dorsi, rhomboid major and minor, infraspinatus, corachobrachialis, biceps brachii, and flexor carpi ulnaris muscles should be examined for the presence of associated TrPs when the serratus anterior muscle is implicated.

Patients with TrPs in the serratus anterior muscle rarely have involvement of only this muscle. Pain from serratus anterior TrPs is most likely only responsible for producing one layer of the patient's symptoms. Muscles of the serratus anterior muscle's functional unit must be considered as possible contributors to the overall pain presentation since they may harbor associated TrPs. Inter-scapular pain that is predominantly unilateral usually involves some combinationn of TrPs in the ipsilateral upper and mid-thoracic paraspinal muscles, the rhomboid muscles, the middle fibers of the trapezius muscle, and possibly the serratus posterior superior and scalene muscles.

Other muscles that may experience overload due to shortening and reduced function of the serratus anterior muscle include the latissimus dorsi muscle, pectoralis minor muscle, and other accessory muscles of inspiration. These muscles may develop TrPs that remain latent for a long period of time. Muscles that can produce a "stitch in the side" (in addition to the serratus anterior muscle) are the diaphragm and the external abdominal oblique muscles.

4.3. Associated Pathology

Differential diagnosis of symptoms caused by TrPs in the serratus anterior muscle should include costochondritis, intercostal nerve entrapment, C7-C8 radicular pain or radiculopathy, and herpes zoster.

Referred pain to the chest from the serratus anterior muscle must be distinguished from a rib fracture or intercostal TrP. In one patient, the stress fracture of a rib was attributed to serratus anterior muscle tension.[29] Referred pain to the chest on the left side must be differentiated from symptoms of cardiac disease. The referred pain to the back from the serratus anterior muscle requires consideration of TrPs in the middle portion of the trapezius, rhomboid, and paraspinal muscles as well as visceral organs such as the pancreas.

Mid-thoracic articular dysfunctions can produce similar symptoms to those of the serratus anterior muscle. Scapular winging may arise due to damage to the long thoracic nerve, most commonly caused by a traction or compression injury.[30] Thus, if scapular winging is observed, the clinician must consider long thoracic nerve damage as well as a C7 radiculopathy as a potential cause of serratus anterior muscle weakness.

In the presence of serratus anterior TrPs, examination of the rib cage can sometimes reveal what appears to be elevation of ribs two through ribs eight or nine. Abnormal tension of the serratus anterior muscle alone can mimic an articular dysfunction of the ribs when, in fact, the apparent articular dysfunction is simply the result of the increased muscle tension caused by the serratus anterior TrPs. In that case, inactivation of the TrPs alleviates whatever apparent articular dysfunction is noted.

5. CORRECTIVE ACTIONS

Patients benefit from avoiding or modifing activities that are likely to activate TrPs in the serratus anterior muscle when possible. If activation of TrPs is due to respiratory disorders or upper respiratory infection, the patients can learn to gently clear the throat and to utlize protective bracing when deep coughing is necessary. Patients should be instructed in and encouraged to utilize diaphragmatic breathing. Sporting activities such as throwing, swimming, rock climbing, and golfing, as well as workout activities such as push-ups, heavy overhead lifting, and chinning should be avoided or modified as they all overload the serratus anterior muscle.

Patients with very irritable TrPs in the serratus anterior muscle are often unable to atttain a comfortable position for sleeping. Lying on the affected side is painful because of pressure on the TrPs, and lying on the other side can be painful as well if the arm of the affected side falls forward onto the bed, placing the muscle in a shortened position. The latter problem is remedied by use of a pillow to support the arm in front of the chest, and to keep it and the scapula from falling forward as illustrated in Figure 22-4A.

Serratus anterior TrPs can be self-treated with pressure release utilizing a tennis ball or other TrP release tools. Trigger point pressure release can be performed in a seated, side-lying, or standing position (Figure 46-4). A seated self-stretch of the muscle can also be used after self-release and to restore healthy function of the muscle. The patient stabilizes the scapula of the involved side by placing the ipsilateral arm behind the chair back. After taking in a deep breath, the patient exhales slowly and turns the thorax toward the contralateral side. In Figure 46-5 the patient rotates the thorax toward the left (turns the front of the chest toward the left) to stretch the right serratus anterior muscle.

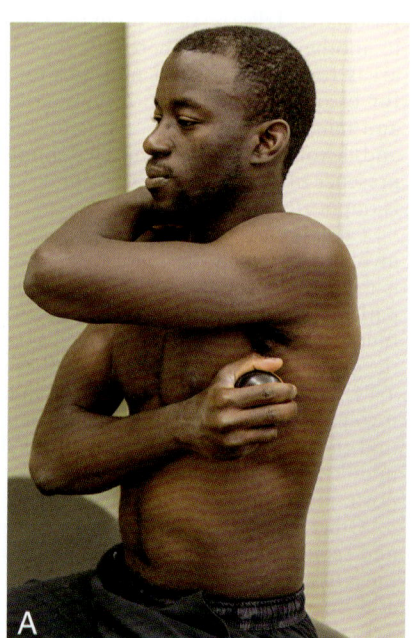
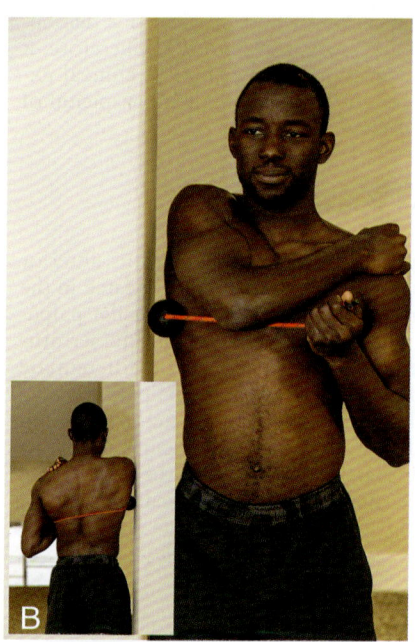
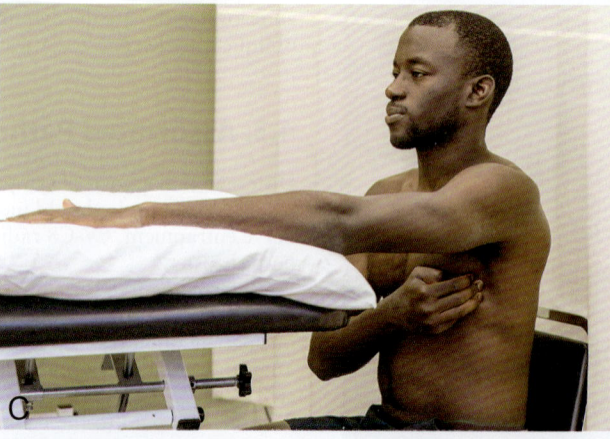

Figure 46-4. Self-pressure release. A and B, Using trigger point pressure release tool. C, Manual self-pressure release.

Chapter 46: Serratus Anterior Muscle

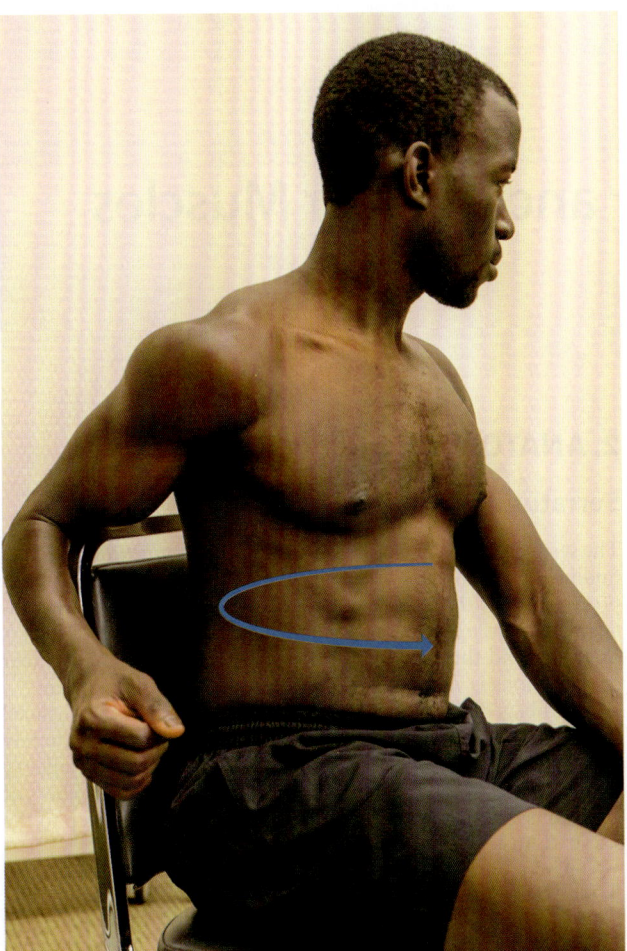

Figure 46-5. Serratus anterior muscle self-stretch.

References

1. Standring S. *Gray's Anatomy: The Anatomical Basis of Clinical Practice*. 41st ed. London, UK: Elsevier; 2015.
2. Webb AL, O'Sullivan E, Stokes M, Mottram S. A novel cadaveric study of the morphometry of the serratus anterior muscle: one part, two parts, three parts, four? *Anat Sci Int*. 2016. doi:10.1007/s12565-016-0379-1.
3. Kaur N, Bhanot K, Brody LT, Bridges J, Berry DC, Ode JJ. Effects of lower extremity and trunk muscles recruitment on serratus anterior muscle activation in healthy male adults. *Int J Sports Phys Ther*. 2014;9(7):924-937.
4. Nasu H, Yamaguchi K, Nimura A, Akita K. An anatomic study of structure and innervation of the serratus anterior muscle. *Surg Radiol Anat*. 2012;34(10):921-928.
5. Smith R Jr, Nyquist-Battie C, Clark M, Rains J. Anatomical characteristics of the upper serratus anterior: cadaver dissection. *J Orthop Sports Phys Ther*. 2003;33(8):449-454.
6. Yazar F, Kilic C, Acar HI, Candir N, Comert A. The long thoracic nerve: its origin, branches, and relationship to the middle scalene muscle. *Clin Anat*. 2009;22(4):476-480.
7. Hamada J, Igarashi E, Akita K, Mochizuki T. A cadaveric study of the serratus anterior muscle and the long thoracic nerve. *J Shoulder Elbow Surg*. 2008;17(5):790-794.
8. Ha SM, Kwon OY, Cynn HS, et al. Comparison of electromyographic activity of the lower trapezius and serratus anterior muscle in different arm-lifting scapular posterior tilt exercises. *Phys Ther Sport*. 2012;13(4):227-232.
9. Kim SH, Kwon OY, Kim SJ, Park KN, Choung SD, Weon JH. Serratus anterior muscle activation during knee push-up plus exercise performed on static stable, static unstable, and oscillating unstable surfaces in healthy subjects. *Phys Ther Sport*. 2014;15(1):20-25.
10. Escamilla RF, Andrews JR. Shoulder muscle recruitment patterns and related biomechanics during upper extremity sports. *Sports Med*. 2009;39(7):569-590.
11. Janda V. Chapter 6. Evaluation of muscular imbalance. In: Liebenson C, ed. *Rehabilitation of the Spine: A Practitioner's Guide*. Baltimore, MD: Williams & Wilkins; 1996:97-112.
12. Seitz AL, McClelland RI, Jones WJ, Jean RA, Kardouni JR. A comparison of change in 3d scapular kinematics with maximal contractions and force production with scapular muscle tests between asymptomatic overhead athletes with and without scapular dyskinesis. *Int J Sports Phys Ther*. 2015;10(3):309-318.
13. Huang TS, Ou HL, Huang CY, Lin JJ. Specific kinematics and associated muscle activation in individuals with scapular dyskinesis. *J Shoulder Elbow Surg*. 2015;24(8):1227-1234.
14. Simons DG, Travell J, Simons L. *Travell & Simon's Myofascial Pain and Dysfunction: The Trigger Point Manual*. Vol 1. 2nd ed. Baltimore, MD: Williams & Wilkins; 1999.
15. Kelly M. Pain in the chest: observations on the use of local anaesthesia in its investigation and treatment. *Med J Aust*. 1944;1:4-7.
16. Travell J, Rinzler SH. The myofascial genesis of pain. *Postgrad Med*. 1952;11(5):425-434.
17. Webber TD. Diagnosis and modification of headache and shoulder-arm-hand syndrome. *J Am Osteopath Assoc*. 1973;72(7):697-710.
18. Travell J. Referred pain from skeletal muscle; the pectoralis major syndrome of breast pain and soreness and the sternomastoid syndrome of headache and dizziness. *N Y State J Med*. 1955;55(3):331-340.
19. Vargas-Schaffer G, Nowakowsky M, Eghtesadi M, Cogan J. Ultrasound-guided trigger point injection for serratus anterior muscle pain syndrome: description of technique and case series. *A A Case Rep*. 2015;5(6):99-102.
20. Rinzler SH, Travell J. Therapy directed at the somatic component of cardiac pain. *Am Heart J*. 1948;35(2):248-268.
21. Torres Lacomba M, Mayoral del Moral O, Coperias Zazo JL, Gerwin RD, Goni AZ. Incidence of myofascial pain syndrome in breast cancer surgery: a prospective study. *Clin J Pain*. 2010;26(4):320-325.
22. Lee ST, Moon J, Lee SH, et al. Changes in activation of serratus anterior, trapezius and latissimus dorsi with slouched posture. *Ann Rehabil Med*. 2016;40(2):318-325.
23. Shamley D, Lascurain-Aguirrebena I, Oskrochi R. Clinical anatomy of the shoulder after treatment for breast cancer. *Clin Anat*. 2014;27(3):467-477.
24. Lucas KR, Rich PA, Polus BI. Muscle activation patterns in the scapular positioning muscles during loaded scapular plane elevation: the effects of latent myofascial trigger points. *Clin Biomech (Bristol, Avon)*. 2010;25(8):765-770.
25. Larsen CM, Sogaard K, Chreiteh SS, Holtermann A, Juul-Kristensen B. Neuromuscular control of scapula muscles during a voluntary task in subjects with subacromial impingement syndrome. A case-control study. *J Electromyogr Kinesiol*. 2013;23(5):1158-1165.
26. McGarvey AC, Osmotherly PG, Hoffman GR, Chiarelli PE. Scapular muscle exercises following neck dissection surgery for head and neck cancer: a comparative electromyographic study. *Phys Ther*. 2013;93(6):786-797.
27. Gerwin RD, Dommerholt J, Shah JP. An expansion of Simons' integrated hypothesis of trigger point formation. *Curr Pain Headache Rep*. 2004;8(6):468-475.
28. Hsieh YL, Kao MJ, Kuan TS, Chen SM, Chen JT, Hong CZ. Dry needling to a key myofascial trigger point may reduce the irritability of satellite MTrPs. *Am J Phys Med Rehabil*. 2007;86(5):397-403.
29. Mintz AC, Albano A, Reisdorff EJ, Choe KA, Lillegard W. Stress fracture of the first rib from serratus anterior tension: an unusual mechanism of injury. *Ann Emerg Med*. 1990;19(4):411-414.
30. Maire N, Abane L, Kempf JF, Clavert P; French Society for Shoulder and Elbow SOFEC. Long thoracic nerve release for scapular winging: clinical study of a continuous series of eight patients. *Orthop Traumatol Surg Res*. 2013;99(6 suppl):S329-S335.

Chapter 47

Serratus Posterior Superior and Inferior Muscles
"Nociception Initiator"

Joseph M. Donnelly and Jennifer L. Freeman

1. INTRODUCTION

The serratus posterior superior muscle is a thin muscle that lies beneath the rhomboid muscles and superficial to the splenii and erector spinae muscles and can be the cause of scapulocostal syndrome and upper extremity symptoms similar to thoracic outlet syndrome. It originates from the lower nuchal ligament, supraspinous ligament, and the spinous processes of C7-T3. It travels inferolaterally to attach to ribs two through five. It has been thought to function during respiration; however, there are no studies that support this notion. Its pain referral pattern is a deep ache below the scapula, proximal up to the cervical spine, and distal to the posterior arm, down to the forearm and hand in a C8-T1 distribution. Patients with serratus posterior superior trigger points (TrPs) may report interference with activities of daily living (ADLs), difficulty holding arms outstretched in front, and trouble sleeping on the affected side. The shoulder girdle and cervical spine should be examined when serratus posterior superior TrPs are suspected. Special attention should be given to the scalene muscles, pectoralis muscle length, scapular position, and any evidence of scapular dyskinesia. Real time ultrasound affords the clinician an opportunity to visualize this muscle and is recommended for TrP injection or dry needling treatment. Differential diagnosis should include scalene TrPs, thoracic outlet syndrome, C7-C8 radicular symptoms, olecranon bursitis, and ulnar neuropathy. Corrective actions should include instruction in proper posture and self-pressure release.

The serratus posterior inferior muscle can be a source of persistent flank pain when all other dysfunctions have been eliminated. It originates from the spinous processes of T11, T12 to L1-L2, and the thoracolumbar fascia. It travels superolaterally to attach to ribs 9 to 12. The function of this muscle has not yet been determined; however, recent research disputes its historically accepted role in respiration. The functional unit is more closely aligned with that of the iliocostalis and longissimus thoracis muscles, as well as the quadratus lumborum muscle. Pain from serratus posterior inferior TrPs is referred to the flank area of the trunk over the ribs and occasionally to the anterior aspect of the trunk. Patients typically report a pain that persists in the flank area following resolution of thoracolumbar musculoskeletal dysfunction. Examination should include postural assessment of the thoracolumbar spine and lower extremity. Somatic dysfunction of the sacroiliac joint should be ruled out. Trigger points may form in this muscle from activities that require prolonged extension and rotation of the trunk or from leg length discrepancy. Erector spinae TrPs and associated articular dysfunctions should be treated prior to addressing TrPs in the serratus posterior inferior muscle. Differential diagnosis should include ruling out renal diseases and lower thoracic radicular pain. Corrective actions include effective sleeping, standing, and sitting postures, along with self-pressure release techniques.

2. ANATOMIC CONSIDERATIONS

Serratus Posterior Superior

The serratus posterior superior muscle originates from the dorsal midline fascia, lower aspect of the nuchal ligament, the spinous processes of C7 through T2 or T3 and their respective supraspinous ligaments.[1] It slopes downward and laterally to the cranial borders of the second through the fifth ribs (Figure 47-1). The number of digitations is variable and the muscle is sometimes absent.[1]

The fibers of the serratus posterior superior muscle are inclined at approximately 45° to the horizontal and lie immediately beneath the fibers of the rhomboid muscles, nearly parallel to them (Figure 47-2). Paraspinally, the vertically aligned fibers of the longissimus thoracis and iliocostalis muscles lie deep to the serratus posterior superior muscle.[2]

Serratus Posterior Inferior

The serratus posterior inferior muscle originates from the thin aponeurosis of the spinous processes of T11,12 and L1-L3 and their respective supraspinous ligaments, and it blends with the lumbar portion of the thoracolumbar fascia.[1] Its fibers travel superolaterally and insert through four digitations to attach to ribs 9-12, just lateral to their angles[1] (Figure 47-3). The digitations to one or more ribs, especially to the ninth and 12th ribs, are sometimes missing. Occasionally, the entire muscle is absent.[1,3]

2.1. Innervation and Vascularization

Serratus Posterior Superior

The serratus posterior superior muscle is innervated by the second through fifth intercostal nerves, which are branches of the anterior primary rami of T2-T5.[1]

Serratus Posterior Inferior

The serratus posterior inferior muscle is innervated by the anterior primary divisions of spinal nerves[1] T9 through T12, unlike the erector spinae muscles which are innervated by the posterior divisions.

2.2. Function

Serratus Posterior Superior

The serratus posterior superior muscle, due to its anatomic alignment of fibers, is thought to raise the ribs to which it is attached, thereby expanding the chest and aiding inhalation; however, there are no electromyographic studies that have validated this assumption.[1,4]

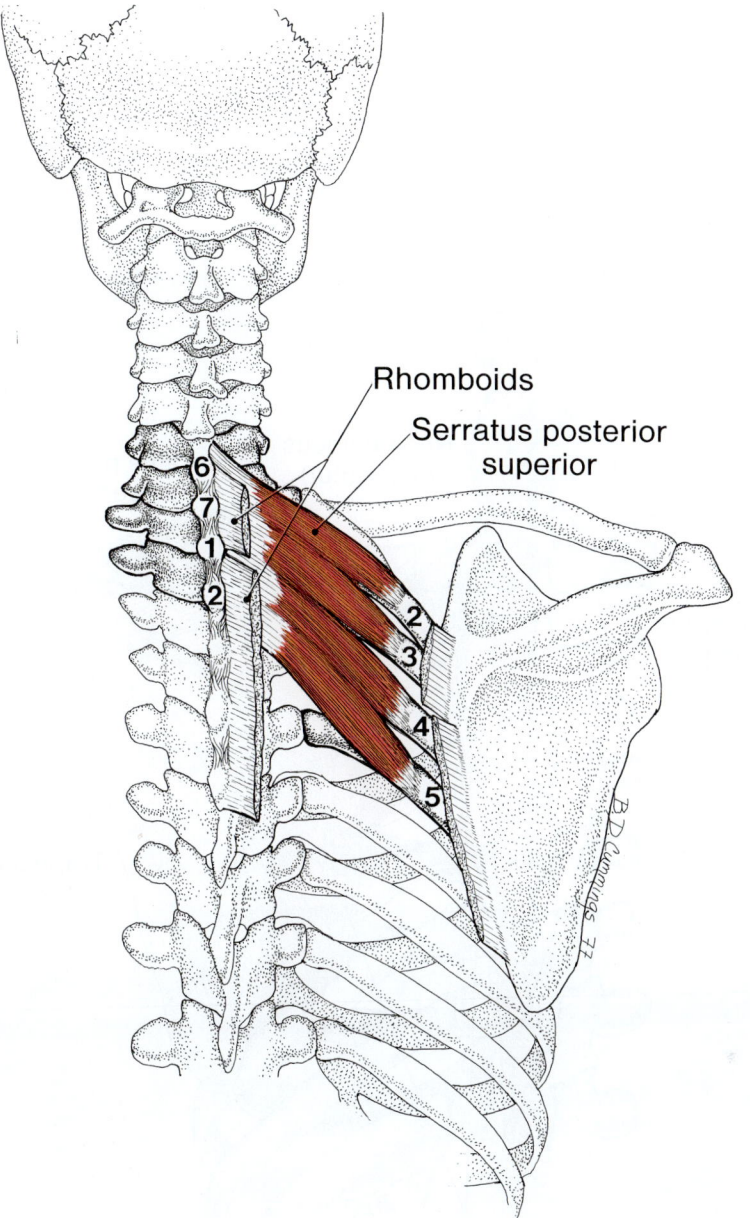

Figure 47-1. Attachments of the serratus posterior superior muscle (*red*) to numbered vertebrae and ribs.

Serratus Posterior Inferior

The serratus posterior inferior muscle attaches to the lower ribs, and due to its anatomic alignment, it has been described as an exhalation muscle or as functioning to pull the lower ribs downwards and backwards.[1] However, one older electromyographic study found no respiratory activity attributable to the muscle.[5]

The functions of the serratus posterior superior or inferior muscles have not been definitively determined in humans, and there is a paucity in the literature regarding their purpose. Vilensky et al[6] suggest that there is no evidence to support the role of the serratus posterior superior or inferior muscles in respiration. They conclude that the clinical importance of these muscles is their ability to generate pain, especially in the shoulder (scapulocostal syndrome) and flank. These muscles may have proprioceptive and postural functions, though to date, no research has been conducted to explore these theories.

In a study by Loukas et al[7] that compared cadavers with a history of chronic obstructive pulmonary disease (COPD) to those without, no difference in the morphology, topography, or morphometry of these muscles was found. Based on these results, the authors concur with Vilensky's[6] suggestion that the serratus posterior superior and inferior muscles do not have a respiratory function.[7]

2.3. Functional Unit

The functional unit to which a muscle belongs includes the muscles that reinforce and counter its actions as well as the joints that the muscle crosses. The interdependence of these structures is functionally reflected in the organization and neural connections of the sensory motor cortex. The functional unit is emphasized because the presence of a TrP in one muscle of the unit increases the likelihood that the other muscles of the unit will also develop TrPs. When inactivating TrPs in a muscle, one must be concerned about TrPs that may develop in muscles that are functionally interdependent.[2]

462 Section 5: Trunk and Pelvis Pain

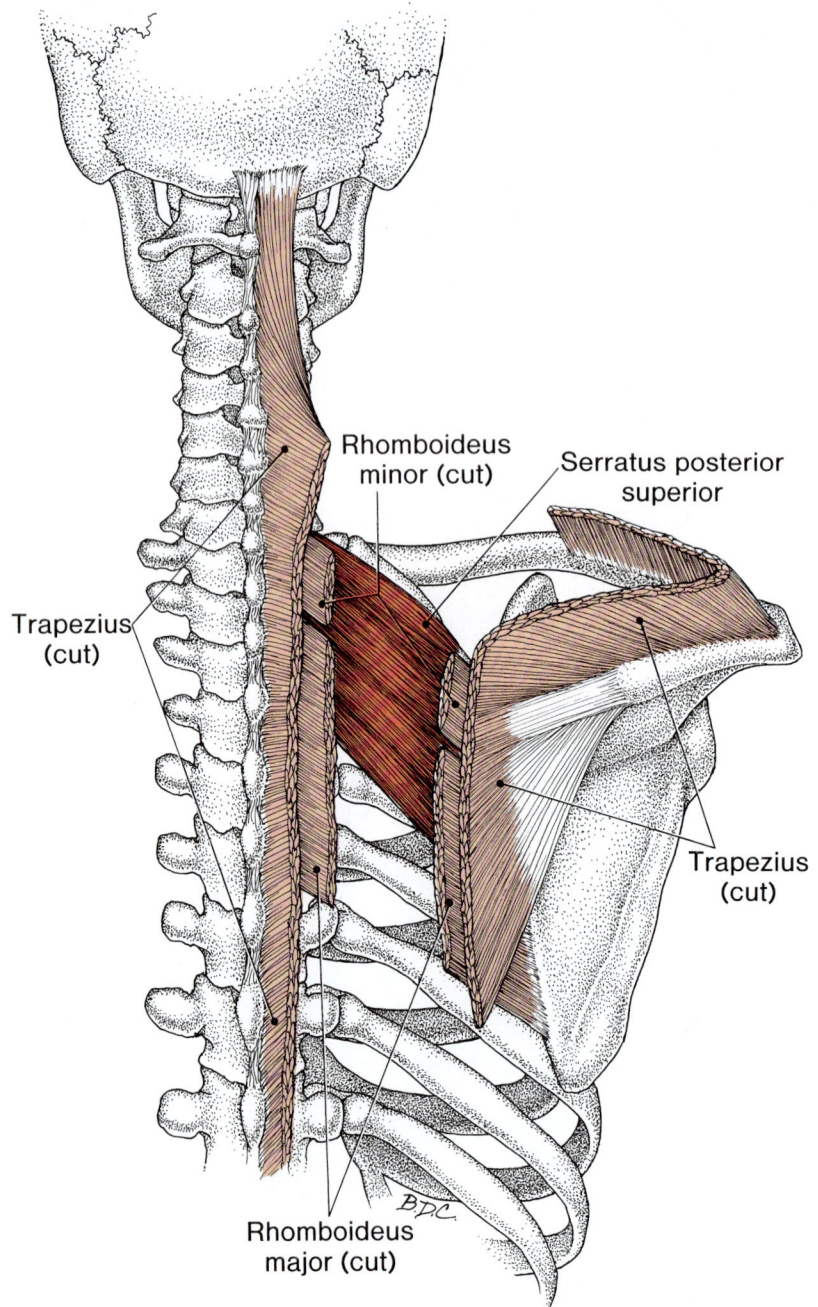

Figure 47-2. Anatomic relations of the serratus posterior superior muscle (*dark red*). The cut trapezius and rhomboid muscles (*light red*) lie over all of the serratus posterior superior muscle, and the iliocostalis and longissimus thoracis muscles (not shown) lie beneath part of this muscle.

Serratus Posterior Superior

If one considers the function of the serratus posterior superior muscle to be a muscle of inspiration then the diaphragm, intercostal, levator costae, and scalene muscles would act synergistically. Muscles of expiration would be considered as its antagonists in this scenario.

Serratus Posterior Inferior

The serratus posterior inferior muscle appears to act synergistically with the ipsilateral iliocostalis and longissimus thoracis muscles, unilaterally for rotation and bilaterally for extension of the spine. As an accessory muscle of exhalation, it would likely act synergistically with the quadratus lumborum muscle.

3. CLINICAL PRESENTATION

3.1. Referred Pain Pattern

Serratus Posterior Superior

The essential pain reference area of this muscle is a deep ache under the upper portion of the scapula (Figure 47-4A). This pain is perceived as deeper than the similar upper back pain that arises from the middle trapezius muscle. Pain is usually felt intensely over the posterior border of the deltoid and over the long head of the triceps brachii muscles.[8-10] It often covers the entire triceps brachii region with an accent on the olecranon process of the ulna and occasionally includes the ulnar side of the forearm, hand, and the entire fifth digit. Anteriorly, the pectoral region

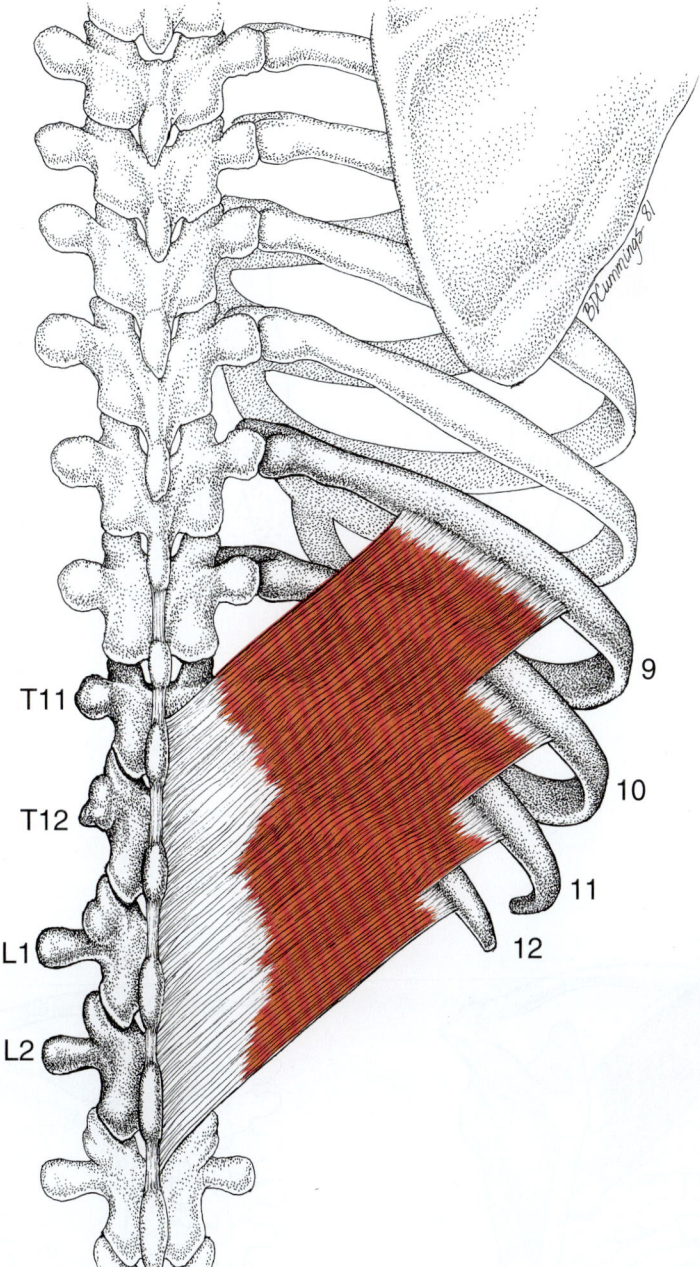

Figure 47-3. Attachments of the serratus posterior inferior muscle laterally to the lowest four ribs and medially to the aponeurosis extending from the spinous processes of the T11 to L2 vertebrae.

may occasionally be painful (Figure 47-4B). Trigger points in the serratus posterior superior muscle often cause numbness into the C8-T1 distribution of the hand.[11]

The most troublesome TrPs in the serratus posterior superior muscle are the ones that lie beneath the scapula. The problem occurs when the scapula compresses the sensitive region of enthesopathy against the underlying rib to which the muscle fibers attach. Among 76 painful shoulders in 58 patients, this muscle was a cause of pain in 98% and the single source of pain in 10%.[9]

Serratus Posterior Inferior

Trigger points in the serratus posterior inferior muscle produces aching discomfort over and around the muscle in the area commonly referred to the flank of the trunk (Figure 47-5). The pain extends across the back and over the lower ribs. Patients may identify this annoying ache as muscular in origin at the thoracolumbar junction. Occasionally, the pain is perceived as extending through the body to the chest.

3.2. Symptoms

Serratus Posterior Superior

The patient may report a deep steady ache under the scapula at rest and with ADLs. Little or no change in the intensity of pain occurs with unloaded movements. However, pain may be increased by lifting objects with outstretched hands or by other activities that cause the scapula to press against TrPs in the muscle, such as lying on the painful side. When asked to

464 Section 5: Trunk and Pelvis Pain

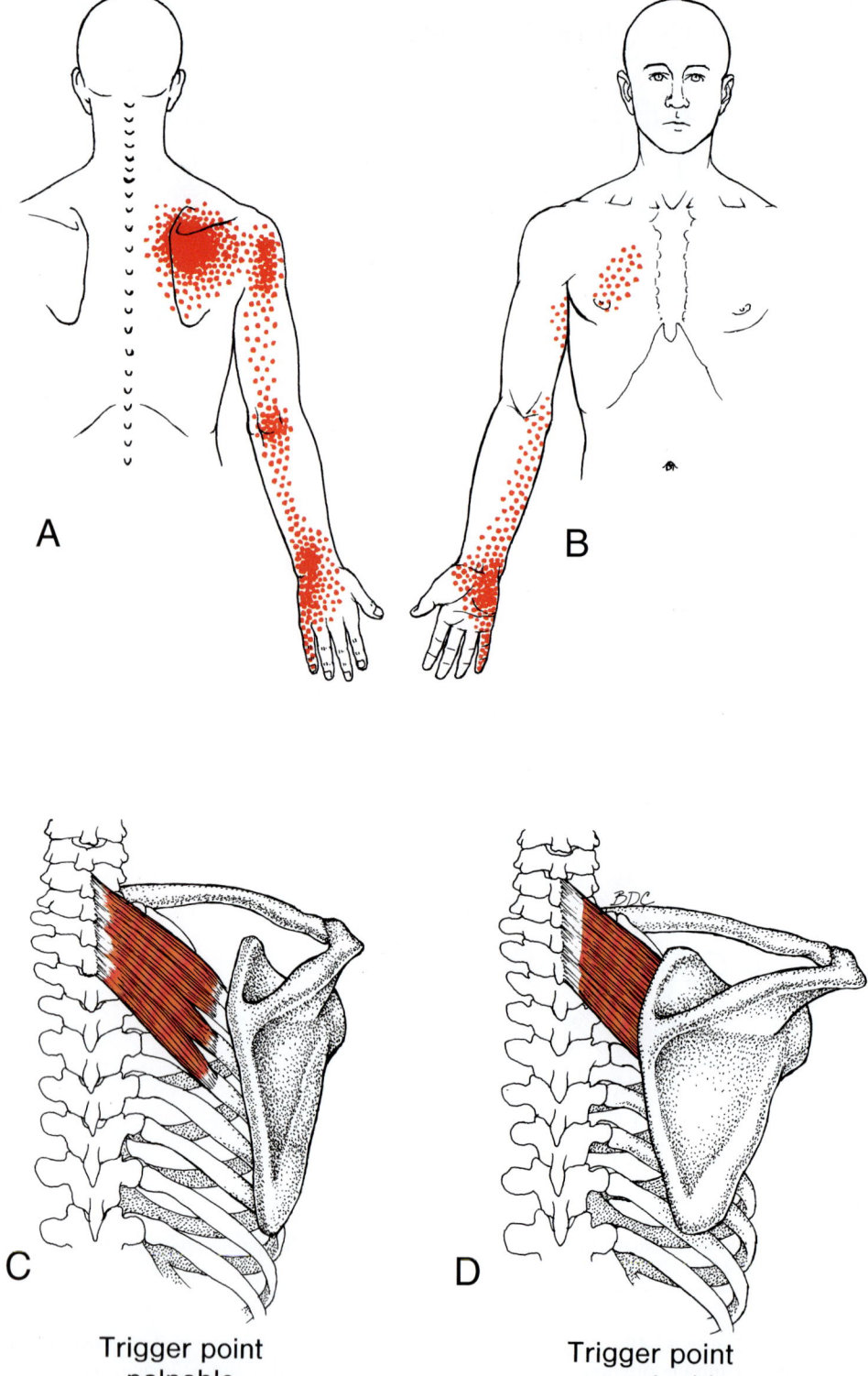

Figure 47-4. Referred pain pattern of a TrP in the right serratus posterior superior muscle. Essential pain is *solid red*, spillover pain is *stippled red*. A, Back view of pain pattern. B, Front view of pain pattern. C, Scapula abducted, making the muscle accessible to palpation and injection/dry needling. D, Scapula in resting position, partially covering the serratus posterior superior muscle.

point to the painful area, patients usually reach back with the opposite arm but are unable to touch the sore area because the shoulder blade covers it.

McCarthy et al[12] identified serratus posterior superior TrPs as a source of symptoms in a 43-year-old woman diagnosed with scapulocostal syndrome who presented with ongoing constant aching pain in the upper subscapular area, which radiated proximally to the cervical spine, and down the posterior aspect of the shoulder and ulnar aspect of the forearm into the fourth and fifth digits. Differential diagnostic tests were unremarkable and the patient failed to progress in physical therapy. The treatment included an ultrasound-guided TrP injection into

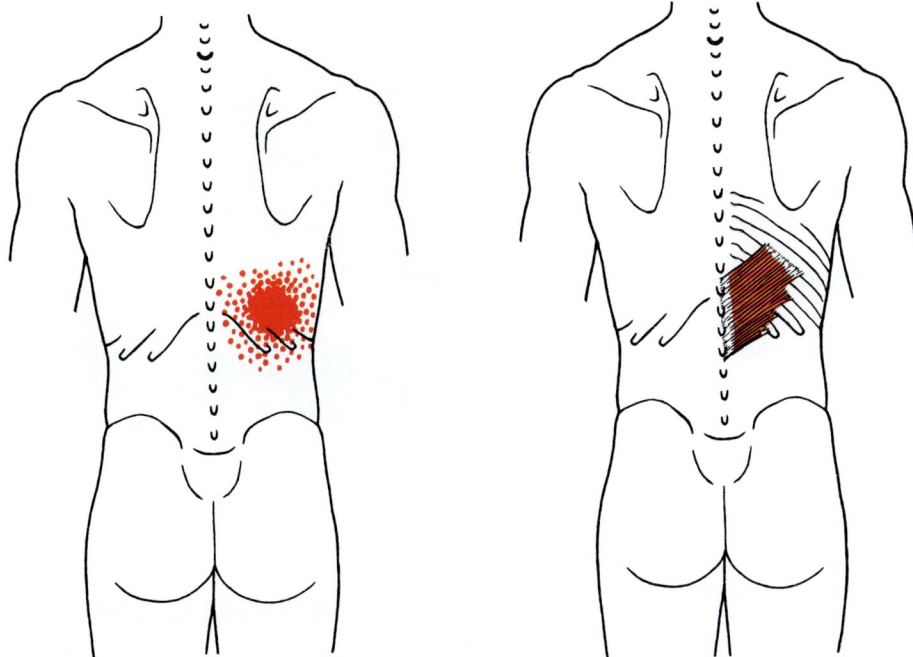

Figure 47-5. Referred pain pattern (essential zone is *solid dark red*, spillover zone is *stippled dark red*) of TrPs in the right serratus posterior inferior muscle (*light red*).

the serratus posterior superior TrPs. At both 30 minutes and 2 weeks post injection, the patient reported relief of her resting symptoms, and was able to perform ADLs including lying on the affected side without pain. The authors therefore conclude that ultrasound-guided TrP injection can confirm a diagnosis of scapulocostal syndrome and be therapeutically beneficial.[12,13]

Serratus Posterior Inferior

Patients may report pain in the flank area of the trunk especially when TrPs of associated major muscles of the back have been eliminated. A patient may be left with a nagging or "annoying" ache in the lower thoracolumbar region that is temporarily relieved with stretching. The onset of the symptoms may be related to activities such as working overhead on a ladder or activities that require combined trunk extension and ipsilateral rotation.

Maximal deep inhalation and coughing usually do not evoke pain from the serratus posterior inferior TrPs as they may from TrPs in the serratus anterior, quadratus lumborum, and deep abdominal wall muscles.

3.3. Patient Examination

After a thorough subjective examination the clinician should make a detailed drawing representing the pain pattern that the patient has described. This depiction will assist in planning the physical examination and can be useful in monitoring the progression of the patient as symptoms improve or change.

Serratus Posterior Superior

For proper examination of the serratus posterior superior muscle, the clinician should observe shoulder girdle posture and scapula position, examine active and passive range of motion of the shoulder girdle, and observe muscle activation patterns, including the scapulo-humeral rhythm. Cervical and thoracic spine active and passive range of motion should also be assessed. The clinician should note when and where pain occurs. When observing the patient from the rear, the clinician may note scapular position and asymmetries. The medial and inferior border of the scapula may be off the rib cage giving the appearance of a "winged scapula." This abnormal resting position will cause scapular dyskinesia during functional upper extremity movements and potentially, increased compression on the serratus posterior superior muscle. Pectoralis minor muscle length should be assessed especially when anterior tipping of the scapula is noted as this may also place abnormal compressive loading of the scapula on the serratus posterior superior muscle.

Accessory joint motion should be tested in the glenohumeral, acromioclavicular, sternoclavicular, and scapulo-thoracic joints, as well as the thoracic rib cage and cervicothoracic vertebrae. Oftentimes, joint hypomobility in the sternoclavicular joint or rib cage can cause impairment in shoulder elevation that contributes to alterations in the normal muscle activation patterns.

Symptoms from TrPs in the serratus posterior superior muscle must be differentiated from scalene TrPs as the pain referral pattern in the scapular region and upper extremity is very similar.

Patients with intrathoracic disease that compromises ventilation, such as emphysema, are in double trouble if they also develop TrPs in this serratus posterior superior muscle. These individuals generally do not exhibit rounded shoulder posture (as compared with those with rhomboid and pectoral muscle involvement), and they have little or no apparent restriction of movement. They often have scoliosis, especially the functional type that results from a leg length discrepancy or small hemipelvis.

Serratus Posterior Inferior

For proper examination of the serratus posterior inferior muscle, the clinician should observe spinal and lower extremity posture, examine active and passive range of motion of the thoracolumbar spine, and observe muscle activation patterns of the thoracolumbar region. The clinician should note when and where pain occurs. Patients may demonstrate slight restriction of thoracolumbar flexion and of spinal extension due to pain, and may be limited in rotating the torso away from the painful side.

Manual examination and palpation of this muscle may be the most definitive examination procedure performed by the clinician.

Accessory joint motion should be assessed in the lower thoracic and upper lumbar inter-vertebral segments, and the lower thoracic rib cage. Iliac crest motion palpation should also be performed due to the related function of the quadratus lumborum.

3.4. Trigger Point Examination

Serratus Posterior Superior

The patient sits and leans forward slightly, with the arm hanging forward and down on the side to be examined (Figure 47-6), or with the ipsilateral hand placed in the opposite axilla, to fully abduct the scapula.[9] The scapula must be abducted and pulled laterally to uncover the serratus posterior superior TrPs beneath the scapula (Figures 47-4C and 47-6). The serratus posterior superior muscle is palpated through the trapezius and rhomboid muscles (Figure 47-2). Cross-fiber flat palpation may elicit local twitch responses of TrPs in the overlying trapezius fibers, which can be identified because of the nearly horizontal orientation of those superficial fibers. However, local twitch responses in the deeper, obliquely oriented rhomboid and serratus posterior superior fibers are not so readily perceived, but may be palpable. Some authors do not believe this muscle can be palpated.[4]

A serratus posterior superior TrP is identified as a spot of deep tenderness when palpated against an underlying rib. It is unlikely that a taut band will be palpable through the two overlying muscles. When manual pressure on a TrP induces the characteristic serratus posterior superior referred pain pattern that the patient recognizes as familiar, it convinces them of the relationship between this TrP and the pain they experience.

Serratus Posterior Inferior

Trigger points in the serratus posterior inferior muscle may be difficult to palpate through, and distinguish from, the overlying latissimus dorsi muscle. However, the mid-fiber TrPs are usually identifiable utilizing a cross-fiber flat palpation technique (Figure 47-7). The TrPs at the lateral attachments of the muscle, close to the muscle's rib attachments, are also readily palpated. Local twitch responses are difficult to elicit and detect by cross-fiber flat palpation in this muscle but may be felt during TrP dry needling or injection.

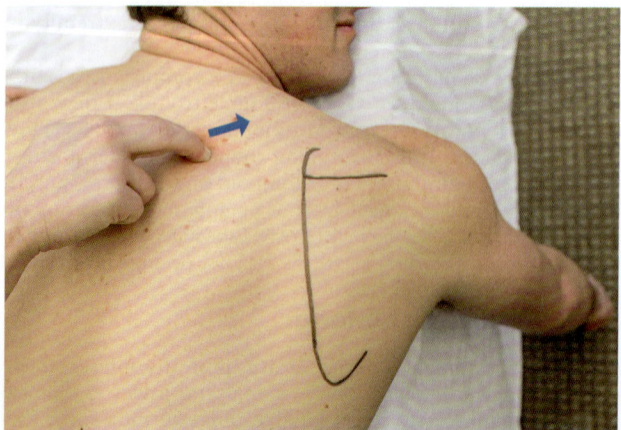

Figure 47-6. Palpation for TrPs in serratus posterior superior muscle using cross-fiber flat palpation. Patient in prone lying with arm off the edge of the table and scapula maximally protracted to gain access to the muscle deep to the rhomboids.

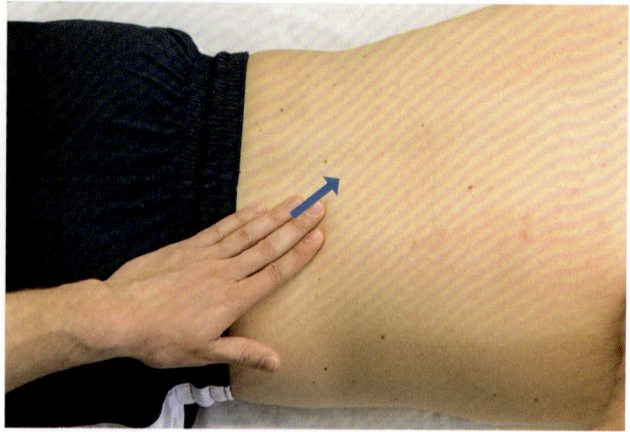

Figure 47-7. Palpation for TrPs in the serratus posterior inferior muscle using cross-fiber flat palpation.

4. DIFFERENTIAL DIAGNOSIS

4.1. Activation and Perpetuation of Trigger Points

In any part of the serratus posterior superior and inferior muscles, TrPs may be activated by compressive loading from the scapula, unaccustomed eccentric loading, eccentric exercise, or maximal or sub-maximal concentric loading.[14] Trigger points may also be activated or aggravated when the muscle is placed in a shortened or lengthened position for an extended period of time.

Serratus Posterior Superior

Movements and postures that stretch and overload the serratus posterior superior muscle may activate TrPs. These situations include prolonged computer use, utilizing an ergonomically inefficient workstation, prolonged overhead activities, repeated forward reaching, and protrusion of the thorax against the scapula by a structural or functional scoliosis.

Serratus Posterior Inferior

The serratus posterior inferior muscle is one of many back muscles that are susceptible to overload during the combined movement of lifting, turning, and reaching. Trigger points in the serratus posterior inferior muscle may develop due to mechanical overload or concurrently with TrPs in associated muscles. Standing on a ladder with the back hyperextended to work overhead may activate TrPs in this muscle, and paradoxical breathing or a leg length discrepancy may perpetuate them.

4.2. Associated Trigger Points

Associated TrPs can develop in the referred pain areas caused by TrPs.[15] Therefore, musculature in the referred pain areas for each muscle should also be considered.

Serratus Posterior Superior

Trigger points in the scalene muscles can induce associated TrPs in the serratus posterior superior muscle[16] and occasionally the relationship occurs in the reverse direction; the serratus posterior superior muscle can be the source of TrPs in the scalene muscles.

Trigger points in the serratus posterior superior muscle lie within the pain reference zone of the scalene muscles. The scalene TrPs may, in part, mimic the pain pattern of the serratus posterior superior muscle. The neck should always be examined for scalene TrPs if a TrP is found in the serratus posterior superior muscle. Other muscles that should be examined for associated TrPs include the rhomboid major and minor, iliocostalis and longissimus thoracis, multifidus, infraspinatus, posterior deltoid, triceps brachii, pectoralis major and minor, and flexor carpi ulnaris muscles as they are in the region of referred pain from the serratus posterior superior muscle.

Serratus Posterior Inferior

Trigger points in the iliocostalis and longissimus thoracis muscles, and in the multifidus muscle have pain referral patterns that overlap that of the serratus posterior inferior muscle and should be addressed prior to attempts to address TrPs in the serratus posterior inferior muscle. The specific area of discomfort associated with TrPs in this muscle is likely to be noticed only after successful treatment of symptoms arising from TrPs in associated muscles.

4.3. Associated Pathology

Serratus Posterior Superior

Differential diagnoses of symptoms caused by TrPs in the serratus posterior superior muscle includes thoracic outlet syndrome, C7-C8 radicular pain, olecranon bursitis, and ulnar neuropathy. The referred pain pattern of this muscle mimics the distribution of pain caused by eighth cervical root compression[17] and this diagnosis must be considered. Confusion is further aggravated by the referred numbness into the C8-T1 distribution of the hand,[11] which may cause a clinician to diagnosis the patient as having C8-T1 radiculopathy, when the symptoms are actually caused by TrPs in the serratus posterior superior muscle.

Fourie[18] described a scapulocostal syndrome associated with myofascial dysfunction. The pain and tenderness was caused by an enthesopathy of the lateral attachments of the serratus posterior superior digitations to the ribs. This syndrome can be diagnosed and managed clinically by utilizing ultrasound-guided TrP injection.[12]

Articular dysfunction associated with this muscle usually occurs at the T1 level. Exquisite tenderness is commonly noted directly over the spinous process of this segment. On inspection, this configuration of articular dysfunctions presents as a regional extension of the upper thoracic spine with inability to flex forward across the involved segments.

Serratus Posterior Inferior

Differential diagnoses of the symptoms caused by TrPs in this muscle include renal diseases (caliectasis, pyelonephritis, or ureteral reflux), and a lower thoracic radicular pain. The most common articular dysfunction associated with serratus posterior inferior TrPs is a neutral dysfunction extending from T10 to L2. Occasionally, one finds a concurrent depression or "exhalation" dysfunction of the lower four ribs.[19]

5. CORRECTIVE ACTIONS

Serratus Posterior Superior

The patient should maintain normal lumbar lordosis during both standing and sitting. When seated, this posture is facilitated by placing an appropriately sized lumbar pillow in the small of the back, then relaxing and leaning against the back of the chair so that the pillow maintains both the normal lumbar and thoracic curves without muscle strain. When sleeping, the patient must avoid compressive loading of the muscle by the shoulder blade. When lying on the back, the corner of the pillow should be tucked between the head and shoulder, not tucked under the shoulder (see Figure 7-5A). A pillow should also be placed between the axilla and chest wall supporting the upper arm so that the arm is in a neutral position. Allowing the arm to fall behind the body will place the pectoral muscles in a prolonged shortened position resulting in a compressive load on the serratus posterior superior muscle and aggravating the TrPs under the scapula (see Figure 22-4B).

It is very important that the patient uses coordinated diaphragmatic breathing, (see Figures 20-12 and 20-13) not paradoxical breathing, to minimize overload of the upper-chest muscles of inspiration, especially the scalene muscles.

While supine, the patient may find it possible to apply pressure release by lying on a tennis ball placed under the interscapular region or using a TrP release tool in sitting (Figure 47-8A), if the shoulder blade can wrap around the side sufficiently. As an alternate strategy, a companion may be taught to apply pressure release.

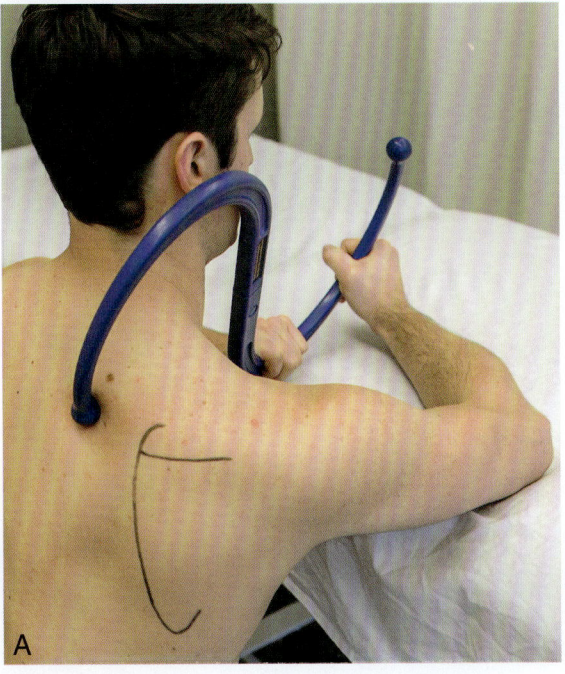
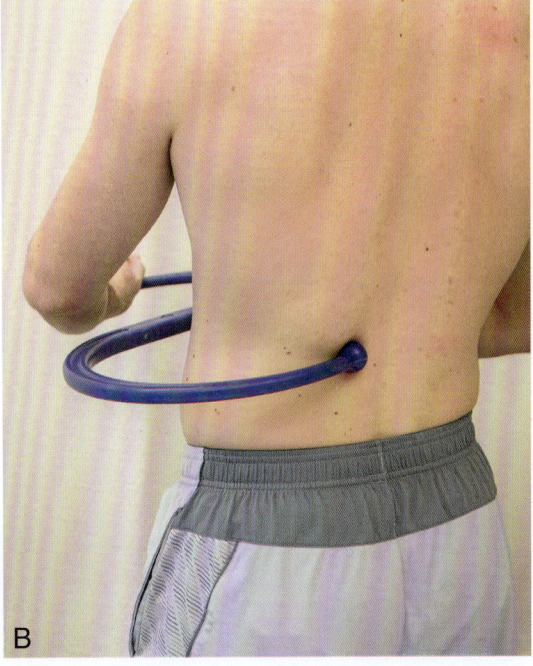

Figure 47-8. Self-pressure release of TrPs using TrP release tool. A, Serratus posterior superior muscle. B, Serratus posterior inferior muscle.

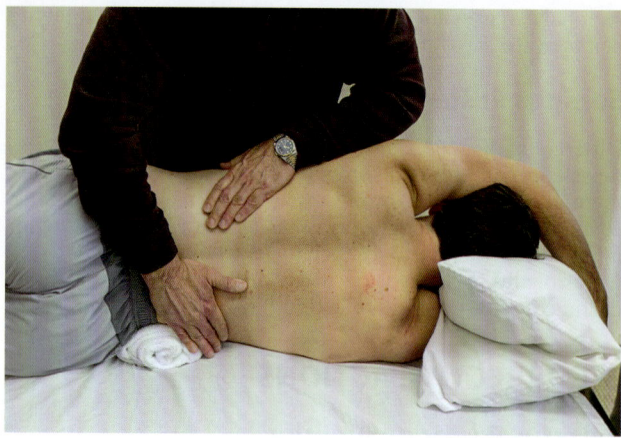

Figure 47-9. Manual stretch of the left serratus posterior inferior muscle. Patient lies on right side with left arm elevated.

Serratus Posterior Inferior

Many of the effective corrective actions for this muscle are covered in other chapters, including the use of lifts to correct the compensatory scoliosis caused by a small hemipelvis when sitting or by a leg length discrepancy when standing; normalization of paradoxical breathing (see Figures 20-12 and 20-13); sitting in well-fitted chairs with adequate lumbar support; standing with a normal lordotic lumbar curve; and sleeping on a firm mattress that supports the natural curves of the spine. Placing a pillow between the legs when sleeping on the side will also keep the spine in a neutral position, thus decreasing abnormal tension on these muscles.

A manual release technique with respiratory augmentation as described and illustrated in Figure 47-9 is recommended. Its effectiveness can often be augmented by post-isometric relaxation. The patient's ipsilateral arm is placed overhead to pull the rib cage upward and the to rotate the torso toward the opposite side to take up slack in the muscle. Similar to the serratus posterior superior muscle, the serratus posterior inferior muscle can also be treated in sitting or standing with a TrP release tool (Figure 47.8B).

References

1. Standring S. *Gray's Anatomy: The Anatomical Basis of Clinical Practice*. 41st ed. London, UK: Elsevier; 2015.
2. Simons DG, Travell J, Simons L. *Travell & Simon's Myofascial Pain and Dysfunction: The Trigger Point Manual*. Vol 1. 2nd ed. Baltimore, MD: Williams & Wilkins; 1999:900.
3. Eisler P. *Die Muskeln des Stammes*. Jena, Germany: Gustav Fischer; 1912.
4. Oatis C. *Kinesiology: The mechanics and Pathomechanics of Human Movement*. Baltimore, MD: Lippinott, Williams & Wilkins; 2009:164, 546.
5. Campbell EJ. Chapter 9. Accessory muscles. In: Campbell EJ, Agostoni E, Davis JN, eds. *The Respiratory Muscles*. 2nd ed. Philadelphia, PA: W.B. Saunders; 1970:181-195.
6. Vilensky JA, Baltes M, Weikel L, Fortin JD, Fourie LJ. Serratus posterior muscles: anatomy, clinical relevance, and function. *Clin Anat*. 2001;14(4):237-241.
7. Loukas M, Louis RG Jr, Wartmann CT, et al. An anatomic investigation of the serratus posterior superior and serratus posterior inferior muscles. *Surg Radiol Anat*. 2008;30(2):119-123.
8. Travell J. Basis for the multiple uses of local block of somatic trigger areas; procaine infiltration and ethyl chloride spray. *Miss Valley Med J*. 1949;71(1):13-21, 18.
9. Travell J, Rinzler SH, Herman M. Pain and disability of the shoulder and arm: treatment by intramuscular infiltration with procaine hydrochloride. *JAMA*. 1942;120:417-422, 418.
10. Travell J, Rinzler SH. Pain syndromes of the chest muscles; resemblance to effort angina and myocardial infarction, and relief by local block. *Can Med Assoc J*. 1948;59(4):333-338, 336.
11. Lynn P. Personal Communication. 1993.
12. McCarthy C, Harmon D. A technical report on ultrasound-guided scapulocostal syndrome injection. *Ir J Med Sci*. 2016;185(3):669-672.
13. Yang CS, Chen HC, Liang CC, et al. Sonographic measurements of the thickness of the soft tissues of the interscapular region in a population of normal young adults. *J Clin Ultrasound*. 2011;39(2):78-82.
14. Gerwin RD, Dommerholt J, Shah JP. An expansion of Simons' integrated hypothesis of trigger point formation. *Curr Pain Headache Rep*. 2004;8(6):468-475.
15. Hsieh YL, Kao MJ, Kuan TS, Chen SM, Chen JT, Hong CZ. Dry needling to a key myofascial trigger point may reduce the irritability of satellite MTrPs. *Am J Phys Med Rehabil*. 2007;86(5):397-403.
16. Hong C-Z. Considerations and recommendations regarding myofascial trigger point injection. *J Musculoskelet Pain*. 1994;2(1):29-59.
17. Reynolds MD. Myofascial trigger point syndromes in the practice of rheumatology. *Arch Phys Med Rehabil*. 1981;62(3):111-114.
18. Fourie LJ. The scapulocostal syndrome. *S Afr Med J*. 1991;79(12):721-724.
19. DeStefano L. *Greenman's Principles of Manual Medicine*. 5th ed. Philadelphia, PA: Wolters Kluwer; 2011:306-308.

Chapter 48

Thoracolumbar Paraspinal Muscles
"Ropey Rivals"

Michelle Finnegan, Margaret M. Gebhardt, and Jennifer L. Freeman

1. INTRODUCTION

The paraspinal muscles are comprised of two layers, a superficial layer of long-fibered extensors (erector spinae), and a deep layer of shorter, more diagonal extensor rotators (spinotransverse muscles). The erector spinae group is comprised of the spinalis, longissimus, and iliocostalis muscles. Within the erector spinae, the longissimus and iliocostalis muscles can be an important source of trigger point (TrP) pain. The spinotransverse group includes the rotatores, multifidus, and semispinalis muscles. Collectively, these back muscles have attachments to C7, the ribs, the thoracic and lumbar spine, and thoracolumbar fascia. They insert to various trunk landmarks including the ribs, lumbar spine, iliac crest, sacrum, and thoracolumbar aponeurosis. Innervation of the erector spinae muscles is provided by the lateral branches of the dorsal rami of the thoracic and lumbar spinal nerves, while the spinotransverse group is innervated by the medial branch of the dorsal rami of the appropriate spinal nerve. The primary functions of the thoracolumbar paraspinals are extension of the thoracic and lumbar spine and lateral trunk flexion. They also function eccentrically to control the trunk as it flexes forward. The iliocostalis muscle refers pain toward the shoulder, chest wall, scapula, abdomen, and down toward the lumbar region. The longissimus muscle refers pain to the lumbar region and buttock. The multifidus muscle refers pain to the region around the spinous process of the adjacent vertebrae, to the abdomen, coccyx, posterior thigh and leg, as well as the anterior thigh. A patient with TrPs in this muscle group will commonly report back pain and have difficulty bending forward. Activation and perpetuation of TrPs in the thoracolumbar paraspinals can result from prolonged awkward postures, quick bending and twisting of the spine, and a leg length discrepancy. Differential diagnosis includes visceral pathology, segmental joint dysfunction, fibromyalgia, radiculopathy, myositis ossificans, fibrodysplasia ossificans progressiva, and acute paraspinal compartment syndrome. Corrective actions should include postural reeducation, a focus on effective ergonomics, proper sleep positions, and elimination of positions and movements that cause recurrent overload on the muscle, self-pressure release of TrPs, and self-stretch exercises.

2. ANATOMIC CONSIDERATIONS

The anatomic complexity of the paraspinal muscles is simplified by classifying them into two layers, a superficial layer of long-fibered extensors (erector spinae) and a deep layer of shorter, more diagonal extensor rotators (spinotransverse muscles) (Figures 48-1 and 48-2). The erector spinae group consists of the spinalis, longissimus, and iliocostalis muscles. The spinotransverse group includes the rotatores, multifidus, and semispinalis muscles.[1] The validity of these traditional classifications is questionable, and recent morphologic evidence suggests that all the epaxial muscles may only be variations of just a few muscles.[2]

Superficial (Erector Spinae)

The erector spinae group is divided into the most medial spinalis muscles, the most lateral iliocostalis muscles, and the longissimus muscles in between. Each muscle may be further divided and discussed relative to the portion of the spine it spans. For example, the iliocostalis thoracis muscle spans a portion of the trunk generally inferior to the iliocostalis cervicis muscle and superior to the iliocostalis lumborum muscle, with some opportunities for overlap. Generally, the more superior components of each of these approximately vertically running muscles are also the most medially located when they overlap, eg, the longissimus capitis muscle is medial to the longissimus cervicis muscle, which is medial to the longissimus thoracis muscle. These classifications are helpful in understanding the anatomy of this complex set of muscles. However, because there is much convergence and interdigitation between them, as well as much morphologic similarity, considering actions and treatment of these muscles as larger functional groups is most effective.[1,2] See anatomy texts for further detail regarding these denominations and relationships. For more information on the superior portions of the erector spinae muscles, see Chapter 16.

The most medial muscle of the erector spinae group is the spinalis muscle. Although it can be absent or hard to distinguish in the cervical and lumbar regions, it is typically evident in the thoracic spine. The fascicles that comprise the spinalis thoracis muscle run from spinous process to spinous process of vertebrae throughout the thoracic spine with a varying number of segments bridged. Fibers from the spinalis muscle often blend with the adjacent longissimus muscle.[1]

The centrally located longissimus muscle is the largest of the erector spinae group (Figure 48-1). It typically has robust lumbar and thoracic components (these are named together as the "longissimus thoracis muscle") that receive the most clinical attention. The thoracic portion consists of fascicles with small, fusiform muscle bellies that have short rostral tendons and longer caudal tendons. As with all the erector spinae muscles, the bellies of the muscle are tiered, with the highest one being the most medial and the lowest one lying most laterally. The upper four fascicles arise from the tips of the first four thoracic transverse processes, whereas subsequent fascicles have bifid tendons that arise from the transverse process and the adjacent rib at each of the lower eight thoracic segments. The long caudal tendons are gathered in parallel to form a wide aponeurosis, allowing them a variety of caudal insertions. The tendons of the uppermost fascicles insert into the lumbar spinous processes and the supraspinous ligament. Those from the first thoracic segment reach the L1-L2 level, whereas fascicles from T6 reach the L5 level. Fascicles from T7-T9 reach the median crest of the sacrum, while whereas those from T10 and T11 attach to the posterior surface of the third segment of the sacrum. The fascicle from T12 attaches to the sacrum and dorsal segment of the iliac crest. The lumbar portion of the longissimus muscle

469

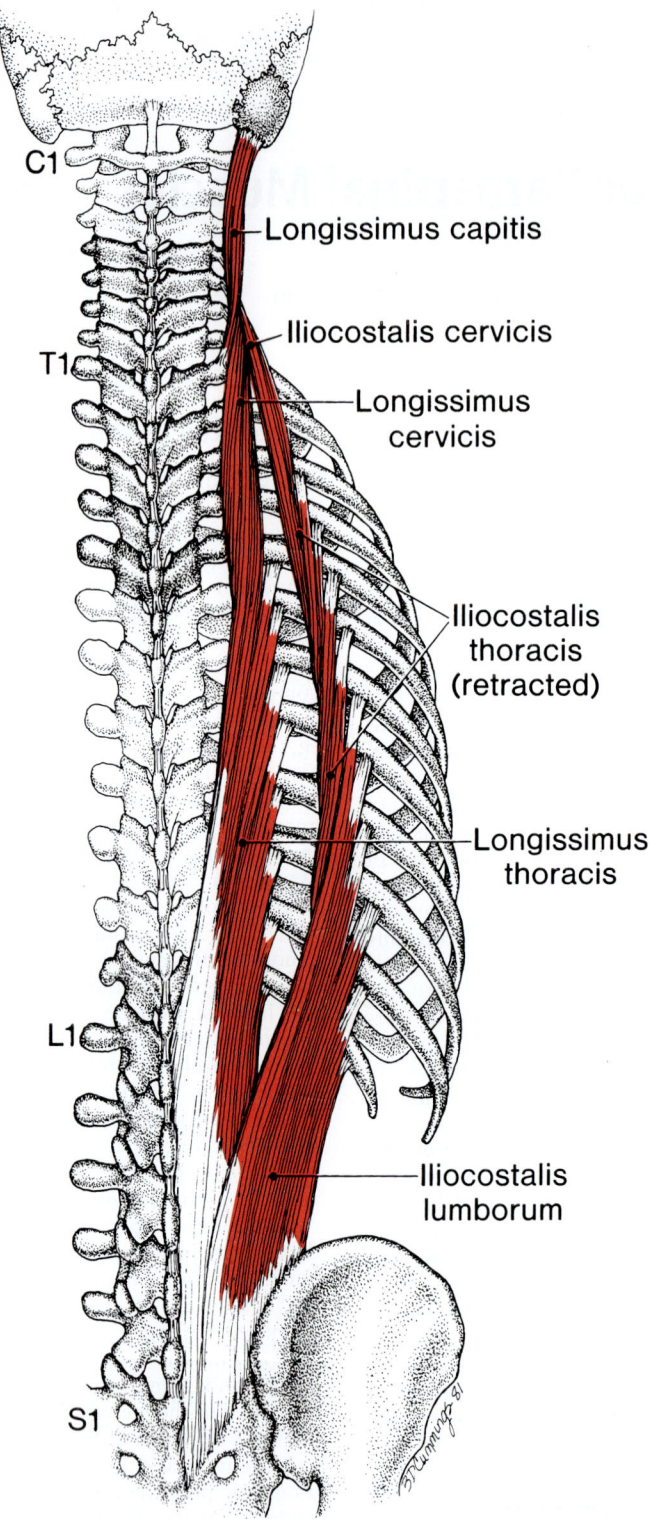

Figure 48-1. Attachments of the superficial (erector spinae muscle) group of paraspinal muscles (red): *medially* the longissimus thoracis muscle, and *laterally* the iliocostalis thoracis and iliocostalis lumborum muscles.

has bundles that arise from the accessory process and medial half of the posterior surface of the transverse process of each of the five lumbar vertebrae. The bundles from the first four lumbar segments converge onto a common flat tendon that covers the lateral surface of the muscle, separating it from the lumbar fibers of the iliocostalis muscle. The fascicle from L1 vertebra attaches rostrally and dorsally to the aponeurosis, whereas successive fascicles attach ventrally and caudally to the aponeurosis. The fascicle from the L5 vertebra inserts deep to the aponeurosis, into the anteromedial aspect of the ilium and upper fibers of the dorsal sacroiliac ligament.[1]

Generally, the iliocostalis muscle is located lateral to the longissimus muscle (Figure 48-1). The thoracic portion is comprised of eight to nine fascicles that arise respectively from the lower eight or nine ribs at their angles, just lateral to the iliocostalis cervicis muscle. The muscle bellies of the fascicles each give rise

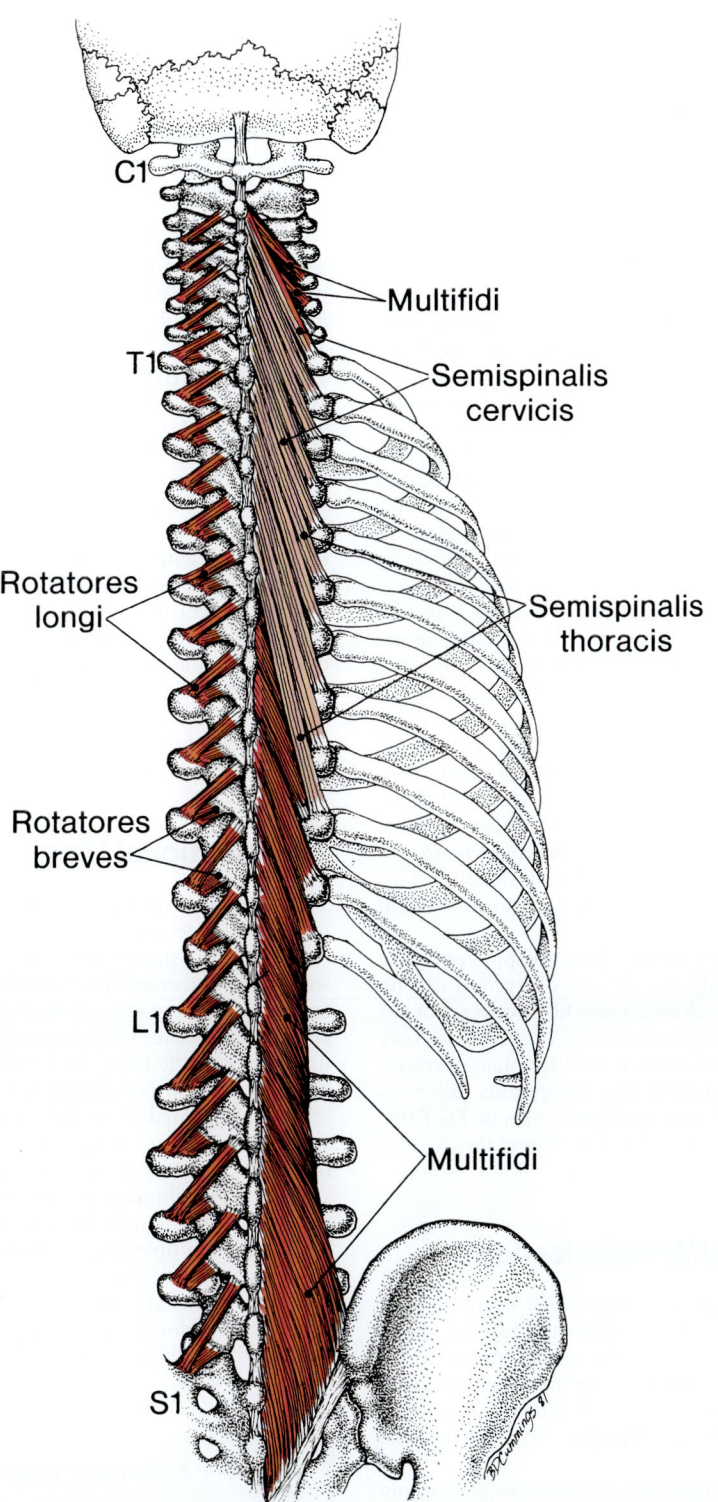

Figure 48-2. Attachments of the deep group of paraspinal muscles. Right, The more superficial of this group is the semispinalis thoracis muscle at the thoracic level (light red), which overlies the multifidi muscles, and the multifidi muscles at the thoracic, lumbar, and sacral levels (dark red). Left, The rotatores muscles form the deepest layer at both the thoracic and lumbar levels. The rotatores muscles occur above the sacral level. Only the multifidi muscles extend across sacral segments.

to a caudal tendon that together form a dorsal aponeurosis that covers the lumbar portion of the iliocostalis muscle and inserts into the medial end of the iliac rest and its dorsal segment.[1] The lumbar portion has fascicles that arise from the tips of the L1-L4 transverse processes and the thoracolumbar fascia, lateral to the tips. They travel inferiorly toward the ilium and insert into the medial end and dorsal segment of the iliac crest. The fascicle from L4 is the most ventral and lateral attachment while the fascicle from L1 is the most dorsal and medial attachment.

Deep Paraspinal (Spinotransverse)

The spinotransverse muscles are a group of muscles comprised of interconnected fascicles that run between spinous and transverse processes of vertebrae throughout the spine. Classical delineations have used different names to subclassify this group into three main categories based on the length of fascicles and proximity to the spine: the smallest and deepest being named the rotatores muscles, the longest and most superficial labeled the semispinalis muscle, and the multifidus muscle having a length and depth between the two. However, recent morphologic studies dispute these classifications on the basis of shared similarity in attachments, fiber alignment, fiber type of these muscles' fascicles, and a lack of separate epimysiums for each fascicle. Discussions of the spinotransverse muscle system may be better informed by an understanding that the categorization of these fascicles into separate muscles is purely nominal and does not represent a functional difference.[2]

The deepest and shortest fascicles of the spinotransverse muscle system (the rotatores muscles) span only one to two segments. There are typically 11 pairs of this type, with the first pair starting between the first and second thoracic vertebrae and the last ending between the 11th and 12th thoracic vertebrae. They connect the lamina and base of the spinous process above to the posterior aspect of the transverse process one to two levels below, respectively.[1]

The middle segments of the spinotransverse muscle system (the multifidus muscle) cover the lamina of the vertebrae in the thoracic and upper lumbar sections; however, at the lumbosacral levels, it expands to also cover the posterior surface of the sacrum. These fascicles typically span two to five segments. Several fascicles arise from the caudal edge of the lateral surface of the spinous process and from the caudal end of its tip, then travel inferiorly to insert into the transverse elements of vertebrae two, three, four, or five levels below. In the thoracic spine, this element is the posterior surface of the transverse processes and in the lumbar spine it is the mammillary processes.[1] This type of fascicle is generally thickest in the lumbar and sacral portions of the spine.

The longest and most superficial fascicles of the spinotransverse muscle group (the semispinalis muscle) are comprised of thin fibers with long tendons on each end. These fibers cover those of the shorter fascicles (the multifidus muscle). Traditionally, they are thought to have a capital, cervical, and thoracic portions, arising from as high as the occiput and the spinous processes of C2-T4 and insert into the transverse processes of T6-T10[1]; however, this layer of long fascicles has been found throughout the lumbar spine as well.[2]

2.1. Innervation and Vascularization

The erector spinae muscle group is innervated by the lateral branches of the dorsal rami of the thoracic and lumbar spinal nerves. At the lumbar levels, the lateral branches innervate the iliocostalis muscle, while the intermediate branches innervate the longissimus. The spinotransverse muscle group is innervated by the medial branches of the dorsal rami of the appropriate spinal nerves.[1]

The intrinsic muscles of the back receive vascular supply from several arteries including the superior intercostal artery via dorsal branches of the upper two posterior intercostal arteries, the posterior intercostal arteries of the lower nine spaces via dorsal branches of the subcostal arteries, dorsal branches of the lumbar arteries, dorsal branches of arteria lumbalis, and dorsal branches of the lateral sacral arteries.[1]

2.2. Function

Superficial Paraspinal (Erector Spinae)

The erector spinae muscles are strong extensors of the spinal column that more commonly act eccentrically than concentrically. Bilaterally, the muscles extend the thoracic and lumbar spine when firing concentrically. Unilaterally, the muscles laterally flex the trunk when firing concentrically. The erector spinae muscles on the contralateral side will eccentrically control lateral trunk motion and, when acting bilaterally, eccentrically control the trunk when bending forward. When fully flexed, most parts of the erector spinae muscles become electromyographically silent.[1]

In individuals with low back pain, the multifidus, paraspinals, external oblique, and rectus abdominis muscles have increased electromyogram (EMG) activity.[3] However, the increase in EMG activity in the paraspinal muscles of individuals with low back pain is not due to guarding; rather, it results from changes in motor control.[4,5]

Deep Paraspinal (Spinotransverse)

The spinotransverse muscles extend the vertebrae from which they arise. They are not able to rotate the spine because of the longitudinal orientation of the fibers.[1] Lee et al[6] found that the multifidus muscle in the thoracic spine is variably active with rotation in either or both directions, thereby contributing to control segmentally or through coupling of motions. The multifidus muscle can control intervertebral shear and torsion without generating torque.[7] It is also part of the feed forward activity during arm movements.[8,9] The lumbar multifidus muscle is activated more during the abdominal bracing maneuver versus the abdominal drawing-in maneuver.[10] The lumbar multifidus muscle is also more active with fast walking,[11,12] with the deep fibers of the multifidus muscle having a greater postural function than the superficial fibers.[12]

2.3. Functional Unit

The functional unit to which a muscle belongs includes the muscles that reinforce and counter its actions as well as the joints that the muscle crosses. The interdependence of these structures is functionally reflected in the organization and neural connections of the sensory motor cortex. The functional unit is emphasized because the presence of a TrP in one muscle of the unit increases the likelihood that the other muscles of the unit will also develop TrPs. When inactivating TrPs in a muscle, one must be concerned about TrPs that may develop in muscles that are functionally interdependent. Box 48-1 grossly represents the functional unit of the thoracolumbar paraspinal muscles.[13]

The thoracolumbar paraspinal muscles function not only to stabilize the spine but also to assist with force transmission. With their multiple angles of origin and insertion, as well as their fascial connections, the paraspinal muscles can work in concert with the abdominal (internal and external oblique and transversus abdominis muscles), latissimus dorsi, gluteal, rhomboid, and middle and lower trapezius muscles. They function

Box 48-1 Functional unit of the paraspinal muscles

Action	Synergists	Antagonists
Thoracic and lumbar extension	Quadratus lumborum, thoracolumbar paraspinals	Rectus abdominus, internal and external oblique
Lateral trunk flexion	Ipsilateral quadratus lumborum, ipsilateral thoracolumbar paraspinals	Contralateral quadratus lumborum, contralateral thoracolumbar paraspinals

to transfer load from the ground into the trunk and vice versa from overhead work. When functioning in a stabilizing role, the paraspinal muscles, along with the transverse abdominis muscle via the paraspinal fascia, assist with stability in the transverse plane.[14]

When there is breakdown in the kinetic chain from injury/trauma, muscle weakness or length/strength imbalances, inhibition, poor biomechanics of the upper or lower quarter, etc, the paraspinal muscles tend to overcompensate in the sagittal plane. They often compensate for weak hip extension or abdominal control when handling heavy loads or with repeated movements in this plane.

3. CLINICAL PRESENTATION

3.1. Referred Pain Pattern

Trigger points in the thoracolumbar paraspinal muscles are one of the most common causes of back pain (see Chapter 53 for more clinical considerations on causes of back pain). The referred pain patterns illustrated for these back muscles at specific segmental levels are common examples, but TrPs may develop at any segmental level.

Superficial Paraspinal (Erector Spinae)

In the thoracic spine, the two muscles that are most likely to develop TrPs are the longissimus thoracis and the iliocostalis thoracis muscles. The iliocostalis thoracis muscle refers pain both cephalad and caudad, while the longissimus thoracis muscle refers pain mainly caudad.[15]

The pattern of referred pain from TrPs in the iliocostalis thoracis muscle at the mid-thoracic level (Figure 48-3A) is up toward the shoulder and laterally to the chest wall. This pain could be mistaken for pleurisy on either side or cardiac angina if present only on the left.[16-18] At the lower thoracic level (Figure 48-3B), iliocostalis thoracis and lumborum TrPs may refer pain upward across the scapula, around to the abdomen, and downward over the lumbar area.[15,19] This pain referred to the abdomen may be mistaken for visceral pain.[18,20,21] Iliocostalis lumborum TrPs at the upper lumbar level (Figure 48-3C) refer pain strongly downward, concentrating on the mid-buttock, and is a frequent source of unilateral posterior hip pain.[15,21,22]

Trigger points in the lower thoracic level of the longissimus thoracis muscle (Figure 48-3D, on right of figure) refer pain strongly low in the buttock.[15,19] This remote source of buttock pain is easily and often overlooked. Longissimus thoracis TrPs in the most caudal portion of the muscle fibers, which are located in the upper lumbar area, usually refer pain several segments caudally but still within the lumbar region (Figure 48-3D, on left of figure).[15,19] This pain is another muscular source of "lumbago."

Kellgren mapped experimentally induced referred pain patterns of the erector spinae muscles by injecting hypertonic saline solution into normal muscles.[23] He reported that the superficial erector spinae muscles at the mid-lumbar level referred pain to the upper part of the buttock. In a similar study, hypertonic saline injection of the structures along the edge of the interspinous ligament at the L1 level referred pain characteristic of renal colic to the loin, inguinal, and scrotal areas, causing retraction of the testicle.[24] At the T9 level, the posteriorly injected hypertonic saline caused palpable rigidity and deep tenderness of the lowest part of the abdominal wall.[25]

Deep Paraspinal (Spinotransverse)

Although the semispinalis thoracis muscle is classified anatomically as the outermost (most superficial) of the deep paraspinal muscles, it is thought that its pain patterns correspond to those of the longissimus fibers at the same segmental level.

The next deeper layer of the deep group of paraspinal muscles, the multifidi muscles, refers pain primarily to the region around the spinous process of the vertebra adjacent to the TrP (Figure 48-4A). Multifidus TrPs located from L1 to L5 may also refer pain anteriorly to the abdomen, which is easily mistaken as visceral in origin (Figure 48-4B on the right).[15,19] The multifidus muscle at L5 can also refer to the posterior thigh and/or leg[23,26] and, less frequently, to the anterior thigh.[26] Multifidus TrPs at the S1 level project pain downward to the coccyx (Figure 48-4B) and render the coccyx hypersensitive to pressure (referred tenderness). The condition is often identified as coccydynia.

When Kellgren injected hypertonic saline experimentally into normal deep paraspinal muscles, he concluded that these deep muscles were more likely than the superficial group to refer pain anteriorly to the abdomen.[23] Pain patterns similar to those observed in adults were reported from TrPs in the longissimus and multifidus muscles of children.[27]

Involvement of the deepest paraspinal muscles, the rotatores muscles, throughout the length of the thoracolumbar spine produces midline pain and referred tenderness to tapping on the spinous process adjacent to a TrP. Only deep palpation of the muscles can determine from which side the midline pain arises. This spine tenderness is used as an osteopathic sign of articular-dysfunction involvement of that vertebra.

3.2. Symptoms

The chief report by patients with active TrPs in the thoracolumbar paraspinal muscles is pain in the back and sometimes in the buttock and abdomen. This pain markedly restricts spinal motion and the patient's activity. The patient will report pain with most spinal motions, especially when controlling forward motion of the trunk against gravity.

When the longissimus muscles are involved bilaterally, often at the L1 level, the patient has difficulty rising from a chair and climbing stairs if he or she faces forward in the usual manner.

When a patient has iliocostalis lumborum TrPs, the patient commonly draws an up-and-down pattern to represent the pain referred from iliocostalis TrPs but a crosswise pattern in the same region of the back to demonstrate the pain referred from TrPs in the lower rectus abdominus muscle.

When the report of "lumbago" is due to TrPs in the deep lumbar paraspinal muscles, patients report the pain usually is a unilateral, extremely aggravating, and steady ache deep in the spine. It becomes bilateral as the muscles on both sides become involved. The patient may point to a one-sided bulging of the long muscles of the lumbar spine. The patient finds little relief by changing position and is often convinced by the way it feels that the pain originates in the bony spine, not in the muscles.

3.3. Patient Examination

After a thorough subjective examination, the clinician should make a detailed drawing representing the pain pattern that the patient has described. This depiction will assist in planning the physical examination and can be useful in monitoring the progression of the patient as symptoms improve or change. The type, quality, and location of the pain should be carefully assessed, and standardized outcome tools should be utilized. A detailed medical screening is also necessary because there are several medical conditions in the cardiovascular, pulmonary, gastrointestinal, hepatic, and biliary and urologic systems that can present with similar types of pain presentations as those from the thoracolumbar paraspinal muscles.[28]

Observation of posture in standing should be carried out with attention to spinal curvature and lower extremity biomechanical alignment. It is important to incorporate assessment for functional and structural scoliosis, presence of a hemipelvis, iliac upslip,[29] and leg length discrepancy. The skin overlying

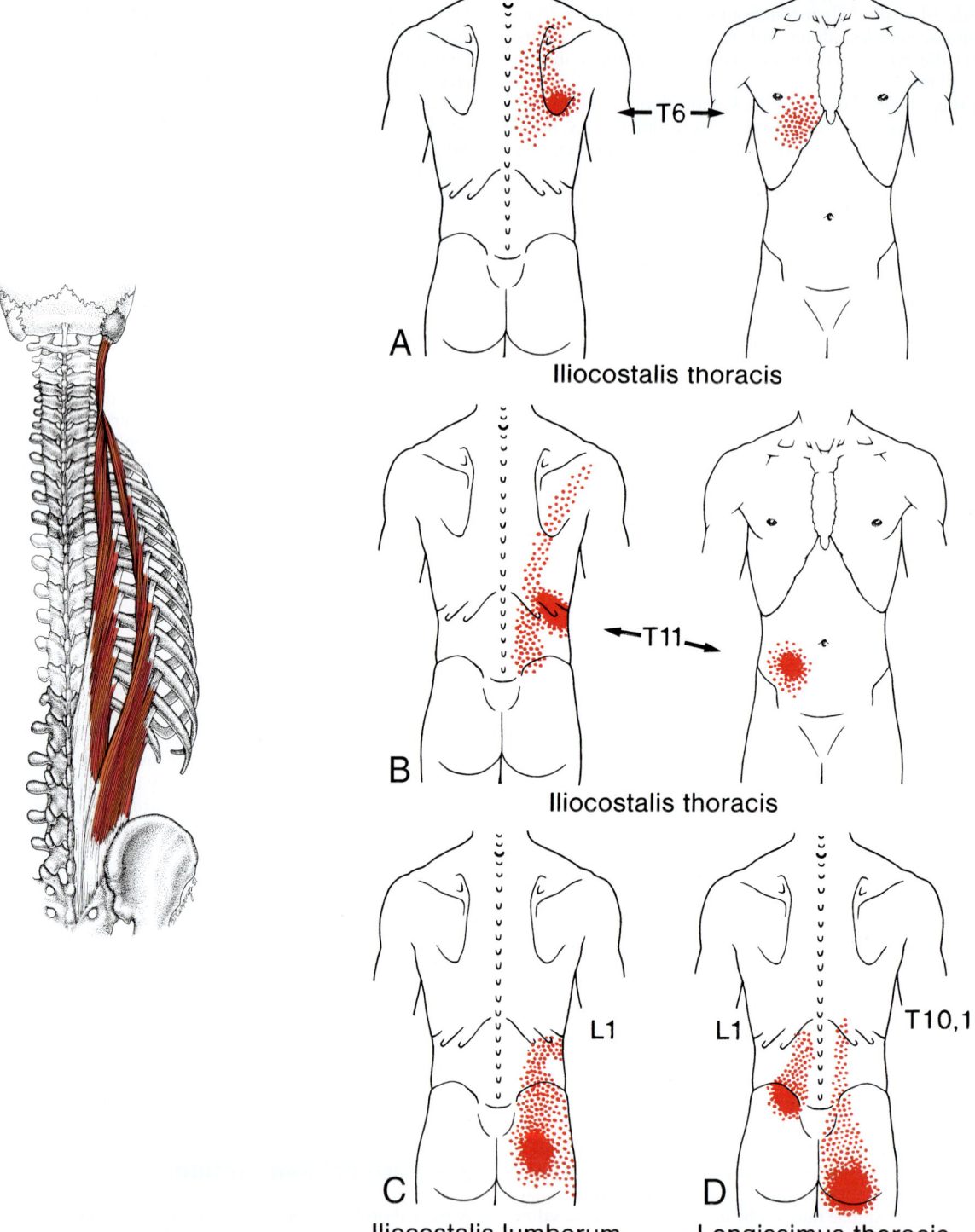

Figure 48-3. Examples of referred pain patterns (essential reference zones are solid red, spillover areas are stippled red) at several levels in the erector spinae muscles. A, The midlevel of the right iliocostalis thoracis muscle. B, The caudal portion of the right iliocostalis thoracis muscle. C, The upper end of the right iliocostalis lumborum muscle. D, The lower thoracic (right) and upper lumbar (left) longissimus thoracis muscles.

involved lumbar paraspinal muscles often exhibits superficial tenderness and resistance to skin rolling (panniculosis) or trophedema, which disappears after therapeutic skin rolling and inactivation of the underlying TrPs.[30,31]

Assessment for a leg length discrepancy is necessary because a difference of 0.6 cm (a quarter of an inch) can place strain on the thoracolumbar muscles. If a discrepancy is found, the corrective lift must be worn whenever the patient is on her feet. Additionally, assessment for a short pelvis (hemipelvis) should also be performed and appropriate corrections made if found. While the patient sits on a flat level wood seat (Figure 48-5B), pelvic tilt is estimated and corrected by placing enough pages or sheets of paper under the ischial tuberosity on the shorter side to level the pelvis exactly (Figure 48-5C). A hard surface requires less correction than a well-padded seat, because the softness of the seat allows the body to tilt to the short side. This shifts more weight to that side and

Chapter 48: Thoracolumbar Paraspinal Muscles 475

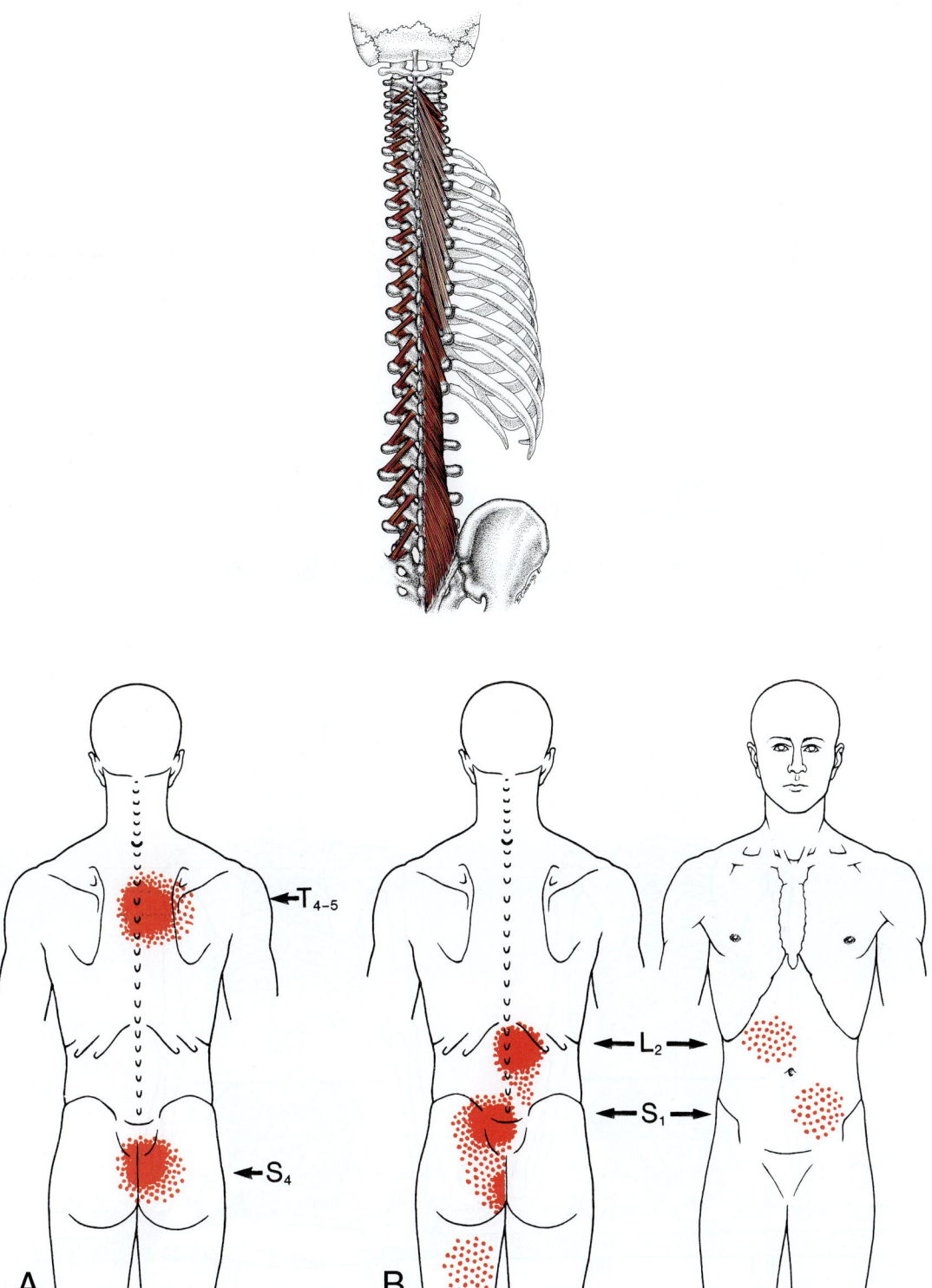

Figure 48-4. Referred pain patterns (red) from the deep paraspinal muscles. Pain referred by the rotatores muscles is felt essentially in the midline. A, Examples of local patterns characteristic of TrPs at the mid-thoracic level and in multifidi muscles at the low sacral level. B, Local and projected pain patterns of TrPs in these muscles at the intermediate L2 and S1 levels, respectively.

increases the pelvic tilt (Figure 48-5D). The patient may also try to compensate for a small hemipelvis by crossing one knee over the other to cantilever up the low side (Figure 48-5A).

Accessory joint motion should be tested in the thoracic spine, lumbar spine, sacroiliac joint, and thoracic rib cage because joint hypomobility is typically present with paraspinal muscle dysfunction. Additionally, sacroiliac and iliosacral movements should be assessed in the standing and seated position.[29] It is important for the clinician to consider the use of the sacroiliac joint special tests cluster developed by Laslett et al.[32] These tests have high clinical utility in identifying sacroiliac joint dysfunction. Clinically, we have found that in the presence of active TrPs in the deep paraspinal muscles, these provocative tests may be false positive due to peripheral sensitization.

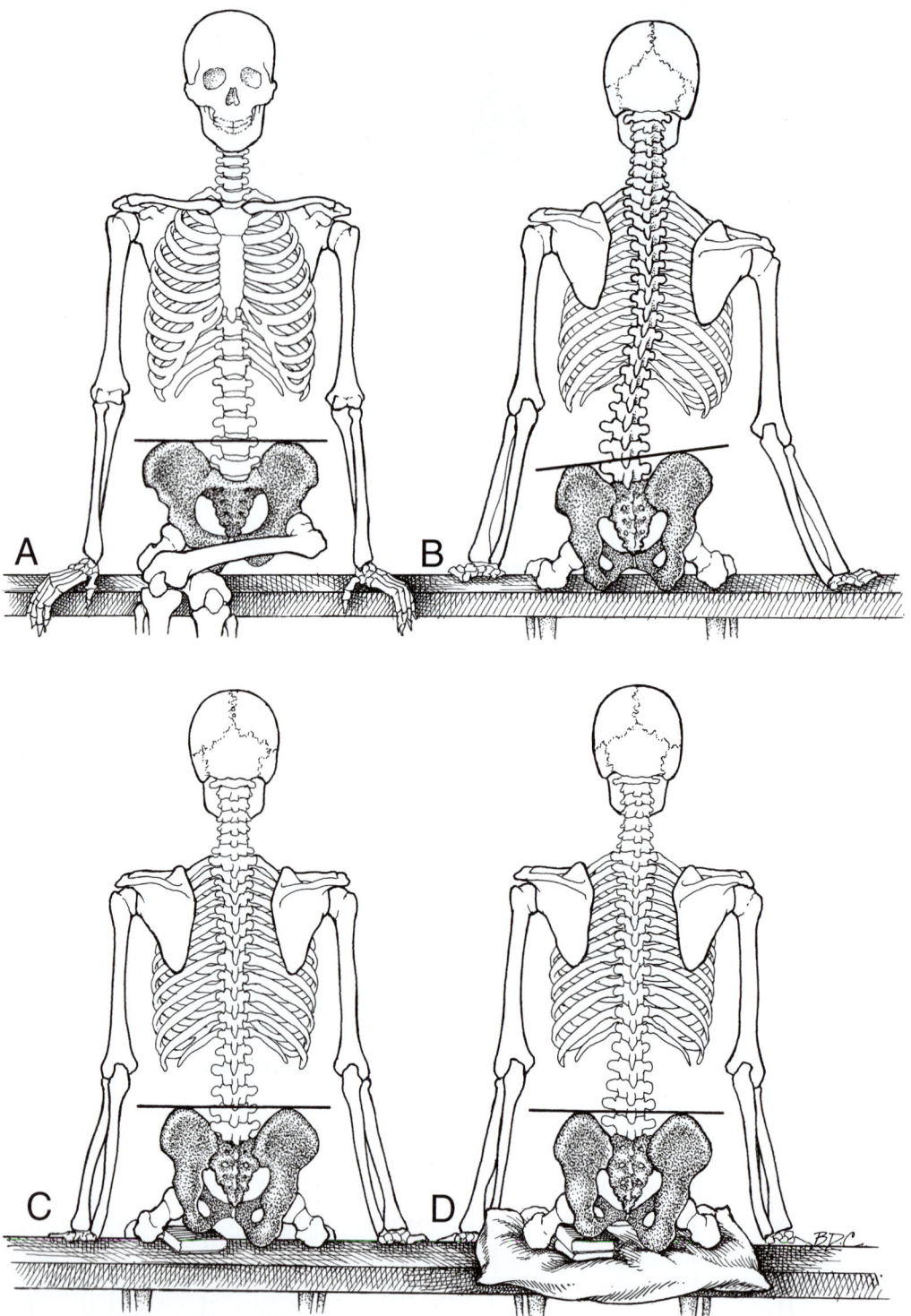

Figure 48-5. Effects of skeletal asymmetry due to a smaller left hemipelvis are demonstrated by sitting on a flat-level wood bench. A, Crossing the leg on the shorter side over the other knee helps level the pelvis. B, The tilted pelvis causes compensatory scoliosis, which tilts the shoulder-girdle axis. C, A small ischial lift levels the pelvis on a hard surface. D, On a soft cushioned surface, a thicker ischial lift is required to provide the same correction as that obtained on a hard surface.

Superficial Paraspinal (Erector Spinae)

Patients with nonspecific low back pain have increased numbers of latent TrPs compared with their healthy counterparts, and those with a greater number of active TrPs have a higher pain intensity. The most prevalent muscles involved include the iliocostalis lumborum, along with the quadratus lumborum, and gluteus medius muscles.[33]

Assessment of active range of motion of the lumbar spine in all planes will give clues of superficial paraspinal (erector spinae) muscle involvement. Frequently, range of motion will be limited in flexion to no more than a few degrees. Functional mobility assessment, as stated previously, will reveal difficulty with transitioning from sit to stand.

Deep Paraspinal (Spinotransverse)

Deep lumbar paraspinal TrPs are likely to occur in patients with either an excessive or absent lumbar lordosis, while deep thoracic paraspinal TrPs tend to occur in patients with marked thoracic kyphosis. Active range of motion testing will commonly be guarded and can restrict all motions of the lumbar spine, especially if involved bilaterally.

Trigger points in the spinotransverse muscles impair movement between two vertebrae during flexion or side bending of the spine. During flexion, a hollow or flat area develops in the smooth curve formed by the spinous processes. The flattening usually spans one to three vertebrae. Involvement of a multifidus muscle or a rotator muscle on either side produces midline tenderness over the adjacent spinous process. This tenderness is easily located by tapping each spinous process in succession. Tenderness disappears after inactivation of the responsible TrPs, which may be located on either or both sides of the spine. Dry needling to the lumbar multifidus muscle has been shown to improve nociceptive sensitivity and increase the contraction of the multifidus muscle.[34]

3.4. Trigger Point Examination

Superficial Paraspinal (Erector Spinae)

Palpation of specific paraspinal muscles is less effective with the patient in standing because of postural muscle tension and protective splinting by normal muscles. The clinician must obtain relaxation of the patient's back muscles so that abnormally taut muscle fibers are distinguishable.

Historically, the reliability of palpating for TrPs in the muscles of the lumbar spine has been accepted as generally poor,[35-37] although it may be minimally improved with modified criteria.[37] These findings are not consistent with more recent studies looking at the reliability of identifying TrPs in muscles in other body regions.[38-42]

To assess the superficial paraspinal (erector spinae) muscles, the patient should be placed in prone (with a pillow under the trunk as needed) and the arms resting comfortably (Figure 48-6A and B). If the patient is unable to lie in prone, the patient can be placed in side-lying with the spine supported in neutral alignment. A small towel roll may be needed to keep the spine aligned (Figure 48-6C and D).

The longissimus thoracis, iliocostalis thoracis, and lumbar iliocostalis muscles are palpated with a cross-fiber flat palpation. The longissimus thoracis muscle is identified by finding the "hill" muscle that is just lateral to the spinous processes on each side (Figure 48-6A). This muscle is frequently "ropey" in nature; therefore, it is essential to compare bilaterally and several segments above and below to ensure proper identification of a TrP. The thoracic iliocostalis muscle is a thinner muscle, lateral to the longissimus thoracis muscle, travelling along the rib angles. The more caudal portion of the muscle travels medially to blend with the iliocostalis lumborum muscle. The iliocostalis lumborum muscle is the "hill" muscle in the lumbar spine, just lateral to the spinous processes (Figure 48-6B).

Deep Paraspinal (Spinotransverse)

With the patient positioned as described above, the clinician taps or presses on the tips of successive spinous processes to elicit tenderness. When a spinous process in the flatter area

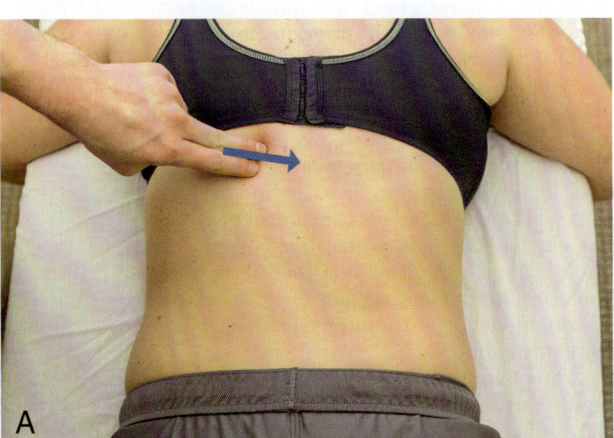
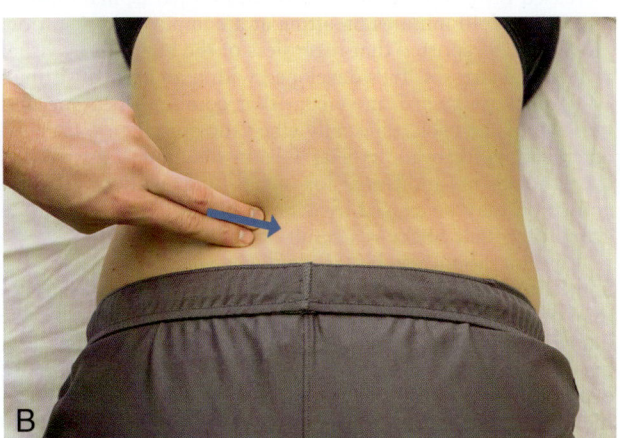
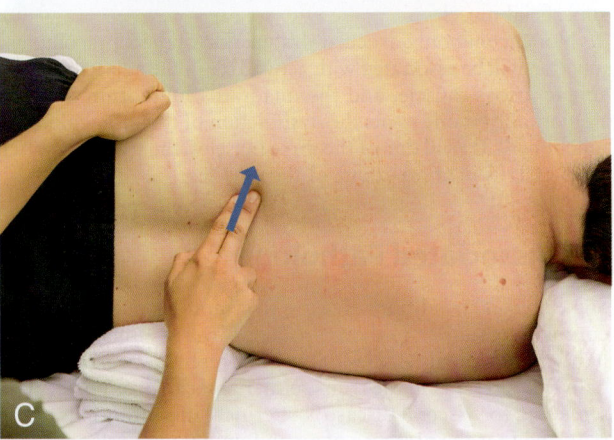
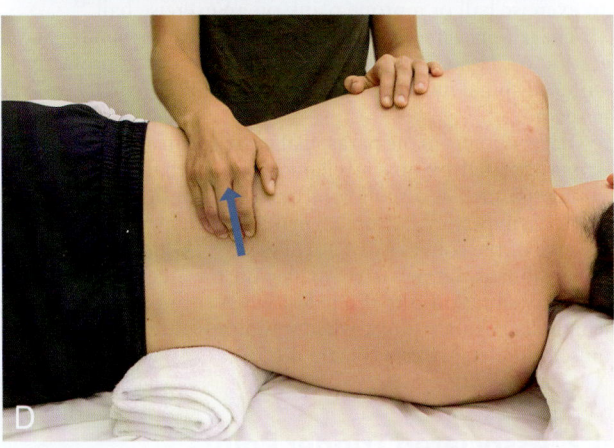

Figure 48-6. Examination of the left erector spinae muscles for TrPs. The longissimus thoracis, iliocostalis thoracis, and iliocostalis lumborum muscles are palpated with a cross-fiber flat palpation. A, The longissimus thoracis muscle. B, Iliocostalis lumborum muscle. C, Palpation of longissimus thoracis muscle with patient side-lying and clinician behind the patient. D, Palpation of iliocostalis lumborum muscle with the patient side-lying and the clinician in front of the patient.

of the spine is hypersensitive, the deep musculature on each side of it is palpated by firm pressure in the groove between the process and the longissimus muscle. A deep cross-fiber flat palpation is directed along the side of the spinous process to exert pressure on the rotatores muscles against the underlying laminae to locate a spot of maximum tenderness. Because of the depth of the muscles in this region, a taut band is rarely found; however, in the area where a TrP is present, the tissue will feel denser than the areas above and below it. If two or three spinous processes are tender, one expects to find adjacent TrPs on at least one side at each level of tenderness. A filiform needle can be utilized to accurately identify a TrP in these deep muscles that can't be reliably manually palpated.

4. DIFFERENTIAL DIAGNOSIS

4.1. Activation and Perpetuation of Trigger Points

In any part of the paraspinal muscles, TrPs may be activated by unaccustomed eccentric loading, eccentric exercise in the unconditioned muscle, or maximal or sub-maximal concentric loading.[43] Trigger points may also be activated or aggravated when the muscle is placed in a shortened or lengthened position for an extended period of time. For example, prolonged immobility, as when sitting for hours in an aircraft or vehicle, may activate TrPs in the paraspinal muscles. Similarly, occupational overload, such as sitting at a computer, can contribute to the development of TrPs. Yoo et al[44] found that there was increased EMG activity in the T10 and L4 paraspinal muscles after 20 and 40 minutes of sitting at a computer workstation. Hoyle et al[45] reported that regardless of the high or low visual or postural stresses, TrPs developed within an hour of sitting.

A quick awkward movement that combines bending and twisting of the back, especially when the muscles are fatigued or chilled, is likely to activate TrPs in the iliocostalis muscle, even though no additional loading (lifting) is involved. This activation may be caused by disproportionate loading of one group of muscle fibers as a result of poor coordination.

Caution should also be exercised when performing exercises. Some exercises are more likely to load the paraspinal muscles than others. Exercises like a bilateral free weight row are more likely to activate the erector spinae muscles than a bilateral machine row or a unilateral free weight row.[46] Additionally, exercises like a side crunch on an exercise ball, side bridge on the toes, and side bridge on the knees are more likely to activate the lumbar paraspinal muscles versus a prone leg extension on an exercise ball or a prone plank on an exercise ball.[47]

The whiplash mechanism of injury that causes sudden acceleration or deceleration is likely to rapidly stretch protectively stiffened spinal muscles, which in turn is likely to activate TrPs in them.

Trigger points in the paraspinal muscles can also be activated or perpetuated by any mechanical factor that disturbs axial symmetry, such as a scoliosis from a leg length discrepancy or pelvic asymmetry.[48] Paraspinal muscle activity will be greater on the side of the convexity of a scoliosis.[49,50] Usually, the vertical dimension of the pelvis is smaller on the side of the shorter leg. This situation tilts the pelvis when sitting, just as the leg length discrepancy tilts it when standing, resulting in the same musculoskeletal effects (Figure 48-5B).

4.2. Associated Trigger Points

Associated TrPs can develop in the referred pain areas of a primary TrP[51]; therefore, muscles in the referred pain areas should also be considered during examination. For TrPs in the iliocostalis thoracis muscle, associated TrPs can develop in several other muscles, including other portions of the iliocostalis muscles, the longissimus, the trunk portion of the latissimus dorsi, serratus posterior inferior, lumbar multifidus, quadratus lumborum, pectoralis major, infraspinatus, supraspinatus, rectus abdominus, abdominal obliques, and psoas major muscles. An iliocostalis thoracis TrP may result from TrPs in the latissimus dorsi, infraspinatus, rhomboid major and minor, serratus posterior superior, scalene, serratus posterior inferior, lower trapezius, middle trapezius, serratus anterior, and/or the rectus abdominus muscles, depending on which portion of the muscle is affected. Therefore, to effectively improve pain from the iliocostalis muscle, these muscles must also be examined and treated.

For TrPs in the iliocostalis lumborum muscle, associated TrPs can develop in the trunk portion of the latissimus dorsi, quadratus lumborum, gluteus maximus, gluteus medius, gluteus minimus, piriformis, and deep hip lateral rotator muscles. A TrP in the iliocostalis lumborum muscle can be caused by a TrP in the rectus abdominus, longissimus thoracis, iliocostalis thoracis, and/or psoas major muscles.

Trigger points in the longissimus thoracis muscle can contribute to the development of associated TrPs in the iliocostalis lumborum, lumbar multifidus, quadratus lumborum, gluteus maximus, piriformis, proximal hamstring, and proximal adductor magnus muscles. A TrP in the longissimus thoracis muscle can result from a TrP in the rectus abdominus, serratus posterior superior, scalenes, rhomboid major and minor, and/or infraspinatus muscles, depending on which portion of the muscle is affected.

Thoracic multifidus TrPs can contribute to associated TrPs in the iliocostalis thoracis and longissimus thoracis muscles. Clinically, this muscle has been seen to refer anteriorly; therefore, the pectoralis major muscle may also develop associated TrPs. A TrP in the thoracic multifidus muscle can be due to a TrP in the rectus abdominus, middle trapezius, and/or iliocostalis thoracis muscles, depending on which region is affected.

Lumbar multifidus TrPs can contribute to associated TrPs in the iliocostalis lumborum, quadratus lumborum, rectus abdominus, abdominal obliques, and psoas major muscles. A TrP in the lumbar multifidus muscle can result from a TrP in the rectus abdominus, longissimus thoracis, and/or psoas major muscles.

Sacral multifidus TrPs can contribute to associated TrPs in the gluteus maximus, gluteus medius, piriformis, hamstrings, psoas major, and abdominal oblique muscles. A TrP in the sacral multifidus muscle can result from a TrP in the rectus abdominus, gluteus maximus, gluteus medius, and or quadratus lumborum muscles.

The spinotransverse muscle group is more likely to demonstrate isolated muscle involvement, whereas the more superficial paraspinal muscles are likely to accumulate associated TrPs in functionally related muscles, especially the contralateral superficial muscles.

Not uncommonly, articular dysfunction of the thoracolumbar junction will be associated with active TrPs in the adjacent erector spinae, psoas muscle, and the quadratus lumborum muscles. Remarkably, if one treats the dysfunction of the thoracolumbar junction, or TrPs in one of the three muscles, the treatment often relieves TrPs in another one of the muscles.[52]

4.3. Associated Pathology

Some medical conditions give rise to symptoms that can appear confusingly similar to those produced by TrPs in the thoracolumbar paraspinal muscles or may be present concurrently. For pain that presents in the trunk, either anteriorly or posteriorly, screening for visceral disease is of critical importance. Jarrell[53] reported that the presence of an abdominal wall TrP predicted evidence of visceral disease in over 90% of subjects, and if a TrP was not present, it was associated with not having visceral disease in 64% of subjects. As a result, if TrPs in the muscles of the trunk continually return, a thorough medical screening and possible referral to the physician may be warranted.

There are several conditions related to the cardiovascular, pulmonary, gastrointestinal, endocrine, hepatic and biliary, and urologic systems that can refer pain to the thoracic region, lumbar region, interscapular, or sacral region, depending on the viscera involved.[28] Knowledge of these pain referrals and symptomology are essential in the differential diagnosis of musculoskeletal pain.

Segmental dysfunction associated with TrPs in the thoracolumbar paraspinal musculature may occur anywhere in this region. The number of segments involved depends on the muscles involved. For example, TrPs in the rotatores muscles can induce a concurrent single level dysfunction. Trigger points in the multifidi muscles are more likely to induce articular dysfunction involving two or three adjacent segmental levels. Semispinalis TrPs at any level will usually be associated with four to six segmental levels of dysfunction. The apex segment is often exquisitely tender to palpation. The most superficial and longest muscles are the iliocostalis and longissimus muscles and their TrPs are associated with group dysfunctions. If the patient compensates proximally to level the shoulders, he or she can present with a double curve (S curve) that is easily misinterpreted as a primary scoliosis. Trigger points in the iliocostalis lumborum muscle are also associated closely with pelvic obliquity secondary to tension applied to the muscle's insertional aponeurosis onto the sacral base.

Schneider[54] emphasized that the symptoms caused by multifidus TrPs mimic those of lumbar facet or sacroiliac syndromes and that an L4-L5 lateral disc herniation produces tightness of the left L4-L5 multifidus muscle, causing a segmental motion block. Clinically, TrPs in the lumbar multifidus muscle have been seen to mimic facet joint dysfunction.

The pain referral patterns of the thoracic zygapophyseal joints[55,56] and costotransverse joints[57] have been established. The referred pain patterns from these joints have overlap with pain referral patterns of the thoracic paraspinal and multifidus muscles.

Any patient with chronic low back pain and additional widespread pain should be examined for central sensitization or fibromyalgia. Trigger points are frequently associated with these conditions,[58-60] with active TrPs reproducing familiar pain of patients.[60] Symptoms of fibromyalgia are also associated with rheumatic diseases such as rheumatoid arthritis, spondyloarthritis, psoriatic arthritis, and connective tissue disorders.[61]

Radicular pain and/or radiculopathy may be caused by pressure on a nerve root from a herniated disc, by encroachment within the spinal foramen as from osteoarthritis, or by a tumor. Lumbar radicular reference of pain usually causes pain that radiates into the lower extremity, paraspinal TrPs alone rarely do. However, when active TrPs in the back muscles induce associated TrPs in the gluteal muscles, the latter TrPs often refer myofascial pain down the lateral or posterior aspect of the thigh or leg, sometimes extending to the foot.[15,22,62-65] Radiculopathy is characterized by neurologic deficits including decreased tendon reflexes, impaired cutaneous sensation, and/or motor weakness with atrophy. Trigger points typically do not cause such neurologic deficits.

Myositis ossificans is a benign condition where heterotopic ossification occurs in muscles, typically in the extremities, rarely in the trunk muscles, and more frequently after trauma.[66] Two cases of myositis ossificans are reported in the literature occurring in the paraspinal muscles, one in the lumbar[67] and one in the thoracic paraspinal muscles.[68]

Another condition to be aware of that causes soft tissue swelling in the paraspinal muscles is fibrodysplasia ossificans progressive.[69-71] It is a rare genetic disease that is autosomal dominant. There is congenital malformation of the great toes, tissue swelling that occurs after a trauma that leads to heterotopic ossification.[72-75]

Another rare condition to consider is acute paraspinal compartment syndrome, which is an increase in interstitial pressure in the paravertebral compartment that typically occurs after some type of strenuous exercise or activity. It typically presents with severe low back pain,[76-79] but may also present with additional symptoms in the abdomen,[76] testicle,[78,79] legs,[79] groin,[78] and flank.[76] Differential diagnosis of this condition is essential because it can mimic an acute lumbar muscle strain, disc herniation, vertebral fracture, inflammatory low back pain, or renal colic.[79] It has also been mistaken as ureteral colic.[76]

5. CORRECTIVE ACTIONS

The patient with paraspinal TrPs should modify activities that induce stress when bending over forward. Bending to pick up heavy items should not be done from bending at the waist but by squatting with the legs. The patient should also avoid holding his or her breath, or twisting while lifting or pulling.

To minimize strain to the thoracolumbar paraspinal muscles, proper mechanics should be utilized when rising from or sitting down to a chair with the "Sit-to-stand" and "Stand-to-sit" Technique (Figure 50-13). To rise from the chair, the hips are moved forward to the front of the chair seat before starting to rise. The body and hips are then turned somewhat to the side and one foot is placed beneath the front edge of the chair. Finally, the torso is held erect while the knees and hips are straightened, lifting the body. The process is reversed in stand-to-sit by turning to the side and placing one foot under the front edge of the chair, keeping the torso erect, and aiming the buttocks at the front edge of the chair seat rather than at the rear of the seat. The person then slides backward on the seat to meet the backrest. This procedure again maintains the back in an erect position and transfers the load from the paraspinal muscles to the hip and thigh muscles.

The paraspinal musculature can be relieved of unnecessary strain by modifying the chair, backrest, armrests, and/or computer so they are ergonomically correct. Refer to Chapter 76 on posture and ergonomics.

When sleeping on the side, a patient with TrPs in the thoracolumbar paraspinal muscles is usually more comfortable with a pillow, or two, placed in between the knees. This prevents the rotary torsion of the lumbar spine that occurs when the knee drops forward onto the bed.

To stretch the thoracolumbar paraspinal muscles, three different types of stretches can be performed. The first is a single knee to chest stretch. In the supine position, the patient draws one knee to the chest while the opposite leg is straight out (Figure 48-7A). Next, the lower extremity is returned to the straight-leg starting position, and the other thigh is flexed to the chest and returned.

A second way to stretch the thoracolumbar paraspinal muscles is with a double knee to chest stretch. In the supine position, both legs are pulled to the chest until a gentle stretch is felt in the back (Figure 48-7B).

A third way to stretch the muscles is in the "prayer position." The patient starts in the quadruped position (Figure 48-7C). While keeping the hands in place, the hips rock back toward the heels as if going to sit on them. The muscles on both sides of the spine will be equally stretched when the arms are directly in front of the patient (Figure 48-7D). To focus the stretch more on one side, the patient should walk the hands away from the side to be stretched, making sure not to lift the hips and buttocks off the heels.

Self-pressure release of the thoracolumbar paraspinal muscles can be performed utilizing a homemade or purchased TrP release tool. With a commercially available rigid tool, the edge of the device can be pressed into the portion of the muscle that refers pain for several seconds (Figure 48-8A). This release can be repeated up and down the muscle group for maximum relief. A homemade tool can also be made with a long sock and a lacrosse or tennis ball (Figure 48-8B top left corner). The patient places the ball in the sock and positions the ball between the wall and his back at the point where pain is referred. Holding the open end of the sock with both hands, the patient may reposition as needed for maximum relief (Figure 48-8B main picture).

70. Subasree R, Panda S, Pal PK, Ravishankar S. An unusual case of rapidly progressive contractures: case report and brief review. *Ann Indian Acad Neurol*. 2008;11(2):119-122.
71. Zaghloul KA, Heuer GG, Guttenberg MD, Shore EM, Kaplan FS, Storm PB. Lumbar puncture and surgical intervention in a child with undiagnosed fibrodysplasia ossificans progressiva. *J Neurosurg Pediatr*. 2008;1(1):91-94.
72. Kaplan FS, Glaser DL, Shore EM, et al. The phenotype of fibrodysplasia ossificans progressiva. *Clinic Rev Bone Miner Metab*. 2005;3(3-4):183-188.
73. Kaplan FS, Tabas JA, Gannon FH, Finkel G, Hahn GV, Zasloff MA. The histopathology of fibrodysplasia ossificans progressiva. An endochondral process. *J Bone Joint Surg Am*. 1993;75(2):220-230.
74. Connor JM, Evans DA. Fibrodysplasia ossificans progressiva. The clinical features and natural history of 34 patients. *J Bone Joint Surg Br*. 1982;64(1):76-83.
75. Connor JM, Evans DA. Genetic aspects of fibrodysplasia ossificans progressiva. *J Med Genet*. 1982;19(1):35-39.
76. Hoyle A, Tang V, Baker A, Blades R. Acute paraspinal compartment syndrome as a rare cause of loin pain. *Ann R Coll Surg Engl*. 2015;97(2):e11-e12.
77. Schreiber VM, Ward WT. Exercise-induced pediatric lumbar paravertebral compartment syndrome: a case report. *J Pediatr Orthop*. 2015;35(6):e49-e51.
78. Vanbrabant P, Moke L, Meersseman W, Vanderschueren G, Knockaert D. Excruciating low back pain after strenuous exertion: beware of lumbar paraspinal compartment syndrome. *J Emerg Med*. 2015;49(5):641-643.
79. Eichner ER, Schnebel B, Anderson S, et al. Acute lumbar paraspinal myonecrosis in football players with sickle cell trait: a case series. *Med Sci Sports Exerc*. 2017;49(4):627-632.

Chapter 49

Abdominal Muscles

"Limbo Limiters"

César Fernández de las Peñas, Joseph M. Donnelly, and Margaret M. Gebhardt

1. INTRODUCTION

The abdominal musculature consists of five different muscles: the rectus abdominis, internal oblique, external oblique, transversus abdominis, and pyramidalis. These muscles perform several functions including flexion, sidebending, and rotation of the trunk, but most important is their role in trunk stability during walking, heavy lifting, and movement of the extremities, particularly the transversus abdominis muscle. In addition, the abdominal muscles protect the abdominal viscera. Trigger points (TrPs) in the abdominal musculature can mimic visceral disease symptomatology (appendicitis, peptic ulcer, gallstone colic, colitis, dysmenorrhea, chronic pelvic pain, and urinary tract disease) because they can refer pain to the abdominal area but also reproduce symptoms such as burning, fullness, bloating, swelling, or gas. It is also possible that TrPs in the abdominal muscles can be related to motor control disturbances in the deep abdominal muscles (transversus abdominis and internal oblique) especially in patients with low back pain. Symptoms from TrPs may be exacerbated by stress, direct trauma, repetitive overload, or most importantly, with visceral pathology. In fact, the activation of TrPs in these muscles can be directly related to viscero-somatic or somato-visceral reflex. Differential diagnosis should include differentiation between abdominal pain from TrP origin or from visceral disease. Careful clinical examination of abdominal wall muscles can assist with differential diagnosis. Corrective actions should include postural reeducation, a progressive strengthening exercise program, self-stretch and TrP self-pressure release, and reeducation of diaphragmatic breathing.

2. ANATOMIC CONSIDERATIONS

The external and internal abdominal oblique muscles, like the external and internal intercostal muscles have a diagonal crisscross arrangement and the two groups of muscles have corresponding orientation. Clinicians should consider which layer runs in which direction (Figure 49-1). Figure 49-2 illustrates a mnemonic for the fiber directions. The fingers of the left hand on the right side of the abdomen against the skin represent the fiber direction of

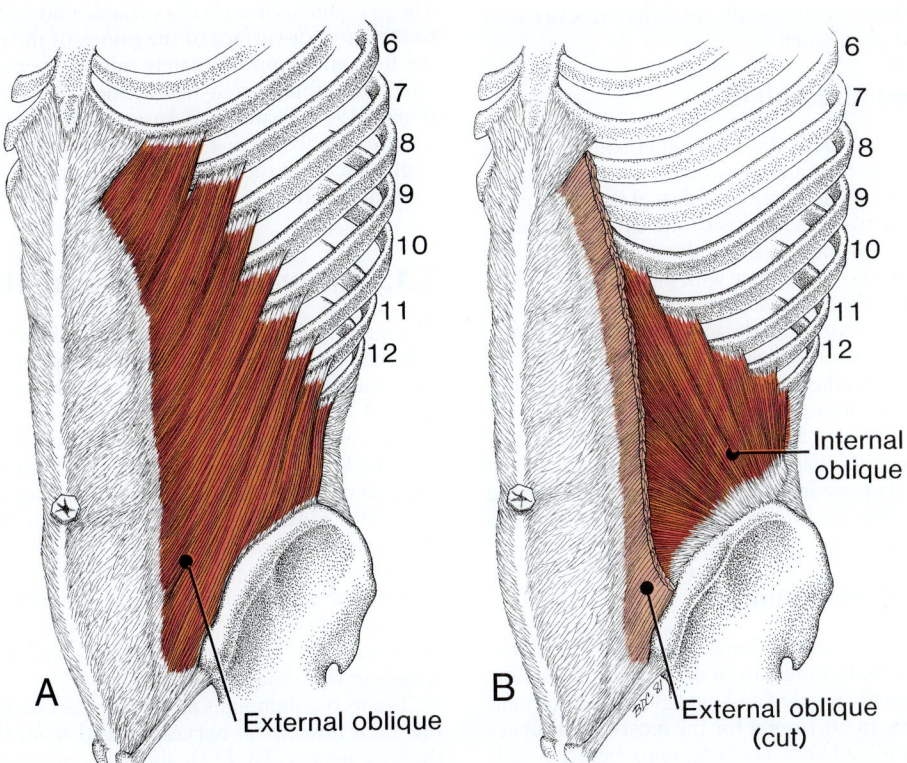

Figure 49-1. Attachments of two lateral abdominal wall muscles. A, External oblique muscle (light red). B, Internal oblique muscle (dark red); the external oblique muscle (light red) is cut.

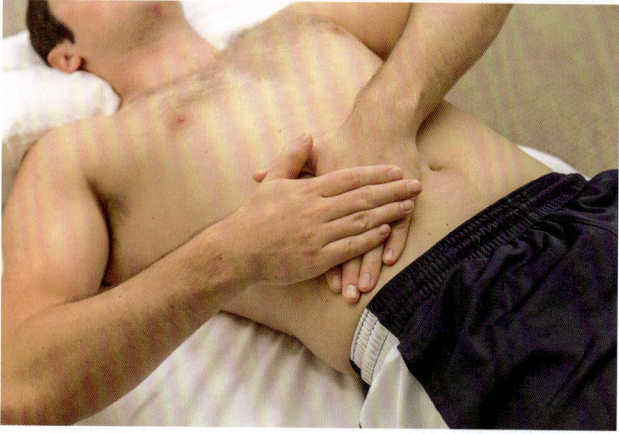

Figure 49-2. Technique for remembering the fiber direction of the oblique abdominal muscles. The top hand represents the fiber direction of the external abdominal oblique and external intercostal muscles. The bottom hand represents fiber direction of the internal abdominal oblique and internal intercostal muscles.

the right internal abdominal oblique (and intercostal) muscles, whereas the right hand on top of the left hand represents the fiber direction of the right external abdominal oblique (and intercostal) muscles. The transversus abdominis fibers run radially around the abdomen as their names imply.

The pattern of relative muscle thickness of abdominal wall muscles is rectus abdominis > internal oblique > external oblique > transversus abdominis.[1] Symmetry for total absolute thickness of all three lateral muscles has been reported to be 8% to 9% (mean), but for individual muscles there was an asymmetry of absolute size from 13% to 24% with a symmetrical relative thickness.[1] In general, men show significantly larger muscles than women,[1] and there are no significant differences between the middle-aged and young men.[2]

External Oblique Abdominis

The external oblique muscle is the most superficial muscle of the abdominal wall. Laterally and proximally, the muscle arises from the external surfaces and inferior borders of the lower eight ribs.[3] The lower three rib attachments of the external oblique muscle interdigitate with the latissimus dorsi muscle, and the upper five rib attachments interdigitate with the serratus anterior muscle. Although these three muscles appear in anatomy books to be quite separate, in dissection, the external oblique muscle appears to form with the other two as an unbroken sheet of muscle. The fasciculi from the lowest two ribs lie nearly vertical and are parallel and adjacent to those fibers of the quadratus lumborum muscle that also connects the iliac crest and the twelfth rib.[3] The fibers run diagonally downward and forward to join the abdominal aponeurosis that attach anteriorly to the linea alba in the midline and to the anterior half of the iliac crest (Figure 49-1A).

Internal Oblique Abdominis

The direction of the fibers in the fan-shaped internal oblique muscle, in the upright body, ranges from nearly vertical posteriorly, through a diagonally upward and medial direction among its intermediate fibers, to horizontal for the most caudal fibers (Figure 49-1B). Laterally, all fibers converge onto the lateral half of the inguinal ligament, the anterior two-thirds of the iliac crest, and the lower portion of the lumbar aponeurosis.[3] Above, the nearly vertical fibers attach to the cartilages of the last three or four ribs. Above and medially, diagonal fibers attach to the linea alba through the anterior and posterior rectus sheath. Medially, the horizontal fibers from the inguinal ligament attach to the arch of the pubis through the conjoined tendon, which this muscle forms with the transversus abdominis muscle.[3]

Transversus Abdominis

Transversus abdominis muscle fibers run nearly horizontal across the abdomen and attach anteriorly to the midline linea alba via the rectus sheath (Figure 49-3), which surrounds the rectus abdominis muscle above the arcuate line and attaches to the pubis through the conjoined tendon.[3] Below that line, the sheath occurs only anterior to the rectus abdominis muscle. Laterally, the transversus muscle attaches to the lateral one-third of the inguinal ligament, the anterior three-quarters of the crest of the ilium, the thoracolumbar fascia, and the inner surface of the cartilages of the last six ribs, where it interdigitates with the fibers of the diaphragm muscle.[3]

Rectus Abdominis

The rectus abdominis muscle attaches along the crest of the pubic bone (Figure 49-4). The fibers of the paired muscles interlace across the symphysis. Above, the muscle attaches to the cartilages of the fifth, sixth, and seventh ribs.[3] The fibers of the rectus abdominis muscle are usually interrupted by three or four, more or less complete, transverse tendinous inscriptions.[4] Of the three most constant tendinous inscriptions, one is found near the tip of the xiphoid process, one close to the level of the umbilicus, and one midway between them.[4] The abdominal section of the pectoralis major muscle (Figure 42-2) may overlap fibers of the upper portion of the rectus abdominis muscle, and thus may account for the occasional reference of pain to the anterior chest from TrPs in this region. The loss of the dorsal half of the rectus sheath below the arcuate line is clear as seen in Figure 49-3.

Pyramidalis

The pyramidalis muscle is a variable muscle that attaches below to the anterior surface of the ramus of the pubis and above to the linea alba approximately midway between the symphysis and the umbilicus.[3] It lies within the anterior rectus sheath (Figure 49-4). Beaton and Anson[5] observed that the pyramidalis muscle was absent in 17.7% when analyzing 430 sides. Anson et al[6] described the usual and variant anatomy of this muscle in great detail.

2.1. Innervation and Vascularization

The lateral abdominal wall muscles, the external and internal obliques, and the transversus abdominis muscles are innervated by branches of the 8th through the 12th intercostal nerves from T8 to T12, showing a segmental innervation.[3] The internal oblique and transversus abdominis muscles are also supplied by branches of the iliohypogastric and ilioinguinal nerves that stem from L1. The ilioinguinal and iliohypogastric nerves emerge through the internal oblique muscle medially and inferiorly to the anterior superior iliac spine.[7]

The external oblique muscle is also innervated by the subcostal nerve.[3] The subcostal nerve lies subcostally and caudal to the rib. The main branches are located between the internal oblique and transversus abdominis muscles. These nerves branches vary widely in the abdominal wall.[8]

The rectus abdominis muscle is innervated by the 7th through the 12th intercostal nerves derived from the corresponding thoracic nerves (T8-T12), and different segmental nerves usually innervate fibers between different tendinous inscriptions, especially in the upper half of the muscle.[3] The nerves pass inferomedially between the internal oblique and transversus abdominis muscles before entering the lateral confluence of the anterior and posterior rectus sheath or in some cases the

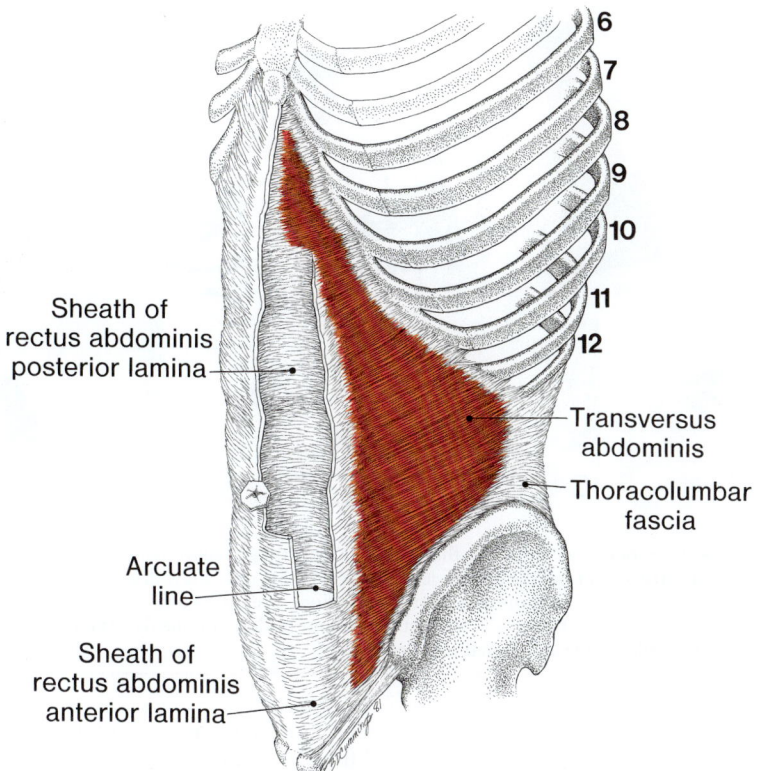

Figure 49-3. Attachments of the transversus abdominis muscle (red), which lie deep to the external and internal oblique muscles.

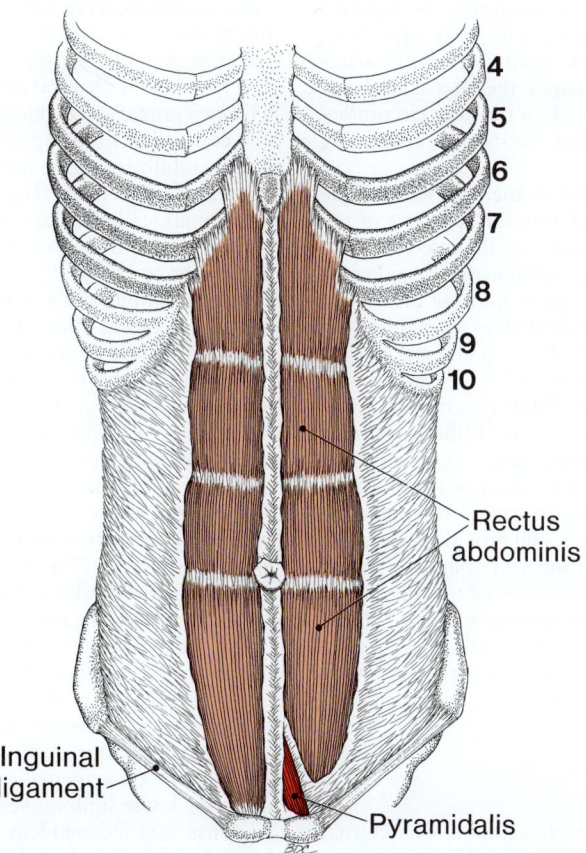

Figure 49-4. Attachments of the rectus abdominis muscle (light red), which connects the anterior rib cage to the pubic bone close to the symphysis, and attachments of the variable pyramidalis muscle (dark red), which lies just above the symphysis pubis within the anterior rectus sheath.

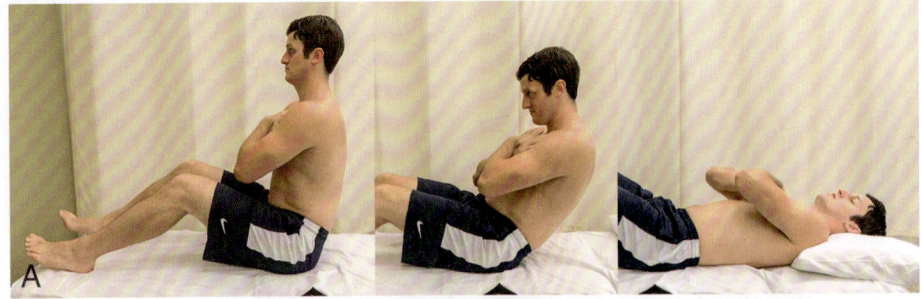
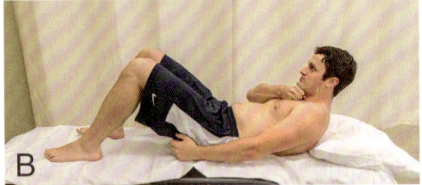
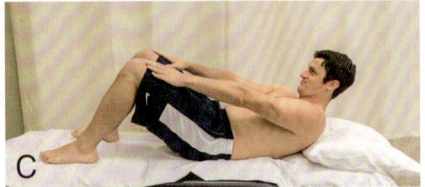
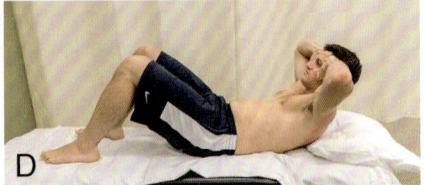

Figure 49-5. A, The sit-back exercise is a progressive uncurling that starts in the sitting position and ends in supine. Knees and hips should be bent and the feet fixed. From this initial sitting position, the patient leans back slightly. After a few degrees of uncurling, the patient returns to the starting position. Progressive uncurling, with assisted return to the starting position, is repeated until uncurling reaches the full supine position. B, Abdominal curl with fist below the chin to support the neck. C, Arm stretched out to decrease the demand on the abdominal muscles. D, Hands placed at side of the head to maximally challenge the abdominal muscles.

posterior rectus sheath.[9] The nerves, which contain varying numbers of sensory, motor, and autonomic fibers, pass under the rectus abdominis muscle and became intramuscular at varying points, with most of them entering into the muscle in the lateral third.[9] Finally, the pyramidalis muscle also receives innervation by a branch of the 12th thoracic nerve.

The internal oblique muscle gets its blood supply from the lower posterior intercostal and subcostal arteries, the superior epigastric artery, the inferior epigastric artery, the superficial and deep circumflex arteries, and the posterior lumbar arteries.[3] Ramasastry et al[10] described a flap in the internal oblique muscle where a single ascending branch of the deep circumflex iliac artery enters the undersurface of the muscle, arborizing within the muscle.

The blood flow of the cranial part of the external oblique muscle is supplied by the lateral and anterior branches of the intercostal arteries.[3] The lateral branches of the intercostal artery run on the surface of the external oblique muscle, whereas the anterior branches of the arteries enter into the muscle. In addition, the caudal part of the muscle derives its main blood supply from one or two branches of the deep circumflex iliac artery (94.7%) or the iliolumbar artery (5.3%).[11] Yang et al[12] reported the presence of a huge variability ranging from 9% to 22% in the vascular supply of the external oblique muscle.

Blood supply for the rectus abdominis muscle is provided by more than one source. Mathes and Nahai[13] describe two pedicles: the inferior epigastric artery runs superiorly on the posterior surface of the muscle, enters the muscle, and provides the supply to the lower part of the muscle; the superior epigastric artery supplies the blood flow to the upper portion of the muscle.[13]

The transversus abdominis muscle receives supply from the following arteries: lower posterior of intercostal and subcostal arteries, superior epigastric artery, inferior epigastric artery, superficial and deep circumflex arteries, and posterior lumbar arteries.[3]

2.2. Function

The four abdominal wall muscles (rectus abdominis, external oblique, internal oblique, and transversus abdominis) play a variety of essential roles in human function. These muscles create the forces necessary to flex, twist, and side-bend spine[14]; stiffen the abdominal cavity and lumbar spine during simple tasks such as standing, sitting, and locomotion[15] as well as during demanding tasks such as dynamic loading and heavy lifting[16,17]; and finally, assist the expiration of air in challenged breathing. Regarding respiratory function, Kim and Kim[18] found that smokers have a higher degree of dependence on internal oblique muscles than transversus abdominis muscles during forceful expiratory conditions as compared with that in nonsmokers. An overreaction of the internal oblique muscle may cause problems in efficiently diffusing loads of the spine. Special functions of the abdominal muscles, particularly as related to respiratory activities, are covered in Chapter 45.

From a biomechanical perspective, the abdominal wall muscles have two primary roles. First, they create movement, both forceful and controlled, of the upper and lower quarters.[19] Second, they play a stabilization role for the thoracic and lumbosacral spine as well as the pelvis.[20] The use of stability generated from the abdominal wall muscles is thought to allow for increased force generation from the extremities. The rectus abdominis muscle is thought to be more a force-producing muscle, whereas the transversus abdominis muscle is the main stabilizing muscle. The external and internal oblique muscles participate in both roles.[19,20] The transversus abdominis, internal and external oblique, and the pelvic floor musculature function together as a unit for stabilization of the lumbosacral spine and pelvic girdle in conjunction with the thoracolumbar fascia.[20,21] In addition, the abdominal wall musculature increases intra-abdominal pressure, an important function for maintaining overall spinal stability.[20] The contraction of the abdominal musculature in conjunction with the contraction of the diaphragm muscle is thought to enhance spinal stability through the production of forces that create a rigid cylinder in the abdominal cavity.

There is scientific evidence supporting a feed-forward action of the lateral abdominal wall muscles in the motor control of the lumbar spine, particularly the transversus abdominis muscle.[22] Several studies have reported that the transversus abdominis (which always starts its contraction first), the internal oblique, the external oblique, rectus abdominis, and the lumbar multifidus muscles are activated in a feed-forward manner before any upper or lower limb movement.[23-25] In fact, this feed-forward response was independent of the movement of the extremity but related to speed of the movement, suggesting that this is not a response to reactive forces but is linked to control of the stability of the spine against potential external perturbations.[25,26] Furthermore, it seems that a codependent mechanism exists involving balanced tension between the transversus abdominis and internal oblique muscles and the lumbar paraspinal muscles throughout the aponeurotic components of the thoracolumbar fascia.[21] This lack of feed-forward can be related to the overload of the superficial trunk muscles. For instance, Ghamkhar and Kahlaee[27] have recently reported that individuals with chronic low back pain had higher global activity of the superficial trunk muscles, such as erector spinae or rectus abdominis muscles.

Lateral Abdominal Wall Muscles

The internal and external oblique muscles function bilaterally to increase intra-abdominal pressure (eg, for urination, defecation, emesis, parturition, and forced exhalation) and to flex the vertebral column. Unilaterally, they bend the vertebral column toward the same side and assist to rotate the vertebral column.[14,28] The external oblique muscle rotates the vertebral column toward the contralateral side, whereas the internal oblique muscle rotates the vertebral column toward the same side. Therefore, the contralateral external oblique and the ipsilateral internal oblique muscles rotating the trunk in the same direction are probably related to the fact that abdominal muscle afferents activate similar pathways to muscles on both sides of the body.[29] An increase in intra-abdominal pressure is also assisted by the contraction of the transversus abdominis muscle.

All lateral abdominal wall muscles help complete exhalation quickly during rapid breathing, and this action is different depending on the position and the presence of load. For instance, activity of the lateral abdominal wall muscle varies depending on the gravity: the internal oblique muscle is more active during both inspiration and expiration in the standing position, whereas the activity of the external oblique muscle is higher in the sitting-with-elbows-on-the-knee position.[30] Similarly, the activation of transversus abdominis, internal oblique, and external oblique musculature was higher with load than without it.[31]

The external and internal oblique muscles show some activity during walking, but they can exhibit a sudden increase in activity with a sudden or sustained increase in intra-abdominal pressure, eg, during an active straight leg raise.[32] In fact, this activity depends on each particular muscle because the activity is increased in the transversus abdominis muscle, but decreased in the external oblique muscles during lifting.[33] The fibers of both transversus abdominis and internal oblique muscles in the region of the inguinal canal are activated continuously during standing because they demonstrate a larger increase in motor unit discharges during activities that would increase intra-abdominal pressure.[32] Selective activation of the internal oblique and transversus abdominis muscles doubles when a sit-back exercise (Figure 49-5A) is performed with the feet unsupported as compared with when the feet are supported, which emphasizes recruitment of other muscles, ie, the iliopsoas.[34]

The cyclical swings in abdominal pressure produced by breathing and by the activity of the abdominal muscles help pump the venous blood out of the abdomen at rest and during exercise. Relaxation of the abdominal wall during inhalation increases blood flow into the abdominal veins from the lower limbs. As the abdominal wall muscles contract for exhalation, the blood is forced upward toward the heart if the valves of the lower extremity veins are competent. A recent study observed that during exercise, the abdominal and diaphragm muscles might play the role of an "auxiliary heart."[35]

Rectus Abdominis

The rectus abdominis muscle is the prime mover for spinal flexion, particularly of the lower thoracic and lumbar spine, and it also tenses the anterior abdominal wall to increase intra-abdominal pressure for trunk stability.[36] Electromyographically, the rectus abdominis muscle is active when a weight is carried on the back but not when the weight is carried anterior to the thigh. In fact, this muscle does not exhibit fatigue during submaximal efforts like the lumbar paraspinal muscles do.[37] Furthermore, the rectus abdominis muscle is inactive during 14 static upright postures.[38] Sit-ups generate much more electrical activity in the rectus abdominis muscle than sit-backs.[39,40] The muscular activity was greatest during the initial phase of the sit-up between 15° and 45° or between scapular lift and hip lift from the floor.[39,40] A small difference was observed in the rectus abdominis muscle electrical activity whether the knees were bent to 65° or were straight.[39] Flexing the knees and anchoring the feet during a sit-up increased the activity of the abdominal muscles as compared with the rectus femoris muscle.[40] Recording of four levels of difficulty of abdominal muscle testing (elevating progressively more of the weight of the lower extremities in the supine position) showed that the lower half of the rectus abdominis muscle was the most active, followed by the upper half of the muscle.[41]

Pyramidalis

The pyramidalis muscle tenses the linea alba.

2.3. Functional Unit

The functional unit to which a muscle belongs includes the muscles that reinforce and counter its actions as well as the joints that the muscle crosses. The functional interdependence of these structures is reflected in the organization and neural connections of the sensory motor cortex. The functional unit is emphasized because the presence of a TrP in one muscle of the unit increases the likelihood that the other muscles of the unit also develops TrPs. When inactivating TrPs in a muscle, one should be concerned about TrPs that may develop in muscles that are functionally interdependent. Box 49-1 grossly represents the functional unit of the abdominal muscles.[42]

Box 49-1 Functional unit of the abdominal muscles

Action	Synergists	Antagonist
Trunk flexion	Rectus abdominis Psoas major	Thoracolumbar paraspinals (longissiumus thoracis)
Trunk rotation	Ipsilateral internal oblique abdominis Contralateral external oblique abdominis Ipsilateral internal intercostals Contralateral external intercostals	Contralateral internal oblique abdominis Ipsilateral external oblique abdominis Contralateral internal intercostals Ipsilateral external intercostals
Trunk sidebending	Ipsilateral internal oblique abdominis Ipsilateral external oblique abdominis Ipsilateral quadratus lumborum Ipsilateral thoracolumbar paraspinals	Contralateral internal oblique abdominis Contralateral external oblique abdominis Contralateral quadratus lumborum Contralateral thoracolumbar paraspinals

For spinal rotation and flexion, the external oblique muscle anatomically appears synergistic with the external intercostals and serratus anterior muscles with which the external oblique also interdigitates, as well as the vertical costal fibers of the latissimus dorsi with which the lower part of the external oblique muscle interdigitates and forms a continuous line of pull.[3]

For lumbar spinal rotation, the external oblique muscle on one side is synergistic with the ipsilateral deepest (diagonal) paraspinal muscles and with the contralateral serratus posterior-inferior and internal oblique muscles.

To increase intra-abdominal pressure for nonrespiratory reasons, the four muscles of the abdominal wall are synergistic with the quadratus lumborum and diaphragm muscles. Functions of the abdominal muscles as related to respiration are covered in Chapter 45.

3. CLINICAL PRESENTATION

3.1. Referred Pain Pattern

Abdominal TrPs may cause as much distress as pain stemming from visceral dysfunction. In fact, symptoms referred from abdominal TrPs commonly confuse the diagnostic process by mimicking visceral abdominal pathology.[43] Muscolino[44] described a patient with a clinical history of Crohn's disease who developed TrP in the abdominal muscles responsible for his pain symptoms. The pain pattern from TrPs in the abdominal musculature, particularly the internal and external oblique muscles, is less consistent from patient to patient than the patterns for most other muscles. Referred pain from abdominal muscles has little respect for the midline; abdominal TrPs on one side frequently cause bilateral pain. In an older study, Gutstein[45] observed that the patient is likely to describe pain caused by abdominal TrPs as "burning," "fullness," "bloating," "swelling," or "gas." The referred pain patterns from abdominal TrPs have been also reported by Melnick.[46]

Abdominal Oblique Muscles

Trigger points in the abdominal oblique muscles have potential referred pain patterns that may reach up into the chest, may travel straight or diagonally across the abdomen, and may extend downward. Whether this variability represents different characteristics of consecutive deeper layers of muscles or less consistency in the patterns of pain referred from TrPs in this musculature, it is not clear. This variability is also possibly related to the fact that the internal oblique muscle is extremely difficult, if not impossible, to palpate directly.

Active TrPs in the external oblique muscle can produce "heartburn" (Figure 49-6A) and other symptoms commonly associated with abdominal hernia. The referred pain from this muscle can also produce deep epigastric pain that occasionally extends to other parts of the abdomen.[47]

Active TrPs located in the musculature of the lower lateral abdominal wall, possibly in any one of the three layers of muscle, refer pain into the groin and testicles and may project pain to other parts of the abdomen (Figure 49-6B). The experimental injection of hypertonic saline into the external oblique muscle near the anterior superior iliac spine induced referred pain over the lower portion of that quadrant of the abdomen, along the inguinal ligament, and into the testicle.[48] An external oblique TrP in a 10-year-old child referred severe pain from the upper quadrant to the inguinal region.[49]

Trigger points in the lower portion of the abdominal muscles, over the pubis or the lateral half of the inguinal ligament, may lie in the internal oblique muscle and possibly in the lower rectus abdominis muscle. These TrPs can increase irritability and spasm of the detrusor and urinary sphincter muscles, producing an increase in urinary frequency, retention of urine, and groin pain. When needled, abdominal wall TrPs often refer pain to the urinary bladder area. Melnick[47] described that TrPs in the lower portion of the abdominal muscles could be a source of chronic diarrhea.

Transversus Abdominis

The transversus abdominis muscle cannot be directly palpated. Trigger points in the transversus abdominis muscle refer pain as a band across the upper abdomen between the anterior costal margins. Sometimes the pain concentrates on the region of the xiphoid process. This pain can be distressing when coughing.

Rectus Abdominis

The symptoms caused by TrPs in this muscle are varied, but largely dependent on the portion of the muscle where they would appear. Symptoms are considered in three groups, those due to TrPs in the upper portion of the muscle (above the umbilical region), those caused by periumbilical TrPs, and those from TrPs in the lower rectus abdominis muscle.

Upper Portion

Trigger points in the upper portion of the rectus abdominis muscle can refer pain to the mid-back bilaterally, which is described by the patient as running horizontally across the back on both sides at the thoracolumbar level (Figure 49-7A).[50-52] Gutstein[45] also noted that treatment of tender spots in abdominal wall muscles relieved back pain. Unilateral backaches at this level, however, more frequently originate in TrPs of the latissimus dorsi muscle. In addition to back pain, TrPs in the upper portion of the rectus abdominis muscle can also refer pain to the xiphoid process. Melnick[47] described symptoms from TrPs in the upper rectus abdominis muscle as abdominal fullness, "heartburn," indigestion, and sometimes nausea or vomiting. These TrPs can also refer pain across the upper abdomen between the costal margins. Injection of hypertonic saline into the rectus abdominis muscle at about 2.5 cm (1 in) above the umbilicus caused brief referred pain throughout the same quadrant of the abdomen and on the same side in the back.[48] It has also been reported in a case report that TrPs in the upper portion of the left rectus abdominis muscle produced precordial pain.[53] When it has been identified that chest pain is myofascial and not cardiac in origin, it can be related to pain from TrPs in the pectoralis major and/or sternalis muscles; a rectus abdominis muscle source of the pain is easily overlooked. Finally, TrPs in the upper portion of the rectus abdominis muscle were observed to refer pain to the same abdominal quadrant and to simulate the symptoms of cholecystitis, gynecological disease, and peptic ulcer.[53]

Periumbilical Portion

Trigger points in the lateral border, periumbilical portion of the rectus abdominis muscle, are likely to produce sensations of abdominal cramping or colic.[47] The patient often bends forward for relief. Application of cold spray to the abdomen has been reported as effective for infants who burp and cry persistently with colic.[54] Lateral TrPs in the rectus abdominis muscle near the umbilicus may evoke diffuse abdominal pain that is accentuated by movement.[55]

Lewis and Kellgren[56] found that experimentally induced irritation of this muscle can mimic pain of intestinal colic. Injection of a hypertonic saline into the rectus abdominis muscle induced a familiar colic-like pain, which was stronger anteriorly than toward the back and extended diffusely over several segments in front.[57]

Lower Portion

Trigger points in the lower part of the rectus abdominis muscle may refer pain bilaterally to the sacroiliac and low back region.[50-52] The patient portrays this pain with a crosswise motion of the hand (Figure 49-7A), rather than the up-and-down pain pattern characteristic of the iliocostalis thoracis muscle, other superficial paraspinal muscles, and psoas major muscle. In some patients, TrPs in the lower rectus abdominis muscle may mimic symptoms associated with dysmenorrhea (Figure 49-7C).

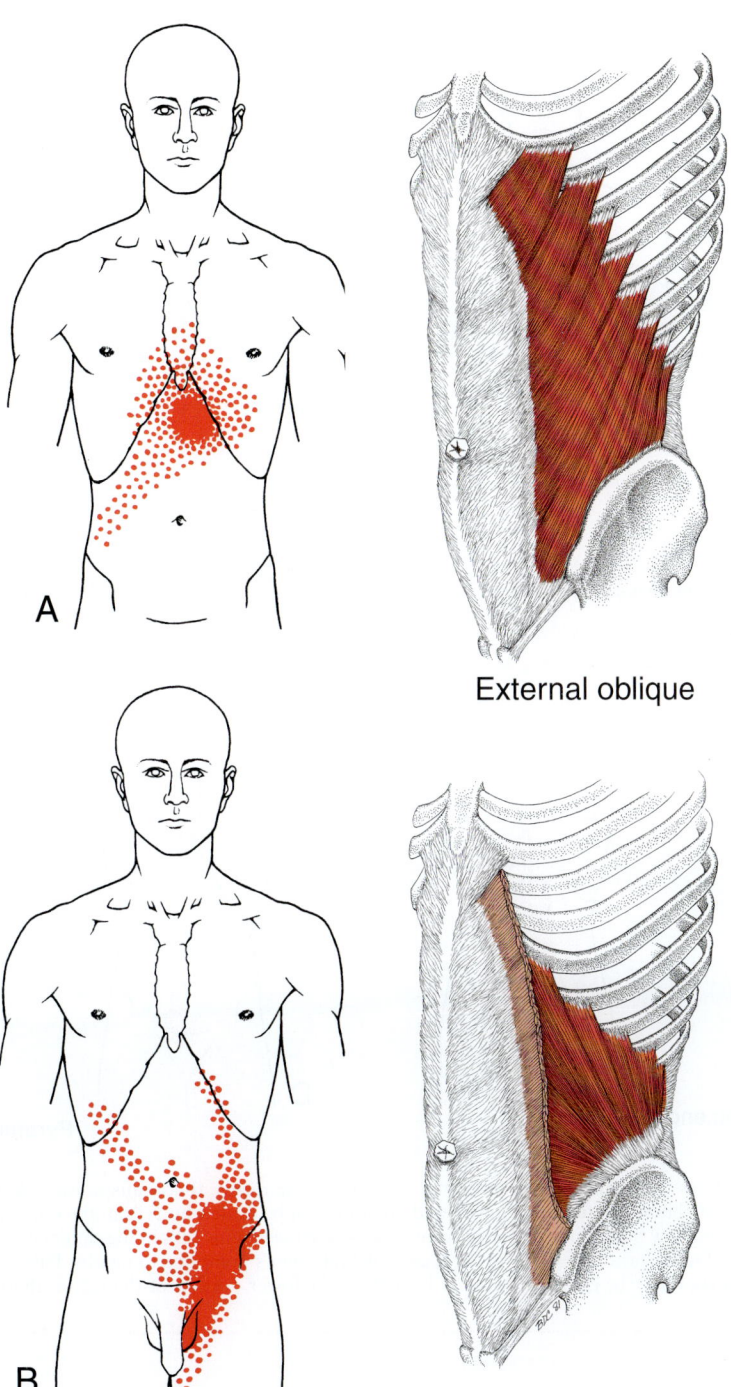

Figure 49-6. Referred pain patterns (red) and visceral symptoms associated with TrPs in the internal and external oblique (and possibly transverse) abdominis muscles. A, "heartburn" associated with external oblique TrPs. B, Groin and/or testicular pain, as well as chiefly lower quadrant abdominal pain, referred from TrPs in the lower lateral abdominal wall musculature, particularly the external oblique muscle.

Several authors have noted that a TrP in the lateral border of the right rectus abdominis muscle in the region of McBurney's point, which is halfway between the anterior superior iliac spine and the umbilicus (Figure 49-7B), is likely to produce symptoms simulating those of acute appendicitis.[58,59] This pain pattern was reported as occurring when the patient was tired, worried, or premenstrual.[60] In one patient, the TrP for this "pseudo-appendicitis" pain was located in the rectus abdominis muscle just above the level of the umbilicus.[58]

Other authors have also observed that TrPs in the region of McBurney's point may refer pain to the same lower quadrant of the abdomen and to the right upper quadrant area.[46,59,60] These TrPs also may refer sharp pain to the iliac fossa, the iliacus muscle, and to the penis.[60]

Pyramidalis

The pyramidalis muscle refers pain close to the midline between the symphysis pubis and the umbilicus (Figure 49-7D).

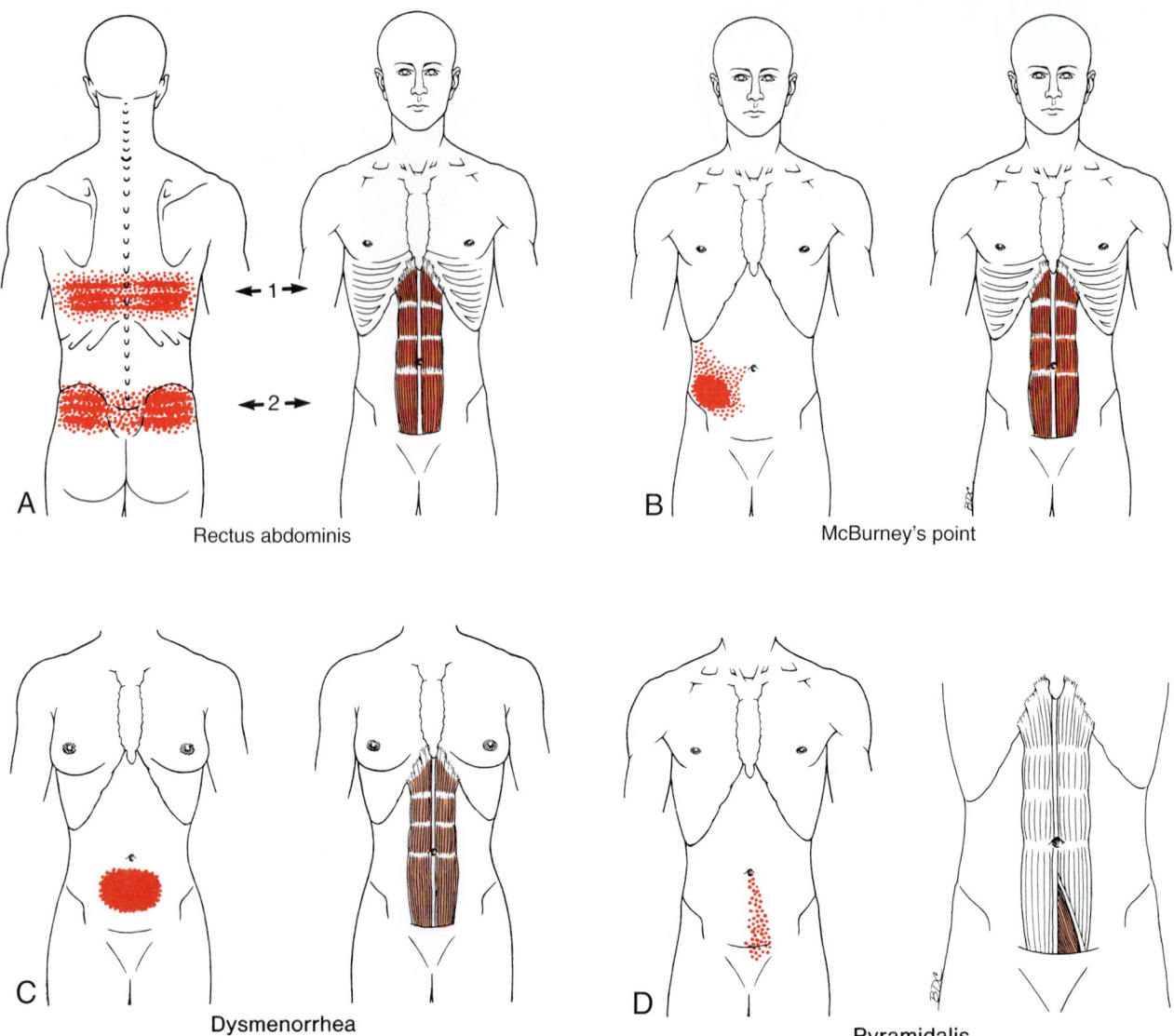

Figure 49-7. Referred pain patterns (red) and visceral symptoms of TrPs in the rectus abdominis muscle. A, Bilateral pain across the back, precordial pain, and/or a feeling of abdominal fullness, nausea, and vomiting can be caused by TrPs in the upper portion of the rectus abdominis muscle. A similar pattern of bilateral low back pain is referred from what is often seen with TrPs in the caudal end of the rectus abdominis muscle. B, Lower right quadrant pain and tenderness may occur in the region of McBurney's point due to nearby TrPs in the lateral border of the rectus abdominis muscle. C, Dysmenorrhea may be greatly intensified by TrPs in the lower portion of the rectus abdominis muscle. D, Referred pain pattern of the pyramidalis muscle.

3.2. Symptoms

It has been recognized since the 1920s that persistent abdominal pain is as likely to originate in the abdominal wall muscles or be referred from chest wall muscles as it is to originate in abdominal viscera.[61] Trigger points in the diaphragm muscle can also cause chest pain.[62] The differential diagnosis of diseases that produce symptoms that are commonly caused by, or may mimic pain caused by, abdominal TrPs includes joint dysfunctions, fibromyalgia, appendicitis, peptic ulcer, gallstone colic, colitis, painful rib syndrome, intractable dysmenorrhea, pelvic pain syndromes, chronic pelvic pain, and urinary tract disease.

Abdominal symptoms are commonly enigmatic and often a source of diagnostic confusion. The pain pattern of a number of abdominal diseases is mimicked by TrPs in the abdominal wall muscles.[63] Montenegro et al[64] have proposed that abdominal myofascial syndrome should be considered in the differential diagnosis of chronic pelvic pain. Trigger points in the abdominal muscles may produce referred abdominal pain and induce visceral disorders (somato-visceral effects). Conversely, visceral disease can also influence somatic sensory perception and can activate TrPs (viscero-somatic effects) that may perpetuate pain and other symptoms long after the patient has recovered from the initiating visceral disease.[65] Understanding the reciprocal somato-visceral and viscero-somatic effects of TrPs helps unravel some of this uncertainty. It has been found that abdominal TrPs have a 93% positive predictive value for visceral disease, particularly chronic pelvic pain syndrome.[66,67] These studies found that the presence of abdominal TrPs, along with abdominal and perineal cutaneous allodynia, discriminated visceral from somatic sources of pain.[67] Furthermore, Anderson et al[68] found that TrPs in the external oblique (80%) and rectus abdominis (75%) muscles were highly prevalent in men with chronic prostatitis or chronic pelvic pain. Different studies have reported the effectiveness of pelvic TrP treatment for relief of abdominal wall and chronic pelvic pain,[69-71] as well as for primary dysmenorrhea.[72] It is important to consider that the European Association of Urology published guidelines suggesting that TrPs should be considered in chronic pelvic pain diagnosis.[73]

Additional differential diagnostic considerations for abdominal wall TrPs should include hiatal hernia (gastroesophageal reflux), gastric carcinoma, chronic cholecystitis or ureteral colic, inguinal hernia, hepatitis, pancreatitis, gynecologic pathology (such as ovarian cysts), diverticulosis, umbilical hernia, thoracic radiculopathy, upper lumbar radiculopathy, costochondritis, ascariasis, epilepsy, and rectus abdominis hematoma.

Melnick[46] has reported the relative frequency of serious symptoms arising from TrP areas in the abdominal muscles among 56 patients (Table 49-1). Long[59] distinguished the "anterior abdominal wall syndrome" from visceral diseases. The syndrome was attributed to TrPs in the abdominal wall muscles. Its distinguishing feature was nearly continuous pain that might relate to movement but not to the ingestion of food or to evacuation. On careful inquiry, some of his patients localized the pain to the abdominal wall. Good[60] observed that referred pain from TrPs in the lateral border of the rectus abdominis muscle was aggravated by bending over when lifting (an activity which shortens and often causes contraction of that muscle). In the experience of the authors of this manual, prolonged vigorous activity that requires forceful abdominal breathing may also increase referred pain from abdominal wall TrPs.

Kelly[74] noted that individuals with myalgic lesions (described like TrPs) of the abdominal wall musculature were likely to report abdominal discomfort or distress, rather than of pain per se. In the authors' experience, active TrPs of the abdominal muscles, especially in the rectus abdominis muscle, may cause a lax, distended abdomen with excessive flatus. Contraction of the abdominal muscles is inhibited by the presence of TrPs; therefore, the patient cannot "pull the stomach in." This apparent distension is readily distinguished from ascites by physical examination.

Feinstein et al[75] injected hypertonic saline into paraspinal musculotendinous tissues 1.3 to 2.5 cm from the midline at each segmental level. The abdominal pain patterns referred from paraspinal muscles at the T7-T12 levels were similar but without the precise degree of segmental correspondence that was previously suggested by Melnick.[46]

Kellgren (along with Lewis in one of their two studies) described referred pain to the abdomen from interspinous ligaments when they injected hypertonic saline.[56,57] Hockaday and Whitty[76] subsequently found that pain was referred from interspinous ligaments only to dorsal areas. The more extensive pain patterns observed by Kellgren[57] may have been due to injection of paraspinal (nonmidline) structures, which Hockaday and Whitty[76] scrupulously avoided.

Abdominal pain in an upper quadrant may be attributed to Tietze's syndrome of the costal cartilages (reported as also affecting the xiphisternal joint) or to abnormal mobility of the lower intercostal joints, which has been variously referred to as the "slipping rib syndrome," or the "rib-tip syndrome".[77,78] These conditions have been diagnosed by the "hooking maneuver," in which the fingers are hooked under the costal margin to pull the ribs forward, demonstrating their abnormal mobility and reproducing the patient's pain.[79] There is a strong likelihood that many of these patients were suffering from enthesitis of muscle attachments to the chondral cartilages. The chondral intercostal muscles, pectoralis major, and transverse abdominal musculature are likely candidates for TrPs that could contribute to the enthesitis.

Right upper quadrant pain due to TrPs in either the internal or external oblique muscles or in the lateral border of the rectus abdominis muscle of the same quadrant is easily confused with the pain of gallbladder disease. Pain simulating appendicitis was projected from "fibrositic nodules" (described like palpable bands and TrPs) in the region covered by the costal portion of the external oblique muscle, and from TrPs in the lateral border of the rectus abdominis muscle in the right lower quadrant.[58]

Abdominal pain, particularly in the lower quadrant of the abdomen, may be referred from TrPs in the para-vertebral muscles (Chapter 48). Trigger points in the lower portion of the rectus abdominis muscle can cause pain in the thoracolumbar region, and a similar pain in that region can also be caused by an avulsion injury of the lumbar multifidus and rotator muscles or from zygapophyseal joints.[50-52,80] Urinary frequency, urinary urgency, and "kidney" pain may be referred from TrPs in the lower abdominal muscles. A TrP high in the adductor muscles of the thigh may refer pain upward into the groin and to the lower lateral abdominal wall as well.[81]

3.3. Patient Examination

The lateral abdominal wall may be injured in a variety of endeavors with occasional acute injuries in the setting of high-energy trauma such as motor vehicle collisions. Injuries to the lateral abdominal wall may result in lumbar hernia formation and also Spigelian hernias.[82] After a thorough subjective examination the clinician should make a detailed drawing representing the pain pattern that the patient has described. This depiction will assist in planning the physical examination and can be useful in monitoring the progression of the patient as symptoms improve or change. Any patient with primary reports of abdominal pain should alert the clinician to perform a thorough systems review. Any concerns regarding the involvement of the cardiovascular, respiratory, or gastrointestinal systems as a source of symptoms should result in an immediate referral to a physician.

The clinician should observe the patient's posture in sitting, standing, walking, and reaching. Articular dysfunctions associated with abdominal muscle TrPs include pubic and innominate dysfunctions, as well as depressed lesions of the lower half of the rib cage. Movement restriction of the thoracolumbar junction is sometimes associated with a shortened rectus abdominis muscle with palpable TrPs. Similar involvement of the psoas and quadratus lumborum muscles is also commonly associated with these joint dysfunctions.[83] All these structures should be carefully examined by the clinician.

Several authors have noted the value of increasing the abdominal muscle tension during examination to help distinguish the pain that is due to TrPs from that due to underlying visceral disease. To conduct the abdominal tension test according to Long,[59] the sensitive area is compressed with sufficient pressure to cause steady pain with the patient in a supine position. When the patient then raises the legs high enough to bring both heels a few inches above the table, the tensed abdominal muscles lift the palpating finger away from the viscera while the digital pressure on the muscle itself is increased. If the pain increases, it suggests that pain may originate from the abdominal wall musculature. If the pain decreases, it more likely originates inside the abdomen. The similar Carnett's technique (the patient is in a supine position, crosses the arms and sits halfway forward) reliably distinguished abdominal wall tenderness from visceral tenderness.[84] Other possibilities for

Table 49-1 Frequency of Serious Complaints among 56 Patients with Abdominal Trigger Points[a]

Symptoms	Number of Patients	Prevalence[b] (%)
Pain	40	71
Pressure and bloating	14	25
Heartburn	6	11
Vomiting	6	11
Diarrhea	2	4

[a]Adapted from Melnick J. Treatment of trigger mechanisms in gastrointestinal disease. NY State J Med. 1954;54:1324-1330.
[b]Percentage and numbers total more than 100% because some patients had more than one symptom.

increasing the contraction of the abdominal wall muscles include asking the patient to lift both heels off the bed alone or in combination with lifting the head. By having patients raise only the head and shoulders free of the table, the test can be performed by those unable to do a sit-up, and they can confirm the test for themselves, assuring themselves of no visceral origin of the pain.[85]

The examiner should observe the displacement of the patient's umbilicus during various activities, such as laughing, coughing, raising one leg up from the bed, or having the patient lift their head off a pillow from a supine position. If there is abdominal muscle imbalance, a umbilicus deviates away from a weaker (or inhibited) muscle and toward a stronger (or more hyperactive) muscle. This deviation indicates a positive Beevor's sign.[86] Simply observing the umbilicus while the patient rests quietly may reveal a deviation toward a muscle with TrP shortening or away from an abdominal muscle that is inhibited by TrPs.

The double leg lowering test and the lower abdominal muscle progression are also two common tests of abdominal muscle performance. A strong association between rectus abdominis muscle activity and external oblique muscle activity was observed with both tests. The association between the internal oblique and transversus abdominis muscles was moderate and weak on each test, respectively.[87]

These tests may measure different qualities of abdominal wall muscle performance. Proper assessment of abdominal wall muscle endurance is clinically significant in these patients because the abdominal muscle fatigue after sustained exercise is primarily due to peripheral mechanisms,[88] suggesting a potential role of TrPs in muscle fatigue.

Abdominal Oblique Muscles

To ensure contraction of the lateral wall abdominal muscles while performing the abdominal tension test, the supine patient should elevate the heels or elevate the head and shoulders high enough to lift both scapulae off any support on the table. When the patient elevates only the head, it is the rectus abdominis muscle that is mainly contracted, not the abdominal oblique muscles. The patient can also rotate the trunk during the head elevation for increasing the diagonal tension of the ipsilateral internal oblique and the contralateral external oblique muscles. Clinical assessment of abdominal oblique muscles is highly relevant in patients with low back pain, because patients with chronic low back pain demonstrated significantly higher activation of the external oblique and rectus abdominis muscles.[89] This overactivity can be a promoting factor for developing TrPs in these muscles.

Transversus Abdominis

There is clear evidence suggesting that patients with low back pain demonstrate a delayed activation of the transversus abdominis muscle; however, this temporal change is not directly associated to related-disability.[22] In fact, patients with low back pain exhibit delayed activation of transversus abdominis and internal oblique muscles, absence of abdominal core muscle coactivation, and impairments in the temporal timing between transversus abdominis and internal oblique muscle onsets.[90] Additionally, the transversus abdominis muscle also exhibits lower activation during weight-bearing tasks.[91] Because direct palpation of the transverse abdominis muscle for the presence of TrPs is difficult, assessment of its function is clinically important in patients with low back or abdominal pain.

Rectus Abdominis

When a patient with TrPs in the rectus abdominis muscle stands, the abdomen is likely to sag and become pendulous. Clinically, TrPs in this muscle inhibit its supportive function. Janda[92] classified the rectus abdominis muscle as prone to inhibition and weakness. The palpable taut band associated with TrPs would shorten only a segment of the rectus abdominis muscle (between fascial delineations) in which it lies. The rectus abdominis muscle has no parallel muscle, except its contralateral partner, that could contract and unload it to provide protective splinting. Nevertheless, recent studies have found increased activation of the rectus abdominis muscle in individuals with chronic low back pain.[27]

If asked to take a deep breath, patients with rectus abdominis TrPs are likely to exhibit paradoxical breathing. Although during quiet respiration, exhalation is essentially performed by the elasticity of the lungs and requires little muscular assistance, the threat of pain due to stretching of the involved rectus abdominis muscle apparently could subconsciously inhibit the normal diaphragmatic contraction on inspiration. This pattern may be a rectus abdominis–diaphragmatic reflex inhibition. When the patient inhales deeply with the diaphragm muscle, protruding the abdomen, referred pain due to rectus abdominis TrPs may be exacerbated. In these patients, the bilateral, transverse, mid-back referred pain from TrPs in the upper portion of the rectus abdominis muscle is usually aggravated by taking a deep breath, especially when the back is arched in marked lumbar lordosis, which further stretches the rectus abdominis muscle. Back pain from paraspinal TrPs is not usually influenced by respiration. Herniation through the abdominal musculature is detected in some cases only when the patient is standing rather than recumbent.

3.4. Trigger Point Examination

Examination of the superficial external oblique and rectus abdominis muscles is easier than examination of the deeper internal oblique and transversus abdominal muscles, because these two are not reliably accessible for diagnostic palpation.

When the abdominal muscles are examined for TrPs, the patient lies supine, taking a deep breath using diaphragmatic (abdominal) breathing and holding the breath to passively stretch the muscles (it helps relax them) and to increase their pressure sensitivity to palpation. To optimize palpation of lateral abdominal TrPs, the patient lies on the contralateral side and holds a similar deep breath.

External Oblique

The external oblique muscle can be examined with a cross-fiber pincer palpation. The most accessible fibers are those located on the lower border of the rib cage and along the line where this muscle attaches to the iliac crest (Figure 49-8A and B). The patient's hips may be flexed to slacken the abdominal muscles; the abdominal wall in the flank area (external and internal oblique and transversus muscles) can then be grasped between the fingers and the thumb. When the TrP or the taut band is strummed with the pincer grasp, the muscle fiber usually responds with a vigorous and visible local twitch response. Cross-fiber flat palpation may also be utilized to identify TrPs in the external oblique muscles (Figure 49-8C).

Internal Oblique

The internal oblique muscle cannot be directly palpated. Tender areas in this muscle can be located along the inferior margins of the tips of the six lower ribs or close to the pubic bone. In our experience, to find them, the clinician should press down against the upper edge of the pubic arch, not on the flat anterior surface of the pubis. These TrPs feel like small buttons or short bands at the region of attachments of the internal oblique muscle.

Rectus Abdominis

Trigger points in the rectus abdominis muscle are easily accessible to a cross-fiber flat palpation. Trigger points can be found in either portion of the muscle (Figure 49-9A and B). The patient's hips may be flexed to slacken the rectus abdominis muscle,

Chapter 49: Abdominal Muscles   493

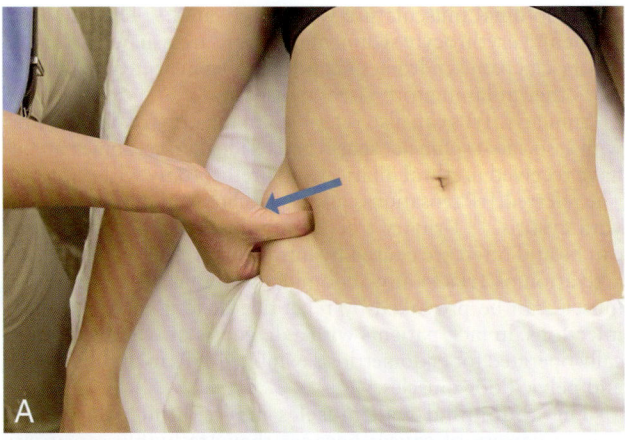
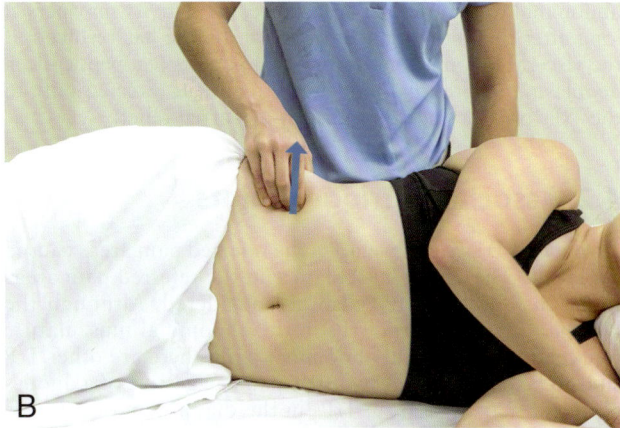
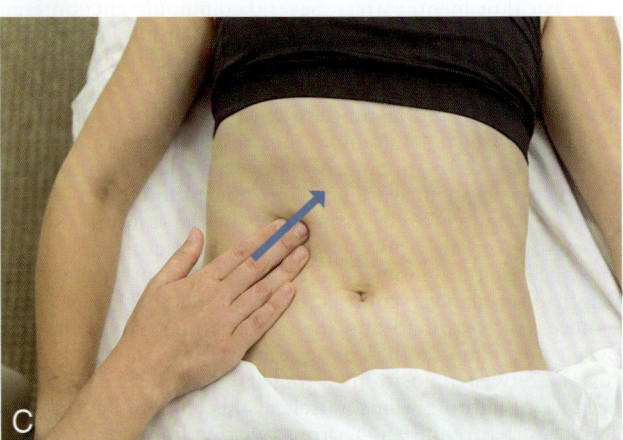

Figure 49-8. Palpation of the right external oblique muscle. A, Cross-fiber pincer palpation with the patient supine; B, Cross-fiber pincer palpation with the patient side-lying. C, Cross-fiber flat palpation.

which is helpful for palpation of the lower portion of the muscle. When the TrP or the taut band is identified with cross-fiber flat palpation, the muscle fiber usually responds with a visible local twitch response.

4. DIFFERENTIAL DIAGNOSIS

4.1. Activation and Perpetuation of Trigger Points

A posture or activity that activates a TrP, if not corrected, can also perpetuate it. In any part of the abdominal muscles, TrPs may be activated by unaccustomed eccentric loading, eccentric exercise in an unconditioned muscle, or maximal or submaximal concentric loading.[93] Trigger points may also be activated or aggravated when the muscle is placed in a shortened or lengthened position for an extended period of time. A posture or activity that activates a TrP, if not corrected or if continued, can also perpetuate it. In addition, many structural and systemic factors (refer to Chapter 3) perpetuate a TrP that has been activated by an acute or chronic overload. Abdominal TrPs are likely to develop in muscles that lie in the zone of pain referral from visceral structures. In general, TrPs may develop in response to visceral disease; direct trauma; and to mechanical, toxic, or emotional stress. These mechanisms are particularly relevant for

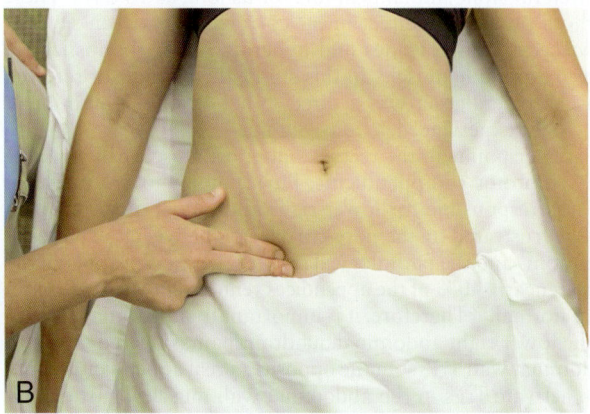

Figure 49-9. Cross-fiber flat palpation of the rectus abdominis muscle with the patient supine. A, Upper portion of the muscle; B, Lower portion of the muscle.

abdominal wall muscles. For instance, TrP activity may persist long after the initiating acute visceral disease has resolved. If the visceral lesion is long-lasting and persists (eg, peptic ulcer, neoplasm, or intestinal parasites), treatment directed only to the TrPs provides merely transient or partial relief.

4.2. Associated Trigger Points

Associated TrPs can develop in the referred pain areas caused by TrPs.[94] Therefore, musculature in the referred pain areas for each muscle should also be considered. Although the clinician first considers TrPs in the abdominal musculature to explain non-visceral abdominal pain, there are other TrP sites to be considered. Epigastric pain suggestive of a duodenal ulcer may arise from TrPs in the diaphragm or serratus anterior muscles.

Trigger points in the lower portion of the lateral abdominal wall muscles are often associated with TrPs high in the adductor muscles of the thigh, which may refer pain upward inside the abdomen. Trigger points in the pelvic floor musculature may often coexist with TrPs in the abdominal wall muscles and can help differentiate pelvic and abdominal pain of visceral versus somatic origin.[66]

Similarly, TrPs in the psoas or iliacus muscles can also refer pain to the abdominal region, contribute to flatulence, or mimic other visceral symptoms.

4.3. Associated Pathology

As mentioned earlier, visceral diseases can be associated with abdominal wall TrPs. Abdominal wall TrPs are especially likely to develop with any inflammatory visceral disease as a result of the viscero-somatic reflex. In fact, the presence of abdominal TrPs and abdominal cutaneous allodynia each had a positive predictive value of 93% for the presence of visceral dysfunction.[67] The relationship between TrPs and visceral problems is bidirectional because modification of the sensory input to the central nervous system in somatic areas of pain referral from visceral nociceptive input can modify the perception of pain. In fact, viscera tissues exhibit similar pain referral areas as TrPs. In healthy subjects, stimulation of the splenic flexure of the small intestine by acute distention induced referred pain to the upper abdomen. In individuals with an irritable colon, this stimulus projected pain also to the precordium, left shoulder, neck, and arm.[95] The upper and lower gastrointestinal tract of 21 patients with "functional" abdominal pain with no organic cause was systematically explored using an inflatable balloon.[96] The authors found referred pain elicited by areas in the esophagus, small intestine, and colon that produced the patients' symptoms. Giamberardino et al[97] studied the responses to ureteral stone implants in rats for as long as 10 days. These authors observed a direct linear correlation between severity of visceral pain episodes and hyperalgesia of the ipsilateral external oblique muscle. In this study, the amount of referred muscle hyperalgesia was a direct function of the amount of colic pain experienced.

Trigger points in the rectus abdominis muscle can simulate the symptoms of appendicitis. Physicians who are unaware of TrPs responsible for lower right abdominal quadrant pain can be frustrated by the poor correlation between the patient's symptoms and the pathological state of the excised appendix.[98] In fact, nearly 40% of the appendices removed in one large series were normal.[99] Therefore, it is important to differentiate if pain in the lower right abdominal quadrant pain is related or not to abdominal wall TrPs. On the opposite, a real appendicitis could also activate TrPs in the abdominal wall muscles, particularly after surgery, provoking persistent pain after the surgery. It has been previously documented that pain responding to medical treatment for a duodenal ulcer became persistent until TrPs in the abdominal musculature were inactivated.[47] The leucocyte count and erythrocyte sedimentation rate are usually normal in myofascial pain syndromes but are elevated in acute appendicitis and other inflammatory visceral diseases.

Similarly, TrPs can also refer pain to the urinary bladder area with associated sphincter spasm and residual urine. Some patients have received urethral dilation and urethrotomy without relief. The referred TrP sensations can also mimic symptoms compatible with cystitis.[100] Urinary tract symptoms indicating prostatitis can be and often are caused by intrapelvic TrPs. Again, somatic activation of TrPs in any abdominal wall muscle or paraspinal muscle can be provoked by repetitive or long-lasting urinary infections. In fact, patients with a diagnosis or who were surgically operated for endometriosis exhibited TrPs in the abdominal and pelvic floor muscles.[101]

The abdominal wall muscles may exhibit dysfunction from a variety of causes because they are highly sensitivity to physical or mental stress. Several commonly encountered stress factors may activate abdominal wall TrPs: fatigue, emotional tension, cold exposure, viral infections, visceral problems, straining due to constipation, and poor posture (such as sitting and leaning forward for hours on a bed or at a desk with the abdominal muscles shortened and tense, with the back not supported). However, some postural disturbances such as forward head or rounded shoulder postures (refer to Chapter 76) can sometimes be the result of the TrP shortening in the upper portion of the rectus abdominis muscle. Structural biomechanical malalignment such as a leg length discrepancy, scoliosis, or small hemipelvis may add unnecessary overload and their effects may be cumulative over time. The external oblique muscle is vulnerable to a sustained twisted position (sitting at a desk, turned sideways because of lighting). This muscle also is vulnerable in sports activities that require a vigorous twisting body motion (ball throwing or racquet swinging).

Acute trauma and chronic occupational strain are important activating factors. Anecdotally, TrPs are likely to occur close to an abdominal scar, as such after an appendectomy or hysterectomy. The initiating stresses during surgery may be the combination of excessive stretch on the muscles by retractors and associated ischemia. The skin and muscles around an incision can be easily infiltrated effectively with procaine at the time of suturing the wound to prevent the development of TrPs following surgery and to reduce postoperative incisional discomfort. In another example, rectus abdominis TrPs may be initiated in conjunction with an abdominal operation and perpetuated by paradoxical breathing that develops as a result of postoperative abdominal soreness. The development of these TrPs also discourages abdominal muscle activity, which could contribute to paradoxical breathing. An unusual source of continuous severe lower abdominal pain is hematoma of the rectus abdominis muscle.[102]

5. CORRECTIVE ACTIONS

When seated, the patient should use a small pillow for lumbar support and should lean against the backrest of the chair. This maintains the natural lumbar lordosis and raises the thoracic cage anteriorly, which places the more longitudinal abdominal wall muscles on gentle stretch. A very tight elastic belt or girdle may compress the abdominal muscles, interfering with their circulation.

Helpful exercises for the abdominal musculature include regular diaphragmatic (abdominal) breathing, the pelvic-tilt and the sit-back/sit-up exercises, and laughter.

Diaphragmatic (Abdominal) Breathing

The most effective active stretch exercise for these muscles is diaphragmatic breathing.[39] Diaphragmatic breathing, with the patient in hook-lying, stretches the lateral abdominal wall muscles (Figure 45-11).

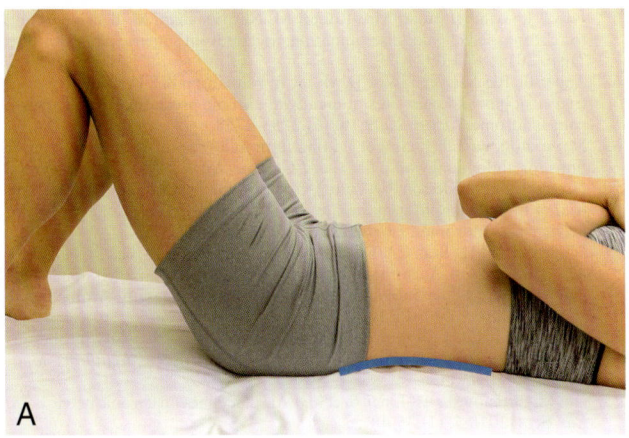 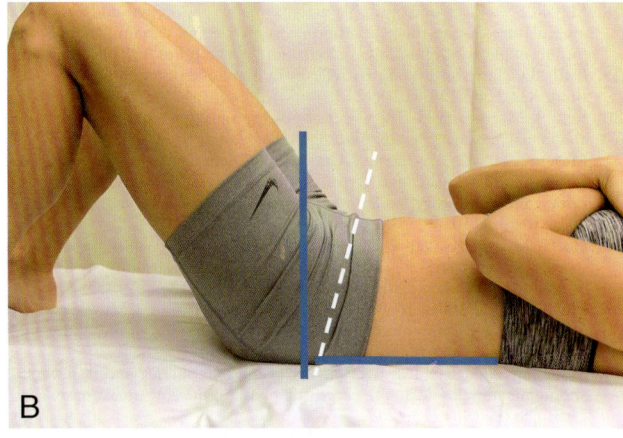

Figure 49-10. The pelvic-tilt exercise engages the abdominal muscles and stretches the lumbar spinal muscles. A, Starting position. B, Patient contracts the abdominal muscles to flatten the lumbar spine against the floor, gently tilting the front of the pelvis toward the nose.

Pelvic Tilt

The pelvic-tilt exercise is a gentle and effective exercise for the lower portion of the rectus abdominis muscle. The exercise is performed as illustrated and described in Figure 49-10.

Sit-back/Abdominal-curl/Sit-up

The sit-back/abdominal-curl/sit-up exercise is the smooth combination of three exercises (Figure 49-5). This combination exercise should always begin with the sit-back exercise. It results in a lengthening, not shortening, contraction of the abdominal musculature. The lengthening contraction of the sit-back places relatively less load on the involved abdominal muscles because of the greater strength and efficiency of a lengthening, as compared with a shortening contraction. First, the patient pushes himself or herself up into the sit-up position with the arms and then does a slow sit-back (Figure 49-5A). The curl-down movement of the sit-back should be made smoothly and slowly, without jerks. The pause between each cycle of the exercise is as important as the movement and should be equally long. A full inspiration and expiration at the end of each sit-back helps reestablish complete relaxation of the muscles and paces the exercise. The patient starts by doing the exercise on alternate days or, if the abdominal muscles are still sore, skipping 2 days. Then, the number of sit-backs is gradually increased to a goal of 10 per daily session. Only when the sit-back goal is reached does the patient proceed to the abdominal curl (Figure 49-5B), which is a partial sit-up. This is done as a "peel-up" with the spine bending forward, so that each successive vertebra leaves the floor in turn (Figure 49-5C and D).

Laughter

Laughter is a vigorous isometric exercise for all the abdominal muscles.

If the exercise program induces fatigue or self-perception of shortening of the muscles, the patient can be also gently stretch the abdominal musculature (Figure 51-5A and B).

References

1. Rankin G, Stokes M, Newham DJ. Abdominal muscle size and symmetry in normal subjects. *Muscle Nerve*. 2006;34(3):320-326.
2. Tanaka NI, Yamada M, Tanaka Y, Fukunaga T, Nishijima T, Kanehisa H. Difference in abdominal muscularity at the umbilicus level between young and middle-aged men. *J Physiol Anthropol*. 2007;26(5):527-532.
3. Standring S. *Gray's Anatomy: The Anatomical Basis of Clinical Practice*. 41st ed. London, UK: Elsevier; 2015.
4. Lange W. On the functional structure of tendinous inscriptions in the human rectus abdominis muscle [in German]. *Gegenbaurs Morphol Jahrb*. 1968;111(3):336-342.
5. Beaton LE, Anson BJ. The pyramidalis muscle: its occurrence and size in American white and negroes. *Am J Phys Anthropol*. 1939;25:261-269.
6. Anson B, Beaton L, McVay C. The pyramidalis muscle. *Anatomical Record*. 1938;72:405-411.
7. Rahn DD, Phelan JN, Roshanravan SM, White AB, Corton MM. Anterior abdominal wall nerve and vessel anatomy: clinical implications for gynecologic surgery. *Am J Obstet Gynecol*. 2010;202(3):234.e1-234.e5.
8. van der Graaf T, Verhagen PC, Kerver AL, Kleinrensink GJ. Surgical anatomy of the 10th and 11th intercostal, and subcostal nerves: prevention of damage during lumbotomy. *J Urol*. 2011;186(2):579-583.
9. Hammond DC, Larson DL, Severinac RN, Marcias M. Rectus abdominis muscle innervation: implications for TRAM flap elevation. *Plast Reconstr Surg*. 1995;96(1):105-110.
10. Ramasastry SS, Granick MS, Futrell JW. Clinical anatomy of the internal oblique muscle. *J Reconstr Microsurg*. 1986;2(2):117-122.
11. Schlenz I, Burggasser G, Kuzbari R, Eichberger H, Gruber H, Holle J. External oblique abdominal muscle: a new look on its blood supply and innervation. *Anat Rec*. 1999;255(4):388-395.
12. Yang D, Morris SF, Geddes CR, Tang M. Neurovascular territories of the external and internal oblique muscles. *Plast Reconstr Surg*. 2003;112(6):1591-1595.
13. Mathes SJ, Nahai F. Classification of the vascular anatomy of muscles: experimental and clinical correlation. *Plast Reconstr Surg*. 1981;67(2):177-187.
14. Arjmand N, Shirazi-Adl A, Parnianpour M. Trunk biomechanics during maximum isometric axial torque exertions in upright standing. *Clin Biomech (Bristol, Avon)*. 2008;23(8):969-978.
15. Masani K, Sin VW, Vette AH, et al. Postural reactions of the trunk muscles to multi-directional perturbations in sitting. *Clin Biomech (Bristol, Avon)*. 2009;24(2):176-182.
16. Hides JA, Wong I, Wilson SJ, Belavy DL, Richardson CA. Assessment of abdominal muscle function during a simulated unilateral weight-bearing task using ultrasound imaging. *J Orthop Sports Phys Ther*. 2007;37(8):467-471.
17. El Ouaaid Z, Arjmand N, Shirazi-Adl A, Parnianpour M. A novel approach to evaluate abdominal coactivities for optimal spinal stability and compression force in lifting. *Comput Methods Biomech Biomed Engin*. 2009;12(6):735-745.
18. Kim LJ, Kim N. Difference in lateral abdominal muscle thickness during forceful exhalation in healthy smokers and non-smokers. *J Back Musculoskelet Rehabil*. 2012;25(4):239-244.
19. Juker D, McGill S, Kropf P, Steffen T. Quantitative intramuscular myoelectric activity of lumbar portions of psoas and the abdominal wall during a wide variety of tasks. *Med Sci Sports Exerc*. 1998;30(2):301-310.
20. Page P, Frank C, Lardner R. *Assessment and Treatment of Muscle Imbalance. The Janda Approach*. Champaign, IL: Human Kinetics; 2010.
21. Vleeming A, Schuenke MD, Danneels L, Willard FH. The functional coupling of the deep abdominal and paraspinal muscles: the effects of simulated paraspinal muscle contraction on force transfer to the middle and posterior layer of the thoracolumbar fascia. *J Anat*. 2014;225(4):447-462.
22. Wong AY, Parent EC, Funabashi M, Kawchuk GN. Do changes in transversus abdominis and lumbar multifidus during conservative treatment explain changes in clinical outcomes related to nonspecific low back pain? A systematic review. *J Pain*. 2014;15(4):377.e1-377.e35.
23. Hodges PW, Richardson CA. Contraction of the abdominal muscles associated with movement of the lower limb. *Phys Ther*. 1997;77(2):132-142; discussion 142-134.
24. Hodges PW, Richardson CA. Delayed postural contraction of transversus abdominis in low back pain associated with movement of the lower limb. *J Spinal Disord*. 1998;11(1):46-56.
25. Hodges PW. Changes in motor planning of feedforward postural responses of the trunk muscles in low back pain. *Exp Brain Res*. 2001;141(2):261-266.
26. Hodges PW, Richardson CA. Relationship between limb movement speed and associated contraction of the trunk muscles. *Ergonomics*. 1997;40(11):1220-1230.
27. Ghamkhar L, Kahlaee AH. Trunk muscles activation pattern during walking in subjects with and without chronic low back pain: a systematic review. *PM R*. 2015;7(5):519-526.

28. McGill SM. Electromyographic activity of the abdominal and low back musculature during the generation of isometric and dynamic axial trunk torque: implications for lumbar mechanics. *J Orthop Res.* 1991;9(1):91-103.
29. Beith ID, Harrison PJ. Stretch reflexes in human abdominal muscles. *Exp Brain Res.* 2004;159(2):206-213.
30. Kera T, Maruyama H. The effect of posture on respiratory activity of the abdominal muscles. *J Physiol Anthropol Appl Human Sci.* 2005;24(4):259-265.
31. Mesquita Montes A, Baptista J, Crasto C, de Melo CA, Santos R, Vilas-Boas JP. Abdominal muscle activity during breathing with and without inspiratory and expiratory loads in healthy subjects. *J Electromyogr Kinesiol.* 2016;30:143-150.
32. Hu H, Meijer OG, van Dieen JH, et al. Muscle activity during the active straight leg raise (ASLR), and the effects of a pelvic belt on the ASLR and on treadmill walking. *J Biomech.* 2010;43(3):532-539.
33. MacKenzie JF, Grimshaw PN, Jones CD, Thoirs K, Petkov J. Muscle activity during lifting: examining the effect of core conditioning of multifidus and transversus abdominis. *Work.* 2014;47(4):453-462.
34. Miller MI, Medeiros JM. Recruitment of internal oblique and transversus abdominis muscles during the eccentric phase of the curl-up exercise. *Phys Ther.* 1987;67(8):1213-1217.
35. Uva B, Aliverti A, Bovio D, Kayser B. The "Abdominal Circulatory Pump": an auxiliary heart during exercise? *Front Physiol.* 2015;6:411.
36. Urquhart DM, Hodges PW, Allen TJ, Story IH. Abdominal muscle recruitment during a range of voluntary exercises. *Man Ther.* 2005;10(2):144-153.
37. Olson MW. Trunk muscle activation during sub-maximal extension efforts. *Man Ther.* 2010;15(1):105-110.
38. Okada M. An electromyographic estimation of the relative muscular load in different human postures. *J Human Ergol.* 1972;1:75-93.
39. Flint MM. An electromyographic comparison of the function of the iliacus and the rectus abdominis muscles. A preliminary report. *Phys Ther.* 1965;45:248-252.
40. Godfrey KE, Kindig LE, Windell EJ. Electromyographic study of duration of muscle activity in sit-up variations. *Arch Phys Med Rehabil.* 1977;58(3):132-135.
41. Gilleard WL, Brown JM. An electromyographic validation of an abdominal muscle test. *Arch Phys Med Rehabil.* 1994;75(9):1002-1007.
42. Simons DG, Travell J, Simons L. *Travell & Simon's Myofascial Pain and Dysfunction: The Trigger Point Manual.* Vol 1. 2nd ed. Baltimore: Williams & Wilkins; 1999.
43. Rivero Fernandez M, Moreira Vicente V, Riesco Lopez JM, Rodrigues Gandia M, Garrido Gomez R, Miliua Salamero J. Pain originating from the abdominal wall: a forgotten diagnostic option [in Spanish]. *Gastroenterol Hepatol.* 2007;30:244-250.
44. Muscolino JE. Abdominal wall trigger point case study. *J Bodyw Mov Ther.* 2013;17(2):151-156.
45. Gutstein RR. The role of abdominal fibrositis in functional indigestion. *Miss Valley Med J.* 1944;66:114-124.
46. Melnick J. Treatment of trigger mechanism in gastrointestinal disease. *N Y State J Med.* 1954;54(9):1324-1330.
47. Melnick J. Trigger areas and refractory pain in duodenal ulcer. *N Y State J Med.* 1957;57(6):1073-1077.
48. Kellgren JH. Observations on referred pain arising from muscle. *Clin Sci.* 1938;3:175-190.
49. Aftimos S. Myofascial pain in children. *N Z Med J.* 1989;102(874):440-441.
50. Simons DG, Travell JG. Myofascial origins of low back pain. 1. Principles of diagnosis and treatment. *Postgrad Med.* 1983;73(2):66, 68-70, 73 passim.
51. Simons DG, Travell JG. Myofascial origins of low back pain. 2. Torso muscles. *Postgrad Med.* 1983;73(2):81-92.
52. Simons DG, Travell JG. Myofascial origins of low back pain. 3. Pelvic and lower extremity muscles. *Postgrad Med.* 1983;73(2):99-105, 108.
53. Mehta M, Ranger I. Persistent abdominal pain. Treatment by nerve block. *Anaesthesia.* 1971;26(3):330-333.
54. Bates T, Grunwaldt E. Myofascial pain in childhood. *J Pediatr.* 1958;53(2):198-209.
55. Travell JG. A trigger point for hiccup. *J Am Osteopath Assoc.* 1977;77(4):308-312.
56. Lewis T, Kellgren JH. Observations relating to referred pain, visceromotor reflexes and other associated phenomena. *Clin Sci.* 1939;4:47-71
57. Kellgren JH. On the distribution of pain arising from deep somatic structures with charts of segmental pain areas. *Clin Sci.* 1939;4:35-46.
58. Good MG. Pseudo-appendicitis. *Acta Med Scand.* 1950;138(5):348-353.
59. Long C, 2nd. Myofascial pain syndromes. III. Some syndromes of the trunk and thigh. *Henry Ford Hosp Med Bull.* 1956;4(2):102-106.
60. Good MG. The role of skeletal muscles in the pathogenesis of diseases. *Acta Med Scand.* 1950;138(4):284-292.
61. Carnett JB. Intercostal neuralgia as a cause of abdominal pain and tenderness. *Surg Gynecol Obstet.* 1926;42:625-632.
62. Ingber RS. Atypical chest pain due to myofascial dysfunction of the diaphragm muscle: a case report. *Arch Phys Med Rehabil.* 1988;69:729.
63. Smith LA. The pattern of pain in the diagnosis of upper abdominal disorders. *J Am Med Assoc.* 1954;156(17):1566-1573.
64. Montenegro ML, Gomide LB, Mateus-Vasconcelos EL, et al. Abdominal myofascial pain syndrome must be considered in the differential diagnosis of chronic pelvic pain. *Eur J Obstet Gynecol Reprod Biol.* 2009;147(1):21-24.
65. Aredo JV, Heyrana KJ, Karp BI, Shah JP, Stratton P. Relating chronic pelvic pain and endometriosis to signs of sensitization and myofascial pain and dysfunction. *Semin Reprod Med.* 2017;35(1):88-97.
66. Jarrell J. Myofascial dysfunction in the pelvis. *Curr Pain Headache Rep.* 2004;8(6):452-456.
67. Jarrell J, Giamberardino MA, Robert M, Nasr-Esfahani M. Bedside testing for chronic pelvic pain: discriminating visceral from somatic pain. *Pain Res Treat.* 2011;2011:692102.
68. Anderson RU, Sawyer T, Wise D, Morey A, Nathanson BH. Painful myofascial trigger points and pain sites in men with chronic prostatitis/chronic pelvic pain syndrome. *J Urol.* 2009;182(6):2753-2758.
69. Nazareno J, Ponich T, Gregor J. Long-term follow-up of trigger point injections for abdominal wall pain. *Can J Gastroenterol.* 2005;19(9):561-565.
70. Fitzgerald MP, Anderson RU, Potts J, et al. Randomized multicenter feasibility trial of myofascial physical therapy for the treatment of urological chronic pelvic pain syndromes. *J Urol.* 2013;189(1 suppl):S75-S85.
71. Montenegro ML, Braz CA, Rosa-e-Silva JC, Candido-dos-Reis FJ, Nogueira AA, Poli-Neto OB. Anaesthetic injection versus ischemic compression for the pain relief of abdominal wall trigger points in women with chronic pelvic pain. *BMC Anesthesiol.* 2015;15:175.
72. Huang QM, Liu L. Wet needling of myofascial trigger points in abdominal muscles for treatment of primary dysmenorrhoea. *Acupunct Med.* 2014;32(4):346-349.
73. Fall M, Baranowski AP, Elneil S, et al. EAU guidelines on chronic pelvic pain. *Eur Urol.* 2010;57(1):35-48.
74. Kelly M. Lumbago and abdominal pain. *Med J Australia.* 1942;1:311-317.
75. Feinstein B, Langton JN, Jameson RM, Schiller F. Experiments on pain referred from deep somatic tissues. *J Bone Joint Surg Am.* 1954;36-A(5):981-997.
76. Hockaday JM, Whitty CW. Patterns of referred pain in the normal subject. *Brain.* 1967;90(3):481-496.
77. Heinz GJ, Zavala DC. Slipping rib syndrome. *JAMA.* 1977;237(8):794-795.
78. Jelenko C III. Tietze's disease predates 'chest wall syndrome'. *JAMA.* 1979;242(23):2556.
79. McBeath AA, Keene JS. The rib-tip syndrome. *J Bone Joint Surg Am.* 1975;57A(6):795-797.
80. Howarth D, Southee A, Cardew P, Front D. SPECT in avulsion injury of the multifidus and rotator muscles of the lumbar region. *Clin Nucl Med.* 1994;19(7):571-574.
81. Travell J. The adductor longus syndrome: a cause of groin pain; Its treatment by local block of trigger areas (procaine infiltration and ethyl chloride spray). *Miss Valley Med J.* 1950;71:13-22.
82. Stensby JD, Baker JC, Fox MG. Athletic injuries of the lateral abdominal wall: review of anatomy and MR imaging appearance. *Skeletal Radiol.* 2016;45(2):155-162.
83. Lewit K. Muscular pattern in thoraco-lumbar lesions. *Manual Med.* 1986;2:105-107.
84. Thomson WH, Dawes RF, Carter SS. Abdominal wall tenderness: a useful sign in chronic abdominal pain. *Br J Surg.* 1991;78(2):223-225.
85. Hall MW, Sowden DS, Gravestock N. Abdominal wall tenderness test [Letter]. *Lancet.* 1991;337:1606.
86. Desai JD. Beevor's sign. *Ann Indian Acad Neurol.* 2012;15(2):94-95.
87. Haladay DE, Denegar CR, Miller SJ, Challis J. Electromyographic and kinetic analysis of two abdominal muscle performance tests. *Physiother Theory Pract.* 2015;31(8):587-593.
88. Taylor BJ, How SC, Romer LM. Exercise-induced abdominal muscle fatigue in healthy humans. *J Appl Physiol (1985).* 2006;100(5):1554-1562.
89. Silfies SP, Squillante D, Maurer P, Westcott S, Karduna AR. Trunk muscle recruitment patterns in specific chronic low back pain populations. *Clin Biomech (Bristol, Avon).* 2005;20(5):465-473.
90. Masse-Alarie H, Flamand VH, Moffet H, Schneider C. Corticomotor control of deep abdominal muscles in chronic low back pain and anticipatory postural adjustments. *Exp Brain Res.* 2012;218(1):99-109.
91. Hides JA, Belavy DL, Cassar L, Williams M, Wilson SJ, Richardson CA. Altered response of the anterolateral abdominal muscles to simulated weight-bearing in subjects with low back pain. *Eur Spine J.* 2009;18(3):410-418.
92. Janda V. Evaluation of muscular imbalance, Chapter 6. In: Liebenson C, ed. *Rehabilitation of the Spine: A Practitioner's Guide.* Baltimore: Williams & Wilkins; 1996:97-112.
93. Gerwin RD, Dommerholt J, Shah JP. An expansion of Simons' integrated hypothesis of trigger point formation. *Curr Pain Headache Rep.* 2004;8(6):468-475.
94. Hsieh YL, Kao MJ, Kuan TS, Chen SM, Chen JT, Hong CZ. Dry needling to a key myofascial trigger point may reduce the irritability of satellite MTrPs. *Am J Phys Med Rehabil.* 2007;86(5):397-403.
95. Dworken HJ, Biel FJ, Machella TE. Supradiaphragmatic reference of pain from the colon. *Gastroenterology.* 1952;22(2):222-243.
96. Moriarty JK, Dawson AM. Functional abdominal pain further evidence that whole gut is affected. *Br Med J.* 1982;284:1670-1672.
97. Giamberardino MA, Valente R, de Bigontina P, Vecchiet L. Artificial ureteral calculosis in rats: behavioural characterization of visceral pain episodes and their relationship with referred lumbar muscle hyperalgesia. *Pain.* 1995;61(3):459-469.
98. Gorrell RL. Appendicitis: failure to correlate clinical and pathologic diagnoses; a surgeon's viewpoint. *Minn Med.* 1951;34(2):137-138; 151 passim.
99. Willauer GJ, O'Neill JF. Late postoperative follow-up studies on patients with recurrent appendicitis. *Am J Med Sci.* 1943;205:334-342.
100. Kelsey MP. Diagnosis of upper abdominal pain. *Tex State J Med.* 1951;47(2):82-85.
101. Stratton P, Khachikyan I, Sinaii N, Ortiz R, Shah J. Association of chronic pelvic pain and endometriosis with signs of sensitization and myofascial pain. *Obstet Gynecol.* 2015;125(3):719-728.
102. Reid JD, Kommareddi S, Lankerani M, Park MC. Chronic expanding hematomas. A clinicopathologic entity. *JAMA.* 1980;244(21):2441-2442.

Chapter 50

Quadratus Lumborum Muscle

"Joker of Low Back Pain"

Joseph M. Donnelly and Deanna Hortman Camilo

1. INTRODUCTION

The quadratus lumborum muscle is a broad, quadrilateral muscle that is located within the posterior abdominal wall. The muscle has a broader attachment at the ilium as compared with its attachment onto the lumbar spine and lower ribs. The three groups of quadratus lumborum muscle fibers consist of nearly vertical fibers that form the posterior portion of the muscle (iliocostal), the diagonal fibers that create the middle muscle layer that travels from the iliac crest to the transverse processes of the lumbar vertebrae (iliotransverse), and the diagonal fibers that form the anterior portion of the muscle that extend from the lumbar vertebrae transverse processes to the lower ribs (costotransverse). It functions to side-bend, extend, and stabilize the lumbar spine. Trigger points (TrPs) in the quadratus lumborum muscle generate local pain in the lateral trunk between the iliac crest and 12th rib. Referred pain extends ipsilaterally to the pelvis or sacroiliac joint (SIJ), buttocks, groin, and anterior thigh. Symptoms may be exacerbated by repetitive activities that involve bending and lifting and compensatory gait mechanics due to gluteal muscle weakness or a leg length discrepency. Due to the location of pain referral, differential diagnosis should include SIJ dysfunction or pathology, greater trochanteric bursitis, and lumbar radicular pain. Corrective actions for quadratus lumborum TrPs should address postural alignment; sleeping positions; ergonomics with bending, lifting, and twisting; self-pressure release techniques; and self-stretching techniques.

2. ANATOMIC CONSIDERATIONS

The quadratus lumborum muscle is a thin flat quadrilateral-shaped muscle located in the posterior aspect of the abdominal wall. It occupies the area of the iliac crest deep to the erector spinae and multifidus muscles.[1,2] The muscle is comprised of an anterior, middle, and posterior layer of intersecting bundles of muscle fibers which vary in size and number.[3,4] The muscle has a broader attachment at the ilium as compared with its attachment onto the lumbar spine and lower ribs.[1] The three groups of quadratus lumborum muscle fibers consist of nearly vertical fibers that form the posterior portion of the muscle (iliocostal), the diagonal fibers that create the middle muscle layer that travels from the iliac crest to the transverse processes of the lumbar vertebrae (iliotransverse), and the diagonal fibers that form the anterior portion of the muscle that extend from the lumbar vertebrae transverse processes to the lower ribs (costotransverse).[1-3]

The iliocostal fibers form the most evident portion of the quadratus lumborum muscle. These fibers travel medially and superiorly from their attachment on the uppermost portion of the posterior iliac crest and iliolumbar ligament toward their attachment on the lower ribs[2] (Figure 50-1).

The iliotransverse and costotransverse portions have more variable diagonal bundles of fibers that attach on the tips of the transverse processes of the upper four lumbar vertebrae. The iliotransverse diagonal fibers connect proximally to the transverse processes of L1-L4 and the lateral aspect of T12 and attach distally to the crest of the ilium and often the iliolumbar ligament. The small costotransverse diagonal fibers, which are often not discernable, attach proximally to the 12th rib and distally to the lumbar transverse processes.[2] Both sets of diagonal fibers of the quadratus lumborum muscle may be thought of as guy wires that provide stabilization forces for the lumbar spine (Figures 50-2 and 50-3).

The iliotransverse diagonal fibers are consistently shown in dorsal view (Figure 50-1).[5,6] This portion of the quadratus lumborum muscle is not under the cover of the erector spinae

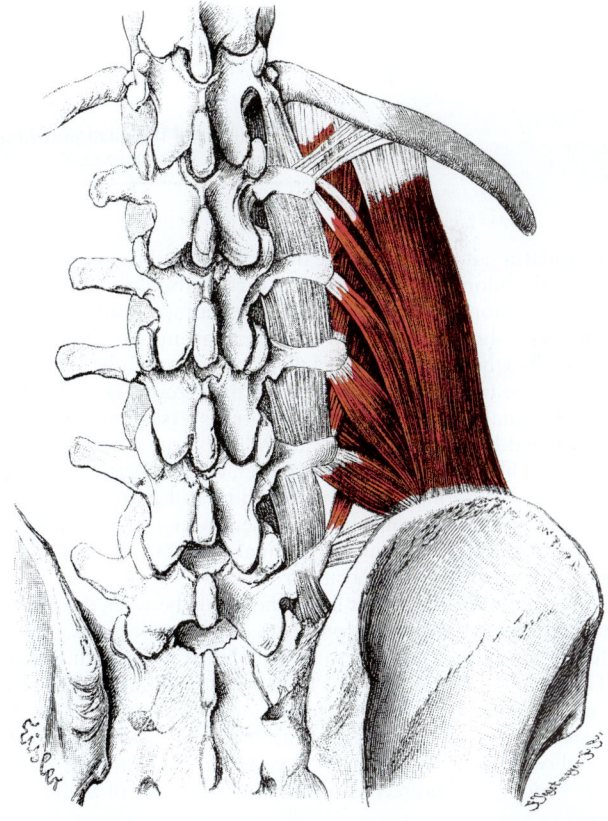

Figure 50-1. Attachments of the quadratus lumborum muscle (red). The intertransversarii lateralis muscle and iliolumbar ligament are uncolored, dorsal view. From Eisler P. *Die Muskeln des Stammes.* Jenna: Gustav Fischer; 1912:654, color added.

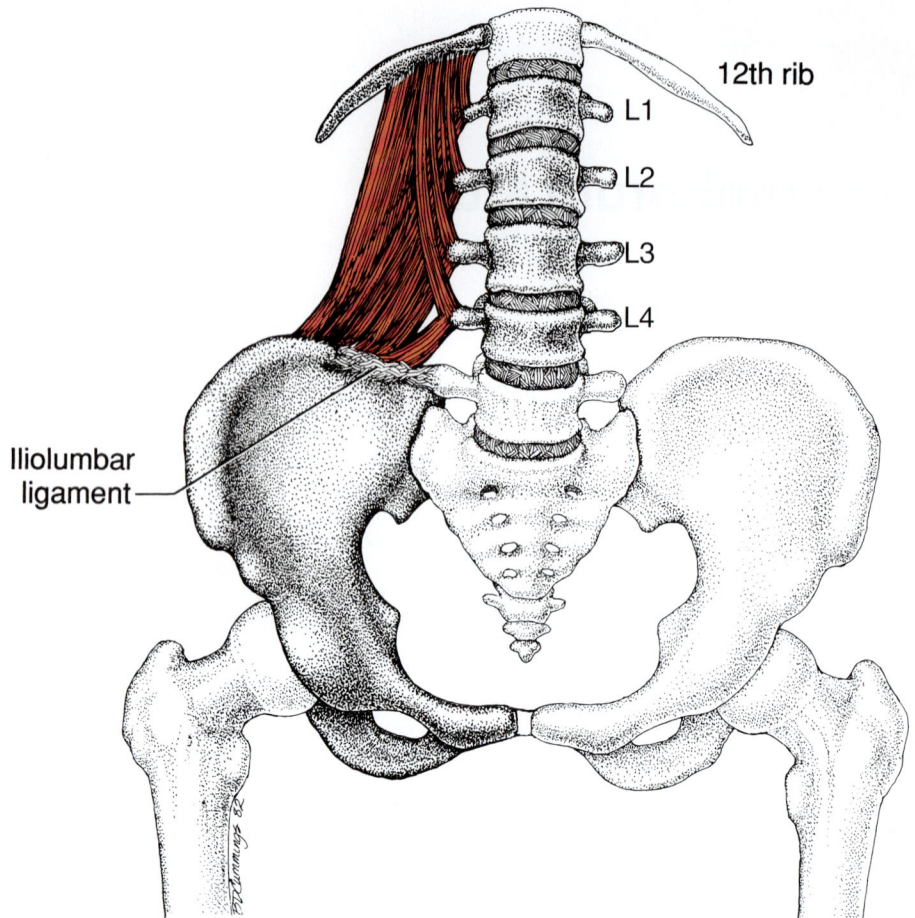

Figure 50-2. Attachments of the quadratus lumborum muscle (red). The iliotransverse, iliocostal, and costotransverse fibers can be visualized, anterior view.

musculature; it lies deep to the thoracolumbar fascia where the internal abdominal oblique, transversus abdominis, and the latissimus dorsi muscles attach to the thoracolumbar fascia.[2] Emphasis should be placed on this anatomic arrangement, especially when palpating for TrPs or muscular tenderness, particularly near the attachments on the iliac crest (Figure 50-4).[2] The diagonal iliotransverse and costotransverse fibers comprise the medial border of the muscle, and the more nearly vertical iliocostal fibers form the lateral border, with increasing overlap and interdigitation as fibers approach their iliac and costal attachments. These diagonal fibers frequently interdigitate between layers of the more lateral longitudinal (vertical) fibers and are most apparent from the posterior view.

The iliolumbar ligament lies in the region between the fourth and fifth lumbar transverse processes and the iliac crests, immediately inferior and medial to the quadratus lumborum muscle (Figures 50-1 and 50-3).[2] The fibers of the iliolumbar ligament blend with the intertransverse ligaments of the lumbar spine and the anterior sacroiliac (SI) ligaments. Together, these ligaments provide stability to the SIJ and the L5-S1 vertebral segment by limiting side-bending and protecting against anterior shear of L5 on S1.[2]

2.1. Innervation and Vascularization

The quadratus lumborum muscle is supplied by branches of the anterior primary rami of T12 and L1-L4.[1]

Vascular supply of the quadratus lumborum muscle is provided by branches of the lumbar arteries, branches from the sacral artery, the iliolumbar artery, and branches from the subcostal artery.[1]

2.2. Function

The quadratus lumborum muscle has, historically, been considered a "hip hiker," elevating the ipsilateral hip during unilateral contraction with a fixed spine. Although the quadratus lumborum muscle does perform this function during ambulation when attempting to compensate for a longer limb,[2] recent research concludes that its primary functions are lateral flexion, extension, and stabilization of the trunk and lumbar spine in the frontal and horizontal planes.[1,2,7-9]

When acting unilaterally with a fixed pelvis, the quadratus lumborum muscle functions as an ipsilateral lateral flexor of the spine (Figure 50-5A and B).[1,7-9] Studies conducted with electromyography (EMG) have shown that the posterior portion of the quadratus lumborum muscle has greater activation during ipsilateral lateral flexion (side-bending) than the anterior portion of the muscle; however, it is during this movement that peak activity of the anterior portion of the quadratus lumborum muscle is achieved.[7,9] Unilateral contraction of the quadratus lumborum muscle has a stabilizing effect on the spine when a person is carrying a load in the contralateral upper extremity.[7] Studies have also shown that the quadratus lumborum muscle is active during contralateral lateral flexion. Thus, the quadratus lumborum muscle on one side of the body serves a stabilizing role, whereas the quadratus lumborum muscle on the contralateral side of the body laterally flexes (side-bends) the spine.[7,9] Lateral trunk motions require both concentric and eccentric contractions between the right and left quadratus lumborum muscles in addition to other trunk muscles to achieve postural stability.

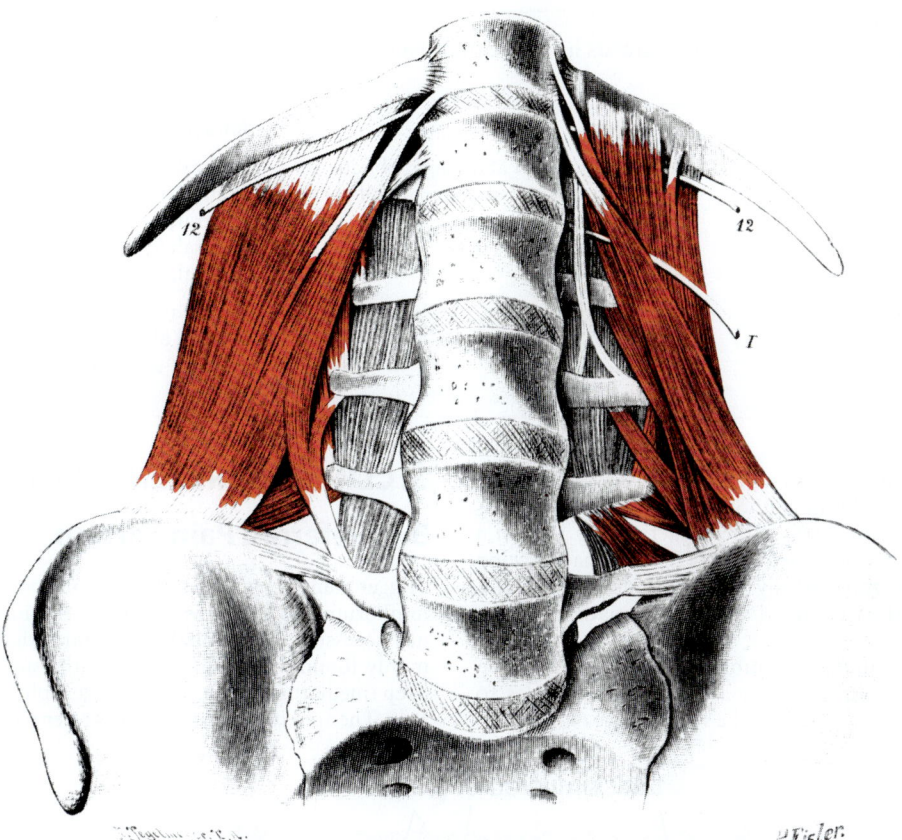

Figure 50-3. Quadratus lumborum (red) and intertransversarii laterales (uncolored) muscles, anterior view. The two halves of the figure are drawn from two different cadaver specimens. *12*, 12th thoracic nerve; *I*, first lumbar nerve. From Eisler P. *Die Muskeln des Stammes*. Jena: Gustav Fischer; 1912:654, 655, color added.

Waters and Morris[10] reported EMG activity in the quadratus lumborum muscle during walking. All recordings were made from the right side of the body. A burst of EMG activity in the right quadratus lumborum muscle occurred in all subjects at moderate and fast walking speeds, preceding and through right and left heel contact.[10] Knapp[11] concluded from clinical observations that, without apparent gluteal muscle weakness, dropping of the pelvis on the swing side when walking in place may be caused by weakness of the oblique fibers of the quadratus lumborum muscle on the opposite side. This supports the biomechanical theory that the quadratus lumborum muscle and the hip abductor muscles serve as guy wires in the frontal plane during the gait cycle.[2]

When contracting bilaterally, the quadratus lumborum muscle extends the spine.[8] In a computer analysis[12] of the lever arms and cross-sectional areas of the regional muscles in two cadavers, the quadratus lumborum muscle was calculated as producing approximately 9% of the muscular force exerted in lateral flexion of the spine and 13% (in one cadaver) or 22% (in the other cadaver) of the extension power of the lumbar spine. This study confirms the extension function deduced from Figure 50-5C, D, and E in all positions of the lumbar spine from full flexion to full extension. In spinal rotation to the contralateral side, the quadratus lumborum muscle was calculated as contributing 9% or 13% of the power.[12]

Bilateral quadratus lumborum muscle contraction also serves a large stabilizing role during spinal compression when the subject is in a standing position,[8] such as when carrying a load with bilateral upper extremities. As the carrying load is increased gradually, the activity of the quadratus lumborum and abdominal oblique muscles increases because more trunk stability is required. To further support the concept of the quadratus lumborum muscle's role in spinal stabilization, researchers have found that stabilization exercises on a Swiss ball in the elderly significantly increases muscle activation in the quadratus lumborum muscle.[13]

Acting bilaterally, the anterior portion of the quadratus lumborum muscle braces the 12th rib and provides support for contraction of the diaphragm muscle, serving as a secondary muscle of inspiration.[1,9] It is also identified as fixing one to two ribs in forced exhalation.[14-16]

The quadratus lumborum muscle can also compensate for a weak gluteus medius muscle during hip abduction. Investigators have studied muscle activation of the quadratus lumborum muscle during hip abduction and found that it compensates for an inadequate gluteus medius muscle, and this compensation is followed with lateral pelvic tilting.[17,18] Recruitment imbalance between the gluteus medius and quadratus lumborum muscles during hip abduction should be considered as a contributing factor to clinical conditions.[17] Recent research has found that utilization of a pelvic compression belt during side-lying hip abduction significantly decreases quadratus lumborum muscle activation and improves gluteus medius muscle activation.[19]

2.3. Functional Unit

The functional unit to which a muscle belongs includes the muscles that reinforce and counter its actions as well as the joints that the muscle crosses. The functional interdependence of these structures is reflected in the organization and neural connections of the sensory motor cortex. The functional unit

Box 50-1 Functional unit of the quadratus lumborum muscle

Action	Synergists	Antagonist
Trunk ipsilateral lateral flexion (side-bending)	Ipsilateral internal abdominal oblique Ipsilateral external abdominal oblique Ipsilateral erector spinae Ipsilateral latissimus dorsi	Contralateral quadratus lumborum Contralateral internal abdominal oblique Contralateral external abdominal oblique Contralateral erector spinae Contralateral latissimus dorsi
Trunk extension	Erector spinae Multifidi Latissiumus dorsi	Rectus abdominis Internal abdominal oblique External abdominal oblique

is emphasized because the presence of a TrP in one muscle of the unit increases the likelihood that the other muscles of the unit also develops TrPs. When inactivating TrPs in a muscle, one should be concerned about TrPs that may develop in muscles that are functionally interdependent. Box 50.1 grossly represents the functional unit of the quadratus lumborum muscle.[20]

During gait, the quadratus lumborum muscle works in conjunction with the hip abductor and adductor muscles to create frontal plane stability during the swing phase of the gait.[2]

3. CLINICAL PRESENTATION

3.1. Referred Pain Pattern

Trigger points may be found within any portion of the quadratus lumborum muscle; however, many portions of the muscle are not accessible by manual palpation. Trigger points are commonly found in four locations: in the superficial (lateral) and deep (medial) portions, each with a cephalad and a caudal TrP area. The superficial (lateral) TrPs refer pain more laterally and

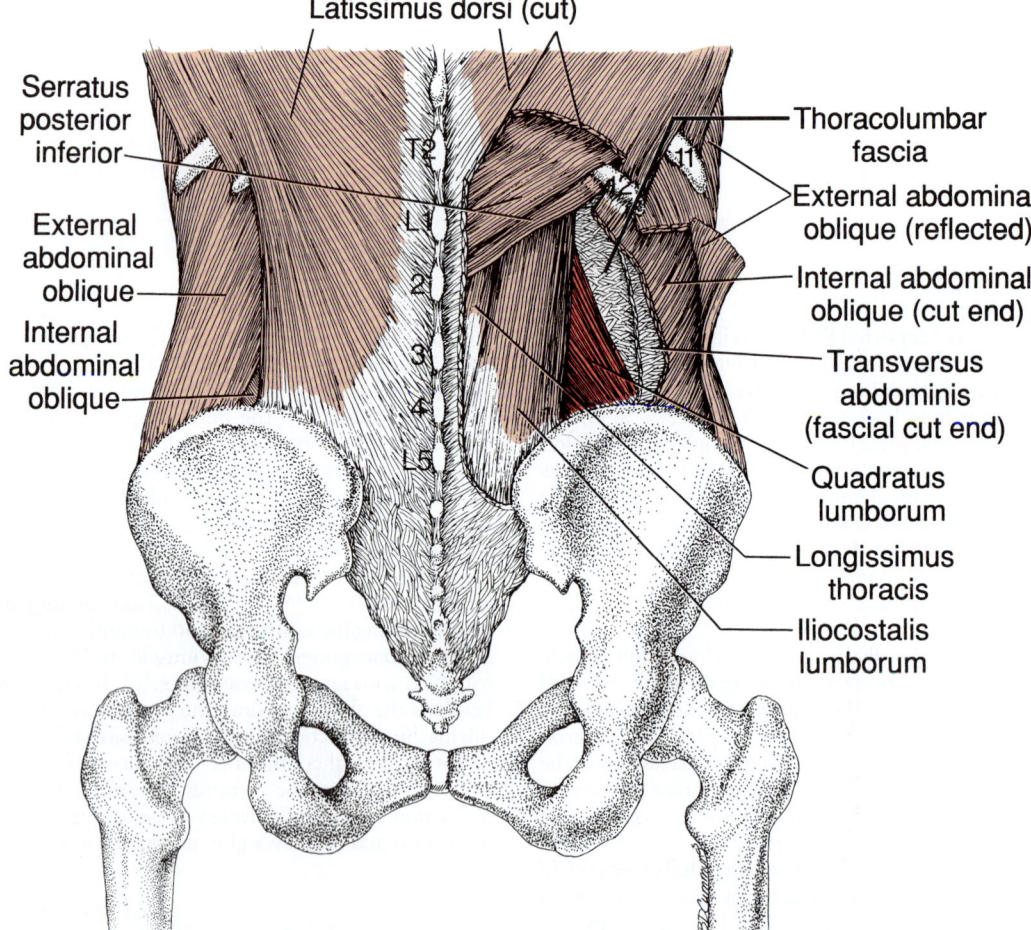

Figure 50-4. Regional anatomy of the right quadratus lumborum muscle (dark red). Neighboring muscles are light red. The thoracolumbar fascia, which lies anterior to (deep to) the quadratus lumborum muscle, is seen between the quadratus lumborum muscle and the cut edge of the transversus abdominis muscle. The transverse abdominis, latissimus dorsi, and internal oblique muscles have been cut and portions removed. The external oblique muscle has also been cut and a portion reflected.

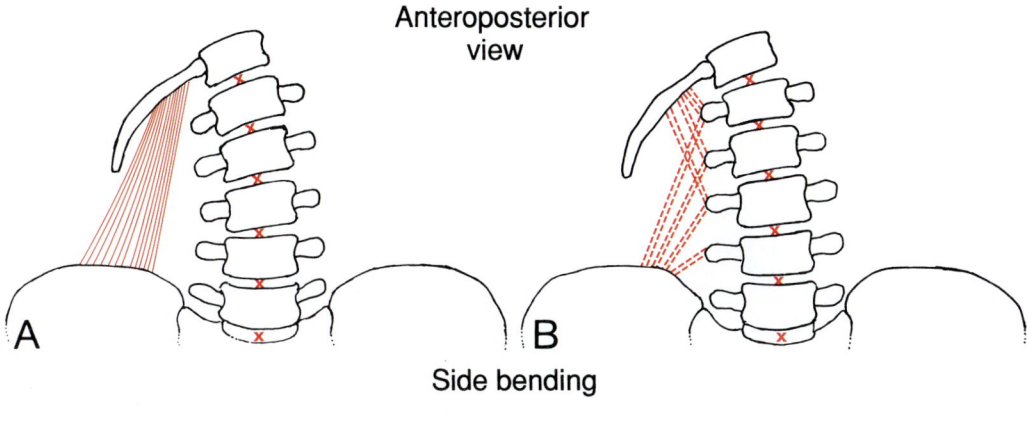
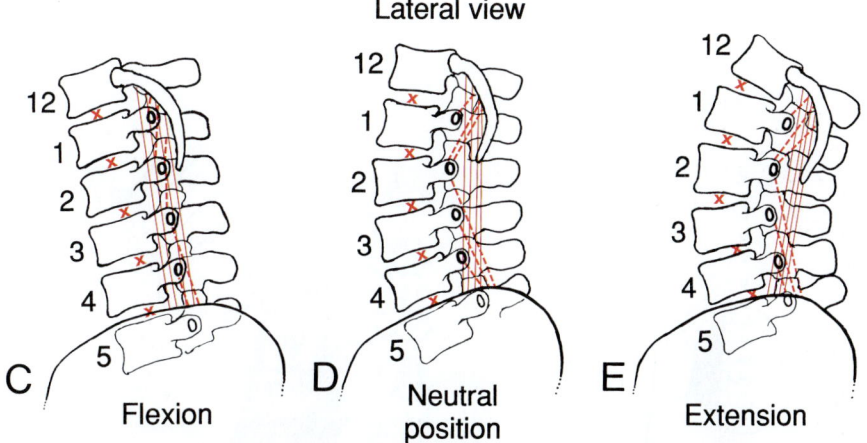

Figure 50-5. Tracings of lumbar radiographs (black) with quadratus lumborum fibers (red lines) added to show their attachments and directions. A and B, Anteroposterior view; C, D, and E, Lateral view. An *X* locates the center of rotation between two vertebrae; an open circle locates the tip of a transverse process. Solid red lines mark the longitudinal iliocostal fibers; dashed red lines indicate the diagonal iliotransverse and costotransverse fibers. A, Superficial lateral iliocostal fibers that laterally flex the lumbar spine toward the same side. B, Medial, deep diagonal iliotransverse, and costotransverse fibers produce the same effect. C, D, and E, All fibers extend the lumbar spine when the subject stands with the lumbar spine in the flexed, neutral, or extended posture, respectively.

anteriorly than the deep TrPs. The caudal TrPs tend to refer pain more distally. The pain from these TrPs is often reported as deep and aching but may be stabbing during movement.

Trigger points in the superficial location (Figure 50-6A) are likely to refer pain along the crest of the ilium and sometimes to the adjacent lower quadrant of the abdomen. The pain may extend to the outer upper aspect of the groin. They are responsible for referred pain to the greater trochanter and outer aspect of the upper thigh. The greater trochanter can be so "sore" (tender to pressure) that the patient cannot tolerate lying on that side, and pain may prevent weight-bearing by the lower extremity on the involved side. The referred pain from these TrPs often result in a misdiagnosis of trochanteric bursitis (Figure 50-6A).

Deep quadratus lumborum TrPs have been shown to refer pain to the front of the thigh, extending from the anterior superior iliac spine to the lateral side of the upper part of the patella in a narrow band about the width of a finger. The more cephalad of the deep TrPs (Figure 50-6B) refer pain strongly to the area of the SIJ; bilaterally, these TrPs frequently may refer pain that extends across the upper sacral region. The caudal deep TrPs refer pain to the lower buttock.

Authors have identified the quadratus lumborum muscle as a source of lumbago,[21-23] backache,[24-28] and lumbar myalgia.[21] More specifically, they have identified the quadratus lumborum muscle as referring pain to the SI region,[29-31] the hip or buttock,[29-31] the greater trochanter,[29-31] the abdomen,[26,27,30,32,33] and the groin.[29,31] Additional areas of pain referral from the quadratus lumborum muscle were reported in the anterior thigh[27] and in the testicles and scrotum.[24]

Tucker et al[34] investigated the nociceptive effects of a hypertonic saline injection into six muscles in the low back. Fifteen subjects were injected with hypertonic saline solution into the longissimus lumborum, quadratus lumborum, and superficial and deep multifidus muscles at L4 and L5. The injections were performed with ultrasound guidance to locate the specific muscles. Participants reported the depth, location, intensity, size, and quality of pain for up to 14 minutes following the injection. The most common descriptors of pain caused by injection of the quadratus lumborum muscle were aching, cramping, dull, sore, and tight. One subject reported paresthesias in the anterolateral thigh that lasted 2 days. The most common referred pain pattern from the quadratus lumborum muscle was to the lateral trunk, lower back, anterior iliac crest, and pelvis, which was very similar to the referred pain pattern from the deep multifidus muscle. The deep and superficial multifidus muscle had an annoying quality and higher cramping and dull ache as compared with the other muscles. The longissimus lumborum muscle was described primarily as aching and annoying. The referred pain patterns were not consistent to that of referred nerve root pain, therefore the authors conclude that there is a diffuse mechanism of referred pain from these six muscles. They also conclude that the individual may not experience pain at

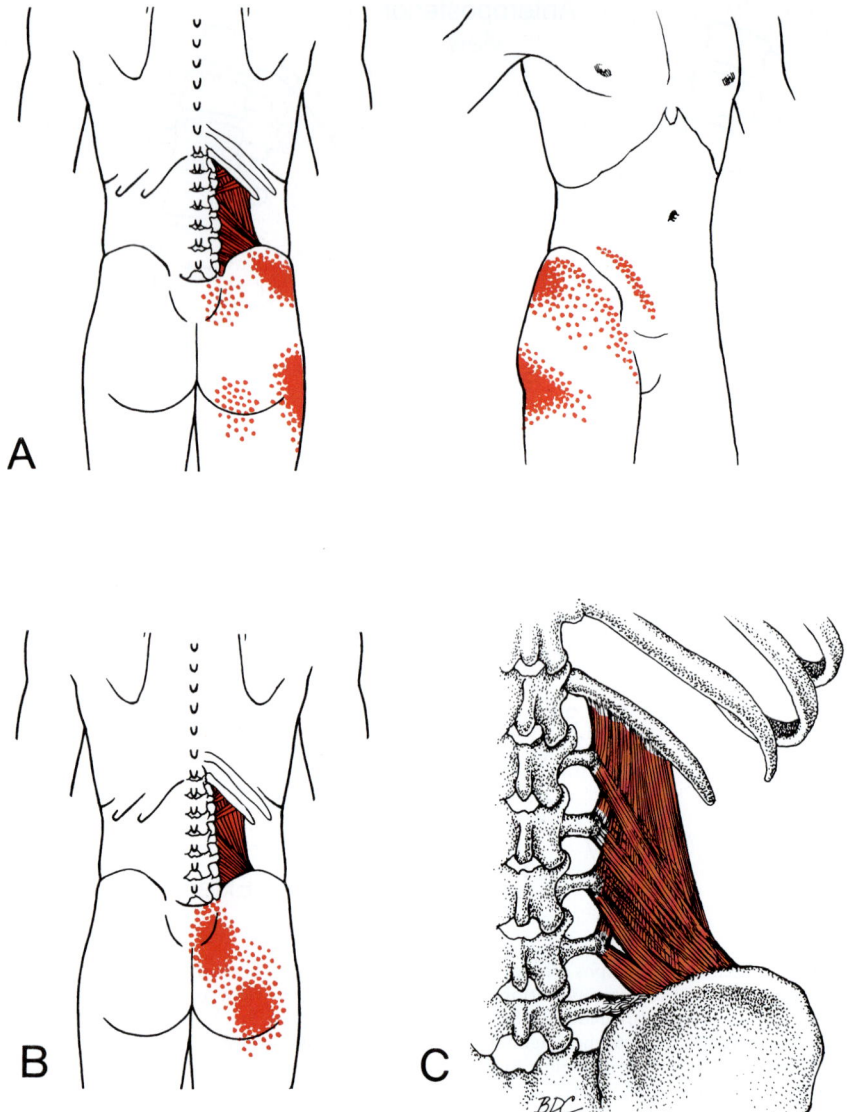

Figure 50-6. Referred pain patterns (bright red) of TrPs in the quadratus lumborum muscle (red). Solid bright red denotes an essential pain pattern, and stippled red, a spillover pattern. A, Pain patterns of superficial (lateral) TrPs that are palpable below and close to the 12th rib and just above the iliac crest. B, Pain patterns of deep (more medial) TrPs close to the transverse processes of the lumbar vertebrae. The more cephalad deep TrPs refer pain to the sacroiliac joint; more caudal TrPs refer pain low in the buttock. C, Trigger points can exist in any part of the muscle. Due to its location, examination may be performed with the use of a filiform needle or with a TrP injection.

the level or location of the nociceptive stimuli.[34] The referred pain pattern noted for the quadratus lumborum muscle in this study was very similar to the referred pain patterns described earlier by Travell and Simons.[35]

3.2. Symptoms

When patients report nonspecific low back pain (LBP), the quadratus lumborum muscle is typically found to be a contributing factor to the patient's report of pain. Trigger points in the quadratus lumborum muscle are common in LBP, but this source is commonly overlooked. Trigger points in the quadratus lumborum muscle should be considered as a potential source of symptoms when the patient reports unilateral LBP, SIJ and buttock pain, pain over the greater trochanter, and groin pain.

Patients with TrPs in the quadratus lumborum muscle may report a persistent, deep, aching pain at rest[29] that increases in the unsupported upright position and in positions that require stabilization of the lumbar spine. Arising from the supine position or getting up out of a chair may be difficult or impossible without help from the upper limbs.

The patient may also experience acute pain over the greater trochanter which is aggravated with sit-to-stand, walking, ascending, and descending stairs. They may also report having significant issues with lying on the affected side, especially at night. These individuals may have had a failed cortisone injection of the greater trochanter bursa.

In addition to back pain distributed in the primary referred patterns of this muscle (Figure 50-6), pain may extend to the groin, testicle, scrotum, or in a sciatic nerve distribution.[24] Patients have reported heaviness of the hips, cramping of the calves, and burning sensations in the legs and feet.[30] The patient may also report increasing difficulty with walking for long periods of time, especially when the strength of the gluteus medius muscle is inadequate to support the pelvis in the mid stance phase of gait.

Utilizing a cross-sectional design, Iglesias-González[36] investigated the difference in the presence of TrPs in 42 patients with nonspecific LBP and 42 age-matched controls. The quadratus lumborum, iliocostalis lumborum, psoas, piriformis, gluteus minimus, and gluteus medius muscles were examined for TrPs. The numeric pain rating scale (NPRS), Roland-Morris Low Back Questionnaire, and the Pittsburgh Sleep Quality Index were used as outcome measures. Patients with nonspecific LBP had a mean of 3.5 active TrPs and two latent TrPs as compared with the control group participants who did not have any active TrPs. Active TrPs in the quadratus lumborum muscle were most prevalent (55%), followed by the gluteus medius muscle (38%), and iliocostalis lumborum muscle (33%) in patients with nonspecific LBP. A greater number of active TrPs was associated with worse sleep quality and higher pain intensity ($P < 0.001$) in the nonspecific LBP group. There was also a significant difference in the presence of latent TrPs in subjects with nonspecific LBP compared with the control group with the quadratus lumborum, iliocostalis lumborum, psoas, piriformis, and gluteus medius muscles being most affected.[36]

3.3. Patient Examination

After a thorough subjective examination, the clinician should make a detailed drawing representing the pain pattern that the patient describes. This depiction will assist in planning the physical examination and can be useful in monitoring the progression of the patient as symptoms improve or change. The type, quality, and location of the pain should be carefully assessed and utilization of standardized outcome tools is imperative while examining patients with LBP and/or lower extremity dysfunctions.

The patient with active TrPs in the quadratus lumborum muscle exhibits muscle guarding that restricts movement between the lumbar vertebrae and the sacrum during walking, lying down, turning over in the bed, getting up from the bed, or when arising from a chair. A vigorous cough may evoke the characteristic pain distribution.

Observation of the posture in standing should be carried out with attention to spinal curvature and lower extremity biomechanical alignment. It is important to incorporate assessment for functional and structural scoliosis, presence of a hemipelvis, iliac upslip,[37] and leg length discrepancy. Due to the quadratus lumborum muscle's attachments to the pelvis and lumbar spine, shortening of the quadratus lumborum muscle can contribute to apparent scoliosis and leg length discrepancies. If there is shortening of the quadratus lumborum muscle (potentially, due to TrPs) in standing, the pelvis is slightly elevated on the affected side or depressed on the side opposite to the affected muscle. The lumbar spine usually exhibits a functional lumbar scoliosis that is convex away from the side of the involved quadratus lumborum muscle.[22] The normal lumbar lordosis is likely to appear flattened due to the vertebral rotation that accompanies the scoliosis, despite the fact that the quadratus lumborum muscle is an extensor and lateral flexor of the spine.

Iliac crest heights and PSIS and ASIS bony landmarks should also be assessed for asymmetry in the seated position.[37] The seated position the patient prefers should also be assessed. Clinically, it is common for the patient to lean toward the affected side while seated when there are active TrPs in the quadratus lumborum muscle. A hemipelvis may be more apparent in this position than in standing.

In supine or prone lying, TrPs may shorten the muscle and can thus distort pelvic alignment, elevating the pelvis on the side of the tense muscle (Figure 50-7). Bony landmarks should also be palpated in this position to differentiate an iliosacral dysfunction[37] from quadratus lumborum TrPs or shortening of the muscle.

Assessment of lumbar spine active range of motion likely reveals limitations in flexion, extension, and lateral flexion (side-bending). Lateral flexion (side-bending) is typically restricted toward the pain-free side and sometimes bilateral restrictions may be noted. Seated or standing rotation of the thoracolumbar spine is usually most restricted toward the side of the involved muscle when its iliocostal fibers are affected.

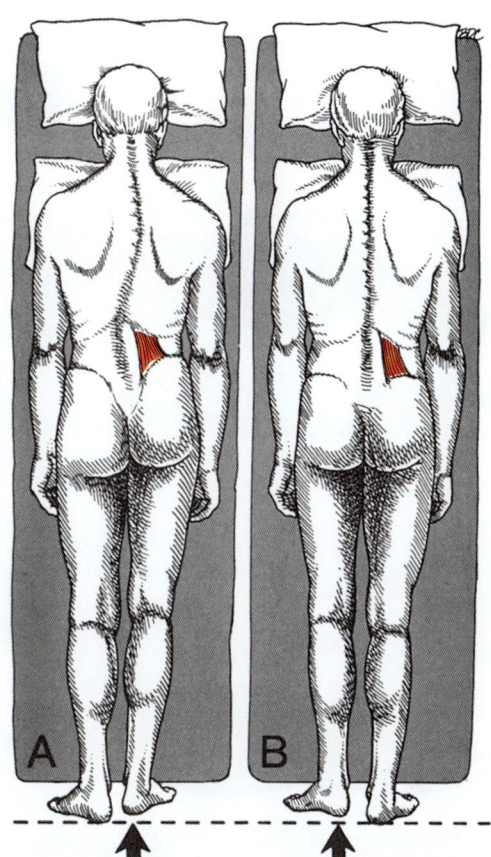

Figure 50-7. Distortion of apparent leg length discrepancy due to a taut quadratus lumborum muscle. A, At the medial malleolus in the prone position, the right lower limb appears shorter than the left due to TrPs and tension in the shortened right quadratus lumborum muscle (dark red). B, True leg length discrepancy becomes apparent when the TrPs in the right quadratus lumborum muscle are eliminated and the muscle returns to its normal resting length (light red). The S-curve functional scoliosis of the spine, seen in A, is also eliminated.

Sacroiliac and iliosacral movements should also be assessed in standing and seated positions.[37] It is important for the clinician to consider the use of the SIJ special tests cluster developed by Laslett et al.[38] These tests have high clinical utility in identifying the SIJ dysfunction. Clinically, however, in the presence of active TrPs in the quadratus lumborum muscle, these provocative tests may be false positive due to peripheral sensitization.

Strength of only the quadratus lumborum muscle is difficult to assess because of the parallel force generated by the lateral portions of the external and internal abdominal oblique muscles. Quadratus lumborum muscle strength may be tested using the side plank position. Figure 50-8A and B depicts two different positions to test the quadratus lumborum muscle. This test position allows the clinician to assess the patient's ability to utilize the quadratus lumborum muscle to stabilize the lumbar spine.

The quadratus lumborum muscle compensates for gluteus medius muscle weakness during gait, and therefore it is important to assess gluteal muscle strength in patients who exhibit quadratus lumborum TrPs or a Trendelenburg gait pattern. The muscle activation pattern and the position of the pelvis during side-lying hip abduction should be observed (Figure 50-9A). Firm stabilization of the pelvis inhibits the quadratus lumborum muscle from compensating for a weak gluteus medius muscle as seen in Figure 50-9B.[19]

Accessory joint motion should be tested in the lumbar spine, SI joint, and lower ribs as joint hypomobility is typically present with quadratus lumborum muscle dysfunction.

504 Section 5: Trunk and Pelvis Pain

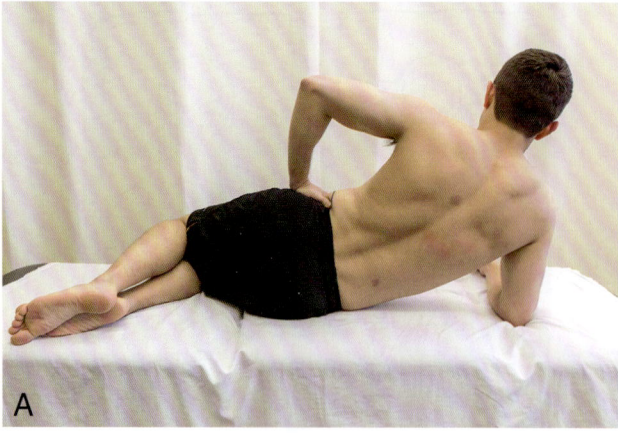 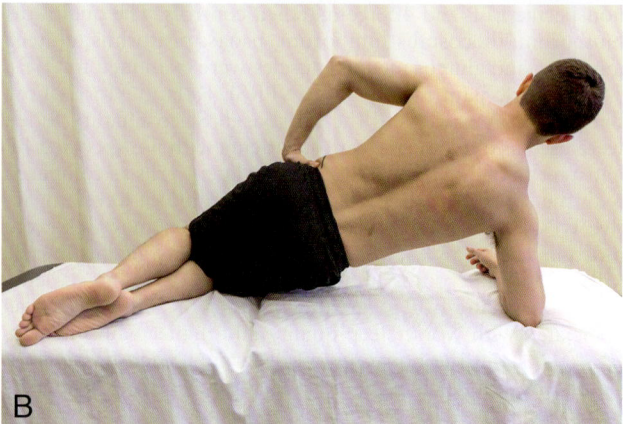
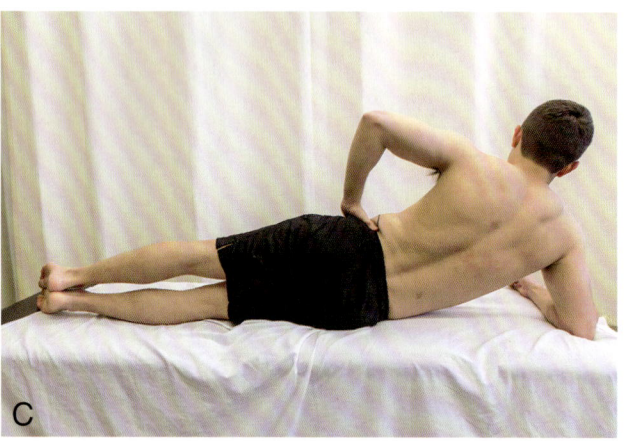 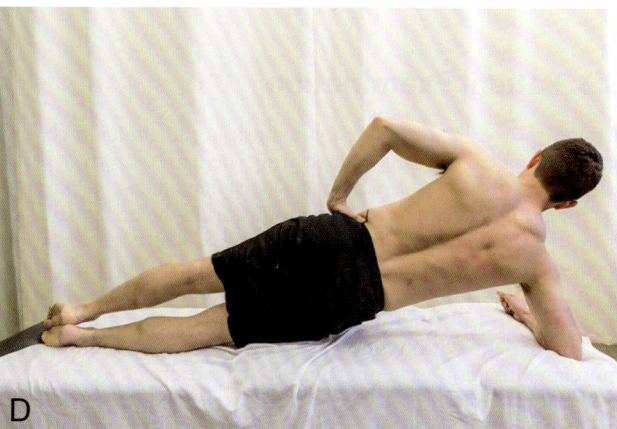

Figure 50-8. Quadratus lumborum muscle strength test using the side plank position. A and B, The knees are bent, giving the patient more stability. C and D, Legs and hips are straight, placing a greater demand on the quadratus lumborum muscle.

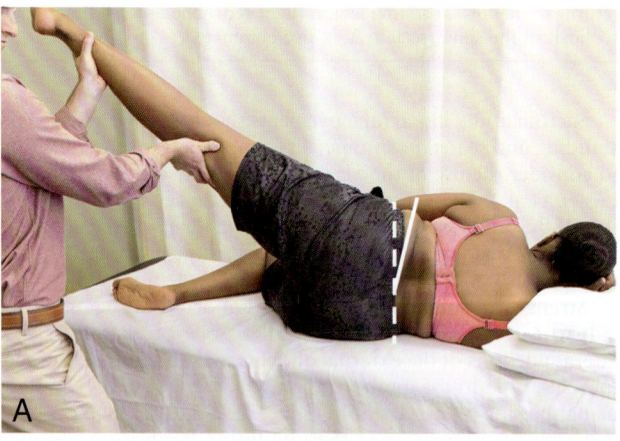 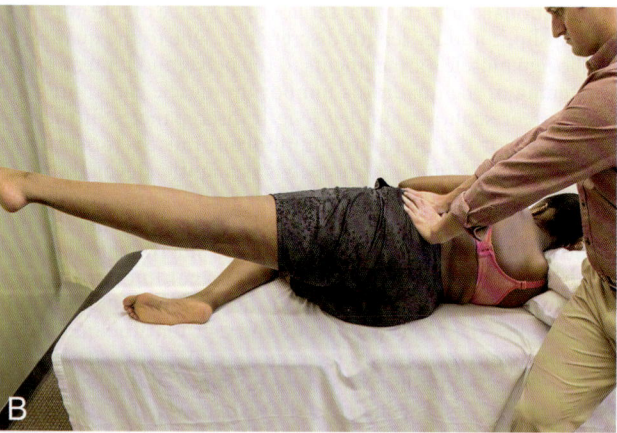

Figure 50-9. Side-lying hip abduction muscle activation pattern and strength test. A, Muscle activation pattern observing hip and pelvic motion. Note elevation of the left iliac crest as indicated by the solid white line demonstrating compensation by the quadratus lumborum muscle for inadequate strength or inhibition of the gluteus medius muscle. B, Stabilization of the pelvis to inhibit the quadratus lumborum muscle for accurate assessment of gluteus medius muscle inhibition or strength deficits. Note the change in the observed hip abduction range of motion.

Lower rib mobility should also be assessed due to the attachment of the quadratus lumborum muscle on the lower ribs and its role in forced respiration such as coughing.

3.4. Trigger Point Examination

Trigger points in the quadratus lumborum muscle are common in patients reporting LBP, SI, or lateral proximal thigh pain.[36]

For examination of TrPs in the quadratus lumborum muscle, positioning is extremely important. Unless the patient is properly positioned lying on the uninvolved side, the TrPs in this muscle are very difficult to palpate.[39-41] The position that the patient ordinarily assumes in side-lying may not permit adequate palpation for deep tenderness of the quadratus lumborum muscle because of inadequate space between the 10th rib and the crest of the ilium.

Raising the arm of the side to be examined onto the top of the table behind the head elevates the thoracic cage (Figure 50-10A).

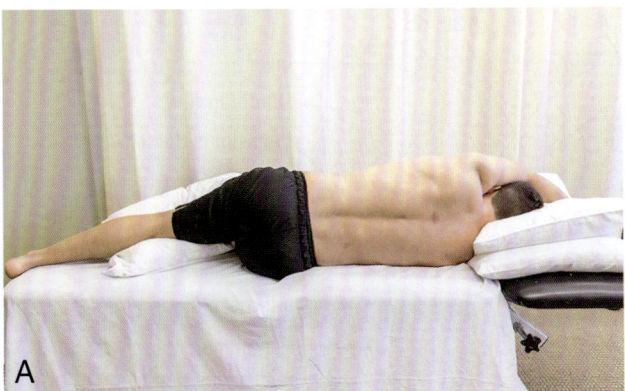
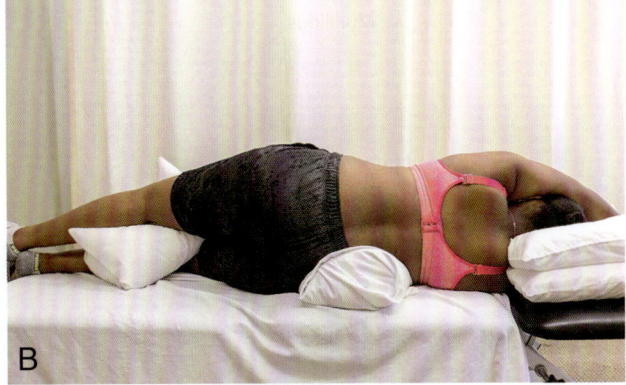
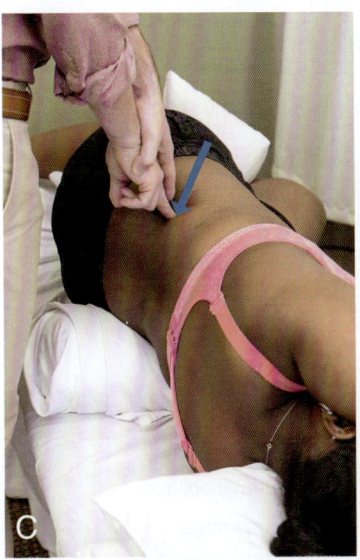
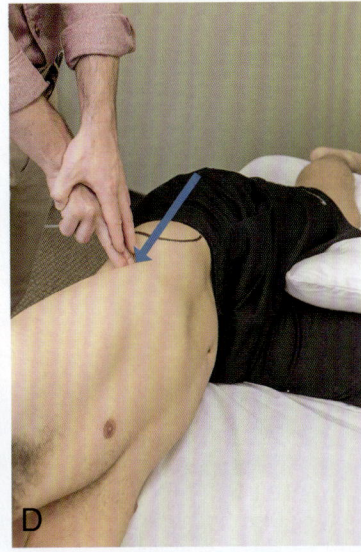
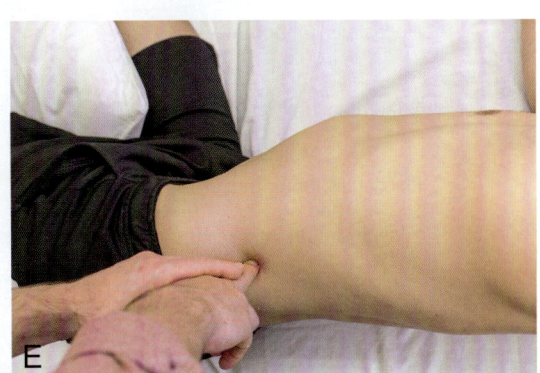

Figure 50-10. Patient positioning for examination of TrPs in the quadratus lumborum muscle. A, Partial opening of the space between the lowest ribs and ilium by having the patient reach overhead with the arm to elevate the rib cage. B, For some patients, especially women, full opening of the space may be provided by the addition of a supporting lumbar roll or pillow. This wider opening permits palpation of the quadratus lumborum muscle. C and D, The arrows indicate the direction in which pressure is applied to elicit spot tenderness. Downward pressure is exerted just above (adjacent to) the crest of the ilium and anterior to the long paraspinal muscle mass at the L4 level. E, To locate the deep, more cephalad TrPs, deep pressure is applied just caudal to the 12th rib and again anterior to the paraspinal muscles.

Dropping the knee of that side toward the examining table behind the other knee, pulls that side of the pelvis distally and lowers the iliac crest. This position creates adequate space for examining the muscle (Figure 50-10A) and adds the tension necessary for palpation. A bolster or towel roll positioned under the waist line may also be utilized to create more access to the quadratus lumborum muscle (Figure 50-10B). However, when the quadratus lumborum muscle is especially tight and tender, this position places the quadratus lumborum muscle under painful tension. The pelvis cannot pull away from the rib cage and the knee on the side being examined does not reach the table. The leg needs to be supported using a pillow placed between the legs or under the leg of the affected side (Figure 50-10A and B).

One reason why TrPs in the quadratus lumborum muscle are so easily overlooked is the location of the muscle, which lies anterior to the paraspinal muscle mass and is inaccessible from the posterior approach (Figure 50-11) of a routine back examination. Examination for quadratus lumborum TrPs begins by palpating for the lateral edge of the paraspinal mass, the 12th rib, and the crest of the ilium. In many patients, the only part of the latissimus dorsi muscle that overlies the quadratus lumborum muscle is its aponeurosis, which presents little obstruction to palpation. In some, however, a thick column of overlying fibers of the latissimus dorsi muscle extends to the crest of the ilium (Figure 50-11).

Three regions in this muscle are examined for TrPs. The first region is deep at the angle where the crest of the ilium meets the paraspinal muscle mass (Figures 50-4 and 50-10C and D). As seen in Figures 50-4 and 50-11, this is the thickest part of the quadratus lumborum muscle, near the level of the L4 transverse process. This location is just cephalad to the point where many vertical iliocostal fibers and diagonal iliotransverse fibers anchor by intertwining with fibers of the iliolumbar ligament. As shown in Figure 50-10C and D, the muscle is examined for tenderness by applying deep pressure superior to the crest of the ilium and anterior to the paraspinal muscles. The pressure is directed toward the tips of the lumbar transverse processes. One should press gently at first because remarkably little pressure on these TrPs can be exquisitely painful. Here, pressure is applied primarily to the diagonal lower iliotransverse fibers of the quadratus lumborum muscle. These fibers are too deep for one to feel their taut bands or to elicit local twitch responses manually.

The second region examined for quadratus lumborum TrPs extends along the inner crest of the ilium where many of the iliocostal fibers attach. The tip of the finger is applied across the direction of the fibers shown in Figure 50-4. This cross-fiber flat palpation locates taut bands with tender spots in those fibers (Figure 50-10E). Local twitch responses are rarely visible

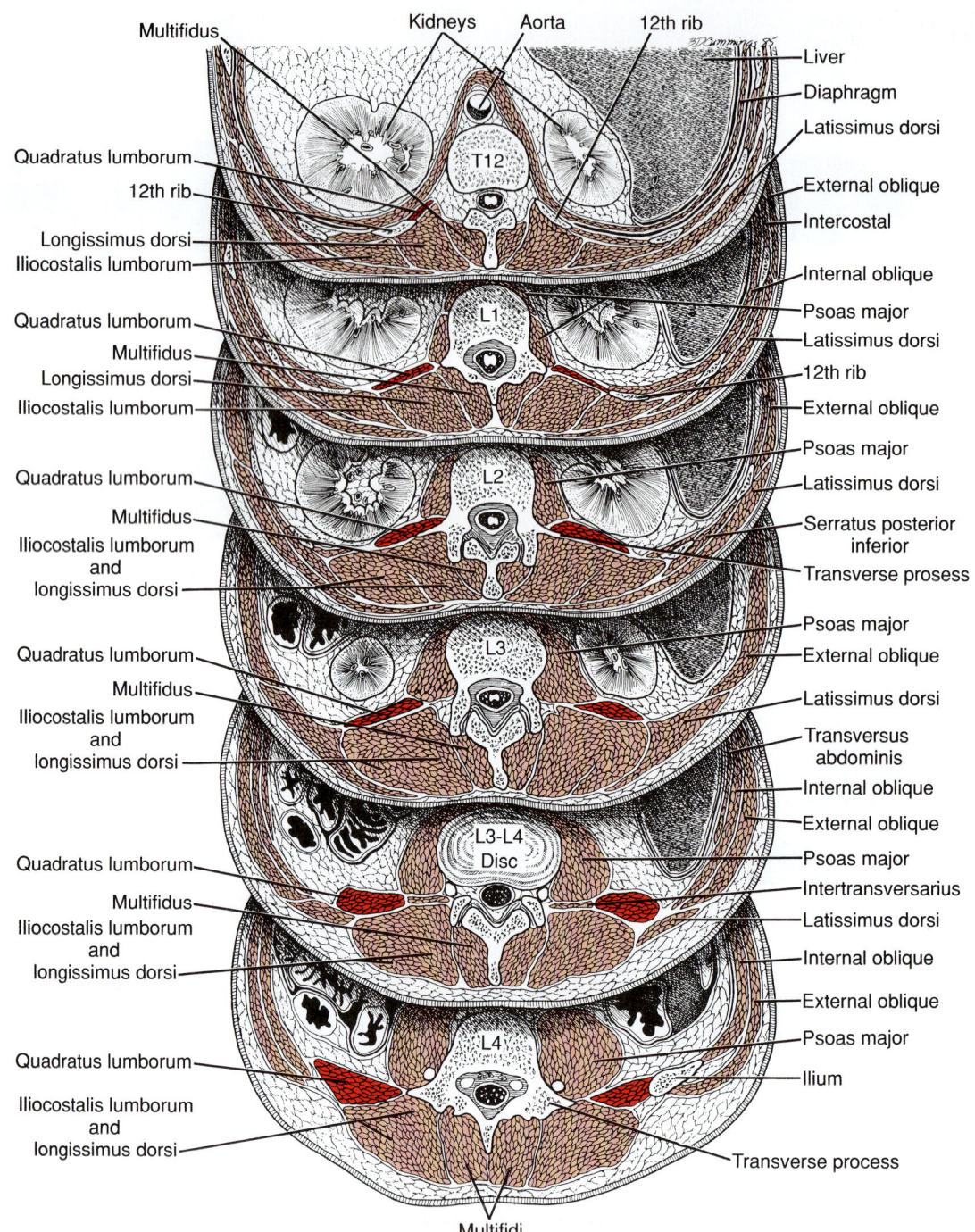

Figure 50-11. Serial cross sections of the quadratus lumborum muscle, dark red; other muscles, light red. Attachment of the muscle to the 12th rib is seen in the T12 and L1 sections; attachment to a transverse process is seen in the L2 section, and attachment to the ilium is seen in the L4 section. The next lower section (not included) would show only the iliolumbar ligament, and no quadratus lumborum muscle. The latissimus dorsi is one muscle usually interposed between the palpating finger and the quadratus lumborum muscle. Only at the L4 level is the muscle directly palpable beneath the skin. Adapted from Carter BL, Morehead, Wolpert SM, et al. *Cross-sectional Anatomy.* New York, NY: Appleton-Century Crofts; 1977:31-34.

unless the individual is thin and has few latissimus dorsi fibers extending this far.

If one progresses too far laterally, the fingers encounter the lateral border of the external abdominal oblique muscle; these fibers run nearly parallel to the lateral iliocostal fibers of the quadratus lumborum muscle. The external abdominal oblique fibers may have taut bands and TrPs that can easily be mistakenly ascribed to the quadratus lumborum muscle (Figure 50-4). Taut bands of the external abdominal oblique muscle angle from the tip of the 12th rib down and forward to the anterior aspect of the crest of the ilium (see Figure 49-1A).[42] The adjacent quadratus lumborum fibers are nearly parallel but are usually at an angle from the middle and posterior portions of the 12th rib to the posterior aspect of the crest of the ilium.

The third region lies in the angle where the paraspinal muscle mass and the 12th rib meet. As seen in Figures 50-2, 50-4, and 50-11, deep fingertip pressure applied in the direction of the L1-L2 transverse processes transmits pressure to the cephalad attachment of the iliocostal and costotransverse fibers of the quadratus lumborum muscle. In some patients, the attachments of the iliocostal fibers extend laterally far enough along the 12th rib to be felt by cross-fiber flat palpation in a manner similar to that described for the second region above. With the patient in the position shown in Figure 50-10C to E one can also apply pressure caudad to L2 seeking tenderness over the L3 transverse process between regions one and three. Only tenderness is elicited because these fibers are too deep to permit palpation of taut bands.

With sustained pressure on any one of these TrPs, one may elicit its pattern of referred pain, although penetration of the TrP with a needle is a more reliable way of eliciting pain referred by TrPs in this muscle.

4. DIFFERENTIAL DIAGNOSIS

4.1. Activation and Perpetuation of Trigger Points

Any posture or activity that activates a TrP, if not corrected, can also perpetuate it. In any part of the quadratus lumborum muscle, TrPs may be activated by unaccustomed eccentric loading, eccentric exercise in unconditioned muscle, or maximal or submaximal concentric loading.[43] Trigger points may also be activated or aggravated when the muscle is placed in a shortened or lengthened position for an extended period of time.

Quadratus lumborum TrPs can be activated acutely by awkward lifting of an unusually heavy load such as a TV set, a child, or a large dog or by a quick bending movement when the torso is twisted or turned somewhat to one side, often to reach for an object on the floor.[31] Another version of the latter stress is that of angling sideways while bending forward to rise from a deep-seated chair, a low bed, or a car seat. Many patients report the onset of pain when putting on pants while standing half stooped and leaning sideways or after losing balance as the feet become entangled in the clothing.

The quadratus lumborum muscle often develops TrPs from an auto accident. Baker[44] investigated the occurrence of TrPs in 34 muscles of 100 occupants (drivers and passengers) who sustained a single motor vehicle impact. The quadratus lumborum muscle was involved more frequently than any other muscle in impacts from the driver's side (81% of subjects) and in impacts from behind (79% of subjects). It was the second most commonly injured muscle (81%) when the impact was from the front and the third most common (63%) when the impact was on the passenger's side. In this study,[44] no distinction could be made between preexisting TrPs that were activated by the accident and TrPs that were initiated by this gross trauma.

Quadratus lumborum TrPs can also be activated by obscure, sustained, or repetitive strain (microtrauma) from activities such as gardening, scrubbing the floor, lifting cement blocks,[25] or by walking or jogging on a slanted surface, as on a beach or along a crowned road. In addition, when one quadratus lumborum muscle becomes involved, the shortening of that muscle at rest tends to overload its contralateral mate and usually results in the development of TrPs in this antagonist but with pain of less intensity.

The introduction of a walking cast or boot can activate quadratus lumborum TrPs, as has been demonstrated experimentally.[32] When quadratus lumborum pain appears immediately after an ankle fracture that required application of a walking cast, the TrP was probably activated by the strain of the fall that also caused the fracture; whereas, if the muscle pain appears a week or two after the application of the cast, the chronic strain of the newly imposed leg length discrepancy most likely activated the TrPs. This pain is relieved (or prevented) by wearing (on the contralateral foot) a shoe with sufficient lift to match the length of the immobilized lower extremity.

Mechanical factors that predispose to the activation of quadratus lumborum TrPs or that perpetuate those TrPs are: a leg length discrepancy,[31] a small hemipelvis,[31] short upper arms,[42] a soft bed with a hammock-like sag, leaning forward with poor elbow support over a desk (frequently caused by wearing eyeglasses with too short a focal length), standing and leaning over a low sink or work surface, and deconditioned or weak abdominal muscles.

The relative importance of a leg length discrepancy and of a small hemipelvis as perpetuating factors in LBP of quadratus lumborum muscle origin is often revealed by a patient's relative tolerance to standing versus sitting and by the way he or she stands. When the patient stands with one foot forward, weight on the other foot (shorter side), or stands with feet wide apart and the pelvis shifted to one side (shorter side), and has pain when standing and walking, the problem is probably due to a leg length discrepancy. When only sitting aggravates the pain, either short upper arms or a small hemipelvis is more likely to be the culprit. When symptoms are present in both positions, a patient may have both a small hemipelvis and a leg length discrepancy on the same side; that is, one side of the body is smaller.

4.2. Associated Trigger Points

It has been shown that associated TrPs can develop in the referred pain areas caused by primary TrPs.[45] Therefore, muscles in the referred pain areas for each muscle should also be considered. Clinically, the muscles most likely to develop associated TrPs due to TrPs in the quadratus lumborum muscle are the contralateral quadratus lumborum, ipsilateral iliopsoas, iliocostalis between T11 and L3, longissimus, piriformis, superficial and deep multifidus,[36] external oblique, and, occasionally, latissimus dorsi muscles.

The two quadratus lumborum muscles work as a team bilaterally to stabilize the lumbar spine, which explains why TrPs on one side are frequently associated with less active TrPs in the quadratus lumborum muscle on the opposite side. The psoas major and lumbar paraspinal muscles help the quadratus lumborum muscle to stabilize the lumbar spine. Both the quadratus lumborum and lumbar paraspinal muscles are spinal extensors. The posterior fibers of the external oblique muscle are nearly parallel to the iliocostal quadratus lumborum fibers, have similar attachments to the rib cage and pelvis, and also are likely to have TrPs if the quadratus lumborum muscle does. In patients with nonspecific LBP in addition to TrPs in the quadratus lumborum muscle, other back muscles, such as the longissimus thoracis and multifidi muscles, can also project pain to the low back, buttock, and SIJ.[42] Iliopsoas TrPs[29] refer LBP that patients describe as radiating unilaterally up and down along the lumbosacral spine rather than horizontally across the back. The TrPs in the lower rectus abdominis muscle[42] refer bilateral LBP, which is described as traveling horizontally at the level of the SIJs. Pain from these other TrPs should be distinguished from quadratus lumborum TrP pain by the history, pain pattern, motions that are restricted and by physical examination and palpation of the muscles.

The gluteus medius and gluteus minimus muscles commonly develop associated TrPs because they lie in the referred pain zones of the quadratus lumborum muscle. Patients sometimes report pain in the reference zones of the gluteus medius and minimus muscles in response to pressure on quadratus lumborum TrPs. With inactivation of the gluteal TrPs, pressure on the quadratus lumborum TrP then refers pain only to its characteristic gluteal and pelvic distribution.

Roach et al[46] examined the prevalence of TrPs in the gluteus medius and quadratus lumborum muscles in patients with patellofemoral pain syndrome (PFPS) in a randomized controlled study with 26 patients with PFPS and 26 matched controls with no history of PFPS. The prevalence of TrPs in the gluteus medius and quadratus lumborum muscles was significantly higher in the PFPS group than in the control group. The prevalence of unilateral TrPs in the quadratus lumborum muscle on the opposite side to the PFPS was 93%. Eighty percent of patients with PFPS had TrPs in the quadratus lumborum muscle bilaterally, whereas the control group had 35% unilaterally and 15% bilaterally. All patients in the PFPS group had at least one quadratus lumborum TrP. They also found a significant decrease in force production in hip abduction strength in the PFPS group as compared with controls. Following one treatment session with pressure release techniques there was no improvement in force production in hip abduction.

Conversely, TrPs can develop in the quadratus lumborum muscle as a consequence of TrPs in other muscles. Jull and Janda[47(pp253-278)] noted that the quadratus lumborum muscle is subject to overload when used to substitute for weak hip abductor muscles in walking. Trigger points in the gluteus medius and gluteus minimus muscles are one of many causes of such weakness.

Lewit[48] related hypomobility at the thoracolumbar junction to TrPs in the iliopsoas, erector spinae, quadratus lumborum, and abdominal muscles. The importance of articular dysfunction as a perpetuating factor for TrPs in these muscles is relatively unexplored and promises to be a fertile area for investigation. However, TrP tension in these muscles can reinforce hypomobility at the thoracolumbar junction.

4.3. Associated Pathology

Differential diagnosis of symptoms caused by TrPs in the quadratus lumborum muscle primarily consists of SIJ dysfunction, trochanteric bursitis, sciatica, spinal stenosis, thoracolumbar (facet joint) articular dysfunction, and lumbar disc derangement. Thoracolumbar articular dysfunction characteristically causes asymmetrical restriction of rotation, side-bending, flexion, or sometimes extension of the thoracolumbar region. Involvement of the quadratus lumborum muscle alone can restrict primarily side-bending away from the involved side, as well as rotation and flexion of the lumbar spine.

In acute LBP with or without radicular symptoms, active TrPs in the quadratus lumborum muscle may present as a flattened lumbar lordosis and/or a lateral shift consistent with the presentation of an acute disc derangement.

Additional diagnoses to consider include spinal tumors; myasthenia gravis; gallstones and liver disease; kidney stones and other urinary tract problems; intra-abdominal infections; intestinal parasites and diverticulitis; abdominal aortic aneurysm; and multiple sclerosis.

5. CORRECTIVE ACTIONS

When major weight-bearing and postural muscles develop TrPs, patients should be instructed in techniques to address the source of symptoms and contributing factors. Often, patients would need to learn to perform their usual activities in a manner that does not stress the implicated muscle. Sleeping conditions such as the mattress and sleeping position can have a profound influence on quadratus lumborum TrPs. A sagging, hammock-like, mattress puts the quadratus lumborum muscle in the shortened position when one lies on the opposite side. If the patient's mattress is too soft or older than 10 years, the patient should consider investing in a new mattress. Sleeping flat on the back with knees straight places the quadratus lumborum muscle in a relatively shortened position by causing the pelvis to tilt forward and lumbar lordosis to increase. This position can be avoided by placing a small pillow or other support under the knees or by sleeping on one side with proper support of the lumbar spine and lower extremities (Figure 50-12A and B). With a pillow

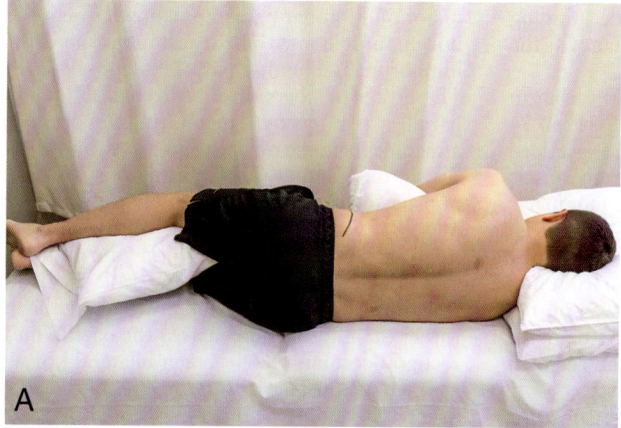
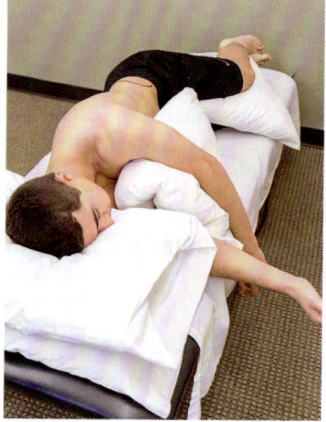
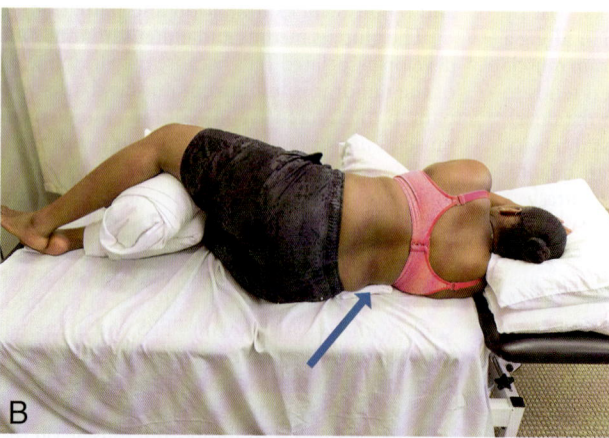
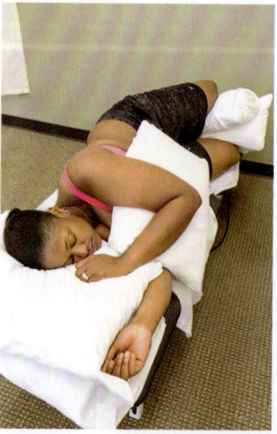

Figure 50-12. Proper sleeping position. A, The patient's uppermost hip is in slight flexion with a pillow between the knees to keep the pelvis level and lumbar spine in a neutral position. A pillow is also placed under the uppermost arm and in front of the trunk to reduce rotation. B, Patient is positioned as previously described in A; however, a towel roll is placed under the waist (arrow) to keep the lumbar spine in a neutral position. Note the increased support between the patient's knees to keep the pelvis in a neutral position.

placed appropriately, the lumbar spine can retain its normal curvature, protecting both the quadratus lumborum muscle and the lumbar discs. (If the patient's problem is one of a posterior disc derangement, the preferred position is prone.) The patient with a persistent quadratus lumborum muscle problem needs to learn how to slide and roll the hips rather than to lift them when turning over in bed at night.

The combined flexion–rotation movement of bending forward and sideways to lift or pull something should be avoided. This is a hazardous maneuver for anyone but especially for the person with quadratus lumborum TrPs. One should turn the entire body to face the task squarely and then perform a pure flexion–extension movement without twisting the trunk. When turning to reach behind, the patient should learn to keep the back erect, avoiding any trunk flexion during rotation.

Sustained flexion and forceful extension of the spine should be avoided. If the lower limb muscles and knees are free of problems, one can lift objects from the floor by bending the knees while keeping the torso erect. Unfortunately, people find this movement difficult; not only does it require additional efforts to lift the entire torso and hip region instead of only the head, neck, and shoulders, but it also throws the load on the quadriceps femoris muscles, which, in this position, are at a mechanical disadvantage.[49]

Learning to avoid unnecessary bending can play a critical role. The importance may not be so much in what is done, but in how it is done. One learns to make up a low bed while kneeling, rather than standing and bending over to reach the bed. Brushing the teeth is done while standing up straight and avoiding leaning over the sink, except to clear the mouth, while supporting the body weight with the free hand or by placing one foot in the vanity shelf or on a stool under the sink if available.

The muscular strain of a near fall, or injury from a fall, is avoided by sitting down to put on socks, pantyhose, skirt or trousers, and so on or by leaning against a wall or heavy furniture so that balance is assured.

A common example of unnecessary forward leaning is the usual way of rising from a chair without arm support (Figure 50-13). When rising with the buttocks at the rear of the chair seat, the body is pitched forward in a stooped position to place the center of gravity over the feet. This heavily loads the extensor muscles of the back as the person straightens up.

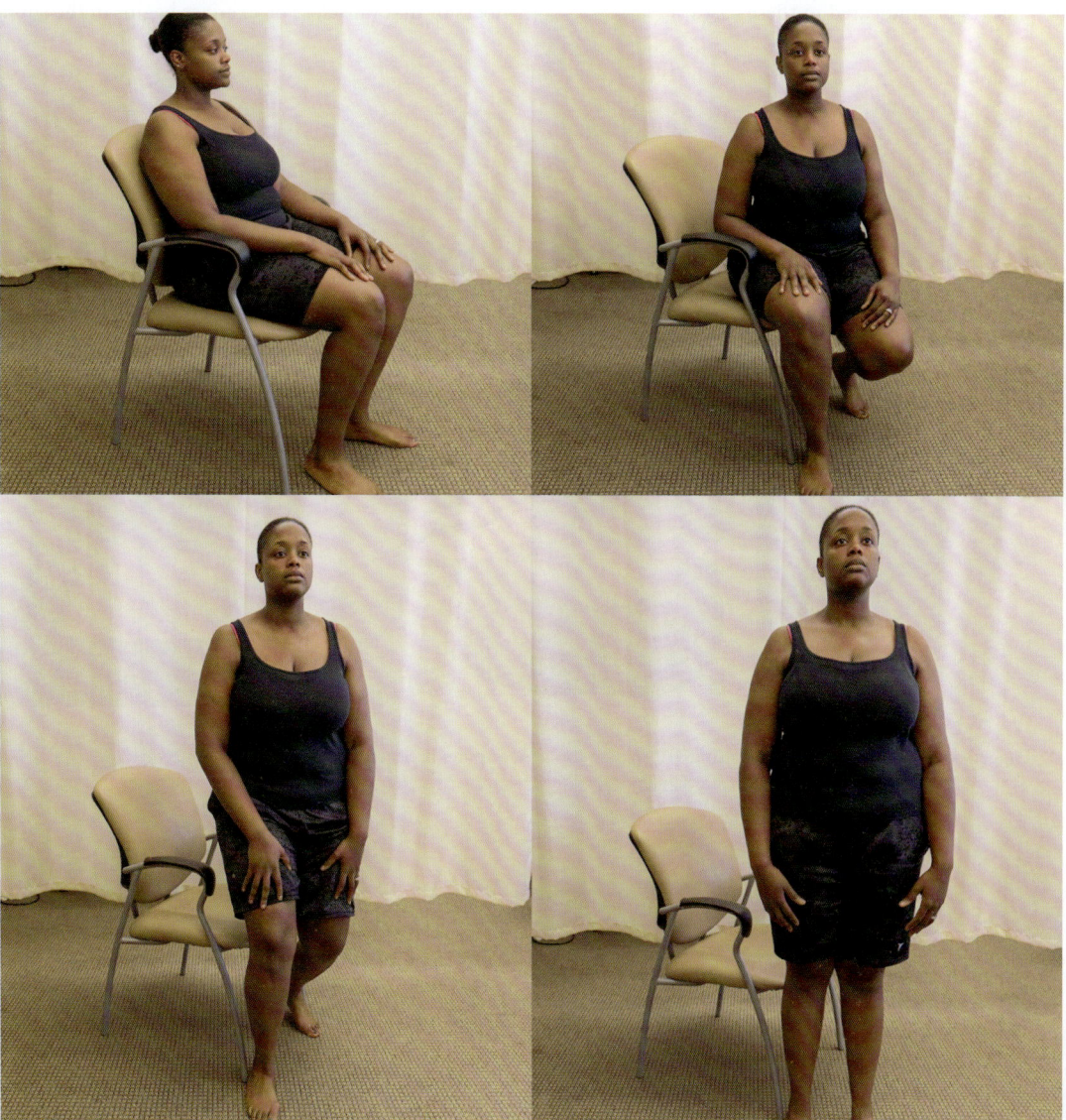

Figure 50-13. The sit-to-stand and stand-to-sit techniques minimize strain on the neck and back muscles and on the intervertebral discs. Start position while seated in a chair, the patient should move the buttocks to the front of the seat and then turn the body to a 45° angle. This positioning permits the spine to stay erect with a neutral lumbar lordosis between sitting to standing. The reverse, stand-to-sit technique, is accomplished by first turning the body, by keeping the trunk erect, if needed using the hands on the thighs to support the trunk while sitting down on the front of the seat, and then sliding the buttocks backward, still keeping the spine erect.

The correct manner of rising from a chair order to spare the back muscles is shown in Figure 50-13. The buttocks are first slid forward to the front of the seat; then, the body is turned sideways about 45° and one foot is placed under the front edge of the seat and under the center of gravity of the body. The body is then lifted with the torso held erect such that the load is placed mainly on the quadriceps femoris muscles. A push by the hands against the thighs assists the lift if the quadriceps muscles are weak. To return to the seated position, the sequence is reversed with the use of the hands on the thighs to lower to the chair.

The same principle applies to walking upstairs or climbing a ladder. If the body is turned 45° to one side, it is much easier to keep the back straight while ascending or descending.

Patients who enjoy gardening activities should sit on a low box or other seat that is 8 to 10 inches high while transplanting and weeding. This low-seated position helps them avoid bending over. In the house, small objects need to be placed on a chair or table rather than on the floor.

Any problem in foot mechanics, such as pronation of the foot and ankle, that produces an asymmetrical gait pattern may contribute to selective muscular overload,[50] including the overuse of the quadratus lumborum muscle. Appropriate corrective shoes or shoe inserts are indicated in these cases.

Asymmetries that produce a painful functional (compensatory) scoliosis that depend on muscular contraction to be maintained should be corrected in patients with a persistent quadratus lumborum myofascial pain syndrome. If appropriate examination has identified a pelvic asymmetry, an effort should be made to level the sacral base. Any existing lower extremity dysfunction, as well as any pelvic torsion and lumbar joint dysfunction, should be corrected to ensure that treatment of quadratus lumborum TrPs last.

The patient may inactivate quadratus lumborum TrPs with the application of TrP self-pressure release by utilizing TrP release tools or a tennis ball. Utilizing a TrP release tool, the patient can lie on their back placing the end of the tool on the muscle and the tool across the body. On the tool, both hands are utilized to provide pressure over the tender area for 15 to 20 seconds and repeat up to six times (Figure 50-14A). The patient can also perform a similar technique in the seated position (Figure 50-14B). Another option is standing against the wall with a TrP release tool or a tennis ball using the same principles above (Figure 50-14C).

The quadratus lumborum supine self-stretch exercise (Figure 50-15) is most effective for the diagonal iliotransverse fibers of that muscle. The exercise begins in the supine position

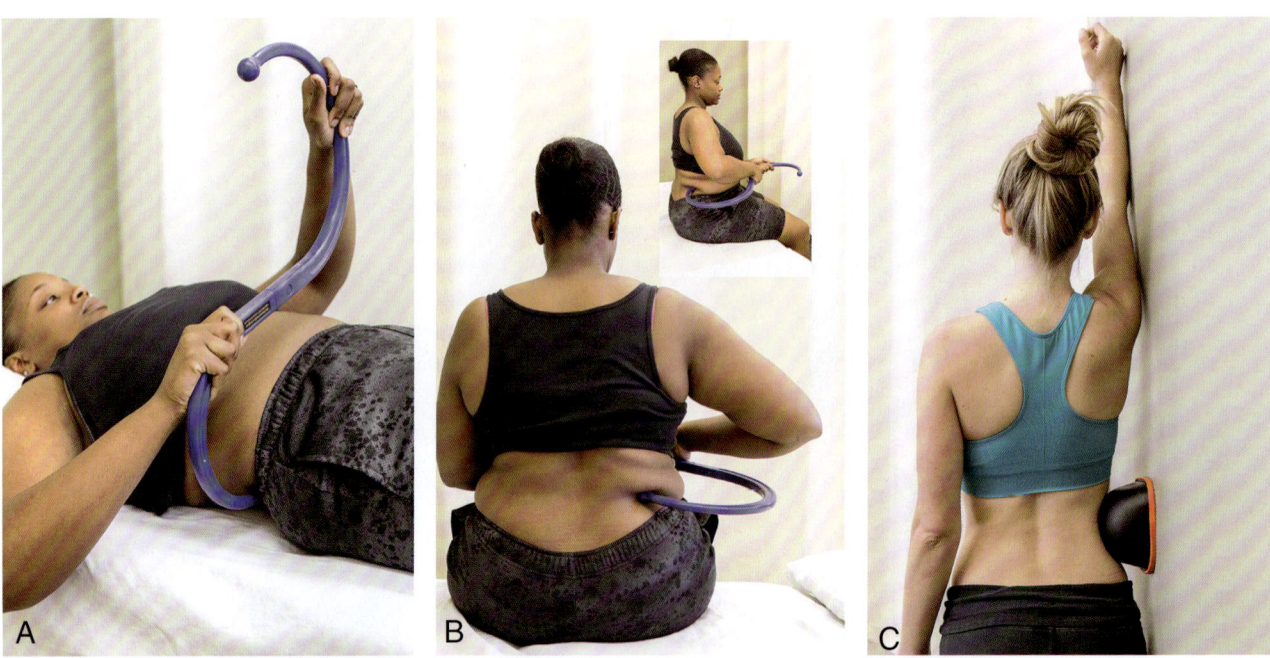

Figure 50-14. Trigger point self-pressure release using TrP release tools. A, Supine. B, Seated. C, Standing.

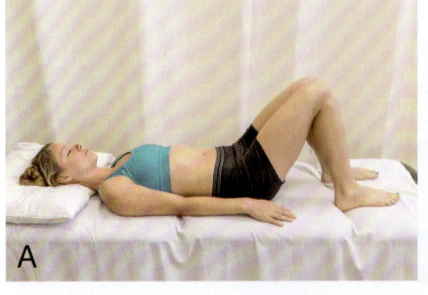 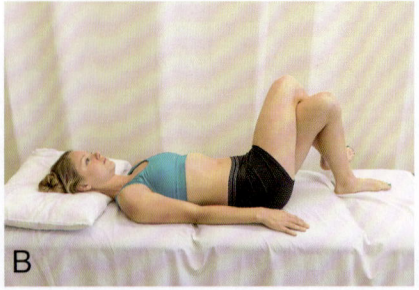 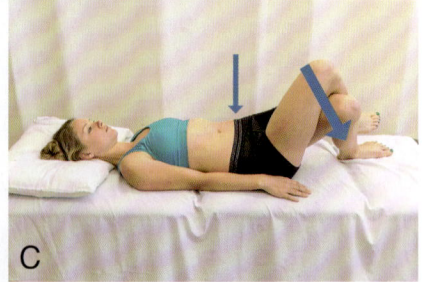

Figure 50-15. Supine self-stretch exercise for the left quadratus lumborum muscle. A, Starting position, supine with the hips and knees bent. B, Preparatory position with the controlling right leg crossed over the left thigh. C, The patient takes a deep breath that contracts the quadratus lumborum muscle and as the patient slowly exhales, the right leg gently pulls the left thigh downward, which rotates the pelvis. Large arrow indicates the direction of applied pressure. Small arrow indicates the pelvic rotation. Steps B and C may be repeated until no further increase in range of motion is achieved. Release the stretch by slipping the controlling (right) leg off the left knee, releasing tension, and assisting the left leg back to the starting position.

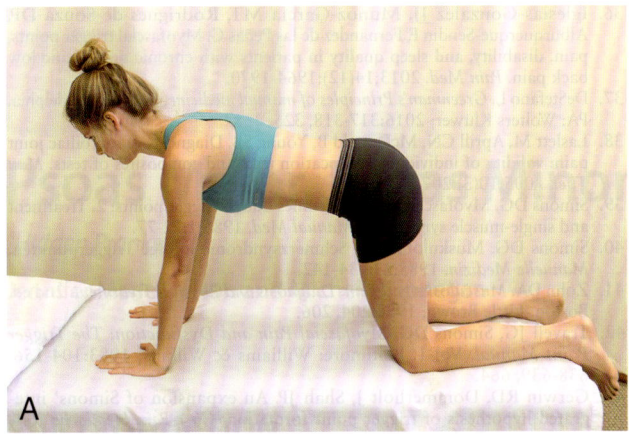
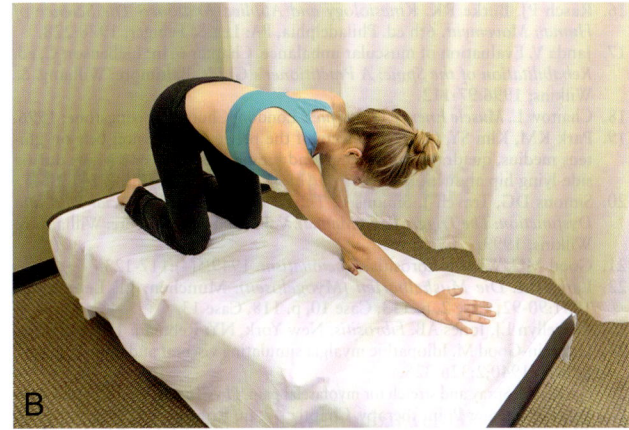
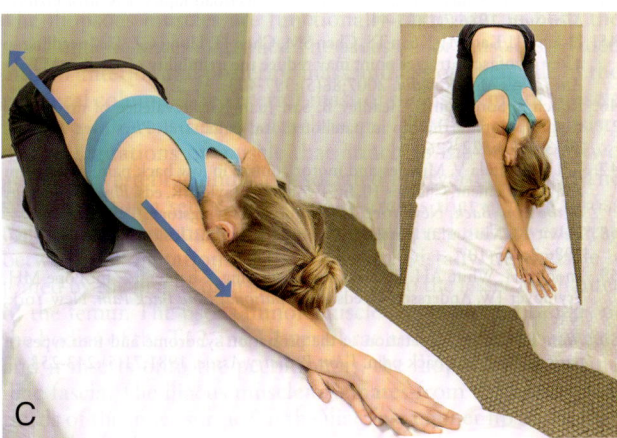

Figure 50-16. Self-stretch of the right quadratus lumborum muscle in the quadruped position ("on all fours"). A, Starting position. B, Preparatory position with the arm forward and across the midline of the body. C, Full stretch with arrows emphasizing the option of reaching the arm forward and pushing the hips down and back to elongate the trunk, further stretching the quadratus lumborum muscle.

with the hips and knees flexed (Figure 50-15A). The thigh on the side of the quadratus lumborum muscle to be stretched is adducted to the point of taking up all the slack in the muscle and the other leg is crossed over the thigh to provide overpressure (Figure 50-15B). The patient then relaxes to allow the pelvis on the involved side to drop down toward the table. With a slow inhalation, the quadratus lumborum muscle contracts isometrically, creating tension. The patient can slowly and gradually stretch the quadratus lumborum muscle by providing a gentle overpressure with the other limb. During slow exhalation, the patient concentrates on relaxing the muscles to be elongated and the uppermost limb helps pull the pelvis caudally by further adducting the thigh on the treatment side to take up all slack that develops (Figure 50-16C). Contraction and relaxation are repeated slowly three to five times until no additional range of motion is achieved. Then, the patient slips the uppermost, assisting limb off the treated limb to help in pushing the latter back to the neutral position. This maneuver avoids overloading the elongated muscles while still under full stretch (a position of vulnerability).

An alternative stretch position for a patient with highly irritable quadratus lumborum TrPs is in the quadruped ("on all fours") position (Figure 50-16A). The arm on the side to be stretched is placed forward and across the midline of the body (Figure 50-16B). The patient shifts the buttocks backward and down toward the heels while keeping the arm across the midline of the body (Figure 50-16C). This position is commonly referred to as the prayer stretch or child's pose position with the modification of the arm placed forward and across the body instead of straight ahead.

References

1. Standring S. *Gray's Anatomy: The Anatomical Basis of Clinical Practice.* 41st ed. London, UK: Elsevier; 2015.
2. Porterfield JA, DeRosa C. *Mechanical Low Back Pain: Perspectives in Functional Anatomy.* 2nd ed. Philadelphia, PA: Saunders; 1998:81-84.
3. Phillips S, Mercer S, Bogduk N. Anatomy and biomechanics of quadratus lumborum. *Proc Inst Mech Eng H.* 2008;222(2):151-159.
4. de Franca GG, Levine LJ. The quadratus lumborum and low back pain. *J Manipulative Physiol Ther.* 1991;14(2):142-149.
5. Eisler P. *Die Muskeln des Stammes.* Jenna: Gustav Fischer; 1912:654.
6. Toldt C. *An Atlas of Human Anatomy.* Vol 1. 2nd ed. New York, NY: Macmillan; 1919:339.
7. Park RJ, Tsao H, Cresswell AG, Hodges PW. Changes in direction-specific activity of psoas major and quadratus lumborum in people with recurring back pain differ between muscle regions and patient groups. *J Electromyogr Kinesiol.* 2013;23(3):734-740.
8. McGill S, Juker D, Kropf P. Quantitative intramuscular myoelectric activity of quadratus lumborum during a wide variety of tasks. *Clin Biomech (Bristol, Avon).* 1996;11(3):170-172.
9. Park RJ, Tsao H, Claus A, Cresswell AG, Hodges PW. Recruitment of discrete regions of the psoas major and quadratus lumborum muscles is changed in specific sitting postures in individuals with recurrent low back pain. *J Orthop Sports Phys Ther.* 2013;43(11):833-840.
10. Waters RL, Morris JM. Electrical activity of muscles of the trunk during walking. *J Anat.* 1972;111(Pt 2):191-199.
11. Knapp ME. Function of the quadratus lumborum. *Arch Phys Med Rehabil.* 1951;32(8):505-507.
12. Rab GT, Chao EY, Stauffer RN. Muscle force analysis of the lumbar spine. *Orthop Clin North Am.* 1977;8(1):193-199.
13. Kim SG, Yong MS, Na SS. The effect of trunk stabilization exercises with a swiss ball on core muscle activation in the elderly. *J Phys Ther Sci.* 2014;26(9):1473-1474.
14. Basmajian J, Deluca C. *Muscles Alive.* 5th ed. Baltimore: Williams & Wilkins; 1985:385-387, 423.
15. Pansky B. *Review of Gross Anatomy.* 4th ed. New York, NY: Macmillan Publishing Co.; 1979:306, 316-317.

and those of the lower levels buried sequentially more deeply within its substance.[3,4] Fibers in the posterior portion are 3 to 5 cm long, and fibers in the anterior portion are 3 to 8 cm long.[2]

As the muscle continues to descend along the pelvic brim, it passes anterior to the sacroiliac joint and is joined by the iliacus muscle. Together, both muscles (together forming the iliopsoas muscle complex) travel posterior to the inguinal ligament, helping to form the floor of the femoral triangle. They then travel anterior to the hip joint capsule and attach onto the lesser trochanter of the femur.[1]

The thickness of the psoas major muscle is reported to vary among different races. Hanson et al[5] examined 21 cadavers that were black and 23 cadavers that were white and found the muscle was approximately twice as thick in black cadavers.

The iliopsoas bursa is a structure that lies beneath the iliopsoas muscle and anterior to the hip joint capsule in 98% of normal individuals. In a small percentage of the population (15%), the bursa can communicate with the hip joint because the tissues between them can be thin and weak.[6]

Early studies on the composition of muscle fiber type of the psoas major muscle suggested a predominance of type I fibers[7-9] or an equal amount of both type I and II fibers.[10] More recently, Arbanas et al[11] found the psoas major muscle to be composed of type I, IIa, and IIx muscles fibers, with type IIa being the most prevalent (49.77%). Type I fibers were the second most common (40.15%) followed by type IIx (10.8%). This data supports the concept of a dynamic function of the muscle. Interestingly, the composition of the fibers were found to change throughout the muscle. The percentage of type IIa and IIx fibers increased from L1 to L4, whereas the percentage of type I fibers decreased from L1 to L4. In light of these trends, it is hypothesized that the cranial portion of the muscle has a more static role (due to a higher percentage of type I fibers) and caudal portion of the muscle has a more dynamic role (due to a higher percentage of type II fibers).

The psoas major muscle also has significant fascial attachments. Superiorly, the psoas fascia forms part of the medial arcuate ligament. Laterally, it blends with the fascia of the upper portion of the quadratus lumborum muscle. More caudally, it continues with the iliac fascia, where it separates the anterior mass of the psoas major muscle from the retroperitoneal structures. The iliac fascia is indistinguishable and continues with the psoas fascia. In the upper retroperitoneum, the fascial blends with the anterior layer of the thoracolumbar fascia over the quadratus lumborum muscle. Caudally, it attaches to the inner aspect of the iliac crest and to the periosteum of the ilium at the pelvic brim.[1]

Psoas Minor

The psoas minor muscle, when present, lies anterior to the psoas major muscle in the lumbar region. It arises from the sides of the bodies of the T12 and L1 vertebrae and the discs between. It has a long flat tendon that inserts onto the pectin pubis, iliopubic ramus, and iliac fascia. The entire muscle is contained within the abdomen and does not attach to the lower extremity.[1] Neumann and Garceau[12] reported that this muscle attached firmly into the iliac fascia in all cadaver hips studied, whereas 90.5% also had a firm bony attachment to the pelvis.

The psoas minor muscle is absent in approximately 40% of people[1]; however, these percentages vary among studies. Maldonado et al[13] reported the psoas minor tendon as absent in 64.7% of unembalmed female cadavers, whereas Neumann and Garceau[12] reported this muscle being absent in 34.4% of cadavers examined. Hanson et al[5] found notable differences in the absence of the psoas minor muscle between races. They found the psoas minor muscle was absent in 91% of black cadavers and 13% of white ones.

Iliacus Muscle

The iliacus muscle originates from the upper two-thirds of the inner surface of the iliac fossa, inner lip of the iliac crest, the iliolumbar and ventral sacroiliac ligaments, and the upper surface of the lateral portion of the sacrum. It travels anteriorly as far as the anterior superior and anterior inferior iliac spines. Most of the fibers of the iliacus muscle join the psoas major tendon, and together they insert onto the lesser trochanter of the femur. Other fibers attach to the femur anterior to the lesser trochanter, including fibers from the upper portion of the hip joint capsule.[1]

Anatomic variations have been reported in the iliacus muscle. D'Costa et al[14] reported a case of an accessory iliacus muscle, covered by a separate fascia, which attached at the middle third of the iliac crest and inserted on the lesser trochanter of the femur with the iliopsoas tendon. Rao et al[15] reported a case of variation in the iliacus muscle bilaterally. On one side, there were two defined variant muscles, an iliacus minimus and an accessory slip of the iliacus muscle. On the other side, there was a single additional slip of the iliacus muscle that fused with the iliopsoas tendon distally. Fabrizio[16] reported a unique variation of the iliacus muscle that originated from the superolateral aspect of the iliac fascia and traveled nearly horizontal to insert into the psoas major muscle, forming a blended iliacus–psoas muscle. Another unique variation of the iliacus muscle, reported by Aleksandrova et al,[17] described slips missing from the middle and anterior parts of the muscle (due to not developing), and the posterior portion of the muscle originated unusually high from the iliolumbar ligament.

There are also reported variations of the iliopsoas tendon at the level of the hip joint. Philippon et al[18] examined 52 cadavers and found more than one tendon present. In only 28% of cadavers were the tendons single-banded. More commonly (64.2%), they were double-banded and there was a small group (7.5%) that were triple-banded.

2.1. Innervation and Vascularization

Innervation of the psoas major muscle is mainly supplied by the ventral rami of L1 and L2, with some contribution from L3.[1] Other variations have been reported. Gibbons et al[2] found through dissection that the posterior fibers of the psoas major muscle were innervated by the ventral rami of spinal nerves T12-L4, whereas the anterior fibers were supplied by branches of the femoral nerve from L2-L4. The lumbar plexus is embedded posteriorly in the substance of the psoas major muscle.[1] Similarly, Kirchmair et al[19] reported that of the 32 embalmed cadavers they dissected, the lumbar plexus was contained in the psoas major muscle in 96.8% of cadavers; however, in 3.2% of the cadavers, the plexus was posterior to the psoas major muscle.

The psoas minor muscle is innervated by a branch of the first lumbar spinal nerve.[1]

The iliacus muscle is innervated by branches of the femoral nerve, L2 and L3.[1] When an accessory iliacus muscle is present, the L4 root of the femoral nerve innervates it.[14]

The vascular supply of the psoas major muscle occurs via several arteries. The lumbar arteries supply the upper portion of the muscle, whereas the anterior branch of the iliolumbar artery supplies the mid portion of the muscle with contributions from the deep circumflex and external iliac arteries. The femoral artery and its branches supply the distal portion of the muscle.[1]

Vascularization of the psoas minor muscle is mainly supplied through the lumbar arteries; however, there could be additional contributions from the arteries that also supply the psoas major muscle.[1]

The primary vascular supply of the iliacus muscle is from the iliac branches of the iliolumbar artery, with additional contributions from the deep circumflex iliac and obturator arteries as well as some branches of the femoral artery.[1]

2.2. Function

Hip Flexion and Stability

The primary function of the psoas major muscle is flexion of the hip.[1,4,20-26] Interestingly, Yoshio et al[27] found that only when the hip was flexed from 45° to 60°, the psoas muscle functioned as a hip flexor.

There is more recent evidence that the psoas major muscle also has a stabilizing function. Yoshio et al[27] analyzed the function of the psoas major muscle using cadavers. They found that when the hip was flexed 0° to 15°, one primary function was to stabilize the femoral head in the acetabulum during hip flexion, another was to maintain an upright position of the lumbar column (discussed further below).

Hip Internal and External Rotation

Contradictory evidence exists exploring the psoas major muscle's ability to externally rotate the hip. Electrophysiologic studies revealed that neither the iliacus nor the psoas muscles are activated during the internal rotation of the hip, but both muscles were often active during external rotation.[28,29] Electrical stimulation of either muscle with the subject in a standing or a supine position produces a slight external rotation.[30] Skyrme et al[26] found that in six cadaveric specimens, hip external rotation was produced only when traction to the iliopsoas was performed with the hip in abduction. Contrary to these studies, Hooper[31] reported that the iliopsoas muscle does not play a significant role in rotation of the normal femur because its tendon is aligned with the axis of rotation in most cases. There is no contemporary electromyographic (EMG) research to support the iliopsoas muscles performing either hip internal or external rotation in adults.[1]

Trunk Movement and Stability

When present, the psoas minor muscle is most likely a weak flexor of the trunk.[1] In a recent cadaveric study, Neumann and Garceau[12] reported that due to the muscle's attachment to the iliac fascia, the psoas minor muscle might partially contribute to control of the position and mechanical stability of the iliopsoas muscles as they cross the femoral head.

The psoas major and iliacus muscles, when acting from below and contracting bilaterally, are able to bend the trunk and pelvis forward against resistance, as when performing a sit-up.[1] Historical studies agree that, after the first 30° of upward movement of a sit-up, the iliacus muscle is vigorously active.[28,32,33] LaBan et al[33] saw no activity in five subjects through the first 30° when the legs were straight but did observe activity when the knees were bent. Flint[32] found mild to moderate activity in three subjects throughout that 30° angle. Interestingly, some individuals depend on the rectus femoris muscle without help from the iliacus muscle, while other individuals use both muscles, when initiating a sit-up. More recent studies of the psoas major muscle, using magnetic resonance diffusion weighted images[34] and EMG,[23] showed that the psoas major muscle is more active in full sit-ups than in curl-ups, but they have not looked at the exact degrees at which the psoas major muscle initiates activation.

Earlier,[4] it was thought that the psoas major muscle was able to produce a small net extensor torque on the three upper lumbar vertebrae, whereas on the lower two vertebrae, the muscle was able to produce a small net flexor torque. More recently, Park et al[35] reported that differences in function exist between two portions of the muscle—the fascicles that arise from the transverse processes and those from the vertebral bodies, not from the higher against the lower levels. The activity of the fascicles of the psoas major muscle that attach to the transverse processes were greater in extension of the trunk against trunk flexion or hip flexion to 90°. The fascicles from the portion of the psoas major muscle attaching to the vertebral bodies had greater activity in hip flexion than flexion of the trunk.

There is growing evidence that the psoas major muscle has a role in stabilization of the trunk. This function stems, in part, from its attachments to the diaphragm and pelvic floor musculature.[2,36]

The role of the psoas major muscle in spinal stability seems to vary on the activity being examined as well as the study setup. Yoshio et al[27] found that the psoas major muscle acts primarily as a spinal stabilizer when the hip is flexed 0° to 45°. Hu et al[20] utilized EMGs to assess activity of the right psoas major, iliacus, rectus femoris, and adductor longus muscles during an active straight leg raise. Interestingly, the iliacus, rectus femoris, and adductor longus muscles activated ipsilaterally before the psoas major muscle. The psoas major muscle activated ipsilaterally and contralaterally at the same time with no difference in amplitude from side to side, supporting the theory that the psoas major muscle acts primarily as a stabilizer.

In sitting, the psoas major muscle acts to balance the trunk.[1] Andersson et al[37] reported that the psoas major muscle was active in sitting with a straight back and when stabilization of the spine in the frontal plane was needed. Similarly, Santaguida and McGill[25] agree that the psoas major muscle is capable of stabilization through bilateral activation. They also reported that changes in lordosis did not have an effect on the mechanical action of the psoas major muscle. This second finding of Santaguida and McGill[25] is not consistent, with recent research. Park et al[35] found that the fascicles of the psoas major muscle that attached to the transverse processes were more active when subjects were in a short lordosis than a flat spine. These fascicles, along with those that attach to the vertebral column, were both active with a flat spine compared with a slumped posture.

2.3. Functional Unit

The functional unit to which a muscle belongs includes the muscles that reinforce and counter its actions as well as the joints that the muscle crosses. The functional interdependence of these structures is reflected in the organization and neural connections of the sensory motor cortex. The functional unit is emphasized because the presence of a TrP in one muscle of the unit increases the likelihood that the other muscles of the unit also develop TrPs. When inactivating TrPs in a muscle, one should be concerned about TrPs that may develop in muscles that are functionally interdependent. Box 51-1 grossly represents the functional unit of the iliopsoas muscle.[38]

Bilaterally, the iliopsoas muscles work to synchronize their activity for functions such as stability of the spine and alternate their activity for functions such as locomotion. As part of the abdominal cylinder, the psoas muscle is also synergistic with the diaphragm, pelvic floor, transversus abdominis, and lumbar multifidus muscles.

During a sit-up, agonists to the psoas major muscle include the rectus abdominus and psoas minor muscles. If the psoas major muscle does provide an anterior shear on the lower lumbar segments, as Hadjipavlou et al[39] and Bogduk et al[4] suggest, then the iliolumbar ligament is ideally situated to provide a counterforce.

3. CLINICAL PRESENTATION

3.1. Referred Pain Pattern

Pain referred from TrPs in the iliopsoas muscles forms a distinctive vertical pattern ipsilaterally along the lumbar spine. It has

---

Box 51-1 Functional unit of the iliopsoas muscles

Action	Synergists	Antagonist
Hip flexion	Rectus femoris Pectineus Sartorius Tensor fasciae latae Gracilis Adductor longus Adductor brevis Adductor magnus (middle portion)	Gluteus maximus Gluteus medius (posterior fibers) Semimembranosus Semitendinosus Biceps femoris

been reported to extend as high as the interscapular region.[40] It extends downward to the sacroiliac region and may continue inferiorly to include the sacrum and proximal medial buttock (Figure 51-2).[41] The referred pain pattern also frequently includes the groin and upper anteromedial aspect of the thigh on the same side. Palpation of TrPs near the attachment of the iliopsoas muscles (mostly iliacus fibers) on the lesser trochanter of the femur may refer pain both to the back and anteriorly to the thigh.

Less frequently, other referred pain patterns have been reported. Stretching the iliopsoas muscles was shown to intensify pain in the scrotum.[42] Pain referral to the medial knee has been reported in the literature[43] and seen several times in clinical practice. The psoas major muscle has also been seen to refer pain into the lower abdomen.

3.2. Symptoms

Patients with unilateral iliopsoas TrPs usually report having vertical low back pain. They frequently run their hand vertically up and down the spine rather than horizontally to demonstrate the location of their pain. When the iliopsoas muscles are involved bilaterally, the patient may perceive the pain as running across the low back, similar to having TrPs in the quadratus lumborum muscle bilaterally. Pain is worse when the patient stands upright but may present as a nagging backache even when recumbent. A frequent additional report is pain in the front of the thigh. Ingber[42] found that patients experienced increased low back pain during antigravity activity and alleviation of the pain when recumbent. The most comfortable recumbent positions were side-lying in a nearly fetal position or lying supine with hips and knees flexed. Patients are likely to have difficulty getting up from a deep-seated chair and are unable to do sit-ups.

Patient's with constipation who also have psoas TrPs may experience referred pain evoked by the passage of a bolus of hard feces that presses against the TrPs. A hypertrophied psoas muscle can compress the neighboring large bowel.[44] Tarsuslu et al[45] utilized iliopsoas muscle release along with sphincter release and bowel mobilizations as an osteopathic treatment technique for chronic constipation in children with cerebral palsy. This intervention was as effective as those who had regular medical care and osteopathic treatment.

3.3. Patient Examination

After a thorough subjective examination the clinician should make a detailed drawing representing the pain pattern that the patient has described. This depiction will assist in planning the physical examination and can be useful in monitoring the progression of the patient as symptoms improve or change. For proper examination of the iliopsoas muscles, the clinician should first start with the observation of the posture in standing. The patient with involvement of the iliopsoas muscle unilaterally demonstrates weight shifting away from the involved side, with the foot of the involved side slightly forward and the torso slightly side bent toward the involved side. Active forward bending of the trunk may reveal a deviation toward the involved side for the first 20° of trunk motion, becoming centered for the rest of the motion.[38] A gait with stooped posture, forward tilt of the pelvis, and hyperlordosis of the lumbar spine is a common finding.

The length of the iliopsoas muscles should be assessed because TrPs in this muscle can cause shortening. Iliopsoas muscle length can be determined with the Thomas test (Figure 51-3).[46] This test can also be utilized to differentiate between iliopsoas, rectus femoris, and/or tensor fascia latae length deficits. To differentiate between muscle tightness and altered neurodynamics, the patient can lift his or her head up in chin tuck position. If there is a change in the patient's symptoms or hip range of motion with cervical motion, it is an indicator there is a femoral nerve involvement.[47-49] The position of the limb to test the tensor fascia latae muscle length also puts more stretch through the saphenous nerve. If dorsiflexion of the foot changes the hip tightness or

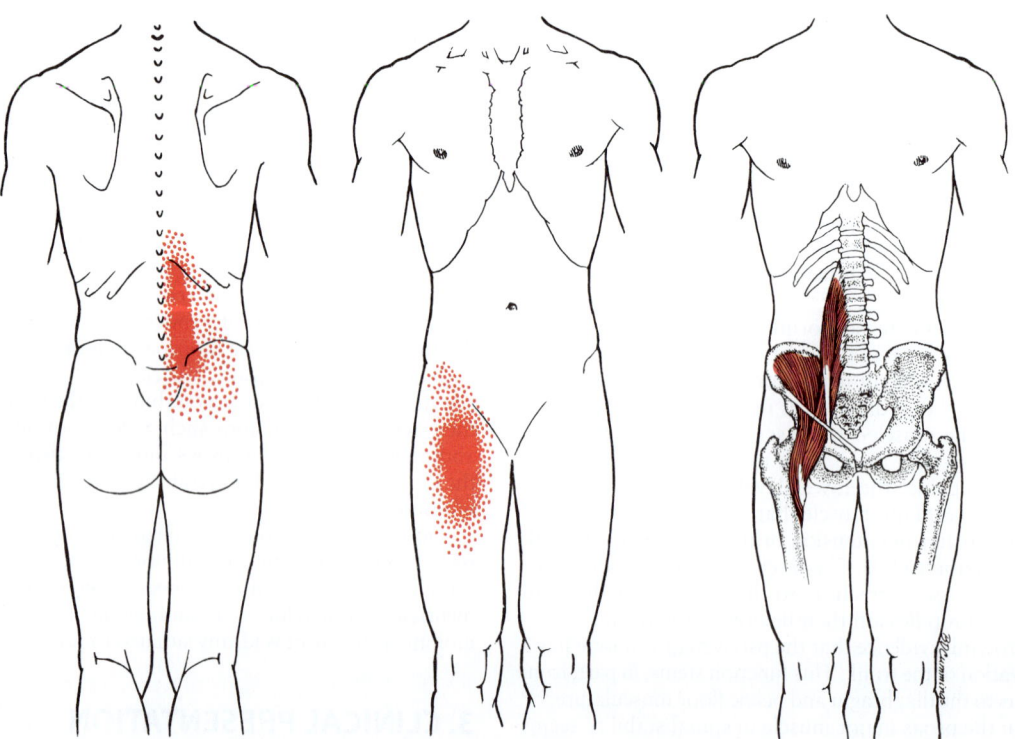

Figure 51-2. Pattern of pain (bright red) referred from palpable myofascial TrPs in the right iliopsoas muscle (darker red). The essential pain reference zone is solid red; the spillover pattern is stippled.

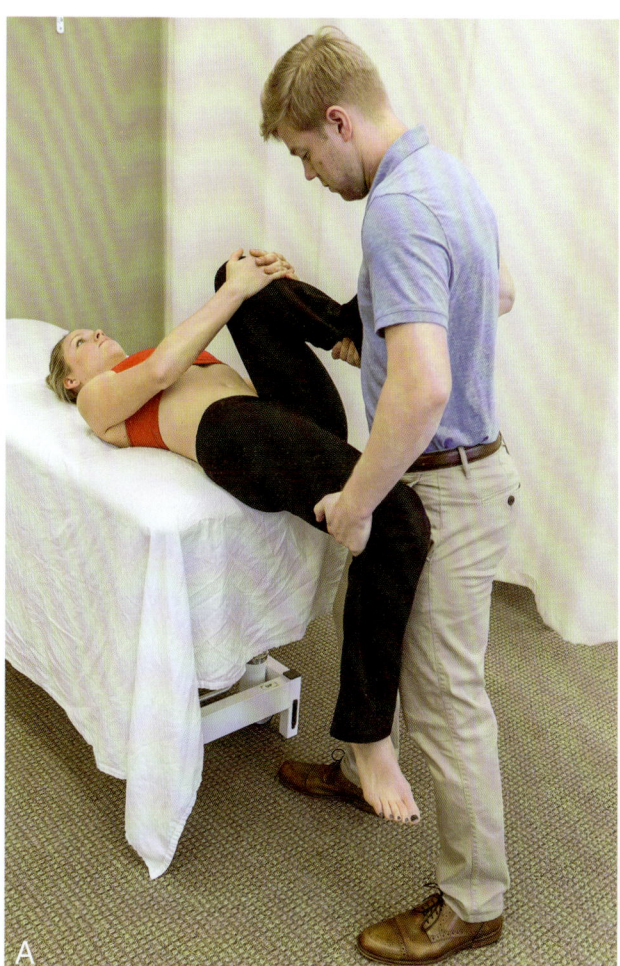 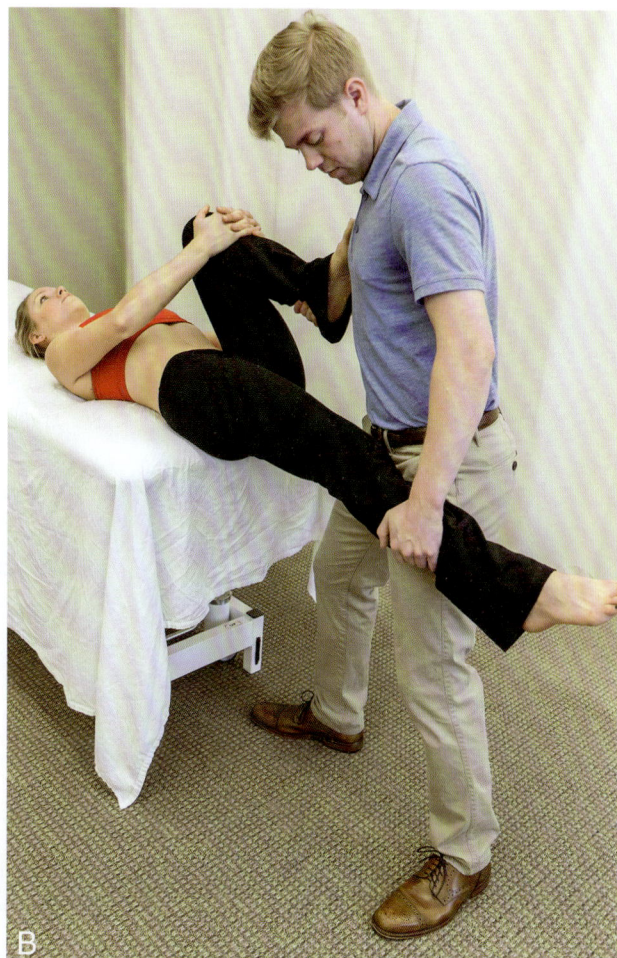

Figure 51-3. Thomas test position for hip flexor length. A, One-joint muscles. B, Two-joint muscle. Adapted from Kendall FP, McCreary EK. *Muscles: Testing and Function, with Posture and Pain.* 5th ed. Baltimore, MD: Lippincott Williams & Wilkins; 2005:376-377.

patient's symptoms, then the saphenous nerve is also likely a contributing factor in the hip range of motion limitation.

Muscle imbalance can change body mechanics. The iliopsoas muscles work in harmony with the rectus abdominus muscle; if this abdominal muscle is weak, the psoas muscle is likely to develop problems trying to compensate. Full function of the abdominal musculature is confirmed if the patient can do a curl-up with the knees bent and without foot support.[50]

Trigger points in a number of muscles other than the iliopsoas muscle refer pain in patterns that may be confused with the pain referral pattern arising from iliopsoas TrPs. Low back pain can also be caused by TrPs in the quadratus lumborum, lowest section of the rectus abdominus, longissimus thoracis, multifidus, and gluteus maximus and medius muscles. Iliopsoas TrPs do not cause pain on coughing and deep breathing as do those in the quadratus lumborum muscle.[41] When the patient reports that pain spreads horizontally across the low back, the pain is much more likely to be referred from TrPs bilaterally in the quadratus lumborum muscles or from the lowest portion of the rectus abdominus muscle (Figure 49-7A).[51] These rectus abdominus TrPs are often associated with TrPs in the iliopsoas muscles. Thigh and groin pain may also be due to TrPs in the tensor fascia latae, pectineus, vastus intermedius, adductor longus and brevis, or the distal parts of the adductor magnus muscles. Of these, only the pectineus muscle and tensor fasciae latae should restrict extension at the hip. Physical examination readily distinguishes the more superficial TrP tenderness of the last two muscles from the deep tenderness of the iliopsoas muscles.

3.4. Trigger Point Examination

Trigger points in the psoas major and iliacus muscles can be detected with a cross-fiber flat palpation in three locations (Figure 51-4). In two of the three locations, the muscle fibers can be palpated beneath the skin without other muscles intervening. To palpate both the psoas major and iliacus muscles, the patient should relax the abdominal muscles. If the patient is ticklish, this task may be difficult. To help the patient relax, place the patient's hand between your two hands as you palpate. Commonly, when TrPs are present in one iliopsoas muscle group, the contralateral iliopsoas muscles need to be examined because they function together. Usually, TrPs are more active in one iliopsoas muscle than in the other, but the contralateral muscle frequently requires treatment as well.

Iliopsoas Common Tendon

With the patient in the supine position and the hip in slight abduction, TrPs can be identified with a cross-fiber flat palpation on the psoas musculotendinous junction and on iliacus muscle fibers against the lateral wall of the femoral triangle, as depicted in Figure 51-4A. If the iliacus muscle is significantly tight, it may be necessary to flex the thigh slightly by supporting it with a pillow. To find the iliopsoas common tendon, the clinician should find the femoral artery within the femoral triangle and then palpate one to two fingers widths laterally over the femoral nerve to the muscle. To confirm that the clinician is palpating the iliopsoas

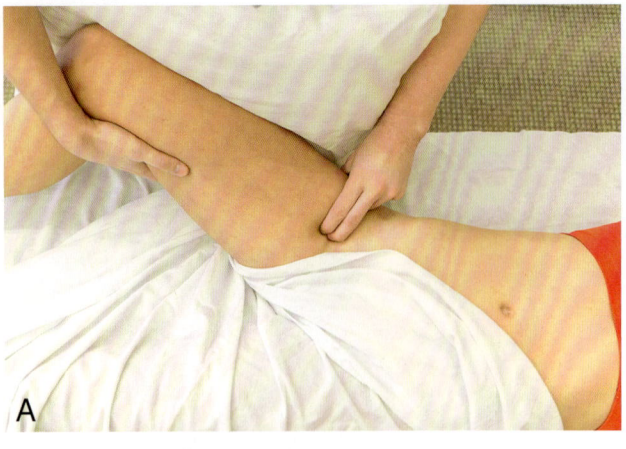
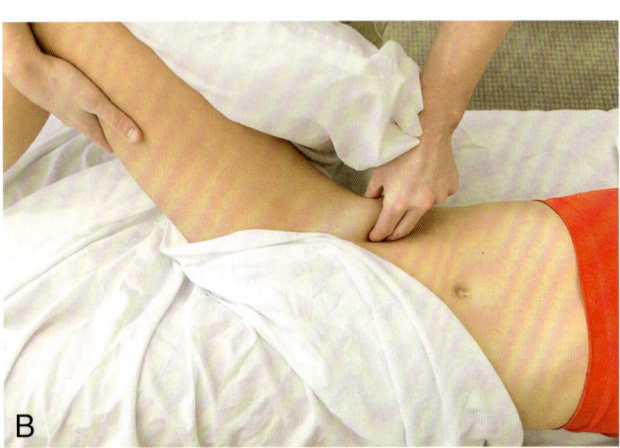
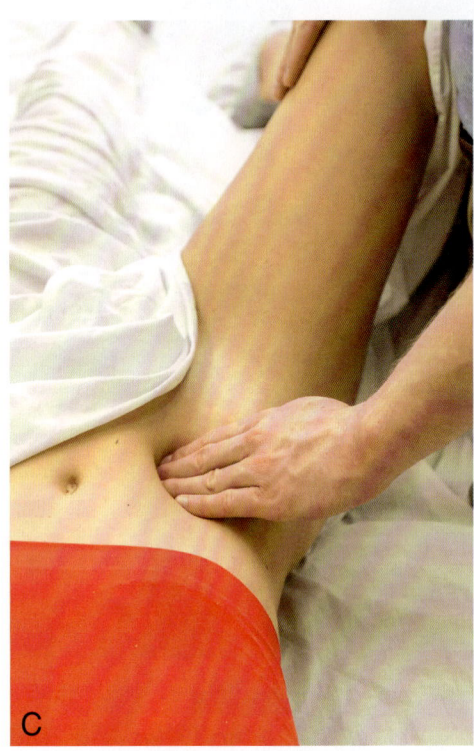

Figure 51-4. Palpation of TrPs in the right iliopsoas muscle at three locations. A, Palpation of the distal iliopsoas TrP region deep along the lateral wall of the femoral triangle, just above the distal attachment of the muscle to the lesser trochanter of the femur. B, Palpation of iliacus TrPs inside the brim of the pelvis behind the anterior superior iliac spine. C, Digital pressure on proximal psoas TrPs applied first downward beside, and then medially, beneath, the rectus abdominis muscle toward the psoas muscle.

muscle, the patient should be asked to think about lifting the leg. If the patient contracts too strongly, it will most likely push the clinician off the TrP, so a gentle contraction is required. A local twitch response is rarely elicited by digital examination at this site and even less frequently at the other two sites.

Iliacus

The proximal fibers of the iliacus muscle can be examined through the aponeurosis of the external oblique muscle using cross-fiber flat palpation along the muscle fibers that lie inside the iliac crest of the pelvis (Figure 51-4B). The fingers reach inside the crest of the ilium starting in the region behind the anterior superior iliac spine and slide back and forth parallel to the iliac crest while pressing against the bone, palpating across the fibers of the iliacus muscle. Occasionally, palpation reveals taut bands and their associated spot tenderness. Pain elicited from these TrPs are more likely to refer to the low back and sacroiliac region than to the thigh. The patient should relax the abdominal muscles in a position that allows the skin of the abdominal wall to slacken.

Psoas Major

Palpation of the psoas major muscle is performed indirectly through the abdominal wall (Figure 51-4C). The patient should be comfortable and the abdominal wall relaxed. With the patient in supine or side-lying, the palpating fingers are placed on the abdominal wall with the fingertips just lateral to the lateral border of the rectus abdominus muscle. Downward pressure is slowly, gradually, and gently exerted to depress the fingers below the level of the rectus abdominus muscle. If the pressure is exerted directly downward with no medial component, it elicits only tenderness of other abdominal contents. Therefore, the clinician exerts slowly increasing pressure medially toward the spinal column. The intervening abdominal contents transmit the pressure to the psoas major muscle against the lumbar spine. The psoas major muscle is examined for tenderness along the entire length of the lumbar spine. If present, tenderness can usually be revealed at approximately the level of the umbilicus or slightly lower. Minimal pressure can elicit a significant amount of pain when the psoas major muscle has TrPs. Pain elicited from this part of the psoas major muscle refers chiefly to the low back.

4. DIFFERENTIAL DIAGNOSIS

4.1. Activation and Perpetuation of Trigger Points

A posture or activity that activates a TrP, if not corrected, can also perpetuate it. In any part of the psoas major, psoas minor, and iliacus muscles, TrPs may be activated by unaccustomed eccentric loading, eccentric exercise in an unconditioned muscle, or maximal or submaximal concentric loading.[52] Trigger points may also be activated or aggravated when the muscle is placed in a shortened and/or lengthened position for an extended period of time.[52] For example, overloading the psoas major muscle by the repetitive vigorous concentric contraction required to perform sit-ups can perpetuate its TrPs. The muscle is more tolerant of the eccentric contraction of slow let-backs or sit-backs.[51]

Tightness of the rectus femoris muscle that prevents full hip extension can also perpetuate TrPs in the iliopsoas muscle.

Trigger points may also be activated when the muscle is placed in a shortened or lengthened position for an extended period of time or activated simultaneously with TrPs in these other muscles by sudden overload during a fall. For example, prolonged sitting with the hips acutely flexed such that the torso leans forward, placing the knees higher than the hips, can place the iliopsoas muscles in a shortened position. This position can occur while driving (or sitting in) a car, sitting at a desk, or sitting on bleachers. Truck drivers and office workers, in particular, are vulnerable to shortening of this muscle.

Sleeping in the fetal position, with the knees drawn up to the chest, can also activate iliopsoas TrPs. Patients often report that their first awareness of pain referred from these TrPs was when they get out of the bed in the morning.

Lewit[53,54] associates TrPs of the psoas major muscle with articular dysfunction in the thoracolumbar region at the levels of T10-L1. Impaired trunk rotation and side bending in this region identify the dysfunction clinically. He associates TrP tenderness of the iliacus muscle with dysfunction of the lumbosacral junction.[53]

A leg length discrepancy or a small hemipelvis can also perpetuate TrPs in the iliopsoas muscles. The involved muscle is most commonly seen on the longer side, but not always. Involvement due to this condition is more likely to be noted when it results from trauma, surgery, or an adaptation then if it is congenital.

4.2. Associated Trigger Points

It has been shown that associated TrPs can develop in the referred pain areas of primary TrPs,[55] therefore, muscles in the referred pain area of the iliopsoas muscle, or muscles referring to the iliopsoas muscle should be considered. Iliopsoas TrPs can contribute to associated TrPs in the quadratus lumborum, multifidi, erector spinae, serratus posterior inferior, gluteus maximus, gluteus medius, adductor longus, adductor brevis, adductor magnus, pectineus, obturator externus, rectus femoris, vastus intermedius, vastus lateralis, vastus medialis, and sartorius muscles. Trigger points in the iliopsoas muscles can be activated by the referred pain from TrPs in the quadratus lumborum, rectus abdominis, pyramidalis, external and internal obliques, multifidi, and erector spinae muscles.

Rarely do the iliopsoas muscles develop TrPs alone; they are commonly involved with other muscles. Its antagonists are likely to develop associated TrPs, including the gluteus maximus, hamstrings, and adductor magnus muscles. Synergistic muscles likely to exhibit TrPs in association with iliopsoas involvement include the rectus abdominis, quadratus lumborum, rectus femoris, tensor fasciae latae, pectineus, lumbar paraspinal, and the contralateral iliopsoas muscles. When the rectus femoris muscle is shortened because of TrPs, the iliopsoas muscle also remain in a shortened position, making it more susceptible to TrPs.

4.3. Associated Pathology

Some medical conditions give rise to symptoms that can appear confusingly similar to those produced by iliopsoas TrPs or may be present concurrently. The psoas major muscle has a close association with lumbar disc pathology. Ingber[42] described several patients with persistent low back pain following a laminectomy for lumbar disc pathology and one with discogenic pain who had not undergone surgery. Injecting the iliopsoas TrPs and initiating extension exercises relieved their symptoms.

The cross-sectional area of the psoas major muscle frequently atrophies in patients with low back pain,[56-60] although this is not consistent in all groups with low back pain.[61-63]

Although a reportedly rare event, the psoas major muscle is susceptible to developing a hematoma in association with an anticoagulation therapy,[64-68] thrombolysis after an acute myocardial infarction,[69] hypertensive emergency,[70] vitamin K antagonist therapy,[65] surgical procedures such as a lateral retroperitoneal transpsoas lumbar interbody fusion,[71] and sometimes following minor trauma in teenagers.[72] The hematoma causes local pain and swelling, difficulty in walking, and often seriously compromises femoral nerve function.

Hematomas in the iliacus muscle are also rare but can develop spontaneously when on an anticoagulation therapy alone,[73] from trauma when on anticoagulant therapy,[74,75] after surgery when on long-term anticoagulants,[76] after a total hip replacement,[77] total hip revision,[78] and in healthy children after a traumatic injury.[79-83]

Iliopsoas bursitis is an inflammation and enlargement of the iliopsoas bursa. It is typically seen in conjunction with underlying conditions such as rheumatoid arthritis,[84-88] chronic arthritis,[89] and less frequently with hip osteoarthritis,[90] calcium pyrophosphate crystal arthritis,[91] after a total hip replacement,[92,93] and secondary to infection.[94] It can also be due to acute trauma or overuse injuries.[95] It can even mimic an iliopsoas abscess.[96] Patients often present with any or all the following symptoms: hip pain,[95,97] groin pain,[98,99] buttock pain,[98] snapping of the hip,[95,97,99] lower limb edema,[92,95] groin mass,[92,95] pain with hyperextension of the hip,[95] and/or pain with flexion/abduction/external rotation.[95,98]

Femoral acetabular impingement is a change in hip morphology that leads to abnormal contact in the joint during movement. It usually presents as a deep ache in the anterior groin, the lateral thigh, or buttocks while sitting. During activity, the pain is often sharp in nature. Weakness and numbness are not common. Pain is increased with activity, especially with those involving high hip flexion angles, sustained flexion loading/rotation in the hip joints, and getting in and out of the car.[100]

The psoas major muscle is not frequently considered part of the pathology of pelvic pain; however; spasms of this muscle have been known to contribute to chronic pelvic pain.[101] In men with a diagnosis of chronic prostatitis, involvement of the iliopsoas muscles[102] and, specifically, the psoas major[103] muscle has been reported. With fascial attachments of the psoas major muscle into the pelvic floor, this muscle should not be overlooked as a potential contributing factor to pelvic pain.

Primary malignant tumors of the iliopsoas muscles are rare and typically have a poor prognosis due to the lack of early diagnosis, large size, and difficulty accessing the tumor surgically.[104] Psoas abscess are primarily reported in a younger population and are most commonly associated with Crohn's disease, appendicitis, colon inflammation, or cancer.[105] Delay in treatment significantly increase mortality rates;[105] thus, it is important to be aware of the possibility of an abscess when assessing the psoas major muscle because they can often mimic TrPs. Ushiyama et al[106] describe the case of an 83-year old with right groin pain, held in a flexed position, and painfully restricted in extension. Movement of the iliopsoas muscles can cause pain when any of the organs it shares a relationship with (kidney, ureter, caecum, appendix, sigmoid colon, pancreas, lumbar lymph nodes, and nerves of the posterior abdominal wall) are diseased.[15]

Trigger points in the iliopsoas muscles can also mimic sports hernias, which are small tears in the lower abdominal walls. The two may occur at the same time, but this author has seen several patients who have undergone sports hernia repairs and continued to have pain. The pain was reproduced and treated by manually treating the TrPs in the psoas major muscle. It is also possible that the symptomatic TrPs were in the abdominal muscles because it is not possible to palpate or treat the psoas major muscle without going through the abdominal oblique muscles.

Because the roots of the lumbar plexus are lodged within the psoas major muscle, with branches of the plexus emerging from the surface and borders of the muscle, there is a possibility of entrapment due to anatomic variations of both the psoas and the iliacus muscles.[107] It is possible for the muscles to entrap the femoral nerve and contribute to symptoms consistent with femoral nerve involvement. In a study of 121 cadavers yielding 242 specimens, D'costa et al[14] found that 7.9% of the time, slips from the iliacus and psoas muscles either pierced or covered the femoral nerve. Tension in this accessory iliacus muscle may lead to strain on the femoral nerve and therefore cause pain to refer into the hip, knee, or L4 dermatome. The obturator nerve arises from the anterior rami of L2, L3, and L4 spinal nerves in the anterior portion of the psoas major muscle and emerges along the medial border of the psoas major muscle before passing into the pelvis. Tightness in the psoas major muscle can lead to tension or entrapment of the obturator nerve in this region.[108]

Several nerves in the region of the psoas major and iliacus muscles can also become entrapped and cause groin, hip, or thigh symptoms for reasons other than muscular involvement. It is important to be able to recognize these symptoms and not assume that they are solely due to TrPs of the psoas major and/or iliacus muscles. The iliohypogastric nerve can become entrapped after an abdominoplasty with plication of the anterior rectus sheath,[109] during pregnancy,[110] after gynecologic laparoscopy,[111,112] or from an external oblique muscle defect because terminal branches travel through it.[113] The ilioinguinal nerve can become entrapped after a hernia surgery,[114-116] laparoscopic gynecologic surgery,[112] or a Cesarean section,[117] and can even be idiopathic.[118] The lateral femoral cutaneous nerve can become entrapped after a laparoscopic hernia repair,[114] at the fascia lata of the thigh,[119] and from a lipoma.[120] The femoral nerve can be entrapped due to an iliopsoas muscular amyloidoma bilaterally in a patient with multiple myeloma[121] from a high-energy knee trauma,[122] an iliopsoas hematoma,[123,124] and/or an iliopsoas bursitis.[125] Finally, the obturator nerve can become entrapped due to fractures of the pelvic ring[126] and acetabulum,[127] endometriosis around the nerve,[128] or can be idiopathic.[129]

5. CORRECTIVE ACTIONS

If a patient has low back pain that does not respond to a directional preference of either flexion or extension and has difficulty ambulating, a cane may be utilized.

When sitting, the patient should maintain an open angle such that the hips are higher than the knees. Raising the seat such that the thigh slopes downward toward the front of the seat assists with this. Leaning back against a slightly reclining backrest is also helpful. If sitting with the hips acutely flexed is unavoidable, then standing up frequently to extend the hips and stretch the iliopsoas muscle helps unload it. If taking a long drive, cruise control provides an opportunity for the driver to shift and change positions slightly to help minimize the load to the iliopsoas muscles.

Poor breathing, as in paradoxical breathing,[51] can impair recovery of the iliopsoas muscles from TrPs. Patients who exhibit paradoxical breathing should practice abdominal breathing until they can regularly breathe in the normal pattern of coordinated chest and abdominal movements during inhalation and exhalation. This style of breathing should be performed in the supine/hook-lying position to provide the best pull on the psoas major muscle by maximal excursion of the fascial attachments of the psoas major muscle to the diaphragm muscle.[2]

For sleeping, the patient may place a small pillow under the knees when lying on the back or under the hips and belly when sleeping prone. This produces a slight hip flexion that lessens the pull of the iliopsoas muscles sufficiently to lie comfortably. The patient should avoid side-lying with the hips flexed excessively because this position shortens the iliopsoas muscles.

To stretch the iliopsoas muscle passively, the thighs and pelvis should be pressed against the table (or floor) because they hyperextend the lumbar spine and hips in a press-up position (Figure 51-5). The muscle can also be stretched in the position utilized for assessment (Figure 51-3A). To increase the stretch further, a post-isometric relaxation technique, which was described and illustrated for this muscle by Lewit,[53] can be effective. The lower extremity on the side of the iliopsoas muscle to be stretched is allowed to hang freely with the knee bent. If the thigh needs more support, the patient may move up on the supporting surface. The pull is increased by pulling the other knee to the chest. This position also loads a sufficiently shortened rectus femoris muscle.

Iliopsoas muscles should not be treated for TrPs by stretching until one identifies any coexisting lumbar spine articular dysfunction. If present, both should be treated because each can prevent recovery of the other. It is important to treat iliopsoas TrPs bilaterally; the muscle on one side rarely develops TrPs without the other also doing so.

Deep massage and hip extension exercises may also be helpful in relieving the pain referred from iliopsoas TrPs.[42,130] Treating the other muscles in the functional unit with massage or stretching may also be beneficial.

To improve the stability function of the psoas major muscle, a consistent low-grade contraction of the muscle can be performed.[2] To stimulate the longitudinal action of the muscle, the patient should gently try to "pull/suck your hip into the socket without moving your back." This is often easier to do if slight distraction of the femur is applied by someone gently pulling on the leg or with the leg dangling off a step. The patient can

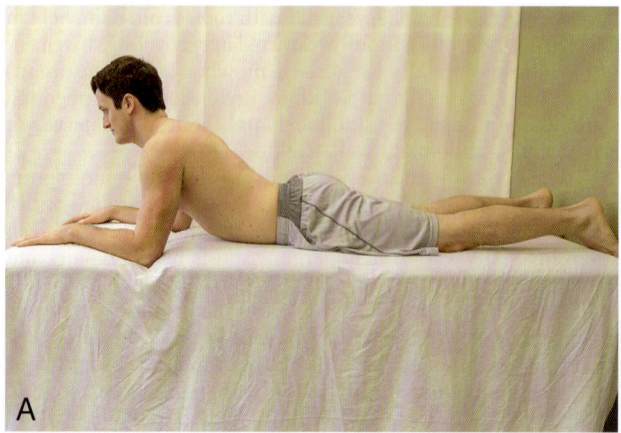
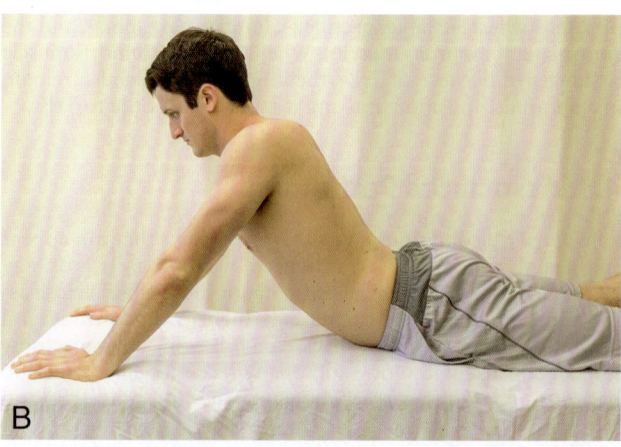

Figure 51-5. Self-stretch of the iliopsoas muscles. A, Initial position for patients with irritable TrPs. B, Progression of iliopsoas stretch.

also lie prone and perform a gentle isometric contraction of the hip into the supporting surface without rotation of the pelvis or spine. In addition, working with a trained clinician on a spinal stabilization program is also helpful, as this has been shown to improve the cross-sectional area of the muscle.[131]

References

1. Standring S. *Gray's Anatomy: The Anatomical Basis of Clinical Practice*. 41st ed: London, UK: Elsevier; 2015.
2. Gibbons S, Comerford MJ, Emerson P. Rehabilitation of the stability function of psoas major. *Orthop Div Rev*. 2002:9-16.
3. Bogduk N, Twomey L. *Clinical Anatomy of the Lumbar Spine*. New York, NY: Churchill Livingstone; 1987.
4. Bogduk N, Pearcy M, Hadfield G. Anatomy and biomechanics of psoas major. *Clin Biomech (Bristol, Avon)*. 1992;7(2):109-119.
5. Hanson P, Magnusson SP, Sorensen H, Simonsen EB. Anatomical differences in the psoas muscles in young black and white men. *J Anat*. 1999;194(Pt 2):303-307.
6. Kim JO, Cho HM. Rapid destruction of the hip joint accompanied by an enlarged iliopsoas bursa in a healthy man. *Hip Pelvis*. 2014;26(3):189-193.
7. Havenith MG, Visser R, Schrijvers-van Schendel JM, Bosman FT. Muscle fiber typing in routinely processed skeletal muscle with monoclonal antibodies. *Histochemistry*. 1990;93(5):497-499.
8. Zheng A, Rahkila P, Vuori J, Rasi S, Takala T, Vaananen HK. Quantification of carbonic anhydrase III and myoglobin in different fiber types of human psoas muscle. *Histochemistry*. 1992;97(1):77-81.
9. Parkkola R, Alanen A, Kalimo H, Lillsunde I, Komu M, Kormano M. MR relaxation times and fiber type predominance of the psoas and multifidus muscle. An autopsy study. *Acta Radiol*. 1993;34(1):16-19.
10. Johnson MA, Polgar J, Weightman D, Appleton D. Data on the distribution of fibre types in thirty-six human muscles. An autopsy study. *J Neurol Sci*. 1973;18(1):111-129.
11. Arbanas J, Klasan GS, Nikolic M, Jerkovic R, Miljanovic I, Malnar D. Fibre type composition of the human psoas major muscle with regard to the level of its origin. *J Anat*. 2009;215(6):636-641.
12. Neumann DA, Garceau LR. A proposed novel function of the psoas minor revealed through cadaver dissection. *Clin Anat*. 2015;28(2):243-252.
13. Maldonado PA, Slocum PD, Chin K, Corton MM. Anatomic relationships of psoas muscle: clinical applications to psoas hitch ureteral reimplantation. *Am J Obstet Gynecol*. 2014;211(5):563.e1-566.e1.
14. D'Costa S, Ramanathan LA, Madhyastha S, et al. An accessory iliacus muscle: a case report. *Rom J Morphol Embryol*. 2008;49(3):407-409.
15. Rao TR, Kanyan PS, Vanishree, Rao S. Bilateral variation of iliacus muscle and splitting of femoral nerve. *Neuroanatomy*. 2008;7:72-75.
16. Fabrizio PA. Anatomic variation of the iliacus and psoas muscles. *Int J Anat Var*. 2011;4:28-30.
17. Aleksandrova JN, Malinova L, Jelev L. Variations of the iliaus muscle: report of two caes and review of the literature. *Int J Anat Var*. 2013;6:149-152.
18. Philippon MJ, Devitt BM, Campbell KJ, et al. Anatomic variance of the iliopsoas tendon. *Am J Sports Med*. 2014;42(4):807-811.
19. Kirchmair L, Lirk P, Colvin J, Mitterschiffthaler G, Moriggl B. Lumbar plexus and psoas major muscle: not always as expected. *Reg Anesth Pain Med*. 2008;33(2):109-114.
20. Hu H, Meijer OG, van Dieen JH, et al. Is the psoas a hip flexor in the active straight leg raise? *Eur Spine J*. 2011;20(5):759-765.
21. Jemmett RS, Macdonald DA, Agur AM. Anatomical relationships between selected segmental muscles of the lumbar spine in the context of multi-planar segmental motion: a preliminary investigation. *Man Ther*. 2004;9(4):203-210.
22. Basmajian JV. Electromyography of iliopsoas. *Anat Rec*. 1958;132(2):127-132.
23. Juker D, McGill S, Kropf P, Steffen T. Quantitative intramuscular myoelectric activity of lumbar portions of psoas and the abdominal wall during a wide variety of tasks. *Med Sci Sports Exerc*. 1998;30(2):301-310.
24. Penning L. Psoas muscle and lumbar spine stability: a concept uniting existing controversies. Critical review and hypothesis. *Eur Spine J*. 2000;9(6):577-585.
25. Santaguida PL, McGill SM. The psoas major muscle: a three-dimensional geometric study. *J Biomech*. 1995;28(3):339-345.
26. Skyrme AD, Cahill DJ, Marsh HP, Ellis H. Psoas major and its controversial rotational action. *Clin Anat*. 1999;12(4):264-265.
27. Yoshio M, Murakami G, Sato T, Sato S, Noriyasu S. The function of the psoas major muscle: passive kinetics and morphological studies using donated cadavers. *J Orthop Sci*. 2002;7(2):199-207.
28. Basmajian J, Deluca C. *Muscles Alive*. 5th ed. Baltimore, MD: Williams & Wilkins; 1985:234-235, 310-313.
29. Basmajian JV, Greenlaw RK. Electromyography of iliacus and psoas with inserted fine-wire electrodes. *Anat Rec*. 1968;160:310-311.
30. Duchenne G. *Physiology of Motion*. Philadelphia, PA: Lippincott; 1949.
31. Hooper AC. The role of the iliopsoas muscle in femoral rotation. *Ir J Med Sci*. 1977;146(4):108-112.
32. Flint MM. An electromyographic comparison of the function of the iliacus and the rectus abdominis muscles. A preliminary report. *Phys Ther*. 1965;45:248-252.
33. LaBan MM, Raptou AD, Johnson EW. Electromyographic study of function of iliopsoas muscle. *Arch Phys Med Rehabil*. 1965;46(10):676-679.
34. Yanagisawa O, Matsunaga N, Okubo Y, Kaneoka K. Noninvasive evaluation of trunk muscle recruitment after trunk exercises using diffusion-weighted MR imaging. *Magn Reson Med Sci*. 2015;14(3):173-181.
35. Park RJ, Tsao H, Claus A, Cresswell AG, Hodges PW. Changes in regional activity of the psoas major and quadratus lumborum with voluntary trunk and hip tasks and different spinal curvatures in sitting. *J Orthop Sports Phys Ther*. 2013;43(2):74-82.
36. Sajko S, Stuber K. Psoas major: a case report and review of its anatomy, biomechanics, and clinical implications. *J Can Chiropr Assoc*. 2009;53(4):311-318.
37. Andersson E, Oddsson L, Grundstrom H, Thorstensson A. The role of the psoas and iliacus muscles for stability and movement of the lumbar spine, pelvis and hip. *Scand J Med Sci Sports*. 1995;5(1):10-16.
38. Simons DG, Travell J, Simons L. *Travell & Simon's Myofascial Pain and Dysfunction: The Trigger Point Manual*. Vol 1. 2nd ed. Baltimore, MD: Williams & Wilkins; 1999.
39. Hadjipavlou AG, Farfan HF, Simmons JW. The functioning spine. In: Farfan HF, Simmons JW, Hadjipavlou AG, eds. *The Sciatic Syndrome*. Thorofare, NJ: Slack; 1996:41-73.
40. Durianova J. Spasm of the m.psoas in the differential diagnosis of pain in the lumbosacral region. *Fysiatr Revmatol Vestn*. 1974;52(4):199-203.
41. Simons DG, Travell JG. Myofascial origins of low back pain. 2. Torso muscles. *Postgrad Med*. 1983;73(2):81-92, 91-92.
42. Ingber RS. Iliopsoas myofascial dysfunction: a treatable cause of "failed" low back syndrome. *Arch Phys Med Rehabil*. 1989;70(5):382-386.
43. Cummings M. Referred knee pain treated with electroacupuncture to iliopsoas. *Acupunct Med*. 2003;21(1-2):32-35.
44. Duprat G Jr, Levesque HP, Seguin R, Nemeeh J, Sylvestre J. Bowel displacement due to psoas muscle hypertrophy. *J Can Assoc Radiol*. 1983;34(1):64-65.
45. Tarsuslu T, Bol H, Simsek IE, Toylan IE, Cam S. The effects of osteopathic treatment on constipation in children with cerebral palsy: a pilot study. *J Manipulative Physiol Ther*. 2009;32(8):648-653.
46. Kendall FP, McCreary EK. *Muscles: Testing and Function, with Posture and Pain*. 5th ed. Baltimore, MD: Lippincott Williams & Wilkins; 2005:376-377.
47. Butler DS, Jones MA. *Mobilisation of the Nervous System*. New York, NY: Churchill Livingstone; 1991.
48. Butler D. *The Sensitive Nervous Systerm*. Adlaide, SA: NOI Group; 2000.
49. Lai WH, Shih YF, Lin PL, Chen WY, Ma HL. Normal neurodynamic responses of the femoral slump test. *Man Ther*. 2012;17(2):126-132.
50. Jull GA, Janda V. Chapter 10, Muscles and motor control in low back pain: assessment and management. In: Twomey L, Taylor JR, eds. *Physical Therapy of the Low Back*. New York, NY: Churchill Livingstone; 1987:253-278.
51. Travell JG, Simons DG. *Myofascial Pain and Dysfunction: The Trigger Point Manual*. Vol 1. Baltimore, MD: Williams & Wilkins; 1983.
52. Gerwin RD, Dommerholt J, Shah JP. An expansion of Simons' integrated hypothesis of trigger point formation. *Curr Pain Headache Rep*. 2004;8(6):468-475.
53. Lewit K. *Manipulative Therapy in Rehabilitation of the Motor System*. London, England: Butterworths; 1985:138, 276, 315 (153, Fig. 4.42).
54. Lewit K. Muscular pattern in thoraco-lumbar lesions. *Man Med*. 1986;2:105-107.
55. Hsieh YL, Kao MJ, Kuan TS, Chen SM, Chen JT, Hong CZ. Dry needling to a key myofascial trigger point may reduce the irritability of satellite MTrPs. *Am J Phys Med Rehabil*. 2007;86(5):397-403.
56. Bok DH, Kim J, Kim TH. Comparison of MRI-defined back muscles volume between patients with ankylosing spondylitis and control patients with chronic back pain: age and spinopelvic alignment matched study. *Eur Spine J*. 2017;26(2):528-537.
57. Wan Q, Lin C, Li X, Zeng W, Ma C. MRI assessment of paraspinal muscles in patients with acute and chronic unilateral low back pain. *Br J Radiol*. 2015;88(1053):20140546.
58. Kamaz M, Kiresi D, Oguz H, Emlik D, Levendoglu F. CT measurement of trunk muscle areas in patients with chronic low back pain. *Diagn Interv Radiol*. 2007;13(3):144-148.
59. Ploumis A, Michailidis N, Christodoulou P, Kalaitzoglou I, Gouvas G, Beris A. Ipsilateral atrophy of paraspinal and psoas muscle in unilateral back pain patients with monosegmental degenerative disc disease. *Br J Radiol*. 2011;84(1004):709-713.
60. Barker KL, Shamley DR, Jackson D. Changes in the cross-sectional area of multifidus and psoas in patients with unilateral back pain: the relationship to pain and disability. *Spine (Phila Pa 1976)*. 2004;29(22):E515-E519.
61. D'Hooge R, Cagnie B, Crombez G, Vanderstraeten G, Dolphens M, Danneels L. Increased intramuscular fatty infiltration without differences in lumbar muscle cross-sectional area during remission of unilateral recurrent low back pain. *Man Ther*. 2012;17(6):584-588.
62. Bouche KG, Vanovermeire O, Stevens VK, et al. Computed tomographic analysis of the quality of trunk muscles in asymptomatic and symptomatic lumbar discectomy patients. *BMC Musculoskelet Disord*. 2011;12:65.
63. Thakar S, Sivaraju L, Aryan S, Mohan D, Sai Kiran NA, Hegde AS. Lumbar paraspinal muscle morphometry and its correlations with demographic and radiological factors in adult isthmic spondylolisthesis: a retrospective review of 120 surgically managed cases. *J Neurosurg Spine*. 2016;24(5):679-685.
64. Conesa X, Ares O, Seijas R. Massive psoas haematoma causing lumbar plexus palsy: a case report. *J Orthop Surg (Hong Kong)*. 2012;20(1):94-97.
65. Llitjos JF, Daviaud F, Grimaldi D, et al. Ilio-psoas hematoma in the intensive care unit: a multicentric study. *Ann Intensive Care*. 2016;6(1):8.
66. Basheer A, Jain R, Anton T, Rock J. Bilateral iliopsoas hematoma: case report and literature review. *Surg Neurol Int*. 2013;4:121.
67. Lee KS, Jeong IS, Oh SG, Ahn BH. Subsequently occurring bilateral iliopsoas hematoma: a case report. *J Cardiothorac Surg*. 2015;10:183.
68. Eltorai AE, Kuris EO, Daniels AH. Psoas haematoma mimicking lumbar radiculopathy. *Postgrad Med J*. 2016;92(1085):182.
69. Abhishek BS, Vijay SC, Avanthi V, Kumar B. Spontaneous psoas hematoma in a case of acute myocardial infarction following streptokinase infusion. *Indian Heart J*. 2016;68(suppl 2):S18-S21.

70. Yogarajah M, Sivasambu B, Jaffe EA. Spontaneous iliopsoas haematoma: a complication of hypertensive urgency. *BMJ Case Rep*. 2015;2015. pii: bcr2014207517.
71. Beckman JM, Vincent B, Park MS, et al. Contralateral psoas hematoma after minimally invasive, lateral retroperitoneal transpsoas lumbar interbody fusion: a multicenter review of 3950 lumbar levels. *J Neurosurg Spine*. 2017;26(1):50-54.
72. Giuliani G, Poppi M, Acciarri N, Forti A. CT scan and surgical treatment of traumatic iliacus hematoma with femoral neuropathy: case report. *J Trauma*. 1990;30(2):229-231.
73. Kong WK, Cho KT, Lee HJ, Choi JS. Femoral neuropathy due to iliacus muscle hematoma in a patient on warfarin therapy. *J Korean Neurosurg Soc*. 2012;51(1):51-53.
74. Spengos K, Anagnostou E, Vassilopoulou S. Subacute proximal leg weakness after a minor traffic accident in a patient treated with anticoagulants. *BMJ Case Rep*. 2012;2012. pii: bcr0220125731.
75. Chan TY. Life-threatening retroperitoneal bleeding due to warfarin-drug interactions. *Pharmacoepidemiol Drug Saf*. 2009;18(5):420-422.
76. Mwipatayi BP, Daneshmand A, Bangash HK, Wong J. Delayed iliacus compartment syndrome following femoral artery puncture: case report and literature review. *J Surg Case Rep*. 2016;2016(6). pii: rjw102.
77. Gogus A, Ozturk C, Sirvanci M, Aydogan M, Hamzaoglu A. Femoral nerve palsy due to iliacus hematoma occurred after primary total hip arthroplasty. *Arch Orthop Trauma Surg*. 2008;128(7):657-660.
78. Nakamura Y, Mitsui H, Toh S, Hayashi Y. Femoral nerve palsy associated with iliacus hematoma following pseudoaneurysm after revision hip arthroplasty. *J Arthroplasty*. 2008;23(8):1240.e1-1240.e4.
79. Chambers S, Berg AJ, Lupu A, Jennings A. Iliacus haematoma causing femoral nerve palsy: an unusual trampolining injury. *BMJ Case Rep*. 2015;2015. pii: bcr2014208758.
80. Khan MA, Whitaker SR, Ibrahim MS, Haddad FS. Late presentation of a subiliacus haematoma after an apophyseal injury of the anterior inferior iliac spine. *BMJ Case Rep*. 2014;2014. pii: bcr2013201071.
81. Yi TI, Yoon TH, Kim JS, Lee GE, Kim BR. Femoral neuropathy and meralgia paresthetica secondary to an iliacus hematoma. *Ann Rehabil Med*. 2012;36(2):273-277.
82. Murray IR, Perks FJ, Beggs I, Moran M. Femoral nerve palsy secondary to traumatic iliacus haematoma—a young athlete's injury. *BMJ Case Rep*. 2010;2010. pii: bcr0520103045.
83. Patel A, Calfee R, Thakur N, Eberson C. Non-operative management of femoral neuropathy secondary to a traumatic iliacus haematoma in an adolescent. *J Bone Joint Surg Br*. 2008;90(10):1380-1381.
84. Iwata T, Nozawa S, Ohashi M, Sakai H, Shimizu K. Giant iliopectineal bursitis presenting as neuropathy and severe edema of the lower limb: case illustration and review of the literature. *Clin Rheumatol*. 2013;32(5):721-725.
85. Tokita A, Ikari K, Tsukahara S, et al. Iliopsoas bursitis-associated femoral neuropathy exacerbated after internal fixation of an intertrochanteric hip fracture in rheumatoid arthritis: a case report. *Mod Rheumatol*. 2008;18(4):394-398.
86. Matsumoto T, Juji T, Mori T. Enlarged psoas muscle and iliopsoas bursitis associated with a rapidly destructive hip in a patient with rheumatoid arthritis. *Mod Rheumatol*. 2006;16(1):52-54.
87. Bianchi S, Martinoli C, Keller A, Bianchi-Zamorani MP. Giant iliopsoas bursitis: sonographic findings with magnetic resonance correlations. *J Clin Ultrasound*. 2002;30(7):437-441.
88. Rodriguez-Gomez M, Willisch A, Fernandez L, Lopez-Barros G, Abel V, Monton E. Bilateral giant iliopsoas bursitis presenting as refractory edema of lower limbs. *J Rheumatol*. 2004;31(7):1452-1454.
89. Murphy CL, Meaney JF, Rana H, McCarthy EM, Howard D, Cunnane G. Giant iliopsoas bursitis: a complication of chronic arthritis. *J Clin Rheumatol*. 2010;16(2):83-85.
90. Tormenta S, Sconfienza LM, Iannessi F, et al. Prevalence study of iliopsoas bursitis in a cohort of 860 patients affected by symptomatic hip osteoarthritis. *Ultrasound Med Biol*. 2012;38(8):1352-1356.
91. Di Carlo M, Draghessi A, Carotti M, Salaffi F. An unusual association: iliopsoas bursitis related to calcium pyrophosphate crystal arthritis. *Case Rep Rheumatol*. 2015;2015:935835.
92. Cheung YM, Gupte CM, Beverly MJ. Iliopsoas bursitis following total hip replacement. *Arch Orthop Trauma Surg*. 2004;124(10):720-723.
93. DeFrancesco CJ, Kamath AF. Abductor muscle necrosis due to iliopsoas bursal mass after total hip arthroplasty. *J Clin Orthop Trauma*. 2015;6(4):288-292.
94. Guiral J, Reverte D, Carrero P. Iliopsoas bursitis due to Brucella melitensis infection—a case report. *Acta Orthop Scand*. 1999;70(5):523-524.
95. Johnston CA, Wiley JP, Lindsay DM, Wiseman DA. Iliopsoas bursitis and tendinitis. A review. *Sports Med*. 1998;25(4):271-283.
96. Fukui S, Iwamoto N, Tsuji S, et al. RS3PE syndrome with iliopsoas bursitis distinguished from an iliopsoas abscess using a CT-guided puncture. *Intern Med*. 2015;54(13):1653-1656.
97. Vaccaro JP, Sauser DD, Beals RK. Iliopsoas bursa imaging: efficacy in depicting abnormal iliopsoas tendon motion in patients with internal snapping hip syndrome. *Radiology*. 1995;197(3):853-856.
98. Parziale JR, O'Donnell CJ, Sandman DN. Iliopsoas bursitis. *Am J Phys Med Rehabil*. 2009;88(8):690-691.
99. Blankenbaker DG, De Smet AA, Keene JS. Sonography of the iliopsoas tendon and injection of the iliopsoas bursa for diagnosis and management of the painful snapping hip. *Skeletal Radiol*. 2006;35(8):565-571.
100. Zhang C, Li L, Forster BB, et al. Femoroacetabular impingement and osteoarthritis of the hip. *Can Fam Physician*. 2015;61(12):1055-1060.
101. Carter JE. *Chronic Pelvic Pain: Diagnosis and Managment*. Golden, CO: Medical Education Collaborative; 1996.
102. Kim DS, Jeong TY, Kim YK, Chang WH, Yoon JG, Lee SC. Usefulness of a myofascial trigger point injection for groin pain in patients with chronic prostatitis/chronic pelvic pain syndrome: a pilot study. *Arch Phys Med Rehabil*. 2013;94(5):930-936.
103. Hetrick DC, Ciol MA, Rothman I, Turner JA, Frest M, Berger RE. Musculoskeletal dysfunction in men with chronic pelvic pain syndrome type III: a case-control study. *J Urol*. 2003;170(3):828-831.
104. Behranwala KA, A'Hern R, Thomas JM. Primary malignant tumors of the iliopsoas compartment. *J Surg Oncol*. 2004;86(2):78-83.
105. Ricci MA, Rose FB, Meyer KK. Pyogenic psoas abscess: worldwide variations in etiology. *World J Surg*. 1986;10(5):834-843.
106. Ushiyama T, Nakajima R, Maeda T, Kawasaki T, Matsusue Y. Perforated appendicitis causing thigh emphysema: a case report. *J Orthop Surg (Hong Kong)*. 2005;13(1):93-95.
107. Vazquez MT, Murillo J, Maranillo E, Parkin IG, Sanudo J. Femoral nerve entrapment: a new insight. *Clin Anat*. 2007;20(2):175-179.
108. Kumka M. Critical sites of entrapment of the posterior division of the obturator nerve: anatomical considerations. *J Can Chiropr Assoc*. 2010;54(1):33-42.
109. Liszka TG, Dellon AL, Manson PN. Iliohypogastric nerve entrapment following abdominoplasty. *Plast Reconstr Surg*. 1994;93(1):181-184.
110. Carter BL, Racz GB. Iliohypogastric nerve entrapment in pregnancy: diagnosis and treatment. *Anesth Analg*. 1994;79(6):1193-1194.
111. El-Minawi AM, Howard FM. Iliohypogastric nerve entrapment following gynecologic operative laparoscopy. *Obstet Gynecol*. 1998;91(5 Pt 2):871.
112. Shin JH, Howard FM. Abdominal wall nerve injury during laparoscopic gynecologic surgery: incidence, risk factors, and treatment outcomes. *J Minim Invasive Gynecol*. 2012;19(4):448-453.
113. Ziprin P, Williams P, Foster ME. External oblique aponeurosis nerve entrapment as a cause of groin pain in the athlete. *Br J Surg*. 1999;86(4):566-568.
114. Lantis JC 2nd, Schwaitzberg SD. Tack entrapment of the ilioinguinal nerve during laparoscopic hernia repair. *J Laparoendosc Adv Surg Tech A*. 1999;9(3):285-289.
115. Hsu W, Chen CS, Lee HC, et al. Preservation versus division of ilioinguinal nerve on open mesh repair of inguinal hernia: a meta-analysis of randomized controlled trials. *World J Surg*. 2012;36(10):2311-2319.
116. Miller JP, Acar F, Kaimaktchiev VB, Gultekin SH, Burchiel KJ. Pathology of ilioinguinal neuropathy produced by mesh entrapment: case report and literature review. *Hernia*. 2008;12(2):213-216.
117. Whiteside JL, Barber MD. Ilioinguinal/iliohypogastric neurectomy for management of intractable right lower quadrant pain after cesarean section: a case report. *J Reprod Med*. 2005;50(11):857-859.
118. ter Meulen BC, Peters EW, Wijsmuller A, Kropman RF, Mosch A, Tavy DL. Acute scrotal pain from idiopathic ilioinguinal neuropathy: diagnosis and treatment with EMG-guided nerve block. *Clin Neurol Neurosurg*. 2007;109(6):535-537.
119. Omichi Y, Tonogai I, Kaji S, Sangawa T, Sairyo K. Meralgia paresthetica caused by entrapment of the lateral femoral subcutaneous nerve at the fascia lata of the thigh: a case report and literature review. *J Med Invest*. 2015;62(3-4):248-250.
120. Rau CS, Hsieh CH, Liu YW, Wang LY, Cheng MH. Meralgia paresthetica secondary to lipoma. *J Neurosurg Spine*. 2010;12(1):103-105.
121. Du X, Zhao L, Chen W, Jiang L, Zhang X. Multiple myeloma-associated iliopsoas muscular amyloidoma first presenting with bilateral femoral nerve entrapment. *Int J Hematol*. 2012;95(6):716-720.
122. Tekin L, Cakar E, Tuncer SK, Dincer U, Kiralp MZ. Femoral nerve entrapment after high energy knee trauma. *J Emerg Med*. 2012;43(2):e145.
123. Kumar S, Pflueger G. Delayed femoral nerve palsy associated with iliopsoas hematoma after primary total hip arthroplasty. *Case Rep Orthop*. 2016;2016:6963542.
124. Podger H, Kent M. Femoral nerve palsy associated with bilateral spontaneous iliopsoas haematomas: a complication of venous thromboembolism therapy. *Age Ageing*. 2016;45(1):175-176.
125. Singh V, Shon WY, Lakhotia D, Kim JH, Kim TW. A rare case of femoral neuropathy associated with ilio-psoas bursitis after 10 years of total hip arthroplasty. *Open Orthop J*. 2015;9:270-273.
126. Barrick EF. Entrapment of the obturator nerve in association with a fracture of the pelvic ring. A case report. *J Bone Joint Surg Am*. 1998;80(2):258-261.
127. Yang KH, Han DY, Park HW, Park SJ. Intraarticular entrapment of the obturator nerve in acetabular fracture. *J Orthop Trauma*. 2001;15(5):361-363.
128. Langebrekke A, Qvigstad E. Endometriosis entrapment of the obturator nerve after previous cervical cancer surgery. *Fertil Steril*. 2009;91(2):622-623.
129. Rigaud J, Labat JJ, Riant T, Bouchot O, Robert R. Obturator nerve entrapment: diagnosis and laparoscopic treatment: technical case report. *Neurosurgery*. 2007;61(1):E175; discussion E175.
130. Saudek CE. Chapter 17, The hip. In: Gould III JA, Davies GJ, eds. *Orthopaedic and Sports Physical Therapy*. Vol II. St. Louis, MO: CV Mosby; 1985:365-407.
131. Kim S, Kim H, Chung J. Effects of spinal stabilization exercise on the cross-sectional areas of the lumbar multifidus and psoas major muscles, pain intensity, and lumbar muscle strength of patients with degenerative disc disease. *J Phys Ther Sci*. 2014;26(4):579-582.

Chapter 52

Pelvic Floor Muscles

"Pain in the Rear"

Timothy Douglas Sawyer and Joseph M. Donnelly

1. INTRODUCTION

The pelvic floor muscles perform multiple functions, including continence and pelvic organ support, sexual function, respiration, spinal stability, and the balancing of intraabdominal pressure. The pelvic floor muscles consist of the levator ani muscle, which has three portions (puborectalis, pubococcygeus, iliococcygeus), the coccygeus, the bulbospongiosus, the ischiocavernosus, the transverse perinei, the sphincter ani, the obturator internus, and the piriformis muscles. Both the pubococcygeus and iliococcygeus portions of the levator ani muscle support and slightly elevate the pelvic floor, resisting increased intraabdominal pressure. The bulbospongiosus, ischiocavernosus, and transversus perinei muscles are responsible for urologic and sexual function. The sphincter ani muscle is in a state of constant tonic contraction and increases its activation during straining, speaking, coughing, laughing, or weight lifting. Symptoms arising from trigger points (TrPs) in one or several of these muscles are very similar to that of coccygodynia, levator ani syndrome, proctalgia fugax, and chronic pelvic pain syndrome (CPPS). Trigger points in the pelvic floor muscles are activated and perpetuated by a severe fall, long periods of prolonged sitting, driving, bicycling, an automobile accident, or by surgery in the pelvic region. A thorough pelvic examination should consist of an external examination and intrapelvic examination both vaginally and rectally. Trigger points of the pelvic floor muscle may be identified in as many as 85% of patients suffering from urologic, colorectal, and gynecologic pelvic pain syndromes and can be responsible for some, if not all, symptoms related to these syndromes. In 2009, the European Association of Urology published guidelines suggesting that TrPs should be considered in the diagnosis of CPPS. Several studies demonstrating the relationship between CPPS and TrPs are highlighted in this chapter.

2. ANATOMIC CONSIDERATIONS

A thorough knowledge of the anatomy of the muscles and their relationship to each other is essential if one is to identify by palpation which muscle is responsible for the patient's report of pain. This knowledge is also valuable for treating TrPs in these muscles and is critically important if one wishes to dry-needle or inject the TrPs to inactivate them. This section first presents the major intrapelvic muscles in the sequence of the physical examination. Then, it reviews the superficial perineal muscles, and lastly, considers variable, but occasionally clinically important, intrapelvic muscles.

Sphincter Ani

The sphincter ani internus and externus muscles consist of four concentric layers or rings of muscle (Figure 52-1). The innermost ring, the sphincter ani internus muscle, comprises autonomically innervated involuntary muscle fibers of the anal wall.[1] The remaining three layers are the deep, superficial, and subcutaneous laminae of the sphincter ani externus muscle. The external sphincter ani muscle is under voluntary control. This sphincter is elliptical in shape, extending three or four times as far anteroposteriorly as it does laterally. It surrounds the last 2 cm of the anal canal. The superficial (middle) lamina of the external sphincter ani muscle contains the bulk of the muscle. This lamina is anchored posteriorly to the tendinous anococcygeal body and anteriorly to the tendinous perineal body, where it is joined by the levator ani, bulbospongiosus, and transversus perinei superficialis muscles (Figure 52-1). The deep layer of the external sphincter ani muscle is closely associated with the sling-like puborectalis portion of the levator ani muscle, which is the most posterior, lateral, and deepest section of the pubococcygeal part of the levator ani muscle (Figure 52-1).[2]

Levator Ani

The paired levator ani muscles meet in the midline to form a muscular sheet, the pelvic diaphragm, across most of the floor of the lesser pelvis. This diaphragm is perforated by the urogenital hiatus and the anal hiatus (Figure 52-2). The levator ani muscle comprises two distinct muscles: the more anterior (lower in the pelvis) pubococcygeus and puborectalis muscles, and the more posterior (higher in the pelvis) iliococcygeus muscle.

The pubococcygeus and puborectalis muscles attach along the dorsal surface of the pubic bone from the symphysis to the obturator canal (Figure 52-2). They form a sling around the anus, prostate gland or vagina, and the urethra. The two halves, pubococcygeus and puborectalis muscles, meet in the midline, some at the perineal body but most at the anococcygeal body (Figures 52-1 and 52-2).[2] Tichy illustrates embryologically how the levator ani muscle develops as a series of telescoping rings and slings.[3] The most anterior (medial) fibers of the pubococcygeus muscle that meet bilaterally at the perineal body in front of the anus are called the levator prostate in men. In women, these anterior fibers are called the pubovaginalis muscle and serve as an important sphincter of the vagina. The more posterior fibers of the pubococcygeus muscle (the puborectalis part) form a sling around the rectum. The closest that any of the pubococcygeus muscle fibers come to the coccyx is usually their attachment to the anococcygeal body.

The posterior section of the levator ani muscle, the iliococcygeus muscle, attaches above to the tendinous arch of the levator ani muscle and to the spine of the ischium. The tendinous arch of the levator ani muscle attaches to the spine of the ischium posteriorly and attaches anteriorly either to the anterior margin of the obturator membrane or to the pubic bone just medial (farther anterior) to the margin of the membrane. This tendinous arch is firmly attached to the fascia covering the obturator

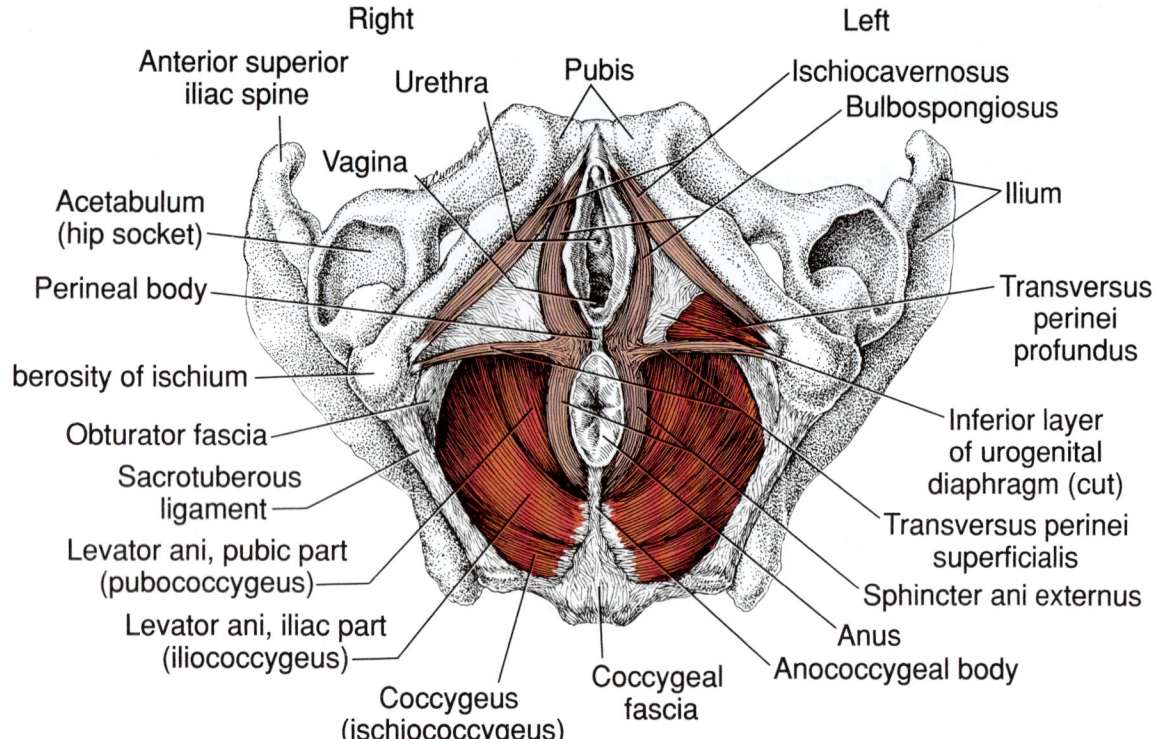

Figure 52-1. Pelvic floor muscles as seen from below in the supine female subject. The muscles of the pelvic diaphragm are dark red, and the associated pelvic muscles are light red. On the subject's left side, part of the deep fascia of the urogenital diaphragm has been cut and removed to reveal the transversus perinei profundus muscle.

internus muscle. As seen from inside the pelvis, the levator ani muscle covers the lower one-half to two-thirds of the obturator internus muscle and essentially all of the obturator foramen.[2]

Below, the iliococcygeus muscle attaches to the anococcygeal muscle body and to the last two segments of the coccyx.[4] The adjacent margins of the pubococcygeus and iliococcygeus muscles may be separated or may overlap. The iliococcygeus muscle may be replaced by fibrous tissue. Its upper border lies adjacent to the sacrospinous ligament and the overlying coccygeus muscle.[2]

Coccygeus

The coccygeus muscle, sometimes called the ischiococcygeus muscle, lies cephalad and adjacent to the iliococcygeus portion of the levator ani muscle. The two muscles often form a continuous plane (Figure 52-1). The coccygeus muscle covers (internally) the sturdy sacrospinous ligament (Figure 52-2). Laterally, the apex of this triangular muscle is attached to the spine of the ischium and to the fibers of the sacrospinous ligament. Medially, it fans out to end on the margin of the coccyx and on the side of the lowest part of the sacrum.[2]

Obturator Internus

Part of the obturator internus muscle that lies outside of the pelvis and attaches to the greater trochanter of the femur is considered in Chapter 57. The intrapelvic portion of the muscle covers the anterolateral wall of the lesser pelvis, where it surrounds and covers the greater part of the obturator foramen (Figure 52-2). The obturator internus muscle is fan-shaped and the direction of its fibers spans an arc of roughly 135°. Its muscle fibers form an anterior and posterior thickening, one in front of and the other behind the obturator canal. This canal allows nerves and vessels to penetrate the obturator membrane along the anterior margin of the obturator foramen, on the side opposite to the lesser sciatic foramen.

Inside the pelvis, the obturator internus muscle attaches to the inner pelvic brim, to the margin of the obturator foramen, and too much of the obturator membrane stretched across that bony foramen. The fibers of the muscle converge toward the lesser sciatic foramen and end in four or five tendinous bands. As the muscle exits the pelvis through the lesser sciatic foramen, it makes a right-angle bend around the grooved surface between the spine and tuberosity of the ischium. This bony pulley is covered with cartilage; the passage of the tendon is also assisted by the ischiadic bursa of the obturator internus muscle.[4] As the tendon crosses the capsule of the hip joint, it is cushioned by the subtendinous bursa of the obturator internus muscle (see Chapter 57). The exit of the obturator internus muscle from the pelvis through the lesser sciatic foramen is marked by palpable ligaments that form two borders of that foramen: the sacrotuberous ligament posteriorly and the sacrospinous ligament above.[2] As the fibers of the two ligaments intermingle, they cross at the upper end of the foramen; the foramen is a tightly enclosed space that leaves no room for expansion of the muscle.[2] The structures forming the lesser sciatic foramen are illustrated in Figure 57-3. This figure serves as a valuable reference throughout this chapter because it clarifies relations of intrapelvic muscles and ligaments.

Piriformis

The piriformis muscle forms part of the posterior wall of the true pelvis and lies posterior to the ischiococcygeus muscle. The lower portion is palpable vaginally but may be difficult depending on the length of the clinician's finger. It is attached from the undersurface of the sacrum at levels S2-S4, gluteal surface of the ilium, sacroiliac joint capsule, and in some individuals, may attach to the sacrotuberous ligament. The piriformis muscle travels inferolaterally and exits the pelvis through the greater sciatic foramen proximal to the sacrospinous ligament and attaches to the greater trochanter of the femur at the hip

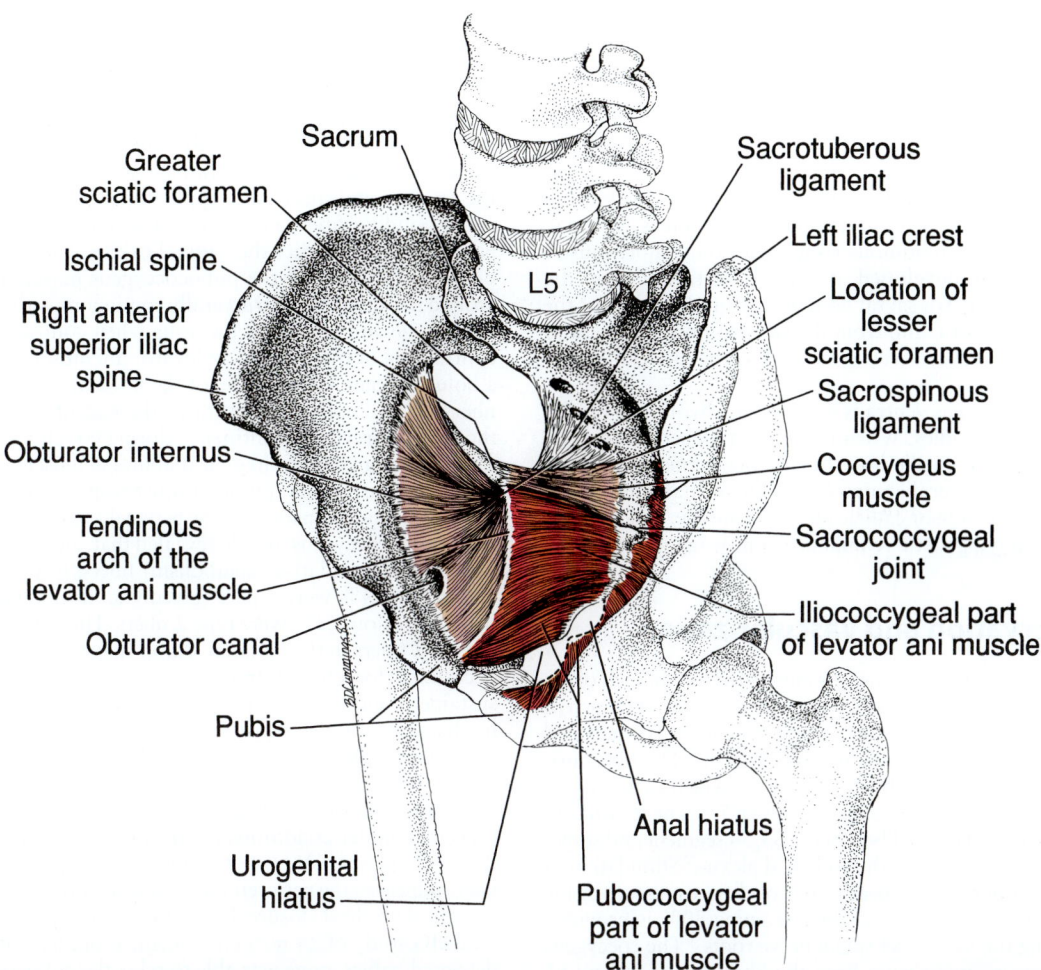

Figure 52-2. The pelvic floor muscles are seen obliquely from above and diagonally from the left side looking down inside the pelvis. The levator ani muscle is dark red. The coccygeus muscle is medium red, and the obturator internus muscle is light red.

joint.[2] This muscle may be palpated with access rectally. See Chapter 57 for more on the piriformis muscle.

Bulbospongiosus, Ischiocavernosus, and Transversus Perinei

Female Anatomy

In women, the bulbospongiosus, ischiocavernosus, and transversus perinei superficialis muscles on each side of the body form a triangle (Figure 52-1). The medial leg of the triangle, the bulbospongiosus muscle (also known as the bulbocavernosus or the sphincter vaginae), surrounds the orifice of the vagina. The muscle attaches anteriorly to the corpora cavernosa of the clitoridis with a muscular fasciculus that also crosses over the body of the clitoris and compresses its deep dorsal vein. Posteriorly, the bulbospongiosus muscle anchors to the perineal body where it blends with the external anal sphincter and the transversus perinei superficialis muscles (Figure 52-2).[2]

The ischiocavernosus muscle in women (formerly called the erector clitoridis) forms the lateral side of the triangle (Figure 52-1). The muscle is located along the lateral boundary of the perineum next to the bony ridge of the anterior pubic ramus, extending between the symphysis pubis and the ischial tuberosity. Above and anteriorly, the ischiocavernosus muscle ends in an aponeurosis that blends with the sides and undersurface of the crus clitoridis. Below and posteriorly, it is attached to the surface of the crus clitoridis and to the ischial tuberosity.[2]

The transversus perinei superficialis muscle forms the base of the triangle. The two muscles together span the perineum laterally between the ischial tuberosities, joining the sphincter ani and bulbospongiosus muscles in the midline at the perineal body (Figure 52-1). The transversus perinei profundus muscle lies deep to the transversus perinei superficialis muscle; it is a broader muscle that courses between the ischial tuberosity and the vagina (Figure 52-2).[2]

Male Anatomy

In men, the bulbospongiosus muscle is more complex than in women and essentially wraps around the corpus spongiosum of the penis, which is the central erectile structure through which the urethra passes. As illustrated, the two symmetrical parts of this muscle begin below at the perineal body and along the median raphe. The fibers extend outward and upward in a pennate fashion to enclose the bulk of the corpus spongiosum penis posteriorly and the corpus cavernosum penis anteriorly. Above, some of the fibers end in a tendinous expansion that covers the dorsal blood vessels of the penis.[2] After 5 months of fetal gestation, this muscle wraps around the bulb of the penis.[5]

The ischiocavernosus muscle in men is similar to that in women but is usually larger. On each side, the muscle attaches posteriorly to the ischial tuberosity and the ischial ramus and angles across the perineum anteriorly toward the crus penis. After coursing lateral to the bulbospongiosus muscle, it ends in an aponeurosis that blends with the sides and undersurface of the crus penis.[1,2,4]

The transversus perinei profundus muscle attaches laterally to the ischial tuberosity as in women, but in men, the muscles interlace in the midline at a tendinous raphe deep to the bulbospongiosus muscle.[1,2]

Sacrococcygeus Ventralis

The sacrococcygeus ventralis (anterior) muscle is variable and was found in 102 of 110 adult bodies. It often is vestigial, consisting mainly of tendinous bands with only short muscle fibers.[6] When well developed, it extends vertically from the sides of the 4th and 5th sacral vertebrae, from the front of the 1st coccygeal vertebra, and from the sacrospinous ligament to the 2nd to 4th coccygeal vertebrae and to the anterior sacrococcygeal ligament.[1,6-8]

The sacrococcygeus ventralis muscle may divide into medial and lateral fiber bundles. When this has happened, the lateral fibers have been identified as the sacrococcygeus ventralis (depressor caudae lateralis) muscle and the medial fibers as the infracoccygeus (depressor caudae medialis) muscle.[6] These fibers are probably phylogenetic remnants of tail-wagging muscles.

2.1. Innervation and Vascularization

The external anal sphincter muscle is innervated by a branch of the 4th sacral nerve and by branches from the inferior rectal branch of the pudendal nerve. The internal sphincter ani muscle is innervated by the fibers of the autonomic nervous system.[2] The obturator internus muscle is supplied by its own nerve, which carries fibers from the L5, S1, and S2 segments[2] (Chapter 57). The levator ani muscle is innervated by the fibers of the S3, S4 segment and sometimes by the S5 segments via the pudendal plexus.[2] Stimulation of the S3 ventral root produces nearly 70% of closure pressure by the external sphincter urethrae and the remaining 30% is provided by stimulating the S2 and S4 spinal nerve roots.[9] The coccygeus muscle derives its innervation from the fibers of the S4 and S5 segments via the pudendal plexus.[2] All of the perineal muscles (including the bulbospongiosus, the ischiocavernosus, and both the superficial and deep transverse perinei muscle) are innervated by the S2, S3, and S4 sacral nerves via the perineal branch of the pudendal nerve.[2] The fibers from the S4 and S5 segments usually innervate the sacrococcygeus ventralis muscle.[6]

The branches of the internal iliac artery constitute the major blood supply to the perineum. The only pelvic organs that don't receive their blood supply from branches of the internal iliac artery are the ovaries and the superior part of the rectum. The lymphatic drainage of the pelvic cavity is mainly to nodes located around the internal iliac vessels.

2.2. Function

The pelvic floor muscles perform multiple functions such as continence and pelvic organ support, sexual function, respiration, spinal stability, and containment of intraabdominal pressure.[10-17] The physiologic mechanisms by which they perform their roles are not clearly understood predominately because of the lack of suitable instrumentation. The pelvic floor muscles remain, particularly from a biomechanical perspective, an understudied region of the body.

Sphincter Ani

Clinical experience shows, and electromyographical (EMG) studies confirm,[18] that the sphincter ani muscle is in a state of constant tonic contraction, which is increased by straining, speaking, coughing, laughing, or weight lifting. The tonic contraction falls to a very low level during sleep and is strongly inhibited during defecation. It is strongly recruited by voluntary effort, which is accompanied by general contraction of the perineal muscles, especially the sphincter urethrae muscle.[18]

Levator Ani

In general, both the pubococcygeus and iliococcygeus portions of the levator ani muscle support and slightly elevate the pelvic floor muscles, resisting increased intraabdominal pressure.[2] In men, the more anterior (medial) pubococcygeal portion, sometimes called the levator prostate muscle, forms a sling around the prostate and specifically applies upward pressure on it. The corresponding fibers in women, also known as the pubovaginal muscle, constrict the vaginal orifice. The more posterior puborectalis fibers of the pubococcygeus muscle form a sling around the anus that is structurally continuous with the sphincter ani muscle and constricts the anus when contracted.[19] Strong contraction of this part of the levator ani muscle can help eject a bolus of feces. Contraction of the more anterior periurethral fibers helps empty the urethra at the end of urination and is thought to prevent incontinence during coughing or sneezing. The levator ani muscle, like the diaphragm muscle, is also active during the inspiration phase of quiet respiration.[2]

A histologic comparison of the perianal and periurethral regions of the pubococcygeus muscle revealed that, although most fibers were type 1 (oxidative metabolism) fibers, in the periurethral region, only 4% were type 2 (glycolytic) fibers, whereas in the perianal region, 23% were type 2 fibers. This higher percentage of type 2 fibers in the perianal region suggests that it is used for occasional forceful contractions, when compared with more sustained contractions in the periurethral region.[19] A later study by this same group[20] reported only type 1 fibers in the external (voluntary) sphincter urethrae muscle.

In a 1989 study,[21] a greater proportion of type 1 (slow-twitch) fibers was associated with improved support of the pelvic viscera, especially under conditions contributing to increased intraabdominal pressure. A greater proportion of type 2 (fast-twitch) fibers improved the periurethral continence mechanism, providing increased urethral closure during mechanical pressure stress. In an EMG study of 24 normal women, about half of whom had delivered babies, none was able to relax the pubococcygeal part of the levator ani muscle in the lithotomy position, whereas some were able to relax the sphincter urethrae muscle completely.[18]

Coccygeus

Anatomically, the coccygeus muscle pulls the coccyx forward and is said to support the pelvic floor muscles against intraabdominal pressure and to play a primary role in achieving rectal and urinary continence.[2] It also stabilizes the sacroiliac joint[22] and has powerful leverage for rotating this joint. Therefore, abnormal tension of the coccygeus muscle could easily hold the sacroiliac joint in a displaced position.

Obturator Internus

The obturator internus muscle is a lower extremity muscle that serves no motor function in the pelvis. As noted in Chapter 57, the obturator internus muscle is most strongly a external rotator of the thigh when the thigh is extended; the muscle becomes increasingly an abductor at the hip as the thigh is flexed.[2]

Piriformis

Like the obturator internus muscle, the piriformis muscle also serves no motor function in the pelvis. The muscle is a external rotator of the hip and assists in abduction of the femur when the hip is flexed (See Chapter 57).

Bulbospongiosus, Ischiocavernosus, and Transversus Perinei

Contraction of the bulbospongiosus muscle in men serves to empty the urethra at the end of urination and contracts during ejaculation.[2] Erection of the penis is primarily a vascular response under autonomic control,[23,24] but the anterior and middle fibers of the bulbospongiosus and ischiocavernosus muscles contribute to erection by reflex and voluntary contraction that compresses the erectile tissue of the bulb of the penis and its dorsal vein.[2,25,26] In women, contraction of this voluntary muscle constricts the orifice of the vagina and contributes to erection of the clitoris by compression of its deep dorsal vein.[2]

In men, contraction of the ischiocavernosus muscle serves to maintain and enhance penile erection by retarding the return of blood through the crus penis. During erection, intracavernous pressure correlated strongly with the duration of voluntary EMG activity in the ischiocavernosus muscle.[27] Change of pressure on the glans reflexively activates the ischiocavernosus muscle. This substantiates the clinical impression that pressure stimulation of the glans penis during coitus contributes to the erectile process.[28]

In women, the ischiocavernosus muscle acts similarly to maintain erection of the clitoris by retarding return flow from the crus clitoridis.[2]

The two pairs of transverse perinei muscles form a muscular sling that cradles the perineal body between the two ischial tuberosities. Bilateral contraction of the superficial and deep transversus perinei muscles serves to fix the perineal body in the midline between the anus and genitalia and to support the pelvic floor muscle. In both men and women, all of these perineal muscles are generally contracted as a unit. EMG studies indicate that selective contraction of individual perineal muscles is difficult, if not impossible.[18]

2.3. Functional Unit

The pelvic floor muscles, especially the anal and urethral sphincters and the levator ani, function closely together. Contractions of the genital bulbospongiosus and ischiocavernosus muscles are scarcely, if at all, voluntarily separable from sphincter activation.

The iliococcygeus and upper pubococcygeus portions of the levator ani muscle are strong flexors of the coccyx. The equally powerful antagonist to this movement is the gluteus maximus muscle; it attaches to the dorsolateral surface of the coccyx[29] with fibers that are directed laterally to form the gluteal cleft. Working together, the levator ani and gluteus maximus muscles provide a more powerful elevation (closure) of the anus than the levator ani muscle could provide independently. When maximum voluntary effort is required to close the anal aperture, the gluteus maximus muscle is powerfully recruited.

The obturator internus and the piriformis muscles function in concert with other external rotators of the thigh, as described in Chapter 57.

3. CLINICAL PRESENTATION

3.1. Referred Pain Pattern

Knowing the location of pain in the pelvic region is helpful in identifying which TrPs could be responsible for it. Trigger points have been associated with urogenital pain with referred pain to the penis, perineum, rectum, suprapubic area, testicles, groin, and coccyx.[17,30] Referred pain from TrPs in the bulbospongiosus, ischiocavernosus, and anterior portions of the levator ani muscles usually project pain or discomfort to the adjacent urogenital structures, perineum, and suprapubic region (Figure 52-3A). Sphincter ani TrPs induce pain in the rectum as well as the immediate surrounding areas of the pelvic floor muscles. Trigger points in the posterior region of the pelvic floor, posterior sphincter ani, iliococcygeus, posterior part of pubococcygeus, and coccygeus muscles are likely to refer pain to the anus, the sacrococcygeal region, coccyx, and perineum (Figure 52-3B).[17] This referred pain pattern is often called coccygodynia, although the coccyx itself is usually normal and not tender.[31,32-34] Because the levator ani muscle is most commonly involved, pain in the region of the coccyx is also called levator ani syndrome.[34] Trigger points in the anterior portion of the levator ani muscle (puborectalis and pubococcygeus) and bulbospongiosus muscle can refer specific pain to the urogenital structures, supra pubic region, and perineum.[17] The levator endopelvic fascia lateral to the prostate represents the most common location of TrPs in men with pelvic pain, often referring pain to the tip of the penis.[35] Vaginal pain has also been reproduced by pressure on the tender sites in the levator ani muscle[32]). Trigger points in the transverse perineal muscles refer to the perineum and the medial side of the ischial tuberosities. The TrPs in the obturator internus muscle refer pain to the urogenital structures, rectum, groin, and hip, with a spillover pattern down the back of the ipsilateral thigh (Figure 52-3C). Goldstein found that injection of obturator internus TrPs relieved pain in the vagina (J. Goldstein, personal communication[36]). The piriformis muscle can also refer into the vagina as well as the hip, ischial tuberosity, and down the back of the thigh.[17]

3.2. Symptoms

Patients with TrPs in the sphincter ani muscle primarily report poorly localized aching pain in the anal region and may experience painful movements or relief after passing their bowels. Depending on where the TrPs are located in the sphincter ani muscle, patients may report specific pain on the side of the TrP. Patients often report that increased physical activity and stress has a direct effect on their symptoms.

In women, TrPs in the bulbospongiosus muscle cause dyspareunia, particularly during entry, and aching pain in the perineal region. In men, these TrPs cause pain in the retroscrotal region, discomfort when sitting erect and forward, and occasionally a degree of impotence, and such people may also report pre- or post–ejaculation penis pain.[17] Ischiocavernosus TrPs likewise cause perineal pain but are less likely to interfere with intercourse. Involvement of the obturator internus muscle can cause pain and a feeling of fullness in the rectum, with occasional referral of pain down the back of the thigh.[37] This muscle may also refer pain into the vagina.[21,22] In women, the piriformis muscle is a common cause of painful intercourse during deep penetration.

The levator ani muscle is the most widely recognized source of referred pain in the perineal region. Patients may report pain in the sacrum,[34] coccyx,[32-34,38] rectum,[34,39,40] pelvic floor or perirectal area,[34,39] vagina,[33] urogenital structures,[17] and low back.[38] Patients will report increased symptoms with sitting and difficulty being comfortable while sitting.[37-40] They may also report increased symptoms while lying supine[32] and with defecation.[40] Patients with TrPs in the posterior region of the pelvic floor, including posterior sphincter ani, iliococcygeus, posterior part of pubococcygeus, and coccygeus muscles, may report a feeling of fullness in the rectum as well as pre– and post–bowel movement pain.[17] Patients with TrPs in the anterior portion of the levator ani (puborectalis and pubococcygeus) and bulbospongiosus muscles often report increased frequency, urgency, bladder discomfort, suprapubic pain, postejaculatory pain, and pain in the tip of the penis.[17,41]

Trigger points in the coccygeus muscle were identified as the cause of pain similar to that ascribed to TrPs in the levator ani muscle and referred to the coccyx, hip, or back. Trigger points in this muscle are likely to cause low back pain late in pregnancy and early in labor. Tenderness and "spasm" (tension) of the coccygeus muscle were usually the key factors responsible for low back pain suffered by 1350 women seen for infertility.[22] The issue of sitting pain has often been described as posterior tail bone discomfort and can also be described as pain in the ischial tuberosities, pain isolated to the soft tissue of the perineum and the rectum (a golf ball in the pelvis), and anterior pain in the perineum and base of the penis in men, and the vulva in women.

3.4. Trigger Point Examination

In 2009, the European Association of Urology published guidelines suggesting that TrPs should be considered in the diagnosis of CPPS, and there are several studies demonstrating the relationship between CPPS and TrPs.[45-48]

Manual examination of TrPs requires adequate manual skills, training, and clinical practice to develop a high degree of reliability in the examination. For the purpose of locating TrPs within the pelvis, the pelvic muscles can be considered in three categories: perineal muscles, pelvic floor muscles, and pelvic wall muscles. Trigger points of the pelvic floor muscles may be identified in as many as 85% of patients suffering from urologic, colorectal, and gynecologic pelvic pain syndromes and can be responsible for some, if not all, symptoms related to these syndromes.[49] Trigger points in the pelvic floor musculature may often coexist with TrPs in the abdominal wall muscles, which can help differentiate pelvic and abdominal pain of visceral versus somatic origin.[50,51]

The external perineal muscles can be examined with both cross-fiber flat palpation and cross-fiber pincer palpation. The intrapelvic muscles are examined through the rectum and the vagina. For the rectal examination, the patient can be placed in a semilateral prone position with pillows under the abdomen. Using a gloved finger, the sphincter ani muscle is examined first. The left internal muscles of the pelvis are then examined with the right hand, and the right pelvis is examined with the left hand, shifting the patient as necessary. The clinician applies a consistent pressure level for tissue palpation. As recommended, when examining patients with fibromyalgia, use an approximate palpation force of 4 kg/cm^2 to assess pain. For each area examined, patients are asked to report the level of pain experienced during palpation from *0 to 3+ (severe)*.[17,52] The patient may also lie supine in the lithotomy position, or if footrests are not available, semi prone in Sims position. It is best to begin the examination with the hand that supinates toward the symptomatic side. If TrPs are found on that side, it is wise to examine the opposite side of the pelvis for comparison, which is most effectively done with the other hand. It is difficult and awkward to perform an adequate rectal examination of the muscles on both sides of the pelvis with one hand.

Pelvic Floor Muscles

The pelvic floor muscles that commonly have TrPs are the sphincter ani, levator ani, coccygeus, and obturator internus muscles. Although the levator ani and coccygeus muscles are over most of the pelvic floor muscles, the intrapelvic rectal digital examination begins with the sphincter ani muscle.

Sphincter Ani

If the patient has TrPs in the anal sphincter muscle, insertion of the finger can be distressing even when done very carefully. First, the clinician should examine the anal orifice for internal hemorrhoids, which can perpetuate TrPs of the anal sphincter muscle. Lubricant is liberally applied to the examining gloved finger and the anal orifice. Ordinarily, as the clinician inserts the finger, he or she would gently apply pressure toward one side of the anus to help relax the sphincter muscle. However, if one inadvertently presses on TrPs in the muscle, it may increase the patient's pain. In the presence of excessive sphincter tension or tenderness, the patient, instead of the clinician applying side pressure, may bear down on the rectum to enhance relaxation of the sphincter ani muscle as the clinician slowly inserts the examining finger directly into the anal orifice. Golfam et al[53] studied the effect of topical nifedipine (a calcium channel blocker) on anal fissures, and it was shown to have a significant effect on pain reduction and improved recovery time in patients with anal fissures and hemorrhoids. Patients in the nifedipine group showed significant healing and relief from pain compared with patients in the control group.[53] This study may lead to an appropriate treatment to reduce sphincter tension and ease the pain of rectal examination of patients with pelvic pain in the future.

By gently flexing the tip of the finger, the clinician can feel when it has passed the sphincter muscles. The finger first encounters the external and then the internal sphincter ani muscle. The finger should be withdrawn to halfway along the sphincter muscles and pressure gently applied to the muscle at every one-eighth of a circle (positions at 12:00, 1:30, 3:00, etc.) to identify tenderness caused from TrPs. When the finger locates tenderness in one direction, the muscle is explored to determine where the spot of maximum tenderness exists. An associated taut band may be identified if the TrP is not too tender and the patient can tolerate the additional pressure. If the muscle is strongly contracted, the patient can relax it by bearing down, making the contrast between the taut band and relaxed fibers more evident. A taut band, when present, usually extends from one-quarter to halfway around the anus. Multiple taut bands are typically identified when TrPs are present.

When an anal sphincter muscle has very active TrPs, their tenderness may preclude further rectal examination of the intrapelvic muscles. The movement and additional pressure of the finger may be intolerable. In women, the vaginal examination may then be substituted. Otherwise, the anal sphincter TrPs must be inactivated before the patient can be examined for intrapelvic TrPs.

Orientation Inside the Pelvis

Establishing relevant bony and ligamentous landmarks for reference, and the prostate gland in men, helps greatly in identifying the intrapelvic muscles by palpation. For orientation purposes, it is helpful in identifying the structures that border the levator ani muscle (Figures 52-1, 52-2, and 52-4).

Usually, there are no muscles found in the midline on the ventral surface of the coccyx and the sacrum. When the patient is examined rectally, only the rectal wall lies between the examining finger and these bones. In the midline below (distal to) the tip of the coccyx, the anococcygeal body (which usually is not distinguishable by palpation) extends to the sphincter ani muscle and serves as the attachment for much of the pubococcygeus portions of the levator ani muscle. Just anterior to the rectum is an analogous structure, the perineal body, to which the bulbospongiosus, transverse perinei, and sphincter ani muscles attach.

It is relatively easy to examine the range of motion of the coccyx. One grasps the coccyx between the finger inside the rectum and the thumb outside to flex, extend, and bend it laterally, testing for tenderness at its articulations. All of the coccygeal joints may be mobile. The most proximal joint that exhibits mobility is usually the sacrococcygeal joint.

A firm, tendinous edge crossing the pelvis at about the level of the sacrococcygeal joint (Figure 52-2) identifies the lower border of the sacrospinous ligament. This border is nearly always sharply delineated. It lies close to the sometimes overlapping borders of the iliococcygeal portion of the levator ani muscle, below, and the coccygeus muscle, above. Laterally, the ligament ends at a palpable, hard, bony prominence, the spine of the ischium, to which the tendinous arch of the levator ani muscle also attaches.[4] The posterior half of this tendinous arch is palpable as it swings around the pelvis to attach anteriorly to the body of the pubis. The arch may become indistinguishable near the anterior margin of the obturator membrane. This arch serves as the lateral attachment of the iliococcygeus portion of the levator ani muscle. Therefore, this portion of the levator ani muscle lies below it. The obturator internus muscle extends above and below the arch of the levator ani muscle. The obturator internus muscle can be palpated directly anywhere above the arch, but below the arch, it can only be palpated through the levator ani (iliococcygeus) muscle. Just caudal to the tip of the ischial spine, a soft spot felt through the levator ani muscle locates the opening of the lesser sciatic foramen.

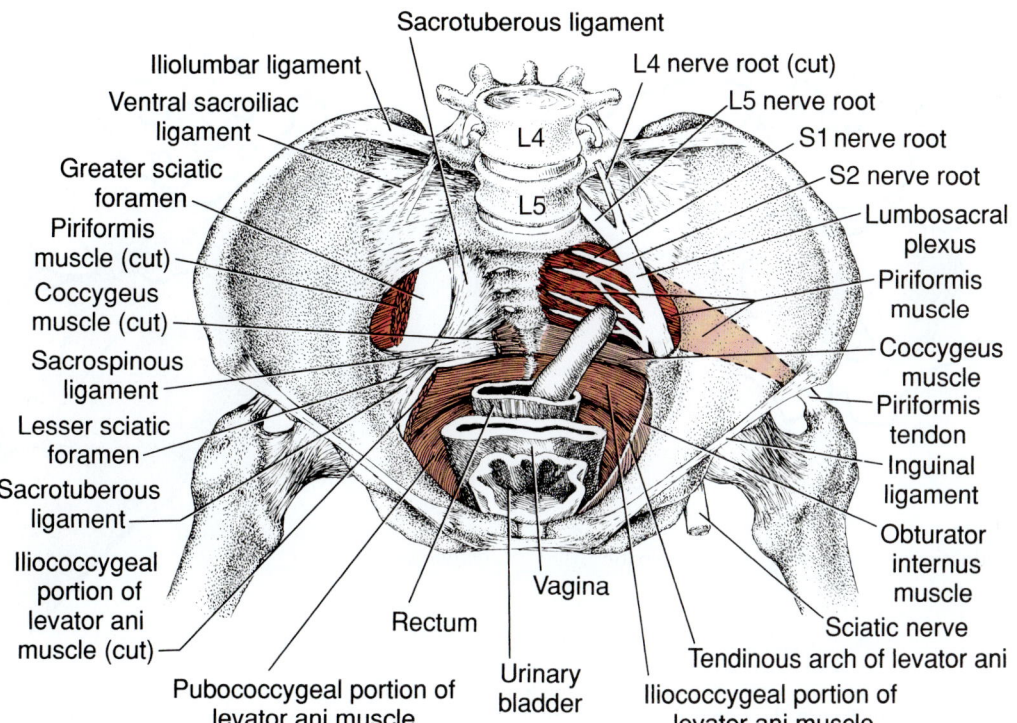

Figure 52-4. Internal palpation of the left piriformis muscle (dark red within the pelvis and light red outside the pelvis) via the rectum, viewed from in front and above. The levator ani muscle is medium red; the coccygeus and obturator internus muscles are light red. The sacrospinous ligament (covered by the coccygeus muscle) is the last major transverse landmark identified by the palpating finger before it reaches the piriformis muscle. The sacrospinous ligament attaches cephalad mainly to the coccyx, which is usually easily palpated and mobile. The posterior wall of the rectum and the S3 and S4 nerve roots lie between the palpating finger and the piriformis muscle.

Levator Ani

Palpation of the most anterior fibers of the levator ani muscle is an important area to check for TrPs that lie alongside the prostate in men, and inserting onto the dorsal surface of the pubis. The pubococcygeus portion of the levator ani muscle is often subdivided into separate parts according to the pelvic viscera to which they relate (puboperinealis, puboprostaticus, pubovaginalis, puboanalis, and puborectalis).[2] These TrPs are associated with the urogenital symptoms mentioned previously. In men, once the finger passes through the anal canal, the clinician first locates the prostate gland central and anterior. With the index finger inserted deep, the knuckles of the hand will come to rest on the ischial tuberosity. This will allow the clinician to examine the deepest fibers of the anterior levator ani muscle (Figure 52-5A and B).

(Note: In women, these deep anterior fibers of the levator ani muscle are much easier palpated vaginally.) Next, the clinician gently slides the finger inferiorly alongside the prostate examining shallower fibers of the muscle until reaching the perineal body. At this location, the clinician can use pincer palpation with the index finger inside and the thumb outside to further examine TrPs in the perineal body and transverse perinei muscle. From this location, the clinician sweeps laterally along the levator ani muscle checking both deep and shallow fibers for TrPs until reaching the middle of the sacrospinous ligament and then the coccyx. Thiele recommended sweeping the finger slowly from side to side through an arc of 180° at successively higher levels, allowing the clinician to palpate all of the fibers of the levator ani, the coccygeus, as well as the obturator internus muscles.[33] He commented on how frequently individual fascicles stood out like tight cords with areas of relaxed muscle between them and reported that sometimes the entire levator ani muscle was tense and felt like a firm sheet of muscle stretched from its tendinous arch to the sacrum, coccyx, and anococcygeal body.[33] A similar examination of the piriformis muscle is illustrated in Figure 52-4 with useful anatomic landmarks. Pressure on levator ani TrPs nearly always reproduces the patient's reported pain, either anteriorly in the urogenital region or posteriorly in the region of the coccyx.[17]

When the clinician finds TrPs that seem to be in the lateral portions of the levator ani muscle below this muscle's tendinous arch, care must be exercised to be sure that the tenderness is not due to TrPs in the underlying obturator internus muscle. The two muscles can be distinguished by palpating while asking the patient to squeeze the finger in the rectum (levator ani muscle activation), relax, and then abduct the flexed thigh or externally rotate the extended thigh on that side against resistance (obturator internus muscle activation). The increase in muscle tension identifies the contracting muscle.

Coccygeus

The coccygeus muscle is palpable usually at the level of the sacrococcygeal joint (Figure 52-2).[4] Much of the muscle lies between the examining finger and the underlying sacrospinous ligament. In some individuals, the muscle is intertwined with the ligament, the caudal border that is usually palpable. Against this firm ligamentous foundation, taut bands and their TrPs are usually readily identified by cross-fiber flat palpation across the coccygeus muscle.

Occasionally, a thick band of coccygeus muscle fibers crosses the midline. Here it is readily palpable against the lowest part of the sacrum or the uppermost region of the coccyx. The gluteus maximus muscle attachment to the outer margins of the sacrum and the coccyx corresponds closely to the coccygeus muscle's attachment on the inner margins of these bones.[29]

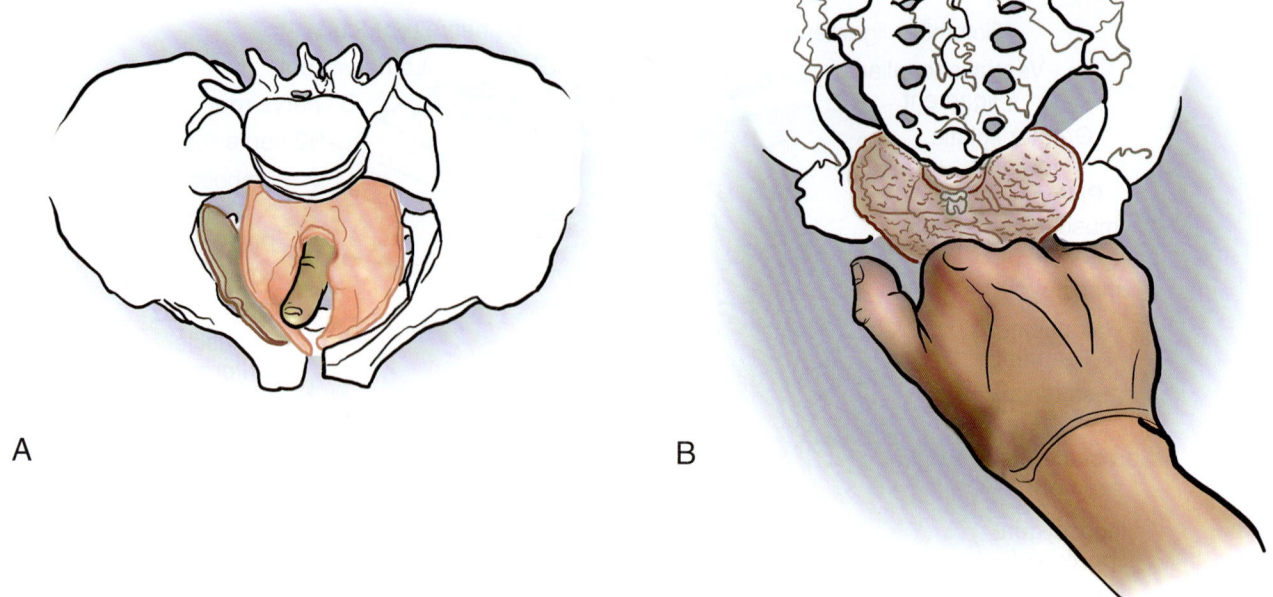

Figure 52-5. A, Anterior view; internal examination of the pelvis, with the index finger palpating internally. B, Posterior view; externally, knuckles rest on the ischial tuberosity. In women, these deep anterior fibers of the levator ani muscle are much easier palpated vaginally.

Pelvic Wall Muscles

One pelvic wall muscle, the obturator internus muscle, covers the anterolateral wall of the lesser pelvis. Looking into the pelvis from above, one sees that much of this muscle is covered by the levator ani muscle (Figure 52-4). The obturator internus muscle exits the pelvis through the lesser sciatic foramen, which is bounded on two sides by the sacrospinous and sacrotuberous ligaments. The sacrotuberous ligament attaches to the externally identifiable ischial tuberosity. The other major intrapelvic muscle, the piriformis muscle, is found cephalad to the sacrospinous ligament, and this is considered in Chapter 57. The sacrococcygeus ventralis muscle, when present, is palpable as longitudinal fibers along the margins of the lower sacrum and the coccyx.

Obturator Internus

A view of the pelvis from above shows that the posterior portion of the obturator internus muscle must be palpated through the levator ani muscle (Figure 52-4).[4] A frontal section[2] likewise illustrates this and shows the relation of these muscles to the tendinous arch. A frontal section and a cross section[54] through the prostate depict how one must palpate the thick posterior part of the obturator internus muscle through a thin layer of the levator ani muscle on either side of the prostate (or vagina).

When running the finger around the lateral wall of the pelvis above the tendinous arch of the levator ani muscle from the ischial spine to the pubis, any observed tender points or taut bands are in the obturator internus muscle. The obturator internus muscle exits the pelvis through the lesser sciatic foramen. This point of exit lies below (caudal to) the tip of the ischial spine beneath the tendinous arch. Because this is an area of musculotendinous junction where most of the obturator internus muscle fibers are represented, it is a critical point to examine for tenderness to determine if TrPs are present anywhere in the muscle. Tenderness at this location is comparable to that in the region of the musculotendinous junction of the psoas major muscle just above its attachment to the lesser trochanter of the femur (see Chapter 51).

Piriformis

See Chapter 57 for a detailed description of the intrapelvic examination of the piriformis muscle. The rectal examination is illustrated in Figure 52-4.

Sacrococcygeus Ventralis

If the sacrococcygeus ventralis muscle (when present) has TrPs, the clinician will find spot tenderness along the lower sacrum or the coccyx in a taut band running parallel to the axis of the spine. The fibers of the levator ani and coccygeus muscles can also cause tenderness at the edge of the coccyx. Pressure on an active sacrococcygeus TrP is likely to reproduce pain in the coccyx.

Vaginal Examination

In women, the bulbospongiosus muscle can be satisfactorily examined for TrPs only by vaginal examination. The patient should be placed in the lithotomy position for this approach. The bulbospongiosus and levator vaginae portions of the levator ani muscle enclose the introitus. They can be located and their strength assessed by having the patient squeeze the clinician's examining finger. Trigger points inhibit these muscles. These muscles are examined for TrPs by gentle cross-fiber pincer palpation at about the middle of each lateral wall of the introitus. When present, the taut bands are clearly delineated, tender, and contain TrPs that, when compressed, usually refer an ache to the vaginal and perineal regions, reproducing the patient's reported pain.

The clinician examines the ischiocavernosus muscle by pressing directly laterally from within the distal vagina against the edge of the pubic arch. This muscle and the crus clitoridis that it covers are normally not tender. When compressed, active TrPs in this muscle refer pain to the perineal region. If the clinician places two fingers against the lateral wall of the pelvis just beyond the inside margin of the pubic arch over the obturator membrane, the upper finger overlies the anterior portion of the obturator internus muscle, whereas the lower finger palpates the levator ani muscle. These muscles can be identified as described previously in the discussion of the levator ani muscle. Furthermore, one can distinguish the backward angulation of the anterior obturator internus muscle fibers from the transverse orientation of the levator ani muscle fibers; this is more difficult to do by rectal examination. Higher in the pelvis, the clinician palpates the bulky posterior portion of the obturator internus muscle anterior to the ischial spine.

The coccygeal region and the coccygeus muscle are more difficult to palpate from the vagina than from the rectum because one must palpate through two layers of rectal mucosa and one of vaginal mucosa. An optimum localization of all the intrapelvic musculoskeletal structures requires both rectal and vaginal examinations.

Perineal Muscles

The perineal muscles (the transverse perinei, bulbospongiosus, and ischiocavernosus) are the most superficial and contribute some support to the pelvic floor muscles. None of these muscles are likely to be identifiable unless they have taut bands that lie parallel to the direction of the muscle fibers. In both sexes, the bilateral ischiocavernosus muscle frames the pubic arch that borders the perineum beneath the symphysis pubis.

External Pelvic Examination: Men

Ideally, the patient should be placed in the lithotomy position with the feet in stirrups. If this is not practical, then he can lie supine, pulling his knees up toward the armpits. The testicles are lifted out of the way with a towel used as a sling.[1,4]

The bulb of the penis is palpable in the midline, between the anus and the base of the shaft of the penis, through the skin of the scrotum between the testicles. The bulbospongiosus muscle fibers angle around the bulb in a pennate fashion, more circumferential than longitudinal. Taut bands and TrP tenderness are most readily detectable if the bulb is at least partially tumescent, so that there is a firmer base against which to perform flat palpation. The ischiocavernosus muscles angle in and upward on either side of the bulb.

The transversus perinei superficialis muscle is not usually distinguishable by palpation unless it contains taut bands. The muscle fibers extend from the ischial tuberosity on each side to the fibrous perineal body that lies between the anus and the bulb of the penis. To feel these taut bands and localize the TrP spot tenderness, it sometimes helps to provide counter pressure against the external palpating finger by one finger in the rectum.

External Pelvic Examination: Women

In woman, the lithotomy position with the feet in stirrups is likewise most satisfactory for examining the superficial pelvic floor muscles. Usually, only the ischiocavernosus and transversus perinei muscles are identifiable by external palpation, and then only if they have taut bands and tender TrPs. The relationships of these muscles are clearly drawn and realistically depicted.[1,2,4]

The ischiocavernosus muscle and its TrPs are more readily located by vaginal examination. The ischiocavernosus muscle lies close to, and along most of the length of, the perineal margin of the pubic bone below the pubic symphysis. On vaginal examination, taut bands become evident when compressed by cross-fiber flat palpation against the margin of the pubic bone at the mid-vaginal level and at right angles to the direction of the muscle fibers.

As in men, the transversus perinei muscle on each side spans the distance between the perineal body centrally and the ischial tuberosity laterally. Palpation must be at right angles to the direction of the fibers, and the muscle must be under slight tension to identify taut bands most effectively.

No nerve entrapments by these pelvic muscles have been demonstrated. However, the situation at the lesser sciatic foramen with regard to potential entrapment of a nerve appears analogous to sciatic nerve compression at the greater sciatic foramen, as discussed in Chapter 57. The lesser sciatic foramen has firm, unyielding boundaries: the bony ischium on one side and heavy ligaments, the sacrotuberous and the sacrospinous, on the other side. As these two ligaments fuse as they pass each other, there is no space available for pressure relief if the foramen becomes completely filled. The pudendal nerve, the internal pudendal vessels, and the obturator internus muscle with its tendon pass through the foramen. At this point, the obturator internus muscle usually has become mainly tendinous, but there may be a sufficient number of muscle fibers passing through the foramen to compress the pudendal nerve and vessels if the muscle develops TrPs, shortens, and bulges. This is a possibility that deserves investigation when perineal pain or dysesthesia is unexplained.

4. DIFFERENTIAL DIAGNOSIS

4.1. Activation and Perpetuation of Trigger Points

In any part of the pelvic floor muscle complex, TrPs may be activated by unaccustomed eccentric loading, eccentric exercise in the unconditioned muscle, or maximal or submaximal concentric loading.[55] Trigger points in the pelvic floor muscles are sometimes activated by a severe fall, long periods of prolonged sitting, driving, bicycling, an automobile accident, or surgery in the pelvic or abdominal region. Often, the patients cannot identify a specific initiating event. However, chronic tension of the pelvic muscles coupled with psychosocial stress and dysfunction can likely contribute to the onset of CPPS and the perpetuation of TrPs in the pelvic floor muscles.[52] Levator ani TrPs are certainly perpetuated, and perhaps activated, by sitting in a slumped posture for prolonged periods of time. Thiele radiographically demonstrated that the acute angulation of the coccygeal joints was caused by sitting on a hard surface in a slumped posture.[33] The compressed gluteus maximus muscle transmits pressure to the coccyx. Thiele attributed coccygodynia to this posture in 32% of 324 patients.[33] Cooper considered prolonged sitting in a slouched position while watching television as the factor responsible for coccygodynia in 14% of 100 patients.[31] Lilius and Valtonen regarded this posture as an important cause of levator ani muscle spasm syndrome.[34] In those patients with no known initiating event, possible causes for the muscle hyperirritability and TrPs are nutritional inadequacies and/or other systemic perpetuating factors.[56,57] Articular dysfunctions of the sacroiliac joints,[41] sacrococcygeal articulation, and the lumbosacral junction may be potent aggravating sources of TrPs in these pelvic floor muscles.

4.2. Associated Trigger Points

Associated TrPs can develop in the musculature within the referred pain areas resultant from an active TrP.[57] Therefore, muscles in the referred pain areas for each muscle should also be considered for examination. Trigger points in the perineal muscles (namely, the bulbospongiosus, ischiocavernosus, and transverse perinei) are likely to present as a single muscle syndrome. On the contrary, pelvic floor muscles (for instance, the sphincter ani, levator ani, and coccygeus) are much more likely to exhibit multiple muscle involvement. Increased tension of the levator ani muscle often occurs in conjunction with increased tension of the gluteus maximus muscle as well as gluteus medius and minimus muscles.[41,58]

The obturator internus and piriformis muscles are lower extremity muscles and, as such, are prone to develop TrPs together, and in association with, other external rotators of the hip (gemelli, obturator externus, and quadratus femoris muscles). Trigger points in the rectus abdominis, external obliques, adductor magnus, gluteus maximus, gluteus minimus, and quadratus lumborum muscles can refer pain to specific pelvic floor areas (Box 52-1).[17]

The rectus abdominis muscle can refer pain to the urogenital structures as well as the rectum and the perineum. The abdominal oblique muscles can refer to the groin, testicles, suprapubic region, and bladder. The quadratus lumborum, psoas, and iliacus muscles can refer to the groin and the adductor magnus muscle to the rectum and the deep pelvic floor muscles.

Numerous authors have used a variety of names to describe what would appear, on thoughtful consideration, to be largely myofascial pain syndromes of the pelvic musculature: tender coccyx,[41] coccygodynia,[31-33,37,59,60] coccygeal spasm,[22] levator syndrome,[39,61-64] levator ani syndrome,[38] levator spasm syndrome,[65] levator ani spasm syndrome,[34,66] tension myalgia of the pelvic floor,[67] pelvic floor syndromes,[68] pelvic pain syndrome,[44] proctalgia fugax,[69-74] and obturator internus spasm.[36]

Coccygodynia

Although the dictionary definition of coccygodynia is "pain in the coccygeal region,"[75] several authors[37,41] draw a sharp distinction between what they consider "true" coccygodynia resulting from traumatic injury to the coccyx and conditions elsewhere that refer pain or tenderness to the coccygeal region. One such condition is a myofascial pain syndrome.

Authors have associated pain in the region of a nontender coccyx (dorsal surface) with abnormal tension and marked tenderness of the levator ani muscle,[32,37,39,41] coccygeus muscle,[22,32,37] and gluteus maximus muscle.[41] Pace and Long explicitly recognized that coccygeal pain is referred from TrPs in the pelvic muscles.[37,68]

Levator Ani Syndromes

The levator ani muscle is associated with several conditions that cause pelvic pain: levator spasm syndrome,[65] levator ani spasm syndrome,[34,66] levator syndrome,[39,61] and pelvic floor syndromes.[68] For example, the levator ani spasm syndrome[34] causes pain in the sacrum, coccyx, rectum, and pelvic diaphragm. It is diagnosed by finding on rectal examination "spastic," tender muscles in the pelvic floor (puborectalis, iliococcygeus, and coccygeus). The piriformis muscle is not included in this group as it refers pain in the buttock and down the thigh.[31,33,34,65,68]

This levator ani syndrome was identified in 31 patients on a physical medicine service. As in other studies, most of the patients with this syndrome were women (90%). The pain was located in the sacrum (100% of patients), pelvic diaphragm (90%), anal region (68%), and in the gluteal region (only 13%). The levator ani muscle was tender and "spastic," and 55% of these signs were bilateral. All patients experienced sharp pain in the sacral area lasting 5 to 10 minutes after digital examination. Of the women who attempted intercourse during the illness, 43% suffered dyspareunia. Forty percent of all patients reported disturbed bowel function (constipation or frequency), but none experienced painful bowel movements. Twenty percent reported pain when sitting. Only 10% of the patients failed to respond to massage therapy of the levator ani muscle, and 74% became symptom-free or had only very slight residual symptoms.[34]

Patients with pelvic floor syndromes experience pain referred in various combinations to the buttock, underneath the sacrum, in the hip laterally, the thigh posteriorly, and from the piriformis, coccygeus, or levator ani muscles.[68] Patients reported pain when seated on hard surfaces and when sitting down or standing up from a chair. Digital examination of an involved muscle revealed trigger areas with local soreness and a tight, fibrous, nodular feel of the involved muscle.

Proctalgia Fugax

Proctalgia fugax is defined as "painful spasm of the muscle about the anus without known cause."[75] It is characterized by paroxysms of anorectal pain in the absence of identifiable local

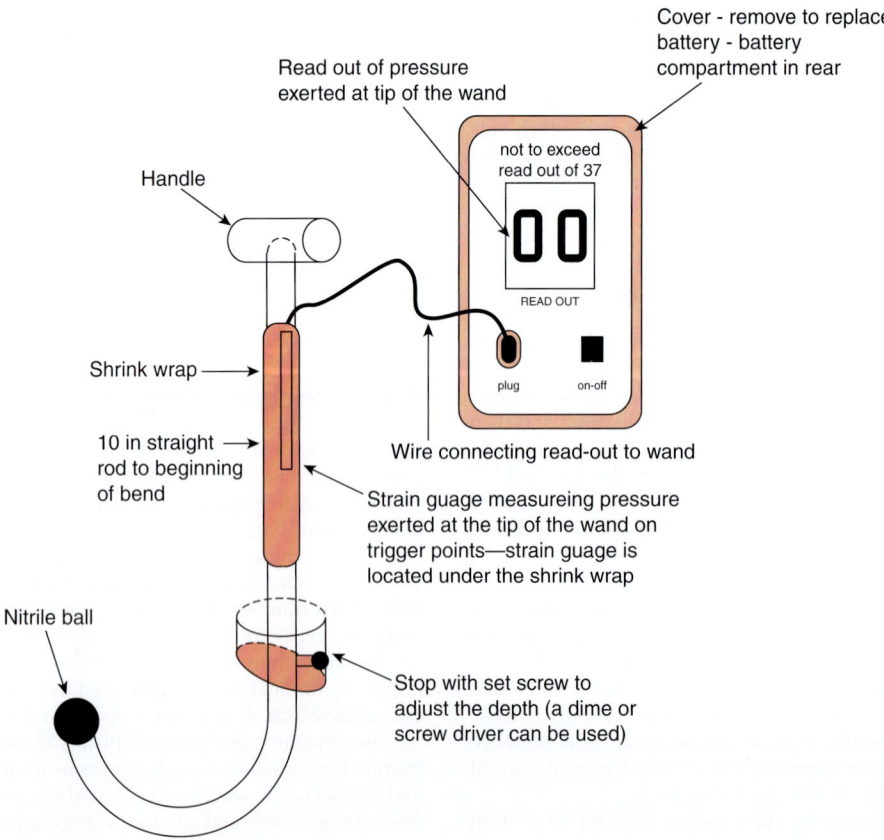

Figure 52-6. Therapeutic wand and instrument for TrP self-pressure release.

lesions. It is not a rare condition, and 13% to 19% of apparently healthy persons surveyed have symptoms of proctalgia fugax, although most experience fewer than seven episodes per year.[71] The pain usually occurs irregularly in bouts that generally show no correlation to activity or to the condition of the patient.[71] Proctalgia can begin as early as 13 years of age.[74] A physician with this condition wrote an eloquent description of it.[72]

As we have learned more about most "idiopathic" diseases, they have turned out to represent a number of conditions lumped together under one rubric. Proctalgia fugax appears to be no exception. The levator ani syndrome, noted previously, and coccygodynia, as described by Thiele,[32,33] bear a remarkable resemblance to proctalgia fugax.

Two studies found evidence of specific causes for proctalgia fugax. One study reported pressures in the rectum and the sigmoid colon measured by inserting instrumented balloons, whereas two patients were experiencing recurrent pain.[70] The small changes in pressure observed in the rectum did not correlate with the episodes of pain, but the intermittent peaks of pressure observed in the sigmoid colon did. The greater the pressure peaks, the more likely the subject was to identify pain, which began a short time before a peak. This study suggested that the pain resulted from muscular contraction of the wall of the sigmoid colon, not from pressure within the lumen.

Trigger points stimulated by tension may exist in smooth muscle, interstitial connective tissue, or the lining of the bowel wall. In the other study, Douthwaite reported 10 physicians who examined themselves during attacks of proctalgia fugax.[69] None detected spasm of the anal sphincter muscle. They did palpate a tense, tender band on one or the other side of the rectum, which they located in the levator ani muscle. These findings are consistent with TrPs in the levator ani muscle. A few patients experience attacks of proctalgia following coitus. Peery postulates that the pain derives from exaggerated or prolonged contraction of the rectal sphincter muscle after orgasm.[71] This pain might also derive from TrPs in the sphincter ani, bulbospongiosus, or ischiocavernosus muscles.

Tension Myalgia of the Pelvic Floor

Sinaki and associates[67] consolidated the various syndromes of the pelvic musculature (piriformis syndrome, coccygodynia, levator ani spasm syndrome, and proctalgia fugax) under one umbrella term: tension myalgia of the pelvic floor muscles.[67] They saw the patients in the Department of Physical Medicine and Rehabilitation at the Mayo Clinic. Nearly all of the 94 patients were between 30 and 70 years of age; most were between 40 and 50 years. Women constituted 83% of the group, which is about the usual percentage of women patients with a levator ani syndrome.[65] Pain in the coccygeal area and a heavy feeling in the rectal or vaginal region were the most prominent symptoms occurring in 82% and 62%, respectively. Defecation caused pain in 33% of the patients. All patients had tenderness of the pelvic floor muscles on rectal examination. This examination elicited localized tenderness of the piriformis, coccygeus, levator ani muscles, sacrococcygeal ligaments, and muscular attachments to the sacrum and coccyx, or some combination of the above. It is likely that many of these patients had TrPs in the tender muscles, but no mention was made of the presence or absence of taut bands or referral of pain when pressure was applied to a tender spot.

Chronic Prostatitis and Chronic Pelvic Pain Syndrome

A recent National Ambulatory Care Survey stated that there may be 20 office visits per 1000 men annually with symptoms consistent with prostatitis, with a high prevalence of 5% to 16%.[76,77] In most instances, the malady is designated chronic prostatitis (CP), and empirical use of antibiotics represents the mainstay of therapy. However, 95% of CP syndromes in men are nonbacterial and idiopathic. They represent a nonspecific pain disorder.[78] The occurrence and persistence of pain described as perineal, testicular, penile, and lower abdominal discomfort with or without voiding symptoms is the primary presenting dilemma. A neurobehavioral perspective to this chronic pain syndrome is now emerging.[79] Pelvic pain manifests as a myofascial pain syndrome, in which abnormal muscular tension could explain much of the discomfort and abnormal urinary dysfunction seen in this disorder.[80,81] Some investigators have evaluated and attempted to treat associated muscular tenderness of chronic pelvic pain, particularly painful TrPs.[17,35,40,82-85] Palpation of specific, painful pelvic TrPs elicits strong association with reported patient description of painful anatomic locations.[17]

4.3. Associated Pathology

Many patients with urogenital dysfunction will present with TrPs in the abdominal and pelvic floor musculature. As mentioned in Chapter 49, visceral diseases can be associated with abdominal wall TrPs. Abdominal wall TrPs are especially likely to develop with any inflammatory visceral disease as a result of the viscerosomatic reflex. In fact, abdominal TrPs had a 93% predictive value for discriminating visceral from somatic pain.[50] The relationship between TrPs and visceral problems is bidirectional because modification of the sensory input to the central nervous system in the somatic areas of pain referral from visceral nociceptive input can modify the perception of pain.

Weiss reported the successful amelioration of symptoms in patients with Bladder Pain syndrome/Interstitial Cystitis (BPS/IC) using TrP release.[86] In 2002, Doggweiler-Wiygul and Wiygul found that inactivation of TrPs in the pelvic floor muscles resolved pain in patients with severe CPPS, BPS/IC, and irritative voiding symptoms.[87] In 2005, Anderson et al demonstrated that the incorporation of TrP inactivation into a multimodal approach for CPPS in men resulted in an effective therapeutic approach, by providing a reduction in pain and urinary symptoms.[35] Later, Anderson et al also found that TrP inactivation was associated with significant improvement in urinary symptoms, libido, and ejaculatory and erectile pain in men with CPPS.[17,35,88] Langford et al demonstrated the effectiveness of TrP inactivation of the levator ani muscles for the management of some patients with CPPS.[89] Fitzgerald et al demonstrated a better response rate of 57% in patients diagnosed with CPPS and who were treated with TrP therapy when compared with the response rate of 21% in those patients receiving global therapeutic massage.[83] In some refractory cases, more aggressive therapy with varied TrP needling techniques, including dry needling, anesthetic injections, or botulinum toxin A injections, can be used, in combination with conservative therapies.[48] Recently, the works of Fitzgerald et al in 2009 and 2012,[83,90] Konkle and Clemens in 2011,[91] and Anderson et al in 2016[92] confirm increasing evidence that internal physical therapy and self-treatment is safe and effective regardless of gender. A neurobehavioral perspective to this chronic pain syndrome is now emerging.[79] Pelvic pain manifests as a myofascial pain syndrome, in which abnormal muscular tension could explain much of the discomfort reported by these individuals.[80,81]

Chronic hemorrhoids and fissures can aggravate symptoms in the related pelvic floor muscles.[34] Chronic inflammatory conditions within the pelvis such as endometritis, adenomyosis, chronic salpingo-oophoritis, chronic prostatovesiculitis,[34] Crohn disease, ulcerative colitis, irritable bowel syndrome, and BPS/IC may evoke referred pain and tenderness of the pelvic floor muscles and have been associated with the levator ani spasm syndrome.[34,93] However, other coexistent pelvic diseases, including ovarian cysts, pelvic adhesions, and fibroids, may have a successful response to local injection of TrPs in the levator ani and coccygeus muscles and in posthysterectomy vaginal cuff scars.[44]

5. CORRECTIVE ACTIONS

When seated, the patient should use a small pillow for lumbar support and should lean against the backrest of the chair. This position maintains the natural lumbar lordosis and raises the thoracic cage anteriorly, which places the lumbopelvic spine in the optimum position. Neutral lumbar spine should be the goal in the seated, supine, prone, and standing positions. In the seated position, the weight should be placed through the "sit" bones and not through the gluteal muscles. Thiele strongly emphasized the therapeutic importance of sitting posture in patients with coccygodynia.[33] He recommended a slow shift of weight from one buttock to another and to avoid placing weight in the middle buttocks, sacrum, or tailbone. He was able to demonstrate acute angulation of the coccyx radiographically when the patient was seated in the slumped posture placing weight through the central buttocks and sacrum. He reports that his patients responded well this postural correction, and he determined this was the cause of the patients' symptoms in 31% of 324 cases.[33] Cooper[31] found that slumped seated posture was responsible for the pain in 14% of 100 cases with a diagnosis of coccygodynia. Other authors have made a point of teaching their patients with coccygodynia who slump while sitting to obtain a more erect seated position.[34] When sleeping on the side, a pillow should be used between the legs to keep the hips and the spine aligned. Proper sleep posture is addressed in Chapter 76.

When patients with TrPs fail to respond to specific local treatment, or when the beneficial results are only transient, the clinician should aggressively investigate the possibility of nutritional inadequacies or other systemic perpetuating factors for the perpetuation of TrPs. For the patient with TrPs in the coccygeus and levator ani muscles, the clinician should identify and, if possible, correct any articular dysfunctions of the sacroiliac joints and sacrococcygeal or lumbosacral articulations. Also in such cases, resolution of any chronic inflammatory condition within the pelvis, such as endometritis, chronic salpingo-oophoritis, chronic prostatovesiculitis, BPS/IC, and urinary tract infections may be critical to pain relief. Recently, a new multimodal approach to treating pelvic TrPs has been documented. Anderson et al have reported successful use of a 6-day intensive treatment protocol for refractory CP and CPPS using TrP release and paradoxical relaxation.[35,51,92]

If an individual experiences pain in the pelvic or coccygeal region, he or she should seek a professional consultation from a clinician who is trained in specific pelvic floor examination and management skills before performing any of the self-treatment techniques described in the following paragraphs.

Patients with TrPs inside the pelvic floor muscles can perform TrP self-pressure release techniques and deactivate their TrPs using their finger or a therapeutic wand.[92,94] Trigger point self-pressure release combined with a self-stretch of external pelvic muscles can also reduce the influence of associated TrPs in the pelvic floor muscles. Anderson et al demonstrated the effectiveness of palpating individual muscle groups, identifying TrPs, and holding pressure for about 60 seconds.[92] Specific physiotherapy techniques that can be used in conjunction with TrP release include voluntary contraction and release, hold-relax, contract-relax, reciprocal inhibition, and deep tissue mobilization, including stripping, strumming, skin rolling, and effleurage. This self-treatment is prescribed weekly for 4 weeks and biweekly for 8 weeks thereafter. Two authors referred to stretching treatment of the levator ani muscle in terms of "stretching the spastic muscles,"[34] and "retropulsion of the coccyx."[22] Dorsal mobilization of the coccyx to stretch the levator ani muscle can be included as part of the self-release procedure.

In conjunction with physiotherapy, a fundamental aspect of the protocol by Anderson is paradoxical relaxation training, which is a method of autonomic self-regulation to reduce pelvic muscle tension.[35] Patients received 1 hour of individual verbal instructions and a supervised practice session at weekly intervals for 8 weeks in paradoxical relaxation exercises devised by Anderson and Wise to achieve specific profound relaxation of the pelvic floor muscles.[88] The word *paradoxical* is used because patients are directed to accept their tension as a way of relaxing/releasing it. Components of the training included a specific breathing technique to quiet anxiety as well as relaxation training sessions directing patients to focus attention on the effortless acceptance of tension in specific areas of the body. Daily home practice relaxation sessions of 1 hour were recommended for a minimum of 6 months using a series of 36 instructional lessons (7-42 minutes each) to accomplish the incremental relaxation of residual tension in specific body areas, aimed at simultaneous relaxation of the pelvic floor muscles. This case study analysis indicates that this protocol was successful in producing a 72% moderate/marked improvement in subject symptoms and it may be an effective treatment approach in patients with CP/CPPS, providing pain and urinary symptom relief with the least downside risk. The treatment that was described is based on the new understanding that certain chronic pelvic pain reflects a self-feeding state of tension in the pelvic floor muscles, perpetuated by cycles of tension, anxiety, and pain. This treatment protocol aims to rehabilitate the pelvic floor muscles, while simultaneously modifying the habit of focusing tension under stress.[35,51,92] Hubbard et al reported that TrPs show a significant increase in EMG activity during psychological stress. Therefore, a major goal in treatment is helping these patients modify their sympathetic response to stress with therapeutic techniques such as paradoxical muscle relaxation, autogenics, imagery, and biofeedback.[95]

Anderson et al studied the effectiveness of an internal pelvic therapeutic wand for self-pressure release and in 2015 conducted a study utilizing the therapeutic wand including both men and women with urologic pelvic pain syndrome.[92,94] The patients were taught the anatomic location of their TrPs that reproduced the patient's reported pain. Brief gentle pressure was applied initially to help the patient make the distinction between the prostate (in men) and the tissue surrounding it in which TrPs typically are found. Patients were assisted in localizing their own TrPs by using the pelvic map specifically generated for them. Figure 52-6 illustrates the therapeutic wand that is made with solid ultem plastic with a distal shepherd's crook curve, a diameter of 3.2 cm, and a nitrile rubber tip that measures 1.9 cm, which allows the patient to insert a predetermined but limited length into the rectum or vagina. A movable guard prevents further advancement. The wand serves as an extended finger that is easily navigated inside the pelvis. It is used to locate and release painful internal TrPs. The algometer sensor is easily visible and allows same-time monitoring of point pressure to prevent excessive or dangerous force. The surface area of the terminal ball that is applied to the tissue surface is 1.91 cm^2 (0.75 in^2), and the pressure gauge integrated with the wand tip provides numerical readings that correspond to applied torque pressure in the range of 0 to 2 kg/cm^2. If a maximum pressure were to be applied, it would equal to 8.7 psi or 0.62 kg/cm^2. Patients were instructed not to exceed read-out values greater than 0.34 kg/cm^2 and were trained to massage their own pelvic musculature without causing rectal or vaginal tissue trauma. They were also instructed to never apply pressure that elicited neurologic stimulation such as tingling, pulsation, or radiated pain such as sciatica. Per protocol, the therapeutic wand manipulations were to be performed on a regular basis, typically 3 to 4 times per week, approximately 5 to 10 minutes during each session to release the pelvic floor TrPs and areas of myofascial tenderness and restriction (Figure 52-6). Patient education included a description of the internal muscles, bladder, cervix, uterus, and prostate anatomy. The physical therapist created individualized drawings to map specific tender TrPs for each patient, the patient insertion, and safe pressure application. Patients used a water-based lubricated, vinyl or nitrile glove over the wand tip. The anus or vaginal introitus were also lubricated with a water-based gel. Care was taken to avoid any tissue dryness or resistance during insertion of the wand.

To palpate anterior TrPs, Figure 52-7A illustrates the recommended patient position, supine, with back and head elevated 45°.

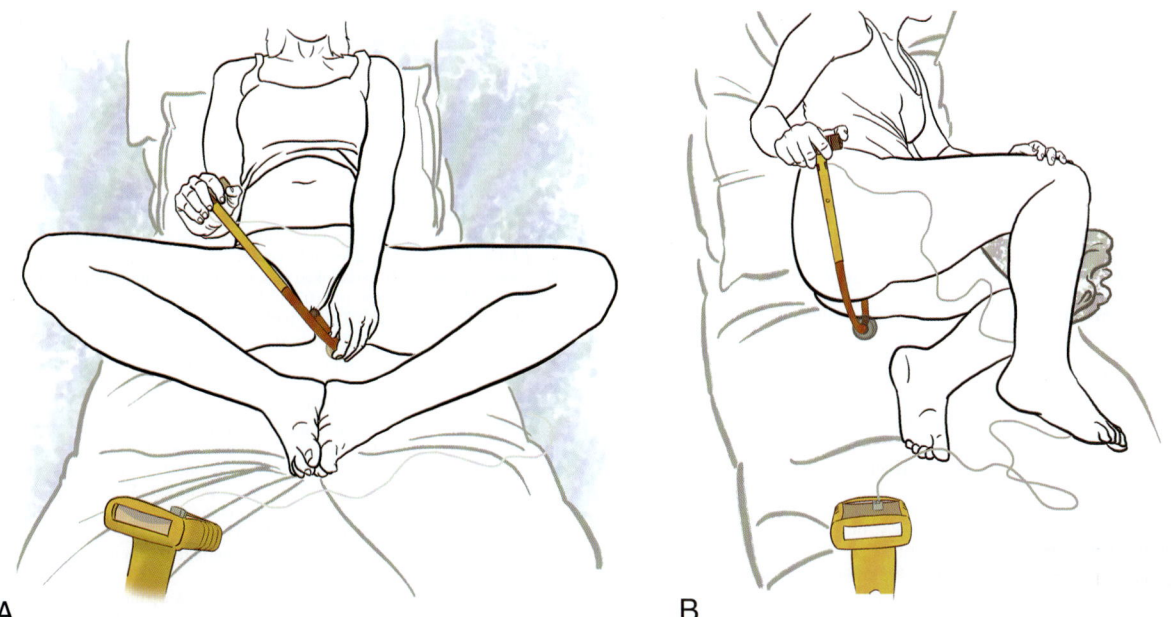

Figure 52-7. Position for TrP self-pressure release with TrP wand. A, Anterior approach. B, Posterior approach.

To palpate posterior and lateral TrPs, the patient is instructed to obtain a side-lying position (Figure 52-7B). Men were taught the anatomic location of the prostate. Brief gentle pressure is applied initially to help the patient make the distinction between the prostate and the tissue surrounding it where TrPs are typically found. Patients were assisted in localizing their own TrPs by using the pelvic map specifically generated for them, beginning at an anterior region and working toward the posterior region. After the identification of deep TrPs, patients were instructed to slowly withdraw the wand in increments of 1 to 2 in in order to recheck at a shallower depth. This was repeated until removal of the wand.

Women were instructed to use both vaginal and rectal wand insertion to determine optimal effectiveness. The glove covering on the tip of the wand was replaced when changing from vaginal to rectal self-pressure release or vice versa. Gradual increased pressure on each TrP started with a 10- to 12-second gentle motion technique to identify the precise TrP and then 15- to 90-second static holding pressure until tenderness around the TrP abated. Acute flare-ups of pain were expected during the initial therapeutic maneuvers as it occurs frequently in manual treatment performed by a physical therapist or physician. However, patients were discouraged from inducing further discomfort or pain beyond a 5 to 7 score on a pain visual analog scale (VAS; 0-10). For continued therapy, patients were instructed to lubricate a gloved finger and gently stretch the rectal or vaginal opening before insertion of the wand. Instruction for home usage of the wand was provided, and patients were checked up to three times for clarifications by the physical therapist or MD before discharge from the clinic. Any trace bleeding was to be promptly reported and the manual therapy discontinued for several days. In the event of continued bleeding, patients were required to have a physician evaluation and follow-up. This study demonstrated that a protocol of proper training, education, and professional supervision provides safety and efficacy for patients with Urological Chronic Pelvic Pain Syndrome (UCPPS) to perform their own internal TrP release using an internal therapeutic wand once the patient has been educated by the clinician. This study also demonstrates that the therapeutic wand is associated with a significant reduction in pelvic muscle sensitivity. The patient's ability to self-administer internal TrP self-pressure release has an obvious benefit by eliminating the need for frequent conventional physical therapy (PT) office visits. In addition, this wand makes internal TrP self-pressure release available for the many individuals suffering from pelvic pain and who do not have access to knowledgeable health care practitioners.[92,94]

Thiele Massage

Thiele presented the classic illustrated description for the examination and treatment by massage of the levator ani and coccygeus muscles via the rectum. He recommended rubbing the muscle fibers along their length, from origin to insertion, with a stripping motion (as when sharpening a straight razor), applying as much pressure as the patient could tolerate with moderate pain. The patient was instructed to "bear down" during massage to relax these muscles. The patient provided the massage motion for 10 to 15 repetitions on each side of the pelvis, and this treatment was repeated daily for 5 or 6 days and then every other day for 7 to 10 days. Massage only once or twice a week was found to be ineffective. Of the 223 patients with coccygodynia who were treated in this way, 64% were "cured" and 27% improved.[33]

Malbohan and associates also reported the successful use of massage of these two muscles in the treatment of nearly 1500 patients with low back pain attributed to coccygeal spasm.[22] Cooper[31] reported that 81% of 62 patients with coccygodynia were relieved of pain by the Thiele type of massage, but careful instruction about proper sitting posture relieved an even higher percentage of 28 other patients.[31] Grant and associates found that two or three levator ani massages spaced 2 to 3 weeks apart, in conjunction with heat and diazepam, provided good results in 63% of patients with the levator syndrome.[61]

Stripping massage is a powerful tool for the inactivation of these accessible TrPs. Massage is painful, but it can be effective when other modalities have failed. One is able to identify the taut bands and TrPs requiring attention and literally place one's finger on the source of the pain, treating its source until the problem is resolved.

Postisometric relaxation is another technique that a patient can utilize to self-treat pain in the coccygeal region. The patient lies on the stomach with the heels rotated outward, which places the gluteus maximus muscle on partial stretch. The patient then squeezes (contract) the buttocks together gently with very little force, and maintains this for 10 seconds, and then relaxes. This is repeated four to five times. The portion of the gluteus maximus muscle that attaches to the coccyx is embryologically separate from the rest of the gluteus maximus muscle; this fact may relate to the effectiveness of the postisometric therapy for this part of the muscle.[3]

References

1. Ferner H, Staubesand J. *Sobotta Atlas of Human Anatomy*. Vol 2. 10th ed. Baltimore, MD: Urban & Schwarzenberg; 1983 (Fig. 152, 292, 329, 404).
2. Standring S. *Gray's Anatomy: The Anatomical Basis of Clinical Practice*. 41st ed. London, UK: Elsevier; 2015.
3. Tichy M. Anatomical basis for relaxation of the muscles attached to the coccyx. *Manual Med*. 1989;4:147-148.
4. Anderson JE. *Grant's Atlas of Anatomy*. 8th ed. Baltimore, MD: Williams & Wilkins; 1983 (pp. 3-39).
5. Netter FH. *Musculoskeletal System. Part 1: Anatomy, Physiology and Metabolic Disorders*. Vol 8. Summit, NJ: Ciba-Geigy Corporation; 1987 (pp. 86, 142-143).
6. Eisler P. *Die Muskeln des Stammes*. Jena, Germany: Gustav Fischer; 1912 (pp. 447-451, Fig. 65).
7. Bardeen C. The musculature, Section 5. In: Jackson CM, ed. *Morris's Human Anatomy*. 6th ed. Philadelphia, PA: Blakiston's Son & Co; 1921 (p. 481, Fig. 424).
8. Pernkopf E. *Atlas of Topographical and Applied Human Anatomy*. Vol 2. Philadelphia, PA: Saunders; 1964 (Fig. 306).
9. Juenemann KP, Lue TF, Schmidt RA, Tanagho EA. Clinical significance of sacral and pudendal nerve anatomy. *J Urol*. 1988;139(1):74-80.
10. DeLancey JO. Anatomy and physiology of urinary continence. *Clin Obstet Gynecol*. 1990;33(2):298-307.
11. Howard D, Miller JM, Delancey JO, Ashton-Miller JA. Differential effects of cough, valsalva, and continence status on vesical neck movement. *Obstet Gynecol*. 2000;95(4):535-540.
12. Baytur YB, Deveci A, Uyar Y, Ozcakir HT, Kizilkaya S, Caglar H. Mode of delivery and pelvic floor muscle strength and sexual function after childbirth. *Int J Gynaecol Obstet*. 2005;88(3):276-280.
13. Hodges PW, Sapsford R, Pengel LH. Postural and respiratory functions of the pelvic floor muscles. *Neurourol Urodyn*. 2007;26(3):362-371.
14. Hemborg B, Moritz U, Lowing H. Intra-abdominal pressure and trunk muscle activity during lifting. IV. The causal factors of the intra-abdominal pressure rise. *Scand J Rehabil Med*. 1985;17(1):25-38.
15. Pool-Goudzwaard A, van Dijke GH, van Gurp M, Mulder P, Snijders C, Stoeckart R. Contribution of pelvic floor muscles to stiffness of the pelvic ring. *Clin Biomech (Bristol, Avon)*. 2004;19(6):564-571.
16. Smith MD, Russell A, Hodges PW. Is there a relationship between parity, pregnancy, back pain and incontinence? *Int Urogynecol J Pelvic Floor Dysfunct*. 2008;19(2):205-211.
17. Anderson RU, Sawyer T, Wise D, Morey A, Nathanson BH. Painful myofascial trigger points and pain sites in men with chronic prostatitis/chronic pelvic pain syndrome. *J Urol*. 2009;182(6):2753-2758.
18. Basmajian J, Deluca C. *Muscles Alive*. 5th ed. Baltimore, MD: Williams & Wilkins; 1985 (pp. 399-403).
19. Critchley HO, Dixon JS, Gosling JA. Comparative study of the periurethral and perianal parts of the human levator ani muscle. *Urol Int*. 1980;35(3):226-232.
20. Gosling JA, Dixon JS, Critchley HO, Thompson SA. A comparative study of the human external sphincter and periurethral levator ani muscles. *Br J Urol*. 1981;53(1):35-41.
21. Koelbl H, Strassegger H, Riss PA, Gruber H. Morphologic and functional aspects of pelvic floor muscles in patients with pelvic relaxation and genuine stress incontinence. *Obstet Gynecol*. 1989;74(5):789-795.
22. Malbohan IM, Mojisova L, Tichy M. The role of coccygeal spasm in low back pain. *J Man Med*. 1989;4:140-141.
23. Bard P. Chapter 10, Control of systemic blood vessels. In: Mountcastle VB, ed. *Medical Physiology*. Vol 1. 12th ed. St. Louis, MO: C.V. Mosby Company; 1968:150-177 (pp. 168-169).
24. Nocenti MR. Chapter 48, Reproduction. In: Mountcastle VB, ed. *Medical Physiology*. Vol 1. 12th ed. St. Louis, MO: C.V. Mosby Company; 1968:992-1028 (pp. 1024-1025).
25. Benoit G, Delmas V, Gillot C, Jardin A. The anatomy of erection. *Surg Radiol Anat*. 1987;9(4):263-272.
26. Karacan I, Hirshkowitz M, Salis PJ, Narter E, Safi MF. Penile blood flow and musculovascular events during sleep-related erections of middle-aged men. *J Urol*. 1987;138(1):177-181.
27. Lavoisier P, Courtois F, Barres D, Blanchard M. Correlation between intracavernous pressure and contraction of the ischiocavernosus muscle in man. *J Urol*. 1986;136(4):936-939.
28. Lavoisier P, Proulx J, Courtois F. Reflex contractions of the ischiocavernosus muscles following electrical and pressure stimulations. *J Urol*. 1988;139(2):396-399.
29. McMinn RMH, Hutchings RT. *Color Atlas of Human Anatomy*. Chicago, IL: Year Book Medical Publishers; 1977:81.
30. Doggweiler-Wiygul R. Urologic myofascial pain syndromes. *Curr Pain Headache Rep*. 2004;8(6):445-451.
31. Cooper WL. Coccygodynia. An analysis of one hundred cases. *J Int Coll Surg*. 1960;33:306-311.
32. Thiele GH. Coccygodynia and pain in the superior gluteal region. *JAMA*. 1937;109:1271-1275.
33. Thiele GH. Coccygodynia: cause and treatment. *Dis Colon Rectum*. 1963;6:422-436.
34. Lilius HG, Valtonen EJ. The levator ani spasm syndrome. A clinical analysis of 31 cases. *Ann Chir Gynaecol Fenn*. 1973;62(2):93-97.
35. Anderson RU, Wise D, Sawyer T, Chan C. Integration of myofascial trigger point release and paradoxical relaxation training treatment of chronic pelvic pain in men. *J Urol*. 2005;174(1):155-160.
36. Simons DG, Travell J, Simons L. *Travell & Simon's Myofascial Pain and Dysfunction: The Trigger Point Manual*. Vol 1. 2nd ed. Baltimore, MD: Williams & Wilkins; 1999 (pp. 178-235).
37. Leigh RE. Obturator internus spasm as a cause of pelvic and sciatic distress. *J Lancet*. 1952;72(6):286-287; passim.
38. Pace JB. Commonly overlooked pain syndromes responsive to simple therapy. *Postgrad Med*. 1975;58(4):107-113.
39. Morris L, Newton RA. Use of high voltage pulsed galvanic stimulation for patients with levator ani syndrome. *Phys Ther*. 1987;67(10):1522-1525.
40. Salvati EP. The levator syndrome and its variant. *Gastroenterol Clin North Am*. 1987;16(1):71-78.
41. Shoskes DA, Nickel JC, Kattan MW. Phenotypically directed multimodal therapy for chronic prostatitis/chronic pelvic pain syndrome: a prospective study using UPOINT. *Urology*. 2010;75(6):1249-1253.
42. Lewit K. *Manipulative Therapy in Rehabilitation of the Motor System*. London, England: Butterworths; 1985 (pp. 113, 174, 223, 278, 306-311).
43. DeStefano L. *Greenman's Principles of Manual Medicine*. 5th ed. Philadelphia, PA: Wolters Kluwer; 2016 (pp. 339-345).
44. Kidd R. Pain localization with the innominate upslip dysfunction. *Manual Med*. 1988;3:103-105.
45. Slocumb JC. Neurological factors in chronic pelvic pain: trigger points and the abdominal pelvic pain syndrome. *Am J Obstet Gynecol*. 1984;149(5):536-543.
46. Fall M, Baranowski AP, Elneil S, et al. EAU guidelines on chronic pelvic pain. *Eur Urol*. 2010;57(1):35-48.
47. Schmidt RA, Vapnek JM. Pelvic floor behavior and interstitial cystitis. *Semin Urol*. 1991;9(2):154-159.
48. Slocumb JC. Chronic somatic, myofascial, and neurogenic abdominal pelvic pain. *Clin Obstet Gynecol*. 1990;33(1):145-153.
49. Moldwin RM, Fariello JY. Myofascial trigger points of the pelvic floor: associations with urological pain syndromes and treatment strategies including injection therapy. *Curr Urol Rep*. 2013;14(5):409-417.
50. Jarrell J. Myofascial dysfunction in the pelvis. *Curr Pain Headache Rep*. 2004;8(6):452-456.
51. Jarrell J, Giamberardino MA, Robert M, Nasr-Esfahani M. Bedside testing for chronic pelvic pain: discriminating visceral from somatic pain. *Pain Res Treat*. 2011;2011:692102.
52. Anderson RU, Wise D, Sawyer T, Glowe P, Orenberg EK. 6-day intensive treatment protocol for refractory chronic prostatitis/chronic pelvic pain syndrome using myofascial release and paradoxical relaxation training. *J Urol*. 2011;185(4):1294-1299.
53. Golfam F, Golfam P, Khalaj A, Sayed Mortaz SS. The effect of topical nifedipine in treatment of chronic anal fissure. *Acta Med Iran*. 2010;48(5):295-299.
54. Rohen JW, Yokochi C. *Color Atlas of Anatomy*. 2nd ed. New York, NY: Igaku-Shoin; 1988 (pp. 311, 316-317).
55. Gerwin RD, Dommerholt J, Shah JP. An expansion of Simons' integrated hypothesis of trigger point formation. *Curr Pain Headache Rep*. 2004;8(6):468-475.
56. Travell JG, Simons DG. *Myofascial Pain and Dysfunction: The Trigger Point Manual*. Vol 1. Baltimore, MD: Williams & Wilkins; 1983.
57. Hsieh YL, Kao MJ, Kuan TS, Chen SM, Chen JT, Hong CZ. Dry needling to a key myofascial trigger point may reduce the irritability of satellite MTrPs. *Am J Phys Med Rehabil*. 2007;86(5):397-403.
58. Lewit K. Postisometric relaxation in combination with other methods of muscular facilitation and inhibition. *Manuelle Medizin*. 1986;2:101-104.
59. Dittrich RJ. Coccygodynia as referred pain. *J Bone Joint Surg Am Vol*. 1951;33-A(3):715-718.
60. Waters EG. A consideration of the types and treatment of coccygodynia. *Am J Obstet Gynecol*. 1937;33:531-535.
61. Grant SR, Salvati EP, Rubin RJ. Levator syndrome: an analysis of 316 cases. *Dis Colon Rectum*. 1975;18(2):161-163.
62. Nicosia JF, Abcarian H. Levator syndrome. A treatment that works. *Dis Colon Rectum*. 1985;28(6):406-408.
63. Oliver GC, Rubin RJ, Salvati EP, Eisenstat TE. Electrogalvanic stimulation in the treatment of levator syndrome. *Dis Colon Rectum*. 1985;28(9):662-663.
64. Sohn N, Weinstein MA, Robbins RD. The levator syndrome and its treatment with high-voltage electrogalvanic stimulation. *Am J Surg*. 1982;144(5):580-582.
65. Smith WT. Levator spasm syndrome. *Minn Med*. 1959;42(8):1076-1079.
66. Wright RR. The levator ani spasm syndrome. *Am J Proctol*. 1969;20(6):447-451.
67. Sinaki M, Merritt JL, Stillwell GK. Tension myalgia of the pelvic floor. *Mayo Clin Proc*. 1977;52(11):717-722.
68. Long C II. Myofascial pain syndromes. III. Some syndromes of the trunk and thigh. *Henry Ford Hosp Med Bull*. 1956;4(2):102-106.
69. Douthwaite AH. Proctalgia fugax. *Br Med J (Clin Res Ed)*. 1962;2(5298):164-165.
70. Harvey RF. Colonic motility in proctalgia fugax. *Lancet*. 1979;2(8145):713-714.
71. Peery WH. Proctalgia fugax: a clinical enigma. *South Med J*. 1988;81(5):621-623.
72. Swain R. Oral clonidine for proctalgia fugax. *Gut*. 1987;28(8):1039-1040.
73. Thompson WG, Heaton KW. Proctalgia fugax. *J R Coll Physicians Lond*. 1980;14(4):247-248.
74. Weizman Z, Binsztok M. Proctalgia fugax in teenagers. *J Pediatr*. 1989;114(5):813-814.
75. Basmajian JV, Burke MD, Burnett GW, et al. *Stedman's Medical Dictionary*. 24nd ed. Baltimore, MD: Williams & Wilkins; 1982 (pp. 293, 1143).

76. Nickel JC, Downey J, Hunter D, Clark J. Prevalence of prostatitis-like symptoms in a population based study using the National Institutes of Health chronic prostatitis symptom index. *J Urol.* 2001;165(3):842-845.
77. Collins MM, Stafford RS, O'Leary MP, Barry MJ. How common is prostatitis? A national survey of physician visits. *J Urol.* 1998;159(4):1224-1228.
78. Nickel JC, Alexander RB, Schaeffer AJ, Landis JR, Knauss JS, Propert KJ; Chronic Prostatitis Collaborative Research Network Study Group. Leukocytes and bacteria in men with chronic prostatitis/chronic pelvic pain syndrome compared to asymptomatic controls. *J Urol.* 2003;170(3):818-822.
79. Miller HC. Stress prostatitis. *Urology.* 1988;32(6):507-510.
80. Barbalias GA, Meares EM Jr, Sant GR. Prostatodynia: clinical and urodynamic characteristics. *J Urol.* 1983;130(3):514-517.
81. Hetrick DC, Ciol MA, Rothman I, Turner JA, Frest M, Berger RE. Musculoskeletal dysfunction in men with chronic pelvic pain syndrome type III: a case-control study. *J Urol.* 2003;170(3):828-831.
82. Berger RE, Ciol MA, Rothman I, Turner JA. Pelvic tenderness is not limited to the prostate in chronic prostatitis/chronic pelvic pain syndrome (CPPS) type IIIA and IIIB: comparison of men with and without CP/CPPS. *BMC Urol.* 2007;7:17.
83. FitzGerald MP, Anderson RU, Potts J, et al. Randomized multicenter feasibility trial of myofascial physical therapy for the treatment of urological chronic pelvic pain syndromes. *J Urol.* 2009;182(2):570-580.
84. Potts JM, O'Dougherty E. Pelvic floor physical therapy for patients with prostatitis. *Curr Urol Rep.* 2000;1(2):155-158.
85. Shoskes DA, Berger R, Elmi A, Landis JR, Propert KJ, Zeitlin S; Chronic Prostatitis Collaborative Research Network Study Group. Muscle tenderness in men with chronic prostatitis/chronic pelvic pain syndrome: the chronic prostatitis cohort study. *J Urol.* 2008;179(2):556-560.
86. Weiss JM. Pelvic floor myofascial trigger points: manual therapy for interstitial cystitis and the urgency-frequency syndrome. *J Urol.* 2001;166(6):2226-2231.
87. Doggweiler-Wiygul R, Wiygul JP. Interstitial cystitis, pelvic pain, and the relationship to myofascial pain and dysfunction: a report on four patients. *World J Urol.* 2002;20(5):310-314.
88. Anderson RU, Wise D, Sawyer T, Chan CA. Sexual dysfunction in men with chronic prostatitis/chronic pelvic pain syndrome: improvement after trigger point release and paradoxical relaxation training. *J Urol.* 2006;176(4, pt 1):1534-1538; discussion 1538-1539.
89. Langford CF, Udvari Nagy S, Ghoniem GM. Levator ani trigger point injections: an underutilized treatment for chronic pelvic pain. *Neurourol Urodyn.* 2007;26(1):59-62.
90. FitzGerald MP, Payne CK, Lukacz ES, et al. Randomized multicenter clinical trial of myofascial physical therapy in women with interstitial cystitis/painful bladder syndrome and pelvic floor tenderness. *J Urol.* 2012;187(6):2113-2118.
91. Konkle KS, Clemens JQ. New paradigms in understanding chronic pelvic pain syndrome. *Curr Urol Rep.* 2011;12(4):278-283.
92. Anderson RU, Wise D, Sawyer T, Nathanson BH, Nevin Smith J. Equal improvement in men and women in the treatment of urologic chronic pelvic pain syndrome using a multi-modal protocol with an internal myofascial trigger point wand. *Appl Psychophysiol Biofeedback.* 2016;41(2):215-224.
93. Lilius HG, Oravisto KJ, Valtonen EJ. Origin of pain in interstitial cystitis. Effect of ultrasound treatment on the concomitant levator ani spasm syndrome. *Scand J Urol Nephrol.* 1973;7(2):150-152.
94. Anderson RU, Wise D, Sawyer T, Nathanson B. Safety and effectiveness of an internal pelvic myofascial trigger point wand for urologic chronic pelvic pain syndrome. *Clin J Pain.* 2011;27(9):764-768.
95. McNulty WH, Gevirtz RN, Hubbard DR, Berkoff GM. Needle electromyographic evaluation of trigger point response to a psychological stressor. *Psychophysiology.* 1994;31(3):313-316.

Chapter 53

Clinical Considerations of Trunk and Pelvic Pain

César Fernández de las Peñas, Joseph M. Donnelly, and Timothy Douglas Sawyer

1. LOW BACK PAIN

1.1. Overview

Back pain is second only to the common cold as a cause of lost time from work and results in more lost productivity than any other medical conditions.[1] It has been estimated to result in 175.8 million days of restricted activity annually in the United States, and at any given time, 2.4 million Americans are disabled secondary to low back pain (LBP). Of these, half are disabled. Data from the National Ambulatory Medical Care Survey from 1989 to 1990 revealed that there were almost 15 million office visits for LBP, ranking this as the fifth reason for all physician visits. The cost of treatment for patients with LBP has a major economic impact worldwide. In the United States, patients with musculoskeletal conditions account for a total annual medical care costs of approximately $240 billion, of which $77 billion is related to musculoskeletal conditions. In 2006, the total costs associated with LBP in the United States exceeded $100 billion per year, with a majority of the costs associated with lost wages and reduced productivity.[2] This figure exceeds the costs for all other musculoskeletal conditions, which total about $77 billion per year.[3] Hoy et al[4] showed that the burden of LBP has increased in the decades since the disability-adjusted life years related to LBP increased from 58.2 million in 1990 to 83.0 million in 2010.

The reported prevalence of LBP ranges from 25% to 75% and depends on the definition used in the epidemiologic study. In a systematic review, Jackson et al[5] found that the prevalence of LBP was 18% for the general adult population, 31% for the elderly general population, and 44% for workers in low-income and middle-income countries. In fact, a recent meta-analysis observed that the prevalence of LBP in standard emergency settings was 4.39%, supporting the high relevance of this condition.[6] Freburger et al[7] examined the trends in the prevalence of chronic LBP in North Carolina comparing a representative sample in 1992 with a sample in 2006. They found the prevalence of chronic LBP for the total population more than doubled over the period, from about 4% to more than 10%. For women of all ages and men aged 45 to 54, the prevalence and incidence nearly tripled. In addition, the number of these individuals seeking health care for treatment also increased from 71% in 1992 to 84% in 2006.[7] Palacios-Ceña et al[8] also found that the prevalence of LBP has slightly increased in recent years in Spain.

These data demonstrate the rising prevalence of chronic LBP in society and the challenge it continues to pose for health care practitioners to find effective treatment and intervention strategies for this condition. Within the population of patients with persistent chronic pain, LBP is one of the most prevalent musculoskeletal disorders, affecting 70% to 85% of the adult population at some point in their life. Twelve months following the onset of an episode of LBP, as many as 45% to 75% of the patients still experience pain, accounting for major expenses in health care and disability systems. Despite extensive global research efforts, persistent chronic pain remains a challenging issue for clinicians and is a huge socioeconomic burden.[9]

LBP is a heterogeneous disorder that includes patients with dominant peripheral nociceptive, neuropathic, and centralized mechanisms of symptoms and may also include autonomic influences. For effective and efficient treatment for patients with LBP, classification systems, clinical practice guidelines, diagnostic procedures, and a proper understanding (subclassification) of pain mechanisms utilized in tandem with a sound clinical reasoning process are showing great promise. Recent research supports the inclusion of the patient's perspectives and biopsychosocial considerations into any classification system or clinical practice guideline related to LBP.[10,11] The neurophysiologic mechanism of the patient's pain report should be classified as predominantly nociceptive, neuropathic, central, or a combination thereof.[10,12] From the authors' perspective, the main observed deficiency in most clinical practice guidelines of LBP is the lack of inclusion of trigger points (TrPs) as a possible source of the patient's symptoms or as a contributing factor to movement impairment and nociceptive pain mechanisms, psychosocial aspects, and the contextual meaning for the patient.

The pathoanatomic approach and the structural lesion model for the treatment of LBP have failed to yield favorable results in regard to effective treatment for LBP. However, they continue to be the preferred and most used medical approaches despite their resulting in clinician and patient frustration. Classification systems have emerged in the past 20 years and are gaining in popularity as they attempt to more effectively manage patients with LBP. Guidelines for LBP developed in 1994 by the Agency for Health Care Policy and Research (AHCPR) are still being utilized by some medical professionals to manage patients with acute LBP.[13] Recent clinical guidelines on the management of LBP in the United Kingdom and the United States have been published by the National Institute for Health and Care Excellence[14] and the American College of Physicians,[15] respectively. These guidelines recommend a combination of pharmacologic drugs, manual therapies, exercise, and education for the management of patients with LBP; no specific reference to TrP therapy is included in any guideline.[14,15] Further and specific to LBP, physicians and physical therapists usually exhibit deficiencies in adhering to the clinical practice guidelines, providing several opportunities for variation in clinical practice. This variation can be related to those findings reported by a recent systematic review where, from more than 20 clinical guidelines on LBP, only 4 can be strongly recommended based on their quality assessed by Appraisal of Guidelines Research and Evaluation score.[16]

There are four primary LBP classification systems that attempt to match a treatment approach to a homogenous population of patients. These four classification systems include the McKenzie mechanical diagnosis and therapy classification,[17] treatment-based classification,[11] movement-systems impairment model,[18] and the mechanism-based classification.[10] However, these four systems each have their own limitations. None is comprehensive in its approach, and they do not fully account for the variability in clinical presentations, the degree to which psychosocial factors are considered, the clinical complexity of utilizing the systems, and the possibility that a patient may be able to independently manage his or her episode of LBP without a formal treatment process. A detailed review of these classification systems is beyond the scope of this book, and readers are referred to other texts for further information. As classification systems are tested for their reliability and treatment efficacy, it is expected that there will be more "convergence of than divergence among the four systems."[11]

Fritz et al[19] compared the effectiveness of treatment-based classification physical therapy with therapy based on AHCPR guidelines for patients with acute work-related LBP. The study included 78 subjects with acute work-related LBP of less than 3 weeks' duration and who were randomly selected to receive therapy based on classification with matched interventions or therapy based on AHCPR guidelines. The use of treatment-based classification therapy approach resulted in improved disability and quality of life as well as return to work status following 4 weeks when compared with those in the AHCPR guideline therapy group. Brennan et al[20] investigated treatment-matched interventions versus nonmatched interventions in 123 individuals presenting with LBP. They found that patients who received matched treatment interventions experienced better short- and long-term reductions in disability than those receiving unmatched interventions. Following a 1-year follow-up, those who received matched treatment interventions continued to have better long-term outcomes. This study supports the use of a treatment-based classification system to treat nonspecific LBP.[20] It is possible that the inclusion of TrP therapy into this treatment-based classification system can lead to the identification of a subgroup of patients with LBP potentially responders to its treatment.

Discogenic Pain

Disc degeneration in humans can begin as early as the third decade of life. Aging, obesity, smoking, awkward or sustained postures, vibration from transportation, excessive axial loads, and other factors accelerate the degeneration of intervertebral discs. At present, most data indicate that chronic LBP is most closely related to the anatomic structure of the intervertebral disc, particularly in patients with no obvious herniation of the nucleus pulposus, representing the clinical pathology of the disease process known as discogenic lower back pain (DLBP). DLBP is believed to be the most common disease of chronic LBP, accounting for 39% of its incidence. Lower disc herniation represents less than 30% of cases, and other causes, such as zygapophysial joint pain, are responsible for an even lower proportion of LBP cases.

The four common classes of disc herniations are as follows: (1) *Disc protrusion* occurs when the nucleus pulposus bulges outward into the annulus fibrosis, but no damage is done to the annulus; (2) *Disc prolapse* occurs when the nucleus pulposus bulges outward into the annulus, and the annular lamina are damaged; (3) *Disc extrusion* occurs when the nucleus pulposus breaks past the outer lamina of the annulus fibrosis and into the space beyond; and (4) *Disc sequestration* occurs when the nucleus pulposus breaks free of the annulus. The mechanism of injury may occur with forward bending with or without rotation, falling onto the buttock with spine flexed, coughing or sneezing, or bearing down for a bowel movement. The disc will commonly refer pain locally into the low back, but in addition to this, the symptoms will commonly extend down posteriorly into the gluteal region. Pain that extends beyond the gluteal region and into the leg is most likely a result of nerve irritation. Symptoms can include referral to the lower thoracic or upper lumbar region, abdomen, flanks, groin, genitals, thighs, knees, calves, ankles, feet, and toes.[21,22]

DLBP results in a loss of lower back function secondary to pain. Although the outer annulus fibrosis of the disc may remain intact, multiple processes (degeneration, end plate injury, inflammation, etc.) can internally stimulate nociception inside the disc without nerve root symptoms. This is mainly due to the outer one-third of the annulus fibrosis having innervation from the recurring meningeal (sinuvertebral) nerve and its vascularization. Additionally, there is no root symptom and no evidence of segmental activities of the radiology. Disc disorders were first documented by Crock in 1970, and the term DLBP was coined in 1979. Since then, many scholars have conducted in-depth studies on this condition. According to epidemiologic data, DLBP is a complex disease with genetic, community, and health care implications. A systematic review looking at magnetic resonance imaging and findings of disc degeneration in adults with LBP found that disc bulge, disc degeneration, disc extrusion, disc protrusion, and spondylolysis were more prevalent in adults presenting with LBP especially at age 50 and over, when compared with asymptomatic adults.[23] Patients with a genetic susceptibility to DLBP are considered high risk and experience changes in the chemical and biologic composition of their intervertebral discs, as well as metabolic changes in their bodies. Abnormal stresses reduce the amount of water in the nucleus pulposus, inducing degeneration of the disc. The disc is then unable to bear stress evenly, and a localized increase in stress can cause structural injuries that lead to a tear or rupture in the annular fibrosis and end plate. Damage to the end plate accelerates the pathologic process of disc degeneration. During this degenerative process, cells of the nucleus generate an inflammatory response, releasing a large number of inflammatory factors or cytokines. Large epidemiologic studies have demonstrated that LBP is commonly associated with lumbar disc degeneration.[24] Studies have also suggested that patients with DLBP have significantly higher levels of released interleukin-1 (IL-1), IL-6, and IL-8 compared with patients with disc herniation. These proinflammatory cytokines travel into the fissure of the end plate or the outer third of the annular fibrosis, stimulate nociception (through free nerve endings), and may produce a pain response. Therefore, DLBP requires two factors to induce pain: the existence of free nerve endings and proinflammatory cytokines. There is a high density of nerves and blood vessels in the outer third of the annulus and end plate area, which is likely the site where nociception is produced. Thus, the inflammatory response is the main pathophysiologic cause of DLBP.[25] Only a small proportion (approximately 20%) of LBP cases can be attributed with reasonable certainty to a pathologic or anatomic entity. Therefore, diagnosing the cause of LBP represents the biggest challenge for medical practitioners. Spinal abnormalities are more common in athletes than in nonathletes in the general population. Spinal injury patterns can be observed in athletes who are subjected to trauma. Athletes are susceptible to degenerative disc changes at an early age due to the repetitive loading activities involved in sports.[25]

Another possible discogenic source of back pain is enthesopathy at the junction of the disc and the vertebral endplate.[26] Sixty-one percent of 67 patients tested experienced back pain when this area was stimulated.[27] Horn et al[28] found that insertion regions that had been exposed to overload tensile forces showed the same changes as those observed in epicondylitis in the elbow. There is a strong possibility that pain from disc tears or disc enthesopathy can cause referred pain and quite likely reflex muscle spasm of the functionally related muscles.

Medical practitioners need to be cautious in determining a cause and effect relationship between degenerative disc disease, disc bulge, and disc prolapse in patients presenting with LBP with or without lower extremity pain. In a systematic review, Brinjikji et al[29] reported that the prevalence of degenerative disc disease, disc bulge, and disc protrusions in asymptomatic individuals increased from 37% at age 20 to 96% at age 80, from 30% at age 20 to 84% at age 80, and from 29% at age 20 to 43% at age 80, respectively. The investigators conclude that many degenerative features identified on diagnostic imaging are more likely not associated with pain but are rather part of the normal aging process, and the results of imaging need to be interpreted in the context of the clinical presentation.[29]

The pain referral from disc dysfunction can be similar to the referred pain from TrPs, and the muscle spasm may be a major activator of TrPs in those same muscles. This connection, however, does not assume that the pain is a result of the muscle spasm itself.

It is very likely that most muscle spasms are of somatic–somatic reflex origin outside of the muscle in spasm. For nearly a century, it has been widely accepted that muscle spasms cause pain and that the pain, in turn, perpetuates muscle spasm. Mense et al[30] completed an extensive review of the error of this theory and concluded that clinical research and neuromuscular physiology make that assumption untenable. Nevertheless, a disc dysfunction can be associated with active TrPs. One study found an association between the presence of TrPs in the muscles innervated by the corresponding segmental level (eg, L4-L5 lesion and tibialis anterior muscle TrPs or L5-S1 lesion with gluteus medius and gastrocnemius TrPs) in individuals with lumbar disc prolapse,[31] supporting this theory. Further, Adelmanesh et al[32] found gluteal TrPs in 75% of patients with lumbar radiculopathy, supporting an association between nerve and muscle pain.

1.2. Initial Evaluation of a Patient With Low Back Pain

The first step when screening a patient with LBP is to determine if he or she is appropriate for conservative care and, in this case, for manual therapy. The clinician must perform a careful historical examination and a motor and sensory examination to establish if the patient has any red flag indicators for referral. Further, clinicians should also be conscious of potential psychosocial factors associated with LBP that the patient can exhibit that may contribute to the patient's persistent pain and related disability. For instance, fear-avoidance beliefs have been associated with poor treatment outcome in patients with LBP of less than 6 months[33]; so, earlier identification is relevant.

Emphasis has been placed on matching the patient to optimal interventions based on the identification of signs and symptoms collected during the interview and physical examination. It is, therefore, important to identify the main pain complaint (eg, numbness, weakness, location of symptoms) of the patient to orientate the examination. A body pain drawing is beneficial to establish a pattern and location of the pain. It helps determine if the pain is mainly located in the lumbar spine or radiates and, if it radiates, the distribution of the symptoms. In addition, the quality of the pain can help identify the main tissue responsible for the symptoms or pain referral. Palpation of those muscles that refer pain to the region, for example, the psoas, iliocostalis lumborum, quadratus lumborum, gluteus medius, piriformis, and other muscles, is extremely important.

The physical examination can include elements of observation (lumbar spine posture), active spinal motion testing, palpation, muscle length, muscle strength, passive physiologic and accessory motion testing, as well as special tests for identifying radiating symptoms. All planes of motion of the lumbar spine should be assessed with active and passive movements. Responses during active movements associated with symptoms or pain noted during the clinical history and presence of aberrant movements should be considered highly relevant. For instance, directional preference (movement reducing the symptomatology—centralization) during lumbar spine range of motion can determine a potential therapeutic line of attack. Specific tests of joint mobility or lumbar spine instability (eg, prone instability test), or other additional tests, such as the straight leg raise test, should also be considered. Motor control examination of abdominal wall musculature, particularly the transversus abdominis and lumbar multifidi muscles, should be included. Finally, clinical examination of the hip, sacroiliac joint, and sometimes thoracic spine may also be warranted to determine their contribution to LBP. For instance, the patient can be examined supine for TrPs in the iliopsoas or abdominal wall muscles. In side-lying, quadratus lumborum, tensor fascia latae, gluteus medius, gluteus maximus, gluteus minimus, and latissimus dorsi muscles can be examined. Once prone, the exanimation continues with the lumbar and thoracic paraspinal, multifidi, and piriformis muscles.

1.3. Trigger Points and Low Back Pain

Several authors suggest a potential role in and importance of TrPs as a contributing factor to LBP.[34-36] Bonica and Sola[37] illustrated 11 specific muscles with TrPs that cause LBP. Rosomoff et al[38] found that 96.7% of 283 patients diagnosed of nonspecific LBP because they had "no objective findings" on routine physical examination exhibited active TrPs. Among 18 patients with lumbago, Dejung[36] found that 14 had TrPs in the gluteal muscles, 13 had TrPs in the abdominal muscles, and 8 had TrPs in the paraspinal muscles; additionally 5 other muscles had also TrPs. Most of the patients had multiple muscles with TrPs. One day following TrP injection therapy, patients experienced a 75% reduction in symptoms, suggesting that TrPs were a potential source of symptoms and a contributing factor. However, a cause and effect relationship could not be proven. Teixera et al[39] identified the presence of active TrPs in the quadratus lumborum and gluteus medius muscles in 85.7% of patients suffering from LBP associated to a postlaminectomy pain syndrome. Chen and Nizar[40] reported that 63.5% of patients with chronic LBP exhibited TrPs in the piriformis and lumbar paravertebral muscles. Patients with nonspecific LBP have increased numbers of latent TrPs compared with their healthy counterparts, and those with a greater number of active TrPs have a higher pain intensity. A more recent study found that the most prevalent muscles involved in nonspecific LBP include the iliocostalis lumborum, quadratus lumborum, and gluteus medius muscles.[41] Controlled research studies critically examining the role of TrPs in LBP are conspicuous by their absence and are urgently needed.

Occasionally, one muscle will be responsible for the symptoms as presented, but it is much more common for several muscles to contribute to overlapping pain patterns and related symptoms. The composite pattern resulting depends upon the extent of muscle involvement. No two patients present exactly the same picture.[42] Therefore, it would be reasonable to suggest that inactivation of active TrPs in patients with LBP could often at least help relieve pain symptoms. There is preliminary evidence of this.[43]

Figure 53-1 illustrates an example of a composite pattern produced by TrPs in four muscles that commonly refer pain to the lumbosacral region. Figure 53-2 illustrates a comparable composite pattern produced by TrPs in four muscles that refer pain to the pelvic region. Thus, it is safe to say that the presence of TrPs is very common in LBP, and that a proper examination and treatment of them will help resolve pain and improve motor control to enable return to functional activities. A significant number of patients with this condition have had multiple treatments of either medical intervention, including steroid injections, nerve blocks, gabapentin, opiates and nonopiate pain relievers, as well as traditional physical therapy, osteopathic or chiropractic manipulation and multiple modalities, including electrical stimulation, ultrasound, or laser therapy with varying outcomes.

2. SACROILIAC JOINT DYSFUNCTION

2.1. Overview

Sacroiliac (SI) joint pathology refers to dysfunction of the innominate articulations that creates pelvic pain. Visser et al[44] found that 41% of patients with LBP and leg pain had mechanical pain of the SI joint. Further, Madani et al[45] observed that 72.3% of subjects who had imaging with confirmed herniated disc pathology also displayed clinical signs and symptoms consistent with SI joint pathology. Nevertheless, the SI joint as a source of LBP is a topic of debate. The gold standard for verifying the SI joint as the source of pain is the use of intra-articular anesthetic injections. The prevalence of intra-articular pain arising from the SI joint has been estimated to be as low as 13% and as high

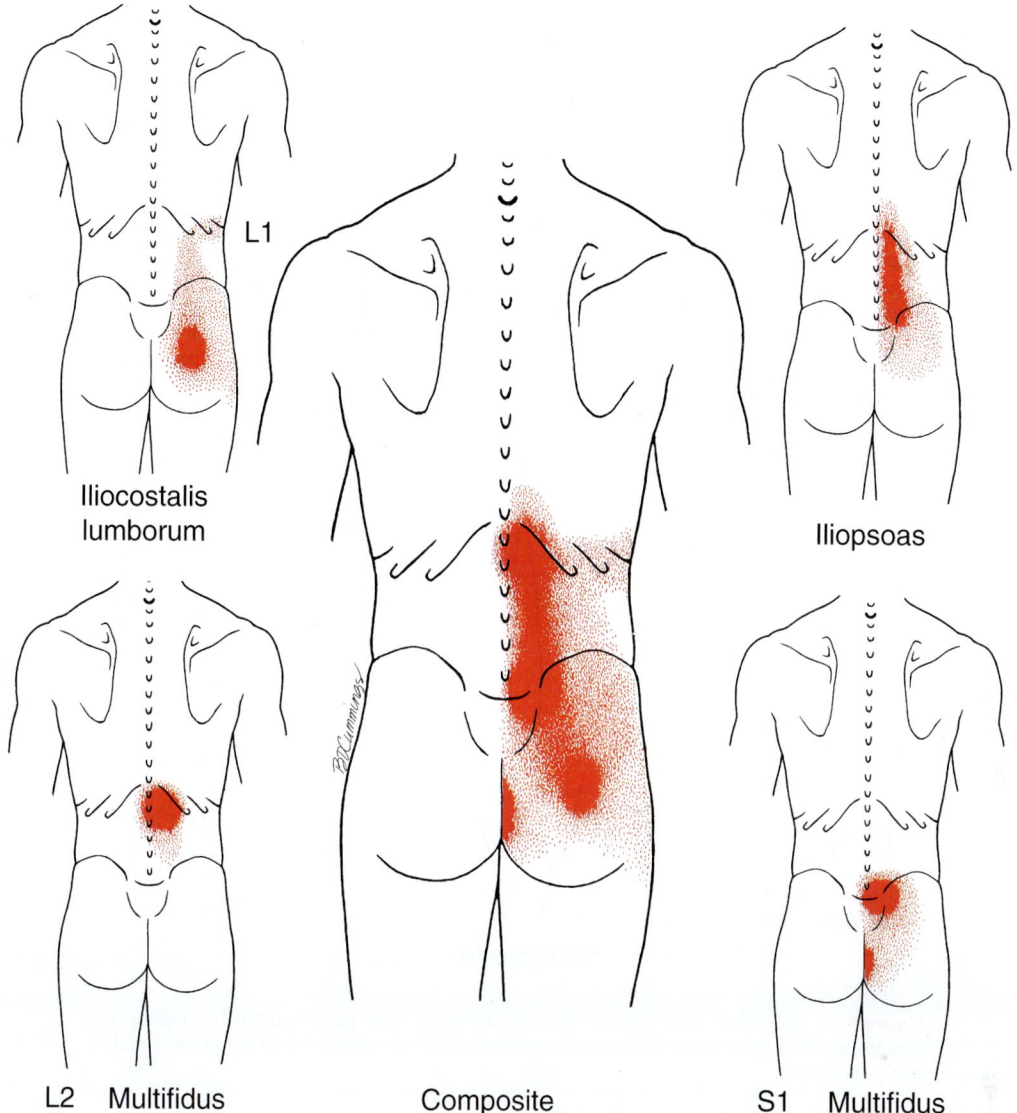

Figure 53-1. Individual referred symptoms of some TrPs that refer pain to the lumbosacral region. The composite pain pattern in the center figure represents the summated referred symptoms a patient may experience.

as 30%.[46-48] Maigne et al[49] found the prevalence to be 18.5% when utilizing double diagnostic anesthetic blocks.

Dreyfuss et al[50] stated that known causes of pain in this region are spondyloarthropathy, crystal and pyogenic arthropathy, fracture of the sacrum and pelvis, and diastasis resulting from pregnancy or childbirth. Other traditionally accepted mechanisms of injury typically include activities that require opposing innominate motion in which one innominate is posteriorly rotated and the other is relatively anteriorly rotated. Falling on to the buttock or heavy lifting may be reported as well. It is important to consider that the SI joint has minimal movement;[48,51] these potential etiologic mechanisms mostly represent changes in compressive forces on the SI joint.

Common signs and symptoms include pain in the region of the sacral sulcus, just medial to the posterior superior iliac spine, and pain that may travel distally into the buttock and posterior thigh. The symptoms generally do not extend beyond the knee or up to the lumbar spine, but Slipman et al[46] noted that occasionally symptoms can travel as far distal as the foot and may also wrap around anteriorly to the groin and sometimes to the abdomen.[46] The symptoms may be aggravated by walking, running, or cycling, movements of sit to stand, twisting activities, rolling over in bed, heavy lifting, and prolonged sitting or standing.

2.2. Initial Evaluation of a Patient With Sacroiliac Joint Dysfunction

Clinical examination of the SI joint is controversial. Pain patterns induced by this joint are debatable, and the ability to detect mobility impairments remains questionable.[48] Pain patterns can help for a first suspicion of associated SI joint pathology. A rectangular pain area just distal to the posterior superior iliac spine has been proposed to be the most often symptomatic pain area for SI joint.[46,52] However, there is high variability in pain referral from SI joint with significant overlap in lumbar pathology, probably due to the complex and variable innervation noted with a proposed contribution of lumbar and sacral roots.[53]

Examination may reveal an apparent leg length discrepancy, thereby affecting both lumbar and thoracic frontal plane curvature. When observed dorsally, there may be the presence of a scoliotic curve. Tests that identify SI joint pathology are classified into the following three categories: motion palpation test, pain provocation tests, and static palpation test for symmetry. The literature shows that pain provocation tests were the most reliable, with palpation being inherently unreliable.[54] Similarly, validity of palpatory and motion symmetry tests for the SI joint has consistently been found to be limited. Therefore, the use of

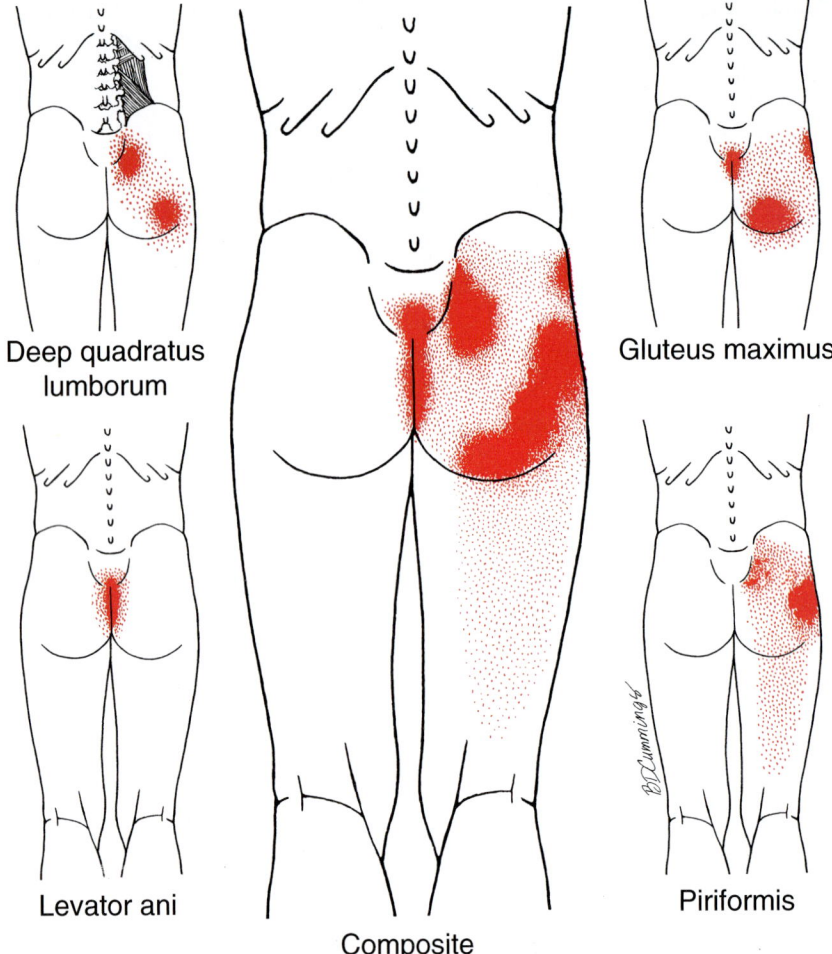

Figure 53-2. Individual pain patterns of some TrPs that refer pain to the pelvic region. The composite pain pattern in the center figure represents the summated referred symptoms a patient may experience.

a cluster of five tests (ie, the thigh thrust test, the compression test, the distraction test, torsional stress test [Gaenslen test], and sacral stress test) emphasizing sacroiliac provocation along with active straight leg raise test and the stork test is an effective evaluation of the SI joint, especially when repeated motions of the lumbopelvic spine have no influence on the symptoms.[55-57] Laslett et al[58] found that the presence of three of these five tests provides a positive likelihood ratio (+LR) of 4.16. Any of these tests is considered positive if they reproduce the patient's comparable sign, that is, familiar symptoms or pain recognition.

2.3. Trigger Points and Sacroiliac Joint Dysfunction

Local pain from SI joint dysfunction could be also mimicked by pain referral from TrPs in some trunk muscles, such as the quadratus lumborum or gluteus medius muscles. When an apparent iliac upslip or innominate shear dysfunction is present, the associated disorder and movement dysfunction at the SI joint may be sustained by inhibition and persistent asymmetrical muscle tension on the pelvis cause by gluteus minimus and medius TrPs. Sacroiliac joint dysfunction can co-exist with piriformis TrPs, and ventral coccygeal tenderness is often associated with a SI joint articular dysfunction.[59] The other muscles likely to be implicated in SI joint dysfunction are the thoracolumbar paraspinals, multifidi, and gluteus maximus muscles. Treatment of SI joint dysfunction requires an effective treatment of associated TrPs, in particular the quadratus lumborum muscle, followed by correction of the articular dysfunction if present or vice versa. In the case of hypermobility, treatment utilizing a stretching technique would be contraindicated. When there are TrPs in muscles that cross hypermobile joints, these TrPs should be inactivated using techniques that do not extend the muscle to its maximum length.

3. LUMBAR STENOSIS

3.1. Overview

Lumbar stenosis may be either central stenosis or lateral stenosis. Central stenosis is a narrowing of the central vertebral canal, and lateral stenosis is a narrowing of the intervertebral foramen. Central stenosis may compromise the cauda equina, whereas lateral stenosis may compromise the spinal nerve roots. Either central or lateral recess stenosis is a degenerative process without a specific history of macro-trauma. It is more common in people with a long history of manual heavy labor jobs and repeat movements of bending or heavy lifting, making the case that stenosis results from micro-trauma. People with lumbar stenosis usually report an insidious onset of LBP.[60] Central stenosis can crowd the lumbar spinal cord or the cauda equine, causing upper motor neuron signs including hyperreflexia, hypertonia, and decreased strength and sensation below the level of pathology. Impingement of the cauda equina can cause lower motor neuron signs, including hyporeflexia, hypotonia, and decreased strength and sensation (saddle anesthesia). Patients with either central or lateral stenosis have low tolerance for trunk extension postures or activities. Patients with lateral stenosis may report pain or sensory changes in one or both lower extremities. Pain may be located below the buttocks or the knees.[61]

3.2. Initial Evaluation of a Patient With Lumbar Stenosis

Physical examination findings include decreased lumbar extension with pain reproduction. Lower extremity pain is reproduced with trunk extension or active hip extension. A positive two-staged treadmill test will show increased time needed to develop symptoms when walking uphill and less recovery time needed when compared with walking on a level surface.[62] Neurologic findings may include an abnormal Romberg test, sensory vibration deficit, lower extremity weakness, and decreased peripheral deep tendon reflexes.[61]

3.3. Trigger Points and Lumbar Stenosis

Because of the degenerative nature of spinal stenosis, symptoms are most likely managed with therapeutic strategies for keeping the intervertebral foramina relatively open by biasing the lumbar spine into a flexion posture combined with mobility exercises to maximize hip and thoracic extension range of motion. Treatment should include abdominal muscle neuromuscular reeducation along with manual therapy to restore lumbar accessory motion, stretching of the one and two joint hip flexors, and progressive body-weight-supported treadmill walking program.[63] If back pain and lower extremity pain are present, TrPs that typically refer to these areas should be specifically assessed. If present, the patient should be taught TrP self-pressure release, instructed in proper resting and active postures, and prescribed a home exercise program. It is highly unlikely that TrP therapy alone will have any long-lasting effect; however, it should be a part of the comprehensive rehabilitation program that may reduce the pain and discomfort associated with the myofascial contributions to the pain presentation.

4. LUMBAR INSTABILITY

4.1. Overview

Identification and management of lumbar spine instability is a challenge for clinicians and their patients. Chronic lumbar instability is presented as a term that can encompass two types of lumbar instability: mechanical (radiographic) and functional (clinical) instability. The components of mechanical and functional instability are presented relative to the development of diagnosis and management. Lumbar segmental instability can be caused by several factors. The excessive intervertebral motion may be due to degenerative changes in the intervertebral disc, spondylolisthesis, fracture, trauma, or a previous surgical procedure. This excessive motion can put pressure on the spinal cord, cauda equina, or nerve roots. Excessive intersegmental motion can also put undue stress on the facet joint capsule or ligaments. The primary age group to experience lumbar instability is 20- to 30-year-olds. Epidemiologic studies using a diagnosis of functional instability are lacking. Puntumetakul et al[64] found the prevalence of clinical lumbar instability in Thai rice farmers to be 13%.

Patients with lumbar segmental instability have been proposed as a unique subgroup of patients with LBP; there have been conflicting studies regarding criteria to define this condition. Hicks et al[65] described a clinical prediction rule for patients with LBP who would be successful with a stabilization classification for treatment (clinical lumbar instability). These authors found that patients who achieve positive outcomes are more than 40 years of age, have a positive prone instability test, the presence of aberrant movements, and a passive straight leg raise test >90°.[65]

4.2. Initial Evaluation of a Patient With Clinical Lumbar Instability

A postural examination can reveal posterior skin creases in the trunk and a limited trunk range of motion in a specific direction, with a possible painful arc of motion. The patient may demonstrate excessive range of motion and abnormal (aberrant) quality of movement with hinging or catching. For instance, an instability catch or hinge in returning from spinal flexion, as well as functional asterisk signs that reproduce the patient's symptoms during such acitivities as going from sit to stand or any other transitional positions, can appear during the active range of motion assessment. In fact, the most common objective factors related to clinical lumbar instability include poor lumbopelvic control such as segmental hinging or pivoting with movement, poor proprioceptive function, poor coordination and neuromuscular control such as juddering or shaking during movement, and decreased strength and endurance of local muscles at a level of segmental instability. Abnormal accessory movement testing, indicating loss of stiffness or increased neutral zone at one segment, is usually present. Passive tests commonly used for clinical lumbar instability include passive accessory intervertebral motion, passive physiologic intervertebral motion, prone instability test, and the prone lumbar extension test.[66] Ferrari et al[67] reported that the prone instability test and the passive lumbar extension test exhibited the highest clinical utility to detect lumbar instability in specific LBP. However, the reliability of these tests has been questioned by others.[68]

4.3. Trigger Points and Lumbar Instability

There may be palpable taut bands indicative of TrPs and facilitation of postural muscles. Therefore, if pain is present, a TrP evaluation should be performed in patients with a suspicion of clinical lumbar instability. However, with this diagnosis, rehabilitation should include proprioceptive training along with specific exercises to facilitate recruitment of the stabilizing muscles, including the deep fibers of the multifidi, transverse abdominus, diaphragm, and pelvic floor muscles as well as TrP therapy. All these muscles should be carefully examined for TrPs, either active or latent, as they could cause dysfunctional muscle activation patterns, early fatigue, and prolonged recovery period. It is possible that TrPs in the local stabilizer muscles can perpetuate muscle imbalance, hence promoting pronounced clinical lumbar instability.

5. LUMBAR LIGAMENT SPRAIN AND STRAIN

5.1. Overview

Lumbar spine sprain and lumbar spine strain are often used interchangeably. A strain refers to injury to a musculotendinous structure, whereas a sprain is a capsuloligamentous injury that arises when ligaments become torn from their attachments, affecting the important relationship between bone and ligament. LBP is sometimes diagnosed as a lumbar spine sprain or muscle strain. Symptoms can be localized to the lumbar spine or they can radiate down into the buttocks. In general, this pain will not spread into the legs, which differentiates lumbar sprain from certain other spinal injuries. Pain will be exacerbated during physical activity and should be reduced during periods of rest. The patient may experience occasional spasms in the lower back. These symptoms are all consistent with lumbar sprain and muscle strain, but if the patient feels weakness in the back, or has poor bowel or bladder control, it may be a more serious injury requiring immediate attention.

The structures of the spine are working almost constantly to maintain strength and balance during innumerable activities and therefore the muscles and ligaments of the lumber spine can be prone to injury through repetitive overuse and micro-trauma. A single incident involving a twisting maneuver or sharp movement can cause injury. There are many other ways with which a sprain can occur, but some recurring contributing factors have been singled out. For instance, unsuitable lifting techniques and sustained awkward postures can cause injury to the lumbar spine. Other risk factors are a lack of sufficient flexibility and strength in the muscles of the back or lower extremities, especially if you rely greatly on the lumbar spine for static and dynamic postures. Additionally, obesity, smoking, deconditioning, poor body mechanics, limited hip flexibility/mobility, and poor trunk strength/dynamic stabilization may be contributing factors.

5.2. Initial Evaluation of a Patient With Lumbar Ligament Sprain

During the physical examination, patients usually present with painful, limited trunk motion in a given direction, whereas other motions may be within normal limits. Active and resistive hip motions may elicit symptoms, and a Gower sign may be present. In cases of complete ligamentous tear, excessive motion may be present but difficult to accurately assess. Clinical diagnosis of lumbar ligament sprain is highly difficult, and it will be based on the presence of a traumatic event as reported in the clinical history. Palpation of the ligament, for example, interspinous or iliolumbar, is usually extremely painful and can elicit pain referral.

5.3. Trigger Points and Lumbar Ligament Sprain

Clinicians should consider that lumbar ligament sprains can also be associated with muscle dysfunctions. Jinkins[69] observed that individuals with lumbosacral interspinous ligament sprain also exhibited associated intrinsic spinal muscle degeneration in the innervated muscles such as multifidi muscles. An important differential diagnosis of symptoms caused by TrPs in thoracolumbar paraspinal muscles includes articular dysfunctions. The chief complaint cause by TrPs in thoracolumbar paraspinal muscles is pain in the back and buttocks. Pain with ligament sprain injury is usually located in the low back and buttocks as well. Trigger points in the following muscles must be considered in a patient with lumbar ligament sprain: thoracolumbar paraspinals, multifidi, lower rectus abdominus, iliopsoas, gluteus medius, gluteus maximus, and quadratus lumborum muscles.

Typical rehabilitation for this condition may begin with exercises in pain-free motions, followed by basic stabilization exercises of the abdominals, hip extensors, hip abductors, and spinal extensors, followed by dynamic and functional stabilization exercises. The only problems that may arise with an exercise regime is that if TrPs have developed in any of the muscles mentioned earlier, the effects of exercise could be limited. Exercises can exacerbate pain due to TrP referral even in the absence of reinjury.

6. SPONDYLOLYSIS AND SPONDYLOLISTHESIS

6.1. Overview

Spondylolysis and spondylolisthesis are common causes of LBP in young athletes where overloading of the posterior elements of the lumbar spine is repetitive or excessive.[70] Spondylolysis is a defect in the pars interarticularis, whereas a spondylolisthesis is a fracture defect that widens and allows the superior segment to slip forward on the inferior segment. The injury most often occurs in children and adolescents who participate in sports that involve repeated stress on the lower back, such as gymnastics, football, and weight lifting. People with this condition have no symptoms. In general, people with spondylolisthesis will report mild-to-moderate back and/or leg pain that is increased with extension positions. The pain may radiate into the buttocks, posterior thighs, or lower legs. Degenerative spondylolisthesis will present with more of a history of lumbar stenosis, and because of instability, patients may complain of catching or shifting in the back with motion. For most patients with these conditions, back pain and other symptoms will improve with conservative treatment. This always begins with a period of rest from sports and other strenuous activities. Patients who have persistent back pain or severe slippage of a vertebra may need surgery to relieve their symptoms and to allow for a return to sports and activities.[71]

6.2. Initial Evaluation of a Patient With Spondylolysis and Spondylolisthesis

The postural examination often reveals an increase in the lumbar lordosis, painful limited trunk extension, hamstring length deficits, weakness/pain in one or both lower extremities, and local pain with posterior–anterior provocation. Neurologic signs may be present depending on the severity of the condition, and in the case of spondylolisthesis, there may be a step-off deformity when palpating the spinous processes. Radiographs in the oblique plane will show a fracture in the region of the pars interarticularis, commonly referred to as "scotty dog collar fracture."

6.3. Trigger Points and Spondylolysis and Spondylolisthesis

Rehabilitation includes avoiding activities that aggravate the symptoms and the administration of anti-inflammatories. Bracing with a thoraco-lumbo-sacral orthosis may be included along with exercises such as muscle strengthening for trunk stabilization biased toward flexion-based exercises and hip and hamstring mobility/flexibility exercises. Trigger points are not common with this condition; however, if pain is persistent in the low back, buttocks, and posterior thighs, then the associated TrPs for those areas should be examined and treated, especially the iliopsoas, quadratus lumborum, and abdominal muscles. In fact, there is evidence supporting that patients with isthmic spondylolisthesis suffer selective atrophy of their lumbar multifidi muscles, whereas their erector spinae muscles undergo a compensatory hypertrophy.[72] This compensatory mechanism could activate TrPs in the paraspinal muscles.

7. ANKYLOSING SPONDYLITIS

7.1. Overview

Ankylosing spondylitis (AS) is a chronic inflammatory disease commonly referred to as one of the spondyloarthritides. Typically, it affects the spine and the SI joints. Occasionally, other joints such as the shoulders or hips are involved. Eye and bowel problems may also occur. Between 0.1% and 1.8% of people are affected.[73] Back pain of inflammatory features and morning stiffness are the characteristic symptoms of AS. Symptoms often have periods of exacerbation and dormancy that can result in a delay in the diagnosis.[74] Stiffness of the affected joints generally worsens over time. There is a 5:1 ratio of men to women affected, and onset is typically between the ages of 30 and 50, though it may occur earlier in life.[74] The cause of AS is currently unknown, but it is believed to involve a combination of genetic and environmental factors. The underlying mechanism is believed to be autoimmune or autoinflammatory. Diagnosis is typically based on the symptoms with support from medical imaging and blood tests. There is no cure for AS, but potential treatments, eg, medication, exercise, and surgery, may improve symptoms and slow the progression of the disease. Medications include nonsteroidal anti-inflammatory drugs (NSAIDs), steroids, disease-modifying anti-rheumatic drugs (DMARDs) such as sulfasalazine, and biologic agents such as infliximab.

Common symptoms are inflammatory lumbar pain rather than mechanically based pain. Patients typically report onset of gluteal pain and stiffness that is often described as dull and hard to localize. Pain may alternate from side to side and is typically intermittent at the onset, and as the pathology progresses, the pain usually affects both gluteal regions and becomes constant. The pain is occasionally referred toward the iliac crest, greater trochanter region, or down the posterior thigh with associated hamstring length deficits. One of the main features of lumbar pain associated with AS is that the pain wakes the patient up at night, and only walking relieves the pain. Lumbar pain and stiffness may occur along with gluteal pain and is usually worse in the AM for approximately 1 to 2 hours after waking. Pain and enthesitis may be present in the Achilles tendon and plantar fascia and may also affect the knees and shoulders.[74] Redness in one eye at a time and photophobia may also be present. Among all therapeutic tools, exercise has been demonstrated to be the most effective for these patients.[75]

7.2. Initial Evaluation of a Patient With Ankylosing Spondylitis

Postural examination typically reveals a flattening of the lumbar lordosis, an increased thoracic kyphosis, upper cervical spine extension with a forward head posture, and knees and hips in slight flexion. As the disease progresses, the intervertebral joints fuse, resulting in a Bamboo Spine.[74] There will be an associated loss of range of motion that correlates with these changes.

7.3. Trigger Points and Ankylosing Spondylitis

Because pain and stiffness can be a significant factor in the progression of the disease, it warrants an examination for the presence of TrPs as a contributing factor to the patient's pain complaints. A pain drawing will be beneficial to assist the clinician in identifying which muscles to examine. Very commonly, the patient may report symptoms in the gluteal region, lateral proximal thigh and down the posterior thigh, to heel and foot. Symptoms in the gluteal region can be induced by TrPs in the iliocostalis lumborum, longissimus thoracis, gluteus medius, minimus and maximus, and quadratus lumborum muscles. Symptoms in the hip and posterior thigh region can be related to TrPs in the quadratus lumborum, tensor fascia latae, hip lateral rotators, and hamstring musculature. Symptoms in the heel and plantar surface of the foot can be reproduced by stimulation of TrPs in the gastrocnemius, soleus, tibialis posterior, and the muscles on the plantar aspect of the foot. Rehabilitation programs should include treatment of those TrPs in conjunction with stretching and strengthening exercises that promote efficient posture and spinal mobility.[75] Diaphragmatic breathing exercises should be incorporated to increase thoracic, rib cage, and chest wall mobility, as well as pulmonary function. Cardiovascular endurance exercises will also help maintain and progress overall fitness. The prognosis for AS is good in the long term.

8. CHRONIC PELVIC PAIN
8.1. Overview

Chronic pelvic pain (CPP) is defined as "non-malignant pain perceived in the structures related to the pelvis of either men or women."[76] CPP has multiple potential etiologic features, and its prevalence ranges from 15% to 20%.[77] Several pain syndromes are included within this term: bladder pain syndrome, endometriosis pain syndrome, interstitial cystitis, prostatic pain syndrome, dysmenorrhea, and vulvodynia are a few examples.[76] Chronic pelvic pain syndrome (CPPS) is relatively poorly understood, even by some specialists in genitourinary dysfunction, and certainly by the general health care community. There is evidence suggesting that CPP can become chronic[78] and that sensitization of the central nervous system is involved in these syndromes[76,79]; therefore, examination and treatment programs should be directed at both biomechanical and neurophysiologic issues.[80]

From a biomechanical point of view, a connection between chronic sacroiliac dysfunction and a wide range of pelvic floor–related problems (CPP) has been suggested, and many patients diagnosed with SI pain also have CPP.[81] In addition, there is evidence supporting an interaction between TrPs and central sensitization in women with CPP associated to endometriosis.[82]

Considering psychological factors is important when treating patients with CPP, because they often exhibit anxiety, depression, alexithymia, catastrophizing beliefs, fear-avoidance behaviors, or hypervigilance.[83,84] These psychological variables may be related to the fact that CPP is usually associated with sexual dysfunction.[85] Treatment of CPP should be biopsychosocial, in nature including physical and psychological approaches.[86,87]

8.2. Initial Evaluation of a Patient With Chronic Pelvic Pain

Clinical examination of a patient with CPP should include active and passive movements of the lumbar spine and the reproduction of symptoms (directional preference) with movement or during a static position, for example, sitting. Symptoms usually appear with prolonged sitting positions when the pelvic floor musculature is under stress. There is not a clear posture of the spine (lordosis, flattened, sideways) associated with CPP. Women with CPP, particularly if they had endometriosis or pain related to the menstrual cycle, can adopt an antalgic posture in lumbar flexion during prolonged static positioning.

One of the most relevant examinations for patients with CPP is evaluation of abdominal wall muscles. In fact, motor control impairments, such as delayed transversus abdominis muscle activation, changes in multifidi muscle morphology, or pelvic floor musculature hypertonicity, can be present. Abdominal TrPs should be explored in all individuals with CPP because they are the most prevalent[88,89] and also predict evidence of visceral disease in 90% of patients with symptoms compatible with CPP.[90] Other muscles that could exhibit TrPs in CPP include the gluteal, adductors, internal and external rotators of the hip, piriformis, iliopsoas, quadratus lumborum, lumbar multifidi, thoracolumbar paraspinals, and obviously, the pelvic floor muscles. In fact, examination of pelvic floor muscles is an important element of the clinical evaluation of women with CPP.[91] The pelvic floor muscles may be hyper or hypotonic in patients with CPP; clinicians should also explore the SI and hip joints to determine any joint impairment that could be involved. Since abdominal TrPs may be perpetuated by paradoxical respiration, the examination of the breathing patterns and diaphragm muscle should also be conducted. Anderson[92] has described palpation and treatment protocols for locating TrPs associated with prostatitis symptoms. Box 53-1 describes TrPs that may be associated with somatovisceral symptoms.

8.3. Trigger Points and Chronic Pelvic Pain

It is important to consider that TrPs may mimic visceral pain and also induce visceral disorders, that is, the somatovisceral effect. Conversely, a visceral disease can also influence somatosensory

Box 53-1 Somatovisceral referred symptoms from trigger points in the abdominal muscles

Referred somatovisceral symptoms from abdominal muscle trigger points	
Muscles	Referred symptoms
External abdominal oblique	Heartburn and symptoms associated with hiatal hernia, deep epigastric pain
Lateral abdominal wall (external and internal abdominal oblique)	Testicular pain, lower quadrant pain
Internal abdominal oblique	Pain in urinary bladder region, urinary frequency or retention, chronic diarrhea
Rectus abdominis (upper portion)	Nausea, epigastric distress, symptoms of cholycystitis, and peptic ulcer.
Rectus abdominis (umbilical level)	Abdominal cramping, abdominal colic
Rectus abdominis (lower portion)	Dysmenorrhea
Right lower abdominal region	Diarrhea, diverticulosis, gynecologic symptoms
Just proximal to pubis	Urinary frequency and retention, detrusor muscle spasm
Region of McBurney point	Ipsilateral lower quadrant and penis

perception and can activate TrPs, that is, the viscerosomatic effect, which may perpetuate pain and other symptoms after the patient has recovered from the initiating visceral disease.[93] Therefore, understanding the reciprocal somatovisceral and viscerosomatic effects regarding TrPs helps unravel some CPPSs. This connection is supported by the fact that abdominal TrPs have a 93% positive predictive value for visceral disease, particularly for CPP.[90,94] Studies have found that the presence of abdominal TrPs along with abdominal and perineal cutaneous allodynia discriminated visceral from somatic sources of pain.[94]

There is clear evidence associating CPP with the presence of TrPs.[95,96] In fact, the clinical guideline published by the European Association of Urology suggests that TrPs should be considered in the diagnosis of CPP as there is evidence demonstrating the relationship between CPP and TrPs.[76] Moldwin and Fariello[97] observed that active TrPs of the pelvic floor muscles were responsible for some, if not all, symptoms related to these pain syndromes in as many as 85% of individuals suffering from urologic, colorectal, and gynecologic pain syndromes. Anderson et al[88] identified the most common location of TrPs in men with CPP: pubococcygeus or puborectalis (90%), external oblique (80%), rectus abdominis (75%), adductors (19%), and gluteus medius (18%) muscles.

Therapeutic approaches aimed at deactivating TrPs, as well as normalizing joint and soft tissue imbalances, together with concomitant postural and breathing pattern retraining, have been shown to be effective for modulating associated symptoms in individuals with various CPPSs, including interstitial cystitis, stress incontinence, irritable bowel syndrome, and chronic prostatitis, among others.[98-103] For that reason, the potential role of TrPs in CPPSs should always be considered when treating these patients.

9. THORACIC AND CHEST PAIN

9.1. Overview

Thoracic and chest pain are common presentations in general practice, which because of diverse and potentially serious causes, particularly related to potential underlying visceral diseases, requires careful and sometimes urgent assessment.[104] Although it is important to rule out life-threatening medical conditions in a primary care setting, musculoskeletal conditions are the most common causes of thoracic and chest pain.[105] Even so, they represent only 6.2% of patients presenting to hospital emergency departments with chest pain.[106] Briggs et al[107] found that the 1-year prevalence of musculoskeletal thoracic spine pain ranged from 3.0% to 55.0% in an adult working population. A systematic review identified that the point prevalence for thoracic pain of musculoskeletal origin ranged from 4% to 72%, the 1-year prevalence from 3.5% to 34.8%, and the lifetime prevalence from 15.6% to 19.5%.[108] The prevalence of thoracic spine pain is higher in women than in men, with a female-to-male ratio of 2:1.[109] Eslick et al[110] found that 35% of individuals reporting noncardiac chest pain also described pain that could be musculoskeletal in origin. Leboeuf-Yde et al[111] reported a 1-year prevalence of radiating pain from the thoracic spine to the chest of 5%. Looking at the clinical features and causes of chest pain in children referred to a pediatric cardiology unit, Sert et al[112] found that the most common causes were musculoskeletal (37.1%), and only 0.3% were cardiac in nature.

It is suggested that the causes of musculoskeletal thoracic and chest wall pain can be grouped into three categories[105]: (1) conditions causing isolated musculoskeletal pain (eg, costochondritis, lower rib pain syndromes, pain from thoracic spine/costovertebral joints, or muscle referred pan from TrPs); (2) rheumatic diseases (eg, fibromyalgia syndrome or rheumatoid arthritis); and (3) systemic nonrheumatologic conditions (eg, osteoporotic fracture, tumors). For instance, costochondritis, an acute and often temporary inflammation of the costal cartilage, is a common cause of chest pain[113] with a prevalence of 13%.[114] The report of symptoms from costochondritis is similar to that of chest pain associated with myocardial infarction.[115] Severe cases of costal cartilage inflammation that also involve painful swelling are sometimes referred to as Tietze syndrome, a term usually used interchangeably with costochondritis. However, some clinicians view costochondritis and Tietze syndrome as separate disease states because of the absence of costal cartilage swelling in costochondritis.[104] Pain may be provoked at rest, during movement of the ribcage, or related to breathing as both syndromes have been associated to repetitive physical activity. For this reason, a differential diagnosis of chest wall pain from other musculoskeletal structures is crucial.

It is also important to consider that several viscera refer to different levels of the thoracic spine, including the heart, aorta, lungs, esophagus, stomach, duodenum, pancreas, gall bladder, liver, kidney, and ureter. For instance, thoracic pain is highly prevalent in patients with chronic obstructive pulmonary disease.[116,117] An association between viscera disease and muscle thoracic pain is the activation of viscerosomatic reflexes, as it has also been commented in the Chronic Pelvic Pain section. Confirming this hypothesis, Bentsen et al[118] postulated that thoracic pain and dyspnea could be related because primary and accessory muscles of breathing in patients with chronic obstructive pulmonary disease are frequently used to manage their breathlessness.

Current evidence suggests that musculoskeletal thoracic and chest pain should be treated with a multimodal program of care, including manual therapy, soft tissue therapy, exercises, heat/ice, advice, and educational sessions,[119] supporting the complexity of the thoracic/chest pain conditions.

9.2. Initial Evaluation of a Patient With Thoracic and Chest Pain

Chest pain needs to be fully characterized by onset, site(s), radiation, and relieving and exacerbating factors (particularly any relationship to posture, specific activities, or acute trauma). Atypical symptoms, such as night pain or severe pain, alert the clinician to look for systemic causes such as fractures, infection, or neoplasm. Proper screening for underlying medical conditions is important to establish accurate diagnosis and develop the optimal plan of care. Localization of the symptoms, the presence of chest wall tenderness, or the reproduction of pain by movements are insufficient to justify ruling out serious nonmusculoskeletal causes.

The musculoskeletal examination includes evaluation of the posture of the ribs; chest wall; and cervical, thoracic, and lumbar musculature and vertebrae. A key point is to identify areas of tenderness in the thoracic spine, chest, and ribs. Muscle tenderness is usually associated with medical pathologies such as costochondritis. Important areas to palpate include costochondral joints, sternum, ribs, thoracic vertebrae, and associated muscles such as intercostals, paraspinal, trapezius, pectoral, and scalene muscles. Pain provocation during active or passive movements of the spine (ie, flexion, extension, lateral flexion, and rotation) should also be assessed.

Another important aspect for clinical evaluation is the assessment of facet joint mobility. The prevalence of thoracic pain from facet joints is reported to range from 34% to 48%.[120,121] In one study including four pain-free individuals, injecting facet joints with contrast caused two participants to report referral patterns toward the sternum.[122] Similarly, injection of the costotransverse joints produced thoracic, but not chest, pain.[123] Segmental dysfunction in the lower cervical (C4-C7) and upper thoracic spine (T1-T8) may cause pain referred to the anterior aspects of the chest. Christensen et al[124] found that 18% of patients with chronic chest pain admitted for coronary angiography at a cardiology department exhibited cervicothoracic and thoracic spine dysfunctions reproducing their symptoms. It should always be considered that the reliability of manual palpation of mobility or tenderness in the chest wall is limited.[125,126]

The pain referral of thoracic interspinous ligaments[127] and paravertebral muscles[128] has also been investigated using injections of hypertonic saline that has shown referred pain to the anterior, lateral, and posterior chest and lower thoracic segments referring lower on the chest. In fact, individuals with costochondritis exhibiting pain during breathing may overactivate accessory muscles such as the scalene muscles secondary to pain, which will prevent expansion of the rib cage. Trigger points located in several muscles of the rib cage and thoracic region can be overloaded, including the lower cervical and thoracic multifidi, thoracic longissimus and iliocostalis, psoas, latissimus dorsi, serratus posterior inferior, rectus abdominus, scalenes, and rhomboid muscles.

9.3. Trigger Points and Thoracic and Chest Pain

The presence of chest pain of myofascial origin was described many years ago.[129] For instance, TrPs in the pectoralis musculature can stimulate the symptoms of angina pectoris. As described in Chapters 42, 43, and 44, the pain patterns of the pectoralis major, sternalis, and pectoralis minor muscles can mimic the pain referral patterns of cardiac ischemia. Lawson et al[130] described a patient with anterior chest pain and normal cardiac examination findings in which active TrPs in the pectoralis minor muscle reproduced the symptoms. After treatment of the TrP, the symptoms disappeared. Although the pain referral elicited by some muscles strongly mimics cardiac pain, TrP pain has a much wider variability in its response to day-to-day activity than the more consistent exercise response on angina pectoris. A definite diagnosis of active TrPs based on their characteristic signs and symptoms and a positive response to local treatment does not exclude cardiac disease. 20% of individuals referred for coronary angiography can also exhibit musculoskeletal chest pain.[124] It is also possible that the small musculature of the thoracic levels related to the affected viscera, including the thoracic multifidi muscles, also develops TrPs. The intercostal muscles have also been implicated in cardiac arrhythmia, and sternalis TrPs can closely mimic the substernal ache of myocardial infarction or angina pectoris.[42] All are examples of different viscerosomatic reflexes.

Abdominal visceral diseases can also produce pain patterns that closely resemble those from TrPs. These include diaphragmatic hernia, peptic ulcer, gastric carcinoma, chronic cholecystitis, gallstone colic, ureteral colic, inguinal hernia, hepatitis, pancreatitis, appendicitis, diverticulitis, colitis, cystitis, and endometriosis. Other common medical conditions include esophagitis, hiatal hernia with reflux, and spastic colon.[42] Some infections, such as postherpetic neuralgia after herpes zoster, can also activate TrPs in the related muscles, like the intercostal muscles.[131] Box 53-1 identifies TrPs that may be associated with somatovisceral symptoms.

Current evidence about the presence of TrPs in the thoracic spine is lacking. Roldan and Huh[132] investigated the pain of myofascial origin in 43 patients who presented to the emergency room with reports of pain in the back, chest, abdomen, or pelvis. The iliocostalis thoracis and lumborum muscles were examined for the presence of TrPs that reproduced the patient's report of pain. They injected the iliocostalis TrPs, and 2 weeks after injection, all patients had satisfactory control of symptoms and no return visits to the emergency room. There is also preliminary evidence suggesting that proper treatment of myofascial tissues is effective for the management of pain in patients with thoracic visceral diseases. Berg et al[133] described that soft tissue treatment was effective in patients with stable coronary heart disease and self-reported chest pain reproduced by the palpation of intercostal TrPs, supporting the role of muscle pain referral in chest pain of noncardiac origin. Fernández de las Peñas et al[134] discussed clinical evidence about the role of TrPs in thoracic spine pain and their management with dry needling. Rock and Rainey[135] reported a case series where the application of dry needling, combined with electrical stimulation on TrPs of the thoracic spine muscles, such as multifidi, longissimus, and iliocostalis muscles, was effective for reducing symptoms of nonspecific thoracic pain.[136]

References

1. GBD 2015 Disease and Injury Incidence and Prevalence Collaborators. Global, regional, and national incidence, prevalence, and years lived with disability for 310 diseases and injuries, 1990-2015: a systematic analysis for the Global Burden of Disease Study 2015. *Lancet*. 2016;388:1545-1602.
2. Katz JN. Lumbar disc disorders and low-back pain: socioeconomic factors and consequences. *J Bone Joint Surg Am*. 2006;88 suppl 2:21-24.
3. Yelin E. Cost of musculoskeletal diseases: impact of work disability and functional decline. *J Rheumatol Suppl*. 2003;68:8-11.
4. Hoy D, March L, Brooks P, et al. The global burden of low back pain: estimates from the Global Burden of Disease 2010 study. *Ann Rheum Dis*. 2014;73(6):968-974.
5. Jackson T, Thomas S, Stabile V, Han X, Shotwell M, McQueen K. Prevalence of chronic pain in low-income and middle-income countries: a systematic review and meta-analysis. *Lancet*. 2015;385 suppl 2:S10.
6. Edwards J, Hayden J, Asbridge M, Gregoire B, Magee K. Prevalence of low back pain in emergency settings: a systematic review and meta-analysis. *BMC Musculoskelet Disord*. 2017;18(1):143.
7. Freburger JK, Holmes GM, Agans RP, et al. The rising prevalence of chronic low back pain. *Arch Intern Med*. 2009;169(3):251-258.
8. Palacios-Ceña D, Alonso-Blanco C, Hernandez-Barrera V, Carrasco-Garrido P, Jimenez-Garcia R, Fernández de las Peñas C. Prevalence of neck and low back

pain in community-dwelling adults in Spain: an updated population-based national study (2009/10-2011/12). *Eur Spine J.* 2015;24(3):482-492.
9. Becker A, Held H, Redaelli M, et al. Low back pain in primary care: costs of care and prediction of future health care utilization. *Spine (Phila Pa 1976).* 2010;35(18):1714-1720.
10. Rabey M, Beales D, Slater H, O'Sullivan P. Multidimensional pain profiles in four cases of chronic non-specific axial low back pain: an examination of the limitations of contemporary classification systems. *Man Ther.* 2015;20(1):138-147.
11. Alrwaily M, Timko M, Schneider M, et al. Treatment-based classification system for low back pain: revision and update. *Phys Ther.* 2016;96(7):1057-1066.
12. Nijs J, Apeldoorn A, Hallegraeff H, et al. Low back pain: guidelines for the clinical classification of predominant neuropathic, nociceptive, or central sensitization pain. *Pain Physician.* 2015;18(3):E333-E346.
13. American Academy of Physical Medicine and Rehabilitation. Academy declines to endorse guideline for low back pain. *Arch Phys Med Rehabil.* 1995;76:294.
14. National Institute for Health and Care Excellence (NICE). Low back pain and sciatica in over 16s: assessment and management. London. 2016. (NG59). https://www.nice.org.uk/guidance/ng59. Accessed September 15, 2017.
15. Qaseem A, Wilt TJ, McLean RM, Forciea MA; Clinical Guidelines Committee of the American College of Physicians. Noninvasive treatments for acute, subacute, and chronic low back pain: a clinical practice guideline from the American College of Physicians. *Ann Intern Med.* 2017;166(7):514-530.
16. Chetty L. A critical review of low back pain guidelines. *Workplace Health Saf.* 2017;65(9):388-394.
17. Flavell CA, Gordon S, Marshman L. Classification characteristics of a chronic low back pain population using a combined McKenzie and patho-anatomical assessment. *Man Ther.* 2016;26:201-207.
18. Van Dillen LR, Sahrmann SA, Norton BJ, Caldwell CA, McDonnell MK, Bloom NJ. Movement system impairment-based categories for low back pain: stage 1 validation. *J Orthop Sports Phys Ther.* 2003;33(3):126-142.
19. Fritz JM, Delitto A, Erhard RE. Comparison of classification-based physical therapy with therapy based on clinical practice guidelines for patients with acute low back pain: a randomized clinical trial. *Spine (Phila Pa 1976).* 2003;28(13):1363-1371; discussion 1372.
20. Brennan GP, Fritz JM, Hunter SJ, Thackeray A, Delitto A, Erhard RE. Identifying subgroups of patients with acute/subacute "nonspecific" low back pain: results of a randomized clinical trial. *Spine (Phila Pa 1976).* 2006;31(6):623-631.
21. Atlas SJ, Keller RB, Wu YA, Deyo RA, Singer DE. Long-term outcomes of surgical and nonsurgical management of sciatica secondary to a lumbar disc herniation: 10 year results from the maine lumbar spine study. *Spine (Phila Pa 1976).* 2005;30(8):927-935.
22. Deville WL, van der Windt DA, Dzaferagic A, Bezemer PD, Bouter LM. The test of Lasegue: systematic review of the accuracy in diagnosing herniated discs. *Spine (Phila Pa 1976).* 2000;25(9):1140-1147.
23. Brinjikji W, Diehn FE, Jarvik JG, et al. MRI findings of disc degeneration are more prevalent in adults with low back pain than in asymptomatic controls: a systematic review and meta-analysis. *AJNR Am J Neuroradiol.* 2015;36(12):2394-2399.
24. Cheung KM, Karppinen J, Chan D, et al. Prevalence and pattern of lumbar magnetic resonance imaging changes in a population study of one thousand forty-three individuals. *Spine (Phila Pa 1976).* 2009;34(9):934-940.
25. Zhang YG, Guo TM, Guo X, Wu SX. Clinical diagnosis for discogenic low back pain. *Int J Biol Sci.* 2009;5(7):647-658.
26. Kuslich SD, Ulstrom CL, Michael CJ. The tissue origin of low back pain and sciatica: a report of pain response to tissue stimulation during operations on the lumbar spine using local anesthesia. *Orthop Clin North Am.* 1991;22(2):181-187.
27. Bogduk N. Lumbar dorsal ramus syndrome. *Med J Aust.* 1980;2:537-541.
28. Horn V, Vlach O, Messner P. Enthesopathy in the vertebral disc region. *Arch Orthop Trauma Surg.* 1991;110(4):187-189.
29. Brinjikji W, Luetmer PH, Comstock B, et al. Systematic literature review of imaging features of spinal degeneration in asymptomatic populations. *AJNR Am J Neuroradiol.* 2015;36(4):811-816.
30. Mense S, Simons DG, Russell IJ. *Muscle Pain: Understanding its Nature, Diagnosis, and Treatment.* Philadelphia, PA: Lippincott Williams & Wilkins; 2001.
31. Samuel AS, Peter AA, Ramanathan K. The association of active trigger points with lumbar disc lesions. *J Musculoskel Pain.* 2007;15(2):11-18.
32. Adelmanesh F, Jalali A, Jazayeri Shooshtari SM, Raissi GR, Ketabchi SM, Shir Y. Is there an association between lumbosacral radiculopathy and painful gluteal trigger points? A cross-sectional study. *Am J Phys Med Rehabil.* 2015;94(10):784-791.
33. Wertli MM, Rasmussen-Barr E, Held U, Weiser S, Bachmann LM, Brunner F. Fear-avoidance beliefs-a moderator of treatment efficacy in patients with low back pain: a systematic review. *Spine J.* 2014;14(11):2658-2678.
34. Gerwin RD. Myofascial aspects of low back pain. *Neurosurg Clin N Am.* 1991;2(4):761-784.
35. Rosen NB. The myofascial pain syndromes. *Phys Med Rehabil Clin N Am.* 1993;4(1):41-63.
36. Dejung B. Manual trigger point treatment in chronic lumbosacral pain [in German]. *Schweiz Med Wochenschr Suppl.* 1994;62:82-87.
37. Bonica J, Sola A. Chapter 72, Other painful disorders of the low back. In: Bonica JJ, Loeser JD, Chapman C, Fordyce WE, eds. *The Management of Pain.* 2nd ed. Philadelphia, PA: Lea & Febiger; 1990:1490-1498.
38. Rosomoff H, Fishbain DA, Goldberg M, Steele-Rosomoff R. Myofascial findings in patients with "chronic intractable benign pain" of the back and neck. *Pain Manag.* 1990;3(2):114-118.
39. Teixeira MJ, Yeng LT, Garcia OG, Fonoff ET, Paiva WS, Araujo JO. Failed back surgery pain syndrome: therapeutic approach descriptive study in 56 patients. *Rev Assoc Med Bras (1992).* 2011;57(3):282-287.
40. Chen CK, Nizar AJ. Myofascial pain syndrome in chronic back pain patients. *Korean J Pain.* 2011;24(2):100-104.
41. Iglesias-Gonzalez JJ, Munoz-Garcia MT, Rodrigues-de-Souza DP, Alburquerque-Sendin F, Fernández de las Peñas C. Myofascial trigger points, pain, disability, and sleep quality in patients with chronic nonspecific low back pain. *Pain Med.* 2013;14(12):1964-1970.
42. Simons DG, Travell J, Simons L. *Travell & Simon's Myofascial Pain and Dysfunction: The Trigger Point Manual.* Vol 1. 2nd ed. Baltimore, MD: Williams & Wilkins; 1999.
43. Itoh K, Katsumi Y, Kitakoji H. Trigger point acupuncture treatment of chronic low back pain in elderly patients—a blinded RCT. *Acupunct Med.* 2004;22(4):170-177.
44. Visser LH, Nijssen PG, Tijssen CC, van Middendorp JJ, Schieving J. Sciatica-like symptoms and the sacroiliac joint: clinical features and differential diagnosis. *Eur Spine J.* 2013;22(7):1657-1664.
45. Madani SP, Dadian M, Firouznia K, Alalawi S. Sacroiliac joint dysfunction in patients with herniated lumbar disc: a cross-sectional study. *J Back Musculoskelet Rehabil.* 2013;26(3):273-278.
46. Slipman CW, Jackson HB, Lipetz JS, Chan KT, Lenrow D, Vresilovic EJ. Sacroiliac joint pain referral zones. *Arch Phys Med Rehabil.* 2000;81(3):334-338.
47. Cohen SP. Sacroiliac joint pain: a comprehensive review of anatomy, diagnosis, and treatment. *Anesth Analg.* 2005;101(5):1440-1453.
48. Laslett M. Evidence-based diagnosis and treatment of the painful sacroiliac joint. *J Man Manip Ther.* 2008;16(3):142-152.
49. Maigne JY, Aivaliklis A, Pfefer F. Results of sacroiliac joint double block and value of sacroiliac pain provocation tests in 54 patients with low back pain. *Spine (Phila Pa 1976).* 1996;21(16):1889-1892.
50. Dreyfuss P, Michaelsen M, Pauza K, McLarty J, Bogduk N. The value of medical history and physical examination in diagnosing sacroiliac joint pain. *Spine (Phila Pa 1976).* 1996;21(22):2594-2602.
51. Goode A, Hegedus EJ, Sizer P, Brismee JM, Linberg A, Cook CE. Three-dimensional movements of the sacroiliac joint: a systematic review of the literature and assessment of clinical utility. *J Man Manip Ther.* 2008;16(1):25-38.
52. Fortin JD, Aprill CN, Ponthieux B, Pier J. Sacroiliac joint: pain referral maps upon applying a new injection/arthrography technique. Part II: Clinical evaluation. *Spine (Phila Pa 1976).* 1994;19(13):1483-1489.
53. Vleeming A, Schuenke MD, Masi AT, Carreiro JE, Danneels L, Willard FH. The sacroiliac joint: an overview of its anatomy, function and potential clinical implications. *J Anat.* 2012;221(6):537-567.
54. van der Wurff P, Hagmeijer RH, Meyne W. Clinical tests of the sacroiliac joint. A systematic methodological review. Part 1: Reliability. *Man Ther.* 2000;5(1):30-36.
55. Cibulka MT. Understanding sacroiliac joint movement as a guide to the management of a patient with unilateral low back pain. *Man Ther.* 2002;7(4):215-221.
56. Laslett M, Aprill CN, McDonald B, Young SB. Diagnosis of sacroiliac joint pain: validity of individual provocation tests and composites of tests. *Man Ther.* 2005;10(3):207-218.
57. Hungerford BA, Gilleard W, Moran M, Emmerson C. Evaluation of the ability of physical therapists to palpate intrapelvic motion with the Stork test on the support side. *Phys Ther.* 2007;87(7):879-887.
58. Laslett M, Young SB, Aprill CN, McDonald B. Diagnosing painful sacroiliac joints: a validity study of a McKenzie evaluation and sacroiliac provocation tests. *Aust J Physiother.* 2003;49(2):89-97.
59. Lewit K. *Manipulative Therapy in Rehabilitation of the Locomotor System.* 2nd ed. Oxford, England: Butterworth Heinemann; 1991.
60. Lurie J, Tomkins-Lane C. Management of lumbar spinal stenosis. *BMJ.* 2016;352:h6234.
61. Govind J. Lumbar radicular pain. *Aust Fam Physician.* 2004;33(6):409-412.
62. Fritz JM, Erhard RE, Delitto A, Welch WC, Nowakowski PE. Preliminary results of the use of a two-stage treadmill test as a clinical diagnostic tool in the differential diagnosis of lumbar spinal stenosis. *J Spinal Disord.* 1997;10(5):410-416.
63. Whitman JM, Flynn TW, Childs JD, et al. A comparison between two physical therapy treatment programs for patients with lumbar spinal stenosis: a randomized clinical trial. *Spine (Phila Pa 1976).* 2006;31(22):2541-2549.
64. Puntumetakul R, Yodchaisarn W, Emasithi A, Keawduangdee P, Chatchawan U, Yamauchi J. Prevalence and individual risk factors associated with clinical lumbar instability in rice farmers with low back pain. *Patient Prefer Adherence.* 2015;9:1-7.
65. Hicks GE, Fritz JM, Delitto A, McGill SM. Preliminary development of a clinical prediction rule for determining which patients with low back pain will respond to a stabilization exercise program. *Arch Phys Med Rehabil.* 2005;86(9):1753-1762.
66. Fritz JM, Piva SR, Childs JD. Accuracy of the clinical examination to predict radiographic instability of the lumbar spine. *Eur Spine J.* 2005;14(8):743-750.
67. Ferrari S, Manni T, Bonetti F, Villafane JH, Vanti C. A literature review of clinical tests for lumbar instability in low back pain: validity and applicability in clinical practice. *Chiropr Man Therap.* 2015;23:14.
68. Ravenna MM, Hoffman SL, Van Dillen LR. Low interrater reliability of examiners performing the prone instability test: a clinical test for lumbar shear instability. *Arch Phys Med Rehabil.* 2011;92(6):913-919.
69. Jinkins JR. Lumbosacral interspinous ligament rupture associated with acute intrinsic spinal muscle degeneration. *Eur Radiol.* 2002;12(9):2370-2376.

70. Lawrence KJ, Elser T, Stromberg R. Lumbar spondylolysis in the adolescent athlete. *Phys Ther Sport.* 2016;20:56-60.
71. Matz PG, Meagher RJ, Lamer T, et al. Guideline summary review: an evidence-based clinical guideline for the diagnosis and treatment of degenerative lumbar spondylolisthesis. *Spine J.* 2016;16(3):439-448.
72. Thakar S, Sivaraju L, Aryan S, Mohan D, Sai Kiran NA, Hegde AS. Lumbar paraspinal muscle morphometry and its correlations with demographic and radiological factors in adult isthmic spondylolisthesis: a retrospective review of 120 surgically managed cases. *J Neurosurg Spine.* 2016;24(5):679-685.
73. Deodhar A, Reveille JD, van den Bosch F, et al. The concept of axial spondyloarthritis: joint statement of the spondyloarthritis research and treatment network and the Assessment of SpondyloArthritis international Society in response to the US Food and Drug Administration's comments and concerns. *Arthritis Rheumatol.* 2014;66(10):2649-2656.
74. Ranganathan V, Gracey E, Brown MA, Inman RD, Haroon N. Pathogenesis of ankylosing spondylitis—recent advances and future directions. *Nat Rev Rheumatol.* 2017;13(6):359-367.
75. Pecourneau V, Degboe Y, Barnetche T, Cantagrel A, Constantin A, Ruyssen-Witrand A. Effectiveness of exercise programs in ankylosing spondylitis: a meta-analysis of randomized controlled trials. *Arch Phys Med Rehabil.* 2017.
76. Fall M, Baranowski AP, Elneil S, et al. EAU guidelines on chronic pelvic pain. *Eur Urol.* 2010;57(1):35-48.
77. Yosef A, Allaire C, Williams C, et al. Multifactorial contributors to the severity of chronic pelvic pain in women. *Am J Obstet Gynecol.* 2016;215(6):760.e1-760.e14.
78. Bajaj P, Bajaj P, Madsen H, Arendt-Nielsen L. Endometriosis is associated with central sensitization: a psychophysical controlled study. *J Pain.* 2003;4(7):372-380.
79. Hoffman D. Central and peripheral pain generators in women with chronic pelvic pain: patient centered assessment and treatment. *Curr Rheumatol Rev.* 2015;11(2):146-166.
80. Samraj GP, Kuritzky L, Curry RW. Chronic pelvic pain in women: evaluation and management in primary care. *Compr Ther.* 2005;31(1):28-39.
81. Vleeming A, Albert HB, Ostgaard HC, Sturesson B, Stuge B. European guidelines for the diagnosis and treatment of pelvic girdle pain. *Eur Spine J.* 2008;17(6):794-819.
82. Stratton P, Khachikyan I, Sinaii N, Ortiz R, Shah J. Association of chronic pelvic pain and endometriosis with signs of sensitization and myofascial pain. *Obstet Gynecol.* 2015;125(3):719-728.
83. Alappattu MJ, Bishop MD. Psychological factors in chronic pelvic pain in women: relevance and application of the fear-avoidance model of pain. *Phys Ther.* 2011;91(10):1542-1550.
84. Cavaggioni G, Lia C, Resta S, et al. Are mood and anxiety disorders and alexithymia associated with endometriosis? A preliminary study. *Biomed Res Int.* 2014;2014:786830.
85. Li HJ, Kang DY. Prevalence of sexual dysfunction in men with chronic prostatitis/chronic pelvic pain syndrome: a meta-analysis. *World J Urol.* 2016;34(7):1009-1017.
86. Ploteau S, Labat JJ, Riant T, Levesque A, Robert R, Nizard J. New concepts on functional chronic pelvic and perineal pain: pathophysiology and multi-disciplinary management. *Discov Med.* 2015;19(104):185-192.
87. Magistro G, Wagenlehner FM, Grabe M, Weidner W, Stief CG, Nickel JC. Contemporary management of chronic prostatitis/chronic pelvic pain syndrome. *Eur Urol.* 2016;69(2):286-297.
88. Anderson RU, Sawyer T, Wise D, Morey A, Nathanson BH. Painful myofascial trigger points and pain sites in men with chronic prostatitis/chronic pelvic pain syndrome. *J Urol.* 2009;182(6):2753-2758.
89. Montenegro ML, Gomide LB, Mateus-Vasconcelos EL, et al. Abdominal myofascial pain syndrome must be considered in the differential diagnosis of chronic pelvic pain. *Eur J Obstet Gynecol Reprod Biol.* 2009;147(1):21-24.
90. Jarrell J. Myofascial dysfunction in the pelvis. *Curr Pain Headache Rep.* 2004;8(6):452-456.
91. Pastore EA, Katzman WB. Recognizing myofascial pelvic pain in the female patient with chronic pelvic pain. *J Obstet Gynecol Neonatal Nurs.* 2012;41(5):680-691.
92. Anderson RU. Management of chronic prostatitis-chronic pelvic pain syndrome. *Urol Clin North Am.* 2002;29(1):235-239.
93. Aredo JV, Heyrana KJ, Karp BI, Shah JP, Stratton P. Relating chronic pelvic pain and endometriosis to signs of sensitization and myofascial pain and dysfunction. *Semin Reprod Med.* 2017;35(1):88-97.
94. Jarrell J, Giamberardino MA, Robert M, Nasr-Esfahani M. Bedside testing for chronic pelvic pain: discriminating visceral from somatic pain. *Pain Res Treat.* 2011;2011:692102.
95. Doggweiler-Wiygul R. Urologic myofascial pain syndromes. *Curr Pain Headache Rep.* 2004;8(6):445-451.
96. Bonder JH, Chi M, Rispoli L. Myofascial pelvic pain and related disorders. *Phys Med Rehabil Clin N Am.* 2017;28(3):501-515.
97. Moldwin RM, Fariello JY. Myofascial trigger points of the pelvic floor: associations with urological pain syndromes and treatment strategies including injection therapy. *Curr Urol Rep.* 2013;14(5):409-417.
98. Weiss JM. Pelvic floor myofascial trigger points: manual therapy for interstitial cystitis and the urgency-frequency syndrome. *J Urol.* 2001;166(6):2226-2231.
99. Doggweiler-Wiygul R, Wiygul JP. Interstitial cystitis, pelvic pain, and the relationship to myofascial pain and dysfunction: a report on four patients. *World J Urol.* 2002;20(5):310-314.
100. Anderson RU, Wise D, Sawyer T, Chan C. Integration of myofascial trigger point release and paradoxical relaxation training treatment of chronic pelvic pain in men. *J Urol.* 2005;174(1):155-160.
101. Anderson RU, Wise D, Sawyer T, Chan CA. Sexual dysfunction in men with chronic prostatitis/chronic pelvic pain syndrome: improvement after trigger point release and paradoxical relaxation training. *J Urol.* 2006;176(4, pt 1):1534-1538; discussion 1538-1539.
102. FitzGerald MP, Anderson RU, Potts J, et al. Randomized multicenter feasibility trial of myofascial physical therapy for the treatment of urological chronic pelvic pain syndromes. *J Urol.* 2009;182(2):570-580.
103. Kim DS, Jeong TY, Kim YK, Chang WH, Yoon JG, Lee SC. Usefulness of a myofascial trigger point injection for groin pain in patients with chronic prostatitis/chronic pelvic pain syndrome: a pilot study. *Arch Phys Med Rehabil.* 2013;94(5):930-936.
104. Stochkendahl MJ, Christensen HW. Chest pain in focal musculoskeletal disorders. *Med Clin North Am.* 2010;94(2):259-273.
105. Winzenberg T, Jones G, Callisaya M. Musculoskeletal chest wall pain. *Aust Fam Physician.* 2015;44(8):540-544.
106. Buntinx F, Knockaert D, Bruyninckx R, et al. Chest pain in general practice or in the hospital emergency department: is it the same? *Fam Pract.* 2001;18(6):586-589.
107. Briggs AM, Bragge P, Smith AJ, Govil D, Straker LM. Prevalence and associated factors for thoracic spine pain in the adult working population: a literature review. *J Occup Health.* 2009;51(3):177-192.
108. Briggs AM, Smith AJ, Straker LM, Bragge P. Thoracic spine pain in the general population: prevalence, incidence and associated factors in children, adolescents and adults. A systematic review. *BMC Musculoskelet Disord.* 2009;10:77.
109. Fouquet N, Bodin J, Descatha A, et al. Prevalence of thoracic spine pain in a surveillance network. *Occup Med (Lond).* 2015;65(2):122-125.
110. Eslick GD, Jones MP, Talley NJ. Non-cardiac chest pain: prevalence, risk factors, impact and consulting—a population-based study. *Aliment Pharmacol Ther.* 2003;17(9):1115-1124.
111. Leboeuf-Yde C, Nielsen J, Kyvik KO, Fejer R, Hartvigsen J. Pain in the lumbar, thoracic or cervical regions: do age and gender matter? A population-based study of 34,902 Danish twins 20-71 years of age. *BMC Musculoskelet Disord.* 2009;10:39.
112. Sert A, Aypar E, Odabas D, Gokcen C. Clinical characteristics and causes of chest pain in 380 children referred to a paediatric cardiology unit. *Cardiol Young.* 2013;23(3):361-367.
113. Proulx AM, Zryd TW. Costochondritis: diagnosis and treatment. *Am Fam Physician.* 2009;80(6):617-620.
114. Klinkman MS, Stevens D, Gorenflo DW. Episodes of care for chest pain: a preliminary report from MIRNET. Michigan Research Network. *J Fam Pract.* 1994;38(4):345-352.
115. Ayloo A, Cvengros T, Marella S. Evaluation and treatment of musculoskeletal chest pain. *Prim Care.* 2013;40(4):863-887, viii.
116. Borge CR, Wahl AK, Moum T. Pain and quality of life with chronic obstructive pulmonary disease. *Heart Lung.* 2011;40(3):e90-e101.
117. Janssen DJ, Wouters EF, Parra YL, Stakenborg K, Franssen FM. Prevalence of thoracic pain in patients with chronic obstructive pulmonary disease and relationship with patient characteristics: a cross-sectional observational study. *BMC Pulm Med.* 2016;16:47.
118. Bentsen SB, Rustoen T, Miaskowski C. Prevalence and characteristics of pain in patients with chronic obstructive pulmonary disease compared to the Norwegian general population. *J Pain.* 2011;12(5):539-545.
119. Southerst D, Marchand AA, Cote P, et al. The effectiveness of noninvasive interventions for musculoskeletal thoracic spine and chest wall pain: a systematic review by the Ontario Protocol for Traffic Injury Management (OPTIMa) collaboration. *J Manipulative Physiol Ther.* 2015;38(7):521-531.
120. Manchikanti L, Boswell MV, Singh V, Pampati V, Damron KS, Beyer CD. Prevalence of facet joint pain in chronic spinal pain of cervical, thoracic, and lumbar regions. *BMC Musculoskelet Disord.* 2004;5:15.
121. Atluri S, Datta S, Falco FJ, Lee M. Systematic review of diagnostic utility and therapeutic effectiveness of thoracic facet joint interventions. *Pain Physician.* 2008;11(5):611-629.
122. Dreyfuss P, Tibiletti C, Dreyer SJ. Thoracic zygapophyseal joint pain patterns. A study in normal volunteers. *Spine (Phila Pa 1976).* 1994;19(7):807-811.
123. Young BA, Gill HE, Wainner RS, Flynn TW. Thoracic costotransverse joint pain patterns: a study in normal volunteers. *BMC Musculoskelet Disord.* 2008;9:140.
124. Christensen HW, Vach W, Gichangi A, Manniche C, Haghfelt T, Hoilund-Carlsen PF. Cervicothoracic angina identified by case history and palpation findings in patients with stable angina pectoris. *J Manipulative Physiol Ther.* 2005;28(5):303-311.
125. Christensen HW, Vach W, Vach K, et al. Palpation of the upper thoracic spine: an observer reliability study. *J Manipulative Physiol Ther.* 2002;25(5):285-292.
126. Christensen HW, Vach W, Manniche C, Haghfelt T, Hartvigsen L, Hoilund-Carlsen PF. Palpation for muscular tenderness in the anterior chest wall: an observer reliability study. *J Manipulative Physiol Ther.* 2003;26(8):469-475.
127. Kellgren JH. On the distribution of pain arising from deep somatic structures with charts of segmental pain areas. *Clin Sci.* 1939;4:35-46.
128. Feinstein B, Langton JN, Jameson RM, Schiller F. Experiments on pain referred from deep somatic tissues. *J Bone Joint Surg Am.* 1954;36-A(5):981-997.
129. Landmann HR. Trigger areas as cause of persistent chest and shoulder pain in myocardial infarction or angina pectoris. *J Kans Med Soc.* 1949;50(2):69-71.

130. Lawson GE, Hung LY, Ko GD, Laframboise MA. A case of pseudo-angina pectoris from a pectoralis minor trigger point caused by cross-country skiing. *J Chiropr Med.* 2011;10(3):173-178.
131. Chen SM, Chen JT, Kuan TS, Hong CZ. Myofascial trigger points in intercostal muscles secondary to herpes zoster infection of the intercostal nerve. *Arch Phys Med Rehabil.* 1998;79(3):336-338.
132. Roldan CJ, Huh BK. Iliocostalis thoracis-lumborum myofascial pain: reviewing a subgroup of a prospective, randomized, blinded trial. A challenging diagnosis with clinical implications. *Pain Physician.* 2016;19(6):363-372.
133. Berg AT, Stafne SN, Hiller A, Slordahl SA, Aamot IL. Physical therapy intervention in patients with non-cardiac chest pain following a recent cardiac event: a randomized controlled trial. *SAGE Open Med.* 2015;3:2050312115580799.
134. Fernández de las Peñas C, Layton M, Dommerholt J. Dry needling for the management of thoracic spine pain. *J Man Manip Ther.* 2015;23(3):147-153.
135. Rock JM, Rainey CE. Treatment of nonspecific thoracic spine pain with trigger point dry needling and intramuscular electrical stimulation: a case series. *Int J Sports Phys Ther.* 2014;9(5):699-711.
136. Lewit K. Muscular pattern in thoraco-lumbar lesions. *Manual Med.* 1986;2:105-107.

Section 6: Hip, Thigh, and Knee Pain

Chapter 54

Gluteus Maximus Muscle

"Swimmers Nemesis"

Joseph M. Donnelly, Paul Thomas, and Jennifer L. Freeman

1. INTRODUCTION

From an evolutionary perspective, the ability to walk bipedally is a uniquely human trait. The gluteus maximus muscle is the largest and most superficial of the gluteal muscles and the largest muscle in the body. The gluteus maximus muscle covers the posterior pelvis from the sacrum, ilium, coccyx, thoracolumbar fascia, lumbar multifidus, distally to the iliotibial tract of the fascia lata, and gluteal tuberosity of the femur. The gluteus maximus muscle primarily attaches to the fascia lata, which suggests a complex biomechanical function across the hip and knee as well as the lumbopelvic region. The gluteus maximus muscle stabilizes the pelvis on the femur and propels the body forward during ambulation. Activities such as walking uphill, swimming freestyle, and sprinting may overload the gluteus maximus muscle, activating and perpetuating trigger points (TrPs). Pain from the gluteus maximus muscle will typically remain in the buttock region, but these symptoms can mimic sacroiliac joint dysfunction, trochanteric bursitis, and high hamstring strain symptoms. Differential diagnosis should include lumbar radicular pain or radiculopathy, lumbar spine and sacroiliac joint dysfunction, piriformis syndrome, hamstring strain, and trochanteric bursitis. Corrective actions should include techniques to improve sitting posture, trunk control, gait mechanics, sleeping position, self-pressure release, and self-stretching techniques. Neuromuscular reeducation and progression to strengthening exercises is key for preventing exacerbation.

2. ANATOMIC CONSIDERATIONS

The gluteus maximus muscle[1] is the most superficial and largest of the three gluteal muscles. The gluteus maximus muscle in humans has a larger cross-sectional area and is much more extensive than in any other primate. This organizational structure of the gluteus maximus muscle supports the upright posture and bipedal walking in human beings. From an evolutionary point of view, upright walking by true bipedal plantigrade progression has been singled out as a unique feature of human locomotion.[2] Humans alone, among mammals, can place the center of gravity of the head, arms, and torso over the hips.[3] This function has been associated with evolutionary changes in the skeleton and gluteus maximus muscle that are uniquely human. These changes include shortening and tilting of the pelvis to permit extension of the thigh at the hip, angulation of gluteus maximus fibers more horizontally,[3] and enlargement of the muscle to more than twice the size of the gluteus medius muscle.[4] These evolutionary changes[5] presumably freed the hands for other activities and were considered[3] to be crucial to the development of the intelligence and unique manual dexterity of humans.

Anatomically, the remarkably large gluteus maximus muscle forms the prominence of the buttock. It is twice as heavy (844 g) as the gluteus medius and gluteus minimus muscles together (421 g),[6] and it often measures more than 2.5 cm (1 in) in thickness. The gluteus maximus muscle originates from the posterior gluteal line of the ilium and the area of bone superior and posterior to it including the iliac crest, the posterolateral surface of the sacrum, and the lateral coccyx. It also has proximal attachments to the sacrotuberous ligament, the fascia covering the gluteus medius muscle, and the dorsal sacroiliac ligaments.[7] Additional slips of muscle may arise from the ischial tuberosity or lumbar aponeurosis

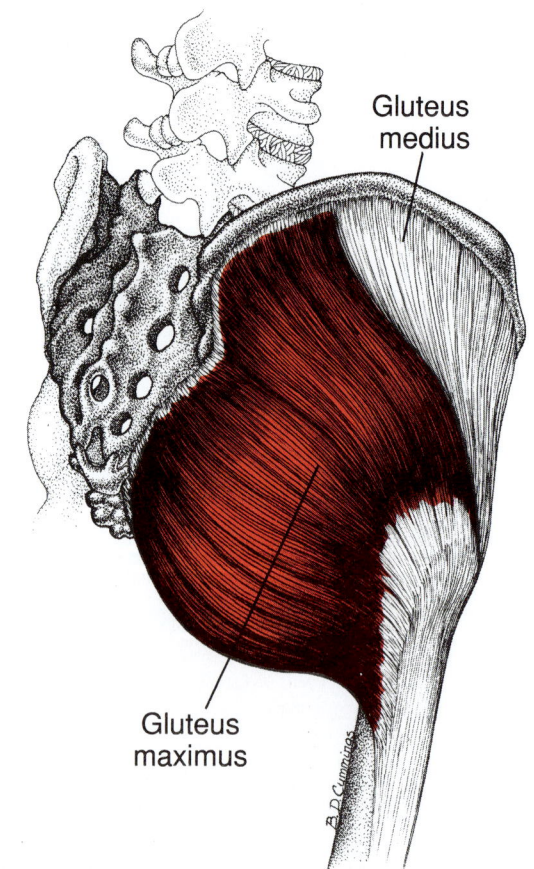

Figure 54-1. Attachments of the right gluteus maximus muscle (red) in the posterolateral view. The gluteus maximus muscle covers the posterior portion of the gluteus medius muscle, but not its anterior portion. Note the expansive insertion into the fascia lata.

(Figure 54-1). The gluteus maximus muscle has attachments to the thoracolumbar fascia and the multifidus muscle at the gluteal raphe, which is located at the superomedial aspect of the gluteus maximus muscle at its attachment to the sacrum.[8] The gluteal raphe serves as an important anatomic convergence joining the multifidus and superficial erector spinae muscles with the gluteus maximus muscle. This area conjoins and converts the three most powerful extensor muscles that cross the lumbar spine, pelvis, and hip on the posterior side of the body.[8]

The gluteus maximus muscle is quadrilateral in shape, and its fibers descend inferolaterally. The superior portion of the muscle, together with the superficial aspect of the lower fibers, terminates in a thick expansive tendinous lamina and inserts into the fascia lata along the iliotibial tract and the lateral intermuscular septum.[9] The majority of the gluteus maximus muscle inserts into the fascia lata.[8] The deep fibers of the inferior portion of the gluteus maximus muscle attach to the gluteal tuberosity between the vastus lateralis and adductor magnus muscles (Figure 54-1).[7,10]

The large trochanteric bursa separates the flat tendon of the gluteus maximus muscle from the greater trochanter.[11,12] An inconstant ischial bursa permits smooth gliding of the muscle over the ischial tuberosity. A third bursa separates the gluteus maximus tendon from that of the vastus lateralis muscle.[7] Other small bursae form as needed throughout the gluteal region to support efficiency of movement.

2.1. Innervation and Vascularization

The gluteus maximus muscle is innervated by the inferior gluteal nerve that arises from the L5, S1, and S2 nerve roots. The inferior gluteal nerve forms from these roots and exits the pelvis through the greater sciatic foramen, inferior to the piriformis muscle and superficial to the sciatic nerve. This nerve usually perforates the inferior part of the gluteus maximus muscle.[13]

Vascularization of the gluteus maximus muscle is primarily supplied through the inferior gluteal artery that supplies approximately two-thirds of the overlying gluteus maximus muscle. The remaining third is supplied mainly by the superior gluteal artery.[7]

2.2. Function

The gluteus maximus muscle is a powerful hip extensor. When the hip is in extension, the gluteus maximus muscle acts as an external rotator. The superior portion of the muscle can contribute to hip abduction, whereas the inferior portion contributes to hip adduction. The superior portion of the muscle is more active during activities that involve hip extension, hip abduction, and/or hip external rotation. The inferior portion contributes to hip adduction, and along with the superior portion they are both active during activities utilizing hip extension.[14] The activity of the gluteus maximus muscle can be enhanced by combining hip extension with abduction and external rotation.[15]

During functional activities, such as descending stairs, squatting, climbing, or transitioning from standing to sitting, the gluteus maximus muscle, contracting eccentrically, controls hip flexion. The gluteus maximus and hamstring muscles act together to bring the trunk from a forward flexed posture back to an upright erect posture.[7,16]

The gluteus maximus muscle stabilizes the pelvis and trunk on the thigh during ambulation and aids in forward propulsion.[17] It is active during both walking and running. It has been found to have a peak muscle activation during lower extremity loading response (foot strike) and remains somewhat active through the stance phase of gait, and again, activation increases at the end of the swing phase to decelerate the lower extremity.[16] As the speed of the lower extremity is increased during gait, and especially when running, the activity of the gluteus maximus muscle increases for both support and propulsion of the lower extremity.[16] It has been shown to act as a control for the transverse plane rotation of the tibia during the gait cycle. Through its action as an external rotator, the gluteus maximus muscle has the capacity to eccentrically control the internal rotation that occurs through the early stance phase of gait. Preece et al demonstrated that higher gluteus maximus muscle activation led to a more rapid deceleration of the tibia.[18] Teng et al[19] found that runners with weak hip extensors utilized a more erect posture during running, resulting in increased demand on their quadriceps muscles to attenuate ground reaction forces, leading to overuse running injuries of the knee.

The gluteus maximus muscle plays a role in the stability of the sacroiliac joint through force closure,[20] both independently and when working in concert with other muscles.[21] One way that this stability is achieved is with the contraction of the biceps femoris muscle, which minimizes motion between the sacrum and the ilium through its attachments on the sacrotuberous ligament. Another mechanism of force closure may occur through the simultaneous contraction of the ipsilateral gluteus maximus and contralateral latissimus dorsi muscles, which increases compression between the sacroiliac joint surfaces because of their influence on the thoracolumbar fascia.[8] Together, their contraction places tension on the posterior layer of the thoracolumbar fascia that crosses the sacroiliac joints perpendicularly, thus creating a compressive force.[10,20,21]

In closed kinetic chain, the gluteus maximus muscle generates a strong influence on the position of the pelvis in the sagittal plane. With the foot fixed on the ground, a bilateral contraction of the gluteus maximus muscle results in a posterior rotary moment of the pelvis that creates a flexion moment at the lumbosacral junction.[8] Through this closed kinetic chain action, the lumbosacral angle is reduced and, in turn, reduces anterior shear forces across the lumbosacral junction. This influence may be a very useful function for those individuals with spinal stenosis or degeneration of the lumbar zygapophyseal joints.[8]

Autopsy samples of normal adult gluteus maximus muscles from individuals under age 44 years have shown that 68% of fibers were slow-twitch (type 1) and 32% were fast-twitch (type 2) muscle fibers. The muscle demonstrated essentially the same composition in two groups of persons older than 44 years: 70% of the fibers were type 1 and 30% were type 2. Although individual variability is great, the percentage of type 1 fibers (those dependent largely on oxidative metabolism) always exceeded the number of type 2 (rapidly fatiguing) fibers that utilize chiefly glycolytic energy pathways.[22] Because of this combination of different muscle fiber types, both low- and high-speed repetitions are necessary for effective training.

2.3. Functional Unit

The functional unit to which a muscle belongs includes the muscles that reinforce and counter its actions as well as the joints that the muscle crosses. The interdependence of these structures functionally is reflected in the organization and neural connections of the sensory motor cortex. The functional unit is emphasized because the presence of a TrP in one muscle of the unit increases the likelihood that the other muscles will develop TrPs. When inactivating TrPs in a muscle, one must be concerned about TrPs that may develop in muscles that are functionally interdependent. Box 54-1 represents the functional unit of the gluteus maximus muscle.[23]

The gluteus maximus muscle works synergistically with the lumbar erector spinae and hamstring muscles to perform extension of the trunk from a forward flexed position in standing. Through acting on the relatively fixed femurs, the muscle works to posteriorly rotate the pelvis raising the trunk.[7]

The gluteus maximus muscle aids in providing stability of the sacroiliac joint and works synergistically with the bicep femoris muscle through attachments on the sacrotuberous ligament. It also works synergistically with the pelvic floor, transversus abdominis, erector spinae, multifidus, and latissimus dorsi muscles to provide force closure of the sacroiliac joints.[20,21]

Box 54-1   Functional unit of the gluteus maximus muscle

Action	Synergists	Antagonists
Trunk extension	Iliocostalis thoracis Iliocostalis lumborum Longissimus thoracis Hamstrings	Iliopsoas Rectus abdominis Internal abdominis oblique External abdominis oblique
Hip extension	Hamstrings Gluteus medius (posterior fibers) Gluteus minimus (posterior fibers) Obturator internus Adductor magnus	Iliopsoas Rectus femoris Tensor fascia lata
Hip abduction	Gluteus medius Gluteus minimis Tensor fascia lata Obturator internus	Adductor magnus Adductor longus Adductor brevis Pectineus Gracilis
Hip external rotation	Piriformis Obturator internus Obturator externus Quadratus femoris Gemelli superior and inferior	Adductor Tensor fascia lata

3. CLINICAL PRESENTATION

3.1. Referred Pain Pattern

Trigger points in the gluteus maximus muscle may refer symptoms, including pain, to the sacrum, inferior buttock, gluteal fold, coccyx, sacrococcygeal region, and laterally, to the area inferior to the iliac crest (Figure 54-2). Trigger points in this muscle refer pain locally in the buttock region and typically do not extend into the lower extremity, unlike the gluteus medius and gluteus minimus muscles that may produce referred symptoms down the lower extremity. Trigger points found along the sacral attachment may refer pain along the gluteal cleft and may extend to the area near the sacroiliac joint or barely into the proximal posterior thigh. Trigger points found just above the ischial tuberosity will usually refer pain to the entire buttock and cause a deep tenderness in the buttock. Trigger points found along the inferomedial fibers of the gluteus maximus muscle will typically cause pain along the coccyx (Figure 54-2).

3.2. Symptoms

Patients with active TrPs in the gluteus maximus muscle may report having pain while sitting. They may try to avoid putting pressure on the area of active TrPs and lean on one side or squirm in their chair because of discomfort. Significant deformation of the inferior gluteus maximus muscle and soft tissues has been observed through positional magnetic resonance imaging in the sitting posture. The gluteus maximus muscle slides away from the ischium along with the subcutaneous fat in a three-directional manner.[24] Whether from ischemic pressure over the muscle itself or from the strain placed on the soft tissue from deformation, pain with sitting can occur when TrPs are present through the inferior aspect of the muscle.[23]

Patients with active TrPs through the gluteus maximus muscle may also report having pain during walking, especially up a hill, as the forward trunk lean places increased demand on the muscle. These symptoms can mimic the symptoms of a sacroiliac joint dysfunction as the aggravating activities are typically the same. Pain from TrPs in this muscle is intensified by vigorous contraction in the shortened position, as when swimming freestyle. This cramp-type pain is more likely to occur in cold water. Sporting activities that require explosive starts such as tennis and sprinting place an increased demand on the gluteus maximus muscle that may result in the patient reporting symptoms similar to those of a proximal hamstring strain.

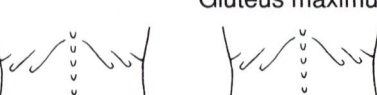

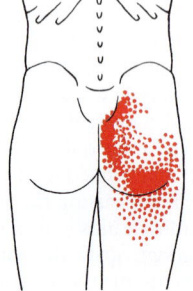 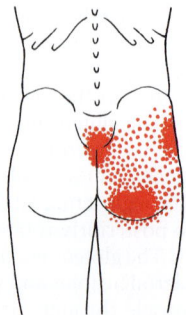 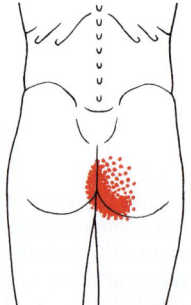 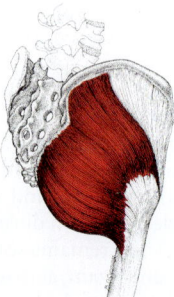

Figure 54-2. Referred pain patterns (solid red and stippled areas) of TrPs in the gluteus maximus muscle.

3.3. Patient Examination

After a thorough subjective examination the clinician should make a detailed drawing representing the pain pattern that the patient has described. This depiction will assist in planning the physical examination and can be useful in monitoring the progression of the patient as symptoms improve or change. The type, quality, and location of the pain should be carefully assessed, and the utilization of standardized outcome tools is imperative when examining patients with low back pain and/or lower extremity dysfunctions.

For proper examination of the gluteus maximus muscle, the clinician should observe sitting and standing postures. Physical examination testing should be conducted to rule out lumbar, sacroiliac, or hip joint pathology. This may include range of motion testing of the hip and lumbar spine; passive accessory motion testing of the hip, sacroiliac joint, and/or lumbar spine; strength testing of the gluteus maximus and other hip muscles; and any appropriate neurologic testing or orthopedic special tests. A careful assessment should be made to rule out referral into the buttock from other muscles, joints, or neural tissues that can refer to the same region.

As the gluteus maximus muscle plays such a large role in maintaining stability of the pelvis over the lower extremity while walking, an observation of the patient's gait pattern is necessary.[17] Common gait deviations include an antalgic gait pattern, an increased lordosis with anterior pelvic tilt,[15] or a decreased stance phase on the affected side and a corresponding brief swing phase on the contralateral side. The regional interdependence of the lumbosacral spine and the hip joint makes it necessary to examine these relationships in a closed and open kinetic chain.

A functional activity that should be assessed in standing is the double-leg squat, which should be observed from a sagittal perspective (Figure 54-3A). The clinician should note any excessive movement in the lumbosacral region or hip joint. During a proper squat, the patient should be able to go through a good range of hip flexion without excessive anterior pelvic tilt or excessive lumbar hyperextension (Figure 54-3B). Movement from a standing to sitting position should be observed to examine eccentric gluteus maximus muscle control during sitting and hip flexion range of motion. Further regional interdependence testing may include quadruped rocking looking at hip flexion range of motion relative to lumbar spine position. The patient attempts to sit back on his or her heels utilizing hip flexion without excessive motion at the lumbosacral spine (Figure 54-4).

The patient should also be observed in an open kinetic prone position. The gluteal skyline may be assessed to determine gluteal atrophy and inhibition that may indicate L5-S2 nerve root or inferior gluteal nerve pathology (Figure 54-5). The patient's muscle bulk is first observed at rest with the patient prone and then the patient is instructed to contract both gluteus maximus muscles, and the clinician assesses these contractions for bilateral symmetry. If asymmetries in gluteus maximus muscle mass or activation are noted, further evaluation to determine if the cause is neurologic or myofascial in origin is warranted.[25] As the gluteus maximus muscle tends to atrophy in women with low back pain, dysfunction of this muscle often requires a more global evaluation.[26]

Gluteus maximus muscle control of hip extension should also be assessed in prone (Figure 54-6A). The clinician passively

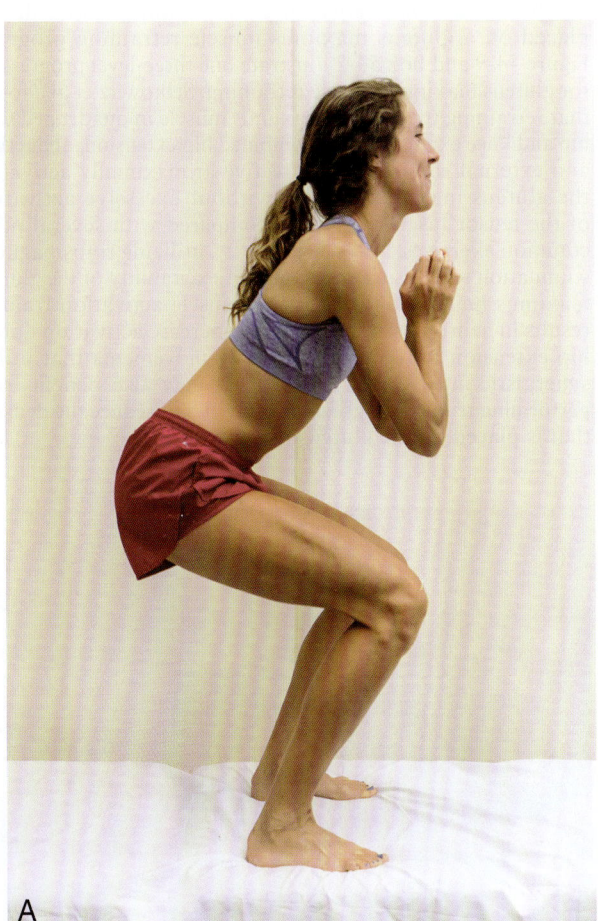 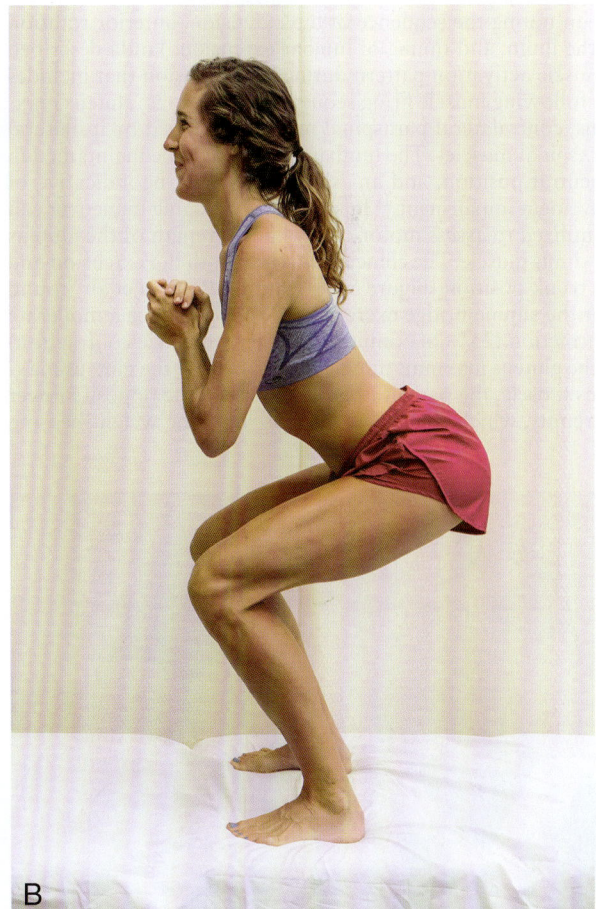

Figure 54-3. Double-leg squat. A, Neutral alignment of lumbar spine with good gluteus maximus muscle control. B, Excessive lumbar lordosis due to inhibited gluteal muscles.

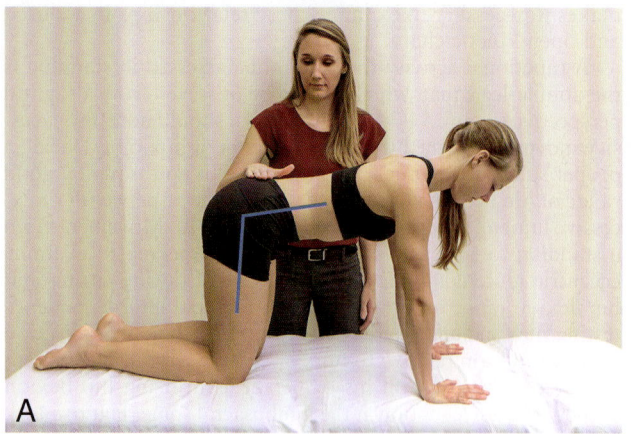 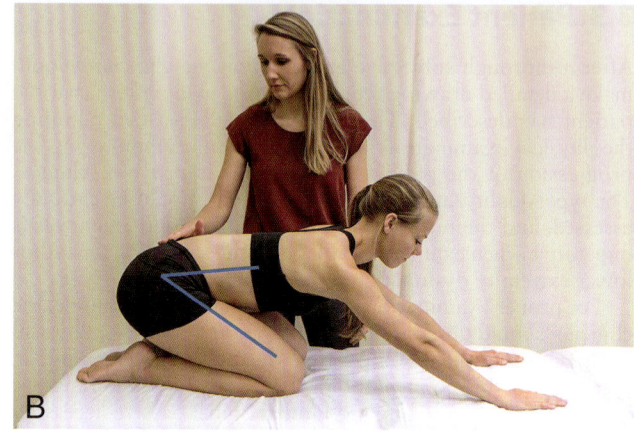

Figure 54-4. Quadruped rocking. A, Starting position with the hip in approximately 90° and lumbar spine in neutral position. B, End position with maximum hip flexion and minimum lumbar flexion.

extends the hip while monitoring the position of the greater trochanter (Figure 54-6B). The clinician then slowly releases the lower extremity while the patient attempts to maintain the hip extension position (Figure 54-6C). The greater trochanter should stay in the same position if the hip extensors are able to maintain the femur in the center of rotation.[27]

Hip range of motion, muscle strength, and muscle activation patterns should be assessed in all planes. Muscle length assessment of one- and two-joint hip flexor muscles should be performed (Figure 54-7). Hip extension range of motion and activation patterns should be assessed in prone, with the clinician noting the sequence of hip extension, anterior rotation of the ilium, and timing of lumbar extension. Janda described a muscle activation pattern during hip extension that includes the following muscle firing sequence: hamstrings, gluteus maximus, contralateral paraspinal muscles followed by ipsilateral paraspinal muscles. The lumbar spine should be maintained in a neutral position, and any deviation would be indicative of movement impairment.[28] In supine, the bridging maneuver can be utilized to assess motor control and strength of the gluteus maximus muscle. The clinician observes both hip extension and the trunk position (Figure 54-8A and B). Reiman et al[29] found that the supine bridge exercise was able to induce a moderate contraction (25% maximum voluntary isometric contraction) of the gluteus maximus muscle. To further test the gluteus maximus muscle, the patient is asked to extend the opposite lower extremity, which challenges the muscle on the weight-bearing side. The clinician watches for the pelvis to drop or raise excessively on the unsupported side, assessing the ability of the gluteus maximus muscle on the weight-bearing side to control the position of the pelvis (Figure 54-8C). This can also be used as a home exercise to increase gluteus maximus muscle control. A traditional manual muscle test can be performed; although, in clinical experience, the gluteus maximus manual muscle may test "good" to "normal," the patient may still demonstrate poor motor control during functional activities.

If the gluteus maximus muscle is found to have impaired muscle activation patterns, the patient should be immediately placed on a gluteus maximus muscle retraining program. Figure 54-9 and Box 54-2 illustrate one three-level progression for gluteus maximus muscle retraining. Selkowitz et al[30] found that retraining the gluteus maximus muscle in quadruped with hip and knee extension, and combined hip extension, abduction, and external rotation was effective at maximally activating the gluteus maximus muscle without excessive activation of the tensor fascia lata when compared with several other common exercises.[30] Researchers[31,32] utilizing transmagnetic stimulation to measure corticomotor excitability of the gluteus maximus muscle found that this muscle activation training results in neuroplastic changes that increase activation during hip extension movements including movements that utilize synergistic muscles.[31,32] Individuals may also benefit from performing trunk strengthening activities to reduce the demand that is placed on the gluteus maximus muscle.

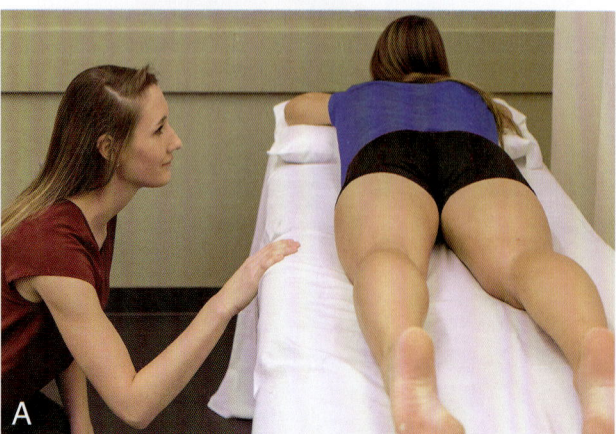 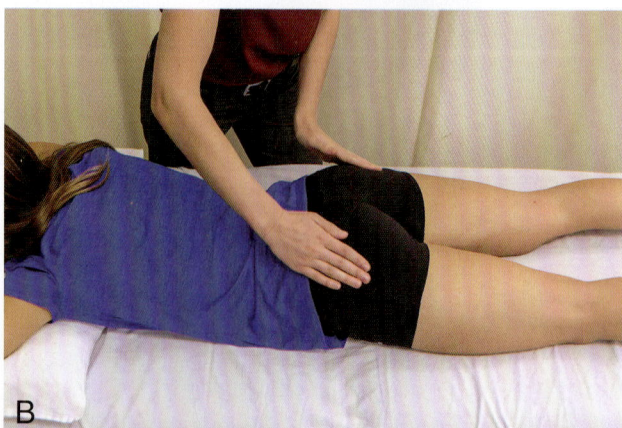

Figure 54-5. Assessment of gluteal skyline. A, First, the gluteal muscles should be assessed for resting symmetry. B, The patient is asked to contract both the left and right gluteus maximus muscles, and the control and strength of the contractions are then assessed for incongruences.

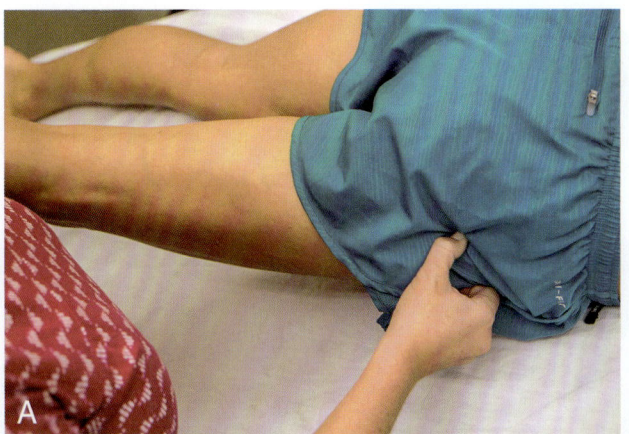
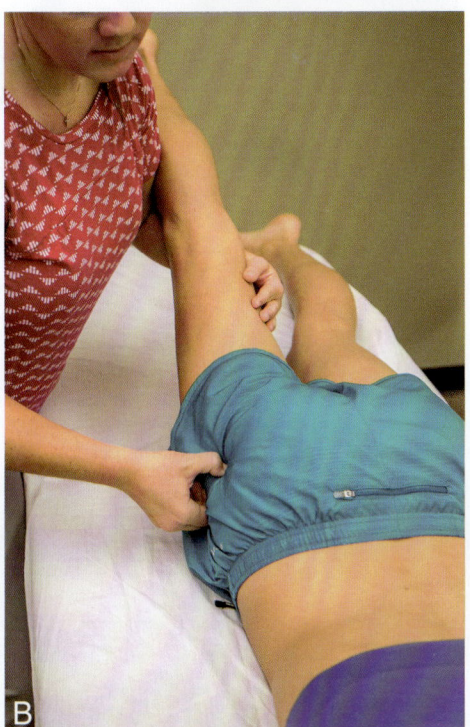
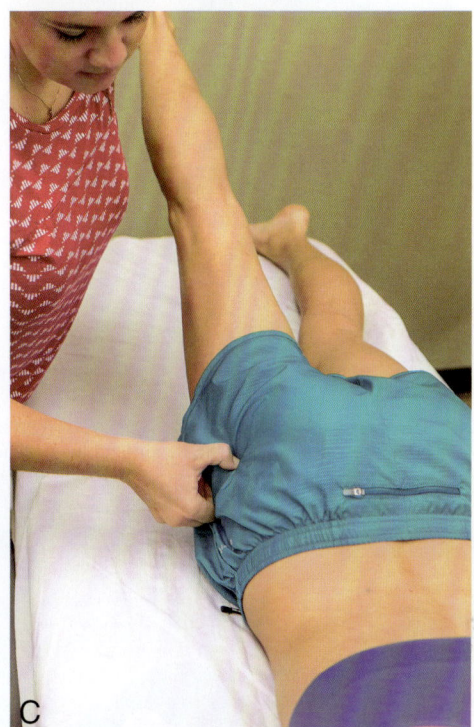

Figure 54-6. Assessment of motor control in prone hip extension. A, Clinician holds greater trochanter with key grip to monitor its position. B, Clinician passively places the hip into end range extension at the hip monitoring the greater trochanter position. C, The clinician releases the leg and monitors the position of the greater trochanter.

3.4. Trigger Point Examination

Trigger point examination requires specific knowledge of fiber direction of the gluteal muscles so that the clinician can be more confident regarding in which muscles the TrPs are found. Figure 54-10 is a depiction of the fiber arrangement of the gluteus maximus, gluteus medius, and gluteus minimus muscles. A cross-fiber flat palpation may be utilized for the examination of TrPs in the gluteus maximus muscle depending on the region of the muscle being examined. The gluteus maximus muscle can be accessed with the patient in the side-lying position (Figure 54-11), with the hips flexed to take up some tissue slack, or in the prone position. The superior fibers can be palpated utilizing a cross-fiber flat palpation (Figure 54-11A and B), whereas the lower fibers may be examined utilizing a cross-fiber pincer palpation (Figure 54-11C). However, all portions of the gluteus maximus muscle can be examined for TrPs using a cross-fiber flat palpation. For some patients, a greater degree of hip flexion may be useful to increase the sensitivity of the TrPs to palpation. Along the inferior and inferolateral aspects of the gluteus maximus muscle, careful examination should be made to differentiate gluteus maximus muscle fiber orientation from the piriformis and hip external rotator muscles. Examination along the lower border of the muscle can be performed using a cross-fiber pincer palpation or a cross-fiber flat palpation against the ischium.

4. DIFFERENTIAL DIAGNOSIS

4.1. Activation and Perpetuation of Trigger Points

A posture or activity that activates a TrP, if not corrected, can also perpetuate it. In any part of the gluteus maximus muscle, TrPs may be activated by unaccustomed eccentric loading, eccentric exercise in an unconditioned muscle, or maximal or submaximal concentric loading.[33] Trigger points may also be activated or aggravated when the muscle is placed in a shortened and/or lengthened position for an extended period of time.

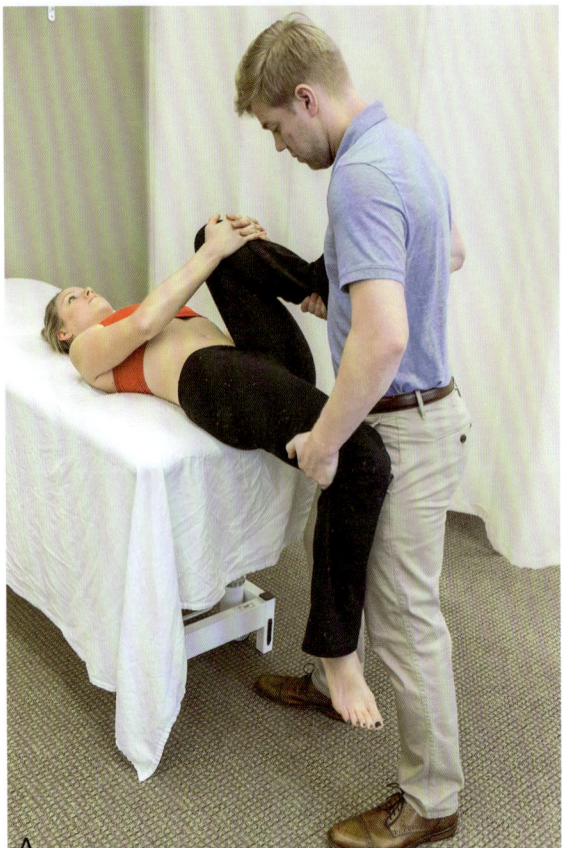
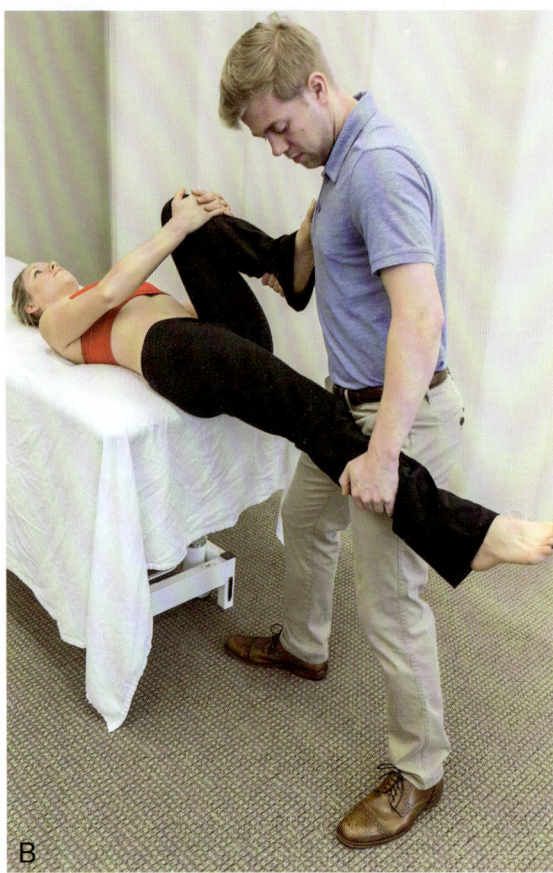

Figure 54-7. Thomas test position for hip flexor length assessment. A, One-joint muscles. B, Two-joint muscle.

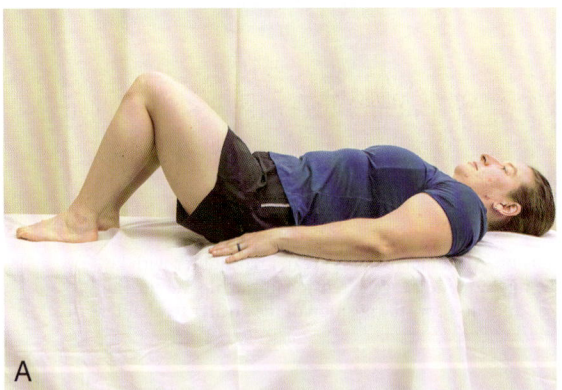
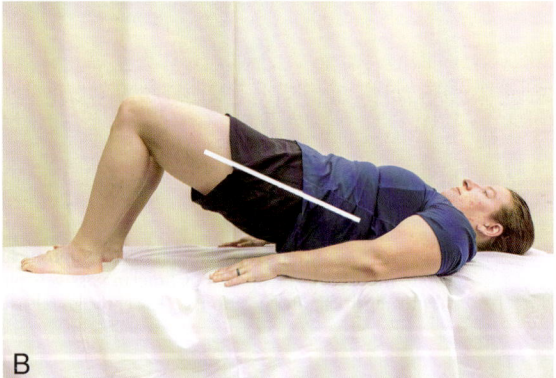
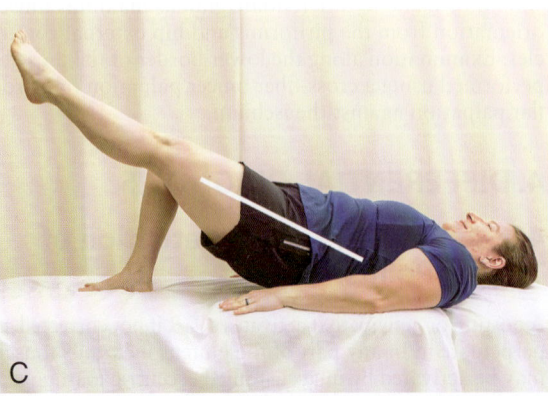

Figure 54-8. Bridging maneuver for assessment of gluteus maximus muscle strength and motor control. A, Starting position. B, End position with trunk and hip in alignment. C, Challenging the right gluteus maximus muscle.

Box 54.2 Gluteus maximus muscle retraining program

Starting position (Figure 54-9A)	A pillow is placed under the abdomen to keep the lumbosacral spine in a neutral position.
Level 1 (Figure 54-9B)	The patient points the toes into the supporting surface and attempts to straighten the knee using the gluteus maximus and hamstring muscles. The clinician should note any substitution with the quadriceps femoris muscles and/or the thoracolumbar paraspinal muscles.
Level 2 (Figure 54-9C)	From the position of level 1, the patient points the toes, so that the lower extremity is no longer supported, and holds this position for 6-10 seconds before slowly placing the toes back down as pictured in level 1. Finally, the patient slowly lowers the knee back to the starting position.
Level 3 (Figure 54-9D)	The patient lifts the leg off the surface leading with the hamstrings, gluteus maximus muscles, and contralateral and ipsilateral paraspinal muscles, with no trunk rotation or excessive motion in the sagittal plane.

Gluteus maximus TrPs may be activated by actions that place the muscle under greater demand and overload its capacity. A fall or a near-fall can cause acute overload of the gluteus maximus muscle especially if the muscle sustains a vigorous eccentric contraction in an effort to prevent the fall. The impact of a direct blow on one buttock, as in a backward fall onto a step or the floor, may be responsible for initiating gluteus maximus TrPs. Sitting on a wallet placed in a back pocket that extends under the buttock can perpetuate and aggravate TrPs in the gluteal muscles by concentrating pressure on them. The resultant low back and buttock pain is likely to be erroneously attributed to nerve pressure and has been called "back pocket sciatica."[34] However, pain referred from TrPs in the gluteus maximus muscle alone would not have a full sciatic nerve distribution. Sleeping on one side with the thigh of the upper lower extremity sharply flexed can overstretch the uppermost gluteus maximus muscle and activate TrPs.

Another common, but avoidable, cause of activation of gluteus maximus or medius TrPs is the injection of an irritant medication intramuscularly into the gluteal area.[35] As the most superficial gluteal muscle, the gluteus maximus muscle is the most likely to be injected. Persons giving such injections should palpate the muscles for TrPs and avoid any hypersensitive spots.

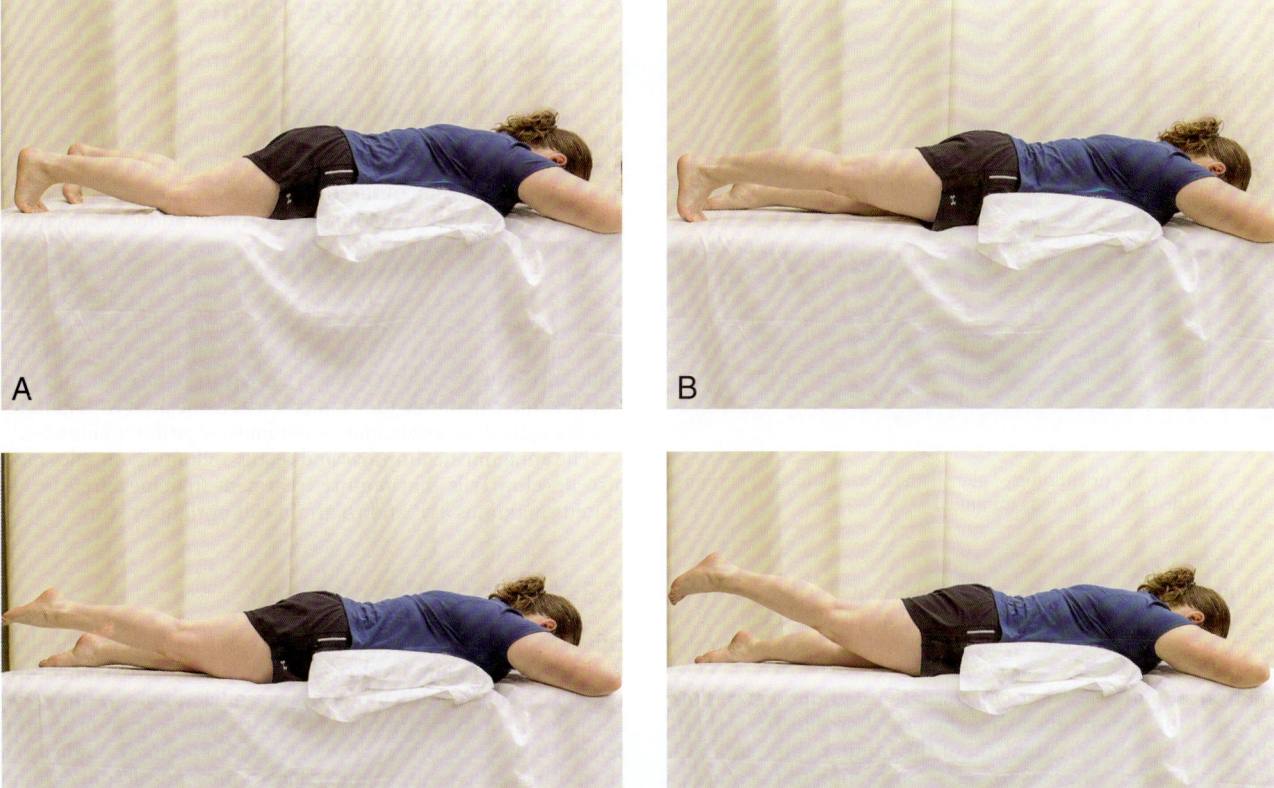

Figure 54-9. Gluteus maximus muscle retraining. A, Starting position. B, Extending the knee with the gluteus maximus and hamstring muscles with the foot on the table. C, Straightening the knee with the gluteus maximus and hamstring muscles, followed by pointing the toes. D, Lifting the leg off the table.

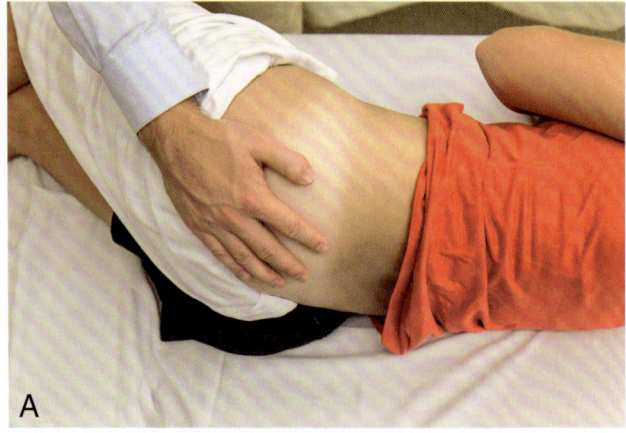
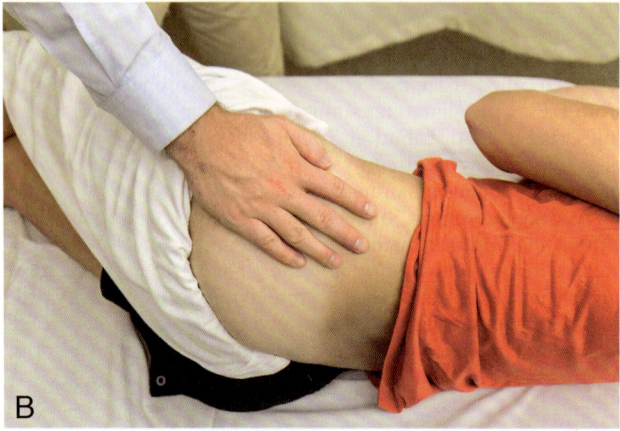
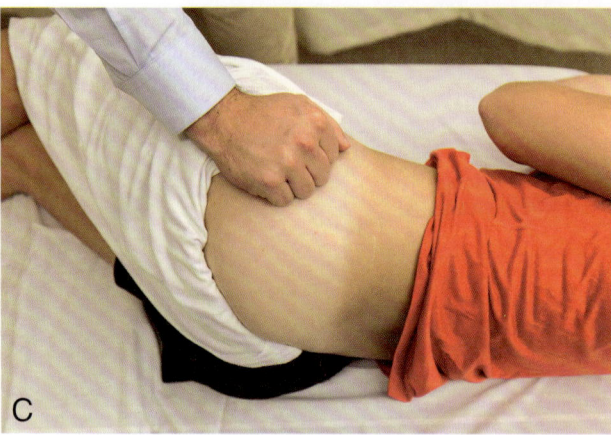

Figure 54-10. Fiber orientation of gluteal muscles. A, Gluteus maximus. B, Gluteus medius. C, Gluteus minimus.

Diluting the material to be injected with an equal quantity of 2% procaine solution may prevent activation of a latent TrP in the event that the medication is accidentally injected into the region of the TrPs.

Physical activities that can perpetuate gluteus maximus TrPs include swimming using the crawl stroke (freestyle), which requires hyperextension of the lumbar spine in addition to hip extension. This forceful contraction of the gluteus maximus and lower paraspinal extensor muscles in a strongly shortened position can activate and perpetuate their TrPs. A similar cause of gluteus maximus muscle overload may be conditioning exercises (leg lifts) that hyperextend the low back and hip, either in the prone or standing position. Repetitious tasks, such as frequently leaning over and lifting a baby out of the playpen or crib, lifting a box from the floor by leaning over, or weeding a garden may perpetuate gluteus maximus TrPs.

The gluteus maximus muscle provides stability of the trunk and pelvis and is innately involved with movement of the hip and lower extremity, ambulation, climbing, lifting, and throwing.[16,21,36] Activities that would potentially perpetuate TrPs may include uphill walking or running, climbing a ladder, or returning to standing from a squatting position.

Biomechanical or motor control changes in the lumbopelvic and hip region can also affect the activation of the gluteus maximus muscle and cause the perpetuation of TrPs. Increased activity of the gluteus maximus muscle has been found to occur in patients with chronic low back pain.[37] Hip pathology has been shown to alter muscle recruitment patterns, either increasing or inhibiting activation of the gluteus maximus muscle.[38-40] Hip arthritis has been demonstrated to cause increased activation of the gluteus maximus muscle during the mid-stance of gait.[39] Changes in foot function that lead to excessive pronation may also lead to activation of TrPs in the gluteal muscles. Abnormal pronation may cause excessive internal rotation of the hip during the stance phase in walking, and this movement is counteracted to some extent by the activity of the horizontal fibers of the gluteus maximus muscle, which may lead to overload of the muscle.

Altered activation patterns of the gluteal muscles and development of TrPs in the gluteus maximus muscle are a common clinical finding present in lower extremity dysfunctions, fibromyalgia,[41] lower back syndromes,[42] and sacroiliac joint dysfunction.[43,44] Adelmanesh et al[42] found associations between TrPs in the gluteal muscles and lumbar radiculopathy in 76.4% of patients when compared with 1.9% of control subjects. Trigger points in the gluteal muscles have also been found in other lower extremity conditions such as patellofemoral pain syndrome.[45]

4.2. Associated Trigger Points

Associated TrPs can develop in the referred pain areas caused by primary TrPs.[46] Therefore, musculature in the referred pain areas for each muscle should also be considered. Examples of muscles in the hip that should be examined include the piriformis, gluteus medius, posterior portion of the gluteus minimus, quadratus lumborum, obturator internus and externus, superior and inferior gemelli, proximal hamstrings, adductor magnus, and coccygeus muscles.[23]

Muscles that can refer into the buttock may also need to be assessed. These muscles include iliocostalis lumborum, longissimus thoracis, quadratus lumborum, semitendinosus, semimembranosus, rectus abdominis, pelvic floor, and soleus muscles.[23] The lumbar multifidus muscle also has been shown to refer pain into the buttock and can mimic the pain patterns associated with gluteus maximus, gluteus medius, gluteus minimus, or piriformis muscles.[47]

The antagonistic iliopsoas and rectus abdominis muscles may also develop TrPs that require treatment to achieve release of gluteus maximus TrP and to attain full upright posture.

4.3. Associated Pathology

Differential diagnosis of clinical conditions should include lumbar pathology (including facet or intervertebral disc dysfunction), radicular pain or radiculopathy, sacroiliac joint dysfunction, coccydynia, or hip pathology. The buttock is a common area of referral from many other pathologies, so a thorough examination should be carried out. Lumbar facet joint and sacroiliac joint dysfunctions frequently will refer pain into the buttock.[48,49] The sacroiliac joint refers pain to the buttock alone and, sometimes, to the buttock and other areas.[50,51] The hip joint has been shown to refer pain into the buttock in as many as 71% of patients presenting with hip dysfunction.[52] Although the most common report with femoroacetabular impingement is groin pain, buttock pain has been found to occur in 29% of patients.[53] Ischiofemoral

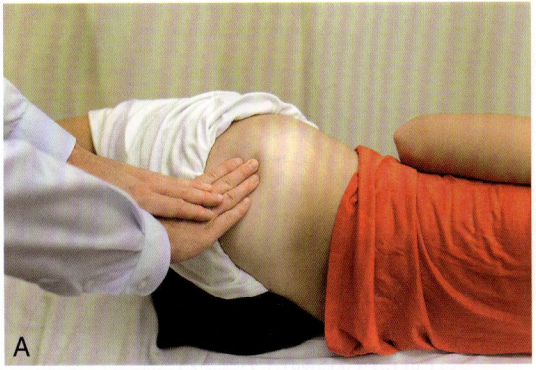
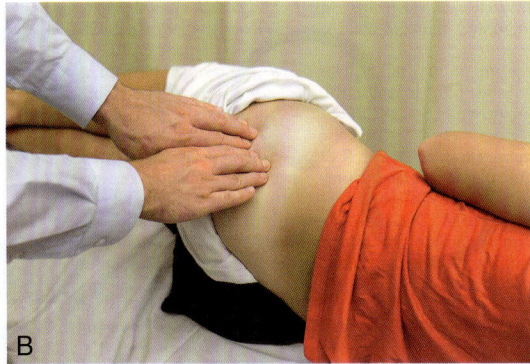
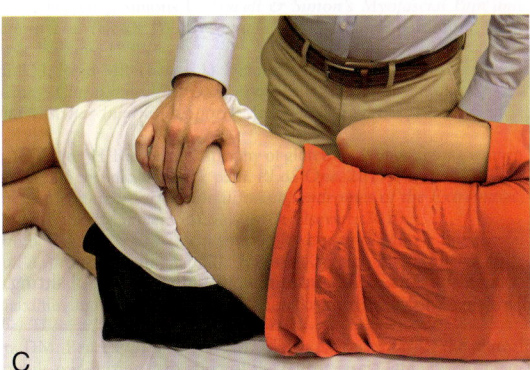

Figure 54-11. Examination for TrPs in the gluteus maximus muscle. A and B, Cross-fiber flat palpation. C, Cross-fiber pincer palpation for lower portion of the gluteus maximus muscle.

ligament impingement may also cause inferior buttock pain mimicking gluteus maximus TrP referral.[54]

Some individuals with greater trochanteric tenderness that is relieved by injection of a local anesthetic have TrPs in the gluteus maximus muscle instead of, or in addition to, bursitis. Subacute trochanteric bursitis has been commonly associated with low back pain, hip disease, and/or leg length discrepancies, conditions often associated with TrPs of the gluteal musculature. However, the location of the bursa is more lateral than the area where gluteus maximus TrPs are usually found. If present, TrPs in this superficial muscle should be detectable by their taut bands, spot tenderness, and referred symptoms.

5. CORRECTIVE ACTIONS

Patients with active TrPs in the gluteus maximus muscle should limit the duration of time spent sitting. Patients who primarily work on a computer should have an ergonomic assessment performed, and adjustments to the workstation should be made as needed. Behavioral modifications including taking short breaks to move, utilizing a standing desk, or improving postural support will also assist in reducing symptoms. Using a timer placed across the room to remind the patient to get up, walk across the room, and reset the device before returning to the chair can be a helpful strategy to encourage movement with minimal distraction from thought. Special consideration should be paid to the design of the chair and the material of the seat because they dictate the amount of pressure and the contact area on the buttocks, as well as the resulting tissue perfusion.[55]

Improvements in posture and postural support may also assist in reducing pain from TrPs in the gluteus maximus muscle. Sleeping side-lying with the painful side up and placing a pillow between the knees may help reduce symptoms and improve sleep quality.

Gluteus maximus TrPs can be treated with self-pressure release techniques utilizing a lacrosse ball or other TrP self-pressure release tools, based on individual preference and general mobility (Figure 54-12A). The patient can place a rounded self-release tool like a ball or dome on the floor and slowly apply pressure to the TrPs by resting the buttocks on the tool and placing weight through the arms to moderate pressure (Figure 54-12B and D). This technique can also be used on a wall (Figure 54-12C). A wrap-around self-release tool can also be utilized in the standing position (Figure 54-12E). For all pressure release techniques, the patient should hold pressure for 15 to 30 seconds, repeating for six repetitions. Self-release can be repeated every 2 to 3 hours as long as relief of symptoms is achieved. Caution is warranted as excessive pressure (more than 4/10 pain scale) on the TrPs can actually cause activation and perpetuation of the TrPs.

Foam rolling can be utilized to help release TrPs in the gluteus maximus muscle and is commonly used by athletes. The patient sits on the foam roller, leans back slightly onto both hands, and works slowly from the bottom of the gluteal region up toward the top. While rolling over the gluteus maximus muscle, the patient should stop and slowly rock over the area of tender spots that are felt to encourage the release of TrPs. Pressure should be mildly uncomfortable but not painful.

Specific stretching of the gluteus maximus muscle is difficult to achieve. To attempt to stretch this muscle, the patient lies face up (Figure 54-13A) or sits on the edge of a chair (Figure 54-13B), bringing the involved knee toward the chest and then crossing the leg over the body. The stretch is held for 30 seconds and repeated a minimum of four times. The patient can also use a hold-relax technique to improve the efficiency of the stretch. While sitting, the individual first pulls the knee toward his or her opposite shoulder in order to flex the hip by grasping the thigh behind the knee (Figure 54-13B). The patient then uses the hands to resist a gentle voluntary effort by the gluteal muscles to push the thigh down toward the floor for 6 to 10 seconds, immediately followed by relaxation. After relaxation, the patient then pulls the thigh a little higher, further stretching the buttocks, and repeats the sequence. This sequence can be repeated three to five times and two to three times per day.

Chapter 55

Gluteus Medius Muscle

"Lumbago Muscle"

Joseph M. Donnelly and Paul Thomas

1. INTRODUCTION

The gluteus medius muscle has been described as an analogist to the deltoid in the shoulder. It is a thick, multipennate muscle that provides most of the strength required for hip abduction. The gluteus medius and gluteus minimus muscles are active throughout the gait cycle and are key to supporting the lower extremity during the mid-stance phase of gait and stabilizing the pelvis in the frontal plane. Trigger points (TrPs) within the gluteus medius muscle can refer pain into the low back just above and below the beltline, the sacrum, the buttock, the lateral hip, and the posterior upper thigh. Patients may report difficulty with rising from a seated position due to the excessive load placed on the gluteus medius muscle, therefore activating and perpetuating its TrPs. Activities that can cause overload of the gluteus medius and gluteus minimus muscles include weight lifting, running, and habitually shifting weight onto one side as in carrying a child or heavy load on the hip. Trigger points in the gluteus medius muscle are commonly associated with other painful conditions of the lower quadrant. Low back pain caused by gluteus medius TrPs can be disabling and interfere with many functional activities. Differential diagnosis should include lumbar radicular pain or radiculopathy, sacroiliac joint dysfunction, greater trochanteric pain syndrome, hip joint pathology or dysfunction, and knee dysfunction. Corrective actions could include techniques to improve sitting and sleeping postures, trunk control, gait mechanics, self-pressure release, and self-stretching techniques. For resolution of symptoms, correction of altered biomechanics in the lower kinetic chain may need to be addressed.

2. ANATOMIC CONSIDERATIONS

The fan-shaped gluteus medius muscle lies deep to the gluteus maximus muscle and superficial to the gluteus minimus muscle. The gluteus medius muscle originates from the external surface of the ilium along the anterior three-fourths of the iliac crest, between the anterior and posterior gluteal lines, and from the gluteal aponeurosis that covers the anterolateral two-thirds of the muscle.[1,2] Figure 55-1 describes the three origins of the gluteus medius muscle. The deep fascicles arise from the gluteal fossa, extending from the posterior sacroiliac ligaments and posterior gluteal line, the body of the ilium above the anterior gluteal line, and the anterior superior iliac spine. The second attachment site is along the deep surface of the gluteal aponeurosis, and the fascia latae. The third site is from the posteroinferior aspect of the iliac crest.[2]

The muscle is multipennate with more fascicles and cross-sectional area in the anterior portion than in the middle or posterior portion.[2] Fibers in the anterior portion of the muscle are directed posterior and inferior, the middle portion fibers are directed vertically, and the posterior portion fibers are directed anteriorly and inferiorly, with some fibers nearly horizontal[2,3] (Figure 55-1). These fibers converge to form a flat tendon that inserts along the lateral surface of the greater trochanter of the femur. Some authors have also described insertions on the superior, posteromedial, anterosuperior, or posterosuperior aspect of the greater trochanter.[1,4,5] At its posterior edge, the gluteus medius muscle may also blend with the piriformis or the gluteus minimus muscle.[1,5]

The trochanteric bursa of the gluteus medius muscle separates the tendon from the surface of the greater trochanter of the femur over which the tendon glides. The bursa lies between the trochanteric attachments of the gluteus minimus muscle proximally and the gluteus medius muscle distally.[1]

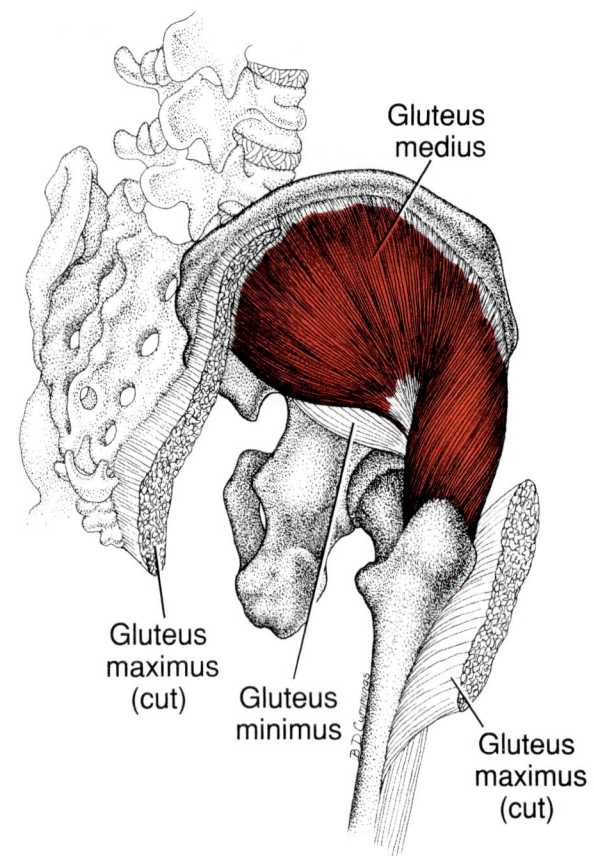

Figure 55-1. Attachments of the right gluteus medius muscle (red) in the posterolateral view. The gluteus maximus muscle has been cut and removed; its distal end is reflected. Note the anteriorly directed posterior fibers and the posteriorly directed anterior fibers.

2.1. Innervation and Vascularization

The gluteus medius muscle is innervated by the superior gluteal nerve, which is mainly derived from the L4, L5, S1 nerve roots. The superior gluteal nerve passes between the gluteus medius and gluteus minimus muscles, sending branches to each muscle, and because of this relationship, it is vulnerable during surgical interventions (lateral or anterolateral approaches) that require splitting the gluteus medius muscle.[1] For instance, the transgluteal approach used for total hip arthroplasty surgery often causes a partially denervated gluteus medius muscle.[6]

The vascular supply of the gluteus medius muscle is provided via the superior gluteal artery, which exits the pelvis through the greater sciatic foramen superior to the piriformis muscle, traveling anterior between the gluteus medius and gluteus minimus muscles along with the superior gluteal nerve.[1,4] The superficial branch of the superior gluteal artery supplies the gluteus maximus muscle, whereas the deep branch of the superior gluteal artery supplies the gluteus medius, gluteus minimus, and tensor fascia latae muscles.[1,7]

2.2. Function

The gluteus medius and gluteus minimus muscles typically function together as primary hip abductors. However, analysis of the moment arms of the gluteus medius muscle suggests that when the hip is flexed above 20°, the entire muscle is responsible for internal rotation and has limited ability to perform hip abduction in this position.[8,9]

The gluteus medius muscle is frequently described as having three divisions. In addition to abduction, the anterior portion of the gluteus medius muscle internally rotates the femur.[1] Retchford et al[10] suggest that the anterior portion of the gluteus medius muscle is active during hip extension in nonweight bearing, which may prevent anterior translation of the femoral head. The primary action of the middle portion of the gluteus medius muscle is hip abduction and hip internal rotation. The large cross-sectional area and vertical fiber orientation of the middle portion of the gluteus medius muscle would suggest that it plays a role in generating strong hip abduction and pelvic stabilization during the gait cycle. The middle portion of the muscle has also been found to be active in hip external rotation, but only at very low levels of intensity.[11] The smaller moment arm and the smaller cross-sectional area of the posterior fibers suggest that it likely plays a role in stabilizing the head of the femur in the acetabulum.[12] With the hip in a neutral and extended position, the posterior portion also boasts a moment arm for external rotation.[8]

One of the main functions of the gluteus medius muscle is to stabilize the pelvis on the femur and help maintain frontal plane alignment with the foot and knee in a closed kinetic chain during the unilateral stance phase of the gait cycle.[12,13] During gait, the anterior fibers of the gluteus medius muscle assist the middle fibers in maintaining pelvic stabilization due to the large cross-sectional area, vertical fiber arrangement, and large moment arm. Also, the anterior fibers are believed to contribute to forward contralateral rotation of the pelvis in the transverse plane during the gait cycle.[12] Studies analyzing the activity of the gluteus medius muscle during gait also suggest a stabilizing effect of the pelvis on the hip by the activation prior to, and after, initial contact of the foot on the ground.

High levels of activation of the gluteus medius muscle take place during the gait cycle but are unaffected by ambulation on a sloped surface. Similar levels of activation occur regardless of walking on flat, inclined, or declined surfaces.[14] The gluteus medius muscle does not show changes in activation with variations in the speed of ambulation.[15,16] During running, peak muscle force of the gluteus medius muscle has been shown to decrease during the stance phase of gait as step rate increases. The opposite is true for the swing phase, when peak force increases in the muscle as the step rate increases.[17]

Using surface electromyography (EMG), Lee et al[18] found that, when the opposite upper extremity was carrying a load greater than 3 kg the posterior portion of the gluteus medius muscle on the opposite side of the load demonstrated significantly more EMG activity as opposed to no load and a 1 kg load.

Autopsy samples[19] of gluteus medius muscles in normal adults under age 44 years showed 58% slow-twitch type 1 fibers and 42% fast-twitch type 2 muscle fibers. A relative (8%) loss of type 2 fibers in the gluteus medius muscle was observed in persons with osteoarthritis of the hip. Another adult group[19] was divided equally between individuals older and younger than 65 years of age (individual variability was great in both groups), and in every subject, the number of slow-twitch type 1 fibers, which depend largely on oxidative metabolism, exceeded the number of fast-twitch type 2 fibers, which utilize glycolytic energy pathways. Therefore, the gluteus medius muscle may respond better to exercises with slow speeds and higher repetitions because a large part of its composition is made up of type 1 fibers.

2.3. Functional Unit

The functional unit to which a muscle belongs includes the muscles that reinforce and counter its actions as well as the joints that the muscle crosses. The functional interdependence of these structures is reflected in the organization and neural connections of the sensory motor cortex. The functional unit is emphasized because the presence of the TrP in one muscle of the unit increases the likelihood that the other muscles will develop TrPs. When inactivating TrPs in a muscle, one must be concerned about TrPs that may develop in muscles that are functionally interdependent. Box 55-1 represents the functional unit of the gluteus medius muscle.[20]

When the hip is flexed, the obturator internus and externus, gemelli superior and inferior, and piriformis muscles also assist with producing hip abduction.[1]

When the hip is positioned in extension, the posterior fibers of the gluteus medius muscle work synergistically with the posterior fibers of the gluteus minimus, gluteus maximus, obturator internus and externus, gemelli superior and inferior, piriformis, and quadratus femoris muscles to produce external rotation of the hip.

The anterior fibers of the gluteus medius muscle in extension, and the entire muscle in flexion, produce internal rotation of the hip. This action is synergistic with the gluteus minimus and tensor fascia latae muscles.

3. CLINICAL PRESENTATION

3.1. Referred Pain Pattern

Trigger points in the gluteus medius muscle refer pain (or other symptoms) into the buttock, lower back, sacrum, posterior crest of the ilium, immediately lateral to the sacroiliac joint, from the lateral buttock to the hip, and to the posterior and lateral upper thigh (Figure 55-2). Any portion of the gluteus medius muscle can refer the symptoms noted. Commonly, TrPs found near the posterior portion of the muscle will refer pain near the sacroiliac joint, sacrum, and buttock. Trigger points found in the middle of the muscle will commonly refer more laterally and to the mid buttock, with occasional referral into the posterior and lateral upper thigh. Trigger points found along the anterior portion of the gluteus medius muscle, where the muscle is more available to palpation, will refer pain and symptoms along the iliac crest, the lower portion of the lumbar spine, and over the sacrum. Trigger points in the gluteus medius muscle can be a commonly overlooked source of pain in the lower back.[20] This hypothesis was demonstrated by Iglesias-Gonzalez et al,[21] who found that active gluteus medius TrPs were highly prevalent in patients with mechanical low back pain.

Box 55-1 Functional unit of the gluteus medius muscle

Action	Synergists	Antagonists
Hip abduction	Gluteus minimus Gluteus maximus Obturator internus Tensor fascia latae Gemelli superior and inferior piriformis Obturator externus (external rotators can abduct the flexed thigh)	Adductor magnus Adductor longus Adductor brevis Gracilis Pectineus
Hip external rotation (hip neutral and extension; posterior fibers)	Gluteus minimus (posterior fibers) Gluteus maximus Obturator internus and externus Gemelli superior and interior quadratus femoris	Gluteus medius (anterior fibers) Gluteus minimus (anterior fibers in extension, all fibers when the hip is flexed) Tensor fascia latae
Hip internal rotation (anterior fibers)	Gluteus minimus Tensor fascia latae	Gluteus medius (posterior fibers) Gluteus maximus Gluteus minimus (posterior fibers when in extension) Obturator internus and externus Gemelli superior and inferior piriformis Quadratus femoris

Other authors illustrate[22-24] or describe[25] similar patterns of referred pain from this muscle. Two older papers describe referral of pain after injection of the gluteus medius muscle with hypertonic saline.[26,27] A more recent study found that the gluteus medius muscle referred pain spread to the greater trochanter, buttock, posterior thigh, lateral thigh, knee, and leg after hypertonic saline injection.[28] Sola[24] described gluteus medius muscle referred pain as extending into the posterior thigh and calf, though it is the opinion of the authors that this pattern of pain probably arises from TrPs in the underlying gluteus minimus muscle (Chapter 56). Sola[24] also notes that the gluteus medius muscle is a frequent cause of hip pain in the later stages of pregnancy. The lateral hip pain pattern has been also noted with rare tear lesions of the proximal attachment of the gluteus medius muscle.[29]

3.2. Symptoms

Patients with active TrPs in the gluteus medius muscle are likely to have a chief report of pain during walking and with weight-bearing activities. As the gluteus medius muscle is most active during weight-bearing activities, the patient will report increased pain and discomfort with walking, running, and stair climbing. It is commonly seen in clinical practice that patients with TrPs in the gluteus medius muscle experience pain during prolonged periods of standing, for example waiting at the bus stop. To avoid the pain in these scenarios, the patient will often change the pelvic stance by shifting weight off the painful lower extremity. Pain with walking on inclines or declines is more commonly reported with gluteus maximus TrPs and is not typically associated with

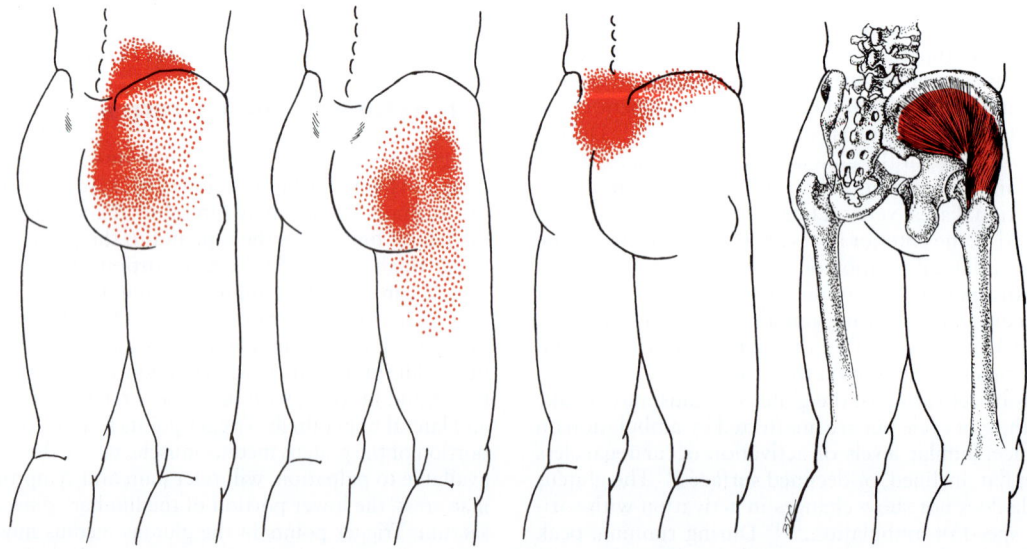

Figure 55-2. Pain patterns (bright red) referred from TrPs in the right gluteus medius muscle. The essential pain pattern is solid red, and the spillover pattern is stippled.

pain from TrPs in this muscle. Getting into and out of the car may be quite painful. The patient may report excruciating pain in the low back along the beltline on the side of the TrPs. Pain from these TrPs can be disabling and interfere with many functional activities. The patient may also report difficulty with rising from a seated position due to the excessive load placed on the gluteus medius muscle during this activity. Difficulty in sleeping may be reported, especially when lying on the involved side, due to pain caused by pressure on the TrPs. Bending and lifting activities will typically not be associated with gluteus medius TrP symptoms. TrPs in the gluteus medius muscles are often the cause of low back and hip pain during the later stages of pregnancy.

3.3. Patient Examination

After a thorough subjective examination the clinician should make a detailed drawing representing the pain pattern that the patient has described. This depiction will assist in planning the physical examination and can be useful in monitoring the progression of the patient as symptoms improve or change. The type, quality, and location of the pain should be carefully assessed, and the utilization of standardized outcome tools is imperative when examining patients with low back pain and lower extremity dysfunctions.

A physical examination should be conducted to rule out lumbar, sacroiliac, or hip joint dysfunctions. Range of motion testing of the hip and lumbar spine; passive accessory motion testing of the hip, sacroiliac joint, and/or lumbar spine; strength testing of the gluteus medius and gluteus minimus and other hip muscles; and any appropriate neurologic testing or orthopedic special tests should be performed. A careful assessment must be made to rule out referral into the buttock from other muscles, joints, or neural tissues.

Both the gluteus medius and gluteus minimus muscles function synergistically to provide frontal plane stability for the lumbopelvic region.[30] It is important to perform a postural examination in standing to identify a structural or functional scoliosis, the presence of an iliac upslip, anterior innominate rotation,[31] and leg length discrepancy. A leg length discrepancy may be identified as a frontal plane asymmetry of the pelvis, with one side of the pelvis elevated and the opposite side depressed. This pelvic deviation could cause TrPs in the gluteus medius and gluteus minimus muscles on either or both sides from muscle overload. Functional activities such as sit-to-stand, single-leg stance, and double- and single-leg squat (Figure 55-3A) should also be examined. The clinician should take note of any frontal plane deviations in the pelvis, hip, and/or knee, and any excessive transverse plane motion at the ankle and foot (Figure 55-3B). The clinician should note gait deviations such as a Trendelenburg sign at mid-stance (Figure 55-4A and B), or forward lean of the trunk at heel strike, both of which indicate gluteus medius and gluteus minimus muscles weakness.[30]

Lee et al[32] investigated static and dynamic single-leg stance postures in 45 recreationally active women between 23 and 34 years of age. They found those with weaker hip abductor muscles demonstrated poor static and dynamic postural stability compared with those with stronger hip abductors. The investigators concluded that in the presence of weak hip abductors, the subjects relied more on their ankle for stability and control when standing on one leg.[32]

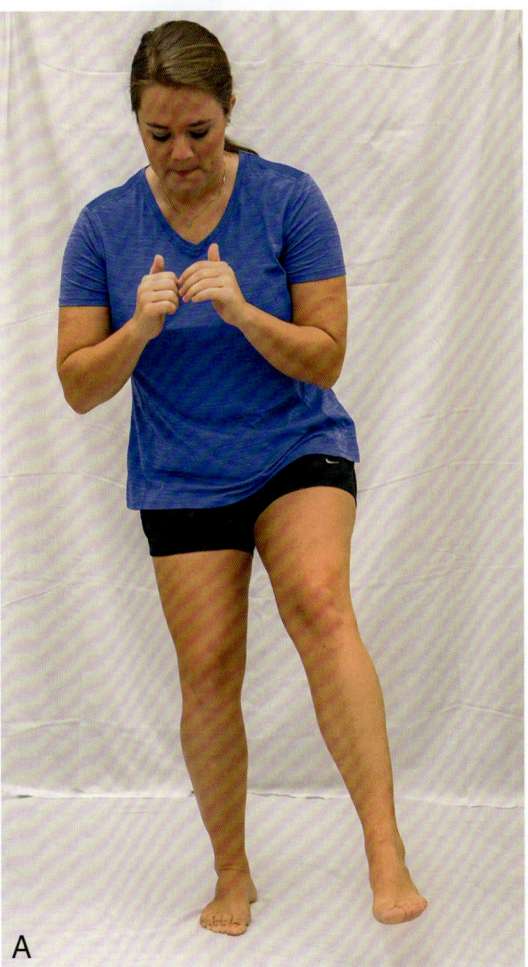 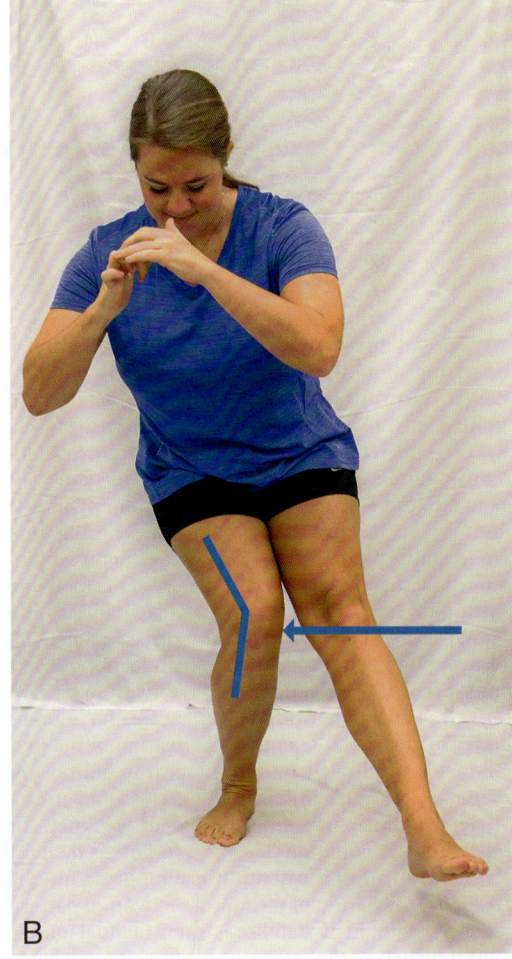

Figure 55-3. Single-leg squat assessment of gluteus medius and gluteus minimus muscle of the knee in the frontal plane. A, Good control. B, Loss of control in the frontal plane with excessive valgus force (line) with increased stress at the medial knee (arrow).

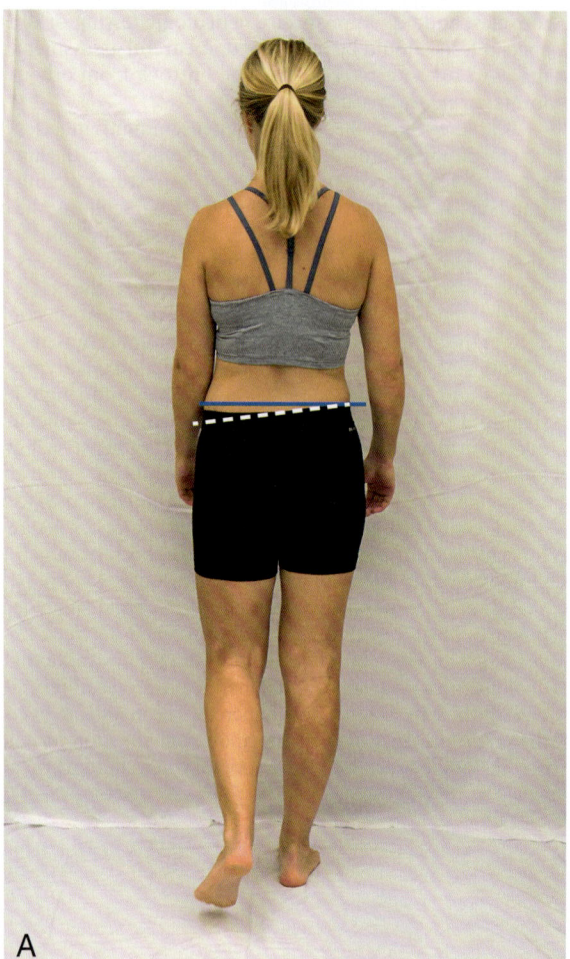 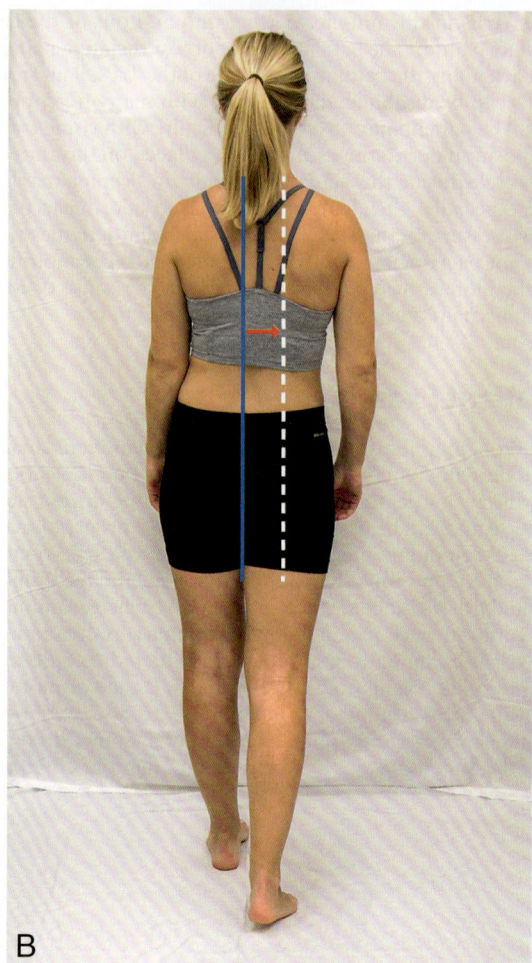

Figure 55-4. Gluteus medius and gluteus minimus muscle weakness. A, Positive Trendelenburg sign. B, Compensated Trendelenburg Sign with shift of the center of gravity over the stance limb.

Because of regional interdependence of the hip and lumbar spine, specific testing should be carried out to identify interactive impairments. The prime movers for efficient hip abduction include the gluteus medius, gluteus minimus, and tensor fascia latae muscles. Oftentimes, the quadratus lumborum muscle compensates for weak gluteus medius or gluteus minimus muscles, which results in excessive forces in the lumbar spine. The role of the quadratus lumborum and abdominal muscles during limb movement are to stabilize the pelvis.[33] To assess the possibility of this compensation, the muscle activation pattern of side-lying hip abduction should be carefully examined. The patient's hip and lumbar spine should be placed and supported in a neutral position prior to examining the side-lying hip abduction muscle activation pattern. The hip abduction muscle activation pattern has been described as beginning with the gluteus medius, gluteus minimus, and tensor fascia latae muscles activating in the first 20° of hip abduction followed by the quadratus lumborum and abdominal muscles.[33] Deviations in this activation pattern, especially pelvic elevation, may indicate gluteal weakness or inhibition due to TrPs. A common deviation to note is facilitation and early recruitment of the quadratus lumborum muscle (Figure 55-5A). If this deviation of the muscle activation pattern is observed, the pelvis should be stabilized during manual muscle testing to accurately assess the strength of the gluteus medius and gluteus minimus muscles (Figure 55-5B).

Hip abductor strength testing should be carried out bilaterally because both sides are responsible for lumbopelvic stability at different times during the gait cycle. If one side tests weaker than the other, excessive frontal plane motion can result in abnormal loading forces in the lumbar spine.

Gluteus medius and gluteus minimus muscle weakness or inhibition (which will present as weakness) can also lead to abnormal loading of the femoral head and cause excessive varus load in the lower extremity secondary to a relatively adducted position of the femur to the pelvis on the stance side.[34] This relative adducted position of the femur can also lead to compressive loading of the greater trochanter of the femur due to tensile loading of the gluteal muscles and may lead to abnormal compressive loading of the trochanteric bursa. The hip adductors should also be examined carefully for length and strength deficits as it is vital that the hip adductors and abductors work synergistically during weight-bearing activities, especially during gait.[30]

If the gluteus medius and gluteus minimus muscles demonstrate impaired muscle activation patterns, release of TrPs should be the first priority for treatment, after which the patient should be placed on a gluteus medius and minimus muscle retraining program. Figure 55-6 and Box 55-2 illustrate a three-level progression for gluteus medius and gluteus minimus muscles retraining.

Effective hip abduction training is essential for athletes because researchers have found that weak hip abductors play a role in anterior knee pain and are correlated to a higher incidence of anterior cruciate ligament ruptures.[35,36] Lower activity of the gluteus medius muscle has been also found in patients after diagnosis of patellofemoral pain[37] or after reconstruction of the anterior cruciate ligament.[38] Additionally, this reduced activity in the gluteus medius muscle is higher in runners with

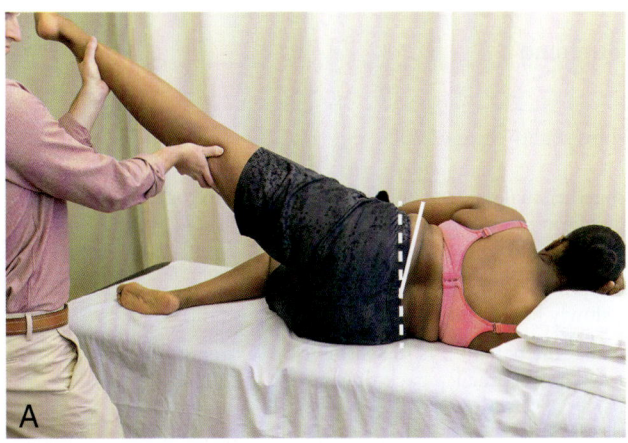
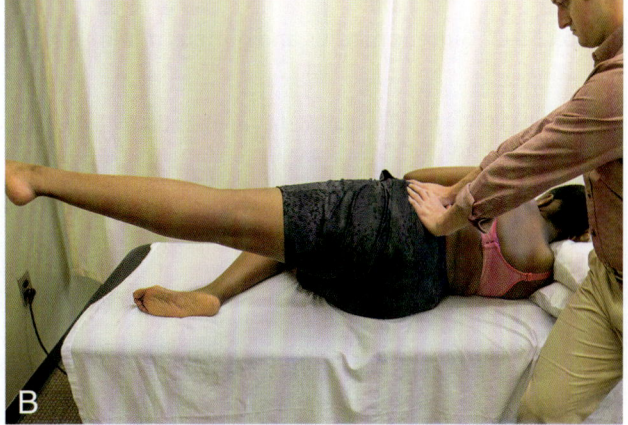

Figure 55-5. Side-lying hip abduction muscle activation pattern and strength test. A, Muscle activation pattern observing hip and pelvic motion. Note elevation of the left iliac crest as indicated by the solid white line demonstrating compensation by the quadratus lumborum muscle for inadequate strength or inhibition of the gluteus medius muscle. B, Stabilization of the pelvis to inhibit the quadratus lumborum muscle for an accurate assessment of gluteus medius muscle inhibition or strength deficits. Note the change in the observed hip abduction range of motion.

rear foot strike and patellofemoral pain syndrome,[39] which suggests that the entire lower extremity should be evaluated. Nevertheless, others have observed that higher gluteus medius muscle activity during running is a risk factor for hamstring injury in football players.[40] Therefore, proper evaluation and treatment of the gluteus medius muscle is essential for athletes as part of a comprehensive lower extremity plan of care.

3.4. Trigger Point Examination

Trigger point examination requires specific knowledge of fiber direction of the gluteal muscles so that the clinician can be confident which muscles contain TrPs. Figure 54-10 illustrates the fiber arrangement and general size of the gluteus maximus, gluteus medius, and gluteus minimus muscles. Trigger points in the gluteus medius muscle are examined with the patient lying on the unaffected side. A pillow is placed between the knees to keep the hip in a neutral position and to avoid an aggravating stretch position. The clinician utilizes a cross-fiber flat palpation to examine the muscle (Figure 55-7A and B). The posterior portion is covered by the gluteus maximus muscle, making it more challenging to differentiate gluteus maximus TrPs from those of the gluteus medius muscle. If TrPs are felt in the gluteus maximus muscle, it may be necessary to inactivate those first to better evaluate the deeper gluteus medius muscle. Trigger points in the superficial fibers of the gluteus maximus muscle are easily palpated and are located just under the skin. Taut bands that feel deeper may be in deeper gluteus maximus muscle fibers or in the underlying gluteus medius muscle.

Figure 55-8 illustrates the borders of each muscle and where the gluteal muscles overlap to better inform palpatory exploration of these muscles. The gluteus medius muscle is limited superiorly by the rim of the pelvis (Figure 55-8A), in front by a

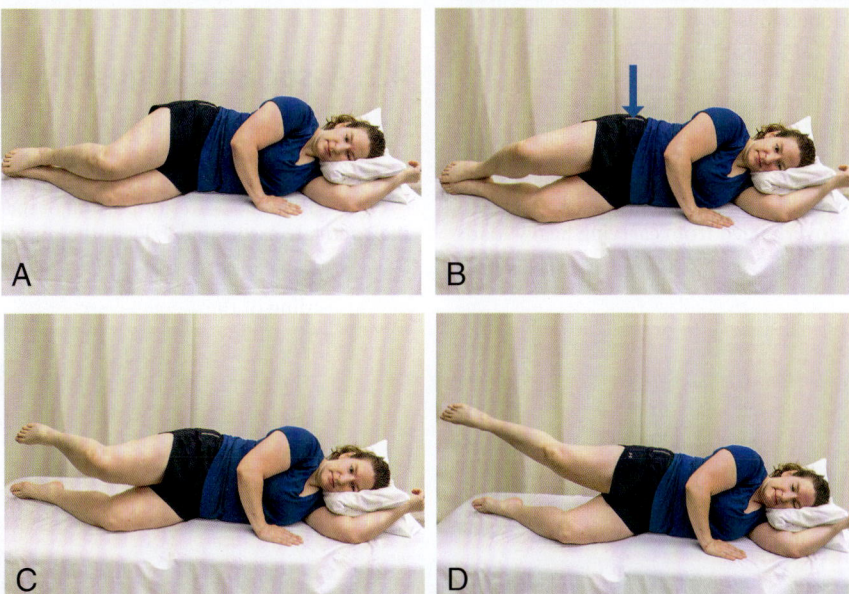

Figure 55-6. Gluteus medius and gluteus minimus muscle retraining. A, Starting position, with the top hip flexed less than 20°. B, The upper hand is pressed into the table to stabilize the trunk. Keeping the feet together, the knee is lifted toward the ceiling by activating the gluteus medius, gluteus minimus, and gluteus maximus muscles (arrow). C, The foot is lifted away from the lower leg until it is parallel with the floor. Attention should be paid so that the foot does not rise above the knee. D, With the knee and hip aligned and straight, the leg is lifted toward the ceiling held for 6 to 10 seconds and lowered slowly.

Box 55-2 Gluteus medius and gluteus minimus muscles retraining

Starting position (Figure 55-6A)	The patient lies on the side, with the knees and hips slightly bent (<20°).
Level 1 (Figure 55-6B)	The patient lifts the knee while keeping the feet together, making sure not to allow the hips to rock back and the lumbar spine to rotate. The hand of the upper arm can press down into the surface to stabilize the trunk.
Level 2 (Figure 55-6C)	From the position of level 1, the patient lifts the top foot to the level of the knee but not above it, and holds this position for 6-10 seconds and then slowly lowers the leg to the starting position.
Level 3 (Figure 55-6D)	Starting with the knee and hip in line with the trunk, the patient lifts the entire lower extremity up without hiking the hip, holds for 6-10 seconds, and slowly lowers the leg back down.

line from slightly behind the anterior superior iliac spine to the greater trochanter, and below (posteriorly) by the piriformis line (Figure 55-8B) that runs along the upper border of the piriformis muscle (Figure 55-8A). The gluteus maximus muscle covers much of the posterior portion of the gluteus medius muscle, and the gluteus minimus muscle lies deep to the distal two-thirds of the gluteus medius muscle. In the region where the gluteus maximus, gluteus medius, and gluteus minimus muscles overlap, the insertion of a monofilament needle into the gluteus medius and gluteus minimus muscles to elicit a local twitch response or reproduce the patient's symptoms may improve accurate differentiation as dry needling can be a helpful diagnostic procedure.

4. DIFFERENTIAL DIAGNOSIS

4.1. Activation and Perpetuation of Trigger Points

A posture or activity that activates a TrP, if not corrected, can also perpetuate it. In any part of the gluteus medius muscle, TrPs may be activated by unaccustomed eccentric loading, eccentric exercise in an unconditioned muscle, or maximal or submaximal concentric loading.[41] Trigger points may also be activated or aggravated when the muscle is placed in a shortened and/or lengthened position for an extended period of time.

Activities that can cause overload of the gluteus medius and gluteus minimus muscles include weight lifting, running, and habitually shifting weight onto one side as in carrying a child or weighted object on the hip. The gluteus medius and gluteus minimus muscles can be overloaded from carrying heavy loads while walking, especially if the load is being handled unilaterally.[18] Another factor to consider is strength imbalance between the gluteus medius and thigh muscles. When the strength ratio of the hip abductors was decreased in comparison with either that of the quadriceps or hamstrings, greater activation of the gluteus medius muscle occured when carrying a moderately intense load in the upper extremities.[42]

Any changes in the lower kinetic chain that place an increase demand on the gluteus medius muscle can activate or perpetuate TrPs. The gluteus medius muscle is active throughout the gait cycle and provides the majority of support through the mid-stance phase of gait.[43] Other abnormal intrinsic factors, such as excessive pronation or hip abductor or external rotator weakness, can contribute to excessive adduction and internal rotation of the hip through the stance phase of gait, resulting in a reduction in efficiency of the gluteus medius muscle in stabilizing the pelvis on the femur. This mechanical disadvantage may result in repetitive micro-trauma and overload of the gluteus medius muscle. Altered activation and reduced recruitment of the gluteus medius muscle has been identified in patients with increased hip joint adduction and internal rotation motion during stair climbing, squatting, and running.[44]

4.2. Associated Trigger Points

Associated TrPs can develop in the referred pain areas caused by primary TrPs.[45] Therefore, musculature in the referred pain areas for each muscle should also be considered.

The TrPs in the posterior portion of the gluteus medius muscle may activate associated TrPs in the piriformis and the posterior

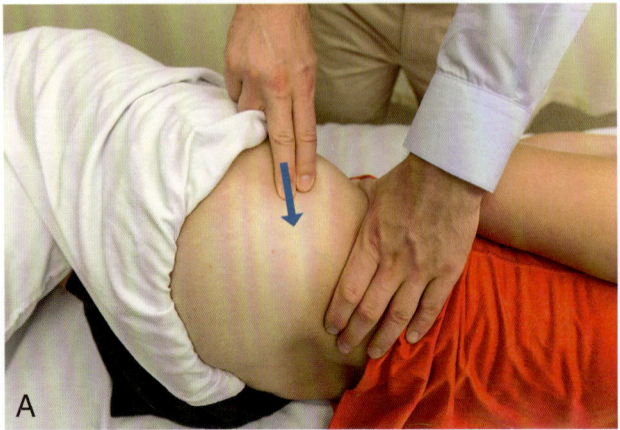 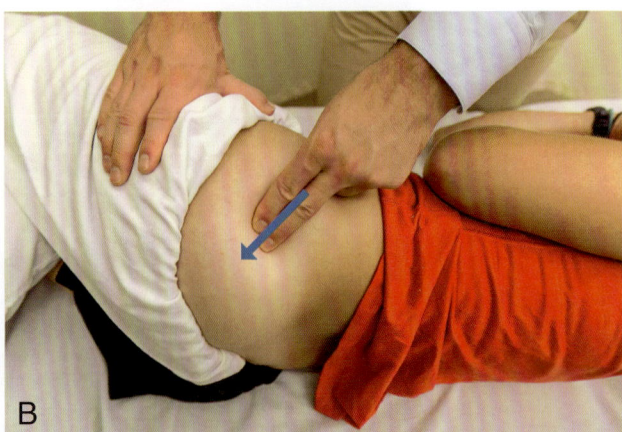

Figure 55-7. Cross-fiber flat palpation for TrPs in the gluteus medius muscle. A, Anterior portion. B, Middle and posterior portion.

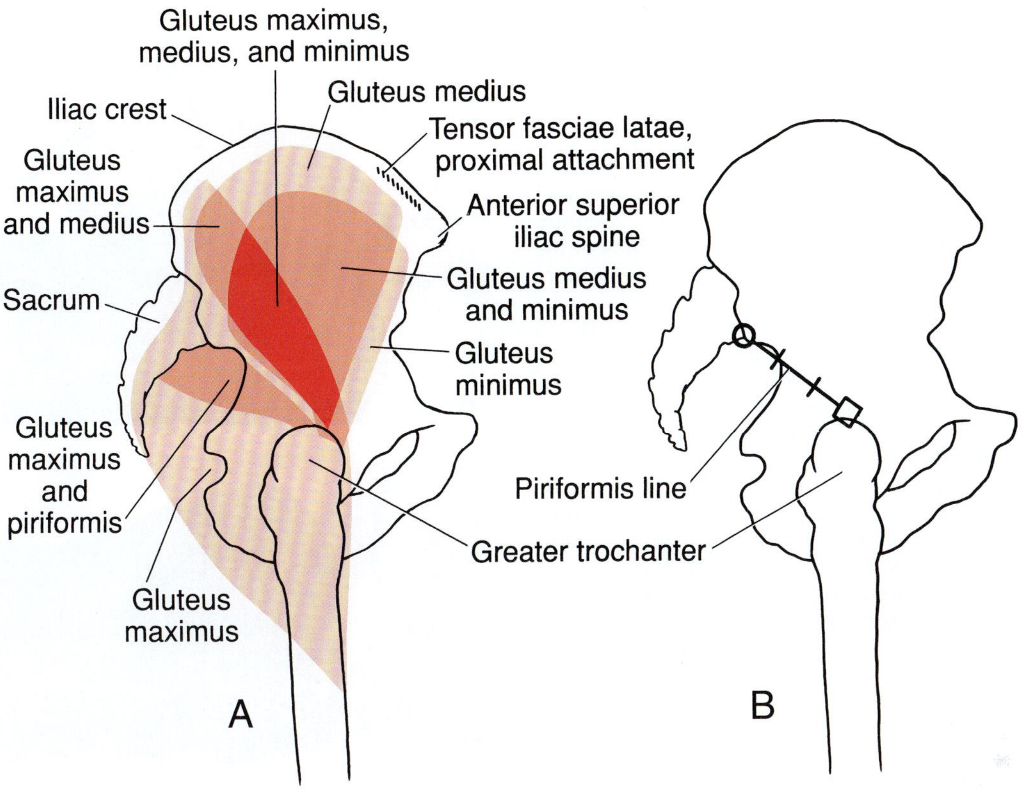

Figure 55-8. Schematic drawing that shows overlap of gluteal and piriformis muscles from a slightly posterior, nearly lateral view. A, light red identifies the areas where only a single gluteal muscle may be palpated, except for the anterior part of the gluteus minimus muscle that is also covered by the tensor fasciae latae muscle (the iliac attachment is marked by a hatched line and is labeled). In these single-muscle areas, there is little likelihood of encountering misleading tenderness from another gluteal muscle or from the piriformis muscle. Medium red on the left side of A illustrates where either the gluteus medius or piriformis muscle may be palpated through the gluteus maximus muscle in an area free of deeper gluteus minimus muscle sensitivity; medium red on the right side of A illustrates where the gluteus medius muscle overlies the gluteus minimus muscle. Dark red shows where three muscle layers—gluteus maximus, gluteus medius, and gluteus minimus muscles—are present. Note that the upper border of the piriformis muscle corresponds closely with the lower borders of the gluteus medius and gluteus minimus muscles. The gluteus medius muscle sometimes overlaps the piriformis muscle. B, The piriformis muscle line that corresponds closely to the upper border of the piriformis muscle runs from the proximal end of the greater trochanter of the femur (open square) to the upper end of the palpable free border of the sacrum where it joins the ilium (open circle). The piriformis muscle line is divided into thirds for convenience in locating TrPs in the posterior part of the gluteus minimus and piriformis muscles.

portion of the gluteus minimus muscle. When TrPs in the anterior portion of the gluteus medius muscle are involved, associated TrPs may develop in the tensor fascia latae as part of the functional unit.

When the quadratus lumborum muscle has active TrPs, the gluteus medius muscle commonly develops associated TrPs as it lies in the pain referral zone of the quadratus lumborum muscle. In the presence of an active TrP in the quadratus lumborum muscle, treatment of the gluteus medius–associated TrP will offer only temporary relief. However, treating the active TrP in the quadratus lumborum muscle will often eliminate the associated TrP in the gluteus medius muscle.

Other muscles that should be evaluated because of the pain referral pattern from the gluteus medius muscle include the gluteus maximus, obturator internus and externus, superior and inferior gemelli, bicep femoris, semitendinosus, semimembranosus, lumbar multifidus, and iliocostalis lumborum muscles. Muscles that refer symptoms to the lateral hip and may activate associated TrPs in the gluteus medius muscle include the piriformis, gluteus maximus, and vastus lateralis muscles.

4.3. Associated Pathology

Differential diagnosis of clinical conditions should include lumbar pathology, sacroiliac dysfunction, and hip pathology. Symptom and pain referral patterns from the lumbar facet or sacroiliac joints overlap with the referred pain from TrPs in the gluteus medius muscle; therefore, examination of the lumbosacral region is indicated. Pain provocation studies looking at the referral zones for the sacroiliac joint have demonstrated referral frequently into the low back, buttock, and occasionally into the posterior or lateral thigh and leg.[46,47] Pain provocation studies mapping the referral zones for the hip joint have also demonstrated referral into the buttock, thigh, or groin in the majority of subjects.[48]

Patients with L4, L5 lumbar radicular symptoms or radiculopathy have been found to have an increased frequency of TrPs in the gluteal muscles. Trigger points were found in 76% of patients with lumbar radiculopathy. The location of the TrPs matched the side of radiculopathy in 75% of subjects.[49] Trigger points in the gluteal muscles were found to be a highly specific indicator for individuals with radiculopathy.[50]

Trigger points in the gluteal muscles have also been found in association with low back pain. Iglesias-Gonzalez et al[21] found an association between active TrPs in the low back and hip muscles in participants with chronic lower back pain. Trigger points in the gluteus medius, iliocostalis lumborum, and quadratus lumborum muscles were the most prevalent. They also demonstrated a correlation between pain intensity and the number of active TrPs present, as well as a correlation between the number of active TrPs and lower sleep quality.[21]

Hip pathology can cause alterations in the patient's biomechanics or motor control, activating TrPs in the gluteus medius muscle. Reduced activation of the gluteus medius muscle has been found in patients with symptomatic labral tears during both concentric and eccentric loading.[51] Weakness of the hip abductor muscles has also been found in patients with femoroacetabular impingement or labral tears.[52]

Altered activation of the gluteus medius muscle has been found with increasing severity of hip osteoarthritis. As the severity of osteoarthritis increases, the activation of the gluteus medius muscle becomes more prolonged between the normal peaks at initial contact and mid stance, leading to repetitive overload of the gluteus medius and gluteus minimus muscles.[53] Uemura et al[54] found that hip osteoarthritis can lead to atrophy of the gluteal muscles, but that the muscle volume can recover more than 2 years after total hip arthroplasty.

Additionally, researchers have found a correlation between weakness of the hip musculature, excessive hip adduction and internal rotation, and patellofemoral pain.[55-59] Roach et al[55] found an increase in the prevalence of TrPs in the bilateral gluteus medius and quadratus lumborum muscles in patients with patellofemoral pain.

Gluteal tendinopathy is considered to be one of the major causes of greater trochanteric pain syndrome (GTPS). Bird et al[60] investigated the presence of gluteus medius tendon pathology in 24 subjects with signs and symptoms consistent with GTPS. They utilized magnetic resonance imaging, positive Trendelenburg sign, and pain with resisted hip abduction and hip internal rotation as predictors of a gluteus medius tendon tear. They found that the Trendelenburg sign had a sensitivity of 0.73 and a specificity of 0.80 in predicting a gluteus medius tendon tear in subjects who failed to respond to conservative care.[60] The recommended intervention for tears of the gluteus medius tendon is trochanteric micropuncture; however, there is a lack of long-term follow-up on this relatively new procedure.[61]

5. CORRECTIVE ACTIONS

Patients with gluteus medius TrPs having difficulty with sleeping may need to modify their sleeping posture. They may benefit from lying supine or sleeping on the opposite side. A pillow between the legs to avoid a painful stretch into adduction of the hip may be necessary if sleeping in side-lying (Figure 55-9). If an individual has TrPs in the posterior portion of the gluteus medius muscle, they may be compressed when lying on the back, resulting in pain in that position.

Self-pressure release of TrPs in the gluteus medius muscle can be achieved with the utilization of a TrP release tool, tennis ball, or a lacrosse ball. To perform TrP self-pressure release with a TrP tool, the affected or painful side is up (Figure 55-10A). The tool can be used to locate a sensitive spot and then to apply light pressure (no more than 4/10 pain) for 15 to 30 seconds

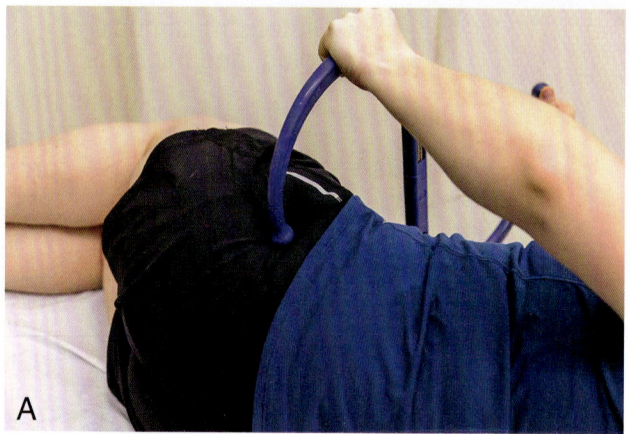

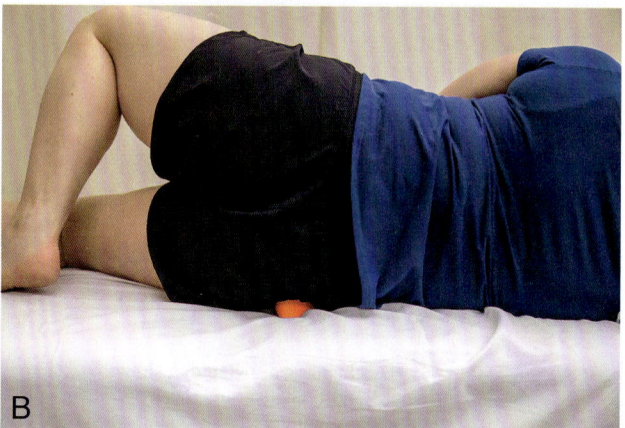

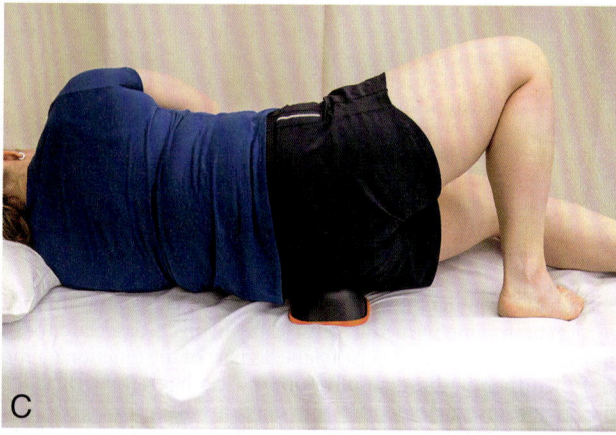

Figure 55-10. Gluteus medius muscle self-pressure release. A, Trigger point pressure-release tool. B, Tennis ball. C, Trigger point pressure-release tool (half round).

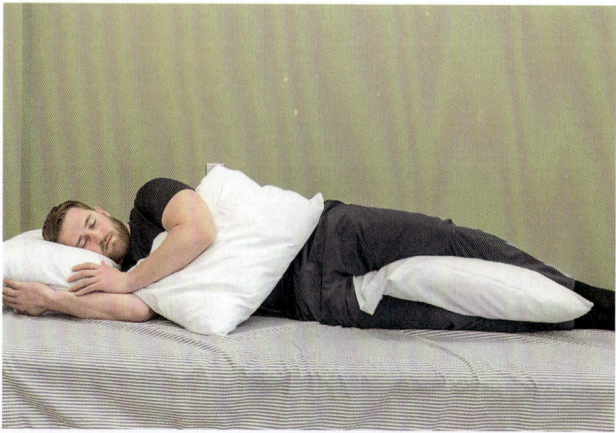

Figure 55-9. Sleeping position for gluteus medius and gluteus minimus muscles. Pillow is placed between the legs to keep the hip aligned with the trunk and shoulder.

or until pain reduces. This release can be repeated five times, several times per day. The patient may also utilize a ball or other handheld tool by gently lying on top of the ball following the same procedure as in Figure 55-10B and C. While rolling over the gluteus medius muscle, attention should be paid to any tender spots. A slow rocking motion or a pause over the area can be used prior to moving to the next area. Pressure should be mildly uncomfortable but not overly painful (Figure 55-10C).

Self-stretch of the gluteus medius muscle can be achieved by lying on the uninvolved side on the edge of a firm surface, flexing the lower hip, so that the lower foot can support the top leg (Figure 55-11A). The top leg can then be lowered until a slight stretch or discomfort is felt over the hip. The lower leg supports the top leg so as not to stretch the TrPs in the gluteus medius muscle too aggressively (Figure 55-11B). The patient

Chapter 55: Gluteus Medius Muscle 575

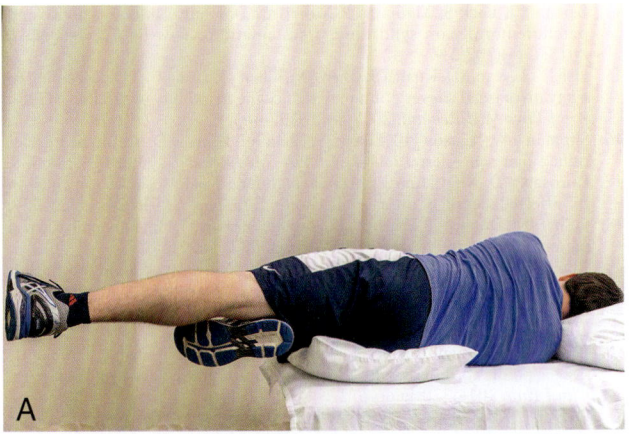
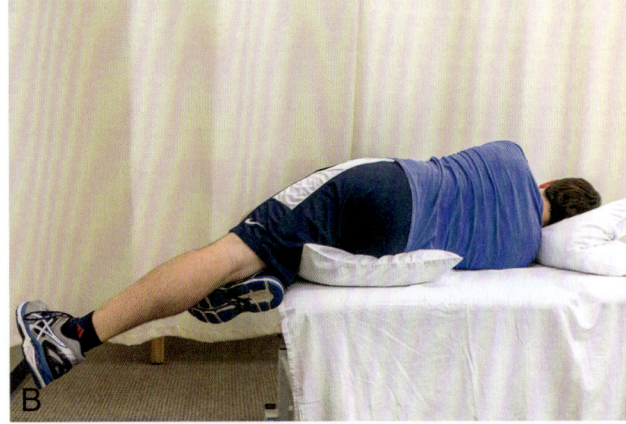
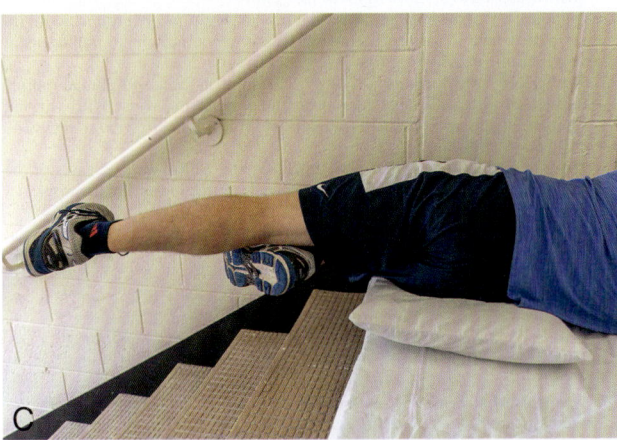
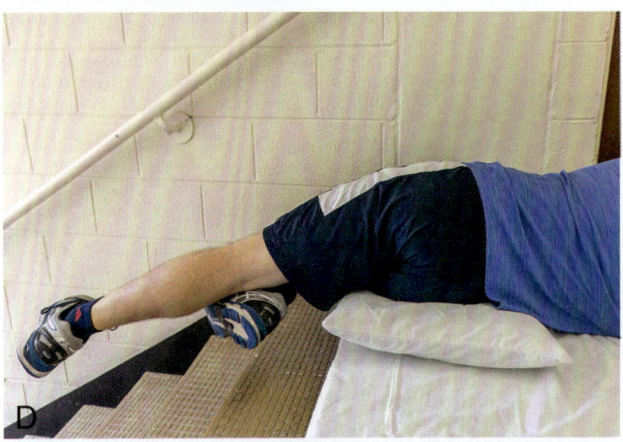

Figure 55-11. Gluteus medius and gluteus minimus muscles self-stretch. A and B, Off the edge of the bed. A, Starting position. B, Ending position. C and D, Off the landing of a staircase. C, Starting position. D, Ending position.

should take a slow inhalation and then relax during exhalation allowing gravity to assist in stretching the gluteus medius muscle (Figure 55-11B). If the bed is too soft, the same stretch maneuver can be performed at the top of a stair landing with a pillow under the bottom hip (Figure 55-11C and D).

Adequate strength of the gluteus medius and gluteus minimus muscles is vital to allow for proper mechanics during walking once the TrPs have been deactivated. Altered mechanics that cause the hip to turn in and/or adduct on the weight-bearing side while walking needs to be corrected. Careful muscle retraining to avoid aggravation of the condition will be beneficial to prevent recurrence. A licensed rehabilitation professional should be consulted for a proper exercise prescription.

References

1. Standring S. *Gray's Anatomy: The Anatomical Basis of Clinical Practice.* 41st ed. London, UK: Elsevier; 2015.
2. Flack NA, Nicholson HD, Woodley SJ. The anatomy of the hip abductor muscles. *Clin Anat.* 2014;27(2):241-253.
3. Gottschalk F, Kourosh S, Leveau B. The functional anatomy of tensor fasciae latae and gluteus medius and minimus. *J Anat.* 1989;166:179-189.
4. Flack NA, Nicholson HD, Woodley SJ. A review of the anatomy of the hip abductor muscles, gluteus medius, gluteus minimus, and tensor fascia lata. *Clin Anat.* 2012;25(6):697-708.
5. Bardeen C. The musculature, Section 5. In: Jackson CM, ed. *Morris's Human Anatomy.* 6th ed. Philadelphia, PA: Blakiston's Son & Co; 1921.
6. Chomiak J, Huracek J, Dvorak J, et al. Lesion of gluteal nerves and muscles in total hip arthroplasty through 3 surgical approaches. An electromyographically controlled study. *Hip Int.* 2015;25(2):176-183.
7. Moore KL, Agur AMR, Dalley AF. *Clinically Oriented Anatomy.* Baltimore, MD: Lippincott Williams & Wilkins; 2014.
8. Delp SL, Hess WE, Hungerford DS, Jones LC. Variation of rotation moment arms with hip flexion. *J Biomech.* 1999;32(5):493-501.
9. Bolgla LA, Uhl TL. Electromyographic analysis of hip rehabilitation exercises in a group of healthy subjects. *J Orthop Sports Phys Ther.* 2005;35(8):487-494.
10. Retchford TH, Crossley KM, Grimaldi A, Kemp JL, Cowan SM. Can local muscles augment stability in the hip? A narrative literature review. *J Musculoskelet Neuronal Interact.* 2013;13(1):1-12.
11. Semciw AI, Neate R, Pizzari T. A comparison of surface and fine wire EMG recordings of gluteus medius during selected maximum isometric voluntary contractions of the hip. *J Electromyogr Kinesiol.* 2014;24(6):835-840.
12. Semciw AI, Pizzari T, Murley GS, Green RA. Gluteus medius: an intramuscular EMG investigation of anterior, middle and posterior segments during gait. *J Electromyogr Kinesiol.* 2013;23(4):858-864.
13. Hollman JH, Kolbeck KE, Hitchcock JL, Koverman JW, Krause DA. Correlations between hip strength and static foot and knee posture. *J Sport Rehabil.* 2006;15:12-23.
14. Alexander N, Schwameder H. Effect of sloped walking on lower limb muscle forces. *Gait Posture.* 2016;47:62-67.
15. Kim TY, Yoo WG, An DH, Shin SJ. The effects of different gait speeds and lower arm weight on the activities of the latissimus dorsi, gluteus medius, and gluteus maximus muscles. *J Phys Ther Sci.* 2013;25:1483-1484.
16. Lee SK, Lee SY, Jung JM. Muscle activity of the gluteus medius at different gait speeds. *J Phys Ther Sci.* 2014;26(12):1915-1917.
17. Lenhart R, Thelen D, Heiderscheit B. Hip muscle loads during running at various step rates. *J Orthop Sports Phys Ther.* 2014;44(10):766-774, A761-A764.
18. Lee JW, Kim YJ, Koo HM. Activation of the gluteus medius according to load during horizontal hip abduction in a one-leg stance. *J Phys Ther Sci.* 2015;27(8):2601-2603.
19. Sirca A, Susec-Michieli M. Selective type II fibre muscular atrophy in patients with osteoarthritis of the hip. *J Neurol Sci.* 1980;44(2-3):149-159.
20. Simons DG, Travell J, Simons L. *Travell & Simon's Myofascial Pain and Dysfunction: The Trigger Point Manual.* Vol 1. 2nd ed. Baltimore, MD: Williams & Wilkins; 1999.
21. Iglesias-Gonzalez JJ, Munoz-Garcia MT, Rodrigues-de-Souza DP, Alburquerque-Sendin F, Fernández de las Peñas C. Myofascial trigger points, pain, disability, and sleep quality in patients with chronic nonspecific low back pain. *Pain Med.* 2013;14(12):1964-1970.
22. Arcangeli P, Digiesi V, Ronchi O, Dorigo B, Bartoli B. Mechanisms of ischemic pain in peripheral occlusive arterial disease. In: Bonica JJ, Albe-Fessard D, eds. *Advances in Pain Research and Therapy.* Vol 1. New York, NY: Raven Press; 1976:965-973.

23. Kellgren JH. A preliminary account of referred pains arising from muscle. *Br Med J.* 1938;1:325-327 (p. 327).
24. Sola AE. Chapter 47, Trigger point therapy. In: Roberts JR, Hedges JR, eds. *Clinical Procedures in Emergency Medicine.* Philadelphia, PA: Saunders; 1985:674-686 (p. 683).
25. Winter Z. Referred pain in fibrositis. *Med Rec.* 1944;157:34-37.
26. Kellgren JH. Observations on referred pain arising from muscle. *Clin Sci.* 1938;3:175-190 (pp. 176, 177).
27. Steinbrocker O, Isenberg SA, Silver M, Neustadt D, Kuhn P, Schittone M. Observations on pain produced by injection of hypertonic saline into muscles and other supportive tissues. *J Clin Invest.* 1953;32(10):1045-1051.
28. Izumi M, Petersen KK, Arendt-Nielsen L, Graven-Nielsen T. Pain referral and regional deep tissue hyperalgesia in experimental human hip pain models. *Pain.* 2014;155(4):792-800.
29. Mehta P, Telhan R, Burge A, Wyss J. Atypical cause of lateral hip pain due to proximal gluteus medius muscle tear: a report of 2 cases. *PM R.* 2015;7(9):1002-1006.
30. Porterfield JA, DeRosa C. *Mechanical Low Back Pain: Perspectives in Functional Anatomy.* 2nd ed. Philadelphia, PA: Saunders; 1998 (pp. 114-117).
31. DeStefano L. *Greenman's Principles of Manual Medicine.* 5th ed. Philadelphia, PA: Wolters Kluwer; 2016 (p. 338).
32. Lee SP, Powers CM. Individuals with diminished hip abductor muscle strength exhibit altered ankle biomechanics and neuromuscular activation during unipedal balance tasks. *Gait Posture.* 2014;39(3):933-938.
33. Page P, Frank C, Lardner R. *Assessment and Treatment of Muscle Imbalance. The Janda Approach.* Champaign, IL: Human Kinetics; 2010 (pp. 80-81).
34. Friberg O. Clinical symptoms and biomechanics of lumbar spine and hip joint in leg length inequality. *Spine.* 1983;8(6):643-651.
35. Khayambashi K, Fallah A, Movahedi A, Bagwell J, Powers C. Posterolateral hip muscle strengthening versus quadriceps strengthening for patellofemoral pain: a comparative control trial. *Arch Phys Med Rehabil.* 2014;95(5):900-907.
36. Khayambashi K, Ghoddosi N, Straub RK, Powers CM. Hip muscle strength predicts noncontact anterior cruciate ligament injury in male and female athletes: a prospective study. *Am J Sports Med.* 2016;44(2):355-361.
37. Goto S, Aminaka N, Gribble PA. Lower extremity muscle activity, kinematics, and dynamic postural control in individuals with patellofemoral pain. *J Sport Rehabil.* 2017:1-29.
38. Harput G, Howard JS, Mattacola C. Comparison of muscle activation levels between healthy individuals and persons who have undergone anterior cruciate ligament reconstruction during different phases of weight-bearing exercises. *J Orthop Sports Phys Ther.* 2016;46(11):984-992.
39. Esculier JF, Roy JS, Bouyer LJ. Lower limb control and strength in runners with and without patellofemoral pain syndrome. *Gait Posture.* 2015;41(3):813-819.
40. Franettovich Smith MM, Bonacci J, Mendis MD, Christie C, Rotstein A, Hides JA. Gluteus medius activation during running is a risk factor for season hamstring injuries in elite footballers. *J Sci Med Sport.* 2017;20(2):159-163.
41. Gerwin RD, Dommerholt J, Shah JP. An expansion of Simons' integrated hypothesis of trigger point formation. *Curr Pain Headache Rep.* 2004;8(6):468-475.
42. Stastny P, Lehnert M, Zaatar A, Svoboda Z, Xaverova Z, Pietraszewski P. The gluteus medius vs. thigh muscles strength ratio and their relation to electromyography amplitude during a farmer's walk exercise. *J Hum Kinet.* 2015;45:157-165.
43. Anderson FC, Pandy MG. Individual muscle contributions to support in normal walking. *Gait Posture.* 2003;17(2):159-169.
44. Barton CJ, Lack S, Malliaras P, Morrissey D. Gluteal muscle activity and patellofemoral pain syndrome: a systematic review. *Br J Sports Med.* 2013;47(4):207-214.
45. Hsieh YL, Kao MJ, Kuan TS, Chen SM, Chen JT, Hong CZ. Dry needling to a key myofascial trigger point may reduce the irritability of satellite MTrPs. *Am J Phys Med Rehabil.* 2007;86(5):397-403.
46. Slipman CW, Jackson HB, Lipetz JS, Chan KT, Lenrow D, Vresilovic EJ. Sacroiliac joint pain referral zones. *Arch Phys Med Rehabil.* 2000;81(3):334-338.
47. Kurosawa D, Murakami E, Aizawa T. Referred pain location depends on the affected section of the sacroiliac joint. *Eur Spine J.* 2015;24(3):521-527.
48. Lesher JM, Dreyfuss P, Hager N, Kaplan M, Furman M. Hip joint pain referral patterns: a descriptive study. *Pain Med.* 2008;9(1):22-25.
49. Adelmanesh F, Jalali A, Jazayeri Shooshtari SM, Raissi GR, Ketabchi SM, Shir Y. Is there an association between lumbosacral radiculopathy and painful gluteal trigger points? A cross-sectional study. *Am J Phys Med Rehabil.* 2015;94(10):784-791.
50. Adelmanesh F, Jalali A, Shirvani A, et al. The diagnostic accuracy of gluteal trigger points to differentiate radicular from nonradicular low back pain. *Clin J Pain.* 2016;32(8):666-672.
51. Dwyer MK, Lewis CL, Hanmer AW, McCarthy JC. Do neuromuscular alterations exist for patients with acetabular labral tears during function? *Arthroscopy.* 2016;32(6):1045-1052.
52. Nepple JJ, Goljan P, Briggs KK, Garvey SE, Ryan M, Philippon MJ. Hip strength deficits in patients with symptomatic femoroacetabular impingement and labral tears. *Arthroscopy.* 2015;31(11):2106-2111.
53. Rutherford DJ, Moreside J, Wong I. Hip joint motion and gluteal muscle activation differences between healthy controls and those with varying degrees of hip osteoarthritis during walking. *J Electromyogr Kinesiol.* 2015;25(6):944-950.
54. Uemura K, Takao M, Sakai T, Nishii T, Sugano N. Volume increases of the gluteus maximus, gluteus medius, and thigh muscles after hip arthroplasty. *J Arthroplasty.* 2016;31(4):906.e1-912.e1.
55. Roach S, Sorenson E, Headley B, San Juan JG. Prevalence of myofascial trigger points in the hip in patellofemoral pain. *Arch Phys Med Rehabil.* 2013;94(3):522-526.
56. Cowan SM, Crossley KM, Bennell KL. Altered hip and trunk muscle function in individuals with patellofemoral pain. *Br J Sports Med.* 2009;43(8):584-588.
57. Rathleff MS, Rathleff CR, Crossley KM, Barton CJ. Is hip strength a risk factor for patellofemoral pain? A systematic review and meta-analysis. *Br J Sports Med.* 2014;48(14):1088.
58. Nakagawa TH, Serrao FV, Maciel CD, Powers CM. Hip and knee kinematics are associated with pain and self-reported functional status in males and females with patellofemoral pain. *Int J Sports Med.* 2013;34(11):997-1002.
59. Wirtz AD, Willson JD, Kernozek TW, Hong DA. Patellofemoral joint stress during running in females with and without patellofemoral pain. *Knee.* 2012;19(5):703-708.
60. Bird PA, Oakley SP, Shnier R, Kirkham BW. Prospective evaluation of magnetic resonance imaging and physical examination findings in patients with greater trochanteric pain syndrome. *Arthritis Rheum.* 2001;44(9):2138-2145.
61. Redmond JM, Cregar WM, Gupta A, Hammarstedt JE, Martin TJ, Domb BG. Trochanteric micropuncture: treatment for gluteus medius tendinopathy. *Arthrosc Tech.* 2015;4(1):e87-e90.

Chapter 56

Gluteus Minimus and Tensor Fasciae Latae Muscles

"Pseudo-Sciatica and Pseudotrochanteric Bursitis"

Paul Thomas, N. Beth Collier, and Joseph M. Donnelly

1. INTRODUCTION

The gluteus minimus muscle is the smallest of the gluteal muscles, but plays an important role in the normal biomechanics of the hip during the gait cycle. It is the deepest of the gluteal muscles and not only shares an intimate attachment with the hip joint capsule but also functions with it. Its primary function is hip abduction with the gluteus medius muscle and is active during several other motions of the hip. It is believed to contribute significantly to the stability of the hip during walking, running, and lateral movements. Individuals with trigger points (TrPs) in the gluteus minimus muscle may report excruciating pain in the hip and lower extremity down to the ankle. The extensive referral pattern of pain into the lower extremity that occurs when TrPs are present in the gluteus minimus muscle makes it necessary to perform a thorough lumbopelvic and hip examination. Differential diagnosis includes lumbar radicular pain or radiculopathy, sacroiliac joint dysfunction, trochanteric bursitis, and hip pathology. Corrective actions should include postural advice to improve sitting and sleeping postures, correction of gait abnormalities, self-pressure release, and self-stretching techniques.

The tensor fasciae latae muscle is a superficial muscle that works with the gluteus medius and minimus muscles to stabilize the pelvis during unilateral standing. It is the smallest of the hip abductors and also contributes to hip flexion and internal rotation. Trigger points in the tensor fasciae latae muscle refer pain to the lateral thigh and can be commonly mistaken for symptoms of trochanteric bursitis. Iliotibial band syndrome should be considered in the differential diagnosis in addition to those identified above for the gluteus minimus muscle. Corrective actions includes postural advice (especially for sitting and sleeping), maximizing efficiency during walking and running activities, self-pressure release, and stretching.

For resolution of symptoms in both the gluteus minimus and tensor fasciae latae muscles, correction of altered biomechanics in the lower kinetic chain will need to be addressed.

2. ANATOMIC CONSIDERATIONS

Gluteus Minimus

The gluteus minimus muscle lies deep to the gluteus medius muscle and is the smallest in length and lightest in weight of the gluteal muscles.[1] Its fan shape corresponds closely to the overlying gluteus medius muscle. The muscle originates along the outer surface of the ilium between the anterior and inferior gluteal lines and approaches the greater sciatic foramen posteriorly (Figure 56-1). Fiber orientation of the muscle can be divided into two portions, with the anterior fascicles arranged more vertically and the posterior fascicles arranged more horizontally[2] (Figure 56-1). The muscle fibers converge into an aponeurosis that terminates in a tendinous attachment along

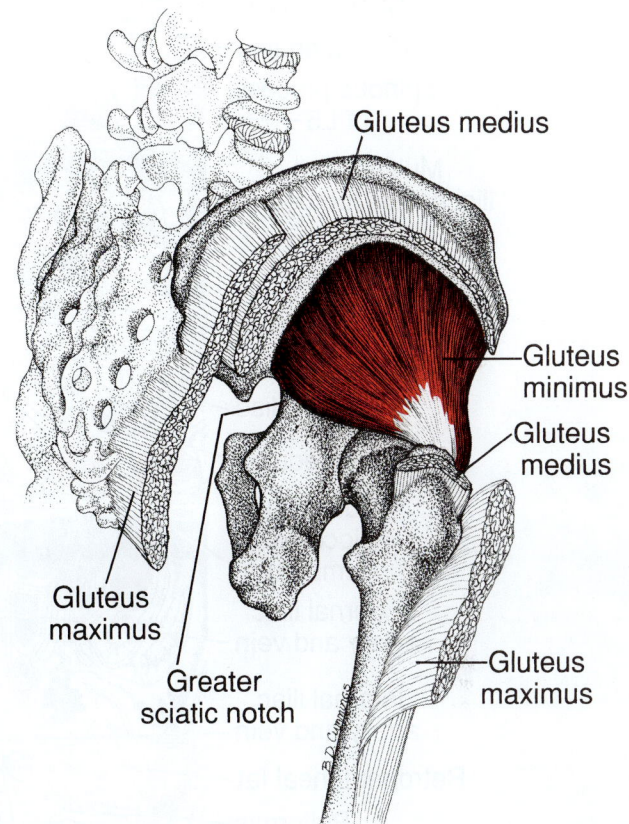

Figure 56-1. Attachments of the right gluteus minimus muscle (red) in the posterolateral view. To a large extent, the overlying gluteus maximus and gluteus medius muscles have been removed.

the anterolateral surface of the greater trochanter, deep and anterior to the piriformis muscle attachment, and contributes a broad insertion superolaterally onto the joint capsule of the hip.[3-6] Additional slips may pass to the piriformis, gemellus superior, or vastus lateralis muscles.[4]

The relative thickness of the gluteus minimus muscle and its anatomic relation to the tensor fasciae latae muscle are shown in the serial cross-sections of Figure 56-2. The greater thickness of the anterior part of the gluteus minimus muscle, when compared with its posterior part, is not generally appreciated. This difference in thickness is seen in the lowest section of Figure 56-2, the plane of which lies approximately midway between the anterior superior iliac spine and the anterior inferior iliac spine. The cross-section also illustrates how the anterior portion of the gluteus minimus muscle can be palpated both

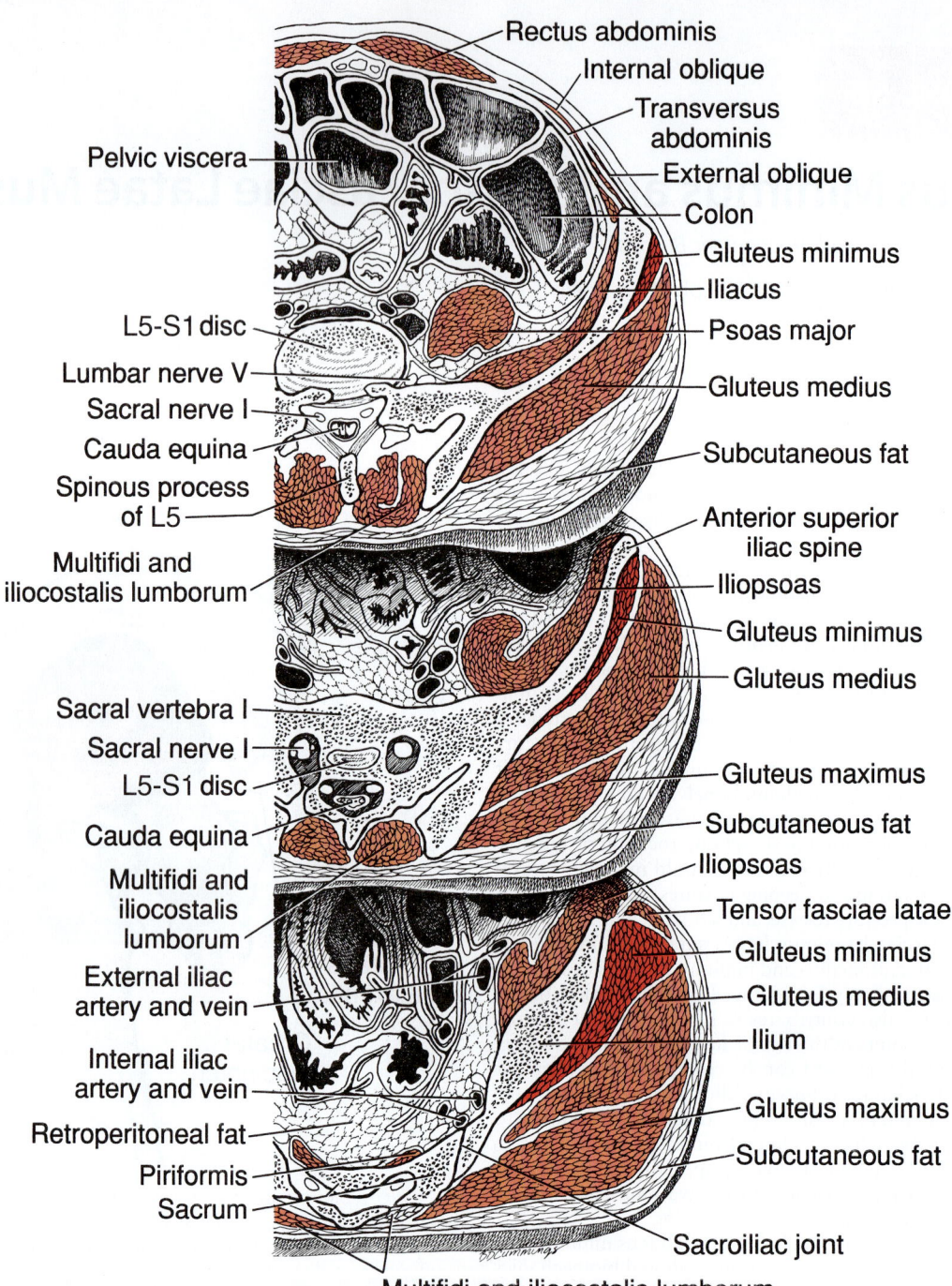

Figure 56-2. Serial cross-sections through the pelvis that show the gluteus minimus muscle (dark red). The three sections show the relation of the anterior portion of this muscle to the ilium, to neighboring muscles (light red), and to the skin. The level of the middle section passes through the anterior superior iliac spine. The plane of the lowest section lies between the anterior superior iliac spine and the anterior inferior iliac spine. At the latter level, the thickest part of the anterior portion of the gluteus minimus muscle may be subcutaneous between the tensor fasciae latae and gluteus medius muscles. This anterior portion is palpated for TrPs along the posterior margin of and deep to the tensor fasciae latae muscle.

behind the posterior margin of the tensor fasciae latae muscle and between the tensor's anterior margin and the anterior border of the ilium.

The trochanteric bursa of the gluteus minimus muscle, which lies between the anterior part of the muscle's tendon and the greater trochanter, facilitates gliding movement of the tendon over the trochanter.[4] This gliding movement of the tendon is necessary for the anterior fibers of the muscle to reach full stretch range of motion.

Tensor Fasciae Latae

The tensor fasciae latae muscle originates from the anterior part of the outer lip of the iliac crest, the lateral aspect of the anterior superior iliac spine, and to the deep surface of the fascia latae.[4] Superiorly, it lies between the gluteus medius and the sartorius muscles. Proximally, the tensor fasciae latae muscle inserts to the aponeurotic fascia superficial to the gluteus medius muscle. It descends and attaches to the two layers of the iliotibial tract

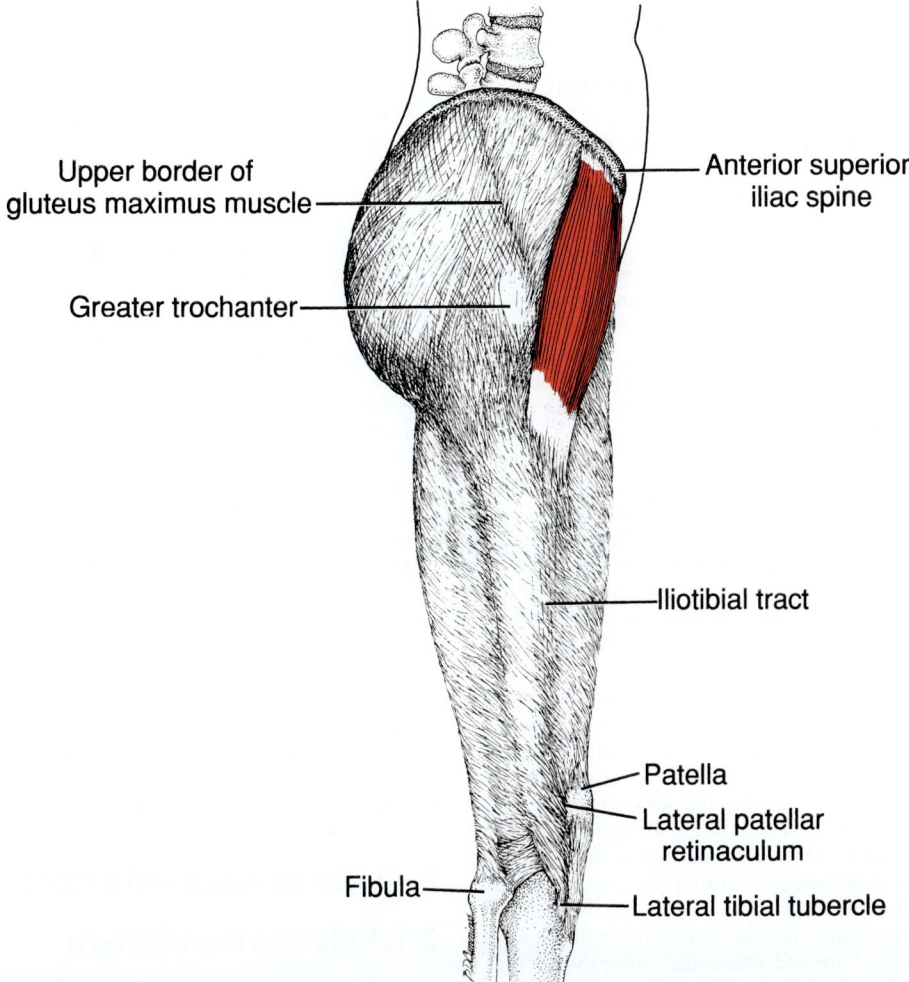

Figure 56-3. Side view of attachments of the right tensor fasciae latae muscle (red, fascia cut). Above, the muscle attaches along and below the crest of the ilium just posterior to the anterior superior iliac spine. Below, the anteromedial tendinous fibers attach to the fascia at the knee, and the posterolateral tendinous fibers anchor to the iliotibial tract, which continues down to the lateral tubercle of the tibia.

and terminates approximately one-third of the way down the thigh, though it may descend as far as the lateral femoral condyle (Figure 56-3).

2.1. Innervation and Vascularization

Gluteus Minimus

The gluteus minimus muscle is innervated by the superior gluteal nerve (L4, L5, and S1).

The gluteus minimus muscle receives its vascularization from the superior gluteal artery which exits the pelvis through the greater sciatic foramen superior to the piriformis muscle, traveling anterior between the gluteus medius and minimus muscles.[2] The superficial branch supplies the gluteus maximus muscle, the deep branch supplies the gluteus medius, gluteus minimus, and tensor fasciae latae muscles.[4,7] The superior gluteal nerve and artery travel between the gluteus medius muscle and the gluteus minimus muscle.[4]

Tensor Fasciae Latae

The tensor fasciae latae muscle is innervated by the superior gluteal nerve, derived from the L4, L5, S1 spinal nerves.

The muscle receives its vascular supply from a large ascending branch of the lateral femoral circumflex artery. The superior aspect of the muscle receives its supply from the superior gluteal artery.[4]

2.2. Function

Gluteus Minimus

The anterior fibers of the gluteus medius and minimus muscles function to abduct the thigh and internally rotate the femur.[4,5] The gluteus minimus muscle may function as a dynamic stabilizer of the hip[6,8] and may retract the hip joint capsule during hip abduction.[5] Biomechanical studies of the gait cycle have shown that muscular forces acting across the hip joint provide 95% of the contact force.[9] Fibers of the gluteus minimus muscle attach to the superoanterior hip joint capsule and may reduce superolateral translation of the head of the femur during gait.[8] Beck et al[10] described the gluteus minimus muscle as a hip abductor and hip flexor but also as a hip internal or external rotator depending on the position of the femur relative to the pelvis.[10] In hip extension, the anterior fibers can produce internal rotation and posterior fibers can produce external rotation.[10] At 90° of hip flexion, all fibers produce hip internal rotation.[10]

When the anterior and posterior fibers contract concurrently, the gluteus minimus muscle also pulls the head of the femur into the acetabulum to increase stability, especially with the hip in extension.[10,11] Tightening of the joint capsule may also aid in stability regardless of position.[6,10]

During the gait cycle, the posterior portion of the gluteus minimus muscle demonstrates a large burst of activity early in the stance phase that may be due to its role as a stabilizer of the femoral head. Both the anterior and posterior portions are active through mid-to-late stance. The role of the anterior gluteus minimus muscle during this phase may minimize forces at the anterior hip joint (acetabulum, capsule, and anterior superior acetabular labrum) through its ability to stabilize the femoral head with the iliopsoas muscle.[12] Anderson et al[13] found that the gluteus medius and gluteus minimus muscles provided nearly all of the support of the pelvis during the mid-stance of the gait cycle.

Tensor Fasciae Latae

The tensor fasciae latae muscle assists flexion, abduction, and internal rotation of the hip.[4] It is considered to be a hip abductor that acts with the gluteus medius and minimus muscles; however, it accounts for only 11% of the total cross-sectional area of the hip abductors.[14] The most posterolateral fibers are also involved in locking the knee in full extension with the hip maintained in internal rotation.[15] Bouillon et al[16] investigated eight muscles utilizing surface electromyography and percent maximum voluntary isometric contractions (%MVIC) during a step down, forward lunge, and side-step lunge. They found that the gluteus maximus and gluteus medius muscles had high %MVIC during the step down, and moderate %MVIC in side step, whereas the tensor fasciae latae (TFL) had low %MVIC during all three activities.

As is the case for most other lower extremity muscles, the tensor fasciae latae muscle functions during the stance phase of gait, more specifically mid-stance, and acts primarily with the gluteus medius and minimus muscles to control frontal plane movement of the pelvis. Paré and associates[15] have shown that the anteromedial half and the posterolateral half of the tensor fasciae latae muscle are active at different times for different reasons. During gait, the most anteromedial fibers were active in the swing limb (mid-swing) and the most posterolateral fibers were activated in the stance limb. The posterolateral fibers assist the gluteus medius and gluteus minimus muscles in stabilizing the pelvis, countering the tendency of a contralateral pelvic drop in mid-stance.[17] The most posterolateral fibers are also involved in stabilizing the knee.[15]

The posterolateral fibers are also active at heel-strike during jogging, running, sprinting,[15,18] stepping up on a platform, and climbing a ladder. The more vigorous is the activity, the more vigorous are the muscle contractions. During bicycling,[19] this muscle was electromyographically active during the period when the hip flexors became active as the pedal progressed upward from horizontal through the top of its stroke.

2.3. Functional Unit

The functional unit to which a muscle belongs includes the muscles that reinforce and counter its actions as well as the joints that the muscle crosses. The interdependence of these structures is functionally reflected in the organization and neural connections of the sensory motor cortex. The functional unit is emphasized because the presence of the TrP in one muscle of the unit increases the likelihood that the other muscles will develop TrPs. When inactivating TrPs in a muscle, one must be concerned about TrPs that may develop in muscles that are functionally interdependent. Box 56-1 represents the functional unit of the gluteus minimus muscle and Box 56-2 represents the functional unit of the tensor fasciae latae muscle.[20]

All fibers of the gluteus minimus muscle are active to produce internal rotation of the hip when it is flexed, and the anterior fibers produce hip internal rotation with the anterior fibers of the gluteus medius muscle when the hip is extended.

3. CLINICAL PRESENTATION
3.1. Referred Pain Pattern

Gluteus Minimus

Pain and symptoms from TrPs in the gluteus minimus muscle can be quite severe and persistent. The pain referral pattern of the gluteus minimus muscle can be extensive, making it

---

Box 56-1 Functional unit of the gluteus minimus muscle

Action	Synergists	Antagonists
Hip abduction	Gluteus medius Gluteus maximus Obturator internus Tensor fasciae latae Gemellus superior and inferior Piriformis Obturator externus	Adductor magnus Adductor longus Adductor brevis Gracilis Pectineus
Hip external rotation (posterior fibers of gluteus minimus when the hip is extended)	Gluteus medius (posterior fibers) Gluteus maximus Obturator internus and externus Gemellus superior and inferior Piriformis Quadratus femoris	Gluteus minimus (anterior fibers in extension, all fibers when the hip is flexed) Tensor fasciae latae
Hip internal rotation (anterior fibers when the hip is extended, all fibers when the hip is flexed)	Tensor fasciae latae Gluteus medius (anterior fibers)	Gluteus minimus (posterior fibers when in extension) Gluteus maximus Gluteus medius (posterior fibers) Obturator internus and externus Gemellus superior and inferior Quadratus femoris Piriformis

Box 56-2 Functional unit of the tensor fasciae latae muscle

Action	Synergists	Antagonists
Hip flexion	Rectus femoris Iliopsoas Pectineus Gluteus medius and minimus (anterior fibers)	Gluteus maximus Hamstring muscles
Hip internal rotation	Gluteus medius (anterior fibers) Gluteus minimus (anterior fibers when the hip is extended, all fibers when the hip is flexed)	Gluteus minimus (posterior fibers when in extension) Gluteus maximus Gluteus medius (posterior fibers) Obturator internus and externus Gemellus superior and inferior Quadratus femoris Piriformis

easy to overlook this muscle as the source of the symptoms. Lower extremity paresthesia and dysesthesia oftentimes accompany the pain referral pattern from TrPs in the gluteus minimus muscle. These symptoms are commonly referred to as "sciatica," which serves as merely a description of pain in the lower extremity and not a diagnosis. Travell in 1946 first distinguished different typical pain referral patterns from the anterior and posterior portions of the gluteus minimus muscle.[21]

Trigger points found within the anterior portion of the gluteus minimus muscle will typically refer pain and tenderness along the lower lateral portion of the buttock, lateral thigh, and lateral leg to the ankle, mimicking L5 radicular symptoms[21] (Figure 56-4).

Trigger points located in the posterior portion of the gluteus minimus muscle will refer pain throughout the buttock, especially the medial lower buttock, into the posterior thigh, posterior knee, and posterior calf, mimicking S1 radicular symptoms[21] (Figure 56-4).

Tensor Fasciae Latae

Patients with TrPs in the tensor fasciae latae muscle often describe pain in the hip joint region spanning inferiorly along

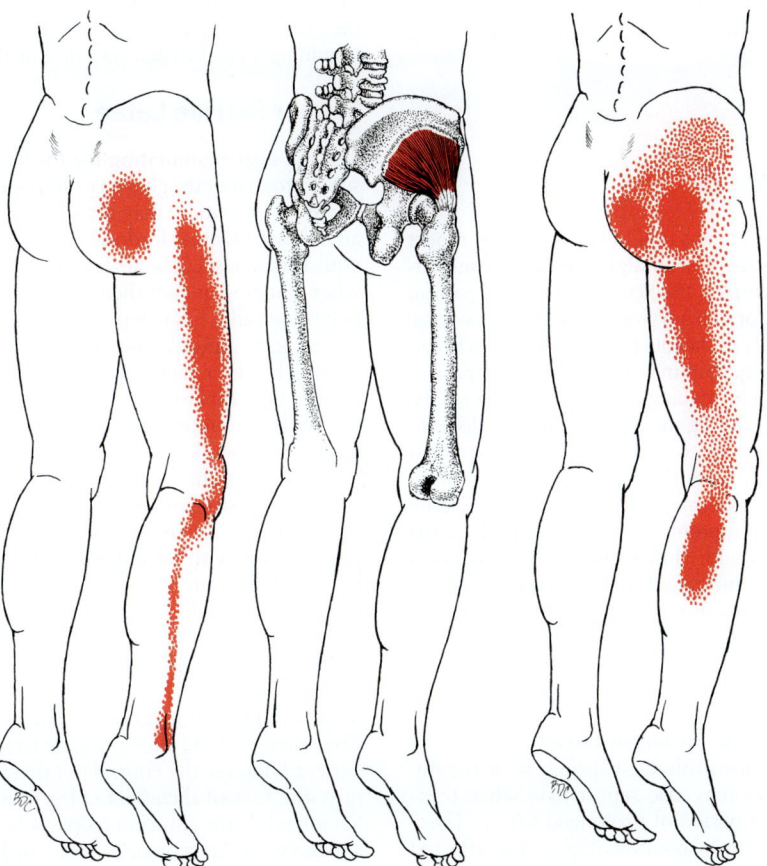

Figure 56-4. Referred pain patterns from TrPs in the gluteus minimus muscle. Referred pain and symptoms can be felt into the buttock, lateral and/or posterior thigh, posterior and/or lateral calf as distal to the lateral malleolus.

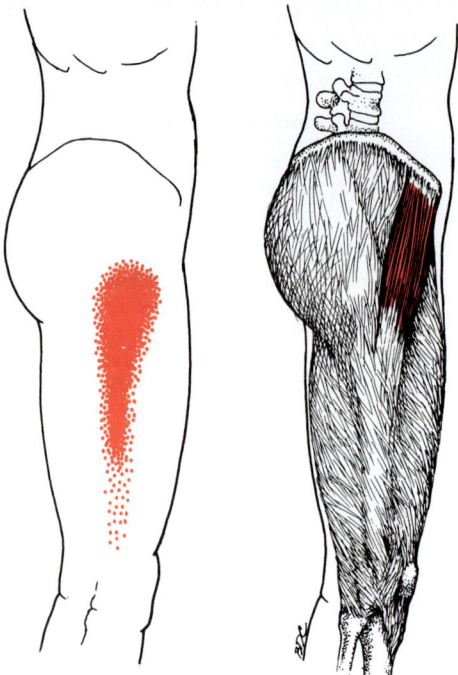

Figure 56-5. Referred pain pattern from TrPs in the tensor fasciae latae muscle (red).

the anterolateral aspect of the thigh, occasionally extending as far as the knee (Figure 56-5). The term "psuedotrochanteric bursitis" often applies to the pain produced by active TrPs in the tensor fasciae latae muscle. The pain is more severe during movement of the hip.[22-24]

3.2. Symptoms

Gluteus Minimus

Individuals with TrPs in the gluteus minimus muscle may report significant hip pain, which causes an antalgic gait pattern and difficulty with weight bearing on the affected side. It may be painful while walking, lying down, or when trying to get up from sitting. Symptoms arising from TrPs in the gluteus minimus muscle can be constant and excruciating. Pain may occur while the patient tries to lie on the affected side, making it necessary to lie on the opposite side or stay awake during the night because of discomfort. The patient may not be able to find a stretching movement or change of position that relieves the pain and can neither lie down comfortably nor walk normally. Coughing and sneezing will typically not aggravate symptoms generated from TrPs in the gluteus minimus muscle. As with gluteus medius TrPs, patients with TrPs in the gluteus minimus muscle usually experience pain during prolonged standing. Patients typically report that they have to shift their weight side to side to avoid pain in their hip and leg.

Tensor Fasciae Latae

Typically, patients with TrPs in the tensor fascial latae muscle will report poor tolerance for prolonged sitting, with the hip flexed to 90° or more. They may also report pain when transitioning to standing after a period of prolonged sitting. These patients are usually unable to lie comfortably on the affected side because of the pressure on the area of referred tenderness over the greater trochanter of the femur as well as directly on the TrPs. They are sometimes unable to lie on the opposite side without a pillow between the knees because of a prolonged stretch on the tensor fasciae latae muscle.

Long-distance runners may report functional limitation because of increased pain in the thigh area from the increased load placed on the tensor fasciae latae muscle during running.

3.3. Patient Examination

After a thorough subjective examination the clinician should make a detailed drawing representing the pain pattern that the patient has described. This depiction will assist in planning the physical examination and can be useful in monitoring the progression of the patient as symptoms improve or change.

Gluteus Minimus

A thorough physical examination of the lumbopelvic and hip regions is indicated when a patient is reporting referred pain and symptoms from TrPs in the gluteus minimus muscle. Because of the extensive referral of symptoms down the lower extremity, the clinician will need to differentiate these symptoms from those of sciatic or radicular origins. Neurodynamic testing should be performed to differentiate signs and symptoms originating from neural tissues from symptoms generated by TrPs in the gluteus minimus muscle. The hip and sacroiliac joints should also be evaluated to determine if there are any biomechanical deviations that could contribute to the activation and perpetuation of TrPs in the gluteus minimus muscle.

The physical examination for the gluteus minimus muscle is the same as that for the gluteus medius muscle, which is detailed in Chapter 55. This assessment includes static and dynamic posture, gait analysis, double- and single-leg squat, muscle activation pattern in side-lying hip abduction, and strength testing of the hip and thigh muscles. Because of the anatomic projection of the gluteus medius and gluteus minimus muscles, confirmation of TrPs in this deep muscle would be feasible with the application of dry needling obtaining a local twitch response or the pain referral pattern.

Tensor Fasciae Latae

The physical examination for the tensor fasciae latae muscle is similar to that of the gluteus medius and gluteus minimus muscles; however, the patient may demonstrate an anterior pelvic tilt and an increased lumbar lordosis while standing. Oftentimes, patients with tensor fasciae latae TrPs may keep the hip slightly flexed when standing or shift their weight to one leg and translate their pelvis laterally. They may demonstrate a lack of hip extension during gait. Ambulation with the hips flexed is typically not painful; however, their pain may prevent the patient from walking rapidly. In a common syndrome of muscle imbalance, tight tensor fasciae latae and quadratus lumborum muscles overpower an inhibited or weak gluteus medius muscle. Trigger points in the facilitated or tight muscles must be released preceding efforts to activate and strengthen the gluteus medius muscle.

The patient may be examined for muscle tightness in a Thomas test position, with the patient at the edge of a table holding one hip in full flexion to maintain a neutral spine and the hip to be inspected lowered into hip extension. In this testing position, the affected thigh can be tested for muscle length restriction by pressing the thigh of the extended limb medially, assessing hip adduction range of motion[25] (Figure 56-6). When the tensor fasciae latae muscle is tight, adduction is limited to a range of less than 15°. Contraction of the tensor fasciae latae muscle is tested with the patient lying on the contralateral side. The patient is asked to raise the foot of the affected leg into abduction and slight hip flexion while the clinician palpates both the gluteus medius and tensor fasciae latae muscles with one hand and tests for strength by applying graded resistance to the limb with the other hand. Loading the muscle during either test is likely to cause pain in the region of the affected hip joint if the muscle has active TrPs.

A tight tensor fasciae latae muscle can contribute to perceived iliotibial band tightness. Iliotibial band restriction can

Chapter 56: Gluteus Minimus and Tensor Fasciae Latae Muscles

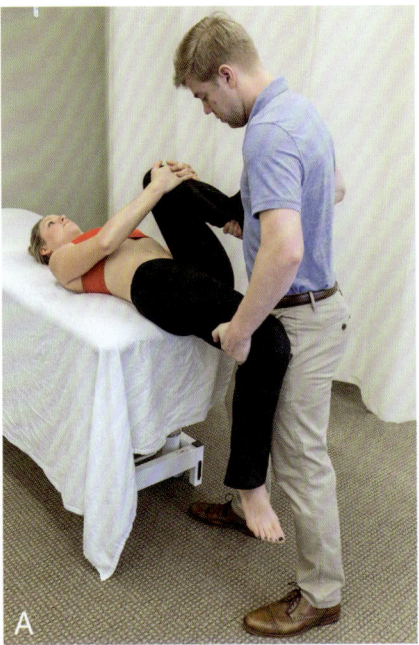
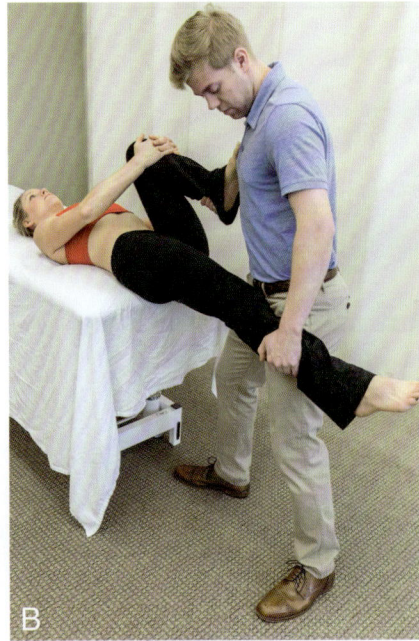

Figure 56-6. Thomas test assessing the length of the tensor fasciae latae muscle. A, Two joint hip flexor muscle length assessment. B, One joint hip flexor muscle length assessmnet.

be assessed with the Ober or modified Ober test.[25] Clinically, a positive Ober test would prompt the clinician to check the length of the gluteus maximus, gluteus medius and tensor fasciae latae muscles as all three of these muscles attach to the fascia latae. Tightness of the tensor fasciae latae muscle can also produce the appearance of a shorter limb on the involved side when the patient is examined in a supine to long sit position.

3.4. Trigger Point Examination

Gluteus Minimus

Trigger points in the gluteus minimus muscle lie deep to the gluteus maximus, gluteus medius, or tensor fasciae latae muscles, making them challenging to palpate. If the superficial muscles are fully relaxed, sometimes the practitioner can palpate some of the TrPs deep in the buttock. Commonly, the taut bands are unlikely to be palpated, but TrP tenderness can be localized. Occasionally, it is possible to reproduce the pain referral pattern with palpation of the TrP, but many times it will be elicited only when stimulated with a filiform or injection needle. The anterior fibers of the gluteus minimus muscle can be palpated with the patient lying supine or in hook-lying (Figure 56-7A). Using deep, cross-fiber flat palpation, the clinician can evaluate the fibers of the gluteus minimus muscle anterior, and then posterior, to the tensor fasciae latae muscle below the level of the anterior superior iliac spine. In some patients, the gluteus medius muscle may lie superficial to the gluteus minimus muscle up to the posterior border of the tensor fasciae latae muscle. To examine the posterior aspect of the gluteus minimus muscle, patients will lie on their side with the hip flexed to about 30° and adducted (Figure 56-7B).

Tensor Fasciae Latae

Trigger points in this superficial muscle can be identified in a supine (Figure 56-8A) or side-lying position with cross-fiber flat palpation (Figure 56-8B). The muscle can be located by palpating its tension while the patient performs a gentle isometric

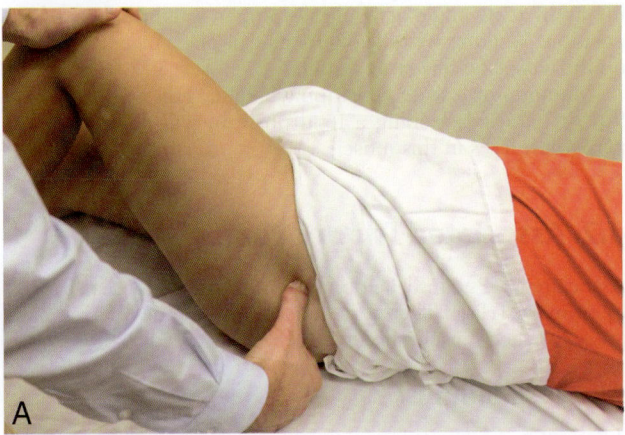
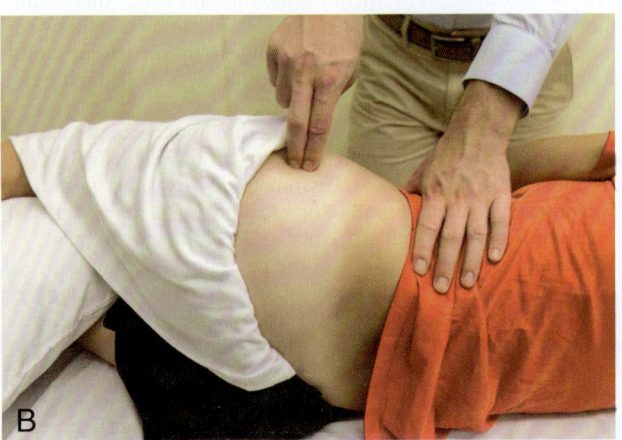

Figure 56-7. Palpation of TrPs in the gluteus minimus muscle using cross-fiber flat palpation. A, Supine anterior portion of the muscle. B, Side-lying through the gluteus medius muscle.

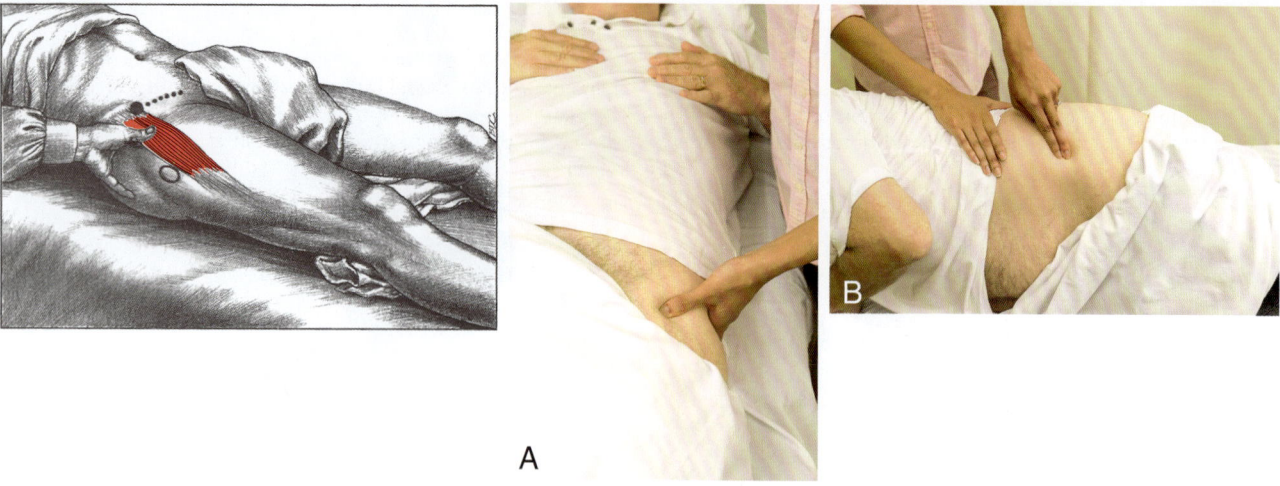

Figure 56-8. Palpation of TrPs in the tensor fasciae latae muscle using cross-fiber flat palpation. A, Supine. B, Side-lying.

contraction of hip abduction and internal rotation. When the patient is fully relaxed and the muscle is placed under slight stretch, the entire muscle belly should be palpated for the presence of TrPs. Trigger points in this muscle may take up to 10 seconds, when compressed, to produce the pain referral pattern into the lateral thigh.

4. DIFFERENTIAL DIAGNOSIS

4.1. Activation and Perpetuation of Trigger Points

A posture or activity that activates a TrP, if not corrected, can also perpetuate it. In any part of the gluteus minimus or tensor fasciae latae muscles, TrPs may be activated by unaccustomed eccentric loading, eccentric exercise in an unconditioned muscle, or maximal or submaximal concentric loading.[26] Trigger points may also be activated or aggravated when the muscle is placed in a shortened and/or lengthened position for an extended period of time.

Gluteus Minimus

Because the gluteus minimus muscle is active throughout the stance phase of gait, any alterations of the mechanics of walking or running gait may play a role in the development of TrPs. Excessive adduction moment on the hip and pelvis due to hip abductor weakness/inhibition, genu valgum, abnormal foot pronation, or gait deviation from an injury to another joint could increase the demand on the gluteus minimus muscle during the stance phase of gait.[27-29]

Trigger points in the gluteus minimus muscle may also be activated by an acute overload due to a fall. Excessive use of the muscles during an unaccustomed activity such as hiking over uneven ground, running, or racquet sports may overload the gluteus minimus muscle, causing development of TrPs.[21]

Sitting on a wallet placed in the back pocket can compress gluteus minimus TrPs and produce referred pain into the lower extremity. Prolonged immobility from standing in line or at a cocktail party, or prolonged sitting while driving, can also aggravate TrPs in the gluteus minimus muscle.

Lumbar radicular pain or radiculopathy in the L4, L5, or S1 nerve roots can activate and perpetuate TrPs in the gluteal muscles. Treatment of the TrPs will give the patient temporary relief of symptoms; however, the source of the radicular symptoms must be treated for long-lasting relief. Following a transforaminal epidural spinal injection or lumbar surgery for the treatment of radicular pain, the intensity of symptoms subsides, but there are often residual symptoms in the referral zones from TrPs in the muscles that are innervated by these nerve roots. Treatment of these TrPs will typically resolve the residual pain and symptoms.

Tensor Fasciae Latae

Activation of tensor fasciae latae TrPs may be due to sudden trauma, as when landing on the feet from a high jump, or chronic overload. Chronic overload may be caused by jogging uphill and downhill without appropriate support for an excessively pronated foot. Similarly, regular walking or running on surfaces that are uneven or sloped to one side, as on the edge of a paved street in a road race, can lead to tensor fasciae latae dysfunction because these slants increase genu varus and supination in one leg and genu valgus and pronation in the other. Poor conditioning and inadequate warm-up stretching exercises can lead to injuries that activate or perpetuate TrPs in runners. Weakness or inhibition from TrPs in the gluteus medius and gluteus minimus muscles may also cause overload to the tensor fasciae latae muscle because of its synergistic role in stabilizing the pelvis in the frontal plane. Allison et al[30] found in individuals with gluteal tendinopathy that the tensor fasciae latae muscle was activated quicker when compared with controls in the early mid-stance phase of gait to assist the gluteal muscles in lateral hip stability.

As in other muscles, TrPs in the tensor fasciae latae muscle are aggravated by immobilization in the shortened position for long periods. This happens during prolonged sitting with the hip at an acute angle or while sleeping in a tightly flexed fetal position. Walking with heavy loads can place increased stress on the tensor fasciae latae muscle.

Maintaining a seated position where the hips are flexed past 90° or habitual sleeping a fetal position will aggravate and perpetuate TrPs in this muscle.

4.2. Associated Trigger Points

Associated TrPs can develop in the referred pain areas caused by primary TrPs.[31] Therefore, musculature in the referred pain areas for each muscle should also be considered.

Gluteus Minimus

Active TrPs in the gluteus minimus muscle rarely present as a single-muscle syndrome. The TrPs in this muscle are most often observed in association with TrPs in the quadratus lumborum, piriformis, gluteus medius, vastus lateralis, and fibularis longus muscles, and sometimes, in the gluteus maximus muscle. The two muscles that are most closely associated functionally with the gluteus minimus muscle (the gluteus medius and the piriformis muscles) are also the most likely to develop associated TrPs. The anterior fibers of the gluteus minimus and the tensor fasciae latae muscles are closely related functionally and may develop associated TrPs.

Trigger points commonly develop in the posterior portion of the gluteus minimus muscle, and less frequently in the anterior portion, as associated to quadratus lumborum TrPs. This coupling can be so strong that pressure exerted on the quadratus lumborum TrPs induces not only the expected referred pain in the buttock but also unexpected pain referred down the back of the lower extremity.[21] This additional pain results from an activation of associated TrPs in the posterior part of the gluteus minimus muscle; pressure applied to these gluteal TrPs elicits the same lower extremity pain. Sometimes, elimination of the quadratus lumborum TrPs inactivates the associated gluteal TrPs. In other patients, TrPs in the two muscles must be inactivated separately.

Similarly, the fibularis longus and fibularis brevis muscles, which lie in the pain reference zone of the anterior part of the gluteus minimus muscle, have been seen to develop associated TrPs. Other muscles that should be evaluated for TrPs for being in the zone of the referred pain pattern from the gluteus minimus muscle include the obturator internus and externus, gemellus superior and inferior, quadratus femoris, bicep femoris, semitendinosus and semimembranosus, gastrocnemius, soleus, popliteus, posterior tibialis, flexor digitorum longus, and flexor halluces longus muscles.[21]

Tensor Fasciae Latae

Pain referred from TrPs in the tensor fasciae latae muscle can easily be mistaken for pain arising from TrPs in the gluteus minimus, gluteus medius, or vastus lateralis muscles. Trigger points in the quadratus lumborum muscle also refer pain and tenderness to the greater trochanter.

Trigger points in the tensor fasciae latae muscle may occur as a single-muscle syndrome or, more commonly, may develop secondary to TrPs in the anterior gluteus minimus and, sometimes, in the rectus femoris, iliopsoas, or sartorius muscles. Tensor fasciae latae TrPs cannot be eliminated if active TrPs remain in the anterior gluteus minimus muscle, which prevent its full stretch range of motion.

4.3. Associated Pathology

Gluteus Minimus

Altered activity of the gluteus minimus muscle has been observed in individuals with hip pain.[32] Earlier onset of activity of the gluteus minimus muscle was observed during step-down activity in a study of participants with hip pain. They also demonstrated increased gluteus minimus muscle activity during swing phase compared with control subjects.[32] Because the gluteus minimus muscle mitigates translation of the hip during the stance phase of gait, overload of the muscle may occur in individuals with instability of the hip.[11] Instability or micro-instability may result from trauma to the ligamentous structures from repetitive loading, bony abnormalities such as anteversion or retroversion, dysplasia, labral tears, sports-related traumas, or connective tissue disorders.[33]

Trigger points in the gluteal and hip muscles have been found in association with lower back pain including the gluteus minimus muscle. Iglesias-Gonzalez et al found an association between active TrPs in the lower back and hip muscles in participants with chronic lower back pain. In their study, they showed a correlation between the intensity of pain and the number of active TrPs and also a correlation between the number of active TrPs and sleep quality.[34]

Adelmanesh et al[35] investigated the prevalence of gluteal TrPs in 271 patients diagnosed with lumbar radiculopathy compared with 152 healthy controls. They found that 76% of patients with unilateral radicular symptoms had gluteal TrPs on the painful side when compared with 2% of the control group. Based on previous work, Adelmanesh et al[36] investigated the diagnostic accuracy of gluteal TrPs to differentiate radicular from nonradicular low back pain. They determined the diagnostic value of identifying gluteal TrPs by manual palpation (gluteal TrP test) in the superior-lateral quadrant in the gluteal region. They found a specificity of 0.91 and a sensitivity of 0.74 of the gluteal TrP test. They conclude that the presence of TrPs in the superolateral quadrant of the gluteal region is a highly specific indicator for individuals with radicular symptoms.[36]

Tensor Fasciae Latae

Radicular pain from the L4 nerve root or the peripheral nerve entrapment of the lateral femoral cutaneous nerve (meralgia paresthetica) may produce symptom distribution confusingly similar to the pattern of pain referred from tensor fasciae latae TrPs. When patients have symptoms of meralgia paresthetica, they may, in addition, have active TrPs in the tensor fasciae latae muscle that contribute to their symptoms.

Patients with tensor fasciae latae TrPs are often misdiagnosed as having trochanteric bursitis. Although patients with TrPs in the tensor fasciae latae muscle do have pain and tenderness over the area of the bursa, the symptoms are referred from the TrPs and are not caused by inflammation of the bursa itself.

Iliotibial tract friction syndrome, or Iliotibial band syndrome, causes diffuse pain and tenderness of the lateral femoral condyle. This condition is common in runners with genu varum and pronated feet and is seen in those who wear shoes with worn lateral soles.[37] Often, TrPs of the tensor fasciae latae, gluteus maximus, and vastus lateralis muscles can mimic or contribute to the pain of this condition.

Alternate minimally invasive total hip arthroplasty (THA) techniques access the hip joint through the interval between the tensor fasciae latae and the gluteus medius muscles, attempting to maintain the integrity of the superior gluteal nerve.[38] Recent investigation of patients' status post THA with an anterior approach reveals that 74% of patients participating in a study ($n = 17$) show signs of denervation injury after surgery, including denervation hypertrophy, atrophy, and fatty infiltration.[38] Likewise, a case report identified similar denervation hypertrophy in a patient with chronic L5 radiculopathy.[39] It is possible that these areas of denervation hypertrophy could be confused with the presence of TrPs in these muscles. Specific palpation to identify a hyperirritable spot tenderness in a taut band within the muscle fibers will aid in determining a specific source of symptoms in these cases.

5. CORRECTIVE ACTIONS

Gluteus Minimus

Patients with gluteus minimus TrPs may need to modify their sleeping posture. Lying supine or sleeping on the opposite side is often more comfortable than sleeping on the painful side. Using a pillow between the legs to avoid a painful stretch into adduction of the hip may be necessary if sleeping in side-lying (see Figure 55-9). Using a cane on the opposite side to offload the gluteus minimus muscle may be helpful if significant pain is experienced with walking and standing. Sitting down when possible to avoid aggravation is beneficial. If prolonged standing is unavoidable, then shifting weight from one foot to the other may help reduce the constant demand on the muscle, and standing with the feet wider than shoulder width may be more comfortable. More vigorous exercise or activities such as running, sports, or hiking should be avoided or slowly progressed with incremental conditioning. Altering training programs for more

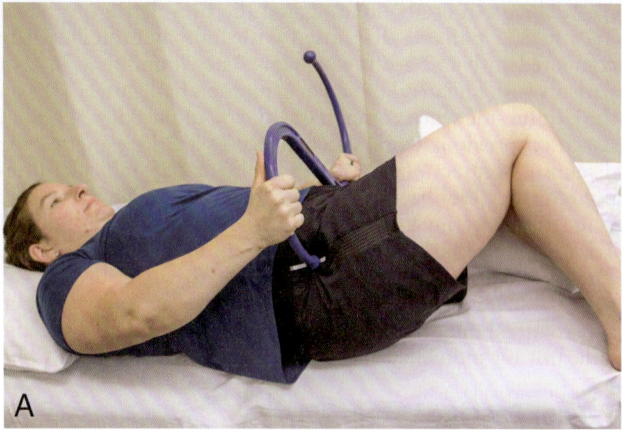
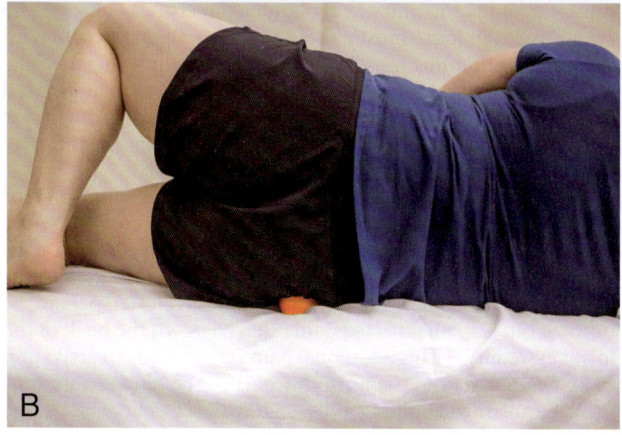

Figure 56-9. Gluteus minimus muscle self-pressure release. A, Using a TrP release tool. B, Utilizing a tennis or lacrosse ball.

mild symptoms may help avoid the need for complete activity cessation. If an individual is experiencing pain from TrPs in the gluteus minimus muscle during walking or running, he or she might benefit from training on sloped terrain because there is reduced demand on the gluteus minimus muscle during walking on an incline or decline surface when compared with a level surface.[40]

Self-pressure release of TrPs in the gluteus minimus muscle can be achieved with utilization of a TrP release tool, tennis ball, or a lacrosse ball. To perform TrP self-pressure release with a TrP tool, the patient lies on the back with a ¼ turn to the opposite side and the hip and knee of the side to be treated bent and supported by a pillow (Figure 56-9A). The sensitive spot is located with the tool and light pressure (no more than 4/10 pain) is applied and held for 15 to 30 seconds until pain reduces. This technique can be repeated five times per session, several times per day. To utilize a ball or other tool, the ball is placed on the floor and the patient gently lies on top of the ball over the tender area of the gluteus minimus muscle and follows the same procedure as Figure 56-9B. While rolling over the gluteus minimus muscle, patients should pay special attention to any tender spot by slowly rocking over the area or pausing to wait for it to release prior to moving to the next area. Pressure should be mildly uncomfortable but not overly painful (Figure 56-9B).

Stretching of the gluteus minimus muscle can be achieved by lying on the uninvolved side on the edge of a firm surface, flexing the lower hip so that the lower foot can support the top leg (see Figure 55-11A). The top leg can be lowered until a slight stretch or discomfort is felt over the hip. The stretch should be held for 30 seconds and be repeated four times. The lower leg supports the top leg so as not to stretch the TrPs in the gluteus minimus muscle too aggressively (see Figure 55-11B). The patient should take a slow inhalation and then relax during exhalation, allowing gravity to apply the stretch to the gluteus minimus muscle (see Figure 55-11B). If the bed is too soft, the same stretch maneuver can be performed at the top of a stair landing with a pillow under the bottom hip (see Figure 55-11C and D). To focus on the back portion of the muscle, the top hip can be moved forward slightly (approximately 30° of hip flexion). Gravity alone should be able to provide adequate stretch to the tight muscle. To focus on the front part of the muscle, the top hip can be moved back so the leg is just behind the pelvis.

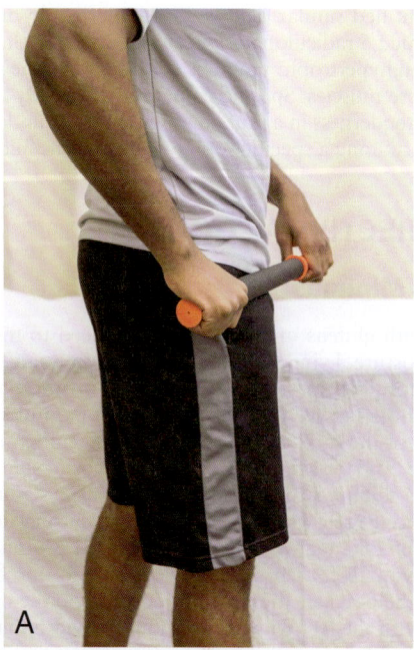
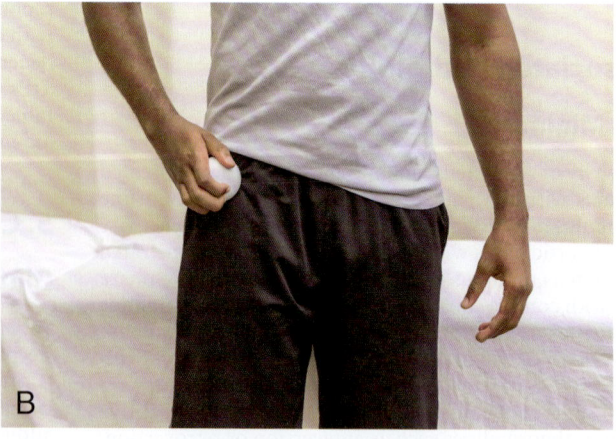

Figure 56-10. Tensor fasciae latae muscle self-pressure release. A, Using a TrP release roller. B, Utilizing a tennis or lacrosse ball.

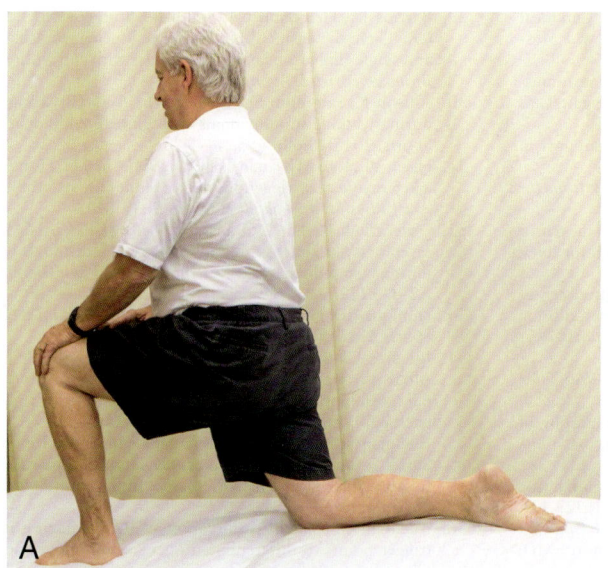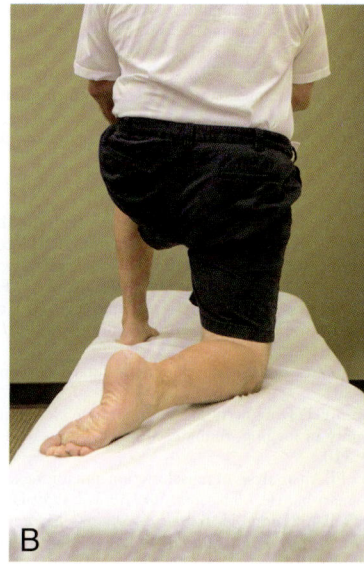

Figure 56-11. Self-stretch of the tensor fasciae latae muscle in half kneeling. A, Starting position. B, The hip and thigh is placed in external rotation and adduction. The patient leans slightly on the affected knee. A stretch should be felt on the front side of the hip.

Tensor Fasciae Latae

Patients with TrPs in the tensor fasciae latae muscle need to avoid prolonged flexion of the hip caused by positions such as sitting in a chair with the knees above the hips, or sleeping in the fetal position with the hips and knees bent up toward the chest. During sleep, the hip should be kept in a position with the leg straight or slightly bent.

Chairs in which the patient sits for any length of time should provide the ability to increase the angle between hips and trunk. Either the backrest should be reclined to allow the patient to lean back against it most of the time or the front of the seat should be downwardly sloped. A firm pillow can be placed across the rear of the seat to achieve this desired slope in a nonadjustable chair.

On long trips in an automobile, cruise control permits change of position of the lower extremities to allow the driver to avoid holding the hip flexor muscles immobilized in a shortened position for long periods. Intermittent breaks during car travel to allow for standing and walking are highly recommended.

To reduce irritability of tensor fasciae latae TrPs, it is important to avoid walking or jogging up hills, which requires leaning forward and flexing the hips. It is also important for a runner to avoid shoes that are excessively worn and to avoid running on surfaces that slope from side to side. Runners with tensor fasciae latae TrPs may benefit from running on a level track, running on one side of the road in one direction and on the same side of the road for the return trip, or running only on the crown of a traffic-free road.

Self-pressure release of TrPs in the tensor fasciae latae muscle can be achieved using a TrP release tool, roller, or ball. To perform TrP self-pressure release with a TrP tool, the patient stands with the affected leg slightly in front of the other (Figure 56-10A). Starting just below the top of the pelvis bone and applying moderate pressure, the patient rolls along the length of the muscle to the outer portion of the thigh. If one spot is more sensitive than other places in the muscle, pausing to apply specific pressure for 10 to 15 seconds, relaxing, and repeating this cycle up to six times may be helpful.

To utilize a ball or other tool, the patient can place the ball on the front of the hip near the top of the pelvis (Figure 56-10B). While rolling over the tensor fasciae latae muscle, patients should pay special attention to any tender spot by slowly rocking over the area or pausing to wait for it to release prior to moving to the next area. Pressure should be mildly uncomfortable but not overly painful (Figure 56-10B).

An ideal stretch for the tensor fasciae latae muscle consists of hip adduction, extension, and knee flexion.[41,42] This combination can be performed independently in a half-kneeling position with the involved knee on the floor and the opposite knee flexed up at least to 90°. The patient should shift the body weight into hip extension and adduction and hold the stretch for 30 seconds, repeating the stretch four times (Figure 56-11).

After successful inactivation of TrPs, strength training of the gluteus medius, gluteus minimus, and tensor fasciae latae muscles is vital for efficient biomechanics during walking and running. Altered mechanics that cause the hip to turn in and/or adduct on the weight-bearing side while walking need to be corrected. Careful muscle retraining to avoid aggravation will be beneficial to prevent recurrence. A licensed rehabilitation professional should be consulted for a proper exercise prescription.

References

1. Weber EF. Ueber die Langenverhaltnisse der Fleischfasern der Muskeln in Allgemeinen. *Berichte uber die Verhandlungen der Koniglich Sachsischen Gesellschaft der Wissenschaften zu Leipzig.* 1851;3:63-86.
2. Flack NA, Nicholson HD, Woodley SJ. A review of the anatomy of the hip abductor muscles, gluteus medius, gluteus minimus, and tensor fascia lata. *Clin Anat.* 2012;25(6):697-708.
3. Cooper HJ, Walters BL, Rodriguez JA. Anatomy of the hip capsule and pericapsular structures: a cadaveric study. *Clin Anat.* 2015;28(5):665-671.
4. Standring S. *Gray's Anatomy: The Anatomical Basis of Clinical Practice.* 41st ed. London, UK: Elsevier; 2015.
5. Flack NA, Nicholson HD, Woodley SJ. The anatomy of the hip abductor muscles. *Clin Anat.* 2014;27(2):241-253.
6. Walters BL, Cooper JH, Rodriguez JA. New findings in hip capsular anatomy: dimensions of capsular thickness and pericapsular contributions. *Arthroscopy.* 2014;30(10):1235-1245.
7. Moore KL, Agur AMR, Dalley AF. *Clinically Oriented Anatomy.* Baltimore, MD: Lippincott Williams & Wilkins; 2014.
8. Semciw A, Pizzari T, Green R. Anterior and posterior gluteus minimus are functionally distinct from anterior and posterior gluteus medius. *J Sci Med Sort.* 2013;16(1):e92.
9. Correa TA, Crossley KM, Kim HJ, Pandy MG. Contributions of individual muscles to hip joint contact force in normal walking. *J Biomech.* 2010;43(8):1618-1622.
10. Beck M, Sledge JB, Gautier E, Dora CF, Ganz R. The anatomy and function of the gluteus minimus muscle. *J Bone Joint Surg Br.* 2000;82(3):358-363.

11. Retchford TH, Crossley KM, Grimaldi A, Kemp JL, Cowan SM. Can local muscles augment stability in the hip? A narrative literature review. *J Musculoskelet Neuronal Interact*. 2013;13(1):1-12.
12. Semciw AI, Green RA, Murley GS, Pizzari T. Gluteus minimus: an intramuscular EMG investigation of anterior and posterior segments during gait. *Gait Posture*. 2014;39(2):822-826.
13. Anderson FC, Pandy MG. Individual muscle contributions to support in normal walking. *Gait Posture*. 2003;17(2):159-169.
14. Neumann DA. *Kinesiology of the Musculoskeletal System: Foundations for Rehabilitaion*. 2nd ed. St. Louis, MO: Mosby; 2010 (p. 495).
15. Paré EB, Stern JT Jr, Schwartz JM. Functional differentiation within the tensor fasciae latae. A telemetered electromyographic analysis of its locomotor roles. *J Bone Joint Surg Am Vol*. 1981;63(9):1457-1471.
16. Bouillon LE, Wilhelm J, Eisel P, Wiesner J, Rachow M, Hatteberg L. Electromyographic assessment of muscle activity between genders during unilateral weight-bearing tasks using adjusted distances. *Int J Sports Phys Ther*. 2012;7(6):595-605.
17. Perry J. The mechanics of walking. A clinical interpretation. *Phys Ther*. 1967;47(9):778-801.
18. Mann RA, Moran GT, Dougherty SE. Comparative electromyography of the lower extremity in jogging, running, and sprinting. *Am J Sports Med*. 1986;14(6):501-510.
19. Houtz SJ, Fischer FJ. An analysis of muscle action and joint excursion during exercise on a stationary bicycle. *J Bone Joint Surg Am Vol*. 1959;41-A(1):123-131.
20. Simons DG, Travell J, Simons L. *Travell & Simon's Myofascial Pain and Dysfunction: The Trigger Point Manual*. Vol 1. 2nd ed. Baltimore, MD: Williams & Wilkins; 1999.
21. Travell J, Simons DG. *Myofascial Pain and Dysfunction: The Trigger Point Manual*. Vol 2. Baltimore, MD: Williams & Wilkins; 1992 (pp. 168-170, 177).
22. Kellgren JH. Observations on referred pain arising from muscle. *Clin Sci*. 1938;3:175-190 (Fig. 8).
23. Kellgren JH. A preliminary account of referred pains arising from muscle. *Br Med J*. 1938;1:325-327 (Case VII).
24. Gutstein M. Diagnosis and treatment of muscular rheumatism. *Br J Phys Med*. 1938;1:302-321.
25. Kendall FP, McCreary EK. *Muscles: Testing and Function, with Posture and Pain*. 5th ed. Baltimore, MD: Lippincott Williams & Wilkins; 2005.
26. Gerwin RD, Dommerholt J, Shah JP. An expansion of Simons' integrated hypothesis of trigger point formation. *Curr Pain Headache Rep*. 2004;8(6):468-475.
27. Roach S, Sorenson E, Headley B, San Juan JG. Prevalence of myofascial trigger points in the hip in patellofemoral pain. *Arch Phys Med Rehabil*. 2013;94(3):522-526.
28. Allison K, Wrigley TV, Vicenzino B, Bennell KL, Grimaldi A, Hodges PW. Kinematics and kinetics during walking in individuals with gluteal tendinopathy. *Clin Biomech (Bristol, Avon)*. 2016;32:56-63.
29. Barrios JA, Heitkamp CA, Smith BP, Sturgeon MM, Suckow DW, Sutton CR. Three-dimensional hip and knee kinematics during walking, running, and single-limb drop landing in females with and without genu valgum. *Clin Biomech (Bristol, Avon)*. 2016;31:7-11.
30. Allison K, Salomoni SE, Bennell KL, et al. Hip abductor muscle activity during walking in individuals with gluteal tendinopathy. *Scand J Med Sci Sports*. 2018;28:686-695.
31. Hsieh YL, Kao MJ, Kuan TS, Chen SM, Chen JT, Hong CZ. Dry needling to a key myofascial trigger point may reduce the irritability of satellite MTrPs. *Am J Phys Med Rehabil*. 2007;86(5):397-403.
32. Dieterich AV, Deshon L, Strauss GR, McKay J, Pickard CM. M-mode ultrasound reveals earlier gluteus minimus activity in individuals with chronic hip pain during a step-down task. *J Orthop Sports Phys Ther*. 2016;46(4):277-285, A271-A272.
33. Dumont GD. Hip instability: current concepts and treatment options. *Clin Sports Med*. 2016;35(3):435-447.
34. Iglesias-Gonzalez JJ, Munoz-Garcia MT, Rodrigues-de-Souza DP, Alburquerque-Sendin F, Fernández de las Peñas C. Myofascial trigger points, pain, disability, and sleep quality in patients with chronic nonspecific low back pain. *Pain Med*. 2013;14(12):1964-1970.
35. Adelmanesh F, Jalali A, Jazayeri Shooshtari SM, Raissi GR, Ketabchi SM, Shir Y. Is there an association between lumbosacral radiculopathy and painful gluteal trigger points? A cross-sectional study. *Am J Phys Med Rehabil*. 2015;94(10):784-791.
36. Adelmanesh F, Jalali A, Shirvani A, et al. The diagnostic accuracy of gluteal trigger points to differentiate radicular from nonradicular low back pain. *Clin J Pain*. 2016;32(8):666-672.
37. Louw M, Deary C. The biomechanical variables involved in the aetiology of iliotibial band syndrome in distance runners—a systematic review of the literature. *Phys Ther Sport*. 2014;15(1):64-75.
38. Unis DB, Hawkins EJ, Alapatt MF, Benitez CL. Postoperative changes in the tensor fascia lata muscle after using the modified anterolateral approach for total hip arthroplasty. *J Arthroplasty*. 2013;28(4):663-665.
39. Soltanzadeh P, Pierce B, Lietman S, Ilaslan H. Unilateral TFL mass as a presentation of lumbosacral radiculopathy. *Neuromuscular Disord*. 2015;25(2):242-243.
40. Alexander N, Schwameder H. Effect of sloped walking on lower limb muscle forces. *Gait Posture*. 2016;47:62-67.
41. Gajdosik RL, Sandler MM, Marr HL. Influence of knee positions and gender on the Ober test for length of the iliotibial band. *Clin Biomech (Bristol, Avon)*. 2003;18(1):77-79.
42. Umehara J, Ikezoe T, Nishishita S, et al. Effect of hip and knee position on tensor fasciae latae elongation during stretching: an ultrasonic shear wave elastography study. *Clin Biomech (Bristol, Avon)*. 2015;30(10):1056-1059.

Chapter 57

Piriformis, Obturator Internus, Gemelli, Obturator Externus, and Quadratus Femoris Muscles

"Double Devils"

Jennifer Marie Nelson and Joseph M. Donnelly

1. INTRODUCTION

Historically, the piriformis muscle has been the star of the short external rotators of the hip, but more recently, the rest of the rotators have been receiving more attention in the literature, most notably, the obturator internus muscle because of its relationship to the pelvic floor. The exact attachments of the deep hip rotator muscles are variable, but generally, the piriformis and the obturator internus muscles attach to the internal side of the pelvis and form the posterolateral, and part of the anterolateral, portion of the true pelvis before attaching to the greater trochanter of the femur. The superior and inferior gemellus as well as the quadratus femoris muscles all attach from the ischium to the greater trochanter of the femur. These muscles have traditionally been thought to be external rotators of the femur; however, more recent research suggests that they are hip stabilizers. The obturator externus muscle is an adductor anatomically and, like the other adductors, it is innervated by the obturator nerve. The referred pain pattern from trigger points (TrPs) in the piriformis and obturator internus muscles are mostly in the gluteal region and down the posterior one-third of the thigh. Studying the pain referral patterns and function of the other deep hip external rotators is complicated because of the depth and proximity to the neurovascular structures. Trigger points in the deep rotators are commonly associated with other conditions. Piriformis syndrome has been used to describe a general distribution of pain but often involves more structures than just the piriformis muscle, and sometimes the piriformis muscle itself is not even involved. Differential diagnosis should include lumbosacral radicular pain or radiculopathy, sacroiliac joint dysfunction, hip and knee dysfunction or pathology. For resolution of symptoms, correction of altered biomechanics in the lower kinetic chain will need to be addressed. Corrective actions should include techniques to improve sitting and sleeping postures, gluteus maximus neuromuscular re-education, self-pressure release, and self-stretching techniques.

2. ANATOMIC CONSIDERATIONS

Piriformis

The name "piriformis" is derived from the Latin *pirum* (pear) and *forma* (shape); it was coined by Adrian Spigelius, a late 16th- and early 17th-century Belgian anatomist.[1] The piriformis muscle can be small with only one or two sacral attachments. Conversely, it can be so broad that it joins with the capsule of the sacroiliac joint above, and also with, the anterior surface of the sacrotuberous and/or sacrospinous ligaments below.[2,3]

Most authors agree that the piriformis muscle has a sacral origin, but the exact attachment sites vary.[4] This muscle originates from the anterior (internal) surface of the sacrum usually by three digitations between the pelvic sacral foramina and anterior sacral foramina (Figures 57-1A and 57-2).[2,4] However, the exact number of digitations can vary.[4] Some fibers may attach to the upper margin of the greater sciatic notch[4] at the capsule of the sacroiliac joint,[2,3,5] the sacrotuberous ligament,[2,4,6] and the posterior inferior iliac spine.[2] The piriformis muscle has no hip joint capsule contribution.[7]

The piriformis muscle inserts laterally and distally via a rounded tendon onto the greater trochanter on the medial side of its superior surface (Figures 57-1B and 57-3).[2] This tendon often blends with the common tendon of the obturator internus and gemelli muscles,[2,4,8,9] and the muscle may fuse with the gluteus medius muscle.[2,4]

Variations of the piriformis muscle can also include two distinct heads of the muscle. In fewer than 20% of cadavers, it is divided into two distinct portions.[4,10,11] However, most variations have to do with where the sciatic nerve passes in relation to the piriformis muscle. Within the pelvis, the piriformis muscle abuts the sacrum, rectum, sacral plexus, and branches of the internal iliac vessels.[2] The piriformis muscle exits the inside of the pelvis through the greater sciatic foramen.[2,8] This rigid opening is formed anteriorly and superiorly by the posterior part of the ilium, posteriorly by the sacrotuberous ligament, and inferiorly by the sacrospinous ligament.[2,8] When the muscle is large enough to fill this space, it has the potential to compress the numerous vessels and nerves that exit the pelvis with it.[2] The piriformis muscle then passes the gluteal region, abutting posteriorly to the gluteus maximus muscle,[2,8] anteriorly to the capsule of the hip joint,[2,9] inferiorly to the gluteus medius muscle and superior gluteal vessels and nerve,[2,9] and superiorly to the coccygeus and gemellus superior muscles. Between the gemellus superior and piriformis muscles run several nerves and vessels.[2] The piriformis muscle then joins the obturator internus/gemelli complex to attach on the upper side of the greater trochanter.[2,4,8,9]

The other short hip external rotators of the thigh, the four GOGO muscles (superior gemellus, obturator internus, inferior gemellus, and obturator externus muscles) and the quadratus femoris muscle, lie distal to the piriformis muscle. They are deep to the gluteus maximus muscle, but in contrast to the usual position of the piriformis muscle, they pass anterior to the sciatic nerve (Figure 57-3).

589

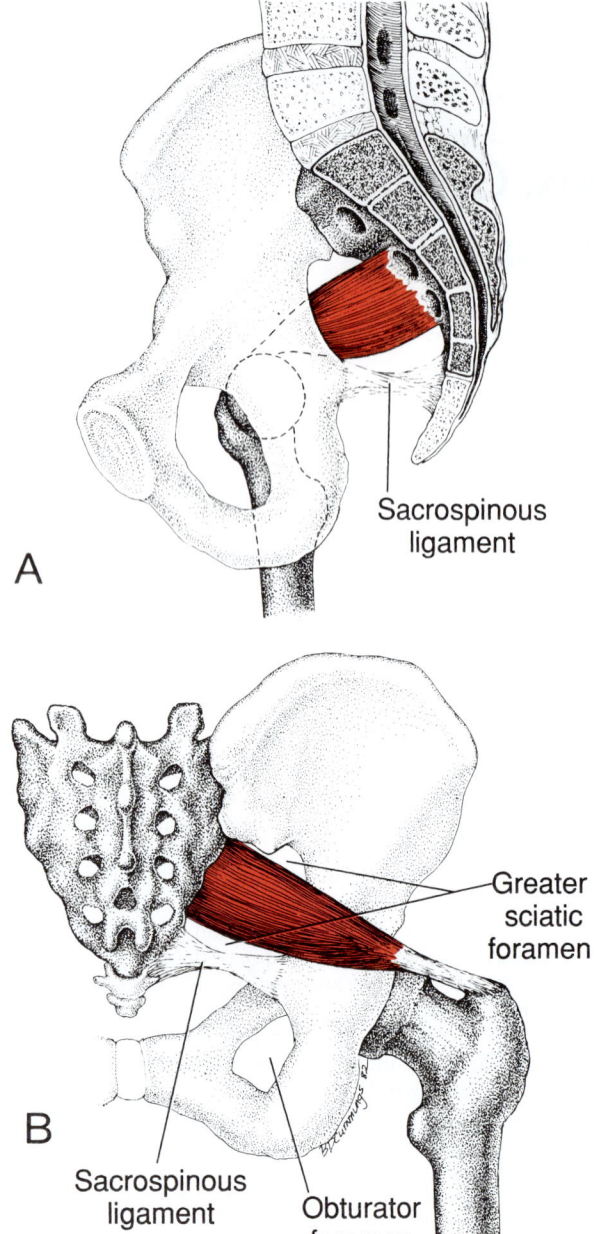

Figure 57-1. Attachments of the right piriformis muscle (red). A, Seen from inside the pelvis in mid-sagittal view showing the attachment of the muscle on the inside of the sacrum, usually between the first four anterior sacral foramina. The fourth foramen is not shown. B, Seen from behind (posterior view). In this figure, a relatively small muscle exits the pelvis through a relatively large sciatic foramen. Its rounded tendon attaches laterally to the superior surface of the greater trochanter. The muscle traverses the greater sciatic foramen just above the sacrospinous ligament. Most of the muscle is accessible to external palpation, and nearly half of the muscle belly is accessible to palpation inside the pelvis.

Obturator Internus

The obturator internus muscle is both an intrapelvic muscle and a hip muscle (Figure 57-3).[2] Within the pelvis, the obturator internus muscle makes contact with the obturator fascia, levator ani muscle, pudendal vessels and nerve, and ischiorectal fossa. It originates medially and proximally and covers the inner surface of the obturator membrane and attaches to the rim of the obturator foramen, except where the obturator nerve and vessels leave the pelvis through the lateral part of the membrane. Specifically, it attaches to the inferior ramus of the pubis, ischial ramus, behind and below the pelvic brim from the greater sciatic notch to the obturator foramen, medial pelvic surface of the obturator membrane, the tendinous arch and the obturator fascia covering the muscle.[2,4] Before the obturator internus muscle exits the pelvis, it heads toward the lesser sciatic foramen and takes a lateral right-angle turn between the ischial spine and the ischial tuberosity.[2,9] As it makes this turn, the obturator internus muscle is separated from the ischium by a bursa and hyaline cartilage.[2] The obturator internus muscle inserts laterally and distally by converging onto a tendon that is usually shared with the gemelli muscles.[2] This tendon inserts on the anterior part of the medial surface of the greater trochanter, proximal to the trochanteric fossa of the femur, and attaches on the greater trochanter near but distal to the piriformis tendon.[2,12] The subtendinous bursa of the obturator internus muscle lies between its tendon and the capsule of the hip joint and may communicate with the ischiadic bursa between the obturator internus muscle and the ischium.[2]

Superior and Inferior Gemelli

The superior and inferior gemelli muscles attach medially/proximally to the ischium and laterally/distally to the medial surface of the upper part of the greater trochanter, proximal to, and nearly parallel with, the quadratus femoris muscle (Figure 57-3). The inferior gemellus muscle attaches below the grove of the obturator internus muscle on the lateral ischial tuberosity[2] and occasionally at the sacrotuberous ligament and lesser sciatic notch.[4] It then joins the extrapelvic obturator internus muscle before inserting into the greater trochanter.[2] The superior gemellus muscle is smaller than the inferior gemellus muscle and is sometimes absent.[2] It originates from the dorsal side of the ischial spine[2] and occasionally from the lesser sciatic foramen and notch[4] before joining superiorly to insert on the medial aspect of the greater trochanter with the obturator internus and inferior gemellus muscles.[2] Accessory gemelli and obturator internus muscles arising from the lesser sciatic notch have also been reported.[4] These three muscles are also called the "triceps coxae," and exactly how much they join together rather than fuse together is a matter of controversy.[4]

Obturator Externus

The obturator externus muscle is considered part of the adductor group by Hollinshead[13]; however, he notes that its primary action would be external rotation, and not adduction, of the thigh. The obturator externus muscle originates medially to the external surface of the anteromedial two-thirds of the obturator membrane, the pubic and ischial rami.[2,4] The fibers run laterally, caudally, and posteriorly, and pass across the distal part of the capsule of the hip joint to insert laterally to the femur at the intertrochanteric fossa[2,4,14] deep to the quadratus femoris muscle. In fact, from the posterior view, it is nearly covered by the quadratus femoris muscle (Figure 57-3).[2,15,16] A bursa often intervenes where the obturator externus muscle crosses the lesser trochanter.[2]

Quadratus Femoris

The quadratus femoris muscle is a rectangular muscle with parallel fibers that originate from the anterolateral surface of the ischial tuberosity, caudad to the inferior gemellus and posterior to the obturator externus muscles. Laterally, it inserts onto the femur on the quadrate tubercle and along the intertrochanteric crest, which extends longitudinally about halfway between the greater and lesser trochanters (Figure 57-3).[2,4] The quadratus femoris muscle is situated between the superior portion of the adductor magnus and gemellus inferior muscles and is in close proximity to the medial circumflex femoral artery.[2] It is

Chapter 57: Piriformis, Obturator Internus, Gemelli, Obturator Externus, and Quadratus Femoris Muscles

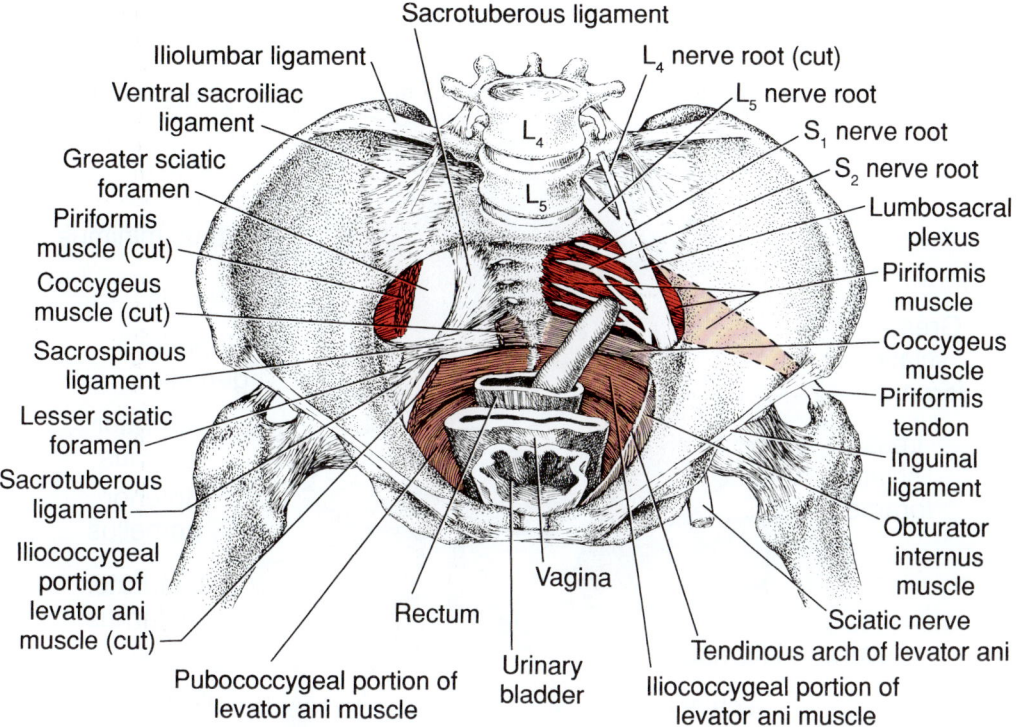

Figure 57-2. Internal palpation of the left piriformis muscle (dark red within the pelvis and light red outside the pelvis) via the rectum, viewed from in front and above. The levator ani muscle is medium red; the coccygeus and obturator internus muscles are light red. The sacrospinous ligament (covered by the coccygeus muscle) is the last major transverse landmark identified by the palpating finger before it reaches the piriformis muscle. The sacrospinous ligament attaches cephalad mainly to the coccyx, which is usually easily palpated and mobile. The posterior wall of the rectum and the S3 and S4 nerve roots lie between the palpating finger and the piriformis muscle.

occasionally missing[2,4] and can be prone to impingement at the ischiofemoral space as well as acute strains.[4,17]

2.1. Innervation and Vascularization

The piriformis muscle is usually innervated by the L5 nerve and S1 and S2 nerves; however, variation of this innervation pattern has been described. It can also be innervated by only one of the sacral nerves as it emerges from the anterior sacral foramina.[2] Other variations described in the literature include branches of the posterior rami of the sacral plexus; nerve to the piriformis muscle from S1 and S2; directly from the anterior rami of S1 and S2; anterior rami of branches from L5, S1, and S2; and from L4, L5, and S1.[4]

The piriformis muscle receives its primary vascularization extrapelvically through the superior gluteal artery and by gemellar branches of the internal pudendal artery. Intrapelvically, the piriformis muscle receives its vascularization from the lateral sacral artery along with the superior and inferior gluteal arteries.[2]

The nerve to the obturator internus muscle innervates the gemellus superior (L5, S1, and S2) and obturator internus (L5 and S1) muscles.[2] However, other variations have been described, including: L5, S1, and S2; S1, S2, and S3[13]; branches of the sacral plexus; nerve to the obturator internus muscle; or branches of L5 and S1.[4]

The extrapelvic portion of the obturator internus muscle receives its vascularization from the gemellar branches of the internal pudendal arteries, whereas the intrapelvic and extrapelvic portions receive vascularization from the branches of the obturator artery. The gemellus superior muscle receives its vascularization from the internal pudendal artery and inferior gluteal artery and occasionally by the superior gluteal artery.[2]

The nerve to the quadratus femoris muscle sends a branch to the inferior gemellus muscle, containing fibers from L4-S1, and to the quadratus femoris muscle, containing fibers from L5 and S1.[2] Other innervations described in the literature include the following: branches of the sacral plexus or nerve to the quadratus femoris muscle alone; nerve to the quadratus femoris muscle or the branches of L4, L5, and S1; and nerve to the quadratus femoris muscle or the branches of L5, S1 (L4 inferior gemellus muscle), L5, S1, and S2.[4]

The quadratus femoris muscle receives its vascularization from the inferior gluteal artery and the medial circumflex femoral artery. The gemellus inferior muscle primarily receives its vascularization by the medial circumflex femoral artery.[2]

Unlike all the other short external rotators, the obturator externus muscle receives its innervation from a posterior branch of the obturator nerve, containing fibers from L3 and L4,[2] but it has also been described as the branches of L2, L3, and L4.[4]

The obturator externus muscle receives its vascularization from the obturator and medial circumflex femoral arteries.[2]

Because of the size of the greater sciatic foramen and the number of structures that pass through it, there is potential for nerves and vessels to become crowded as they pass through it. The superior gluteal nerve and blood vessels usually pass between the superior border of the piriformis muscle and the upper (sacroiliac) rim of the foramen. This nerve supplies the gluteus medius, gluteus minimus, and tensor fasciae latae muscles.[18] The sciatic nerve usually exits between the piriformis muscle and the rim of the greater sciatic foramen (Figure 57-3). It supplies the skin and muscles of the posterior thigh and most of the leg and foot. Numerous variations of how the sciatic nerve courses from the pelvis down the leg have been described in the literature.[10,19-22] Recent studies have shown that anatomic variations of the sciatic nerve around the piriformis muscle are present in around 6% to 11% of individuals.[23,24] The relationship between the sciatic nerve and the piriformis muscle follows the typical anatomic pattern of an undivided

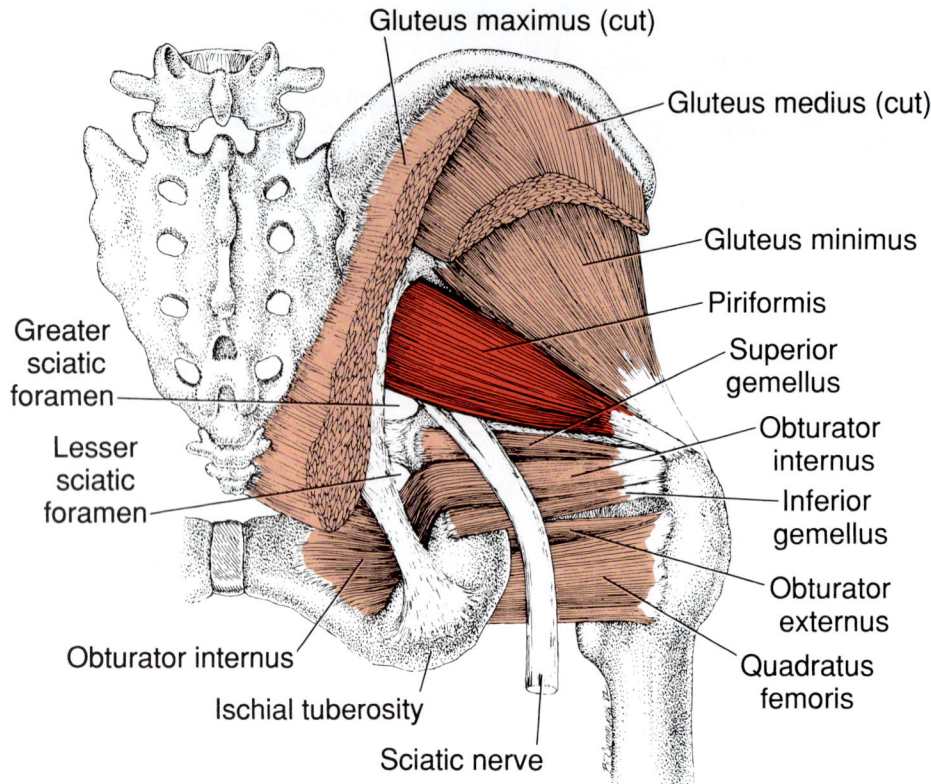

Figure 57-3. Piriformis muscle, regional anatomy: posterior view of anatomic relations of the right piriformis muscle (dark red) to neighboring muscles (light red). The gluteus maximus and gluteus medius muscles have been cut and removed; the distal cut ends of these gluteal muscles are not shown because they would obscure the attachment of the piriformis muscle to the femur.

sciatic nerve passing below the muscle, in around 90% of the subjects. Other anatomic variations are as follows: the common fibular nerve passed through and the tibial nerve below a double piriformis muscle (4%-10%); the common fibular nerve coursed superior and the tibial nerve below the piriformis muscle (0.5%), or both nerves penetrated the piriformis muscle (0.5%).[23,24] These anatomic variations are described in Figure 57-4 and Table 57-1.

Also exiting the pelvis along the lower border of the piriformis muscle are the pudendal nerve and vessels. The pudendal nerve then crosses the spine of the ischium and re-enters the pelvis through the lesser sciatic foramen (Figure 57-3). It supplies the external anal sphincter muscle and helps supply the skin of the posterior thigh and scrotum or labia majora. Innervation of the pelvic floor muscles by the pudendal nerve is presented in Chapter 52. The inferior gluteal nerve, which exclusively supplies the gluteus maximus muscle, the posterior femoral cutaneous nerve, and the nerves to the gemelli, obturator internus, and quadratus femoris muscles, also passes through the greater sciatic foramen with the piriformis muscle.[25] Collectively, these nerves are responsible for all gluteal muscle sensation and function, anterior perineal sensory and motor function, and nearly all of the sensation and motor function in the posterior thigh and calf. These symptoms are described as deep gluteal pain syndromes.[26] It is apparent that chronic compression of these nerves would cause buttock, inguinal, and posterior thigh pain, as well as pain lower in the limb.[2]

2.2. Function

The six "short external rotators" are the piriformis, the superior and inferior gemelli, the obturator internus and externus, and the quadratus femoris muscles.[27]

The piriformis muscle is primarily an external rotator when the hip is in a neutral or extended position. It is also considered a secondary hip abductor, and this function increases as the hip moves toward 90° of hip flexion. Giphart et al[28] found the piriformis muscle to be most active during prone heel squeezes and single-leg bridges.

In weight-bearing activities, the piriformis muscle is often needed to restrain (control) vigorous and/or rapid internal rotation of the thigh, especially during the early-stance phase of walking and running. The piriformis muscle is also thought to stabilize the hip joint and to assist in holding the femoral head in the acetabulum.[4]

The remaining five short external rotator muscles have been traditionally thought of almost exclusively as external rotators[29] in either hip flexion or extension. However, more recently, it is being suggested that they are more postural stabilizers of the hip than primary movers[2,28,30] and that hip flexion and extension may change the function of the muscles.[2,30-34] Examination of an articulated skeleton theoretically demonstrates that the degree of flexion of the thigh profoundly affects the function of the piriformis muscle: at 90° of flexion, it produces horizontal abduction of the thigh.[13,35] The obturator internus muscle's primary function in a closed kinetic chain when the foot is firmly planted on the ground is to rotate the pelvis and trunk relative to the femoral head (relative hip external rotation on the stance side). This force compresses the hip joint surfaces, resulting in a portion of dynamic stability to the hip joint. All of the external rotators act with the gluteus maximus muscle to change directions by rotating the trunk and pelvis backward on a fixed femur when the foot is planted.[27]

Electromyographic (EMG) study of the functional kinesiology of any of these muscles has been difficult to perform because of the depth and close proximity to neurovascular structures. However, recent research using fine-wire EMG has produced

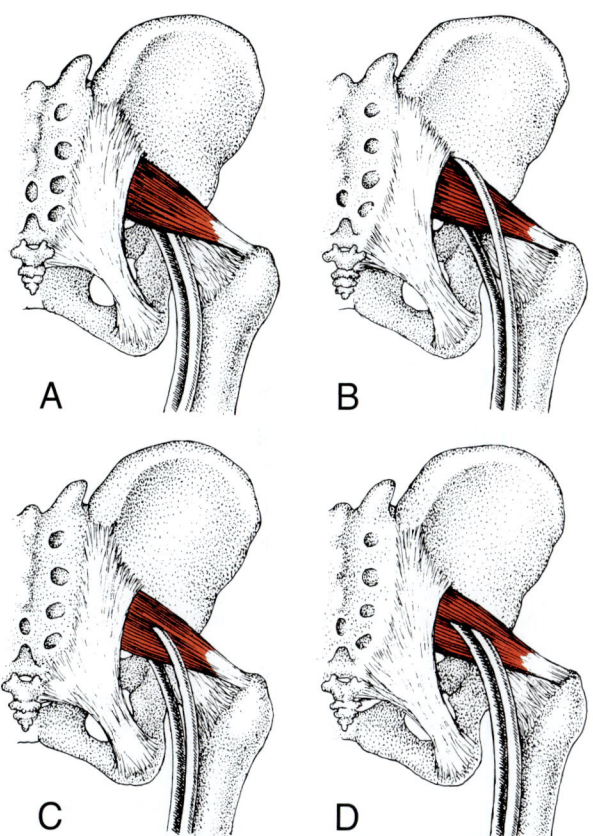

Figure 57-4. Four routes by which portions of the sciatic nerve may exit the pelvis: A, The usual route, in which all fibers of the nerve pass anterior to the piriformis muscle between the muscle (red) and the rim of the greater sciatic foramen, seen in about 85% of cadavers; B, The peroneal portion of the nerve passes through the piriformis muscle and the tibial portion travels anterior to the muscle, as seen in more than 10% of cadavers; C, The peroneal portion of the sciatic nerve loops above and then posterior to the muscle and the tibial portion passes anterior to it; both portions lie between the muscle and the upper or lower rim of the greater sciatic foramen, as seen in 2% to 3% of cadavers; D, An undivided sciatic nerve penetrates the piriformis muscle in less than 1% of cadavers. (After Beaton LE, Anson BJ. The sciatic nerve and the piriformis muscle: their relationship a possible cause of coccygodynia. J Bone Joint Surg(Br). 1938;20:686-688, with permission.)

when the hip was in slight extension and during activities that required hip stabilization. The investigators conclude that the piriformis muscle has more of a hip stabilizer function than a primary mover function.[28]

Hodges et al[31] investigated fine-wire EMG with ultrasound guidance into the right obturator internus, quadratus femoris, piriformis, and gluteus maximus muscles of 10 human subjects during maximum isometric hip flexion, extension, external rotation, internal rotation, abduction, and adduction, with the hip in neutral and at 60° of flexion. They found that the obturator internus muscle was activated first during abduction and external rotation when compared with the other muscles, regardless of position. However, all four muscles were most active with extension and least active during hip flexion, adduction, and internal rotation. When comparing external rotation and abduction activation, they found that the obturator internus and quadratus femoris muscles were more active with external rotation than the piriformis muscle. The piriformis muscle was the most active muscle during abduction. The quadratus femoris muscle was the most active during extension. They also demonstrated that the amount of activation changed depending on if the hip was in neutral or flexed. When the hip was flexed to 60°, there was increased obturator internus and quadratus femoris muscle activation during external rotation but decreased activation of the piriformis muscle. The opposite happened during hip abduction.

String models have been a popular way to investigate the function of these muscles because EMG studies are difficult. Gudena et al[30] used 18 hips from 22 cadavers and found that the obturator externus muscle was an external rotator when the hip was flexed and a hip stabilizer in extension and internal rotation. Vaarbakken et al[32] looked at three cadavers and found the motion arm switched from external rotation to internal rotation at 95° of hip flexion for the obturator internus muscle and 65° hip flexion for the piriformis muscle. When looking at the function of the quadratus femoris and obturator externus muscles, Vaarbakken et al[33] found that the quadratus femoris muscle is primarily a hip extensor from a flexed position and the obturator externus muscle flexed and adducted an extended hip.

Three-dimensional computer models have also been used to help understand the function of the hip muscles. Delp et al[34] looked at the hip muscles' moment arms as the hip was flexed from 0° to 90°. They found that the obturator externus, quadratus femoris, and obturator internus muscles did not become internal rotators; however, the obturator internus muscle significantly reduced its external rotation moment arm in flexion. The piriformis muscle, however, did become an internal rotator based on their computer model.[34]

The obturator internus muscle also plays a role in pelvic floor function. This function is discussed in detail in Chapter 52. Strengthening the hip external rotators, and specifically targeting the obturator internus muscle, has been shown to increased pelvic floor muscle strength measured with peak vaginal squeeze

some varying results. Giphart et al[28] looked at the EMG activity of 10 volunteers performing 13 hip exercises (only 6 produced acceptable EMG signals). They found that the piriformis muscle was most active during static external rotation and abduction

| Table 57-1 | How Often the Peroneal and Tibial Portions of the Sciatic Nerve Go Around or Through the Piriformis Muscle (Percent of Limbs) |

Authors	Both[a] Below Muscle (%)	Peroneal[b] Through Tibial Below (%)	Peroneal[c] Above, Tibial Below (%)	Both[d] Through (%)	Both Above (%)	Peroneal Above, Tibial Through (%)	Number of limbs
Anderson[36]	87.3	12.2	0.5	0	0	0	640
Beaton and Anson[37]	90	7.1	2.1	0.8	0	0	240
Beaton and Anson[38]	89.3	9.8	0.7	0.2	0	0	2250
Lee and Tsai[39]	70.2	19.6	1.5	1.8	3	1.2	168
Pećina[40]	78.5	20.7	0.8	0	0	0	130

[a] Illustrated in Figure 57-4A.
[b] Illustrated in Figure 57-4B.
[c] Illustrated in Figure 57-4C.
[d] Illustrated in Figure 57-4D.

> **Box 57-1** Functional unit of the piriformis and external rotator muscles
>
> | Action | Synergists | Antagonists |
> |---|---|---|
> | Hip external rotation | Gluteus maximus
Long head of biceps femoris
Sartorius | Semitendinosus
Semimembranosus
Tensor fasciae latae
Anterior fibers of gluteus medius and minimus
Psoas major
Gracilis (with knee flexion) |

pressure[41] and produces a greater decrease in stress urinary incontinence[42] compared with the control group. However, no studies have looked at how much the pelvic floor is active during hip external rotation exercises and therefore a question arises whether the external rotation exercises were effective or whether the pelvic floor was actually trained more because it was active during the additional exercises.[41] Hip abduction strength has been shown to have no correlation in women with or without stress urinary incontinence.[43] However, the obturator internus muscle is more of an external rotator and stabilizer than a hip abductor, which may be why no correlation was found.

2.3. Functional Unit

The functional unit to which a muscle belongs includes the muscles that reinforce and counter its actions as well as the joints that the muscle crosses. The interdependence of these structures is functionally reflected in the organization and neural connections of the sensory motor cortex. The functional unit is emphasized because the presence of a TrP in one muscle of the unit increases the likelihood that the other muscles of the unit will also develop TrPs. When inactivating TrPs in a muscle, one must be concerned about TrPs that may develop in muscles that are functionally interdependent. Box 57-1 grossly represents the functional unit of the piriformis and external rotator muscles.[44]

The piriformis muscle and the other five short external rotator muscles, together with the gluteus maximus muscle, are the prime external rotators of the thigh.[2,13,29,45] The short external rotator muscles also aid in stabilization of the hip joint.

3. CLINICAL PRESENTATION

3.1. Referred Pain Pattern

Piriformis TrPs frequently contribute significantly to complex myofascial pain syndromes of the pelvis and hip regions. The myofascial pain syndrome of the piriformis muscle is well recognized[46-51] and can sometimes overlap with signs and symptoms associated with piriformis pain syndrome. Trigger points in the piriformis muscle refer pain primarily to the sacroiliac region, to the buttock generally, and over the hip joint posteriorly. The referred pain and symptoms can also extend over the proximal two-thirds of the posterior thigh (Figure 57-5). Additional pain referred from TrPs in the adjacent members of this external rotator group may be difficult to distinguish from pain originating in the piriformis TrPs.

Trigger points in the obturator internus refer to the coccyx region and the posterior middle thigh (see Figure 52-3). A case study in a person with a strain to the obturator internus muscle showed that this muscle can produce pain in the groin.[52] George et al[53] found that dry needling the gluteal and pelvic floor muscles with focus on the obturator internus muscle reduced pelvic pain. Dalmau-Carolà[54] found that TrP injections to the piriformis muscle reduced trochanteric gluteal pain by 50%, adding that injection of the obturator internus muscle abolished the rest of

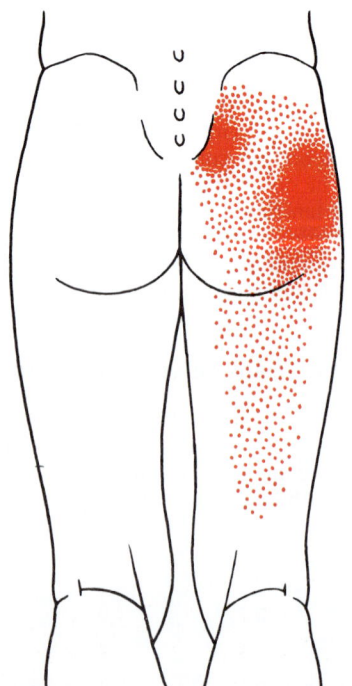
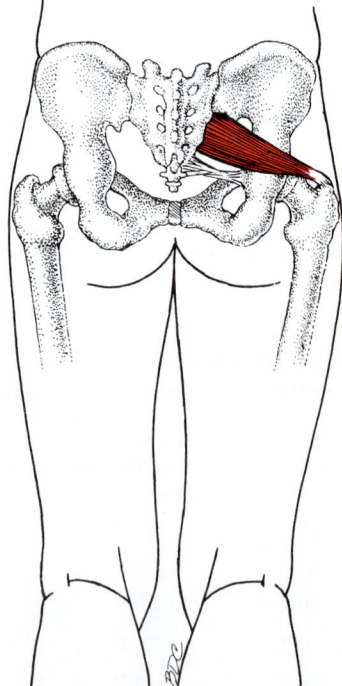

Figure 57-5. Composite pattern of pain referred from TrPs in the right piriformis muscle medial to sacrum and lateral buttock (darker red) and proximal one-third of the posterior thigh (stippled).

the pain, and additionally, the reported cold feeling the patient had in the ipsilateral foot was also abolished. Clinically, TrPs in both the obturator internus and piriformis muscles have been seen to refer into the dorsum of the foot with and without pain down the back of the thigh and into the calf. These symptoms were only produced by intravaginal palpation.

The referral pattern of TrPs in the quadratus femoris muscle was not described by Travell and Simons[44]; however, case studies[55-57] have shown that tears and strains to the quadratus femoris muscle can refer to the gluteal region, groin, posterior thigh, or hip with the posterior thigh being the most common. There has also been one case study that showed that a strain to both the obturator internus and externus muscles can produce sharp pain deep in the buttocks and a constant ache radiating into the hip; however, it is not clear which muscles were referring pain to which areas.[58]

3.2. Symptoms

Patients with TrPs and injuries in the deep hip external rotators will often report pain in the gluteal region[17,52,56] but may also describe pain in the low back, groin,[17,52,56] perineum, hip,[56,58] and posterior thigh.[17,52,55,56] Patients may report sharp pain on occasion, but often they describe their symptoms as an ache.[58] Because of the area and behavior of their pain, patients may think they have injured a hamstring or adductor muscle, or that they have a groin strain or sciatica.

Patients may also report a loss in their hip range of motion or flexibility[55,58] into internal rotation and adduction. Often, they would have identified tenderness in the area of the ischial tuberosity, and the symptoms are aggravated in the seated position.[55,58] A recent review has reported that the four most common symptoms of piriformis muscle syndrome are buttock pain, pain aggravated on sitting, external tenderness near the greater sciatic notch, pain on any maneuver that increases piriformis muscle tension, and limitation of straight leg raising.[59]

3.3. Patient Examination

After a thorough subjective examination, and establishing the event(s) associated with the onset of reported symptoms, the clinician should make a detailed drawing representing the pain pattern that the patient has described. This depiction will assist in planning the physical examination and can be useful in monitoring the progression of the patient as symptoms improve or change. Prior to beginning a physical examination, the clinician should do a thorough medical screening, and any concerns regarding the involvement of the gastrointestinal or urogenital systems as a source of symptoms should result in an immediate referral to a physician. All potential perpetuating factors should be noted and mechanical factors considered.

Because of the close association these external hip rotator muscles have with the nerves in the sciatic foramen, a thorough and careful neurologic examination of the lower extremity neural tissue is indicated. The clinician should perform a screening examination of the lumbosacral spine, the knee, foot, and ankle, as well as an assessment of the patient's posture and gait. Several neurodynamic tests can be used for assessing mechanical nerve sensitivity. Specifically, the slump test has been found to be sensitive for diagnosis of neuropathic pain in the lower extremity.[60] A careful assessment should be made to rule out referral into the buttock from other tissues, including muscles and joints that can refer to the same region.

In standing, the clinician should observe the pelvis for symmetry in the frontal and sagittal planes. Functional activities such as sit to stand, single-leg stance, and double- and single-leg squat (see Figure 55-3A) should be examined. The clinician should take note of any frontal plane deviations in the pelvis, hip and/or knee, and any excessive transverse plane motion at the ankle and foot (see Figure 55-3B). Deviations in the frontal plane at the knee and transverse plane at the foot and ankle may indicate gluteal and external hip rotator muscle weakness because the activation of the piriformis and obturator internus muscles as hip abductors increases as hip flexion increases.[31]

During examination of the patient's gait, the clinician should note any deviations such as a Trendelenburg sign at mid-stance (see Figure 55-4A and B). This is a sign of weakness in the hip abductor muscles. The patient may also have pain with unilateral stance during gait and with static standing on one leg because of the increased use of the external hip rotator muscles for static stability.

In sitting, the patient may sit with external rotation or abduction of the hip because of shortening of the hip external rotator muscles and frequently shift in the seat to take pressure off the piriformis and/or obturator internus muscles.

Because of the varying muscle activation patterns of the external hip rotators, a thorough examination of hip muscle activation patterns and strength should be carried out. All six of the deep hip rotators are tested as one for strength in hip external rotation. The obturator internus and piriformis muscles differ in activation of external rotation and abduction depending on the position of the hip in flexion or extension. Increased pain or weakness during hip external rotation while the hip is flexed would be indicative of obturator internus TrPs or dysfunction because it is most active when the hip is in flexion. The piriformis muscle is a secondary hip abductor and increases activation significantly with the hip in 90° of flexion. The Pace Abduction Test is effective in testing hip abduction strength and activation when the hip is flexed.[51,61,62] While the patient is in the seated position with the hips flexed to 90°, the clinician places the hands on the lateral aspects of the knees and asks the patient to push the hands apart. Pain and/or weakness will be observed on the affected side if the test is positive.[48] The muscle activation patterns of hip extension and hip abduction should also be examined to identify inhibition or weakness of the gluteal muscles.

Hip abduction and external rotation strength testing should be carried out bilaterally as both sides are responsible for lumbopelvic stability at different times during the gait cycle. If one side is weaker than the other, excessive frontal plane motion results, which can cause abnormal loading forces in the lumbar spine and hip musculature.

Muscle length of the deep hip rotators can be tested with the patient in supine. Pain and limitation of passive internal rotation of the affected thigh with the hip in neutral and the patient in the supine position was first described by Freiberg. This test was illustrated by TePoorten, and is frequently referred to[35,48,51,63-65] as Freiberg's sign. The movement of the test increases the tension on an already tight piriformis muscle. More recently, the flexion adduction internal rotation (FAIR) test has been identified as one of the special tests to confirm a diagnosis of piriformis muscle syndrome. None of the investigators mention or examine the piriformis muscle for the presence of TrPs; however, all patients responded favorably to anesthetic injection of the piriformis muscle,[66,67] leading us to believe that the investigators were treating TrPs in the piriformis muscle.

Fishman et al[66] investigated the diagnostic utility of the FAIR to identify an operational definition of piriformis muscle syndrome and found it to have a sensitivity of 0.81 and a specificity of 0.83. They concluded that piriformis muscle syndrome is accurately identified by the FAIR test and effectively treated with injection coupled with physical therapy.

Chen and Nizar[67] investigated the prevalence of piriformis muscle syndrome in patients with chronic low back pain (LBP) utilizing a combination of the FAIR test with the Laseque sign (tenderness in the gluteal region near the piriformis muscle) to diagnose piriformis syndrome. They found that 17% of patients presenting with chronic LBP had a positive combined FAIR and Laseque sign, indicating the presence of piriformis muscle syndrome. These individuals received a piriformis muscle injection with an anesthetic under fluoroscopic guidance into the most tender point in the muscle.[67] The investigators did not attempt to identify the presence of TrPs in the piriformis muscle, but they did identify the most tender region of the piriformis muscle (which could have, in the authors' opinion, been a TrP) to determine placement of the injection, with 100% of patients having 50% reduction of their symptoms immediately post injection.[67]

3.4. Trigger Point Examination

To locate the hip external rotator muscles in patients, it is helpful to note that the piriformis and the upper three GOGO muscles form a fanlike arrangement spreading out from the upper end of the greater trochanter. Manual examination of this group of external rotator muscles for TrPs is complicated by the fact that all of them lie deep to the gluteus maximus muscle, as seen in Figure 57-3. The piriformis muscle can be examined through a relaxed gluteus maximus muscle for most of its length. Its medial end is accessible to nearly direct palpation by rectal or vaginal examination. The femoral (lateral) ends of the gemelli and obturator internus muscles are not individually distinguishable by external palpation, but much of the intrapelvic obturator internus and piriformis muscles is directly palpable from inside the pelvis (Figure 57-2). Tenderness in the femoral end of the quadratus femoris muscle may be palpable through the gluteus maximus muscle. Using this approach, tenderness is less likely to be palpable in the underlying obturator externus muscle. Obturator externus muscle tenderness is best located by palpating between and deep to the pectineus and adductor brevis muscles in the groin. Though this muscle cannot be readily palpated, tenderness in the pectineus muscle may be due to TrPs in the pectineus or underlying obturator externus muscles. Diagnosis of TrPs may be determined by the use of a filiform or injection needle when a local twitch response or pain referral is elicited.

Piriformis

The location of the piriformis muscle is determined for external examination by drawing a line from the uppermost border of the greater trochanter through the sacroiliac (cephalad) end of the greater sciatic foramen (Figure 57-6). When the gluteus maximus muscle is relaxed, the greater trochanter may be located by circular deep palpation with the flat of the hand over the hip laterally, revealing the underlying bony prominence. The crescent-shaped medial boundary of the sciatic foramen along the lateral border of the sacrum (dotted line, Figure 57-6) is palpable inferior to the posterior inferior iliac spine through the relaxed gluteus maximus muscle.

Cross-fiber flat palpation is used to locate TrPs in the piriformis muscle (Figure 57-7A). The outline of a tense piriformis muscle is sometimes palpable along the piriformis line, and the muscle may show marked tenderness throughout its length.[64,68] Figure 57-3 illustrates how closely the lower borders of the gluteus medius and gluteus minimus muscles approximate the upper border of the piriformis muscle, permitting palpation of the piriformis muscle without interference from them. If one palpates too far cephalad, the gluteus medius and minimus muscles, and not the piriformis muscle, will be palpated deep to the gluteus maximus muscle.

Kipervas et al[69] established the location for palpating the piriformis muscle through the skin somewhat differently. They selected the junction of the middle and lower thirds of a line drawn between the anterior superior iliac spine and the ischiococcygeus muscle.

If any doubt exists as to the cause of tenderness over the greater sciatic foramen, the medial end of the piriformis muscle should be palpated within the pelvis by the rectal or vaginal route.[47,48,61,65,69] This examination is performed most effectively with the clinician's longest finger and may not be possible for a clinician with smaller than average hands (Figure 57-2). The technique is also illustrated by Thiele.[65] The patient is placed side-lying with the affected side uppermost and with that knee and hip flexed. The transversely oriented sacrospinous ligament is felt as a firm band stretching between the sacrum and the ischial spine and is normally covered by the fibers of the coccygeus muscle[51] that can also have TrPs. The piriformis muscle lies just cephalad to this ligament and, if involved, is tender and feels tense.[48,50,65,69,70]

Clinicians can often examine the muscle bimanually, with one hand pressing externally on the buttock while the other hand palpates internally. The greater sciatic foramen presents an unmistakable soft spot through which palpation pressure from one finger outside the pelvis can be transmitted to another finger inside the pelvis. To confirm identification of the piriformis muscle, the clinician palpates for contractile tension in the muscle while having the patient attempt to abduct the thigh by trying to lift the uppermost knee.

The sacral nerve roots lie between the clinician finger and the piriformis muscle (Figure 57-2). If the nerve roots are irritated by entrapment at the greater sciatic foramen, they may also be tender and are likely to project pain in a sciatic distribution.

Gemelli and Obturator Internus

Figure 57-3 shows that, in the anatomic position, all of the piriformis muscle lies above the level of its attachment to the uppermost part of the greater trochanter. Cross-fiber flat palpation at the level of, and medial to, the upper one-third of the greater trochanter (Figure 57-7B) is used to identify TrPs in the gemelli and obturator internus muscles. Deep tenderness (deep to the gluteus maximus muscle) inferior to the piriformis muscle is most likely tenderness of one of the gemelli or of the obturator internus muscles. If TrPs in the obturator internus muscle are responsible for this tenderness, it can be palpated directly by rectal or vaginal examination, as described in Chapter 52. The obturator internus muscle can also be palpated along the medial border of the obturator foramen utilizing cross-fiber flat palpation (Figure 57-8).

Figure 57-3 reminds clinicians that the sciatic nerve is also compressed as pressure is applied medial to a point midway between the greater trochanter and the ischial tuberosity. The nerve usually emerges between the piriformis and superior

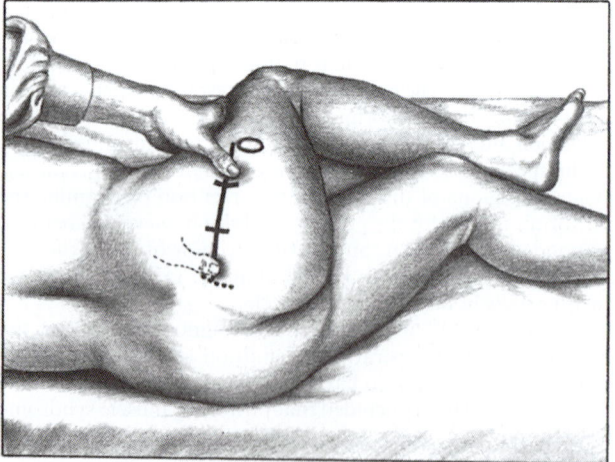

Figure 57-6. External cross-fiber flat palpation to identify TrPs in the right piriformis muscle through a relaxed gluteus maximus muscle. The solid line (piriformis line) overlies the superior border of the piriformis muscle and extends from immediately above the greater trochanter to the cephalic border of the greater sciatic foramen at the sacrum. The line is divided into equal thirds. The dotted line marks the palpable edge along the lateral border of the sacrum, which corresponds closely to the medial margin of the greater sciatic foramen.

Chapter 57: Piriformis, Obturator Internus, Gemelli, Obturator Externus, and Quadratus Femoris Muscles

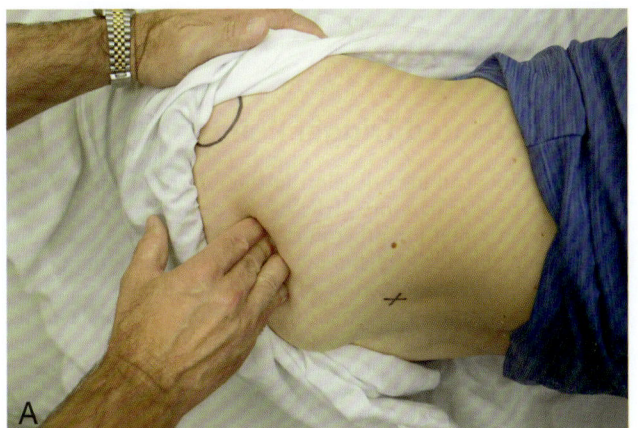
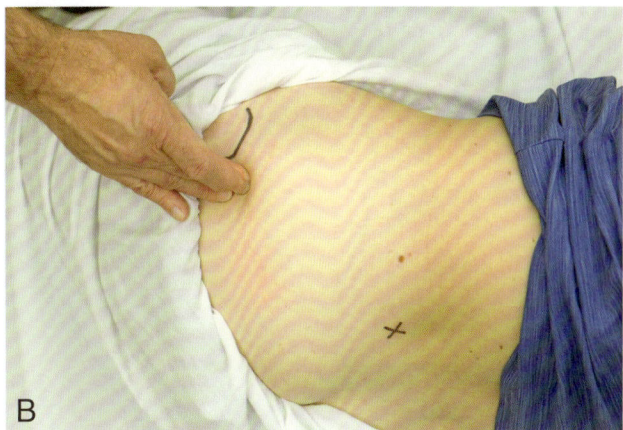
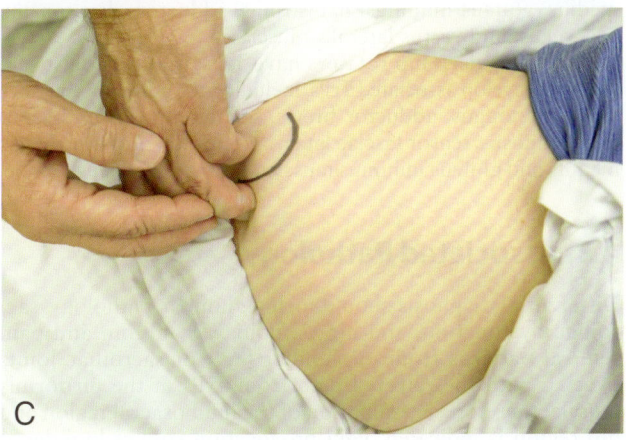

Figure 57-7. Palpation for TrPs in the external rotator muscles of the hip. The X represents the posterior superior iliac spine (PSIS) and the half moon represents the greater trochanter of the femur. A, Cross-fiber flat palpation for TrPs in the piriformis muscle. B, Cross-fiber flat palpation for TrPs in the gemelli and obturator internus muscles along the upper one-third of the greater trochanter. C, Cross-fiber flat palpation of the quadratus femoris and obturator externus muscles along the lower two-thirds of the greater trochanter.

gemellus muscles and continues its course superficial to the superior gemellus, obturator internus, inferior gemellus, obturator externus, and quadratus femoris muscles.

Quadratus Femoris and Obturator Externus

Cross-fiber flat palpation is utilized at the lower two-thirds of the greater trochanter to locate TrPs in these muscles. Deep tenderness probably arises in the quadratus femoris muscle or, possibly, in the even deeper obturator externus muscle (Figure 57-7C). Trigger points in the quadratus femoris muscle can also be palpated along the lateral side of the ischial tuberosity.

Tenderness due to TrPs in the obturator externus muscle may also be detected in the groin. One must first palpate the pectineus and adductor brevis muscles to confirm that they do not have TrPs that would obscure a deeper source of tenderness. Deep pressure is then applied between the pectineus and adductor brevis muscles against the outer surface of the obturator membrane that is covered by the obturator externus muscle (Figure 57-9). This muscle cannot be directly palpated and therefore a monofilament needle or injection needle may be necessary to elicit a local twitch response or reproduce the pain or pain referral pattern of these muscles.

4. DIFFERENTIAL DIAGNOSIS

4.1. Activation and Perpetuation of Trigger Points

A posture or activity that activates a TrP, if not corrected, can also perpetuate it. In any part of the gluteus maximus muscle, TrPs may be activated by unaccustomed eccentric loading, eccentric exercise in an unconditioned muscle, or maximal or submaximal concentric loading.[71] Trigger points may also be activated or aggravated when the muscle is placed

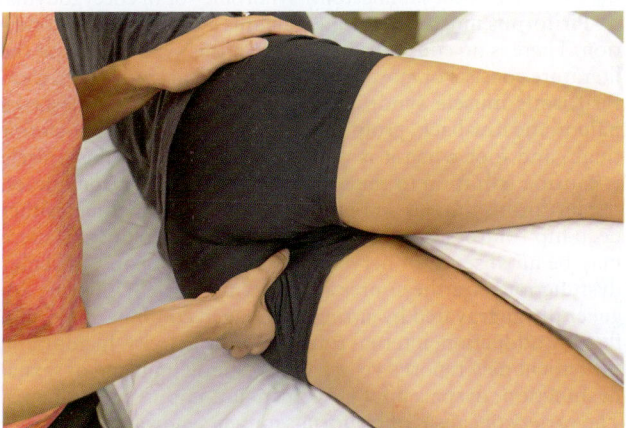

Figure 57-8. Cross-fiber flat palpation of the obturator internus muscle at the medial aspect of the right ischial tuberosity and the obturator foramen muscle.

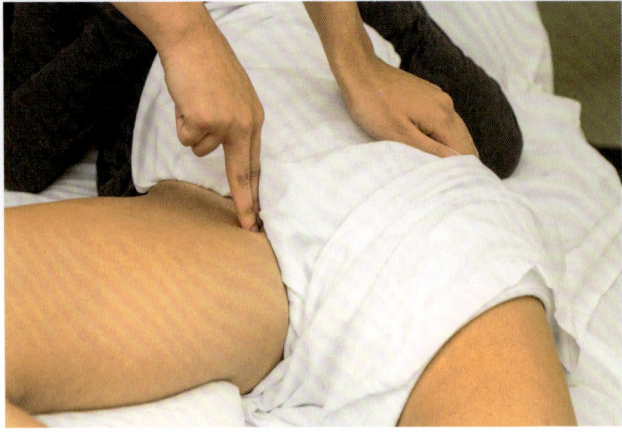

Figure 57-9. Cross-fiber flat palpation of obturator externus muscle through the pectineus and adductor brevis muscles. This muscle can't be directly palpated.

in a shortened and/or lengthened position for an extended period of time.

The deep hip rotators can become overloaded when they undergo a strong lengthening contraction to restrain vigorous and/or rapid internal rotation of the weight-bearing limb such as with running and walking and especially if the gluteal muscles are weak or inhibited. The gluteus maximus muscle is the strongest of the external rotators of the hip; therefore, if it is weak or inhibited, it will place an overload on the smaller hip external rotator muscles.

Overload can also occur in the piriformis muscle when one catches oneself from falling when the foot slips,[48] with lifting or lowering heavy objects with the legs in a wide base of support,[48] twisting sideways while bending and lifting an object,[72] or forceful rotation while standing on one leg.[48,68] These are common movements in many athletic and sporting activities and can also occur with yard and housework. Activities that would potentially perpetuate TrPs may include uphill walking or running, climbing a ladder, or returning from a squatting position especially if the lower extremities are placed in a wide base of support and the gluteus maximus muscle is weak and or inhibited.

Sitting on a wallet placed in a back pocket that extends under the buttock can perpetuate and aggravate TrPs in the hip external rotators, especially the piriformis muscle, by concentrating pressure on them. The resultant low back and buttock pain is likely to be erroneously attributed to nerve pressure and has been called "back pocket sciatica."[73] However, pain referral from TrPs in the piriformis muscle or other external rotator muscles alone would not have a full sciatic nerve distribution.

Flexing the thighs at the hips with the knees spread apart for sitting, as in driving a car with the foot on the accelerator for long periods or sitting on one foot[68] are activities that can perpetuate piriformis TrPs. These positions, which combine a shortened position of the piriformis muscle, with the sciatic nerve held in a lengthened or stretched position, along with a lack of mobility, create a vulnerability for piriformis muscle syndrome. Obstetric or urologic procedures, as well as coitus, also put the piriformis muscle in a shortened position that has been associated with onset of the piriformis muscle syndrome.[68,72]

Chronic infections are known to perpetuate TrPs. Specifically, chronic pelvic inflammatory disease[74] and infectious sacroiliitis[72] have been identified in piriformis muscle syndrome. Other conditions that may perpetuate piriformis TrPs include arthritis of the hip joint, sciatica, chronic LBP, and conditions that lead to total hip arthroplasty.[48]

4.2. Associated Trigger Points

Trigger points can also develop in the referred pain areas of primary TrPs.[75] Therefore, TrPs in the deep hip rotators can be due to active TrPs in other muscles, including the quadratus lumborum, multifidi, longissimus thoracis, iliocostalis lumborum coccygeus, levator ani, tensor fasciae latae, gluteus maximus, gluteus medius, gluteus minimus, hamstrings, vastus lateralis, and soleus muscles. In addition, active TrPs in the pectineus, external and internal oblique, and psoas major muscles can produce TrPs in the obturator externus muscle. Active TrPs in the deep hip external rotators can also contribute to associated TrPs in other muscles including the gluteus maximus, gluteus medius, gluteus minimus, hamstrings, adductors, levator ani, coccygeus, and vastus lateralis muscles.

When the deep hip rotators have TrPs, the antagonists are likely to develop associated TrPs, including the adductor magnus, adductor longus, adductor brevis, semitendinosus and semimembranosus, tensor fasciae latae, anterior fibers of the gluteus medius and gluteus minimus muscles, and the pectineus muscle.

4.3. Associated Pathology

Differential diagnosis should include lumbar pathology, sacroiliac dysfunction, and hip pathology. Symptom and pain referral patterns from the lumbar facet or sacroiliac joints overlap with the referred pain from TrPs in the piriformis muscle; therefore, examination of the lumbosacral region and hip region is indicated. Pain provocation studies looking at the referral zones for the sacroiliac joint have demonstrated referral frequently into the low back, buttock, and occasionally into the posterior or lateral thigh.[76,77] Pain provocation studies mapping the referral zones for the hip joint have also demonstrated referral into the buttock, thigh, or groin in the majority of subjects.[78]

Some medical conditions give rise to symptoms that can appear similar to those produced by TrPs in the piriformis, GOGOs, and quadratus femoris muscles or may be present concurrently. Piriformis myofascial pain syndrome is recognized by the characteristic pain pattern projected by its TrPs, by pain and weakness on resisted abduction of the thigh with the hip flexed 90°, by eliciting tenderness of the piriformis muscle using external palpation, and by palpating taut bands and tenderness via intrapelvic examination. Piriformis muscle syndrome may be the cause of a "post-laminectomy syndrome" or of coccygodynia.

Piriformis muscle syndrome remains a controversial condition. There is no constant definition for this syndrome, and the literature consists of mostly case studies and narrative reviews.[79] Piriformis muscle syndrome is commonly used to describe pain in the low back, groin, perineum, buttocks, hip, posterior thigh, and foot when it is thought that the piriformis muscle is causing irritation to the sciatic nerve. However, sometimes, the piriformis muscle is not involved at all.[79] Sometimes, other deep hip rotators cause the nerve irritation or pain, and there may be an absence of nerve irritation. Occasionally, articular dysfunctions are the source of the symptoms. Symptoms are generally aggravated by sitting, prolonged combination of hip flexion, adduction, internal rotation, or by activity. In addition, the patient may report swelling in the painful limb and of sexual dysfunction, dyspareunia in women and impotence in men.[80] The variety of causes of piriformis muscle syndrome are further discussed in Chapter 62.

Nerve entrapment is suggested by paresthesias and dysesthesias in the distribution of nerves passing through the greater sciatic foramen and by sensory disturbance extending well beyond midthigh. Malignant neoplasm, neurogenic tumors, and local infection[81-85] can compress the sciatic nerve at the greater sciatic foramen. These conditions have been identified by computed tomography scanning.[86]

Another source of pain referred to the buttock and lateral thigh is an episacroiliac lipoma.[87] These herniated nodules of fat are exquisitely tender to palpation and are responsive to injection of a local anesthetic. Sometimes they require surgical removal under local anesthesia for lasting relief.

Symptoms of piriformis TrPs or syndrome are easily confused with radicular pain from compression of the lower lumbar and sacral nerve roots. Absence or marked weakness of the Achilles tendon reflex[88] and motor denervation shown by EMG, suggest a radiculopathy. Conversely, slowing of conduction velocity in the sciatic nerve through the pelvis suggests piriformis muscle entrapment. Palpation for piriformis muscle tenderness is essential to confirm or rule out entrapment and should be performed in all cases of "sciatica." Incidental radiographic reports of "narrowing of the disc space" or "degenerative changes with spur formation" or "disc herniation" are not by themselves sufficient to account for the pain characteristic of piriformis muscle syndrome or LBP. Degenerative changes occur in the spine with aging and do not correlate well with clinical symptoms.[89-91]

Symptoms of a facet syndrome with LBP and sciatica may be difficult to distinguish from a myofascial piriformis muscle syndrome until the muscle is examined.[61] A facet block may relieve the back pain of a facet syndrome, but only successful inactivation of piriformis TrPs relieves the antalgic gait pattern and the buttock and posterior thigh pain of myofascial and related entrapment origin.[48] Huang et al[92] looked at 52 patients with chronic myofascial pain in the piriformis muscle who received a facet injection at L5/S1. Eighty-eight percent of the patients had a reduction in their pain or complete relief of symptoms. At the 6-month follow-up, 35 patients had lasting results.

Piriformis muscle syndrome may develop secondary to sacroiliitis (sacroiliac arthritis). The diagnosis of sacroiliitis is confirmed by radiography. Sacroiliitis affects one or both SI joints and may cause pain and tenderness in the low back, buttock, and lateral thigh that may also extend as far as the ankle on one or both sides. Patients with sacroiliitis are usually young people who are HLA-B27 positive and may have ankylosing spondylitis (see Chapter 53),[93] usually bilaterally symmetric sacroiliitis,[94] psoriatic arthritis or Reiter disease (usually asymmetric sacroiliitis),[94] or arthritis related to inflammatory bowel disease.[94,95]

A venous thrombosis can also present as a myofascial syndrome of the piriformis or gluteus medius muscles. At least one case has been presented in the literature of an 18-year-old woman with pain in the left lumbosacral region and referral into the posterior thigh. The pain was of insidious onset in the buttock and thigh without a report of paresthesias or dysesthesias. There was tenderness with palpation in the left piriformis and gluteus medius muscles. Two days following treatment, the patient developed severe abdominal pain with heaviness in the leg and swelling in the calf.[96] Venous thrombosis is more common in women of childbearing age, but after age 60, it is more common in men and yet most common over the age of 70 and slightly more common in the left leg than in the right.[97] Risk factors for a venous thrombosis include a trauma or surgery (the more major the trauma or surgery the greater the risk),[97,98] active cancer,[97] chemotherapy,[98] oral contraceptives,[97,98] marked immobility,[97,98] pregnancy,[98] central venous line,[98] obesity,[98] and varicose veins.[98] A venous thrombosis is diagnosed by a venous Doppler ultrasound. It is important to diagnose these quickly because proximal deep vein thrombosis is more likely to cause a pulmonary embolism than a distal vein thrombosis.[98]

In patients with chronic kidney disease who are undergoing dialysis, calcium phosphate can be deposited into the muscles and form calcification near the larger joints.[99] This condition is called tumoral calcinosis and is rare, but when it does occur around the hip joint, it can produce pain in the buttocks, pain in the lateral hip, and tenderness at the piriformis muscle and greater trochanter.[99] The calcium phosphate deposits can be seen on ultrasound, radiographs, and magnetic resonance imaging (MRI).[99]

Surgeries such as transvaginal tape or total hip arthroplasty can also have an effect on the hip external rotator muscles. TVT ABBREVO tape is used for urinary stress incontinence, and it is supposed to use less foreign material in hopes of reducing groin pain.[100] It is attached to the obturator membrane on both sides of the pelvis.[100] However, when investigating where the insertion points actually ended up on eight embalmed female cadavers who had received this procedure by very experienced surgeons, the tape attached only to the obturator membrane 50% of the time.[100] It attached to the obturator internus muscle one time, went through the obturator membrane and onto the obturator externus muscle five times, and through the obturator internus muscle, obturator membrane, and the obturator externus muscle onto the adductor muscles two times.[100] Total hip arthroplasty can also contact or change the course of the obturator externus muscle. In MRI of 40 patients with total hip replacement, 13 showed contact with the obturator externus muscle and 9 showed clear displacement of the muscle's course. However, these findings were not correlated to visual analog pain scores or patient satisfaction scores.[101]

Ischiofemoral impingement is a crowding of the quadratus femoris between the lesser trochanter and the ischial tuberosity or ischium-hamstring tendon.[102,103] It can cause damage to the quadratus femoris musle and mimic TrPs in the quadratus femoris muscle. Ischiofemoral impingement can be diagnosed with MRI.[102] There is also an association of femoroacetabular impingement and TrPs in the deep hip external rotators. When there is a dysfunction in the deep hip external rotators, the muscles lose the ability to dynamically stabilize the hip especially in a closed kinetic chain. This loss of stability can lead to maltracking of the hip joint and possible anterior impingement. If this maltracking persists, it can lead to increased friction on the labrum, which makes it more vulnerable to increased micro-trauma and subsequent tears.

5. CORRECTIVE ACTIONS

Patients with TrPs in the piriformis and deep external rotator muscles of the hip will have to modify their sitting and sleeping postures. While sitting, the knees should be kept in alignment with the hips and shoulders. Keeping the knees placed in or out for prolonged periods of time should be avoided. When sitting, patients should be encouraged to move as much as possible. Sitting in a rocking chair or using a foot rest helps encourage movement. A patient who tends to sit with the knees rotated outward (abducted) can occasionally pull the legs inward (adduct) by squeezing knees together and rotating the feet outward. When sleeping, pillows can be used as described in Figure 57-10 to help keep the hips and spine in a neutral position and reduce pressure on the lower hip.

Because the deep hip external rotator muscles are also hip stabilizers, activities, such as standing on one leg, that require hip stabilization may need to be avoided if the TrPs are too irritable. However, exercises to target these muscles and the gluteus maximus muscle should be started as soon as tolerable.

A TrP self-pressure release tool or tennis ball may be used for self-treatment of the piriformis and deep external rotator muscles of the hip (Figure 57-11). These techniques should be employed cautiously because of the muscles' proximity, and therefore the potential to cause irritation of the nerve tissue. This treatment can be helpful for lateral piriformis TrPs and for the other five short external rotator muscles. The tennis ball must be placed far enough laterally to avoid the sciatic nerve where pressure causes numbness and tingling below the knee. The patient should use the TrP self-pressure release tool or tennis ball to rub the area and provide friction instead of just sustained pressure.

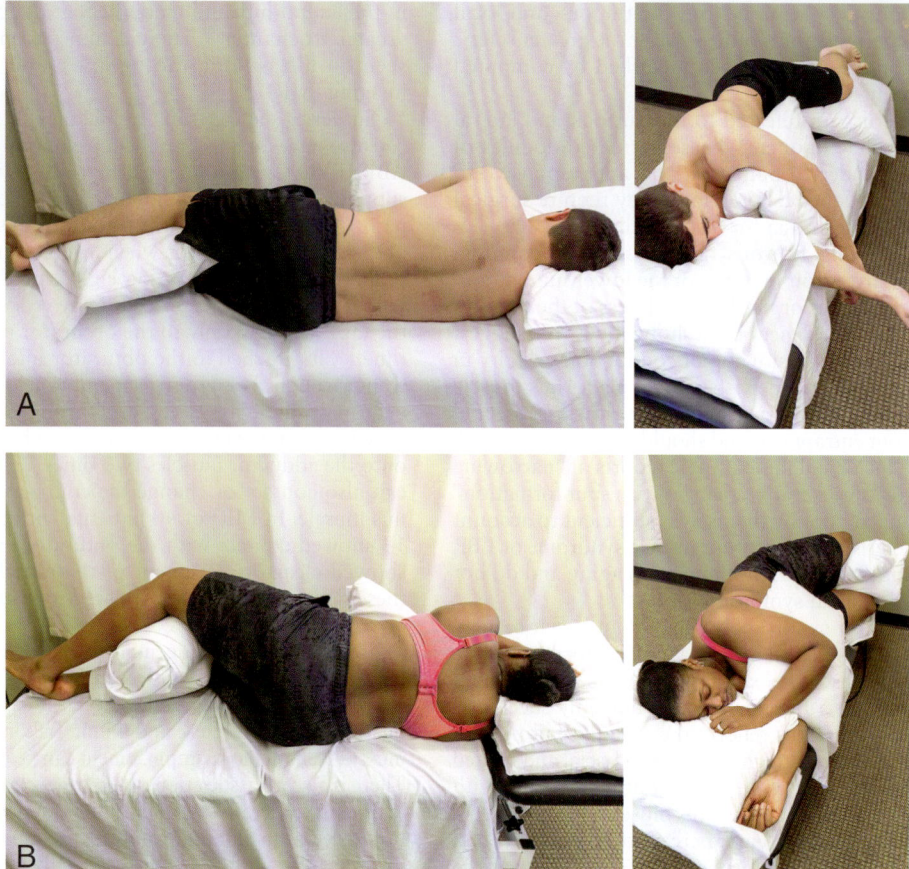

Figure 57-10. Proper positions to improve sleep when lying on the unaffected side. A, A pillow is placed between the knees and ankles in order to avoid adduction of the uppermost thigh at the hip. B, A small pillow or folded towel under the waist line can prevent side bending away from the hip on against the bed and reduce the pressure on the lower hip.

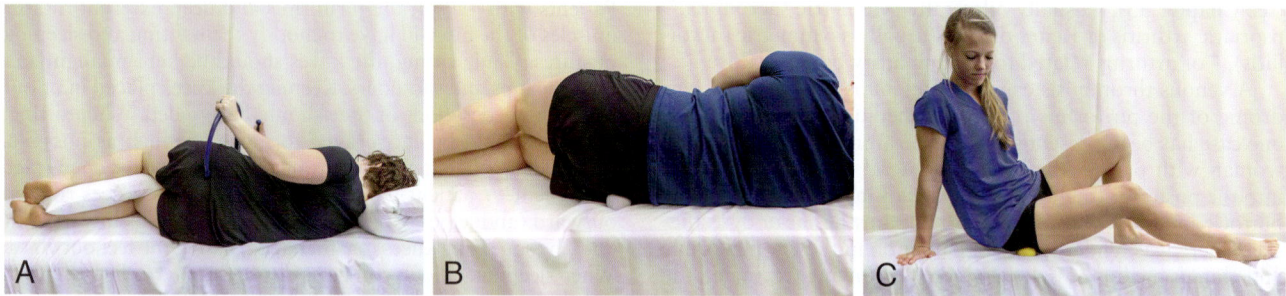

Figure 57-11. Piriformis muscle self-pressure release. A, Using a TrP release tool. B, Using a tennis ball. C, Self-pressure release of other deep external rotator muscles.

To perform the piriformis muscle self-stretch, the patient lies supine (Figure 57-12), crosses the leg of the involved side over the opposite thigh, and flexes the hip up to about 90°, resting the opposite hand on the knee of the uppermost affected limb. This hand is used to assist bringing the involved thigh across midline. The patient stabilizes the hip on the involved side by pressing down on the pelvis with the ipsilateral hand. Release of muscle tension is augmented by the patient "thinking" of gently lifting the weight of the affected leg (but not actually moving it) during slow inhalation and then, during slow exhalation, having the muscle relax and slowly allowing the piriformis muscle to stretch.

A more dynamic stretch, such as the seated hip internal rotation stretch, may be more appropriate if there is any nerve involvement because nerves do not respond well to sustained "stretching"[104] or sustained pressure.[105] The patient sits on a firm surface with an erect posture and places a small towel roll under the back of the thigh near the knee to place the hip at 90° or more of flexion (Figure 57-13A). Rotate the foot on the affected side outward so the femur internally rotates, hold for 3 to 5 seconds, then slowly lower the leg back to the starting position (Figure 57-13B). To keep the body better aligned, this motion can be performed with both legs at the same time (Figure 57-13C). Flexing the hip past 90° may also augment the stretch.[106]

Chapter 57: Piriformis, Obturator Internus, Gemelli, Obturator Externus, and Quadratus Femoris Muscles 601

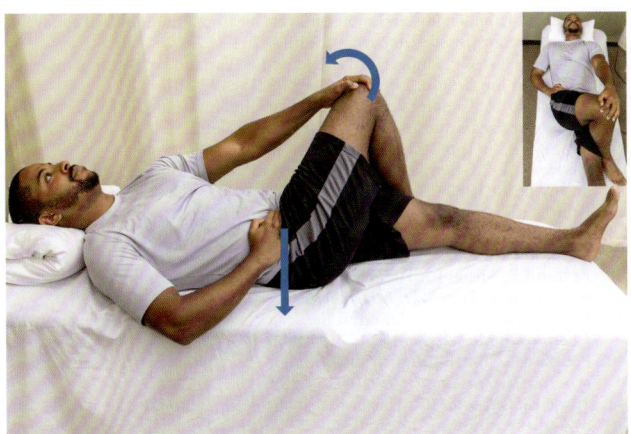

Figure 57-12. Self-stretch of the right piriformis muscle. The right thigh is flexed nearly 90° at the hip with the right foot on the treatment table. To adduct the thigh at the hip, pressure is exerted downward with both hands (large arrows), one on the thigh and the other on the pelvis, pulling against each other. To perform postisometric relaxation, the individual then attempts to abduct the thigh by pressing it *gently* against the resisting left hand for a few seconds (isometric contraction of abductors), then relaxes and gently moves the thigh into adduction, which gradually lengthens the piriformis muscle.

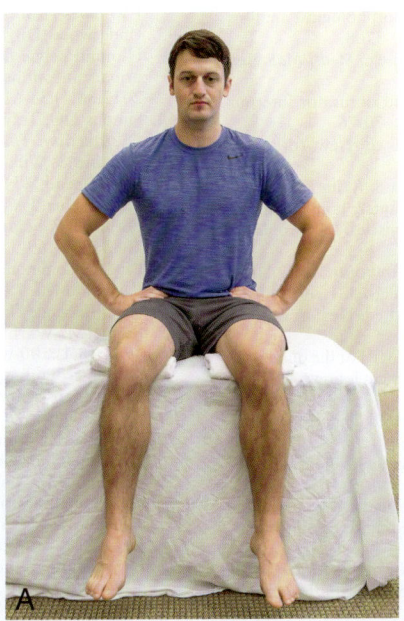

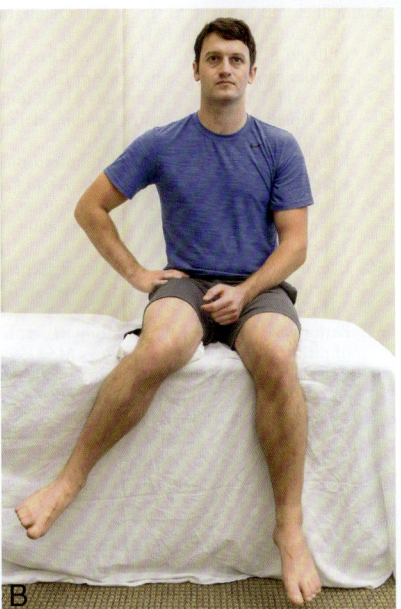 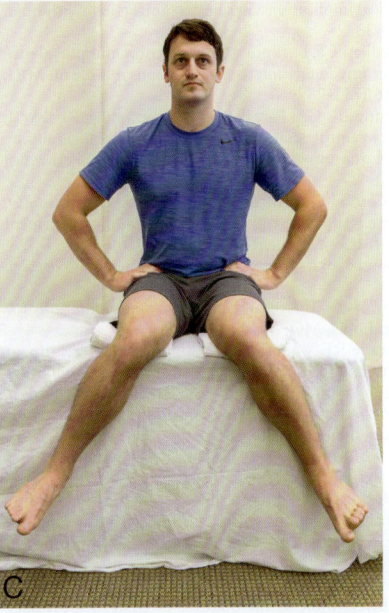

Figure 57-13. Reciprocal inhibition of external rotator muscles. A, Sit with knees aligned with the hips and shoulders. B, Rotate the foot outward on the affected side so the femurs internally rotate, hold and slowly lower leg to starting position. C, Rotate the feet outward so the femur internally rotates, hold and slowly lower legs to starting position.

References

1. Dye SF, van Dam BE, Westin GW. Eponyms and etymons in orthopaedics. *Contemp Orthop.* 1983;6:92-96.
2. Standring S. *Gray's Anatomy: The Anatomical Basis of Clinical Practice.* 41st ed. London, UK: Elsevier; 2015.
3. Freiberg AH, Vinke TH. Sciatica and the sacroiliac joint. *J Bone Joint Surg Am.* 1934;16:126-136.
4. Yoo S, Dedova I, Pather N. An appraisal of the short lateral rotators of the hip joint. *Clin Anat.* 2015;28(6):800-812.
5. Freiberg AH. Sciatic pain and its relief by operations on muscle and fascia. *Arch Surg.* 1937;34:337-350.
6. Ravindranath Y, Manjunath KY, Ravindranath R. Accessory origin of the piriformis muscle. *Singapore Med J.* 2008;49(8):e217-e218.
7. Cooper HJ, Walters BL, Rodriguez JA. Anatomy of the hip capsule and pericapsular structures: a cadaveric study. *Clin Anat.* 2015;28(5):665-671.
8. Michel F, Decavel P, Toussirot E, et al. The piriformis muscle syndrome: an exploration of anatomical context, pathophysiological hypotheses and diagnostic criteria. *Ann Phys Rehabil Med.* 2013;56(4):300-311.
9. Solomon LB, Lee YC, Callary SA, Beck M, Howie DW. Anatomy of piriformis, obturator internus and obturator externus: implications for the posterior surgical approach to the hip. *J Bone Joint Surg Br.* 2010;92(9):1317-1324.
10. Haladaj R, Pingot M, Polguj M, Wysiadecki G, Topol M. Anthropometric study of the piriformis muscle and sciatic nerve: a morphological analysis in a Polish population. *Med Sci Monit.* 2015;21:3760-3768.
11. Myint K. Nerve compression due to an abnormal muscle. *Med J Malaysia.* 1981;36:227-229.
12. Pine J, Binns M, Wright P, Soames R. Piriformis and obturator internus morphology: a cadaveric study. *Clin Anat.* 2011;24(1):70-76.
13. Hollinshead WH. *Anatomy for Surgeons.* Vol 3. 3rd ed. New York, NY: Harper & Row; 1982 (pp. 666-668, 702).
14. Tamaki T, Nimura A, Oinuma K, Shiratsuchi H, Iida S, Akita K. An anatomic study of the impressions on the greater trochanter: bony geometry indicates the alignment of the short external rotator muscles. *J Arthroplasty.* 2014;29(12):2473-2477.
15. Ferner H, Staubesand J. *Sobotta Atlas of Human Anatomy.* Vol 2. 10th ed. Baltimore, MD: Urban & Schwarzenberg; 1983 (Figs. 331, 403, 406).
16. Rohen JW, Yokochi C. *Color Atlas of Anatomy.* 2nd ed. New York, NY: Igaku-Shoin; 1988 (pp. 418, 419).
17. Kassarjian A, Tomas X, Cerezal L, Canga A, Llopis E. MRI of the quadratus femoris muscle: anatomic considerations and pathologic lesions. *AJR Am J Roentgenol.* 2011;197(1):170-174.
18. Clemente C. *Gray's Anatomy of the Human Body.* 30th ed. Philadelphia, PA: Lea & Febiger; 1985 (pp. 568-571).
19. Smoll NR. Variations of the piriformis and sciatic nerve with clinical consequence: a review. *Clin Anat.* 2010;23(1):8-17.
20. Butz JJ, Raman DV, Viswanath S. A unique case of bilateral sciatic nerve variation within the gluteal compartment and associated clinical ramifications. *Australas Med J.* 2015;8(1):24-27.
21. Patil J, Swamy RS, Rao MK, Kumar N, Somayaji SN. Unique formation of sciatic nerve below the piriformis muscle—a case report. *J Clin Diagn Res.* 2014;8(1):148-149.
22. Berihu BA, Debeb YG. Anatomical variation in bifurcation and trifurcations of sciatic nerve and its clinical implications: in selected university in Ethiopia. *BMC Res Notes.* 2015;8:633.
23. Varenika V, Lutz AM, Beaulieu CF, Bucknor MD. Detection and prevalence of variant sciatic nerve anatomy in relation to the piriformis muscle on MRI. *Skeletal Radiol.* 2017;46(6):751-757.
24. Natsis K, Totlis T, Konstantinidis GA, Paraskevas G, Piagkou M, Koebke J. Anatomical variations between the sciatic nerve and the piriformis muscle: a contribution to surgical anatomy in piriformis syndrome. *Surg Radiol Anat.* 2014;36(3):273-280.
25. Carro LP, Hernando MF, Cerezal L, Navarro IS, Fernandez AA, Castillo AO. Deep gluteal space problems: piriformis syndrome, ischiofemoral impingement and sciatic nerve release. *Muscles Ligaments Tendons J.* 2016;6(3):384-396.
26. Martin HD, Reddy M, Gomez-Hoyos J. Deep gluteal syndrome. *J Hip Preserv Surg.* 2015;2(2):99-107.
27. Neumann DA. *Kinesiology of the Musculoskeletal System: Foundations for Rehabilitation.* 2nd ed. St. Louis, MO: Mosby; 2010.
28. Giphart JE, Stull JD, Laprade RF, Wahoff MS, Philippon MJ. Recruitment and activity of the pectineus and piriformis muscles during hip rehabilitation exercises: an electromyography study. *Am J Sports Med.* 2012;40(7):1654-1663.
29. Rasch PJ, Burke RK. *Kinesiology and Applied Anatomy: The Science of Human Movement.* 6th ed. Philadelphia, PA: Lea & Febiger; 1978 (p. 278).
30. Gudena R, Alzahrani A, Railton P, Powell J, Ganz R. The anatomy and function of the obturator externus. *Hip Int.* 2015;25(5):424-427.
31. Hodges PW, McLean L, Hodder J. Insight into the function of the obturator internus muscle in humans: observations with development and validation of an electromyography recording technique. *J Electromyogr Kinesiol.* 2014;24(4):489-496.
32. Vaarbakken K, Steen H, Samuelsen G, et al. Lengths of the external hip rotators in mobilized cadavers indicate the quadriceps coxa as a primary abductor and extensor of the flexed hip. *Clin Biomech (Bristol, Avon).* 2014;29(7):794-802.
33. Vaarbakken K, Steen H, Samuelsen G, Dahl HA, Leergaard TB, Stuge B. Primary functions of the quadratus femoris and obturator externus muscles indicated from lengths and moment arms measured in mobilized cadavers. *Clin Biomech (Bristol, Avon).* 2015;30(3):231-237.
34. Delp SL, Hess WE, Hungerford DS, Jones LC. Variation of rotation moment arms with hip flexion. *J Biomech.* 1999;32(5):493-501.
35. Porterfield JA. Chapter 23, The sacroiliac joint. In: Gould III JA, Davies GJ, eds. *Orthopaedic and Sports Physical Therapy.* Vol II. St. Louis, MO: Mosby; 1985:550-580 (pp. 553, 565-566).
36. Anderson FE. *Grants Atlas of Anatomy.* 8th ed. Baltimore, MD: Williams and Wilkins; 1983:26.
37. Beaton LE, Anson BJ. The sciatic nerve and the piriformis muscle: their relationship a possible cause of coccygodynia. *J Bone Joint Surg(Br).* 1938;20:686-688.
38. Beaton LE, Anson BJ. The relation of the sciatic nerve and its subdivisions to the piriformis muscle. *Anat Rec.* 1937;70(suppl):1-5.
39. Lee CS, Tsai TL. The relation of the sciatic nerve to the piriformis muscle. *J Formosan Med Assoc.* 1974;73:75-80.
40. Pećina M. Contribution to the etiological explanation of the piriformis syndrome. *Acta Anat.* 1979;105:181-187.
41. Tuttle LJ, DeLozier ER, Harter KA, Johnson SA, Plotts CN, Swartz JL. The role of the obturator internus muscle in pelvic floor function. *J Womens Health Phys Ther.* 2016;40(1):15-19.
42. Jordre B, Schweinle W. Comparing resisted hip rotation with pelvic floor muscle training in women with stress urinary incontinence: a pilot study. *J Womens Health Phys Ther.* 2014;38(2):81-89.
43. Underwood DB, Calteaux TH, Cranston AR, Novotny SA, Hollman JH. Hip and pelvic floor muscle strength in women with and without stress urinary incontinence: a case-control study. *J Womens Health Phys Ther.* 2012;36(1):55-61.
44. Simons DG, Travell J, Simons L. *Travell & Simon's Myofascial Pain and Dysfunction: The Trigger Point Manual.* Vol 1. 2nd ed. Baltimore, MD: Williams & Wilkins; 1999 (p. 104).
45. Hollinshead WH. *Functional Anatomy of the Limbs and Back.* 4th ed. Philadelphia, PA: Saunders; 1976 (pp. 299-301).
46. Hallin RP. Sciatic pain and the piriformis muscle. *Postgrad Med.* 1983;74(2):69-72.
47. Pace JB. Commonly overlooked pain syndromes responsive to simple therapy. *Postgrad Med.* 1975;58(4):107-113.
48. Pace JB, Nagle D. Piriform syndrome. *West J Med.* 1976;124(6):435-439.
49. Stein JM, Warfield CA. Two entrapment neuropathies. *Hosp Pract.* 1983;18(1):100A, 100E, 100H passim.
50. Steiner C, Staubs C, Ganon M, Buhlinger C. Piriformis syndrome: pathogenesis, diagnosis, and treatment. *J Am Osteopath Assoc.* 1987;87(4):318-323 (p. 322, Fig. 3).
51. Wyant GM. Chronic pain syndromes and their treatment. III. The piriformis syndrome. *Can Anaesth Soc J.* 1979;26(4):305-308.
52. Velleman MD, Jansen Van Rensburg A, Janse Van Rensburg DC, Strauss O. Acute obturator internus muscle strain in a rugby player: a case report. *J Sports Med Phys Fitness.* 2015;55(12):1544-1546.
53. George AR, VanEtten L, Briggs MS. 2016 combined sections meeting poster: dry needling of the obturator internus for female pelvic pain: a case series. *J Womens Health Phys Ther.* 2016;40(1):38-51.
54. Dalmau-Carolà J. Myofascial pain syndrome affecting the piriformis and the obturator internus muscle. *Pain Pract.* 2005;5(4):361-363.
55. Willick SE, Lazarus M, Press JM. Quadratus femoris strain. *Clin J Sport Med.* 2002;12(2):130-131.
56. O'Brien SD, Bui-Mansfield LT. MRI of quadratus femoris muscle tear: another cause of hip pain. *AJR Am J Roentgenol.* 2007;189(5):1185-1189.
57. Zibis AH, Fyllos AH, Karantanas AH, Raoulis V, Karachalios TS, Arvanitis DL. Quadratus femoris tear as an unusual cause of hip pain: a case report. *Hip Int.* 2016;26(1):e7-e9.
58. Khodaee M, Jones D, Spittler J. Obturator internus and obturator externus strain in a high school quarterback. *Asian J Sports Med.* 2015;6(3):e23481.
59. Hopayian K, Danielyan A. Four symptoms define the piriformis syndrome: an updated systematic review of its clinical features. *Eur J Orthop Surg Traumatol.* 2018;28:155-164.
60. Urban LM, MacNeil BJ. Diagnostic accuracy of the slump test for identifying neuropathic pain in the lower limb. *J Orthop Sports Phys Ther.* 2015;45(8):596-603.
61. Barton PM, Grainger RW, Nicholson RL, et al. Toward a rational management of piriformis syndrome. *Arch Phys Med Rehabil.* 1988;69:784.
62. Reichel G, Gaerisch F Jr. Piriformis syndrome. A contribution to the differential diagnosis of lumbago and coccygodynia [in German]. *Zentralblatt fur Neurochirurgie.* 1988;49(3):178-184.
63. Evjenth O, Hamberg J. *Muscle Stretching in Manual Therapy: A Clinical Manual.* Vol 1. Alfta, Sweden: Alfta Rehab Forlag; 1984 (pp. 97, 122, 172).
64. TePoorten BA. The piriformis muscle. *J Am Osteopath Assoc.* 1969;69:150-160.
65. Thiele GH. Coccygodynia and pain in the superior gluteal region. *JAMA.* 1937;109:1271-1275.
66. Fishman LM, Dombi GW, Michaelsen C, et al. Piriformis syndrome: diagnosis, treatment, and outcome—a 10-year study. *Arch Phys Med Rehabil.* 2002;83(3):295-301.
67. Kean Chen C, Nizar AJ. Prevalence of piriformis syndrome in chronic low back pain patients. A clinical diagnosis with modified FAIR test. *Pain Pract.* 2013;13(4):276-281.
68. Retzlaff EW, Berry AH, Haight AS, et al. The piriformis muscle syndrome. *J Am Osteopath Assoc.* 1974;73(10):799-807.

69. Kipervas IP, Ivanov LA, Urikh EA, Pakhomov SK. Clinico-electromyographic characteristics of piriform muscle syndromes [in Russian]. *Zh Nevropatol Psikhiatr Im S S Korsakova*. 1976;76(9):1289-1292.
70. Mirman MJ. Sciatic pain: two more tips. *Postgrad Med*. 1983;74(5):50.
71. Gerwin RD, Dommerholt J, Shah JP. An expansion of Simons' integrated hypothesis of trigger point formation. *Curr Pain Headache Rep*. 2004;8(6):468-475.
72. Namey TC, An HS. Emergency diagnosis and management of sciatica: differentiating the nondiskogenic causes. *Emergency Med Reports*. 1985;6:101-109.
73. Gould N. Letter: back-pocket sciatica. *N Engl J Med*. 1974;290(11):633.
74. Shordania JF. Die chronischer Entzundung des Musculus piriformis—die piriformitis—alseine der Ursachen von Kreuzschmerzen bei Frauen. *Die Medizinische Welt*. 1936;10:999-1001.
75. Hsieh YL, Kao MJ, Kuan TS, Chen SM, Chen JT, Hong CZ. Dry needling to a key myofascial trigger point may reduce the irritability of satellite MTrPs. *Am J Phys Med Rehabil*. 2007;86(5):397-403.
76. Slipman CW, Jackson HB, Lipetz JS, Chan KT, Lenrow D, Vresilovic EJ. Sacroiliac joint pain referral zones. *Arch Phys Med Rehabil*. 2000;81(3):334-338.
77. Kurosawa D, Murakami E, Aizawa T. Referred pain location depends on the affected section of the sacroiliac joint. *Eur Spine J*. 2015;24(3):521-527.
78. Lesher JM, Dreyfuss P, Hager N, Kaplan M, Furman M. Hip joint pain referral patterns: a descriptive study. *Pain Med*. 2008;9(1):22-25.
79. Hopayian K, Song F, Riera R, Sambandan S. The clinical features of the piriformis syndrome: a systematic review. *Eur Spine J*. 2010;19(12):2095-2109.
80. Cass SP. Piriformis syndrome: a cause of nondiscogenic sciatica. *Curr Sports Med Rep*. 2015;14(1):41-44.
81. Toda T, Koda M, Rokkaku T, et al. Sciatica caused by pyomyositis of the piriformis muscle in a pediatric patient. *Orthopedics*. 2013;36(2):e257-e259.
82. Koda M, Mannoji C, Watanabe H, et al. Sciatica caused by pyomyositis of the piriformis muscle. *Neurol India*. 2013;61(6):668-669.
83. Sharma PR, McEvoy HC, Floyd DC. Streptococcal necrotising myositis of obturator internus and piriformis in a type 2 diabetic patient presenting as sepsis of unknown origin. *Ann R Coll Surg Engl*. 2011;93(6):e99-e101.
84. King RJ, Laugharne D, Kerslake RW, Holdsworth BJ. Primary obturator pyomyositis: a diagnostic challenge. *J Bone Joint Surg Br*. 2003;85(6):895-898.
85. Hsu WC, Hsu JY, Chen MY, Liang CC. Obturator internus pyomyositis manifested as sciatica in a patient with subacute bacterial endocarditis: a rare case report. *Medicine (Baltimore)*. 2016;95(30):e4340.
86. Cohen BA, Lanzieri CF, Mendelson DS, et al. CT evaluation of the greater sciatic foramen in patients with sciatica. *AJNR Am J Neuroradiol*. 1986;7(2):337-342.
87. Pace JB, Henning C. Episacroiliac lipoma. *Am Fam Physician*. 1972;6(3):70-73.
88. Freiberg AH. The fascial elements in associated low-back and sciatic pain. *J Bone Joint Surg [AM]*. 1941;23:478-480.
89. Stimson BB. The low back problem. *Psychosom Med*. 1947;9(3):210-212.
90. Brinjikji W, Diehn FE, Jarvik JG, et al. MRI findings of disc degeneration are more prevalent in adults with low back pain than in asymptomatic controls: a systematic review and meta-analysis. *AJNR Am J Neuroradiol*. 2015;36(12):2394-2399.
91. Cheung KM, Karppinen J, Chan D, et al. Prevalence and pattern of lumbar magnetic resonance imaging changes in a population study of one thousand forty-three individuals. *Spine (Phila Pa 1976)*. 2009;34(9):934-940.
92. Huang JT, Chen HY, Hong CZ, et al. Lumbar facet injection for the treatment of chronic piriformis myofascial pain syndrome: 52 case studies. *Patient Prefer Adherence*. 2014;8:1105-1111.
93. Ehrlich GE. Early diagnosis of ankylosing spondylitis: role of history and presence of HLA-B27 Antigen. *Intern Med Spec*. 1982;3(3):112-116.
94. Rodnan GP. *Primer on the Rheumatic Diseases*. Atlanta, GA: Arthritis Foundation; 1983 (pp. 87, 179, 181).
95. Pope MH, Frymoyer JW, Anderson G. *Occupational Low Back Pain*. New York, NY: Praegar; 1984.
96. Marchand AA, Boucher JA, O'Shaughnessy J. Multiple venous thromboses presenting as mechanical low back pain in an 18-year-old woman. *J Chiropr Med*. 2015;14(2):83-89.
97. Naess IA, Christiansen SC, Romundstad P, Cannegieter SC, Rosendaal FR, Hammerstrom J. Incidence and mortality of venous thromboembolism: a population-based study. *J Thromb Haemost*. 2007;5(4):692-699.
98. Riddle DL, Wells PS. Diagnosis of lower-extremity deep vein thrombosis in outpatients. *Phys Ther*. 2004;84(8):729-735.
99. Baek D, Lee SE, Kim WJ, et al. Greater trochanteric pain syndrome due to tumoral calcinosis in a patient with chronic kidney disease. *Pain Physician*. 2014;17(6):E775-E782.
100. Hubka P, Nanka O, Masata J, Martan A, Svabik K. TVT ABBREVO: cadaveric study of tape position in foramen obturatum and adductor region. *Int Urogynecol J*. 2016;27(7):1047-1050.
101. Muller M, Dewey M, Springer I, Perka C, Tohtz S. Relationship between cup position and obturator externus muscle in total hip arthroplasty. *J Orthop Surg Res*. 2010;5:44.
102. Tosun O, Algin O, Yalcin N, Cay N, Ocakoglu G, Karaoglanoglu M. Ischiofemoral impingement: evaluation with new MRI parameters and assessment of their reliability. *Skeletal Radiol*. 2012;41(5):575-587.
103. Ali AM, Teh J, Whitwell D, Ostlere S. Ischiofemoral impingement: a retrospective analysis of cases in a specialist orthopaedic centre over a four-year period. *Hip Int*. 2013;23(3):263-268.
104. Watanabe M, Yamaga M, Kato T, Ide J, Kitamura T, Takagi K. The implication of repeated versus continuous strain on nerve function in a rat forelimb model. *J Hand Surg Am*. 2001;26(4):663-669.
105. Dyck PJ, Lais AC, Giannini C, Engelstad JK. Structural alterations of nerve during cuff compression. *Proc Natl Acad Sci U S A*. 1990;87(24):9828-9832.
106. Gulledge BM, Marcellin-Little DJ, Levine D, et al. Comparison of two stretching methods and optimization of stretching protocol for the piriformis muscle. *Med Eng Phys*. 2014;36(2):212-218.

Chapter 58

Quadriceps Femoris and Sartorius Muscles

"Four-Faced Troublemaker and Surreptitious Accomplice"

N. Beth Collier and Joseph M. Donnelly

1. INTRODUCTION

The muscles of the anterior compartment of the thigh are informally termed the "quadriceps" when discussed as a group. The main four muscles that make up the quadriceps femoris muscles are the rectus femoris, vastus lateralis, vastus medialis, and vastus intermedius muscles. The quadriceps femoris muscles merge into a common tendon that attaches to the patella that then attaches to the tibial tuberosity by the patellar ligament and allows for knee extension. The three vasti muscles only cross the knee joint and act to extend the knee. As the rectus femoris muscle crosses both the hip and knee joint, it also contributes to hip flexion. The sartorius muscle also lies in the anterior compartment of the thigh and contributes to hip flexion, abduction, and external rotation as well as knee flexion. Trigger points (TrPs) in the quadriceps femoris and sartorius muscles can refer pain to the thigh anteriorly, laterally, and to the knee region medially, laterally, and posterolaterally. Trigger points in the quadriceps femoris muscle can be debilitating and can cause buckling or giving way of the knee during walking or descending stairs. Clinicians should consider TrPs in these muscles when patients present with a diagnosis of L4 radicular pain or radiculopathy, patellofemoral pain syndrome, knee osteoarthritis, iliotibial band syndrome, patellar tendinopathy, or greater trochanteric bursitis. To treat TrPs in the quadriceps femoris and sartorius muscles, patients may perform self-pressure release techniques and self-stretching of the involved muscles. Patients may also benefit from improving or supporting static and dynamic postures that contribute to overuse or shortening of these muscles.

2. ANATOMIC CONSIDERATIONS

Rectus Femoris

The two-joint rectus femoris muscle lies between the vastus medialis and vastus lateralis muscles and covers the vastus intermedius muscle. The rectus femoris muscle originates from the pelvis by two tendons, one attached to the anterior inferior iliac spine and the other to a groove above the posterior brim of the acetabulum. It then inserts to the proximal border of the patella and through the patellar ligament to the tuberosity of the tibia (Figure 58-1). Proximally, the rectus femoris muscle is covered by the sartorius muscle at, and just inferior to, the anterior inferior iliac spine.[1]

Vastus Intermedius

The vastus intermedius muscle lies deep to the rectus femoris and vastus lateralis muscles. It originates from the anterior and the lateral surfaces of the upper two-thirds of the shaft of the femur and from the distal aspect of the lateral intermuscular

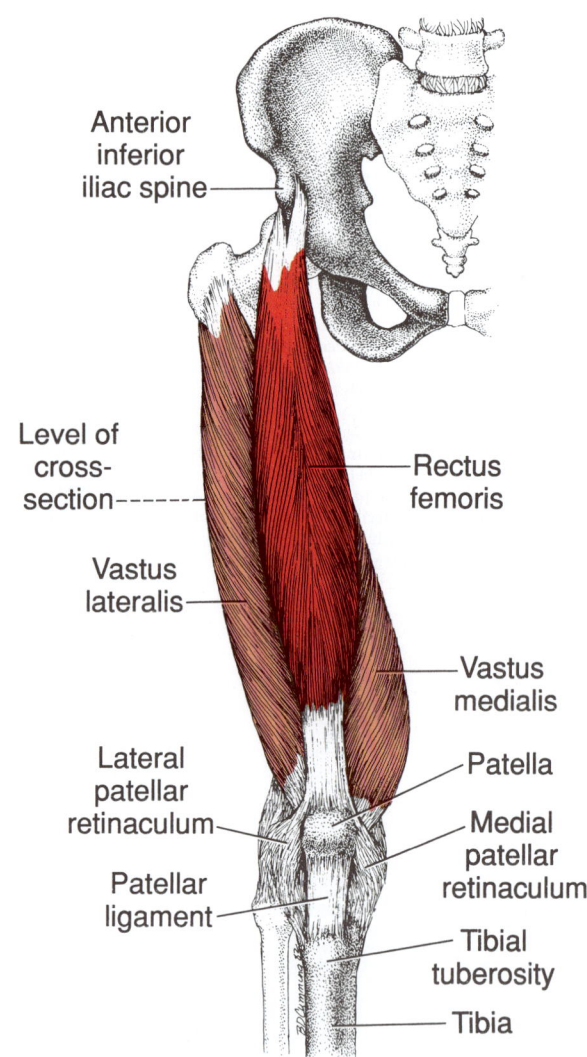

Figure 58-1. Attachments (anterior view) of the right rectus femoris muscle (dark red) in relation to the vastus lateralis and vastus medialis muscles (light red).

septum. It inserts on the lateral border of the patella, the lateral condyle of the tibia and through the patellar ligament to the tibial tuberosity (Figure 58-2). The vastus intermedius muscle is clearly separated on its medial side from the vastus medialis muscle, but laterally, the vastus intermedius fibers merge with those of the vastus lateralis muscle.[1]

Vastus Medialis

The vastus medialis muscle originates from the distal half of the intertrochanteric line, the medial lip of the linea aspera, and the upper part of the medial supracondylar line of the femur.[1] The vastus medialis muscle attaches to the aponeurosis of the quadriceps femoris tendon with the vastus intermedius muscle, and its fibers wrap around the femur angling anteriorly and inferiorly from its posterior attachments. The vastus medialis muscle inserts on the medial border of the patella and through the patellar ligament to the tibial tuberosity. It also inserts by a slip of muscle to the medial patellar retinaculum that reinforces the capsule of the knee joint, and it ultimately terminates at the medial tibial condyle[1] (Figure 58-2).

The distal fibers of the vastus medialis muscle are markedly angulated in the region of the patella and can be clearly separated from the rest of the vastus medialis muscle by fiber direction and also by a fascial plane. These distal angulated fibers often attach chiefly to the adductor magnus muscle, partly to the adductor longus muscle, and to the medial intermuscular septum. These obliquely oriented fibers are often referred to as the vastus medialis obliquus (VMO).[1,2] In fact, the insertion of these fibers is variable and changes significantly with advancing age and the presence of knee degeneration.[3] Some authors, who deem the VMO a separate muscle, have proposed the term "vastus medialis longus" for those fibers with a more vertical orientation that originate from the medial lip of the linea aspera and the medial intramuscular septum and travel to the medial margin and anterior surface of a quadriceps tendon aponeurosis. Controversy continues as to whether the vastus medialis muscle should be classified as one or two muscles.[4]

Vastus Lateralis

The vastus lateralis muscle is the largest component of the quadriceps femoris muscle group. It originates by way of a broad aponeurosis from the superior portion of the intertrochanteric line, the anterior and inferior borders of the greater trochanter, the lateral lip of the gluteal tuberosity, and the proximal half of the lateral lip of the linea aspera of the femur[1] (Figure 58-3). Some fibers also originate from the tendon of the gluteus maximus muscle as well as the lateral intermuscular septum between vastus lateralis muscle and the short head of biceps femoris muscle.

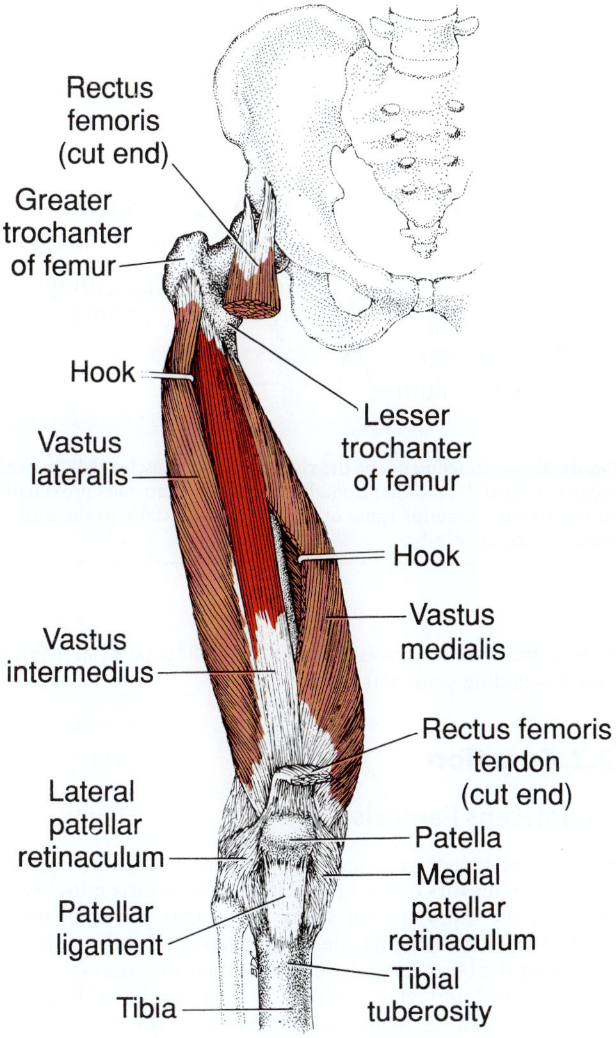

Figure 58-2. Attachments (anterior view) of the right vastus medialis (light red), vastus intermedius (dark red), and vastus lateralis (light red) muscles of the quadriceps femoris muscle group. The bulk of the overlying rectus femoris muscle has been cut and removed. Part of the anterior attachment of the vastus medialis muscle to the aponeurosis of the quadriceps femoris tendon along the medial edge of the vastus intermedius muscle has been cut and pulled aside by the lower hook. This reveals the deeper fibers of the vastus medialis muscle as they disappear to attach behind the femur, and it exposes the bone deep to the fibers anteriorly. The upper hook pulls the vastus lateralis muscle aside to show the underlying portion of the vastus intermedius muscle.

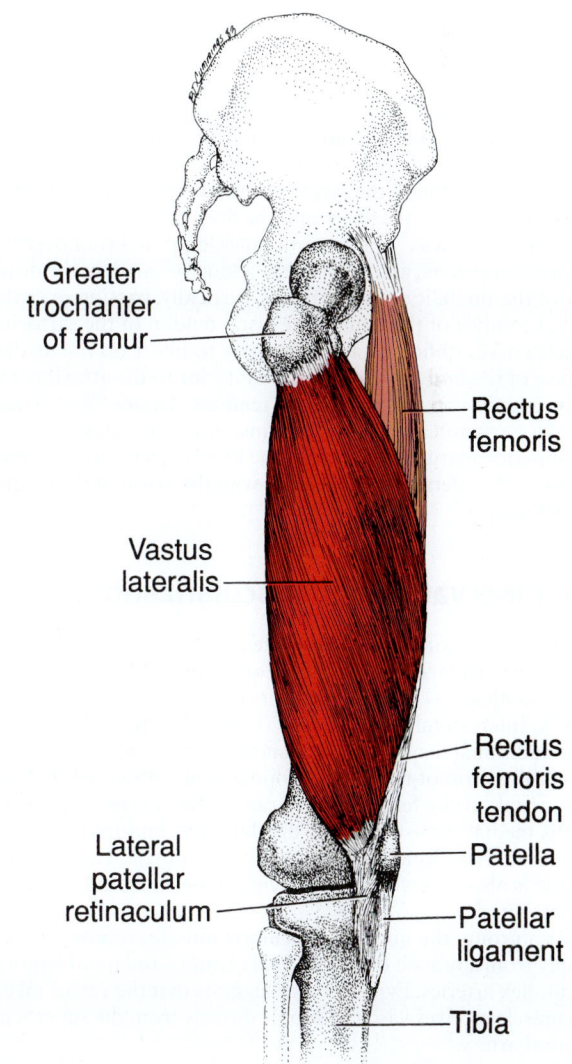

Figure 58-3. Attachments (lateral view) of the right vastus lateralis muscle (dark red) in relation to the rectus femoris muscle (light red).

The aponeurosis deep to the muscle inserts on the lateral border of the patella and blends into the common quadriceps femoris tendon. It also contributes to the capsule of the knee joint that descends to the lateral condyle of the tibia and the iliotibial band.[1] However, the gross anatomy of the vastus lateralis muscle described in the literature is inconsistent.[5]

Tensor of the Vastus Intermedius

Recent cadaveric research has identified a fifth major contribution to the quadriceps femoris muscle group, termed the tensor of the vastus intermedius (TVI) muscle. Specific dissection of 26 specimens identified a separate TVI muscle in all cases that received separate nervous and vascular supply from the femoral nerve and lateral femoral circumflex artery. The TVI muscle is a separate muscle that lies between the vastus intermedius and the vastus lateralis muscles and attaches distally to the medial aspect of the patella by way of its own aponeurosis that adjoins the quadriceps femoris tendon.[6] The TVI muscle has also been demonstrated via magnetic resonance imaging (MRI) to blend with fibers of the vastus lateralis and vastus medialis muscles dorsally into its attachment at the lateral lip of the linea aspera.[7]

The articularis genu muscle is a tiny, deep muscle that occasionally blends with the vastus intermedius muscle but is often separate. It originates from the anterior surface of the distal femoral shaft and attaches to the proximal aspect of the synovial membrane of the knee joint.[1]

Sartorius

The sartorius, a narrow strap muscle, is the longest muscle in the body. It originates from the anterior superior iliac spine and descends obliquely across the front of the thigh, lateral to medial. The tendon of the sartorius muscle forms an additional aponeurosis that sends fibers into the deep fascia of the quadriceps femoris muscle.[8] The sartorius muscle forms a roof over the femoral artery, vein, and nerve in the adductor canal. In the distal part of the thigh, it descends nearly vertically, passing over the medial condyle of the femur. The distal tendon of the sartorius muscle curves obliquely and anteriorly to insert on the medial surface of the body of the tibia just anterior to the attachments of the gracilis and semitendinosus tendons (Figure 58-4). Thus, it is the most anterior of the "pes anserinus" muscles. A slip of the superior margin blends with the knee capsule and another slip from the inferior margin blends with the fascia of the medial side of the leg.[1]

2.1. Innervation and Vascularization

All the muscles of the quadriceps femoris group, including the TVI and articularis genu muscles, are supplied by branches of the femoral nerve composed of fibers from L2, L3, and L4 spinal nerves. Interestingly, Günal et al[9] found that the VMO fibers have additional femoral nerve branches, explaining its relevance for stabilization of the patella. Jojima et al[10] observed that the main trunk of the femoral nerve ran in the mid-portion of the vastus medialis muscle before dividing into multiple branches that entered the distal oblique fibers of the muscle. The sartorius muscle is also innervated by the femoral nerve from L2 and L3 nerve roots.[1]

As a group, the quadriceps femoris muscles receive arterial supply from a branch of the profunda femoris or lateral femoral circumflex arteries. Evidence also suggests that the vastus medialis muscle receives vascular supply directly from the superficial femoral artery.[11]

The proximal third of the sartorius muscle receives its arterial supply from the common femoral, the profunda femoris, and the lateral circumflex femoral arteries, as well as the artery to the quadriceps femoris muscle. The middle third of the muscle receives its supply from the superficial femoral artery. The distal

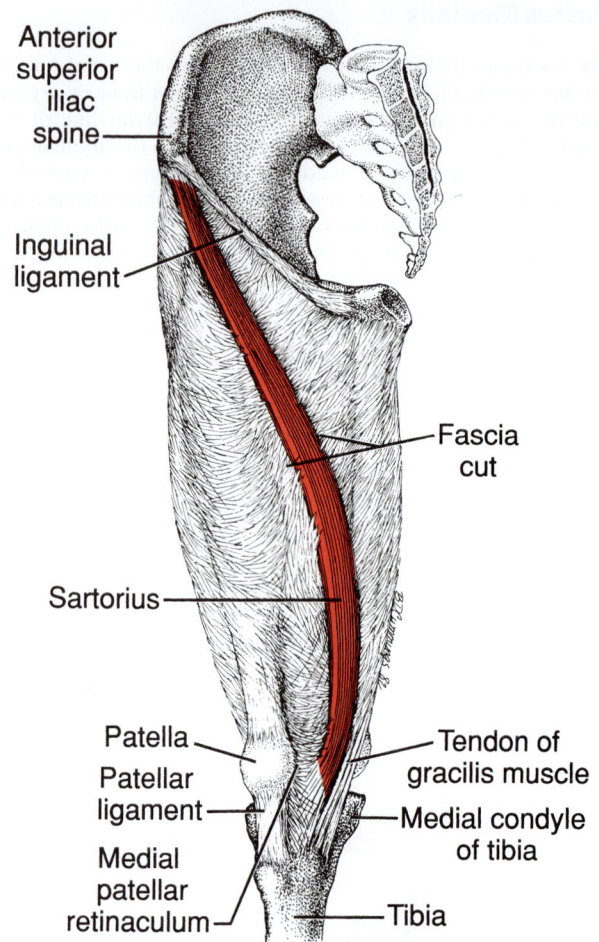

Figure 58-4. Attachments of the right sartorius muscle (red), viewed from in front and somewhat from the medial side. It attaches proximally to the anterior superior spine of the ilium and distally to the medial aspect of the upper tibia.

third of the muscle receives its supply from the superficial femoral and descending genicular arteries.[1]

2.2. Function

Quadriceps Femoris

In open kinetic chain, the quadriceps femoris muscles act together as prime extensors of the knee. The rectus femoris muscle can also flex the hip. A recent study found that proximal fibers of the rectus femoris muscle can be activated independently from distal fibers. Therefore, the activation succession between fibers could change direction (from proximal to distal, or inversely) and depends on the context of the movement.[12] Collectively, the vastus medialis, vastus lateralis, and vastus intermedius muscles respond simultaneously to vigorous effort[13]; however, contributions from the rectus femoris muscle depend on demands at the hip joint. The four main muscles of the quadriceps femoris group trade-off among themselves in variable ways during slow increase of knee extension force to a maximum effort.[14] Balanced tension on the patella between the vastus medialis and vastus lateralis muscles maintains normal positioning and tracking of the patella.[15-17] Nevertheless, some authors have suggested that the main medial stabilizer of the patella is the VMO muscle as it reduces lateral pressure of the patella cartilage.[18]

In weight-bearing positions, the quadriceps femoris muscle group functions to control trunk extension and knee flexion as with squatting, sitting down from the standing position, and descending stairs. However, the quadriceps femoris muscles are not active in static standing.[13,19,20] During gait, the quadriceps femoris muscles are active immediately after heel strike to control knee flexion during weight acceptance and again at toe off to stabilize the knee in extension. They are not active during the period that the knee is extending during stance. The quadriceps femoris muscle group is not active in extension of the leg during the early swing phase, but it is active in the last part of the swing phase, in preparation for weight bearing. Stance phase quadriceps femoris muscle activity is either prolonged or increased (or both) under certain circumstances, such as when there is significant loss of function in the plantar flexors, when heavy loads are carried on the back, when walking speed is increased, and when one wears high heels.[13,21-25] The quadriceps femoris muscle also serves an important function during rising from sitting and in ascending stairs.[19] A strong peak of activity appears in the middle of the down stroke during upright cycling.[26,27]

Sartorius

The sartorius muscle earned its name as the muscle that assists the hip movements necessary to assume the position of a cross-legged tailor. This muscle, like the tensor fasciae latae muscle, is a flexor and abductor of the thigh, but the sartorius muscle rotates the thigh externally instead of internally.[1] Activation of this muscle by knee flexion or extension is highly variable.[28,29] It is more likely to assist knee flexion when the hip is also flexed.[29]

During the swing phase of gait, sartorius muscle activity peaks to assist the iliacus and tensor fasciae latae muscles in hip flexion, and the muscle assists the short head of the biceps femoris muscle in knee flexion. It may assist the vastus medialis, gracilis, and semitendinosus muscles in supporting the knee medially against the valgus thrust that occurs during single limb balance.[30] During bicycling, the sartorius muscle is active as a hip flexor.

2.3. Functional Unit

The functional unit to which a muscle belongs includes the muscles that reinforce and counter its actions as well as the joints that the muscle crosses. The interdependence of these structures is functionally reflected in the organization and neural connections of the sensory motor cortex. The functional unit is emphasized because the presence of a TrP in one muscle of the unit increases the likelihood that the other muscles of the unit will also develop TrPs. When inactivating TrPs in a muscle, one must be concerned about TrPs that may develop in muscles that are functionally interdependent. Box 58-1 grossly represents the functional unit of the quadriceps muscle group and the sartorius muscle.[31]

3. CLINICAL PRESENTATION

3.1. Referred Pain Pattern

Trigger points in all four main muscles of the quadriceps femoris muscle group refer pain to the thigh and knee region. Rectus femoris and vastus medialis TrPs produce anterior and medial knee pain. The referred pain from rectus femoris TrPs is more likely to be felt deep in the knee joint than is the knee pain referred from the vastus medialis or vastus lateralis muscles. Trigger points in the vastus lateralis muscle cause hip, lateral thigh, and posterolateral knee pain.

Rectus Femoris (Two-jointed Puzzler)

Trigger points in the rectus femoris muscle are extremely common and frequently overlooked. This muscle rarely undergoes full stretch in daily activities. The rectus femoris muscle is a two-joint puzzler because TrPs are commonly identified proximally, just below the anterior inferior iliac spine. However, the pain is typically felt at the anterior knee in and around the patella and sometimes deep in the knee joint (Figure 58-5). Patients with TrPs in the rectus femoris muscle often have severe deep aching pain at night over the distal thigh above the knee anteriorly. They are typically unable to find a position or movement that provides relief until they learn how to fully stretch this muscle. Trigger points can occasionally be found in the distal end of the rectus femoris muscle just proximal to the patella and may refer pain deep into the knee joint.

Vastus Intermedius (Frustrator)

The vastus intermedius muscle is a "frustrator" because it develops TrPs that cannot be palpated directly due to coverage from the more superficial rectus femoris muscle. The pain from these TrPs extends over the anterior aspect of the thigh nearly to the knee but is most intense at the mid-thigh. Trigger points at the vastus intermedius muscle may refer pain and tenderness that extends over the upper thigh anterolaterally (Figure 58-6). Kellgren[32] reported that 0.1 mL of 6% hypertonic saline solution injected into the vastus intermedius muscle caused pain in the knee joint.

Vastus Medialis (Buckling Knee Muscle)

Trigger points in the vastus medialis muscle more commonly occur distally in the muscle and refer pain to the anterior knee area. Proximal vastus medialis TrPs commonly refer an aching pain in a linear distribution over the anteromedial aspect of the knee and lower thigh (Figure 58-7).

Trigger points in this muscle are easily overlooked because the taut muscle fibers only minimally restrict knee flexion range of motion and the TrPs may not produce intense pain. Commonly, TrPs of the vastus medialis muscle tend to produce more motor dysfunction (inhibition weakness) after the initial acute pain phase. The pain from TrPs in the muscle may be replaced

Box 58-1 Functional unit of the quadriceps femoris muscle group and sartorius muscle

Action	Synergists	Antagonists
Knee extension	Rectus femoris Vastus medialis Vastus intermedius Vastus lateralis Tensor of the vastus intermedius	Semimembranosus Semitendinosus Biceps femoris Gastrocnemius Popliteus Gracilis Sartorius
Hip flexion (rectus femoris, sartorius)	Iliopsoas Pectineus Tensor fascia latae Hip adductors Anterior fibers of gluteus medius and minimus	Gluteus maximus Semimembranosus Semitendinosus Biceps femoris Adductor magnus (ischiocondylar portion)
Hip abduction (sartorius)	Piriformis Gluteus medius Gluteus minimus	Pectineus Adductor longus Adductor brevis Adductor magnus Gracilis

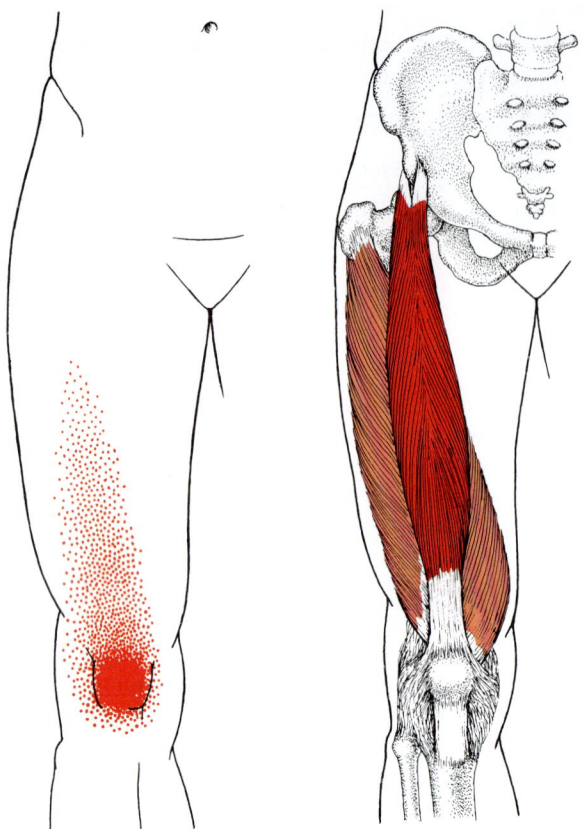

Figure 58-5. Referred pain patterns from TrPs in the rectus femoris muscle. Solid bright red denotes the essential pattern of pain from TrPs in the rectus femoris muscle. Red stippling indicates the occasional extension of its essential referred pain pattern.

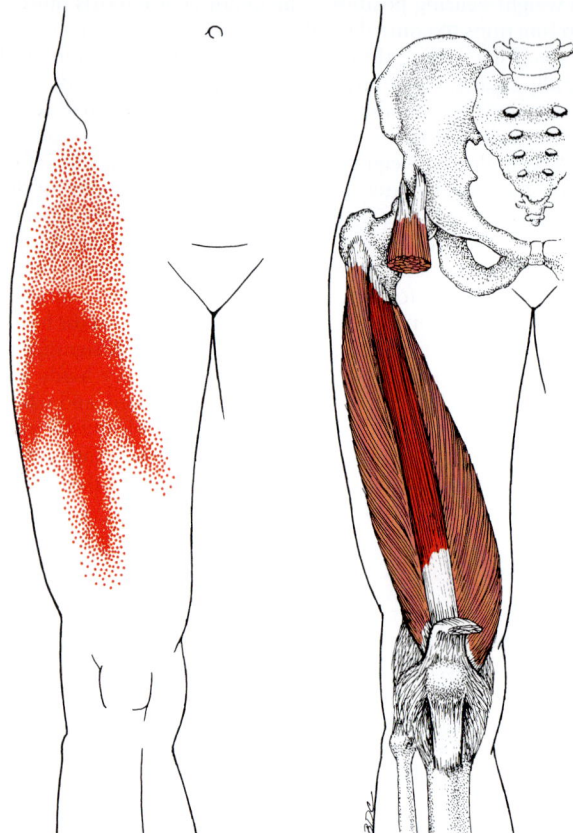

Figure 58-6. Referred pain pattern from TrPs in the vastus intermedius muscle. Dark solid red denotes the essential pattern of pain felt with TrPs in the vastus intermedius muscle. Red stippling indicates occasional extension of the essential referred pain pattern.

by unexpected episodes of quadriceps femoris inhibition that result in buckling of the knee. This sudden perceived weakness may cause the individual to fall, often inflicting injury. Vastus medialis TrPs are frequently seen in adults and children. Nguyen[33] proposed a hypothetical pain model in which TrPs in the knee muscles can cause muscle tightness, pain, and weakness leading to early pathologic neuromuscular changes including knee instability and consequently, falls. In this hypothetical model, long-lasting TrPs may promote knee instability and therefore facilitate degenerative changes in the knee, which will, in turn, present as typical arthrogenic muscle inhibition seen in patients with knee osteoarthritis.[33] However, there is no research supporting this hypothesis.

Vastus Lateralis (Stuck Patella Muscle)

The vastus lateralis muscle characteristically develops multiple TrPs along the lateral aspect of the thigh. This muscle has the largest mass of the four heads of the quadriceps femoris muscle group. TrPs in this muscle can refer pain throughout the full length of the thigh laterally and to the posterolateral aspect of the knee (Figure 58-8). Occasionally, the referred lateral thigh pain extends as high as the pelvic crest. Superficial TrPs in this muscle are more likely to have a local pattern, whereas TrPs located deep in the muscle usually produce a widespread pain throughout the thigh. When vastus lateralis TrPs refer pain and tenderness to the proximal thigh region, the patient may be unable to lie on that side, disturbing restful sleep. In an older report, Good[34] found that "myalgic spots" (probably TrPs) in the lateral edge of the vastus lateralis muscle referred pain to the knee.

A distinctive feature of TrPs in the distal portion of the vastus lateralis muscle is the feeling of a "stuck patella" in addition to pain around the lateral border of the patella that sometimes extends upward over the lateral region of the thigh (Figure 58-8). Trigger points located in the more posterior distal portion of the vastus lateralis muscle also cause pain lateral to the patella, but these TrPs refer pain more extensively up to the lateral aspect of the thigh and sometimes down the lateral aspect of the leg. Trigger points commonly located posterolaterally at the mid-thigh level refer pain that travels the entire length of the posterolateral region of the thigh and includes the lateral half of the popliteal space. It is the one quadriceps femoris TrP area that can produce posterior knee pain.

Trigger points located at mid-thigh level in the anterior portion of the muscle, just above the iliotibial band, are common and likely to cause severe pain over the entire length of the lateral thigh, slightly anterior to the iliotibial band, and extending upward almost to the pelvic crest. Distally, the pain referred from this area of the muscle can refer pain anteriorly around the lateral border of the patella rather than posteriorly to the popliteal space. Trigger points in the proximal area of the vastus lateralis muscle refer pain and tenderness only in its immediate vicinity (Figure 58-8).

Sartorius

Trigger points in the sartorius muscle produce superficial, sharp, or tingling symptoms or pain along the anterior and medial thigh, as well as to the medial knee. These TrPs are commonly mistaken for knee pathology (Figure 58-9).

Chapter 58: Quadriceps Femoris and Sartorius Muscles 609

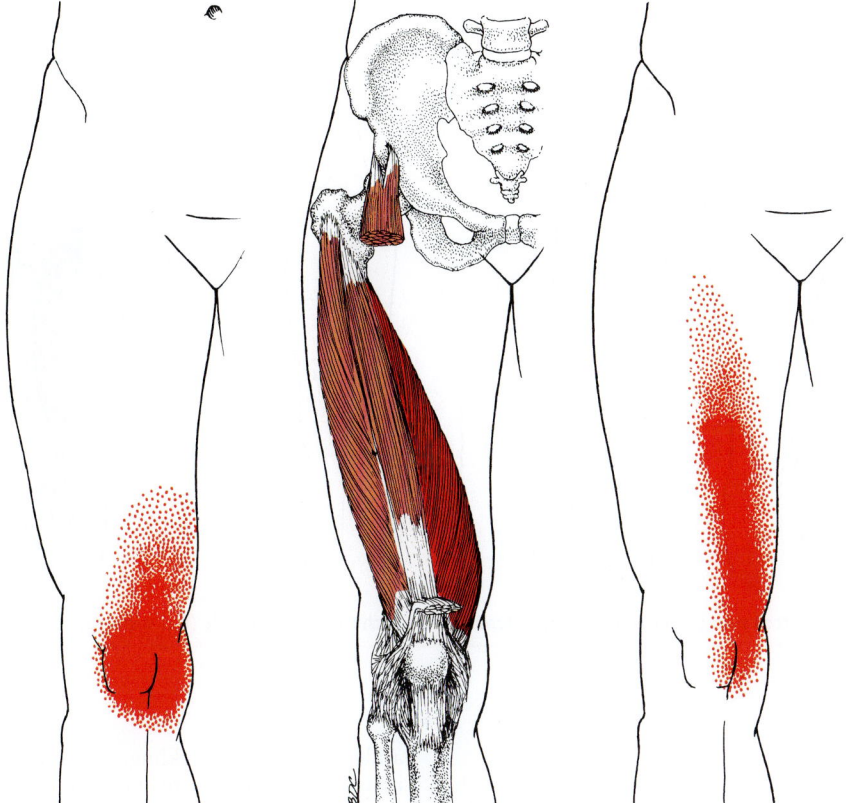

Figure 58-7. Referred pain patterns from TrPs in the vastus medialis muscle. Solid dark red depicts the essential pattern of pain experienced with TrPs in the vastus medialis muscle. Red stippling indicates the occasional extension of the essential referred pain pattern.

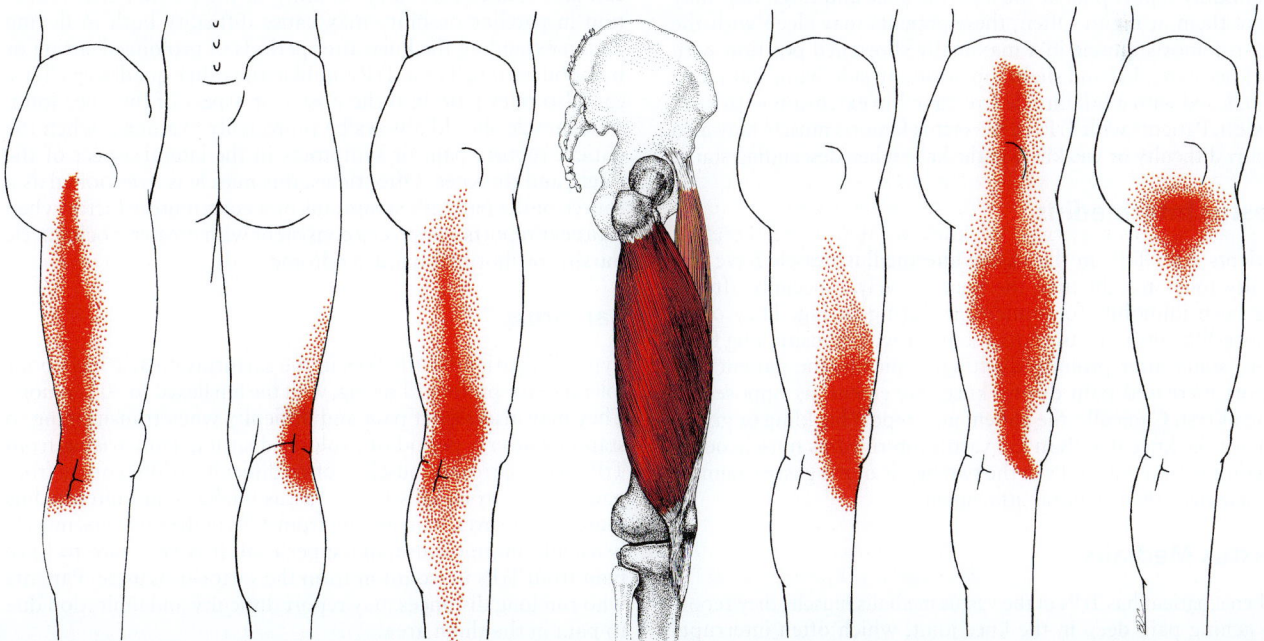

Figure 58-8. Referred pain pattern from TrPs in the vastus lateralis muscle. Solid bright red denotes the basic pain experienced by nearly everyone with TrPs in the vastus lateralis muscle. Red stippling indicates the occasional extension of the essential referred pain pattern.

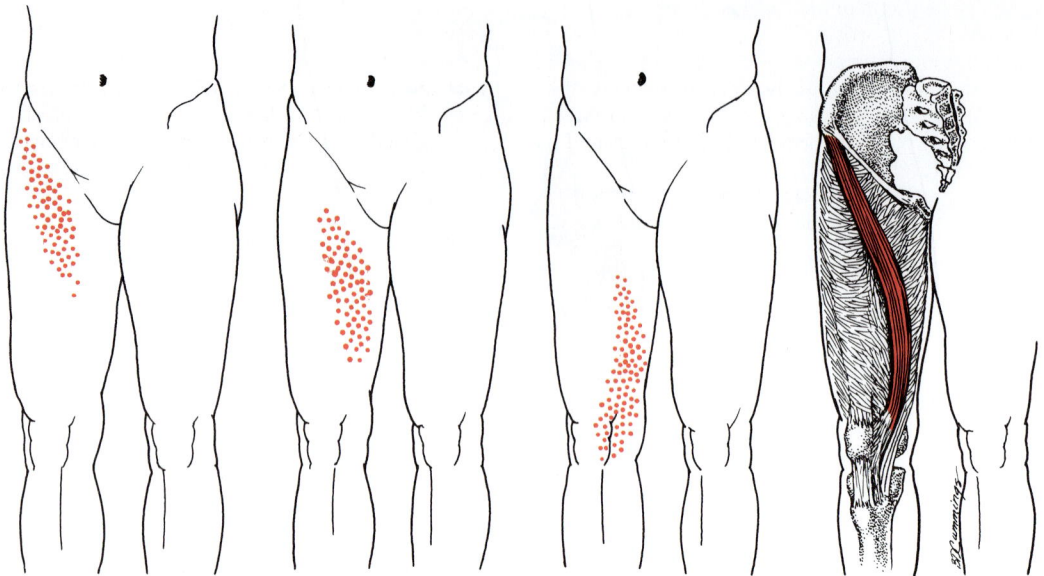

Figure 58-9. Referred pain patterns of TrPs at different levels in the sartorius muscle (red stippled), anteromedial view.

3.2. Symptoms

Referred pain is commonly the presenting symptom of the quadriceps femoris muscle group with two exceptions, muscle inhibition of the vastus medialis muscle causing buckling (giving way) of the knee and restricted patellar mobility from the vastus lateralis muscle.

Rectus Femoris

Patients who experience TrPs in the rectus femoris muscle commonly report pain at the anterior knee and thigh that may wake them at night. Often, these patients may sleep with the rectus femoris muscle in a maximally shortened position with the knee extended and slight hip flexion in side-lying. Pain may be relieved with a full muscle stretch in hip extension with knee flexion. Patients with TrPs in the rectus femoris muscle may also report difficulty or weakness in the knee when descending stairs.

Vastus Intermedius

Patients with TrPs in the vastus intermedius muscle have difficulty fully straightening the knee actively, especially after it has been immobile for some time during sitting. They often report difficulty with ascending stairs or with transitioning from sit-to-stand after prolonged sitting. Typically, the patient will report increased pain during knee movement, as opposed to pain at rest. Clinically, the patient may report buckling or giving way of the knee if TrPs in the vastus intermedius muscle occur in conjunction with TrPs in the two heads of the gastrocnemius muscle near their femoral attachments.

Vastus Medialis

When a patient has TrPs in the vastus medialis muscle, they report an aching pain deep in the knee joint, which often interrupts their sleep pattern. It may be misinterpreted as being due to inflammation of the knee joint.[35] Over time, the concerning knee pain will fade and the patient will instead experience episodic inhibition of quadriceps femoris muscle function that causes unexpected buckling (inhibition weakness) of the knee during walking.[36] This buckling response may cause the individual to fall. Baker[36] cites the case of an incapacitated 12-year-old athlete with knee buckling, which completely resolved upon inactivation of the vastus medialis TrPs.

Vastus Lateralis

Patients who have TrPs in the vastus lateralis muscle exhibit pain with walking that extends along the lateral aspect of the thigh including the knee. Patients with TrPs in the vastus lateralis may report difficulty lying on the involved side, and pain may disturb their sleep. The patient may also report a feeling of "stiffness" in the knee as TrPs in the distal end of the vastus lateralis muscle can also reduce accessory mobility of the patella. This reduction in patellar mobility may cause difficulty both in flexing and in extending the knee after periods of prolonged sitting or immobilization. These TrPs, unlike any other quadriceps TrPs, can also refer pain into the posterior aspect of the knee joint. This muscle should always be thoroughly examined when the patient reports pain or symptoms in the lateral aspect of the thigh, and the knee. Oftentimes, this muscle is overlooked as a source of the patient's symptoms or a contributing factor when a patient reports symptoms consistent with greater trochanteric bursitis or iliotibial band syndrome.

Sartorius

Typically, patients with TrPs in the sartorius muscle have poor tolerance for prolonged sitting, with the hip flexed to 90° or more. They may also report pain and difficulty when transitioning to standing after a period of prolonged sitting. Pain arising from TrPs in the sartorius muscle is often difficult to differentiate from pain arising from TrPs in the vastus medialis and intermedius muscles; however, pain arising from TrPs in the sartorius muscle is usually more diffuse and superficial. It is very rare to have pain from TrPs in isolation from the sartorius muscle. Patients who run long distances may report difficulty and limitation due to pain in the thigh area.

3.3. Patient Examination

After a thorough subjective examination the clinician should make a detailed drawing representing the pain pattern the patient has described. This depiction will assist in planning the physical examination and can be useful in monitoring the progression of the patient as symptoms improve or change. If TrPs in any of the quadriceps femoris muscles are suspected, clinicians should perform a thorough examination of the knee, hip, foot, ankle, and possibly the pelvis if the rectus femoris muscle is involved. Accessory motion of the patellofemoral and tibiofemoral joints should be carefully assessed.

Functional activities such as sit-to-stand, stair descent, single-leg stance, double-leg squat, and single-leg squat (Figure 55-3A) should be examined. The clinician should take note of any frontal or sagittal plane deviations noted in the pelvis, hip and/or knee, and any excessive transverse plane motion at the ankle and foot (Figure 55-3B). The clinician should note any gait deviations such as a Trendelenburg sign at mid-stance (Figure 55-4A and B), or forward lean of the trunk at heel strike.[37] These deviations could be indicative of gluteal muscle weakness or lower extremity biomechanical faults. The quadriceps femoris muscle group can be overloaded in the presence of gluteal muscle weakness or lower extremity biomechanical malalignment, especially during sit-to-stand and single- and double-leg squat activities.[38]

With the patient supine, knee flexion range of motion can be assessed by bringing the heel toward the buttock with the hip flexed. Trigger points in the vastus intermedius muscle can significantly restrict flexion range of motion at the knee. Typically, the heel does not reach the buttock by several fingerbreadths. However, TrPs in the vastus lateralis muscle also cause this restriction if the patella is hypomobile. Trigger points in the vastus medialis muscle cause minor restrictions of knee flexion range of motion. In order to fully assess the extensibility of the rectus femoris muscle, the patient must demonstrate simultaneous hip extension and knee flexion, as in the Thomas test (see Figure 56-6) or Ely test. Restriction of this range from muscle length deficits caused by TrPs in the rectus femoris muscle occurs commonly. A tight iliopsoas muscle group restricts extension at the hip, but does not affect flexion at the knee.

Hip abduction and adduction strength should be evaluated bilaterally as both sides are responsible for lumbopelvic stability at different times during the gait cycle. The strength of the quadriceps femoris muscles should be tested and compared to the unaffected side. Trigger points induce intermittent weakness inhibition of knee extension without muscle atrophy.[39] The presence of marked quadriceps femoris muscle atrophy is usually associated with knee joint pathology. Patients with patellofemoral pain syndrome exhibit quadriceps femoris muscle atrophy, though it is not clear if this atrophy is mostly related to the vastus medialis,[40] the vastus lateralis, or all the quadriceps femoris muscles.[41]

Clinicians may also consider performing isokinetic testing of the quadriceps femoris and hamstring muscles within the same limb to identify the hamstring:quadriceps femoris ratio. Aagaard et al[42] proposed considering functional ratios of strength in which eccentric hamstring:concentric quadriceps femoris identifies functional extension ratios, and concentric hamstrings:eccentric quadriceps femoris identifies functional flexion ratios. Increased muscle activity of the hamstring muscles, as well as coactivity of the quadriceps femoris and hamstring muscles, has been identified as factors for those with knee osteoarthritis.[43]

During accessory mobility testing of the patella, the knee should be fully extended and the quadriceps femoris muscle completely relaxed, as tension from the quadriceps femoris muscle can restrict passive accessory movement of the patella. Before examining for patellar mobility, the clinician should observe and palpate the resting position of the patella.[44] Trigger point–induced tension in the vastus medialis muscle can restrict lateral mobility of the patella. Trigger points in the distal portion of the vastus lateralis muscle reduces all normal accessory movement of the patella, including the inferior glide of at least 1 cm that occurs during effective knee flexion.

Sartorius TrPs are typically associated with quadriceps femoris TrPs. Patients with TrPs in the sartorius muscle may report having pain in the anterior and medial thigh and/or about the medial knee area. Trigger points in this muscle typically do not limit movement or cause mechanical dysfunction; therefore, range of motion is not restricted. Weakness and pain on loading the sartorius muscle can be tested with the patient in a seated position with the knee flexed to 90° while asking the patient to perform external rotation of the thigh at the hip against resistance. The pain caused by TrPs in the sartorius muscle is typically vague and more superficial than the pain caused by quadriceps TrPs.

3.4. Trigger Point Examination

Rectus Femoris

In most individuals, a cleft is palpable between the vastus medialis muscle and the medial border of the rectus femoris muscle. The lateral border of the rectus femoris muscle is usually palpable along the length of the anterolateral thigh. Borders of the muscle can be defined by asking the patient to perform a submaximal isometric contraction into knee extension.

Trigger points in the rectus femoris muscle are commonly located proximally in the muscle, close to the anterior inferior iliac spine, and can be identified with cross-fiber flat palpation (Figure 58-10A). The rectus femoris muscle is distinguished from the sartorius muscle by having the patient perform isometric knee extension without hip flexion. Of these two muscles, only the rectus femoris muscle extends the knee, whereas the sartorius becomes active with knee flexion. Trigger points may also be identified along the distal aspect of the rectus femoris muscle, not less than about 10 cm (4 in) above the superior border of the patella.

Vastus Intermedius

It is nearly impossible to palpate the individual taut bands of TrPs in the deep muscle mass of the vastus intermedius muscle, and the entire muscle feels tense deep to the rectus femoris muscle. When it is possible to palpate its TrPs, they are found by first locating the superior lateral border of the rectus femoris muscle and following it a short distance distally until the fingers feel a space that permits cross-fiber flat palpation very deep, close to the femur (Figure 58-10B). However, it is common that digital pressure on the muscle does not reproduce the TrP referred pain, whereas needle penetration of the TrP does reproduce it. Therefore, the role of these TrPs is easily underestimated. Because of the overlying fascia and muscle, what appear to be TrPs of only slight or moderate tenderness on palpation often prove very painful when penetrated by a filiform needle.

When both the rectus femoris and vastus intermedius muscles contain TrPs, inactivating those in the former makes it easier to locate those in the latter. The vastus intermedius muscle is more likely than the rectus femoris muscle to have TrPs located in the distal part of the muscle.

Vastus Medialis

For examination of the vastus medialis muscle, the patient should lie supine with the thigh of the symptomatic side placed in moderate abduction and the knee supported at about 30° of flexion. A pad or pillow under the knee improves the patient's comfort. Cross-fiber flat palpation is used to identify TrPs that are most commonly found close to the medial border of the muscle (Figure 58-10C). Distal TrPs can be the most troublesome and the ones most likely to cause buckling of the knee (Figure 58-10C). The adductor muscles are commonly involved when distal TrPs in the vastus medialis muscle are present.

A cluster of TrPs may also be located along the medial border of the muscle approximately where the transition to oblique fibers would be expected. The more proximal TrPs are likely to evoke referred pain and not buckling or giving way of the knee. These pain producers are commonly found at about mid-thigh near the medial border of the vastus medialis muscle next to the adductor muscles. Occasionally, a taut band can be palpated close to the

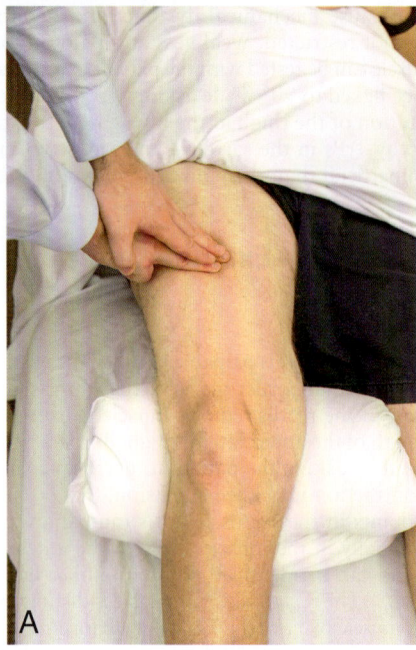
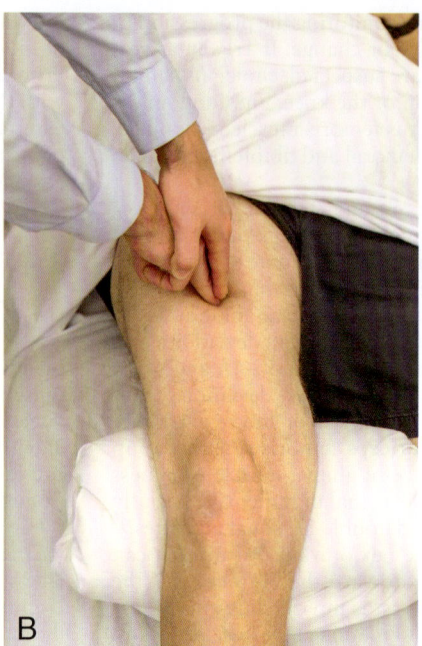
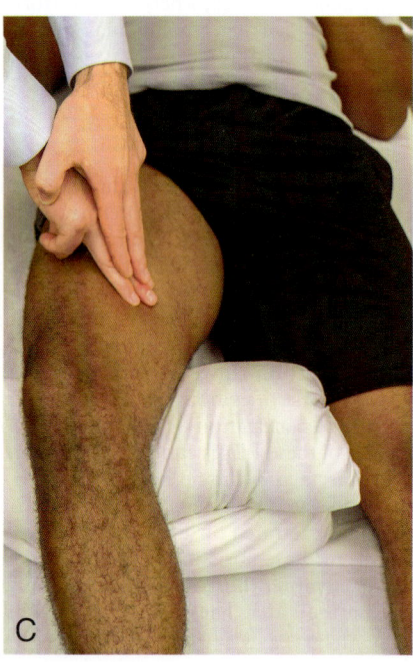
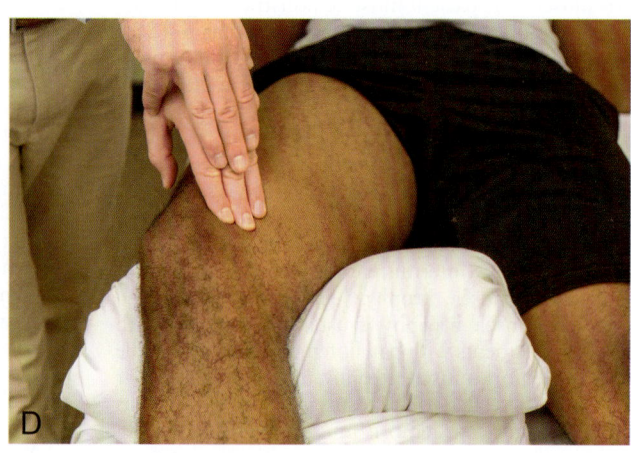

Figure 58-10. Cross-fiber flat palpation for trigger points in the quadriceps femoris muscle group. A, Rectus femoris muscle. B, Vastus intermedius muscle. C, Vastus medialis muscle (proximal). D, Vastus medialis muscle (distal).

linea aspera where the adductor magnus muscle also attaches. During palpation, pressure should be directed toward the femur to locate the taut band and to evoke a pattern of referred pain. Rozenfeld et al[45] have recently reported that examination of the vastus medialis muscle is reliable for the presence of latent and active TrPs showing kappa values ranging from 0.53 to 0.72.

Vastus Lateralis

For examination of the vastus lateralis muscle, the patient should assume the side-lying position with a pillow placed between the knees to keep the hip in neutral with the knees slightly flexed (Figure 58-11A to D). The vastus lateralis muscle, like the vastus intermedius muscle, usually has multiple TrPs, and many of them lie deep in the muscle. The taut bands of these TrPs can be located by cross-fiber flat palpation directly against the underlying bone (Figure 58-11A-C and E) or with a cross-fiber pincer palpation with the patient in side-lying or ¼ turned toward prone (Figure 58-11D and F). Taut bands of the vastus lateralis muscle are accessible from the anterior and posterior aspect of the iliotibial band (Figure 58-11B and C).

Trigger points in the distal aspect of the muscle can be identified while the patient lies with a relaxed, extended knee. The clinician may also depress the patella inferiorly and medially to palpate the vastus lateralis muscle in line with, and close to, the lateral border of the patella, in an area that the patella had covered before being depressed. Trigger points here often feel like an exquisitely tender hard knot.[39]

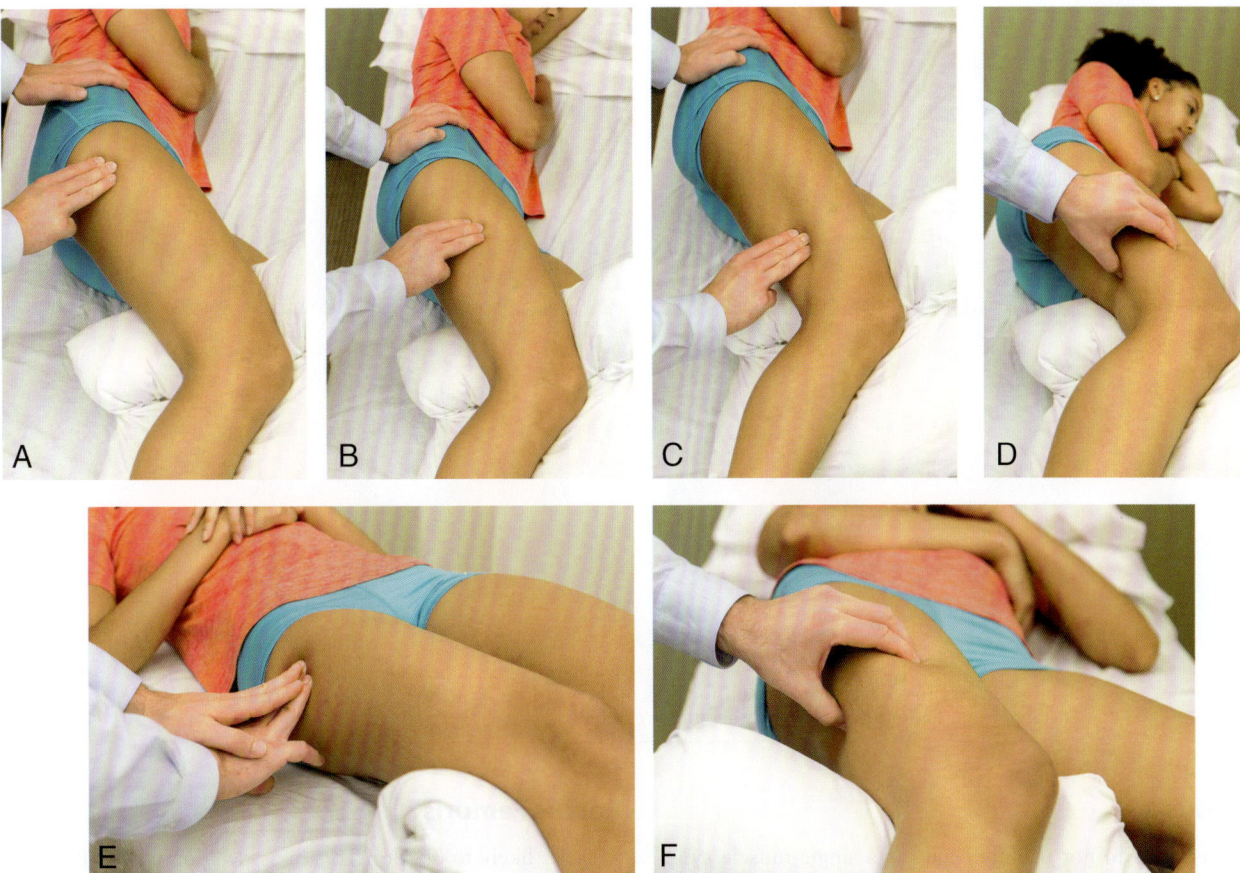

Figure 58-11. Palpation for TrPs in the vastus lateralis muscle. A, Side-lying cross-fiber flat palpation, proximal portion. B, Side-lying cross-fiber flat palpation, mid-portion anterior to iliotibial band (ITB). C, Side-lying cross-fiber flat palpation, distal portion posterior to ITB. D, Side-lying cross-fiber pincer palpation. E, Supine cross-fiber flat palpation mid-thigh. F, Supine ¼ turned pincer palpation.

Sartorius

The TrPs of the sartorius muscle are very superficial and easily missed. With the patient in a supine position, TrPs can be identified with cross-fiber flat palpation along the entire length of the muscle (Figure 58-12A and B). Local twitch responses elicited by snapping palpation at the TrP are often visible in this muscle. Confirmation of muscle location can be achieved by asking the patient to perform a gentle isometric hip external rotation and flexion contraction.

4. DIFFERENTIAL DIAGNOSIS

4.1. Activation and Perpetuation of Trigger Points

A posture or activity that activates a TrP, if not corrected, can also perpetuate it. In any part of the quadriceps femoris or sartorius muscles, TrPs may be activated by unaccustomed eccentric loading, eccentric exercise in an unconditioned muscle, or maximal or submaximal concentric loading.[46] Trigger points may also be activated or aggravated when the muscle is placed in a shortened and/or lengthened position for an extended period of time.

Quadriceps Femoris

The quadriceps femoris group is susceptible to activation of TrPs by an acute overload from a sudden vigorous eccentric contraction, such as stepping into a hole, stepping off the curb, or from stumbling (tripping). Direct trauma by impact against the femur can activate TrPs in any head of the quadriceps femoris muscle, most likely in the vastus lateralis muscle and least likely in the vastus intermedius muscle. Walking in high heel shoes or shoes with wedged-soles can also activate and perpetuate TrPs in the quadriceps femoris muscle group.

Acute or chronic overload can occur in an exercise program that includes deep squats. This exercise perpetuates quadriceps femoris TrPs, especially those in the vastus intermedius muscle. Another exercise that is likely to perpetuate TrPs in the quadriceps femoris muscle group is an attempt to strengthen the muscle utilizing open chain knee extension with a load at the ankles when TrPs are already present in the muscle. Other activities that can perpetuate TrPs in the quadriceps femoris muscles include skiing, sprinting, ascending/descending stairs, and walking downhill. Sporting activities such as kicking a football or soccer ball can overload the rectus femoris and sartorius muscles.

Immobilization is often an integral part of therapy for orthopedic problems of the lower extremity, such as knee or hip surgery. Often, after such surgeries or when in pain, patients will self-immobilize, holding the limb in a guarded position. Patients should be checked for TrPs before and after immobilization, especially if they are experiencing unexpected pain afterward. Prolonged sitting postures can also exacerbate TrPs of the quadriceps femoris muscles, such as sitting with one foot tucked under the buttock, sitting with a child sitting on the lap, or prolonged kneeling.

Indirectly, any traumatic event into the knee, such as surgery, can also activate TrPs in the quadriceps femoris muscle. In fact, it has been found that patients after a meniscectomy[47] or after reconstruction of an anterior cruciate ligament (ACL)[48] develop TrPs.

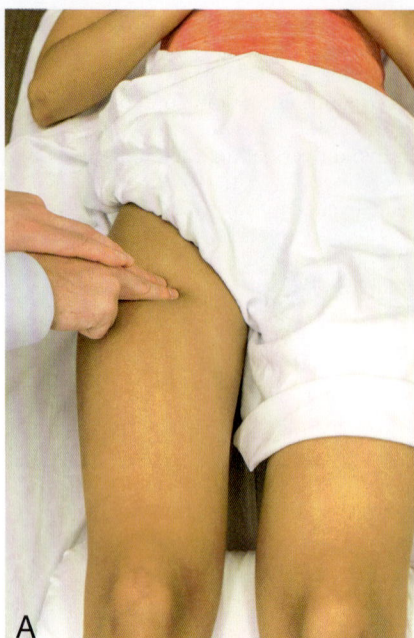 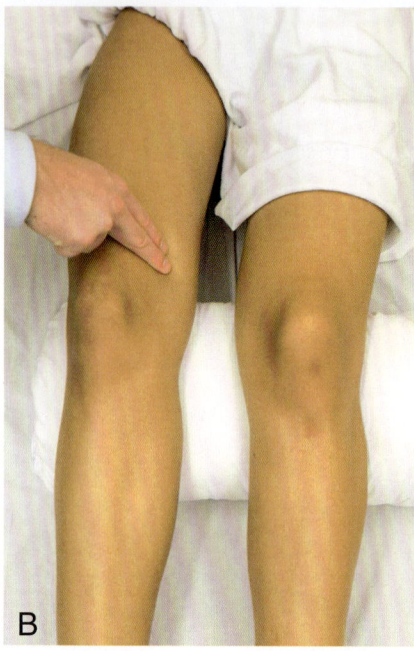

Figure 58-12. Cross-fiber flat palpation for TrPs in the sartorius muscle. A, Proximal portion. B, Distal portion. The entire muscle belly should be examined.

Sartorius

Sartorius TrPs do not usually occur as a single-muscle syndrome, but rather occur in conjunction with TrP involvement of related muscles especially the iliopsoas, tensor fasciae latae, gluteus medius, gluteus minimus, piriformis, adductors, and quadriceps femoris muscles. Sartorius TrPs usually develop when TrPs in other muscles of its functional unit are present. Occasionally, these TrPs may be initiated by an acute overload strain in a twisting fall or during activities that require the foot to be planted while the leg and trunk are rotated in the opposite direction. More often, TrPs in this muscle are activated from overload that occurs when walking with an excessively pronated foot.

4.2. Associated Trigger Points

Associated TrPs can develop in the referred pain areas caused by TrPs.[49] Therefore, musculature in the referred pain areas for each muscle should also be considered. Limitation of knee flexion due to TrPs in any one vastus muscle encourages the development of TrPs in the other two vasti muscles as well as the rectus femoris muscle. Shortening of the hamstring muscles due to TrPs, especially in the biceps femoris muscle, overloads the antagonistic quadriceps femoris muscle; when the hamstring muscles have TrPs, usually the quadriceps femoris group will also have associated TrPs. The quadriceps femoris muscle group cannot recover until the hamstring TrPs are alleviated or hamstring length deficits are addressed. The patient may report pain referred from the quadriceps femoris TrPs, not from the hamstring TrPs that are the perpetuating factor. Quadriceps femoris TrPs are also perpetuated by overload resulting from TrPs in the soleus muscle. Soleus TrPs restrict ankle dorsiflexion, and this limitation can overload the quadriceps femoris muscles, especially when lifting with a sound squat form. Trigger points in the gluteus minimus, tensor fasciae latae, iliopsoas, and adductor muscles can also cause associated TrPs in the quadriceps femoris and sartorius muscles as these muscles lie within their referred pain pattern zone.

Rectus Femoris

Muscles likely to develop TrPs in association with TrPs in the rectus femoris muscle include the three vasti and iliopsoas muscles. The vastus intermedius muscle is the muscle most likely to be involved, and the vastus medialis muscle is the least likely. Proximal TrPs in the sartorius muscle may also appear.

Vastus Intermedius

The rectus femoris and vastus lateralis muscles of the quadriceps femoris group are the agonists most likely also to be involved when the vastus intermedius muscle develops TrPs.

Vastus Medialis

The vastus medialis muscle is the member of the quadriceps femoris muscle group that is most likely to develop TrPs in the absence of TrPs in the other three heads. Such TrPs are often associated with a Morton foot structure that may also lead to the development of TrPs in the peroneus longus and gluteus medius muscles.

Trigger points in the vastus medialis muscle are often associated with TrPs in the hip adductor and tensor fasciae latae muscles.

Vastus Lateralis

Trigger points in the vastus lateralis muscle are often associated with TrPs in the gluteus medius or tensor fasciae latae muscles.

Sartorius

Sartorius TrPs are likely to be observed in conjunction with TrPs in other muscles of the functional unit, such as the rectus femoris and vastus medialis muscles. Sartorius TrPs may also be associated with TrPs in its antagonists, the hip adductor muscles.

4.3. Associated Pathology

Patellofemoral pain syndrome refers to anterior knee pain localized around the patella and has been otherwise identified in previous research as chondromalacia patellae, patellar tracking dysfunction, patellar tendinopathy, and anterior knee pain syndrome. This pathology is characterized by pain around or behind the patella that is aggravated by activities that increase flexion and/or loading of the knee. Patellofemoral pain syndrome is commonly found in women, sedentary individuals, athletes, and young adults. There are several contributing factors that have been identified in patellofemoral pain syndrome, such as weak quadriceps femoris muscles (especially vastus medialis muscle), weak hip external rotators, hyperpronation or pes planus, increased Q-angle, and anteversion of the femoral head.[50,51] Some literature identifies weakness and dysfunction of the quadriceps femoris muscles found in patellofemoral pain syndrome and relates these findings to the presence of TrPs that cause muscle inhibition and reduced strength and flexibility.[52,53] With referred pain patterns similar to those experienced with patellofemoral pain syndrome, TrPs in the quadriceps femoris muscles, particularly those from the vastus medialis muscle, should also be considered as a potential source of the patient's pain and dysfunction.

The clinical features of patellar tendinopathy are pain with quadriceps femoris muscle loading and pain located at the inferior pole of the patella. A thorough clinical examination is required as patients can have a positive MRI indicating patellar tendinopathy and experience no pain. In light of these false positives, the clinical examination and patient reported symptoms are essential for making this diagnosis. This condition is best managed through close monitoring of knee extensor tendon loading, which has a very slow rehabilitation process and may be complicated by lower extremity biomechanical faults and muscle imbalances.[54]

Knee osteoarthritis can lead to early changes in knee extensor muscle function possibly because of TrP activity in the quadriceps femoris muscle group. Kemnitz et al[55] investigated changes in thigh muscle strength prior to, and concurrent with, symptomatic and radiographic evidence of knee osteoarthritis progression in both men and women. The results of their study revealed a loss of both knee extensor and flexor strength concurrent with the progression of symptoms in women but not in men. This loss of strength that occurs with the progression of knee osteoarthritis seems specific to women.[55] In this population of patients, it is important to examine for the presence of TrPs in the quadriceps femoris, hip adductors, sartorius, hamstrings, gastrocnemius, soleus, and popliteus muscles. In fact, there is evidence to support the role of active TrPs in pain and disability related to knee osteoarthritis.[56]

Lateral thigh pain characteristic of proximal vastus lateralis TrPs is commonly misdiagnosed as trochanteric bursitis because of referred pain and referred tenderness in the area of the greater trochanter. A similar pain pattern may also be caused by TrPs in the anterior portion of the gluteus minimus muscle or by TrPs in the tensor fasciae latae muscle. Further, the referred pain pattern of vastus lateralis muscle may mimic the pain of iliotibial band dysfunction that commonly occurs at the lateral knee.[57]

Many patients with diabetes mellitus are taught to inject insulin into the lateral aspect or midline of the thigh, and patients can develop TrPs in the rectus femoris or vastus lateralis muscles where they inject themselves. Injection of insulin or other drugs in the region of a latent TrP can activate it. Quadriceps femoris myofibrosis can result from repeated intramuscular injections.[58]

Sartorius

A sartorius TrP can be discovered serendipitously during injection or dry needling of a vastus medialis TrP deep to the sartorius muscle. When the needle encounters superficial sartorius TrPs, the patient reports a sharp or tingling pain felt diffusely over the adjacent thigh. The pain from sartorius TrPs referred to the knee may also be mistaken for pathology of that joint.[35]

5. CORRECTIVE ACTIONS

In patients with quadriceps femoris TrPs, two guiding principles require attention: to avoid shortening and/or prolonged immobilization of the quadriceps femoris muscle group and to avoid overloading these muscles. Deep squatting should be prohibited for patients with quadriceps femoris TrPs. These maneuvers can cause serious overload of the quadriceps femoris muscles during the initial effort to rise unassisted. In the squatting position, the quadriceps femoris muscle has a poor mechanical advantage. A partial squat, or a partial knee-bend, is relatively safe and recommended.[20] Until TrPs and pain in the quadriceps femoris muscle group have resolved, it is important for the patient to avoid overloading these muscles when rising from a seated position. To accomplish this, the patient can use the upper limbs to assist by pushing against an armrest of the chair with one hand and against the distal thigh with the other hand; if no armrests are available, the hands push against both thighs distally. An alternate strategy for sit-to-stand is illustrated in Figure 58-13. The buttocks are first slid forward to the front of the seat. Then the body is turned sideways about 45° and the affected side foot is placed under the front edge of the seat and under the center of gravity of the body. The body is then lifted with the torso slightly flexed forward, so that the load is placed mainly on the gluteus maximus muscle of the forward leg. A push by the hands against the thighs assists the lift if the quadriceps femoris muscles are weak. To return to the seated position, the sequence would be reversed with the use of the hands on the thighs to lower to the chair.

During sitting, one should avoid hip flexion with the knees extended, as occurs in many automobiles with tall seats or when resting feet on an ottoman or in a recliner. Automatic cruise control can be helpful by permitting more flexibility in positioning the right foot on the accelerator pedal during long car trips. Any long trip should be split up by a rest and stretch stop at least every hour. Conversely, habitually sitting with one foot flexed under the other buttock immobilizes the quadriceps femoris and sartorius muscles for long periods. When patients have TrPs in the vastus medialis muscle, they should avoid kneeling on the floor, but rather they should sit on a low bench or box.

To avoid maintaining the quadriceps femoris and sartorius muscles in a shortened position at night, it is important to avoid marked hip flexion with full knee flexion or extension. When in the side-lying position, a pillow should be placed between the knees. This can reduce pressure on the area of referred tenderness over the knee as well as on the muscle itself when there are TrPs in the vastus medialis or sartorius muscles. This position also avoids putting the vastus lateralis muscle in a stretch position. Patients with vastus lateralis TrPs should avoid sleeping on their affected side because the resulting pressure can be enough to irritate or activate the TrPs. For sleeping on the back, a pillow may be placed under the entire leg, but placing a pillow under the knee alone should be avoided.

The self-pressure release of TrPs in the quadriceps femoris muscles can be achieved with the utilization of a TrP release tool, tennis ball, or a lacrosse ball. To perform TrP self-pressure release with a TrP tool, the patient is seated (Figure 58-14A to E). Finding the sensitive spot with the tool, the patient should apply light pressure (no more than 4/10 pain), hold for 15 to 30 seconds until pain reduces, and repeat five times. This technique can be repeated several times per day. When using a TrP release roller, the patient can work from the top part of the muscle and slowly roll down the muscle until a tender point is felt. When one is encountered, one should stop and slowly rock over the area or pause to wait for it to release prior to moving to the next area. Pressure should be mildly uncomfortable but not overly painful (Figure 58-14A, C, and E).

A tennis or lacrosse ball can be used on the vastus lateralis muscle in side-lying with a pillow between the knees and the

618 Section 6: Hip, Thigh, and Knee Pain

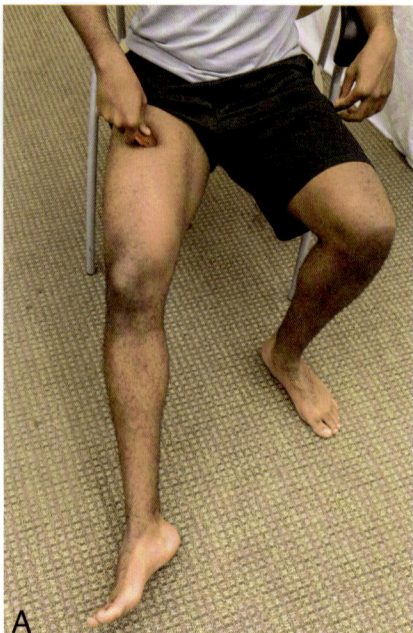
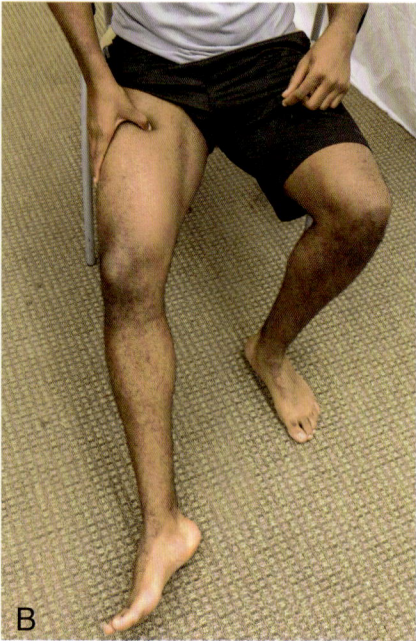

Figure 58-15. Trigger point self-pressure release of the sartorius muscle. A, Trigger point release tool. B, Self-manual release with thumb.

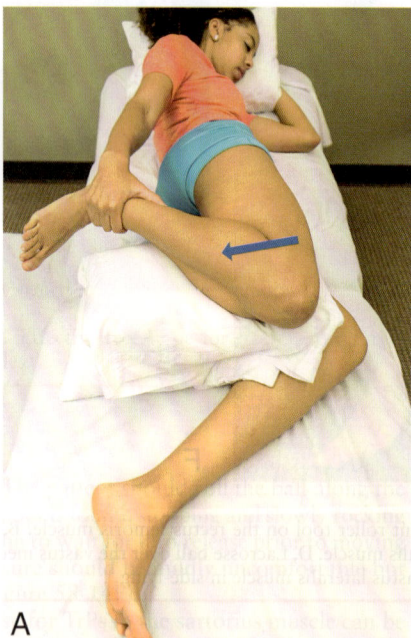
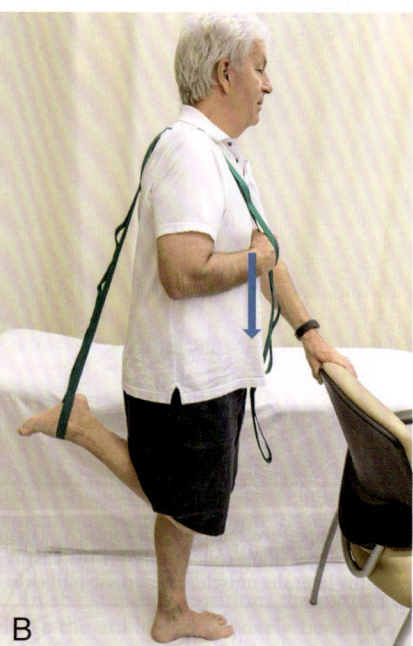

Figure 58-16. Self-stretch of the quadriceps femoris muscle group. A, Side-lying self-stretch for the rectus femoris muscle. The unaffected leg should be placed in hip flexion to stabilize the pelvis. The patient passively brings the heel of the affected leg toward the buttock while maintaining and then increasing hip extension; the hand holds the ankle. B, Standing self-stretch for the quadriceps femoris muscle using a strap around the ankle to assist in maintaining an erect posture.

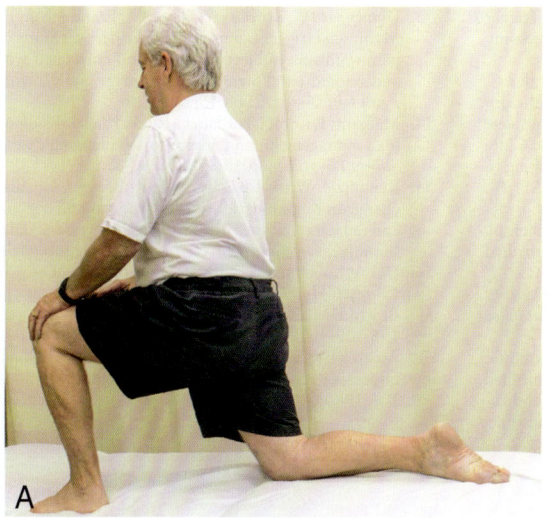
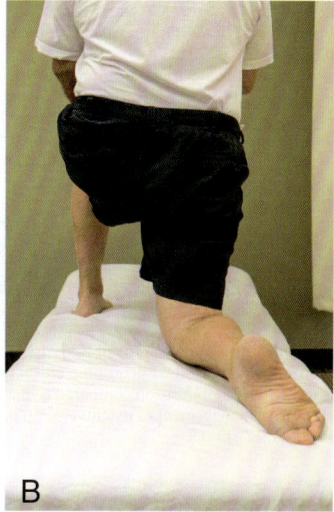

Figure 58-17. Self-stretch of the sartorius muscle in half-kneeling. A, Starting position. B, The hip and thigh are placed in internal rotation and adduction. The patient leans slightly on the affected knee. A stretch should be felt on the front side of the hip.

References

1. Standring S. *Gray's Anatomy: The Anatomical Basis of Clinical Practice.* 41st ed. London, UK: Elsevier; 2015.
2. Travnik L, Pernus F, Erzen I. Histochemical and morphometric characteristics of the normal human vastus medialis longus and vastus medialis obliquus muscles. *J Anat.* 1995;187(pt 2):403-411.
3. Roberts VI, Mereddy PK, Donnachie NJ, Hakkalamani S. Anatomical variations in vastus medialis obliquus and its implications in minimally-invasive total knee replacement. An MRI study. *J Bone Joint Surg Br.* 2007;89(11):1462-1465.
4. Smith TO, Nichols R, Harle D, Donell ST. Do the vastus medialis obliquus and vastus medialis longus really exist? A systematic review. *Clin Anat.* 2009;22(2):183-199.
5. Becker I, Woodley SJ, Baxter GD. Gross morphology of the vastus lateralis muscle: an anatomical review. *Clin Anat.* 2009;22(4):436-450.
6. Grob K, Ackland T, Kuster MS, Manestar M, Filgueira L. A newly discovered muscle: the tensor of the vastus intermedius. *Clin Anat.* 2016;29(2):256-263.
7. Grob K, Manestar M, Gascho D, et al. Magnetic resonance imaging of the tensor vastus intermedius: a topographic study based on anatomical dissections. *Clin Anat.* 2017;30(8):1096-1102.
8. Dziedzic D, Bogacka U, Ciszek B. Anatomy of sartorius muscle. *Folia Morphol (Warsz).* 2014;73(3):359-362.
9. Günal I, Arac S, Sahinoglu K, Birvar K. The innervation of vastus medialis obliquus. *J Bone Joint Surg Br.* 1992;74(4):624.
10. Jojima H, Whiteside LA, Ogata K. Anatomic consideration of nerve supply to the vastus medialis in knee surgery. *Clin Orthop Relat Res.* 2004(423):157-160.
11. Taylor GI, Razaboni RM. *Michael Salmon: Anatomic Studies. Book 1, Arteries of the Muscles of the Extremities and the Trunk.* St Louis, MO: Quality Medical Publishing; 1994.
12. von Lassberg C, Schneid JA, Graf D, Finger F, Rapp W, Stutzig N. Longitudinal sequencing in intramuscular coordination: a new hypothesis of dynamic functions in the human rectus femoris muscle. *PLoS One.* 2017;12(8):e0183204.
13. Duarte Cintra AI, Furlani J. Electromyographic study of quadriceps femoris in man. *Electromyogr Clin Neurophysiol.* 1981;21(6):539-554.
14. Deutsch H, Lin DC. Quadriceps kinesiology (emg) with varying hip joint flexion and resistance. *Arch Phys Med Rehabil.* 1978;59(5):231-236.
15. Peeler J, Cooper J, Porter MM, Thliveris JA, Anderson JE. Structural parameters of the vastus medialis muscle. *Clin Anat.* 2005;18(4):281-289.
16. Waligora AC, Johanson NA, Hirsch BE. Clinical anatomy of the quadriceps femoris and extensor apparatus of the knee. *Clin Orthop Relat Res.* 2009;467(12):3297-3306.
17. Ng GY, Zhang AQ, Li CK. Biofeedback exercise improved the EMG activity ratio of the medial and lateral vasti muscles in subjects with patellofemoral pain syndrome. *J Electromyogr Kinesiol.* 2008;18(1):128-133.
18. Elias JJ, Kilambi S, Goerke DR, Cosgarea AJ. Improving vastus medialis obliquus function reduces pressure applied to lateral patellofemoral cartilage. *J Orthop Res.* 2009;27(5):578-583.
19. Townsend MA, Lainhart SP, Shiavi R, Caylor J. Variability and biomechanics of synergy patterns of some lower-limb muscles during ascending and descending stairs and level walking. *Med Biol Eng Comput.* 1978;16(6):681-688.
20. Jaberzadeh S, Yeo D, Zoghi M. The effect of altering knee position and squat depth on VMO: VL EMG ratio during squat exercises. *Physiother Res Int.* 2016;21(3):164-173.
21. Ghori GM, Luckwill RG. Responses of the lower limb to load carrying in walking man. *Eur J Appl Physiol Occup Physiol.* 1985;54(2):145-150.
22. Milner M, Basmajian JV, Quanbury AO. Multifactorial analysis of walking by electromyography and computer. *Am J Phys Med.* 1971;50(5):235-258.
23. Yang JF, Winter DA. Surface EMG profiles during different walking cadences in humans. *Electroencephalogr Clin Neurophysiol.* 1985;60(6):485-491.
24. Joseph J. The pattern of activity of some muscles in women walking on high heels. *Ann Phys Med.* 1968;9(7):295-299.
25. Sutherland DH, Cooper L, Daniel D. The role of the ankle plantar flexors in normal walking. *J Bone Joint Surg Am Vol.* 1980;62(3):354-363.
26. Ericson MO, Nisell R, Arborelius UP, Ekholm J. Muscular activity during ergometer cycling. *Scand J Rehabil Med.* 1985;17(2):53-61.
27. Ericson M. On the biomechanics of cycling. A study of joint and muscle load during exercise on the bicycle ergometer. *Scand J Rehabil Med Suppl.* 1986;16:1-43.
28. Andriacchi TP, Andersson GB, Ortengren R, Mikosz RP. A study of factors influencing muscle activity about the knee joint. *J Orthop Res.* 1984;1(3):266-275.
29. Johnson CE, Basmajian JV, Dasher W. Electromyography of sartorius muscle. *Anat Rec.* 1972;173(2):127-130.
30. Perry J, Burnfield JM. *Hip. Gait Analysis: Normal and Pathological Function.* 2nd ed. Thorofare, NJ: SLACK; 2010.
31. Simons DG, Travell J, Simons L. *Travell & Simon's Myofascial Pain and Dysfunction: The Trigger Point Manual.* Vol 1. 2nd ed. Baltimore, MD: Williams & Wilkins; 1999 (p. 104).
32. Kellgren JH. Observations on referred pain arising from muscle. *Clin Sci.* 1938;3:175-190.
33. Nguyen BM. Myofascial trigger point, falls in the elderly, idiopathic knee pain and osteoarthritis: an alternative concept. *Med Hypotheses.* 2013;80(6):806-809.
34. Good MG. What is fibrositis? *Rheumatism.* 1949;5(4):117-123.
35. Reynolds MD. Myofascial trigger point syndromes in the practice of rheumatology. *Arch Phys Med Rehabil.* 1981;62(3):111-114.
36. Baker BA. Myofascial pain syndromes: ten single muscle cases. *J Neurol Orthop Med Surg.* 1989;10:129-131.
37. Porterfield JA, DeRosa C. *Mechanical Low Back Pain: Perspectives in Functional Anatomy.* 2nd ed. Philadelphia, PA: Saunders; 1998.
38. Slater LV, Hart JM. Muscle activation patterns during different squat techniques. *J Strength Cond Res.* 2017;31(3):667-676.
39. Nielsen AJ. Spray and stretch for myofascial pain. *Phys Ther.* 1978;58(5):567-569.
40. Pattyn E, Verdonk P, Steyaert A, et al. Vastus medialis obliquus atrophy: does it exist in patellofemoral pain syndrome? *Am J Sports Med.* 2011;39(7):1450-1455.
41. Giles LS, Webster KE, McClelland JA, Cook J. Does quadriceps atrophy exist in individuals with patellofemoral pain? A systematic literature review with meta-analysis. *J Orthop Sports Phys Ther.* 2013;43(11):766-776.
42. Aagaard P, Simonsen EB, Magnusson SP, Larsson B, Dyhre-Poulsen P. A new concept for isokinetic hamstring: quadriceps muscle strength ratio. *Am J Sports Med.* 1998;26(2):231-237.
43. Hortobagyi T, Westerkamp L, Beam S, et al. Altered hamstring-quadriceps muscle balance in patients with knee osteoarthritis. *Clin Biomech (Bristol, Avon).* 2005;20(1):97-104.
44. Miller GM. Resident review #24: subluxation of the patella. *Orthop Rev.* 1980;9:65-76.
45. Rozenfeld E, Finestone AS, Moran U, Damri E, Kalichman L. Test-retest reliability of myofascial trigger point detection in hip and thigh areas. *J Bodyw Mov Ther.* 2017;21(4):914-919.
46. Gerwin RD, Dommerholt J, Shah JP. An expansion of Simons' integrated hypothesis of trigger point formation. *Curr Pain Headache Rep.* 2004;8(6):468-475.

47. Torres-Chica B, Nunez-Samper-Pizarroso C, Ortega-Santiago R, et al. Trigger points and pressure pain hypersensitivity in people with postmeniscectomy pain. *Clin J Pain*. 2015;31(3):265-272.
48. Velazquez-Saornil J, Ruiz-Ruiz B, Rodriguez-Sanz D, Romero-Morales C, Lopez-Lopez D, Calvo-Lobo C. Efficacy of quadriceps vastus medialis dry needling in a rehabilitation protocol after surgical reconstruction of complete anterior cruciate ligament rupture. *Medicine (Baltimore)*. 2017;96(17):e6726.
49. Hsieh YL, Kao MJ, Kuan TS, Chen SM, Chen JT, Hong CZ. Dry needling to a key myofascial trigger point may reduce the irritability of satellite MTrPs. *Am J Phys Med Rehabil*. 2007;86(5):397-403.
50. Crossley K, Bennell K, Green S, Cowan S, McConnell J. Physical therapy for patellofemoral pain: a randomized, double-blinded, placebo-controlled trial. *Am J Sports Med*. 2002;30(6):857-865.
51. Heintjes E, Berger MY, Bierma-Zeinstra SM, Bernsen RM, Verhaar JA, Koes BW. Exercise therapy for patellofemoral pain syndrome. *Cochrane Database Syst Rev*. 2003(4):CD003472.
52. Stakes N, Myburgh C, Brantingham J, Moyer R, Jensen M, Globe G. A prospective randomized clinical trial to determine efficacy of combined spinal manipulation and patella mobilization compared to patella mobilization alone in the conservative management of patellofemoral pain syndrome. *J Amer Chir Assoc*. 2006;43(7):11-18.
53. Dippenaar DL, Korporaal C, Jones A, Brantingham JW, Globe G, Snyder WR. Myofascial trigger points in the quadriceps femoris muscle of patellofemoral pain syndrome subjects assessed and correlated with NRS-101, algometry, and piloted patellofemoral pain severity and myofascial diagnostic scales *J Am Chir Assoc*. 2008;45(2):16-18.
54. Malliaras P, Cook J, Purdam C, Rio E. Patellar tendinopathy: clinical diagnosis, load management, and advice for challenging case presentations. *J Orthop Sports Phys Ther*. 2015;45(11):887-898.
55. Kemnitz J, Wirth W, Eckstein F, Ruhdorfer A, Culvenor AG. Longitudinal change in thigh muscle strength prior to and concurrent with symptomatic and radiographic knee osteoarthritis progression: data from the Osteoarthritis Initiative. *Osteoarthritis Cartilage*. 2017;25(10):1633-1640.
56. Dor A, Kalichman L. A myofascial component of pain in knee osteoarthritis. *J Bodyw Mov Ther*. 2017;21(3):642-647.
57. Brody DM. Running injuries. Prevention and management. *Clin Symp*. 1987;39(3):1-36.
58. Alvarez EV, Munters M, Lavine LS, Manes H, Waxman J. Quadriceps myofibrosis. A complication of intramuscular injections. *J Bone Joint Surg Am Vol*. 1980;62(1):58-60.

Chapter 59

Adductor Longus, Adductor Brevis, Adductor Magnus, Pectineus, and Gracilis Muscles

"Obvious Problem Makers"

N. Beth Collier and Joseph M. Donnelly

1. INTRODUCTION

The adductor muscles lie in the medial thigh between the quadriceps femoris muscle group anteriorly and the hamstring muscles posteriorly. The most anterior of the three major adductor muscles is the adductor longus muscle; the adductor brevis muscle is intermediate, and the adductor magnus muscle is the most posterior. The pectineus muscle lies partly anterior and superior to the adductor brevis muscle. The gracilis muscle is the only one of this muscle group that crosses two joints—the hip and the knee. Trigger points (TrPs) in these muscles can present as medial thigh pain, groin pain, pelvic pain, and/or anterior-medial knee pain. Activities that cause the adductor muscles to be overstretched will activate TrPs in this muscle group in addition to activities such as hiking up hill, horseback riding, and gymnastics. Clinicians should consider TrPs in the adductor muscles when suspecting a diagnosis of hip osteoarthritis, inguinal or sports hernia, pubic bone stress injury (osteitis pubis), or a hip labral tear. In treating TrPs in the adductor muscle group, patients may find relief in performing self-pressure release, self-stretch of the involved muscle, and correcting faulty static and dynamic postures that contribute to overuse or shortening of these muscles.

2. ANATOMIC CONSIDERATIONS

Adductor Longus

The adductor longus muscle is the most superficial and prominent of the three major adductor muscles in the anteromedial aspect of the thigh. It attaches proximally by a narrow flat tendon to a relatively small spot on the outer surface of the pelvis between the symphysis pubis and the obturator foramen (Figure 59-1).[1] Its fibers angle inferolaterally and posteriorly to anchor to its insertion at the linea aspera on the middle third of the femur. The fibers of the adductor longus muscle often blend with those of the vastus medialis muscle distally at their femoral attachment. The adductor longus muscle may unite superiorly with the pectineus muscle, in which case they completely cover the adductor brevis muscle. Superiorly, there appears to be secondary anatomic continuity between the proximal anterior fibers of the adductor longus tendon and the distal attachment of the rectus abdominis muscle as well as the capsule of the pubic symphysis.[2,3]

Adductor Brevis

Viewed from the front, the adductor brevis muscle is partially covered by the pectineus muscle proximally and by the adductor longus muscle distally (Figure 59-2). It is sandwiched between these two adductor muscles anteriorly and the adductor magnus muscle posteriorly. The adductor brevis muscle attaches proximally to the inferior ramus of the pubis and distally to the linea aspera just posterolateral to the adductor longus muscle. Often, the adductor brevis muscle has multiple separate parts or may blend with the adductor magnus muscle.[1]

Adductor Magnus

The adductor magnus muscle is a large, triangular, and a deeply located muscle that has three parts: the most anterior and superior part, the middle part, and the posteriorly positioned, largely ischiocondylar, third part (Figure 59-3). The most superior of the three parts of the adductor magnus muscle, often known as the adductor minimus muscle, attaches to the inferior pubic ramus of the pelvis, anterior to the attachment of the middle part. Its fibers are the most horizontal as they angle toward its lateral attachment to the femur just inferior to the lesser trochanter of the femur and extending down along the linea aspera. The adductor minimus muscle usually constitutes its own muscle belly.[1]

The middle part is fan shaped and may overlap the adductor minimus muscle posteriorly. If so, these intermediate fibers run more diagonally from the ischial ramus to the linea aspera to the tendinous (adductor) hiatus, through which the femoral vessels pass. An upward extension of this hiatus often clearly separates the middle and posterior parts of the adductor magnus muscle.

Proximally, the bulk of the third (most posterior or ischiocondylar) portion attaches to the ischial tuberosity and along the ischial ramus, largely posterior to the other two portions of the muscle. Distally, most of the ischiocondylar part inserts by a thick tendon to the adductor tubercle on the medial condyle of the femur. A few fibers attach to a fibrous expansion that completes the space between the adductor tubercle and the tendinous (adductor) hiatus.[1] This part of the adductor magnus muscle is similar to a hamstring muscle except that it does not cross the knee joint. The vastus medialis muscle attaches medially to all of the adductor muscles, thus covering the lower part of the adductor longus and adductor magnus muscles anteriorly.

The adductor canal (Hunter's canal) is an intermuscular tunnel spanning the distal two-thirds of the medial aspect of the thigh. The adductor hiatus marks the distal (outlet) of the adductor canal that begins proximally at the apex of the femoral triangle. The adductor canal is covered by a fascial layer deep to the sartorius muscle and is bounded anteriorly and laterally by the vastus medialis muscle and posteriorly by the adductor longus and adductor magnus muscles. The canal contains the femoral artery, femoral vein, and the saphenous nerve.[1]

Pectineus

The pectineus muscle is a flat, quadrangular muscle that comprises most of the medial floor of the femoral triangle. It attaches proximally to the pectin pubis deep to the inguinal ligament and

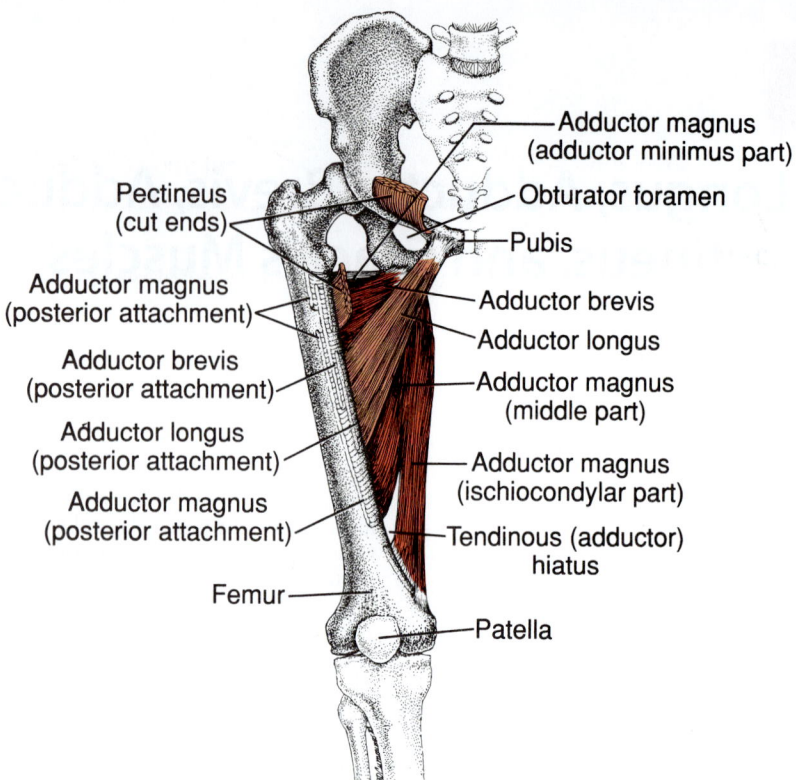

Figure 59-1. Attachments of the right adductor muscle group, anterior view. The pectineus muscle is cut and largely removed (light red). The most superficial adductor muscle, the adductor longus muscle, is also light red. The adductor brevis muscle (medium red) extends distally only to the middle section of the femoral attachment of the adductor longus muscle and deep to it. The adductor magnus muscle (dark red) is the deepest (most posterior) and the largest of the adductor muscles.

may be wholly or partially attached to the hip capsule. Its fibers descend posteromedially and then posterolaterally to eventually attach in a line from the lesser trochanter to the linea aspera on the femur. The pectineus muscle covers the proximal fibers of the adductor brevis muscle (Figure 59-4). The pectineus muscle may be bilaminar, consisting of a ventral and dorsal layer that may be separately innervated and may include the pectineus muscle in the anterior compartment of the thigh.[1]

Gracilis

The gracilis muscle is superficial and extends the length of the medial aspect of the thigh, crossing two joints, the hip, and the knee (Figure 59-5). It attaches proximally to the lower rim of the outside of the pelvis at the junction of the body of the pubis and the inferior pubic ramus as well as the adjoining part of the ischial ramus.[1] The gracilis muscle inserts distal to the medial tibial condyle on the medial surface of the tibia. Here, its tendon joins the sartorius and semitendinosus tendons to form the pes anserinus. The pes anserine bursa lies between these tendons and the tibia. Some fibers from the distal tendon extend and are continuous with the deep fascia of the leg and can blend with the medial head of the gastrocnemius muscle.[1]

2.1. Innervation and Vascularization

Adductor Longus

The adductor longus muscle is supplied by the anterior division of the obturator nerve from the L2, L3, and L4 spinal nerves. Its vascular supply consists of the "artery to the adductors" of the profunda artery. Additionally, the proximal portion receives a supply from the medial circumflex femoral artery and a distal supply from the femoral artery.[1]

Adductor Brevis

The adductor brevis muscle is innervated by the obturator nerve from the L2 and L3 spinal nerves. Its vascular supply is from the obturator artery at the deep surface, the profunda femoris artery distally, and the "artery to the adductors" more proximally. There may be an additional proximal supply from the medial circumflex femoral artery.[1]

Adductor Magnus

The superior (adductor minimus muscle) and middle parts of the adductor magnus muscle are supplied by the anterior division of the obturator nerve, and the ischiocondylar part is supplied by the tibial division of the sciatic nerve, both from the L2, L3, and L4 spinal nerves.[1] The vascular supply of the adductor magnus muscle is also divided into anterior and posterior aspects. Anteriorly, the obturator, profunda femoris, and femoral arteries all contribute to the primary supply coming directly from the distal part of the profunda femoris artery. There may also be vascular contributions to the distal aspect of the adductor magnus muscle from the femoral and descending genicular arteries. The medial circumflex femoral, the first and second perforating, and the popliteal arteries supply the adductor magnus muscle posteriorly.[1]

Pectineus

The pectineus muscle is innervated by the femoral nerve from L2 and L3 and the accessory obturator nerve, L3. If the pectineus

Chapter 59: Adductor Longus, Adductor Brevis, Adductor Magnus, Pectineus, and Gracilis Muscles   **623**

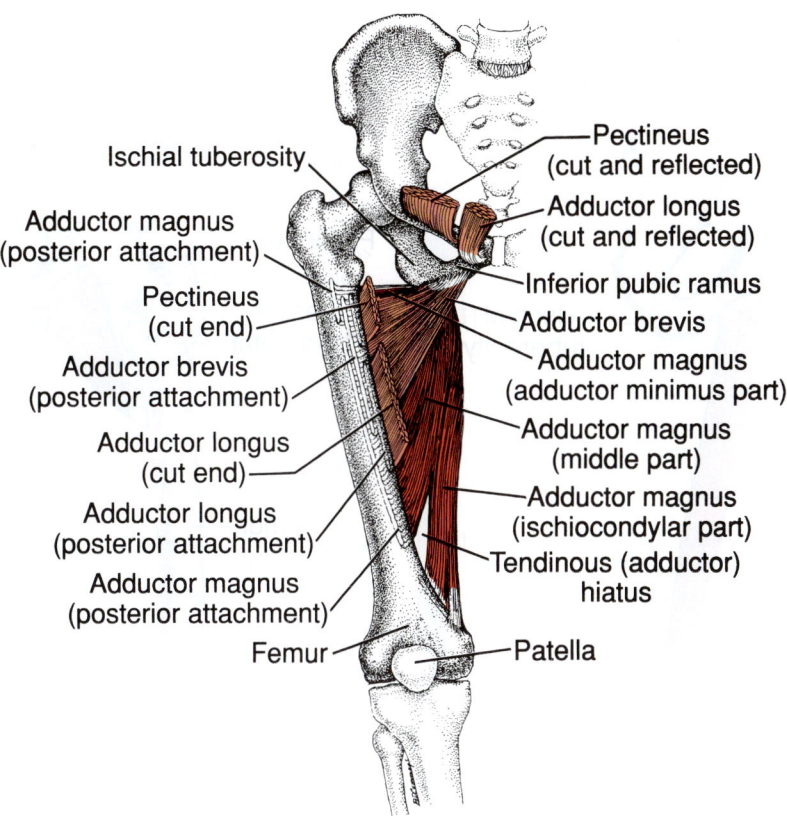

Figure 59-2. Attachments of the right deep adductor muscles, anterior view. The overlying pectineus and adductor longus muscles have been cut and the ends reflected (light red). The adductor brevis muscle (medium red) lies anterior to the larger adductor magnus muscle (dark red). Attachments of the adductor muscles to the posterior aspect of the femur, not in view, are rendered schematically.

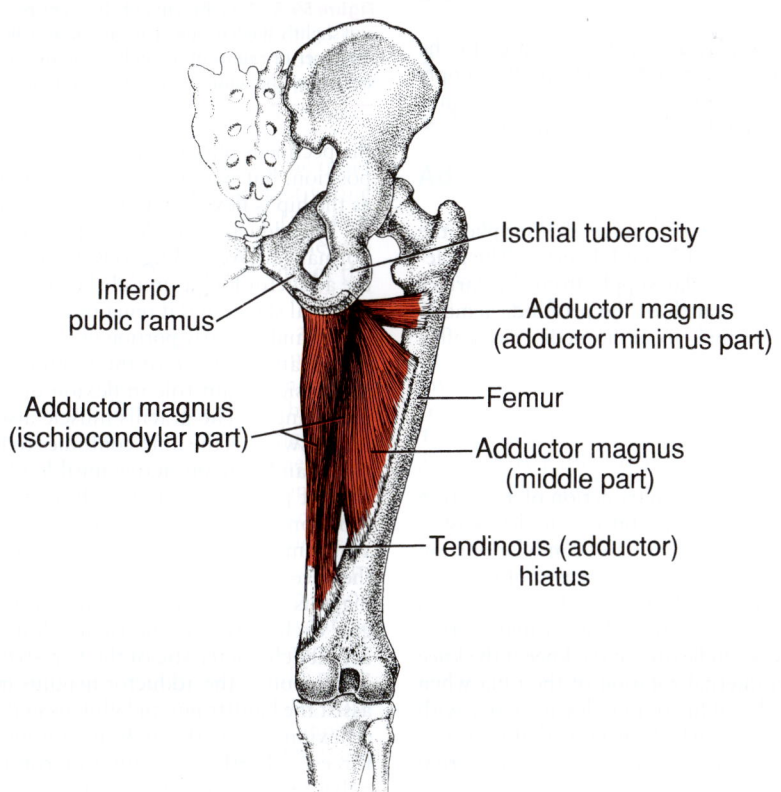

Figure 59-3. Attachments (posterior view) of the right adductor magnus muscle (red) showing the distinctions among its three parts.

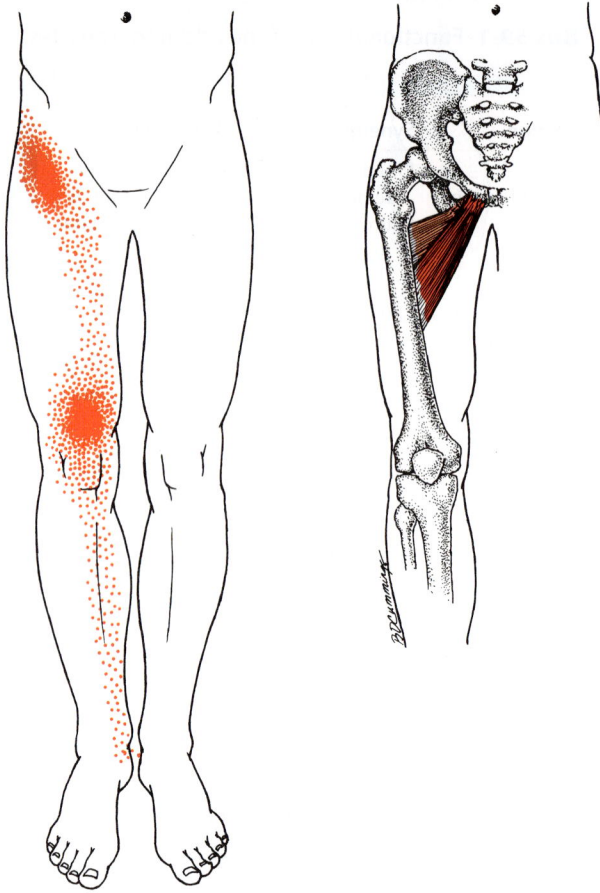

Figure 59-6. Anterior view of the right adductor longus and adductor brevis muscles and the composite pain pattern (dark red) referred from TrPs in these two muscles (light red). The essential pain pattern is solid red; red stippling indicates occasional extension to a spillover pain pattern.

In children,[24] the essential referred pain from adductor longus TrPs was illustrated distal to the inguinal ligament; its secondary pattern covered the anteromedial thigh, medial knee, and upper two-thirds of the medial aspect of the leg. Fine[25] reported inguinal pain in a 10-year-old boy caused by TrPs in the adductors muscles of the thigh.

Adductor Magnus

The relatively common TrP location in the mid-muscle belly of the adductor magnus muscle refers pain superiorly into the groin below the inguinal ligament and also inferiorly over the anteromedial aspect of the thigh to the knee (Figure 59-7). This groin pain is described as deep, almost as if it might be in the pelvis, but the patient is unable to identify pain in any specific pelvic structure.

Pain referred from TrPs in the more proximal region of the adductor magnus muscle is usually described as a generalized internal pelvic pain but may be identified as including the pubic bone, vagina, rectum, or (less often) the bladder. The pain may also be described as shooting up inside the pelvis and exploding like a firecracker.

Pectineus

Trigger points in the pectineus muscle produce deep-seated aching pain in the groin immediately distal to the inguinal ligament. The pain may also cover the upper part of the anteromedial aspect of the thigh. The deep groin pain may extend medially to the region where the adductor magnus muscle attaches to the pelvis (Figure 59-8).

Gracilis

The TrPs in the gracilis muscle produce a local, hot, stinging, superficial pain that travels along the medial aspect of the thigh (Figure 59-9).

3.2. Symptoms

Adductor Longus and Adductor Brevis

Patients with TrPs in these two adductor muscles are frequently aware of the pain in the groin and medial thigh only during vigorous activity or muscular overload, rather than at rest. The reported pain is typically increased by weight bearing and by sudden twists of the hip.[22] The patients usually do not recognize that abduction of the thigh is severely restricted, but occasionally, they note restricted external rotation of the thigh.

Adductor Magnus

Patients with TrPs in the proximal end of the adductor magnus muscle may report intrapelvic pain that may be specifically localized to the vagina, penis, or rectum or may be diffuse and described only as somewhere "deep inside." In some patients, symptoms occur only during sexual intercourse. When TrPs along the mid-muscle belly are active, the patient may report primarily of anteromedial thigh and groin pain.

Patients with adductor magnus TrPs frequently report having difficulty positioning the lower extremity comfortably at night. They usually prefer to lie on the opposite side with a pillow placed between the knees and legs.

Pectineus

Patients with pectineus TrPs report pain locally in the region of the muscle and may also be aware of limited abduction at the hip, especially when seated in the lotus or criss-cross position. Among the muscles that act as adductors, TrPs in the pectineus muscle restrict the range of abduction the least. Clinically, TrPs in the pectineus muscle may present with limited hip flexion range of motion with a springy or muscle guarding end feel.

Gracilis

Patients with active TrPs in the gracilis muscle typically present with a chief report of a superficial, hot, stinging pain in the medial thigh. It may be constant at rest, and changing position or stretching typically does not reduce the pain. Walking, however, tends to relieve it.

3.3. Patient Examination

After a thorough subjective examination the clinician should make a detailed drawing representing the pain pattern that the patient described. This depiction will assist in planning the physical examination and can be useful in monitoring the progression of the patient as symptoms improve or change. The type, quality, and location of the pain should be carefully assessed, and the utilization of standardized outcome tools is imperative when examining patients with lower extremity dysfunctions.

A physical examination should be conducted to rule out lumbar, iliosacral, hip, and knee joint dysfunctions. This includes range-of-motion testing of the lumbar spine, hip, and knee; passive accessory motion testing of the hip, iliosacral joint, knee, and/or lumbar spine; strength testing of the adductor muscles and other hip muscles; and any appropriate neurologic testing or orthopedic special tests. A careful assessment should be made

Chapter 59: Adductor Longus, Adductor Brevis, Adductor Magnus, Pectineus, and Gracilis Muscles

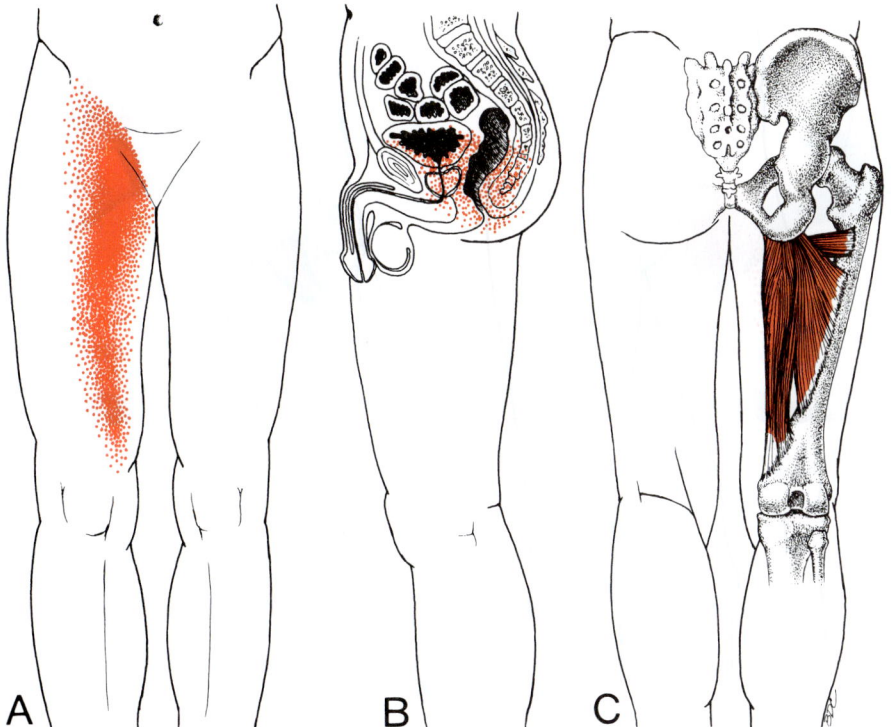

Figure 59-7. Pain pattern (dark red) referred from TrPs in the right adductor magnus muscle (light red). The essential pain pattern is solid red; red stippling locates occasional extension of the referred pain in a spillover pattern. A, Anterior view of the referred pain pattern from the midthigh region. B, Mid-sagittal view showing the intrapelvic pain pattern. These TrPs are found in the most proximal portion of the ischiocondylar part of the adductor magnus muscle medial to, or deep to, the gluteus maximus muscle. C, Adductor muscles on the right from behind.

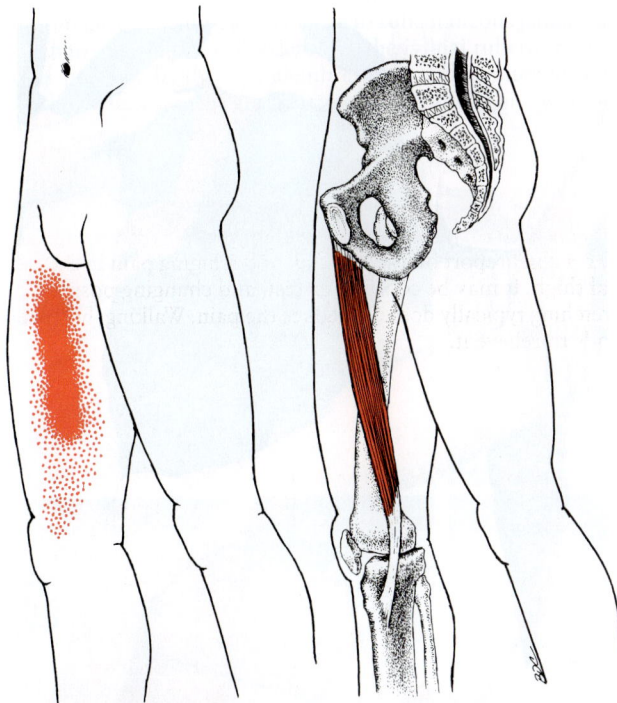

Figure 59-8. Medial view of the composite pain pattern (dark red) referred from TrPs in the right gracilis muscle (light red). Solid red denotes the essential pain pattern, and red stippling indicates the occasional spillover pain pattern.

to rule out referral into the medial thigh from other muscles, joints, or neural tissues that can refer to the same region.

It is important to perform a postural examination in standing to identify a structural or functional scoliosis, the presence of a hemipelvis, iliac upslip, anterior innominate rotation or pubic symphysis dysfunction,[26] and leg length discrepancy. A leg length discrepancy will be identified as a frontal plane asymmetry of the pelvis with one side of the pelvis elevated and the opposite side depressed. This pelvic deviation could cause TrPs in the adductor muscle on either or both sides from muscle overload. Functional activities such as sit to stand, single leg stance, and double- and single-leg squat (see Figure 55-3A) should be examined. The clinician should take note of any frontal plane deviations noted in the pelvis, hip and/or knee, and any excessive transverse plane motion at the ankle and foot (see Figure 55-3B) A deviation in the frontal plane as described may lead to overload in the adductor muscles because of an increase in the adductor moment secondary to hip abductor muscle weakness. This relative adducted position of the femur can also lead to compressive loading of the greater trochanter of the femur because of tensile loading of the gluteal muscles and may lead to abnormal compressive loading of the trochanteric bursa. The presence of hip adductor TrPs or length and strength deficits may lead to inhibition weakness of the hip abductor muscles. The hip adductors should be examined carefully for length and strength deficits as it is vital that the hip adductors and abductors work together during weight-bearing activities such as gait to stabilize the lower extremity.[27]

Because of regional interdependence of the hip and lumbosacral spine and hip and knee, specific testing should be carried out to identify interactive impairments. Patients with adductor TrPs typically do not exhibit an abnormal gait pattern unless the pain from the TrPs is so severe that it causes an antalgic gait with a reduced duration of stance phase on the affected

Pectineus

With the patient in a supine hook-lying position, the proximal aspect of the pectineus muscle can be palpated just lateral to the pubic tubercle. Taut bands may be palpable when strumming parallel to the pubic ramus just distal to the muscle's insertion (Figure 59-12E). The distal end of the muscle is deep to the femoral neurovascular bundle and difficult to palpate; however, it is readily accessible by needle penetration.

Gracilis

Trigger points in the gracilis muscle may be located by cross-fiber pincer palpation in patients who are thin or have relatively loose skin, but examination often requires superficial cross-fiber flat palpation (Figure 59-12D).

4. DIFFERENTIAL DIAGNOSIS

4.1. Activation and Perpetuation of Trigger Points

A posture or activity that activates a TrP, if not corrected, can also perpetuate it. In any part of the adductor muscles, TrPs may be activated by unaccustomed eccentric loading, eccentric exercise in an unconditioned muscle, or maximal or submaximal concentric loading.[28] Trigger points may also be activated or aggravated when the muscle is placed in a shortened and/or lengthened position for an extended period of time.

Trigger points in the adductor muscle group are likely to be activated by sudden overload, as when someone slips on ice and resists spreading the legs apart while trying to recover balance. Adductor TrPs may also be activated by osteoarthritis of the hip or after hip surgery.

Adductor magnus TrPs are often activated by skiing or by taking a long bicycle trip. Running uphill or downhill may also perpetuate adductor TrPs. Patients with TrPs from the larger adductor muscles are more likely to identify the onset of symptoms with a specific event than are patients with pectineus TrPs. Adductor TrPs may also be perpetuated by sitting in a fixed position while riding in a car or plane or while sitting for long periods in a chair with the hips acutely flexed and one thigh or leg crossed over the opposite knee.

4.2. Associated Trigger Points

Associated TrPs can develop in the referred pain areas caused by TrPs.[29] Therefore, musculature in the referred pain areas for each muscle should also be considered. Trigger points in the adductor longus and adductor brevis muscles may be associated with TrPs in the adductor magnus muscle and occasionally with TrPs in the pectineus muscle. Involvement of the adductor longus and adductor magnus muscles may be associated with TrPs in the most medial fibers of the vastus medialis muscle. Anatomically, they are literally fused. The fascial coverings of these muscles form a thick bridge between them above the knee that helps establish a medial pull on the patella that counters the lateral pull of the vastus lateralis muscle.

Pectineus TrPs are frequently discovered in association with TrPs in the iliopsoas muscle group, the three adductors, and the gracilis muscles. If the pectineus muscle has TrPs, the other adductor muscles almost always will as well; therefore, they need to be addressed first. When these associated TrPs have been inactivated, a search for the cause of the residual tenderness and deep groin pain reveals the pectineus muscle TrPs. For this reason, it is important to always check for residual pain-producing TrPs in the pectineus muscle after eliminating any TrPs in the iliopsoas and adductor muscles.

Surprisingly, TrPs in the gracilis muscle are rarely associated with TrPs in the primary adductors, but these may be associated with TrPs in the lower end of the sartorius muscle.

4.3. Associated Pathology

In patients with persistent chronic pain, one must expect that multiple etiologies are responsible. Ekberg and associates[30] employed a multidisciplinary approach to manage long-standing unexplained groin pain in 21 male athletes. The diagnostic medical team evaluated the athletes for inguinal hernia, neuralgia, adductor tenoperiostitis, symphysitis, and prostatitis. The evaluation included radiographs of the pelvis and radioisotope studies of the pubic symphysis. Only two patients had just one condition, namely, symphysitis. Ten patients had two conditions, six patients had three conditions, and three patients had four conditions. The authors did not explore the additional possibility of myofascial pain caused by TrPs. Holmich[31] proposed diagnostic categorization of groin pain based on five clinical entities: adductor-related pain, iliopsoas-related pain, abdominal wall–related/hernia, hip joint pathology, and pubic bone stress injury (formerly osteitis pubis).

Typical signs of adductor-related pain include pain with palpation of adductor muscle origin and pain with passive stretch.[32]

Pain of iliopsoas muscle origin is typically provoked with palpation of the muscle as well as resisted hip flexion. During a modified Thomas test, pain will likely be reproduced during a hip extension stretch.[32] In a review of 894 patient cases, iliopsoas pathology was most commonly seen in female patients. Women with ligamentous laxity tend to demonstrate excessive use of and myofascial tightness in the iliopsoas muscle.[32] Iliopsoas muscle pain is also prevalent among runners. The iliopsoas muscle plays an important role in running as a hip flexor and, as such, is at risk for being overused.[33]

A sports hernia is a deficiency of the posterior wall of the inguinal canal secondary to dysfunction of the conjoint tendon. Patients typically report pain in the lower abdomen or groin.[34] Pain is typically exacerbated with palpation of the rectus abdominis muscle and the conjoint tendon. Pain is further provoked during a resisted situp. A femoral or inguinal hernia may be visible upon inspection or display a cough impulse.[32]

Intra-articular dysfunction is characterized by pain and restriction reproduced during hip range of motion.[32] Multiple sources[22,35] warn that the referred pain from adductor longus TrPs may be mistaken for the pain of osteoarthritis of the hip. It is easy to attribute all the pain to osteoarthritis and not consider the potential role of hip adductor TrPs. Inactivating the adductor TrPs provides satisfactory pain relief to some patients with osteoarthritis of the hip joint.[17] Clinically, the pain of osteoarthritis is usually deeper in the groin and is more likely to be referred laterally rather than medially.[22]

The concept that part of the disability associated with osteoarthritis of the hip is of muscular origin was substantiated by a study[36] in which patients with osteoarthritis of the hip were given stretching exercises for the adductor musculature. The mean increase of 8.3° in the range of hip abduction and the increase in the cross-sectional area of type 1 and type 2 fibers in the adductor muscles was significant.[36]

Rold and Rold[37] emphasized that pubic stress symphysitis of athletes must be distinguished from adductor tendon avulsion at the pelvis, from fractures of the pubic or ischial rami, and from local septic conditions. Pubic stress symphysitis usually has a gradual insidious onset of groin or lower abdominal pain with acute exacerbation during stressful sports activity.[38] Examination reveals focal tenderness of the pubic symphysis bilaterally and pain on abduction and extension of the thighs.[37,39] Symphysitis sometimes is accompanied by adductor TrPs. In this situation, abduction and extension are more restricted on the side of the TrPs. The most anterior adductor muscles, the pectineus and adductor longus muscles, are the most likely to be involved.

This situation is understandable because these two adductor muscles have the most effective leverage for putting asymmetric stress on the pubic symphysis. Radiographic evidence of sclerosis and irregularity of the pubic bones at the symphysis, as well as scintigraphic evidence of increased radionuclide uptake at the symphysis, are confirmatory findings.[37,40] The tendency for the pelvis to seesaw up and down is aggravated by tension of the adductor muscles.[40] Further, the tension of the adductor muscles may lead to disruption of the fibrocartilaginous symphyseal disc.[41]

The obturator and genitofemoral nerves may cause pain or tingling in the groin or in the medial thigh when they become entrapped. The genitofemoral nerve may be involved by TrPs or shortness in the iliopsoas muscle group.

About half of the patients who have an obturator hernia (usually elderly women) develop symptoms of entrapment of the obturator nerve including pain and paresthesias down the medial surface of the thigh to the knee (Howship-Romberg sign).[42-46] Extension of the thigh increases the pain,[43] and the adductor deep tendon reflex is diminished or absent. (This reflex is elicited with a reflex hammer by tapping a finger placed across the musculotendinous junction of the adductor magnus muscle about 5 cm [2 in] above the medial epicondyle).[42]

Entrapment of the genitofemoral nerve is often caused by excessively tight clothing over the inguinal ligament. Patients with entrapment of this nerve experience pain and/or numbness in an elliptic area on the anterior aspect of the thigh immediately below the middle of the inguinal ligament. This area also shows reduced perception of pinprick and touch. Appendectomy, psoas muscle infection, and local trauma are predisposing factors.[47]

Although tension due to TrPs in the adductor longus, adductor brevis, and gracilis muscles are not known to cause nerve entrapment, TrPs in the adductor magnus muscle can lead to compression of vascular structures. A taut adductor magnus muscle can compress the femoral vessels at their exit through the adductor (tendinous) hiatus. Sometimes, the middle and posterior parts of the adductor magnus muscle are fused, which greatly reduces the size of the hiatus. A patient who lacks a palpable dorsalis pedis pulse can experience a return of the pulse immediately after inactivation of a TrP in the adductor magnus muscle. This unusual result may be due to an atypical anatomic structure that facilitated compression of the femoral artery combined with a taut band of adductor magnus fibers at the adductor hiatus.

Three cases of thrombosis of the superficial femoral artery at the outlet of the adductor canal were reported in association with athletic activities.[48] The arterial injury and thrombosis were attributed in two cases to a scissor-like compression by the vastus medialis and adductor magnus tendons at this location and, in another case, to compression by a constricting tendinous band extending across the femoral artery from the adductor magnus muscle to the vastus medialis tendon at the

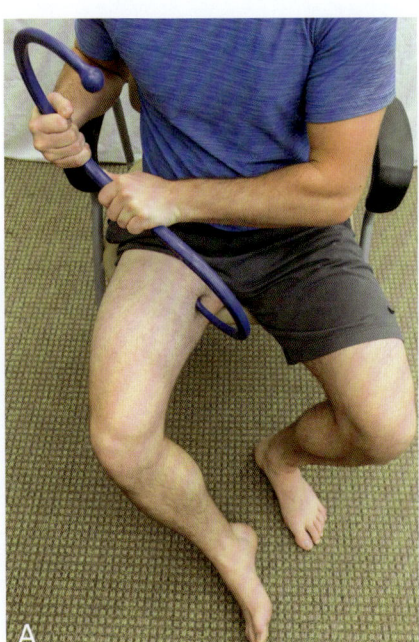
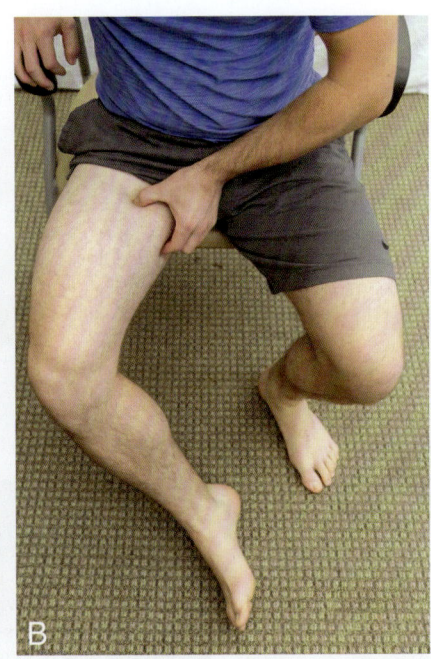
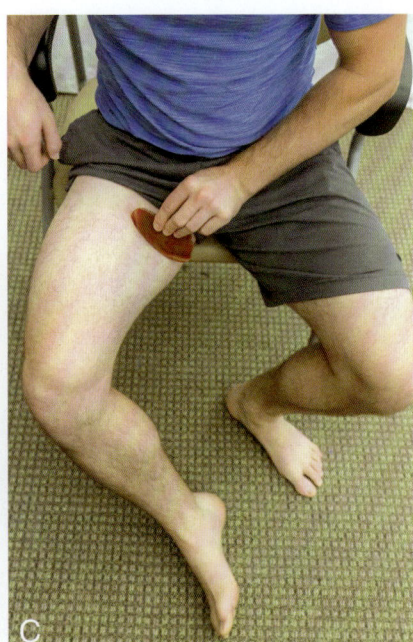
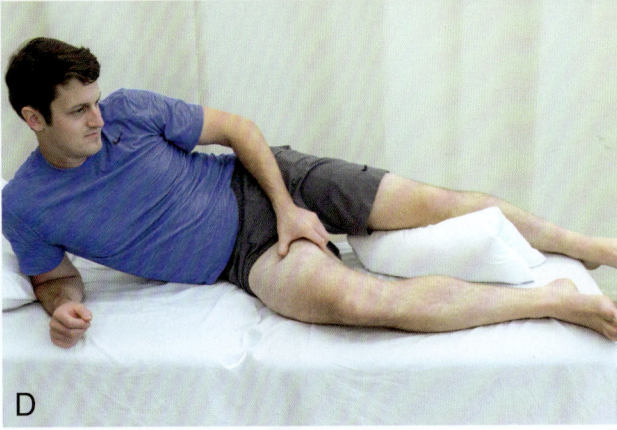

Figure 59-13. Self-pressure release of TrPs in the adductor muscles. A, TrP release tool for TrPs in the adductor longus and adductor brevis muscles. B, Manual release using pincer grasp. C, Using a small tool. D, Side-lying manual release of the gracilis and adductor magnus muscles.

level of the adductor canal outlet. These observations suggest that, in some adductor canal configurations, taut-band tension on the tendons forming the margins of the canal might cause at least venous compression at this site.

When adductor longus TrPs develop bilaterally, as may occur with strenuous horseback riding, the symmetric distribution of referred pain can simulate a mid-lumbar spinal dysfunction.[18]

5. CORRECTIVE ACTIONS

Patients with TrPs in the adductor muscles should limit the time they spend sitting with one knee crossed over the other. If patients feel the need to cross their legs, they should opt for crossing the affected leg's ankle over the other ankle. Crossing the legs at the ankle will leave the thigh and adductor muscles in a better resting position. Taking intermittent breaks during long periods of sitting to walk and stretch are also encouraged. For all the hip adductor muscles, it is important to avoid leaving the muscle in a shortened position for a long period of time. This shortened position is avoided when the patient is sleeping on one side by placing a pillow between the knees and legs. Excessive prolonged hip flexion should also be avoided.

Self-treatment of the adductor muscles can be achieved with the utilization of a TrP self-pressure release tool or with manual (hands-on) release. To perform TrP self-pressure release with a tool or manually, the patient is seated or side-lying (Figure 59-13A to D). Finding the sensitive spot with the tool, by pincer grasp, or with digital pressure, the patient applies light force (no more than 4/10 pain), holds for 15 to 30 seconds until pain reduces, and repeats five times. This release can be repeated several times per day. Pressure should be mildly uncomfortable but not overly painful.

Patients with a strong upper body can utilize a foam roller along the adductor muscles. In a side-lying position, the bottom leg should be placed in maximal hip flexion so that the medial aspect of the affected leg can rest on the foam roller. The patient can roll along the foam roller until identifying the tender TrP, at which point the patient should hold constant isolated pressure for up to 90 seconds or until the tenderness reduces. For patients who are unable to attain this position, a similar technique may be utilized in sitting using a hand-held roller.

Following pressure release, a self-stretch of the adductor muscles should be performed as long as the stretch does not increase symptoms. A clinician should instruct the patient in a home-stretch program to maintain full adductor muscle length.

The patient can perform bent-knee fallouts with post-isometric relaxation to reduce the activity of TrPs in the adductor muscles. The patient lies on the back with the hips and knees flexed (Figure 59-14). For TrPs that are irritable, the patient supports the affected leg with the hand on the outside of the

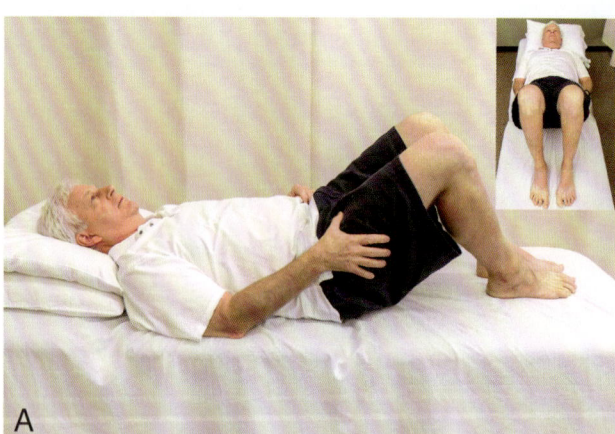

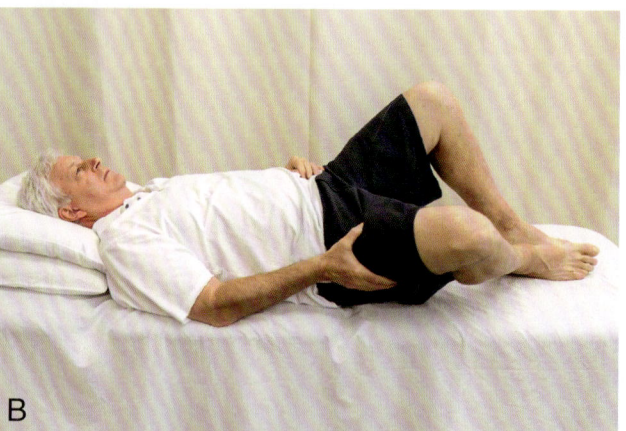

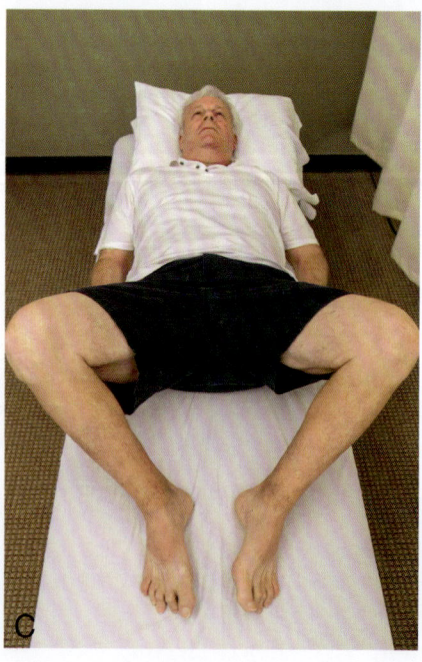

Figure 59-14. Bent-knee fall out. A, Starting position. B, With manual support to control the stretch in the adductor muscles for irritable TrPs. C, Bilateral bent-knee fall out to increase stretch and to maintain symmetry between both hip adductor muscle groups.

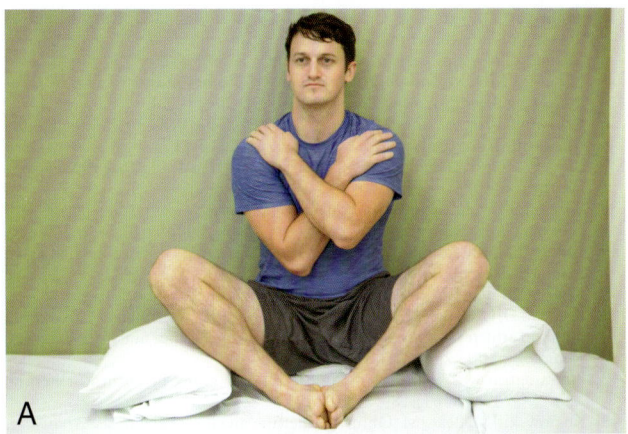
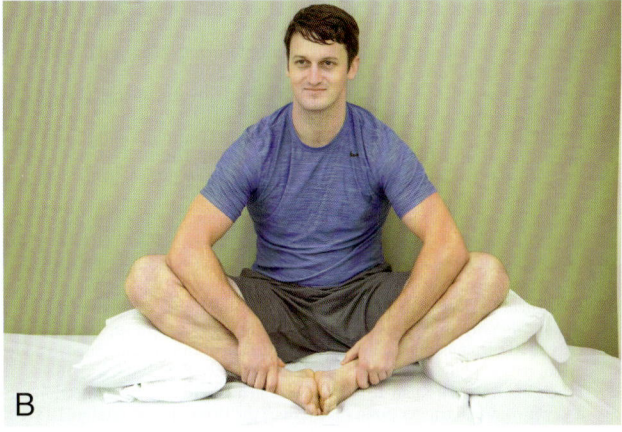
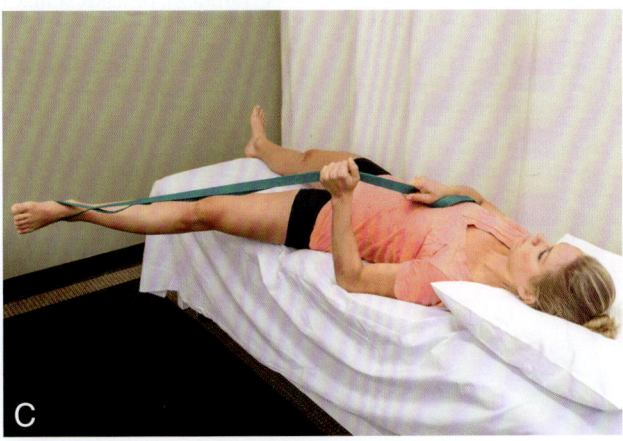

Figure 59-15. Self-stretch of the adductor muscles. A, Gravity assisted stretch of the adductors if TrPs are irritable. B, Gentle overpressure to enhance the stretch. C, Yoga strap–assisted stretch for stretch of the gracilis muscle.

knee (Figure 59-14A). The patient keeps the opposite lower extremity in this position while slowly lowering the affected knee down toward the bed until a slight stretch is felt on the inner thigh (Figure 59-14B). Once the stretch is felt, the patient can take a deep breath that causes a slight contraction in the adductor muscles, holding the breath for 6 to 10 seconds and then breathing slowly out. At the end of the exhalation, the patient relaxes the adductor muscle until a stretch is felt again on the inner thigh. This cycle can be repeated three to five times as long as there is no increase in pain or symptoms. To enhance the stretch and achieve balance in the adductor muscle length, this can be performed on both sides at the same time (Figure 59-14C).

Patients can also stretch the adductor muscles by sitting with their back against a wall with both hips flexed, externally rotated, and abducted using a pillow under the outside of the knees and thighs to support this position (Figure 59-15A). Patients can also be instructed in a contract-relax technique to stretch the adductor muscles (Figure 59-15B). Möller and associates[49] found that the contract-relax adductor muscle stretch was one of the most effective (Figure 59-15B). The stretch techniques described for the adductor muscle group do not stretch the gracilis muscle because bending the knee shortens the gracilis muscle. A stretch of the gracillis muscle can be accomplished with the assistance of a stretch strap (Figure 59-15C).

References

1. Standring S. *Gray's Anatomy: The Anatomical Basis of Clinical Practice.* 41st ed. London, UK: Elsevier; 2015.
2. Norton-Old KJ, Schache AG, Barker PJ, Clark RA, Harrison SM, Briggs CA. Anatomical and mechanical relationship between the proximal attachment of adductor longus and the distal rectus sheath. *Clin Anat.* 2013;26(4):522-530.
3. Davis JA, Stringer MD, Woodley SJ. New insights into the proximal tendons of adductor longus, adductor brevis and gracilis. *Br J Sports Med.* 2012;46(12):871-876.
4. Jonsson B, Steen B. Function of the gracilis muscle. An electromyographic study. *Acta Morphol Neerl Scand.* 1966;6(4):325-341.
5. Freedman AD, Ross SE, Gayle RC. Teaching "Not So Exact" science: the controversial pectineus. *Am Biol Teach.* 2008;70(7):34-36.
6. Ranchos Los Amigos National Rehabilitation Center. *Observational Gait Analysis.* 4th ed. Downey, CA: Los Amigos Research and Education Institute; 2001.
7. Green DL, Morris JM. Role of adductor longus and adductor magnus in postural movements and in ambulation. *Am J Phys Med.* 1970;49(4):223-240.
8. Lyons K, Perry J, Gronley JK, Barnes L, Antonelli D. Timing and relative intensity of hip extensor and abductor muscle action during level and stair ambulation. An EMG study. *Phys Ther.* 1983;63(10):1597-1605.
9. Perry J. The mechanics of walking. A clinical interpretation. *Phys Ther.* 1967;47(9):778-801.
10. Leighton RD. A functional model to describe the action of the adductor muscles at the hip in the transverse plane. *Physiother Theory Pract.* 2006;22(5):251-262.
11. Markhede G, Stener B. Function after removal of various hip and thigh muscles for extirpation of tumors. *Acta Orthop Scand.* 1981;52(4):373-395.
12. Mann RA, Moran GT, Dougherty SE. Comparative electromyography of the lower extremity in jogging, running, and sprinting. *Am J Sports Med.* 1986;14(6):501-510.
13. Delmore RJ, Laudner KG, Torry MR. Adductor longus activation during common hip exercises. *J Sport Rehabil.* 2014;23(2):79-87.
14. Serner A, Jakobsen MD, Andersen LL, Holmich P, Sundstrup E, Thorborg K. EMG evaluation of hip adduction exercises for soccer players: implications for exercise selection in prevention and treatment of groin injuries. *Br J Sports Med.* 2014;48(14):1108-1114.
15. Broer M, Houtz S. *Patterns of Muscular Activity in Selected Sports Skills: An Electromyographic Study.* Springfield, IL: Charles C. Thomas; 1967.
16. Simons DG, Travell J, Simons L. *Travell & Simon's Myofascial Pain and Dysfunction: The Trigger Point Manual.* Vol 1. 2nd ed. Baltimore, MD: Williams & Wilkins; 1999 (p. 104).
17. Travell J. The adductor longus syndrome: a cause of groin pain: its treatment by local block of trigger areas (procaine infiltration and ethyl chloride spray). *Miss Valley Med J.* 1950;71:13-22.
18. Travell J. Symposium on mechanism and management of pain syndromes. *Proc Rudolf Virchow Med Soc.* 1957;16:126-136.

19. Travell J, Rinzler SH. The myofascial genesis of pain. *Postgrad Med.* 1952;11(5):425-434.
20. Kelly M. Some rules for the employment of local analgesic in the treatment of somatic pain. *Med J Austral.* 1947;1:235-239.
21. Kelly M. The relief of facial pain by procaine (Novocaine) injections. *J Am Geriatr Soc.* 1963;11:586-596.
22. Long C II. Myofascial pain syndromes. III. Some syndromes of the trunk and thigh. *Henry Ford Hosp Med Bull.* 1956;4(2):102-106.
23. Kellgren JH. Observations on referred pain arising from muscle. *Clin Sci.* 1938;3:175-190 (p. 186).
24. Bates T, Grunwaldt E. Myofascial pain in childhood. *J Pediatr.* 1958;53(2):198-209.
25. Fine PG. Myofascial trigger point pain in children. *J Pediatr.* 1987;111(4):547-548.
26. DeStefano L. *Greenman's Principles of Manual Medicine.* 5th ed. Philadelphia, PA: Wolters Kluwer; 2016 (p. 338).
27. Porterfield JA, DeRosa C. *Mechanical Low Back Pain: Perspectives in Functional Anatomy.* 2nd ed. Philadelphia, PA: Saunders; 1998 (pp. 114-117).
28. Gerwin RD, Dommerholt J, Shah JP. An expansion of Simons' integrated hypothesis of trigger point formation. *Curr Pain Headache Rep.* 2004;8(6):468-475.
29. Hsieh YL, Kao MJ, Kuan TS, Chen SM, Chen JT, Hong CZ. Dry needling to a key myofascial trigger point may reduce the irritability of satellite MTrPs. *Am J Phys Med Rehabil.* 2007;86(5):397-403.
30. Ekberg O, Persson NH, Abrahamsson PA, Westlin NE, Lilja B. Longstanding groin pain in athletes. A multidisciplinary approach. *Sports Med.* 1988;6(1):56-61.
31. Holmich P, Bradshaw C. Groin pain. In: Brukner PD, Khank, eds. *Clinical Sports Medicine.* Sydney, Australia: McGraw-Hill; 2012:545-578.
32. Rankin AT, Bleakley CM, Cullen M. Hip joint pathology as a leading cause of groin pain in the sporting population: a 6-year review of 894 cases. *Am J Sports Med.* 2015;43(7):1698-1703.
33. Holmich P. Long-standing groin pain in sportspeople falls into three primary patterns, a "clinical entity" approach: a prospective study of 207 patients. *Br J Sports Med.* 2007;41(4):247-252; discussion 252.
34. Munegato D, Bigoni M, Gridavilla G, Olmi S, Cesana G, Zatti G. Sports hernia and femoroacetabular impingement in athletes: a systematic review. *World J Clin Cases.* 2015;3(9):823-830.
35. Reynolds MD. Myofascial trigger point syndromes in the practice of rheumatology. *Arch Phys Med Rehabil.* 1981;62(3):111-114.
36. Leivseth G, Torstensson J, Reikeras O. Effect of passive muscle stretching in osteoarthritis of the hip. *Clin Sci.* 1989;76(1):113-117.
37. Rold JF, Rold BA. Pubic stress symphysitis in a female distance runner. *Phys Sportsmed.* 1986;14:61-65.
38. Avrahami D, Choudur HN. Adductor tendinopathy in a hockey player with persistent groin pain: a case report. *J Can Chiropr Assoc.* 2010;54(4):264-270.
39. Nelson EN, Kassarjian A, Palmer WE. MR imaging of sports-related groin pain. *Magn Reson Imaging Clin N Am.* 2005;13(4):727-742.
40. Brody DM. Running injuries. *Clin Symp.* 1980;32(4):1-36.
41. Brennan D, O'Connell MJ, Ryan M, et al. Secondary cleft sign as a marker of injury in athletes with groin pain: MR image appearance and interpretation. *Radiology.* 2005;235(1):162-167.
42. Hannington-Kiff JG. Absent thigh adductor reflex in obturator hernia. *Lancet.* 1980;1(8161):180.
43. Kozlowski JM, Beal JM. Obturator hernia: an elusive diagnosis. *Arch Surg.* 1977;112(8):1001-1002.
44. Larrieu AJ, DeMarco SJ III. Obturator hernia: report of a case and brief review of its status. *Am Surg.* 1976;42(4):273-277.
45. Martin NC, Welch TP. Obturator hernia. *Br J Surg.* 1974;61(7):547-548.
46. Somell A, Ljungdahl I, Spangen L. Thigh neuralgia as a symptom of obturator hernia. *Acta Chir Scand.* 1976;142(6):457-459.
47. Rischbieth RH. Genito-femoral neuropathy. *Clin Exp Neurol.* 1986;22:145-147.
48. Balaji MR, DeWeese JA. Adductor canal outlet syndrome. *JAMA.* 1981;245(2):167-170.
49. Möller M, Ekstrand J, Oberg B, Gillquist J. Duration of stretching effect on range of motion in lower extremities. *Arch Phys Med Rehabil.* 1985;66(3):171-173.

Chapter 60

Hamstring Muscles
Semitendinosus, Semimembranosus, and Biceps Femoris

"Chair Seat Victims"

N. Beth Collier

1. INTRODUCTION

The muscles of the posterior compartment of the thigh are informally termed the "hamstrings" when discussed as a group. Individually, this group includes the true hamstring muscles, the semitendinosus, semimembranosus, and the long head of the biceps femoris muscles. The true hamstring muscles cross the hip and knee joint and contribute to both hip extension and knee flexion. The short head of the biceps femoris muscle acts only in knee flexion. Trigger points (TrPs) in these muscles refer pain as widespread posterior thigh and/or knee pain and often mimic knee joint pathology. They can be activated by inactivity, especially by prolonged sitting with the hips and knees flexed or from an ill-fitting chair. Sporting activities such as football, basketball, and soccer can overload the hamstring muscles because of the combined hip flexion and knee extension that is required. Differential diagnosis should include hamstring muscle strain, proximal hamstring tendinopathy, lumbosacral radicular pain or radiculopathy, ischial bursitis, and pes anserine bursitis. Corrective actions should include techniques to improve sitting posture, gait mechanics, self-pressure release, and self-stretching techniques.

2. ANATOMIC CONSIDERATIONS

Semitendinosus

The semitendinosus muscle originates proximally from the posterior aspect of the ischial tuberosity by a common tendon with the long head of the biceps femoris muscle.[1] The belly of the semitendinosus muscle becomes tendinous below mid-thigh and travels distally, superficial to the semimembranosus muscle. Its tendon curves around the posteromedial aspect of the medial condyle of the tibia passes superficial to the tibial collateral ligament and inserts into the medial aspect of the tibia (Figure 60-1). Of the three tendons that insert together at this site, called the "pes anserinus," the semitendinosus tendon inserts most distally. The sartorius and gracilis muscles also attach at the pes anserinus. The pes anserine bursa separates the three tendons of the pes anserinus from the underlying tibial collateral ligament of the knee joint. This distal tendon attachment is considerably farther from the axis of rotation of the knee joint than is that of the other hamstring muscles. This gives the semitendinosus strong leverage to flex the knee after the knee is partially bent. This leverage becomes apparent when one bends the knee to a right angle, contracts the hamstring muscles, and palpates the relative prominence of the semitendinosus tendon. Furthermore, at the distal attachment, there is a blending with the tendon of the gracilis muscle, the deep fascia of the leg, and the medial head of the gastrocnemius muscle. These multiple extra fascial connections with the semitendinosus muscle can cause difficulty when harvesting the tendon surgically for a graft, but it increases its functional influence at the knee.

The division of the semitendinosus muscle into two tandem segments by the tendinous inscription across the midline of the muscled is apparently related to its phylogenic origin. Two distinct end plate bands are found in the semitendinosus muscle, one above and one below the inscription (Figure 60-1).

Semimembranosus

The relatively broad semimembranosus muscle originates proximally on the posterior aspect of the ischial tuberosity and lateral and deep to the common tendon of the semitendinosus and biceps femoris muscles. This anatomic arrangement places the semimembranosus muscle deep to the semitendinosus muscle on the medial aspect of the posterior compartment of the thigh (Figure 60-2). In fact, the semimembranosus muscle has the longest proximal tendon and the greatest muscle-tendon

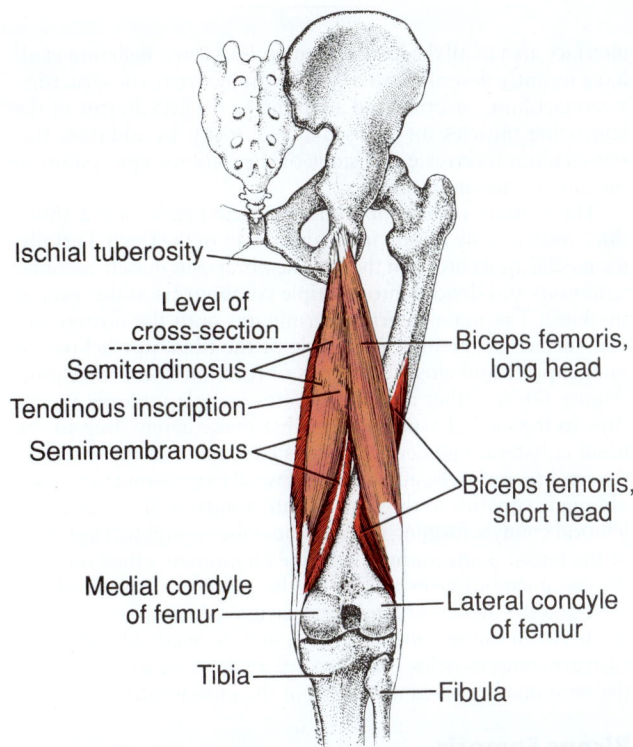

Figure 60-1. Attachments of the right superficial hamstring muscles, posterior view. The semitendinosus and long head of the biceps femoris muscles are light red. The underlying semimembranosus and short head of the biceps femoris muscles are dark red.

635

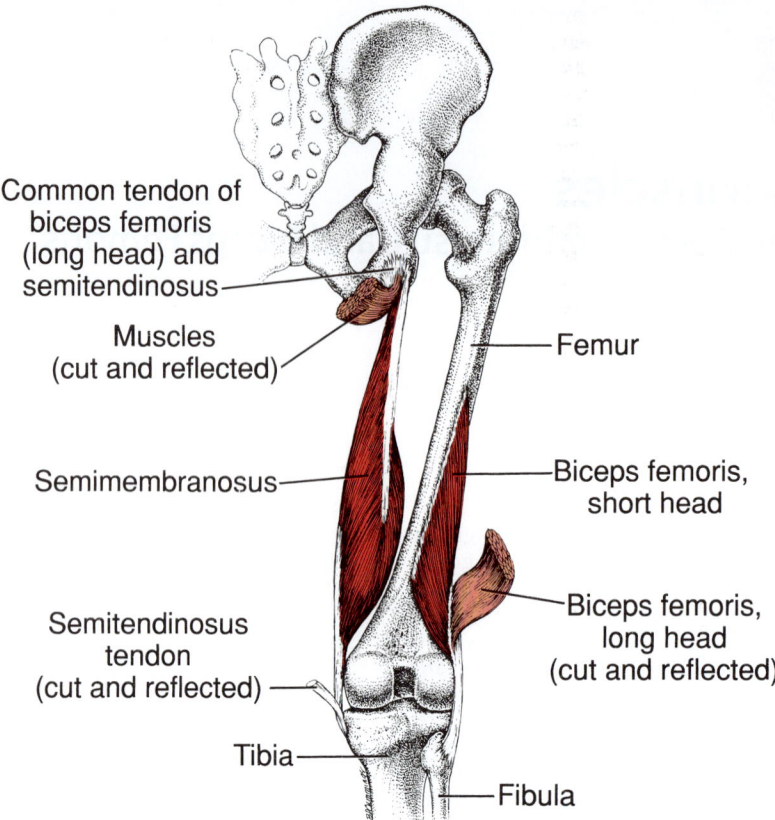

Figure 60-2. Attachments of the deep layer of right hamstring muscles, posterior view. The semimembranosus and short head of the biceps femoris muscles are dark red. The cut ends of the superficial layer of hamstring muscles are light red.

interface area of all the hamstring muscles.[2] Pérez-Bellmunt et al[3] have recently described an annular connective tissue structure, a retinaculum, covering and adapting to the attachment of the hamstring muscles on the ischial tuberosity. In addition, this retinaculum receives expansions of the anterior epimysium of the gluteus maximus muscle.[3]

The oblique semimembranosus muscle fibers form a short, thick muscle belly mostly in the distal half of the thigh. Distally, the medial aponeurosis of the semimembranosus muscle becomes tendinous and divides into multiple components at the level of the knee. The main insertion terminates onto the posteromedial surface of the medial condyle of the tibia, just below the joint capsule and close to the axis of rotation of the knee joint (Figure 60-3). Other attachment sites include multiple fascial slips to the medial aspect of the tibia immediately deep to the tibial collateral ligament; a fibrous expansion to the fascia of the popliteus muscle; and a strong fascial expansion that passes obliquely superior to the femoral intercondylar line and lateral femoral condyle forming much of the oblique popliteal ligament of the knee.[1] Some authors describe an intimate attachment of the semimembranosus tendon to the posterior capsule of the knee and the medial or lateral meniscus.[4-7] An important bursa lies between the semimembranosus and the medial head of the gastrocnemius muscles, and a secondary bursa exists to separate the semimembranosus muscle from the knee joint.[1]

Biceps Femoris

The biceps femoris muscle, in the posterolateral compartment of the thigh, is comprised of a long head and a short head. The long head crosses both the hip and knee joints, but the short head crosses only the knee joint.

The long head of the biceps femoris muscle originates proximally at the posterior aspect of the ischial tuberosity from a common tendon with the semitendinosus muscle and at the inferior portion of the sacrotuberous ligament[8] (Figure 60-1). Frequently, the superior bursa of the biceps femoris muscle separates this common tendon from the deeper tendon of the semimembranosus muscle. The short head of the biceps femoris muscle originates proximally from the lateral lip of the linea aspera, between the adductor magnus and vastus lateralis muscles, extending from approximately the gluteus maximus muscle distally along the lateral supracondylar line to just superior to the lateral femoral condyle. Distally, the short head joins the long head in a common tendon that inserts into the posterolateral aspect of the head of the fibula (Figure 60-2). The biceps femoris muscle also has attachments to the fibular collateral ligament and the lateral tibial condyle.[1] Tosovic et al[9] have recently described a nonuniform architecture of the muscle in which the distal portion of the long head of the biceps femoris muscle has significantly shorter fascicles and larger pennation angles than its proximal sites.

There are several anatomic variations of the hamstring muscles. For instance, the long head of the biceps femoris and the semimembranosus muscles can have hemipennate architecture, and their fiber length can be shorter than that of semitendinosus and short head of biceps femoris muscles.[10] On some occasions, the short head of biceps femoris muscle may be absent. Also, additional attachment sites may include the ischial tuberosity, linea aspera, or medial supracondylar line.

Throughout the posterior thigh, the sciatic nerve lies deep to a hamstring muscle. In the upper thigh, it lies deep to the gluteus maximus muscle and the lateral side of the long head of the biceps femoris muscle, resting on the adductor magnus muscle. As it descends through the upper half of the thigh, the nerve crosses deep to the long head of the biceps femoris muscle from its lateral side to its medial side. At mid-thigh, the nerve lies deep to the biceps femoris muscle and between it and the semimembranosus muscle, still resting on the adductor magnus muscle.

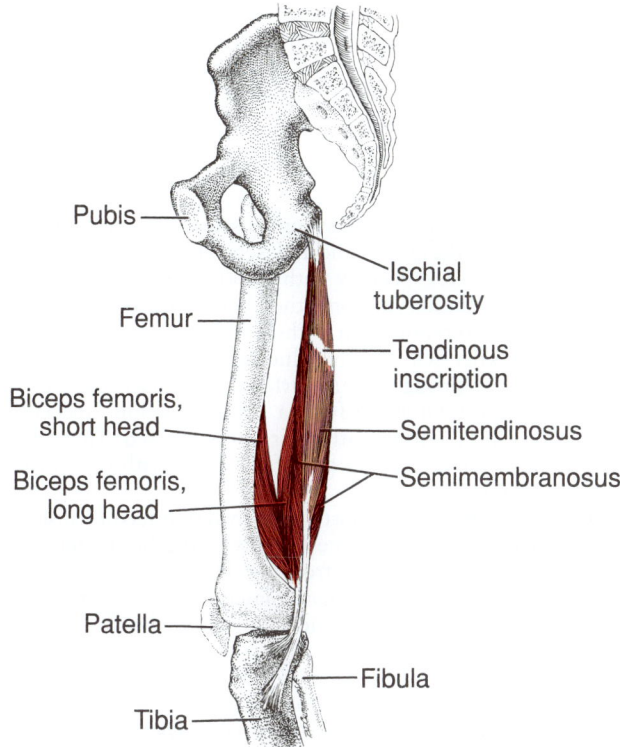

Figure 60-3. Attachments of the right hamstring muscles, medial view. The superficial semitendinosus muscle is light red, and the deeper semimembranosus muscle is dark red. The two heads of the biceps femoris muscle are intermediate red.

In the distal thigh, the tibial and peroneal branches of the sciatic nerve lie deep in the space between the semimembranosus muscle and the tendon of the long head of the biceps femoris muscle, lateral to the popliteal vessels.[1]

2.1. Innervation and Vascularization

The semitendinosus, semimembranosus, and long head of the biceps femoris muscles are supplied by branches from the tibial portion of the sciatic nerve containing fibers of the L5, S1, S2 nerve roots. The short head of the biceps femoris muscle is supplied by branches of the common fibular division of the sciatic nerve, which also receives fibers from the L5, S1, S2 nerves.[1] Additionally, it has been observed that the hamstring muscles demonstrate an intramuscular arborization innervation.[11]

The hamstring muscles receive their vascularization from the perforating arteries. The semitendinosus and biceps femoris muscles are also supplied superiorly by the medial circumflex femoral artery. Each hamstring muscle may receive some accessory vascularization from the inferior gluteal artery at the ischial tuberosity. Distally, at the tibial attachment, there may be an accessory vascularization from the superior lateral and medial genicular or popliteal arteries.[1]

2.2. Function

The three true hamstring muscles (semitendinosus, semimembranosus, and long head of the biceps femoris) act primarily as hip extensors and knee flexors when the thigh and leg are free to move. The hamstring muscles provide between 30% and 50% of hip extensor strength.[12] During standing and forward bending, they control flexion at the hip. All the hamstring muscles are involved in knee flexion. The medial hamstring muscles (semitendinosus and semimembranosus) assist with internal rotation of the thigh at the hip, and the long head of the biceps femoris muscle assists external rotation of the thigh at the hip when the hip is extended. When the knee is flexed, the semitendinosus and semimembranosus muscles also internally rotate the leg, and both heads of the biceps femoris muscle externally rotate it. The short head of the biceps femoris muscle is primarily a flexor of the knee joint.

All three of the true hamstring muscles are electromyographically quiescent during static standing, as is the case with the quadriceps femoris, adductor magnus, and gluteus maximus muscles. However, in contrast to the gluteus maximus muscle, any action that takes the center of gravity in front of a medial-lateral axis at the hip joint, such as reaching or bending forward, is accompanied by a vigorous eccentric contraction of the hamstring muscles. As the forward trunk lean increases, the hip extensor moment arm of the hamstring muscles increases, whereas the hip extensor moment arm of the gluteus maximus muscle decreases.[13] Because of the increased moment arm of the hamstring muscles, their activation in the forward trunk lean provides an important contribution to the lumbopelvic rhythm in forward flexion of the trunk.[14]

In gait, the hamstrings muscles function indirectly to keep the trunk erect during stance (directly restraining the tendency toward hip flexion that is produced by body weight) and to decelerate the forward-moving limb at terminal swing, regardless of speed.[15,16] During the last half of swing, the hamstring musculature is active, lengthened, and absorbing energy from decelerating the limb in preparation for foot contact.[16,17] The biceps femoris muscle experiences the greatest musculotendinous muscle stretch during terminal swing, which may contribute to its greater likelihood to be strained when compared with the other two hamstring muscles.[18] Additionally, significant differences in the activation patterns between the biceps femoris and semitendinosus muscles were observed. With higher running speed, the biceps femoris muscle was more activated during the late-swing phase, whereas the semitendinosus muscle was significantly more activated during the middle-swing phase.[19] The hamstring muscles also help extend the hip during late-stance to pre-swing phase of gait. The individual hamstring muscles do not act consistently in flexing the knee during gait, though the short head of the biceps femoris muscle is active in knee flexion for toe clearance.

Ericson[20] calculated that, together, all of the hip extensor muscles produce 27% of the total positive mechanical work during ergometer cycling. An average of surface electrode activity through 25 cycles of pedaling in 11 subjects[21] showed that the electromyographic (EMG) activity of the biceps femoris muscle peaked at the beginning of the backward motion of the pedal. In contrast, the combination of semitendinosus and semimembranosus muscles EMG activity peaked near the end of this period. Activity of the biceps femoris muscle increased with increased pedaling rate and with increased seat height.[21]

The hamstring muscles also provide dynamic stability for the knee joint because of their distal medial and lateral attachments at the knee. This function is supported by the anatomy of the popliteus muscle and the presence of a three-layered retinaculum acting as kinematic sustentation for the hamstring muscles.[22] The hamstring muscles also lend active resistance to the anterior glide of the tibia on the femur, providing the anterior cruciate ligament with dynamic support.[12]

2.3. Functional Unit

The functional unit to which a muscle belongs includes the muscles that reinforce and counter its actions as well as the joints that the muscle crosses. The interdependence of these structures is functionally reflected in the organization and neural connections of the sensory motor cortex. The functional unit is emphasized because the presence of a TrP in one muscle of the unit increases the likelihood that the other muscles of the unit will also develop TrPs. When inactivating TrPs in a muscle, one

Box 60-1 Functional unit of the hamstring muscle group

Action	Synergists	Antagonists
Hip extension	Gluteus maximus Adductor magnus (ischiocondylar portion)	Iliopsoas Tensor fascia latae Rectus femoris Sartorius
Knee flexion	Sartorius Gracilis Gastrocnemius Plantaris	Quadriceps femoris

must be concerned about TrPs that may develop in muscles that are functionally interdependent. Box 60-1 grossly represents the functional unit of the hamstring muscle group.[23]

3. CLINICAL PRESENTATION

3.1. Referred Pain Pattern

The referred pain pattern of TrPs in the semitendinosus and semimembranosus muscles usually projects upward to the ischial tuberosity and gluteal fold. Referred pain can also extend inferiorly to the medial posterior thigh, posterior knee, and occasionally to the medial calf, often with a sharpness that is less commonly felt from the other hamstring muscles (Figure 60-4A).

The pain pattern referred from TrPs in either or both heads of the biceps femoris muscle often projects distally to the posterior lateral knee. Chan et al[24] described a case report where a calcific tendinitis of the biceps femoris muscle was a cause of acute knee pain. The referred pain can also spread inferiorly below the knee into the calf and may also extend upward in the posterior thigh as high as the gluteal fold (Figure 60-4B).

3.2. Symptoms

Patients with TrPs in the hamstring muscles will report pain in the buttock near the gluteal fold and ischial tuberosity, posterior thigh and/or knee, especially with walking or running. Some authors called these symptoms the "hamstring syndrome."[25] Patients can also report pain in the buttock, upper thigh, and back of the knee when sitting due to pressure on the TrPs, especially when sitting on hard surfaces. They may also report increased pain upon rising from a seated position especially if they have been sitting with their knees crossed. They may tend to push themselves up out of the chair with their arms because of pain.

The patient may also report a disturbed or interrupted sleep pattern that is commonly due to TrPs in the biceps femoris muscle. Pain and symptoms from the biceps femoris muscle are typically located in the posterolateral aspect of the knee, and pain can be focused around the head of the fibula at its attachment.

Patients can also experience a wide distribution of symptoms and pain in the posterior thigh that may lead to a diagnosis of "sciatica." Even when the patient may have experienced a traumatic injury resulting in a hamstring muscle strain, examination for TrPs is necessary to help control painful symptoms caused by the associated TrPs.

3.3. Patient Examination

After a thorough subjective examination the clinician should make a detailed drawing representing the pain pattern that the patient

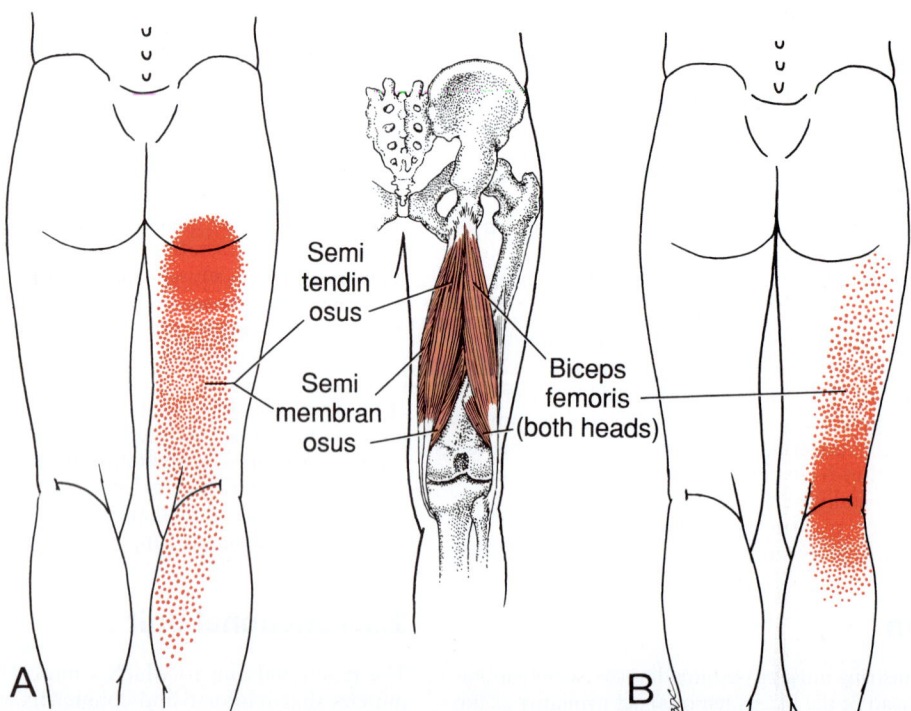

Figure 60-4. Composite pain patterns (dark red) referred from TrPs in the hamstring muscles. Solid red denotes the essential pain distribution referred from these TrPs. Red stippling locates the occasional extension of the pattern in some patients. A, Semitendinosus and semimembranosus muscles. B, Long and short heads of the biceps femoris muscle.

has described. This depiction will assist in planning the physical examination and can be useful in monitoring the progression of the patient as symptoms improve or change. In assessing posture, persons with short or stiff hamstring muscles may present with a posterior pelvic tilt and a reduced lumbar lordosis. A typical swayback posture, as could be seen in this population, would also include a forward head posture. The importance of a thorough examination, even when all muscular symptoms are limited to one half of the body, cannot be overemphasized.

For proper examination of the hamstring muscles, the clinician should observe sitting and standing postures. In sitting, posture and environmental setup should also be assessed. The clinician should watch for potential compression of the posterior thighs by the front of a chair seat that may occur if the patient's legs are not long enough to rest fully on the floor. A tendency for the patient to cross the knees in sitting could also contribute to the presence of TrPs in the hamstring muscles. Further, when the patient is seated, he or she may lean forward to reduce the load on the ischial tuberosities, thus placing an increased load in the mid-thigh region of the hamstring muscles.

Physical examination should be conducted to rule out lumbar, sacroiliac, hip, or knee joint pathology. This evaluation may include range of motion testing of the lumbar spine, hip, and knee; passive accessory motion testing of the hip, sacroiliac joint, or knee; strength testing of the hip (especially in extension, adduction, and knee flexion) and other associated muscles or movement; and any appropriate neurologic testing or orthopedic special tests. A careful assessment should be made to rule out pain or symptom referral into the buttock or posterior thigh from other muscles, joints, or neural tissues that can also refer pain to the same region.

It is also important to observe the patient's gait pattern with close attention to terminal swing phase and early-stance phase as this is when the hamstring muscles are most active during the gait pattern. The knee may be held in a flexed position throughout the stance phase due to pain in the hamstring region from TrPs. Gluteus maximus muscle weakness may also lead to overload of the hamstring musculature during gait, and observation of the lumbar spine and innominate positions during the stance phase is warranted.

The regional interdependence of the lumbosacral spine and hip, as well as the hip and knee joints, makes it necessary to examine these relationships in a closed and open kinetic chain. A functional activity that should be assessed in standing is the double-leg squat, which should be observed from a sagittal perspective (see Figure 54-3A). The clinician should note any excessive movement in the lumbosacral region or hip joint. During a proper squat, the patient should be able to demonstrate a good range of hip flexion without an excessive anterior pelvic tilt, excessive lumbar hyperextension, or a major shift of the knee in front of the foot in the sagittal plane (see Figure 54-3B). Movement from a standing to sitting position should be observed to examine gluteus maximus and hamstring muscle control during sitting along with hip and knee flexion range of motion.

Hip and knee range of motion, muscle strength, and activation patterns should be assessed in all planes. Muscle length assessment of one and two joint hip flexor muscles should be performed (see Figure 54-7). Hip extension muscle activation patterns should be assessed in the prone position. Janda described a muscle activation pattern during hip extension that includes the following muscle firing sequence: hamstrings, gluteus maximus, and contralateral paraspinal muscles, followed by ipsilateral paraspinal muscles. The lumbar spine should be maintained in a neutral position and the knee in extension; any deviation would be indicative of movement impairment.[26] Hamstring muscle strength should be tested both for its role in hip extension and knee flexion.

Muscle length assessment should be differentiated from the altered neurodynamics of the sciatic nerve. Hamstring muscle tightness or stiffness is the most frequent reason why an individual may have limited forward bending or excessive lumbar flexion when attempting to touch one's toes with the knees extended,[27] though the tightness does not restrict flexion at the hip when the knees are bent. Hamstring extensibility can be assessed utilizing the 90/90 test, in which the hip is flexed to 90° and the knee is passively moved from 90° of knee flexion toward full extension (Figure 60-5).

Trigger points in the hamstring muscles markedly limit motion during the Straight Leg Raise Test (Figure 60-6). The pain that TrPs cause at the limit of hip flexion may be felt in the lower buttock, the back of the thigh, or behind the knee. Structural differentiation with ankle dorsiflexion would still be necessary to determine the relative contributions of neural tension and myofascial tension. The addition of dorsiflexion at the end of their range of motion during the straight leg test should not further provoke TrPs in the hamstring muscles, and thus no change in pain in the buttock or posterior thigh should increase with this differentiating maneuver. In some muscles, active TrPs cause pain when the muscle is maximally shortened, so that they restrict both the shortened range of motion and the stretch range of motion. Active TrPs in the hamstring muscles may slightly restrict the combination of active extension at the hip with combined flexion at the knee, giving the impression that a tight rectus femoris muscle is responsible. In this situation, inactivation of the hamstring TrPs restores active range of motion. However, this hypothesis is not supported by two studies showing that dry needling combined with stretching of hamstring muscles was not more effective than stretching alone for improving their length.[28;29]

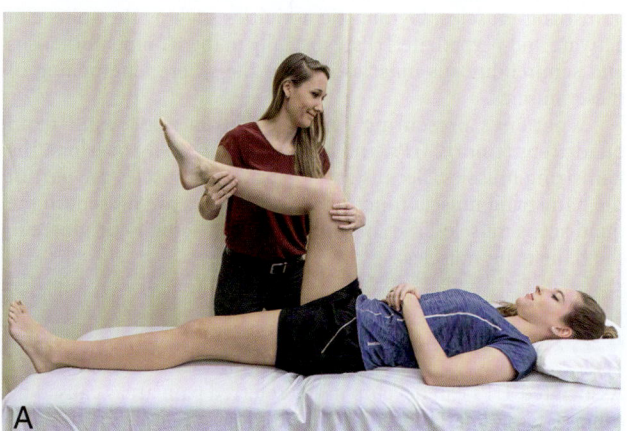 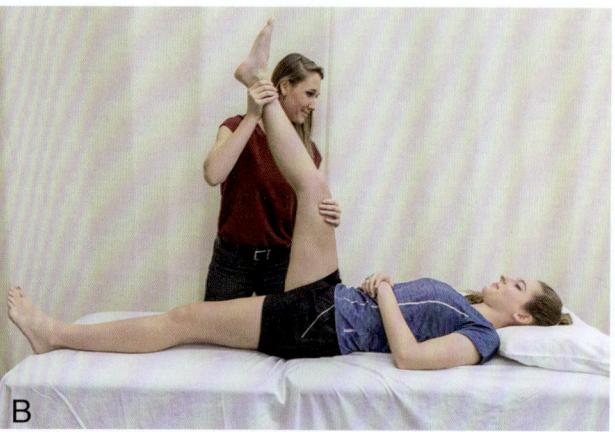

Figure 60-5. Hamstring muscle length test using 90-90 position. A, Starting position. B, End position demonstrating hamstring muscle length deficit.

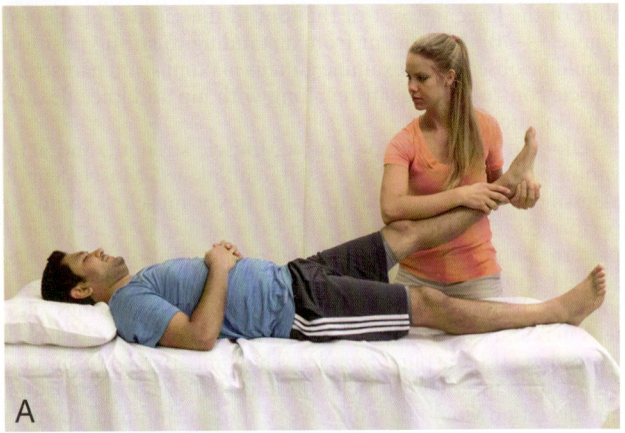 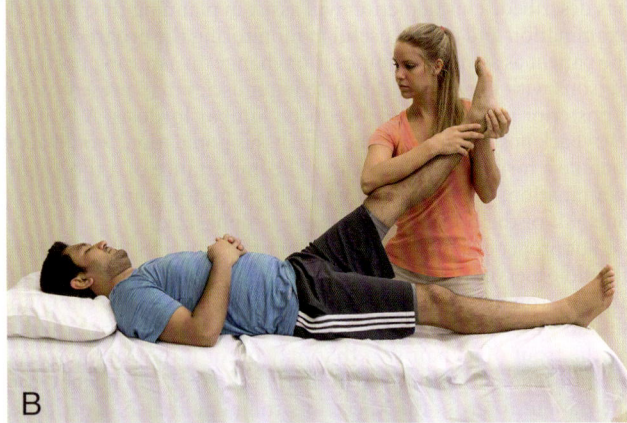

Figure 60-6. Hamstring muscle length assessment using the straight leg raise. A, Starting position. B, End position demonstrating hamstring muscle length deficit.

3.4. Trigger Point Examination

The semitendinosus muscle is easily identified by locating its prominent tendon behind the medial aspect of the knee when the knee is flexed against resistance and then by following the tendon superiorly into the thigh. The semimembranosus muscle lies deep to the semitendinosus muscle and is muscular in the distal thigh. Its muscle fibers can be palpated on each side of the semitendinosus tendon. The semimembranosus muscle forms the medial border of the hamstrings and is adjacent to the gracilis muscle in the lower half of the thigh.

To palpate TrPs in the semitendinosus or semimembranosus muscles, the patient can lie prone, side-lying, or supine, though prone is preferred. To locate TrPs in the semitendinosus or semimembranosus muscles, the patient lies in the prone position, with the involved thigh in a slightly abducted position and the knee slightly flexed with the ankle resting on a pillow. Cross-fiber flat palpation can be used for examination of the distal medial hamstring muscles (Figure 60-7A) by applying direct pressure on the muscle against the underlying femur. Cross-fiber flat palpation can also be used to palpate TrPs in the proximal portion of the medial hamstring muscles (Figure 60-7B). With the patient side-lying with the affected side down, cross-fiber pincer palpation can be used to identify TrPs in the semitendinosus muscle (Figure 60-7C). While the patient is lying supine with the hip slightly flexed, abducted, and externally rotated and a pillow placed under the knee and upper lower leg, cross-fiber pincer palpation can be used to identify TrPs in the semitendinosus and semimembranosus muscles (Figure 60-7D).

When examining the biceps femoris muscle for TrPs, it is best to approach it from the posterior and lateral aspect of the thigh. The short head of the biceps femoris muscle lies deep to the long head in the distal half of the thigh. The two heads can be distinguished by palpation as the long head becomes tense when the patient tries to extend the hip, whereas the short head does not change tension. Cross-fiber flat palpation is utilized to identify TrPs in the short head of the biceps femoris muscle (Figure 60-8A). To palpate for TrPs in the long head of the biceps femoris muscle, cross-fiber flat palpation should be used by applying direct pressure on the muscle against the underlying femur with the patient in prone with a pillow placed under the ankle to place the knee in slight flexion (Figure 60-7B). Trigger points can also be located in side-lying utilizing cross-fiber flat palpation (Figure 60-7C).

4. DIFFERENTIAL DIAGNOSIS

4.1. Activation and Perpetuation of Trigger Points

Any posture or activity that activates a TrP, if not corrected, can also perpetuate it. In any part of the hamstring muscles, TrPs may be activated by unaccustomed eccentric loading, eccentric exercise in an unconditioned muscle, or maximal or submaximal concentric loading.[30] Trigger points may also be activated or aggravated when the muscle is placed in a shortened and/or lengthened position for an extended period of time.

Hamstring TrPs are often activated and perpetuated by a sedentary lifestyle or by immobility where the knees and hips are frequently kept in a flexed position for a prolonged period of time. Under-thigh compression by an ill-fitting chair can both activate and perpetuate TrPs in the hamstring muscles. Short-statured individuals with hamstring TrPs who sit in customary chairs, or patients of average stature who sit in chairs with a high seat, can experience aggravation of pain due to excess pressure on hamstring TrPs as a result of the weight of the dangling legs. In addition, they may experience the tingling and numbness of neurapraxia due to pressure on the sciatic nerve. To address this problem of under-thigh compression by the chair seat, the seat should be lowered to allow the feet to rest on the ground if possible, or the patient can utilize a footstool that supports the heels and lifts the thighs. As seen in the younger population, many school chairs present this same problem because chairs of one size are used for children of widely different heights.

Sporting activities such as football, basketball, and soccer can result in hamstring muscle injuries, especially in unconditioned or poorly trained athletes. Kicking motions often require simultaneous flexion at the hip and extension at the knee placing the muscle in a passively insufficient position while performing an eccentric contraction to decelerate the leg. This scenario can easily overload the hamstring muscles. Other exercise activities such as swimming or cycling may also lead to an overload of the hamstring muscles. Gymnastic activities such as the splits can activate and perpetuate TrPs, especially in the semimembranosus and semitendinosus muscles, due to the severe lengthening of these muscles.

A patient's presenting thigh condition may result from quadriceps femoris TrPs, and a clinician can easily overlook the hamstring muscles. Because the quadriceps muscles are part of the hamstring muscle functional unit, if TrPs are present in the quadriceps muscles, the dysfunction could actually originate in the hamstring muscles.

4.2. Associated Trigger Points

Associated TrPs can develop in the referred pain areas caused by other TrPs.[31] Therefore, musculature in the referred pain areas for each muscle should also be considered.

In association with TrPs in the hamstring muscles, TrPs are likely to develop in the posterior (ischiocondylar) part of the adductor magnus muscle, which helps extend the hip as part of

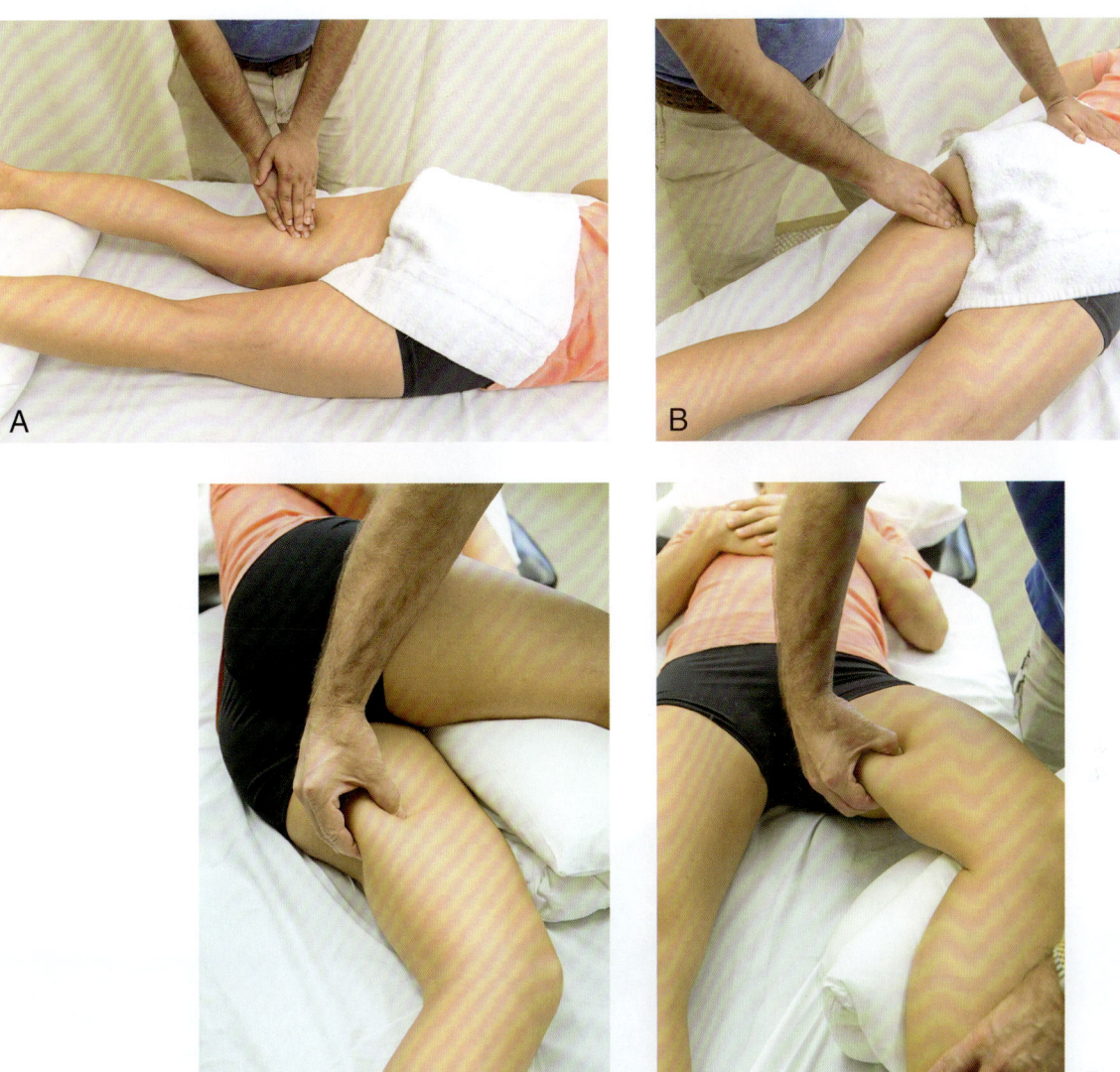

Figure 60-7. Palpation for TrPs in the medial hamstring muscles. A, Cross-fiber flat palpation of distal medial hamstring muscles. B, Cross-fiber flat palpation proximal medial hamstring muscles. C, Side-lying cross-fiber pincer palpation. D, Supine cross-fiber pincer palpation.

the hamstring muscle functional unit. The gastrocnemius muscle also tends to develop TrPs in association with hamstring TrPs. The vastus lateralis muscle is prone to developing TrPs when TrPs exist in the long head of the biceps femoris muscle.

Antagonists to the hamstrings may also develop associated TrPs, especially the iliopsoas muscle and the quadriceps femoris muscles. The patient may only report symptoms of quadriceps femoris TrPs even when there is dysfunction in the hamstring muscles. Shortening of the hamstring muscles caused by TrPs is likely to overload the quadriceps femoris muscles. This overload can activate TrPs in the quadriceps femoris muscles. In this case, the quadriceps femoris muscle symptoms will not resolve until the TrPs in the hamstring muscles have been eliminated.

Hamstring muscle length deficits or tension caused by TrPs produces a posterior tilt of the pelvis that causes associated flattening of the lumbar spine that can result in thoracic kyphosis and a forward head position. This postural dysfunction imposes compensatory overload on a number of muscles of the trunk, including the periscapular and neck muscles, thoracic paraspinal muscles, and quadratus lumborum and rectus abdominis muscles. Hamstring muscle tension caused by TrPs and/or muscle length deficits is often a key to low back pain of myofascial origin. Clinically, starting treatment by releasing the hamstring muscles, even though the iliopsoas or quadratus lumborum muscles seem to be involved, will provide improved results as TrPs in the proximal muscles are typically associated with the TrPs in the hamstring muscles.

Several other muscles whose pain referral patterns overlap those of the hamstring muscles and could have associated TrPs include the obturator internus, piriformis, gluteus medius, gluteus minimus, vastus lateralis, popliteus, and gastrocnemius muscles.

4.3. Associated Pathology

A hamstring muscle strain is defined as posterior thigh pain where direct contact to the area is excluded as the mechanism of injury. Detection of hyperintense signals on magnetic resonance imaging (MRI) within the hamstring muscles is indicative of a hamstring muscle strain.[32] Hamstring muscle strains commonly occur in athletes who employ high-speed kicking and sprinting, such as football and soccer.[33] Athletes may describe an audible pop as part of the mechanism of injury when the proximal hamstring tendon is involved and are likely not able to continue with sport activity immediately after the injury.[34] With proximal tendon

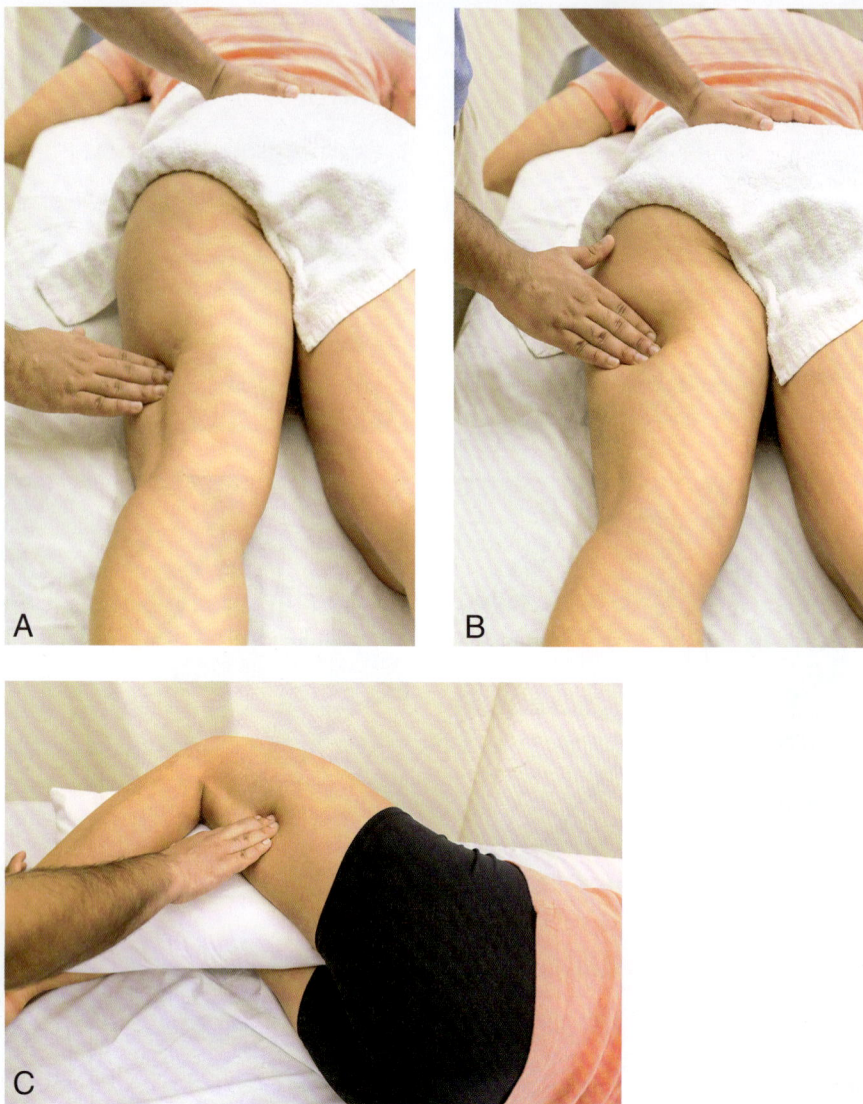

Figure 60-8. Palpation for TrPs in the lateral hamstring muscles. A, Cross-fiber flat palpation of the short head of the biceps femoris muscle in prone. B, Cross-fiber flat palpation of the long head of biceps femoris muscle in prone. C, Cross-fiber flat palpation side-lying.

involvement, the patient may report pain while sitting on the ischial tuberosity,[35] swelling, weakness, and a loss of range of motion at the hip and at the knee.[36] Clinically, palpation typically reveals local area tenderness and a possible apparent defect in the affected muscle.[36] However, it is important to consider that pathology of the hamstring muscles is also prevalent in asymptomatic people. Thompson et al[37] demonstrated that 15% of individuals without symptoms had bilateral partial tears, and 2% had bilateral complete tears of hamstring muscle insertion, with the semimembranosus muscle most often affected.

Puranen and Orava[38] were the first to describe "hamstring syndrome" as pain in the lower gluteal area that radiated down the posterior thigh to the popliteal space. Contemporary medicine refers to this diagnosis as "proximal hamstring tendinopathy" or, in lay terms, "high hamstring" tendinopathy. This pathology is characterized by pain as described previously that is easily aggravated during sports activities, specifically running at a faster pace. Often, the pain can be so intense that the athlete is not able to sprint at all. Pain can also be exacerbated with prolonged sitting and made worse with continued exercise and stretching of the hamstring muscles. Because of the complex nature of diagnosing pain in the gluteal region and posterior thigh, MRI is often used to confirm or negate the diagnosis of hamstring tendinopathy and exclude other potential sources of pain.[39]

Proximal hamstring tendinopathy is an insertional disease that can affect athletic and nonathletic populations. Pain is typically reported as deep buttock pain about the ischial tuberosity and common hamstring tendon. The onset of pain may occur from training errors, especially in runners introducing sprinting, lunging, hurdles, and/or hill training; prolonged static stretch positions, as may occur in participation in yoga or Pilates; or compressive loading from prolonged sitting, particularly on a firm surface.[40] Proximal hamstring tendinopathy is assessed by adding compressive or tensile load to the common hamstring attachment at the ischial tuberosity. Tensile loading assessment from a 90/90 hamstring muscle length test or straight leg raise may provoke local pain symptoms (Lasegue sign). Compressive loading can be assessed by asking the patient to perform active hamstring muscles exercises, such as a low-level bridge and gradually increasing load on the hamstring muscles up to a single-leg deadlift.[40]

Proximal hamstring tendinopathy and hamstring TrPs present very similarly. In both cases, pain is exacerbated by sitting postures, hamstring muscle length is decreased, and taut bands can be palpated. The thickening or fibrosing of the common proximal hamstring tendon that occurs with tendinopathy produces a taut band with palpation. Trigger points and tendinopathy can occur together. Two case reports of runners with proximal hamstring tendinopathy showed improved pain reports with TrP dry needling to the hamstrings and adductor magnus muscles. The authors propose that release of the involved TrPs may reduce tension on the tendinous insertion to the ischial tuberosity.[41] After TrP dry needling, treatment progressed to eccentric training of the hamstring muscles following recommendations for achilles tendinopathy rehabilitation.

Typical MRI findings of hamstring tendinopathy include increased tendon girth, intrasubstance signal heterogeneity, and asymmetric involvement of hamstring tendons (in unilateral cases).[42] Martin et al[25] proposed that diagnosis in a patient with posterior hip pain should differentiate deep gluteal syndrome, hamstrings syndrome, and ischiofemoral impingement. Clinically, the fibrotic bands of hamstring tendinopathy should be distinguished from taut bands of TrPs by the fact that they are connective and not muscle tissue, and should not produce local twitch responses on snapping palpation.

Ischial or ischiogluteal bursitis is an inflammation of the ischiogluteal bursae due to excessive or ineffective form with physical activity such as running, jumping, kicking, or prolonged sitting.[43] Patients with ischiogluteal bursitis typically present with buttock pain that is exacerbated by any activity that recruits the hamstring muscles, that stretches the hamstring muscles, or that requires sitting on the ischial tuberosity. Pain and tenderness is typically identified with palpation over the ischial tuberosity.[44] Ischial bursitis is rare and an infrequently recognized pathology that requires diagnostic imaging to differentiate from other soft tissue pathologies and local area tumors.[45] Ultrasound and MRI are best for visualization of the ischial bursae.[46]

Distally, the pes anserine refers to the tendons of the sartorius, gracilis, and semitendinosus muscles along the insertions into the proximal medial aspect of the tibia. In pes anserine bursitis, the bursa separating these three tendons becomes inflamed and causes pain. Patients experiencing pes anserine bursitis may report of vague medial knee pain and may experience swelling and tenderness along the medial proximal tibia. Pes anserine bursitis is commonly associated with degenerative joint disease, obesity, genu valgum, pes planus, and sport activities.[47,48]

5. CORRECTIVE ACTIONS

Patients with TrPs in the hamstring muscles should limit the duration of time spent sitting. If they are employed in a desk job where the majority of the day is spent sitting, assessment and education for proper ergonomics and sitting postures would be beneficial. Taking short breaks to stand, utilizing a standing desk, or improving postural support will assist in reducing symptoms. A timer placed across the room can remind the patient to get up, walk across the room, reset the device, and return to the chair with minimal distraction from thought. The design of the chair that the individual uses and the materials that the seat are made of change the amount of pressure, contact area, and tissue perfusion.[49] Under-thigh compression can be avoided by selecting or adjusting chairs to match the leg length of the individual, or by propping the feet up on a footrest placed a short distance in front of the chair.

When selecting a chair for home, one should ensure that the front edge of its seat is rounded and well-padded. When driving on long automobile trips, prolonged immobilization and excessive pressure on the hamstring muscles can be alleviated by using automatic cruise control. This function permits alteration in the leg position and allows frequent "stretch" breaks. Sleeping on the side with a pillow between the legs to keep the hip in a neutral position and knees closer to being fully straightened may assist in addressing hamstring TrP activation and perpetuation especially in the biceps femoris muscle. Patients should avoid placing a pillow under the knee while sleeping on their back, as this will keep the hamstring muscles in a prolonged shortened position that can activate and perpetuate TrPs in the hamstring muscles.

Hamstring TrPs can be self-treated with self-pressure release techniques utilizing a TrP release tool, tennis or lacrosse ball, or a foam roller based on personal preference and abilities. Utilizing a TrP release tool, the patient lies on the unaffected side and the tool is placed on a tender point in the hamstring muscle (Figure 60-9A). The patient can also use a pincer grasp while seated to perform self-release by finding the most tender

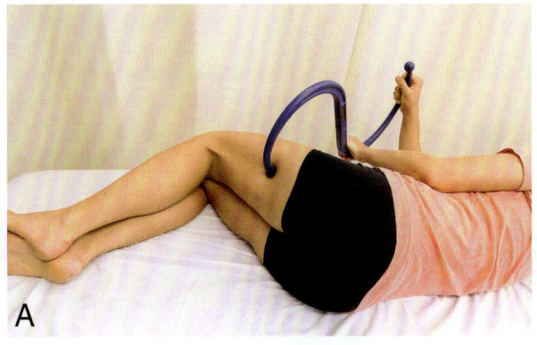 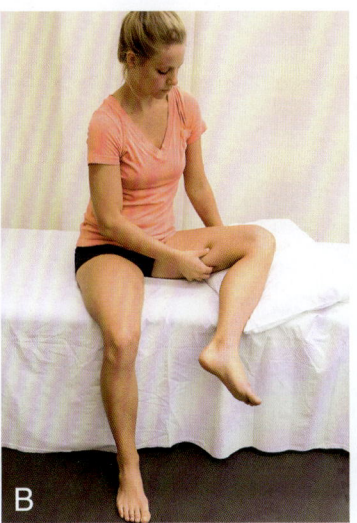 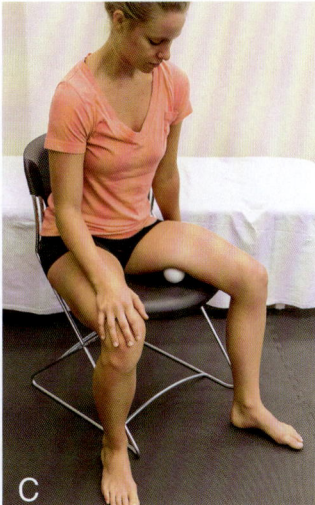

Figure 60-9. Trigger point self-pressure release. A, Lateral hamstring muscles. B, Manual self-release medial hamstring muscles. C, Tennis ball under hamstring muscles.

spot and applying a light pressure to the area (Figure 60-9B). A ball can be used by placing it under the thigh for pressure on the tender area (Figure 60-9C). In all pressure-release techniques, pressure should be held for 15 to 30 seconds and repeated six times. This sequence can be repeated every 2 to 3 hours as long as relief of symptoms is achieved. Too much pressure (no more than 4/10 pain scale) on the TrPs should be avoided, as excessive pressure can actually cause activation and perpetuation of the TrPs.

Foam rolling can be utilized to help release TrPs in the hamstring muscles and is commonly used by athletes. In a long sitting position, the unaffected leg should be placed in knee flexion with the foot planted on the floor and the posterior aspect of the affected leg resting on the foam roller. The patient can roll along the foam roller until identifying the tender TrP, at which point the patient should hold constant isolated pressure for 15 to 30 seconds or until the tenderness reduces, as instructed earlier.

Assuming that patients have no neural tension (no numbness, tingling with stretch), a basic stretch that those with hamstring TrPs should perform at home is the single-leg long-sit stretch. The patient should sit at the edge of a table with one leg on the table with the knee extended and the ankle in a neutral relaxed position (Figure 60-10A). The opposite limb should be firmly planted on the ground to provide stability during the stretch. Ensuring a neutral or slight anterior tilt of the pelvis and neutral lumbar spine, the patient should flex forward in an attempt to touch the belly button to the thigh (Figure 60-10B).

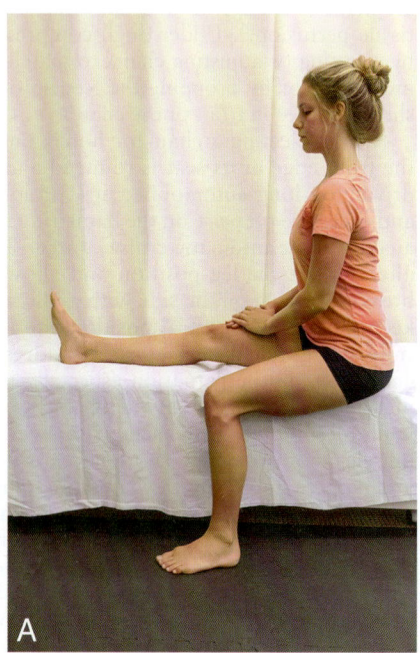
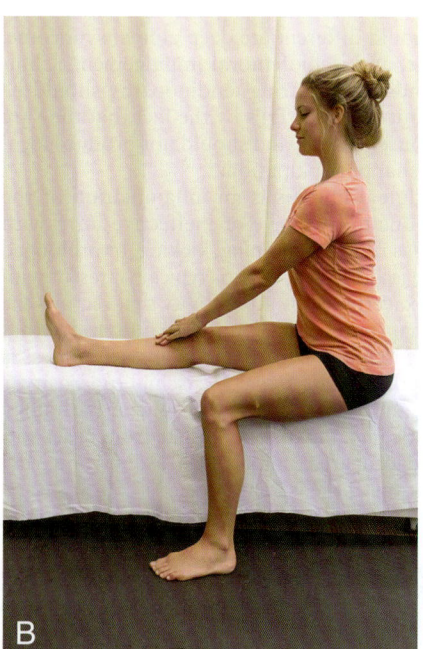
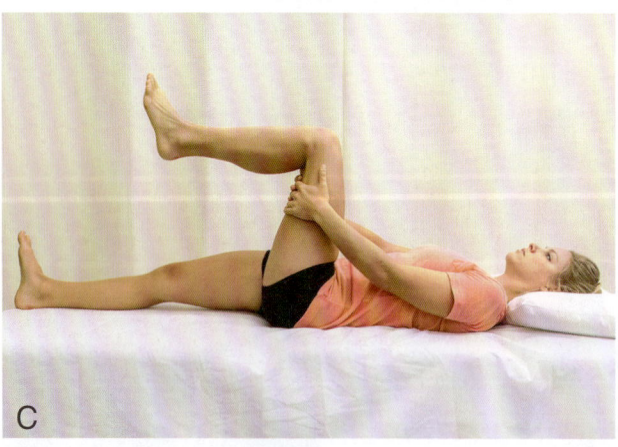
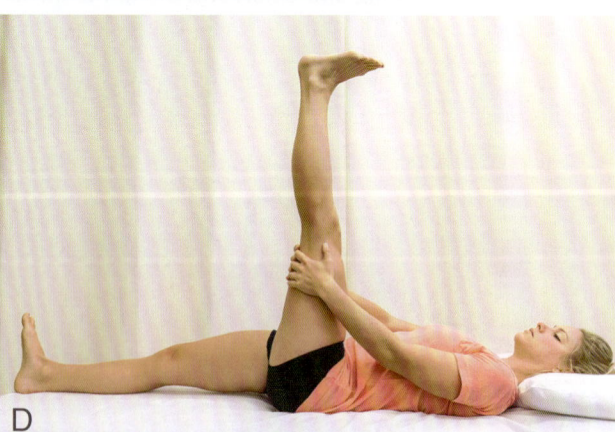

Figure 60-10. Hamstring muscles self-stretch. A, Start position in erect posture with neutral lumbar spine. B, Leaning forward maintaining neutral lumbar spine until a stretch is felt behind the thigh. C, Starting position for supine 90-90 stretch. D, Actively straightening the knee until a gentle stretch is felt behind the thigh.

Chapter 60: Hamstring Muscles 645

The stretch should be maintained for a 30-second hold followed by relaxation and repeated four times as long as the symptoms are resolving. This sequence can be repeated two to three times per day.

If the patient has neural tension with hamstring TrPs (numbness, tingling), he or she can perform a supine active hamstring muscle stretch from the 90/90 position (Figure 60-10C), in which the patient stabilizes the thigh at 90° of hip flexion with the hands placed behind the thigh and actively extends the knee to the point of stretch behind the thigh and knee but prior to the onset of pain of neural provocation (Figure 60-10D).

When the patient or athlete requires a prolonged stretch, the doorway stretch can be utilized (Figure 60-11). The patient lies on the floor with the unaffected leg through the doorway and the affected side up on the door jamb. The patient should not start with the hip at greater than a 45° angle. A slight stretch should be felt in the back of the thigh and knee; no numbness or tingling should be experienced in the back of the thigh, calf, or foot. This stretch is commonly used for true muscle length deficits and performed following the elimination of TrPs.

A yoga strap can be used to assist and augment a hamstring muscle stretch through a full range of hip motions (Figure 60-12). The yoga strap should be secured around the foot just below the bottom of the heel of the foot. The leg is then placed out to the side, and the stretch should be felt along the inner thigh and behind the knee (Figure 60-12A). Using the hands and arms, the leg is pulled up into hip flexion while slightly out to the side and held in the position of a firm stretch (Figure 60-12B). The leg is positioned so that it is aligned with the trunk (Figure 60-12C) and then placed across midline (Figure 60-12D). Each stretch position should be held for 15 to 30 seconds with a minimum of four stops through the range. The patient should not experience numbness or tingling in the leg or foot at any time. If these sensations are felt, the stretch should be stopped immediately.

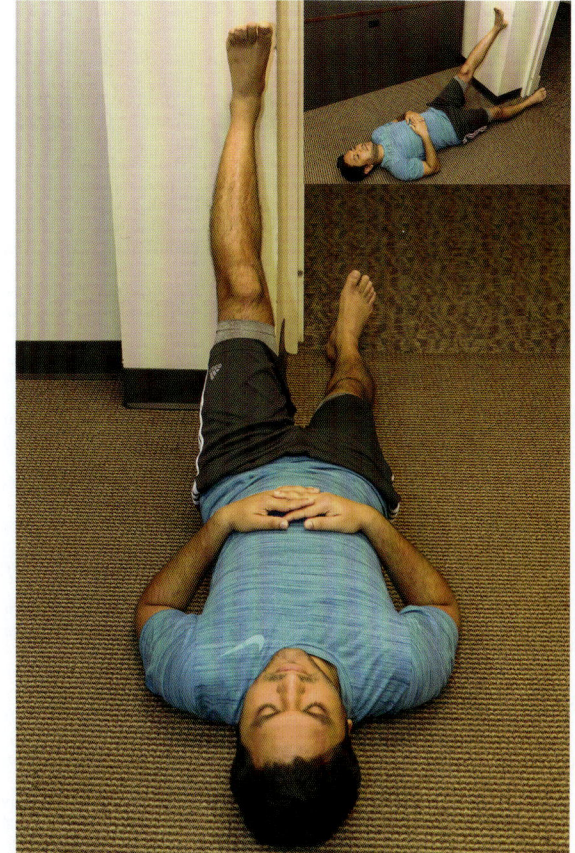

Figure 60-11. Hamstring stretch in the doorway.

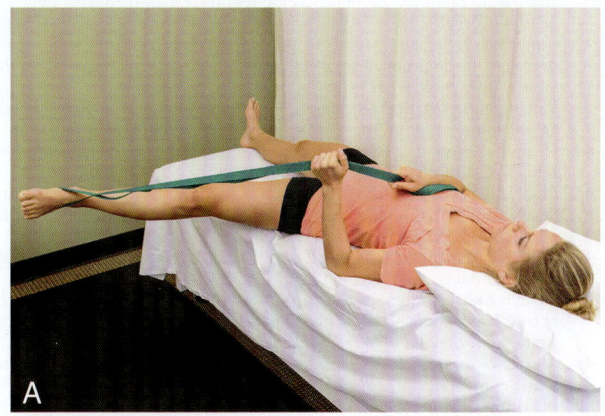

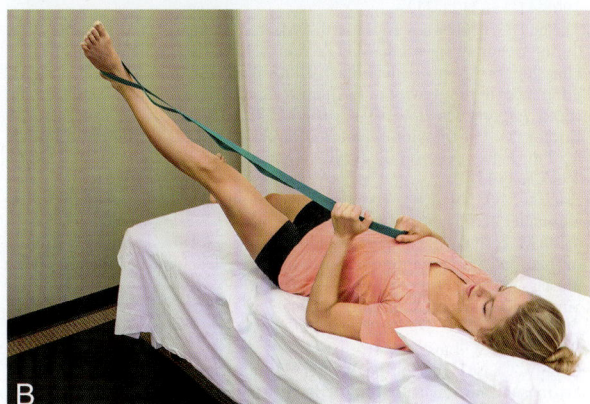

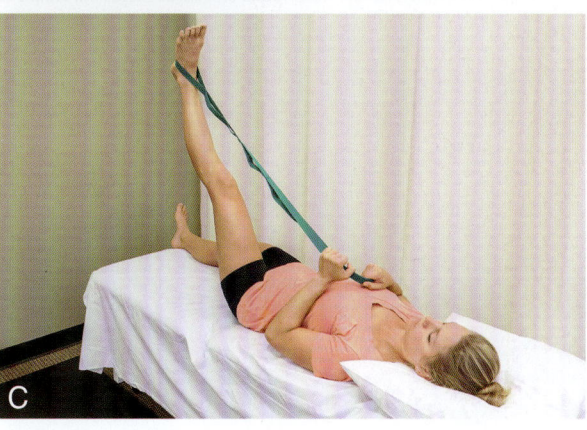

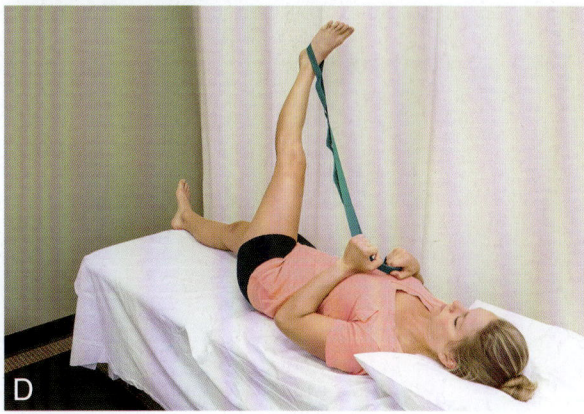

Figure 60-12. Hamstring muscle stretch utilizing yoga strap through full range of hip motion. A, Staring position. B, Medial hamstring muscle stretch. C, Medial and lateral hamstring muscle stretch. D, Lateral hamstring and hip abductor muscle stretch.

References

1. Standring S. *Gray's Anatomy: The Anatomical Basis of Clinical Practice.* 41st ed. London, UK: Elsevier; 2015.
2. Storey RN, Meikle GR, Stringer MD, Woodley SJ. Proximal hamstring morphology and morphometry in men: an anatomic and MRI investigation. *Scand J Med Sci Sports.* 2016;26(12):1480-1489.
3. Pérez-Bellmunt A, Miguel-Perez M, Brugue MB, et al. An anatomical and histological study of the structures surrounding the proximal attachment of the hamstring muscles. *Man Ther.* 2015;20(3):445-450.
4. Kim YC, Yoo WK, Chung IH, Seo JS, Tanaka S. Tendinous insertion of semimembranosus muscle into the lateral meniscus. *Surg Radiol Anat.* 1997;19(6):365-369.
5. LaPrade RF, Engebretsen AH, Ly TV, Johansen S, Wentorf FA, Engebretsen L. The anatomy of the medial part of the knee. *J Bone Joint Surg Am.* 2007;89(9):2000-2010.
6. LaPrade RF, Morgan PM, Wentorf FA, Johansen S, Engebretsen L. The anatomy of the posterior aspect of the knee. An anatomic study. *J Bone Joint Surg Am.* 2007;89(4):758-764.
7. Beltran J, Matityahu A, Hwang K, et al. The distal semimembranosus complex: normal MR anatomy, variants, biomechanics and pathology. *Skeletal Radiol.* 2003;32(8):435-445.
8. Sato K, Nimura A, Yamaguchi K, Akita K. Anatomical study of the proximal origin of hamstring muscles. *J Orthop Sci.* 2012;17(5):614-618.
9. Tosovic D, Muirhead JC, Brown JM, Woodley SJ. Anatomy of the long head of biceps femoris: an ultrasound study. *Clin Anat.* 2016;29(6):738-745.
10. Kumazaki T, Ehara Y, Sakai T. Anatomy and physiology of hamstring injury. *Int J Sports Med.* 2012;33(12):950-954.
11. Rha DW, Yi KH, Park ES, Park C, Kim HJ. Intramuscular nerve distribution of the hamstring muscles: application to treating spasticity. *Clin Anat.* 2016;29(6):746-751.
12. Oatis C. *Kinesiology: The Mechanics and Patho Mechanics of Human Movement.* 2nd ed. Baltimore, MD: Lippinott, Williams & Wilkins; 2009 (pp. 776-777).
13. Neumann DA. *Kinesiology of the Musculoskeletal System: Foundations for Rehabilitation.* 2nd ed. St. Louis, MO: Mosby; 2010 (p. 493).
14. Porterfield JA, DeRosa C. *Mechanical Low Back Pain: Perspectives in Functional Anatomy.* 2nd ed. Philadelphia, PA: Saunders; 1998 (p. 110).
15. Lyons K, Perry J, Gronley JK, Barnes L, Antonelli D. Timing and relative intensity of hip extensor and abductor muscle action during level and stair ambulation. An EMG study. *Phys Ther.* 1983;63(10):1597-1605.
16. Chumanov ES, Heiderscheit BC, Thelen DG. The effect of speed and influence of individual muscles on hamstring mechanics during the swing phase of sprinting. *J Biomech.* 2007;40(16):3555-3562.
17. Yu B, Queen RM, Abbey AN, Liu Y, Moorman CT, Garrett WE. Hamstring muscle kinematics and activation during overground sprinting. *J Biomech.* 2008;41(15):3121-3126.
18. Thelen DG, Chumanov ES, Hoerth DM, et al. Hamstring muscle kinematics during treadmill sprinting. *Med Sci Sports Exerc.* 2005;37(1):108-114.
19. Higashihara A, Ono T, Kubota J, Okuwaki T, Fukubayashi T. Functional differences in the activity of the hamstring muscles with increasing running speed. *J Sports Sci.* 2010;28(10):1085-1092.
20. Ericson M. On the biomechanics of cycling. A study of joint and muscle load during exercise on the bicycle ergometer. *Scand J Rehabil Med Suppl.* 1986;16:1-43.
21. Ericson MO, Nisell R, Arborelius UP, Ekholm J. Muscular activity during ergometer cycling. *Scand J Rehabil Med.* 1985;17(2):53-61.
22. Satoh M, Yoshino H, Fujimura A, Hitomi Y, Isogai S. Three-layered architecture of the popliteal fascia that acts as a kinetic retinaculum for the hamstring muscles. *Anat Sci Int.* 2016;91(4):341-349.
23. Simons DG, Travell J, Simons L. *Travell & Simon's Myofascial Pain and Dysfunction: The Trigger Point Manual.* Vol 1. 2nd ed. Baltimore, MD: Williams & Wilkins; 1999 (p. 104).
24. Chan W, Chase HE, Cahir JG, Walton NP. Calcific tendinitis of biceps femoris: an unusual site and cause for lateral knee pain. *BMJ Case Rep.* 2016;2016.
25. Martin HD, Khoury A, Schroder R, Palmer IJ. Ischiofemoral impingement and hamstring syndrome as causes of posterior hip pain: where do we go next? *Clin Sports Med.* 2016;35(3):469-486.
26. Page P, Frank C, Lardner R. *Assessment and Treatment of Muscle Imbalance. The Janda Approach.* Champaign, IL: Human Kinetics; 2010.
27. Lewit K. Postisometric relaxation in combination with other methods of muscular facilitation and inhibition. *Manuelle Medizin.* 1986;2:101-104.
28. Geist K, Bradley C, Hofman A, et al. Clinical effects of dry needling among asymptomatic individuals with hamstring tightness: a randomized controlled trial. *J Sport Rehabil.* 2016:1-31.
29. Mason JS, Crowell M, Dolbeer J, et al. The effectiveness of dry needling and stretching vs. stretching alone on hamstring flexibility in patients with knee pain: a randomized controlled trial. *Int J Sports Phys Ther.* 2016;11(5):672-683.
30. Gerwin RD, Dommerholt J, Shah JP. An expansion of Simons' integrated hypothesis of trigger point formation. *Curr Pain Headache Rep.* 2004;8(6):468-475.
31. Hsieh YL, Kao MJ, Kuan TS, Chen SM, Chen JT, Hong CZ. Dry needling to a key myofascial trigger point may reduce the irritability of satellite MTrPs. *Am J Phys Med Rehabil.* 2007;86(5):397-403.
32. Verrall GM, Slavotinek JP, Barnes PG. The effect of sports specific training on reducing the incidence of hamstring injuries in professional Australian Rules football players. *Br J Sports Med.* 2005;39(6):363-368.
33. Liu H, Garrett W, Moorman C, Yu B. Injury rate, mechanism, and risk factors of hamstring strain injuries in sport: a literature review. *J Sport Health Sci.* 2012;1:92-101.
34. Askling CM, Tengvar M, Saartok T, Thorstensson A. Proximal hamstring strains of stretching type in different sports: injury situations, clinical and magnetic resonance imaging characteristics, and return to sport. *Am J Sports Med.* 2008;36(9):1799-1804.
35. Cohen S, Bradley J. Acute proximal hamstring rupture. *J Am Acad Orthop Surg.* 2007;15(6):350-355.
36. Heiderscheit BC, Sherry MA, Silder A, Chumanov ES, Thelen DG. Hamstring strain injuries: recommendations for diagnosis, rehabilitation, and injury prevention. *J Orthop Sports Phys Ther.* 2010;40(2):67-81.
37. Thompson SM, Fung S, Wood DG. The prevalence of proximal hamstring pathology on MRI in the asymptomatic population. *Knee Surg Sports Traumatol Arthrosc.* 2017;25(1):108-111.
38. Puranen J, Orava S. The hamstring syndrome. A new diagnosis of gluteal sciatic pain. *Am J Sports Med.* 1988;16(5):517-521.
39. Fredericson M, Moore W, Guillet M, Beaulieu C. High hamstring tendinopathy in runners: meeting the challenges of diagnosis, treatment, and rehabilitation. *Phys Sportsmed.* 2005;33(5):32-43.
40. Goom TS, Malliaras P, Reiman MP, Purdam CR. Proximal hamstring tendinopathy: clinical aspects of assessment and management. *J Orthop Sports Phys Ther.* 2016;46(6):483-493.
41. Jayaseelan DJ, Moats N, Ricardo CR. Rehabilitation of proximal hamstring tendinopathy utilizing eccentric training, lumbopelvic stabilization, and trigger point dry needling: 2 case reports. *J Orthop Sports Phys Ther.* 2014;44(3):198-205.
42. Lempainen L, Sarimo J, Mattila K, Orava S. Proximal hamstring tendinopathy: overview of the problem with emphasis on surgical treatment. *Oper Tech Sports Med.* 2009;17:225-228.
43. Van Mieghem IM, Boets A, Sciot R, Van Breuseghem I. Ischiogluteal bursitis: an uncommon type of bursitis. *Skeletal Radiol.* 2004;33(7):413-416.
44. Hitora T, Kawaguchi Y, Mori M, et al. Ischiogluteal bursitis: a report of three cases with MR findings. *Rheumatol Int.* 2009;29(4):455-458.
45. Ekiz T, Bicici V, Hatioglu C, Yalcin S, Cingoz K. Ischial pain and sitting disability due to ischiogluteal bursitis: visual vignette. *Pain Physician.* 2015;18(4):E657-E658.
46. Akisue T, Yamamoto T, Marui T, et al. Ischiogluteal bursitis: multimodality imaging findings. *Clin Orthop Relat Res.* 2003(406):214-217.
47. Uysal F, Akbal A, Gokmen F, Adam G, Resorlu M. Prevalence of pes anserine bursitis in symptomatic osteoarthritis patients: an ultrasonographic prospective study. *Clin Rheumatol.* 2015;34(3):529-533.
48. Alvarez-Nemegyei J. Risk factors for pes anserinus tendinitis/bursitis syndrome: a case control study. *J Clin Rheumatol.* 2007;13(2):63-65.
49. Makhsous M, Lin F, Hanawalt D, Kruger SL, LaMantia A. The effect of chair designs on sitting pressure distribution and tissue perfusion. *Hum Factors.* 2012;54(6):1066-1074.

Chapter 61

Popliteus Muscle
"Bent Knee Troublemaker"

Orlando Mayoral del Moral, Óscar Sánchez Méndez, María Torres-Lacomba, and Michelle Finnegan

1. INTRODUCTION

The popliteus muscle is a deeply located triangular muscle that attaches proximally to the lateral condyle of the femur and distally to the posterior aspect of the medial tibia. The main function of the popliteus muscle appears to be to "unlock" the knee at the start of weight bearing by externally rotating the femur on a fixed tibia. Activity of this muscle prevents forward displacement of the femur on the tibia when a person squats, and places weight on the bent knee. The pain referred from trigger points (TrPs) in the popliteus muscle normally concentrates in the back of the knee proximal to the location of the TrP. It can also include the posteromedial and medial sides of the tibia, projecting to the pes anserine area. Symptoms mainly appear when squatting, running, walking downhill, when going downstairs, as well as standing up after prolonged sitting. Popliteus myofascial pain syndrome can readily be misdiagnosed as popliteus tendinopathy. Other diagnoses that can appear confusingly similar include a Baker cyst, anteromedial and posterolateral instability of the knee joint, and avulsion of the popliteus tendon. For TrP examination, the popliteus muscle is most accessible close to the lower (medial) and upper (lateral) ends of its muscle belly. Trigger points in the popliteus muscle may be activated while the person plays soccer or football, runs, twists, or slides and can be perpetuated by knee joint conditions; by associated TrPs in biceps femoris, gastrocnemius, and vastus lateralis muscles; by prolonged immobilization; or by excessive pronation of the foot. Corrective actions for the treatment of TrPs in the popliteus muscle include dynamic and static postural education, self-pressure release, and self-stretching exercises.

2. ANATOMIC CONSIDERATIONS

The popliteus is a thin, flat muscle with the shape of an obtuse triangle that forms the lower part of the popliteal fossa behind the knee (Figure 61-1).[1,2] It originates proximally and laterally by a strong tendon that is inserted in a depression on the outer side of the lateral condyle of the femur (Figure 61-2). This tendinous attachment lies anteroinferior to the proximal attachment of the lateral collateral ligament on the lateral epicondyle of the femur.[2] Some variations of the proximal attachments of the popliteus muscle have been reported. These include attachments to the lateral femoral condyle (100%), posterior horn of the lateral meniscus (63%), or fibular head (52.1%).[3] The popliteus muscle is the only muscle that attaches posteriorly within the joint capsule of the knee. The popliteus tendon crosses the knee joint in a posteroinferior direction beneath the lateral collateral ligament and the tendon of biceps femoris muscle.[4] It then passes through the popliteal hiatus and is joined by collagenous fibers arising from the arcuate popliteal ligament, the fibrous capsule adjacent to the lateral meniscus, and the outer margin of the meniscus.[1] In the posterolateral part of the knee, the popliteus muscle has another important attachment to the fibula by a short and strong structure named the popliteofibular ligament (PFL).[1,5] It is one of the strongest lateral stabilizers of the knee joint.[2] The PFL has the shape of an inverted Y; the anterior limb originates from the anterior aspect of the fibular head, and the posterior limb arises from the posterosuperior aspect of the fibular head. Both insert proximally into the musculotendinous junction of the popliteus muscle and into the popliteomeniscal fascicle.[5,6]

Fleshy fibers expand from the inferior limit of the tendon to form a triangular muscle that descends distally and medially to insert into the medial two-thirds of the triangular area above the soleal line on the posterior surface of the tibia and into the tendinous expansion that covers its surface (Figure 61-1).[1]

The PFL is the single most important stabilizer of the posterolateral corner of the knee. It prevents posterior translation, varus angulation, and external rotation of the tibia on the femur.[1,6,7] Murthy[8] found the attachment to the fibular head to be missing bilaterally in 4 out of 30 cadavers. Other studies have shown that the PFL is present in 100% of the population.[6,7,9,10] The most plausible explanation for these criteria differences among the authors is that the shallow layer of the PFL is close to the arcuate ligament in terms of its direction and position making its identification in prior studies inconsistent.[10]

Regarding the meniscus, different authors have found, clearly delineated but highly variable, three popliteomeniscal fascicles attaching into the lateral meniscus.[5,11-14] Tria et al[15] found no strong connection in 45% of subjects. Only 17.5% of subjects had that strong connection to the lateral meniscus as described by others. Unquestionably, this meniscal attachment is of importance in some, and possibly many, individuals.

The popliteal bursa is an extra-articular extension of the synovial membrane of the knee joint. The course of the bursa extends from the popliteal hiatus along the proximal part of the popliteus tendon in order to separate this tendon from the lateral condyle of the femur above the head of the fibula.[2]

The popliteus muscle is analogous to the deep portion of the pronator teres muscle in the forearm and is rarely absent.[16] There are several anatomic variants for the popliteus complex, such as variations of the medial portion and on the aponeurotic extension of the muscle.[17,18] Morphologic alterations of the popliteus tendon have also been described, such as the possibility of bifurcation[19,20] or a three-bundle form.[21] Benthien and Brunner[22] reported a case of posterolateral knee pain caused by the presence of a sesamoid bone named cyamella located between the popliteal tendon and the femur. Also, the sesamoid bone has been found as a proximal attachment to an accessory muscle.[23] Occasionally, two other muscles may be found deep in the posterior aspect of the knee: the popliteus minor muscle, a small muscle situated above the popliteus muscle that runs from the posterior surface of the lateral tibial condyle, medial to the plantaris muscle, to the oblique popliteal ligament, and the peroneotibialis muscle, located deeper than the popliteus muscle and running from the medial side of the fibular head to the upper end of the soleal line.[1]

647

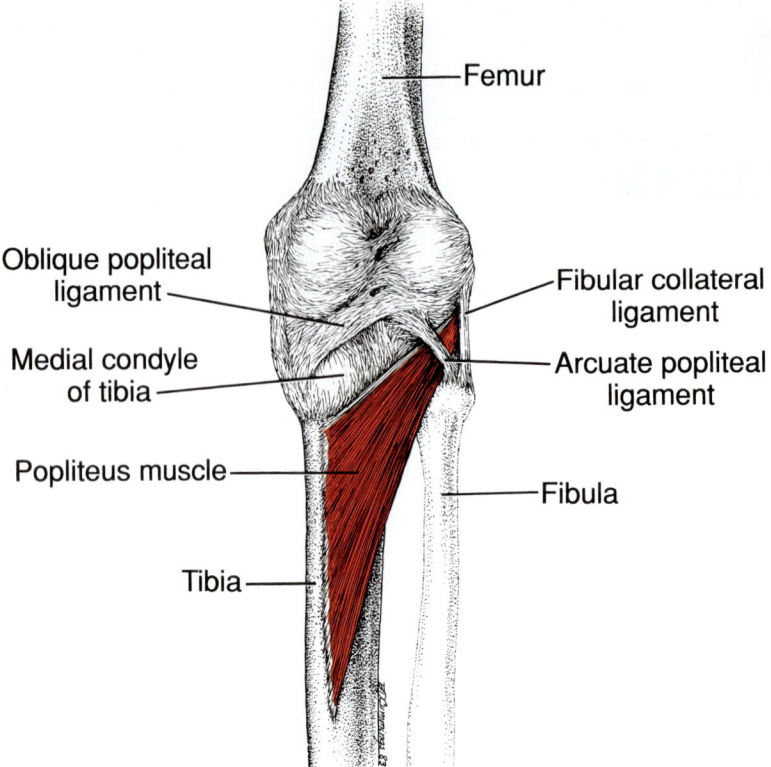

Figure 61-1. Attachments of the right popliteus muscle (red), from a posterior view. Its attachment to the femur is shown in Figure 61-2. Not shown in this figure because of the complexity of the popliteus muscle attachments: popliteofibular ligament, popliteal meniscal ligament, and fabellofibular ligament.[5,6,13]

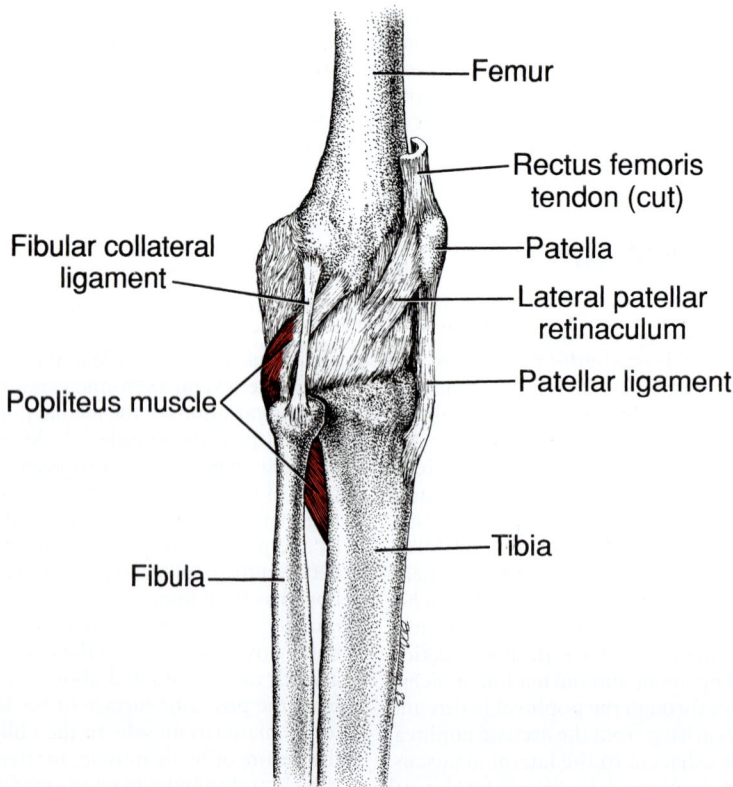

Figure 61-2. Proximal attachment of the right popliteus muscle (red) to the femur, from the lateral view.

2.1. Innervation and Vascularization

The popliteus muscle is innervated by two to three parallel branches of the tibial nerve that arise from the L4, L5, and S1 spinal nerves.[1,24] These branches descend obliquely across the popliteal vessels, wind around the distal border of the muscle, and enter through its anterior surface. The nerve entry point is approximately 3 cm below the fibular head.[24] These nerve branches further separate into the left, right, and anterior branches so as to innervate different parts of the muscle.[24]

Vascularization to the popliteus muscle is supplied by the inferior medial and lateral genicular arteries, two branches that originate from the popliteal artery deep to the gastrocnemius muscle. The course of the lateral inferior genicular artery is on the surface of, through, or underneath the arcuate ligament.[10] It is possible that the muscle has additional supplies from the nutrient artery of the tibia, the proximal part of the posterior tibial artery, and the posterior tibial recurrent artery.[1]

2.2. Function

The popliteus muscle rotates the tibia internally on the femur when the thigh is fixed and the leg is free to move, as when sitting erect.[1,25] When the tibia is fixed, as happens in a standing position, the popliteus muscle is capable of rotating the femur externally on the tibia, thus "unlocking" the knee joint at the beginning of the flexion movement.[1,26,27] This muscle also acts as a dynamic stabilizer of the knee.[2,12,28,29] Its role as a stabilizer can be related to the presence of the high density of Ruffini endings at its tendon.[30]

Basmajian and Lovejoy[31] studied this muscle electromyographically using fine-wire electrodes in 20 subjects. These investigators found that, with the leg free to move, the popliteus muscle was activated by voluntary effort to produce internal rotation of the leg at various knee angles between knee straight and 90° of flexion in the sitting and prone positions.[31]

Several authors[31-34] have reported that, when the person stood in semicrouched bent-knee position between 30° and 50° of knee flexion, the popliteus muscle showed continuous motor unit activity. In this typical "ready" position, normally adopted in sport activities that involve sudden stopping, such as running with directional changes,[35] the noncontractile tissue structures are relaxed and the body weight tends to slide the femur downward and forward on the slope of the tibia. This contraction of the popliteus and quadriceps femoris muscles assists the posterior cruciate ligament in preventing forward dislocation of the femur[33] on the knee and acts as a dynamic knee joint guidance.

Basmajian and Lovejoy[31] reported that during walking, the greatest electromyography occurs during initial contact and mid-stance. Mann and Hagy[25] found that the highest activity of the muscle develops at the early part of the stance phase. Perry[36] reported that popliteus muscle activity occurs during all the gait phases, except on initial swing and mid-swing, with great variability between subjects. Davis et al[37] reported a strong activation of the popliteus muscle during downhill walking at the mid-stance gait phase. Nevertheless, the muscle is inactive when the person quietly stands erect.[38]

According to Amonoo-Kuofi,[39] human fetal popliteus muscles contained many muscle spindles arranged in complex and tandem forms. The author concluded that these spindles could provide a major part of the kinesthesia needed to monitor locking and unlocking of the human knee joint.[38]

2.3. Functional Unit

The functional unit to which a muscle belongs includes the muscles that reinforce and counter its actions as well as the joints that the muscle crosses. The interdependence of these structures is functionally reflected in the organization and neural connections of the sensory motor cortex. The functional unit is emphasized because the presence of a TrP in one muscle of the unit increases the likelihood that the other muscles of the unit will also develop TrPs. When inactivating TrPs in a muscle, one must be concerned about TrPs that may develop in muscles that are functionally interdependent. Box 61-1 grossly represents the functional unit of the popliteus muscle.[40]

Box 61-1 Functional unit of the popliteus muscle

Action	Synergist	Antagonist
Internal rotation of the leg	Semimembranosus Semitendinosus Sartorious Gracilis	Biceps femoris

3. CLINICAL PRESENTATION

3.1. Referred Pain Pattern

Trigger points in the popliteus muscle refer pain primarily to the back of the knee joint (Figure 61-3). Mayoral et al[41] has clinically observed a variant in this pain pattern including the posteromedial and medial sides of the tibia and, projecting to the pes anserinus area.

Patients rarely report pain in the knee solely due to TrPs in the popliteus muscle. Initially, the source of knee pain is identified as coming from TrPs in other muscles, such as the gastrocnemius or biceps femoris muscles. On first examination, the latter appears to account for the patient's report of pain; however, after the TrPs in these other muscles have been inactivated, the patient becomes more aware of back-of-the-knee pain that examination then identifies as originating in the

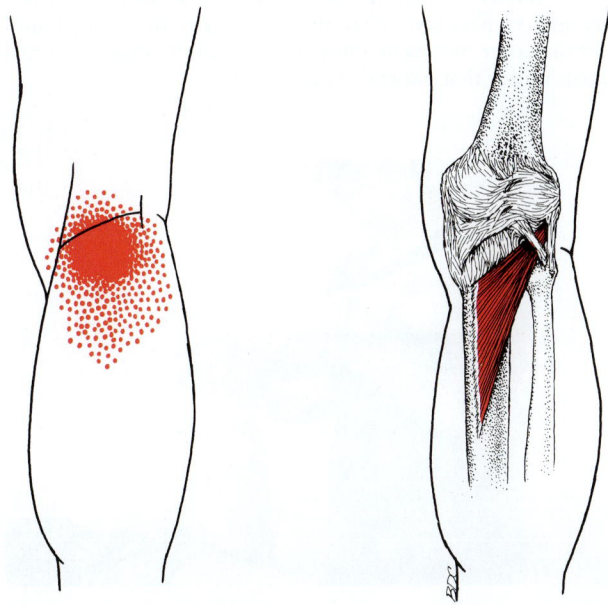

Figure 61-3. Referred pain pattern (dark red) of a TrP in the right popliteus muscle (light red) seen in posterior view. The essential pain pattern is solid red. Red stippling indicates occasional spillover of the essential pattern.

popliteus muscle. Deep pain felt within the posterior area of the knee joint can alert the clinician to examine for TrPs in the popliteus muscle from the outset.

3.2. Symptoms

The chief report of pain in patients with TrPs in the popliteus muscle is pain in the back of the knee when crouching, running, or walking, especially while going downstairs, downhill, or wearing high heels. Trigger points in the popliteus muscle may produce stiffness that could make it painful and difficult to extend the knee when getting out of bed in the morning or standing up following a long period of sitting.[41] Patients with popliteal TrPs rarely report of knee pain at night and are frequently not aware of their relatively slight decrease in range of motion at the knee or weakness of internal rotation of the tibia.

3.3. Patient Examination

If the popliteus muscle has TrPs, the knee is painful when the patient attempts to fully extend or flex it. The tibial attachment and tendon of the popliteus muscle should be examined for tenderness. The position described and illustrated to examine the knee for popliteus tendinitis[25,42] may also be used for examining the femoral end of the muscle and its tendon. The seated patient places the leg of the affected limb on the opposite knee, leaving the foot to hang relaxed. The proximal attachment of the popliteus tendon on the lateral side of the femoral condyle is examined for tenderness, and the tendon is palpated along the 2-cm distance proximal to the point where it passes posteriorly deep to the fibular collateral ligament that is a well-defined landmark (Figure 61-2).[25] The TrP tightness of the popliteus muscle restricts the range of passive external rotation and weakens the active internal rotation of the leg with the knee flexed nearly 90°. To assess the popliteus muscle with an active functional test, the patient lies in the supine position with 90° of hip and knee flexion and is asked to resist the examiner's external rotation force on the tibia. If the maneuver reproduces the posterolateral pain of the patient, the test is considered positive suggesting popliteus tendinopathy[43] (Figure 61-4).

The relatively small restriction of full knee extension (usually only 5°, possibly 10°) is often not clearly appreciated until retesting after treatment. Only then is the full range of normal extension for that patient's knee identified.

3.4. Trigger Point Examination

The popliteus muscle is palpated for TrPs with the patient lying on the affected side and the knee slightly flexed (Figure 61-5A) or with the patient positioned in hook-lying with the knee supported by the clinician (Figure 61-5B). Alternatively, the patient can lie supine with the hip in flexion and external rotation and the knee flexed comfortably. The slight flexion of the knee slackens the overlying gastrocnemius muscle, whereas a plantar-flexed foot further slackens the gastrocnemius and plantaris muscles, and the external rotation of the leg places the popliteus muscle on a slight stretch that can be adjusted to increase tenderness of the popliteus TrPs for examination.

The medial side of the mid-part of the muscle is approachable between the semitendinosus tendon and the medial head of the gastrocnemius muscle along its attachment to the tibia.[1] The most distal portion of the tibial attachment of the popliteus muscle is covered by the soleus muscle[1] that can usually be displaced laterally to partially uncover the popliteus muscle. This medial, distal end of the popliteus muscle is examined for TrPs, as illustrated in Figure 61-5. It is important to displace the overlying muscles laterally as part of the examination.

In the popliteal space, the upper lateral end of the popliteus muscle is covered by the plantaris muscle and the lateral head

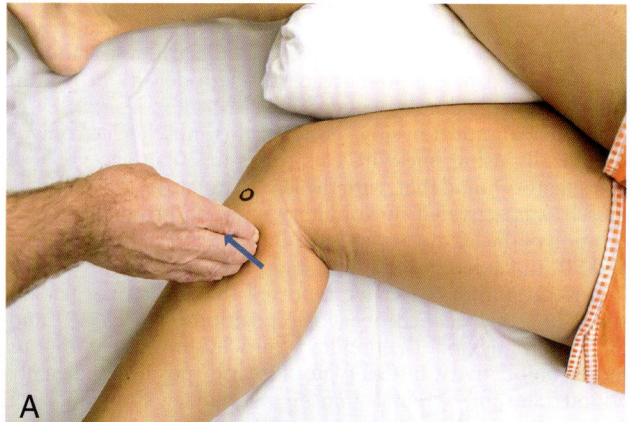

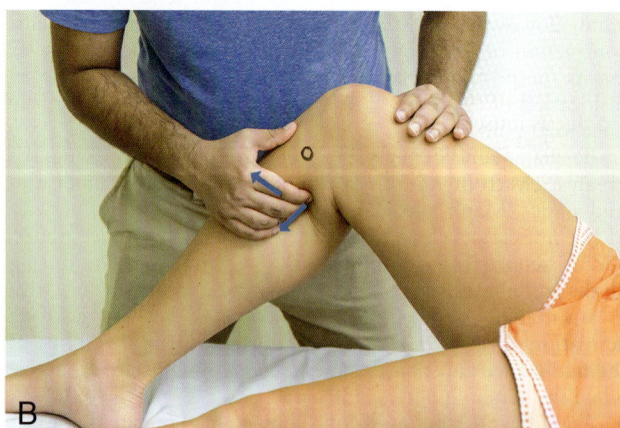

Figure 61-5. Palpation for TrPs in the lower medial part of the right popliteus muscle. The circle marks the medial condyle of the tibia. The patient lies on the affected side with the knee flexed, and the foot plantar is flexed at the ankle to place the gastrocnemius and plantaris muscles on slack. A, Cross-fiber flat palpation of the tibial attachment of the popliteus muscle is performed in a superior to inferior direction. The clinician also applies anterior pressure against the posterior surface of the tibia. B, Hook-lying cross-fiber flat palpation for TrPs in the popliteus muscle, as described in A. This position allows gravitational pull of the gastrocnemius muscle away from the tibia.

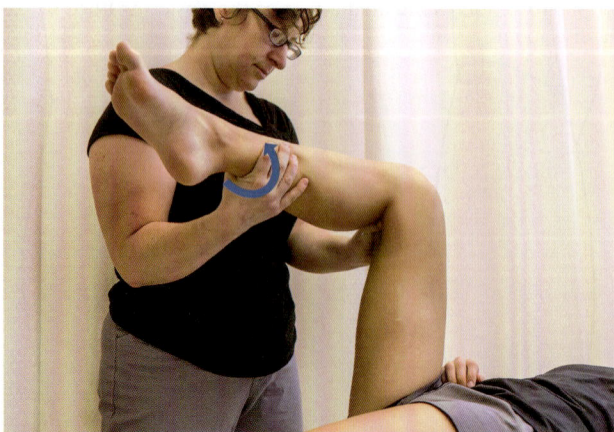

Figure 61-4. Popliteus tendinopathy assessment. The clinician, while palpating the popliteus muscle, provides an external rotation force to the tibia while the patient attempts to resist the movement. Production of symptoms in the posterolateral aspect of the knee may be indicative of popliteus tendinopathy.

of the gastrocnemius muscle. However, as the popliteus muscle crosses the leg diagonally just above the head of the fibula (Figure 61-2), it can be reached by palpating between the tendon of the biceps femoris muscle laterally and the lateral head of the gastrocnemius muscle and the plantaris muscle medially.[44] With the patient in one of the positions of Figure 61-5, these overlying muscles can be displaced to the side with one hand while palpating for TrPs with the other as needed. If the popliteus muscle has active TrPs, this spot will be painful, and pressure on it will cause diffuse pain referred throughout the back of the knee. The region of attachment of the popliteus tendon onto the tibia will also be painful.

If popliteus TrPs are sufficiently irritable, pain may be elicited by pressure exerted straight into the belly of the popliteus muscle through the overlying soleus muscle. The proximal end of the soleus muscle runs nearly parallel with the popliteus muscle fibers and covers the distal half of them.[45] It is difficult to distinguish TrPs unambiguously in the intermediate portions of the popliteus muscle from TrPs in the intervening musculature.

4. DIFFERENTIAL DIAGNOSIS

4.1. Activation and Perpetuation of Trigger Points

A posture or activity that activates a TrP, if not corrected, can also perpetuate it. In the popliteus muscle, TrPs may be activated by unaccustomed eccentric loading, eccentric exercise in an unconditioned muscle, or maximal or submaximal concentric loading.[46] Specifically, TrPs may be activated in the popliteus muscle due to an overload produced by an eccentric contraction that takes place when there is internal rotation of the femur on the tibia in a closed kinematic chain,[41] for example, when an individual plays soccer or football, runs, twists, slides, and especially, runs or skis downhill. This muscle is also specifically overloaded by breaking the forward motion of the femur on the tibia during a twisting turn with the body weight on a slightly bent knee of the side toward which the body is turning. Overload that causes a tear of the plantaris muscle may also activate TrPs in the popliteus muscle.

A trauma or strain that tears the posterior cruciate ligament of the knee can also overload and strain the popliteus muscle,[47,48] which can then lead to the development of TrPs in the muscle.

Knee joint conditions such as meniscus tears, osteoarthritis, or hydrarthrosis can also activate and perpetuate TrPs in the popliteus muscle.[41]

Brody[42] reported an association between an excessively pronated foot during weight-bearing activities and aggravation of popliteus tendinitis symptoms. The added stress from excessive pronation could also perpetuate TrPs in the popliteus muscle.

4.2. Associated Trigger Points

Associated TrPs can develop in the referred pain areas caused by TrPs.[49] Therefore, musculature in the referred pain areas for each muscle should also be considered. The TrPs in the proximal portion of either or both heads of the gastrocnemius muscle are the ones most commonly associated with TrPs in the popliteus muscle. Other muscles associated with TrPs in the popliteus muscle are the biceps femoris and vastus lateralis muscles.[41] In a few patients, popliteus TrPs have been associated with a tear of the plantaris muscle and may have been activated when the plantaris muscle was torn.

With the foot dorsiflexed, the degree of pain in the popliteal fossa and restriction of motion at the knee caused by TrPs in the lateral head of the gastrocnemius muscle is comparable to that caused by TrPs in the popliteus muscle.

4.3. Associated Pathology

Popliteus TrPs are easily overlooked when a diagnosis of popliteus tendinitis or tenosynovitis is the focus of attention. Other conditions to consider in the differential diagnosis of posterior knee pain include Baker cyst, thrombosis of the popliteal vein, anteromedial and posterolateral instability of the knee, avulsion of the popliteus tendon, and tear of a meniscus or of the posterior capsule of the knee joint.

One should be wary of blaming pain in the back of the knee on a torn plantaris muscle months or years after injury. In that case, the muscle should have healed. Such residual pain is more likely to be caused by TrPs in the popliteus muscle.

Popliteus tendinopathy and popliteus tenosynovitis are closely associated with activities that would overload an inadequately conditioned popliteus muscle. Mayfield[50] reported on 30 patients seen with the diagnosis of tenosynovitis in a 5-year period. The findings leading to this diagnosis are apparently more common than is generally appreciated.[50,51] The characteristic symptom is pain in the lateral aspect of the knee on weight bearing with the knee flexed 15° to 30°, as when running or walking downhill.[50] Anterolateral knee pain has also been reported,[51] as well as pain in the lateral knee after a direct hit to the knee in 90° of flexion, causing intermittent pain with running and short-distance walking.[51] Backpacking enthusiasts reportedly spent days ascending into the mountains without symptoms until the end of the journey, but during a rapid descent out of the mountains, the symptoms developed.[50] Sometimes, pain is also experienced during the early part of the swing phase of gait and on attempting to rise from the cross-legged sitting position.[50] Brody[42] also noted that symptoms were aggravated more readily when the patient walked on a slanted surface or performed some other activity that excessively pronated the foot during weight bearing.

The visualization of tenosynovitis through the use of ultrasonography has been well-documented.[52] Ultrasound characterizations of this condition include increased size of the tendon, loss of homogeneity, and a hypoechogenic area surrounding the tendon due to inflammatory fluid.

Calcific tendonitis of the popliteus tendon is another condition that can present with lateral knee pain,[53-56] mimicking popliteal tendinopathy or popliteal TrPs. It can also mimic symptoms of tear of the lateral meniscus.[55] The calcifications can be visualized with radiographs,[53,54,56] ultrasound,[53] or magnetic resonance imaging (MRI).[53,54]

In one study,[57] MRI of the normal popliteus tendon was sometimes mistaken for a tear in the posterior horn of the lateral meniscus. In another study of 200 knees,[58] the bursa of the popliteus tendon simulated a tear of the posterior horn of the lateral meniscus in 27.5% of the knees studied by MRI. This bursa can also be confused with a tear of the popliteus tendon or of the posterior capsule.[2]

Trigger points in the popliteus muscle can mimic the symptoms of a popliteal (Baker) cyst that produces pain in much of the same posterior region of the knee joint. The cyst produces a swelling, often painful, in the popliteal space that is caused by an enlargement of the bursa that lies deep to the medial head of the gastrocnemius muscle and/or an enlargement of the semimembranosus bursa, both of which normally communicate with the synovial cavity of the knee joint. The swelling may be more prominent in the standing patient than in the recumbent one. Flexion of the knee increases discomfort. The swelling (effusion) is usually due to disease or injury of the knee joint, such as rheumatoid arthritis or a meniscal tear in adults, but not in children. If appropriate treatment does not relieve the swelling and pain, surgery may be considered directed to the intra-articular cause of the joint fluid production, not to the popliteal cyst, unless it is unduly large and highly symptomatic.[59] Although TrPs in the popliteus muscle may elicit deep tenderness in much the same region as a Baker cyst, the TrPs do not produce visible or palpable swelling. For differential diagnosis, MRI is the gold standard as it allows differentiation from other conditions. Ultrasound is also an option for diagnosis as its ability to detect Baker cyst is nearly 100%, although it lacks the specificity for differentiating it from other conditions.[59]

Rupture of a Baker cyst may closely simulate thrombophlebitis. If the rupture of the Baker cyst is thought to be very likely, further imaging with a venogram, ultrasound, or arthrogram clearly shows the entry of dye from the knee joint into the region of the calf muscles should be considered before placement of antithrombotics.[59]

The popliteus muscle is a major contributor to rotational stability of the knee joint. Together, the popliteus tendon and PFL are the primary stabilizers for external rotation of the knee at both 60° and 90° of flexion.[60-62] These two structures can contribute to varus stability at 30° of knee flexion and also have a role of providing static stabilization of the knee in extension.[62] Because of the important stabilizing function at the knee, tears in the popliteus tendon or other structures of the posterolateral corner of the knee can contribute to instability.[63]

Surgical treatment typically has positive outcomes for the improvement of stability.[63] In cadavers, structures of the posterolateral corner have been resected, thereby demonstrating increased instability of the knee and altered kinematics. After reconstruction, kinematics improved.

Surgically shortening the popliteus muscle-tendon unit that was elongated or torn in eight patients, resulted in static and dynamic stability and return to full function in seven of them. None of the eight experienced any loss of power in the popliteus muscle.[64] Depending on which ligaments are lax or torn, excessive internal rotation of the femur on the tibia produces either rotary anteromedial instability[64] or rotary posterolateral instability.[65,66] In either condition, surgical relocation of the tibial attachment of the popliteus muscle in order to shorten it increases its tension, improves its dynamic function, and corrects the problem.

Several cases of avulsion or rupture of the popliteus tendon have been reported.[67] Radiographs are commonly used initially, frequently showing the avulsion.[68,69] However, in one case, it was reportedly normal.[67] As a result, MRI is better to evaluate the nature of the knee injury.[67-69] The diagnosis can also be confirmed by an arthroscopic examination.[67]

This injury may be treated conservatively or surgically by repairing the rupture and/or fixating the bone avulsion.[67] Satisfactory outcomes have been reported for both the surgical treatment[70,71] and the nonsurgical treatment[68,71]; however, the latter type of treatment was not as successful in one subject.[71]

5. CORRECTIVE ACTIONS

The patient may wear a properly fitted, elastic sleeve brace (knee support) with an opening in front for the patella that extends from above the knee to below it. This device is consistently helpful and worth using as long as symptoms persist. It applies counter pressure over the region of the TrPs, reducing their sensitivity, and it reminds the patient that the knee should be protected.

Splinting or immobilizing the knee and leg with a stiff brace or cast tends to aggravate popliteus TrPs. When popliteus TrPs present a problem, immobilization should be avoided, or the period of immobilization be minimized, to prevent worsening of symptoms.[72]

Before the patient can get back to participation in sports, it is best to gradually condition the muscle, starting with nonweight-bearing exercises and moving on to dynamic weight-bearing exercises.[12]

Individuals prone to popliteus TrPs should avoid a sudden increase in the amount of downhill running or walking because this change in activity could overload the muscle.[50] Additionally, high heels should be avoided, as wearing them is tantamount to continuously walking downhill.

Effort should be made to limit walking or running on laterally sloped surfaces, such as on the sides of paved roads designed for water drainage (the grade of which increases pronation of the foot and the effect of a longer lower extremity on the high side). Running can be performed on a track, on the crown of an empty road, or on the same side of the road for both directions of the trip. Appropriate shoe inserts should be utilized if indicated.

Trigger point self-pressure release may be performed in the seated position, as demonstrated in Figure 61-6. A patient should locate the popliteus muscle on the inside of the leg, just under the knee, by shifting the bulk of the calf muscle toward the outside of the knee and placing either a thumb, or two fingers along the backside of the shin to find a tender point. The patient should be careful not to place pressure on the popliteal vessels by gently feeling for a pulse behind the knee and avoiding it when locating the popliteus muscle. Firm pressure may be held on a TrP of the popliteus muscle for up to 30 seconds or until a decrease in tenderness is felt. This technique may be repeated several times until an adequate release is obtained.

Self-stretch of the popliteus muscle may be very difficult for a patient to perform independently without specific instructions and observation of the technique by a proper professional. The self-stretch is performed in the prone or seated position. In each position, the knee is flexed 15° to 20°. If no one is available to be instructed as an assistant at home, reciprocal inhibition can be used instead of a passive stretch.

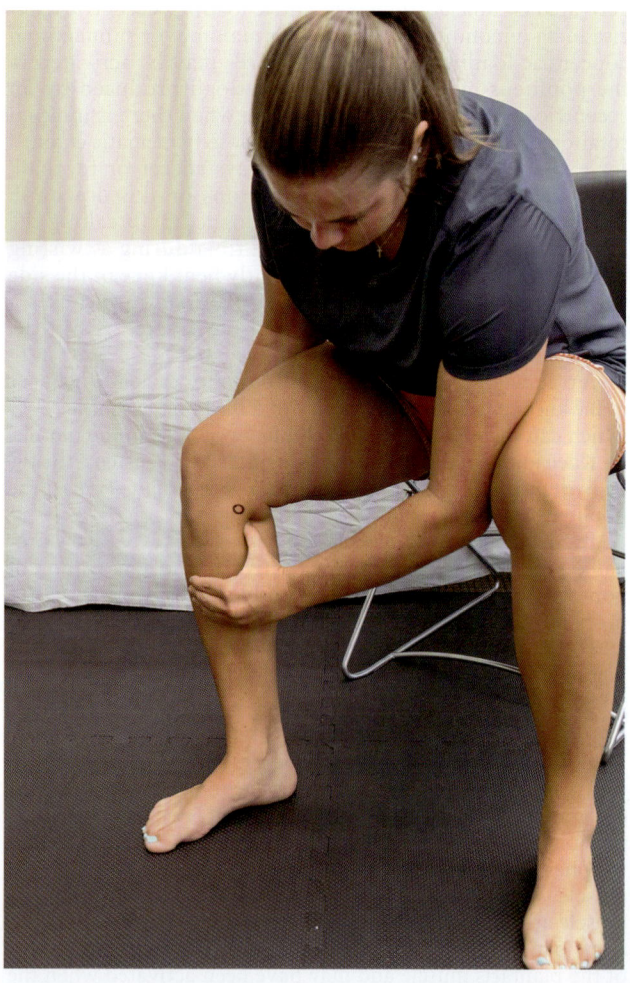

Figure 61-6. Self-pressure release of the popliteus muscle. The patient sits with the foot of the leg to be treated resting on the floor. The thumbs or the fingers may be used to locate the popliteus muscle on the inside of the calf underneath the bulk of the gastrocnemius muscle.

Chapter 61: Popliteus Muscle 653

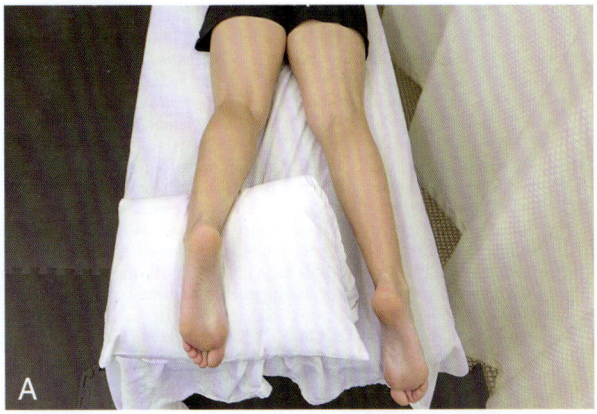
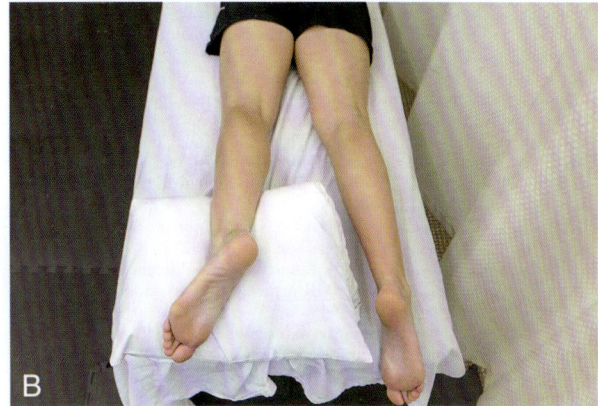
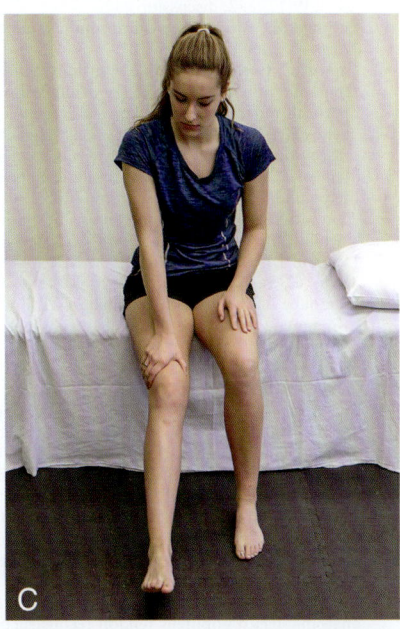
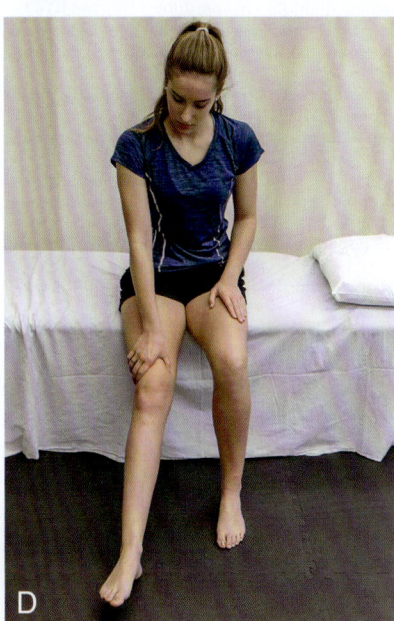

Figure 61-7. Self-stretch of the popliteus muscle. A, Prone starting position with pillow under the ankle to place the knee in slight flexion. B, Prone turning foot out to stretch the popliteus muscle. C, Sitting start position with the knee in slight flexion and weight of the leg is resting on the floor. D, Sitting foot turned outward to stretch the popliteus muscle. The hand above the knee ensures the thigh does not move.

For the prone position, the patient lies on his or her stomach with enough blanket roll or pillow under the distal leg to flex the knee 15° to 20° (Figure 61-7A,B). The patient tries to rotate the leg externally for several seconds (reciprocally inhibiting the popliteus) and then relaxes fully. The cycle is repeated a few times. The advantage of this position is that the thigh is stabilized so that the leg, rather than the thigh, rotates. If the blanket roll or pillow touches the foot, friction may help maintain external rotation during relaxation. Otherwise, gravity pulls the foot and leg back into neutral position.

For relaxation of the popliteus muscle in the sitting position, the seated patient places the leg forward with the heel on the floor and the knee flexed 15° to 20° (Figure 61-7C,D). A low-seated bench or chair may be required. As thigh rotation is often substituted for leg rotation in this position, special care must be taken to ensure that the patient knows the difference and achieves external rotation of the leg at the knee. After a maximal external rotation effort for several seconds, the patient relaxes fully while gravity tends to maintain the external rotation. This cycle is repeated at least three times with a pause between each cycle.

Each stretching session is completed with a full active range of motion through internal and external rotation of the leg and then through knee flexion and extension.

References

1. Standring S. *Gray's Anatomy. The Anatomical Basis of Clinical Practice*. 41st ed. London, UK: Elsevier; 2016.
2. Jadhav SP, More SR, Riascos RF, Lemos DF, Swischuk LE. Comprehensive review of the anatomy, function, and imaging of the popliteus and associated pathologic conditions. *Radiographics*. 2014;34(2):496-513.
3. Chuncharunee A, Chanthong P, Lucksanasombool P. The patterns of proximal attachments of the popliteus muscle: form and function. *Med Hypotheses*. 2012;78(2):221-224.
4. Lovejoy JF Jr, Harden TP. Popliteus muscle in man. *Anat Rec*. 1971;169(4):727-730.
5. Staubli HU, Birrer S. The popliteus tendon and its fascicles at the popliteal hiatus: gross anatomy and functional arthroscopic evaluation with and without anterior cruciate ligament deficiency. *Arthroscopy*. 1990;6(3):209-220.
6. Shahane SA, Ibbotson C, Strachan R, Bickerstaff DR. The popliteofibular ligament. An anatomical study of the posterolateral corner of the knee. *J Bone Joint Surg Br*. 1999;81(4):636-642.
7. Maynard MJ, Deng X, Wickiewicz TL, Warren RF. The popliteofibular ligament. Rediscovery of a key element in posterolateral stability. *Am J Sports Med*. 1996;24(3):311-316.
8. Murthy CK. Origin of popliteus muscle in man. *J Indian Med Assoc*. 1976;67(4):97-99.
9. Aronowitz ER, Parker RD, Gatt CJ. Arthroscopic identification of the popliteofibular ligament. *Arthroscopy*. 2001;17(9):932-939.
10. Ishigooka H, Sugihara T, Shimizu K, Aoki H, Hirata K. Anatomical study of the popliteofibular ligament and surrounding structures. *J Orthop Sci*. 2004;9(1):51-58.
11. Kimura M, Shirakura K, Hasegawa A, Kobayashi Y, Udagawa E. Anatomy and pathophysiology of the popliteal tendon area in the lateral meniscus: 2. Clinical investigation. *Arthroscopy*. 1992;8(4):424-427.

12. Nyland J, Lachman N, Kocabey Y, Brosky J, Altun R, Caborn D. Anatomy, function, and rehabilitation of the popliteus musculotendinous complex. *J Orthop Sports Phys Ther*. 2005;35(3):165-179.
13. Recondo JA, Salvador E, Villanua JA, Barrera MC, Gervas C, Alustiza JM. Lateral stabilizing structures of the knee: functional anatomy and injuries assessed with MR imaging. *Radiographics*. 2000;20 Spec No:S91-S102.
14. Watanabe Y, Moriya H, Takahashi K, et al. Functional anatomy of the posterolateral structures of the knee. *Arthroscopy*. 1993;9(1):57-62.
15. Tria AJ Jr, Johnson CD, Zawadsky JP. The popliteus tendon. *J Bone Joint Surg Am Vol*. 1989;71(5):714-716.
16. Bardeen CR. The musculature. In: Jackson CM, ed. *Morris's Human Anatomy*. 6th ed. Philadelphia, PA: Blakiston's Son & Co.; 1921.
17. Peduto AJ, Nguyen A, Trudell DJ, Resnick DL. Popliteomeniscal fascicles: anatomic considerations using MR arthrography in cadavers. *AJR Am J Roentgenol*. 2008;190(2):442-448.
18. Bartonicek J. Rare bilateral variation of the popliteus muscle: anatomical case report and review of the literature. *Surg Radiol Anat*. 2005;27(4):347-350.
19. Perez Carro L, Sumillera Garcia M, Sunye Gracia C. Bifurcate popliteus tendon. *Arthroscopy*. 1999;15(6):638-639.
20. Leal-Blanquet J, Gines-Cespedosa A, Monllau JC. Bifurcated popliteus tendon: a descriptive arthroscopic study. *Int Orthop*. 2009;33(6):1633-1635.
21. Doral MN, Atay AO, Bozkurt M, Ayvaz M, Tetik O, Leblebicioglu G. Three-bundle popliteus tendon: a nonsymptomatic anatomical variation. *Knee*. 2006;13(4):342-343.
22. Benthien JP, Brunner A. A symptomatic sesamoid bone in the popliteus muscle (cyamella). *Musculoskelet Surg*. 2010;94(3):141-144.
23. Wagstaffe WW. Description of an accessory muscle in connection with the popliteus. *J Anat Physiol*. 1871;6(pt 1):214-215.
24. Yu D, Yin H, Han T, Jiang H, Cao X. Intramuscular innervations of lower leg skeletal muscles: applications in their clinical use in functional muscular transfer. *Surg Radiol Anat*. 2016;38:675-685.
25. Mann RA, Hagy JL. The popliteus muscle. *J Bone Joint Surg Am Vol*. 1977;59(7):924-927.
26. Last RJ. The popliteus muscle and the lateral meniscus. *Bone Joint J*. 1950;32-B(1):93-99.
27. Paraskevas G, Papaziogas B, Kitsoulis P, Spanidou S. A study on the morphology of the popliteus muscle and arcuate popliteal ligament. *Folia Morphol (Warsz)*. 2006;65(4):381-384.
28. Schinhan M, Bijak M, Unger E, Nau T. Electromyographic study of the popliteus muscle in the dynamic stabilization of the posterolateral corner structures of the knee. *Am J Sports Med*. 2011;39(1):173-179.
29. LaPrade RF, Wozniczka JK, Stellmaker MP, Wijdicks CA. Analysis of the static function of the popliteus tendon and evaluation of an anatomic reconstruction: the "fifth ligament" of the knee. *Am J Sports Med*. 2010;38(3):543-549.
30. Cabuk H, Kusku Cabuk F. Mechanoreceptors of the ligaments and tendons around the knee. *Clin Anat*. 2016;29(6):789-795.
31. Basmajian JV, Lovejoy JF Jr. Functions of the popliteus muscle in man. A multifactorial electromyographic study. *J Bone Joint Surg Am Vol*. 1971;53(3):557-562.
32. Prado Reis F, Ferraz de Carvalho CD. Electromyographic study of the popliteus muscle. *Electromyogr Clin Neurophysiol*. 1973;13(4):445-455.
33. Barnett CH, Richardson AT. The postural function of the popliteus muscle. *Ann Phys Med*. 1953;1(5):177-179.
34. Buford WL Jr, Ivey FM Jr, Nakamura T, Patterson RM, Nguyen DK. Internal/external rotation moment arms of muscles at the knee: moment arms for the normal knee and the ACL-deficient knee. *Knee*. 2001;8(4):293-303.
35. Malinzak RA, Colby SM, Kirkendall DT, Yu B, Garrett WE. A comparison of knee joint motion patterns between men and women in selected athletic tasks. *Clin Biomech (Bristol, Avon)*. 2001;16(5):438-445.
36. Perry J. *Gait Analysis: Normal and Pathological Function*. Thorofare, NJ: SLACK Incorporated; 1992.
37. Davis M, Newsam CJ, Perry J. Electromyograph analysis of the popliteus muscle in level and downhill walking. *Clin Orthop Relat Res*. 1995(310):211-217.
38. Basmajian JV, Deluca CJ. *Muscles Alive*. 5th ed. Baltimore, MD: Williams & Wilkins; 1985.
39. Amonoo-Kuofi HS. Morphology of muscle spindles in the human popliteus muscle. Evidence of a possible monitoring role of the popliteus muscle in the locked knee joint? *Acta Anat (Basel)*. 1989;134(1):48-53.
40. Simons DG, Travell J, Simons L. *Travell & Simon's Myofascial Pain and Dysfunction: The Trigger Point Manual*. Vol 1. 2nd ed. Baltimore, MD: Williams & Wilkins; 1999 (p. 104).
41. Mayoral del Moral O, Torres-Lacomba I, Sánchez Méndez Ó. Punción seca de músculos y otras estructuras de la pierna y el pie. In: Mayoral del Moral O, Salvat Salvat I, eds. *Fisioterapia Invasiva del Síndrome de Dolor Miofascial*. Editorial Médica Panamericana; 2016.
42. Brody DM. Running injuries. *Clin Symp*. 1980;32(4):1-36.
43. Petsche TS, Selesnick FH. Popliteus tendinitis: tips for diagnosis and management. *Phys Sportsmed*. Toledo, Spain: 2002;30(8):27-31.
44. Ferner H, Staubesand J. *Sobotta Atlas of Human Anatomy*. Vol 2. 10 ed. Baltimore, MD: Urban & Schwarzenberg; 1983 (Fig. 436).
45. Netter FH. *The Ciba Collection of Medical Illustrations. Vol. 8, Musculoskeletal System. Part I: Anatomy, Physiology and Metabolic Disorders*. Summit, NJ: Ciba-Geigy Corporation; 1987 (pp. 85, 101).
46. Gerwin RD, Dommerholt J, Shah JP. An expansion of Simons' integrated hypothesis of trigger point formation. *Curr Pain Headache Rep*. 2004;8(6):468-475.
47. Kang KT, Koh YG, Jung M, et al. The effects of posterior cruciate ligament deficiency on posterolateral corner structures under gait- and squat-loading conditions: a computational knee model. *Bone Joint Res*. 2017;6(1):31-42.
48. Kozanek M, Fu EC, Van de Velde SK, Gill TJ, Li G. Posterolateral structures of the knee in posterior cruciate ligament deficiency. *Am J Sports Med*. 2009;37(3):534-541.
49. Hsieh YL, Kao MJ, Kuan TS, Chen SM, Chen JT, Hong CZ. Dry needling to a key myofascial trigger point may reduce the irritability of satellite MTrPs. *Am J Phys Med Rehabil*. 2007;86(5):397-403.
50. Mayfield GW. Popliteus tendon tenosynovitis. *Am J Sports Med*. 1977;5(1):31-36.
51. Blake SM, Treble NJ. Popliteus tendon tenosynovitis. *Br J Sports Med*. 2005;39(12):e42; discussion e42.
52. Fornage BD, Rifkin MD. Ultrasound examination of tendons. *Radiol Clin North Am*. 1988;26(1):87-107.
53. Doucet C, Gotra A, Reddy SMV, Boily M. Acute calcific tendinopathy of the popliteus tendon: a rare case diagnosed using a multimodality imaging approach and treated conservatively. *Skeletal Radiol*. 2017;46(7):1003-1006.
54. Shenoy PM, Kim DH, Wang KH, et al. Calcific tendinitis of popliteus tendon: arthroscopic excision and biopsy. *Orthopedics*. 2009;32(2):127.
55. Tennent TD, Goradia VK. Arthroscopic management of calcific tendinitis of the popliteus tendon. *Arthroscopy*. 2003;19(4):E35.
56. Tibrewal SB. Acute calcific tendinitis of the popliteus tendon—an unusual site and clinical syndrome. *Ann R Coll Surg Engl*. 2002;84(5):338-341.
57. Herman LJ, Beltran J. Pitfalls in MR imaging of the knee. *Radiology*. 1988;167(3):775-781.
58. Watanabe AT, Carter BC, Teitelbaum GP, Bradley WG Jr. Common pitfalls in magnetic resonance imaging of the knee. *J Bone Joint Surg Am Vol*. 1989;71(6):857-862.
59. Frush TJ, Noyes FR. Baker's cyst: diagnostic and surgical considerations. *Sports Health*. 2015;7(4):359-365.
60. Vap AR, Schon JM, Moatshe G, et al. The role of the peripheral passive rotation stabilizers of the knee with intact collateral and cruciate ligaments: a biomechanical study. *Orthop J Sports Med*. 2017;5(5):2325967117708190.
61. Domnick C, Frosch KH, Raschke MJ, et al. Kinematics of different components of the posterolateral corner of the knee in the lateral collateral ligament-intact state: a human cadaveric study. *Arthroscopy*. 2017;33(10):1821.e1-1830.e1.
62. Plaweski S, Belvisi B, Moreau-Gaudry A. Reconstruction of the posterolateral corner after sequential sectioning restores knee kinematics. *Orthop J Sports Med*. 2015;3(2):2325967115570560.
63. Chahla J, James EW, Cinque ME, LaPrade RF. Midterm outcomes following anatomic-based popliteus tendon reconstructions. *Knee Surg Sports Traumatol Arthrosc*. 2017.
64. Southmayd W, Quigley TB. The forgotten popliteus muscle. Its usefulness in correction of anteromedial rotatory instability of the knee. A preliminary report. *Clin Orthop Relat Res*. 1978(130):218-222.
65. Fleming RE Jr, Blatz DJ, McCarroll JR. Posterior problems in the knee. Posterior cruciate insufficiency and posterolateral rotatory insufficiency. *Am J Sports Med*. 1981;9(2):107-113.
66. Shino K, Horibe S, Ono K. The voluntarily evoked posterolateral drawer sign in the knee with posterolateral instability. *Clin Orthop Relat Res*. 1987(215):179-186.
67. Guha AR, Gorgees KA, Walker DI. Popliteus tendon rupture: a case report and review of the literature. *Br J Sports Med*. 2003;37(4):358-360.
68. McKay SD, Holt A, Stout T, Hysa VQ. Successful nonoperative treatment of isolated popliteus tendon avulsion fractures in two adolescents. *Case Rep Orthop*. 2014;2014:759419.
69. Wheeler LD, Lee EY, Lloyd DC. Isolated popliteus tendon avulsion in skeletally immature patients. *Clin Radiol*. 2008;63(7):824-828.
70. Liu JN, Rebolledo BJ, Warren RF, Green DW. Surgical management of isolated popliteus tendon injuries in paediatric patients. *Knee Surg Sports Traumatol Arthrosc*. 2016;24(3):788-791.
71. von Heideken J, Mikkelsson C, Bostrom Windhamre H, Janarv PM. Acute injuries to the posterolateral corner of the knee in children: a case series of 6 patients. *Am J Sports Med*. 2011;39(10):2199-2205.
72. Mason JS, Tansey KA, Westrick RB. Treatment of subacute posterior knee pain in an adolescent ballet dancer utilizing trigger point dry needling: a case report. *Int J Sports Phys Ther*. 2014;9(1):116-124.

Chapter 62

Clinical Considerations of Hip, Thigh, and Knee Pain

César Fernández de las Peñas and N. Beth Collier

1. HIP OSTEOARTHRITIS

1.1. Overview

Osteoarthritis (OA) of the hip is a common cause of hip pain and dysfunction in older adults. Hip and knee OA was ranked as the 11th highest contributor to global disability and 38th highest in affecting quality of life.[1] Dagenais et al[2] reported an overall prevalence for hip OA ranging from 0.9% to 27%. Prevalence data on lower extremity OA is variable depending on the utilization of radiographic changes as a criterion for a diagnosis of OA.[3] The American College of Rheumatology (ACR) has established criteria that are commonly used for the diagnosis of hip OA in clinical practice.[4] However, because clinical criteria are usually combined with radiologic findings of hip degeneration, it is important to consider that there is little correlation between the presence of hip pain and radiologic evidence of degenerative changes. Patients with hip pain do not always exhibit radiographic changes associated with hip OA.[5]

Osteoarthritis is a metabolically active, dynamic process that involves all synovial joint tissues (cartilage, bone, synovium/capsule, ligaments, and muscles) and is characterized mainly by focal areas of loss of articular cartilage within the synovial joints associated with hypertrophy of the bone (osteophytes and subchondral bone sclerosis) and thickening of the joint capsule. Hip OA can result in hip capsular changes, cartilage degeneration, osteophyte formation, sclerosis of subchondral bone, and muscle weakness.[6]

Hip OA is considered to be a multifactorial condition where genetic, constitutional, and biomechanical factors occur at the same time. Among the constitutional factors, age is probably the most common predisposing factor for hip OA because this condition affects mainly individuals over 60 years of age.[4,7] Other risk factors associated with the development of hip OA include a history of hip dysplasia,[8,9] a previous hip injury,[10] and an increased body mass index.[11]

Individuals with hip OA usually will experience debilitating pain. In fact, some people with minimal radiographic changes exhibit severe symptoms, whereas other people with radiographic evidence of advanced joint degeneration have minimal symptoms.[5] This inconsistency between symptoms and imaging findings should lead the clinician to consider the presence of nociceptive sensitization mechanisms in patients with hip OA. Although symptoms of pain in patients with hip OA can have mainly musculoskeletal origins, a recent systematic review has reported a prevalence of 23% of neuropathic pain in patients with knee or hip OA.[12] In fact, several studies have confirmed that individuals with hip OA exhibit central sensitization,[13,14] and when the nociceptive afferent input was removed (hip replacement), this process reversed.[15] A recent study has reported that central sensitization may be a determinant of how much patients with hip or knee OA benefit from joint replacement, but the effect varies by the severity of structural changes in the joint.[16] Therefore, current evidence supports the role of periarticular tissues surrounding the hip (eg, muscles) as a source of neuroplastic changes.

Most international clinical practice guidelines on hip and knee OA advocate for nonpharmacologic treatments as the first line of management, followed by pharmacologic treatment, and finally (if needed) surgery. The recommendations of the OA Research Society International include education, exercise, acupuncture, and weight reduction as nonpharmacologic therapies that are effective for hip OA.[17] The European League Against Rheumatism produced an evidence-based clinical guideline for nonpharmacologic management of people with hip or knee OA that suggests a combined treatment approach including[18] (1) education regarding OA, (2) regular individualized exercise programs, and (3) addressing weight loss if overweight or obese. Further, the UK clinical guidelines for management of hip OA also recommend the inclusion of manual therapy,[19] although its effectiveness is questioned by others.[20] Similarly, the clinical practice guideline proposed by the ACR recommends the use of multimodal treatment, including manual therapy, for the management of hip and knee OA.[21]

1.2. Initial Evaluation of a Patient With Hip Osteoarthritis

The clinical presentation of hip OA is characterized by pain, stiffness, reduced movement or function, and variable degrees of local inflammation. A clinical diagnosis of hip OA is confirmed when patients present with one of the following clusters of clinical findings: (1) hip pain, hip flexion less than 115°, and hip internal rotation less than 15°; or (2) pain with hip internal rotation, duration of morning stiffness of the hip less than or equal to 60 minutes, and age over 50 years.[4] These clinical criteria have shown a sensitivity of 86% and a specificity of 75%.[4] A radiographic diagnosis of hip OA is made by viewing a narrowed joint space, osteophyte formation, or subchondral sclerosis on plain film radiographs.[4,22,23] Sutlive et al[24] identified five possible clinical predictors for a diagnosis of hip OA, as defined by a Kellgren and Lawrence score of ≥2: pain with squatting, a positive scour test, pain with active hip flexion, pain with active hip extension, and passive range of motion of hip internal rotation less than 25°. The presence of symptoms potentially associated with hip OA diagnosis should alert the clinician to perform a thorough examination.

The clinician must perform a thorough subjective and physical examination that includes motor and sensory testing to establish whether the patient is appropriate for manual therapy or has any red flags indicating the need for referral to a physician. A human body pain drawing is beneficial to establish the location and area of the reported pain or symptoms. A pain drawing helps determine whether the reported pain is located mainly in the anterior, lateral, or posterior part of the hip or extends into the lower extremity. This drawing can be useful in monitoring the progression of the patient as symptoms improve and/or change. In addition, a report of the quality of the pain can help incriminate the main tissue responsible for the symptoms or pain referral.

Hip OA can lead to activity limitations, participation restrictions, or disabilities associated with walking, climbing stairs, getting in and out of a car, cycling, putting on shoes, and social participation. Therefore, it is essential that the clinical physical examination include the entire lower extremity, the pelvis, and the lumbar spine (see Chapter 53). The physical examination should include observation of posture, gait, active and passive range of motion testing, muscle length testing, muscle weakness, passive physiologic or accessory motion testing, palpation, and special tests to rule in or rule out OA and other conditions. All planes of motion of the hip should be assessed with active and passive movement testing. A patient with hip OA will present with restricted and painful hip range of motion, particularly in internal rotation and flexion.[25] Of particular interest is limitation of hip internal rotation because it is a predictive factor for the development of low back pain (LBP) in patients with hip OA.[26] The Flexion Abduction External Rotation (FABER) and scour tests can be used to further support a diagnosis of hip OA,[25,27] although it should be recognized that the sensitivity and specificity of these tests are low.

Patients with hip OA exhibit a generalized muscle strength deficit of 20% in the affected lower extremity.[28] Of particular interest is gluteus medius muscle weakness. Patients with hip OA also demonstrate limited ranges of coordinated motion of the pelvis, femur, and hip joint, especially in deeply flexed and rotated positions.[29] Therefore, a comprehensive examination of the soft tissue surrounding the hip is essential, including the examination for trigger points (TrPs) in the tensor fasciae latae, gluteus medius, gluteus minimus, gluteus maximus, piriformis, pectineus, adductor longus, adductor brevis, adductor magnus, quadriceps femoris group, quadratus lumborum, iliopsoas, and other lumbopelvic muscles as indicated.

1.3. Trigger Points in Hip Osteoarthritis

The pain of hip OA is perceived as deep in the hip and/or groin area, and it is more likely to refer laterally than medially. Several muscles can refer pain to this area, mimicking symptoms of hip OA; however, most studies investigating TrPs in the hip musculature, eg, gluteus medius muscle, have been conducted in patients with LBP[30] or patellofemoral pain.[31] Clinically, patients with hip OA present with weakness of the hip abductor muscles compared to the unaffected side and to healthy controls,[28] although the muscle morphology is significantly different.[32] Trigger points within the gluteus medius muscle can lead to inhibition weakness with no changes in the muscle cross-sectional area.

Older publications suggested that the referred pain from adductor longus TrPs may be mistaken for the pain of hip OA.[33,34] Inactivation of the adductor longus TrPs provides satisfactory pain relief to some patients with hip OA.[35] Nevertheless, a more recent experimentally induced pain study has observed that hypertonic saline injection of the adductor longus caused regionalized pain distribution with pain in the groin.[36]

Functionally, hip flexion and abduction range of motion, as seen in the FABER test position, can result from TrPs in the adductor muscles. Similarly, internal rotation of the hip can be limited by the presence of TrPs in the hip external rotation muscles, particularly the piriformis muscle. In fact, Izumi et al[36] found that hypertonic saline injections into the hip muscles led to a positive FABER test, suggesting that the test can be positive because of muscle pain and not just hip OA. Finally, the role of TrPs in hip OA is supported by the goals of the therapeutic management of hip OA because the objective is to increase the hip range of motion and strengthen both the hip and the knee musculature to reduce the excess load absorbed by the joint when hip/knee musculature is weak.

2. NONARTHRITIC HIP PAIN

2.1. Overview

Femoral Acetabular Impingement

Femoral acetabular impingement (FAI) is caused by repetitive approximation of an abnormally shaped femoral head and/or acetabulum at the end range of hip motion.[37] This process eventually leads to damage to the acetabular labrum and acetabular cartilage.[37] Osseous deformity of the femoral head/neck, or cam impingement, is most commonly seen in men aged 20 to 30 years and is the most common form of isolated FAI; osseous deformity of the acetabulum, or pincer impingement, is most commonly seen in women aged 30 to 40 years.[38-40] However, the most common form of FAI is a combined impingement that has components of both cam and pincer impingement.[38] Eijer and Hogervorst[41] have recently hypothesized that migration of the femoral head occurring in patients with cam or pincer impingement can lead to hip OA. These authors suggest that the impingement caused by femoral head migration can lead to hip joint cartilage damage.

Labral Tear

Acetabular labral tear is the most common intra-articular hip disorder and is commonly associated with other hip pathologies that may contribute to a patient's symptoms, such as FAI.[42] It is commonly found in an athletic population because acetabular labral tears are often the result of repetitive microtraumas.[43] Patients with a symptomatic labral tear report anterior groin pain that may radiate medially, laterally, or posteriorly in the hip.[44] The patient may report clicking or "locking" of the hip, and symptoms are exacerbated with activity.[42] There is also a clinical overlap between symptoms from FAI and labral tears.

Athletic Pubalgia (Groin Pain)

Historically referred to as "sports hernia," athletic pubalgia is defined as lower abdominal or groin pain without the presence of a hernia.[45] Other terms used to describe this condition include footballer hernia, inguinal insufficiency, conjoined tendon tear, hockey player's groin, or Gilmore groin.[46] Typically experienced while performing athletic sport activities involving hyperextension or rotation, athletic pubalgia is thought to occur when the adductor longus muscle pulls on its insertion in the pubic symphysis in an unopposed fashion, as would occur with a weak or inhibited rectus abdominis muscle.[45] This pathogenic mechanism may explain why osteitis pubis and adductor tenoperiostitis coexist in these patients. Muscular imbalances and decreased hip range of motion may increase the risk of injury in the groin area.[47] Athletic pubalgia is more common in men because of the narrower and less stable nature of the male pelvis.[48] Proper management of athletic pubalgia includes strengthening exercises for the adductor and abdominal muscles.[49] Therefore, a careful examination of soft tissues surrounding the hip seems to be crucial in all these nonarthritic conditions.

2.2. Initial Evaluation of a Patient With Nonarthritic Hip Pain

The clinician must perform a thorough subjective and physical examination that includes motor and sensory testing to establish whether the patient is appropriate for manual therapy or has any red flags indicating the need for referral to a physician. A human body pain drawing is beneficial to establish the location and area of the reported pain or symptoms. A pain drawing helps determine whether the reported pain is located mainly in the anterior, lateral, or posterior part of the hip or extends into the lower extremity. This drawing can be useful in monitoring the progression of the patient as symptoms improve and/or change. In addition, a report of the quality of the pain can help incriminate the main tissue responsible for the symptoms or pain referral.

In FAI, symptoms are more common in the anterior area of the hip and sometimes spread to the medial area (groin pain). In labral tears, the groin and greater trochanter areas are the most common locations of referred pain.[44] Patients with athletic pubalgia report unilateral deep groin pain, lower abdominal pain, or pubic pain that are more proximal and deeper than a hip flexor or adductor muscle strain.[50]

Westermann et al[51] have recently observed that patient factors, including mental health, activity level, gender, and smoking, were more predictive of hip pain and function than were intra-articular findings during hip arthroscopy in subjects with FAI; therefore, a thorough clinical examination is crucial for these patients. The physical examination of a patient with nonarthritic hip pain should include observation of hip and pelvic posture and gait, active and passive hip range of motion, muscle length testing, muscle strength testing, passive physiologic or accessory motion testing, palpation, as well as special tests to rule in or rule out FAI, labral tear, or other conditions. All planes of motion of the hip should be assessed with active and passive movements. The flexion, adduction, and internal rotation (FADIR) test, also called the impingement test, has been used for assessment of intra-articular pathologies such as labral tears and FAI. The meta-analysis conducted by Reiman et al[52] found that the FADIR and the flexion-internal rotation tests accurately screen for diagnosis of FAI or labral tears. Similarly, subjects with athletic pubalgia and those who had recurrent symptoms compared with those who had recovered from their groin pain episode also exhibit reduction of internal and external hip range of motion.[53] Typically, a patient with nonarthritic hip pain will present with less than 20° of hip internal rotation measured at 90° of hip flexion; this clinical finding is also common in patients with hip OA and patients with LBP. Further diagnostic imaging may be indicated and should include radiography or magnetic resonance arthrography to visualize bony structures, joint integrity, and other surrounding soft tissue structures.[54]

Patients with nonarthritic hip pain also exhibit weakness of the surrounding musculature, particularly the gluteal and adductor muscles. Therefore, a comprehensive examination of the following muscles should be performed for TrPs: gluteus medius, gluteus minimus, gluteus maximus, piriformis, adductors, pectineus, rectus abdominis, rectus femoris, and iliopsoas muscles.

2.3. Trigger Points and Nonarthritic Hip Pain

Similar to hip OA, as described previously, there is no study investigating the prevalence of TrPs in patients with FAI, labral tear, or athletic pubalgia. The patient's pain and symptom reports should dictate which muscles need to be examined for the presence of TrPs and their contribution to the patient's clinical presentation. For instance, in a patient with FAI, the pectineus, iliopsoas, and tensor fasciae latae muscles can be more relevant; whereas in a patient with athletic pubalgia, the rectus abdominis or adductor longus muscles might be more relevant.

3. GREATER TROCHANTERIC PAIN SYNDROME

3.1. Overview

Greater trochanteric pain syndrome (GTPS) refers to pain originating from any of the multiple structures that relate to the greater trochanter of the femur, including tendons and bursae. The tendons of gluteus medius, gluteus minimus, piriformis, obturator internus, obturator externus, and superior and inferior gemelli muscles all insert in some capacity to the greater trochanter and thus may cause pain if in an inflammatory state.[55] There are also multiple bursae in the area that lie between each layer of muscle in the region. Pathology of these bursae has historically been called trochanteric bursitis; however, recent diagnostic testing has revealed that the presence of inflammation in the bursa may be much less common than once believed.[56,57] The incidence peaks between the fourth and sixth decades of life, with women more affected than men.

Gluteal tendinopathy, which encompasses overuse injuries to the gluteus medius or gluteus minimus tendons, commonly causes pain in the greater trochanteric area.[58] Muscle imbalances caused by weakness or abnormal tightness throughout the hip can predispose the tendons that attach to the greater trochanter to overload and thereby cause injury. A commonly observed muscle imbalance or altered muscle activation pattern in those patients with GTPS is an overcompensation by the tensor fasciae latae muscle in hip abduction leading to weakness and atrophy of the posterior portion of the gluteus medius muscle.[59] Therefore, conservative management of GTPS includes rest during the acute phase, followed by physical therapy, corticosteroid injections, and other analgesic modalities.[60,61]

3.2. Initial Evaluation of a Patient With Greater Trochanteric Pain Syndrome

The clinician must perform a thorough subjective and physical examination that includes motor and sensory testing to establish whether the patient is appropriate for manual therapy or has any red flags indicating the need for referral to a physician. A human body pain drawing is beneficial to establish the location and area of the reported pain or symptoms. A pain drawing helps determine whether the reported pain is located mainly in the anterior, lateral, or posterior part of the hip or whether it extends into the lower extremity. This drawing can be useful in monitoring the progression of the patient as symptoms improve and/or change. In addition, a report of the quality of the pain can help incriminate the main tissue responsible for the symptoms or pain referral.

Patients with GTPS may report pain with lying on the affected side, walking, and bearing weight on the affected leg. Pain is typically reported along the lateral hip and sometimes along the lateral thigh; the pain rarely spreads below the knee area.[56]

The hip should be inspected for local visible signs of inflammation, particularly around the greater trochanter. Careful palpation should be performed in an attempt to identify anatomical structures responsible for the patient's clinical presentation.[56] In fact, palpation of the greater trochanter has been reported to be the most provocative test included in clinical exam for lateral hip pain.[62] In the presence of gluteus medius tendinopathy, pain will be reproduced with resisted hip abduction and external or internal rotation, and the patient may exhibit a positive Trendelenburg sign. Lequesne et al[63] found that if single-leg stance can be held for less than 30 seconds, it has a sensitivity and specificity of 100% and 97.3%, respectively, for the diagnosis of gluteus medius tendinopathy.

Other factors that have been linked to lateral hip pain in the athlete include a wide pelvis, leg length discrepancy, excessive foot pronation, and poor running surfaces. Therefore, a thorough examination of the entire lower extremity should be carried out. Active hip range of motion, muscle length and strength testing, and passive physiologic or accessory motion testing should be conducted. Passive external rotation of the hip with the hip in 90° of flexion is typically the only painful provocative movement for patients with GTPS during hip range of motion assessment.[63]

3.3. Trigger Points and Greater Trochanteric Pain Syndrome

There are several muscles that may refer pain to the greater trochanteric area when dysfunctional, including the following muscles: tensor fasciae latae, vastus lateralis, gluteus medius, gluteus minimus, gluteus maximus, piriformis, gemelli, and quadratus lumborum muscles. Differential diagnosis of specific source tissues can be difficult in GTPS, and palpation to implicate a bursa may be specific only with an acute inflammatory presentation of trochanteric bursitis. A recent randomized control trial reported that patients with GTPS who received either cortisone injection to the trochanteric bursae or deep dry needling to surrounding musculature obtained similar results in pain reduction and functional outcome measures.[64] Similarly, Jacobson et al[65] found that the application of tendon fenestration, a technique similar to dry needling, was equally effective as platelet-rich plasma injection for patients with GTPS. These studies would suggest that regardless of identifying the specific anatomical source of symptoms, treatment of TrPs in the surrounding area in a patient with suspected GTPS may be sufficient to relieve pain.

4. PIRIFORMIS SYNDROME

4.1. Overview

Piriformis syndrome describes a neuromuscular disorder in which the piriformis muscle compresses the sciatic nerve, inducing sciatic-type pain, paresthesias, and numbness in the buttocks and along the sciatic nerve pathway down to the lower thigh and into the leg. Patients with piriformis syndrome typically report pain deep in the buttock that may or may not have correlating symptoms of radiating pain down the leg and dysesthesias associated with the sciatic nerve. Onset of piriformis syndrome is most common in the fourth or fifth decade of life and can be associated with both sedentary and active lifestyles.[66] However, sometimes the piriformis muscle is not involved at all.[67]

4.2. Initial Evaluation of a Patient With Piriformis Syndrome

It has been recently reported that the four most common symptoms of piriformis syndrome include buttock pain, pain aggravated on sitting, external tenderness near the greater sciatic notch, pain with any maneuver that increases piriformis muscle tension, and limitation in straight leg raising.[68] The patient may also report a loss in his or her hip range of motion or flexibility into internal rotation and adduction. Fishman et al[69] investigated the diagnostic utility of the flexion adduction internal rotation test (FAIR) to identify an operational definition of piriformis syndrome and found it to have a sensitivity of 0.81 and a specificity of 0.83. Therefore, a careful examination of the hip and pelvic regions should be conducted. Because the tissue source of symptoms in piriformis syndrome can be difficult to discern (muscle or sciatic nerve), neurodynamic tests can be used for assessing mechanical nerve sensitivity. The slump test is sensitive for diagnosing neuropathic pain in the lower extremity.[70] The entire lower extremity should be examined when a patient presents with symptoms consistent with piriformis syndrome because other conditions can also mimic these symptoms, as previously discussed.

4.3. Trigger Points and Piriformis Syndrome

All symptoms associated with piriformis syndrome can be directly related to the presence of TrPs in the piriformis muscle; however, there is no study that has explicitly investigated this association. Differentiating symptoms from compression of the sciatic nerve caused by a tight piriformis muscle, or sensory symptoms elicited by the pain referral associated with piriformis TrPs, is extremely difficult. Manual palpation of the muscle and exclusion of contribution from neural components by utilizing neurodynamic tests are key for differential diagnosis.

5. PATELLOFEMORAL PAIN SYNDROME

5.1. Overview

Patellofemoral pain syndrome (PFPS) is a condition causing pain at the anterior and/or medial knee during activities that load or compress the patella, such as prolonged sitting and climbing stairs. Importantly, PFPS is an "umbrella" term to describe pain in and around the patella in the absence of other pathologies. Although the prevalence of PFPS has been estimated to be as high as 40%, the annual incidence and prevalence of this condition are unknown.[71] The pathophysiology of PFPS is not well understood, and the general consensus is that the etiology is multifactorial, including repeated knee microtrauma, muscle imbalances of the knee extensors, biomechanical dysfunctions in the lower extremity, and changes in nociceptive pain processing.[72,73] For instance, biomechanical factors involved in PFPS include muscle strength imbalance between the activity of the vastus medialis muscle in relation to the vastus lateralis muscle, reduced flexibility, patellar tracking, altered quadriceps angle, and altered patellofemoral joint morphology.[74] In their review, Lankhorst et al[75] identified the following variables associated with PFPS: larger Q-angle, sulcus angle, patellar tilt, reduced hip abduction strength, weaker hip external rotation, and reduced knee extension peak torque. Pain from PFPS is also influenced by confounding psychosocial factors, such as fear-avoidance behaviors.[76]

There is a plethora of treatments proposed for the management of PFPS. Barton et al[77] concluded that the treatment of PFPS should include gluteal and quadriceps femoris muscle strengthening, patellar taping, neuromuscular control exercises, education, and activity modification. The review conducted by Cochrane concluded that there is consistent, but low-quality, evidence regarding the effectiveness of exercise for patients with PFPS, but no data exists to determine the best form of exercise.[78] Historical therapeutic strategies for PFPS targeted the knee muscles, but research supports focus on the hip abductors and external rotators.[79] It would be reasonable to consider a potential role of TrPs as part of a rehabilitation plan of care.

5.2. Initial Evaluation of a Patient With Patellofemoral Pain Syndrome

Symptoms of PFPS usually include pain around the patella or surrounding areas (most commonly in the anterior or medial areas), swelling, crepitus, and catching of the knee. Symptom behavior often includes aggravation with loading of the joint during activities such as climbing stairs, squatting (especially beyond 20°–30° of knee flexion), and sitting with knee flexion for a prolonged period of time. Hallmark clinical features of PFPS include quadriceps femoris and hip muscle strength deficit, particularly in the vastus medialis,[80] hip abductor, and hip external rotator muscles.[79] Patients with PFPS also exhibit quadriceps femoris muscle atrophy, which may primarily affect vastus medialis[81] or the vastus lateralis muscles, or it may impact all the quadriceps femoris muscles.[82]

Clinical assessment of a patient with PFPS should include provocative tests for pain from surrounding structures, assessment of kinetic chain influences, functional tests, and assessment of patellar mobility and palpatory tests.[83] A comprehensive manual exploration should be performed of the lower extremity musculature, including the following muscles: gluteus medius,[31] gluteus minimus, piriformis, iliopsoas, pectineus, rectus femoris, vastus medialis, vastus lateralis, hamstrings, and gastrocnemius muscles. Additionally, the patient should undergo a thorough biomechanical analysis of weight-bearing activities, such as gait, running, and jumping, as pain allows. Patients with PFPS usually display excessive hip adduction and internal rotation, as well as contralateral pelvic drop during single-limb tasks when compared with healthy individuals.[84] If these impairments are identified, evaluation of hip and foot function and structure should be conducted to determine the source of biomechanical inefficiencies.

5.3. Trigger Points and Patellofemoral Pain Syndrome

Knee extensor musculature weakness with PFPS may be a result of inhibition of quadriceps femoris muscles or altered timing of muscle activation during functional activities caused by the presence of TrPs.[85] Referral pain patterns from several muscles (vastus medialis, rectus femoris, vastus lateralis, or vastus intermedius) can mimic the symptoms experienced by patients with PFPS; however, there is no epidemiologic study investigating the prevalence of TrPs in this population. Roach et al[31] reported the presence of latent TrPs in the hip muscles (gluteus medius and quadratum lumborum) in patients with PFPS. In this study, reduced hip abduction strength was associated with the presence of latent TrPs. There is preliminary evidence suggesting that manual compression of TrPs surrounding the knee area, mostly applied to the vastus medialis muscle, is effective in the short and medium term for reducing symptoms in patients with PFPS.[86,87]

6. KNEE OSTEOARTHRITIS

6.1. Overview

Knee OA is a multifactorial degenerative disease influenced by age, genetics, and history of repetitive microtrauma of the knee. Hip and knee OA were ranked together as the 11th highest contributor to global disability and 38th highest in affecting quality of life.[1] The clinical diagnosis of knee OA is typically made using the ACR clinical criteria developed by Altman that has been found to be 89% sensitive and 88% specific.[88] These criteria are age older than 50 years, less than 30 minutes of morning stiffness, crepitus on active motion, bony tenderness, and bony enlargement and/or no palpable warmth of synovium.[88] Clinical criteria are usually combined with radiologic findings of degeneration, although as with hip OA, pain in knee OA is highly individual, and no radiologic changes have demonstrated a robust correlation with pain manifestation.

Many structural features of the joint have been suggested to be involved in knee OA related–pain, including, but not limited to, the presence of osteophytes in the knee, focal or diffuse cartilaginous abnormalities, subchondral cysts, bone marrow edema, subluxation of the meniscus, meniscal tears, or Baker cysts.[89] The fact that no association exists between degenerative changes and symptoms has inspired researchers to investigate the presence of sensitization pain mechanisms in knee OA.[90,91] Therefore, multimodal management of individuals with knee OA should include manual therapy, exercises, cognitive-behavioral therapy, neuroscience education, and pharmacologic drugs.[92] The clinical practice guideline proposed by the ACR strongly recommends nonpharmacologic interventions for individuals with knee OA, including aerobic, aquatic, and/or resistance exercise as well as weight loss for individuals who are overweight.[21] It has also been demonstrated that the addition of manual therapy and/or exercise can improve the cost-effectiveness of the management of patients with knee OA.[93]

An important feature in knee OA is arthrogenic muscle inhibition caused mainly by a change in the discharge of articular sensory receptors arising from factors such as swelling, inflammation, joint laxity, and damage to joint afferents.[94] Interestingly, the presence of symptomatic, radiographic changes is not associated with deficits in the temporal recruitment of the vastus medialis and vastus lateralis muscles during stair climbing in subjects with knee OA.[95] This supports the notion that arthrogenic muscle inhibition is not the main cause of muscle pain and inhibition in this population.

6.2. Initial Evaluation of a Patient With Knee Osteoarthritis

The main clinical features in patients with knee OA are joint pain, stiffness in the morning or after rest, limited joint motion, night pain, and/or joint deformity. Although pain symptoms are located mainly in the knee area, the presence of diffuse pain distribution has also been found in this population as a result of sensitization mechanisms.[92] Therefore, a thorough clinical examination and the use of pain-body diagrams can be helpful in determining the pain pattern in a patient with knee OA.

Abnormal knee loading is a key factor in OA progression[96]; therefore, a comprehensive examination of the lower extremity is required. Biomechanically, knee OA is influenced by body weight, knee range of motion, and excessive varus or valgus moments during gait.[96,97] Clinicians should explore the pelvis, hip, knee, and ankle joints for identification of dysfunctions that could contribute to increased loading in the knee. Active and passive range of motion (with and without overpressure), mobility tests, and muscle length in the lower extremity should be assessed.

Assessment of muscle strength and endurance is a key component of the clinical examination in patients with knee OA and should guide the rehabilitation program. In fact, quadriceps femoris muscle power[98] and strength[99] are predictive factors of radiographic and symptomatic knee OA. In this scenario, identification of active and latent TrPs in the musculature of the lower extremity should precede a therapeutic exercise program. Muscles that should be examined are gluteus medius, gluteus minimus, piriformis, iliopsoas, rectus femoris, vastus medialis, vastus lateralis, adductors, hamstrings, tibialis anterior, and gastrocnemius muscles.

6.3. Trigger Points and Knee Osteoarthritis

Evidence supports the role of myofascial pain and of TrPs in individuals with knee OA.[100] Studies describe patients with painful knee OA who also had active TrPs in the muscles surrounding the knee that reproduced the patient's symptoms.[101-104] In these studies, the number of active TrPs was associated with the intensity of persistent pain, and the intensity of knee pain was inversely related to the physical function of the patients, meaning that patients with more intense pain experienced reduced physical function. Alburquerque-García et al[101] found that the vastus medialis, vastus lateralis, and gastrocnemius muscles were the most affected by active TrPs. Bajaj et al[104] found that the rectus femoris, gastrocnemius, and vastus medialis muscles were the most affected. And Itoh et al[103] found that the quadriceps femoris, the iliopsoas, sartorius, hip adductors, and hamstring muscles were the most affected. In addition, referred pain areas evoked by intramuscular injection of hypertonic saline were also significantly larger in patients with knee OA.[104] Henry et al[102] observed that patients with painful knee OA who were waitlisted for total knee arthroplasty surgery had active TrPs in the quadriceps femoris, hamstrings, and gastrocnemius muscles and experienced a significant reduction in pain reports 8 weeks after TrP treatment. Similarly, treatment of TrPs by different electrotherapy and manual therapy modalities has also been found to be effective in addressing pain in patients with knee OA.[105]

When patients with knee OA undergo a total knee arthroplasty procedure, increased pain is typically experienced within the first month postsurgery, and TrPs have been found in patients following total knee arthroplasty. In a study of 40 subjects undergoing total knee arthroplasty as a knee OA intervention, Mayoral et al[106] investigated the effect of TrP dry needling on postoperative pain. Dry needling was performed after administration of anesthesia in the group assigned to treatment. Postoperative pain levels were compared between the group that received dry needling prior to surgery and the group that did not. Results showed reduced pain in the treatment group immediately after surgery and 1 month postsurgery, but no difference was found at 3 and 6 months postsurgery. This study demonstrates that in patients with knee OA who undergo total knee arthroplasty, TrPs likely play a role in a patient's pain experienced postoperatively.[106] Núñez-Cortés et al[107] described a case series of patients with pain following total knee arthroplasty in whom dry needling combined with therapeutic exercise was effective for improving pain, range of motion, and function; however, the lack of a control group limits the extrapolation of the results. Nguyen[108] has proposed a hypothetical pain model where TrPs in the knee muscles can provoke muscle tightness, pain, and weakness leading to early pathologic neuromuscular changes including knee instability and, consequently, falls in older adults. In this model, long-term TrPs may promote knee instability and can facilitate degenerative changes in the knee joint, which will in turn, cause arthrogenous muscle inhibition typical of knee OA.[108] There is no study supporting this hypothesis, so further studies are warranted.

7. ILIOTIBIAL BAND SYNDROME

7.1. Overview

Iliotibial Band Syndrome (ITBS) typically presents with an insidious onset of lateral knee pain from functional overuse and is commonly seen in athletes, particularly runners.[109] The mechanism underlying ITBS is questioned in the scientific literature. The historically accepted theory of ITBS described friction occurring between the distal iliotibial band (IT band) and the lateral femoral epicondyle during repetitive knee flexion and extension activities.[110] More recent research shows that the distal end of the IT band actually compresses against the lateral femoral epicondyle at 30° of knee flexion and is likely not flexible enough to move over the lateral femoral epicondyle as the friction theory suggests.[111] This conclusion may be related to the fact that the IT band is a thickening of the fasciae latae system of the thigh and is firmly connected to the linea aspera of the femur rather than being a separate, mobile band.[112]

Factors contributing to ITBS include downhill running, wearing worn-out or old shoes, leg length discrepancy, repetitive running on the same side of a road, excessive pronation of the foot, weakness of the gluteus medius muscle, and an increased Q-angle.[109]

7.2. Initial Evaluation of a Patient With Iliotibial Band Syndrome

A body pain drawing is beneficial to establish a pattern and location of the pain. A pain drawing helps determine whether the pain is located mainly in the anterior, lateral, or posterior aspect of the knee or if the distribution of symptoms radiates to the leg. Patients affected by ITBS often report sharp and occasionally burning pain localized to the lateral aspect of the knee. These symptoms are exacerbated mostly by physical activity, particularly running, hiking, or jumping. A thorough examination of the lower extremity should be carried out to identify contributing factors such as pes planus that can contribute to the development of ITBS from increasing strain on the IT band caused by increased internal rotation of the leg during walking and running gait.[110] The physical examination should include observation of the lower extremity during gait; active motion testing of the knee, hips, and ankle; manual palpation of muscles and structures; muscle length and strength assessment; passive physiologic or accessory motion testing; and any indicated orthopedic special tests. Symptoms may be provoked with the Noble Compression test that compresses the IT band at the lateral femoral condyle as the patient performs active knee extension from an initial position of 90° of flexion.[113] The Ober test or Modified Ober test may be used to assess for IT band length;[114] however, this test may actually be assessing muscle length deficits of the tensor fasciae latae, gluteus maximus, and gluteus medius muscles, given the extensive attachments of these muscles to the IT band. The Thomas test may also be used to identify muscle length deficits of the iliopsoas, rectus femoris, and/or the tensor fasciae latae muscles. Of particular relevance would be the examination of myofascial restrictions or TrPs in the vastus lateralis, tensor fasciae latae, gluteus maximus, gluteus medius, piriformis, and distal biceps femoris muscles.

Because runners with ITBS show reduced hip abductor muscle strength in their affected lower extremity as compared with their nonaffected lower extremity and as compared with a control group,[115] a functional assessment of muscle strength of the hip musculature is also crucial. Additionally, some patients with ITBS may also exhibit imbalances between the posterior fibers of the gluteus medius and tensor fasciae latae and/or the gluteus maximus and hamstring muscles.[114] Therefore, assessment of hip function and strength is vital in order to design a comprehensive rehabilitation program for individuals with ITBS.

7.3. Trigger Points and Iliotibial Band Syndrome

Treatment of ITBS includes flexibility exercises targeting muscles that have an attachment to the IT band and strengthening exercises that avoid exacerbation of symptoms.[110,114] However, the strengthening phase should be initiated only once myofascial restrictions and/or TrPs have been addressed and normal flexibility has been established.[113,114] Therefore, identification and inactivation of TrPs is crucial for the proper management of patients with ITBS. However, the literature on this topic is scant. Pavkovich[116] described a case report of a patient with a diagnosis of ITBS in whom the application of dry needling to the vastus lateralis and other thigh muscles was effective for reducing pain and improving function.

Clinically, it has been noted that TrPs in the vastus lateralis and tensor fasciae latae muscles directly refer pain in a pattern similar to that of ITBS. Dysfunction of these muscles, typically from overuse or sometimes direct trauma (in the case of the vastus lateralis muscle), can be the source of lateral knee pain symptoms. Given the anatomical relationship between the vastus lateralis muscle and the IT band, a hypertrophied or tonic vastus lateralis muscle will result in increased approximation to the overlying IT band, potentially resulting in a general lack of mobility and perhaps increased compression on the lateral aspect of the knee.

Additionally, the imbalance between the gluteus maximus, the posterior fibers of the gluteus medius, and the tensor fasciae latae muscles present in many patients with ITBS[114] can also be related to the presence of TrPs in these muscles. Treating TrPs inhibiting the gluteus medius and minimus muscles could help improve stability to the pelvis during single limb-stance activity, as is required in running. Treatment aimed at TrPs and neuromuscular retraining of the tensor fasciae latae muscle and inhibition of the gluteus maximus muscle, both of which share an attachment to the IT band, can restore normal biomechanical function of the IT band.

8. INJURIES OF THE KNEE

8.1. Overview

Articular structures of the knee, including ligaments and menisci, are commonly damaged during knee joint trauma. The anterior cruciate ligament (ACL) and the menisci are the structures most commonly affected, although injury or tears on the collateral ligaments are also highly prevalent. Globally, the annual incidence of ACL injuries is estimated to be 0.01% to 0.05%[117], although these rates are higher in athletes.[118] Medial collateral ligament injury is usually associated with an injury in the ACL and has an annual incidence of 0.24 per 1000 people roughly.[119] Nevertheless, meniscal injuries are the most common intra-articular knee lesions and are the most frequent cause of orthopedic surgery.[120] Meniscal tears occur more frequently in the firmly attached medial meniscus but can also occur in the lateral meniscus.[121] Injuries to the knee typically occur when a patient performs an abrupt or uncontrolled twisting maneuver with the foot planted, commonly referred to as a "noncontact injury." The patient may report a "tearing" sensation or an audible "pop" at the time of injury, with later complaints of "locking" or "catching" in the knee in the case of meniscal damage or instability in the case of ACL injury. The patient typically presents with delayed effusion at the knee joint 6 to 24 hours after injury; immediate onset of a joint effusion is indicative of multistructural injury.

Different risk factors have been associated with knee injuries. In a meta-analysis, Snoeker et al[122] reported strong evidence that age over 60 years, male gender, work-related kneeling or squatting, and climbing stairs were risk factors for degenerative meniscal tears. Additionally, strong evidence for associated acute meniscal injuries in soccer and rugby players was reported. This meta-analysis also concluded that waiting longer than 12 months between an ACL injury and a reconstructive surgery was a strong risk factor for a medial, but not lateral, meniscal tear.[122]

Knee injuries, including ACL and meniscal tears, can be managed with conservative or surgical treatment, and the data is inconclusive on the best therapeutic options following ACL or meniscus injury. The Cochrane review concluded that there is insufficient evidence from randomized clinical trials to determine whether surgery or conservative management is best following ACL injury at 2 and 5 years postinjury.[123] Further, the incidence of radiologic knee OA is similar between patients treated conservatively and those who underwent surgical treatment and is also independent of the preoperative grade of laxity and the functional status of the patients.[124] Nevertheless, some authors suggest that the menisci should be repaired in patients with residual laxity on clinical assessment after ACL reconstruction because of a potential risk of failure of the ACL reconstruction.[125]

Most clinicians support the implementation of exercise programs for management and also for prevention of knee injuries. This suggestion is based on the fact that scientific and clinical research notes that the knee musculature demonstrates deleterious effects following a knee injury. A recent meta-analysis found that both the quadriceps femoris and hamstring muscles demonstrated reduced strength in patients with an ACL tear, but the reduction in quadriceps femoris strength was 3-fold greater than that in the hamstrings.[126] In fact, there is also evidence that neuromuscular and proprioceptive training reduces knee injury in general and ACL injury in particular, confirming the role of the dynamic knee stabilizer muscles in traumatic knee events.[127] Swart et al[128] concluded that exercise and meniscectomy yielded comparable results on pain and function; however, there is no evidence supporting one form of exercise over another.[129] In fact, quadriceps femoris muscle strengthening is an important milestone in the rehabilitation of knee injuries and is achieved through a combination of open and closed kinetic chain exercises. The clinical practice guidelines on ACL injury from the Dutch Orthopaedic Association and from the Orthopaedic Section of the American Physical Therapy Association (APTA) have found moderate to strong evidence that open and closed chain strength training had a positive effect on the strength of both the quadriceps femoris and hamstring muscles along with functional recovery in patients following knee injury.[130,131]

8.2. Initial Evaluation of a Patient after an Injury of the Knee

In any patient with a history of knee injury, clinicians must perform a thorough subjective and physical examination to establish whether the patient is appropriate for manual therapy or has any red flags indicating serious structural damage. In fact, current recommendations suggest the use of diagnostic imaging only when fracture is suspected based on the Ottawa Knee rules or when the physical examination is positive for meniscal or ligamentous knee damage.[132] These guidelines are confirmed by the American College of Radiology Appropriateness Criteria for acute knee injury.[133]

Patients with a meniscal tear typically experience joint line pain on the medial or lateral aspect of the knee, usually with maximum passive knee flexion and/or extension range of motion. Furthermore, these patients can also report the presence of "locking or blocking events," mostly in maximum knee flexion. Patients with an ACL tear can experience deep pain inside the knee or sometimes pain at the insertion of the ligament; however, the main clinical symptom of an ACL tear is an anterior-to-posterior instability. Clinical assessment should include provocative tests of knee structures, active and passive range of motion, functional testing, assessment of patellar mobility, and palpatory examination of knee structures and associated musculature. Of particular interest is identification of aberrant knee joint movement, including hypo- or hypermobility. Several tests can be used to identify ACL tear (the Lachman test is the most sensitive [87.1%], whereas the pivot shift test is the most specific [97.5%])[134] and meniscus tear (McMurray test: sensitivity 61%, specificity 84%; joint interline pain tenderness: sensitivity 83%, specificity 83%; Thessaly test: sensitivity 75%, specificity 87%).[135]

Altered quadriceps femoris and hamstring muscle activation patterns may change anterior shear forces and knee extensor moments, making the individual more susceptible to an ACL injury. Hewett et al[136] reported altered quadriceps femoris and lowered hamstring muscle activation strategies, along with lowered hamstring muscle to quadriceps femoris torque ratios after ACL rupture. Therefore, examination of knee injuries should include muscle strength, power, endurance, and flexibility assessment. All musculature of the lower extremity should be examined, including gluteus medius, gluteus minimus, hip external rotator, hip adductor, rectus femoris, vastus medialis, vastus lateralis, hamstrings, and gastrocnemius muscles. Other factors, including psychosocial elements, such as hypervigilance, catastrophization, and fear avoidance behaviors should also be identified.

8.3. Trigger Points and Injuries of the Knee

Although research is lacking on the relationship between ACL or meniscal tears and TrPs, it is commonly seen in clinical practice that pain referral from the vastus medialis, vastus lateralis, rectus femoris, sartorius, adductor longus, and adductor brevis muscles can mimic similar symptoms of a medial or lateral meniscal tear, and therefore, they should be considered in the differential diagnosis of a patient presenting with knee pain after an injury. Similarly, active TrPs in the knee musculature can be activated after a knee injury, with or without an associated ACL injury. Torres-Chica et al[137] found a higher number of active TrPs in the quadriceps femoris muscle, but particularly within the vastus medialis muscle, in individuals experiencing pain following a meniscectomy. Additionally, the number of active TrPs was associated with the intensity of knee pain after surgery. These authors hypothesize that TrPs could have developed from dynamic mobility changes that commonly occur after a meniscal tear or from the physiologic changes produced by the surgery itself.[137] Velázquez-Saornil et al[138] have recently observed that the inclusion of dry needling of active TrPs in the vastus medialis muscle into a rehabilitation protocol was effective for increasing range of motion and function in patients after surgical reconstruction of complete ACL rupture. Because the vastus medialis muscle is the main stabilizing muscle of the medial aspect of the knee, it seems that this muscle is the most affected by TrPs in patients after they experience a knee injury. Therefore, the presence of active TrPs in the knee muscles could be related to deficits in muscle strength (inhibition weakness) and proprioception.

9. HIP AND KNEE NERVE ENTRAPMENTS

9.1. Overview

Radicular pain typically extends from the lumbar spine into the lower extremity and generally distal to the knee in the case of lumbar or sacral nerve root compression or inflammation. Pain that extends beyond the gluteal region and into the leg is often a result of nerve irritation. Symptoms can include referral to the lower thoracic or upper lumbar region, abdomen, flanks, groin, genitals, thighs, knees, calves, ankles, feet, and toes. Lumbar radicular pain is considered a subclassification of LBP and is often characterized by a radiating pain in one or more lumbar dermatomes that may or may not be accompanied by other radicular irritation symptoms.[139,140] Symptoms of radiculopathy may include numbness, motor loss, muscle wasting, weakness, and loss of reflexes. Prognostic indicators of successful recovery in cases of radicular pain or radiculopathy include patients with higher education levels, working full-time, and with low fear avoidance; predictors of nonsuccess include higher patient age and the presence of reflex impairments.[141]

In a systematic review, Hahne et al[142] found moderate evidence that stabilization exercises are better than no treatment at short-term follow-up and that manipulation is better than sham manipulation at short-term and intermediate-term follow-up for people with acute lumbar disc herniation and radicular symptoms who had an intact annulus.

9.2. Initial Evaluation of a Patient with Nerve Entrapment

The presence of discogenic pain has also been discussed in Chapter 53 of this textbook. Therefore, in this chapter, we will focus on diagnosis differentiation with other hip and thigh conditions that cause pain or other symptoms in this region. Symptoms associated with radicular pain or nerve entrapment include pain in dermatomal patterns. The most common affected nerves are the femoral (anterior hip or thigh pain) and sciatic (posterior thigh, knee, or leg pain) nerves. Therefore, proper examination should differentiate between radicular, peripheral nerve, and myofascial pain symptoms. The presence of urinary retention, saddle anesthesia, or bilateral neurologic symptoms represents potential red flags, and the patient should be referred to a physician.

In common nerve entrapment clinical presentations, the LBP clinical practice guideline from the Academy of Orthopaedic Physical Therapy, of the APTA classifies patient presentations as LBP with radiating pain.[143] Initial evaluation of patients within this clinical classification should include movement testing to assess for specific directional movements of lumbar active range of motion that may provoke or relieve symptoms; nerve mobility testing such as a straight leg raise and/or slump test; and neurologic testing, including sensory, motor, and reflex testing.[143] Forward trunk flexion is usually accompanied by peripheralization of pain symptoms toward the legs or buttocks. Repeated movement into flexion often worsens the nature of the symptoms. The straight leg raise is a common provocation test used when differentially diagnosing lumbar radicular pain or radiculopathy from other neurogenic causes. Other neurodynamic tests that can be used are the slump test or the femoral nerve slump test.[144] Once radicular pain or other nerve involvement has been excluded or identified, TrPs should be investigated.

9.3. Trigger Points and Hip and Knee Nerve Entrapment

Referred pain from TrPs can be easily mistaken for common reports of radicular pain. In addition, TrPs can also be activated on account of nerve root irritation. In fact, the presence of gluteal TrPs showed a high specificity (91.4%) of predicting lumbar radiculopathy, as confirmed with diagnostic magnetic resonance imaging.[145] Active TrPs in the gluteal muscles were significantly correlated with the same side as reported radiating pain.[146] Therefore, examination of those muscles innervated by the nerve root affected (eg, gastrocnemius with L5, S1 nerve root involvement, rectus femoris with L2, L3 nerve root involvement) is crucial because active TrPs could be the source of, or a contributing factor to, the patient's symptoms. Additionally, patients who failed spinal surgery for lumbar nerve root decompression have been found, on multiple occasions, to present with active TrPs in the piriformis and other muscles of the back and hip, suggesting that TrPs in associated muscles can serve as persistent pain generators, even after decompression of nervous tissue in this patient population.[147]

References

1. Cross M, Smith E, Hoy D, et al. The global burden of hip and knee osteoarthritis: estimates from the global burden of disease 2010 study. *Ann Rheum Dis.* 2014;73(7):1323-1330.
2. Dagenais S, Garbedian S, Wai EK. Systematic review of the prevalence of radiographic primary hip osteoarthritis. *Clin Orthop Relat Res.* 2009;467(3):623-637.
3. Pereira D, Peleteiro B, Araujo J, Branco J, Santos RA, Ramos E. The effect of osteoarthritis definition on prevalence and incidence estimates: a systematic review. *Osteoarthritis Cartilage.* 2011;19(11):1270-1285.
4. Altman R, Alarcon G, Appelrouth D, et al. The American College of Rheumatology criteria for the classification and reporting of osteoarthritis of the hip. *Arthritis Rheum.* 1991;34(5):505-514.
5. Kim C, Nevitt MC, Niu J, et al. Association of hip pain with radiographic evidence of hip osteoarthritis: diagnostic test study. *BMJ.* 2015;351:h5983.
6. Murphy NJ, Eyles JP, Hunter DJ. Hip osteoarthritis: etiopathogenesis and implications for management. *Adv Ther.* 2016;33(11):1921-1946.
7. Quintana JM, Arostegui I, Escobar A, Azkarate J, Goenaga JI, Lafuente I. Prevalence of knee and hip osteoarthritis and the appropriateness of joint replacement in an older population. *Arch Intern Med.* 2008;168(14):1576-1584.
8. Jacobsen S, Sonne-Holm S. Hip dysplasia: a significant risk factor for the development of hip osteoarthritis. A cross-sectional survey. *Rheumatology (Oxford).* 2005;44(2):211-218.
9. Felson DT, Lawrence RC, Dieppe PA, et al. Osteoarthritis: new insights. Part 1: the disease and its risk factors. *Ann Intern Med.* 2000;133(8):635-646.
10. Richmond SA, Fukuchi RK, Ezzat A, Schneider K, Schneider G, Emery CA. Are joint injury, sport activity, physical activity, obesity, or occupational activities predictors for osteoarthritis? A systematic review. *J Orthop Sports Phys Ther.* 2013;43(8):515-519.
11. Jiang L, Rong J, Wang Y, et al. The relationship between body mass index and hip osteoarthritis: a systematic review and meta-analysis. *Joint Bone Spine.* 2011;78(2):150-155.
12. French HP, Smart KM, Doyle F. Prevalence of neuropathic pain in knee or hip osteoarthritis: a systematic review and meta-analysis. *Semin Arthritis Rheum.* 2017;47(1):1-8.
13. Gwilym SE, Keltner JR, Warnaby CE, et al. Psychophysical and functional imaging evidence supporting the presence of central sensitization in a cohort of osteoarthritis patients. *Arthritis Rheum.* 2009;61(9):1226-1234.
14. Kuni B, Wang H, Rickert M, Ewerbeck V, Schiltenwolf M. Pain threshold correlates with functional scores in osteoarthritis patients. *Acta Orthop.* 2015;86(2):215-219.
15. Aranda-Villalobos P, Fernández de las Peñas C, Navarro-Espigares JL, et al. Normalization of widespread pressure pain hypersensitivity after total hip replacement in patients with hip osteoarthritis is associated with clinical and functional improvements. *Arthritis Rheum.* 2013;65(5):1262-1270.
16. Wylde V, Sayers A, Odutola A, Gooberman-Hill R, Dieppe P, Blom AW. Central sensitization as a determinant of patients' benefit from total hip and knee replacement. *Eur J Pain.* 2017;21(2):357-365.
17. Zhang W, Nuki G, Moskowitz RW, et al. OARSI recommendations for the management of hip and knee osteoarthritis: part III: changes in evidence following systematic cumulative update of research published through January 2009. *Osteoarthritis Cartilage.* 2010;18(4):476-499.
18. Fernandes L, Hagen KB, Bijlsma JW, et al. EULAR recommendations for the non-pharmacological core management of hip and knee osteoarthritis. *Ann Rheum Dis.* 2013;72(7):1125-1135.
19. National Institute for Health and Clinical Excellence (NICE). Osteoarthritis: the care and management of osteoarthritis in adults. 2008.
20. Wang Q, Wang TT, Qi XF, et al. Manual therapy for hip osteoarthritis: a systematic review and meta-analysis. *Pain Physician.* 2015;18(6):E1005-E1020.
21. Hochberg MC, Altman RD, April KT, et al. American College of Rheumatology 2012 recommendations for the use of nonpharmacologic and pharmacologic therapies in osteoarthritis of the hand, hip, and knee. *Arthritis Care Res (Hoboken).* 2012;64(4):465-474.
22. Bierma-Zeinstra SM, Oster JD, Bernsen RM, Verhaar JA, Ginai AZ, Bohnen AM. Joint space narrowing and relationship with symptoms and signs in adults consulting for hip pain in primary care. *J Rheumatol.* 2002;29(8):1713-1718.

23. Birrell F, Croft P, Cooper C, Hosie G, Macfarlane G, Silman A; PCR Hip Study Group. Predicting radiographic hip osteoarthritis from range of movement. *Rheumatology (Oxford).* 2001;40(5):506-512.
24. Sutlive TG, Lopez HP, Schnitker DE, et al. Development of a clinical prediction rule for diagnosing hip osteoarthritis in individuals with unilateral hip pain. *J Orthop Sports Phys Ther.* 2008;38(9):542-550.
25. Cibulka MT, White DM, Woehrle J, et al. Hip pain and mobility deficits—hip osteoarthritis: clinical practice guidelines linked to the international classification of functioning, disability, and health from the orthopaedic section of the American Physical Therapy Association. *J Orthop Sports Phys Ther.* 2009;39(4):A1-A25.
26. Tanaka S, Matsumoto S, Fujii K, Tamari K, Mitani S, Tsubahara A. Factors related to low back pain in patients with hip osteoarthritis. *J Back Musculoskelet Rehabil.* 2015;28(2):409-414.
27. Maslowski E, Sullivan W, Forster Harwood J, et al. The diagnostic validity of hip provocation maneuvers to detect intra-articular hip pathology. *PM R.* 2010;2(3):174-181.
28. Loureiro A, Mills PM, Barrett RS. Muscle weakness in hip osteoarthritis: a systematic review. *Arthritis Care Res (Hoboken).* 2013;65(3):340-352.
29. Hara D, Nakashima Y, Hamai S, et al. Dynamic hip kinematics in patients with hip osteoarthritis during weight-bearing activities. *Clin Biomech (Bristol, Avon).* 2016;32:150-156.
30. Iglesias-Gonzalez JJ, Munoz-Garcia MT, Rodrigues-de-Souza DP, Alburquerque-Sendin F, Fernández de las Peñas C. Myofascial trigger points, pain, disability, and sleep quality in patients with chronic nonspecific low back pain. *Pain Med.* 2013;14(12):1964-1970.
31. Roach S, Sorenson E, Headley B, San Juan JG. Prevalence of myofascial trigger points in the hip in patellofemoral pain. *Arch Phys Med Rehabil.* 2013;94(3):522-526.
32. Marshall AR, Noronha M, Zacharias A, Kapakoulakis T, Green R. Structure and function of the abductors in patients with hip osteoarthritis: systematic review and meta-analysis. *J Back Musculoskelet Rehabil.* 2016;29(2):191-204.
33. Long C II. Myofascial pain syndromes. III. Some syndromes of the trunk and thigh. *Henry Ford Hosp Med Bull.* 1956;4(2):102-106.
34. Reynolds MD. Myofascial trigger point syndromes in the practice of rheumatology. *Arch Phys Med Rehabil.* 1981;62(3):111-114.
35. Travell J. The adductor longus syndrome: a cause of groin pain. Its treatment by local block of trigger areas (procaine infiltration and ethyl chloride spray). *Miss Valley Med J.* 1950;71:13-22.
36. Izumi M, Petersen KK, Arendt-Nielsen L, Graven-Nielsen T. Pain referral and regional deep tissue hyperalgesia in experimental human hip pain models. *Pain.* 2014;155(4):792-800.
37. Ganz R, Parvizi J, Beck M, Leunig M, Notzli H, Siebenrock KA. Femoroacetabular impingement: a cause for osteoarthritis of the hip. *Clin Orthop Relat Res.* 2003(417):112-120.
38. Beck M, Kalhor M, Leunig M, Ganz R. Hip morphology influences the pattern of damage to the acetabular cartilage: femoroacetabular impingement as a cause of early osteoarthritis of the hip. *J Bone Joint Surg Br.* 2005;87(7):1012-1018.
39. Ganz R, Leunig M, Leunig-Ganz K, Harris WH. The etiology of osteoarthritis of the hip: an integrated mechanical concept. *Clin Orthop Relat Res.* 2008;466(2):264-272.
40. Banerjee P, McLean CR. Femoroacetabular impingement: a review of diagnosis and management. *Curr Rev Musculoskelet Med.* 2011;4(1):23-32.
41. Eijer H, Hogervorst T. Femoroacetabular impingement causes osteoarthritis of the hip by migration and micro-instability of the femoral head. *Med Hypotheses.* 2017;104:93-96.
42. Bharam S, Philippon M. Diagnosis and management of acetabular labral tears in the athlete. *Int Sport Med J.* 2008;9:1-11.
43. Narvani AA, Tsiridis E, Kendall S, Chaudhuri R, Thomas P. A preliminary report on prevalence of acetabular labrum tears in sports patients with groin pain. *Knee Surg Sports Traumatol Arthrosc.* 2003;11(6):403-408.
44. Arnold DR, Keene JS, Blankenbaker DG, Desmet AA. Hip pain referral patterns in patients with labral tears: analysis based on intra-articular anesthetic injections, hip arthroscopy, and a new pain "circle" diagram. *Phys Sportsmed.* 2011;39(1):29-35.
45. Cohen B, Kleinhenz D, Schiller J, Tabaddor R. Understanding athletic pubalgia: a review. *R I Med J (2013).* 2016;99(10):31-35.
46. Unverzagt CA, Schuemann T, Mathisen J. Differential diagnosis of a sports hernia in a high-school athlete. *J Orthop Sports Phys Ther.* 2008;38(2):63-70.
47. Verrall GM, Slavotinek JP, Barnes PG, Esterman A, Oakeshott RD, Spriggins AJ. Hip joint range of motion restriction precedes athletic chronic groin injury. *J Sci Med Sport.* 2007;10(6):463-466.
48. Meyers WC, Greenleaf R, Saad A. Anatomic basis for evaluation of abdominal and groin pain in athletes. *Oper Tech Sports Med.* 2005;13(1):55-61.
49. Valent A, Frizziero A, Bressan S, Zanella E, Giannotti E, Masiero S. Insertional tendinopathy of the adductors and rectus abdominis in athletes: a review. *Muscles Ligaments Tendons J.* 2012;2(2):142-148.
50. Kachingwe AF, Grech S. Proposed algorithm for the management of athletes with athletic pubalgia (sports hernia): a case series. *J Orthop Sports Phys Ther.* 2008;38(12):768-781.
51. Westermann RW, Lynch TS, Jones MH, et al. Predictors of hip pain and function in femoroacetabular impingement: a prospective cohort analysis. *Orthop J Sports Med.* 2017;5(9):2325967117726521.
52. Reiman MP, Goode AP, Cook CE, Holmich P, Thorborg K. Diagnostic accuracy of clinical tests for the diagnosis of hip femoroacetabular impingement/labral tear: a systematic review with meta-analysis. *Br J Sports Med.* 2015;49(12):811.
53. Verrall GM, Hamilton IA, Slavotinek JP, et al. Hip joint range of motion reduction in sports-related chronic groin injury diagnosed as pubic bone stress injury. *J Sci Med Sport.* 2005;8(1):77-84.
54. Enseki K, Harris-Hayes M, White DM, et al. Nonarthritic hip joint pain. *J Orthop Sports Phys Ther.* 2014;44(6):A1-A32.
55. Ho GW, Howard TM. Greater trochanteric pain syndrome: more than bursitis and iliotibial tract friction. *Curr Sports Med Rep.* 2012;11(5):232-238.
56. Mallow M, Nazarian LN. Greater trochanteric pain syndrome diagnosis and treatment. *Phys Med Rehabil Clin N Am.* 2014;25(2):279-289.
57. Redmond JM, Chen AW, Domb BG. Greater trochanteric pain syndrome. *J Am Acad Orthop Surg.* 2016;24(4):231-240.
58. Klauser AS, Martinoli C, Tagliafico A, et al. Greater trochanteric pain syndrome. *Semin Musculoskelet Radiol.* 2013;17(1):43-48.
59. Bewyer DC, Bewyer KJ. Rationale for treatment of hip abductor pain syndrome. *Iowa Orthop J.* 2003;23:57-60.
60. Lustenberger DP, Ng VY, Best TM, Ellis TJ. Efficacy of treatment of trochanteric bursitis: a systematic review. *Clin J Sport Med.* 2011;21(5):447-453.
61. Barratt PA, Brookes N, Newson A. Conservative treatments for greater trochanteric pain syndrome: a systematic review. *Br J Sports Med.* 2017;51(2):97-104.
62. Woodley SJ, Nicholson HD, Livingstone V, et al. Lateral hip pain: findings from magnetic resonance imaging and clinical examination. *J Orthop Sports Phys Ther.* 2008;38(6):313-328.
63. Lequesne M, Mathieu P, Vuillemin-Bodaghi V, Bard H, Djian P. Gluteal tendinopathy in refractory greater trochanter pain syndrome: diagnostic value of two clinical tests. *Arthritis Rheum.* 2008;59(2):241-246.
64. Brennan KL, Allen BC, Maldonado YM. Dry needling versus cortisone injection in the treatment of greater trochanteric pain syndrome: a noninferiority randomized clinical trial. *J Orthop Sports Phys Ther.* 2017;47(4):232-239.
65. Jacobson JA, Yablon CM, Henning PT, et al. Greater trochanteric pain syndrome: percutaneous tendon fenestration versus platelet-rich plasma injection for treatment of gluteal tendinosis. *J Ultrasound Med.* 2016;35(11):2413-2420.
66. Kean Chen C, Nizar AJ. Prevalence of piriformis syndrome in chronic low back pain patients. A clinical diagnosis with modified FAIR test. *Pain Pract.* 2013;13(4):276-281.
67. Hopayian K, Song F, Riera R, Sambandan S. The clinical features of the piriformis syndrome: a systematic review. *Eur Spine J.* 2010;19(12):2095-2109.
68. Hopayian K, Danielyan A. Four symptoms define the piriformis syndrome: an updated systematic review of its clinical features. *Eur J Orthop Surg Traumatol.* 2018;28:155-164.
69. Fishman LM, Dombi GW, Michaelsen C, et al. Piriformis syndrome: diagnosis, treatment, and outcome—a 10-year study. *Arch Phys Med Rehabil.* 2002;83(3):295-301.
70. Urban LM, MacNeil BJ. Diagnostic accuracy of the slump test for identifying neuropathic pain in the lower limb. *J Orthop Sports Phys Ther.* 2015;45(8):596-603.
71. Rothermich MA, Glaviano NR, Li J, Hart JM. Patellofemoral pain: epidemiology, pathophysiology, and treatment options. *Clin Sports Med.* 2015;34(2):313-327.
72. Powers CM, Bolgla LA, Callaghan MJ, Collins N, Sheehan FT. Patellofemoral pain: proximal, distal, and local factors, 2nd International Research Retreat. *J Orthop Sports Phys Ther.* 2012;42(6):A1-A54.
73. Lankhorst NE, Bierma-Zeinstra SM, van Middelkoop M. Risk factors for patellofemoral pain syndrome: a systematic review. *J Orthop Sports Phys Ther.* 2012;42(2):81-94.
74. Willy RW, Meira EP. Current concepts in biomechanical interventions for patellofemoral pain. *Int J Sports Phys Ther.* 2016;11(6):877-890.
75. Lankhorst NE, Bierma-Zeinstra SM, van Middelkoop M. Factors associated with patellofemoral pain syndrome: a systematic review. *Br J Sports Med.* 2013;47(4):193-206.
76. Piva SR, Fitzgerald GK, Wisniewski S, Delitto A. Predictors of pain and function outcome after rehabilitation in patients with patellofemoral pain syndrome. *J Rehabil Med.* 2009;41(8):604-612.
77. Barton CJ, Lack S, Hemmings S, Tufail S, Morrissey D. The 'Best Practice Guide to Conservative Management of Patellofemoral Pain': incorporating level 1 evidence with expert clinical reasoning. *Br J Sports Med.* 2015;49(14):923-934.
78. van der Heijden RA, Lankhorst NE, van Linschoten R, Bierma-Zeinstra SM, van Middelkoop M. Exercise for treating patellofemoral pain syndrome. *Cochrane Database Syst Rev.* 2015;1:CD010387.
79. Khayambashi K, Fallah A, Movahedi A, Bagwell J, Powers C. Posterolateral hip muscle strengthening versus quadriceps strengthening for patellofemoral pain: a comparative control trial. *Arch Phys Med Rehabil.* 2014;95(5):900-907.
80. Botanlioglu H, Kantarci F, Kaynak G, et al. Shear wave elastography properties of vastus lateralis and vastus medialis obliquus muscles in normal subjects and female patients with patellofemoral pain syndrome. *Skeletal Radiol.* 2013;42(5):659-666.
81. Pattyn E, Verdonk P, Steyaert A, et al. Vastus medialis obliquus atrophy: does it exist in patellofemoral pain syndrome? *Am J Sports Med.* 2011;39(7):1450-1455.
82. Giles LS, Webster KE, McClelland JA, Cook J. Does quadriceps atrophy exist in individuals with patellofemoral pain? A systematic literature review with meta-analysis. *J Orthop Sports Phys Ther.* 2013;43(11):766-776.
83. Cook C, Mabry L, Reiman MP, Hegedus EJ. Best tests/clinical findings for screening and diagnosis of patellofemoral pain syndrome: a systematic review. *Physiotherapy.* 2012;98(2):93-100.
84. Powers CM. The influence of abnormal hip mechanics on knee injury: a biomechanical perspective. *J Orthop Sports Phys Ther.* 2010;40(2):42-51.
85. Lucas KR. The impact of latent trigger points on regional muscle function. *Curr Pain Headache Rep.* 2008;12(5):344-349.
86. Hains G, Hains F. Patellofemoral pain syndrome managed by ischemic compression to the trigger points located in the peri-patellar and retro-patellar areas: a randomized clinical trial. *Clin Chiropractic.* 2010;13(3):201-209.

87. Behrangrad S, Kamali F. Comparison of ischemic compression and lumbopelvic manipulation as trigger point therapy for patellofemoral pain syndrome in young adults: a double-blind randomized clinical trial. *J Bodyw Mov Ther.* 2017;21(3):554-564.
88. Altman R, Asch E, Bloch D, et al. Development of criteria for the classification and reporting of osteoarthritis. Classification of osteoarthritis of the knee. Diagnostic and Therapeutic Criteria Committee of the American Rheumatism Association. *Arthritis Rheum.* 1986;29(8):1039-1049.
89. Read SJ, Dray A. Osteoarthritic pain: a review of current, theoretical and emerging therapeutics. *Expert Opin Investig Drugs.* 2008;17(5):619-640.
90. Arendt-Nielsen L. Pain sensitisation in osteoarthritis. *Clin Exp Rheumatol.* 2017;35 suppl 107(5):68-74.
91. Fingleton C, Smart K, Moloney N, Fullen BM, Doody C. Pain sensitization in people with knee osteoarthritis: a systematic review and meta-analysis. *Osteoarthritis Cartilage.* 2015;23(7):1043-1056.
92. Lluch Girbes E, Duenas L, Barbero M, et al. Expanded Distribution of Pain as a Sign of Central Sensitization in Individuals With Symptomatic Knee Osteoarthritis. *Phys Ther.* 2016;96(8):1196-1207.
93. Pinto D, Robertson MC, Abbott JH, Hansen P, Campbell AJ, MOA Trial Team. Manual therapy, exercise therapy, or both, in addition to usual care, for osteoarthritis of the hip or knee. 2: economic evaluation alongside a randomized controlled trial. *Osteoarthritis Cartilage.* 2013;21(10):1504-1513.
94. Rice DA, McNair PJ. Quadriceps arthrogenic muscle inhibition: neural mechanisms and treatment perspectives. *Semin Arthritis Rheum.* 2010;40(3):250-266.
95. Hinman RS, Bennell KL, Metcalf BR, Crossley KM. Temporal activity of vastus medialis obliquus and vastus lateralis in symptomatic knee osteoarthritis. *Am J Phys Med Rehabil.* 2002;81(9):684-690.
96. Farrokhi S, Voycheck CA, Gustafson JA, Fitzgerald GK, Tashman S. Knee joint contact mechanics during downhill gait and its relationship with varus/valgus motion and muscle strength in patients with knee osteoarthritis. *Knee.* 2016;23(1):49-56.
97. Hanada M, Hoshino H, Koyama H, Matsuyama Y. Relationship between severity of knee osteoarthritis and radiography findings of lower limbs: a cross-sectional study from the TOEI survey. *J Orthop.* 2017;14(4):484-488.
98. Davison MJ, Maly MR, Keir PJ, et al. Lean muscle volume of the thigh has a stronger relationship with muscle power than muscle strength in women with knee osteoarthritis. *Clin Biomech (Bristol, Avon).* 2017;41:92-97.
99. Segal NA, Glass NA. Is quadriceps muscle weakness a risk factor for incident or progressive knee osteoarthritis? *Phys Sportsmed.* 2011;39(4):44-50.
100. Dor A, Kalichman L. A myofascial component of pain in knee osteoarthritis. *J Bodyw Mov Ther.* 2017;21(3):642-647.
101. Alburquerque-García A, Rodrigues-de-Souza DP, Fernández de las Peñas C, Alburquerque-Sendin F. Association between muscle trigger points, ongoing pain, function, and sleep quality in elderly women with bilateral painful knee osteoarthritis. *J Manipulative Physiol Ther.* 2015;38(4):262-268.
102. Henry R, Cahill CM, Wood G, et al. Myofascial pain in patients waitlisted for total knee arthroplasty. *Pain Res Manag.* 2012;17(5):321-327.
103. Itoh K, Hirota S, Katsumi Y, Ochi H, Kitakoji H. Trigger point acupuncture for treatment of knee osteoarthritis—a preliminary RCT for a pragmatic trial. *Acupunct Med.* 2008;26(1):17-26.
104. Bajaj P, Bajaj P, Graven-Nielsen T, Arendt-Nielsen L. Osteoarthritis and its association with muscle hyperalgesia: an experimental controlled study. *Pain.* 2001;93(2):107-114.
105. Rahbar M, Toopchizadeh V, Eftekharsadat B, Ganjeifar V. Therapeutic efficacy of myofascial trigger point therapy in patients with bilateral knee osteoarthritis: a randomized clinical trial. *Life Sci J.* 2013;10(6s):472-478.
106. Mayoral O, Salvat I, Martin MT, et al. Efficacy of myofascial trigger point dry needling in the prevention of pain after total knee arthroplasty: a randomized, double-blinded, placebo-controlled trial. *Evid Based Complement Alternat Med.* 2013;2013:694941.
107. Núñez-Cortés R, Cruz-Montecinos C, Vasquez-Rosel A, Paredes-Molina O, Cuesta-Vargas A. Dry needling combined with physical therapy in patients with chronic postsurgical pain following total knee arthroplasty: a case series. *J Orthop Sports Phys Ther.* 2017;47(3):209-216.
108. Nguyen BM. Myofascial trigger point, falls in the elderly, idiopathic knee pain and osteoarthritis: an alternative concept. *Med Hypotheses.* 2013;80(6):806-809.
109. Louw M, Deary C. The biomechanical variables involved in the aetiology of iliotibial band syndrome in distance runners—A systematic review of the literature. *Phys Ther Sport.* 2014;15(1):64-75.
110. Fredericson M, Wolf C. Iliotibial band syndrome in runners: innovations in treatment. *Sports Med.* 2005;35(5):451-459.
111. Fairclough J, Hayashi K, Toumi H, et al. The functional anatomy of the iliotibial band during flexion and extension of the knee: implications for understanding iliotibial band syndrome. *J Anat.* 2006;208(3):309-316.
112. Fairclough J, Hayashi K, Toumi H, et al. Is iliotibial band syndrome really a friction syndrome? *J Sci Med Sport.* 2007;10(2):74-76; discussion 77-78.
113. Fredericson M, Weir A. Practical management of iliotibial band friction syndrome in runners. *Clin J Sport Med.* 2006;16(3):261-268.
114. Baker RL, Souza RB, Fredericson M. Iliotibial band syndrome: soft tissue and biomechanical factors in evaluation and treatment. *PM R.* 2011;3(6):550-561.
115. Mucha MD, Caldwell W, Schlueter EL, Walters C, Hassen A. Hip abductor strength and lower extremity running related injury in distance runners: a systematic review. *J Sci Med Sport.* 2017;20(4):349-355.
116. Pavkovich R. The use of dry needling for a subject with chronic lateral hip and thigh pain: a case report. *Int J Sports Phys Ther.* 2015;10(2):246-255.
117. Moses B, Orchard J, Orchard J. Systematic review: annual incidence of ACL injury and surgery in various populations. *Res Sports Med.* 2012;20(3-4):157-179.
118. Fernandez WG, Yard EE, Comstock RD. Epidemiology of lower extremity injuries among U.S. high school athletes. *Acad Emerg Med.* 2007;14(7):641-645.
119. Schein A, Matcuk G, Patel D, et al. Structure and function, injury, pathology, and treatment of the medial collateral ligament of the knee. *Emerg Radiol.* 2012;19(6):489-498.
120. Salata MJ, Gibbs AE, Sekiya JK. A systematic review of clinical outcomes in patients undergoing meniscectomy. *Am J Sports Med.* 2010;38(9):1907-1916.
121. Jones JC, Burks R, Owens BD, Sturdivant RX, Svoboda SJ, Cameron KL. Incidence and risk factors associated with meniscal injuries among active-duty US military service members. *J Athl Train.* 2012;47(1):67-73.
122. Snoeker BA, Bakker EW, Kegel CA, Lucas C. Risk factors for meniscal tears: a systematic review including meta-analysis. *J Orthop Sports Phys Ther.* 2013;43(6):352-367.
123. Monk AP, Davies LJ, Hopewell S, Harris K, Beard DJ, Price AJ. Surgical versus conservative interventions for treating anterior cruciate ligament injuries. *Cochrane Database Syst Rev.* 2016;4:CD011166.
124. Tsoukas D, Fotopoulos V, Basdekis G, Makridis KG. No difference in osteoarthritis after surgical and non-surgical treatment of ACL-injured knees after 10 years. *Knee Surg Sports Traumatol Arthrosc.* 2016;24(9):2953-2959.
125. Alessio-Mazzola M, Formica M, Coviello M, Basso M, Felli L. Conservative treatment of meniscal tears in anterior cruciate ligament reconstruction. *Knee.* 2016;23(4):642-646.
126. Kim HJ, Lee JH, Ahn SE, Park MJ, Lee DH. Influence of anterior cruciate ligament tear on thigh muscle strength and hamstring-to-quadriceps ratio: a meta-analysis. *PLoS One.* 2016;11(1):e0146234.
127. Donnell-Fink LA, Klara K, Collins JE, et al. Effectiveness of knee injury and anterior cruciate ligament tear prevention programs: a meta-analysis. *PLoS One.* 2015;10(12):e0144063.
128. Swart NM, van Oudenaarde K, Reijnierse M, et al. Effectiveness of exercise therapy for meniscal lesions in adults: a systematic review and meta-analysis. *J Sci Med Sport.* 2016;19(12):990-998.
129. Trees AH, Howe TE, Grant M, Gray HG. WITHDRAWN: exercise for treating anterior cruciate ligament injuries in combination with collateral ligament and meniscal damage of the knee in adults. *Cochrane Database Syst Rev.* 2011(5):CD005961.
130. Meuffels DE, Poldervaart MT, Diercks RL, et al. Guideline on anterior cruciate ligament injury. *Acta Orthop.* 2012;83(4):379-386.
131. Logerstedt DS, Scalzitti D, Risberg MA, et al. Knee stability and movement coordination impairments: knee ligament sprain revision 2017. *J Orthop Sports Phys Ther.* 2017;47(11):A1-A47.
132. Jackson JL, O'Malley PG, Kroenke K. Evaluation of acute knee pain in primary care. *Ann Intern Med.* 2003;139(7):575-588.
133. Tuite MJ, Daffner RH, Weissman BN, et al. ACR appropriateness criteria((R)) acute trauma to the knee. *J Am Coll Radiol.* 2012;9(2):96-103.
134. Huang W, Zhang Y, Yao Z, Ma L. Clinical examination of anterior cruciate ligament rupture: a systematic review and meta-analysis. *Acta Orthop Traumatol Turc.* 2016;50(1):22-31.
135. Smith BE, Thacker D, Crewesmith A, Hall M. Special tests for assessing meniscal tears within the knee: a systematic review and meta-analysis. *Evid Based Med.* 2015;20(3):88-97.
136. Hewett TE, Myer GD, Ford KR, Paterno MV, Quatman CE. The 2012 ABJS Nicolas Andry Award: the sequence of prevention: a systematic approach to prevent anterior cruciate ligament injury. *Clin Orthop Relat Res.* 2012;470(10):2930-2940.
137. Torres-Chica B, Nunez-Samper-Pizarroso C, Ortega-Santiago R, et al. Trigger points and pressure pain hypersensitivity in people with postmeniscectomy pain. *Clin J Pain.* 2015;31(3):265-272.
138. Velázquez-Saornil J, Ruiz-Ruiz B, Rodriguez-Sanz D, Romero-Morales C, Lopez-Lopez D, Calvo-Lobo C. Efficacy of quadriceps vastus medialis dry needling in a rehabilitation protocol after surgical reconstruction of complete anterior cruciate ligament rupture. *Medicine (Baltimore).* 2017;96(17):e6726.
139. Murphy DR, Hurwitz EL, Gerrard JK, Clary R. Pain patterns and descriptions in patients with radicular pain: does the pain necessarily follow a specific dermatome? *Chiropr Osteopat.* 2009;17:9.
140. Van Boxem K, Cheng J, Patijn J, et al. 11. Lumbosacral radicular pain. *Pain Pract.* 2010;10(4):339-358.
141. Iversen T, Solberg TK, Wilsgaard T, Waterloo K, Brox JI, Ingebrigtsen T. Outcome prediction in chronic unilateral lumbar radiculopathy: prospective cohort study. *BMC Musculoskelet Disord.* 2015;16:17.
142. Hahne AJ, Ford JJ, McMeeken JM. Conservative management of lumbar disc herniation with associated radiculopathy: a systematic review. *Spine (Phila Pa 1976).* 2010;35(11):E488-E504.
143. Delitto A, George SZ, Van Dillen LR, et al. Low back pain. *J Orthop Sports Phys Ther.* 2012;42(4):A1-A57.
144. Lai WH, Shih YF, Lin PL, Chen WY, Ma HL. Normal neurodynamic responses of the femoral slump test. *Man Ther.* 2012;17(2):126-132.
145. Adelmanesh F, Jalali A, Shirvani A, et al. The diagnostic accuracy of gluteal trigger points to differentiate radicular from nonradicular low back pain. *Clin J Pain.* 2016;32(8):666-672.
146. Adelmanesh F, Jalali A, Jazayeri Shooshtari SM, Raissi GR, Ketabchi SM, Shir Y. Is there an association between lumbosacral radiculopathy and painful gluteal trigger points? A cross-sectional study. *Am J Phys Med Rehabil.* 2015;94(10):784-791.
147. Rigoard P, Blond S, David R, Mertens P. Pathophysiological characterisation of back pain generators in failed back surgery syndrome (part B). *Neurochirurgie.* 2015;61 suppl 1:S35-S44.

Section 7

Leg, Ankle, and Foot Pain

Chapter 63

Tibialis Anterior Muscle

"Foot Drop Muscle"

Wesley J. Wedewer

1. INTRODUCTION

As the strongest dorsiflexor of the ankle, the tibialis anterior muscle is one of the main muscles of ambulation. It commonly develops trigger points (TrPs) and produces pain over the anteromedial ankle and the dorsal and medial surfaces of the great toe. On occasion, pain may refer to the anterior leg and dorsal ankle. This muscle is important for force absorption and foot clearance during ambulation and plays a key role in dynamic standing balance. Trigger points in the tibialis anterior muscle can be caused by strenuous walking, running, and climbing. Walking down hill, or on rough or uneven terrain can also activate TrPs in the tibialis anterior muscle. The differential diagnosis should include L5 radicular pain and/or radiculopathy, chronic exertional compartment syndrome, shin splints, and herniation of the tibialis anterior muscle. Corrective actions are self-pressure release, self-stretching tight antagonist gastrocnemius-soleus muscles and the tibialis anterior muscle, and activity modification to reduce recurrent overload of the muscle.

2. ANATOMIC CONSIDERATIONS

The tibialis anterior muscle is subcutaneous just lateral to the anterior sharp edge of the tibia. It is thick and fleshy at its upper portion and becomes tendinous in the lower third of the leg (Figure 63-1). It originates proximally from the lateral condyle of the tibia, the superior half or two-thirds of the lateral surface of the tibia, the deep surface of the deep fascia, the adjacent interosseous membrane, and the intermuscular septum between itself and the extensor digitorum longus muscle.[1] The fibers of the tibialis anterior muscle converge on their aponeurosis and tendon in circumpennate form, like the spokes of a wheel, and insert into an internal axial tendon that extends the length of the muscle.[2,3] The tendon descends and crosses in front of the tibia to the medial side of the foot where it inserts distally on the medial and plantar surfaces of the medial cuneiform and the base of the 1st metatarsal.[1,4] Brenner[4] found variations in the attachment of the tibialis anterior muscle in the dissection of 156 feet. In the typical presentation, 96.2% inserted on both the 1st metatarsal and medial cuneiform, 1.9% had a single insertion at the 1st metatarsal base, and 1.3% had an insertion at the medial cuneiform. A subtendinous bursa was detected in 17.3% of cases. In a separate cadaveric study, the majority of specimens showed a larger overall area of the tendon footprint (3:2) at the medial cuneiform compared with the 1st metatarsal. Additional tendon slips were observed in 4.8% of specimens; inserting at the proximal 1st metatarsal shaft and at the distal metatarsal shaft.[5]

The distribution of motor endplates was studied by staining longitudinal cryosections of whole tibialis anterior muscles for cholinesterase. The neuromuscular junctions were diffusely distributed, with the greatest concentration found toward the periphery and toward the proximal end of the muscle.[6]

A cross-section at the lower part of the middle third of the leg (Figure 63-2) shows the unyielding fascial structures and bones that form the anterior compartment. The tibialis anterior muscle shares this relatively small compartment with the extensor digitorum longus, extensor hallucis longus, and fibularis tertius muscles, the deep fibular nerve, and the anterior tibial artery and vein. The deep fibular nerve and anterior tibial vessels lie on the interosseous membrane deep to the tibialis anterior muscle.[1]

2.1. Innervation and Vascularization

The deep fibular nerve supplies the tibialis anterior muscle with fibers from ventral rami of the L4 and L5 spinal nerves[1,7] and sometimes[7] the S1 spinal nerve of the sacral plexus.

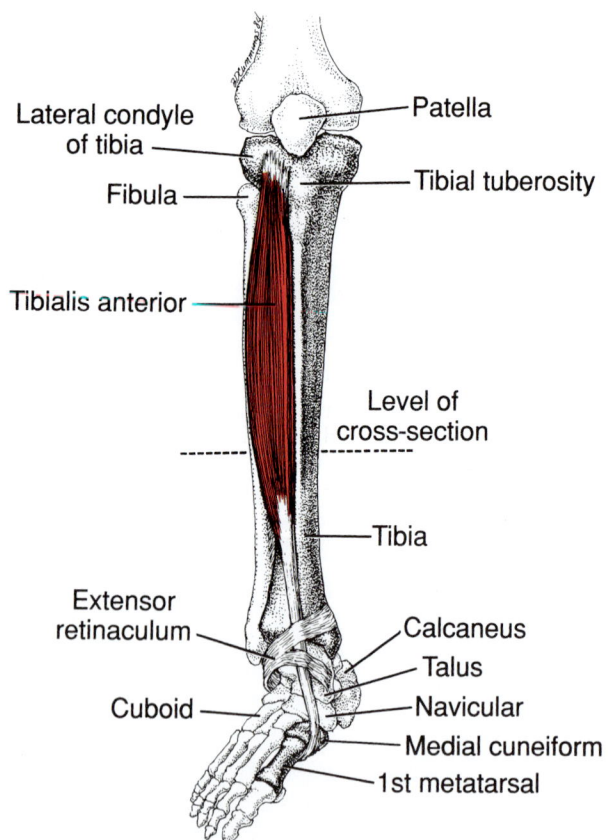

Figure 63-1. Attachments of the right tibialis anterior muscle (red), anterior view. The foot is turned outward to show the distal attachments to the medial cuneiform and 1st metatarsal bones.

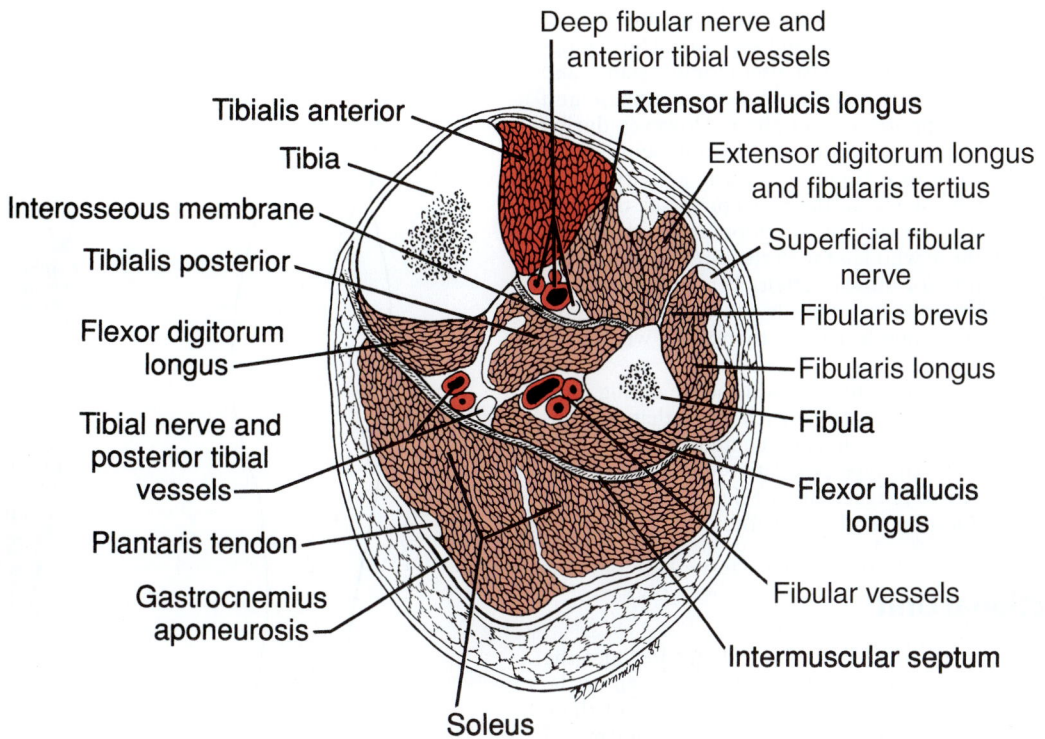

Figure 63-2. Cross-section outlining the compartments of the middle third of the right leg, viewed from above. The anterior compartment is located anterior to the interosseous membrane, medial to the shaft of the fibula, and lateral to the shaft of the tibia, and it is bound anteriorly by the deep fascia of the leg. (After Figure 4-72 in Anderson JE. *Grant's Atlas of Anatomy*. 8th ed. Baltimore, MA: Williams and Wilkins; 1983 [p. 107]).

The vascularization of the inextensible anterior compartment of the leg is supplied by a series of medial and anterior branches of the anterior tibial artery. Proximally, there is an accessory supply from the anterior tibial recurrent artery. The tibialis anterior tendon is supplied by the anterior medial malleolar artery, dorsalis pedis artery, medial tarsal arteries, and by the medial malleolar and calcaneal branches of the posterior tibial artery.[1,8]

2.2. Function

The tibialis anterior muscle has important functions in posture and gait. It maintains standing balance by controlling excessive posterior postural sway and assists in keeping the leg vertical over the fixed foot.[9-12] The tibialis anterior muscle functions eccentrically in gait for force absorption to control lowering of the foot following initial contact[13-16] and functions concentrically for foot clearance in the swing phase of gait.[14,15]

In the nonweight-bearing limb, the tibialis anterior muscle dorsiflexes the foot at the talocrural joint and supinates (inverts and adducts) the foot at the subtalar and transverse tarsal joints[1,17]; however, it is not active as an invertor during plantar flexion.[18] In standing, the tibialis anterior muscle becomes more active with leaning backward, and activity ceases when leaning forward, at any rate of movement.[9,10] The further one leans back, and the closer the center of pressure moved toward the heel, the greater the electromyographic (EMG) activity of the tibialis anterior muscle.[11] Additionally, this muscle contributes to lateral sway control for narrower stances, such as feet together and tandem stance.[19] Di Giulio et al[12] identified the deep compartment of the tibialis anterior muscle as the best mechanical source of proprioceptive information among the ankle muscles in maintaining human upright posture.

The potential active role of the tibialis anterior muscle during standing has relevant implications for fall prevention in the elderly. Middle-aged adults exhibit impaired mediolateral postural control at the ankle compared with young adults.[20] Reduced ankle strength and rate of torque development of ankle dorsiflexor muscles have been suggested as key factors that distinguish those individuals who fall from those who do not.[21]

The primary peak of EMG activity in the tibialis anterior muscle occurs at initial contact[14,15,22] during all speeds of ambulation.[23] More specifically, the ankle dorsiflexors (tibialis anterior and long extensor muscles of the toes) prevent foot slap just after initial contact; they undergo a lengthening contraction as they control the descent of the foot to the floor. The secondary peak, during walking, appears at terminal stance[14,15,22] at all speeds of ambulation.[23] Dragging of the toes at the beginning of the swing phase is commonly due to inadequate hip and knee flexion; later in swing, as the limb moves forward, toe dragging results from inadequate dorsiflexion.[24]

In healthy children, aged 6 to 11 years old, a third of the activation pattern is present during mid-stance, likely due to the tibialis anterior muscle controlling balance during single limb support.[25] In a similar study of healthy children, greater than 80% of the gait cycle resulted in cocontractions of the gastrocnemius muscle lateral head and tibialis anterior muscle. This increased complexity in muscle recruitment strategy beyond pure activation suggests that cocontractions are likely functional to further physiologic tasks such as balance improvement and joint stability.[26]

In comparison with level and upslope walking, downslope treadmill walking imposes increased demands on the tibialis anterior muscle. For instance, during downslope walking, there is increased displacement of the center of mass anteriorly and increased foot deceleration moments at initial contact.[27] The deceleration moment is produced by a significant eccentric tibialis anterior muscle contraction to control the lowering of the foot from initial contact to the loading response.[28] This eccentric effort leads to delayed onset muscle soreness that is unique to downslope walking,[29] and it may also contribute to the formation of TrPs in the tibialis anterior muscle.

The pattern of EMG activity of the tibialis anterior muscle changes between jogging, running, and sprinting. During jogging and running, activity begins just after terminal stance and continues throughout the remainder of the swing phase and the first half of the support (stance) phase. However, during sprinting, EMG activity ceases briefly at mid-swing when plantar flexion of the foot begins.[30] Muscle activity varies between runners who strike on the rearfoot versus the forefoot. Runners who strike with the rearfoot land with greater dorsiflexion than those who land with the forefoot, and there is greater tibialis anterior muscle activity before foot contact. In contrast, runners striking primarily on the forefoot have greater gastrocnemius muscle activity than those who strike on the rearfoot.[31,32]

This muscle is moderately to vigorously active during most sports activities.[33,34] Its type 1 (slow-twitch) fibers that predominate, whereas type 2 (fast-twitch) fibers compose, at most, only one-third of the muscle. The type 2 oxidative muscle fibers, with an inherent resistance to fatigue, support the muscle's primary function for long-duration aerobic activities.[35-37]

2.3. Functional Unit

The functional unit to which a muscle belongs includes the muscles that reinforce and counter its actions as well as the joints that the muscle crosses. The interdependence of these structures is reflected functionally in the organization and neural connections of the sensory motor cortex. The functional unit is emphasized because the presence of a TrP in one muscle of the unit increases the likelihood that the other muscles of the unit will also develop TrPs. When inactivating TrPs in a muscle, one must be concerned about TrPs that may develop in muscles that are functionally interdependent. Box 63-1 grossly represents the functional unit of the tibialis anterior muscle.[38]

3. CLINICAL PRESENTATION

3.1. Referred Pain Pattern

The tibialis anterior muscle can exhibit TrPs in any part of the muscle. Commonly, TrPs found in the upper third of the muscle refer pain and tenderness primarily to the anteromedial aspect of the ankle and over the dorsal and medial surfaces of the great toe (Figure 63-3).[39,40] In addition, sometimes, the pain may extend downward over the shin to the ankle and foot anteromedially.[39,41,42] Other authors reported that tibialis anterior

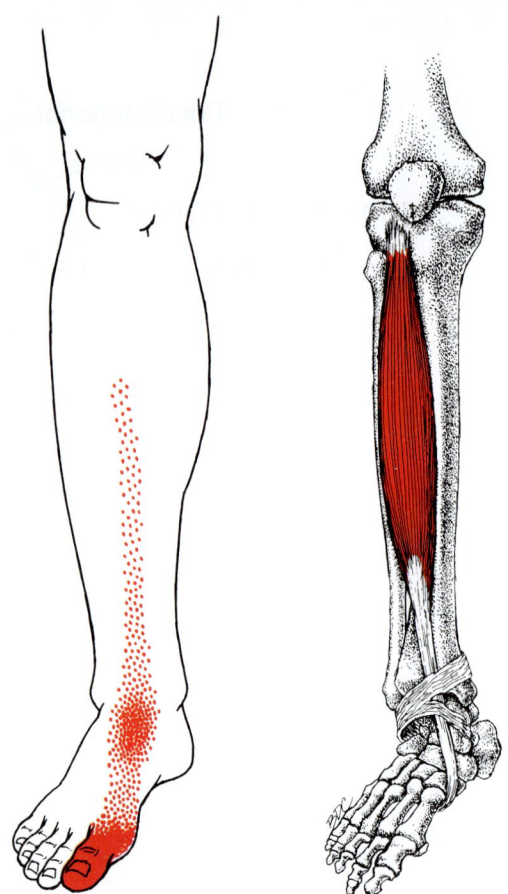

Figure 63-3. Pain pattern (dark red) referred from a TrP in the right tibialis anterior muscle (light red), as seen in the anterior view with the foot slightly abducted. The essential pain pattern is solid red; the red stippling indicates occasional extension of the essential pattern.

TrPs referred pain to the anterior leg and dorsal ankle[43,44]; dorsal ankle and dorsal region of the great toe[45]; to the leg, ankle, and foot; or specifically, to the dorsal surface of the great toe.[46,47] Occasionally, a taut band with spot tenderness occurs distally along the lower half of the muscle near the musculotendinous junction. The referral pattern in the latter case is severe burning pain in the foot and knee that is exacerbated with long periods of standing.[48] Tibialis anterior TrPs are occasionally the source of the chief report of pain in children. The referred pain pattern is similar to that seen in adults.[49]

In 15 subjects, Rubin and colleagues[50] injected the tibialis anterior muscle with 0.5 mL of 5% hypertonic saline solution. The injection caused a deep, dull ache in the muscle belly, and often referred pain to the front of the ankle and dorsum of the medial foot. Several subjects had pain only referred to the ankle, whereas others had pain only in the leg. Additionally, one subject reported pain internal to the medial and dorsal surface of the knee, another reported pain in the medial gastrocnemius muscle, and a third reported pain proximal to the ankle joint. After injection of lignocaine, pain disappeared in all but two subjects, where the mean total pain intensity of primary and referred pain declined in parallel by 74%, suggesting that referred muscle pain usually depends on ongoing noxious inputs from the site of primary pain.[50]

The typical referral outlined earlier is similar to the pattern Kellgren described.[51] Gibson also found the same referral patterns induced by injection of hypertonic saline into the tibialis anterior muscle belly, proximal tendon-bone junction, and tendon. Several of the subjects also noted referral into the toes as well.[52]

Box 63-1 Functional unit of the tibialis anterior muscle

Action	Synergists	Antagonists
Dorsiflexion of the foot	Extensor digitorum longus Extensor hallucis longus Fibularis tertius	Gastrocnemius Soleus Fibularis longus and brevis Long flexors of the toes Tibialis posterior
Inversion of the foot	Tibialis posterior Extensor hallucis longus	Fibularis longus and brevis Fibularis tertius Extensor digitorum longus

3.2. Symptoms

Patients with TrPs in the tibialis anterior muscle primarily report pain on the anteromedial aspect of the ankle and in the great toe. Other reports of symptoms may include the following: weakness of dorsiflexion that can present as falling or tripping due to insufficient toe clearance during gait, as well as general weakness of the ankle. Painful motion of the ankle may bother the patient in the absence of any evidence of joint injury.[39] Loss of function is especially evident when TrPs in the long extensor muscles of the toes contribute to additional dorsiflexion weakness.

Usually, patients with tibialis anterior TrPs do not report nocturnal pain, and a plantar flexed position of the ankle throughout the night does not bother this muscle unless its TrPs are sufficiently active to cause some degree of constant referred pain. Tibialis anterior myofascial pain syndrome occasionally presents alone as a single-muscle syndrome, but more commonly occurs in association with TrPs in other leg muscles.

3.3. Patient Examination

After a thorough subjective examination, the clinician should make a detailed drawing representing the pain pattern that the patient has described. This depiction will assist in planning the physical examination and can be useful in monitoring the progression of the patient as symptoms improve or change. The type, quality, and location of the pain should be carefully assessed, and the utilization of standardized outcome tools is imperative when examining patients with lower extremity dysfunctions.

Observation of static and dynamic posture is essential due to the role of the tibialis anterior muscle in postural stability. Functional testing such as double- and single-leg squat will allow a quick assessment of hip and knee control, as well as a quick assessment of dorsiflexion range of motion. Functional dorsiflexion is best tested by asking the subject to walk on the heels.[1] Timed single-leg stance with eyes open and closed will give a quantitative measure of balance and will allow the clinician to observe foot and ankle strategies related to balance and control.

Examination of the talocrural joint is necessary to identify a tight Achilles tendon or muscle length deficits in the gastrocnemius/soleus muscle complex, reduced accessory motion, or excessive pronation evident at the subtalar joint. These impairments can be significant contributing factors in tibialis anterior muscle overload during weight-bearing activities.[53] A thorough gait analysis will assist in identifying compensatory patterns if the tibialis anterior muscle is weak or painful including the following: waddling gait (demonstrated by a lean to the contralateral side and "hiking" the hip), swing-out gait (in which the dysfunctional leg is circumducted laterally), or high-stepping, steppage gait (with excessive flexion at the hip and knee) to clear the toes in the swing phase.[54]

Trigger points in this muscle cause some degree of inhibition weakness. This weakness is easily masked by compensatory contraction of the long extensor muscles of the toes or the fibularis tertius muscle. To test the tibialis anterior muscle for strength, the seated patient first inverts and then dorsiflexes the foot against resistance without extension of the great toe.[55] The clinician should observe the patient for foot slap and/or foot drop during ambulation. Foot slap occurs when the forefoot slaps to the floor immediately following heel strike. Foot drop is a failure to dorsiflex the foot sufficiently to provide adequate clearance between the toes and the floor, particularly during late swing.

Active or latent TrPs in the tibialis anterior muscle restrict the stretch range of motion into plantar flexion and eversion because of pain and muscle tightness. Deep palpation over the ankle and great toe may provoke pain in a patient with TrPs of the tibialis anterior muscle secondary to its pain referral pattern.[39]

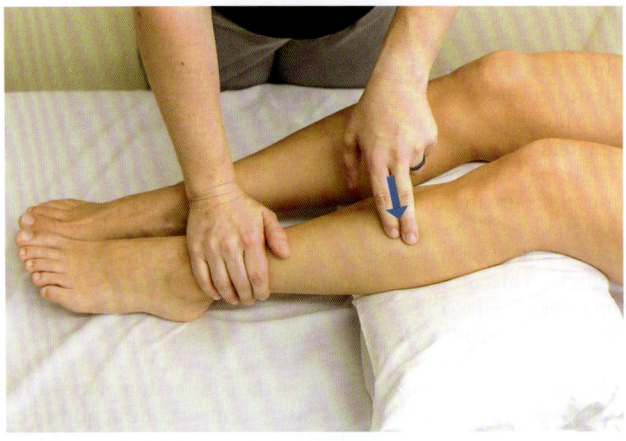

Figure 63-4. Cross-fiber flat palpation of TrPs in the left tibialis anterior muscle.

3.4. Trigger Point Examination

For examination of the tibialis anterior muscle, the patient may be positioned in long sitting or preferably supine (Figure 63-4). A pillow or bolster may be placed under the patient's knees to ensure relaxation. The most common TrP region is located at the sharp edge of the tibia at the junction of the proximal and middle third of the leg, approximately;[44] however, the entire muscle should always be thoroughly examined. Cross-fiber flat palpation reveals taut bands and TrP spot tenderness in the muscle mass lateral to the tibia (Figure 63-4). The taut bands in this muscle are parallel to the tibia. Digital pressure applied to a TrP will usually evoke or intensify the pain referred to the anterior ankle[39] and dorsum of the foot.

A recent study examined three ankle muscles, one of which was the tibialis anterior muscle, and found fair to moderate reliability for the presence or absence of TrPs (agreement 70%-85% and kappa 0.25-0.48), the presence of referred pain (agreement 63%-78% and kappa 0.26-0.51), and the palpation of a nodule in a taut band in the tibialis anterior muscle (agreement 65%-90% and kappa 0.25-0.43). The identification of a local twitch response and a jump sign by manual palpation was unreliable in this muscle.[40]

4. DIFFERENTIAL DIAGNOSIS

4.1. Activation and Perpetuation of Trigger Points

A posture or activity that activates a TrP, if not corrected, can also perpetuate it. In any part of the tibialis anterior muscle, TrPs may be activated by unaccustomed eccentric loading, eccentric exercise in an unconditioned muscle, or maximal or submaximal concentric loading.[56] Trigger points may also be activated or aggravated when the muscle is placed in a shortened and/or lengthened position for an extended period of time.

Trigger points of the tibialis anterior muscle are likely to be activated by similar mechanisms as those that could result in other significant ankle injuries. Any force that could cause an ankle sprain or fracture or exertional overload sufficient to induce anterior compartment syndrome could also result in TrPs of the tibialis anterior muscle.

The TrPs of the tibialis anterior muscle are often the result of serious gross trauma but can also occur from overuse (repetitive, micromechanical trauma) injuries. Walking or running downhill can increase eccentric load placed on the anterior compartment muscles and activate tibialis anterior TrPs. Additionally, wearing shoes with an elevated heel, such as cowboy boots or high heels, will further increase the demand of the ankle dorsiflexor muscles. Untrained persons ambulating on rough terrain, hard surfaces, or unusually soft surfaces (such as sand) for extended distances may also be predisposed to developing myofascial dysfunctions of the lower extremity.

Maximum angular velocity of the ankle joint during kicking in amateur soccer players is as high as 1720° per second in men and 1520° per second in women.[57] Activation of the tibialis anterior muscle is greater during the side-foot kick compared with the instep kick.[34] These forceful contractions can contribute to the development of TrPs and associated pain in the tibialis anterior muscle. This situation is commonly seen in athletes who are unaccustomed to the task or who quickly increase their training load, such as in the transition from offseason to preseason.

Catching the toe on an obstruction during the early-swing phase (tripping or stumbling during the contraction phase of the tibialis anterior muscle) can cause eccentric contraction overload that activates or perpetuates TrPs in this muscle. Athletes participating on artificial turf versus grass are more likely to experience this event, and it may occur simultaneously with a turf toe injury.[58] The overload is aggravated by a proportional increase in the reflex response to sudden stretch, a response that ranges from 0% to 40% of maximum voluntary contraction.[59]

4.2. Associated Trigger Points

Associated TrPs can develop in the referred pain areas caused by TrPs.[60] Therefore, musculature in the referred pain areas for each muscle should also be considered. The fibularis longus and tibialis anterior muscles often become involved together; they operate as a pair of well-matched antagonists for achieving stabilization and balance of the foot. The extensor hallucis longus and, to a lesser degree, extensor digitorum longus muscles may also develop TrPs as agonists to the tibialis anterior muscle. Tibialis posterior TrPs are not usually identified as related to TrPs in the tibialis anterior muscle. The muscles of the functional unit of the tibialis anterior muscle should be examined for the presence of TrPs as these associated TrPs can perpetuate TrPs in the tibialis anterior muscle.

4.3. Associated Pathology

Lumbar radicular pain or radiculopathy from the L5 nerve root often results in the formation of TrPs in those muscles innervated by the same nerve root. Often, patients with L5 radicular pain will report having lateral thigh, lateral calf, and great toe pain, with or without paresthesias on the dorsal ankle and foot, and with radiculopathy weakness in ankle dorsiflexion.[61] The presence of the tendon reflex of the tibialis anterior muscle reduces the likelihood of an L5 radicular compression as a contributing cause of the patient's pain. This reflex[62] was absent bilaterally in 11%, and missing on only one side an additional 6%, of 70 healthy subjects. A hand-held reflex hammer elicited the reflex response and surface electrodes recorded it electromyographically. However, the reflex was absent on the affected side in 72% of 18 patients with L5 nerve root compression. Patients presenting with leg paresthesias, sensory changes, reports of weakness, or signs of central nervous system disorders (excessive muscle tone or clonus) should receive a thorough neurologic examination including assessment of sensation, reflexes, muscle power, motor control, and movement coordination. If a potential serious medical condition is suspected, the patient should be referred to an appropriate medical practitioner.[63]

The sciatic nerve divides into the common fibular and tibial nerves proximal to the popliteal fossa. The posterior divisions of the ventral rami ultimately form the common fibular nerve. The common fibular nerve then travels across the lateral head of the gastrocnemius muscle and courses laterally and just distal to the head of the fibula where the nerve becomes subcutaneous. It continues between the fibularis longus muscle and the fibula. At this point, it divides into two main branches, deep and superficial fibular nerves.[7,64]

The deep fibular nerve innervates the anterior muscles of the leg by traveling deep to the fibularis longus muscle and passing into the anterior compartment by piercing the interosseous membrane between the tibia and the fibula. In the foot, the nerve remains in close proximity to the interosseous membrane with the anterior tibial artery. Finally, it terminates in a cutaneous branch that innervates the web space between the first and second toes.[1,7]

The common fibular nerve is susceptible to injury because it has a superficial location near the fibula. Compromise has been reported due to numerous traumatic and insidious causes. Traumatic causes occur in association with musculoskeletal injury or with isolated nerve traction, compression, or laceration. Examples of traumatic injury to the common fibular nerve include proximal fibular fracture,[65] tibial plateau fracture,[66] traumatic knee dislocation,[67] ligamentous knee injury,[68] ligamentous or bony injury of the ankle,[65] improper casting after ankle injury,[69] or laceration.[70,71] Other less common causes include osteoarthritis,[72] tumors,[71] and iatrogenic injury experienced during orthopedic surgery.[69]

Exertional compartment syndromes of the leg are a common form of overuse injury. Compartment syndromes are characterized by increased pressure within a muscular compartment sufficient to compromise the circulation of the muscles within it. The increased pressure obstructs venous outflow, which causes further swelling and more pressure. If prolonged, the resultant ischemia can lead to necrosis of the muscles and nerves within the compartment. When following a traumatic injury, it is most important that this condition be recognized immediately and managed properly to avoid possibly catastrophic consequences. Anterior compartment syndromes are recognized more commonly, followed by lateral, deep posterior and superficial posterior compartment syndromes.[73,74] Diffuse tightness and tenderness over the entire muscle belly of tibialis anterior muscle suggests an anterior compartment syndrome. The patients with this condition exhibit pain, paresthesias, and tenderness both in the ischemic muscles and in the region supplied by the deep fibular nerve. The muscles are sensitive to passive stretch and active contraction of the muscles increases symptoms.

Chronic exertional compartment syndrome is caused by abnormally high intramuscular pressure during exercise or sports participation such as running and weight lifting.[75] Among athletes and military service members, symptoms may develop over a period of time.[73,74] Tight, shortened calf muscles overload weakened anterior compartment muscles and predispose athletes to developing an anterior compartment syndrome.[76] In non-traumatic acute cases, a brief period of rest and cryotherapy to reduce pain, swelling, and metabolic demand can be tried with close monitoring before further measures are considered. One case series investigated the effect of massage, exercise, and avoidance of exacerbating activities over 5 weeks and concluded that it was effective in reducing symptoms upon reinitiation of activities.[77] Diebal published a case series of 10 patients who underwent 6 weeks of therapy with a focus on changing subjects' running technique to promote a forefoot running pattern, decreased stride length, and increased cadence. This intervention led to reduced postrunning leg intracompartmental pressures and significantly reduced pain and disability for up to 1 year after intervention.[78]

Shin splints is a common injury in runners and military personnel. This condition is the result of mechanical inflammation induced by repetitive stress of the broad proximal portion of any of the musculotendinous units originating from the lower part of the tibia during weight bearing.[79] Shin splints can be anterolateral or posteromedial. Anterolateral shin splints result from microtrauma and acute myositis of the tibialis anterior, extensor hallucis longus, and extensor digitorum longus muscles. Trigger points can develop in these muscles and exacerbate the patient's symptoms. Pain and tenderness will be present over the muscles of the anterior compartment.

Commonly, muscle imbalance between weak dorsiflexor muscle groups and tight gastrocnemius-soleus muscles is noted.[53] The soleus muscle and excessive foot pronation have been reported as likely contributors to posteromedial shin splints, also known as medial tibial stress syndrome.[80-82] Reinking et al[81] found female gender, increased weight, greater navicular drop, previous running injury, and greater hip external rotation with the hip in flexion as risk factors in the development of medial tibial stress syndrome.[81]

Subcutaneous herniation of the tibialis anterior muscle through its investing fascia may be painful during standing and walking, or it may be of cosmetic concern.[83] Magnetic resonance imaging, unlike computed tomography, unequivocally identifies the extent of fascial splitting and the size of muscle herniation because it distinguishes more clearly between these two soft-tissue structures.[84,85] The herniation will be pronounced with dorsiflexion of the foot, and if palpable and reducible, the outlined fascial defect may be appreciated.[86]

5. CORRECTIVE ACTIONS

Pulling the foot up and maintaining that position for an extensive period of time, as when driving a car with a steeply angled pedal, can cause sustained shortening of the tibialis anterior muscle, which will, in turn, activate and perpetuate TrPs in it. The use of a cruise control provides an opportunity for the driver to change foot position and obtain periodic relief from immobility. When a person is seated for a prolonged period of time, the ankle pump exercise usually provides welcome relief as it stretches the tibialis anterior muscle as well as the soleus muscle.

In general, the leg muscles feel better if the ankle is maintained in a neutral position throughout the night; therefore, adjusting a patient's sleeping posture may be necessary. This position is facilitated by having the bed sheets at the foot of the bed untucked to reduce external weight pulling the ankle into excessive plantar flexion. When side-lying, placing a pillow between the legs and knees will position the foot and ankle into a more restful position.

A major source of overload of the tibialis anterior muscle can be the result of increased tension or shortening of the calf musculature. An essential first step in the treatment of the tibialis anterior muscle is to reduce gastrocnemius-soleus (calf musculature) tightness and inactivate any responsible TrPs. When stretching the gastrocnemius/soleus muscle complex ("heel cord" or Achilles tendon), care should be taken to ensure that the subtalar joint (rear foot) is maintained in a neutral position and is not tilted in or out. Using the forefoot as a lever for stretching will result in additional dorsiflexion of the transverse tarsal joint, which may add further tendency toward pronation of the foot (flattening of the arch). To control this flattening of the foot, the patient should place a small towel under the medial aspect (inside border) of the bare foot during the standing stretch (see Figure 65-8). If the anterior compartment muscles are weak, a strengthening program consisting of both eccentric and concentric exercises for the tibialis anterior and other dorsiflexor muscles of the foot may be necessary to restore muscular balance at the ankle.[53]

Walking on flat surfaces is preferred instead of uneven ground such as bricks, cracked pavement, grass, or sand. In addition, a surface that is level from side to side and not tilted laterally, as is the edge of a crowned road or a slanted beach, is optimal.

Self-pressure release for TrPs in the tibialis anterior muscle can be performed in long sitting by placing the heel of the unaffected side on a tender spot in the affected tibialis anterior muscle (Figure 63-5A), manually with the thumbs (Figure 63-5B), or with a TrP release tool (Figure 63-5C). Finding the sensitive spot with the opposite heel, thumbs, or a tool, light pressure (no more than 4/10 pain) should be applied and held for 15 to 30 seconds or until the pain reduces. This release can be repeated five times per session, several times per day.

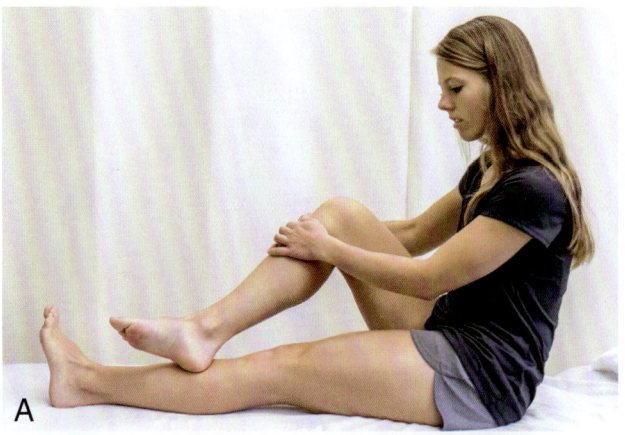
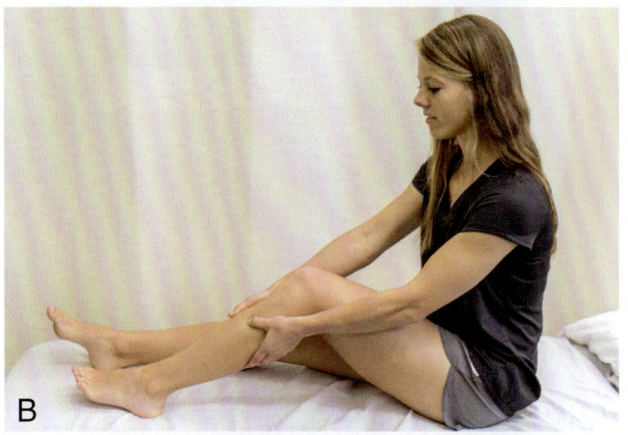
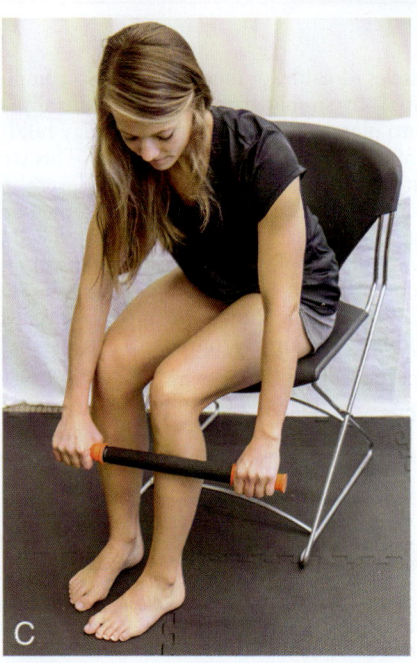

Figure 63-5. Trigger point self-pressure release of the tibialis anterior muscle. A, Using the heel of the opposite leg. B, Using the thumb. C, TrP self-release tool (roller).

The patient can perform self-stretch of the tibialis anterior muscle by crossing the involved foot over the other thigh and using a hand to passively plantar flex and pronate (abduct and evert) the foot in a down and back motion (Figure 63-6A). Additional stretching of the extensor digitorum longus and extensor hallucis

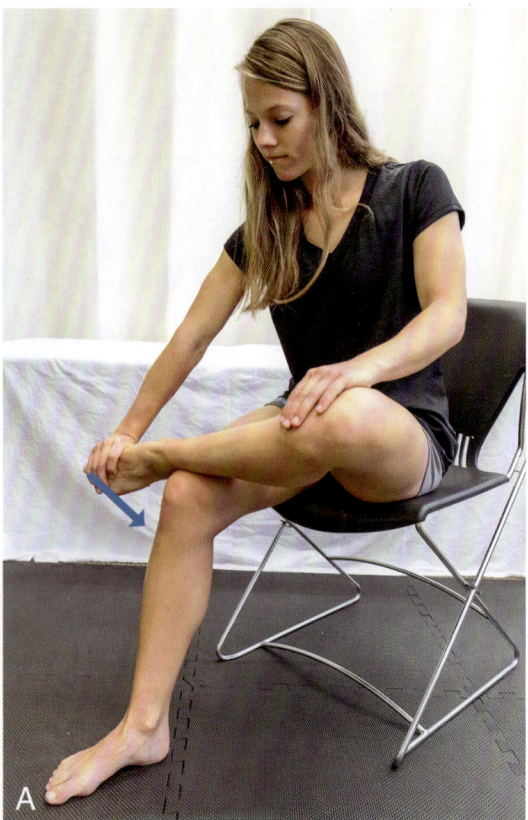 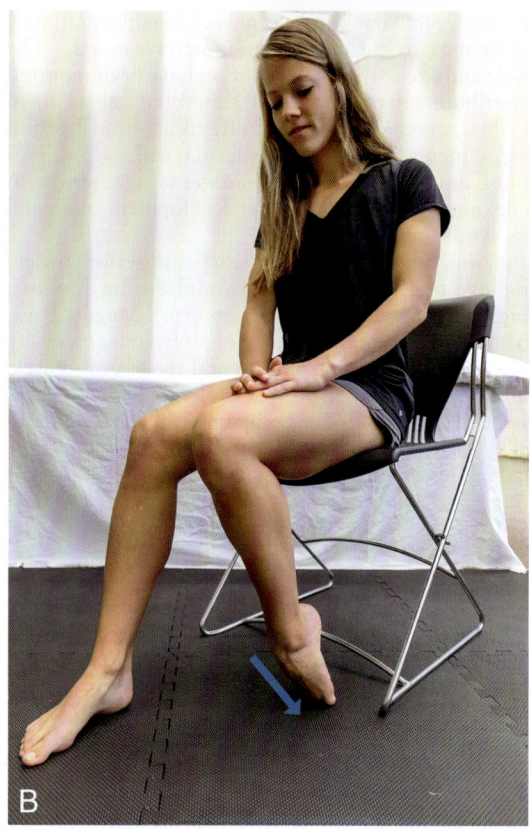

Figure 63-6. Self-stretch of the tibialis anterior muscle. A, Overpressure pulling the foot back and down toward the floor. B, Top of the toes on the floor positioning the foot with more pressure on the great toe side. A stretch should be felt on the shin.

longus muscles (dorsiflexor muscles) can be accomplished in the same position by simply sliding the hand distally and pulling the toes into plantar flexion. The patient may hold the stretch for up to 30 seconds and repeat four times. This stretch of the tibialis anterior muscle can be performed several times daily. An alternate stretch can be performed with the patient sitting forward on a chair with the foot of the leg stretched back under the chair and placing the foot in plantar flexion and eversion with the top of the toes on the ground (Figure 63-6B). Adding a gentle calf muscle contraction to enhance plantar flexion during the stretch phase (reciprocal inhibition) can also be helpful.

References

1. Standring S. *Gray's Anatomy: The Anatomical Basis of Clinical Practice*. 41st ed. London, UK: Elsevier; 2015.
2. Mathes SJ, Nahai F. *Reconstructive Surgery: Principles, Anatomy & Technique*. New York, NY; St. Louis, MO: Churchill Livingstone; 1997.
3. Hirshowitz B, Moscona R, Kaufman T, Har-Shai Y. External longitudinal splitting of the tibialis anterior muscle for coverage of compound fractures of the middle third of the tibia. *Plast Reconstr Surg*. 1987;79(3):407-414.
4. Brenner E. Insertion of the tendon of the tibialis anterior muscle in feet with and without hallux valgus. *Clin Anat*. 2002;15(3):217-223.
5. Willegger M, Seyidova N, Schuh R, Windhager R, Hirtler L. Anatomical footprint of the tibialis anterior tendon: surgical implications for foot and ankle reconstructions. *Biomed Res Int*. 2017;2017:9542125.
6. Aquilonius SM, Askmark H, Gillberg PG, Nandedkar S, Olsson Y, Stalberg E. Topographical localization of motor endplates in cryosections of whole human muscles. *Muscle Nerve*. 1984;7(4):287-293.
7. Baima J, Krivickas L. Evaluation and treatment of peroneal neuropathy. *Curr Rev Musculoskelet Med*. 2008;1(2):147-153.
8. Pillet J, Cronier P, Mercier P, et al. The anterior tibial artery and vascularization of the muscles of the anterior compartment of the leg. Application to the anterior compartment syndrome of the leg [in French]. *Bull Assoc Anat (Nancy)*. 1984;68(201):223-231.
9. Gantchev GN, Draganova N. Muscular synergies during different conditions of postural activity. *Acta Physiol Pharmacol Bulg*. 1986;12(4):58-65.
10. Oddsson L. Motor patterns of a fast voluntary postural task in man: trunk extension in standing. *Acta Physiol Scand*. 1989;136(1):47-58.
11. Okada M, Fujiwara K. Muscle activity around the ankle joint as correlated with the center of foot pressure in an upright stance. In: Matsui M, Kobayashi K, eds. *Biomechanics 8A*. Champaign, IL: Human Kinetics Publishers; 1983: 209-216.
12. Di Giulio I, Maganaris CN, Baltzopoulos V, Loram ID. The proprioceptive and agonist roles of gastrocnemius, soleus and tibialis anterior muscles in maintaining human upright posture. *J Physiol*. 2009;587(pt 10):2399-2416.
13. Duquette AM, Andrews DM. Tibialis anterior muscle fatigue leads to changes in tibial axial acceleration after impact when ankle dorsiflexion angles are visually controlled. *Hum Mov Sci*. 2010;29(4):567-577.
14. Basmajian J, Deluca C. *Muscles Alive*. 5th ed. Baltimore, MD: Williams & Wilkins; 1985 (pp. 256-257).
15. Townsend MA, Shiavi R, Lainhart SP, Caylor J. Variability in synergy patterns of leg muscles during climbing, descending and level walking of highly-trained athletes and normal males. *Electromyogr Clin Neurophysiol*. 1978;18(1):69-80.
16. Gray EG, Basmajian JV. Electromyography and cinematography of leg and foot ("normal" and flat) during walking. *Anat Rec*. 1968;161(1):1-15.
17. Basmajian JV, Slonecker CE. *Grant's Method of Anatomy*. 11th ed. Baltimore, MD: Williams & Wilkins; 1989 (p. 332).
18. Rasch PJ, Burke RK. *Kinesiology and Applied Anatomy: The Science of Human Movement*. 6th ed. Philadelphia, PA: Lea & Febiger; 1978 (pp. 317-330).
19. Lemos T, Imbiriba LA, Vargas CD, Vieira TM. Modulation of tibialis anterior muscle activity changes with upright stance width. *J Electromyogr Kinesiol*. 2015;25(1):168-174.
20. Bonnet CT, Mercier M, Szaffarczyk S. Impaired mediolateral postural control at the ankle in healthy, middle-aged adults. *J Mot Behav*. 2013;45(4):333-342.
21. LaRoche DP, Cremin KA, Greenleaf B, Croce RV. Rapid torque development in older female fallers and nonfallers: a comparison across lower-extremity muscles. *J Electromyogr Kinesiol*. 2010;20(3):482-488.
22. Di Nardo F, Ghetti G, Fioretti S. Assessment of the activation modalities of gastrocnemius lateralis and tibialis anterior during gait: a statistical analysis. *J Electromyogr Kinesiol*. 2013;23(6):1428-1433.
23. Yang JF, Winter DA. Surface EMG profiles during different walking cadences in humans. *Electroencephalogr Clin Neurophysiol*. 1985;60(6):485-491.
24. Perry J. The mechanics of walking. A clinical interpretation. *Phys Ther*. 1967;47(9):778-801.
25. Agostini V, Nascimbeni A, Gaffuri A, Imazio P, Benedetti MG, Knaflitz M. Normative EMG activation patterns of school-age children during gait. *Gait Posture*. 2010;32(3):285-289.
26. Di Nardo F, Mengarelli A, Burattini L, et al. Normative EMG patterns of ankle muscle co-contractions in school-age children during gait. *Gait Posture*. 2016;46:161-166.

27. Kuster M, Sakurai S, Wood GA. Kinematic and kinetic comparison of downhill and level walking. *Clin Biomech (Bristol, Avon)*. 1995;10(2):79-84.
28. Lay AN, Hass CJ, Richard Nichols T, Gregor RJ. The effects of sloped surfaces on locomotion: an electromyographic analysis. *J Biomech*. 2007;40(6):1276-1285.
29. Sabatier MJ, Wedewer W, Barton B, Henderson E, Murphy JT, Ou K. Slope walking causes short-term changes in soleus H-reflex excitability. *Physiol Rep*. 2015;3(3).
30. Mann RA, Moran GT, Dougherty SE. Comparative electromyography of the lower extremity in jogging, running, and sprinting. *Am J Sports Med*. 1986;14(6):501-510.
31. Yong JR, Silder A, Delp SL. Differences in muscle activity between natural forefoot and rearfoot strikers during running. *J Biomech*. 2014;47(15):3593-3597.
32. Shih Y, Lin KL, Shiang TY. Is the foot striking pattern more important than barefoot or shod conditions in running? *Gait Posture*. 2013;38(3):490-494.
33. Broer M, Houtz S. *Patterns of Muscular Activity in Selected Sports Skills, an Electromyographic Study*. Springfield, IL: Charles C. Thomas; 1967.
34. Brophy RH, Backus SI, Pansy BS, Lyman S, Williams RJ. Lower extremity muscle activation and alignment during the soccer instep and side-foot kicks. *J Orthop Sports Phys Ther*. 2007;37(5):260-268.
35. Henriksson-Larsen KB, Lexell J, Sjostrom M. Distribution of different fibre types in human skeletal muscles. I. Method for the preparation and analysis of cross-sections of whole tibialis anterior. *Histochem J*. 1983;15(2):167-178.
36. Henriksson-Larsen K. Distribution, number and size of different types of fibres in whole cross-sections of female m tibialis anterior. An enzyme histochemical study. *Acta Physiol Scand*. 1985;123(3):229-235.
37. Helliwell TR, Coakley J, Smith PE, Edwards RH. The morphology and morphometry of the normal human tibialis anterior muscle. *Neuropathol Appl Neurobiol*. 1987;13(4):297-307.
38. Simons DG, Travell J, Simons L. *Travell & Simon's Myofascial Pain and Dysfunction: The Trigger Point Manual*. Vol 1. 2nd ed. Baltimore, MD: Williams & Wilkins; 1999 (p. 104).
39. Travell J, Rinzler SH. The myofascial genesis of pain. *Postgrad Med*. 1952;11(5):425-434.
40. Sanz DR, Lobo CC, Lopez DL, Morales CR, Marin CS, Corbalan IS. Interrater reliability in the clinical evaluation of myofascial trigger points in three ankle muscles. *J Manipulative Physiol Ther*. 2016;39(9):623-634.
41. Simons DG. *Chapter 45, Myofascial Pain Syndrome Due to Trigger Points*. St. Louis, MO: Mosby; 1988:710-711.
42. Simons DG, Travell J. Chapter 25, Myofascial pain syndromes. In: Wall PD, Melzack R, Bonica JJ, eds. *Textbook of Pain*. Edinburgh, Scotland; New York, NY: Churchill Livingstone; 1989:368-385.
43. Sola AE. Treatment of myofascial pain syndromes. In: Benedetti C, Chapman C, Moricca G, eds. *Recent Advances in the Management of Pain*. Vol 7. New York, NY: Raven Press; 1984:467-485.
44. Sola AE. Chapter 47, Trigger Point therapy. In: Roberts JR, Hedges JR, eds. *Clinical Procedures in Emergency Medicine*. Philadelphia, PA: Saunders; 1985:674-686.
45. Jacobsen S. Myofascial pain syndrome [in Danish]. *Ugeskrift for laeger*. 1987;149(9):600-601.
46. Sola AE, Williams RL. Myofascial pain syndromes. *Neurology*. 1956;6(2):91-95.
47. Arcangeli P, Digiesi V, Ronchi O, Dorigo B, Bartoli B. Mechanisms of ischemic pain in peripheral occlusive arterial disease. In: Bonica JJ, Albe-Fessard D, eds. *Advances in Pain Research and Therapy*. Vol 1. New York, NY: Raven Press; 1976:965-973.
48. Gutstein M. Common rheumatism and physiotherapy. *Br J Phys Med*. 1940;3:46-50.
49. Bates T, Grunwald E. Myofascial pain in childhood. *J Pediatr*. 1958;53(2):198-209.
50. Rubin TK, Gandevia SC, Henderson LA, Macefield VG. Effects of intramuscular anesthesia on the expression of primary and referred pain induced by intramuscular injection of hypertonic saline. *J Pain*. 2009;10(8):829-835.
51. Kellgren JH. Observations on referred pain arising from muscle. *Clin Sci*. 1938;3:175-190.
52. Gibson W, Arendt-Nielsen L, Graven-Nielsen T. Referred pain and hyperalgesia in human tendon and muscle belly tissue. *Pain*. 2006;120(1-2):113-123.
53. Hertling D. *Management of Common Musculoskeletal Disorders: Physical Therapy Principles and Methods*. 4th ed. Philadelphia, PA: LWW; 2005 (pp. 573-611).
54. Moore KL, Dalley AF, Agur AMR. *Clinically Oriented Anatomy*. 6th ed. Philadelphia, PA: Lippincott Williams and Wilkins; 2009 (pp. 588-608).
55. Kendall FP, McCreary EK. *Muscles: Testing and Function, with Posture and Pain*. 5th ed. Baltimore, MD: Lippincott Williams & Wilkins; 2005.
56. Gerwin RD, Dommerholt J, Shah JP. An expansion of Simons' integrated hypothesis of trigger point formation. *Curr Pain Headache Rep*. 2004;8(6):468-475.
57. Katis A, Kellis E, Lees A. Age and gender differences in kinematics of powerful instep kicks in soccer. *Sports Biomech*. 2015;14(3):287-299.
58. Drakos MC, Taylor SA, Fabricant PD, Haleem AM. Synthetic playing surfaces and athlete health. *J Am Acad Orthop Surg*. 2013;21(5):293-302.
59. Toft E, Sinkjaer T, Andreassen S. Mechanical and electromyographic responses to stretch of the human anterior tibial muscle at different levels of contraction. *Exp Brain Res*. 1989;74(1):213-219.
60. Hsieh YL, Kao MJ, Kuan TS, Chen SM, Chen JT, Hong CZ. Dry needling to a key myofascial trigger point may reduce the irritability of satellite MTrPs. *Am J Phys Med Rehabil*. 2007;86(5):397-403.
61. Kreiner DS, Hwang SW, Easa JE, et al. An evidence-based clinical guideline for the diagnosis and treatment of lumbar disc herniation with radiculopathy. *Spine J*. 2014;14(1):180-191.
62. Stam J. The tibialis anterior reflex in healthy subjects and in L5 radicular compression. *J Neurol Neurosurg Psychiatry*. 1988;51(3):397-402.
63. Delitto A, George SZ, Van Dillen LR, et al. Low back pain. *J Orthop Sports Phys Ther*. 2012;42(4):A1-A57.
64. Anderson JC. Common fibular nerve compression: anatomy, symptoms, clinical evaluation, and surgical decompression. *Clin Podiatr Med Surg*. 2016;33(2):283-291.
65. Kim YC, Jung TD. Peroneal neuropathy after tibio-fibular fracture. *Ann Rehabil Med*. 2011;35(5):648-657.
66. Khatri K, Sharma V, Goyal D, Farooque K. Complications in the management of closed high-energy proximal tibial plateau fractures. *Chin J Traumatol*. 2016;19(6):342-347.
67. Woodmass JM, Romatowski NP, Esposito JG, Mohtadi NG, Longino PD. A systematic review of peroneal nerve palsy and recovery following traumatic knee dislocation. *Knee Surg Sports Traumatol Arthrosc*. 2015;23(10):2992-3002.
68. Mook WR, Ligh CA, Moorman CT III, Leversedge FJ. Nerve injury complicating multiligament knee injury: current concepts and treatment algorithm. *J Am Acad Orthop Surg*. 2013;21(6):343-354.
69. Kretschmer T, Antoniadis G, Braun V, Rath SA, Richter HP. Evaluation of iatrogenic lesions in 722 surgically treated cases of peripheral nerve trauma. *J Neurosurg*. 2001;94(6):905-912.
70. Seidel JA, Koenig R, Antoniadis G, Richter HP, Kretschmer T. Surgical treatment of traumatic peroneal nerve lesions. *Neurosurgery*. 2008;62(3):664-673; discussion 664-673.
71. Kim DH, Murovic JA, Tiel RL, Kline DG. Management and outcomes in 318 operative common peroneal nerve lesions at the Louisiana State University Health Sciences Center. *Neurosurgery*. 2004;54(6):1421-1428; discussion 1428-1429.
72. Fetzer GB, Prather H, Gelberman RH, Clohisy JC. Progressive peroneal nerve palsy in a varus arthritic knee. A case report. *J Bone Joint Surg Am*. 2004;86-A(7):1538-1540.
73. Rajasekaran S, Hall MM. Nonoperative management of chronic exertional compartment syndrome: a systematic review. *Curr Sports Med Rep*. 2016;15(3):191-198.
74. Campano D, Robaina JA, Kusnezov N, Dunn JC, Waterman BR. Surgical management for chronic exertional compartment syndrome of the leg: a systematic review of the literature. *Arthroscopy*. 2016;32(7):1478-1486.
75. Buschbacher M, Ralph M. *Practical Guide to Musculoskeletal Disorders: Diagnosis and Rehabilitation*. 2nd ed. Boston, MA: Butterworth-Heinemann; 2002.
76. Mirkin G. Keeping pace with new problems when your patients exercise. *Mod Med NZ*. 1980:6-14.
77. Blackman PG, Simmons LR, Crossley KM. Treatment of chronic exertional anterior compartment syndrome with massage: a pilot study. *Clin J Sport Med*. 1998;8(1):14-17.
78. Diebal AR, Gregory R, Alitz C, Gerber JP. Forefoot running improves pain and disability associated with chronic exertional compartment syndrome. *Am J Sports Med*. 2012;40(5):1060-1067.
79. Jones DC, James SL. Overuse injuries of the lower extremity: shin splints, iliotibial band friction syndrome, and exertional compartment syndromes. *Clin Sports Med*. 1987;6(2):273-290.
80. Galbraith RM, Lavallee ME. Medial tibial stress syndrome: conservative treatment options. *Curr Rev Musculoskelet Med*. 2009;2(3):127-133.
81. Reinking MF, Austin TM, Richter RR, Krieger MM. Medial tibial stress syndrome in active individuals: a systematic review and meta-analysis of risk factors. *Sports Health*. 2017;9(3):252-261.
82. Hamstra-Wright KL, Bliven KC, Bay C. Risk factors for medial tibial stress syndrome in physically active individuals such as runners and military personnel: a systematic review and meta-analysis. *Br J Sports Med*. 2015;49(6):362-369.
83. Harrington AC, Mellette JR Jr. Hernias of the anterior tibialis muscle: case report and review of the literature. *J Am Acad Dermatol*. 1990;22(1):123-124.
84. Govindarajan A, Inigo A. Tibialis anterior muscle hernia: a rare differential of a soft tissue tumour. *BMJ Case Rep*. 2015;2015.
85. Zeiss J, Ebraheim NA, Woldenberg LS. Magnetic resonance imaging in the diagnosis of anterior tibialis muscle herniation. *Clin Orthop Relat Res*. 1989;(244):249-253.
86. Nguyen JT, Nguyen JL, Wheatley MJ, Nguyen TA. Muscle hernias of the leg: a case report and comprehensive review of the literature. *Can J Plast Surg*. 2013;21(4):243-247.

Chapter 64

Fibularis Longus, Brevis, and Tertius Muscles

"Weak Ankle Muscles"

Wesley J. Wedewer

1. INTRODUCTION

Note: Following revised anatomic terminology published in 1998, the peroneal muscles are now known as the fibularis muscles, to prevent confusion of these muscles with those regions with similar names. "Perone" is another term for fibular and, thus, the revised terminology for these muscles, and related nerve and its branches, is based on language describing the location. Although both fibular and peroneal are considered acceptable terms, "fibular" and its related terminology is preferred and therefore will be used throughout this text.[1,2]

The fibularis longus and brevis muscles, along with the superficial fibular nerve, occupy the lateral compartment of the leg. The fibular muscles are important in foot and ankle function and are commonly seen in clinical practice to have trigger points (TrPs). They mainly control motion during gait and aid in proprioception of the foot and ankle. The collective group is responsible for ankle eversion; the fibularis longus and brevis muscles contribute to plantar flexion, whereas the fibularis tertius muscle assists in dorsiflexion. Trigger points in the fibularis muscles produce pain over the lateral malleolus of the ankle, above, behind, and below it. Pain can also extend a short distance along the lateral aspect of the heel and foot. On occasion, pain may cover the lateral aspect of the middle third of the leg. Trigger points in these muscles may be activated or perpetuated by excessive or vigorous running, walking, and jumping. Trigger points in these muscles are very common following an inversion ankle sprain or fibular fracture. Differential diagnosis should include fibular nerve entrapment, lumbar radicular pain or radiculopathy, compartment syndromes, ankle sprain, rupture of fibularis longus or brevis tendons, and an abnormal foot structure. Corrective actions include correcting or supporting abnormal foot posture and mechanics, modification of sitting and sleeping posture, self-pressure release techniques, self-stretch exercises, activity modification, and implementing lower extremity proprioceptive and motor control exercise programs.

2. ANATOMIC CONSIDERATIONS

The fibularis longus and fibularis brevis muscles, along with the superficial fibular nerve, occupy the lateral compartment of the leg (Figure 64-1). They evert the foot and plantar flex the ankle. The fibularis tertius muscle lies in the anterior compartment with the tibialis anterior muscle and the deep fibular nerve. It also everts the foot but additionally produces dorsiflexion of the ankle.[3] The cross-section of the middle third of the leg, see Figure 63-2 in the previous chapter, shows the compartmental relationships.

Anatomists report many variations of the fibular muscle group. The fibularis tertius muscle was absent in 5.0% to 8.2% of specimens.[4,5] A bifid fibularis brevis muscle was reported as the cause of symptoms that required surgical correction.[6] A commonly noted but rare (2%)[4] muscle, the fibularis digiti minimi muscle, arises from the distal quarter of the fibula and attaches to the extensor aponeurosis of the fifth toe.[7,8] Also, a fibularis quartus muscle was identified using magnetic resonance imaging in 7.6% to 10%[9,10] of subjects. Incidence rates of the fibularis quartus muscle on cadaver specimens varied from 13% to 23%.[10] It attaches proximally onto the back of the fibula between the fibularis brevis and flexor hallucis longus muscles, and distally to either the calcaneus or the cuboid.

Fibularis Longus

The fibularis longus muscle is located at the upper part of the outside leg and is the longer and more superficial of the fibularis muscles (Figure 64-1A). Proximally, it originates from the head and proximal two-thirds of the lateral surface of the fibula, the deep surface of the deep fascia, the anterior and posterior intermuscular septa, and occasionally by a few fibers from the lateral condyle of the tibia. Distally, it becomes tendinous in the middle third of the leg. The long tendon curves behind the lateral malleolus and passes in a groove it shares with the tendon of the fibularis brevis muscle. The groove is converted into a canal by the superior fibular retinaculum, so that the tendon of the fibularis longus muscle and that of the fibularis brevis muscle, which lies in front of the fibularis longus tendon, are contained in a common synovial sheath. If the fibular retinaculum is ruptured by injury and fails to heal, the tendons can dislocate from the groove. On the lateral side of the calcaneus, these tendons occupy separate osseoaponeurotic canals. The tendon of the fibularis longus muscle again curves sharply and runs in a groove on the anteroinferior aspect of the cuboid bone. It then crosses the sole of the foot obliquely and inserts by two slips, one to the lateral side of the base of the 1st metatarsal and one to the lateral aspect of the medial cuneiform (Figure 64-1B); occasionally, a third slip is attached to the base of the 2nd metatarsal. The long tendon of the fibularis longus muscle attaches opposite to the tendon of the tibialis anterior muscle on the medial aspect of the base of the 1st metatarsal bone.[3,11,12] Tendinous slips from the fibularis longus muscle may extend to the base of the 3rd, 4th, or 5th metatarsals or to the adductor hallucis muscle.[3]

The tendon changes direction below the lateral malleolus and on the cuboid bone. At both sites, it is thickened, and at the second site, a sesamoid fibrocartilage is present.[3] Some sesamoids ossify, whereas others remain fibrous or cartilaginous. When this fibrocartilage ossifies, it becomes the os peroneum. The os peroneum has an irregular shape and is visible in approximately 20%[13,14] of foot radiographs in mature individuals. In a cadaver study, 30% of tendons displayed an os peroneum both radiographically and histologically. The results of the study also suggested that the presence of os peroneum does not appear to be associated with increased endochondral ossification or degenerative joint disease. The bone formation may be associated with biomechanical functions within the foot.[15] The origin of the os peroneum has given rise to much controversy. Its presence may stem from a response to the intense mechanical stresses involved at the angulated part of the fibularis longus tendon, and it may assist the tendon to glide without getting caught or impinged.[16,17] Phylogenetically, it may be in the process of

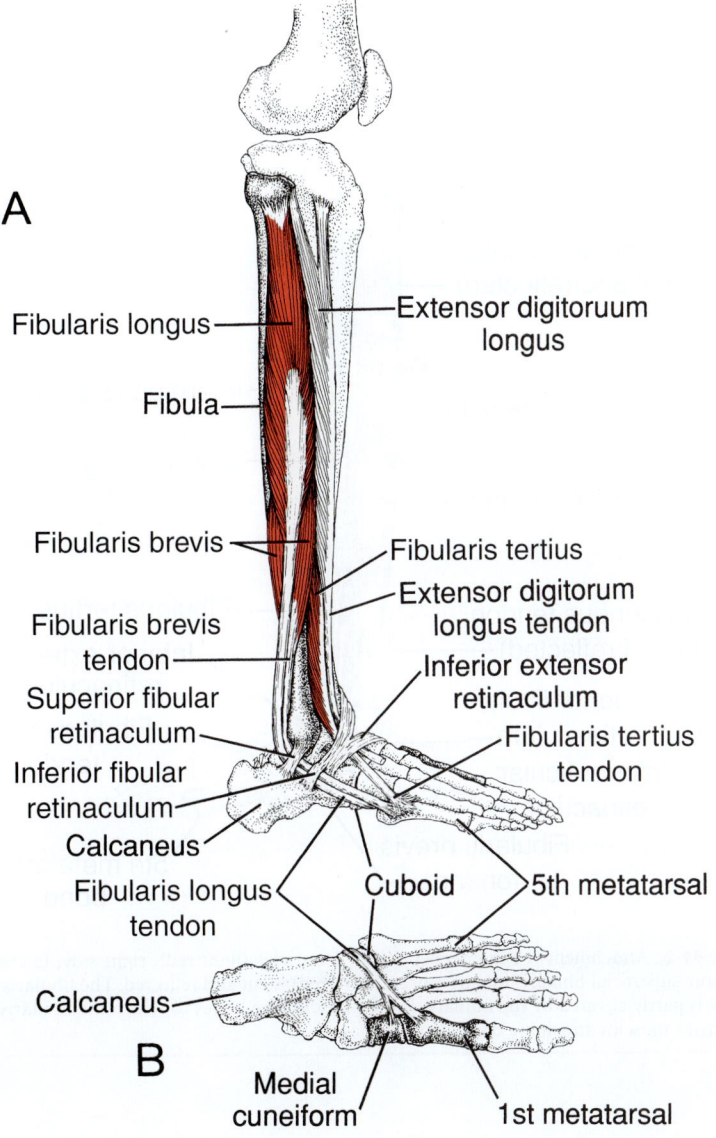

Figure 64-1. Anatomical relations and attachments of the right fibularis muscles. A, Lateral view. B, Plantar view of the right foot. The bones to which the fibularis longus muscle attaches are darkened.

disappearing from the human race due to loss of its functional importance for hallux opposability.[14]

Fibularis Brevis

The fibularis brevis muscle is shorter and smaller than the fibularis longus muscle and lies deep to it. The belly of fibularis brevis muscle extends distally beyond that of the fibularis longus muscle (Figures 64-1A and 64-2). Proximally, fibularis brevis muscle originates from the distal two-thirds of the lateral surface of the fibula, anterior to the fibularis longus muscle, and adjacent to the intermuscular septa (Figure 64-2). The tendon of this muscle travels with that of the fibularis longus muscle within a common synovial sheath as it curves behind the lateral malleolus under the superior fibular retinaculum (Figures 64-1 and 64-2). Farther distally, these tendons have separate synovial sheaths. The fibularis brevis tendon then runs forward on the lateral side of the calcaneus above the tendon of the fibularis longus muscle and inserts distally to the tuberosity on the dorsolateral aspect of the base of the 5th metatarsal (Figure 64-1A). Fusion of the fibularis longus and brevis muscles has been reported, but is rare.[3]

Fibularis Tertius

The fibularis tertius muscle (Figure 64-2) differs anatomically and functionally from the other two fibularis muscles. This muscle is absent in hominoid apes and is hypothesized to have emerged as a recent addition of the human foot with the acquisition of the bipedal gait to support the relatively weak human mid-foot and make the bipedal gait more effective and efficient.[18,19] Although the fibularis tertius muscle is located just lateral and runs parallel in close proximity to the extensor digitorum longus muscle, it is usually anatomically distinct from the extensor digitorum longus muscle.[4] Some describe the fibularis tertius muscle to be part of the extensor digitorum longus muscle and might label it as its "fifth tendon."[3] A recent meta-analysis including 3628 legs demonstrated that the fibularis tertius muscle is highly prevalent in humans (93.2%). It originates on the distal half of the fibula (70.2%), distal third of the fibula (13%), or from the extensor digitorum longus muscle itself (15.8%).[18] Additionally, it attaches to the adjoining anterior surface of the interosseous membrane and the anterior intermuscular septum.[3] The two lateral fibularis muscles attach to the other side of this septum. The fibularis

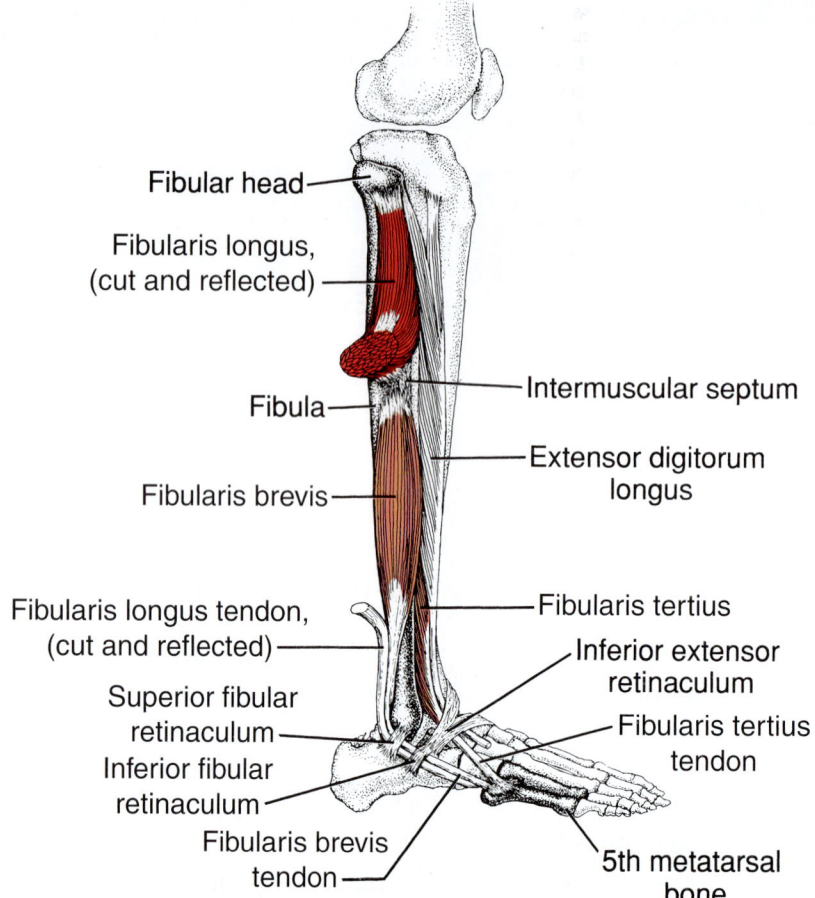

Figure 64-2. Attachments of the deeper fibularis muscles (light red), right side, lateral view. The more superficial fibularis longus muscle (dark red) is cut and reflected. The fibularis tertius muscle is partly covered by the fibularis brevis muscle. The bones to which the fibularis brevis and tertius muscles attach are darkened.

tertius muscle is usually as large as, or larger than, the extensor digitorum longus muscle. Distally, the fibularis tertius tendon inserts broadly on the tubercle along the mediodorsal surface of the base of the 5th metatarsal, unlike the extensor digitorum longus tendon, which attaches to the lateral four proximal phalanges.[3,4] Insertional points in addition to the 5th metatarsal have been observed on the fascia covering the 4th interosseous space (16.7%) and the base of the 4th metatarsal (11.9%).[18,20] These tendinous projections spiral and tighten during passive inversion of the foot or straighten and relax during passive eversion.[4]

2.1. Innervation and Vascularization

Branches of the superficial fibular nerve supply the fibularis longus and fibularis brevis muscles. This nerve contains fibers from the L4, L5, and S1 spinal nerves. The deep fibular nerve supplies the fibularis tertius muscle in the anterior compartment with fibers from only the L5 and S1 spinal nerves. Branches of the anterior tibial artery primarily provide vascularization to the three fibularis muscles.[3]

Fibularis Longus and Fibularis Brevis

Branches of the superficial fibular nerve supply the fibularis longus and fibularis brevis muscles as well as the skin of the leg. The segmental innervation comes from the L5, S1,[3,12] and sometimes from the S2 spinal nerves.[12] The superficial fibular nerve begins at the bifurcation of the common fibular nerve. It passes anteroinferiorly between the fibularis longus, fibularis brevis, and extensor digitorum longus muscles, and pierces the deep fascia in the distal third of the leg. Cutaneous branches supply the distal third of the anterior leg and skin of the dorsum of all toes except that of the fifth toe, supplied by the sural nerve, and the adjoining sides of the great and second toes, supplied by the deep fibular nerve.[3]

The vascularization of the fibularis longus and brevis muscles is derived from superior and inferior branches of the anterior tibial artery. There is also a lesser, variable contribution from the fibular artery in the distal part of the leg. Distally, the tendons are supplied by the fibular perforating, anterior lateral malleolar, lateral calcaneal, lateral tarsal, arcuate, lateral plantar, and medial plantar arteries.[3]

Fibularis Tertius

The deep fibular nerve supplies the fibularis tertius muscle in the anterior compartment with fibers from the L5 and S1 spinal nerves.[3] The deep fibular nerve innervates the anterior muscles of the leg by traveling deep to the fibularis longus muscle. In the foot, the nerve remains in close proximity to the interosseous membrane with the anterior tibial artery. Finally, it terminates in a cutaneous branch, which innervates the web space between the first and second toes.[3,21]

The vascularization of the fibularis tertius muscle is derived from anteriorly and laterally placed branches of the anterior tibial artery, supplemented distally from the perforating branch of the fibular artery. The tendon is supplied at the ankle and in the foot by the anterior lateral malleolar artery and malleolar network, and by lateral tarsal, metatarsal, plantar, and digital arteries. In the foot, it receives an additional supply from the termination of the arcuate artery and the 4th dorsal metatarsal artery.[3]

2.2. Function

The fibularis longus, brevis, and tertius muscles function as dynamic stabilizers of the ankle and are important in proprioception, independent of the status of the lateral ankle ligaments. Poor fibularis muscle function can give patients a sense of instability, even in a mechanically stable ankle.[22] The fibularis muscles all act to evert the nonweight-bearing foot. A major difference in these muscles is that the fibularis tertius muscle dorsiflexes the foot because its tendon crosses in front of the ankle joint, whereas the fibularis longus and fibularis brevis muscles plantar flex the foot because their tendons pass behind the ankle joint.[3]

The fibularis muscles, like most other lower extremity muscles, frequently function to control movement rather than to produce it. This function is particularly evident for the fibularis longus and brevis muscles when the foot is fixed in the stance phase during jogging, standing, and walking. At this time, these muscles often function through eccentric contractions. In contrast, the fibularis tertius muscle is thought to work primarily during the swing phase in conjunction with extensor digitorum longus and tibialis anterior muscles to clear the foot.[23]

Fibularis Longus and Fibularis Brevis

The primary function of the fibularis longus and fibularis brevis muscles is not to elevate the lateral margin of the foot as commonly thought. Instead, they appear to act during weight-bearing activities and sports to depress or fix the medial margin of the foot to the contact surface in order to resist inadvertent or excessive inversion of the foot, which is the most vulnerable position of the ankle.[12,24] Because they attach to opposite sides of the 1st metatarsal, the tibialis anterior and fibularis longus muscles form an effective sling for control of inversion and eversion of the foot.[11] The protective mechanisms, in an event of excessive ankle inversion, involve fibularis longus and fibularis brevis muscle contractions guided by central reflexes and mediated by spinal and cortical centers.[25,26]

In the nonweight-bearing position, the fibularis longus and fibularis brevis muscles cause the foot to abduct (toe out) and to evert (elevate its lateral side); together, these two movements act at the subtalar and transverse tarsal joints to produce pronation.[3] Basmajian and Deluca[27] established that during level walking, the fibularis longus muscle helps stabilize the leg and foot in mid-stance. The fibularis longus and the tibialis posterior muscles, working in concert, control the shift from inversion during early stance to a neutral position at mid-stance. The fibularis brevis muscle acts synchronously with the fibularis longus muscle during ordinary walking. Throughout most of the stance phase, the fibularis longus muscle is generally more active in individuals with hypermobile feet ("flatfooted") than in individuals with more typical foot flexibility.

The control of mediolateral balance of the foot was studied during walking in 11 normal adults.[28] When the force plate measured a large lateral component of ground reaction force, electromyographic (EMG) activity of the fibularis longus muscle was marked during the mid-stance phase of gait, whereas the amount of pronation (eversion and abduction) of the foot was small. The researchers suggest that the fibularis longus muscle was active during the mid-stance phase to prevent medial inclination of the leg of the fixed foot, moreover to stabilize the head of the 1st metatarsal because this muscle inserts on the 1st metatarsal. Matsusaka concluded that the fibularis muscles (as well as the tibialis posterior and flexor digitorum longus muscles) contribute to the control of mediolateral balance during ambulation.[28]

Tropp and Odenrick[29] studied postural control in single-leg stance using surface EMG and force plate recordings of 30 physically active men. They found that the ankle played a central role in minor corrections of postural balance. Fibularis longus muscle EMG activity and the location of the center of pressure on the force plate correlated closely with ankle position. When the body experienced major disequilibrium, however, subjects made corrections at the hip. The subject's internal strategy of maintaining balance changed from an inverted pendulum model (at the ankle) to a multisegmental chain model when adjustments at the ankle were no longer able to maintain adequate postural control.

Landry and colleagues[30] compared healthy subjects' postural sway and muscle activity in an unstable shoe with standing barefoot and in a traditional shoe with stability and support features. Standing in an unstable shoe increased postural sway and EMG activity of the fibularis longus, flexor digitorum longus, and anterior compartment muscles in comparison with standing barefoot or wearing stability controlled shoes. Interestingly, no differences were noted in activity of the soleus muscle. Postural sway while standing in the unstable shoe also reduced over a 6-week period.

Patients with ankle instability, when tested by standing on one foot following an ankle inversion injury, showed no significant inversion or eversion weakness compared with the unaffected ankle.[31] The problem was apparently one of impaired muscle control and balance rather than one of muscle weakness. In a more recent study, subjects with chronic ankle instability demonstrated significantly slower reaction time for ankle eversion on the affected side than the control group, because of slower onset of muscle activity to movement (motor time) for the fibularis longus muscle.[32]

Konradsen and colleagues[26] investigated the role of a muscular defense in the stabilization and protection of the ankle joint against sudden forced inversion. Ten volunteers with mechanically stable ankles were tested in different standing and walking situations. Standing on a custom platform with a secret trap door under the examined foot, the trap door was able to tilt 30°, in approximately 80 msec, in the frontal plane and provide a sudden ankle inversion perturbation to the subject. EMG activity of the fibularis longus and brevis muscles were detected, prior to the quadriceps and hamstring muscles, at approximately 54 msec from the start of ankle inversion. The time for the neuromuscular system to perceive the sudden inversion and generate a protective goniometric subtalar eversion muscular response was after 176 msec. The fibularis muscles' reflex alone during standing or walking does not appear to be fast enough to protect the ankle from injury in the case of sudden inversion (less than 100 msec).[26,33] The potential for ligamentous injury to the ankle is high whenever the rate and magnitude of ankle loading exceeds the response time for the neuromuscular system.[34]

Fibularis Tertius

The function and significance of the fibularis tertius muscle is not well studied, and there is limited data to suggest the importance of this phylogenetically young structure. There is consensus that it dorsiflexes the foot and assists in eversion at the ankle.[3,8,35,36] Duchenne observed that when there is absent or weak development of the fibularis tertius muscle, the extensor digitorum longus muscle substitutes for the fibularis tertius muscle in dorsiflexion, abduction, and eversion.[36] Some authors theorize that the fibularis tertius muscle may also play a special proprioceptive role in sensing sudden inversion and then contracting reflexively to protect the anterior talofibular ligament, the most commonly sprained ligament of the body.[12] In contrast, Witvrouw et al[37] performed a prospective study on 100 students and concluded that congenital absence of the fibularis tertius muscle does not increase risk for an ankle ligament injury.

Krammer and associates[4] concluded that the fibularis tertius muscle evolves in bipedal posture for the purpose of shifting the line of body weight toward the medial margin of the foot. This shift from lateral to medial develops in infant standing balance and with the onset of walking, and it occurs in each walking cycle of an adult human.

Conversely, Jungers et al[23] used EMG to test the fibularis tertius muscle, among other muscles, for recruitment and function in human bipedal walking and running and compared it with the data of three species of nonhuman primates typically lacking fibularis tertius muscles. In humans, both walking and running elicited highly predictable recruitment of the fibularis longus and fibularis brevis muscles only during stance phase, peaking just after mid-stance. The recruitment of the fibularis tertius muscle occurred predominantly during the swing phase. It functions in concert with tibialis anterior and extensor digitorum longus muscles, likely assisting to dorsiflex the foot at the ankle, so that the toes clear the ground in anticipation of the next stance phase. In doing so, the inverting effect of the tibialis anterior muscle is balanced by the everting component of the fibularis tertius muscle and the sole of the foot is leveled prior to initial contact. In nonhuman primates lacking a fibularis tertius muscle, the fibularis longus or brevis muscle is active during the swing phase. Although these muscles are evertors of the foot, they are also plantar flexors. A more economical way to counter the inverting effect of the tibialis anterior muscle is to recruit a dorsiflexor/evertor, which may explain the evolution of the fibularis tertius muscle in humans as an adaptation to insure functional efficiency.

2.3. Functional Unit

The functional unit to which a muscle belongs includes the muscles that reinforce and counter its actions as well as the joints that the muscle crosses. The interdependence of these structures is functionally reflected in the organization and neural connections of the sensory motor cortex. The functional unit is emphasized because the presence of a TrP in one muscle of the unit increases the likelihood that the other muscles of the unit will also develop TrPs. When inactivating TrPs in a muscle, one must be concerned about TrPs that may develop in muscles that are functionally interdependent. Boxes 64-1 and 64-2 grossly represent the functional unit of the fibularis longus and brevis muscles, and the fibularis tertius muscle, respectively.[38]

3. CLINICAL PRESENTATION

3.1. Referred Pain Pattern

The fibularis muscles can exhibit TrPs in any part of the muscle. Fibularis longus and fibularis brevis TrPs project pain and tenderness primarily to the region over the lateral malleolus of

Box 64-1 Functional unit of the fibularis longus and brevis muscles

Action	Synergists	Antagonists
Eversion of the foot	Extensor digitorum longus Fibularis tertius	Tibialis anterior Tibialis posterior Extensor hallucis longus Flexor hallucis longus
Plantar flexion of the foot	Gastrocnemius Soleus Plantaris Flexor digitorum longus Flexor hallucis longus Tibialis posterior	Fibularis tertius Tibialis anterior Extensor digitorum longus Extensor hallucis longus

Box 64-2 Functional unit of the fibularis tertius muscle

Action	Synergists	Antagonists
Eversion of the foot	Extensor digitorum longus Fibularis longus and brevis	Tibialis anterior Tibialis posterior Extensor hallucis longus Flexor hallucis longus
Dorsiflexion of the foot	Tibialis anterior Extensor digitorum longus Extensor hallucis longus	Gastrocnemius Soleus Plantaris Fibularis longus and brevis Flexor digitorum longus Flexor hallucis longus Tibialis posterior

the ankle, above, behind, and below it; they also extend a short distance along the lateral aspect of the foot (Figure 64-3A).[39-41] A pain pattern of fibularis longus TrPs may cover the lateral aspect of the middle third of the leg as well.[39,40]

Jacobsen[42] reported a pain pattern referred from fibularis longus and fibularis brevis TrPs as going around the back of the lateral malleolus. Bates and Grunwaldt[43] reported that, in children, the referred pain pattern of the fibularis longus muscle also concentrates behind the lateral malleolus but tends to extend up to the side of the leg rather than along the side of the foot. Good[44] attributed the symptoms in 15 of 100 patients with painful feet to myalgic spots in the fibularis brevis muscle. Kellgren[45] reported that the injection of 6% hypertonic saline solution into the fibularis longus muscle evoked pain referred to the lateral ankle.

Fibularis tertius TrPs refer pain and tenderness along the anterolateral aspect of the ankle and project downward behind the lateral malleolus to the lateral aspect of the heel (Figure 64-3B). A less commonly referred pain pattern runs distally over the dorsum of the foot.

3.2. Symptoms

Weakness of any of the three fibularis muscles can contribute to a patient report of "weak ankles." Patients with fibularis TrPs report pain and tenderness behind the ankle and over the lateral malleolus, especially after an inversion sprain of the ankle. These patients often report spraining their ankles frequently. Ankle instability limits performance during higher-level activities in sports such as basketball, soccer, gymnastics,[46] or hockey.

Patients with fibularis TrPs, in addition to inverting and spraining their ankles potentially because of inadequate fibularis muscle support, are also prone to ankle fractures. Treatment of the fracture by a cast on the ankle, which immobilizes the fibularis muscles, may aggravate and perpetuate fibularis TrPs that cause ankle pain. In this situation, the fracture can be healing, or fully healed, and not be the cause of the patient's reported and continuous ankle pain.

3.3. Patient Examination

After a thorough subjective examination, the clinician should make a detailed drawing representing the pain pattern described by the patient. This depiction will assist in planning the physical examination and can be useful in monitoring the progression of

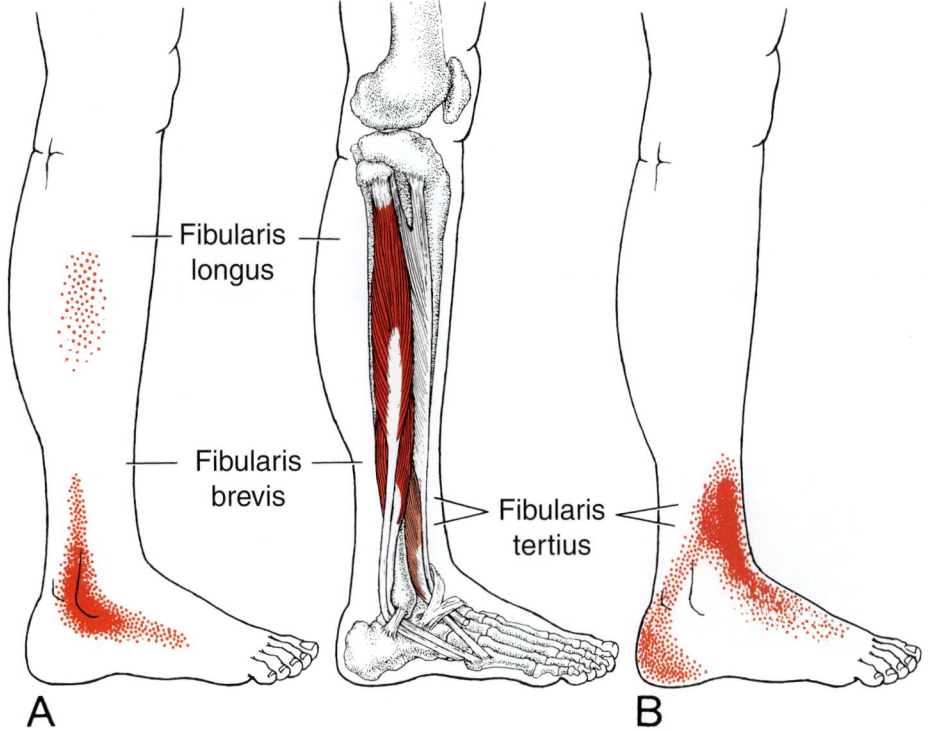

Figure 64-3. Pain patterns (dark red) referred from TrP locations in the fibularis muscles. The essential patterns of referred pain and tenderness are solid red, and the red stippling shows the less common extension of pain. These TrPs all refer pain distally. A, Composite pain pattern for the fibularis longus and fibularis brevis muscles (medium red). The stippled pattern proximally applies only to the fibularis longus TrP. B, Pain pattern of the fibularis tertius muscle (light red).

the patient as symptoms improve or change. The type, quality, and location of the pain should be carefully assessed, and the utilization of standardized outcome tools is imperative when examining patients with lower extremity dysfunctions.

Observation of static and dynamic posture is essential, given the role of the fibularis muscles in postural stability. Functional testing such as double- and single-leg squat will allow a quick assessment of hip and knee control, as well as a quick assessment of talocrural, subtalar, and mid-foot range of motion. Timed single-leg stance with eyes open and closed will give a quantitative measure of balance and will allow the clinician to observe foot and ankle strategies related to balance and control.

The clinician should observe the patient's gait pattern from behind to note excessive pronation of the foot or other related deviations. A mediolaterally rocking foot with associated fibularis longus TrPs can produce a sense of ankle weakness severe enough to convince some patients to use an assistive device or ambulate with an antalgic gait where stride length of the uninvolved leg is notably decreased due to perceived instability of the stance leg. Patients with latent TrPs in the fibularis longus muscle are asymptomatic with regard to pain but, for years, these latent TrPs may cause characteristic calluses and inhibition weakness of the ankles.[47]

For proper assessment and examination of the fibularis muscles, the clinician should assess bilateral ankle and foot posture, range of motion, and accessory motion of the talocrural, subtalar, transverse tarsal, talon naviculocuneiform, and cuboid-fifth metatarsal joints. Examination may identify underlying dysfunction contributing to joint hypermobility and/or hypomobility and can lead to a mechanically or functionally unstable ankle. The clinician should also examine the patient's shoes for proper fit and for abnormal wearing patterns.

To examine for fibularis longus and fibularis brevis muscle weakness, the patient lies on the side not being tested.

The clinician stabilizes the uppermost leg and places the foot in plantar flexion and eversion; with the toes relaxed, the patient then holds the foot in that position against resistance supplied by the clinician, who presses against the lateral border of the foot in the direction of inversion and dorsiflexion.[48,49] While applying resistance, the tendons are visualized at the lateral ankle and in the foot. The calf muscles and long flexors of the toes can also produce powerful plantar flexion, but the fibularis longus and brevis muscles are the chief force for eversion of the foot in plantar flexion. The fibularis tertius and extensor digitorum longus muscles also produce eversion, but they dorsiflex, rather than plantar flex the foot. Patients with fibularis longus and fibularis brevis TrPs have difficulty holding the foot in eversion and plantar flexion against resistance when compared with the uninvolved side. Baker[46] describes a ratchety resistance to movement as "breakaway" weakness. The more active the TrPs, the more marked is this weakness.

Active fibularis longus and fibularis brevis TrPs cause pain on eversion effort with the foot already everted, and they also painfully restrict passive inversion range of motion. Fibularis tertius TrPs cause pain on active dorsiflexion in the dorsiflexed (shortened) position and limit passive plantar flexion.

3.4. Trigger Point Examination

Fibularis Longus

For examination of the fibularis muscles for TrPs, the patient lies side-lying or supine with the foot free to move (Figure 64-4). Although the most common TrP location in the fibularis longus muscle is about 2 to 4 cm (approximately an inch or slightly more) distal to the head of the fibula over the shaft of the fibula, the entire muscle should be examined for TrPs (Figure 64-4A). Taut bands are clearly delineated by cross-fiber flat palpation

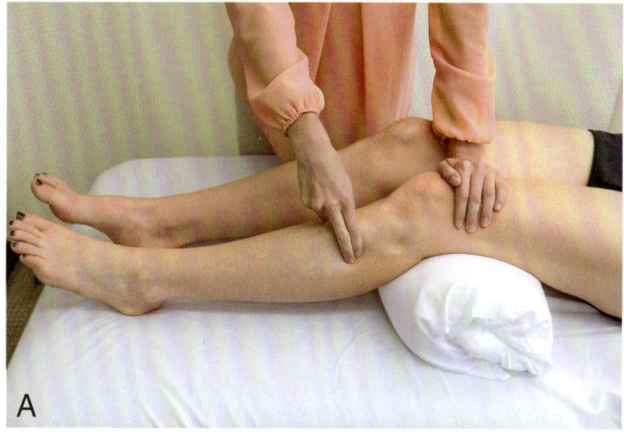
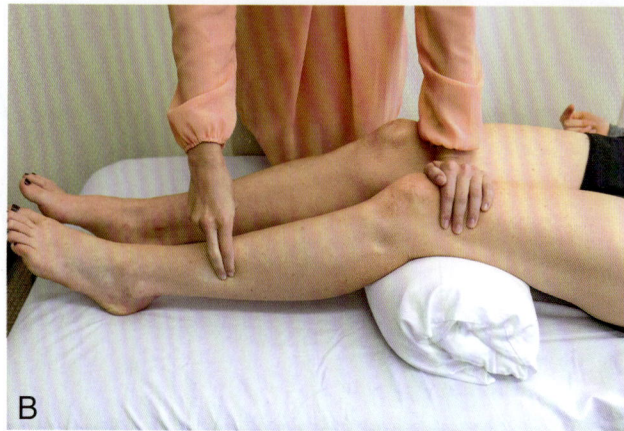
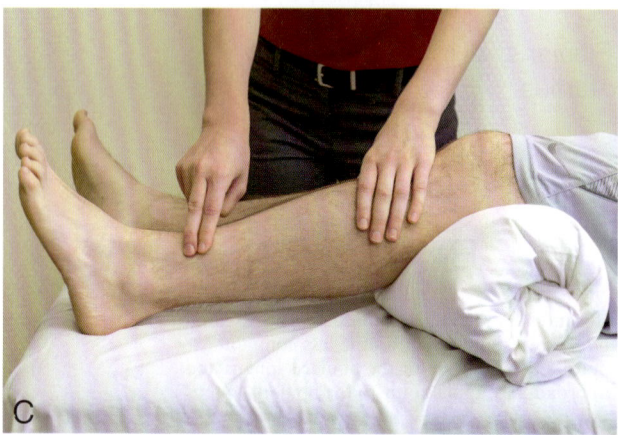

Figure 64-4. Cross-fiber flat palpation of A, Fibularis longus muscle. B, Fibularis brevis muscle. C, Fibularis tertius muscle.

against the underlying bone. The common fibular nerve crosses diagonally over the neck of the fibula just below the fibular head and has a cordlike consistency. The nerve is distinguished from a taut band by its proximal position and a course running across the muscle rather than running the length of the muscle nearly parallel to the shaft of the fibula.[50] Excessive pressure on the nerve may cause painful tingling sensations (dysesthesias) over the lateral side of the leg and the foot.

Fibularis Brevis

For clinical examination of fibularis brevis TrPs, the patient is side-lying or supine so that the muscle is relaxed. Trigger points in the fibularis brevis muscle can be found on either side of, and deep to, the fibularis longus tendon near the junction of the middle and lower third of the leg (Figure 64-4B). These TrPs also are palpable against the shaft of the fibula utilizing a cross-fiber flat palpation. Pressure on TrPs in either of these muscles characteristically elicits referred pain in, behind, and distal to the lateral malleolus, and this area also exhibits referred tenderness.

Fibularis Tertius

Trigger points in the fibularis tertius muscle (Figure 64-4C) are identified using cross-fiber flat palpation slightly distal and anterior to the fibularis brevis muscle and proximal and anterior to the lateral malleolus. The tendon of this muscle stands out and is readily palpable in the anterolateral aspect of the ankle and foot (lateral to the extensor digitorum longus tendons) when the patient attempts to evert the foot by lifting the 5th metatarsal up and out (dorsiflexion with eversion). Taut bands in this muscle are often difficult to delineate by palpation, but pressure on the sensitive TrP usually refers pain to the anterolateral ankle and sometimes to the lateral side of the heel and dorsum of the foot (Figure 64-3B).

4. DIFFERENTIAL DIAGNOSIS

4.1. Activation and Perpetuation of Trigger Points

A posture or activity that activates a TrP, if not corrected, can perpetuate it. In any part of the fibularis muscles, TrPs may be activated by unaccustomed eccentric loading, eccentric exercise in an unconditioned muscle, or maximal or submaximal concentric loading.[51] Trigger points may also be activated or aggravated when the muscle is placed in a shortened or lengthened position for an extended period of time. For instance, a fall with twisting and inversion of the ankle can activate TrPs by overloading the fibularis longus and fibularis brevis muscles. Weakness or inhibition induced by prolonged immobilization, as by an ankle cast, predisposes these muscles to developing TrPs.

Sleeping with the foot strongly plantar flexed places the fibularis longus and fibularis brevis muscles in the shortened position for prolonged periods. This common position aggravates fibularis TrPs.

A tight elastic top of a long sock can constrict circulation in the fibularis longus, extensor digitorum longus, and gastrocnemius muscles by direct compression, like a tourniquet, and thus perpetuate their TrPs. An indented red line or marking around the leg indicates a high probability of this constriction. The soleus muscle usually is too deep to be affected.

Wearing high heels perpetuates fibularis TrPs by shifting the body weight forward onto the ball of the foot during standing, which reduces the base of support, thus increasing the length of the lever arm against which the muscles must operate. The resultant functional instability overloads the fibularis longus and fibularis brevis muscles. A shoe with a spike heel of any height provides an unstable base of support that can overload the fibularis muscles.

Clinically, individuals with flat feet and unsupported arches are likely to have spot tenderness and taut bands in the fibularis longus and fibularis brevis muscles,[52] as these muscles are more active during the stance phase of gait.[23,27]

4.2. Associated Trigger Points

Associated TrPs can develop in the referred pain areas of other TrPs.[53] Therefore, muscles in the referred pain areas for each muscle should also be considered for examination. The fibularis longus muscle is almost always involved when either of the other two fibularis muscles has TrPs. Not surprisingly, the muscle that most commonly develops TrPs associated with TrP-weakened fibularis muscles is their prime agonist for eversion, the extensor digitorum longus muscle. The fact that the extensor digitorum longus muscle also serves as a prime antagonist to the fibularis longus muscle can account for the likelihood of both muscles developing TrPs. Fibularis longus TrPs are also likely to occur in association with tibialis posterior TrPs as these two muscles are specific antagonists in regard to inversion-eversion, but they are synergistic in regard to plantar flexion and to stabilizing the weight-bearing foot.

Although the fibularis longus and fibularis brevis muscles are weak assistants to the prime plantar flexors, TrPs in the powerful gastrocnemius and soleus muscles are not likely to induce associated TrPs in the fibularis muscles. The function of the triceps surae muscle is also not likely to be compromised because of TrPs in the fibularis muscles.

Gluteus minimus TrPs refer pain to the lateral aspect of the leg and can induce associated TrPs in the fibularis muscles. The extensor digitorum longus and fibularis tertius muscles work closely together as synergists and TrPs in one can induce associated TrPs in the other. Five extensor muscles of the leg project referred pain in patterns that might be confused with those of the fibularis muscles: the tibialis anterior muscle, the long and short extensor muscles of the hallux, and the long and short extensor muscles of the lesser toes. However, TrPs in these other muscles do not refer pain behind the lateral malleolus, to the heel, or to the lateral side of the leg.

The lateral heel pain referred from fibularis tertius TrPs contrasts from the soleus muscle referral pain pattern, as it does not include the entire Achilles tendon or the plantar surface of the heel. Because of the local tenderness associated with the pain referred to the ankle by TrPs in the fibularis muscles, these myofascial pain symptoms are easily mistaken for arthritis of the ankle joint.[54]

4.3. Associated Pathology

Trigger points in the fibularis muscles are associated with, and can mimic, many different conditions; therefore, a thorough medical screening and examination with possible referral to another healthcare practitioner may be necessary. Fibular nerve entrapment,[2] lumbar radiculopathy,[55] Morton foot structure,[56,57] acute or chronic exertional compartment syndrome,[58] ankle sprains or fractures,[59] and rupture of fibularis longus or brevis muscles[22,60] can all be associated with TrPs in the fibularis muscles.

Fibular neuropathy is the most frequent mononeuropathy encountered in the lower extremity and the third most common focal neuropathy encountered overall, after median and ulnar neuropathies.[2,61,62] In children, the common fibular nerve was the most often injured (59%), as opposed to the deep (12%), superficial (5%), or a nonlocalizable level of injury (24%). These findings are similar to those of adults.[63] Entrapment of the common fibular nerve, the superficial fibular nerve, or the deep fibular nerve can produce symptoms of pain and paresthesias in the anterolateral ankle and dorsum of the foot with concomitant weakness of the ankle,[2] which can be suggestive of fibularis myofascial pain syndromes.

Numbness and tingling caused by entrapment of the common fibular nerve appears on the lateral part of the posterior aspect of the proximal leg, distal third of the anterior surface of leg, and dorsum of the foot. The superficial branch supplies the anterolateral leg and dorsum of the foot, except for the triangular area of the first interdigital web space that is supplied by the deep fibular nerve (Figure 64-5B). The Achilles reflex will be preserved in the presence of nerve entrapment.[3,12]

The superficial fibular nerve emerges through the deep fascia in the lower third of the leg[3] where it is vulnerable to acute or chronic trauma and subject to entrapment by the fascia. The pain and altered sensation without motor deficit in the distribution of this nerve appears confusingly like a combination of tibialis anterior and fibularis tertius muscle myofascial pain syndromes. This entrapment, however, is not dependent on TrPs in these muscles.

Taut bands caused by TrPs in the fibularis longus muscle increase the tension of the muscle and can cause entrapment of the common fibular nerve and/or the superficial and deep fibular[47] nerves, if the nerve branches far enough proximally (Figure 64-5A). The nerve compression may occur against the fibula, or it may result from compression of the nerve by muscle tension on the bands of fascia that surround the nerve.[64,65] The compression of motor fibers in the common fibular nerve or in the deep fibular nerve by taut bands in the fibularis longus muscle can cause significant foot drop.[39,40] Foot drop and changes in sensation caused by entrapment of the fibular nerve may result from residual fibularis TrPs that originated during an L4, L5 radiculopathy that was later resolved.

Reported causes of fibular nerve palsy in the leg include proximal fibular fracture,[66] tibial plateau fracture,[67] traumatic knee dislocation,[68] ligamentous knee injury,[69] ligament or bony injury of the ankle,[66] improper casting after ankle injury[70] or laceration.[71,72] Other less common causes include osteoarthritis,[73] tumors,[72] and iatrogenic injury suffered during orthopedic surgery.[70]

Two common tests were evaluated for their diagnostic accuracy of fibular nerve compression neuropathy. The scratch collapse test showed a sensitivity of 0.77 and a specificity of 0.99, whereas the Tinel sign showed 0.65 and 0.99, respectively. Both are sensitive and specific provocative tests that aid in the diagnosis of common fibular neuropathy.[74]

Together, the symptoms of common fibular nerve entrapment and the referred pain of fibularis TrPs may suggest a radicular source of pain which, if present, can also activate fibularis TrPs in a segmental distribution. Therefore, patients with such symptoms may have a myofascial pain syndrome with or without neurologic symptoms and signs; or their symptoms may be due to a combination of radicular pain, fibular nerve entrapment, and referred myofascial pain.

The Morton foot structure (relatively short first and long second metatarsal) with a mediolaterally rocking foot may perpetuate TrPs primarily in the fibularis longus[39,40,47] and also fibularis brevis muscles but rarely in the fibularis tertius muscle. Individuals may have an equally marked Morton foot structure bilaterally but have pain only on one side, usually the side of a shorter lower extremity. Similarly, bunions may appear the same on both feet but may be painful on only one foot. Even with the same foot structure bilaterally, pain may be present in one foot if there is a leg length discrepancy that results in unequal force distribution.

The Morton foot structure must be distinguished from Morton neuroma (Morton metatarsalgia). The latter is generally thought to result from interdigital nerve entrapment in the region of the transverse metatarsal ligament.[75] The Morton foot structure is a variation in skeletal structure[57] that is usually not painful but can cause problems for muscles and other structures. Indeed, abnormal pressures caused by the structure could be a factor in development of the neuroma. The foot squeeze test and web space tenderness between the 2nd and 3rd metatarsals are sensitive tests that can be performed easily in the clinic to identify a potential interdigital neuroma.[56]

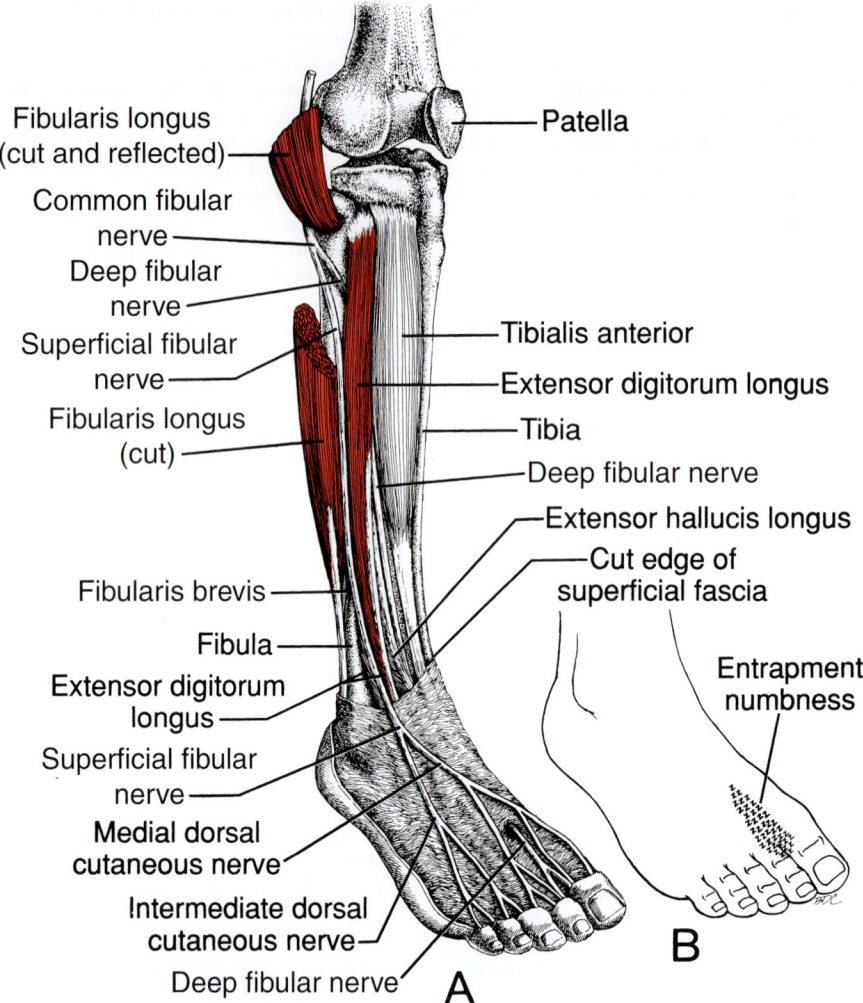

Figure 64-5. Entrapment of the common, deep, or superficial fibular nerve. A, By a tense fibularis longus muscle (dark red) that is reflected. Entrapment of the deep fibular nerve can be caused by a tense extensor digitorum longus muscle (medium red). Both the deep and superficial branches of the fibular nerve pass between the fibularis longus muscle and the underlying fibula where taut bands associated with TrPs in the fibularis longus muscle can compress the nerve and cause neurapraxia. B, Deep fibular nerve zone of entrapment numbness (Zs) on the dorsum of the first and second toes due to taut TrP bands in the fibularis longus muscle.

Acute or chronic exertional lateral compartment syndrome with pain along the lateral side of the leg that is aggravated by activity can be suggestive of fibularis longus and fibularis brevis TrP pain, but the tenderness and tension of the musculature in the compartment syndrome is diffuse, not localized, as in the myofascial syndromes. Immediate referral to a physician is warranted when acute compartment syndrome is suspected after major trauma and/or a fracture. The subject may present with one or all of the five Ps: pain, pallor, paresthesias, paralysis, and pulselessness. Time is of the essence in referral to a specialist, as an emergency fasciotomy may be indicated, with tissue necrosis occurring after only 4 to 6 hours of ischemia.[76]

Chronic exertional or exercise induced compartment syndrome is likely to develop in runners, military personnel, or endurance athletes.[58,77] It occurs with repetitive activity and microtrauma, which increases intramuscular pressure causing transient ischemia. Unlike acute compartment syndrome, tissue necrosis does not occur because symptoms typically resolve when the aggravating activity is stopped and the patient rests.[59] Conservative treatment addressing biomechanical issues, soft tissue restriction, and activity modification with proper progression of load and exercise can manage this condition in some athletes.[78] Diebal[79] published a case series of 10 patients who underwent 6 weeks of therapy with a focus on changing subjects running technique to promote a forefoot running pattern, decreased stride length, and increased cadence. This intervention led to reduced post–running leg intracompartmental pressures, and significantly reduced pain and disability for up to 1 year following intervention.[79] When conservative treatment fails, an open fasciotomy is successful in approximately two-thirds of the athletic population.[58]

The trauma that causes a lateral ankle sprain can also readily activate fibularis TrPs that refer pain and tenderness to the ankle. Examination of the fibularis muscles for TrPs reveals this source of the symptoms; however, other causes of the pain should be ruled out. Usually, injury to the lateral ligaments of the ankle results from an inversion-plantar flexion sprain. The first structures to tear are the anterior lateral joint capsule and the anterior talofibular ligament.[80] The immediate region of the torn ligament is tender and swollen. Tenderness referred from TrPs usually includes a larger area without such marked swelling.

Patients sustaining a plantar flexion and inversion ankle sprain, or who have an unstable foot, are at risk for a subluxation or misalignment of the cuboid in an inferomedial direction. This condition can potentially irritate the surrounding joint capsule, ligaments, and the fibularis longus tendon. The fibularis longus muscle's strength and function depends on proper position and stability of the cuboid.[59] Jennings and Davies[81] found 7 of 104 (6.7%) patients with lateral ankle sprains had subluxed cuboids. In ballet dancers, 17% of foot injuries involve the cuboid.[82] One or two treatment sessions of manual (cuboid squeeze) or manipulative (cuboid whip) therapy prove to be extremely effective in treating this poorly recognized condition.[81,82] The fibularis longus muscle should be examined for TrPs and, if present, they should be released prior to treating the cuboid dysfunction.

An acute fibularis tendon dislocation or tearing occurs when the ankle sustains a sudden forced dorsiflexion accompanied by a concomitant reflexive contraction of the fibularis muscles. Fibularis brevis longitudinal tendon tears are more frequent than fibularis longus tendon tears and are present in up to 30% of patients undergoing surgery for ankle instability.[22,83] Squires et al[22] identified six findings that are key to diagnosis of tendon tears: swelling posterolaterally along the course of the tendons, pain on palpation along the course of the tendon, pain exacerbated by compression of the superior fibular retinaculum as the patient actively everts the ankle, crepitation or squeaking of the tendons, pain with extreme active dorsiflexion, difficulty maintaining stability on single-stance heel rise, and retro malleolar pain with anterior drawer testing. Conservative treatment consists of anti-inflammatory medication, lateral heel wedge, bracing, and physical therapy. Treatment of an established tear has a high failure rate and often requires operative management.

Fibularis tendon subluxation can also be the result of ankle sprains, contributing to prolonged pain and dysfunction. The integrity of the fibularis retinaculum can be tested with the patient in prone with the knee bent to 90° (Figure 64-6). While stabilizing the leg, the foot is placed in dorsiflexion with eversion while palpating gently over the lateral malleolus and heel. The patient then moves through plantar flexion and dorsiflexion of the ankle while maintaining eversion. The clinician will see and/or feel for sliding of the fibularis tendon over the lateral malleolus. Surgical repair is often required if the fibularis retinaculum is disrupted.[84]

The os peroneum is a sesamoid bone of the fibularis longus tendon that develops in about 10% of individuals. When it has suffered trauma and becomes painful, it can be treated successfully either surgically[60] or conservatively.[85] The os peroneum may fracture and rupture the fibularis longus tendon[60] when the individual tries to prevent a fall[86] or imposes sudden inversion stress on the ankle, often with an audible snap.[85]

5. CORRECTIVE ACTIONS

Adjusting posture can decrease prolonged shortening of these muscles especially if the individual's feet do not rest firmly on the floor when seated. For correction of under thigh compression caused by too high of a chair seat, possible solutions include a footstool to raise the feet, shortening of the chair legs, or tilting the seat pan downward at the front of the seat.

In general, the leg muscles feel better if the ankle is maintained in a neutral position throughout the night; therefore, adjusting the patient's sleeping posture may be necessary. This position is facilitated by having the bed sheets at the foot of the bed untucked as this will reduce external stresses of the ankle into excessive plantar flexion (see Figure 65-6). When side-lying, placing a pillow between the legs and knee will place the foot and ankle into a more restful position. Patients with irritable TrPs should avoid lying on the affected side as the pressure from the bed may perpetuate TrP activity.

Shoes that provide good arch and foot support, such as some sneakers, jogging shoes, and boots that are snug, effectively reduce strain on the fibularis muscles, thus making specific TrP therapy more effective. High heels, and especially stiletto heels, should be avoided. For exercise such as walking, the individual is encouraged to walk on flat surfaces instead of uneven ground such as uneven bricks, cracks, grass, or sand. In addition, a surface that is level from side to side and not tilted laterally, as is the edge of a crowned road or a slanted beach, is optimal. The patient with TrPs and weakness of the fibularis longus and fibularis brevis muscles should avoid walking on a slanted sidewalk or running on a laterally slanted track, which contributes to overload of those muscles.

Self-pressure release for TrPs in the fibularis muscles can be performed in long sitting, or while seated in a chair (Figure 64-7A, B, and C). Pressure can be provided manually with the thumbs (Figure 64-7A and B), with a TrP release tool, or with a lacrosse or tennis ball (Figure 64-7C). Finding the sensitive spot with the thumbs or a tool, light pressure (no more than 4/10 pain) should be applied and held for 15 to 30 seconds until pain reduces. This technique may be repeated five times per session, several times per day (Figure 64-7A, B, and C).

Gentle passive self-stretch of the fibularis longus and fibularis brevis muscles can be performed in the sitting position. The patient grasps the forefoot and gently pulls the foot up and toward the nose until a stretch is felt on the outside of the leg (inversion, adduction, and dorsiflexion) (Figure 64-8). Postisometric relaxation can facilitate a painless stretch. For this technique, the patient uses one hand to stabilize the leg just above the ankle and the other hand to resist an active effort to evert and plantar flex the foot gently while slowly taking in a deep breath. Then, while exhaling slowly and fully relaxing the leg and foot, the patient takes up any slack that develops by maintaining a steady pull up toward the nose (inversion and dorsiflexion). After a pause, this cycle should be repeated until no further gain in the range of inversion and dorsiflexion occurs.

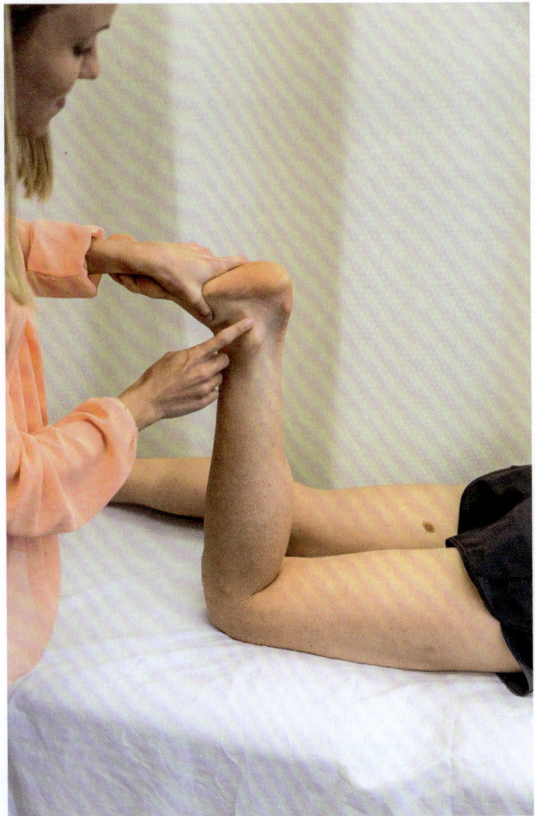

Figure 64-6. Test for subluxation of the fibularis tendons. The patient's foot is placed in dorsiflexion with eversion. The clinician maintains eversion while the patient performs plantar flexion and dorsiflexion. The clinician palpates the tendons to monitor if the tendons sublux over the lateral malleolus.

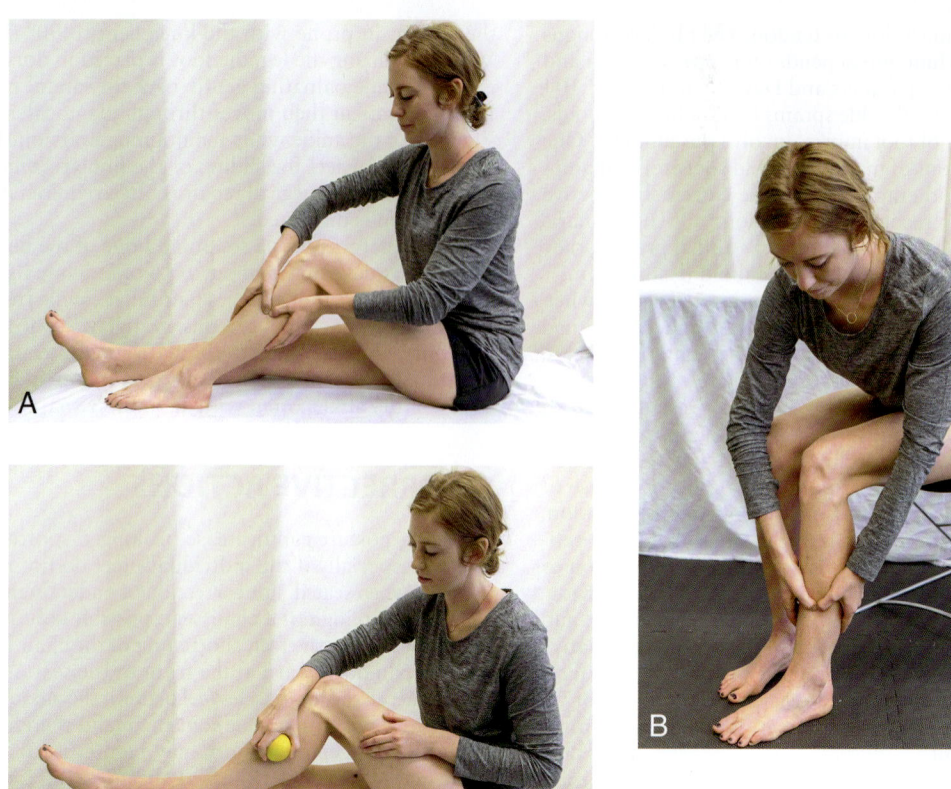

Figure 64-7. Trigger point self-pressure release. A and B, Manual release using thumbs. C, Using a lacrosse ball.

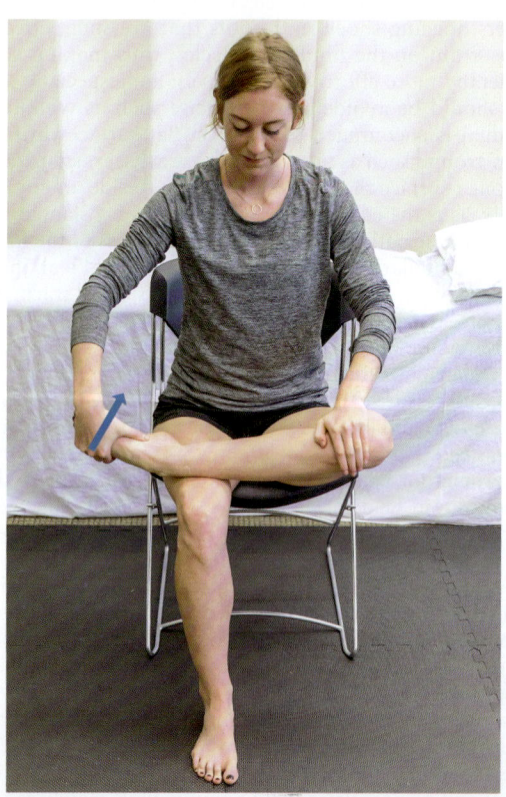

Figure 64-8. Self-stretch of the fibularis longus and fibularis brevis muscles. The arrow identifies the direction of pull: inversion first with plantar flexion, then dorsiflexion of the fully inverted foot. This stretch can be effectively combined with postisometric relaxation.

For patients able to handle the additional complexity, voluntarily trying to invert and dorsiflex the foot while using the hand to assist moving it in the same direction may increase further gains. This contraction activates the tibialis anterior and posterior muscles, and the antagonists of the fibularis longus and fibularis brevis muscles, reciprocally inhibiting them and thereby increasing their relaxation and tolerance to stretch.

It is important to avoid stretching to their full range of motion those muscles that cross hypermobile joints, especially after an acute lateral ankle sprain or fracture. Care should be taken to avoid stretching into inversion for the first several weeks after injury, as this could cause pain, apprehension, and further injury.

References

1. Federative Committee on Anatomical Terminology. *Terminologia anatomica*. Stuttgart, Germany: Thieme; 1998 (p. 140).
2. Marciniak C. Fibular (peroneal) neuropathy: electrodiagnostic features and clinical correlates. *Phys Med Rehabil Clin N Am*. 2013;24(1):121-137.
3. Standring S. *Gray's Anatomy: The Anatomical Basis of Clinical Practice*. 41st ed. London, UK: Elsevier; 2015.
4. Krammer EB, Lischka MF, Gruber H. Gross anatomy and evolutionary significance of the human peroneus III. *Anat Embryol (Berl)*. 1979;155(3):291-302.
5. Stevens K, Platt A, Ellis H. A cadaveric study of the peroneus tertius muscle. *Clin Anat*. 1993;6(2):106-110.
6. Hammerschlag WA, Goldner JL. Chronic peroneal tendon subluxation produced by an anomalous peroneus brevis: case report and literature review. *Foot Ankle*. 1989;10(1):45-47.
7. Bardeen C. The musculature, Section 5. In: Jackson CM, ed. *Morris's Human Anatomy*. 6th ed. Philadelphia, PA: Blakiston's Son & Co; 1921.
8. Clemente C. *Gray's Anatomy of the Human Body*. 30th ed. Philadelphia, PA: Lea & Febiger; 1985.
9. Rios Nascimento SR, Watanabe Costa R, Ruiz CR, Wafae N. Analysis on the incidence of the fibularis quartus muscle using magnetic resonance imaging. *Anat Res Int*. 2012;2012:485149.
10. Sookur PA, Naraghi AM, Bleakney RR, Jalan R, Chan O, White LM. Accessory muscles: anatomy, symptoms, and radiologic evaluation. *Radiographics*. 2008;28(2):481-499.

11. Netter FH. *Musculoskeletal System. Part 1: Anatomy, Physiology and Metabolic Disorders.* Vol 8. Summit, NJ: Ciba-Geigy Corporation; 1987.
12. Moore KL, Dalley AF, Agur AMR. *Clinically Oriented Anatomy.* 6th ed. Philadelphia, PA: Lippincott Williams and Wilkins; 2009 (pp. 589-652).
13. Wang X-T, Rosenberg ZS, Mechlin MB, Schweitzer ME. Normal variants and diseases of the peroneal tendons and superior peroneal retinaculum: MR imaging features. *Radiographics.* 2005;25(3):587-602.
14. Le Minor JM. Comparative anatomy and significance of the sesamoid bone of the peroneus longus muscle (os peroneum). *J Anat.* 1987;151:85-99.
15. Muehleman C, Williams J, Bareither ML. A radiologic and histologic study of the os peroneum: prevalence, morphology, and relationship to degenerative joint disease of the foot and ankle in a cadaveric sample. *Clin Anat.* 2009;22(6):747-754.
16. Patil V, Frisch NC, Ebraheim NA. Anatomical variations in the insertion of the peroneus (fibularis) longus tendon. *Foot Ankle Int.* 2007;28(11):1179-1182.
17. Mittal PS, Joshi SS, Chhaparwal R, Joshi SD. Prevalence and mophometry of os peroneum amongst Central Indians. *J Clin Diagn Res.* 2014;8(11):AC08-AC10.
18. Yammine K, Eric M. The fibularis (peroneus) tertius muscle in humans: a meta-analysis of anatomical studies with clinical and evolutionary implications. *Biomed Res Int.* 2017;2017:6021707.
19. Jana R, Roy TS. Variant insertion of the fibularis tertius muscle is an evidence of the progressive evolutionary adaptation for the bipedal gait. *Clin Pract.* 2011;1(4):e81.
20. Ercikti N, Apaydin N, Kocabiyik N, Yazar F. Insertional characteristics of the peroneus tertius tendon: revisiting the anatomy of an underestimated muscle. *J Foot Ankle Surg.* 2016;55(4):709-713.
21. Baima J, Krivickas L. Evaluation and treatment of peroneal neuropathy. *Curr Rev Musculoskelet Med.* 2008;1(2):147-153.
22. Squires N, Myerson MS, Gamba C. Surgical treatment of peroneal tendon tears. *Foot Ankle Clin.* 2007;12(4):675-695, vii.
23. Jungers WL, Meldrum DJ, Stern JT. The functional and evolutionary significance of the human peroneus tertius muscle. *J Hum Evol.* 1993;25(5):377-386.
24. Linford CW, Hopkins JT, Schulthies SS, Freland B, Draper DO, Hunter I. Effects of neuromuscular training on the reaction time and electromechanical delay of the peroneus longus muscle. *Arch Phys Med Rehabil.* 2006;87(3):395-401.
25. Menacho Mde O, Pereira HM, Oliveira BI, Chagas LM, Toyohara MT, Cardoso JR. The peroneus reaction time during sudden inversion test: systematic review. *J Electromyogr Kinesiol.* 2010;20(4):559-565.
26. Konradsen L, Voigt M, Højsgaard C. Ankle inversion injuries. The role of the dynamic defense mechanism. *Am J Sports Med.* 1997;25(1):54-58.
27. Basmajian J, Deluca C. *Muscles Alive.* 5th ed. Baltimore, MD: Williams & Wilkins; 1985.
28. Matsusaka N. Control of the medial-lateral balance in walking. *Acta Orthop Scand.* 1986;57(6):555-559.
29. Tropp H, Odenrick P. Postural control in single-limb stance. *J Orthop Res.* 1992;6(6):833-839.
30. Landry SC, Nigg BM, Tecante KE. Standing in an unstable shoe increases postural sway and muscle activity of selected smaller extrinsic foot muscles. *Gait Posture.* 2010;32(2):215-219.
31. Baker B. The muscle trigger: evidence of overload injury. *J Neurol Orthop Med Surg.* 1986;7(1):35-44.
32. Kavanagh JJ, Bisset LM, Tsao H. Deficits in reaction time due to increased motor time of peroneus longus in people with chronic ankle instability. *J Biomech.* 2012;45(3):605-608.
33. Hung YJ. Neuromuscular control and rehabilitation of the unstable ankle. *World J Orthop.* 2015;6(5):434-438.
34. Ricard MD, Schulties SS, Saret JJ. Effects of high-top and low-top shoes on ankle inversion. *J Athl Train.* 2000;35(1):38-43.
35. Sutherland DH. An electromyographic study of the plantar flexors of the ankle in normal walking on the level. *J Bone Joint Surg Am.* 1966;48(1):66-71.
36. Duchenne G. *Physiology of Motion.* Philadelphia, PA: Lippincott; 1949.
37. Witvrouw E, Borre KV, Willems TM, Huysmans J, Broos E, De Clercq D. The significance of peroneus tertius muscle in ankle injuries: a prospective study. *Am J Sports Med.* 2006;34(7):1159-1163.
38. Simons DG, Travell J, Simons L. *Travell & Simon's Myofascial Pain and Dysfunction: The Trigger Point Manual.* Vol 1. 2nd ed. Baltimore, MD: Williams & Wilkins; 1999 (p. 104).
39. Simons DG. *Chapter 45, Myofascial Pain Syndrome Due to Trigger Points.* St. Louis, MO: Mosby; 1988.
40. Simons DG, Travell J. Chapter 25, Myofascial pain syndromes. In: Wall PD, Melzack R, Bonica JJ, eds. *Textbook of Pain.* 2nd ed. Edinburgh, Scotland; New York, NY: Churchill Livingstone; 1989:368-385.
41. Travell J, Rinzler SH. The myofascial genesis of pain. *Postgrad Med.* 1952;11(5):425-434.
42. Jacobsen S. Myofascial pain syndrome [in Danish]. *Ugeskrift for laeger.* 1987;149(9):600-601.
43. Bates T, Grunwaldt E. Myofascial pain in childhood. *J Pediatr.* 1958;53(2):198-209.
44. Good MG. Painful feet. *Practitioner.* 1949;163(975):229-232.
45. Kellgren JH. Observations on referred pain arising from muscle. *Clin Sci.* 1938;3:175-190.
46. Baker BA. Myofascial pain syndromes: ten single muscle cases. *J Neurol Orthop Med Surg.* 1989;10:129-131.
47. Travell J. Low back pain and the Dudley J. Morton foot (long second toe). *Arch Phys Med Rehabil.* 1975;56:566.
48. Janda V. *Muscle Function Testing.* London, England: Butterworths; 1983.
49. Kendall FP, McCreary EK. *Muscles: Testing and Function, with Posture and Pain.* 5th ed. Baltimore, MD: Lippincott Williams & Wilkins; 2005.
50. McMinn RMH, Hutchings RT. *Color Atlas of Human Anatomy.* Chicago, IL: Year Book Medical Publishers; 1977.
51. Gerwin RD, Dommerholt J, Shah JP. An expansion of Simons' integrated hypothesis of trigger point formation. *Curr Pain Headache Rep.* 2004;8(6):468-475.
52. Lange M. *Die Muskelharten (Myogelosen).* Munich, Germany: J.F. Lehmanns; 1931.
53. Hsieh YL, Kao MJ, Kuan TS, Chen SM, Chen JT, Hong CZ. Dry needling to a key myofascial trigger point may reduce the irritability of satellite MTrPs. *Am J Phys Med Rehabil.* 2007;86(5):397-403.
54. Reynolds MD. Myofascial trigger point syndromes in the practice of rheumatology. *Arch Phys Med Rehabil.* 1981;62(3):111-114.
55. Urban LM, MacNeil BJ. Diagnostic accuracy of the slump test for identifying neuropathic pain in the lower limb. *J Orthop Sports Phys Ther.* 2015;45(8):596-603.
56. Owens R, Gougoulias N, Guthrie H, Sakellariou A. Morton's neuroma: clinical testing and imaging in 76 feet, compared to a control group. *Foot Ankle Surg.* 2011;17(3):197-200.
57. Morton DJ. *The Human Foot.* New York, NY: Columbia University Press; 1935.
58. Campano D, Robaina JA, Kusnezov N, Dunn JC, Waterman BR. Surgical management for chronic exertional compartment syndrome of the leg: a systematic review of the literature. *Arthroscopy.* 2016;32(7):1478-1486.
59. Sueki D, Brechter J. *Orthopedic Rehabilitation Clinical Advisor.* 1st ed. Maryland Heights, MO: Mosby; 2009.
60. Stockton KG, Brodsky JW. Peroneus longus tears associated with pathology of the os peroneum. *Foot Ankle Int.* 2014;35(4):346-352.
61. Cruz-Martinez A, Arpa J, Palau F. Peroneal neuropathy after weight loss. *J Peripher Nerv Syst.* 2000;5(2):101-105.
62. Katirji MB, Wilbourn AJ. Common peroneal mononeuropathy: a clinical and electrophysiologic study of 116 lesions. *Neurology.* 1988;38(11):1723-1728.
63. Jones HR Jr, Felice KJ, Gross PT. Pediatric peroneal mononeuropathy: a clinical and electromyographic study. *Muscle Nerve.* 1993;16(11):1167-1173.
64. Jeyaseelan N. Anatomical basis of compression of common peroneal nerve. *Anat Anz.* 1989;169(1):49-51.
65. Mitra A, Stern JD, Perrotta VJ, Moyer RA. Peroneal nerve entrapment in athletes. *Ann Plast Surg.* 1995;35(4):366-368.
66. Kim YC, Jung TD. Peroneal neuropathy after tibio-fibular fracture. *Ann Rehabil Med.* 2011;35(5):648-657.
67. Khatri K, Sharma V, Goyal D, Farooque K. Complications in the management of closed high-energy proximal tibial plateau fractures. *Chin J Traumatol.* 2016;19(6):342-347.
68. Woodmass JM, Romatowski NP, Esposito JG, Mohtadi NG, Longino PD. A systematic review of peroneal nerve palsy and recovery following traumatic knee dislocation. *Knee Surg Sports Traumatol Arthrosc.* 2015;23(10):2992-3002.
69. Mook WR, Ligh CA, Moorman CT III, Leversedge FJ. Nerve injury complicating multiligament knee injury: current concepts and treatment algorithm. *J Am Acad Orthop Surg.* 2013;21(6):343-354.
70. Kretschmer T, Antoniadis G, Braun V, Rath SA, Richter HP. Evaluation of iatrogenic lesions in 722 surgically treated cases of peripheral nerve trauma. *J Neurosurg.* 2001;94(6):905-912.
71. Seidel JA, Koenig R, Antoniadis G, Richter HP, Kretschmer T. Surgical treatment of traumatic peroneal nerve lesions. *Neurosurgery.* 2008;62(3):664-673; discussion 664-673.
72. Kim DH, Murovic JA, Tiel RL, Kline DG. Management and outcomes in 318 operative common peroneal nerve lesions at the Louisiana State University Health Sciences Center. *Neurosurgery.* 2004;54(6):1421-1428; discussion 1428-1429.
73. Fetzer GB, Prather H, Gelberman RH, Clohisy JC. Progressive peroneal nerve palsy in a varus arthritic knee. A case report. *J Bone Joint Surg Am.* 2004;86-A(7):1538-1540.
74. Gillenwater J, Cheng J, Mackinnon SE. Evaluation of the scratch collapse test in peroneal nerve compression. *Plast Reconstr Surg.* 2011;128(4):933-939.
75. Alexander IJ, Johnson KA, Parr JW. Morton's neuroma: a review of recent concepts. *Orthopedics.* 1987;10(1):103-106.
76. Schwartz JT Jr, Brumback RJ, Lakatos R, Poka A, Bathon GH, Burgess AR. Acute compartment syndrome of the thigh. A spectrum of injury. *J Bone Joint Surg Am.* 1989;71(3):392-400.
77. Rajasekaran S, Hall MM. Nonoperative management of chronic exertional compartment syndrome: a systematic review. *Curr Sports Med Rep.* 2016;15(3):191-198.
78. Blackman PG, Simmons LR, Crossley KM. Treatment of chronic exertional anterior compartment syndrome with massage: a pilot study. *Clin J Sport Med.* 1998;8(1):14-17.
79. Diebal AR, Gregory R, Alitz C, Gerber JP. Forefoot running improves pain and disability associated with chronic exertional compartment syndrome. *Am J Sports Med.* 2012;40(5):1060-1067.
80. Cox JS, Brand RL. Evaluation and treatment of lateral ankle sprains. *Phys Sportsmed.* 1977;5:51-55.
81. Jennings J, Davies GJ. Treatment of cuboid syndrome secondary to lateral ankle sprains: a case series. *J Orthop Sports Phys Ther.* 2005;35(7):409-415.

82. Marshall P, Hamilton WG. Cuboid subluxation in ballet dancers. *Am J Sports Med*. 1992;20(2):169-175.
83. Dombek MF, Orsini R, Mendicino RW, Saltrick K. Peroneus brevis tendon tears. *Clin Podiatr Med Surg*. 2001;18(3):409-427.
84. Safran MR, O'Malley D Jr, Fu FH. Peroneal tendon subluxation in athletes: new exam technique, case reports, and review. *Med Sci Sports Exerc*. 1999;31(7 suppl):S487-S492.
85. Cachia VV, Grumbine NA, Santoro JP, Sullivan JD. Spontaneous rupture of the peroneus longus tendon with fracture of the os peroneum. *J Foot Surg*. 1988;27(4):328-333.
86. Peacock KC, Resnick EJ, Thoder JJ. Fracture of the os peroneum with rupture of the peroneus longus tendon. A case report and review of the literature. *Clin Orthop Relat Res*. 1986(202):223-226.

Chapter 65

Gastrocnemius Muscle

"Calf Cramp Muscle"

Kathleen Geist, Jennifer L. Freeman, and Jeffrey Gervais Ebert

1. INTRODUCTION

The gastrocnemius muscle is a bipennate muscle located in the posterior compartment of the leg that, along with the soleus and plantaris muscles, comprises the muscle group known as the triceps surae muscles. The primary function of the gastrocnemius muscle is plantar flexion of the ankle and flexion of the knee joint at the end range. The gastrocnemius muscle creates quick dynamic force activity such as jumping and running with a high percentage of type 2 fast twitch muscle fibers. Trigger points (TrPs) are commonly identified in the mid-portion of the medial or lateral muscle belly. Trigger points in the gastrocnemius muscle can refer pain proximally to the posterior aspect of the knee joint or distally into the foot. Active TrPs identified in the medial head of the gastrocnemius muscle commonly refer pain into the medial longitudinal aspect of the foot. Symptoms may be exacerbated by walking, especially uphill, and can cause nocturnal calf cramps. Nocturnal calf cramps are described as a painful stimulus from a sudden, involuntary contraction of the gastrocnemius muscle that can disrupt the quality and duration of sleep. Symptoms of TrPs in the gastrocnemius muscle include posterior knee or calf pain and range-of-motion restrictions in the knee and ankle during a single-leg squat. Differential diagnosis should include assessment of ligamentous injury of the knee, muscle strain of the hamstring and popliteus, common fibularis nerve injury, meniscal or bone injury, Baker or ganglion cysts, neurovascular injury, or an S1 radiculopathy from the lumbar spine. Additionally, TrPs in the gastrocnemius muscle can also be present in individuals with Achilles tendinopathy. Corrective actions include postural education, especially sleeping and sitting positions, activity and footwear modifications, TrP self-pressure release, and self-stretching techniques.

2. ANATOMIC CONSIDERATIONS

The gastrocnemius muscle comprises a medial and lateral head and is the most superficial muscle in the posterior compartment of the leg. The medial head originates from the popliteal surface of the femur, posterior to the medial supracondylar line, and the posterior aspect of the adductor tubercle of the femur.[1-3] The lateral head originates from the posterolateral aspect of the lateral femoral condyle and the inferior aspect of the supracondylar line (Figure 65-1).[2,3] Several cadaveric and human studies have reported differences in the structural characteristics between the medial and the lateral heads of the gastrocnemius muscle.[4,5] For instance, the muscle belly of the medial head has a unipennate structure and is larger than that of the lateral head, which has a bipennate structure.[6] The medial and the lateral heads of the gastrocnemius muscle cross the tibiofemoral joint, and fibers from the posterior aspect of the knee capsule blend into both heads along with a contribution of the popliteal ligament blending into the lateral head of the gastrocnemius muscle.[7] The medial and the lateral heads of the gastrocnemius muscle descend inferiorly, with the medial head muscle fibers extending below the lateral head muscle fibers, and both muscle bellies stay separate until they blend into a broad aponeurosis that, in turn, blends with the soleus muscle to form the calcaneal (Achilles) tendon and cross the talocrural and subtalar joints.[2,3,8] The Achilles tendon inserts into the calcaneal tuberosity on the posterior surface of the calcaneus.[2] The insertion of each muscle of the triceps surae into the Achilles tendon is not uniform as the largest component comes from the subtendon of the lateral gastrocnemius muscle (44.4%), followed by the soleus muscle (27.9%), and the medial gastrocnemius muscle (27.7%).[9]

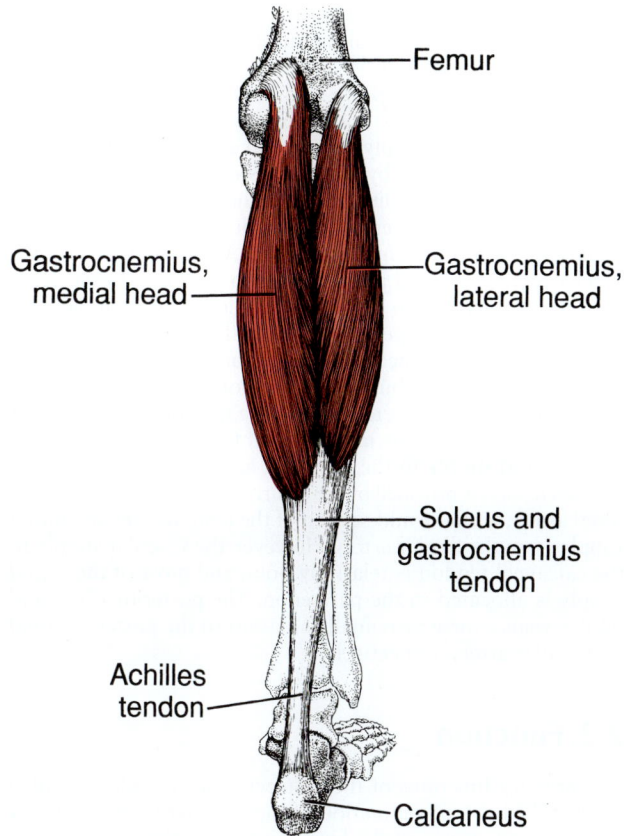

Figure 65-1. Attachments of the right gastrocnemius muscle (red) seen from the rear. The distal (deep) aponeurosis of the gastrocnemius muscle merges with the superficial soleus aponeurosis to form the Achilles tendon.

2.1. Innervation and Vascularization

The gastrocnemius muscle is innervated by the tibial nerve from the S1 and S2 nerve roots of the lumbosacral plexus. The tibial nerve branches off the sciatic nerve in the posterior aspect of the thigh and descends through the popliteal fossa into the posterior compartment of the leg. The tibial nerve innervates the superficial and deep muscles of the posterior aspect of the leg. The tibial nerve continues distally through the posterior compartment of the leg and courses between the flexor digitorum and flexor hallucis longus tendons posterior to the medial malleolus of the tibia.[3] The sural nerve is a cutaneous nerve, consisting of branches from the tibial and common fibular nerve, that courses lateral to the Achilles tendon in the posterior-lateral compartment of the leg.[1] The sural nerve crosses the Achilles tendon approximately 3.5 cm distal to the myotendinous junction and approximately 11 cm proximal to the calcaneal tuberosity.[1] Anatomic variations in the formation and course of the sural nerve are quite common in the general population.[10]

The arterial supply to the medial and the lateral heads of the gastrocnemius muscle course distally into the muscle bellies following the nerve supply. The medial and the lateral heads of the muscle are supplied by individual sural arteries that branch from the proximal popliteal artery. The sural arteries usually enter the medial and lateral heads of the gastrocnemius muscle at the level of the tibiofemoral joint line. Additionally, the medial sural artery has several perforators into the medial gastrocnemius muscle that run to the subfascial plexus through the deep fascia and nourish the perforator-based flaps.[11] The sural artery supplying the medial head of the gastrocnemius muscle enters proximal to the tibiofibular joint line compared with the sural artery supplying the lateral head of the gastrocnemius muscle, which usually enters the muscle distal to the tibiofibular joint line. Arterial supply to the proximal and distal portion of the Achilles tendon is provided by the recurring branch of the posterior tibial artery, with the mid-section of the tendon receiving blood supply from the fibular artery. However, the vascular supply to the calcaneal tendon is relatively poor, and most of the blood supply is allocated to the paratenon. The posterior tibial and fibular veins course proximally adjacent to the posterior tibial and fibular artery, respectively.[3]

2.2. Function

The primary functions of the gastrocnemius muscle are ankle plantar flexion and supination of the subtalar joint as well as flexion or extension of the knee joint, depending if the lower extremity is in a weight-bearing position or not, respectively.[12]

The gastrocnemius muscle crosses the knee joint and, collectively with the rectus femoris and hamstring muscles, make up approximately 98% of the total cross-sectional area of the musculature surrounding the knee.[13] When the lower extremity is in a nonweight-bearing position, the gastrocnemius muscle can function as a knee flexor along with the hamstring muscles. In a weight-bearing position, when the knee is in full extension, the gastrocnemius muscle provides an increased amount of torque into knee flexion.[14] It prevents hyperextension of the knee and excessive strain on the posterior capsule due to the anatomic connections between the capsule and the medial and the lateral heads of the muscle. As the knee joint moves into flexion, the gastrocnemius muscle is unable to generate a sufficient amount of torque into flexion.[14] The rectus femoris and gastrocnemius muscles work synergistically as dynamic stabilizers of the knee in weight-bearing positions.[15]

The gastrocnemius muscle is active during the stance and pre-swing phase of gait. Most authors agree that a role of the gastrocnemius muscle is providing vertical support of the lower extremity during the stance phase of gait; however, there is current debate as to the propulsive role of the gastrocnemius muscle during the mid-stance phase of gait. Toward the end of the loading response during the gait cycle, the gastrocnemius muscle provides stability and support of the knee joint to prevent excessive hyperextension.[16] The gastrocnemius and soleus muscles are also considered to be strong supinators of the subtalar and talocalcaneonavicular joint during ambulation.

Research suggests that the gastrocnemius muscle serves as an antagonist to prevent excessive strain on the anterior cruciate ligament (ACL) and may be important to consider during the rehabilitation process. Oeffinger et al[17] demonstrated that a latency in the gastrocnemius muscle demonstrated a significant amount of angular displacement of the tibia during sudden perturbations in patients with ACL repair. Fleming et al[16] studied the amount of translatory strain on the anteromedial bundle of the ACL through the individual electrical stimulation of the gastrocnemius, quadriceps, and hamstrings muscles and measured the strain rates based upon a paired combination of the muscles. The results demonstrated that when the knee joint was positioned in 15° and 30°, the simulataneous stimulation of the gastrocnemius and hamstrings muscles resulted in a reduction in strain on the ACL compared with gastrocnemius muscle stimulation alone.[16]

2.3. Functional Unit

The functional unit to which a muscle belongs includes the muscles that reinforce and counter its actions as well as the joints that the muscle crosses. The interdependence of these structures functionally is reflected in the organization and neural connections of the sensory motor cortex. The functional unit is emphasized because the presence of a TrP in one muscle of the unit increases the likelihood that the other muscles of the unit will also develop TrPs. When inactivating TrPs in a muscle, one must be concerned about TrPs that may develop in muscles that are functionally interdependent. Box 65-1 grossly represents the functional unit of the gastrocnemius muscle.[18]

3. CLINICAL PRESENTATION

3.1. Referred Pain Pattern

An individual with TrPs in the gastrocnemius muscle may present with posterior knee, calf, or plantar heel pain (Figure 65-2).[19] Trigger points in the lateral head of the gastrocnemius muscle may refer pain to the posterior and lateral aspect of the calf. Trigger points in the medial head of the gastrocnemius muscle can refer pain into the posteromedial aspect of the leg and

---

Box 65-1 Functional unit of the gastrocnemius muscle

Action	Synergists	Antagonists
Plantar flexion	Soleus Plantaris Fibularis longus Fibularis brevis Flexor digitorum longus Tibialis posterior	Extensor hallucis longus Extensor digitorum longus Tibialis anterior Fibularis tertius
Knee flexion	Hamstrings Popliteus Plantaris Gracilis Sartorius	Rectus femoris Vastus medialis Vastus lateralis Vastus intermedius

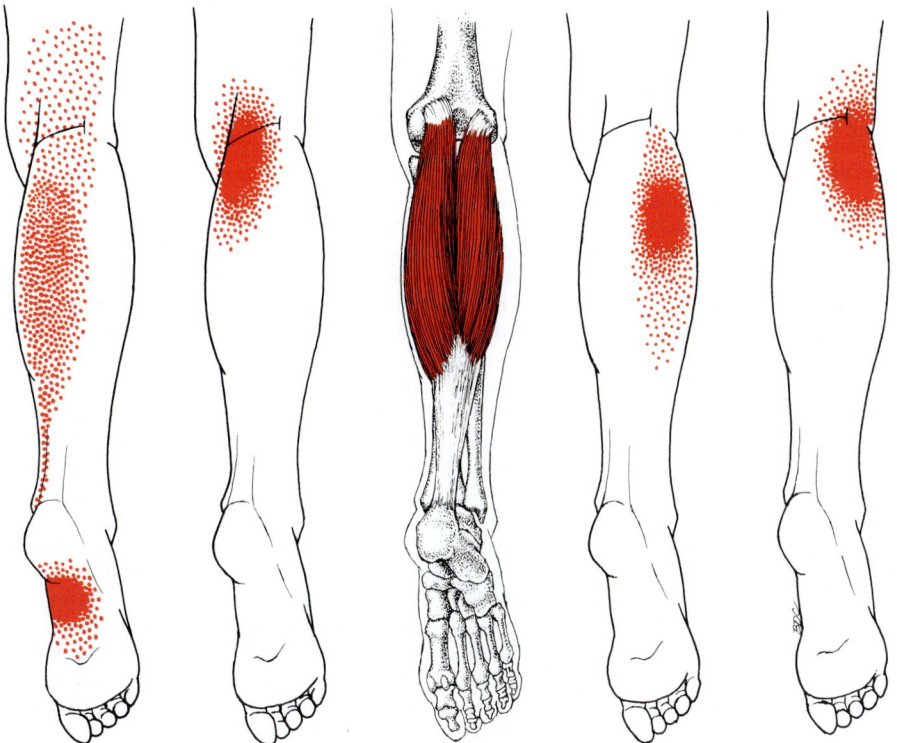

Figure 65-2. Pain (dark red) referred from TrPs in the right gastrocnemius muscle (light red). The essential pain pattern is solid red. Red stippling indicates the extension of the essential pattern. Trigger point in the belly of the medial head, and to a lesser extent TrPs in the belly of the lateral head, are likely to be present when the patient has painful nocturnal calf cramps.

the medial longitudinal arch of the foot or can cause painful muscle cramps in the posterior leg.[18] Individuals with TrPs in the gastrocnemius muscle may report sharp pain along the plantar surface of the heel upon weight-bearing activities with the first few steps upon waking in the morning and heel pain with weight-bearing activity following a period of nonweight bearing such as prolonged sitting.[20] Activities such as walking on inclines or stair climbing may also be painful with TrPs in the gastrocnemius muscle.

3.2. Symptoms

Individuals with TrPs in the gastrocnemius muscle primarily report pain located in the medial longitudinal arch especially with walking and stair climbing. The patient may report pain in the back of the knee on effort, as when climbing up steep slopes, over rocks, or when walking along a slanted surface, such as a beach or the side of a domed street. Patients with gastrocnemius TrPs rarely report weakness or restricted range of motion even when dorsiflexion of the ankle is found to be limited upon testing. The individual may also report calf or plantar heel pain and nocturnal calf cramping.[18,21] The presence of latent TrPs in the gastrocnemius muscle can give rise to painful, involuntary muscle cramps in the calf region. Muscle cramps can occur as part of a myopathic or pathoneurologic process but can also occur in healthy individuals during pregnancy, sport activities, and sleep.[22]

Latent TrPs are more commonly found in the medial head of the gastrocnemius muscle and can cause nocturnal calf cramps, negatively impacting sleep quality. Several studies evaluated the effects of TrP injections in the gastrocnemius muscle and found that using a local anesthetic both reduced the intensity and the frequency of pain associated with nocturnal calf cramps and appears to lessen the severity of insomnia during the night.[22,23]

The pathophysiologic effects of latent TrPs causing nocturnal calf cramps are not clearly understood; however, several theories, including spontaneous discharges or abnormal excitability from motor nerves and overexcitability of the motor unit in the presence of spinal disinhibition, have been suggested.[22] In a study conducted by Ge et al[21] glutamate injection into a latent TrP in the gastrocnemius muscle reproduced the onset of muscle cramps in the calf. The authors suggest that there may be an association between excitation of the afferent muscle fibers and a subsequent increase in nociceptive sensitivity that elicits muscle cramping.[21] The authors propose that there may be a relationship between the presence of TrPs and the development of muscle cramps.

3.3. Patient Examination

After a thorough subjective examination, the clinician should make a detailed drawing representing the pain pattern described by the patient. This depiction will assist in planning the physical examination and can be useful in monitoring the progression of the patient as symptoms improve or change. The type, quality, and location of the pain should be carefully assessed, and the utilization of standardized outcome tools is imperative when examining patients with lower extremity dysfunctions.

Observation of static and dynamic posture is essential due to the role of the gastrocnemius muscles in postural stability. During an observation of static standing posture, the patient may be unable to fully extend the involved extremity when keeping the heel on the floor.[18] Functional testing such as double- and single-leg squat will allow a quick assessment of hip and knee control, as well as a quick assessment of talocrural, subtalar, and mid-foot range of motion. Timed single-leg stance with eyes open and closed will give a quantitative measure of balance and will afford the clinician to observe foot and ankle strategies related to balance and control.

Restricted active or passive range of motion in ankle dorsiflexion may be identified during the clinical examination.[24,25] A reduction in the amount of passive ankle dorsiflexion when the knee is extended, and an increase with the knee flexed, suggests that the motion restriction is related to tightness of the gastrocnemius muscle rather than a joint or capsular restriction of the talocrural joint.[15] The clinician should maintain the rearfoot in a varus position to accurately measure the amount of dorsiflexion at the talocrural joint. Passive dorsiflexion of the talocrural joint with the rearfoot in valgus allows excessive motion to occur at the mid-foot and subtalar joint.[26] Patients with TrPs in the gastrocnemius muscle may display alterations in their gait, exhibiting a flat-footed or a stiff-legged gait pattern.

Examination of the extensibility of the gastrocnemius muscle is performed with the individual in a supine or prone nonweight-bearing position (Figure 65-3). A lack of dorsiflexion of the talocrural joint by >10° is known as a talipes equinus.[27] A common cause of restricted ankle dorsiflexion is adaptive shortening of the triceps surae muscles. Restricted passive ankle dorsiflexion with the knee extended and an increase in passive ankle dorsiflexion with the knee flexed is known as the Silfverskiold sign[26] (Figure 65-3A and B). To date, the psychometric properties of the Silfverskiold sign are not known. A reduction in the amount of passive ankle dorsiflexion when the knee is extended and an increase with the knee flexed suggest that the motion restriction is related to tightness of the gastrocnemius muscle rather than a joint or capsular restriction of the talocrural joint.[14] To test for the presence of talipes equinus, a 2 kg force should be placed under the forefoot while providing a passive dorsiflexion force to minimize a false-positive test.[26]

Passive accessory motion of the talocrural joint, as well as the distal and proximal tibiofibular joints, should be examined. Passive accessory motion of the tibiofemoral joint should be examined when the patient reports posterior knee pain and loss of knee extension range of motion that may be associated with gastrocnemius TrPs.

The results on the effects of the gastrocnemius muscle stretching on ankle dorsiflexion range of motion remain equivocal. A systematic review by Young et al[28] evaluated the efficacy of the gastrocnemius muscle stretching alone compared with a multimodal approach. A meta-analysis of 8 studies showed that passive gastrocnemius muscle stretching had a significant effect on an increase in ankle dorsiflexion, whereas 12 other studies demonstrated no significant effect of the gastrocnemius muscle stretching on ankle dorsiflexion compared with a control group.[28] The results of a 3-week gastrocnemius stretching program were shown to be effective in increasing passive ankle dorsiflexion range of motion; however, the increases in range of motion did not translate to an increase in time-to-heel off during gait.[29] Edama et al[6] investigated on cadavers the best position for stretching the medial gastrocnemius muscle and reported that knee extension, with dorsiflexion and inversion of the ankle, induced the greatest tension in the medial head. However, none of these studies investigated the presence of TrPs in the gastrocnemius muscle prior to the stretching program, which could account for the equivocal findings.

There is moderate to strong evidence that supports the utilization of manual TrP release to relieve muscle pain associated with active and latent TrPs.[30] A study by Grieve et al[25] assessed the effect of manual TrP release of latent TrPs and passive stretching of the triceps surae muscles in healthy, recreational runners. Following combined treatment of manual TrP release and passive stretching of the triceps surae muscles, the runners demonstrated an improvement in the extensibility of both the soleus and gastrocnemius muscles. Based on a paired *t*-test, the participants showed a statistically significant increase in muscle extensibility of the soleus and gastrocnemius muscles.[25]

A multimodal approach that includes TrP release techniques and stretching for the triceps surae muscle is an effective treatment for the management of plantar heel and foot pain. Grieve et al[24] reported on the effects of a multimodal treatment approach for participants with calf pain. All participants received an initial evaluation for an assessment of the independent variables including pain scale, pain pressure threshold (PPT), functional status on the lower extremity functional scale (LEFS), and ankle dorsiflexion range of motion. Ten participants received TrP release to the tricep surae muscles, instructed in a self-pressure TrP release technique, and a home-stretching program. Nine of the participants demonstrated an increase in ankle dorsiflexion range of motion and an increase in the individual LEFS scores.[24] Ordine et al[20] found that manual TrP release directed over TrPs identified in either muscle bellies of the gastrocnemius muscle, in addition to a self-stretching exercise for the triceps surae muscles and plantar fascia, resulted in a significant decrease in pain and a significant improvement in the Short-Form (SF)-36 Questionnaire and the PPT over the gastrocnemius and soleus muscles.[20]

3.4. Trigger Point Examination

A suspicion of the presence of the TrP is usually made based on a combination of subjective and objective physical examination findings.[18] A cross-fiber flat or pincer palpation is effective in identifying TrPs within the medial or lateral heads of the gastrocnemius muscle. A cross-fiber flat palpation approach is selected when the subcutaneous soft tissue of the posterior calf is tight and nonmobile. For those patients who have pliable and mobile subcutaneous soft tissue of the calf, a cross-fiber pincer palpation

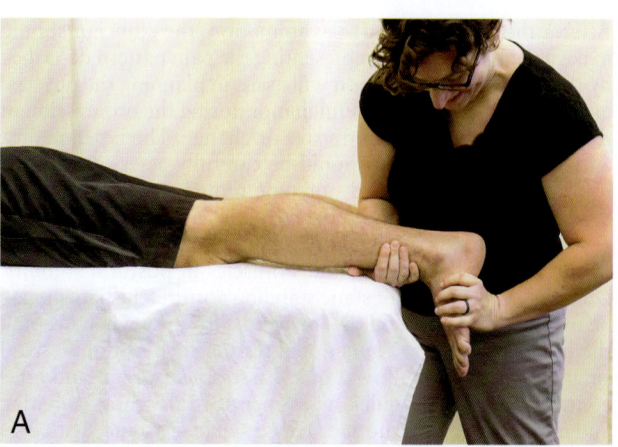
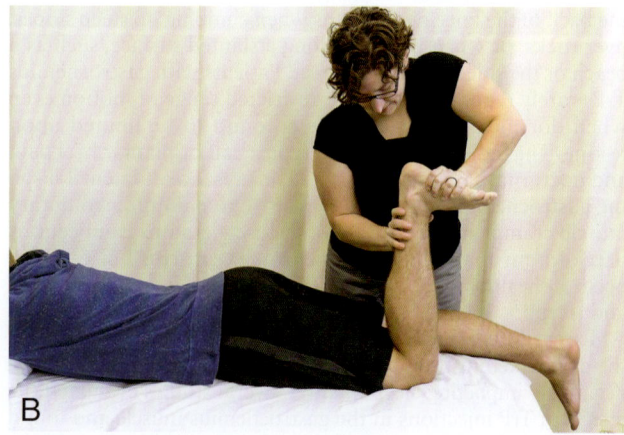

Figure 65-3. Muscle length testing. A, Gastrocnemius muscle. B, Soleus muscle. Note the change in dorsiflexion with the knee flexed.

may be used. Manual palpation of the gastrocnemius muscle can be performed with the patient prone, side-lying, or hook-lying (Figures 65-4 and 65-5). When examining the gastrocnemius muscle in side-lying, the patient should lie on the side with the involved extremity to be treated uppermost. When examining the patient in a prone position, a pillow should be placed under the patient's feet to maintain knee flexion of approximately 20° and to allow some slack in the gastrocnemius muscle.[18]

Cross-fiber pincer palpation to identify TrPs in the lateral head of the gastrocnemius muscle can be performed in side-lying (Figure 65-4A), prone (Figure 65-4B), or hook-lying (Figure 65-4C). Cross-fiber flat palpation is utilized to identify TrPs in the proximal portion of the lateral head or the entire muscle belly if the tissue on the posterior calf is immobile or too taut.

Cross-fiber pincer palpation of the medial head of the gastrocnemius muscle is performed in the prone or side-lying position (Figure 65-5A and B). Cross-fiber flat palpation is utilized to identify TrPs in the proximal portion of the medial head or the entire muscle belly if the tissue on the posterior calf is immobile or too taut.

4. DIFFERENTIAL DIAGNOSIS

4.1. Activation and Perpetuation of Trigger Points

A posture or activity that activates a TrP, if not corrected, can also perpetuate it. In any part of the gastrocnemius muscle, TrPs may be activated by unaccustomed eccentric loading, eccentric exercise in an unconditioned muscle, or maximal or submaximal concentric loading.[31] Trigger points may also be activated or aggravated when the muscle is placed in a shortened and/or lengthened position for an extended period of time.

Trigger points can develop in the gastrocnemius muscle from mechanical overload or activity that involves forceful plantar flexion of the ankle when the knee is in a flexed position. Activity that involves cycling, walking, running on inclined surfaces, or climbing steep terrain can promote the development of TrPs within the gastrocnemius muscle that produces posterior knee pain. Other causes of muscle overload include swimming with the toes pointed in a flutter kick, wearing high heeled shoes, or sitting with prolonged pressure on the back of the thigh or calf. Sleeping supine with the feet held in plantar flexion by tucked in blankets may also perpetuate TrPs.

Immobilization of the lower extremity after an injury, such as a fracture, can facilitate the development of TrPs in the gastrocnemius muscle from the resultant trauma. During the immobilization period, the gastrocnemius muscle can become atrophied and deconditioned and once weight bearing is initiated, the individual may report a painful and stiff calf muscle.

Perpetuation of TrPs in the gastrocnemius muscle can occur from sustained external compression of the leg that creates a localized ischemic event. External compression of the gastrocnemius muscle that may contribute to the perpetuation of TrPs can occur from tight socks or elastic bands around the leg, from sustained compression of a chair seat or from maintaining knee flexion and ankle plantar-flexion during prolonged sitting tasks.[18]

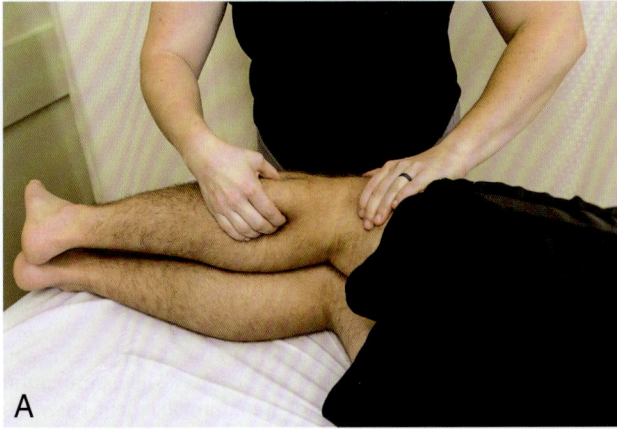
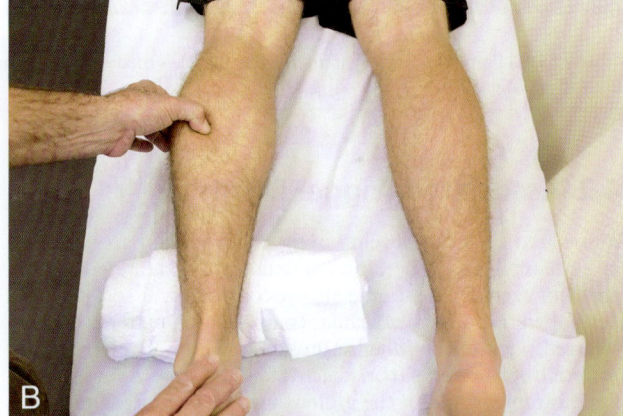
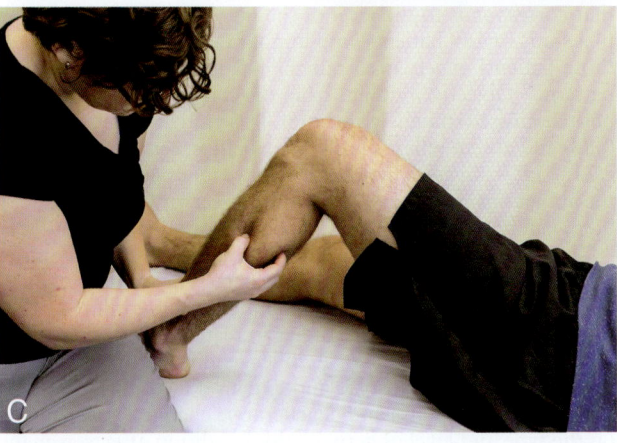
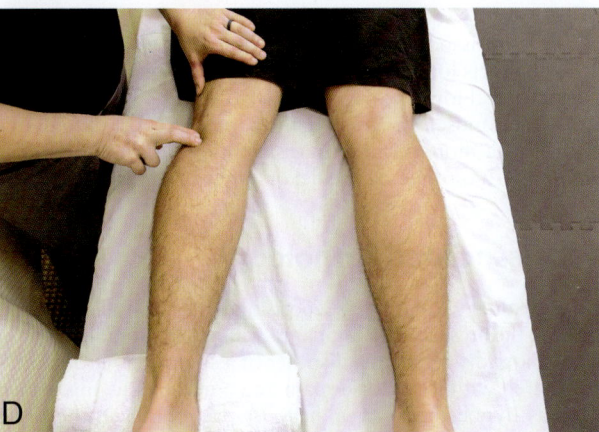

Figure 65-4. Palpation of the gastrocnemius muscle's lateral head. Cross-fiber pincer palpation. A, Side-lying. B, Prone. C, Hook-lying. D, Cross-fiber flat palpation proximal portion.

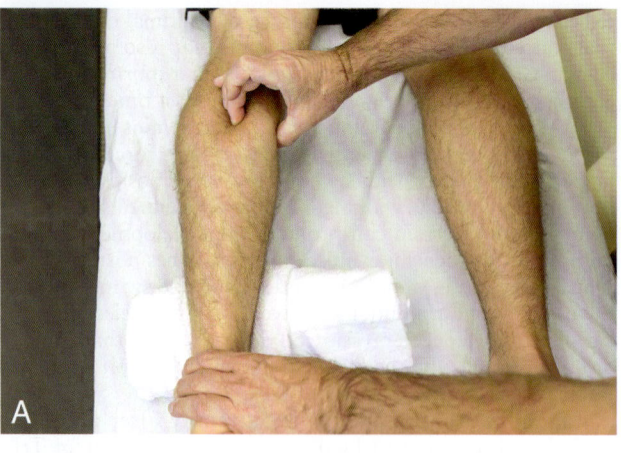
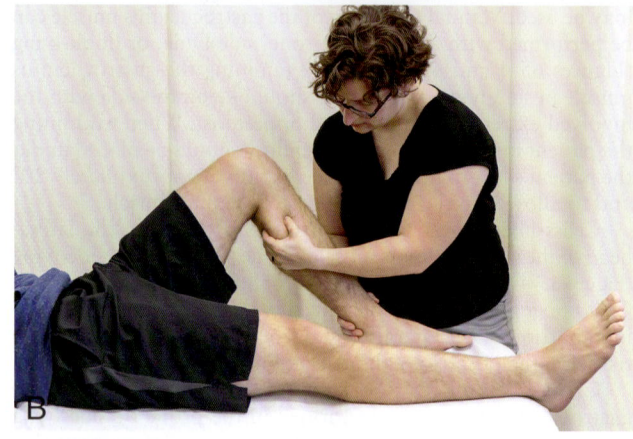
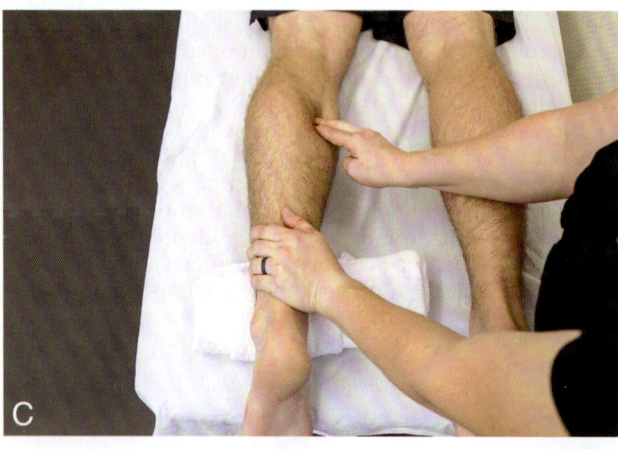
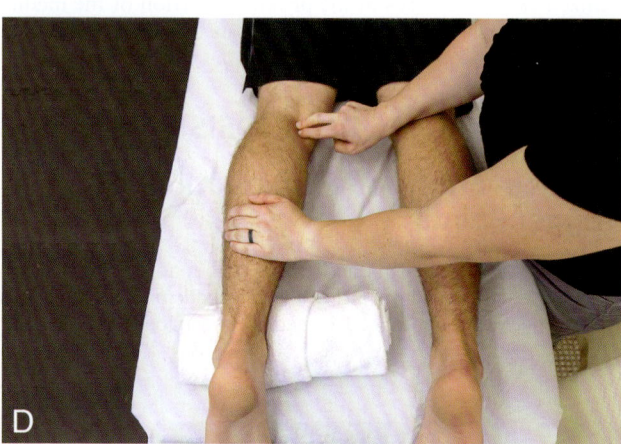

Figure 65-5. Palpation of the gastrocnemius muscle's medial head. Cross-fiber pincer palpation. A, Prone. B, Hook-lying. Cross-fiber flat palpation. C, Mid-muscle belly. D, Proximal portion.

4.2. Associated Trigger Points

Associated TrPs can develop in the referred pain areas caused by primary TrPs.[32] Therefore, musculature in the referred pain areas for each muscle should also be considered. Associated TrPs develop in response to muscular compensation patterns or from referred phenomena when a muscle is within a referred pain pattern from a proximal or adjacent to the gastrocnemius muscle. For example, a TrP in the gluteus medius or gluteus minimus muscles can refer pain into the proximal region of the calf, and an associated TrP can develop in the gastrocnemius muscle.[18]

Patients who develop active TrPs in the gastrocnemius muscle can develop associated TrPs in the hamstring, popliteus, soleus, flexor hallucis longus, and flexor digitorum longus muscles on the ipsilateral lower extremity. Once the active TrPs in the gastrocnemius muscle are treated, the patient's report of pain may change to a more distal pain distribution due to the referred pain pattern of the long toe flexors or soleus muscles.[18]

4.3. Associated Pathology

An individual with primary reports of calf pain should be evaluated for the presence of a lumbar radicular pain or radiculopathy. Radiculopathy refers to a disorder of a spinal nerve root and is associated with leg or back pain and a neurologic impairment such as hypoesthesia, weakness, or paresthesia in the lower extremity.[33] A neurologic examination should be performed in the lower extremities to assess for the presence of dermatomal, myotomal, or reflex changes. This examination should also assess for the presence of a nerve root irritation or compression of the L5 nerve root that can give rise to pain along the lateral aspect of the leg with weakness of the ankle plantar flexors or a diminished or absent Achilles reflex. Lumbar radiculopathy associated with an S1 nerve root can result in pain along the lateral border of the foot, weakness of the ankle plantar flexors, and a diminished or absent Achilles reflex.[34]

Radicular pain originating from a spinal nerve root can cause sharp, shooting pain distal to the knee. The examination cannot always deduce the level of spinal involvement based on the pattern of sensory deficits or pain. There is little evidence to support that radicular pain follows a specific dermatomal pattern that corresponds to the level of the involved spinal nerve root. In a study of 169 patients with lumbar radiculopathy, 64.1% of those patients experienced radicular pain in a nondermatomal pattern.[35] Objective findings from the clinical exam including a positive crossed straight leg raise (SLR) (sensitivity 0.29, specificity 0.88) and absent reflexes (sensitivity 0.14, specificity 0.93, +LR 2.21, −LR 0.78) assist in ruling in a nerve root syndrome, whereas the absence of symptoms with a SLR (sensitivity 0.91, specificity 0.26) can be used to rule out a diagnosis of radiculopathy.[36,37]

Pain in the posterior aspect of the calf can include injuries from repeated overload, mechanical stress, or trauma. Achilles tendinopathy is one of the most common overuse injuries of the foot and ankle, particularly among recreational and competitive athletes.[38-42] The etiology of Achilles tendinopathy is multifactorial and includes intrinsic and extrinsic factors leading to a failed healing response and degenerative changes.[43] Depending on the type and level of activity, this condition affects as many as 9% to 40% of athletes,[44,45] especially runners.[45-47] Although athletes tend to be at greatest risk of developing this condition, it can affect relatively sedentary individuals as well.[48,49] Achilles tendinopathy can generally be classified into two categories: insertional tendinopathy and noninsertional, or mid-portion, tendinopathy. Noninsertional tendinopathy is the most commonly occurring classification.[44] Achilles tendinopathy is typically a noninflammatory condition and instead involves degenerative changes within the substance of the tendon, especially in chronic presentations that make up the majority of cases.[50-53] The incidence of Achilles tendinopathy tends to increase with age,[54,55] with an average age range of 30 to 50 years of age.[42,56,57] This condition appears to affect men more than women.[40,57,58]

Several risk factors for Achilles tendinopathy have been documented. These risk factors include limited ankle dorsiflexion range of motion,[59] excessive pronation,[40,60] reduced ankle plantar flexion strength,[60,61] abnormal subtalar range of motion,[40,59] obesity,[48] diabetes,[48] training errors,[39] and medication usage—specifically, the antibiotic fluoroquinolone.[62,63]

Patients with chronic Achilles tendinopathy will most commonly report increased pain with activity[64] and ankle stiffness after periods of prolonged inactivity[65] that diminishes with continued activity.[66] In mild to moderate cases, patients may experience pain only at the end of their recreational activity[65] and, as the condition becomes more severe, they may experience pain throughout the activity and may need to discontinue the activity completely.[66] Typical findings utilized in the diagnosis of Achilles tendinopathy include local tenderness with palpation of the mid-portion of the tendon (approximately 2-6 cm proximal to its insertion) with noninsertional tendinopathy[67] and at the bone-tendon junction with insertional tendinopathy[60]; a positive arc sign[67]; reduced ankle plantar flexion strength[68,69]; and a positive Royal London Hospital Test.[67] Reiman et al[70] found that the presence of morning stiffness and local pain with palpation for crepitus showed high sensitivity and specificity for clinical diagnosis of Achilles tendinopathy.

In cases in which a diagnosis of Achilles tendinopathy is uncertain following the history and physical examination, magnetic resonance imaging (MRI) and/or diagnostic ultrasound can be utilized to rule in or rule out the condition more definitively[64,71,72] if needed to change the clinical plan of care.

An acute onset of pain and swelling in the posterior aspect of the leg can be caused by localized inflammation in tendons or an acute tear of the muscle or tendon. Ruptures of the medial head of the gastrocnemius muscle, known as "tennis leg," can occur with eccentric lengthening of the gastrocnemius muscle as the foot moves into dorsiflexion and the knee moves into extension following a serve in tennis.[18] In fact, strain in the medial gastrocnemius muscle represents the most common injury of the posterior compartment of the lower extremity. Two-thirds of calf injuries occur at the junction of the fascia between the medial head of the gastrocnemius and the soleus muscles.[73]

Muscles overlying the posterior compartment of the knee that are commonly subject to injury include the hamstring and popliteus muscles. The hamstring muscles can be injured during sprinting activity and may cause posterolateral knee pain with tenderness to palpation inferior to the joint. Resisted testing of the hamstring muscles with the knee flexed and the tibia rotated internally or externally can assist in the diagnosis of injury to the semimembranosus, semitendinosus, and biceps femoris muscles, respectively.[14] Clinical findings of a tear within a muscle include the presence of swelling, tenderness, or a palpable defect within the muscle belly. A rupture of the popliteus muscle can occur with ligamentous injury to the posterior cruciate ligament. An acute tear of the plantaris tendon can often occur in association with a tear of the gastrocnemius muscle. A rapid diagnosis of an acute musculotendinous lesion can be identified by the utilization of musculoskeletal ultrasound from the localization of hypoechoic changes (<2 cm) for a partial tear or the presence of a hypoechoic hematoma formation in the presence of a full tear.[74] Days following the injury, a hematoma can form around the area of injury. Acute traumatic injuries associated with swelling or hematoma formation should also be screened for associated nerve injury to the common fibular nerve.[75]

Additional causes of pain in the posterior aspect of the calf include Baker cysts, tumors, infections, arterial insufficiency, or deep vein thrombosis. A Baker cyst forms in the popliteal region from herniation and leaking of synovial fluid from the posterior knee capsule as a result of internal derangement within the knee joint.[75] The presence of a Baker cyst can be identified through palpation of a painful or tender nodule between the semimembranosus and medial head of the gastrocnemius muscles. The use of MRI is the best imaging modality used to diagnose the presence of a Baker cyst because an MRI can identify the presence of an intra-articular derangement and adjacent relationship of the anatomic structures.[75]

Complications from Baker cysts include infection, rupture with concomitant compression of surrounding anatomic structures, and hemorrhage.[74,75] The presence of an infection should be suspected in the presence of a systemic illness, presence of a cyst with posterior knee pain, and swelling with local signs of warmth and erythema. A Baker cyst can cause deep venous thrombosis and ischemia. The associated symptoms from a ruptured cyst can mimic the clinical examination findings of thrombophlebitis. Diagnosis of vascular injuries associated with posterior knee pain can be established with MRI or computerized tomography angiography.[75]

5. CORRECTIVE ACTIONS

An individual with TrPs in the gastrocnemius muscle should avoid postures or activities with sustained active or passive ankle plantar flexion. Positions that should be avoided include sitting in high chairs in which the feet are not completely supported on the floor and prolonged driving activity with the ankle held in sustained plantar flexion. Patients should adjust sitting surfaces to allow their feet and ankles to rest in a neutral ankle position, and cruise control use during prolonged driving activities can prevent the perpetuation of TrPs in the triceps surae muscles. Other helpful activity modifications may include walking on level surfaces instead of inclined surfaces, avoiding tight or elastic materials around the calf, avoiding prolonged ankle plantar flexion with swimming activities, and avoiding wearing shoes with a heel greater than 2 in. Electromyographic assessment of the gastrocnemius muscle in individuals wearing a small heel lift demonstrates reduced activity of the gastrocnemius muscle during walking activity.[76] Therefore, the use of a small heel lift may be beneficial for temporary off-loading of the gastrocnemius muscle after an acute injury or after surgical repair of the Achilles tendon.

Nocturnal (nighttime) calf cramps are often associated with TrPs in the gastrocnemius muscle. Warming the calf with an electric blanket or heating pad for a few minutes prior to bed can help reduce the irritability of TrPs, and maintaining the ankles in a neutral position while sleeping can help reduce nocturnal night cramps. To prevent the onset of nocturnal muscle cramps, one can alternate full active range of motion in ankle dorsiflexion and plantar flexion. Active range of motion while sitting helps minimize immobility and promotes blood flow to the lower extremities.[18]

In general, the leg muscles feel better if the ankle is maintained in a neutral position throughout the night; therefore, adjusting the patients' sleeping posture may be necessary. This position is facilitated by having the bed sheets at the foot of the bed untucked to reduce external force into excessive plantar flexion (Figure 65-6). Using a pillow between the legs and knees in side-lying to place the foot and ankle in a neutral position may also be beneficial. Patients with irritable TrPs should avoid lying on the affected side as the pressure from the bed may perpetuate TrP activity.

Gastrocnemius TrP self-pressure release can be performed in the seated and long sitting positions (Figure 65-7). Pressure may be applied manually with a pincer grasp (Figure 65-7A), with a TrP release tool or firm ball (Figure 65-7B), or with a TrP

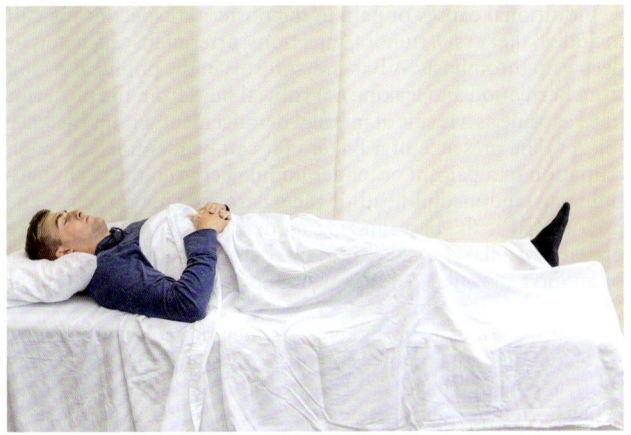

Figure 65-6. Sleeping posture with the foot of the affected side outside the covers to avoid the weight of the covers pulling the foot and ankle down and placing the muscle in a prolonged shortened position.

release roller tool (Figure 65-7C). Finding the sensitive spot with the hands or a tool, light pressure (no more than 4/10 pain) is applied and held for 15 to 30 seconds until pain reduces. This technique can be repeated up to five times, several times per day (Figure 65-7A, B, and C).

Gastrocnemius muscle self-stretching can be performed in a sitting or standing position. Self-stretching of the gastrocnemius muscle in a sitting position requires the patient to maintain a long sitting position with the involved knee fully extended. A long strap is placed under the forefoot, while maintaining the knee in an extended position, and a prolonged passive stretch into dorsiflexion is applied at the foot and ankle (Figure 65-8A). Self-stretching of the gastrocnemius muscle in standing is performed with the individual in a stride-stance facing a wall, with both feet placed in a neutral position and their hands on the wall at shoulder height or on a chair (Figure 65-8B). With the affected leg behind, the foot should be placed in slight supination using a small wedge along the entire inside edge of the foot (Figure 65-6B, small pic) to emphasize dorsiflexion through the rear foot and prevent excessive forces into dorsiflexion through the mid-foot.[77] The individual should lean the trunk forward

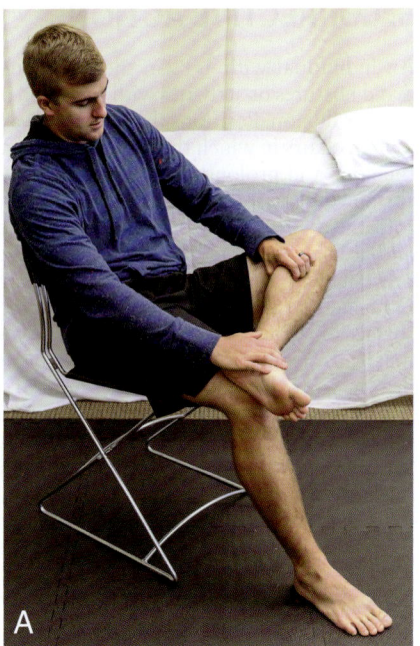
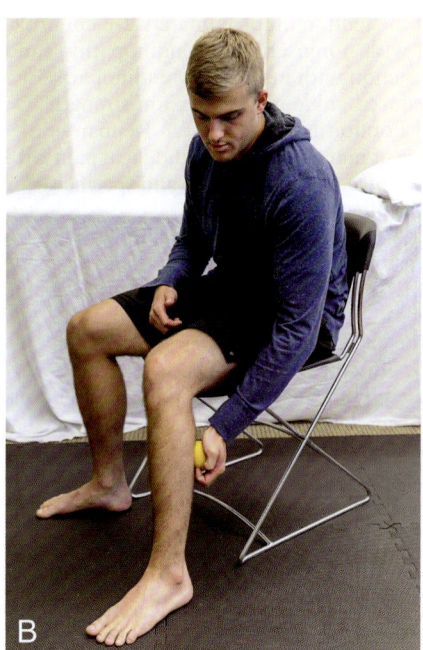
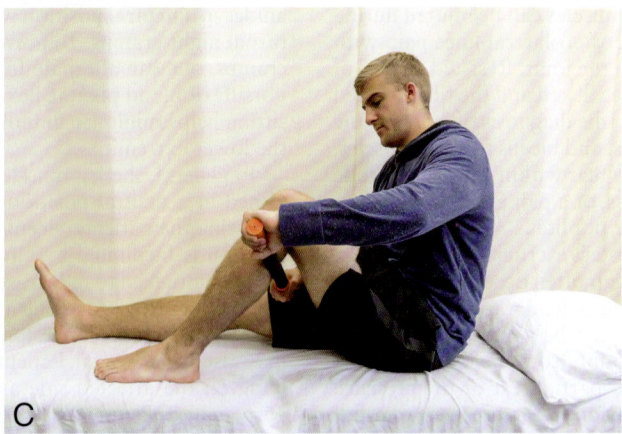

Figure 65-7. Trigger point self-pressure release. A, Manual release. B, Using a lacrosse ball. C, Using a TrP self-release roller.

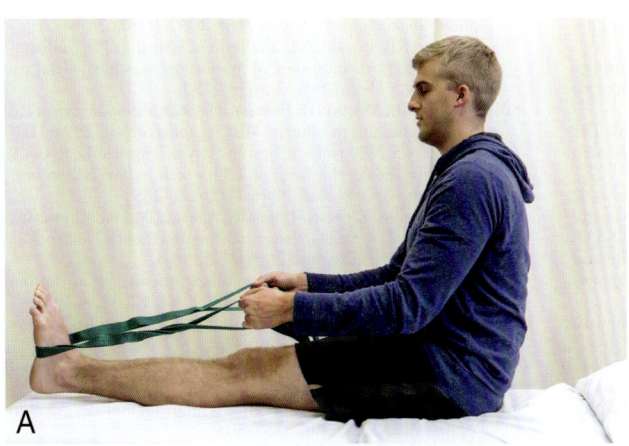
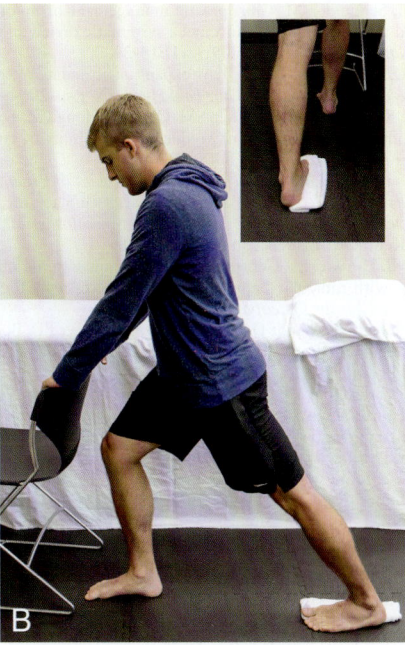

Figure 65-8. Self-stretch of the gastrocnemius muscle. A, Gentle stretch with a strap or sheet for irritable TrPs in the gastrocnemius muscle. B, Runners stretch. A flat towel is placed along the inside of the foot to prevent flattening of the arch while stretching.

while maintaining the heels on the floor and shifting weight toward the lead foot, maintaining the knee in a fully extended position. This stretch may be augmented by postisometric relaxation. At the first onset of a stretch in the calf, the ball of the foot is pushed into the floor with a slight contraction of the calf muscles, but the heel or foot remains on the floor. Holding the contraction for 6 to 10 seconds, a deep inhalation is performed. Then, during a slow exhale though the mouth, the calf muscle is allowed to relax and another slight lean forward can be performed until a stretch is felt once again in the calf. This procedure can be repeated three to five times and can be performed three times daily.

References

1. Doral MN, Alam M, Bozkurt M, et al. Functional anatomy of the Achilles tendon. *Knee Surg Sports Traumatol Arthrosc.* 2010;18(5):638-643.
2. Parson S. *Clinically Oriented Anatomy.* 6th ed. Baltimore, MD: Lippincott Williams and Wilkins; 2010.
3. Standring S. *Gray's Anatomy: The Anatomical Basis of Clinical Practice.* 41st ed. London, UK: Elsevier; 2015.
4. Ward SR, Eng CM, Smallwood LH, Lieber RL. Are current measurements of lower extremity muscle architecture accurate? *Clin Orthop Relat Res.* 2009;467(4):1074-1082.
5. Abellaneda S, Guissard N, Duchateau J. The relative lengthening of the myotendinous structures in the medial gastrocnemius during passive stretching differs among individuals. *J Appl Physiol (1985).* 2009;106(1):169-177.
6. Edama M, Onishi H, Kumaki K, Kageyama I, Watanabe H, Nashimoto S. Effective and selective stretching of the medial head of the gastrocnemius. *Scand J Med Sci Sports.* 2015;25(2):242-250.
7. Watanabe Y, Moriya H, Takahashi K, et al. Functional anatomy of the posterolateral structures of the knee. *Arthroscopy.* 1993;9(1):57-62.
8. Chazan IM. Achilles tendinitis part I: anatomy, histology, classification, etiology, and pathomechanics. *J Man Manip Ther.* 1998;6:63-69.
9. Pekala PA, Henry BM, Ochala A, et al. The twisted structure of the Achilles tendon unraveled: a detailed quantitative and qualitative anatomical investigation. *Scand J Med Sci Sports.* 2017;27(12):1705-1715.
10. Ramakrishnan PK, Henry BM, Vikse J, et al. Anatomical variations of the formation and course of the sural nerve: a systematic review and meta-analysis. *Ann Anat.* 2015;202:36-44.
11. Xie XT, Chai YM. Medial sural artery perforator flap. *Ann Plast Surg.* 2012;68(1):105-110.
12. Kisner C, Colby L. *Therapeutic Exercise: Foundations and Techniques.* 6th ed. Philadelphia, PA: FA Davis; 2012.
13. Wickiewicz TL, Roy RR, Powell PL, Edgerton VR. Muscle architecture of the human lower limb. *Clin Orthop Relat Res.* 1983(179):275-283.
14. Levangie PK, Norkin CC. *Joint Structure and Function: A Comprehensive Analysis.* 5th ed. Philadelphia, PA: FA Davis; 2011.
15. Kvist J, Gillquist J. Anterior positioning of tibia during motion after anterior cruciate ligament injury. *Med Sci Sports Exerc.* 2001;33(7):1063-1072.
16. Fleming BC, Renstrom PA, Ohlen G, et al. The gastrocnemius muscle is an antagonist of the anterior cruciate ligament. *J Orthop Res.* 2001;19(6):1178-1184.
17. Oeffinger DJ, Shapiro R, Nyland J, Pienkowski D, Caborn DN. Delayed gastrocnemius muscle response to sudden perturbation in rehabilitated patients with anterior cruciate ligament reconstruction. *Knee Surg Sports Traumatol Arthrosc.* 2001;9(1):19-27.
18. Simons DG, Travell J, Simons L. *Travell & Simon's Myofascial Pain and Dysfunction: The Trigger Point Manual.* Vol 1. 2nd ed. Baltimore, MD: Williams & Wilkins; 1999 (p. 104).
19. DeLisa JA, Gans BM, Walsh NE. *Physical Medicine and Rehabilitation: Principles and Practice.* Vol 1. 4th ed. Philadelphia, PA: Lippincott Williams & Wilkins; 2005.
20. Renan-Ordine R, Alburquerque-Sendin F, de Souza DP, Cleland JA, Fernández de las Peñas C. Effectiveness of myofascial trigger point manual therapy combined with a self-stretching protocol for the management of plantar heel pain: a randomized controlled trial. *J Orthop Sports Phys Ther.* 2011;41(2):43-50.
21. Ge HY, Zhang Y, Boudreau S, Yue SW, Arendt-Nielsen L. Induction of muscle cramps by nociceptive stimulation of latent myofascial trigger points. *Exp Brain Res.* 2008;187(4):623-629.
22. Kim DH, Yoon DM, Yoon KB. The effects of myofascial trigger point injections on nocturnal calf cramps. *J Am Board Fam Med.* 2015;28(1):21-27.
23. Prateepavanich P, Kupniratsaikul V, Charoensak T. The relationship between myofascial trigger points of gastrocnemius muscle and nocturnal calf cramps. *J Med Assoc Thai.* 1999;82(5):451-459.
24. Grieve R, Barnett S, Coghill N, Cramp F. Myofascial trigger point therapy for triceps surae dysfunction: a case series. *Man Ther.* 2013;18(6):519-525.
25. Grieve R, Cranston A, Henderson A, John R, Malone G, Mayall C. The immediate effect of triceps surae myofascial trigger point therapy on restricted active ankle joint dorsiflexion in recreational runners: a crossover randomised controlled trial. *J Bodyw Mov Ther.* 2013;17(4):453-461.
26. Barouk P, Barouk LS. Clinical diagnosis of gastrocnemius tightness. *Foot Ankle Clin.* 2014;19(4):659-667.
27. Vaes PH, Duquet W, Casteleyn PP, Handelberg F, Opdecam P. Static and dynamic roentgenographic analysis of ankle stability in braced and nonbraced stable and functionally unstable ankles. *Am J Sports Med.* 1998;26(5):692-702.
28. Young R, Nix S, Wholohan A, Bradhurst R, Reed L. Interventions for increasing ankle joint dorsiflexion: a systematic review and meta-analysis. *J Foot Ankle Res.* 2013;6(1):46.
29. Johanson MA, Wooden M, Catlin PA, et al. Effects of gastrocnemius stretching on ankle dorsiflexion and time-to-heel off during the stance phase of gait. *Phys Ther Sport.* 2006;7(2):93-100.

30. Vernon H, Schneider M. Chiropractic management of myofascial trigger points and myofascial pain syndrome: a systematic review of the literature. *J Manipulative Physiol Ther.* 2009;32(1):14-24.
31. Gerwin RD, Dommerholt J, Shah JP. An expansion of Simons' integrated hypothesis of trigger point formation. *Curr Pain Headache Rep.* 2004;8(6):468-475.
32. Hsieh YL, Kao MJ, Kuan TS, Chen SM, Chen JT, Hong CZ. Dry needling to a key myofascial trigger point may reduce the irritability of satellite MTrPs. *Am J Phys Med Rehabil.* 2007;86(5):397-403.
33. Stetts D, Carpenter J. *Physical Therapy Management of Patients with Spinal Pain: An Evidence Based Approach.* Thorofare, NJ: Slack Inc; 2014.
34. Flynn T, Cleland J, Whitman J. *User's Guide to Musculoskeletal Examination.* Buckner, Kentucky: Evidence in Motion; 2008.
35. Murphy DR, Hurwitz EL, Gerrard JK, Clary R. Pain patterns and descriptions in patients with radicular pain: does the pain necessarily follow a specific dermatome? *Chiropr Osteopat.* 2009;17:9.
36. Deville WL, van der Windt DA, Dzaferagic A, Bezemer PD, Bouter LM. The test of Lasegue: systematic review of the accuracy in diagnosing herniated discs. *Spine (Phila Pa 1976).* 2000;25(9):1140-1147.
37. Vroomen PC, de Krom MC, Wilmink JT, Kester AD, Knottnerus JA. Diagnostic value of history and physical examination in patients suspected of lumbosacral nerve root compression. *J Neurol Neurosurg Psychiatry.* 2002;72(5):630-634.
38. Sobhani S, Dekker R, Postema K, Dijkstra PU. Epidemiology of ankle and foot overuse injuries in sports: a systematic review. *Scand J Med Sci Sports.* 2013;23(6):669-686.
39. Clement DB, Taunton JE, Smart GW. Achilles tendinitis and peritendinitis: etiology and treatment. *Am J Sports Med.* 1984;12(3):179-184.
40. Kvist M. Achilles tendon injuries in athletes. *Ann Chir Gynaecol.* 1991;80(2):188-201.
41. Maffulli N, Wong J, Almekinders LC. Types and epidemiology of tendinopathy. *Clin Sports Med.* 2003;22(4):675-692.
42. Magnussen RA, Dunn WR, Thomson AB. Nonoperative treatment of midportion Achilles tendinopathy: a systematic review. *Clin J Sport Med.* 2009;19(1):54-64.
43. Li HY, Hua YH. Achilles tendinopathy: current concepts about the basic science and clinical treatments. *Biomed Res Int.* 2016;2016:6492597.
44. Kvist M. Achilles tendon injuries in athletes. *Sports Med.* 1994;18(3):173-201.
45. Kujala UM, Sarna S, Kaprio J. Cumulative incidence of achilles tendon rupture and tendinopathy in male former elite athletes. *Clin J Sport Med.* 2005;15(3):133-135.
46. Johansson C. Injuries in elite orienteers. *Am J Sports Med.* 1986;14(5):410-415.
47. Lysholm J, Wiklander J. Injuries in runners. *Am J Sports Med.* 1987;15(2):168-171.
48. Holmes GB, Lin J. Etiologic factors associated with symptomatic achilles tendinopathy. *Foot Ankle Int.* 2006;27(11):952-959.
49. Rolf C, Movin T. Etiology, histopathology, and outcome of surgery in achillodynia. *Foot Ankle Int.* 1997;18(9):565-569.
50. Kader D, Saxena A, Movin T, Maffulli N. Achilles tendinopathy: some aspects of basic science and clinical management. *Br J Sports Med.* 2002;36(4):239-249.
51. Alfredson H, Lorentzon R. Chronic tendon pain: no signs of chemical inflammation but high concentrations of the neurotransmitter glutamate. Implications for treatment? *Curr Drug Targets.* 2003;3(1):43-54.
52. Jarvinen M, Jozsa L, Kannus P, Jarvinen TL, Kvist M, Leadbetter W. Histopathological findings in chronic tendon disorders. *Scand J Med Sci Sports.* 1997;7(2):86-95.
53. Khan KM, Cook JL, Taunton JE, Bonar F. Overuse tendinosis, not tendinitis part 1: a new paradigm for a difficult clinical problem. *Phys Sportsmed.* 2000;28(5):38-48.
54. Fahlstrom M, Lorentzon R, Alfredson H. Painful conditions in the Achilles tendon region in elite badminton players. *Am J Sports Med.* 2002;30(1):51-54.
55. Krolo I, Viskovic K, Ikic D, Klaric-Custovic R, Marotti M, Cicvara T. The risk of sports activities—the injuries of the Achilles tendon in sportsmen. *Coll Antropol.* 2007;31(1):275-278.
56. Petersen W, Welp R, Rosenbaum D. Chronic Achilles tendinopathy: a prospective randomized study comparing the therapeutic effect of eccentric training, the AirHeel brace, and a combination of both. *Am J Sports Med.* 2007;35(10):1659-1667.
57. Rompe JD, Nafe B, Furia JP, Maffulli N. Eccentric loading, shock-wave treatment, or a wait-and-see policy for tendinopathy of the main body of tendo Achillis: a randomized controlled trial. *Am J Sports Med.* 2007;35(3):374-383.
58. Paavola M, Kannus P, Paakkala T, Pasanen M, Jarvinen M. Long-term prognosis of patients with Achilles tendinopathy. An observational 8-year follow-up study. *Am J Sports Med.* 2000;28(5):634-642.
59. Kaufman KR, Brodine SK, Shaffer RA, Johnson CW, Cullison TR. The effect of foot structure and range of motion on musculoskeletal overuse injuries. *Am J Sports Med.* 1999;27(5):585-593.
60. McCrory JL, Martin DF, Lowery RB, et al. Etiologic factors associated with Achilles tendinitis in runners. *Med Sci Sports Exerc.* 1999;31(10):1374-1381.
61. Mahieu NN, Witvrouw E, Stevens V, Van Tiggelen D, Roget P. Intrinsic risk factors for the development of Achilles tendon overuse injury: a prospective study. *Am J Sports Med.* 2006;34(2):226-235.
62. Barge-Caballero E, Crespo-Leiro MG, Paniagua-Martin MJ, et al. Quinolone-related Achilles tendinopathy in heart transplant patients: incidence and risk factors. *J Heart Lung Transplant.* 2008;27(1):46-51.
63. Greene BL. Physical therapist management of fluoroquinolone-induced Achilles tendinopathy. *Phys Ther.* 2002;82(12):1224-1231.
64. Maffulli N, Kader D. Tendinopathy of tendo achillis. *J Bone Joint Surg Br.* 2002;84(1):1-8.
65. Leach RE, James S, Wasilewski S. Achilles tendinitis. *Am J Sports Med.* 1981;9(2):93-98.
66. Schepsis AA, Jones H, Haas AL. Achilles tendon disorders in athletes. *Am J Sports Med.* 2002;30(2):287-305.
67. Maffulli N, Kenward MG, Testa V, Capasso G, Regine R, King JB. Clinical diagnosis of Achilles tendinopathy with tendinosis. *Clin J Sport Med.* 2003;13(1):11-15.
68. MacLellan GE, Vyvyan B. Management of pain beneath the heel and Achilles tendonitis with visco-elastic heel inserts. *Br J Sports Med.* 1981;15(2):117-121.
69. Silbernagel KG, Gustavsson A, Thomee R, Karlsson J. Evaluation of lower leg function in patients with Achilles tendinopathy. *Knee Surg Sports Traumatol Arthrosc.* 2006;14(11):1207-1217.
70. Reiman M, Burgi C, Strube E, et al. The utility of clinical measures for the diagnosis of Achilles tendon injuries: a systematic review with meta-analysis. *J Athl Train.* 2014;49(6):820-829.
71. Bleakney RR, White LM. Imaging of the Achilles tendon. *Foot Ankle Clin.* 2005;10(2):239-254.
72. Neuhold A, Stiskal M, Kainberger F, Schwaighofer B. Degenerative Achilles tendon disease: assessment by magnetic resonance and ultrasonography. *Eur J Radiol.* 1992;14(3):213-220.
73. Bright JM, Fields KB, Draper R. Ultrasound diagnosis of calf injuries. *Sports Health.* 2017;9(4):352-355.
74. Kane D, Balint PV, Gibney R, Bresnihan B, Sturrock RD. Differential diagnosis of calf pain with musculoskeletal ultrasound imaging. *Ann Rheum Dis.* 2004;63(1):11-14.
75. English S, Perret D. Posterior knee pain. *Curr Rev Musculoskelet Med.* 2010;3(1-4):3-10.
76. Lee KH, Matteliano A, Medige J, Smiehorowski T. Electromyographic changes of leg muscles with heel lift: therapeutic implications. *Arch Phys Med Rehabil.* 1987;68(5, pt 1):298-301.
77. Johanson MA, DeArment A, Hines K, et al. The effect of subtalar joint position on dorsiflexion of the ankle/rearfoot versus midfoot/forefoot during gastrocnemius stretching. *Foot Ankle Int.* 2014;35(1):63-70.

Chapter 66

Soleus and Plantaris Muscles

"Jogger's Heel"

Kathleen Geist and Joseph M. Donnelly

1. INTRODUCTION

The soleus and plantaris muscles are located in the superficial posterior compartment of the leg along with the gastrocnemius muscle. The primary function of the soleus muscle is plantar flexion of the ankle joint, inversion of the subtalar joint, and postural control. It is also an essential component of the lower extremity musculovenous pump. The plantaris muscle is thought to have a primary proprioceptive role at the foot and ankle. Trigger points (TrPs) in the soleus and plantaris muscles can cause posterior knee, calf, Achilles tendon, and heel pain. In rare instances, a TrP in the soleus muscle refers pain proximally to the ipsilateral posterior superior iliac spine. Trigger points in the soleus muscle can restrict active and passive ankle dorsiflexion with the knee flexed. Symptoms associated with TrPs in the soleus muscle include pain over the posterior aspect of the lower leg, posterior and inferior aspect of the heel, and arch of the foot, which is exacerbated by walking on inclined surfaces, stair climbing, or running. Differential diagnosis of soleus TrPs should include screening for lumbar radicular pain or radiculopathy, referred pain from the sacroiliac joint, Achilles tendinopathy, exertional compartment syndrome, and Haglund syndrome. Corrective actions for soleus TrPs include postural education, self-stretching, and TrP self-pressure release.

2. ANATOMIC CONSIDERATIONS

Soleus

The soleus muscle is a bipennate muscle located in the superficial posterior compartment of the leg and makes up the triceps surae muscle group together with the gastrocnemius and plantaris muscles. The soleus muscle lies deep to the gastrocnemius muscle in the posterior compartment of the leg (Figure 66-1).[1,2] The proximal attachment of the soleus muscle originates from the soleal line and middle third of the posterior aspect of the tibia, the proximal fourth of the posterior surface of the fibula, and the posterior aspect of the fibular head. A fibrous band forms between the proximal medial and lateral origin of the soleus muscle in which the popliteal artery, popliteal vein, and tibial nerve pass distally into the leg (Figures 66-2 and 66-3).[3] The soleus muscle fibers attach to the underside of the aponeurosis that also provides an attachment for the gastrocnemius muscle. This aponeurosis forms the Achilles tendon and inserts into the posterior aspect of the calcaneus.[1,4]

Morphologic three-dimensional studies demonstrate the separation of the soleus muscle into marginal, anterior, and posterior divisions based on fiber direction and location of the aponeurosis attachment. The anterior aspect of the soleus muscle gives rise from medial and lateral proximal aponeuroses that blend to form the anterior epimysium. A central tendon emerges from the anterior aponeurosis of the soleus muscle and

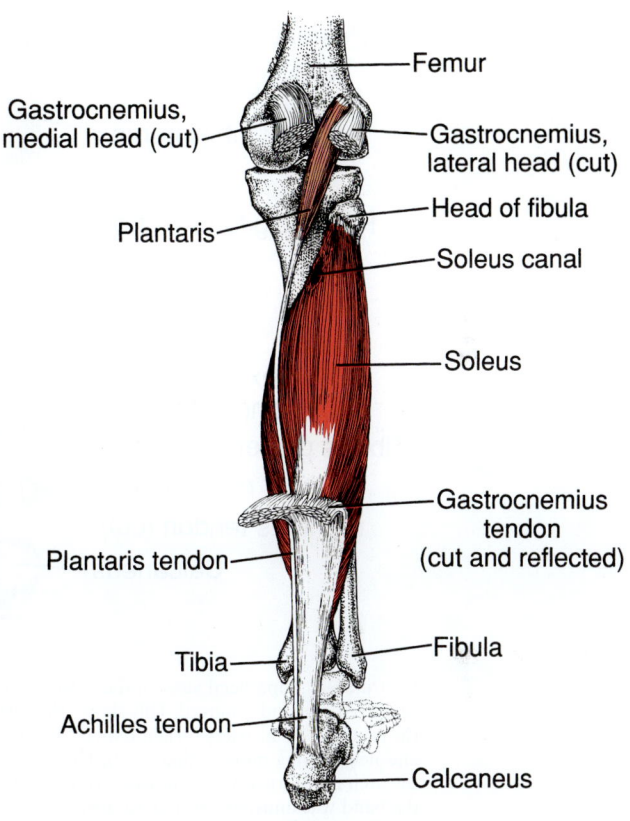

Figure 66-1. The proximal aspect of the soleus muscle arises from the head of the fibula, proximal 1/3 and mid-shaft of the posterior tibia and soleal line and inserts into the posterior aspect of the calcaneus. The plantaris muscle takes origin from the lateral supracondylar line of the femur and inserts on the posterior aspect of the calcaneus.

extends distally to blend into the anterior and central aspect of the Achilles tendon.[2] The distal attachment of the soleus muscle is blended with the gastrocnemius muscle to form the calcaneal, or Achilles, tendon, which inserts on the posterior surface of the calcaneus.[2,4] The fibers of the Achilles tendon twist approximately 90° before insertion. The tendinous fibers from the soleus muscle attach to the medial one-third of the calcaneus (Figure 66-4), and the fibers from the gastrocnemius muscle attach to the lateral two-thirds.[5] In fact, the soleus muscle represents only 28% of the insertion of the triceps surae into the Achilles tendon.[6]

The marginal soleus muscle is located at the periphery of the soleus muscle and has direct attachments to the anterior and posterior aponeuroses of the posterior leg. The direction

697

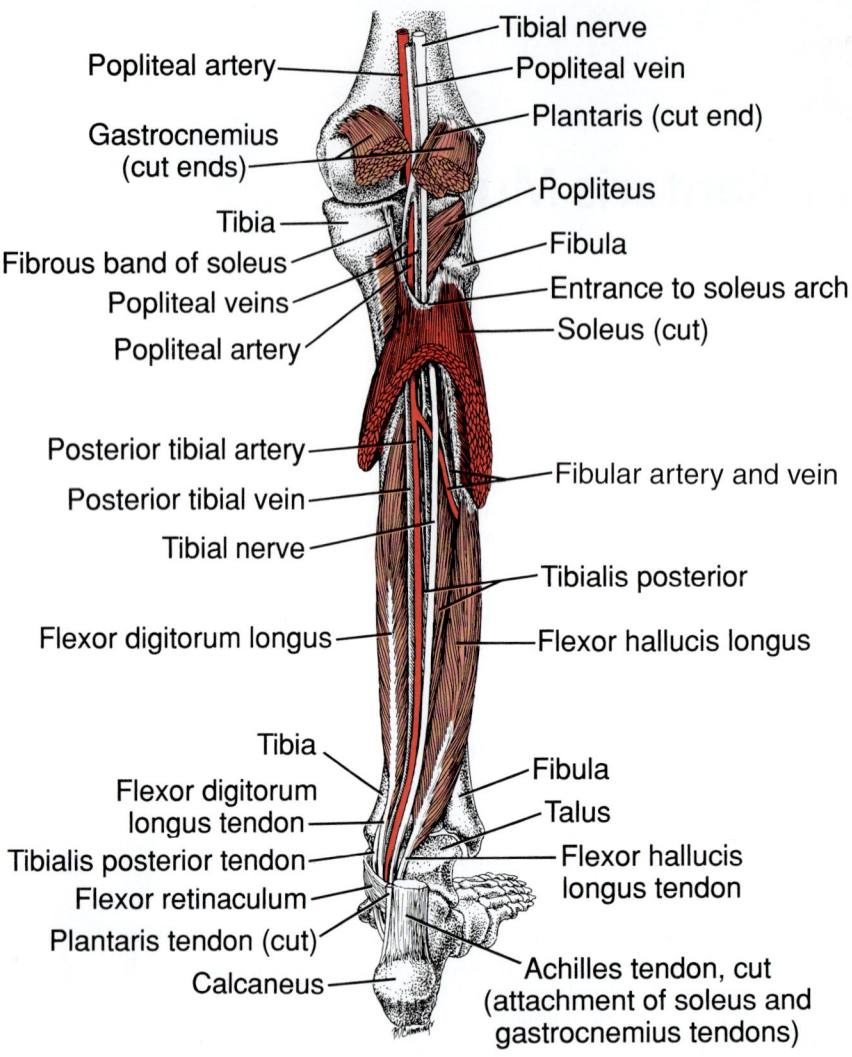

Figure 66-2. Superficial view of the soleus canal with the major portion of the right soleus muscle (dark red) cut and removed. This shows the relations of the soleus tendinous arch and the muscle to the posterior tibial artery (bright red), posterior tibial veins (black cross hatching), tibial nerve (white), and neighboring muscles (light red). The fibrous band that extends upward from the medial side of the arch that forms the soleus canal is drawn from a photograph of an anatomic specimen in which the band was unusually well developed.

of the fiber bundles of the marginal region of the soleus muscle facilitates a tightening of the anterior and posterior aponeuroses, improving the efficiency of muscle contraction.

The presence of an accessory soleus muscle is an atypical anatomic variant and is believed to occur from an early splitting of a soleus fascicle during embryologic development. An accessory soleus muscle is usually identified from incidental findings on magnetic resonance imaging (MRI) and can be an uncommon source of exertional compartment syndrome with concomitant tarsal tunnel syndrome. The anatomic variant is present in 0.7% to 5.6% of the general population.[7] The origin of an accessory soleus muscle can arise posteriorly from the distal aspect of the tibia or from the ventral aspect of the soleus muscle. The distal attachments of an accessory soleus muscle can insert on the superior aspect of the calcaneus or on anteromedial aspect of the Achilles tendon.[7] Others have reported that the accessory soleus muscle has three possible attachments: (1) a distal attachment to the medial aspect of the calcaneus by a separate tendon (26.1%), (2) a distal tendinous attachment to the calcaneal tendon (3.5%), and (3) a distal fleshy attachment to the medial surface of the calcaneus (4.3%).[8]

Plantaris

The plantaris muscle is located in the superficial posterior compartment of the leg and together with the gastrocnemius and soleus muscles are known as the tricep surae muscles. The plantaris muscle is considered to be an accessory to the lateral head of the gastrocnemius muscle. It is a small, thin muscle originating from the inferior aspect of the lateral supracondylar line of the femur and fibers of the oblique popliteal ligament that courses proximally in an inferior and medial direction in the popliteal fossa. The length of the plantaris muscle belly varies in size from 7 to 13 cm in length from the origin on the femur. The myotendinous junction of the plantaris muscle occurs in the proximal one-third of the leg at the level of the superior attachment of the soleus muscle on the tibia. The plantaris tendon travels along the medial aspect of the muscle belly and descends distally as the tendon courses between the soleus muscle and the medial head of the gastrocnemius muscle at the mid-portion of the leg. The tendon continues in an inferomedial direction along the medial aspect of the Achilles tendon and inserts on the calcaneal tuberosity[3,9] (Figure 66-1).

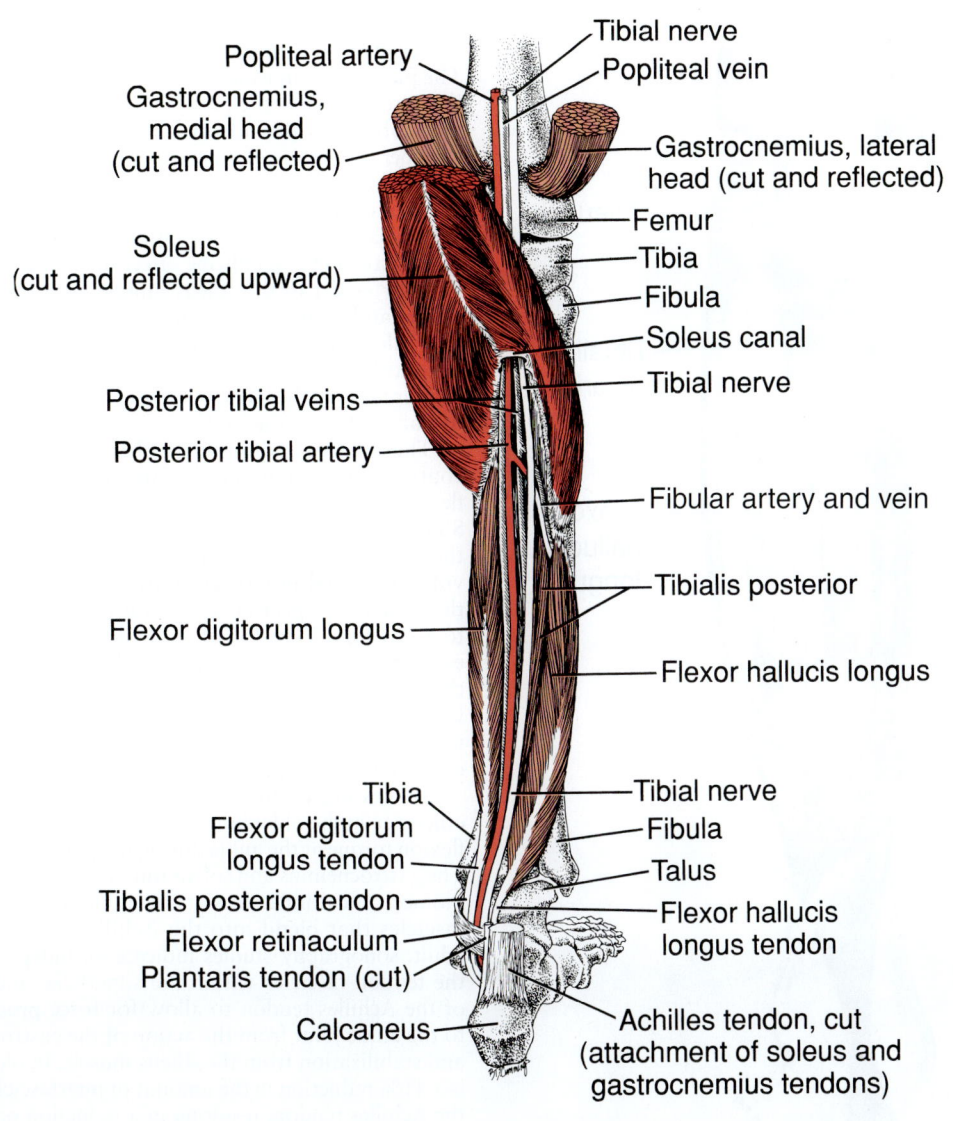

Figure 66-3. The soleus muscle (dark red) has been reflected upward showing the distal opening of the soleus canal and its relation to the tibial nerve (white), to the posterior tibial artery (bright red), to the posterior tibial veins (black cross hatching), and to the adjacent musculature (light red). This is an artist's reconstruction of what the canal would look like if it were possible to reflect the muscle without cutting its proximal attachments to the tibia and fibula. The gastrocnemius muscle is cut and reflected.

A retrospective review was performed establishing the prevalence of an accessory plantaris muscle on routine MRI of 1000 individuals with acute or chronic knee pain.[10] An accessory plantaris muscle was identified in 63 of the 1000 individuals, with the origin of 62 accessory plantaris muscles merging with the origin of the plantaris muscle and one accessory plantaris muscle merging with the lateral head of the gastrocnemius muscle and inserting distally to the insertion site of the vastus lateralis muscle. There was variability among the insertion sites of 43 individuals including the lateral patellar retinaculum and the iliotibial band.[10]

2.1. Innervation and Vascularization

The soleus and plantaris muscles are innervated by the tibial nerve from the L5, S1, and S2 nerve roots of the lumbosacral plexus. The soleus muscle receives most of its innervation from S1 and S2 and the plantaris muscle mostly from L5 and S1 nerve roots.[3] The tibial nerve continues distally through the posterior compartment of the leg and courses between the flexor digitorum and flexor hallucis longus tendons posterior to the medial malleolus of the tibia at the tarsal tunnel.[3]

The popliteal artery descends inferiorly to the knee joint, giving rise to the posterior tibial artery that supplies the soleus, plantaris, and flexor digitorum muscles in the posterior compartment of the leg. As the posterior tibial artery courses distally, the fibular artery provides a muscular branch to the soleus, tibialis posterior, and flexor hallucis longus muscles.[4]

2.2. Function

Soleus

The soleus muscle has the largest cross-sectional area of any muscle in the leg and is comprised of primarily slow-twitch, type I muscle fibers that are responsible for postural control and activities that require slower speeds of motion such as walking.[2,11] The predominance of type I muscle fibers in the soleus muscle suggests that the role of the soleus muscle is to

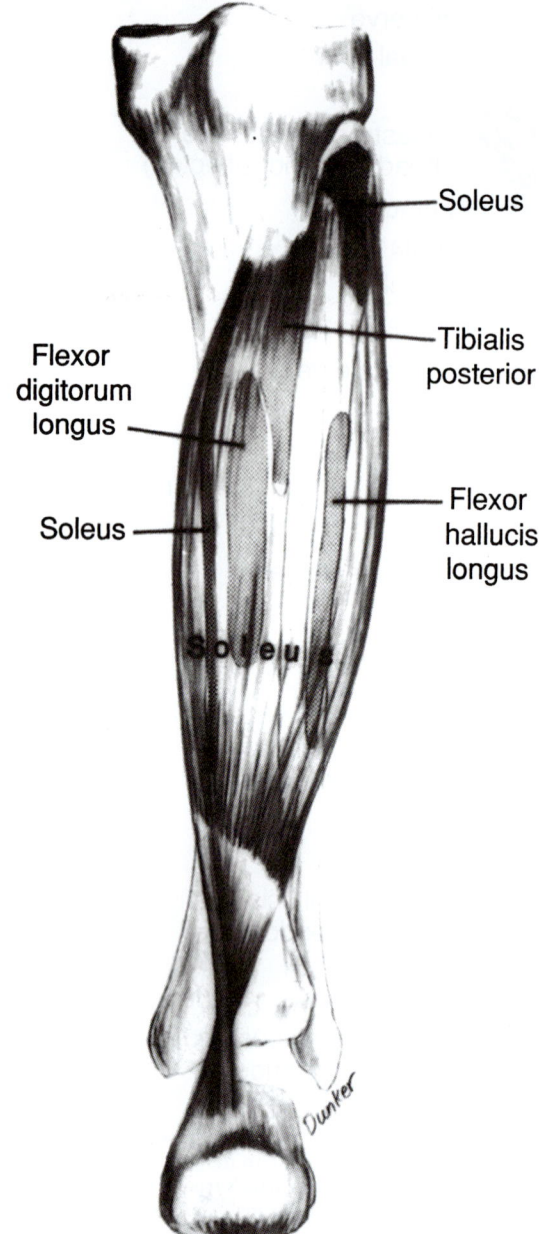

Figure 66-4. Attachment of the soleus portion of the right Achilles tendon to the os calcis, posterior view. Note the tendon's rotation of 90° and attachment to the medial one-third of the calcaneus. The gastrocnemius portion of the tendon (not shown) attaches to the lateral two-thirds of the os calcis. Reproduced with permission from Michael RH, Holder LE. The soleus syndrome. A cause of medial tibial stress (shin splints). *Am J Sports Med.* 1985;13:87-94.

provide tonic postural control of the limb in weight bearing and lower intensity muscle contractions in ankle plantar flexion.[12]

Because of the close proximity of the vascular structures to the soleus muscle, the gentle muscle contractions that occur in the soleus muscle with postural control suggest a secondary role with facilitation of venous blood return from the lower leg. The soleus muscle provides a major pumping action to return blood from the lower extremity to the heart. Venous sinuses in the soleus muscle are compressed by the muscle's strong contractions, so that its venous blood is forced upward toward the heart. This pumping action (the body's second heart) depends on competent valves in the popliteal veins. Valves in the veins to prevent reflux of the blood are most numerous in the veins of the lower extremities where the vessels must return blood against high hydrostatic pressure. The popliteal vein usually contains four valves.[3] Deeper veins that are subject to the pumping action of muscle contraction are more richly provided with valves.

Fiber orientation of the soleus muscle has distinct implications for the different biomechanical influences during movement. The fibers of the posterior aspect of the soleus muscle are of shorter length, have an oblique orientation, and serve to generate higher forces, creating a stabilizing effect at the leg. The fibers of the anterior aspect of the soleus muscle are longer on the lateral aspect and shorter on the medial aspect. The longer muscle fibers along the lateral aspect of the anterior surface are thought to contribute to generating ankle plantar flexion forces, and the shorter fibers of the medial aspect of the soleus muscle contribute to stabilization of the leg.[13]

The anterior and posterior fibers of the soleus muscle may contribute to variation in function by providing ankle plantar flexion and stabilization of the leg in weight-bearing positions. Some authors suggest that the variation of fiber sizes within the medial and lateral aspect of the soleus muscle may provide functional differences during activity.[13] The muscles in the posterior aspect of the leg must have sufficient flexibility to allow for 10° to 15° of ankle dorsiflexion while providing eccentric control of the leg over the foot and stabilization of the knee joint during the early-stance phase of gait. During the late-stance and push-off phase of gait, the soleus and plantaris muscles contract concentrically to assist in forward propulsion of the lower extremity.

Studies suggest that age-related changes affect the muscular efficiency in the older adult and result in a reduction of plantar flexion torque at the ankle during the push-off phase of gait.[14,15] The gastrocnemius and soleus muscles can have complimentary biomechanical influences at the ankle through shared tendon fascicles that blend into the Achilles tendon. In a younger adult, sonography studies indicate an independent gliding of the tendon fascicles within the superficial and deep portions of the Achilles tendon to allow for force production transfer to the ankle joint from the action of the gastrocnemius muscle and stabilization from the soleus muscle. In older adults, there is a 41% reduction in the amount of interfascicle gliding within the Achilles tendon, resulting in a reduction of plantar flexion torque at the ankle during gait, in turn, resulting in less peak ankle power during the push-off phase of gait.[14,15]

Plantaris

The anatomic location and cross-sectional size of the plantaris muscle suggests that it may be a very weak flexor of the knee with minimal biomechanical influence at the foot and ankle.[11] Although the plantaris muscle is not a significant contributor to knee flexion or ankle plantar flexion, it is considered to have a large contribution to proprioception at the foot and ankle due to the higher proportion of high-density muscle spindles within the musculotendinous unit.[9]

2.3. Functional Unit

The functional unit to which a muscle belongs includes the muscles that reinforce and counter its actions as well as the joints that the muscle crosses. The interdependence of these structures is functionally reflected in the organization and neural connections of the sensory motor cortex. The functional unit is emphasized because the presence of a TrP in one muscle of the unit increases the likelihood that the other muscles of the unit will also develop TrPs. When inactivating TrPs in a muscle, one must be concerned about TrPs that may develop in muscles that are functionally interdependent. Box 66-1 grossly represents the functional unit of the soleus and plantaris muscles.[16]

Chapter 66: Soleus and Plantaris Muscles 701

Box 66-1 Functional unit of the soleus and plantaris muscles

Action	Synergists	Antagonists
Plantar flexion	Gastrocnemius Flexor hallucis longus Flexor digitorum longus Tibialis posterior Fibularis longus Fibularis brevis	Tibialis anterior Extensor digitorum longus Extensor hallucis longus Fibularis tertius

3. CLINICAL PRESENTATION

3.1. Referred Pain Pattern

Soleus

An individual presenting with TrPs in the soleus muscle may report pain in the posterior aspect of the calf, plantar heel, and the ipsilateral sacroiliac joint (Figure 66-5A). Trigger points in the soleus muscle can be developed in any portion of the muscle; however, it has been clinically observed that there are three common areas. The most common area for the development of TrPs is distal within the muscle belly, medial to the Achilles tendon, with referred pain along the Achilles tendon and into the posterior and inferior aspects of the calcaneus. This clinical pattern may be related to the fact that this area of the soleus muscle receives the highest stress from the Achilles tendon. A second common location for TrP development is approximately 1 to 2 in inferior to the proximal attachment of the soleus muscle to the tibia and fibula. The common referred pain pattern is along the midline of the posterior aspect of the calf, inferior to the popliteal crease, and superior to the Achilles tendon. The least common area for TrP development is along the distal aspect of the soleus muscle lateral to the Achilles tendon. The referred pain pattern for a TrP in this area can be located on the ipsilateral sacroiliac joint (Figure 66-5A).

An exceptional pain pattern referred to the jaw from the TrP in the soleus muscle has been observed twice (Figure 66-5B). In one patient, this TrP referred pain to the ipsilateral face deep in the jaw and temporomandibular joint with malocclusion ("Now my teeth don't meet," she said) whenever the ankle on that side was actively or passively dorsiflexed, but with no pain that is usually characteristic of the soleus muscle. The jaw pain and spasm were eliminated immediately by injecting the soleus TrPs. Occasionally, such totally unexpected patterns of pain referred from TrPs may be noted with other muscles, which emphasizes the importance of obtaining a detailed and comprehensive pain history.[17]

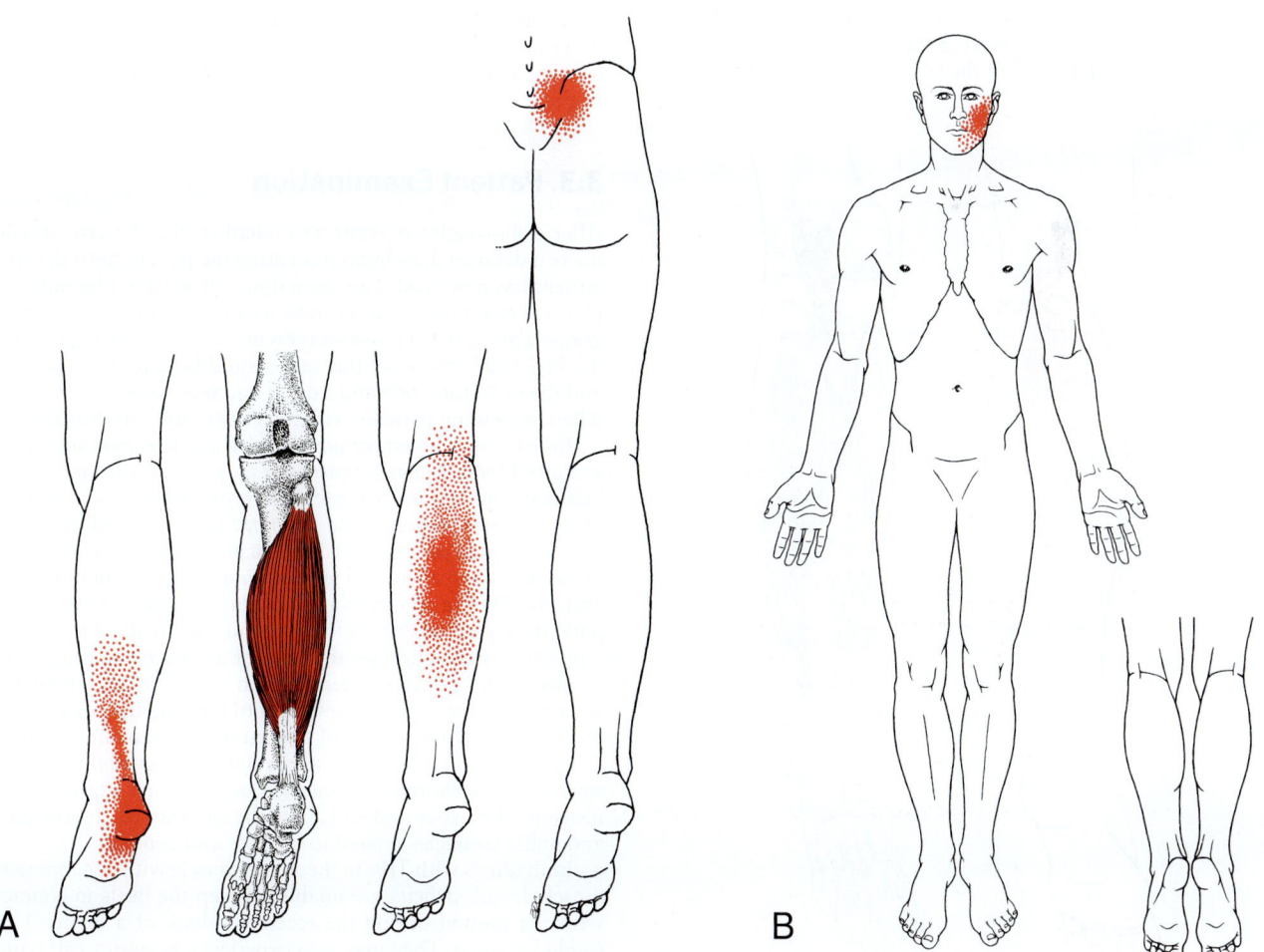

Figure 66-5. Referred pain patterns of the soleus muscle. A, More common pain referral symptoms. B, Exceptional pain pattern.

Plantaris

Referred pain from TrPs in the plantaris muscle refers to the midline of the posterior aspect of the knee and proximal leg (Figure 66-6).

3.2. Symptoms

An individual with TrPs in the soleus muscle will report pain along the Achilles tendon, both medially and laterally, extending down to the heel and to the plantar aspect of the heel. Additionally, TrPs located in the soleus muscle can reproduce an isolated sharp pain into the plantar aspect of the heel. The patient may report unbearable pain in the plantar aspect of the heel upon the first step in the morning or after prolonged periods of rest. These symptoms are compatible with a clinical diagnosis of plantar heel pain or plantar fasciitis. Heel pain is one of the most common reports of pain in recreational runners. These athletes may present with a previous diagnosis of heel spurs or plantar fasciitis when the issue is actually arising from TrPs in the soleus muscle. A Delphi study reported that most physical therapists considered the soleus as a relevant muscle for the management of plantar heel pain.[18] Renan-Ordine et al[19] found that multimodal treatment intervention including TrP release, neuromuscular soft-tissue release, and stretching to the gastrocnemius and soleus muscles was effective for reducing pain and improving physical function in individuals with plantar heel pain. Nevertheless, no epidemiologic study has investigated the prevalence of soleus muscle TrPs in this population. The patient may also report nocturnal heel pain; however, reports of nocturnal calf cramping are more related to gastrocnemius TrPs.

Trigger points in the soleus muscle may also contribute to reports of pain and discomfort in the ipsilateral sacroiliac joint. The presence of TrPs within the soleus muscle can reproduce a "pulling" or aching sensation in the posterior aspect of the leg, especially with resisted ankle plantar flexion or with passive dorsiflexion range of motion with the knee flexed. Patients may also experience hypersensitivity to manual palpation or mechanical hyperalgesia.[20] In fact, pain referral from soleus TrPs is felt deep within the posterior part of the leg, which could help differentiate between more superficial symptoms induced by gastrocnemius TrPs.

Soleus TrPs often restrict ankle dorsiflexion; therefore, the patient may report difficulty with performing a squat because of the limitation in ankle dorsiflexion with the knee flexed. Individuals with soleus TrPs are prone to develop low back pain because the restriction of ankle dorsiflexion leads them to lean over and lift improperly or inefficiently. If soleus TrPs are highly irritable, the patient may also report increased difficulty with walking uphill or on an incline or with ascending and descending stairs. Different studies have demonstrated significant improvements in ankle dorsiflexion range of motion following one manual TrP release[21,22] or multimodal treatment intervention including TrP release and stretching of gastrocnemius and soleus muscles in individuals with triceps surae dysfunction.[23] A case report has described the benefit of dry needling to the triceps surae muscles in a ballet dancer with chief reports of right posterior knee pain with jumping, pivoting, walking, and running activities. Following two sessions of dry needling of TrPs to the triceps surae muscles, the dancer was able to return to full dance activity without pain or activity limitations.[20] The randomized clinical trial conducted by Cotchett et al[18] found that TrP dry needling of several muscles, including the soleus, was effective for the management of plantar heel pain; although its clinical significance was small. Finally, the application of extracorporeal shock wave therapy over TrPs in the soleus muscle has also been effective for patients with plantar heel pain.[24]

Soleus TrPs located in the proximal portion of the muscle are more likely to interfere with the soleus musculovenous pump, causing symptoms of calf and foot pain together with edema of the foot and ankle.

3.3. Patient Examination

After a thorough subjective examination, the clinician should make a detailed drawing representing the pain pattern that the patient has described. This depiction will assist in planning the physical examination and can be useful in monitoring the progression of the patient as symptoms improve or change. The type, quality, and location of the pain should be carefully assessed, and the utilization of standardized outcome tools is imperative when examining patients with lower extremity dysfunctions.

Individuals who report posterior leg and heel pain should be examined for radicular symptoms or radiculopathy from the lumbosacral spine and referred pain from proximal joints and muscles of the posterior aspect of the sacroiliac joint, hip, and thigh.[20]

Observation of static and dynamic posture is essential because of the role of the soleus and plantaris muscles in postural stability and gait. During an observation of static standing posture, the patient may be unable to fully extend the involved extremity when keeping the heel on the floor or a genu recurvatum may be observed.[16] Functional testing such as double- and single-leg squat will allow a quick assessment of hip and knee control, as well as a quick assessment of talocrural, subtalar, and midfoot range of motion along with soleus muscle extensibility. Timed single-leg stance with eyes open and closed will give a quantitative measure of balance and will allow the clinician to observe foot and ankle strategies related to balance and control.

Individuals with TrPs in the soleus muscle with concomitant muscle length deficits are unable to keep the heels in contact with the ground during the eccentric phase of a bilateral or single-leg squat. They may also experience posterior calf pain, demonstrate a weight shift to the uninvolved side to unload the involved extremity, and avoid ankle plantar flexion with the concentric phase of a double-leg squatting task.[20]

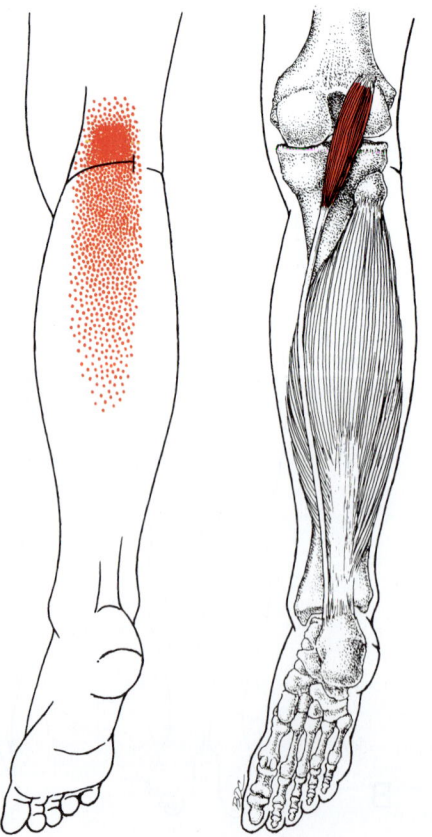

Figure 66-6. Referred pain pattern of the plantaris muscle.

Trigger points in the soleus muscle can cause a limitation of ankle dorsiflexion resulting in a postural alteration in standing, thus creating genu recurvatum at the knee joint. A limitation in soleus muscle extensibility limits the forward progression of the tibia over the foot during the stance phase of gait with a resultant early heel rise during the late-stance and push-off phases of gait.[11] Ankle dorsiflexion of 10° is required for tibial advancement over the foot during walking and 15° to 20° with running tasks.[25] The presence of TrPs in the soleus muscle can limit passive ankle dorsiflexion during gait, causing changes in the biomechanics of the knee, ankle, and subtalar joints that can predispose an individual to injury.[26] An analysis of kinetic and kinematic data of an individual with chronic myofascial dysfunction demonstrated increased knee flexion and an increase in the vertical ground reaction force during the early-and late-stance phases of gait.[27]

To differentiate gastrocnemius muscle from soleus muscle length restrictions, the clinician passively dorsiflexes the talocrural joint first with the knee straight and then flexed to 90°. If range of motion in dorsiflexion increases with the knee flexed to 90°, more than likely there is a length deficit in the gastrocnemius muscle. Further, structural differentiation of the foot and ankle can direct the practitioner to evaluate if a restriction in ankle dorsiflexion is attributable either to limited extensibility of the soleus muscle or joint hypomobility of the talocrural joint. With the patient in the prone position with the knee flexed to 90°, the clinician passively dorsiflexes the ankle, and if the clinician feels a muscular end feel and the patient reports a feeling of stretch over the posterior aspect of the lower leg, a soleus muscle length deficit is implicated. However, if a capsular end feel is experienced by the clinician and the patient reports a feeling of tightness over the anterior joint line of the talocrural joint, the talocrural joint is implicated (Figure 66-7).

Soleus muscle weakness is tested by having the patient stand on the ball of one foot with the knee flexed to 10° to 15° with adequate stabilization. During this test, a strong tendency for the foot to invert indicates substitution by the tibialis posterior muscle and/or the long flexor muscles of the toes, whereas a strong tendency for it to evert indicates substitution by the fibularis longus and brevis muscles. These substitutions suggest soleus muscle weakness. Also, with normal triceps surae strength, the subject should be able to jump at least 10 times on the ball of the foot without heel contact on the floor.[28]

In addition to talocrural joint testing, passive accessory motion of the distal and proximal tibiofibular joints should be examined, especially when the patient reports posterior knee pain and loss of knee extension range of motion that may be associated with soleus and/or plantaris TrPs.

Neurodynamic assessment should also be conducted to rule in or out symptoms caused by nervous tissue in the tibial, fibular, or sural nerves, which can give rise to symptoms in the posterior leg, ankle, and foot.

3.4. Trigger Point Examination

Trigger points in the soleus muscle contribute to limitations in joint range of motion, postural changes, alterations in muscular activation, and modifications in functional movement patterns.[20] Studies assessing the prevalence of TrPs have demonstrated a greater occurrence of latent TrPs within the soleus muscle.[26] Two hundred and twenty research participants were evaluated for the presence of latent TrPs. The results indicated that 33% of healthy, asymptomatic individuals had latent TrPs in one or both of the triceps surae muscles, with the identification of latent TrPs in the left soleus muscle more common than in the right.[26] The most common diagnostic criteria for the identification of latent TrPs in the soleus muscle were the presence of a taut band and a localized, tender spot upon palpation. Similarly, Zuil-Escobar et al[29] also reported that 30% of an asymptomatic sample of 206 individuals exhibited latent TrPs in the soleus muscle. This study also reported an average number of 7.5 latent TrPs in the lower extremity musculature in asymptomatic people.

Soleus

The soleus muscle can be palpated with an individual in a prone, side-lying or hook-lying position. In prone, the knee joint is flexed to 10° to 15° by placing a pillow under the ankle to ease muscular tension from the gastrocnemius (Figure 66-8). In side-lying, the knees are held in flexion to place the gastrocnemius muscle on slack. The soleus muscle can be palpated inferior to the medial and lateral heads of the gastrocnemius muscle and lateral to the Achilles tendon when an individual actively plantar-flexes the ankle joint.[30] Cross-fiber flat palpation is used to identify TrPs within the soleus muscle in the prone and side-lying positions (Figure 66-8A and B). A cross-fiber pincer palpation can also be used to identify TrPs in the soleus muscle in side-lying with the affected leg up or in hook-lying position (Figure 66-8C and D).

Plantaris

The plantaris muscle can be palpated in the popliteal fossa with an individual in the prone position with the knee flexed to 90°. Palpation of the proximal aspect of the plantaris muscle can be performed medial and superior to the lateral head of the gastrocnemius muscle (Figure 66-9). With the patient in prone and the knee passively flexed to 90°, the clinician asks the patient to perform a gentle contraction into knee flexion and ankle plantar flexion while maintaining palpation of the proximal insertion of the plantaris muscle with the cranial hand[9] (Figure 66-9).

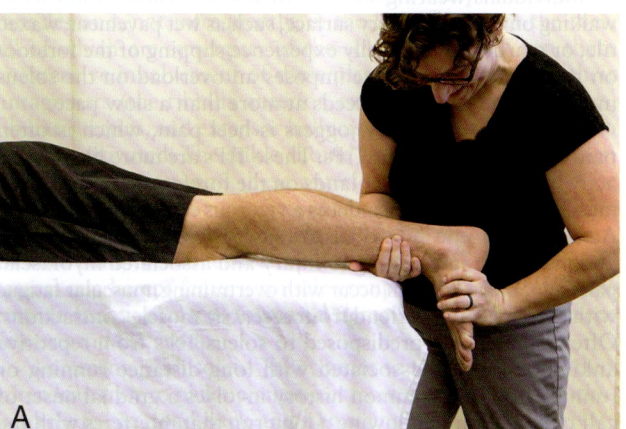
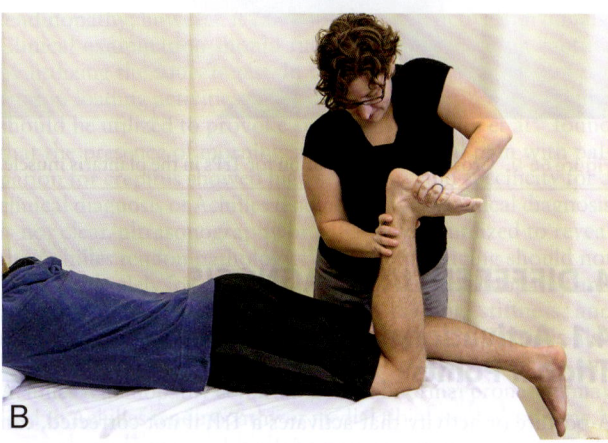

Figure 66-7. Muscle length testing. A, Gastrocnemius muscle. B, Soleus muscle. Note the change in dorsiflexion with the knee flexed.

present, it is commonly associated with Achilles tendinopathy. It often presents as a painful mass at the posteromedial ankle and is associated with exercise-induced pain.[43,44]

If pain and tenderness are referred to the tendon by active soleus TrPs, they can be distinguished from the symptoms of tendinopathy through treatment of the soleus TrPs. Inactivation of the soleus TrPs relieves the pain and tenderness immediately if these symptoms are referred and not due to tendinopathy.

Haglund syndrome is associated with posterior heel pain with or without a visible and palpable haglund deformity, or "pump bump."[45] In this syndrome, there is a thickening of the soft tissues at the insertion of the Achilles tendon. It is seen in those who wear stiff shoes with a shallow heel while engaging in strenuous activity. Haglund syndrome is characterized by a radiographically prominent calcaneal enlargement at the insertion of the Achilles tendon, retrocalcaneal bursitis, thickening of the Achilles tendon, and a convexity of the superficial soft tissues at the level of the Achilles tendon insertion. The degree of enlargement is measurable by radiography.[45]

Singh et al[46] investigated the progression of isolated calf deep vein thrombosis in 156 patients and 180 limbs. There were no gender differences identified, and 15% had bilateral deep vein thrombosis with the soleal vein most commonly involved, followed by the fibular, posterior tibial, and gastrocnemius veins. Propagation to a proximal vein was found in 11 patients, and pulmonary embolism was found in 9 patients within the 1 to 3-month follow-up period. The investigators concluded that isolated calf deep vein thrombosis can be safely observed without anticoagulation therapy. However, if patients have comorbidities such as immobilization or status-postorthopedic surgery, anticoagulation therapy is recommended until they are fully ambulating and the follow-up duplex scan is negative.[46] Other investigators found that exercises intended to strengthen the muscular component of the musculovenous pump (posterior calf muscles) and correction of the step cycle during gait lead to clinical improvements in the course of varicose vein disease.[47] This finding supports the essential function of the triceps surae muscles as a musculovenous pump to improve limb circulation, and this function is dependent on talocrural joint accessory mobility and adequate extensibility of the gastrocnemius and soleus muscles.

Exertional compartment syndromes of the leg are a common form of overuse injury. Compartment syndromes are characterized by increased pressure within a muscular compartment sufficient to compromise the circulation of the muscles within it. The increased pressure obstructs venous flow, which causes further swelling and more pressure. If prolonged, the resultant ischemia can lead to necrosis of the muscles and nerves within the compartment. Following a traumatic injury, it is vital that this condition be recognized immediately and managed properly to avoid possibly catastrophic consequences. Anterior compartment syndromes are most common, followed by lateral, deep posterior, and finally superficial posterior compartment syndromes.[48,49]

Deep posterior chronic exertional compartment syndrome (dp-CECS) of the leg is usually gradually induced by exercise in young endurance athletes. It produces a sense of tightness, dull aching and cramping, and diminished sensibility of the involved muscles. As the condition intensifies, pain persists for longer periods following exercise. Posterior compartment syndromes are commonly bilateral, usually fail to respond to conservative therapy, are often relieved by prolonged periods of rest, and often require fasciotomy.[50] On examination, dp-CECS demonstrates tenderness deep in the calf in the muscle tissue itself. The diagnosis of dp-CECS is confirmed by finding elevated intracompartmental pressure within the deep posterior compartment. However, diagnostic techniques and surgical interventions are highly subjective and lack standardization.[50]

The precise etiology of the posterior compartment syndromes has not yet been established. An initiating trauma or hypertrophy of the muscle has been postulated. The role of TrPs as part of this process is unknown, but there is a strong possibility that, in muscles prone to developing a compartment syndrome, TrPs may make a significant contribution. Chapter 63 (Section 4.3) contains additional information on chronic exertional compartment syndrome.

5. CORRECTIVE ACTIONS

Individuals with TrPs in the soleus muscle may benefit from adopting sitting or standing postures that place the ankle in a small degree of plantar flexion. While sitting, an individual can sit with his or her knees in 50° or 60° of knee flexion allowing the foot to contact the floor for lower extremity support, while providing ankle plantar flexion to place more slack on the soleus muscle. A common perpetuating cause of TrPs in the soleus muscle is an improperly designed or improperly used leg rest that causes calf compression. People who sit in reclining chairs with built-in leg rests that concentrate weight on a portion of the calf may require additional pillows or may need to restrict elevation of the leg rest. If an ottoman is used for leg support, it should be designed and arranged, so that part of the weight is carried by the heels and not by the bulk of the calf muscle. In standing postures, individuals can place a wedge under the shoe insert to provide ankle plantar flexion and take tension off the Achilles tendon, or they can wear a running shoe with a higher inclination under the posterior aspect of the shoe.

In general, the leg muscles feel better if the ankle is maintained in a neutral position throughout the night; therefore, adjusting the patient's sleeping posture may be necessary. This position is facilitated by having the bed sheets at the foot of the bed untucked to reduce external force into excessive plantar flexion (see Figure 66-6). Using a pillow between the legs and knees in side-lying to place the foot and ankle in a neutral position may also be beneficial. Patients with irritable TrPs should avoid lying on the affected side because the pressure from the bed may perpetuate TrP activity.

Other activities that should be modified include walking on level surfaces instead of inclined surfaces, avoiding tight or elastic materials around the calf, avoiding prolonged or excessive ankle plantar flexion (toes pointed) with swimming activities, and avoiding wearing shoes with a heel greater than 2 in. During walking, the patient may be encouraged to facilitate an early heel off to prevent excessive stretching of the soleus muscle during late-stance phase of gait. Soleus muscle overload can be avoided by limiting walking in soft sand, unless the calf muscles are conditioned for it, and by not walking long distances on a sidewalk or beach slanted to one side.

Patients with soleus TrPs often experience pain when walking upstairs facing forward as usual. This problem may be corrected by approaching the stairway with the body erect and angled 45°, placing the entire foot flat on the step above without markedly pulling the toes and foot up toward the ceiling. This technique avoids painful strain and stretch of the soleus muscle by minimizing ankle plantar flexion and dorsiflexion. Keeping the body erect minimizes strain on the back muscles and gives the strong quadriceps femoris muscle a larger share of the load. This angling technique works equally well on a ladder. It can also be used when ascending a steep slope by turning the body and feet to one side and climbing sideways or by following a zigzag course up the hill. When driving on a long trip, one should make frequent stops to walk around for a few minutes to restore circulation; cruise control also provides an opportunity to change positions.

Soleus TrP self-pressure release can be performed in the supine and seated positions (Figure 66-10A and B). Pressure can be provided by placing the affected soleus muscle on top of the opposite knee (Figure 66-10A). Moving the leg down over the knee along the back of the calf starting at the back of the ankle and moving slowly toward the knee, the patient stops and holds light pressure over the area of discomfort (no more than 4/10 pain) for 15 to 30 seconds. This can be repeated five times. Trigger point self-pressure release can also be performed with a manual technique (Figure 66-10B). Finding the most tender spot, light pressure (no more than 4/10 pain) is applied with a pincer grasp (Figure 66-10B), with a TrP release tool or ball (see Figure 65-7B), or with a TrP release roller

Chapter 66: Soleus and Plantaris Muscles 707

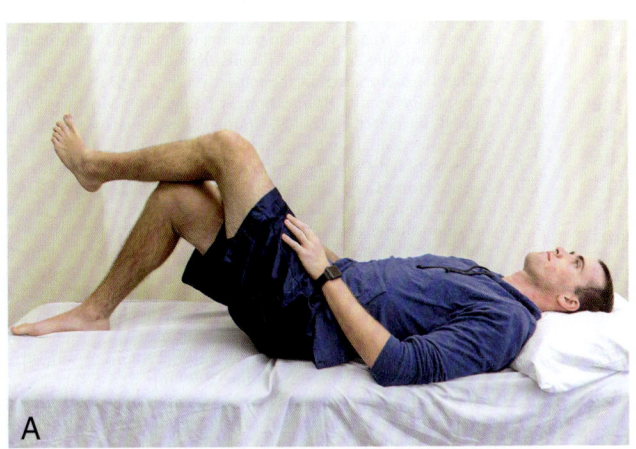
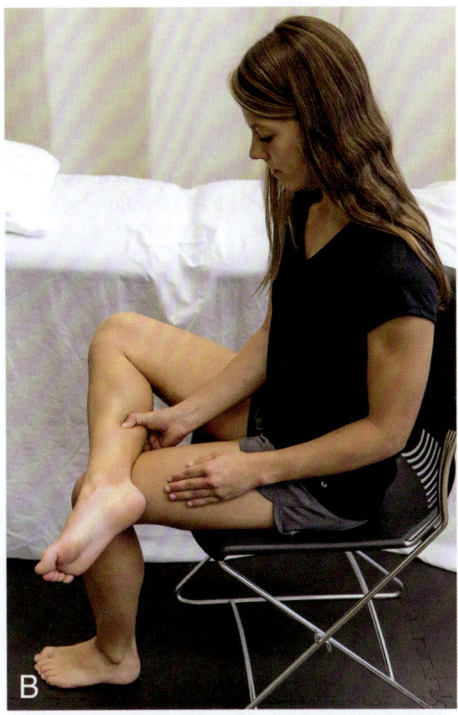

Figure 66-10. Trigger point self-pressure release. A, The patient uses the knee of the opposite side to apply pressure on the TrPs. B, Manual release with pincer grasp.

tool (see Figure 65-7C). Pressure is held for 15 to 30 seconds or until pain reduces, and this technique can be repeated five times, several times per day (Figure 66-10A and B).

Soleus muscle self-stretching can be performed in a sitting or standing position. Self-stretching of the soleus muscle in a sitting position requires the patient to maintain a long sitting position with the involved knee flexed to 70°. A long strap is placed under the forefoot, while maintaining the knee in a flexed position to place the gastrocnemius muscle on slack, and a prolonged passive stretch is applied to the foot and ankle into dorsiflexion (Figure 66-11A). Self-stretching of the soleus muscle in standing is performed with the individual in a stride stance facing a wall, with both feet placed in a neutral position and the hands on the wall at shoulder height or on a chair (Figure 66-11B).

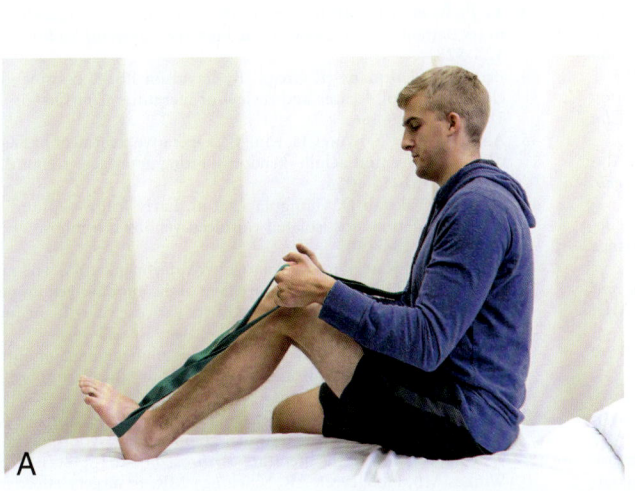
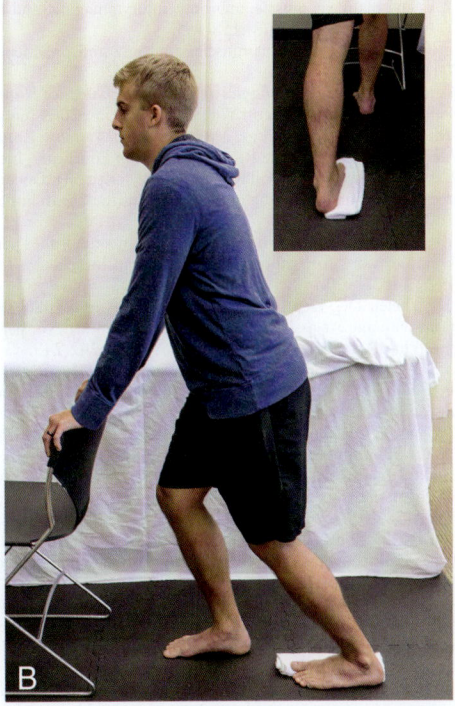

Figure 66-11. Self-stretch of the soleus muscle. A, Gentle stretch with a strap or sheet for irritable TrPs. B, Runners stretch. A flat towel is placed along the inside of the foot to prevent flattening of the arch while stretching.

With the affected leg behind, the foot should be placed in slight supination using a small wedge along the entire inside edge of the foot (Figure 68-6B, small pic) to emphasize dorsiflexion through the hindfoot and prevent excessive forces into dorsiflexion through the midfoot.[51] While maintaining the knee in a slightly flexed position and the heel on the floor, the individual leans forward until he or she feels a stretch in the lower aspect of the calf region. This stretch may be augmented by postisometric relaxation. At the first onset of a stretch in the calf, the ball of the foot is pushed into the floor with a slight contraction of the calf muscles, but the heel or foot remains on the floor. Holding the contraction for 6 to 10 seconds, a deep inhalation is performed. Then, during a slow exhale though the mouth, the calf muscle is allowed to relax, and another slight lean forward can be performed until a stretch is felt once again in the calf. This procedure can be repeated three to five times and can be performed three times daily. Although there is debate regarding the value of static stretching alone on pain and range of motion in the long term for individuals with plantar fasciitis, a majority of the literature supports the inclusion of stretching as part of a multimodal treatment plan.[19,52]

References

1. Doral MN, Alam M, Bozkurt M, et al. Functional anatomy of the Achilles tendon. *Knee Surg Sports Traumatol Arthrosc.* 2010;18(5):638-643.
2. Balius R, Alomar X, Rodas G, et al. The soleus muscle: MRI, anatomic and histologic findings in cadavers with clinical correlation of strain injury distribution. *Skeletal Radiol.* 2013;42(4):521-530.
3. Standring S. *Gray's Anatomy: The Anatomical Basis of Clinical Practice.* 41st ed. London, UK: Elsevier; 2015.
4. Moses K, Banks J, Nava P, Peterson D. *Atlas of Clinical Gross Anatomy.* 2nd ed. Philadelphia, PA: Elsevier Saunders; 2013.
5. Michael RH, Holder LE. The soleus syndrome. A cause of medial tibial stress (shin splints). *Am J Sports Med.* 1985;13(2):87-94.
6. Pekala PA, Henry BM, Ochala A, et al. The twisted structure of the Achilles tendon unraveled: a detailed quantitative and qualitative anatomical investigation. *Scand J Med Sci Sports.* 2017;27(12):1705-1715.
7. Carrington SC, Stone P, Kruse D. Accessory soleus: a case report of exertional compartment and tarsal tunnel syndrome associated with an accessory soleus muscle. *J Foot Ankle Surg.* 2016;55(5):1076-1078.
8. Hatzantonis C, Agur A, Naraghi A, Gautier S, McKee N. Dissecting the accessory soleus muscle: a literature review, cadaveric study, and imaging study. *Clin Anat.* 2011;24(7):903-910.
9. Spina AA. The plantaris muscle: anatomy, injury, imaging, and treatment. *J Can Chiropr Assoc.* 2007;51(3):158-165.
10. Herzog RJ. Accessory plantaris muscle: anatomy and prevalence. *HSS J.* 2011;7(1):52-56.
11. Oatis C. *Kinesiology: The Mechanics and Pathomechanics of Human Movement.* Philadelphia, PA: Lippincott Williams & Wilkins; 2004 (pp. 812-814).
12. Foster M. *Therapeutic Kinesiology: Musculoskeletal Systems, Palpation, and Body Mechanics.* Upper Saddle River, NJ: Pearson Education, Inc; 2013.
13. Agur AM, Ng-Thow-Hing V, Ball KA, Fiume E, McKee NH. Documentation and three-dimensional modelling of human soleus muscle architecture. *Clin Anat.* 2003;16(4):285-293.
14. Franz JR, Thelen DG. Imaging and simulation of Achilles tendon dynamics: implications for walking performance in the elderly. *J Biomech.* 2016;49(9):1403-1410.
15. Franz JR, Thelen DG. Depth-dependent variations in Achilles tendon deformations with age are associated with reduced plantarflexor performance during walking. *J Appl Physiol (1985).* 2015;119(3):242-249.
16. Simons DG, Travell J, Simons L. *Travell & Simons's Myofascial Pain and Dysfunction: The Trigger Point Manual.* Vol 1. 2nd ed. Baltimore, MD: Williams & Wilkins; 1999 (p. 104).
17. Travell J, Simons DG. *Myofascial Pain and Dysfunction: The Trigger Point Manual.* Vol 2. Baltimore, MD: Williams & Wilkins; 1992 (p. 429).
18. Cotchett MP, Landorf KB, Munteanu SE, Raspovic AM. Consensus for dry needling for plantar heel pain (plantar fasciitis): a modified Delphi study. *Acupunct Med.* 2011;29(3):193-202.
19. Renan-Ordine R, Alburquerque-Sendin F, de Souza DP, Cleland JA, Fernández de las Peñas C. Effectiveness of myofascial trigger point manual therapy combined with a self-stretching protocol for the management of plantar heel pain: a randomized controlled trial. *J Orthop Sports Phys Ther.* 2011;41(2):43-50.
20. Mason JS, Tansey KA, Westrick RB. Treatment of subacute posterior knee pain in an adolescent ballet dancer utilizing trigger point dry needling: a case report. *Int J Sports Phys Ther.* 2014;9(1):116-124.
21. Grieve R, Clark J, Pearson E, Bullock S, Boyer C, Jarrett A. The immediate effect of soleus trigger point pressure release on restricted ankle joint dorsiflexion: a pilot randomised controlled trial. *J Bodyw Mov Ther.* 2011;15(1):42-49.
22. Grieve R, Cranston A, Henderson A, John R, Malone G, Mayall C. The immediate effect of triceps surae myofascial trigger point therapy on restricted active ankle joint dorsiflexion in recreational runners: a crossover randomised controlled trial. *J Bodyw Mov Ther.* 2013;17(4):453-461.
23. Grieve R, Barnett S, Coghill N, Cramp F. Myofascial trigger point therapy for triceps surae dysfunction: a case series. *Man Ther.* 2013;18(6):519-525.
24. Moghtaderi A, Khosrawi S, Dehghan F. Extracorporeal shock wave therapy of gastroc-soleus trigger points in patients with plantar fasciitis: a randomized, placebo-controlled trial. *Adv Biomed Res.* 2014;3:99.
25. McClay IS. A biomechanical perspective. In: Craik RL, Oatis CS, eds. *Gait Analysis: Theory and Application.* St Louis, MO: Mosby; 1995 (p. 399).
26. Grieve R, Barnett S, Coghill N, Cramp F. The prevalence of latent myofascial trigger points and diagnostic criteria of the triceps surae and upper trapezius: a cross sectional study. *Physiotherapy.* 2013;99(4):278-284.
27. Wu S-K, Hong C-Z, You J-Y, Chen C-L, Wang L-H, Su F-C. Therapeutic effect on the change of gait performance in chronic calf myofascial pain syndrome: a time series case study. *J Musculoske Pain.* 2005;13(3):33-43.
28. Kendall FP, McCreary EK. *Muscles: Testing and Function, with Posture and Pain.* 5th ed. Baltimore, MD: Lippincott Williams & Wilkins; 2005.
29. Zuil-Escobar JC, Martinez-Cepa CB, Martin-Urrialde JA, Gomez-Conesa A. The prevalence of latent trigger points in lower limb muscles in asymptomatic subjects. *PM R.* 2016;8(11):1055-1064.
30. Moore KL, Dalley AF. *Clinically Orientated Anatomy.* 4th ed. New York, NY: Lippincott Williams & Wilkins; 1999 (pp. 586-587).
31. Gerwin RD, Dommerholt J, Shah JP. An expansion of Simons' integrated hypothesis of trigger point formation. *Curr Pain Headache Rep.* 2004;8(6):468-475.
32. Fields KB, Rigby MD. Muscular calf injuries in runners. *Curr Sports Med Rep.* 2016;15(5):320-324.
33. Arcangeli P, Digiesi V, Ronchi O, Dorigo B, Bartoli B. Mechanisms of ischemic pain in peripheral occlusive arterial disease. In: Bonica JJ, Albe-Fessard D, eds. *Advances in Pain Research and Therapy.* Vol 1. New York, NY: Raven Press; 1976:965-973.
34. Hsieh YL, Kao MJ, Kuan TS, Chen SM, Chen JT, Hong CZ. Dry needling to a key myofascial trigger point may reduce the irritability of satellite MTrPs. *Am J Phys Med Rehabil.* 2007;86(5):397-403.
35. Bright JM, Fields KB, Draper R. Ultrasound diagnosis of calf injuries. *Sports Health.* 2017;9(4):352-355.
36. Harwin JR, Richardson ML. "Tennis leg": gastrocnemius injury is a far more common cause than plantaris rupture. *Radiol Case Rep.* 2017;12(1):120-123.
37. Li HY, Hua YH. Achilles tendinopathy: current concepts about the basic science and clinical treatments. *Biomed Res Int.* 2016;2016:6492597.
38. Reiman M, Burgi C, Strube E, et al. The utility of clinical measures for the diagnosis of achilles tendon injuries: a systematic review with meta-analysis. *J Athl Train.* 2014;49(6):820-829.
39. Campbell RS, Grainger AJ. Current concepts in imaging of tendinopathy. *Clin Radiol.* 2001;56(4):253-267.
40. Khan KM, Forster BB, Robinson J, et al. Are ultrasound and magnetic resonance imaging of value in assessment of Achilles tendon disorders? A two year prospective study. *Br J Sports Med.* 2003;37(2):149-153.
41. Becker J, James S, Wayner R, Osternig L, Chou LS. Biomechanical factors associated with achilles tendinopathy and medial tibial stress syndrome in runners. *Am J Sports Med.* 2017;45(11):2614-2621.
42. Luck MD, Gordon AG, Blebea JS, Dalinka MK. High association between accessory soleus muscle and Achilles tendonopathy. *Skeletal Radiol.* 2008;37(12):1129-1133.
43. Yu JS, Resnick D. MR imaging of the accessory soleus muscle appearance in six patients and a review of the literature. *Skeletal Radiol.* 1994;23(7):525-528.
44. Brodie JT, Dormans JP, Gregg JR, Davidson RS. Accessory soleus muscle. A report of 4 cases and review of literature. *Clin Orthop Relat Res.* 1997;(337):180-186.
45. Ahn JH, Ahn CY, Byun CH, Kim YC. Operative treatment of Haglund syndrome with central achilles tendon-splitting approach. *J Foot Ankle Surg.* 2015;54(6):1053-1056.
46. Singh K, Yakoub D, Giangola P, et al. Early follow-up and treatment recommendations for isolated calf deep venous thrombosis. *J Vasc Surg.* 2012;55(1):136-140.
47. Kravtsov PF, Katorkin SA, Volkovoy VV, Sizonenko YV. The influence of the training of the muscular component of the musculo-venous pump in the lower extremities on the clinical course of varicose vein disease [in Russian]. *Vopr Kurortol Fizioter Lech Fiz Kult.* 2016;93(6):33-36.
48. Rajasekaran S, Hall MM. Nonoperative management of chronic exertional compartment syndrome: a systematic review. *Curr Sports Med Rep.* 2016;15(3):191-198.
49. Campano D, Robaina JA, Kusnezov N, Dunn JC, Waterman BR. Surgical management for chronic exertional compartment syndrome of the leg: a systematic review of the literature. *Arthroscopy.* 2016;32(7):1478-1486.
50. Winkes MB, Hoogeveen AR, Scheltinga MR. Is surgery effective for deep posterior compartment syndrome of the leg? A systematic review. *Br J Sports Med.* 2014;48(22):1592-1598.
51. Johanson MA, DeArment A, Hines K, et al. The effect of subtalar joint position on dorsiflexion of the ankle/rearfoot versus midfoot/forefoot during gastrocnemius stretching. *Foot Ankle Int.* 2014;35(1):63-70.
52. Radford JA, Landorf KB, Buchbinder R, Cook C. Effectiveness of calf muscle stretching for the short-term treatment of plantar heel pain: a randomised trial. *BMC Musculoskelet Disord.* 2007;8:36.

Chapter 67

Tibialis Posterior Muscle
"Runner's Nemesis"

Orlando Mayoral del Moral, Isabel Salvat, and Joseph M. Donnelly

1. INTRODUCTION

The tibialis posterior muscle is a deep bipennate muscle with a proximal attachment consisting of three tapered portions: two medial portions from the interosseous membrane and tibia, and one lateral portion from the fibula and the intermuscular septa. Distally, it inserts into the navicular tuberosity, all of the tarsal bones except for the talus, and the 1st through 4th metatarsals. It is a strong invertor and an adductor of the foot, and it assists in ankle plantar flexion. In weight bearing, and especially during gait, the tibialis posterior muscle functions to distribute body weight among the heads of the metatarsals and prevent excessive pronation of the foot, thus contributing to ankle stability. Trigger points (TrPs) in the tibialis posterior muscle will produce pain over the Achilles tendon that can extend through the midcalf down to the heel and over the entire plantar surface of the foot. Activation and perpetuation of TrPs usually results from walking, running, or jogging, especially on uneven ground or on laterally slanted surfaces. Ill-fitting shoes or worn footwear that promote eversion and rocking of the foot, along with excessive pronation, can contribute to the activation and perpetuation of TrPs in the tibialis posterior muscle. Differential diagnosis should include tibialis posterior tendon dysfunction, medial tibial stress syndrome, and deep posterior chronic exertional compartment syndrome. Corrective actions include proper sitting and sleeping postures along with self-pressure release techniques. Early recognition and treatment of tibialis posterior TrPs or muscle/tendon dysfunction is critical to slow the progression to a tendon tear or rupture and prevent surgical intervention.

2. ANATOMIC CONSIDERATIONS

The tibialis posterior muscle is the deepest muscle in the posterior calf. It lies between the interosseous membrane anteriorly and the posterior tibial vessels and soleus muscle posteriorly, in between the flexor hallucis longus and flexor digitorum longus muscles (Figure 67-1). Proximally, its attachment consists of three portions separated by an interval traversed by the anterior tibial vessels. The two medial portions attach to the interosseous membrane and to a lateral area of the posterior surface of the body of the tibia. The lateral portion attaches to the medial surface of the fibula, from the transverse intermuscular septum, and from the intermuscular septa of adjacent muscles.[1] The tibial attachment of the muscle commonly continues into the distal third of the leg as far as, or more distal than, the crossing of the tibialis posterior tendon with that of the flexor digitorum longus muscle. The attachment to the fibula usually includes an intramuscular septum, in which case the muscle is multipennate.[2] In the distal quarter of the leg, its tendon passes anterior to the tendon of the flexor digitorum longus muscle, behind the medial malleolus. To enter the foot, it passes deep to the flexor retinaculum and superficial to the deltoid ligament. In the foot, it divides into anterior, middle, and posterior components just proximal to the navicular bone. The anterior component is the most superficial and largest, and this component is a direct continuation of the main tendon that inserts into the navicular tuberosity and the medial cuneiform. The middle portion of the tendon extends to the second and third cuneiforms, the cuboid bone, and the bases of the 2nd, 3rd, and 4th metatarsals. The posterior component is recurrent, arises from the main tendon, proximal to the navicular bone, and inserts as a band into the anterior aspect of the sustentaculum tali of the calcaneus[3] (Figure 67-2). Occasionally, a sesamoid bone occurs in the tendon of the tibialis posterior muscle on the plantar aspect of the navicular tuberosity.[1]

The tibialis secundus muscle, an uncommon, anatomic variant muscle of small size, has been described as arising from the back of the tibia and inserting into the capsule of the ankle joint.[1] An anomalous muscle has also been described as running close to the tibialis posterior muscle and presenting with compression neuropathy. It arises from the posterior compartment and inserts into the posteromedial portion of the calcaneus.[4] Occasionally, the tibialis posterior muscle may have an anomalous insertion of its tendon to an enlarged navicular tuberosity.[3]

2.1. Innervation and Vascularization

The tibial nerve supplies the tibialis posterior muscle with contributions from L4 and L5.[1] The mean distance of the nerve entry point was located at a 75% of the distance from the lateral malleolus to the fibular head. The intramuscular branching demonstrates a minimum of one and a maximum of four intramuscular branches, located at 80% to 90% of the muscle length. The arborization patterns appear as these fine branches extended distally. The most distally located intramuscular nerve ending may be observed at around 30% to 40% of the muscle length.[5]

The tibial nerve, after emerging from the sciatic nerve, passes anterior to the arch of the soleus muscle to continue into the leg with the posterior tibial vessels. Its muscular branches supply all of the muscles in the posterior compartment of the leg. Proximally, the tibial nerve is located deep to the gastrocnemius and soleus muscles and then becomes overlapped by the flexor hallucis longus muscle. The tibial nerve demonstrates a wide range of variation in branching, but in all the cases, the tibialis posterior muscle was innervated by both proximal and distal branches that arise from the fibular side of the main nerve.[6]

Vascularization of the tibialis posterior muscle is provided by the posterior tibial and fibular arteries. Distally, the tendon is supplied by arteries of the medial malleolar network and by the medial plantar artery.[1] The middle portion of the tibialis posterior tendon between the proximal musculotendinous junction and the distal tenoperiosteal junction is commonly referred to as the watershed zone, which is a zone of hypovascularity. This zone of the tendon is where tendinopathy is commonly observed.[7]

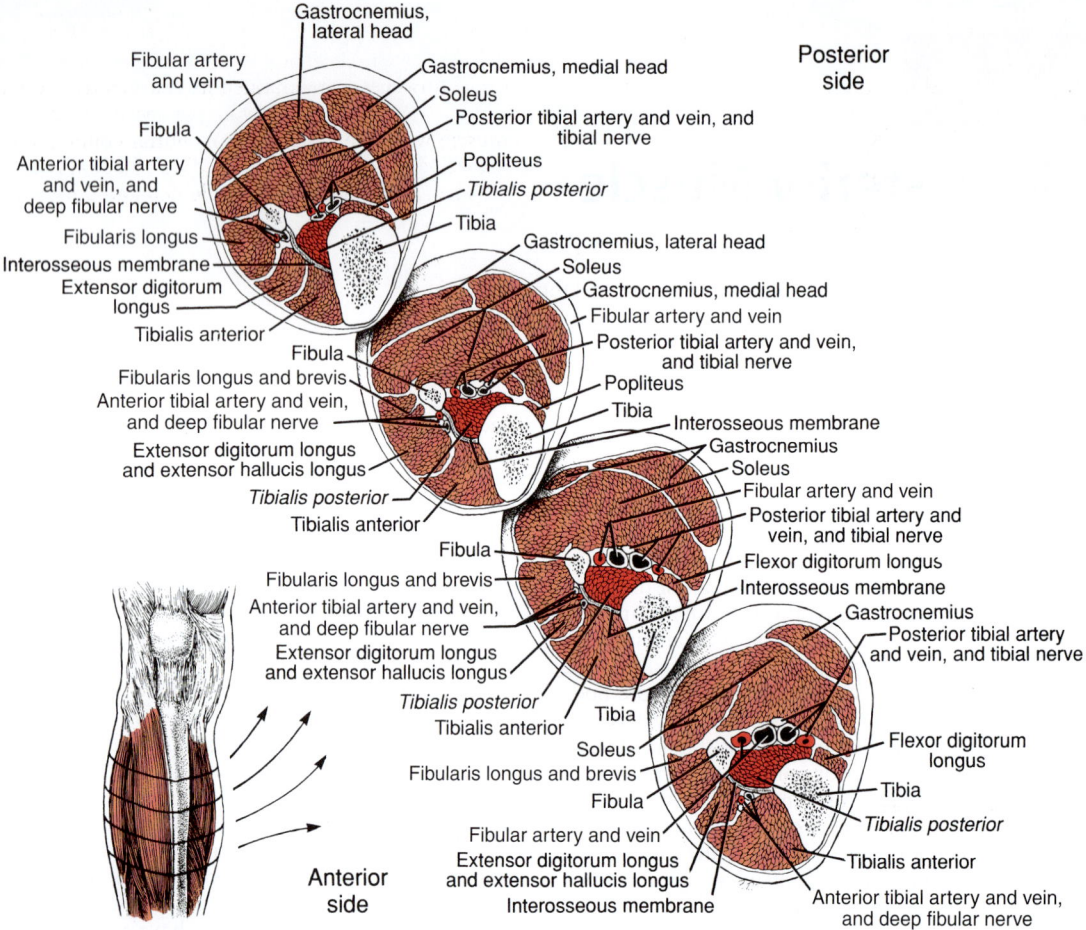

Figure 67-1. Four serial cross-sections of the right tibialis posterior muscle (medium red), in relation to other muscles of the leg (light red), viewed from above. Arteries are bright red, veins are black surrounded by uncolored walls, and nerves are uncolored. These sections are oriented as one palpates the calf of the prone patient. The levels of the cross-section are identified in the lower left corner. The flexor hallucis longus muscle is not distinguished from the soleus muscle in the distal section. Adapted from A Cross-Section Anatomy, by Eycleshymer and Schoemaker, published by D. Appleton Company, 1911.

2.2. Function

The tibialis posterior muscle acts to invert and strongly adduct (supinate) the hindfoot and midfoot, and it assists in plantar flexion of the ankle.[2] It is a powerful muscle and is the principal invertor of the foot.[1] The tibialis posterior muscle, along with the flexor digitorum longus and flexor hallucis muscles, is the primary supinators of the foot, with the tibialis posterior muscle producing the greatest force in supination in both the hindfoot and midfoot.[8] The tibialis posterior muscle's moment arm is advantageous for ankle inversion, whereas the moment arm for the tibialis anterior muscle is small for inversion.[9]

Under bodyweight, the medial longitudinal arch of the foot tends to be lowered to the ground and the hindfoot pronated, which induces pronation of the subtalar joint and midfoot. In this regard, the tibialis posterior muscle has a better counteraction force in supination than any other muscle, and it has classically been considered the major dynamic supporting structure maintaining the medial longitudinal arch during weight bearing.[9,10] Based on electromyographic (EMG) activity, the tibialis posterior muscle does not contribute significantly to arch support under static load conditions.[1,11,12] However, the changes in the foot that occur in the absence of the force exerted by the tibialis posterior muscle show that it is essential for maintenance of normal foot configuration and posture.[13] Co-contractions of the tibialis posterior and the fibularis longus muscles may help support the medial arch to prevent hyperpronation of the foot, especially during fast walking and running.[2,14] The tibialis posterior muscle also assists in distributing bodyweight on the heads of the metatarsals, helping shift weight toward the lateral side of the foot that has strong plantar ligaments that equip it to bear bodyweight.[12,15]

Regarding the role of the tibialis posterior muscle in plantar flexion, the previous edition of this text[2] pointed out a controversy because some authors considered the tibialis posterior muscle as a major plantar flexor,[16-18] whereas others did not.[19,20] Perry et al[21] investigated the role of the tibialis posterior muscle in plantar flexion utilizing EMG and reported that during plantar flexion, the force created by the tibialis posterior muscle was equal to the force created by the flexor digitorum longus and the fibularis brevis muscles; however, it was much less than the force created by the other plantar flexor muscles. They concluded that the relative plantar flexor force of the tibialis posterior muscle is 1.8% of the force that is exerted by the soleus muscle.[21] Sutherland[22] reported that the tibialis posterior muscle is potentially the third most powerful plantar flexor; however, it could exert only 6% of the moment of force contributed by the gastrocnemius and soleus muscles combined.

During gait, the function of the tibialis posterior muscle is to prevent excessive foot pronation during the contact phase and to supinate the hindfoot and midfoot to provide increased stiffness in the forefoot for the propulsion phase.[23,24] The tibialis posterior muscle is the strongest supinator of the midfoot and hindfoot. It is active in the first 55% of the gait cycle. During the initial 35% of the gait cycle, it controls or decelerates pronation of the foot,

Chapter 67: Tibialis Posterior Muscle   711

when compared with normal and slower gait speeds. At faster gait speeds, the tibialis posterior muscle showed a significant delay in time to peak amplitude which occurred later in the gait cycle; however, it maintained its characteristic biphasic amplitude.[29,30] At subject-preferred gait speeds, the tibialis posterior muscle was active just prior to initial contact and hit its first peak EMG activity at limb loading and again at mid-stance.[30]

The tibialis posterior muscle demand and action increases at initial contact and mid-stance at increased gait speeds.[29,30] During the entire stance phase, the tibialis posterior muscle tendon unit lengthens, whereas the muscle fascicle shortens and functions almost isometrically.[30]

Akuzawa et al[27] investigated calf muscle activation during the stance phase of gait during barefoot walking, walking with footwear, and walking with an orthosis that supported the medial longitudinal arch, transverse arch, and lateral arch. Utilizing fine-wire EMG, they studied the tibialis posterior, peroneus longus, and flexor digitorum longus muscles during all three conditions at initial contact, mid-stance, and at propulsion phases of gait. The percent of maximum volitional isometric contraction (%MVIC) of the tibialis posterior muscle was significantly reduced in walking with an orthosis when compared with barefoot walking during the mid-stance and propulsion phase of gait. There was also a difference between %MVIC of the tibialis posterior muscle under all three conditions during the initial contact and mid-stance phase of gait. They concluded that an orthosis that supports all three arches of the foot may be beneficial to offload the tibialis posterior muscle for individuals with muscle and/or tendon dysfunction.[27]

2.3. Functional Unit

The functional unit to which a muscle belongs includes the muscles that reinforce and counter its actions as well as the joints that the muscle crosses. The interdependence of these structures is functionally reflected in the organization and neural connections of the sensory motor cortex. The functional unit is emphasized because the presence of a TrP in one muscle of the unit increases the likelihood that the other muscles of the unit will also develop TrPs. When inactivating TrPs in a muscle, one must be concerned about TrPs that may develop in muscles that are functionally interdependent. Box 67-1 grossly represents the functional unit of the tibialis posterior muscle.[31]

The long toe flexors are also agonists for the weight-bearing function of assisting transverse plane balance.

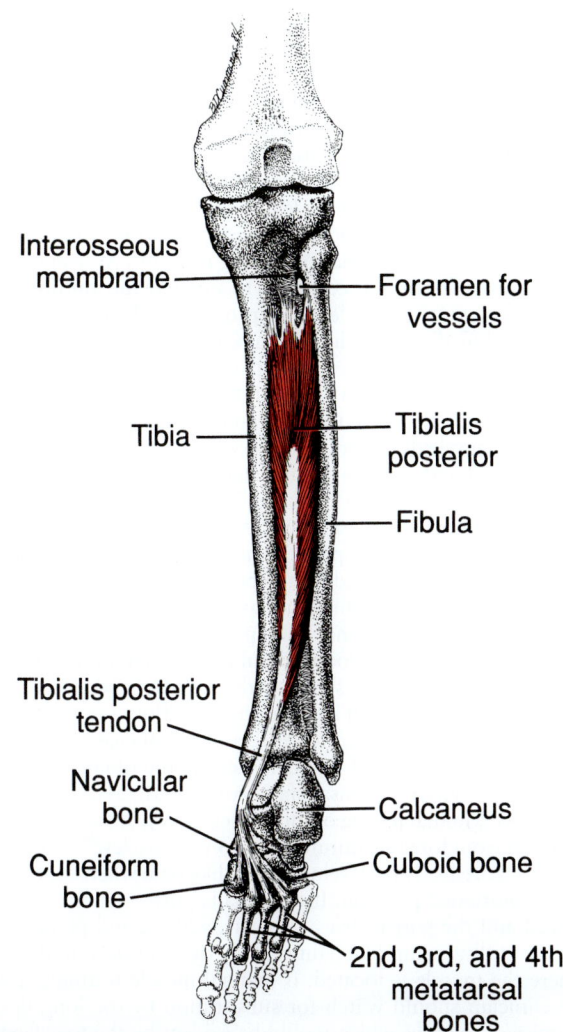

Figure 67-2. Attachments of the right tibialis posterior muscle (red). The bones to which this muscle attaches are darkened.

followed by supination of the hindfoot and midfoot along with external rotation of the tibia, which is a necessary coupled motion from mid-stance to toe off to create a rigid lever that improves the efficiency of force transmission to the forefoot for propulsion.[13,25,26]

In the gait cycle, the tibialis posterior muscle has biphasic activity and activates just prior to initial contact (as the first muscle to activate), peaks at initial contact, and peaks again during the propulsive phase[21,24,27]; however, these results are inconsistent among subjects.[24] The tibialis posterior muscle restrains the pronation forces that occur during the limb-loading response and early-stance phase of gait. During mid-stance, it prevents excessive pronation and provides transverse plane balance and control. Sutherland[22] concluded that the plantar flexors, including the tibialis posterior muscle, also decelerate the forward movement of the tibia over the fixed foot during stance, thus indirectly providing knee stabilization. This deceleration function is also supported by recent research.[27]

Perry et al[28] compared the EMG activity of the tibialis posterior muscle during slow, free, and fast gait with the amount of activity generated by various degrees of voluntary effort graded according to muscle-testing criteria. Results showed that EMG activity increased directly as more muscular force was required during the different manual muscle test levels and with increased walking speeds. Investigators[29,30] utilizing fine-wire EMG examined the effects of different gait speeds on the function of the tibialis posterior muscle. They found that this muscle had a significant increase in peak EMG amplitude at faster gait speeds

Box 67-1 Functional unit of the tibialis posterior muscle

Action	Synergists	Antagonist
Plantar flexion of the foot	Gastrocnemius Soleus Fibularis longus and brevis Flexor digitorum longus Flexor hallucis longus	Extensor digitorum longus Extensor hallucis longus Fibularis tertius
Inversion of the foot	Tibialis anterior Flexor digitorum longus Flexor hallucis longus Extensor hallucis longus	Fibularis longus and brevis Fibularis tertius Extensor digitorum longus

3. CLINICAL PRESENTATION

3.1. Referred Pain Pattern

The tibialis posterior muscle can exhibit TrPs in any part of the muscle. The referred pain concentrates primarily over the Achilles tendon, proximal to the calcaneus, and can extend through the midcalf down to the heel and over the entire plantar surface of the foot and toes (Figure 67-3). Pain due to TrPs in the tibialis posterior muscle is not likely to present as a single-muscle syndrome.[2]

3.2. Symptoms

An individual with TrPs in the tibialis posterior muscle is likely to report pain in the foot when running or walking. The pain may be felt quite severely in the plantar surface of the foot and Achilles tendon, and to a lesser degree in the midcalf and heel. The patient will report increasing difficulty with walking or running, especially on uneven surfaces, for example, on gravel or cobblestones that are sufficiently irregular as to require additional stabilization of the foot.[2]

3.3. Patient Examination

After a thorough subjective examination, the clinician should make a detailed drawing representing the pain pattern that the patient has described. This depiction will assist in planning the physical examination and can be useful in monitoring the progression of the patient as symptoms improve or change. The type, quality, and location of the pain should be carefully assessed, and the utilization of standardized outcome tools is imperative when examining patients with lower extremity dysfunctions.

Observation of static and dynamic posture is essential because of the role of the tibialis posterior muscle in postural stability and gait. If the tibialis posterior TrPs are active or have been present for some time, the patient may walk with the foot partly everted and abducted, in a flatfooted gait. The patient should be observed walking barefoot to identify relevant gait deviations such as early excessive pronation, excessive pronation at mid-stance (pes planus), or late pronation during push-off. At heel off, the tibialis posterior muscle contracts to supinate the hindfoot and midfoot to create a rigid lever for propulsion. Tibialis posterior and/or flexor digitorum longus muscle weakness may be indicated if the calcaneus does not move into inversion at heel-off.

A collapse of the medial longitudinal arch or a midfoot posture with forefoot abduction is commonly observed with tibialis posterior muscle dysfunction. Observation of the ankle and foot from behind with a focus on the relationship of the hindfoot to forefoot may reveal a "too many toes" sign on one side that may be indicative of tibialis posterior muscle dysfunction. Static measures such as the navicular drop test[32] and the windlass mechanism[33] should be assessed in standing as a predictor of dynamic function of the foot. Functional testing, such as double- and single-leg squat, will allow a quick assessment of hip and knee control, as well as a quick assessment of talocrural, subtalar, and midfoot range of motion. Timed single-leg stance with eyes open and closed gives a quantitative measure of balance and will afford the clinician to observe foot and ankle strategies related to balance and control.

The usual method of manually testing the tibialis posterior muscle for strength[34] is unsatisfactory to identify relatively slight weakness. Manual testing of this muscle poorly discriminates its function from force substituted by agonist muscles.[28,35] Muscles with TrPs are likely to develop cramp-like pain when contracted in the shortened position. If the tibialis posterior muscle is involved and the patient tries to invert, adduct, and plantar-flex the foot fully, cramp-like pain is likely to occur deep in the calf, where the muscle is located. If manual muscle testing is used, the clinician should watch for substitution by the long flexor muscles of the toes which would be evident by the toes flexing during the test. The single-heel-rise test is the recommended test to assess function of the tibialis posterior muscle in a functional position.[35] The patient tries to perform the single-heel-rise test while standing on one foot in an attempt to achieve 8 to 10 repetitions.[36] Normally, the tibialis posterior muscle first inverts the foot and locks the calcaneus to provide a rigid structure that permits transfer of weight to the forefoot. In the event of tibialis posterior muscle weakness or dysfunction, initial heel inversion is weak and the patient either raises the heel incompletely without locking the hindfoot or fails to rise onto the ball of the foot. Pain and tenderness may be experienced along the path of the tendon, mainly behind the medial malleolus and medial to its primary insertion on the navicular tuberosity. Unfortunately, patients do not usually present with this dysfunction as a chief report, but it is at this early stage that the condition should be fully correctable, often with conservative measures. Active TrPs in this muscle cause a perceptible degree of functional inhibition weakness.

To test this muscle for restricted range of motion, the patient may be supine or seated. The clinician first fully everts and abducts the foot and then attempts to place it into dorsiflexion. Tibialis posterior TrPs painfully restrict this movement. Restriction of this movement can also be caused by tightness of the flexor digitorum longus and flexor hallucis longus muscles. If, at the limit of the restricted range of motion, the clinician can extend all five toes without pain, the restriction is caused by the tibialis posterior muscle and not by either of the long toe flexors.

Passive physiologic and accessory motion should be tested in the talocrural, subtalar, midtarsal, and forefoot joints. It is also imperative to assess for great toe and first ray range of motion in dorsiflexion, as limitation in this motion may cause abnormal pronation of the foot during the propulsive phase of gait, placing an abnormal tensile load on the tibialis posterior muscle.

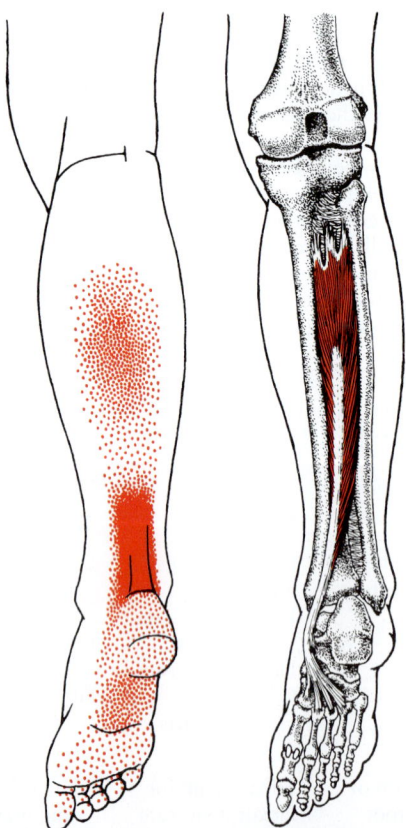

Figure 67-3. Composite pain pattern (bright red) referred from TrPs in the right tibialis posterior muscle (darker red). The essential pain pattern (solid dark red) denotes where pain is usually experienced when these TrPs are active. Red stippling indicates the occasional extension of the essential pain pattern.

The clinician should identify abnormal foot structure by examining the patient's feet and shoes and analyzing the role of abnormal foot structure in observed and tested function. By the time patients with tibialis posterior TrPs are seen for their persistent foot pain, they usually have tried one or more corrective devices. One device frequently used is an insert that adds support to the foot but often ends short of the head of the 1st metatarsal. A total contact foot orthoses, extending past the metatarsal heads to maximize foot function, is preferred over this common, shorter orthosis. However, people with tibialis posterior TrPs frequently find that wearing a corrective orthotic device is painful because it presses on the region of tenderness referred from the TrPs to the sole of the foot. This referred tenderness disappears promptly with inactivation of the responsible TrPs in the tibialis posterior muscle.

3.4. Trigger Point Examination

The tibialis posterior muscle lies deep in the posterior leg and its TrPs are accessible to examination by palpation only indirectly through other muscles with the patient side-lying with the affected side down and the knee flexed to place the gastrocnemius muscle on slack (Figure 67-4). At most, one can determine only a direction of deep tenderness. Interpreting this tenderness that is caused by tibialis posterior TrPs depends on the preceding examination having established evidence of this muscle's involvement and on having reason to believe that the intervening muscles are free of TrPs. As shown in Figure 67-1, the tibialis posterior muscle is inaccessible to digital examination anteriorly because of the intervening tibialis anterior muscle and interosseous membrane.

From behind, one can usually elicit tenderness of tibialis posterior TrPs and tenderness of that muscle's tibial attachment by pressing deeply between the posterior border of the tibia and the soleus muscle, which can be partially displaced posteriorly (Figure 67-4). The muscle should be examined for tenderness, as illustrated in Figure 67-4, proximal to the midleg by cross-fiber deep flat palpation. As one palpates from the location illustrated distally, the flexor digitorum longus muscle will also be encountered behind the tibia. Occasionally, on the lateral side, tenderness of the tibialis posterior muscle through the soleus and the flexor hallucis longus muscles can be elicited. Discerning which muscle may be involved is a very difficult task.

No neural or vascular entrapments by this muscle have been observed, nor are any expected, because it lies deep to the vessels and nerves. A monofilament or injection needle may be used to identify the tibialis posterior TrPs; however, one should proceed very cautiously because of the extensive neurovascular bundle that lies between the soleus and tibialis posterior muscles.

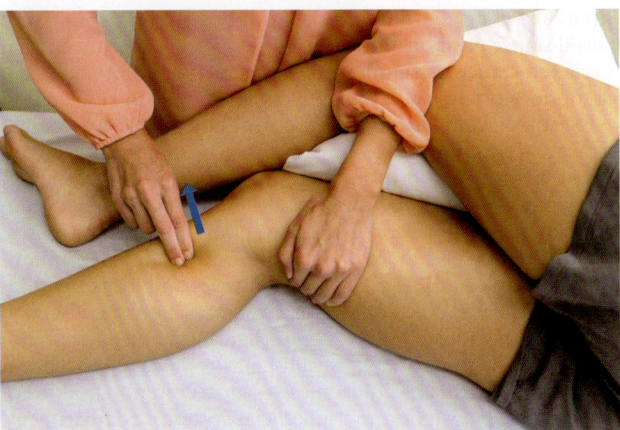

Figure 67-4. Cross-fiber flat palpation for TrPs in the tibialis posterior muscle. Arrow depicts the anteriorly directed force against the posterior surface of the tibia.

4. DIFFERENTIAL DIAGNOSIS

4.1. Activation and Perpetuation of Trigger Points

In any part of the tibialis posterior muscle, TrPs may be activated by unaccustomed eccentric loading, eccentric exercise in unconditioned tibialis posterior muscle, or maximal or submaximal concentric loading.[37] Trigger points may also be activated or aggravated when the muscle is placed in a shortened or lengthened position for an extended period of time.

Mechanical stresses from running can cause the formation of TrPs in the tibialis posterior muscle, especially running on uneven or laterally slanted surfaces. Interestingly, tibialis posterior TrPs are not commonly observed in tennis players who characteristically train on smooth, level surfaces and wear shoes that provide ample foot support; however, footwear that is worn down and that encourages eversion and rocking of the foot contribute to TrPs in this muscle.

Although pronation in early stance is normal to accommodate the weight-bearing surface and for lower extremity shock absorption, excessive pronation can overload the tibialis posterior muscle and may contribute to the activation of, and certainly to the perpetuation of, TrPs in it. The foot may excessively pronate because of a hypomobile hindfoot, hypermobile midfoot, ankle equinus, loss of great toe dorsiflexion, muscular imbalance, or some other structural or functional cause.

4.2. Associated Trigger Points

Associated TrPs can develop in the referred pain areas caused by TrPs.[38] Therefore, musculature in the referred pain areas for each muscle should also be considered. The two long toe flexors that also invert and plantar-flex the foot, the flexor digitorum longus and flexor hallucis longus muscles, are commonly involved with the tibialis posterior muscle. The primary foot plantar flexors, the gastrocnemius and soleus muscles, are not prone to develop TrPs in association with the tibialis posterior muscle; however, it has been clinically observed.

Trigger points in the fibularis muscles, especially in patients with abnormal foot structure, are commonly associated with TrPs in the tibialis posterior muscle. The fibularis longus and fibularis brevis muscles are primary antagonists to the inversion action of the tibialis posterior muscle but are agonists to its roles in plantar flexion and stabilization of the foot.

Tibialis posterior TrPs could develop in response to TrPs in gluteus minimus, hamstrings, gastrocnemius, soleus, and flexor digitorum longus muscles. In addition, the plantar intrinsic foot muscles should also be considered for examination, because they are within the referred pain area of tibialis posterior TrPs. Imamura et al[39] studied the effects of treatment for myofascial pain components in individuals with plantar fasciitis with very good results.[39] In this study, 30% of the patients were found to have TrPs in the tibialis posterior muscle and were successfully treated. In a modified Delphi study attempting to elucidate the best dry needling protocol for the treatment of plantar heel pain (commonly diagnosed as plantar fasciitis), the tibialis posterior muscle was included as one of the muscles that should be assessed for the presence of TrPs as a possible source of the patient's pain and was included in the dry needling treatment.[40] A randomized controlled trial following the indications of the modified Delphi study described previously reported good results in the reduction of plantar heel pain.[41]

4.3. Associated Pathology

Serious dysfunction of the tibialis posterior muscle and/or tendon is not unusual and deserves careful consideration in the differential diagnosis of ankle and foot pain. Some common conditions include dysfunction of the tibialis posterior muscle-tendon complex, medial tibial stress syndrome ("shin splints"), and deep posterior chronic exertional compartment syndrome. Tibialis posterior TrPs are thought to be a contributing factor to these leg, ankle, and foot conditions, although there is no solid scientific evidence to support this notion.

Tibialis posterior tendon dysfunction is thought to be a progressive disorder and is believed to lead to altered foot biomechanics. Johnson and Strom developed a scheme in 1989 to explain the successive stages of tibialis posterior tendon dysfunction,[35] and this has since been modified by Bluman and Myerson to include a Stage IV.[42] The first two stages are isolated to soft-tissue changes, and the third and fourth stages have associated arthritic changes[43]: *Stage I: tendon length is normal* and inflamed with minimal pain and dysfunction; *Stage II: tendon elongated*, acquired pes planus but passively correctable, commonly unable to perform a heel raise; *Stage III: tendon elongated, hindfoot deformed and stiff* with lateral foot pain and marked eversion of the foot when bearing weight. Subtalar joint arthropathy and degeneration are noted; *Stage IV*: end-stage disease with a fixed valgus angulation of the talus, midfoot planus, and early degeneration of the ankle joint.[42,44] In Stage 1, the tibialis posterior muscle strength and function are mildly decreased. When the patient attempts to perform the single-heel-rise test, reduced endurance may be noted with an inability to perform multiple attempts.[36] Normally, the tibialis posterior muscle first everts and locks the calcaneus to provide a rigid structure that permits transfer of weight to the forefoot. In stage 1, initial calcaneal inversion is weak, and the patient either raises the heel incompletely without locking the hindfoot or fails to rise onto the ball of the foot. Pain and tenderness are found along the path of the tendon, chiefly just before it passes behind the medial malleolus and medial to its insertion on the navicular. Unfortunately, patients do not usually present with this dysfunction as a chief report, but it is at this early stage that the condition should be fully correctable, often with conservative measures. Radiographs are typically unremarkable and magnetic resonance imaging (MRI) revealing a tenosynovitis is the gold standard for diagnosis in this stage.[43]

With progression to stage 2, pain increases in severity and distribution, and the patient has serious difficulty with walking. The single-heel-rise test is more abnormal, and the patient stands with the foot everted and abducted sufficiently to display "too many toes" when viewed from behind. This is a simple, reproducible, and recordable measure of foot posture. Routine radiographs from the anteroposterior view show the forefoot abducted in relation to the hindfoot, because the calcaneus and navicular are subluxed laterally off the head of the talus. In the lateral view, the talus is tipped forward in relation to the calcaneus. This stage has been subdivided into 2a, which identifies tendon changes with elongation, and 2b, in which the tendon has ruptured. This latter stage requires surgical repair of the tendon.[43]

In stage 3, there is evidence of subtalar joint arthropathy and degeneration[43] along with associated damage to the static supporting structures of the foot that have resulted in fixed flatfoot and requires realignment of the foot structures and arthrodesis. An isolated subtalar arthrodesis suffices in most cases; however, a triple arthrodesis may be required.[35,43]

In stage 4, the rigid hindfoot and the valgus angulation of the talus usually require a tibiotalocalcaneal arthrodesis and deltoid ligament reconstruction.[44]

Muscles with TrPs are under continuous increased tension because of taut bands; thus, TrPs in the tibialis posterior muscle is one condition that could possibly account for Johnson and Strom's stage 1 findings: a detectable muscle weakness under high-load conditions, and degenerative changes of the tendon exposed to abnormal sustained tension caused by muscle length deficits. Subsequent stages could follow failure to correct the condition in its initial stage.

A number of authors[45-52] and one comprehensive review[53] discuss rupture of the tibialis posterior tendon as a separate entity (stages 2 and 3 of Johnson and Strom). The patient presents with a report that may include the following: "My foot is becoming flat," "My shoe is running over," "I can't walk like I used to," or "I have trouble going up and down stairs." Frequently, the absence of the displaced tendon is noted on palpation when compared with the normal side. The discontinuity of the tendon has been imaged by ultrasound[47,54] and by MRI.[47,55] Duchenne noted that, in patients with tibialis posterior musculotendinous deficit, the foot turned outward when they were walking or standing.[19] EMG data obtained by Ringleb et al[56] suggest that tibialis posterior tendon dysfunction is associated with compensatory activity in the fibularis, tibialis anterior, and gastrocnemius muscles. Weakness of the tibialis posterior muscle can lead to an excessively pronated foot, unlocking of the midtarsal joint that allows plantar subluxation of the hindfoot on the forefoot, and development of a severe pes planus deformity.[57] Tendon rupture or weakness of the tibialis posterior muscle caused by slippage of the tendon around the medial malleolus will quickly cause a flexible pes valgus deformity.[58] Loss of tibialis posterior muscle function may result in progressive and dramatic pes planus deformity with a marked abduction component. If uncorrected within months of loss, tendon transfer alone will no longer suffice and arthrodesis will be required.[59]

Rupture of the tibialis posterior tendon due to rheumatoid arthritis can cause a sag in the medial longitudinal arch on weight bearing within 10 days. In one patient, examination 2.5 years after rupture revealed a collapsed, but mobile, longitudinal arch. Radiographs of the foot showed marked osteopenia, a calcaneal valgus angle, and an anterior and inferior displacement of the talar head.[35,47]

Medial tibial stress syndrome is defined as painful symptoms on the medial aspect of the tibia, often located at the middle or distal portion.[60] Onset usually occurs with running or impact loading of the lower extremity, and the resulting pain will typically limit running activity. Variation in nomenclature such as "shin splint syndrome" and "soleus enthesopathy" is evident in the historic and current literature, and it is likely that such has contributed to the current lack of understanding of the condition.[61] Some authors attributed it to the tibialis posterior muscle, but cadaveric studies of the myofascial anatomy are inconsistent as to which myofascial element is involved because there is large variation in the site of attachment of tibialis posterior, soleus, and flexor digitorum longus muscles.[61,62] However, posteromedial muscular tenderness is a consistent clinical feature of the syndrome. Whether this tenderness is a primary cause or an effect of the condition remains unclear.[61]

It is probable that a combination of structures is involved in medial tibial stress syndrome, and some authors have suggested grading systems based on this premise.[62] Increased navicular drop (difference in height of the navicular tuberosity in the subtalar neutral stance position and the height of the navicular tuberosity in relaxed stance) is significantly associated with an increased risk of developing medial tibial stress syndrome in runners.

Exertional compartment syndromes of the leg are a common form of overuse injury. Compartment syndromes are characterized by increased pressure within a muscular compartment sufficient to compromise the circulation of the muscles within it. The increased pressure obstructs venous outflow that causes further swelling and more pressure. If prolonged, the resultant ischemia can lead to necrosis of the muscles and nerves within the compartment. When following a traumatic injury, it is vitally important that this condition be recognized immediately and managed properly to avoid possibly catastrophic consequences. Anterior compartment syndromes are most common, followed by lateral, deep posterior, and superficial posterior compartment syndromes.[63,64]

The superficial posterior compartment contains the soleus and gastrocnemius muscle bellies. The deep posterior compartment encloses the flexor digitorum longus, flexor hallucis longus, popliteus, and tibialis posterior muscle bellies.[1]

Deep posterior chronic exertional compartment syndrome (dp-CECS) of the leg is usually gradually induced by exercise in young endurance athletes. It produces a sense of tightness, dull aching and cramping, and diminished sensibility of the involved muscles. As the condition intensifies, pain persists for longer periods following exercise. Posterior compartment syndromes are commonly bilateral, usually fail to respond to conservative therapy, are often relieved by prolonged periods of rest, and often require fasciotomy.[65] On examination, dp-CECS demonstrates tenderness deep in the calf in the muscle tissue itself. The diagnosis of dp-CECS is confirmed by finding elevated intracompartmental pressure within the deep posterior compartment. However, diagnostic techniques and surgical interventions are highly subjective and lack standardization.[65]

The precise etiology of the posterior compartment syndromes has not yet been established. An initiating trauma or hypertrophy of the muscle has been postulated. The role of TrPs as part of this process is unknown, but there is a strong possibility that, in muscles prone to developing a compartment syndrome, TrPs may make a significant contribution. Chapter 63 contains additional information on chronic exertional compartment syndrome.

Surgical intervention to relieve symptoms identified as resulting from a chronic compartment syndrome is controversial. One group of surgeons reported an 88% success rate on 26 legs of patients with compartment syndromes, performing the operation only after conservative measures failed but without measuring intramuscular pressures.[66] Other surgeons who performed a fasciotomy of the deep posterior compartment based on intramuscular pressure criteria did not achieve results that were as good as those obtained when treating the anterior compartment syndrome surgically.[67] In this series of eight patients, a deep posterior compartment syndrome was diagnosed if intramuscular pressure was more than 15 mm Hg at rest, if it increased during exercise, and if it demonstrated a delayed return to the pre-exercise level.[67] A more recent systematic review on the effectiveness of surgery for the deep posterior compartment syndrome of the leg reported a modest success rate (ranging from 30% to 65%) after fasciotomy and argued for an optimization of diagnostic criteria and a standardization of treatment modalities for the condition.[65] Another recent review showed a success rate of 61% of surgical treatment for deep posterior compartment syndrome.[64]

5. CORRECTIVE ACTIONS

Individuals with TrPs in the tibialis posterior muscle may benefit from adopting sitting or standing postures that place the ankle in some degree of plantar flexion. While seated, an individual can sit with his or her knees in 50° or 60° of flexion, allowing the foot to contact the floor for lower extremity support, while providing ankle plantar flexion to place more slack on the tibialis posterior muscle. A common perpetuating cause of TrPs in the tibialis posterior muscle is an improperly designed or improperly used leg rest that causes calf compression. People who sit in reclining chairs with built-in leg rests that concentrate weight on a portion of the calf may require additional pillows or may need to restrict elevation of the leg rest.

A patient with tibialis posterior TrPs who walks or runs for exercise should do so on a flat surface and always wear shoes with adequate support. Excessive pronation due to a hypermobile midfoot should be corrected with a good medial longitudinal arch support. Initially, corrections made by the insert of the shoe may be uncomfortable due to referred tenderness from the TrPs, but with resolution of the tibialis posterior TrPs, this related tenderness of the sole of the foot disappears. Whether or not the individual walks, runs, or jogs, he or she should always wear well-fitted shoes with high-enough sides to enhance lateral stability of the foot. Proper footwear should be recommended by a clinician with knowledge of the structure and function of the foot and ankle and its relationship to the entire lower extremity, pelvis, and spine.

If the TrP activity responds poorly to treatment, running as a form of exercise could be replaced by swimming or cycling. High heels and stilettos must be avoided. High top shoes may be necessary if other measures do not suffice.

In general, the leg muscles feel better if the ankle is maintained in a neutral position throughout the night; therefore, adjusting the patients' sleeping posture may be necessary. This position is facilitated by having the bed sheets at the foot of the bed untucked to reduce external force into excessive plantar flexion (see Figure 66-6). Using a pillow between the legs and knees in side-lying to place the foot and ankle in a neutral position may also be beneficial.

Tibialis posterior TrP self-pressure release can be performed in the seated position with the affected leg crossed over the opposite leg at the ankle (Figure 67-5). Manual TrP self-pressure release

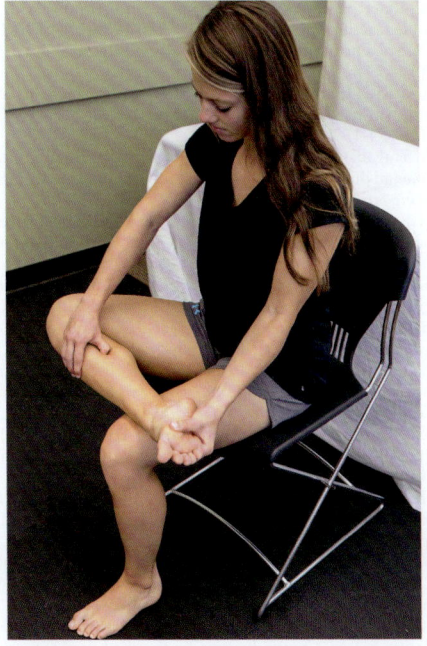
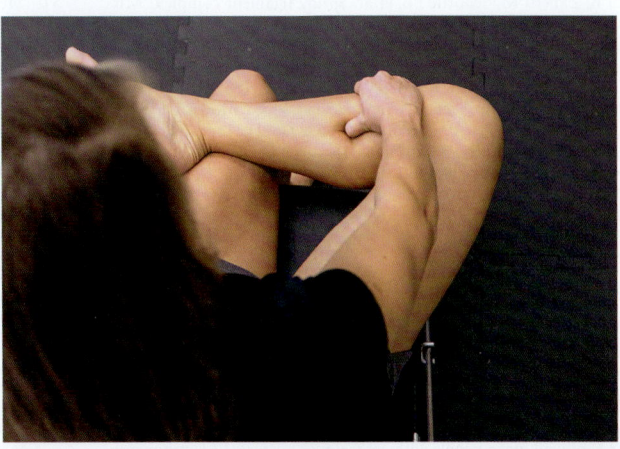

Figure 67-5. Self-pressure release of TrPs in the tibialis posterior muscle.

can be provided with the thumb on the undersurface of the tibia (Figure 67-5). Finding the most sensitive spot along the posterior surface of the tibia, often about a hand width below the knee, and gentle light pressure (no more than 4/10 pain) is applied manually with a thumb or fingers. A TrP release tool should be used with caution because of its proximity to the bone and neurovascular structures as well as the depth of the tibialis posterior muscle (Figure 67-5). If tingling or numbness is felt with self-pressure release of TrPs, the technique should be discontinued.

Self-stretch of the tibialis posterior muscle is typically not recommended because of the potential of tibialis posterior tendon dysfunction. Stretching the tibialis tendon may be more harmful than helpful due to the watershed (hypovascular) zone of the tendon between the medial malleolus and its insertion on the navicular bone in the midfoot. Consultation with a clinician who treats patients with lower extremity, ankle, and foot dysfunctions is highly recommended.

References

1. Standring S. *Gray's Anatomy: The Anatomical Basis of Clinical Practice*. 41st ed. London, UK: Elsevier; 2015.
2. Travell J, Simons DG. *Myofascial Pain and Dysfunction: The Trigger Point Manual*. Vol 2. Baltimore, MD: Williams & Wilkins; 1992.
3. Pastore D, Dirim B, Wangwinyuvirat M, et al. Complex distal insertions of the tibialis posterior tendon: detailed anatomic and MR imaging investigation in cadavers. *Skeletal Radiol*. 2008;37(9):849-855.
4. Ollivere BJ, Ellahee N, Sikdar T, Nairn DS. Anomalous tibialis posterior muscle, functional or functionless? *Foot*. 2006;16(4):218-220.
5. Yi KH, Rha DW, Lee SC, et al. Intramuscular nerve distribution pattern of ankle invertor muscles in human cadaver using sihler stain. *Muscle Nerve*. 2016;53(5):742-747.
6. Apaydin N, Loukas M, Kendir S, et al. The precise localization of distal motor branches of the tibial nerve in the deep posterior compartment of the leg. *Surg Radiol Anat*. 2008;30(4):291-295.
7. Frey C, Shereff M, Greenidge N. Vascularity of the posterior tibial tendon. *J Bone Joint Surg Am*. 1990;72(6):884-888.
8. Kulig K, Burnfield JM, Reischl S, Requejo SM, Blanco CE, Thordarson DB. Effect of foot orthoses on tibialis posterior activation in persons with pes planus. *Med Sci Sports Exerc*. 2005;37(1):24-29.
9. Klein P, Mattys S, Rooze M. Moment arm length variations of selected muscles acting on talocrural and subtalar joints during movement: an in vitro study. *J Biomech*. 1996;29(1):21-30.
10. Kamiya T, Uchiyama E, Watanabe K, Suzuki D, Fujimiya M, Yamashita T. Dynamic effect of the tibialis posterior muscle on the arch of the foot during cyclic axial loading. *Clin Biomech (Bristol, Avon)*. 2012;27(9):962-966.
11. Basmajian JV, Stecko G. The role of muscles in arch support of the foot. *J Bone Joint Surg Am Vol*. 1963;45:1184-1190.
12. Basmajian J, Deluca C. *Muscles Alive*. 5th ed. Baltimore, MD: Williams & Wilkins; 1985.
13. Kaye RA, Jahss MH. Tibialis posterior: a review of anatomy and biomechanics in relation to support of the medial longitudinal arch. *Foot Ankle*. 1991;11(4):244-247.
14. Mengiardi B, Zanetti M, Schottle PB, et al. Spring ligament complex: MR imaging-anatomic correlation and findings in asymptomatic subjects. *Radiology*. 2005;237(1):242-249.
15. Netter FH. *Musculoskeletal System. Part 1: Anatomy, Physiology and Metabolic Disorders*. Vol 8. Summit, NJ: Ciba-Geigy Corporation; 1987.
16. Bardeen C. The musculature, Section 5. In: Jackson CM, ed. *Morris's Human Anatomy*. 6th ed. Philadelphia, PA: Blakiston's Son & Co; 1921 (pp. 522, 523).
17. Rasch PJ, Burke RK. *Kinesiology and Applied Anatomy: The Science of Human Movement*. 6th ed. Philadelphia, PA: Lea & Febiger; 1978.
18. Janda V. *Muscle Function Testing*. London, England: Butterworths; 1983.
19. Duchenne G. *Physiology of Motion*. Philadelphia, PA: Lippincott; 1949.
20. Clemente C. *Gray's Anatomy of the Human Body*. 30th ed. Philadelphia, PA: Lea & Febiger; 1985.
21. Perry J, Burnfield JM. *Hip. Gait Analysis: Normal and Pathological Function*. 2nd ed. Thorofare, NJ: SLACK; 2010.
22. Sutherland DH. An electromyographic study of the plantar flexors of the ankle in normal walking on the level. *J Bone Joint Surg Am*. 1966;48(1):66-71.
23. Kokubo T, Hashimoto T, Nagura T, et al. Effect of the posterior tibial and peroneal longus on the mechanical properties of the foot arch. *Foot Ankle Int*. 2012;33(4):320-325.
24. Murley GS, Buldt AK, Trump PJ, Wickham JB. Tibialis posterior EMG activity during barefoot walking in people with neutral foot posture. *J Electromyogr Kinesiol*. 2009;19(2):e69-e77.
25. Okita N, Meyers SA, Challis JH, Sharkey NA. Midtarsal joint locking: new perspectives on an old paradigm. *J Orthop Res*. 2014;32(1):110-115.
26. Neumann DA. *Kinesiology of the Musculoskeletal System: Foundations for Rehabilitation*. 2nd ed. St. Louis, MO: Mosby; 2010.
27. Akuzawa H, Imai A, Iizuka S, Matsunaga N, Kaneoka K. Calf muscle activity alteration with foot orthoses insertion during walking measured by fine-wire electromyography. *J Phys Ther Sci*. 2016;28(12):3458-3462.
28. Perry J, Ireland ML, Gronley J, Hoffer MM. Predictive value of manual muscle testing and gait analysis in normal ankles by dynamic electromyography. *Foot Ankle*. 1986;6(5):254-259.
29. Murley GS, Menz HB, Landorf KB. Electromyographic patterns of tibialis posterior and related muscles when walking at different speeds. *Gait Posture*. 2014;39(4):1080-1085.
30. Maharaj JN, Cresswell AG, Lichtwark GA. The mechanical function of the tibialis posterior muscle and its tendon during locomotion. *J Biomech*. 2016;49(14):3238-3243.
31. Simons DG, Travell J, Simons L. *Travell & Simon's Myofascial Pain and Dysfunction: The Trigger Point Manual*. Vol 1. 2nd ed. Baltimore, MD: Williams & Wilkins; 1999 (p. 104).
32. Reinking MF, Austin TM, Richter RR, Krieger MM. Medial tibial stress syndrome in active individuals: a systematic review and meta-analysis of risk factors. *Sports Health*. 2017;9(3):252-261.
33. Aquino A, Payne C. Function of the windlass mechanism in excessively pronated feet. *J Am Podiatr Med Assoc*. 2001;91(5):245-250.
34. Kendall FP, McCreary EK. *Muscles: Testing and Function, with Posture and Pain*. 5th ed. Baltimore, MD: Lippincott Williams & Wilkins; 2005.
35. Johnson KA, Strom DE. Tibialis posterior tendon dysfunction. *Clin Orthop Relat Res*. 1989(239):196-206.
36. Bubra PS, Keighley G, Rateesh S, Carmody D. Posterior tibial tendon dysfunction: an overlooked cause of foot deformity. *J Family Med Prim Care*. 2015;4(1):26-29.
37. Gerwin RD, Dommerholt J, Shah JP. An expansion of Simons' integrated hypothesis of trigger point formation. *Curr Pain Headache Rep*. 2004;8(6):468-475.
38. Hsieh YL, Kao MJ, Kuan TS, Chen SM, Chen JT, Hong CZ. Dry needling to a key myofascial trigger point may reduce the irritability of satellite MTrPs. *Am J Phys Med Rehabil*. 2007;86(5):397-403.
39. Imamura M, Fischer AA, Imamura ST, Kaziyama HS, Carvalho AE, Salomao O. Treatment of myofascial pain components in plantar fasciitis speeds up recovery: documentation by algometry. *J Musculoske Pain*. 1998;6(1):91-110.
40. Cotchett MP, Landorf KB, Munteanu SE, Raspovic AM. Consensus for dry needling for plantar heel pain (plantar fasciitis): a modified Delphi study. *Acupunct Med*. 2011;29(3):193-202.
41. Cotchett MP, Munteanu SE, Landorf KB. Effectiveness of trigger point dry needling for plantar heel pain: a randomized controlled trial. *Phys Ther*. 2014;94(8):1083-1094.
42. Bluman EM, Myerson MS. Stage IV posterior tibial tendon rupture. *Foot Ankle Clin*. 2007;12(2):341-362, viii.
43. Ling SK, Lui TH. Posterior tibial tendon dysfunction: an overview. *Open Orthop J*. 2017;11:714-723.
44. Myerson MS. Adult acquired flatfoot deformity: treatment of dysfunction of the posterior tibial tendon. *J Bone Joint Surg*. 1996;78(5):780-792.
45. Lipsman S, Frankel JP, Count GW. Spontaneous rupture of the tibialis posterior tendon. A case report and review of the literature. *J Am Podiatry Assoc*. 1980;70(1):34-39.
46. Banks AS, McGlamry ED. Tibialis posterior tendon rupture. *J Am Podiatric Med Assoc*. 1987;77(4):170-176.
47. Downey DJ, Simkin PA, Mack LA, Richardson ML, Kilcoyne RF, Hansen ST. Tibialis posterior tendon rupture: a cause of rheumatoid flat foot. *Arthritis Rheum*. 1988;31(3):441-446.
48. Sammarco GJ, DiRaimondo CV. Surgical treatment of lateral ankle instability syndrome. *Am J Sports Med*. 1988;16(5):501-511.
49. Soballe K, Kjaersgaard-Andersen P. Ruptured tibialis posterior tendon in a closed ankle fracture. *Clin Orthop Relat Res*. 1988(231):140-143.
50. Helal B. Tibialis posterior tendon synovitis and rupture. *Acta Orthop Belg*. 1989;55(3):457-460.
51. Mendicino SS, Quinn M. Tibialis posterior dysfunction: an overview with a surgical case report using a flexor tendon transfer. *J Foot Surg*. 1989;28(2):154-157.
52. West MA, Sangani C, Toh E. Tibialis posterior tendon rupture associated with a closed medial malleolar fracture: a case report and review of the literature. *J Foot Ankle Surg*. 2010;49(6):565.e9-512.e9.
53. Holmes GB Jr, Cracchiolo A III, Goldner JL, Mann RA. Current practices in the management of posterior tibial tendon rupture. *Contemp Orthop*. 1990;20:79-108.
54. Bruyn GA, Hanova P, Iagnocco A, et al. Ultrasound definition of tendon damage in patients with rheumatoid arthritis. Results of a OMERACT consensus-based ultrasound score focussing on the diagnostic reliability. *Ann Rheum Dis*. 2014;73(11):1929-1934.
55. Ikoma K, Ohashi S, Maki M, Kido M, Hara Y, Kubo T. Diagnostic characteristics of standard radiographs and magnetic resonance imaging of ruptures of the tibialis posterior tendon. *J Foot Ankle Surg*. 2016;55(3):542-546.
56. Ringleb SI, Kavros SJ, Kotajarvi BR, Hansen DK, Kitaoka HB, Kaufman KR. Changes in gait associated with acute stage II posterior tibial tendon dysfunction. *Gait Posture*. 2007;25(4):555-564.
57. Green DR, Lepow GM, Smith TF. Chapter 8, Pes cavus. In: McGlamry ED, ed. *Comprehensive Textbook of Foot Surgery*. Vol 1. Baltimore, MD: Williams & Wilkins; 1987:287-323.
58. McGlamry ED, Mahan KT, Green DR. Chapter 12, Pes valgo planus deformity. In: McGlamry ED, ed. *Comprehensive Textbook of Foot Surgery*. Vol 1. Baltimore, MD: Williams & Wilkins; 1987:403-465.
59. Miller S. Chapter 23, Principles of muscle-tendon surgery and tendon transfers. In: McGlamry ED, ed. *Comprehensive Textbook of Foot Surgery*. Baltimore, MD: Williams & Wilkins; 1987:714-755.
60. Reshef N, Guelich DR. Medial tibial stress syndrome. *Clin Sports Med*. 2012;31(2):273-290.

61. Newman P, Witchalls J, Waddington G, Adams R. Risk factors associated with medial tibial stress syndrome in runners: a systematic review and meta-analysis. *Open Access J Sports Med*. 2013;4:229-241.
62. Hamstra-Wright KL, Bliven KC, Bay C. Risk factors for medial tibial stress syndrome in physically active individuals such as runners and military personnel: a systematic review and meta-analysis. *Br J Sports Med*. 2015;49(6):362-369.
63. Rajasekaran S, Hall MM. Nonoperative management of chronic exertional compartment syndrome: a systematic review. *Curr Sports Med Rep*. 2016;15(3):191-198.
64. Campano D, Robaina JA, Kusnezov N, Dunn JC, Waterman BR. Surgical management for chronic exertional compartment syndrome of the leg: a systematic review of the literature. *Arthroscopy*. 2016;32(7):1478-1486.
65. Winkes MB, Hoogeveen AR, Scheltinga MR. Is surgery effective for deep posterior compartment syndrome of the leg? A systematic review. *Br J Sports Med*. 2014;48(22):1592-1598.
66. Wiley JP, Clement DB, Doyle DL, Taunton JE. A primary care perspective of chronic compartment syndrome of the leg. *Phys Sportsmed*. 1987;15:111-120.
67. Rorabeck CH, Fowler PJ, Nott L. The results of fasciotomy in the management of chronic exertional compartment syndrome. *Am J Sports Med*. 1988;16(3):224-227.

Chapter 68

Long Toe Extensor Muscles
Extensor Digitorum Longus and Extensor Hallucis Longus

"Muscles of Classic Hammer Toes"

Carol A. Courtney and Dhinu J. Jayaseelan

1. INTRODUCTION

The extensor hallucis longus (EHL) and extensor digitorum longus (EDL) muscles are considered long toe extensor muscles. Together with the tibialis anterior muscle, they inhabit the anterior compartment of the leg. These muscles are primarily active during gait and functionally provide dynamic stability for balance. Dysfunction in these muscles, or other muscles involved in gait (such as the tibialis anterior or fibularis muscles), could contribute to the development of trigger points (TrPs). Trigger points in these muscles contribute to a patient report of "sore feet" focused on the dorsal aspect of the ankle and foot, anterior leg, and spreading to the related great and lesser toes. Activities such as walking, climbing, and running can activate TrPs in these muscles. Kicking a ball or stubbing a toe as in a "turf toe" injury may also overload the long toe extensor muscles. Differential diagnosis should include tibial stress fractures, compartment syndrome, lumbar spine radicular pain or radiculopathy, hammer toe, claw toe, or mallet toe deformity. Corrective actions include TrP self-pressure release, self-stretching of the long toe extensor muscles and the gastrocnemius/soleus muscle complex, and activity and shoe modification to reduce recurrent overload of these muscles.

2. ANATOMIC CONSIDERATIONS

The long toe extensor muscles, the EDL and EHL muscles, share their position at the anterior compartment of the leg with the tibialis anterior and fibularis tertius muscles. Given their origin proximal to the ankle, and insertion within the foot itself, the EDL and EHL muscles are considered extrinsic toe extensor muscles.[1]

Extensor Digitorum Longus

The EDL muscle is a penniform muscle that originates proximally on the lateral surface of the lateral condyle of the tibia, the proximal two-thirds to three-quarters of the medial surface of the fibula, deep surface of the deep fascia, and adjacent anterior surface of the interosseous membrane above the EHL muscle (Figure 68-1). The part of the muscle that originates from the tibial condyle and head of the fibula covers the deep fibular nerve as it courses around the neck of the fibula to reach the intermuscular septum. The deep fibular nerve and the anterior tibial vessels lie between the EDL and tibialis anterior muscles. At the ankle, the tendon passes deep to the superior and inferior extensor retinacula that prevent bowstringing of the tendon. Distally, the EDL tendon inserts into the extensor hood mechanism on the dorsum of the metatarsophalangeal joints and the proximal phalanges of the lateral four toes. A central slip inserts to the base of the middle phalanx, and two collateral slips insert to the base of the distal phalanx.[1] The EDL muscle has the second largest cross-sectional area of the anterior compartment muscles, second to the tibialis anterior muscle. The mean width of the EDL muscle is 12.4 mm in a cadaveric dissection of 68 feet.[2]

Extensor Hallucis Longus

The EHL muscle originates on the middle half of the medial surface of the fibula and the adjacent anterior surface of the interosseous membrane. It lies between the tibialis anterior and the EDL muscles and is also partially overlapped by these two muscles (Figure 68-1). The deep fibular nerve and anterior tibial vessels lie between the EHL and the tibialis anterior muscles. After coursing distally, beneath the extensor retinaculum at the anterior aspect of the talocrural joint, the EHL muscle inserts at the dorsal aspect of the base of the distal phalanx of the first toe.[1] In comparison with other muscles occupying the anterior compartment of the leg, the EHL muscle has the third largest cross-sectional area, behind the tibialis anterior and the EDL muscles, respectively. In the same cadaveric study by Solomon and colleagues, the mean width of the EHL muscle was 7.5 mm.[2]

Interestingly, cadaveric and operative studies have demonstrated different insertion patterns of the EHL muscle. One study performed found three different insertional patterns in 60 cadavers: 65% had a single tendinous insertion, 26.7% had two tendinous insertions, and 8.3% had three insertional tendon slips.[3] However, when evaluating 60 cases presenting for correction of severe hallux valgus and interphalangeus, in 98.3% of cases (all but one), there was an accessory medial EHL tendon inserting at the dorsomedial aspect of the metatarsophalangeal joint capsule. The authors referred to this tendon as the extensor hallucis capsularis, which was consistent with previous research.[4] In fact, a recent study has found that 26% of cadavers show an accessory tendon that inserts on the dorsomedial side of the 1st metatarsophalangeal joint capsule of the EHL muscle.[5]

Although the EDL and EHL muscles are distinctly different in their form and function, their anatomic relationship is strong. Solomon et al[2] reported that the space between the EDL and EHL muscles was, on average, 3.7 mm. In 14 cases, there was no space between the EDL and EHL muscles, and in 3 cases, these muscles overlapped up to 2 mm. Given their intimate anatomic relationship, it can be difficult for clinicians to examine or treat either in isolation. Consequently, clinicians, researchers, and educators are reminded to understand anatomic variations exist and to consider how these variations may affect typical motion.

Chapter 68: Long Toe Extensor Muscles

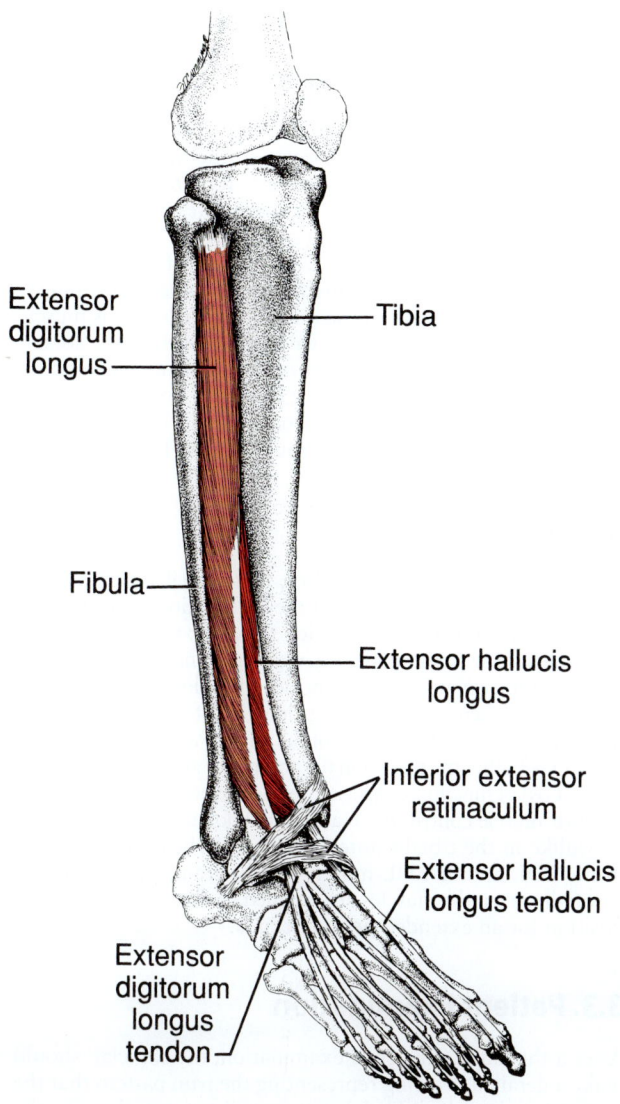

Figure 68-1. Attachments of the right long extensor muscles of the toes, anterolateral view. The extensor digitorum longus muscle is medium red, and the extensor hallucis longus muscle is dark red. The superior extensor retinaculum is not pictured.

2.1. Innervation and Vascularization

The lumbosacral plexus provides innervation to the long toe extensor muscles via the L4, L5, and S1 spinal nerve root levels. The common fibular nerve branches off the sciatic nerve laterally in the posterior aspect of the knee, wrapping anteriorly to lie just inferior and posterior to the fibular head. The common fibular nerve then divides into the superficial and deep fibular nerve. The deep fibular nerve goes on to provide motor supply to the EDL and EHL muscles and also provides cutaneous sensory input to the dorsal aspect of the space between the first and second toes. Although anatomic variations will occur, a recent cadaveric study elucidated common nerve distribution patterns.[6]

For the EDL muscle, after entering the posterosuperior aspect of the muscle, two branching patterns were seen: (1) the deep fibular nerve branches into two components, supplying the anterosuperior and posteroinferior compartments, and then it further divides into 1 to 2 branches distally and (2) just before or after entering the EDL muscle, the deep fibular nerve separates into 2 to 3 branches and travels parallel to the tendon distally.[6]

For the EHL muscle, the deep fibular nerve enters the anterior surface nearly 5 in inferior to the fibular head and divides into 1 to 3 more branches. In most cases, two nerve branches continue distally in parallel to supply the anterosuperior and posteroinferior compartments.[6]

Proximal vascular supply to the EDL and EHL muscles is provided by the anterior tibial artery, with perforating branches of the fibular artery. Distally, closer to the ankle, the anterior lateral and medial malleolar arteries supply the EDL and EHL muscles, respectively. Additional arterial branches are present to ensure adequate perfusion and oxygenation.

2.2. Function

Given their location on the leg, the EDL and EHL muscles are active during many functional activities. Proper coordination of the extrinsic and intrinsic foot and ankle muscles allows for functional gait and sport-based movement. In the presence of muscle performance or length impairments, movement abnormalities will be present. The tibialis anterior, EDL, and EHL muscles have primary weight-bearing functions. They maintain standing balance by controlling excessive posterior postural sway and assist in keeping the leg vertical over the fixed foot.[7-10]

Working as a unit, the long toe extensor muscles assist the tibialis anterior muscle in producing dorsiflexion at the talocrural joint. Adequate ankle dorsiflexion is integral to a functional gait cycle. Typical dorsiflexor muscle activity during gait is biphasic, with peak intensity noted during initial swing and loading response. The muscle activity starts in the preswing phase, as the foot prepares to clear the ground, and ends after the loading response. At initial contact, the pretibial muscles are active eccentrically to combat the rotational demand of the forefoot. Progressing into the loading response, the ankle dorsiflexors contract concentrically to facilitate anterior translation of the tibia.

During pre- and initial swing, the anterior compartment muscles are again active concentrically to clear the foot. During mid- and terminal swing, these muscles function isometrically to resist the downward force of gravity. These muscles are generally not active during mid- and terminal stance, as the heel rocker facilitates forward momentum, and the gastrocnemius muscle eccentrically controls anterior tibial translation.[11]

Although the tibialis anterior, EDL, and EHL muscles work in coordination during ankle dorsiflexion, weakness of any or all of these muscles will lead to muscle and joint compensation. Unopposed tibialis anterior muscle activity during swing, for example, secondary to EDL muscle weakness or paralysis, would lead to excessive inversion and a cavus appearing foot. Subsequently, without further compensation, this reaction would likely lead to excessive loading of the lateral border of the foot during initial contact and loading response and, subsequently, inadequate force absorption.[11]

Although the function of the long toe extensor muscles is primarily described in the context of gait, clinicians should consider the role of the EDL and EHL muscles in sport and functional activities as well. For example, dynamic multiplanar activities such as soccer, football, or basketball all require rapid directional changes. Although the long toe extensor muscles function primarily to extend the toes and dorsiflex the ankle, they work in conjunction with other soft tissues around the foot. In activities requiring active eversion, the EDL muscle should be examined separately from the fibularis muscles, which perform the same action. The EHL muscle is also thought to help the foot adapt to the ground during walking.

Extensor Digitorum Longus

The EDL muscle has multiple actions. Proximally, it acts to dorsiflex the ankle, and because its tendon runs lateral to the axis of the subtalar joint, it everts the foot as well.[11] This eversion action is thought to balance the inversion pull of the tibialis anterior muscle. The EDL muscle also provides primary extension of the lateral four metatarsophalangeal joints and contributes to extension of those proximal and distal interphalangeal joints in conjunction with the foot intrinsic muscles.

Extensor Hallucis Longus

The EHL muscle assists the tibialis anterior and EDL muscles in ankle dorsiflexion. Although it has been reported that the EHL muscles assist with inversion,[11] the muscle crosses the subtalar joint close to its axis, making its role in moving the subtalar joint questionable.[12,13] One study examining both cadavers and live subjects reported an ability of the EHL muscle to slightly supinate the foot. Electromyographic activity of the EHL muscle was noted during supination tasks, such as lifting the medial border of the foot when in weight bearing.[11] Additionally, the EHL muscle serves an important function in providing the only active extension to the great toe interphalangeal joint and the primary active extension force of the 1st metatarsophalangeal joint. This extension movement is crucial for the beginning of the swing phase of the gait cycle when action of the EHL muscle is required for great toe extension to clear the supporting surface.

2.3. Functional Unit

The functional unit to which a muscle belongs includes the muscles that reinforce and counter its actions as well as the joints that the muscle crosses. The interdependence of these structures is functionally reflected in the organization and neural connections of the sensory motor cortex. The functional unit is emphasized because the presence of a TrP in one muscle of the unit increases the likelihood that the other muscles of the unit will also develop TrPs. When inactivating TrPs in a muscle, one must be concerned about TrPs that may develop in muscles that are functionally interdependent. Box 68-1 grossly represents the functional unit of the EDL and EHL muscles.[14]

Box 68-1 Functional unit of the EDL and EHL muscles

Action	Synergists	Antagonists
Dorsiflexion of the foot	Fibularis tertius Tibialis anterior	Gastrocnemius Soleus Fibularis longus and brevis Flexor digitorum longus Flexor hallucis longus Tibialis posterior
Inversion of the foot (EHL)	Tibialis posterior Tibialis anterior Flexor digitorum longus Flexor hallucis longus	Fibularis longus and brevis Fibularis tertius Extensor digitorum longus
Eversion of the Foot (EDL)	Fibularis longus and brevis Fibularis tertius	Tibialis posterior Tibialis anterior Flexor digitorum longus Flexor hallucis longus

3. CLINICAL PRESENTATION

3.1. Referred Pain Pattern

Extensor digitorum longus TrPs refer pain primarily over the dorsum of the foot and toes, nearly to the tips of the middle three toes (Figure 68-2A), as previously reported.[15] Sometimes, the pain referred from EDL TrPs concentrates more strongly at the ankle than over the dorsum of the foot. The pain pattern may extend halfway up the leg from the ankle toward the muscle belly (Figure 68-2A). Jacobsen[16] reported pain spreading to the anterolateral region of the ankle from TrPs in this muscle. Extensor hallucis longus TrPs refer pain primarily to the dorsum of the foot over the distal aspect of the 1st metatarsal and the base of the great toe. The pain may extend downward to the tip of the great toe and upward over the dorsum of the foot and leg, sometimes as far as the muscle belly (Figure 68-1B).

3.2. Symptoms

Patients with TrPs in the EDL or EHL muscles will typically report pain along the anterior aspect of the leg and dorsum of the foot with or without activity. In addition to pain, patients may report tenderness in the front of their leg, weakness, and possibly reduced function. Other symptoms may include the following: weakness of dorsiflexion when walking, falling, dragging of the foot that causes tripping, and general weakness of the ankle. Painful motion of the ankle may bother the patient in the absence of any evidence of joint injury. Loss of function is especially evident when TrPs in the tibialis anterior muscle contribute to additional dorsiflexion weakness.

Unlike in the tibialis anterior muscle, when there are TrPs in the EDL and/or EHL muscles, night cramps are common, especially when the muscles are fatigued or placed in a shortened position for an extended period of time.

3.3. Patient Examination

After a thorough subjective examination, the clinician should make a detailed drawing representing the pain pattern that the patient has described. This depiction will assist in planning the physical examination and can be useful in monitoring the progression of the patient as symptoms improve or change. The type, quality, and location of the pain should be carefully assessed, and the utilization of standardized outcome tools is imperative when examining patients with lower extremity dysfunctions.

The objective examination should identify a symptom provoking functional movement such as ascending/descending stairs, walking, squatting, or climbing. Typically, the clinician will ascertain a functional movement that provokes symptoms. Finding this movement early can provide the clinician an important reassessment sign and provide an opportunity to differentiate the source of symptoms early in the examination.

Observation of static and dynamic posture is essential because of the role of the EDL and EHL muscles in postural stability. Functional testing such as double- and single-leg squat will allow a quick assessment of hip and knee control, as well as a quick assessment of talocrural, subtalar, and midfoot range of motion. Timed single-leg stance with eyes open and closed will give a quantitative measure of balance and will allow the clinician to observe foot and ankle strategies related to balance and control.

The position of the toes should be examined because these muscles often contribute to hammertoe and/or claw toe. If these abnormalities are noted, each toe should be examined to determine if the abnormality is flexible or rigid. The clinician should assess active range of motion with passive overpressure in all planes of motion. In addition, the assessment of physiologic and/or accessory joint movement of the ankle, hindfoot, midfoot, and forefoot is often valuable because TrPs and joint dysfunction are often found concurrently.

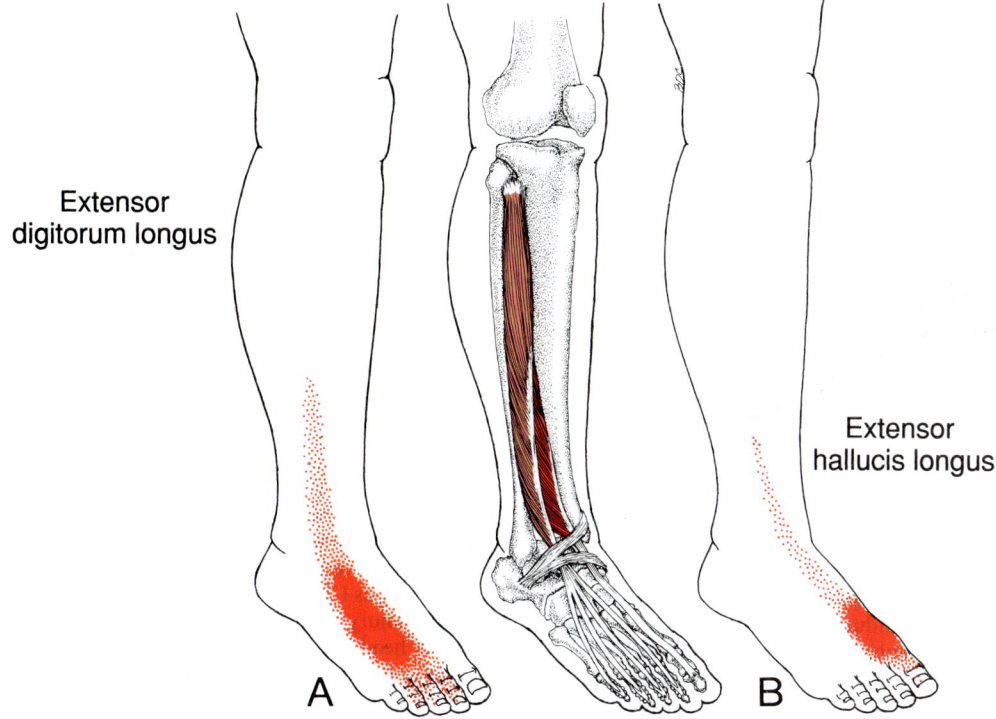

Figure 68-2. Pain patterns (bright red) referred from TrPs in the right long extensor muscles of the toes. The essential pain pattern (solid bright red) denotes the pain experienced by nearly everyone with TrPs. Red stippling indicates occasional spreading of the essential pattern. A, Extensor digitorum longus muscle (light red). B, Extensor hallucis longus muscle (dark red).

A thorough gait analysis will assist in identifying compensatory patterns if the EDL and/or EHL muscles are weak or painful. Common compensations include waddling gait (a lean to the contralateral side and "hiking" the hip), swing-out gait (in which the dysfunctional leg is circumducted laterally), or high-stepping/steppage gait (in which extra flexion is utilized at the hip and knee) to clear the toes in swing phase.[17]

The long toe extensor muscles receive their innervation via deep fibular nerve branches that contain fibers from the L4, L5, and S1 spinal nerves, though L5 is the primary contributor.[18] Injury to these nerves may occur subtly, with only pain or sensory signs and symptoms. With progression or persistence of nerve injury, symptoms may include muscle weakness. Functionally, the patient may describe catching a toe or a subtle foot slap, indicating L5 myotomal weakness.[19]

3.4. Trigger Point Examination

For examination of the EDL and EHL muscles, the patient may be in long sitting or, preferably, supine (Figure 68-3). A pillow or bolster may be put under the patient's knees to ensure relaxation. A cross-fiber flat palpation technique should be utilized to identify taut bands and TrPs in the EDL and EHL muscles. Focal bands of taut muscle tissue should be evaluated with firm pressure to determine if the patient's familiar symptoms are reproduced, if there is referral of symptoms, or if symptoms are reduced. As it is common for multiple TrPs to exist in the same muscle, palpatory examination should not terminate after finding a single TrP. However, as both EDL and EHL muscles are covered by the tibialis anterior muscle, direct palpation of these muscles is not possible. A recent study has reported that palpation of TrPs in the EDL muscle exhibits moderate to substantial reliability.[20]

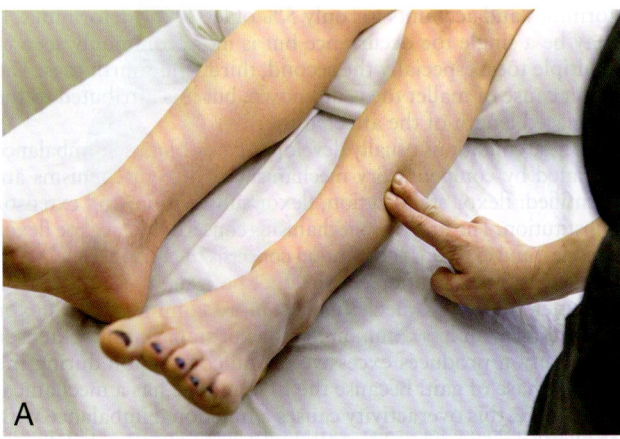
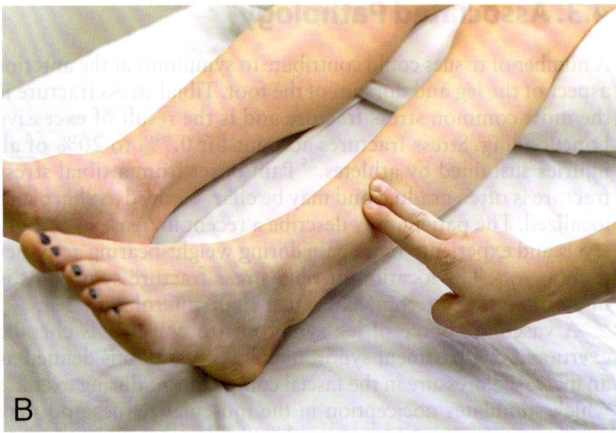

Figure 68-3. Cross-fiber flat palpation of long toe extensor muscles. A, Extensor digitorum longus muscle. B, Extensor hallucis longus muscle.

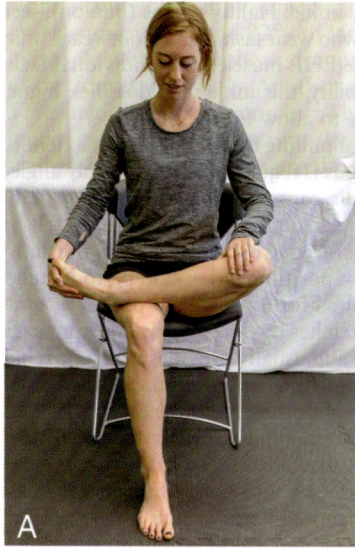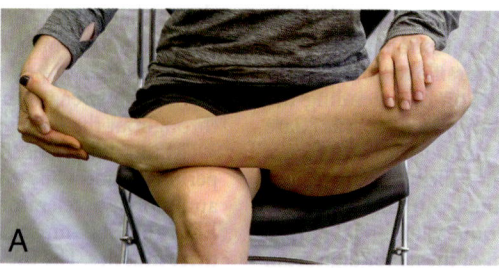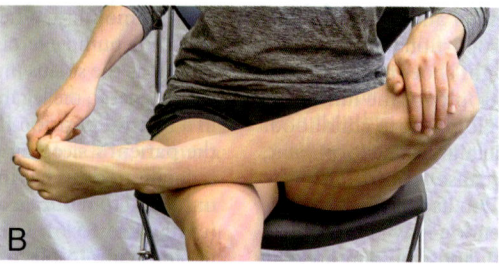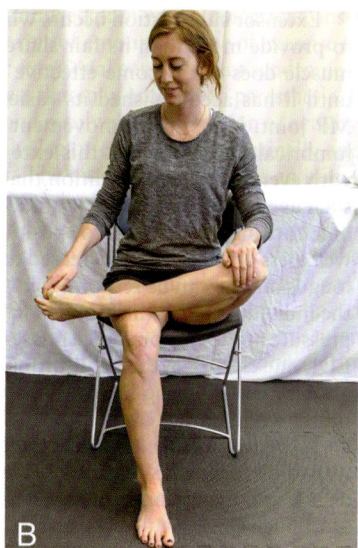

Figure 68-5. Self-stretch. A, Extensor digitorum longus muscle. B, Extensor hallucis longus muscle.

manually with the thumbs (Figure 68-4B), or with a TrP release tool (Figure 68-4C). Finding the sensitive spot with the heel, thumbs, or a tool light pressure (no more than 4/10 pain) is applied and held for 15 to 30 seconds or until pain reduces. This technique can be repeated five times, several times per day. Also, patients could perform self-massage along the length of the involved soft tissues to enhance soft-tissue mobility.

In cases where the toe extensor muscles are adaptively shortened, self-stretching exercises should be incorporated. One way to stretch the EDL (Figure 68-5A) and EHL (Figure 68-5B) muscles is in a seated position with the involved leg crossed over the opposite thigh. In this position, one hand can passively move the toes into flexion, then gradually pull the ankle down toward plantar flexion until a stretch is felt on the top of the foot/ankle. The opposite hand can be used to stabilize the distal tibiofibular joint complex as needed. The patient should hold the stretch for up to 30 seconds and repeat this stretch four times.

In cases where muscle strength is impaired, individuals may strengthen the long toe extensor muscles in a variety of ways. To activate the EHL and EDL muscles in relative isolation, patients may lift all the toes off the ground without allowing ball of the foot to come off the ground—a task performed with minimal contribution from the tibialis anterior muscle because the ankle should stay stationary. Because these muscles work in conjunction with the tibialis anterior muscle, performing ankle dorsiflexion can also improve muscle performance.

References

1. Standring S. *Gray's Anatomy: The Anatomical Basis of Clinical Practice.* 41st ed. London, UK: Elsevier; 2015.
2. Solomon LB, Ferris L, Henneberg M. Anatomical study of the ankle with view to the anterior arthroscopic portals. *ANZ J Surg.* 2006;76(10):932-936.
3. Al-saggaf S. Variations in the insertion of the extensor hallucis longus muscle. *Folia Morphol (Warsz).* 2003;62(2):147-155.
4. Bayer T, Kolodziejski N, Flueckiger G. The extensor hallucis capsularis tendon—a prospective study of its occurrence and function. *Foot Ankle Surg.* 2014;20(3):192-194.
5. Natsis K, Konstantinidis GA, Symeonidis PD, Totlis T, Anastasopoulos N, Stavrou P. The accessory tendon of extensor hallucis longus muscle and its correlation to hallux valgus deformity: a cadaveric study. *Surg Radiol Anat.* 2017;39(12):1343-1347.
6. Yu D, Yin H, Han T, Jiang H, Cao X. Intramuscular innervations of lower leg skeletal muscles: applications in their clinical use in functional muscular transfer. *Surg Radiol Anat.* 2016;38(6):675-685.
7. Gantchev GN, Draganova N. Muscular synergies during different conditions of postural activity. *Acta Physiol Pharmacol Bulg.* 1986;12(4):58-65.
8. Oddsson L. Motor patterns of a fast voluntary postural task in man: trunk extension in standing. *Acta Physiol Scand.* 1989;136(1):47-58.
9. Okada M, Fujiwara K. Muscle activity around the ankle joint as correlated with the center of foot pressure in an upright stance. In: Matsui M, Kobayashi K, eds. *Biomechanics 8A*. Champaign, IL: Human Kinetics Publishers; 1983:209-216.
10. Di Giulio I, Maganaris CN, Baltzopoulos V, Loram ID. The proprioceptive and agonist roles of gastrocnemius, soleus and tibialis anterior muscles in maintaining human upright posture. *J Physiol.* 2009;587(pt 10):2399-2416.
11. Perry J, Burnfield JM. *Hip. Gait Analysis: Normal and Pathological Function.* 2nd ed. Thorofare, NJ: SLACK; 2010.
12. Oatis C. *Kinesiology: The Mechanics and Pathomechanics of Human Movement.* 2nd ed. Baltimore, MD: Lippinott, Williams & Wilkins; 2009.
13. Neumann DA. *Kinesiology of the Musculoskeletal System: Foundations for Rehabilitaion.* 2nd ed. St. Louis, MO: Mosby; 2010.
14. Simons DG, Travell J, Simons L. *Travell & Simon's Myofascial Pain and Dysfunction: The Trigger Point Manual.* Vol 1. 2nd ed. Baltimore, MD: Williams & Wilkins; 1999 (p. 104).
15. Simons DG, Travell J. Chapter 25, Myofascial pain syndromes. In: Wall PD, Melzack R, Bonica JJ, eds. *Textbook of Pain.* 2nd ed. Edinburgh, Scotland: Churchill Livingstone; 1989:368-385 (p. 378, Fig. 25.9G).
16. Jacobsen S. Myofascial pain syndrome [in Danish]. *Ugeskrift for laeger.* 1987;149(9):600-601.
17. Moore KL, Dalley AF, Agur AMR. *Clinically Oriented Anatomy.* 6th ed. Philadelphia, PA: Lippincott Williams and Wilkins; 2009 (pp. 588-608).
18. Barr K. Electrodiagnosis of lumbar radiculopathy. *Phys Med Rehabil Clin N Am.* 2013;24(1):79-91.
19. Freynhagen R, Baron R, Gockel U, Tolle TR. painDETECT: a new screening questionnaire to identify neuropathic components in patients with back pain. *Curr Med Res Opin.* 2006;22(10):1911-1920.
20. Sanz DR, Lobo CC, Lopez DL, Morales CR, Marin CS, Corbalan IS. Interrater reliability in the clinical evaluation of myofascial trigger points in three ankle muscles. *J Manipulative Physiol Ther.* 2016;39(9):623-634.
21. Zuil-Escobar JC, Martínez-Cepa CB, Martín-Urrialde JA, Gómez-Conesa A. Prevalence of myofascial trigger points and diagnostic criteria of different muscles in function of the medial longitudinal arch. *Arch Phys Med Rehabil.* 2015;96(6):1123-1130.
22. Zuil-Escobar JC, Martínez-Cepa CB, Martín-Urrialde JA, Gómez-Conesa A. The prevalence of latent trigger points in lower limb muscles in asymptomatic subjects. *PM R.* 2016;8(11):1055-1064.
23. Gerwin RD, Dommerholt J, Shah JP. An expansion of Simons' integrated hypothesis of trigger point formation. *Curr Pain Headache Rep.* 2004;8(6):468-475.
24. Hsieh YL, Kao MJ, Kuan TS, Chen SM, Chen JT, Hong CZ. Dry needling to a key myofascial trigger point may reduce the irritability of satellite MTrPs. *Am J Phys Med Rehabil.* 2007;86(5):397-403.
25. Fredericson M, Jennings F, Beaulieu C, Matheson GO. Stress fractures in athletes. *Top Magn Reson Imaging.* 2006;17(5):309-325.
26. Brewer RB, Gregory AJ. Chronic lower leg pain in athletes: a guide for the differential diagnosis, evaluation, and treatment. *Sports Health.* 2012;4(2):121-127.
27. Williams GN, Allen EJ. Rehabilitation of syndesmotic (high) ankle sprains. *Sports Health.* 2010;2(6):460-470.
28. Williams GN, Jones MH, Amendola A. Syndesmotic ankle sprains in athletes. *Am J Sports Med.* 2007;35(7):1197-1207.
29. Iversen T, Solberg TK, Romner B, et al. Accuracy of physical examination for chronic lumbar radiculopathy. *BMC Musculoskelet Disord.* 2013;14:206.
30. Reife MD, Coulis CM. Peroneal neuropathy misdiagnosed as L5 radiculopathy: a case report. *Chiropr Man Therap.* 2013;21:12.
31. Craig A. Entrapment neuropathies of the lower extremity. *PM R.* 2013; 5(5 suppl):S31-S40.

32. Jimenez AL, McGlamry ED, Green DR. Chapter 3, Lesser ray deformities. In: McGlamry ED, ed. *Comprehensive Textbook of Foot Surgery*. Vol 1. Baltimore, MD: Williams & Wilkins; 1987:57-113 (pp. 57-58, 66-71).
33. Kwon JY, De Asla RJ. The use of flexor to extensor transfers for the correction of the flexible hammer toe deformity. *Foot Ankle Clin*. 2011;16(4):573-582.
34. Errichiello C, Marcarelli M, Pisani PC, Parino E. Treatment of dynamic claw toe deformity flexor digitorum brevis tendon transfer to interosseous and lumbrical muscles: a literature survey. *Foot Ankle Surg*. 2012;18(4):229-232.
35. Molloy A, Shariff R. Mallet toe deformity. *Foot Ankle Clin*. 2011;16(4):537-546.
36. Marchetti DC, Chang A, Ferrari M, Clanton TO. Turf toe: 40 years later and still a problem. *Op Tech Sports Med*. 2017;25(2):99-107.
37. Smith TF. Chapter 6, Common pedal prominences. In: McGlamry ED, ed. *Comprehensive Textbook of Foot Surgery*. Vol 1. Baltimore, MD: Williams & Wilkins; 1987:252-263 (p. 260).
38. Nix SE, Vicenzino BT, Collins NJ, Smith MD. Characteristics of foot structure and footwear associated with hallux valgus: a systematic review. *Osteoarthritis Cartilage*. 2012;20(10):1059-1074.

Chapter 69

Long Toe Flexor Muscles
Flexor Digitorum Longus and Flexor Hallucis Longus

"Clawtoe Muscles"

Thomas L. Christ, John Sharkey, and Joseph M. Donnelly

1. INTRODUCTION

The flexor digitorum longus (FDL) and flexor hallucis longus (FHL) muscles are located in the deep compartment of the posterior leg along with the popliteus and tibialis posterior muscles. Both the FDL and FHL muscles are innervated by the tibial nerve. They each function together to plantar flex the talocrural joint, invert the subtalar joint, support the longitudinal arch of the foot, and flex the metatarsophalangeal and interphalangeal joints. Trigger points (TrPs) in the FDL muscle primarily refer pain to the plantar surface of the forefoot, proximal to toes 2 to 5. Trigger points in the FHL muscle primarily refer pain to the plantar surface of the great toe and head of the 1st metatarsal. Symptoms often include pain on the sole of the forefoot and plantar surfaces of the toes that is noticed while walking. Activation and perpetuation of TrPs in the FDL and FHL muscles usually results from overload during weight-bearing activities such as beginning a walking or jogging exercise program or long-distance running without proper training. Differential diagnosis should include assessment for nerve irritation or entrapment (tibial nerve, L5 nerve root); FHL tendon dysfunction; hallux valgus; claw, mallet and hammer toe abnormality; media tibial stress syndrome; and chronic exertional compartment syndrome. Corrective actions include education and assessment of proper footwear, activity modification, modification of sitting and sleeping postures, TrP self-pressure release, and self-stretching exercises.

2. ANATOMIC CONSIDERATIONS

The two long (extrinsic) toe flexor muscles share the deep posterior compartment of the leg with the tibialis posterior and popliteus muscles.[1]

Flexor Digitorum Longus

The thinly veiled FDL muscle is the smaller of the two muscles and originates below the soleal line, just medial to the tibialis posterior muscle from the medial aspect of the posterior tibia and the tibialis posterior fascia.[1] The muscle is narrow at its proximal attachment and widens as it descends in the leg. The fibers of this pennate muscle converge on the tendon that passes behind the medial malleolus in a groove shared with the tendon of the tibialis posterior muscle, passing deep to the flexor retinaculum but in a separate compartment and in a separate synovial sheath. The tendon crosses the medial aspect of the sustentaculum tali of the calcaneus, and as the tendon approaches the navicular bone and passes into the sole of the foot, it crosses superficial to the FHL tendon, from which it receives a strong tendinous slip.[1] At approximately midsole, the flexor accessories (quadratus plantae) muscle joins the FDL tendon that then divides into four tendons, each of which passes through an opening in the corresponding tendon of the flexor digitorum brevis muscle. The four tendons insert into the base of the distal phalanges of digits 2 to 5 (Figure 69-1).

The FDL muscle has a smaller cross-sectional area than the FHL muscle and similarly maintains a short fiber to muscle length ratio (0.16 ± 0.09).[2] Variations are common. The FDL muscle may be more or less divided into separate fasciculi for the individual toes.[3] One of the more common anomalous muscles of the leg is the flexor accessorius longus digitorum muscle that spans from the fibula or tibia to the tendon of the FDL muscle or to the flexor accessories (quadratus plantae) muscle and may send slips to the FHL and tibialis anterior muscles.[1,4-6] A sesamoid bone may develop in the tendon of the FHL muscle where it passes over the talus and the calcaneus.[3]

Flexor Hallucis Longus

The FHL muscle is a strong, large, multiarticular muscle contained within the deep posterior compartment of the leg. This pennate muscle is located distal and lateral to the FDL and tibialis posterior muscles. The FHL muscle sits predominantly over the posterior surface of the lower two-thirds of the posterior fibula attaching proximally to the interosseous membrane and to the intermuscular septa shared with associated muscles on both sides of it. The fibers of this muscle continue to converge on its tendon as it crosses the posterior surface of the lower end of the tibia. The tendon then crosses the posterior surface of the talus and the inferior surface of the sustentaculum tali of the calcaneus—deep to the tendon of the FDL muscle. Marginally, distal to the common tendon sheath, the lateral aspect of the FHL tendon attaches by two slips to the medial two tendons of the FDL muscle, forming a conjoined tendon. At this juncture, both tendons merge to attach to the cupola of the foot's arch by the knot of Henry or the common tendon sheath and binds to the medial surface of the navicular.

In the sole of the foot, the FHL tendon courses forward between the two heads of the flexor hallucis brevis muscle, passing between the medial and lateral sesamoid bones under the metatarsophalangeal joint to insert into the base of the terminal phalanx of the great (first) toe[1] (Figure 69-1).

According to Friederich and Brand[7] (and later confirmed by Kura et al[8] and Ward et al[2]), the cross-sectional area of the FHL muscle is the largest of all the short and long toe flexor muscles. Ward et al[2] also demonstrated that the FHL muscle presents a short fiber length to muscle length ratio (0.20 ± 0.5).

The dense fibrous fascia located within the compartments of the leg act to provide both connection and disconnection by means of fascial (septal) thickening. The deep fasciae take the form of interweaving, interlacing fibers, creating continuity receives innervation from the level L5, S1, and S2 spinal nerves. The FDL muscle receives its vascularization from ever-smaller branches of the posterior tibial artery entering its lateral side. Several branches of the fibular artery supply the muscle belly of the FHL muscle, whereas the tendon is supplied by the arteries of the ankle and foot.

2.2. Function

The FDL and FHL muscles act together in plantar flexion of the metatarsophalangeal and interphalangeal joints. During the swing phase of gait, both of these muscles assist in plantar flexion and inversion of the foot. During mid-to-late stance of gait, these muscles stabilize the foot to ensure mediolateral balance and to maintain stability of the longitudinal arches of the foot. During forefoot push-off, these muscles pull the toes into flexion, decelerating passive dorsiflexion of the distal phalanges. The FHL muscle contributes to plantar flexion at the ankle and inversion at the subtalar joint. The FDL muscle flexes the distal phalanx of each of the four lessor toes, whereas the FHL muscle flexes the distal phalanx of the great toe.

The small fiber length to muscle length ratio of both the FDL and FHL muscles proposes an architectural design favoring isometric function of these muscles.[2] This hypothesis has been supported both in vivo and with cadaveric specimens. Hofmann et al[10] used a robotic dynamic activity simulator to replicate gait in cadaveric lower extremities while measuring the FDL and FHL tendon excursions during the stance phase of gait. Both muscles showed minimal tendon length excursions, suggesting isometric functions. Peter et al[11] supported this conclusion in vivo by using ultrasound to measure FHL fascicle length at different gait speeds and found that the FHL fascicle length is relatively constant throughout the stance phase of gait, regardless of speed.

This relatively isometric nature of the FDL and FHL muscles may be due to their role in stabilizing the arches of the foot. The FDL and FHL muscles are active from the mid-stance to the push-off phase of gait as the body's center of mass rotates over the arch of the foot. Researchers found that force under the great toe increased when gait speed increased from increased FHL muscle activity, but no significant changes in fascicle length were noted. These data support the notion that, as walking speed increases, the reliance on the FHL muscle to maintain the longitudinal arch also increases.[12] Isometric contractions also require less energy output than eccentric or concentric contractions; therefore, the nature of the FDL and FHL muscles' isometric function may also conserve energy.[10]

The FDL and FHL muscles are activated during the stance phase and into the push-off phase of gait.[13,14] Zelik et al[14] showed a sequential order of lower extremity muscle activation during the gait cycle that works proximally to distally. The FHL and FDL muscles reach their peak activation 3% to 11% later in the gait cycle than the gastrocnemius and soleus muscles and 25% earlier than the ankle dorsiflexor muscles in normal linear gait.

2.3. Functional Unit

The functional unit to which a muscle belongs includes the muscles that reinforce and counter its actions as well as the joints that the muscle crosses. The interdependence of these structures is functionally reflected in the organization and neural connections of the sensory motor cortex. The functional unit is emphasized because the presence of a TrP in one muscle of the unit increases the likelihood that the other muscles of the unit will also develop TrPs. When inactivating TrPs in a muscle, one must be concerned about TrPs that may develop in muscles that are functionally interdependent. Box 69-1 grossly represents the functional unit of the FHL and FDL muscles.[15]

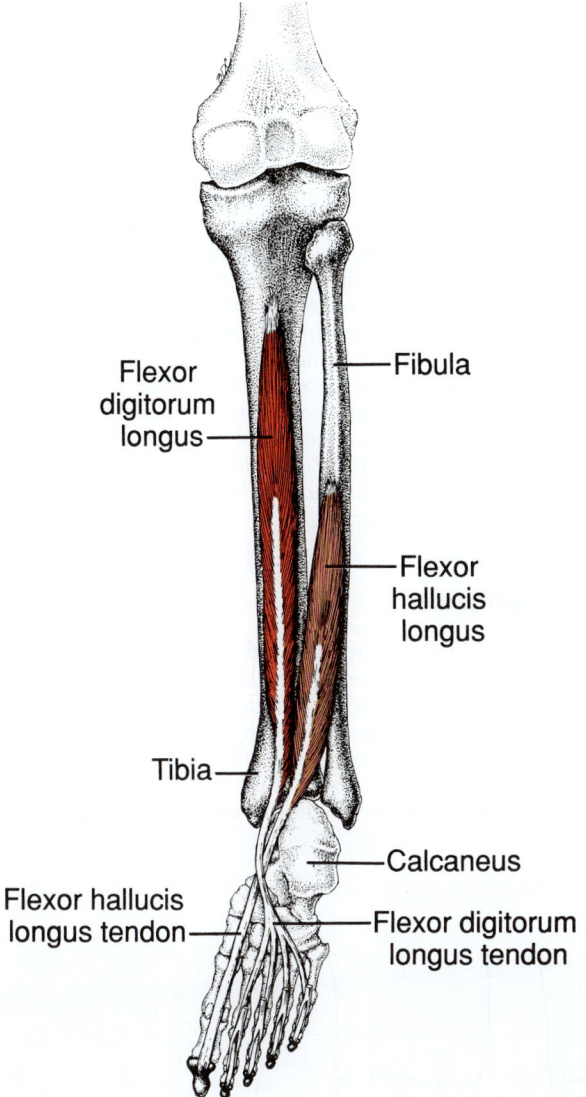

Figure 69-1. The FDL muscle (dark red) originates proximally just below the soleal lone of the posterior tibia and travels distally posterior to the medial malleolus and through the flexor retinaculum into the sole of the foot where it divides into four tendons, each attaching to the distal phalanges of digits 2 to 5. The FHL muscle (light red) attaches proximally to the interosseous membrane and the intermuscular septa and extends distally passing between the medial and lateral sesamoid bones to insert into the distal phalanx of the great toe.

through the various aponeuroses, sheaths, and epimysium surrounding and enveloping the muscle fibers and the associated neurovascular structures. Connective tissue is continuous from the skin and superficial fascia (sub cutis) to the deep fascia (profundus), providing a continuity that allows the expression of muscle fibers (ie, force production) to have a direct effect locally and at some distance. The translation of muscular forces into mechanical expression (such as movement) and physiologic activity (such as cellular metabolism) occurs by means of force transmission.[9]

2.1. Innervation and Vascularization

The tibial nerve, with specific spinal nerve contribution, innervates all the superficial and deep muscles of the posterior compartment of the leg. The FDL muscle receives innervation from the level L5 and S1 spinal nerves, and the FHL muscle

Box 69-1 Functional unit of the flexor hallucis longus and flexor digitorum longus muscles		
Action	Synergists	Antagonists
Plantar flexion	Gastrocnemius Soleus Tibialis posterior Fibularis longus	Tibialis anterior Extensor digitorum longus Extensor hallucis longus Fibularis tertius
Subtalar inversion	Tibialis anterior Tibialis posterior	Fibularis longus Fibularis brevis Fibularis tertius
1st toe flexion	Flexor hallucis brevis	Extensor hallucis longus Extensor hallucis brevis
2nd-5th toe flexion	Flexor digitorum brevis Flexor digiti minimi brevis Interossei Flexor accessorius (Quadratus plantae)	Extensor digitorum longus Extensor digitorum brevis Lumbricals Interossei

3. CLINICAL PRESENTATION

3.1. Referred Pain Pattern

Typically, with FDL and FHL TrPs, patients will report pain in the foot and ankle, including the great toe. Pain and other sensations are reported on the sole of the foot as well as the plantar surfaces of the smaller digits and great toe. Trigger points in the FDL muscle refer pain and tenderness primarily to the middle of the plantar forefoot, proximal to the four lesser toes and, sometimes, with spreading to the toes (Figure 69-2). Occasionally, these TrPs refer pain to the medial side of the ankle and calf; however, they do not refer pain to the heel. Thus, when patients report that the sole of the forefoot is painful and tender, clinicians must consider the calf as a source of the patient's symptoms. Trigger points in the FHL muscle refer pain intensely to the plantar surface of the great toe and the head of the 1st metatarsal (Figure 69-2). Pain may occasionally radiate proximally for a short distance on the plantar surface but does not extend to the heel or leg.

3.2. Symptoms

Patients with TrPs in the FDL and/or FHL muscles typically report that their feet hurt when they walk. A chief report is pain that occurs in the sole of the forefoot and on the plantar surfaces of the toes especially with weight-bearing activities. Although pain in the foot may result from a problem within the foot itself, this is not always the case. Extrinsic and intrinsic foot muscles can be painful as a direct or indirect result from

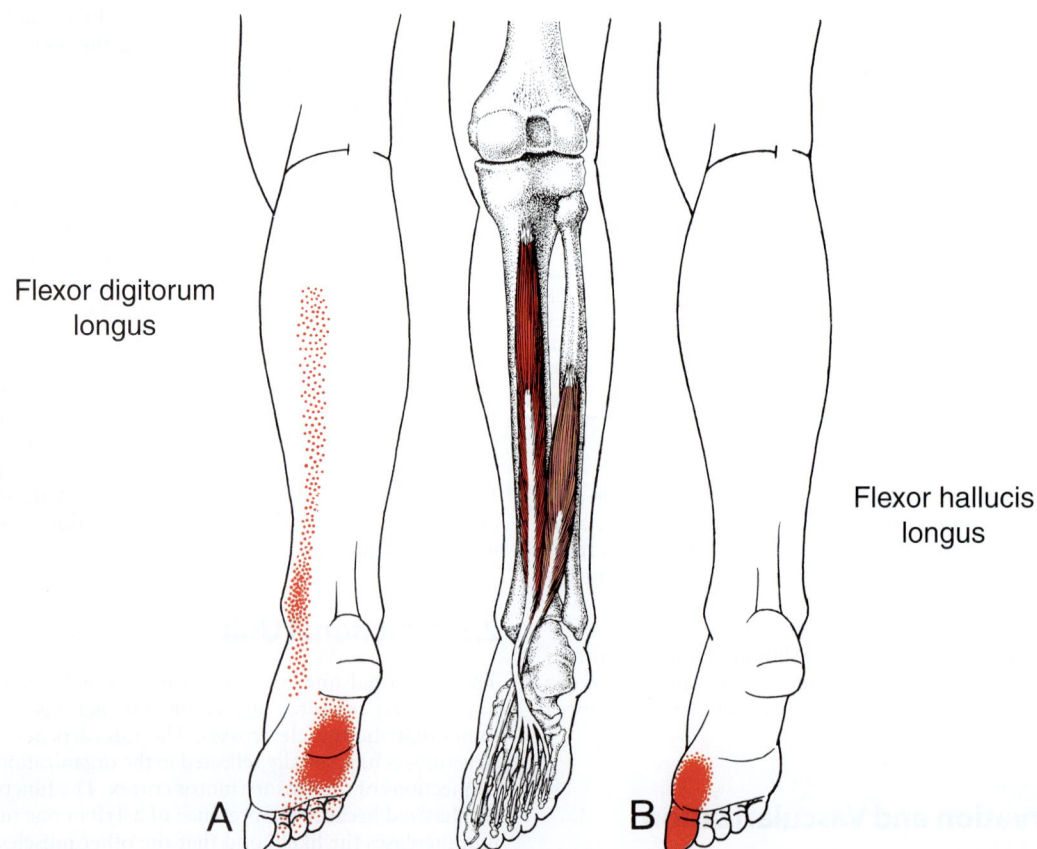

Figure 69-2. Referred pain pattern of TrPs. A, Flexor digitorum longus muscle (dark red). B, Flexor hallucis longus muscle (light red).

insults to neural, fascial, visceral, or other tissues. Symptoms of pain or other sensations in the feet can be a direct result of pelvic organ dysfunction or low back pathology. Pathology other than TrPs should always be ruled out. Custom inserts (orthoses) to reduce stress on the foot are useful in managing foot pain. Patients may also report a feeling of cramping in the toes or calf. Trigger points in the long extrinsic toe flexors may occasionally cause painful contraction of these muscles similar to the calf cramps of gastrocnemius TrPs. However, toe flexor "cramping" is more likely to be caused by TrPs of the intrinsic flexors of the toes.

3.3. Patient Examination

After a thorough subjective examination, the clinician should make a detailed drawing representing the pain pattern that the patient has described. This depiction will assist in planning the physical examination and can be useful in monitoring the progression of the patient as symptoms improve or change. The type, quality, and location of the pain should be carefully assessed, and the utilization of standardized outcome tools is imperative when examining patients with lower extremity dysfunctions.

Observation of static and dynamic posture is essential given the role of the FDL and FHL muscles in postural stability and gait. The toes should be examined for any abnormalities such as claw toe, hammer toe, and hallux valgus. These abnormalities should be assessed to determine if they are flexible or rigid and then addressed appropriately. The presence of deviations, such as ankle equinus, pes planus, or pes cavus, should be noted. The patient should be observed walking barefoot, with the clinician noting any relevant gait deviations such as early excessive pronation, excessive pronation at mid-stance (pes planus), or late pronation during push-off. Excessive flexion of the toes during the stance and push-off phases of gait may indicate joint hypomobility of the foot and ankle as well as muscle imbalances. At heel-off, the FDL, FHL, and tibialis posterior muscles contract to supinate the hindfoot and midfoot, creating a rigid lever for propulsion. If the calcaneus does not move into inversion at heel-off, tibialis posterior and/or FDL muscle weakness may be indicated.

A collapse of the medial longitudinal arch, or a midfoot posture with forefoot abduction, is commonly observed with tibialis posterior muscle dysfunction as discussed in Chapter 67. This deviation may lead to excessive overload and abnormal tensile loading of the extensor digitorum longus and extensor hallucis longus muscles. Measures such as the navicular drop test[16] and the windlass mechanism[17] should be assessed in standing as a predictor of dynamic function of the foot. Functional testing such as double- and single-leg squat will allow a quick assessment of hip and knee control, as well as a quick assessment of talocrural, subtalar, and midfoot range of motion. Timed single-leg stance with eyes open and closed will give a quantitative measure of balance and will allow the clinician to observe foot and ankle strategies related to balance and control.

The patient's feet should be examined for muscular imbalances, and passive physiologic and accessory motion should be tested in the talocrural, subtalar, midtarsal, and forefoot joints. Assessment for great toe and first ray range of motion in dorsiflexion is vital, because limitation in this motion may cause abnormal pronation of the foot during the propulsive phases of gait, placing an abnormal tensile load on the FDL and FHL muscles.

Examination should include the distal phalanges of all toes for flexion weakness, as described by Kendall and McCreary.[18] Weakness of the FDL and FHL muscles affects flexion of the distal phalanx of the lesser toes, whereas weakness of the flexor digitorum brevis muscle affects flexion of the middle phalanx in the lesser toes. Maximum flexion effort of the great toe or four lesser toes with the foot in the plantar flexed position is likely to be particularly painful for the patient with TrPs in the corresponding flexor muscle. Passive extension range of motion of the great toe is restricted with FHL muscle involvement,[19] and passive extension of the four lesser toes is restricted when the FDL muscle has TrPs.

The patient's shoe may show a wear pattern characteristic of an abnormal foot structure or evidence of excessive wear. Indications of excessive wear are as follows: asymmetry between the two shoes, cracks between the midsole and edge of the shoe, a definite lean of the shoe either inward or outward when set on a level surface, loss of the sole pattern in sports shoes, and a flattened or expanded heel pattern of the shoe.

3.4. Trigger Point Examination

Trigger points can form at any point along the length of the FDL and FHL muscles.

Palpation for TrPs in the FDL and FHL muscles is achieved by placing the patient in a prone or side-lying position, with the leg to be treated supported appropriately. For palpation of TrPs in the FDL muscle, the patient lies on the involved side and the clinician uses cross-fiber flat palpation to exert pressure between the tibia and the soleus/gastrocnemius muscles on the medial side of the leg (Figure 69-3A).

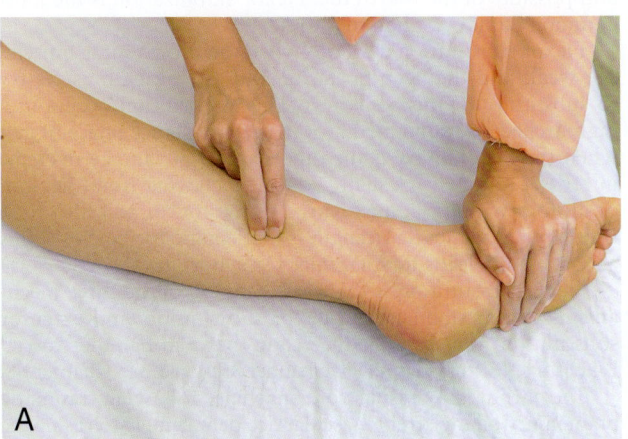 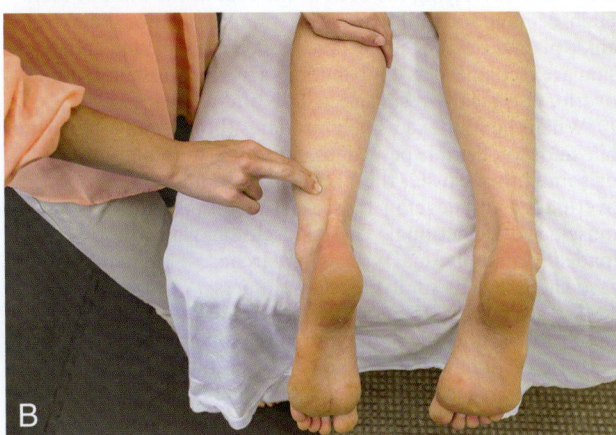

Figure 69-3. Cross-fiber flat palpation for TrPs. A, Flexor digitorum longus muscle. B, Flexor hallucis longus muscle.

An alternate method is performed with the knee flexed to 90° and the foot plantar flexed so that the gastrocnemius muscle can be pressed posteriorly away from the tibia to expose the FDL muscle for more effective palpation. The clinician first exerts pressure toward the back of the tibia and then laterally against the FDL muscle belly with a cross-fiber flat palpation technique.

For examination of TrPs in the FHL muscle, the patient lies prone and the clinician uses cross-fiber flat palpation, applying deep pressure at the junction of the middle and lower thirds of the calf, just lateral to the midline, against the posterior aspect of the fibula (Figure 69-3B). The pressure of palpation must be projected through the soleus muscle, as well as through the thick aponeuroses that becomes the achilles tendon. Tenderness can be attributed to the FHL muscle only if the clinician is sure that the overlying muscles are free of TrPs.

For clinicians with appropriate training, safe use of a solid filiform or injection needle, from the lateral or medial aspect of the muscles, makes these structures more easily accessible and identifiable through reproduction of their referred pain patterns.

4. DIFFERENTIAL DIAGNOSIS

4.1. Activation and Perpetuation of Trigger Points

A posture or activity that activates a TrP, if not corrected, can also perpetuate it. In any part of the FHL or FDL muscles, TrPs may be activated by unaccustomed eccentric loading, eccentric exercise in an unconditioned muscle, or maximal or submaximal concentric loading.[20] Trigger points may also be activated or aggravated when the muscle is placed in a shortened and/or lengthened position for an extended period of time. FDL and FHL TrPs are activated by overload during weight-bearing activities. When initiating a walking or running exercise program, individuals should gradually ease into the exercise routine. Excessive frequency, intensity, and/or duration in the early stages of a weight-bearing exercise program may result in overload and, consequently, TrP development in the untrained FDL and FHL muscles. Acute overload, such as running a half marathon without proper training, can also lead to TrP development. Additionally, TrPs can be activated, and are then perpetuated, by running or jogging on uneven ground or on laterally slanted or cantilevered surfaces. Clinically, common ballet foot postures such as relevé, during which the individual maintains extreme angles of ankle plantar flexion, require excessive isometric contractions of the FDL and FHL muscles, and these can lead to muscle overload and TrP development.

Therapeutic success involves controlling perpetuating factors such as poorly fitted orthotics that can lead to irritation of soft tissues overlying the arch of the foot at the knot of Henry. High-demand forceful repetitive actions in positions of extreme ankle plantar flexion and metatarsophalangeal flexion and extension are recognized as contributing factors in musculotendinous overload, typically resulting in TrPs and tendinosis.

When the foot excessively pronates (because of a hypermobile midfoot, flexible pes valgus deformity, muscular imbalance, or some other cause), the FDL and FHL muscles can become overloaded and develop TrPs, especially if the tibialis posterior muscle is dysfunctional. These muscles may also become overloaded in an individual with a high-arched, supinated foot with associated triceps surae muscle weakness.

Trigger points are more often than not the result of a functional adaptation due to impairment in joint mobility or muscle performance. Impaired mobility of the joints of the foot can perpetuate TrPs in these muscles. A common mistake committed by joggers and runners is to continue using a shoe after it has developed excessive wear on the sole and heel. Loss of cushioning and flexibility produces excessive strain on the joints and muscles, including the long flexor muscles of the toes. Walking and running on soft sand, especially barefoot, heavily loads the FDL muscle and can perpetuate, or activate, TrPs in this muscle.

4.2. Associated Trigger Points

Associated TrPs can develop in the referred pain areas caused by TrPs.[21] Therefore, musculature in the referred pain areas for each muscle should also be considered. The muscles most likely to have associated TrPs, when one finds them in the long toe flexors, are muscles of the functional unit including the tibialis posterior, extensor hallucis longus and brevis, and extensor digitorum brevis muscles. The short (intrinsic) toe flexors, the flexor hallucis, and digitorum brevis muscles may also develop associated TrPs as part of the functional unit and because they are in the referred pain area of the muscles. Additionally, the adductor hallucis and flexor accessories (quadratus plantae) muscles can develop TrPs because the muscles are located in the referred pain area of the FHL and FDL muscles.

4.3. Associated Pathology

Injury and insult can occur along the entire FHL tendon. A common source of insult is repetitive, high-demand forces exceeding physiologic parameters resulting in tendinopathy or stenosing tenosynovitis. Hallux trigger or claw toe is a common sign of stenosing tenosynovitis of the FHL tendon. Tendon adhesions with accompanied nodules develop within the tendon sheath, thus reducing the ability of tendon gliding. Tendinopathy, a less-associated inflammatory condition in the leg, can involve partial tears of the deeper internal tissues leading to mucinoid degradation and nodule development.[22]

Spontaneous rupture of the FHL tendon can occur during overload without evidence of previous disease or injury.[23] Even though surgical repair does not always restore function of the great toe, the authors concluded that, in cases of laceration or rupture, surgical repair seems justified.[23]

Classic hammer toe, mallet toe, and claw toe deformities are presented in Section 4.3 in Chapter 68. Flexor stabilization most commonly occurs when the long flexor muscles of the toes attempt to stabilize the osseous structures of the foot in the presence of a flexible pes planus (flat foot) deformity. Pronation of the subtalar joint allows hypermobility and unlocking of the midtarsal joint, which, in turn, leads to hypermobility of the forefoot.[24] The long toe flexor muscles then act earlier and longer than in normal gait.[25] Instead of stabilizing the forefoot, this abnormal activity usually overpowers the smaller intrinsic lumbrical and interossous muscles, as well as the flexor accessories (quadratus plantae) muscle. Loss of flexor accessories (quadratus plantae) muscle function allows adductovarus deviation of the fifth toe and possibly of the fourth toe. Flexor stabilization is the most common etiology of hammer toes.[24,26]

Flexor substitution develops when the triceps surae muscles are weak and the deep posterior and lateral leg muscles try to substitute for this weakness. This substitution occurs in a high-arched and supinated foot in the late-stance phase of gait when the flexors have gained mechanical advantage over the interossei muscles; it usually produces clawing (total flexion) of all toes without adductovarus of the fourth and fifth toes. If triceps surae muscle strength is inadequate for push-off, this action readily leads to a hammer toe syndrome.[26]

Flexor substitution is the least common of the three mechanisms (flexor stabilization, flexor substitution, and extensor substitution) that can produce claw toes and hammer toes.[24] Extensor substitution is reviewed under Section 4.3 in Chapter 68.

Toe curling may result from spasticity following traumatic brain injury or any cerebrovascular accident. Simply releasing the FHL and FDL tendons provided satisfactory relief in only about one-fourth of 41 feet. Additional release of the flexor digitorum brevis tendon often achieved a more functional result.[27] Kwon

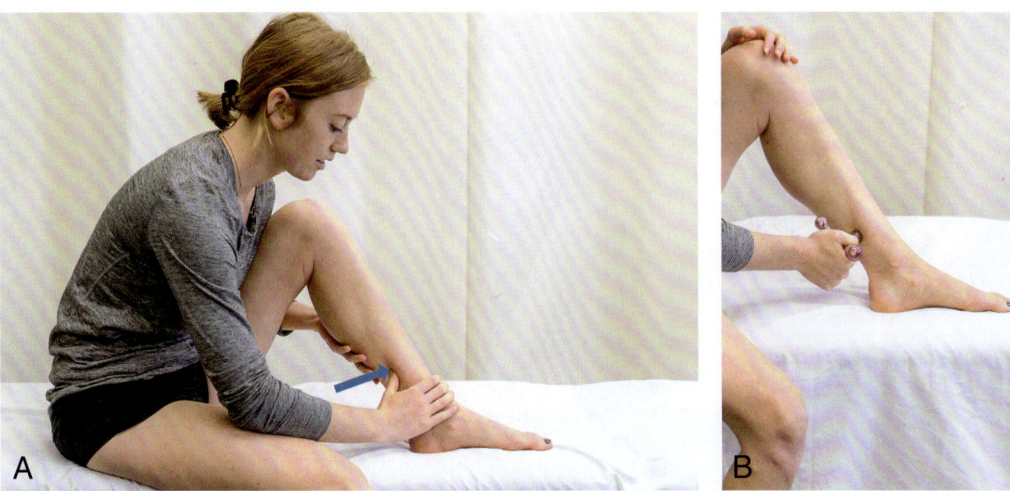

Figure 69-4. Self-pressure release of TrPs in the flexor digitorum longus muscle. A, Manual release with thumb. B, TrP release tool.

and DeAsla[26] describe a technique utilizing a flexor to extensor transfer for correction of a flexible hammer toe deformity.[26]

Hallux valgus is more commonly known as a "bunion" and is the most common forefoot deformity, affecting women more than men. The cause of hallux valgus is thought to be attributed to ill-fitting shoes, genetic predisposition, pronated feet, and asymmetry of the bones and joints of the feet.[28] Bunions are typically caused by an imbalance between both extrinsic and intrinsic muscles of the great toe and forefoot and ligamentous structures in the great toe and forefoot.[29] There may be subluxation of the 1st metatarsophalangeal joint with an associated medial deviation of the proximal and distal phalanx of the great toe leading to arthritic changes in the joint.[30] This angulation can change the angle of pull on the FHL muscle and overload it, leading to the formation of TrPs, thus increasing pain in the region of the great toe.

Bouché and Johnson[31] suggest that medial tibial stress syndrome is due to a "tenting" of the tibial fascia resulting from eccentric contraction of the deep leg flexor muscles including the gastrocnemius, soleus, tibialis posterior, FDL, and FHL muscles. In a pilot study using cadaveric specimens, these researchers demonstrated a linear increase in tension applied to the tibialis posterior, FDL, and soleus tendons and strain on the tibial fascia. Because the tibial fascia inserts directly into the medial tibial crest, the repetitive eccentric contractions of these muscles to prevent excessive pronation at the midtarsal and subtalar joints during the stance phase of gait may cause the medial tibial stress syndrome pathology. A follow-up study by Brown[32] found that in all of the studied 22 cadaveric legs, the FDL muscle was attached to the middle third of the posterior tibia, and in all but one specimen, the soleus muscle attached to the middle third of the posterior tibia, the common site of pain in medial tibial stress syndrome (MTSS).

Garth and Miller[33] examined 17 athletes who presented for treatment of incapacitating pain and soreness located posteromedially along the middle third of the tibia (over the attachment and belly of the FDL muscle). Symptoms were provoked and aggravated by repetitive weight bearing. Similar symptoms may be diagnosed as shin splints, MTSS,[33] and chronic exertional compartment syndrome.[34] Seventeen asymptomatic athletes served as controls. The symptomatic athletes consistently demonstrated a mild claw toe deformity of the second toe, with abnormal displacement of its arc of motion toward extension of the metatarsophalangeal joint, as well as weakness of the lumbrical muscles. It appears as if the relatively stronger FDL muscle became overloaded because of inadequate metatarsophalangeal joint stabilization due to lumbrical muscle weakness that resulted in clawing of the lesser toes rather than in effective stabilization. Symptoms were relieved by a treatment regimen consisting of toe flexion exercises, reduced athletic activity, and metatarsal and arch pads to compensate for the weak lumbrical muscle action.[33]

Exertional compartment syndromes of the leg are a common form of overuse injury. Compartment syndromes are characterized by increased pressure within a muscular compartment sufficient to compromise the circulation of the muscles within it. The increased pressure obstructs venous outflow, which causes further swelling and more pressure. If prolonged, the resultant ischemia can lead to necrosis of the muscles and nerves within the compartment. When following a traumatic injury, it is vitally important that this condition be recognized immediately and managed properly to avoid possibly catastrophic consequences. Anterior compartment syndromes are recognized more commonly, followed by lateral, deep posterior, and superficial posterior compartment syndromes.[35,36] Deep posterior chronic exertional compartment syndrome is discussed in Section 4.3 of Chapter 67.

5. CORRECTIVE ACTIONS

Individuals with TrPs in the FDL or FHL muscles may benefit from adopting sitting or standing postures that place the ankle in some degree of plantar flexion. While seated, an individual

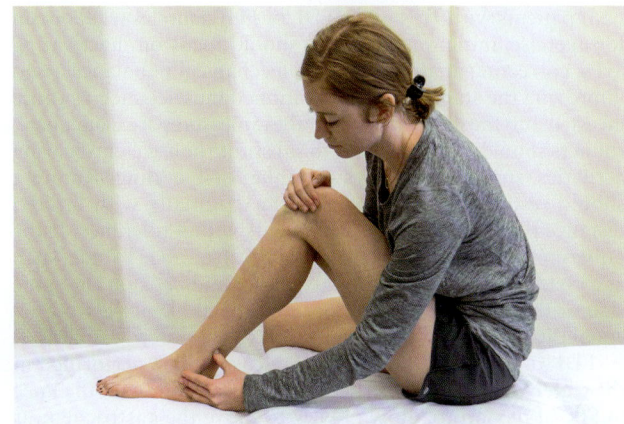

Figure 69-5. Self-pressure release of TrPs in the flexor hallucis longus muscle.

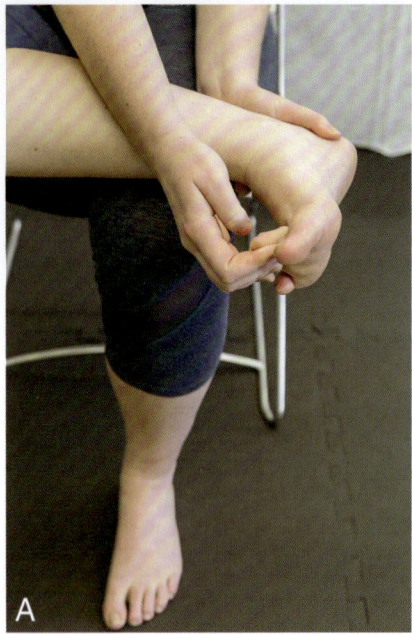 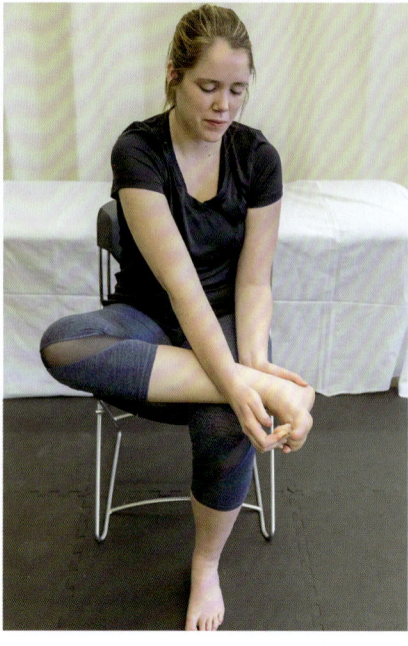 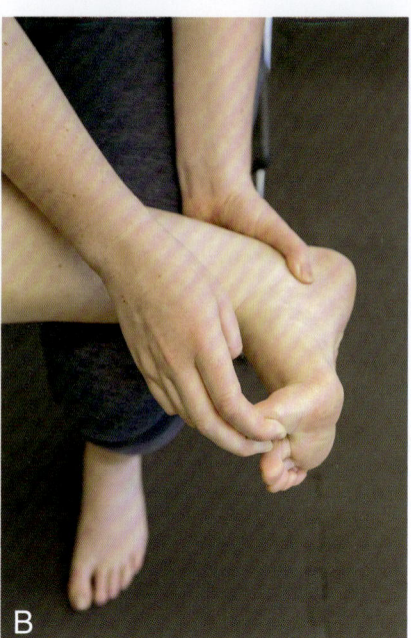

Figure 69-6. Self-stretch. A, Flexor digitorum longus muscle. B, Flexor hallucis longus muscle.

can sit with the knees in 50° or 60° of flexion, allowing the foot to contact the floor for lower extremity support, while providing ankle plantar flexion to place more slack on the long toe flexor muscles.

In general, the leg muscles feel better if the ankle is maintained in a neutral position throughout the night; therefore, adjusting the patient's sleeping posture may be necessary. This position is facilitated by having the bed sheets at the foot of the bed untucked to reduce external force into excessive plantar flexion (see Figure 65-6). Using a pillow between the legs and knees in side-lying to place the foot and ankle in a neutral position may also be beneficial.

Individuals with TrPs in the FDL and/or FHL muscles should wear comfortable shoes that have adequate shock absorption and flexibility of the sole, especially under the ball of the foot. New shoes should be tested at the time of purchase to ensure they have enough space in the toe box to allow for an insert, as needed. Worn-out shoes and those with poor flexibility of the distal sole must be replaced. An extremely stiff sole that prevents extension of the metatarsophalangeal joint of the great toe should be avoided. Also, high heels and stiletto heels should be avoided completely (see Chapter 77).

If patients with TrPs in the FDL or FHL muscles walk or run for exercise, initial management should focus on inactivating TrPs, correcting anatomic and biomechanical imbalances, and improving the stamina of deconditioned muscles such as those invested into the iliotibial band. If these measures are inadequate, runners should be encouraged to substitute non-weight-bearing activities, such as rowing, swimming, or bicycling. Running should resume on a flat, even surface, initially with limited distance that progresses by increments within tolerance. If the only running surface available is slanted from side to side, such as a road, the individual should run out and back on the same side of the road so that the foot and the ankle are getting an equal distribution of extrinsic forces.

FDL or FHL TrP self-pressure release can be performed in the seated position on the edge of the bed or floor with the knee in 90° of flexion to allow gravity to move the gastrocnemius and soleus muscles out of the way. Manual TrP self-pressure release of the FDL muscle can be performed with the thumb on the undersurface of the tibia (Figure 69-4). Finding the most tender spot along the posterior surface of the tibia, light pressure (no more than 4/10 pain) should be gently applied below the muscle bulk of the gastrocnemius muscle (Figure 69-4A). A TrP self-release tool should be used with caution because of the proximity of the bone (Figure 69-4B). For self-pressure release of the FHL muscle, pressure is applied on the undersurface of the outer part of the leg, over the fibula (Figure 69-5). Finding the sensitive spot with the thumb, light pressure (no more than 4/10 pain) should be applied and held for 15 to 30 seconds or until pain reduces. These techniques may be repeated five times, several times per day. Also, patients may perform self-massage along the length of the involved soft tissues to enhance soft-tissue mobility.

In cases where the long toe flexor muscles are adaptively shortened, self-stretching exercises may be helpful. One way to stretch the FDL (Figure 69-6A) and FHL muscles (Figure 69-6B) is in a seated position with the involved leg crossed over the opposite thigh. In this position, one hand can passively move the toes into extension, and with distal extension sustained, gradually move the ankle toward dorsiflexion, until a stretch on the back of the foot/ankle is felt. The opposite hand can be used to stabilize the distal tibiofibular joint complex as needed. The stretch is held for up to 30 seconds and repeated four times.

References

1. Standring S. *Gray's Anatomy: The Anatomical Basis of Clinical Practice.* 41st ed. London, UK: Elsevier; 2015.
2. Ward SR, Eng CM, Smallwood LH, Lieber RL. Are current measurements of lower extremity muscle architecture accurate? *Clin Orthop Relat Res.* 2009;467(4):1074-1082.
3. Bardeen C. Section 5, The musculature. In: Jackson CM, ed. *Morris's Human Anatomy.* 6th ed. Philadelphia, PA: Blakiston's Son & Co; 1921 (pp. 521-523).
4. Hollinshead WH. *Anatomy for Surgeons.* Vol 3. 3rd ed. New York, NY: Harper & Row; 1982 (p. 783).
5. Sammarco GJ, Stephens MM. Tarsal tunnel syndrome caused by the flexor digitorum accessorius longus. A case report. *J Bone Joint Surg Am Vol.* 1990;72(3):453-454.
6. Wood J. On some varieties in human myology. *Proc Roy Soc Lond.* 1864;13:299-303.
7. Friederich JA, Brand RA. Muscle fiber architecture in the human lower limb. *J Biomech.* 1990;23(1):91-95.
8. Kura H, Luo ZP, Kitaoka HB, An KN. Quantitative analysis of the intrinsic muscles of the foot. *Anat Rec.* 1997;249(1):143-151.
9. Langevin HM. Connective tissue: a body-wide signaling network? *Med Hypotheses.* 2006;66(6):1074-1077.

10. Hofmann CL, Okita N, Sharkey NA. Experimental evidence supporting isometric functioning of the extrinsic toe flexors during gait. *Clin Biomech (Bristol, Avon)*. 2013;28(6):686-691.
11. Peter A, Hegyi A, Finni T, Cronin NJ. In vivo fascicle behavior of the flexor hallucis longus muscle at different walking speeds. *Scand J Med Sci Sports*. 2017;27(12):1716-1723.
12. Peter A, Hegyi A, Stenroth L, Finni T, Cronin NJ. EMG and force production of the flexor hallucis longus muscle in isometric plantarflexion and the push-off phase of walking. *J Biomech*. 2015;48(12):3413-3419.
13. Akuzawa H, Imai A, Iizuka S, Matsunaga N, Kaneoka K. Calf muscle activity alteration with foot orthoses insertion during walking measured by fine-wire electromyography. *J Phys Ther Sci*. 2016;28(12):3458-3462.
14. Zelik KE, La Scaleia V, Ivanenko YP, Lacquaniti F. Coordination of intrinsic and extrinsic foot muscles during walking. *Eur J Appl Physiol*. 2015;115(4):691-701.
15. Simons DG, Travell J, Simons L. *Travell & Simon's Myofascial Pain and Dysfunction: The Trigger Point Manual*. Vol 1. 2nd ed. Baltimore, MD: Williams & Wilkins; 1999 (p. 104).
16. Reinking MF, Austin TM, Richter RR, Krieger MM. Medial tibial stress syndrome in active individuals: a systematic review and meta-analysis of risk factors. *Sports Health*. 2017;9(3):252-261.
17. Aquino A, Payne C. Function of the windlass mechanism in excessively pronated feet. *J Am Podiatr Med Assoc*. 2001;91(5):245-250.
18. Kendall FP, McCreary EK. *Muscles: Testing and Function, with Posture and Pain*. 5th ed. Baltimore, MD: Lippincott Williams & Wilkins; 2005.
19. Macdonald AJ. Abnormally tender muscle regions and associated painful movements. *Pain*. 1980;8(2):197-205.
20. Gerwin RD, Dommerholt J, Shah JP. An expansion of Simons' integrated hypothesis of trigger point formation. *Curr Pain Headache Rep*. 2004;8(6):468-475.
21. Hsieh YL, Kao MJ, Kuan TS, Chen SM, Chen JT, Hong CZ. Dry needling to a key myofascial trigger point may reduce the irritability of satellite MTrPs. *Am J Phys Med Rehabil*. 2007;86(5):397-403.
22. Hur MS, Kim JH, Gil YC, Kim HJ, Lee KS. New insights into the origin of the lumbrical muscles of the foot: tendinous slip of the flexor hallucis longus muscle. *Surg Radiol Anat*. 2015;37(10):1161-1167.
23. Rasmussen RB, Thyssen EP. Rupture of the flexor hallucis longus tendon: case report. *Foot Ankle*. 1990;10(5):288-289.
24. Jimenez AL, McGlamry ED, Green DR. Chapter 3, Lesser ray deformities. In: McGlamry ED, ed. *Comprehensive Textbook of Foot Surgery*. Vol 1. Baltimore, MD: Williams & Wilkins; 1987:57-113 (pp. 66-68).
25. Gray EG, Basmajian JV. Electromyography and cinematography of leg and foot ("normal" and flat) during walking. *Anat Rec*. 1968;161(1):1-15.
26. Kwon JY, De Asla RJ. The use of flexor to extensor transfers for the correction of the flexible hammer toe deformity. *Foot Ankle Clin*. 2011;16(4):573-582.
27. Keenan MA, Gorai AP, Smith CW, Garland DE. Intrinsic toe flexion deformity following correction of spastic equinovarus deformity in adults. *Foot Ankle*. 1987;7(6):333-337.
28. Neumann DA. *Kinesiology of the Musculoskeletal System: Foundations for Rehabilitation*. 2nd ed. St. Louis, MO: Mosby; 2010.
29. Nguyen US, Hillstrom HJ, Li W, et al. Factors associated with hallux valgus in a population-based study of older women and men: the MOBILIZE Boston Study. *Osteoarthritis Cartilage*. 2010;18(1):41-46.
30. Singh SK, Jayasekera N, Nazir S, Sharif K, Kashif F. Use of a simple suture to stabilize the chevron osteotomy: a prospective study. *J Foot Ankle Surg*. 2004;43(5):307-311.
31. Bouché RT, Johnson CH. Medial tibial stress syndrome (tibial fasciitis): a proposed pathomechanical model involving fascial traction. *J Am Podiatr Med Assoc*. 2007;97(1):31-36.
32. Brown AA. Medial tibial stress syndrome: muscles located at the site of pain. *Scientifica (Cairo)*. 2016;2016:7097489.
33. Garth WP Jr, Miller ST. Evaluation of claw toe deformity, weakness of the foot intrinsics, and posteromedial shin pain. *Am J Sports Med*. 1989;17(6):821-827.
34. Wiley JP, Clement DB, Doyle DL, Taunton JE. A primary care perspective of chronic compartment syndrome of the leg. *Phys Sportsmed*. 1987;15:111-120.
35. Rajasekaran S, Hall MM. Nonoperative management of chronic exertional compartment syndrome: a systematic review. *Curr Sports Med Rep*. 2016;15(3):191-198.
36. Campano D, Robaina JA, Kusnezov N, Dunn JC, Waterman BR. Surgical management for chronic exertional compartment syndrome of the leg: a systematic review of the literature. *Arthroscopy*. 2016;32(7):1478-1486.

Chapter 70

Intrinsic Muscles of the Foot
"Sore Foot Muscles and Viper's Nest"

Jeffrey Gervais Ebert

1. INTRODUCTION

There are approximately 20 relatively small muscles that make up the intrinsic muscles of the foot, depending on anatomic variations and classifications. Although each muscle has its own particular action, many of the intrinsic foot muscles work collectively to help support and stabilize the foot, especially during gait. Trigger points (TrPs) in these muscles often result in plantar foot pain. Activation and perpetuation of TrPs in the intrinsic foot muscles often result from an acute overload due to walking or running over soft or uneven terrain, from ill-fitting footwear, or from structural issues within the foot. Differential diagnosis should include assessment for plantar heel pain due to plantar fasciitis or entrapment of the lateral plantar nerve, structural issues including navicular drop or hallux valgus, and metatarsalgia. Corrective actions should include education regarding proper sleeping position, elimination of positions and activities that cause recurrent overload of the muscle, TrP self-pressure release, self-stretch exercises, and strengthening exercises.

2. ANATOMIC CONSIDERATIONS

The intrinsic muscles of the foot include flexors, located on the plantar aspect of the foot, and extensors, located on the dorsum of the foot. The plantar muscles are customarily divided into four groups or layers, from superficial to deep. The first, and most superficial, layer consists of the abductor hallucis, abductor digit minimi, and flexor digitorum brevis muscles. The second layer includes the flexor accessorius (quadratus plantae) muscle and the four lumbrical muscles. The third layer contains the flexor hallucis brevis, adductor hallucis, and flexor digiti minimi brevis muscles. The fourth, and deepest, layer consists of the plantar and dorsal interosseous muscles. The dorsally located extensor muscles include the extensor digitorum brevis and extensor hallucis brevis muscles.[1]

Plantar Muscles

First Layer

The abductor hallucis muscle originates primarily from the flexor retinaculum but also from the medial aspect of the calcaneal tuberosity and the plantar aponeurosis. It inserts, along with the medial tendon of the flexor hallucis brevis muscle, onto the medial aspect of the base of the proximal phalanx of the great toe (Figure 70-1B). In some instances, fibers are attached to the medial sesamoid bone of the great toe.[1]

The flexor digitorum brevis muscle originates via a narrow tendon from the medial aspect of the calcaneal tuberosity and from the central part of the plantar aponeurosis. It divides into four tendons, each of which enters tendinous sheaths along with the tendons of the flexor digitorum longus muscle, which lie deep to them. They ultimately insert onto the shafts of the middle phalanges of the 2nd through 5th digits (Figure 70-1B).[1]

The abductor digiti minimi muscle originates from both processes of the calcaneal tuberosity and from the plantar aponeurosis. Its tendon lies in a groove on the plantar surface of the base of the 5th metatarsal and inserts, along with the flexor digiti minimi brevis muscle, onto the lateral side of the base of the proximal phalanx of the fifth toe (Figure 70-1B).[1]

Second Layer

The flexor accessorius (quadratus plantae) muscle consists of two heads, with the long plantar ligament located deeply between them. The larger medial head originates from the medial surface of the calcaneus. The flat and tendinous lateral head originates from the calcaneus distal to the lateral process of the tuberosity and from the long plantar ligament. The muscle inserts into the flexor digitorum longus tendon at the point where it divides into its four tendons (Figure 70-2A). In some instances, this muscle may be absent.[1]

The lumbrical muscles (numbered beginning at the medial side of the foot) are four small muscles that arise from the terminal flexor digitorum longus tendons. Their tendons pass distally on the medial sides of the lateral four toes and insert into the dorsal digital expansions on the proximal phalanges (Figure 70-2A).[1]

Third Layer

The flexor hallucis brevis muscle originates from two locations. A lateral branch of its tendon originates from the medial aspect of the plantar surface of the cuboid and from the adjacent part of the lateral cuneiform. The medial tendon branch has an attachment that is continuous with the lateral division of the tendon of the tibialis posterior muscle. The muscle belly itself also divides into medial and lateral parts, the tendons of which are attached to the sides of the base of the proximal phalanx of the great toe. The medial attachment blends with the tendon of the abductor hallucis muscle and the lateral attachment with that of the adductor hallucis muscle (Figure 70-2B).[1]

The adductor hallucis muscle consists of two heads: oblique and transverse. The oblique head originates from the bases of the 2nd, 3rd, and 4th metatarsals and from the sheath of the tendon of the fibularis longus muscle. The transverse head originates from the plantar metatarsophalangeal ligaments of the third, fourth, and fifth toes and from the deep transverse metatarsal ligaments between them. The oblique head is further divided into medial and lateral portions. The medial portion blends with the lateral part of the flexor hallucis brevis muscle and is attached to the lateral sesamoid bone of the great toe. The lateral part attaches to the transverse head, the base of the proximal phalanx of the great toe, and to the lateral sesamoid bone of the great toe[2] (Figure 70-2B). The oblique head is significantly larger than the transverse head,[3] and the transverse portion of the adductor hallucis muscle is sometimes absent.[4]

The flexor digiti minimi brevis muscle originates from the medial aspect of the plantar surface of the base of the 5th

Chapter 70: Intrinsic Muscles of the Foot 735

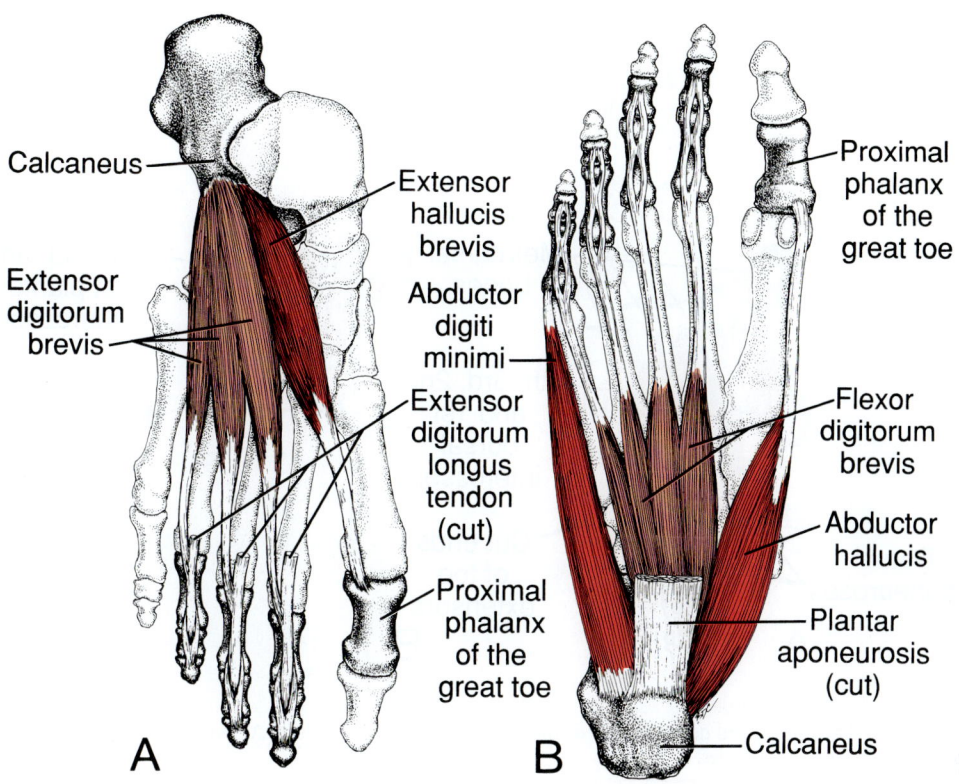

Figure 70-1. A, The dorsal intrinsic muscles of the foot. B, The first, and most superficial, layer of the plantar intrinsic muscles of the foot.

metatarsal and from the tendon sheath of the fibularis longus muscle. It inserts onto the lateral aspect of the base of the proximal phalanx of the fifth toe (Figure 70-2B). Periodically, some of its deeper fibers extend to the lateral part of the distal half of the 5th metatarsal, forming what is sometimes described as a separate muscle known as the opponens digiti minimi muscle.[1]

Fourth Layer

The dorsal interosseous muscles are located between the metatarsals. They consist of four bipennate muscles, each originating by two heads from the adjacent metatarsals. The first inserts onto the medial aspect of the base of the proximal phalanx of the second toe. The remaining three insert onto the lateral aspect

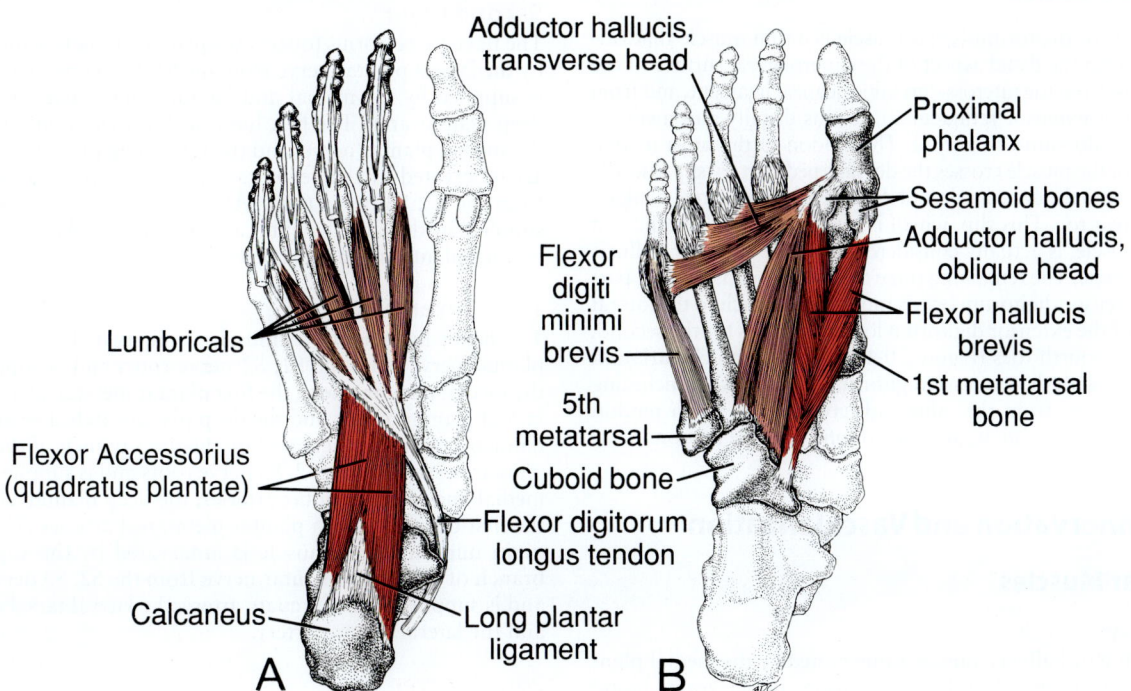

Figure 70-2. A, The second layer of the plantar intrinsic muscles of the foot. B, The third layer of the plantar intrinsic muscles of the foot.

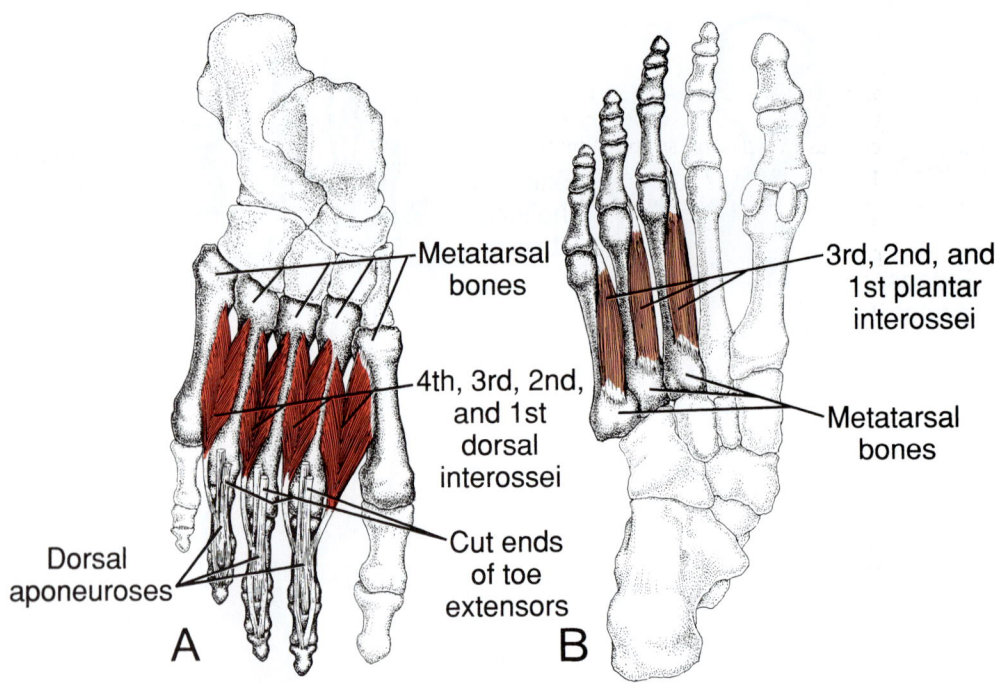

Figure 70-3. The fourth, and deepest, layer of the intrinsic muscles of the foot. A, Dorsal interosseous muscles. B, Plantar interosseous muscles.

of the proximal phalanges of the second, third, and fourth toes (Figure 70-3A).[1]

There are three plantar interosseous muscles. Unlike the dorsal interosseous muscles, these muscles are located under the metatarsals rather than between them, and each muscle is attached to only one metatarsal. They are unipennate. They originate from the bases and medial aspects of the 3rd, 4th, and 5th metatarsals, and they insert onto the medial aspect of the bases of the proximal phalanges of the third, fourth, and fifth toes (Figure 70-3B).

Dorsal Muscles

The extensor digitorum brevis muscle is a thin muscle that originates from the distal aspect of the superolateral surface of the calcaneus, from the interosseous talocalcaneal ligament, and from the inferior extensor retinaculum. It runs distally and medially across the dorsum of the foot. The tendon of the most medial portion of the muscle crosses the dorsalis pedis artery superficially to insert onto the dorsal aspect of the base of the proximal phalanx of the great toe. This slip, which is rather distinct from the rest of the muscle, is actually considered to be the extensor hallucis brevis muscle. The remaining three tendons are considered a part of the extensor digitorum brevis muscle and attach to the lateral aspects of the extensor digitorum longus tendons for the second, third, and fourth toes (Figure 70-1A). There is much variation associated with the extensor digitorum brevis muscle, including accessory slips from the talus and navicular, an extra tendon running to the 5th digit, or a lack of one or more tendons.[1]

2.1. Innervation and Vascularization

Plantar Muscles

First Layer
The abductor hallucis muscle is innervated by the medial plantar nerve from the S1 and S2 nerve roots. It receives its blood supply from the medial malleolar network, the medial calcaneal branches of the lateral plantar artery, the medial plantar artery (directly and via superficial and deep branches), the first plantar metatarsal artery, and the plantar arterial arch. The flexor digitorum brevis muscle is also innervated by the medial plantar nerve from the S1, S2 nerve roots and is supplied by the lateral and medial plantar arteries, the plantar metatarsal arteries, and the plantar digital arteries of the lateral four toes. The abductor digiti minimi muscle is innervated by the lateral plantar nerve from the S1, S2, S3 nerve roots and is supplied by the medial and lateral plantar arteries, the plantar digital artery, branches from the deep plantar arch, the fourth plantar metatarsal artery, and the arcuate and lateral tarsal arteries.[1]

Second Layer
The flexor accessorius (quadratus plantae) muscle is innervated by the lateral plantar nerve from the S1, S2, S3 nerve roots and is supplied by the medial and lateral plantar arteries and the deep plantar arch. The first lumbrical muscle is innervated by the medial plantar nerve, and the remaining lumbrical muscles are innervated by the deep branch of the lateral plantar nerve from the S2, S3 nerve roots. All of the lumbrical muscles are supplied by the lateral plantar artery and deep plantar arch and by four plantar metatarsal arteries.[1]

Third Layer
The flexor hallucis brevis muscle is innervated by the medial plantar nerve from the S1, S2 nerve roots and is supplied by the medial plantar artery, the first plantar metatarsal artery, the lateral plantar artery, and the deep plantar arch. The adductor hallucis muscle is innervated by the deep branch of the lateral plantar nerve from the S2, S3 nerve roots and is supplied by the medial and lateral plantar arteries, the deep plantar arch, and the first through fourth plantar metatarsal arteries. The flexor digiti minimi brevis muscle is innervated by the superficial branch of the lateral plantar nerve from the S2, S3 nerve roots and is supplied by the arcuate artery, the lateral tarsal arteries, and the lateral plantar artery.

Fourth Layer
The first three dorsal interosseous muscles are innervated by the deep branch of the lateral plantar nerve from the S2, S3 nerve roots. The fourth is innervated by the superficial branch

of the lateral plantar nerve, also from the S2, S3 nerve roots. The dorsal interosseous muscles are supplied by the arcuate artery, the lateral and medial tarsal arteries, the first through fourth plantar arteries, the first through fourth dorsal metatarsal arteries, and the dorsal digital arteries of the lateral four toes. The first two plantar interosseous muscles are supplied by the deep branch of the lateral plantar nerve from the S2, S3 nerve roots, and the third is innervated by the superficial branch of the lateral plantar nerve (S2, S3). The plantar interosseous muscles are supplied by the lateral plantar artery, the deep plantar arch, the second through fourth plantar metatarsal arteries, and the dorsal digital arteries of the lateral three toes.[1]

Dorsal Muscles

The extensor digitorum brevis and extensor hallucis brevis muscles are innervated by the deep fibular nerve from the L5, S1 nerve roots and are supplied by the fibular artery, the anterior lateral malleolar artery, the lateral tarsal arteries, the dorsalis pedis artery, the arcuate artery, the first through third dorsal metatarsal arteries, the proximal and distal perforating arteries, and the dorsal digital arteries of the first four toes.

2.2. Function

Many of the intrinsic muscles of the foot, particularly the plantar muscles, work collectively, along with the extrinsic muscles of the foot, to aid in effective gait by maintaining medial longitudinal arch height,[5-9] controlling the extent and speed of arch deformation,[10] and assisting in dynamic postural control.[9,11-13] Contrary to previous belief, Kelly et al have shown that intrinsic foot muscles are also active during quiet stance.[11] The intrinsic foot muscles that demonstrate the most involvement in maintaining foot stability during gait and during static and dynamic posture include the abductor hallucis, abductor digiti minimi, flexor digitorum brevis, flexor hallucis brevis, flexor accessorius (quadratus plantae), lumbrical, and interosseous muscles.[9,11]

In addition to this collective function, each muscle has its own individual action(s). These individual actions, along with specific contributions to foot static and dynamic stability, if known, are described as follows:

Plantar Muscles

First Layer
The abductor hallucis muscle creates abduction, and often flexion, of the great toe at the metatarsophalangeal joint.[1] The abductor hallucis muscle is particularly important, along with the extrinsic tibialis posterior muscle, for supporting and elevating the medial longitudinal arch.[6,8,14] The flexor digitorum brevis muscle flexes toes 2 to 5 at their proximal interphalangeal joints. It performs this action equally effectively regardless of ankle joint position.[1] The abductor digiti minimi muscle acts on the fifth toe by, despite its name, flexing it at the metatarsophalangeal joint more than it abducts it.[1]

Second Layer
The flexor accessorius (quadratus plantae) muscle creates pure flexion of digits 2 to 4 from the posteromedial pull of the flexor digitorum longus muscle.[15,16] This action can be performed regardless of the ankle position.[1] It is also believed that the flexor accessorius muscle is a muscle that acts as a "truss" for the longitudinal arches by actively resisting bending forces during ambulation.[15] The lumbrical muscles help maintain interphalangeal joint extension of digits 2 to 4.[1]

Third Layer
The flexor hallucis brevis muscle, as its name implies, flexes the great toe at the metatarsophalangeal joint.[1] The adductor hallucis muscle assists with flexion of the metatarsophalangeal joint of the great toe. It also works to stabilize the metatarsal heads.[1] The flexor digiti minimi brevis muscle flexes the metatarsophalangeal joint of the fifth toe.[1]

Fourth Layer
The dorsal interosseous muscles abduct digits 2 to 4. They also contribute to flexion of the metatarsophalangeal joint and extension of the interphalangeal joints of digits 2 to 4.[1] The plantar interosseous muscles adduct digits 3 to 5, and they flex the metatarsophalangeal joints and extend the interphalangeal joints of the same digits. Together, the dorsal and plantar interosseous muscles also stabilize the tarsometatarsal joints late in the stance phase of gait, contributing to foot rigidity at push-off.[17]

Dorsal Muscles

The extensor digitorum brevis muscle aids in extension of digits 2 to 4 via the extensor digitorum longus tendons. The extensor hallucis brevis muscle aids in extension of the great toe. The recruitment pattern of these muscles during ambulation has been shown to vary significantly among individuals, and their contribution to additional functions in the foot remains, for the most part, unknown.[18,19]

2.3. Functional Unit

The functional unit to which a muscle belongs includes the muscles that reinforce and counter its actions as well as the joints that the muscle crosses. The interdependence of these structures is functionally reflected in the organization and neural connections of the sensory motor cortex. The functional unit is emphasized because the presence of a TrP in one muscle of the unit increases the likelihood that the other muscles of the unit will also develop TrPs. When inactivating TrPs in a muscle, one must be concerned about TrPs that may develop in muscles that are functionally interdependent. Box 70-1 grossly represents the functional unit of the plantar intrinsic foot muscles and Box 70-2 represents the functional unit of the dorsal intrinsic foot muscles.[20]

3. CLINICAL PRESENTATION

3.1. Referred Pain Pattern

With the possible exception of the dorsal and plantar interosseous muscles, the intrinsic muscles of the foot do not refer pain proximally to the foot.[20] Although referral patterns for many muscles of the body have been studied extensively, very few published reports exist that document the referred pain patterns of the intrinsic foot muscles. Much of what does exist comes from the original work of Janet G. Travell, MD and David G. Simons, MD.

Box 70-1 Functional unit of the plantar intrinsic foot muscles

Action	Synergists	Antagonists
Toe flexion 2-5	Flexor digitorum longus	Dorsal interossei 2-4 Extensor digitorum longus Extensor digitorum brevis
Great toe flexion	Flexor hallucis longus	Extensor hallucis longus Extensor hallucis brevis

Box 70-2 Functional unit of the dorsal intrinsic foot muscles

Action	Synergists	Antagonists
Toe extension 2-5	Extensor digitorum longus Lumbricals	Flexor digitorum longus Flexor digitorum brevis Flexor digiti minimi brevis Abductor digiti minimi Flexor accessorius (quadratus plantae)
Great toe extension	Extensor hallucis longus	Flexor hallucis longus Flexor hallucis brevis Abductor hallucis

Plantar Muscles

First Layer
The abductor hallucis muscle refers pain primarily to the medial aspect of the heel, with some extension to the posteromedial heel and along the medial longitudinal arch[20] (Figure 70-4). The abductor digit minimi muscle refers pain to the plantar aspect of the 5th metatarsal head, occasionally extending onto the lateral aspect of the distal forefoot[20] (Figure 70-5A). The flexor digitorum brevis muscle refers pain to the plantar surface of the foot over the 2nd to 4th metatarsal heads. It can sometimes refer pain to the 5th metatarsal head as well[20] (Figure 70-5B).

Second Layer
The flexor accessorius (quadratus plantae) muscle tends to refer pain to the plantar aspect of the heel[20] (Figure 70-6). A referred pain pattern for the lumbrical muscles has not been well established but is believed to follow a pattern similar to that of the interosseous muscles (see Figure 70-8).[20]

Third Layer
The flexor hallucis brevis muscle refers pain to the plantar and medial aspects of the 1st metatarsal head. It can occasionally extend to all of the great toe and part of the second toe[20] (Figure 70-7B). Good reported that the flexor hallucis brevis muscle (along with some contribution from the flexor digitorum brevis muscle) was found to be responsible for more than half of the 100 cases of patients with painful feet due to muscle-related pain.[21] The adductor hallucis muscle refers pain to the plantar aspect of the 1st through 4th metatarsal heads, with the transverse head sometimes causing a sensation of numbness and/or swelling over the same region[20] (Figure 70-7A). A referred pain pattern for the flexor digiti minimi brevis muscle has not been well established but is believed to follow a pattern similar to that of the abductor digiti minimi muscle (see Figure 70-5A).[20]

Fourth Layer
The dorsal and plantar interosseous muscles are believed to produce similar pain referral patterns.[20] Typically, TrPs in an interosseous muscle refer pain primarily to the side of the digit to which the tendon is attached, along with referral to the dorsal and plantar aspects of the foot along the corresponding metatarsal[20] (Figure 70-8). The first dorsal interosseous muscle can sometimes produce tingling in the great toe.[20] Kellgren discovered potential pain referral of the interosseous muscles into the lateral ankle and calf.[22]

Dorsal Muscles
The combined referred pain pattern of the extensor digitorum brevis and extensor hallucis brevis muscles is to the dorsal aspect of the midfoot[20] (Figure 70-9). The extensor digitorum brevis muscle can also refer pain to the area over the medial longitudinal arch.[23]

3.2. Symptoms
Patients with TrPs in the abductor hallucis brevis, flexor digitorum brevis, and abductor digiti minimi muscles often report having very sore feet.[20] Typically, they have experimented with

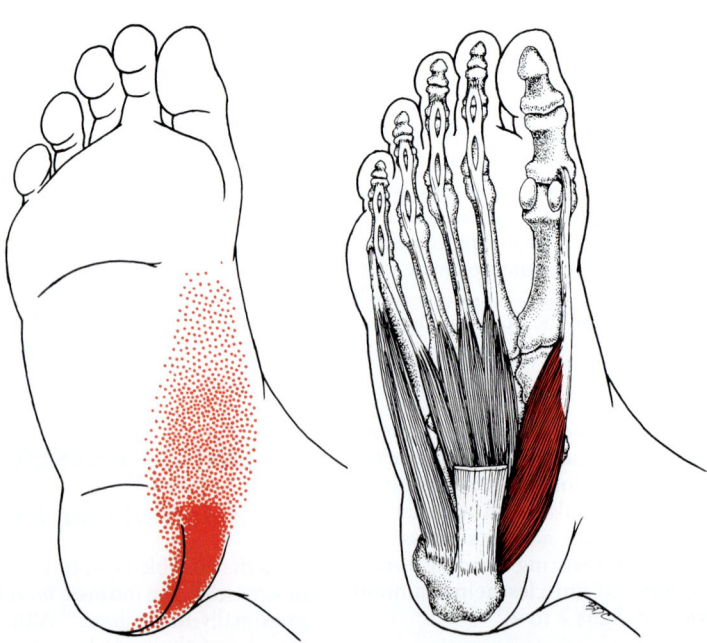

Figure 70-4. Referred pain patterns (red), in the right abductor hallucis muscle (shown in dark red). Solid red shows essential referred pain zones; stippled red areas show spillover zones.

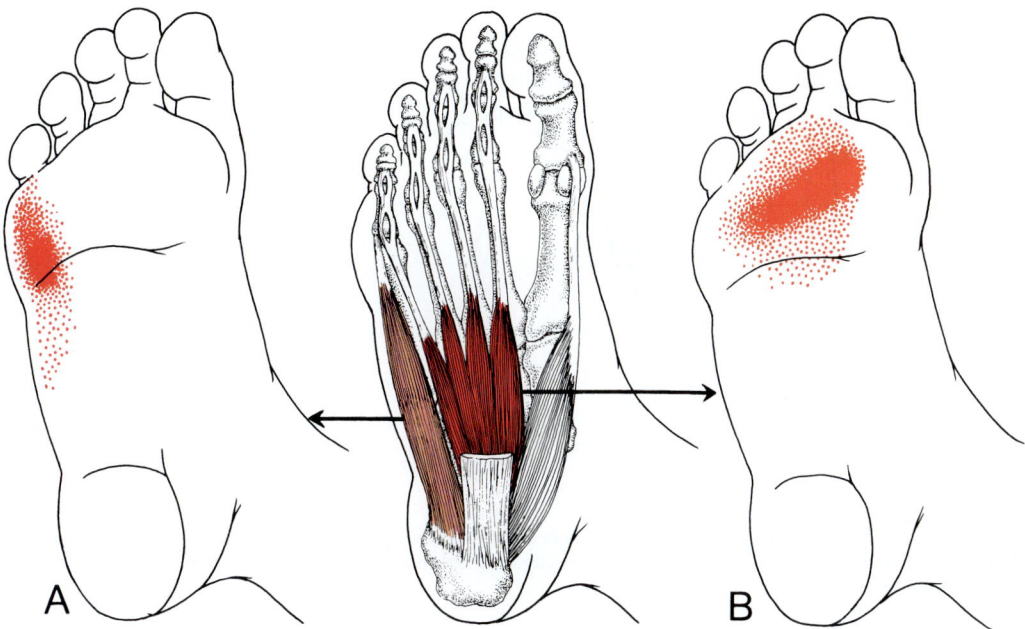

Figure 70-5. A, Referred pain pattern (red) in the right abductor digit minimi muscle (shown in light red). B, Referred pain pattern (red) in the right flexor digitorum brevis muscle (shown in dark red). Solid red shows essential referred pain zones; stippled red areas show spillover zones.

a variety of different shoe types and shoe inserts. Inserts are often uncomfortable because they press against the areas of muscle pain. Some of these patients may also report having "fallen arches" or "flat feet." They may have a limited range of ambulation, and they might even exhibit a limp due to pain and soreness in their feet.

In addition to the symptoms described previously, patients with TrPs in the muscles of the deeper layers of the foot may have significant walking limitations resulting from pain. They may report numbness in the foot and a sensation of swelling. Some patients even report the feeling of a "bunched-up" sock under the foot causing them to check inside their shoe. Trigger points in the interosseous muscles may also contribute to a hammer toe deformity as their function to extend the proximal and distal interphalangeal joints may be inhibited.

3.3. Patient Examination

After a thorough subjective examination, the clinician should make a detailed drawing representing the pain pattern that the patient has described. This depiction will assist in planning the physical examination and can be useful in monitoring the progression of the patient as symptoms improve or change. The type, quality, and location of the pain should be carefully assessed, and the utilization of standardized outcome tools is imperative when examining patients with ankle and foot dysfunctions.

For proper examination of the ankle, foot, and intrinsic foot muscles, the clinician should observe the patient during ambulation, both with and without shoes. The clinician should note any sign of excessive supination or pronation. A patient with TrPs in the deeper muscles of the forefoot may be unable to hop on the involved foot.

Passive range of motion should be examined in the foot and all of the toes as TrPs often painfully restrict range of motion when the involved muscle is stretched. If pain limits flexion of the great toe and/or the lesser toes, the extensor hallucis brevis and/or extensor digitorum brevis muscle(s) may be adaptively shortened or as a result of TrPs in these muscles.[24] If pain limits passive extension of the 5th digit, the abductor digiti minimi muscle may be shortened due to TrPs. Painful limitation of passive extension of digits 2 to 4 may be the result of adaptive shortening of the flexor digitorum brevis muscle or as a result of the presence of TrPs.[24] Similar findings with passive extension of the great toe at the proximal phalanx may implicate the flexor hallucis brevis and/or abductor hallucis brevis muscle(s).[24]

Palpation is important to help establish whether the pain is potentially referred from TrPs or joint structures in the foot. Because chronic TrPs can result in pain at the attachment sites of a muscle, patients with TrPs in the intrinsic toe flexor muscles are likely to be tender to palpation at the anterior aspect of the calcaneus where the plantar fascia attaches.

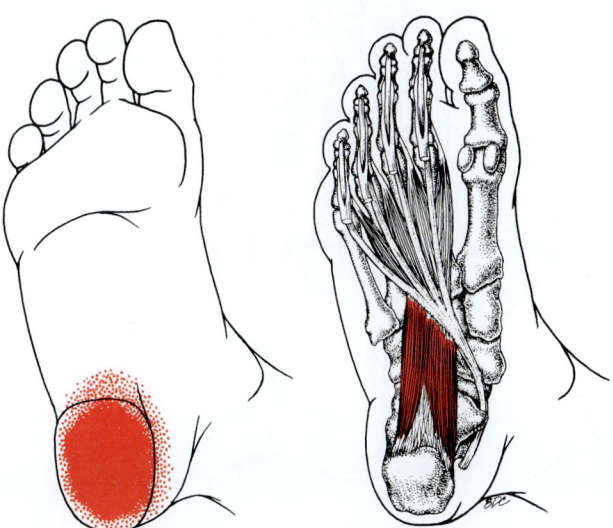

Figure 70-6. Referred pain pattern (red) in the right flexor accessorius (quadratus plantae) muscle. Solid red shows essential referred pain zones; stippled red areas show spillover zones.

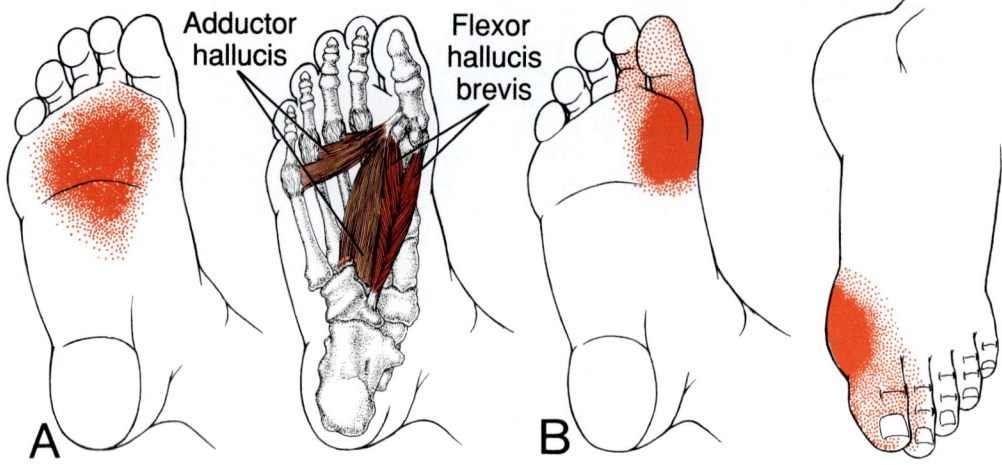

Figure 70-7. A, Referred pain patterns in the oblique and transverse heads of the right adductor hallucis muscle. B, Referred patterns in the flexor hallucis brevis muscle. Solid red shows essential referred pain zones; stippled red areas show spillover zones.

Joint mobility, including accessory motions, of the ankle, hindfoot, midfoot, forefoot, and phalanges should be examined for restriction or for hypermobility. Careful biomechanical examination should be performed for structural deviations such as hindfoot varus/valgus, forefoot varus/valgus, pes equinus, long 2nd metatarsal, pes cavus, hallux valgus, and hammer or claw toes. The presence and thickness of calluses should be noted, and the patient's shoes should be examined for abnormal wear patterns that may indicate altered foot mechanics.

Strength of involved muscles and active contraction in the shortened position are also often limited by pain. Examination of strength of great toe metatarsophalangeal flexion is performed by stabilizing the forefoot and resisting flexion at the proximal phalanx, which tests the flexor hallucis brevis muscle and, to a degree, the abductor hallucis and adductor hallucis muscles. Strength examination of the interosseous and lumbrical muscles is performed by resisting the patient's effort to extend the interphalangeal joints of digits 2 to 5, while stabilizing the metatarsophalangeal joints with the foot in 20° to 30° of plantar flexion.[24,25]

The dorsalis pedis and posterior tibial pulses should be palpated to assess the status of arterial circulation. The skin and nails should be examined for lesions, and the skin of the foot should be examined for color, temperature, and edema. Patients' feet should be screened for insensation with a 5.7 Semmes Weinstein monofilament as an early indicator of diabetes mellitus.

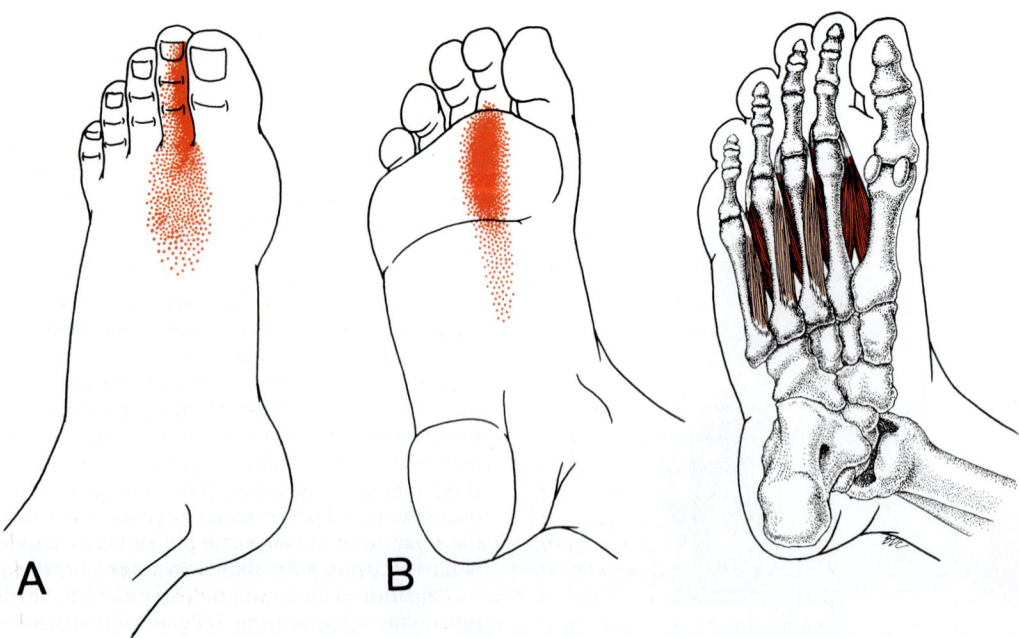

Figure 70-8. Referred pain pattern in the right first dorsal interosseous muscle. A, Dorsal view. B, Plantar view. Solid red shows essential referred pain zones; stippled red areas show spillover zones.

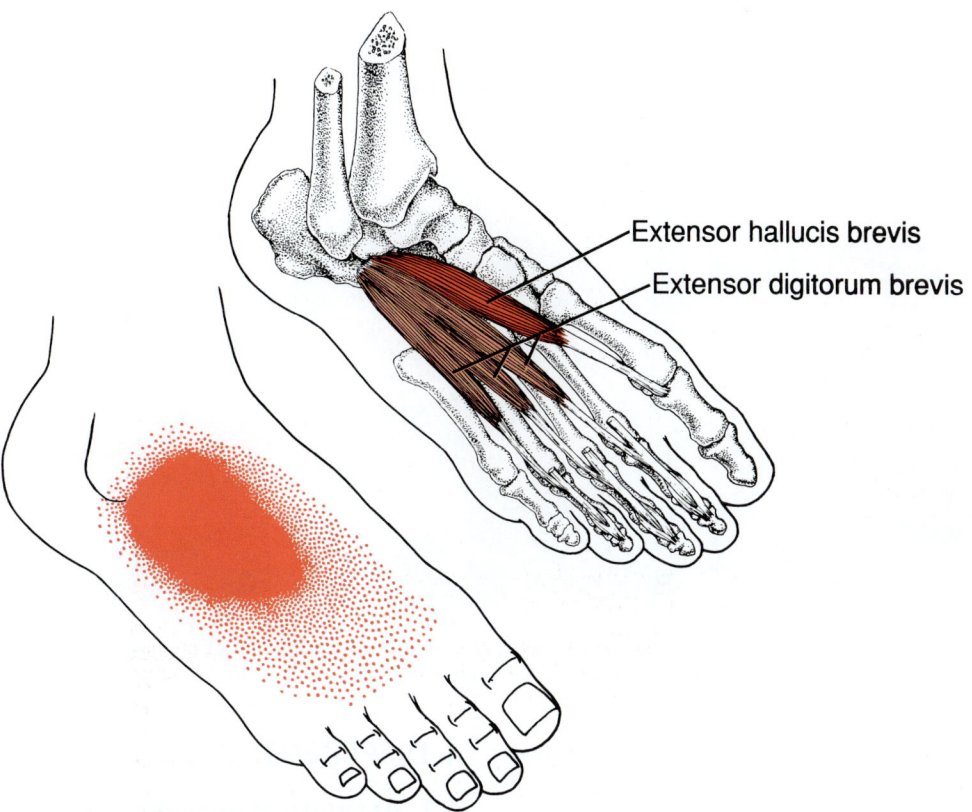

Figure 70-9. Referred pain patterns in the right extensor digitorum brevis and extensor hallucis brevis muscles. Solid red shows essential referred pain zones; stippled red areas show spillover zones.

Any patient with painful intrinsic foot muscles, especially if associated with inflammation of the 1st metatarsophalangeal joint, should be examined for gout or other arthritides.

3.4. Trigger Point Examination

Examination of TrPs of the intrinsic muscles of the foot is most easily accomplished by positioning the patient in prone, supine, or long sitting, with the patient's feet just off the end of the examination table.

Plantar Muscles

First Layer

Trigger points in the first layer of intrinsic muscles of the plantar aspect of the foot are usually examined by cross-fiber flat palpation against underlying structures. The flexor digitorum brevis muscle lies deep to the thick plantar aponeurosis, potentially requiring deeper palpation (Figure 70-10A). The abductor hallucis muscle is a remarkably thick muscle for its size. This thickness makes its deeper fibers relatively inaccessible and may require strong, deep cross-fiber flat palpation rather than gentler cross-fiber flat palpation to elicit pain from deeper TrPs (Figure 70-10B). Typically, the abductor digiti minimi muscle is most effectively examined through cross-fiber pincer palpation along the length of the muscle at the lateral edge of the sole of the foot (Figure 70-10C). The clinician should explore both distal to, and proximal to, the base of the 5th metatarsal for taut bands and TrP pain.

Second Layer

Deep palpation must be utilized to examine the flexor accessories (quadratus plantae) muscle for TrPs. The clinician must apply enough pressure to palpate deep to the plantar aponeurosis, with the toes slightly extended (Figure 70-11A). Local areas of pain are often detectable, but the clinician will likely not feel a taut band in this muscle. The lumbrical muscles are palpated with the interosseous muscles (Figure 70-11B).

Third Layer

The flexor hallucis brevis muscle is largely covered by the plantar aponeurosis; therefore, the medial head of this muscle is best palpated by cross-fiber flat palpation through the thinner skin along the medial edge of bottom of the foot. A TrP in this head of the muscle may be palpable against the underlying 1st metatarsal. Trigger points in the lateral head must be examined for pain by deep palpation through the plantar surface of the foot. The clinician must be careful not to mistake the tendon of the abductor hallucis muscle for a taut band in the flexor hallucis brevis muscle. The adductor hallucis muscle is examined by first abducting the great toe to create a stretch in the muscle. It is then palpated through the plantar aponeurosis in the distal forefoot, just proximal to the metatarsal heads. Taut bands are rarely palpable, but pain can be elicited (Figure 70-12B and C). The flexor digiti minimi brevis muscle can rarely be differentiated from the abductor digiti minimi muscle and is palpated at the same time using the same technique (Figure 70-10C).

Fourth Layer

The dorsal and plantar interosseous muscles are palpated using both hands to gently separate adjacent metatarsals and apply a stretch to the muscles. The dorsal interosseous muscles are palpated with the finger of one hand and counter pressure to the plantar surface of the foot with a finger of the other hand (Figure 70-12D). Pain in the plantar interosseous and lumbrical muscles can be elicited by deep palpation through the plantar aponeurosis against counter pressure to the dorsal aspect of the foot (Figure 70-12E). It is usually possible to palpate taut bands of TrPs in a dorsal interosseous muscle against its adjacent metatarsal bone, eliciting a local twitch response. One cannot

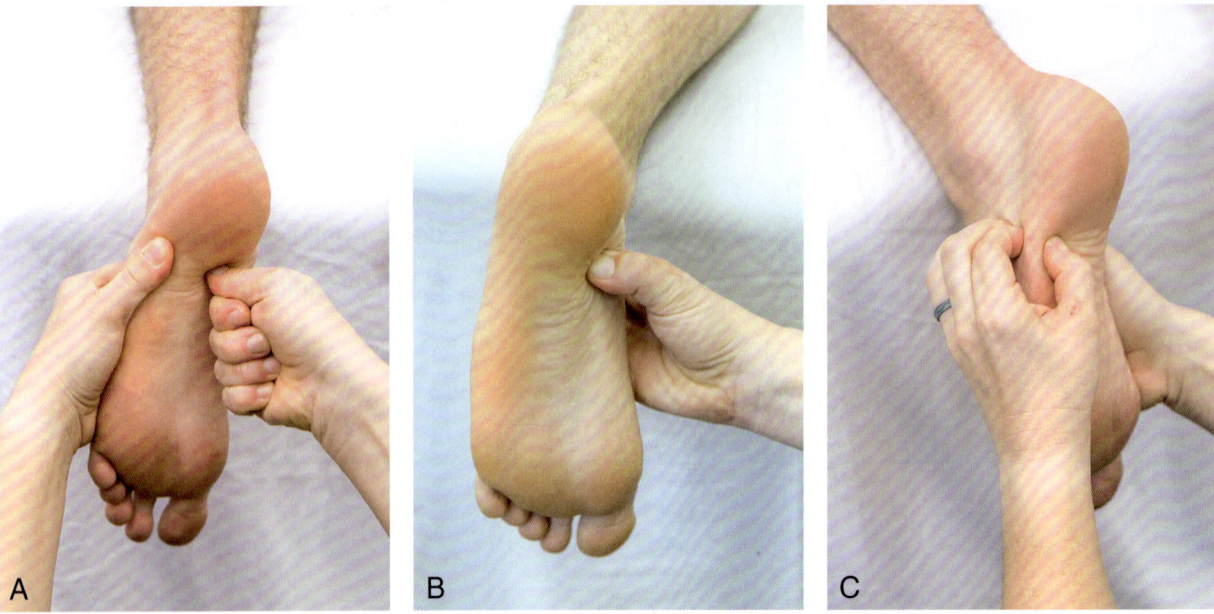

Figure 70-10. Palpation of the first layer of plantar foot muscles. A, Cross-fiber flat palpation of the flexor digitorum brevis muscle. B, Cross-fiber flat palpation of the abductor hallucis muscle. C, Cross-fiber pincer palpation of the abductor digiti minimi muscle.

differentiate between palpation of the lumbrical and plantar interosseous muscles through the plantar aponeurosis.

Dorsal Muscles

The extensor digitorum brevis and extensor hallucis brevis muscles are palpated on the dorsal aspect of the foot using flat palpation, but the overlying tendons of extrinsic foot muscles can sometimes complicate the examination (Figure 70-13).

4. DIFFERENTIAL DIAGNOSIS

4.1. Activation and Perpetuation of Trigger Points

A posture or activity that activates a TrP, if not corrected, can also perpetuate it. In any part of the intrinsic foot muscles, TrPs may be activated by unaccustomed eccentric loading, eccentric exercise in an unconditioned muscle, or maximal or submaximal

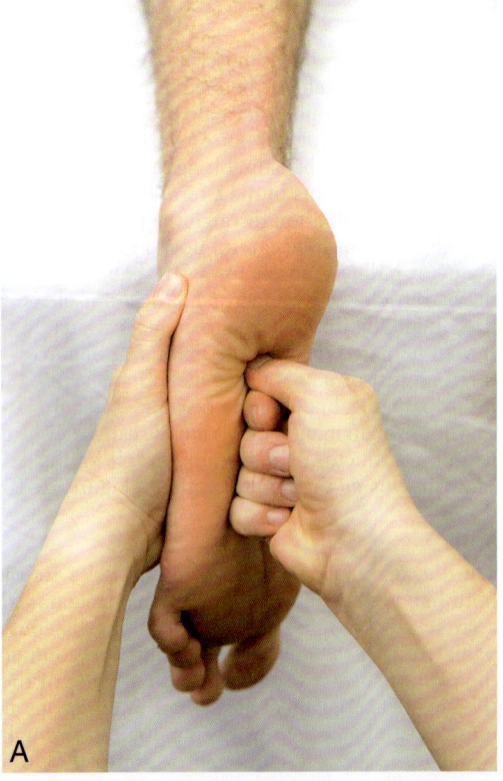 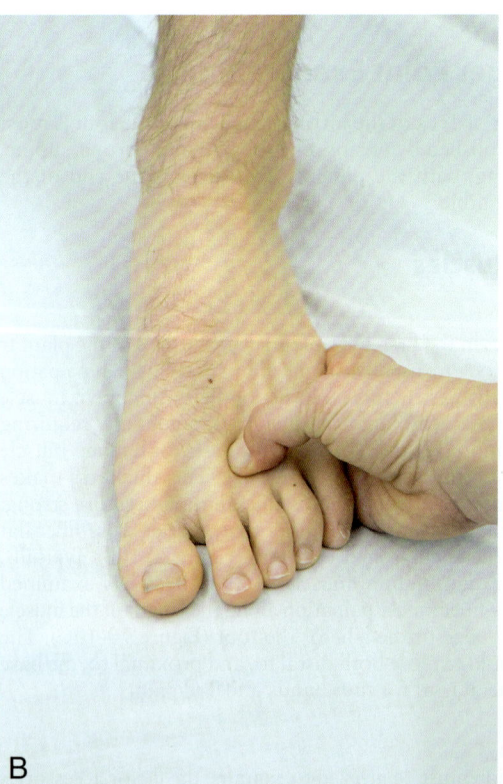

Figure 70-11. Palpation of the second layer of plantar foot muscles. A, Cross-fiber flat palpation of the flexor accessorius muscle (quadratus plantae). B, Lumbrical muscles.

Chapter 70: Intrinsic Muscles of the Foot   743

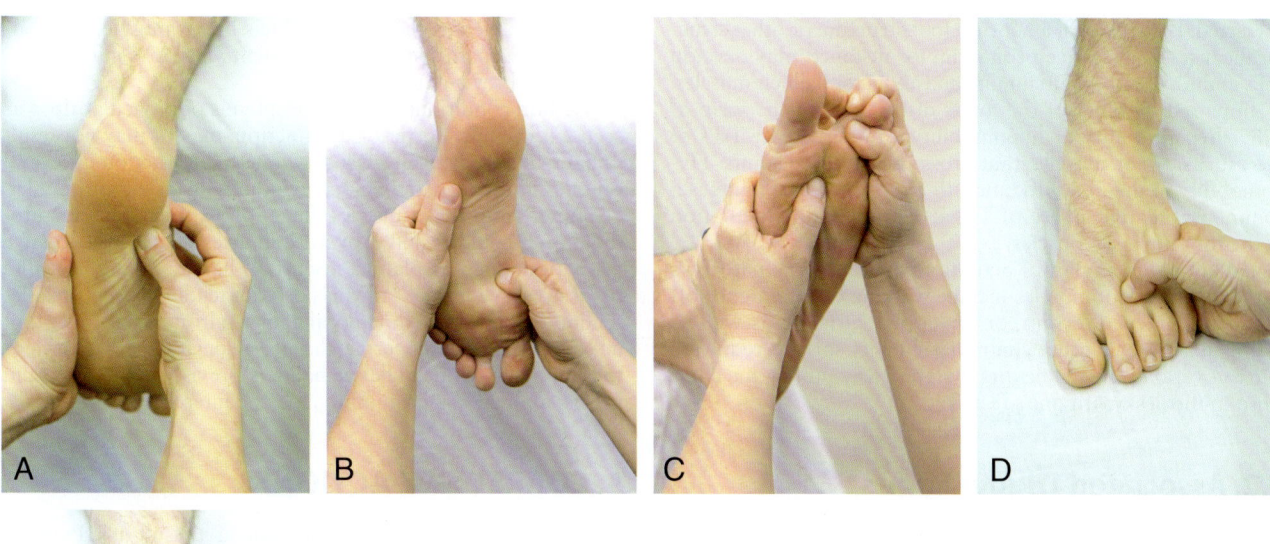

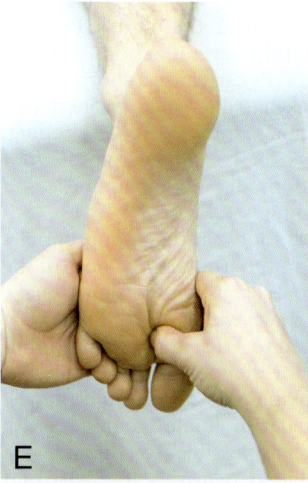

Figure 70-12. Cross-fiber flat palpation of the third layer of plantar foot muscles. A, Flexor hallucis brevis muscle. B, Adductor hallucis muscle. C, Adductor hallucis muscle (transverse head). D, Dorsal interosseous muscles. E, Plantar interosseous muscles.

concentric loading.[26] Trigger points may also be activated or aggravated when the muscle is placed in a shortened and/or lengthened position for an extended period of time.

Tight-fitting shoes and shoes with an inflexible sole can restrict toe movement, which can lead to overload of the intrinsic foot muscles and activate TrPs in them. Once activated, the continued use of restrictive footwear perpetuates the TrPs. A similar pattern can occur following a fracture of the foot or ankle bones, especially when prolonged immobilization is involved. Trigger points in the interosseous muscles are more likely to be activated and perpetuated by footwear that is too short (see Chapter 77).

Injuries to the foot intrinsic muscles in the form of trauma, such as bruising, banging, stubbing the toes, and falling, can initiate TrPs in them. Although pronation of the foot during the early stance phase of gait is normal, excessive pronation can activate and perpetuate TrPs in the intrinsic foot muscles if not

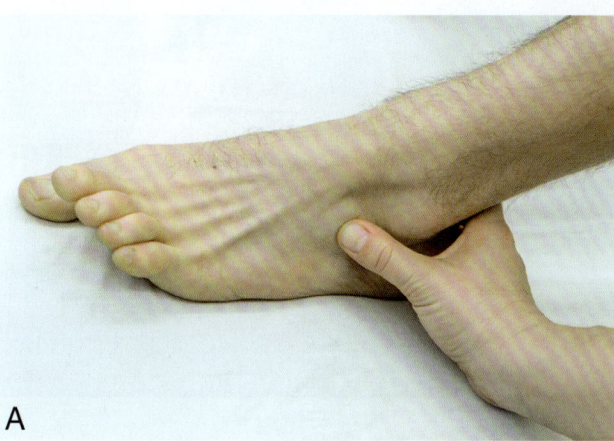
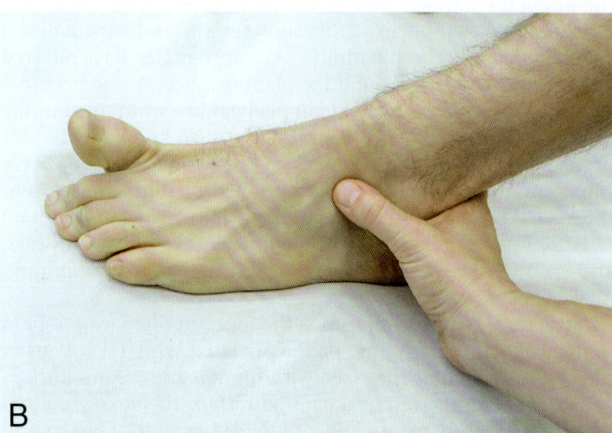

Figure 70-13. Cross-fiber flat palpation of dorsal intrinsic foot muscles. A, Extensor digitorum brevis muscle. B, Extensor hallucis brevis muscle.

corrected. Patients with a Morton foot structure or other structural causes of excessive pronation, for instance, may develop TrPs in the abductor digiti minimi and abductor hallucis muscles.

Impaired mobility of the joints of the foot, in the form of either hypermobility or hypomobility, can perpetuate TrPs of the intrinsic foot muscles that cross the involved joints. Hypomobility in the 2nd, 3rd, and 4th tarsometatarsal joints is a common potential source of TrP activation and perpetuation in the foot intrinsic muscles.[27]

Additional examples of activities that can perpetuate TrPs in the intrinsic foot muscles include walking or running in soft sand, over uneven terrain, or on sloped surfaces, as well as sitting in a wheeled office chair on a slippery surface, requiring one to overload the toe flexors by repeatedly pulling the chair close to the desk with one's feet.

4.2. Associated Trigger Points

Associated TrPs can develop in the referred pain areas caused by primary TrPs.[28] Therefore, musculature in the referred pain areas for each muscle should also be considered.

Trigger points in the extensor digitorum brevis and extensor hallucis brevis muscles are typically associated with TrPs in the corresponding long toe extensor muscles. Trigger points in the abductor hallucis muscle tend to coincide with those in the nearby deep intrinsic muscles, resulting in soreness throughout the entire foot, particularly the distal plantar surface. Similarly, flexor digitorum brevis TrPs are often associated with those in the long toe flexor muscles and, occasionally, with the deeper flexor hallucis brevis muscle. Conversely, the abductor digiti minimi muscle tends to appear as a single-muscle syndrome, usually as the result of ill-fitting shoes. The interosseous muscles are another example of muscles that present as single-muscle myofascial pain syndrome.

4.3. Associated Pathology

Several conditions exist that can potentially mimic the pain associated with TrPs in the intrinsic muscles of the foot or that can lead to and/or exacerbate TrPs in those muscles.

Plantar heel pain is a rather common source of pain, with a prevalence rate estimated at 3.6% to 7.5%.[29-31] Plantar heel pain primarily affects middle-age and older adults[30] and is believed to account for roughly 8% of running-related injuries.[32]

There are several factors and mechanisms believed to contribute to plantar heel pain, including reduced ankle dorsiflexion range of motion, obesity, and prolonged standing.[33,34] There is some evidence that TrPs can also be involved in plantar heel pain. Trigger points have been found to be prevalent in some intrinsic muscles of the foot in patients with plantar heel pain, including the abductor hallucis and flexor digitorum brevis muscles.[35] Furthermore, two intrinsic foot muscles, the abductor hallucis and flexor accessorius (quadratus plantae) muscles, have referred pain patterns at and around the plantar aspect of the heel.[20]

An additional cause of plantar heel pain is entrapment of the first branch of the lateral plantar nerve, also known as Baxter nerve or the inferior calcaneal nerve.[36,37] Entrapment of this nerve can occur as it passes between the abductor hallucis muscle and the medial border of the flexor accessorius (quadratus plantae) muscle,[38] potentially resulting in plantar heel pain, paresthesia, and even weakness and atrophy of the abductor digiti minimi muscle.[37,39]

Structural issues or injuries in the foot can often lead to pain that can potentially mimic pain associated with TrPs. Pain in the great toe such as that seen with bunion and sesamoiditis is consistent with the referred pain pattern of the flexor hallucis brevis muscle. Turf-toe, an injury of the 1st metatarsal phalangeal joint resulting from hyperextension of the joint, can result in pain that is consistent with TrPs in the first dorsal interosseous muscle[40] as well as the flexor hallucis brevis muscle. Metatarsalgia shares pain symptoms consistent with TrPs in the flexor digitorum brevis muscle.

Certain conditions, such as pes planus or navicular drop as seen with tibialis posterior dysfunction, may or may not result in pain, but are typically associated with dysfunction of several muscles in the foot and ankle, including intrinsic foot muscles. Dysfunction in these muscles that support the medial longitudinal arch could result in overuse injuries related to excessive pronation[8] such as plantar fasciitis,[41] hallux valgus,[42] medial tibial stress syndrome,[43] tibialis posterior tendinopathy,[44] achilles tendonitis,[45] and patellofemoral pain syndrome.[46] Intrinsic foot muscles involved in supporting the medial longitudinal arch include the abductor hallucis, flexor hallucis brevis, flexor digitorum brevis, abductor digiti minimi, and the interosseous muscles.[9]

5. CORRECTIVE ACTIONS

Patients experiencing plantar foot pain as a result of TrPs in the intrinsic muscles of the foot can take several actions to try to address their symptoms. Because TrPs can cause a shortening of involved muscles, care should be taken to discourage positions that promote a shortened position of these muscles. When sleeping, patients should be sure to untuck the bedsheets from the foot of the bed to help minimize the foot and ankle plantar flexion positioning caused by tight bedding (see Figure 65-6).

Patients should be sure to select footwear that is appropriate. There should be plenty of room in the front, or toe box, of the shoe. For plantar pain related to TrPs, it is important to have room for the toes to move up and down within the shoe. For great toe and 1st metatarsal pain related to TrPs, it is also important that there is at least some room for the toes to move from side to side. Shoes should have a flexible sole and should be well cushioned. Patients with TrP-related pain should avoid shoes with heels and/or pointed toes as much as possible (see Chapter 77).

Various products are available at relatively low cost that may prove beneficial for certain conditions. Off-the-shelf shoe orthoses with arch support can sometimes be helpful for patients with TrP-related plantar pain by reducing stress on involved muscles. For patients with TrPs in the adductor hallucis muscle related to a bunion deformity, a toe spacer may be beneficial to prevent shortening of the muscle and perpetuation of the TrP (Figure 70-14). Metatarsal pads may be helpful for patients with forefoot plantar pain related to TrPs.

There are exercises and soft-tissue mobilization techniques that patients with plantar foot pain related to TrPs in the intrinsic foot muscles can try. Stretching of the gastrocnemius and soleus muscles of the calf can increase the amount of ankle dorsiflexion

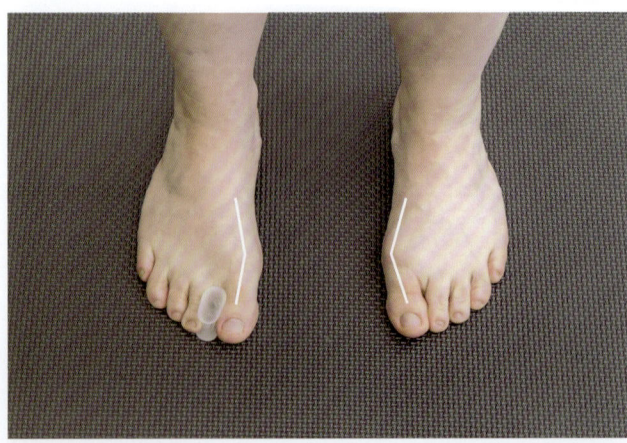

Figure 70-14. Toe spacer for trigger points in the adductor hallucis muscle related to a bunion.

Chapter 70: Intrinsic Muscles of the Foot   **745**

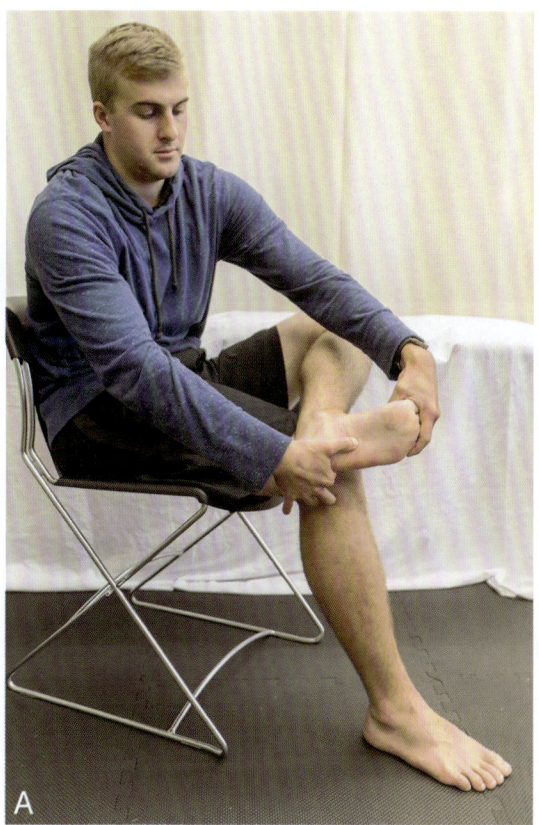 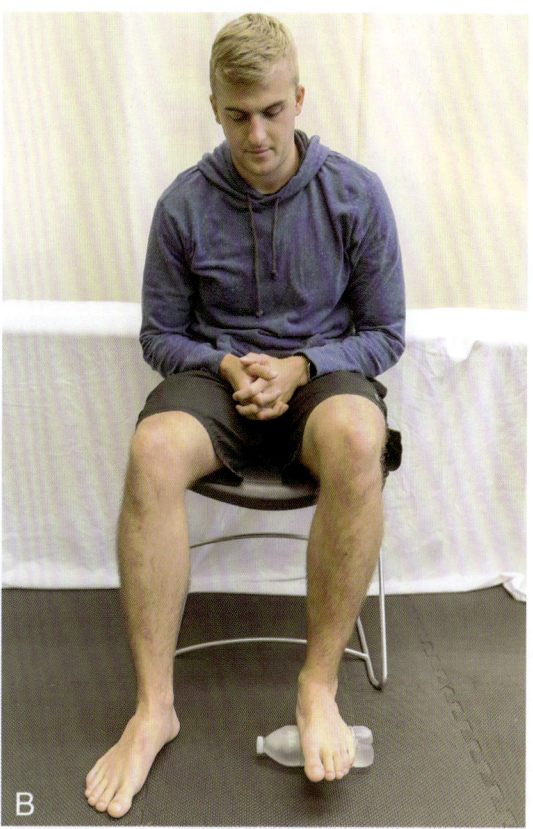

Figure 70-15. Trigger point self-pressure release of plantar foot muscles. A, Manual pressure with stretch. B, Frozen water bottle.

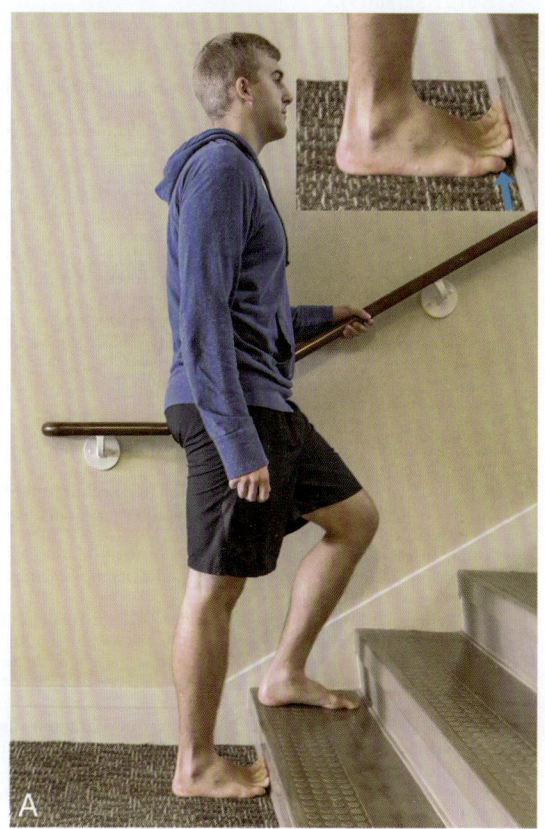 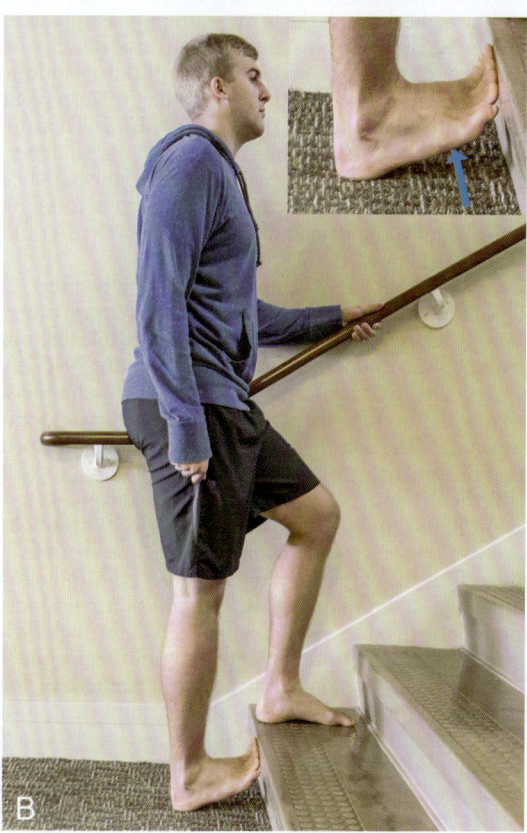

Figure 70-16. Self-stretch of foot intrinsic muscles and plantar fascia. A, Toe flexors. B, Plantar fascia.

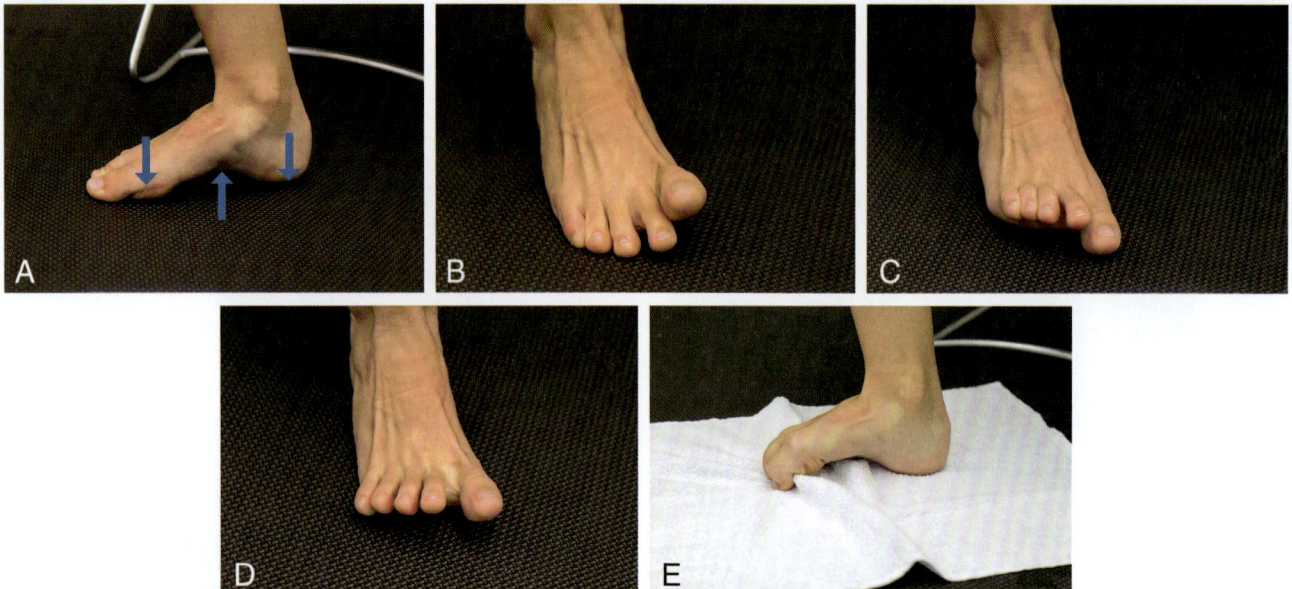

Figure 70-17. Exercises to strengthen the intrinsic muscles of the foot. A, Short-foot exercise. B, First-toe extension exercise. C, Second-to-fifth-toe extension exercise. D, Toes-spread-out exercise. E, Towel scrunches.

and thereby lessen the stress applied to the involved muscles during walking and running. There are multiple methods to perform this stretch (see Figures 65-8 and 66-11).

Extending the great toe in order to put a stretch on the plantar fascia and the flexor hallucis brevis muscle can be helpful as well. Combining this stretch while performing a deep stroking massage of the plantar fascia and short toe flexors can be even more beneficial (Figure 70-15A). Other self-pressure release techniques include placing a golf ball under the foot and applying as much body weight through the lower extremity as tolerated while rolling the ball over tender areas in the intrinsic muscles on the plantar aspect of the foot. A modification of this technique involves filling a textured soda bottle and freezing it. The patient then rolls the bottle under the foot (Figure 70-15B). The texture and contour of the bottle address the TrPs in much the same way as the golf ball technique, and the ice can help ease the patient's discomfort. Additional techniques can be performed in standing to stretch the plantar foot intrinsic muscles (Figure 70-16A) and the plantar fascia (Figure 70-16B).

Specific exercises that have been shown to strengthen several of the intrinsic foot muscles exist. The short-foot exercise is performed by trying to accentuate the arch of the foot while the foot is on the ground but without flexing the toes[47] (Figure 70-17A). This exercise is effective for targeting the abductor hallucis, flexor accessorius (quadratus plantae), and abductor digiti minimi muscles.[47,48] The first-toe extension exercise is performed by extending the great toe, while keeping all remaining toes in contact with the ground[47] (Figure 70-17B). This exercise targets the flexor digitorum brevis muscle as it works to keep toes two through five on the ground, while the great toe extends.[47] The second-to-fifth-toe extension exercise targets the abductor digiti minimi, flexor hallucis brevis, and adductor hallucis muscles and is performed by extending the second through fifth toes, while keeping the great toe in contact with the ground[47] (Figure 70-17C). The toes-spread-out exercise is effective for targeting the abductor hallucis, interosseous, lumbrical, and adductor digiti minimi muscles.[47,49] This exercise is performed by first extending all toes and then abducting all toes while simultaneously flexing the first and fifth toes and maintaining extension of the second through fourth toes[47] (Figure 70-17D).

Another exercise commonly performed to try to strengthen the intrinsic foot muscles is toe curling. This exercise can be performed using a variety of techniques, including picking up marbles with the toes and grasping a towel with the toes in an effort to "scrunch" the towel (Figure 70-17E).

References

1. Standring S. *Gray's Anatomy: The Anatomical Basis of Clinical Practice.* 41st ed. London, UK: Elsevier; 2015.
2. Owens S, Thordarson DB. The adductor hallucis revisited. *Foot Ankle Int.* 2001;22(3):186-191.
3. Arakawa T, Tokita K, Miki A, Terashima T. Anatomical study of human adductor hallucis muscle with respect to its origin and insertion. *Ann Anat.* 2003;185(6):585-592.
4. Cralley JC, Schuberth JM. The transverse head of adductor hallucis. *Anat Anz.* 1979;146(4):400-409.
5. Chang R, Kent-Braun JA, Hamill J. Use of MRI for volume estimation of tibialis posterior and plantar intrinsic foot muscles in healthy and chronic plantar fasciitis limbs. *Clin Biomech (Bristol, Avon).* 2012;27(5):500-505.
6. Fiolkowski P, Brunt D, Bishop M, Woo R, Horodyski M. Intrinsic pedal musculature support of the medial longitudinal arch: an electromyography study. *J Foot Ankle Surg.* 2003;42(6):327-333.
7. Kelly LA, Cresswell AG, Racinais S, Whiteley R, Lichtwark G. Intrinsic foot muscles have the capacity to control deformation of the longitudinal arch. *J R Soc Interface.* 2014;11(93):20131188.
8. Headlee DL, Leonard JL, Hart JM, Ingersoll CD, Hertel J. Fatigue of the plantar intrinsic foot muscles increases navicular drop. *J Electromyogr Kinesiol.* 2008;18(3):420-425.
9. Mann R, Inman VT. Phasic activity of intrinsic muscles of the foot. *J Bone Joint Surg Am.* 1964;46:469-481.
10. Lees A, Lake M, Klenerman L. Shock absorption during forefoot running and its relationship to medial longitudinal arch height. *Foot Ankle Int.* 2005;26(12):1081-1088.
11. Kelly LA, Kuitunen S, Racinais S, Cresswell AG. Recruitment of the plantar intrinsic foot muscles with increasing postural demand. *Clin Biomech (Bristol, Avon).* 2012;27(1):46-51.
12. Mulligan EP, Cook PG. Effect of plantar intrinsic muscle training on medial longitudinal arch morphology and dynamic function. *Man Ther.* 2013;18(5):425-430.
13. Grey T, Redguard D, Wengle R, Wegsheider P. Effect of plantar flexor muscle fatigue on postural control. *WURJ: Health Nat Sci.* 2013;4(1):1.
14. Wong YS. Influence of the abductor hallucis muscle on the medial arch of the foot: a kinematic and anatomical cadaver study. *Foot Ankle Int.* 2007;28(5):617-620.
15. Reeser LA, Susman RL, Stern JT Jr. Electromyographic studies of the human foot: experimental approaches to hominid evolution. *Foot Ankle.* 1983;3(6):391-407.
16. Hollinshead WH. *Anatomy for Surgeons.* Vol 3. 3rd ed. New York, NY: Harper & Row; 1982.
17. Kalin PJ, Hirsch BE. The origins and function of the interosseous muscles of the foot. *J Anat.* 1987;152:83-91.
18. Basmajian J, Deluca C. *Muscles Alive.* 5th ed. Baltimore, MD: Williams & Wilkins; 1985.

19. de Carvalho CA, Konig B Jr, Vitti M. Electromyographic study of the muscles "extensor digitorum brevis" and "extensor hallucis brevis". *Rev Hosp Clin Fac Med Sao Paulo.* 1967;22(2):65-72.
20. Simons DG, Travell J, Simons L. *Travell & Simon's Myofascial Pain and Dysfunction: The Trigger Point Manual.* Vol 1. 2nd ed. Baltimore, MD: Williams & Wilkins; 1999 (p. 104).
21. Good MG. Painful feet. *Practitioner.* 1949;163(975):229-232.
22. Kellgren JH. Observations on referred pain arising from muscle. *Clin Sci.* 1938;3:175-190.
23. Kelly M. The relief of facial pain by procaine (Novocaine) injections. *J Am Geriatr Soc.* 1963;11:586-596.
24. Kendall FP, McCreary EK. *Muscles: Testing and Function, with Posture and Pain.* 5th ed. Baltimore, MD: Lippincott Williams & Wilkins; 2005.
25. Jarret BA, Manzi JA, Green DR. Interossei and lumbricales muscles of the foot: an anatomical and function study. *J Am Podiatr Assoc.* 1980;70:1-13.
26. Gerwin RD, Dommerholt J, Shah JP. An expansion of Simons' integrated hypothesis of trigger point formation. *Curr Pain Headache Rep.* 2004;8(6):468-475.
27. Lewit K. *Manipulative Therapy in Rehabilitation of the Motor System.* London, England: Butterworths; 1985.
28. Hsieh YL, Kao MJ, Kuan TS, Chen SM, Chen JT, Hong CZ. Dry needling to a key myofascial trigger point may reduce the irritability of satellite MTrPs. *Am J Phys Med Rehabil.* 2007;86(5):397-403.
29. Hill CL, Gill TK, Menz HB, Taylor AW. Prevalence and correlates of foot pain in a population-based study: the North West Adelaide health study. *J Foot Ankle Res.* 2008;1(1):2.
30. Dunn JE, Link CL, Felson DT, Crincoli MG, Keysor JJ, McKinlay JB. Prevalence of foot and ankle conditions in a multiethnic community sample of older adults. *Am J Epidemiol.* 2004;159(5):491-498.
31. Menz HB, Tiedemann A, Kwan MM, Plumb K, Lord SR. Foot pain in community-dwelling older people: an evaluation of the Manchester Foot Pain and Disability Index. *Rheumatology (Oxford).* 2006;45(7):863-867.
32. Taunton JE, Ryan MB, Clement DB, McKenzie DC, Lloyd-Smith DR, Zumbo BD. A retrospective case-control analysis of 2002 running injuries. *Br J Sports Med.* 2002;36(2):95-101.
33. Irving DB, Cook JL, Menz HB. Factors associated with chronic plantar heel pain: a systematic review. *J Sci Med Sport.* 2006;9(1-2):11-22; discussion 23-14.
34. Irving DB, Cook JL, Young MA, Menz HB. Obesity and pronated foot type may increase the risk of chronic plantar heel pain: a matched case-control study. *BMC Musculoskelet Disord.* 2007;8:41.
35. Imamura M, Fischer AA, Imamura ST, Kaziyama HS, Carvalho AE, Salomao O. Treatment of myofascial pain components in plantar fasciitis speeds up recovery: documentation by algometry. *J Musculoske Pain.* 1998;6(1):91-110.
36. Saggini R, Bellomo RG, Affaitati G, Lapenna D, Giamberardino MA. Sensory and biomechanical characterization of two painful syndromes in the heel. *J Pain.* 2007;8(3):215-222.
37. Recht MP, Grooff P, Ilaslan H, Recht HS, Sferra J, Donley BG. Selective atrophy of the abductor digiti quinti: an MRI study. *AJR Am J Roentgenol.* 2007;189(3):W123-W127.
38. Rondhuis JJ, Huson A. The first branch of the lateral plantar nerve and heel pain. *Acta Morphol Neerl Scand.* 1986;24(4):269-279.
39. del Sol M, Olave E, Gabrielli C, Mandiola E, Prates JC. Innervation of the abductor digiti minimi muscle of the human foot: anatomical basis of the entrapment of the abductor digiti minimi nerve. *Surg Radiol Anat.* 2002;24(1):18-22.
40. Pajaczkowski JA. Mimicking turf-toe: myofasopathy of the first dorsal interosseous muscle treated with ART. *J Can Chiropr Assoc.* 2003;47(1):28-32.
41. Wearing SC, Smeathers JE, Urry SR, Hennig EM, Hills AP. The pathomechanics of plantar fasciitis. *Sports Med.* 2006;36(7):585-611.
42. Arinci Incel N, Genc H, Erdem HR, Yorgancioglu ZR. Muscle imbalance in hallux valgus: an electromyographic study. *Am J Phys Med Rehabil.* 2003;82(5):345-349.
43. Senda M, Takahara Y, Yagata Y, et al. Measurement of the muscle power of the toes in female marathon runners using a toe dynamometer. *Acta Med Okayama.* 1999;53(4):189-191.
44. Tome J, Nawoczenski DA, Flemister A, Houck J. Comparison of foot kinematics between subjects with posterior tibialis tendon dysfunction and healthy controls. *J Orthop Sports Phys Ther.* 2006;36(9):635-644.
45. Ryan M, Grau S, Krauss I, Maiwald C, Taunton J, Horstmann T. Kinematic analysis of runners with achilles mid-portion tendinopathy. *Foot Ankle Int.* 2009;30(12):1190-1195.
46. Powers CM, Maffucci R, Hampton S. Rearfoot posture in subjects with patellofemoral pain. *J Orthop Sports Phys Ther.* 1995;22(4):155-160.
47. Gooding TM, Feger MA, Hart JM, Hertel J. Intrinsic foot muscle activation during specific exercises: a t2 time magnetic resonance imaging study. *J Athl Train.* 2016;51(8):644-650.
48. Jung DY, Kim MH, Koh EK, Kwon OY, Cynn HS, Lee WH. A comparison in the muscle activity of the abductor hallucis and the medial longitudinal arch angle during toe curl and short foot exercises. *Phys Ther Sport.* 2011;12(1):30-35.
49. Kim MH, Kwon OY, Kim SH, Jung DY. Comparison of muscle activities of abductor hallucis and adductor hallucis between the short foot and toe-spread-out exercises in subjects with mild hallux valgus. *J Back Musculoskelet Rehabil.* 2013;26(2):163-168.

Chapter 71

Clinical Considerations of Leg, Ankle, and Foot Pain

Jeffrey Gervais Ebert, Stella Fuensalida-Novo, and César Fernández de las Peñas

1. ANKLE SPRAIN—ANKLE INSTABILITY

1.1. Overview

Ankle sprains represent one of the most common lesions of the leg. Doherty et al[1] found a higher incidence of ankle sprains in women than in men, and in children and adolescents than in adults. The sport category with the highest incidence of ankle sprain was indoor/court sports, and lateral ankle sprain was much more prevalent than medial ankle sprain.[1] Acute ankle sprains are often described according to the severity of the injury and classified as grade I, II, or III depending on the extent and severity of ligament damage (grade I is the least involved and grade III the most severe type of injury).[2] Conservative management is the initial treatment option for ankle sprains; however, the most appropriate treatment strategy is unclear. A recent meta-analysis revealed significant immediate benefits of joint mobilization for improving dynamic balance and weight-bearing ankle dorsiflexion range of motion in patients with ankle sprains; however, long-term effects are still unknown.[3] Another recent meta-analysis found strong evidence for nonsteroidal anti-inflammatory drugs (NSAIDs) and early mobilization and moderate evidence for exercise and manual therapies for improving pain and function in acute ankle sprain.[4]

It should be considered that ankle sprains may be a self-limited condition in around 50% of individuals; however, when symptoms continue after an ankle injury, mostly associated with lateral ankle sprains, patients are commonly diagnosed as having ankle instability. Chronic ankle instability has been defined as the presence of persistent postacute symptoms such as occasional swelling, impaired strength, instability, and impaired balance responses for greater than 6 months following the initial ankle injury.[5] Doherty et al[6] identified an inability to complete jumping and landing tasks within 2 weeks of a first-time lateral ankle sprain, poorer dynamic postural control, and lower self-reported function 6 months after a first-time lateral ankle sprain as being predictive of eventual chronic ankle instability. Functional ankle instability can be defined as recurrent ankle sprains or ongoing sensations of the ankle giving way with normal ankle motion and the absence of objective joint laxity. Some studies have reported that manual therapy, including joint mobilization techniques, is effective for the management of ankle instability[7-9]; however, the quality of these studies is low.[10]

It seems that neuromuscular/proprioceptive interventions are the most appropriate for the treatment of ankle instability,[11] which suggests that the targeted structure for the management of ankle instability is the musculature. In fact, factors that contribute to functional ankle instability include muscle weakness, impaired muscle recruitment patterns, reduced ankle range of motion, balance deficits, and impaired joint proprioception. There is evidence demonstrating that subjects with ankle instability exhibit delayed fibularis muscle reaction time when compared with the contralateral uninvolved limb or a healthy control group.[12] These findings support a potential role of trigger points (TrPs) in the leg musculature in patients with ankle sprain or functional ankle instability.

1.2. Initial Evaluation of a Patient With Ankle Sprain

Initial examination of a patient with an ankle sprain starts with assessment of the injury mechanism because it can assist in determining the likelihood of the presence of a fracture. The Ottawa Ankle Rules were developed in 1992 to reduce the frequency of radiographic imaging following ankle sprain. These rules dictate that in the presence of a traumatic injury to the ankle, there is a need for an ankle radiographic series if a patient exhibits the following: (1) tenderness at the posterior edge or tip of the lateral malleolus, (2) tenderness at the posterior edge or tip of the medial malleolus, and/or (3) inability to bear weight both immediately postinjury and in the emergency room for four steps (including limping).[13]

Pain distribution or the presence of paresthesias can help differentiate comorbid conditions such as osteochondritis dissecans of the subtalar joint or ankle anterior impingement. Clinical examination of the ankle and foot should include palpation of the ligaments of the ankle and foot, passive and active ankle range of motion in both nonweight- and weight-bearing positions, assessment of passive physiologic movements of the ankle and foot joints, and specific orthopedic special tests. For instance, the anterior drawer test can be used for assessing the integrity of the anterior inferior tibiofibular ligament,[14] whereas the medial talar tilt test can be used to assess the amount of talar inversion occurring within the ankle mortise, testing the integrity of the calcaneofibular ligament.[15] Trigger points in the fibularis longus or fibularis brevis, tibialis anterior, gastrocnemius, and soleus muscles can be related to symptoms associated with ankle sprains or ankle instability. Finally, it is important to evaluate the stability of the entire lower extremity with functional tests such as single limb balance or the Star Excursion Balance Test.[16]

1.3. Trigger Points and Ankle Sprain

Trigger points in the fibularis muscles can refer pain to the lateral aspect of the ankle, mimicking the symptoms experienced after an ankle sprain.[17] Additionally, TrPs in these muscles could contribute to motor disturbances and delayed activation in the fibularis muscles found in individuals with functional ankle instability. Nevertheless, there are no epidemiologic studies published on this topic. Salom-Moreno et al[18] found that subjects with functional ankle instability who received TrP dry needling into the fibularis longus muscle before application of a proprioceptive and strengthening exercise program exhibited better improvements in pain and function than those receiving proprioceptive and strengthening exercise program in isolation. The greatest benefits found with application of dry needling were in functional outcomes, supporting the hypothesis that TrPs in the fibularis muscles could be related to motor disturbances observed in these patients.[18]

2. TIBIALIS POSTERIOR TENDON DYSFUNCTION

2.1. Overview

The tibialis posterior muscle is one of the dynamic stabilizers active during the late midstance and push-off phases of gait.[19] Therefore, tibialis posterior tendon dysfunction, also known as tibialis posterior tendinopathy, involves the progressive loss of this stabilization function. Although this condition can be present at any age, it is commonly seen in middle-aged women who are overweight.[20] It also tends to affect the athletic population, particularly runners and those involved in sports that require rapid changes in direction, such as basketball or soccer.[21] The etiology of this syndrome includes inflammatory, degenerative, functional, and traumatic processes often secondary to systemic inflammatory diseases. Tibialis posterior tendon dysfunction secondary to chronic overuse and subsequent tendon degeneration occurs more frequently in late middle-aged women.[21] Tibialis posterior tendon dysfunction has been described using a four-stage classification system ranging from mild signs and symptoms consistent with tendinopathy to a fixed hindfoot valgus deformity.[22-24]

There is no agreement regarding the efficacy of conservative treatment approaches for tibialis posterior tendinopathy.[25] General recommendations include relative rest, pain medication, physical therapy, and walking cast or ankle foot orthosis in stage I, referral to an orthopedic surgeon in stage II, or surgical repair in stage III or IV.[26,27] Exercises to strengthen the weakened tibialis posterior musculotendinous complex, albeit in the presence of painful tendon dysfunction, are strongly recommended.[27]

2.2. Initial Evaluation of a Patient With Tibialis Posterior Tendon Dysfunction

In stage I, patients with tibialis posterior tendon dysfunction may report mild pain over the medial aspect of the ankle and along the path of the posterior tibialis tendon that is aggravated by activity. Physical examination reveals tenderness and possible swelling over the course of the tendon. Tendon length is typically normal.[28] In this stage, pathologic examination of the tendon reveals tenosynovial proliferation.[29] Additional findings may include normal foot and ankle alignment and mild weakness on a single-leg heel raise test. No bony structural changes are expected on radiographic images.[28]

In stage II, pain is moderate and typically becomes more debilitating, and swelling and tenderness with palpation are more pronounced. The posterior tibial tendon is lengthened, resulting in a pes planus deformity.[28] Pathologic examination indicates degenerative changes with longitudinal tears within the tendon.[29] There is significant weakness with a single-leg heel raise test, and there is a visible, yet mobile, valgus deformity of the hindfoot. The "too many toes" sign (sensitivity 65%-80%) is evident. Radiographs reveal forefoot abduction relative to the hindfoot, and a talonavicular subluxation is likely present.[28]

In stages III and IV, the pain can become severe and may present over the lateral aspect of the ankle in addition to the medial aspect. There is pronounced lengthening and disruption of the tendon. Physical examination often reveals less swelling, but the deformity is more severe.[28] Pathologic examination indicates tendon disruption with visible tearing.[29] There is significant pain and weakness with a single-leg heel raise test. The hindfoot valgus and forefoot abduction deformities are now typically fixed, and the "too many toes" sign is still evident. Radiographs reveal the same changes seen in stage II along with degenerative changes in the subtalar, talonavicular, and calcaneocuboid joints.[28] Deltoid ligament insufficiency resulting in a lateral talar tilt indicates the progression to stage IV.[23] The 1st-metatarsal rise test, which has demonstrated excellent sensitivity, can also be used in the examination.

Examination of a patient with tibialis posterior tendon dysfunction, independent of the stage, should include postural analysis of gait behaviors and an exhaustive clinical evaluation of the lower extremity. Passive and active range of motion of the foot, ankle, knee, and hip, with or without overpressure should be included. Because the tibialis posterior tendon runs closer to the tibialis posterior nerve in the tarsal tunnel, a differential diagnosis with a potential neuropathy should include neurodynamic test of this nerve.[30] All musculature of the lower extremity should be palpated for the presence of TrPs, especially the tibialis posterior, tibialis anterior, gastrocnemius, and soleus muscles.

2.3. Trigger Points in Tibialis Posterior Tendon Dysfunction

Examination for the presence of TrPs is important with a potential diagnosis of tibialis posterior tendon dysfunction. There are several muscles whose TrPs refer pain to the medial ankle region, where tibialis posterior tendon dysfunction symptoms are most prevalent. Trigger points in the flexor digitorum longus muscle can refer pain to the medial aspect of the ankle.[17] Abductor hallucis TrPs can also result in pain in the same region.[17] Therefore, it is important to look for TrPs in these muscles as alternate sources of, or as contributors to, tibialis posterior tendon dysfunction pain.

Trigger points in the tibialis posterior muscle can, on occasion, refer pain symptoms along the course of its own tendon[17]; however, it is more likely a contributor to the development of tibialis posterior tendon dysfunction. The presence of TrPs in the tibialis posterior muscle can lead to medial arch collapse because of impaired function of the muscle.[17,31,32]

3. TARSAL TUNNEL SYNDROME

3.1. Overview

Tarsal tunnel syndrome is an entrapment neuropathy of the posterior tibial nerve and/or one or more of its associated terminal branches, including the medial plantar, lateral plantar, and calcaneal nerves.[33,34] The tarsal tunnel runs deep to the fascia and the flexor retinaculum, and within the abductor hallucis muscle, a nerve entrapment can occur at any of these points along the tunnel.[35] A particular cause of tarsal tunnel syndrome can be identified in 60% to 80% of cases, with the remaining ones being idiopathic.[36,37]

Intrinsic factors that can cause tarsal tunnel syndrome include osteophytes, hypertrophic retinaculum tendinopathy, hypertrophy of the extensor hallucis brevis muscle, lipoma, ganglion cysts, venous varicosities, pseudoaneurysms,[34,38] tumors, accessory muscles,[39,40] and other space-occupying lesions. In addition, the fascial septa and the flexor retinaculum themselves have been identified as sources of entrapment.[41] Entrapment of the lateral plantar nerve as it passes through the abductor hallucis muscle[42] or between the abductor hallucis and flexor accessorius (quadratus plantae) muscles can result in plantar heel pain[43] and is often associated with, or mistaken for, plantar fasciitis.[44,45] In fact, tarsal tunnel syndrome has also been associated with an accessory soleus[46] or flexor digitorum longus[47] muscle.

Extrinsic factors can include trauma, tight-fitting shoes, hindfoot varus or valgus, lower extremity edema, systemic inflammatory arthropathy, mucolipidoses, and diabetes.[34] The incidence of tarsal tunnel syndrome is unknown but is believed to occur primarily in adults and affects women more than men.[48-50] Tarsal tunnel syndrome is a relatively rare condition with a variable presentation and symptom severity depending on the specific nerve(s) involved,[51] and consequently, it can often be misdiagnosed if a clinician does not consider it a likely diagnosis.[52,53]

3.2. Initial Evaluation of a Patient With Tarsal Tunnel Syndrome

Although specific symptoms of an entrapment neuropathy will vary based on the nerve(s) involved, patients with tarsal tunnel syndrome will typically report burning, tingling, and pain along the plantar aspect of the foot. Occasionally, pain can extend proximally to the medial aspect or midcalf region of the leg.[54,55] Sensory changes are limited to the distribution of the terminal branches of the posterior tibial nerve. As a result, the dorsal aspect of the foot is not usually involved. Symptoms tend to worsen with walking, prolonged standing, or wearing high-heeled shoes, and patients will often report that their symptoms are worst at night. Symptoms are typically unilateral, so in patients with bilateral symptoms, underlying systemic illness and polyneuropathy should be ruled out.[54] Symptoms are often alleviated by rest and elevation of the leg.[56]

Palpation and visual inspection should be utilized to locate soft-tissue masses on the tibial nerve course, varicosities, or hindfoot misalignment.[57] In severe or chronic cases, muscles innervated by the tibial nerve, distal to the site of entrapment, may show atrophy and motor deficit, although these manifestations rarely interfere with function.[52,57]

Patients may demonstrate a positive Tinel sign.[56] Neural tension with selective targeting of the tibial nerve can reproduce symptoms by positioning the foot and ankle in a combination of dorsiflexion and eversion.[30,58-60]

Nerve conduction testing and electromyography (EMG) can be helpful in diagnosing tarsal tunnel syndrome[61,62]; however, nerve conduction studies for this condition have a high false-negative rate, whereas EMG has been shown to have a high false-positive rate.[61] Therefore, negative nerve conduction studies do not necessarily rule out a diagnosis of tarsal tunnel syndrome.[37,56,62] Pain and paresthesia in the foot, a positive Tinel sign, and positive electrodiagnostic studies are considered strong indicators for the presence of tarsal tunnel syndrome when all three are present.[63,64]

Clinicians should inquire about the presence of low back pain to help rule out a lumbar spine condition as a source of the patient's foot and ankle symptoms. Reflex testing and determining the distribution of sensory and motor deficits are essential in making a differential diagnosis.[65]

Similarly to evaluating a patient with tibialis posterior tendon dysfunction, clinical examination of a patient with tarsal tunnel syndrome should include postural analysis of gait behaviors and an exhaustive clinical evaluation of the lower extremity. Passive and active range of motion of the foot, ankle, knee, and hip, with or without overpressure, should be included. Musculature of the leg and foot related to the tibial nerve, such as the tibialis posterior, gastrocnemius, soleus, abductor hallucis, flexor accessories (quadratus plantae) muscles, should be examined for the presence of TrPs.

3.3. Trigger Points in Tarsal Tunnel Syndrome

There is no epidemiologic study on tarsal tunnel syndrome and the presence of TrPs. Trigger point referral patterns themselves are not always implicated by the burning and tingling symptoms often reported by patients with tarsal tunnel syndrome.[17] However, TrPs in the abductor hallucis muscle could mimic or contribute to the painful symptoms associated with a particular form of tarsal tunnel syndrome. Trigger points in the abductor hallucis muscle can contribute to shortening of the muscle and increase the likelihood of entrapment of the lateral plantar nerve as it passes through the abductor hallucis muscle or between abductor hallucis and flexor accessorius (quadratus plantae) muscles, potentially resulting in pain and paresthesias.[45] Trigger points in the tibialis posterior or soleus muscles could also contribute to potential entrapment of the tibial nerve through its course in the lower extremity.

4. PLANTAR HEEL PAIN OR PLANTAR FASCIITIS

4.1. Overview

Plantar fasciitis, also referred to as plantar fasciosis or plantar heel pain, consists of a sharp pain at the insertion of the plantar fascia at the medial tuberosity of the calcaneus and along the medial border of the plantar fascia. Previously believed to involve inflammation of the plantar fascia aponeurosis, current evidence indicates that this condition is the result of microscopic degeneration of collagen with subsequent thickening of the plantar fascia caused by chronic overload.[66-69] Pathologic changes within the foot intrinsic musculature, that is, atrophy of the abductor digiti minimi muscle[70] or forefoot intrinsic muscles,[71] have also been reported in people with plantar heel pain.

Plantar heel pain affects 10% of the population at some point in their lifetime.[72] It is the most common foot condition seen by healthcare practitioners[72] and tends to affect middle-aged people who are sedentary. It is also commonly seen in people who engage in activities such as running and dancing that require significant ankle plantar flexion and metatarsophalangeal joint extension.[73] Several factors have been identified that put patients at greater risk for developing plantar heel pain. These include increased body mass index, particularly in a sedentary population,[74-76] increased age, occupations requiring prolonged standing on hard surfaces,[77] reduced ankle dorsiflexion range of motion, reduced 1st metatarsophalangeal extension range of motion, prolonged standing,[75] and tightness of the calf and hamstring muscles.[78] Weakness or atrophy of the ankle plantar flexors and toe flexor muscles has also been observed in individuals with plantar heel pain.[71,79-81]

Management of plantar heel pain is controversial because numerous interventions are used such as strapping, stretching, foot orthoses, shoe modifications, NSAIDs, corticoid injections, education, exercise, modalities, manual therapy, weight reduction, and laser therapy.[82,83] A recent meta-analysis has found that TrP dry needling is effective for reducing pain compared with placebo in plantar fasciitis.[84] These findings would suggest that TrPs in the foot musculature can play a relevant role in this condition.

4.2. Initial Evaluation of a Patient With Plantar Heel Pain

Patients with plantar heel pain typically present with insidious pain at the insertion of the plantar fascia on the calcaneus and often report pain along the length of the plantar fascia medially. A classic symptom of plantar fasciitis is a pronounced increase in pain with the first step after a period of inactivity.[72,85] The onset of plantar heel pain often coincides with a change in the type and level of activity or a change in footwear. As the condition progresses, these symptoms can become more severe and can impact the patient's ability to bear weight. According to the updated clinical practice guidelines from the Academy of Orthopaedic Physical Therapy of the American Physical Therapy Association, the signs and symptoms fitting the diagnosis of plantar heel pain or plantar fasciitis include the following: medial plantar heel pain with initial steps after inactivity, increased heel pain with weight-bearing activity, pain with palpation of the calcaneal insertion of the plantar fascia, reduced ankle dorsiflexion range of motion, an abnormal foot posture index score, a high body mass index in a nonathlete, a positive windlass test, and negative tarsal tunnel tests.[72]

Although imaging is typically not necessary for diagnosis of plantar heel pain, diagnostic ultrasound may be useful in some cases.[72] Diagnostic ultrasound can be used to assess the thickness of the plantar fascia. A reduction in plantar fascia thickness has been linked to a reduction in plantar heel pain.[68,86]

Clinical examination of a patient with plantar heel pain should include palpation of the soft-tissue structures of the ankle and foot, passive and active ankle and foot range of motion in both nonweight- and weight-bearing positions, and evaluation of accessory motion of the ankle and foot joints. Trigger points in the soleus, gastrocnemius, quadratus plantae, abductor hallucis, and flexor digitorum brevis muscles are considered relevant for the management of plantar heel pain.[87]

4.3. Trigger Points and Plantar Heel Pain

Trigger points are a significant potential source of or contributor to plantar heel pain, including those of several intrinsic and extrinsic muscles of the foot.[17] Trigger points in the abductor hallucis muscle refer pain at or near the plantar aspect of the heel that can mimic plantar heel pain.[17] Trigger points in the abductor hallucis muscle can result in entrapment of the lateral plantar nerve, which can also result in plantar heel pain.[45] Extrinsic foot muscles, including the tibialis posterior and flexor digitorum longus muscles, can also have TrPs that mimic pain associated with plantar heel pain.[17]

Trigger points in the gastrocnemius muscle not only have a referral pattern that includes the plantar heel region, but they can also mimic many of the "classic" signs and symptoms of plantar fasciitis very closely. Individuals with TrPs in the gastrocnemius muscle may report sharp pain along the plantar surface of the heel with weight-bearing activities, especially with the first few steps upon waking in the morning or after a prolonged period of nonweight bearing. In fact, treatment of TrPs in the gastrocnemius muscle was effective for the management of patients with plantar heel pain.[88] Saban et al[89] found that deep massage of the calf muscles, neural mobilization exercises, and a self-stretch program were also effective for plantar fasciitis. These results support the role of muscle TrPs in this condition.

Although they are not a direct source of plantar heel pain, TrPs in muscles that support the medial longitudinal arch and/or contribute to foot stability during gait, such as the flexor digitorum brevis muscle,[90] have been shown to be prevalent with many cases of plantar heel pain.[91,92] Trigger points in these muscles can lead to dysfunction that results in overuse injuries related to excessive pronation, including plantar heel pain.[92,93] Nevertheless, TrPs in the flexor accessorius (quadratus plantae) muscle would probably be the most relevant in plantar fasciitis because taut bands in this muscle can increase tension in the plantar fascia at the calcaneal tuberosity.[17]

5. METATARSAL STRESS FRACTURE

5.1. Overview

Repetitive loading of bone without sufficient opportunity for the bone tissue to adapt can result in structural changes and reduced ability to withstand loading at the site(s) of maximal stress.[94,95] Stress fractures of the metatarsals are one of the most common overuse injuries in athletes, making up nearly 4% of all sport-related injuries.[96] Metatarsal stress fractures account for nearly 10% to 20% of all stress fractures,[97-101] and fractures of the 2nd and 3rd metatarsals comprise as many as 90% of metatarsal stress fractures.[96,102,103] The 2nd through 4th metatarsals are the least resistant to bending stresses but sustain the highest peak loading forces during weight-bearing activity, especially running.[101,104] The incidence of metatarsal stress fractures in women is 1.5 to 12 times greater than that in men.[105-111]

5.2. Initial Evaluation of a Patient With Metatarsal Stress Fracture

Patients with metatarsal stress fracture often report a dull aching pain in the forefoot with weight-bearing activity and increased pain with palpation of the involved bone. There may be swelling and erythema in the surrounding soft tissue.[112,113] Clinicians should examine patients for structural foot abnormalities such as pes cavus or hypomobility of the first ray.[112,114] Misdiagnosis of arthritis or tendinopathy is common, so a careful history will typically reveal recent changes in the type, duration, and/or frequency of walking or running activity without a specific traumatic event.[113] Early diagnosis is important to prevent progression to a complete fracture.[115]

Radiography in the early stages of metatarsal stress fracture may not reveal pathology. It can take 3 to 6 weeks following the initial fracture before any findings will be evident on a radiograph.[116] Early diagnosis of stress fracture is often based on magnetic resonance imaging, which is expensive.[117] More recently, diagnostic ultrasound has shown good reliability for early diagnosis of stress fracture at a significantly lower cost.[115]

Once the fracture has been stabilized, clinical examination of the hindfoot and forefoot joint passive accessory movements, with and without overpressure, should be conducted. Further, palpation of the intrinsic foot muscles, such as the dorsal interosseous and lumbrical muscles, is also recommended.

5.3. Trigger Points and Metatarsal Stress Fracture

Trigger points can produce pain that refers to the plantar aspect of the forefoot and mimics the symptoms associated with metatarsal stress fracture. Intrinsic foot muscles associated with this pain referral pattern include the flexor digitorum brevis, flexor digitorum longus, flexor hallucis brevis, extensor digitorum brevis, abductor hallucis, abductor digiti minimi, and the interosseous muscles.[118] Extrinsic foot muscles that can create pain at or around the metatarsal heads include the extensor hallucis longus, tibialis posterior, flexor digitorum longus, and flexor hallucis longus muscles.[118]

6. MORTON NEUROMA

6.1. Overview

Morton neuroma is a benign but painful mechanical entrapment neuropathy involving a common digital nerve in the forefoot.[119] Its name is a misnomer as it is not a true neuroma but rather a fibrosis of the perineurium.[120] Morton neuroma most commonly occurs between the 3rd and 4th metatarsals.[121] No data currently exist regarding the prevalence of Morton neuroma in the general population; however, women are affected more often than men.[121,122] The average age of those affected is between 45 and 50 years old.[122] It can occur bilaterally but rarely involves more than one site within the same foot.[121] Approximately one-third of people who have a Morton neuroma are asymptomatic, with the likelihood of pain increasing as the size of the fibrous tissue formation increases.[123]

Although the exact cause of Morton neuroma is unknown, several factors have been described that may contribute to the condition. It is believed, in part, to affect women more than men because women's shoes more often have a tight-fitting toe box and/or high heels.[124] Runners and dancers are more prone to the condition because of hyperextension of the metatarsophalangeal joints and repetitive trauma to the metatarsals.[124] Age-related structural changes are believed to increase the risk of developing a Morton neuroma.[125,126] Biomechanical factors such as overpronation, pes cavus, and equinus deformity are often associated with the condition. It is proposed that overpronation causes forefoot instability during gait, resulting in excessive traction and strain of the plantar digital nerves.[127] Pes cavus and equinus deformity are believed to be a factor because of the increased strain on the plantar fascia and transverse intermetatarsal ligament.[128] A Cochrane review concluded that there is insufficient evidence to determine the effectiveness of either surgical or nonsurgical interventions for Morton neuroma.[129]

6.2. Initial Evaluation of a Patient With Morton Neuroma

Patients with Morton neuroma often report the insidious onset of a burning pain in the ball of the foot, worsened by activity and tight footwear and relieved by rest.[123,130] The pain is occasionally described as dull and cramping with brief episodes of sharp pain, or it may be described as numb and tingly.[121] Patients may report a sensation of having a small rock in their shoe when walking.[130]

Several examination procedures can help reach a diagnosis of Morton neuroma. Reproduction of the patient's symptoms with direct pressure applied at the 3rd intermetatarsal space is indicative of the condition, especially if combined with compression of the five metatarsal heads together.[119] If a click is elicited during compression of the metatarsal heads, this is known as Mulder sign and is also indicative of Morton neuroma.[119,121,131,132]

Although usually unnecessary, imaging in the form of magnetic resonance[123,131,133] or ultrasonography[119,134-136] has shown good validity and reliability data for the diagnosis of Morton neuroma. Utilization of a nerve block has been advocated for diagnosis. If the block provides symptom relief, it is considered indicative of Morton neuroma.[132,137,138]

Clinical examination of the hindfoot and forefoot joint passive accessory movements, with and without overpressure, should be conducted. Further, palpation of the intrinsic foot muscles, such as the dorsal interosseous and lumbrical muscles, is also recommended.

6.3. Trigger Points and Morton Neuroma

Trigger points of several muscles can result in pain in the forefoot and metatarsal region, as in the case of pain experienced with Morton neuroma. The muscle(s) involved depend on the exact symptom location. Intrinsic foot muscles associated with this pain referral pattern are the flexor digitorum brevis, flexor digitorum longus, flexor hallucis brevis, extensor digitorum brevis, abductor hallucis, abductor digiti minimi, and the interosseous muscles.[17] Extrinsic foot muscles that can create pain at or around the metatarsal heads are the extensor hallucis longus, tibialis posterior, flexor digitorum longus, and flexor hallucis longus muscles.[17]

7. HALLUX VALGUS

7.1. Overview

Hallux valgus, one of the most common structural deformities of the foot, is a lateral displacement of the great toe.[139-141] It is a progressive, irreversible condition[142] involving lateral, or valgus, displacement of the great toe with a medial, or varus, displacement of the 1st metatarsal.[139,142-144] Hallux valgus deformity also usually involves an overgrowth of bone—called exostosis—and other tissue that forms on the dorsomedial aspect of the 1st metatarsal head, commonly known as a "bunion."[143,145] It is believed to affect 12% to 70% of the general population,[140,146,147] with a larger prevalence in women (as much as 30%-58%) than in men.[146,148] It is especially prevalent in women during the third through sixth decades of life.[139,140]

There is no single definitive cause for hallux valgus; rather, there exist a multitude of factors involved in the development of the deformity.[139,142] These factors include tight or high-heeled footwear,[139,149] abnormalities in foot anatomy and/or foot mechanics,[150-152] leg length discrepancy,[139] inflammatory conditions,[153,154] occupational demands,[139] and genetics.[155-157]

7.2. Initial Evaluation of a Patient With Hallux Valgus

Diagnosis of hallux valgus is based largely on visual inspection, as the deformity is typically evident on observation. Patients with hallux valgus will typically report pain over the dorsomedial aspect of the 1st metatarsophalangeal joint and often present with callus formation or bunion deformity.[139,158] Patients may also report pain where the great toe and second toe overlap, or they may experience midfoot pain.[158] Additional alignment issues or structural deformities may also be observed, including pronation of the great toe, lateral shift of the sesamoid bones, medial arch collapse,[143,145] and leg length discrepancy.[139] Patients should be examined for intrinsic foot muscle weakness, as this is believed to play a role in the development and/or exacerbation of hallux valgus.[159,160] In addition, TrPs of the great toe can be involved.[118]

A thorough history should include questions about footwear, because shoes with a narrow toe box or high heels can increase the progression of hallux valgus.[149] The clinician should also inquire about occupational requirements[139] and family history of foot problems.[139,155-157]

Clinical examination of the hindfoot and forefoot joint passive accessory movements, with and without overpressure, should be conducted. Further, palpation of the intrinsic foot muscles, such as dorsal interosseous and lumbrical muscles, is also recommended.

7.3. Trigger Points and Hallux Valgus

Several muscles can refer pain to the region of the great toe and 1st metatarsal head. The flexor hallucis longus, flexor hallucis brevis, tibialis posterior, first dorsal interosseous,[17] and tibialis anterior muscles[118] have all been implicated in pain in this region. Trigger points in the intrinsic muscles of the foot, such as the abductor hallucis muscle, can result in weakness or dysfunction of those muscles. As mentioned earlier, this type of dysfunction may be involved in the development or progression of hallux valgus.[159,160]

In addition, according to Travell & Simons, ill-fitting footwear can activate or perpetuate TrPs in muscles of the foot.[17] Given the link between tightly fitting or high-heeled shoes and the development or exacerbation of hallux valgus,[149] it is important to strongly consider the role of footwear when it comes to pain at or around the great toe.

8. SESAMOIDITIS

8.1. Overview

Sesamoiditis is a condition involving pain and inflammation of the sesamoid bones of the first ray of the foot and their associated peritendinous structures.[161-163] It most commonly affects the medial sesamoid and is often associated with a previous history of trauma.[161,163] The prevalence of this condition is higher in teenagers and young adults,[162,164] and it is most commonly seen in dancers and runners. Prevalence rates for dancers are unknown, but for runners, sesamoid disorders, in general, make up 12% of great toe injuries, 4% to 9% of foot and ankle injuries, and 1.2% of all running-related injuries.[165-167]

Factors that may predispose individuals to sesamoiditis include a cavus foot posture with a plantar flexed first ray, asymmetry between medial and lateral sesamoid size, rotational malalignment, and enlargement of both sesamoids.[162] Footwear, particularly high-heeled shoes, can contribute to this condition.[164]

8.2. Initial Evaluation of a Patient With Sesamoiditis

Patients with sesamoiditis will report pain localized under the 1st metatarsal head during weight-bearing activity. Patients will often recall a single incident that started their symptoms, but some cases will not be associated with a traumatic event.[161] Patients will typically experience pain with direct palpation of the sesamoids and the plantar aspect of the 1st metatarsophalangeal joint,[164,168] and crepitus may be felt along the distal path of the flexor hallucis longus tendon.[165,169] Because of the proximity of the sesamoid bones to the flexor hallucis longus tendon, palpation alone cannot be relied on to make a definitive diagnosis.[161] Motion at the 1st metatarsophalangeal joint is often painful and limited,[164,168] and patients may exhibit swelling around the joint. Plantar flexion and dorsiflexion strength of the great toe are likely to be reduced. In some cases, callus formation may be present under the sesamoids.[164] Patients should be assessed for postural or alignment issues such as pes cavus and a plantar flexed first ray.[162]

True sesamoiditis does not result in radiographic changes, which can be helpful in distinguishing it from other sesamoid pathologies such as fracture or osteochondritis.[161,162]

Clinical examination of the hindfoot and forefoot joint passive accessory movements, with and without overpressure, should be conducted. Further, palpation of the intrinsic foot muscles, such as dorsal interosseous and lumbrical muscles, is also recommended.

8.3. Trigger Points and Sesamoiditis

Trigger point involvement for sesamoiditis is quite similar to that of hallux valgus,[17] and the flexor hallucis longus, flexor hallucis brevis, tibialis posterior, first dorsal interosseous, and tibialis anterior muscles need to be considered.[118]

As mentioned in the hallux valgus section, ill-fitting footwear can activate or perpetuate TrPs in muscles of the foot, resulting in pain in the region of the great toe.[17] Consequently, it is important to consider the role of footwear when it comes to pain at or around this region (see Chapter 77 Footwear Considerations).

References

1. Doherty C, Delahunt E, Caulfield B, Hertel J, Ryan J, Bleakley C. The incidence and prevalence of ankle sprain injury: a systematic review and meta-analysis of prospective epidemiological studies. *Sports Med.* 2014;44(1):123-140.
2. Martin RL, Davenport TE, Paulseth S, Wukich DK, Godges JJ; Orthopaedic Section American Physical Therapy Association. Ankle stability and movement coordination impairments: ankle ligament sprains. *J Orthop Sports Phys Ther.* 2013;43(9):A1-A40.
3. Weerasekara I, Osmotherly P, Snodgrass S, Marquez J, de Zoete R, Rivett DA. Clinical benefits of joint mobilization on ankle sprains: a systematic review and meta-analysis. *Arch Phys Med Rehabil.* 2017.
4. Doherty C, Bleakley C, Delahunt E, Holden S. Treatment and prevention of acute and recurrent ankle sprain: an overview of systematic reviews with meta-analysis. *Br J Sports Med.* 2017;51(2):113-125.
5. O'Loughlin PF, Murawski CD, Egan C, Kennedy JG. Ankle instability in sports. *Phys Sportsmed.* 2009;37(2):93-103.
6. Doherty C, Bleakley C, Hertel J, Caulfield B, Ryan J, Delahunt E. Recovery from a first-time lateral ankle sprain and the predictors of chronic ankle instability: a prospective cohort analysis. *Am J Sports Med.* 2016;44(4):995-1003.
7. van der Wees PJ, Lenssen AF, Hendriks EJ, Stomp DJ, Dekker J, de Bie RA. Effectiveness of exercise therapy and manual mobilisation in ankle sprain and functional instability: a systematic review. *Aust J Physiother.* 2006;52(1):27-37.
8. Harkey M, McLeod M, Van Scoit A, et al. The immediate effects of an anterior-to-posterior talar mobilization on neural excitability, dorsiflexion range of motion, and dynamic balance in patients with chronic ankle instability. *J Sport Rehabil.* 2014;23(4):351-359.
9. Cruz-Diaz D, Lomas Vega R, Osuna-Perez MC, Hita-Contreras F, Martinez-Amat A. Effects of joint mobilization on chronic ankle instability: a randomized controlled trial. *Disabil Rehabil.* 2015;37(7):601-610.
10. Kosik KB, Gribble PA. The effect of joint mobilization on dynamic postural control in patients with chronic ankle instability: a critically appraised topic. *J Sport Rehabil.* 2016:1-15.
11. de Vries JS, Krips R, Sierevelt IN, Blankevoort L, van Dijk CN. Interventions for treating chronic ankle instability. *Cochrane Database Syst Rev.* 2011(8):CD004124.
12. Hoch MC, McKeon PO. Peroneal reaction time after ankle sprain: a systematic review and meta-analysis. *Med Sci Sports Exerc.* 2014;46(3):546-556.
13. Bachmann LM, Kolb E, Koller MT, Steurer J, ter Riet G. Accuracy of Ottawa ankle rules to exclude fractures of the ankle and mid-foot: systematic review. *BMJ.* 2003;326(7386):417.
14. Croy T, Koppenhaver S, Saliba S, Hertel J. Anterior talocrural joint laxity: diagnostic accuracy of the anterior drawer test of the ankle. *J Orthop Sports Phys Ther.* 2013;43(12):911-919.
15. Hertel J, Denegar CR, Monroe MM, Stokes WL. Talocrural and subtalar joint instability after lateral ankle sprain. *Med Sci Sports Exerc.* 1999;31(11):1501-1508.
16. Hertel J, Braham RA, Hale SA, Olmsted-Kramer LC. Simplifying the star excursion balance test: analyses of subjects with and without chronic ankle instability. *J Orthop Sports Phys Ther.* 2006;36(3):131-137.
17. Simons DG, Travell J, Simons L. *Travell & Simon's Myofascial Pain and Dysfunction: The Trigger Point Manual.* Vol 1. 2nd ed. Baltimore, MD: Williams & Wilkins; 1999.
18. Salom-Moreno J, Ayuso-Casado B, Tamaral-Costa B, Sanchez-Mila Z, Fernández de las Peñas C, Alburquerque-Sendin F. Trigger point dry needling and proprioceptive exercises for the management of chronic ankle instability: a randomized clinical trial. *Evid Based Complement Alternat Med.* 2015;2015:790209.
19. Otis JC, Gage T. Function of the posterior tibial tendon muscle. *Foot Ankle Clin.* 2001;6(1):1-14, v.
20. Trnka HJ. Dysfunction of the tendon of tibialis posterior. *J Bone Joint Surg Br.* 2004;86(7):939-946.
21. Yao K, Yang TX, Yew WP. Posterior tibialis tendon dysfunction: overview of evaluation and management. *Orthopedics.* 2015;38(6):385-391.
22. Bluman EM, Title CI, Myerson MS. Posterior tibial tendon rupture: a refined classification system. *Foot Ankle Clin.* 2007;12(2):233-249, v.
23. Myerson MS. Adult acquired flatfoot deformity: treatment of dysfunction of the posterior tibial tendon. *Instr Course Lect.* 1997;46:393-405.
24. Ling SK, Lui TH. Posterior tibial tendon dysfunction: an overview. *Open Orthop J.* 2017;11:714-723.
25. Bowring B, Chockalingam N. Conservative treatment of tibialis posterior tendon dysfunction—a review. *Foot (Edinb).* 2010;20(1):18-26.
26. Kulig K, Reischl SF, Pomrantz AB, et al. Nonsurgical management of posterior tibial tendon dysfunction with orthoses and resistive exercise: a randomized controlled trial. *Phys Ther.* 2009;89(1):26-37.
27. Simpson MR, Howard TM. Tendinopathies of the foot and ankle. *Am Fam Physician.* 2009;80(10):1107-1114.
28. Johnson KA, Strom DE. Tibialis posterior tendon dysfunction. *Clin Orthop Relat Res.* 1989;(239):196-206.
29. Mueller TJ. Ruptures and lacerations of the tibialis posterior tendon. *J Am Podiatry Assoc.* 1984;74(3):109-119.
30. Boyd BS, Topp KS, Coppieters MW. Impact of movement sequencing on sciatic and tibial nerve strain and excursion during the straight leg raise test in embalmed cadavers. *J Orthop Sports Phys Ther.* 2013;43(6):398-403.
31. Zuil-Escobar JC, Martínez-Cepa CB, Martín-Urrialde JA, Gómez-Conesa A. Prevalence of myofascial trigger points and diagnostic criteria of different muscles in function of the medial longitudinal arch. *Arch Phys Med Rehabil.* 2015;96(6):1123-1130.
32. Tome J, Nawoczenski DA, Flemister A, Houck J. Comparison of foot kinematics between subjects with posterior tibialis tendon dysfunction and healthy controls. *J Orthop Sports Phys Ther.* 2006;36(9):635-644.
33. Abouelela AA, Zohiery AK. The triple compression stress test for diagnosis of tarsal tunnel syndrome. *Foot (Edinb).* 2012;22(3):146-149.
34. Doneddu PE, Coraci D, Loreti C, Piccinini G, Padua L. Tarsal tunnel syndrome: still more opinions than evidence. Status of the art. *Neurol Sci.* 2017;38(10):1735-1739.
35. Kohno M, Takahashi H, Segawa H, Sano K. Neurovascular decompression for idiopathic tarsal tunnel syndrome: technical note. *J Neurol Neurosurg Psychiatry.* 2000;69(1):87-90.
36. Lopez-Ben R. Imaging of nerve entrapment in the foot and ankle. *Foot Ankle Clin.* 2011;16(2):213-224.
37. Franson J, Baravarian B. Tarsal tunnel syndrome: a compression neuropathy involving four distinct tunnels. *Clin Podiatr Med Surg.* 2006;23(3):597-609.
38. Park SE, Kim JC, Ji JH, Kim YY, Lee HH, Jeong JJ. Post-traumatic pseudoaneurysm of the medial plantar artery combined with tarsal tunnel syndrome: two case reports. *Arch Orthop Trauma Surg.* 2013;133(3):357-360.
39. Deleu PA, Bevernage BD, Birch I, Maldague P, Gombault V, Leemrijse T. Anatomical characteristics of the flexor digitorum accessorius longus muscle

and their relevance to tarsal tunnel syndrome a systematic review. *J Am Podiatr Med Assoc.* 2015;105(4):344-355.
40. Molloy AP, Lyons R, Bergin D, Kearns SR. Flexor digitorum accessorius causing tarsal tunnel syndrome in a paediatric patient: a case report and review of the literature. *Foot Ankle Surg.* 2015;21(2):e48-e50.
41. Ferkel E, Davis WH, Ellington JK. Entrapment neuropathies of the foot and ankle. *Clin Sports Med.* 2015;34(4):791-801.
42. Kurashige T. Hypertrophy of the abductor hallucis muscle: a case report and review of the literature. *SAGE Open Med Case Rep.* 2017;5:2050313X17727638.
43. Rondhuis JJ, Huson A. The first branch of the lateral plantar nerve and heel pain. *Acta Morphol Neerl Scand.* 1986;24(4):269-279.
44. Alshami AM, Souvlis T, Coppieters MW. A review of plantar heel pain of neural origin: differential diagnosis and management. *Man Ther.* 2008;13(2):103-111.
45. Gould JS. Tarsal tunnel syndrome. *Foot Ankle Clin.* 2011;16(2):275-286.
46. Carrington SC, Stone P, Kruse D. Accessory soleus: a case report of exertional compartment and tarsal tunnel syndrome associated with an accessory soleus muscle. *J Foot Ankle Surg.* 2016;55(5):1076-1078.
47. Saar WE, Bell J. Accessory flexor digitorum longus presenting as tarsal tunnel syndrome: a case report. *Foot Ankle Spec.* 2011;4(6):379-382.
48. Lau JT, Daniels TR. Tarsal tunnel syndrome: a review of the literature. *Foot Ankle Int.* 1999;20(3):201-209.
49. Llanos L, Vila J, Nunez-Samper M. Clinical symptoms and treatment of the foot and ankle nerve entrapment syndromes. *Foot Ankle Surg.* 1999;5:211-218.
50. Joshi SS, Joshi SD, Athavale SA. Anatomy of tarsal tunnel and its applied significance. *J Anat Soc India.* 2006;55(1):52-56.
51. Lee MF, Chan PT, Chau LF, Yu KS. Tarsal tunnel syndrome caused by talocalcaneal coalition. *Clin Imaging.* 2002;26(2):140-143.
52. Antoniadis G, Scheglmann K. Posterior tarsal tunnel syndrome: diagnosis and treatment. *Dtsch Arztebl Int.* 2008;105(45):776-781.
53. Oh SJ, Meyer RD. Entrapment neuropathies of the tibial (posterior tibial) nerve. *Neurol Clin.* 1999;17(3):593-615, vii.
54. Merriman L, Turner W. *Assessment of the Lower Limb.* 2nd ed. London, England: Churchill Livingstone; 2002.
55. Tu P, Bytomski JR. Diagnosis of heel pain. *Am Fam Physician.* 2011;84(8):909-916.
56. Ahmad M, Tsang K, Mackenney PJ, Adedapo AO. Tarsal tunnel syndrome: a literature review. *Foot Ankle Surg.* 2012;18(3):149-152.
57. Campbell WW, Landau ME. Controversial entrapment neuropathies. *Neurosurg Clin N Am.* 2008;19(4):597-608, vi-vii.
58. Kinoshita M, Okuda R, Morikawa J, Jotoku T, Abe M. The dorsiflexion-eversion test for diagnosis of tarsal tunnel syndrome. *J Bone Joint Surg Am.* 2001;83-A(12):1835-1839.
59. Daniels TR, Lau JT, Hearn TC. The effects of foot position and load on tibial nerve tension. *Foot Ankle Int.* 1998;19(2):73-78.
60. Lau JT, Daniels TR. Effects of tarsal tunnel release and stabilization procedures on tibial nerve tension in a surgically created pes planus foot. *Foot Ankle Int.* 1998;19(11):770-777.
61. Pomeroy G, Wilton J, Anthony S. Entrapment neuropathy about the foot and ankle: an update. *J Am Acad Orthop Surg.* 2015;23(1):58-66.
62. Buxton WG, Dominick JE. Electromyography and nerve conduction studies of the lower extremity: uses and limitations. *Clin Podiatr Med Surg.* 2006;23(3):531-543.
63. Mann RA, Baxter DE. Diseases of the nerve. In: Mann RA, Coughlin JO, eds. *Surgery of the Foot and Ankle.* Vol 1. 6th ed. St Louis, MO: Mosby-Year Book; 1993:554-558.
64. Galardi G, Amadio S, Maderna L, et al. Electrophysiologic studies in tarsal tunnel syndrome. Diagnostic reliability of motor distal latency, mixed nerve and sensory nerve conduction studies. *Am J Phys Med Rehabil.* 1994;73(3):193-198.
65. McSweeney SC, Cichero M. Tarsal tunnel syndrome-A narrative literature review. *Foot (Edinb).* 2015;25(4):244-250.
66. Schwartz EN, Su J. Plantar fasciitis: a concise review. *Perm J.* 2014;18(1):e105-e107.
67. Chen H, Ho HM, Ying M, Fu SN. Association between plantar fascia vascularity and morphology and foot dysfunction in individuals with chronic plantar fasciitis. *J Orthop Sports Phys Ther.* 2013;43(10):727-734.
68. Fabrikant JM, Park TS. Plantar fasciitis (fasciosis) treatment outcome study: plantar fascia thickness measured by ultrasound and correlated with patient self-reported improvement. *Foot (Edinb).* 2011;21(2):79-83.
69. Lemont H, Ammirati KM, Usen N. Plantar fasciitis: a degenerative process (fasciosis) without inflammation. *J Am Podiatr Med Assoc.* 2003;93(3):234-237.
70. Chundru U, Liebeskind A, Seidelmann F, Fogel J, Franklin P, Beltran J. Plantar fasciitis and calcaneal spur formation are associated with abductor digiti minimi atrophy on MRI of the foot. *Skeletal Radiol.* 2008;37(6):505-510.
71. Chang R, Kent-Braun JA, Hamill J. Use of MRI for volume estimation of tibialis posterior and plantar intrinsic foot muscles in healthy and chronic plantar fasciitis limbs. *Clin Biomech (Bristol, Avon).* 2012;27(5):500-505.
72. Martin RL, Davenport TE, Reischl SF, et al. Heel pain-plantar fasciitis: revision 2014. *J Orthop Sports Phys Ther.* 2014;44(11):A1-A33.
73. Pohl MB, Hamill J, Davis IS. Biomechanical and anatomic factors associated with a history of plantar fasciitis in female runners. *Clin J Sport Med.* 2009;19(5):372-376.
74. Butterworth PA, Landorf KB, Smith SE, Menz HB. The association between body mass index and musculoskeletal foot disorders: a systematic review. *Obes Rev.* 2012;13(7):630-642.
75. Irving DB, Cook JL, Menz HB. Factors associated with chronic plantar heel pain: a systematic review. *J Sci Med Sport.* 2006;9(1-2):11-22; discussion 23-14.
76. Irving DB, Cook JL, Young MA, Menz HB. Obesity and pronated foot type may increase the risk of chronic plantar heel pain: a matched case-control study. *BMC Musculoskelet Disord.* 2007;8:41.
77. Werner RA, Gell N, Hartigan A, Wiggerman N, Keyserling WM. Risk factors for plantar fasciitis among assembly plant workers. *PM R.* 2010;2(2):110-116; quiz 1 p following 167.
78. Bolivar YA, Munuera PV, Padillo JP. Relationship between tightness of the posterior muscles of the lower limb and plantar fasciitis. *Foot Ankle Int.* 2013;34(1):42-48.
79. Allen RH, Gross MT. Toe flexors strength and passive extension range of motion of the first metatarsophalangeal joint in individuals with plantar fasciitis. *J Orthop Sports Phys Ther.* 2003;33(8):468-478.
80. Kibler WB, Goldberg C, Chandler TJ. Functional biomechanical deficits in running athletes with plantar fasciitis. *Am J Sports Med.* 1991;19(1):66-71.
81. Sullivan J, Burns J, Adams R, Pappas E, Crosbie J. Musculoskeletal and activity-related factors associated with plantar heel pain. *Foot Ankle Int.* 2015;36(1):37-45.
82. Grieve R, Palmer S. Physiotherapy for plantar fasciitis: a UK-wide survey of current practice. *Physiotherapy.* 2017;103(2):193-200.
83. Salvioli S, Guidi M, Marcotulli G. The effectiveness of conservative, non-pharmacological treatment, of plantar heel pain: a systematic review with meta-analysis. *Foot (Edinb).* 2017;33:57-67.
84. He C, Ma H. Effectiveness of trigger point dry needling for plantar heel pain: a meta-analysis of seven randomized controlled trials. *J Pain Res.* 2017;10:1933-1942.
85. Thing J, Maruthappu M, Rogers J. Diagnosis and management of plantar fasciitis in primary care. *Br J Gen Pract.* 2012;62(601):443-444.
86. Mahowald S, Legge BS, Grady JF. The correlation between plantar fascia thickness and symptoms of plantar fasciitis. *J Am Podiatr Med Assoc.* 2011;101(5):385-389.
87. Cotchett MP, Landorf KB, Munteanu SE, Raspovic AM. Consensus for dry needling for plantar heel pain (plantar fasciitis): a modified Delphi study. *Acupunct Med.* 2011;29(3):193-202.
88. Renan-Ordine R, Alburquerque-Sendin F, de Souza DP, Cleland JA, Fernández de las Peñas C. Effectiveness of myofascial trigger point manual therapy combined with a self-stretching protocol for the management of plantar heel pain: a randomized controlled trial. *J Orthop Sports Phys Ther.* 2011;41(2):43-50.
89. Saban B, Deutscher D, Ziv T. Deep massage to posterior calf muscles in combination with neural mobilization exercises as a treatment for heel pain: a pilot randomized clinical trial. *Man Ther.* 2014;19(2):102-108.
90. Mann R, Inman VT. Phasic activity of intrinsic muscles of the foot. *J Bone Joint Surg Am Vol.* 1964;46:469-481.
91. Imamura M, Fischer AA, Imamura ST, Kaziyama HS, Carvalho AE, Salomao O. Treatment of myofascial pain components in plantar fasciitis speeds up recovery: documentation by algometry. *J Musculoske Pain.* 1998;6(1):91-110.
92. Headlee DL, Leonard JL, Hart JM, Ingersoll CD, Hertel J. Fatigue of the plantar intrinsic foot muscles increases navicular drop. *J Electromyogr Kinesiol.* 2008;18(3):420-425.
93. Wearing SC, Smeathers JE, Urry SR, Hennig EM, Hills AP. The pathomechanics of plantar fasciitis. *Sports Med.* 2006;36(7):585-611.
94. Wolff R. Stressfraktur-Ermudungsbruch-Stressreaktion. *Dtsch Z Sportmed.* 2001;52(4):124-128.
95. Weist R, Eils E, Rosenbaum D. The influence of muscle fatigue on electromyogram and plantar pressure patterns as an explanation for the incidence of metatarsal stress fractures. *Am J Sports Med.* 2004;32(8):1893-1898.
96. Iwamoto J, Takeda T. Stress fractures in athletes: review of 196 cases. *J Orthop Sci.* 2003;8(3):273-278.
97. McBryde AM Jr. Stress fractures in athletes. *J Sports Med.* 1975;3(5):212-217.
98. McBryde AM Jr. Stress fractures in runners. *Clin Sports Med.* 1985;4(4):737-752.
99. Orava S. Stress fractures. *Br J Sports Med.* 1980;14(1):40-44.
100. Sullivan D, Warren RF, Pavlov H, Kelman G. Stress fractures in 51 runners. *Clin Orthop Relat Res.* 1984(187):188-192.
101. Gross TS, Bunch RP. A mechanical model of metatarsal stress fracture during distance running. *Am J Sports Med.* 1989;17(5):669-674.
102. Fetzer GB, Wright RW. Metatarsal shaft fractures and fractures of the proximal fifth metatarsal. *Clin Sports Med.* 2006;25(1):139-150, x.
103. Weinfeld S, Haddad S, Myerson M. Stress fractures. *Clin Sports Med.* 1997;16:319-338.
104. Griffin NL, Richmond BG. Cross-sectional geometry of the human forefoot. *Bone.* 2005;37(2):253-260.
105. Bennell KL, Brukner PD. Epidemiology and site specificity of stress fractures. *Clin Sports Med.* 1997;16(2):179-196.
106. Burr DB. Bone, exercise, and stress fractures. *Exerc Sport Sci Rev.* 1997;25:171-194.
107. Callahan LR. Stress fractures in women. *Clin Sports Med.* 2000;19(2):303-314.
108. Greaney RB, Gerber FH, Laughlin RL, et al. Distribution and natural history of stress fractures in U.S. Marine recruits. *Radiology.* 1983;146(2):339-346.
109. Kadel NJ, Teitz CC, Kronmal RA. Stress fractures in ballet dancers. *Am J Sports Med.* 1992;20(4):445-449.
110. Nattiv A, Armsey TD Jr. Stress injury to bone in the female athlete. *Clin Sports Med.* 1997;16(2):197-224.
111. Reeder MT, Dick BH, Atkins JK, Pribis AB, Martinez JM. Stress fractures. Current concepts of diagnosis and treatment. *Sports Med.* 1996;22(3):198-212.
112. Hunt KJ, McCormick JJ, Anderson RB. Management of forefoot injuries in the athlete. *Oper Tech Sports Med.* 2010;18:34-45.
113. Peris P. Stress fractures. *Best Pract Res Clin Rheumatol.* 2003;17(6):1043-1061.
114. Glasoe WM, Allen MK, Kepros T, Stonewall L, Ludewig PM. Dorsal first ray mobility in women athletes with a history of stress fracture of the second or third metatarsal. *J Orthop Sports Phys Ther.* 2002;32(11):560-565; discussion 565-567.
115. Banal F, Gandjbakhch F, Foltz V, et al. Sensitivity and specificity of ultrasonography in early diagnosis of metatarsal bone stress fractures: a pilot study of 37 patients. *J Rheumatol.* 2009;36(8):1715-1719.

116. Devas M. Stress fractures. In: Helal B, Rowley DI, Caracchiolo A, eds. *Surgery of Disorders of the Foot*. London, England: Martin Dunitz; 1996:761-773.
117. Sofka CM. Imaging of stress fractures. *Clin Sports Med*. 2006;25(1):53-62, viii.
118. Travell J, Simons DG. *Myofascial Pain and Dysfunction: The Trigger Point Manual*. Vol 2. Baltimore, MD: Williams & Wilkins; 1992.
119. Wu KK. Morton's interdigital neuroma: a clinical review of its etiology, treatment, and results. *J Foot Ankle Surg*. 1996;35(2):112-119; discussion 187-118.
120. Espinosa N. Peripheral nerve entrapment around the foot and ankle. In: Miller MD, Thompson SR, DeLee J, et al, eds. *DeLee & Drez's Orthopaedic Sports Medicine: Principles and Practice*. 4th ed. Philadelphia, PA: Elsevier/Saunders; 2014:1351-1368.
121. Mollica MB. Morton's neuroma: getting patients back on track. *Phys Sportsmed*. 1997;25(5):76-82.
122. Jain S, Mannan K. The diagnosis and management of Morton's neuroma: a literature review. *Foot Ankle Spec*. 2013;6(4):307-317.
123. Bencardino J, Rosenberg ZS, Beltran J, Liu X, Marty-Delfaut E. Morton's neuroma: is it always symptomatic? *AJR Am J Roentgenol*. 2000;175(3):649-653.
124. Balalis K, Topalidan A, Balali C, Tzagarakis G, Katonis P. The treatment of Morton's neuroma, a significant cause of metatarsalgia for people who exercise. *Int J Clin Med*. 2013;4(1):19-24.
125. Adams WR II. Morton's neuroma. *Clin Podiatr Med Surg*. 2010;27(4):535-545.
126. Bowling FL, Metcalfe SA, Wu S, Boulton AJ, Armstrong DG. Liquid silicone to mitigate plantar pedal pressure: a literature review. *J Diabetes Sci Technol*. 2010;4(4):846-852.
127. Giannini S, Bacchini P, Ceccarelli F, Vannini F. Interdigital neuroma: clinical examination and histopathologic results in 63 cases treated with excision. *Foot Ankle Int*. 2004;25(2):79-84.
128. Barrett SL, Jarvis J. Equinus deformity as a factor in forefoot nerve entrapment: treatment with endoscopic gastrocnemius recession. *J Am Podiatr Med Assoc*. 2005;95(5):464-468.
129. Thomson CE, Gibson JN, Martin D. Interventions for the treatment of Morton's neuroma. *Cochrane Database Syst Rev*. 2004(3):CD003118.
130. Willick SE, Herring SA. Common lower extremity neuropathies in athletes. *J Musculoskeletal Med*. 1998;15:48-58.
131. Biasca N, Zanetti M, Zollinger H. Outcomes after partial neurectomy of Morton's neuroma related to preoperative case histories, clinical findings, and findings on magnetic resonance imaging scans. *Foot Ankle Int*. 1999;20(9):568-575.
132. Rosenberg GA, Sferra JJ. Morton's neuroma: primary, recurrent, and their treatment. *Foot Ankle Clin*. 1998:473-484.
133. Zanetti M, Strehle JK, Kundert HP, Zollinger H, Hodler J. Morton neuroma: effect of MR imaging findings on diagnostic thinking and therapeutic decisions. *Radiology*. 1999;213(2):583-588.
134. Mendicino SS, Rockett MS. Morton's neuroma. Update on diagnosis and imaging. *Clin Podiatr Med Surg*. 1997;14(2):303-311.
135. Shapiro PP, Shapiro SL. Sonographic evaluation of interdigital neuromas. *Foot Ankle Int*. 1995;16(10):604-606.
136. Kaminsky S, Griffin L, Milsap J, Page D. Is ultrasonography a reliable way to confirm the diagnosis of Morton's neuroma? *Orthopedics*. 1997;20(1):37-39.
137. Basadonna PT, Rucco V, Gasparini D, Onorato A. Plantar fat pad atrophy after corticosteroid injection for an interdigital neuroma: a case report. *Am J Phys Med Rehabil*. 1999;78(3):283-285.
138. Younger AS, Claridge RJ. The role of diagnostic block in the management of Morton's neuroma. *Can J Surg*. 1998;41(2):127-130.
139. Pique-Vidal C, Sole MT, Antich J. Hallux valgus inheritance: pedigree research in 350 patients with bunion deformity. *J Foot Ankle Surg*. 2007;46(3):149-154.
140. Roddy E, Zhang W, Doherty M. Prevalence and associations of hallux valgus in a primary care population. *Arthritis Rheum*. 2008;59(6):857-862.
141. Mortka K, Lisinski P. Hallux valgus—a case for a physiotherapist or only for a surgeon? Literature review. *J Phys Ther Sci*. 2015;27(10):3303-3307.
142. Nix SE, Vicenzino BT, Collins NJ, Smith MD. Characteristics of foot structure and footwear associated with hallux valgus: a systematic review. *Osteoarthritis Cartilage*. 2012;20(10):1059-1074.
143. Glasoe WM, Nuckley DJ, Ludewig PM. Hallux valgus and the first metatarsal arch segment: a theoretical biomechanical perspective. *Phys Ther*. 2010;90(1):110-120.
144. Ferrari J. Bunions. *BMJ Clin Evid*. 2009;2009.
145. Perera AM, Mason L, Stephens MM. The pathogenesis of hallux valgus. *J Bone Joint Surg Am*. 2011;93(17):1650-1661.
146. Nix S, Smith M, Vicenzino B. Prevalence of hallux valgus in the general population: a systematic review and meta-analysis. *J Foot Ankle Res*. 2010;3:21.
147. Menz HB, Lord SR. Gait instability in older people with hallux valgus. *Foot Ankle Int*. 2005;26(6):483-489.
148. Nguyen US, Hillstrom HJ, Li W, et al. Factors associated with hallux valgus in a population-based study of older women and men: the MOBILIZE Boston Study. *Osteoarthritis Cartilage*. 2010;18(1):41-46.
149. Coughlin MJ. Roger A. Mann Award. Juvenile hallux valgus: etiology and treatment. *Foot Ankle Int*. 1995;16(11):682-697.
150. Glasoe WM, Phadke V, Pena FA, Nuckley DJ, Ludewig PM. An image-based gait simulation study of tarsal kinematics in women with hallux valgus. *Phys Ther*. 2013;93(11):1551-1562.
151. Glasoe WM, Jensen DD, Kampa BB, et al. First ray kinematics in women with rheumatoid arthritis and bunion deformity: a gait simulation imaging study. *Arthritis Care Res (Hoboken)*. 2014;66(6):837-843.
152. Steinberg N, Finestone A, Noff M, Zeev A, Dar G. Relationship between lower extremity alignment and hallux valgus in women. *Foot Ankle Int*. 2013;34(6):824-831.
153. Haas C, Kladny B, Lott S, Weseloh G, Swoboda B. Progression of foot deformities in rheumatoid arthritis—a radiologic follow-up study over 5 years [in German]. *Z Rheumatol*. 1999;58(6):351-357.
154. Shi K, Tomita T, Hayashida K, Owaki H, Ochi T. Foot deformities in rheumatoid arthritis and relevance of disease severity. *J Rheumatol*. 2000;27(1):84-89.
155. Pontious J, Mahan KT, Carter S. Characteristics of adolescent hallux abducto valgus. A retrospective review. *J Am Podiatr Med Assoc*. 1994;84(5):208-218.
156. Barouk LS, Diebold P. Hallux valgus congenital. *Med Chir Pied*. 1991;7:65-112.
157. Kilmartin TE, Barrington RL, Wallace WA. Metatarsus primus varus. A statistical study. *J Bone Joint Surg Br*. 1991;73(6):937-940.
158. Easley ME, Trnka HJ. Current concepts review: hallux valgus part 1: pathomechanics, clinical assessment, and nonoperative management. *Foot Ankle Int*. 2007;28(5):654-659.
159. Rao S, Song J, Kraszewski A, et al. The effect of foot structure on 1st metatarsophalangeal joint flexibility and hallucal loading. *Gait Posture*. 2011;34(1):131-137.
160. Hurn SE, Vicenzino B, Smith MD. Functional impairments characterizing mild, moderate, and severe hallux valgus. *Arthritis Care Res (Hoboken)*. 2015;67(1):80-88.
161. Beaman DN, Nigo LJ. Hallucal sesamoid injury. *Operative Tech Sports Med*. 1999;7(1):7-13.
162. Boike A, Schnirring-Judge M, McMillin S. Sesamoid disorders of the first metatarsophalangeal joint. *Clin Podiatr Med Surg*. 2011;28(2):269-285, vii.
163. Dobas DC, Silvers MD. The frequency of partite sesamoids of the first metatarsophalangeal joint. *J Am Podiatry Assoc*. 1977;67(12):880-882.
164. Anwar R, Anjum SN, Nicholl JE. Sesamoids of the foot. *Curr Orthop*. 2005;19:40-48.
165. Dedmond BT, Cory JW, McBryde A Jr. The hallucal sesamoid complex. *J Am Acad Orthop Surg*. 2006;14(13):745-753.
166. Knuttzen K, Hart L. Running. In: Caine DJ, Caine CG, Lindner KJ, eds. *Epidemiology of Sports Injuries*. Champaign, IL: Human Kinetics; 1996.
167. McBryde AM Jr, Anderson RB. Sesamoid foot problems in the athlete. *Clin Sports Med*. 1988;7(1):51-60.
168. Hockenbury RT. Forefoot problems in athletes. *Med Sci Sports Exerc*. 1999;31(7 suppl):S448-S458.
169. Cohen BE. Hallux sesamoid disorders. *Foot Ankle Clin*. 2009;14(1):91-104.

for treatment failure, seen clinically, is the lack of postneedling treatment care and instructions or failure to recognize or address systemic perpetuating factors (see Chapter 4).

3. WET NEEDLING OR DRY NEEDLING

Clinicians may consider the potential risks and benefits of utilizing TrPI with solutions versus application of DN techniques. Trigger point injections are administered using hypodermic needles, a hollow needle through which a solution is injected at the TrP site.

Local anesthetics, corticosteroids, and neurolytics are substances commonly used in pain management[7] and are also used in solutions for TrP management. Trigger point injection involves depositing approximately 0.2 mL of solution at the TrP.[2] Some studies have used larger volumes up to several milliliters. For example, Ay et al[8] used 2 mL of 1% lidocaine injection for comparison with DN in conjunction with exercise and found no significant differences between the groups relative to pain level, cervical range of motion, and depressive mood; both groups benefited.

Hypodermic needles used for TrPI have a beveled, cutting edge. Filiform needles have a conical point. This difference should be considered when treating areas close to visceral anatomy such as pleural, vascular, or neural structures. The use of a noncutting needle may reduce the risk of laceration of these tissues that could lead to complications such as bleeding, pneumothorax, or nerve injury. DN may be preferable if injecting close to a nerve to avoid possible anesthetic block. Also, the use of DN prevents inadvertent intervascular deposition of treatment solution. It is prudent to aspirate, especially in the vicinity of large vessels, prior to injecting to assess that the needle has not entered a vessel. Accurate injection at deep sites, near neurovascular structures, or in patients who are obese may be improved by the use of ultrasonic or electromyography (EMG) guidance.[9,10]

As with DN, the goal is to accurately locate and deactivate the TrP loci. Obtaining LTRs is similarly desirable. Mechanical disruption of the TrPs is effective by DN as well as needling in conjunction with TrPI of solution. Good technique and provocation of an LTR are important in obtaining a positive result, whether using DN or TrPI of a local anesthetic.[11] Nevertheless, the topic of the LTR during DN is currently under debate.[12]

Myofascial pain often has a chronic component, frequently requiring serial treatments. Clinicians may adjust their approach, including needle or solution options, at subsequent sessions to assess the best individualized treatment approach. Adequate treatment adjustment trials are appropriate prior to determining that TrPI or DN is not effective for a particular patient as long as effective postneedling care and home self-management is employed.

Practical considerations may also drive the decision to use DN rather than TrPI solutions. Some clinicians may not have the option to utilize injection therapy within professional licensing parameters. Reimbursement issues and price point of supplies may also bias the clinician's choice.

Studies of TrPI have been limited by heterogeneity of subject groups and small sample sizes. Pain is complex, and multiple factors can affect fluctuations in pain intensity, quality-of-life measures, and perceived relief. Limited high-quality randomized controlled trials (RCTs) are available for review. A majority of the studies available involve treatment of the neck and upper quadrant.[13] Additional research would be helpful in assessing optimal treatment approach and response to specific patient types. Huang and Liu[14] found that abdominal muscle TrPI with lidocaine 2 weeks prior to menstruation yielded improvement in primary dysmenorrhea. However, no comparison with DN treatment was included in this study.[14]

There is little consensus regarding the superiority of either DN or TrPI. A meta-analysis demonstrated that both wet needling and DN were effective for neck and shoulder myofascial pain without clear differences between the needling therapies.[13]

Another systematic review found no differences between DN and wet needling using lidocaine after treatment or at follow-up intervals of 1 month or at 3 to 6 months.[15] Nevertheless, some studies showed evidence that lidocaine injection may be more effective for pain reduction than DN at 4 weeks.[16,17] An older randomized, double-blind crossover study compared the use of 0.5% bupivacaine, 1% etidocaine, or physiologic saline. Pain categories measured prior to treatment and 15 minutes, 24 hours, and 7 days after treatment indicated the use of the local anesthetic injections to be preferable over saline.[18] Although the sample size was small (n = 15), the crossover component of this study limits heterogeneity of the comparison groups and compares response of different treatment solutions on the same patients.[18]

In clinical practice, patients are generally treated with more than one session. A double-blinded study of individuals with episodic tension-type headache compared TrPI using saline to 0.5% lidocaine and compared single injection with a series of five injections.[19] The results indicated that repeated lidocaine injections showed improvement at 2, 4, and 6 months, but only the group treated with a series of lidocaine injections showed significant changes at 6 months, suggesting multiple lidocaine injections may be more effective than a single treatment.[19] Treatment frequency and duration may be factors to consider when reviewing comparative studies.

4. SELECTION OF NEEDLE GAUGE

The clinician must determine an appropriate needle gauge and length to access the target tissue. Choice may vary greatly, from 30-gauge ½ in to treat the anterior border of the upper trapezius to ultrasound-guided 20-gauge 3.5-in spinal needle to address the piriformis muscle. In thick subcutaneous muscles, such as the gluteus maximus or paraspinal muscles, a 21-gauge, 5-cm (2-in) hypodermic needle, or 0.30×50 mm filiform needle is usually necessary. For TrPI or DN technique, the needle should be long enough to reach the TrP without inserting the needle to its hub. A 21-gauge, 6.4-cm (2.5-in) hypodermic needle or a 0.30×60 to 75 mm filiform needle is generally long enough to reach TrPs in the deepest muscles, such as the gluteus minimus, quadratus lumborum, and psoas muscles. The spinal needle is not as effective for TrP injection as the hypodermic type needle because the spinal needle may push the TrP aside, rather than penetrating it because of its flexibility and diamond-shaped tip.

It would seem intuitive that a smaller gauge needle would be less painful for the patient. When initiating TrPI, patients will often ask, "how big is the needle?" Some authors, including Simons, hypothesize that a larger gauge allows for more accurate localization and improved mechanical disruption in treatment of TrPs with TrPI or DN. There is limited data on response as related to needle gauge. Yoon et al[20] measured treatment efficacy comparing 21, 23, and 25 gauge hypodermic needles in individuals with TrPs in the upper trapezius muscle followed up to 14 days after treatment. All the groups improved and, interestingly, there was no difference in the pain perception of injection needle size. Nevertheless, although no difference in pain relief scores was noted, 21 or 23 gauge needles were more effective in SF-36 health survey scores.[20]

A knowledge of anatomy, the depth of target tissue, and the clinical status of the patient are all factors to be considered by clinicians when choosing needle gauge and length for TrPI or DN. Larger gauge needles may offer less flexibility and possibly more accurate localization and treatment of TrPs. Muscles that are deep or in close proximity to neurovascular structures may best be accessed utilizing ultrasound guidance. Consideration may be given to using a smaller gauge in patients being treated with capillary fragility, platelet disorders, or anticoagulant agents such as warfarin or novel oral anticoagulants.

Coagulopathy may be inherent or medically induced and should be included in patient evaluation prior to embarking on TrP management by invasive techniques, such as needling or even with some manual therapy techniques. It is prudent for patients on warfarin to check for current monitoring and stability of international normalized ratio (INR) within range. Consider consultation with the patient's hematologist in the setting of coagulopathy, such as platelet dysfunction. Also, consider the anatomy of the target site to assess that the treatment area is readily compressible (hemostasis) to limit bruising or bleeding.

Clinically, a 30-gauge needle is effective for TrPI with the effect of obtaining LTR and clinical response with less bleeding noted. A 30-gauge needle has a nominal outer diameter or 0.30 mm that corresponds to a fairly common filiform needle diameter choice for use in DN techniques. Ga et al[21] compared the efficacy of treatment with a 0.30 mm DN compared to TrPI using 0.5% lidocaine administered 25-gauge needle in elderly patients. Although the with a 25-gauge needle has a greater diameter, there was no significant difference in postinjection soreness or in improvement of cervical range or motion or myofascial pain.

5. CLINICAL GUIDELINE FOR APPLICATION OF NEEDLING THERAPIES

Prior to performing any needling technique (TrPI or DN), the clinician should consider patient positioning, medical history with regard to possible increased bleeding tendency, needle selection, proper cleansing, painless skin penetration, and the value of preinjection blocks.

The patient should be positioned in recumbence (supine, semisupine, side-lying, prone, or semiprone) for any TrPI or DN technique to avoid falling associated with psychogenic syncope. When the patient sits on a chair or is standing, needle therapies can be hazardous in susceptible individuals.[22,23] Recumbence also facilitates manual palpation of the TrPs because the patient is typically more comfortable and relaxed. It is also easier to adjust muscle tension so that the bands containing TrPs stand out in a background of relaxed muscle fibers.

Trigger point injection and DN are not sterile techniques. The area to be needled should be properly cleaned with alcohol or soap and water. The needles used are sterile, single use, and disposable. Nevertheless, there is an ongoing debate whether disinfection of the skin or the use of gloves is necessary or not, and guidelines vary in different countries and regions.[24,25]

Some patients are afraid of the skin pain caused by needle penetration. This fear of the needle is usually acquired in childhood and creates obstacles to the therapeutic alliance.[26] Most patients find the sharp skin pain more threatening than the deep aching and more severe pain of the needle contact with the TrPs. The skin pain is avoidable with the use of cold anesthesia for TrPI or in the case of DN holding the tube firmly against the patient's skin prior to tapping the needle through the skin.

In adults, vapocoolant spray can provide cold anesthesia[27,28] to effectively block nerve conduction when the skin temperature falls to 10°C (50°F). After carefully disinfecting the skin with alcohol, vapocoolant spray is applied from a distance of about 45 cm (18 in) for 5 or 6 seconds, and then the needle is inserted quickly after the spray has evaporated leaving the skin dry.[26,29] For young children who dislike the sudden cold impact of the vapocoolant jet stream, a sterile, fluffy, small cotton ball is saturated with vapocoolant until it is dripping wet. The wet cotton is held *lightly* against the skin for about 10 seconds and then removed. At the instant the skin dries, the needle is inserted painlessly.

Three less reliable, but more convenient, techniques that can be combined are to (1) insert the needle *very quickly* through the skin with a flick of the wrist or with a very firm tap with a DN, (2) place the skin under tension so that the additional tension of the needle penetration is hardly noticeable (this can be done by the clinician strongly spreading the fingers apart against the skin and inserting a needle between them), and (3) increase skin tension by pinching a fold of the skin between the thumb and fingers and inserting the needle through the tightly folded skin. When the skin has been cleansed with an alcohol wipe, a film of liquid alcohol can remain for seconds. If the needle is inserted through the wet alcohol, it produces a stinging sensation because the needle carries some of it into the skin. This can be avoided by simply waiting until the alcohol dries. The particular technique used is less important than the communication to the patient that the clinician cares and knows how to insert the needle painlessly.

Prior to TrPI or DN, the patient should be warned that successful needle contact with TrPs may produce a flash of distant pain and likely will cause the muscle to twitch. The patient should be asked to note where that pain is felt, permitting an accurate description afterward of the pattern of pain referred by the TrPs. In this way, the clinician can confirm the referred pain pattern of that TrP, and the patient can realize the connection between the pain and the TrP in that muscle (pain recognition or not). This reassures both the clinician and the patient as to the importance of inactivating it. Patients learn to welcome this painful harbinger of a successful TrPI or DN treatment and future relief.

A preinjection block may be used prior to the TrPI procedure. It is now well established that even brief exposure to considerable pain can cause neuroplastic changes in the spinal cord that tend to enhance sensitization and pain. For patients who are particularly pain-sensitive, or who have found the pain produced by needle encounter with TrPs seriously distressing, a preinjection block can be helpful. This procedure must be adopted with due caution. It is described in detail by Fischer[30] who presents two methods: one involves diffuse infiltration of a local anesthetic proximal to the area to be injected and the other involves infiltration of the entire TrP area with a local anesthetic before needling individual active loci. It is important, if a clinician does these infiltrations, to use 0.5% procaine because of its lower myotoxicity, its relative innocuousness if a vessel were accidently injected, and the more rapid recovery of normal nerve function.[30]

Although there are a number of alternate TrPI and DN techniques now in use, the following precision technique is the one that was presented by Simons et al.[2] It is a basic technique that is applicable to TrPs in any muscle location that can be reached with a needle.

Localization of a TrP is done mainly by the practitioner's sense of feel, assisted by patient expressions of pain, and by visual observation of LTRs.

The two methods of palpation (cross-fiber flat or pincer palpation) are utilized to identify TrPs. The more precisely the TrP is localized, the more effective the needling technique will be. When flat palpation is used to locate the TrP for needling, its position can be confirmed precisely by pushing the nodular TrP back and forth between two fingers (Figure 72-1A and B). The TrP can be fixed for needling by pinning it down midway between the index and middle finger tips (Figure 72-1C). This identifies for the clinician the plane that passes through the TrP perpendicular to the skin. The needle can be aimed and directed half way between the fingers precisely in that plane and angled to whatever depth is necessary to reach the TrP. The needle should be considered as an extension of the clinician's finger; the clinician, therefore, palpates the TrP with the tip of the needle and penetrates it. When pincer palpation is used to locate the TrP, the degree of tension placed on the muscle fibers can be fine-tuned by varying the distance that the muscle is pulled away from underlying tissues. The nodule is located by rolling sequential portions of the taut band between the clinician's digits (Figure 72-2). For needling, the TrPs are held tightly between the thumb, index, and middle fingertips; the needle is typically directed toward the TrPs; and the clinician's fingers on the underside of the tissue. The needling procedures for both flat and pincer palpation should

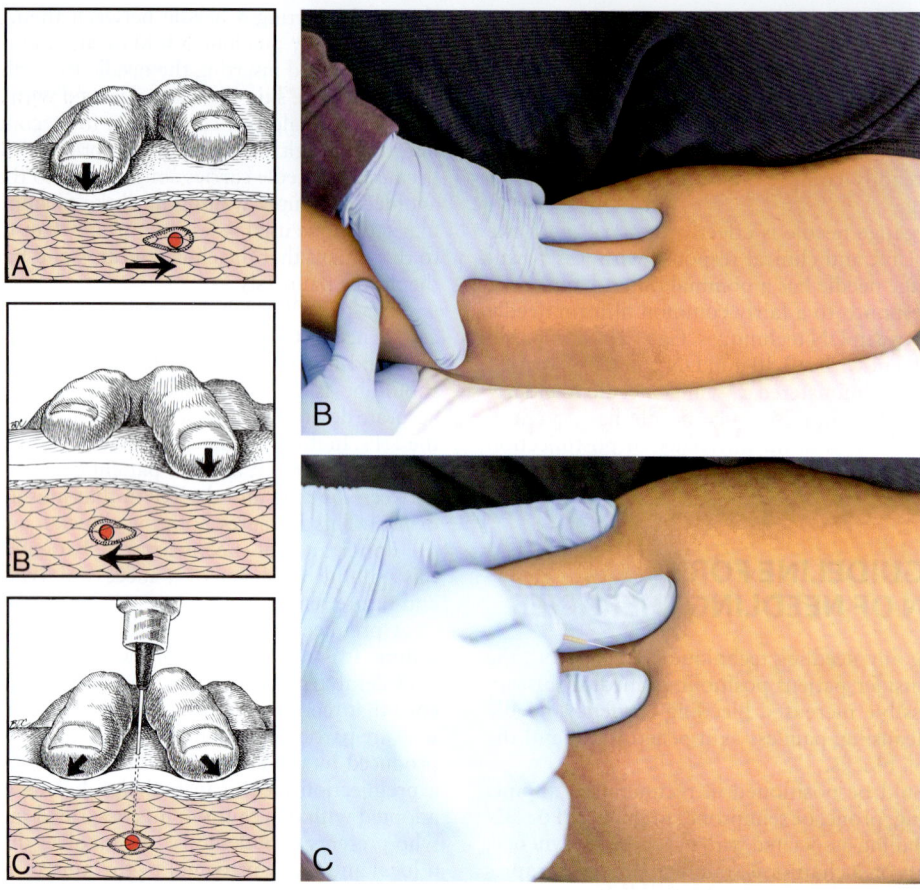

Figure 72-1. Cross-sectional schematic drawing of flat palpation to localize and hold the TrP (dark red spot) for TrP injections or dry needle. A and B, Use of alternating pressure between two fingers to confirm the location of the palpable TrP. C, Positioning of the TrP half way between the fingers to keep it from sliding to one side during the needling.

be conducted similar to manual palpation techniques for the identification of TrPs.

For TrPI or DN of TrPs when employing any method of palpation, the muscle fibers of the taut band are placed on sufficient stretch to take up any slack but not enough stretch to cause additional pain. This tautness is necessary to help hold the TrP in position. If the muscle is slack, there is a tendency for the dense contracture knots of the TrP to slide to one side as the needle tip encounters them.

To needle TrPs in superficial layers of muscle close to the skin, the needle tip can be brought precisely to the TrP by first carefully locating TrP with the finger and then, after inserting the needle subcutaneously, pressing it against the finger through the skin to accurately localize the TrPs. Finally, the needle tip is directed into the TrP by means of this "tactile vision" provided by palpating both the needle and the TrP at the same time.

The same technique is useful for TrPI or DN in the area of the muscle opposite the needling site when using a pincer grasp. The location of the needle and the TrP can be identified by palpation as the needle approaches the skin after penetrating most of the muscle.

Trigger point injection or DN TrPs is a full-time job for both hands of the clinician. The needling hand is busy placing the needle and controlling the plunger of the syringe for TrPI. The palpating hand constantly maintains hemostasis and often must fix the TrP to help the needle penetrate it. It also must be ready to detect any palpable LTRs. Hemostasis is important. Local bleeding irritates the muscle, causes postinjection soreness, and can produce unsightly ecchymosis. Ecchymosis is usually preventable; when it occurs, only time eradicates it.

To prevent bleeding, the fingers of the palpating hand of the clinician should be spread apart, maintaining tension on the skin (Figure 72-3A) to reduce the likelihood of subcutaneous bleeding where the needle has penetrated during TrPI. Bleeding is considered a minor adverse event when performing DN. Also, during TrPI or DN, the fingers exert pressure around the needle tip to provide hemostasis in deeper tissues. When the angle of the needle is changed, the direction of the pressure changes with it. The pressure should be applied throughout the needling procedure. As the needle is withdrawn, one finger slides over the track of the needle and instantly applies pressure where the needle was. If visible bleeding develops, prolonged hemostasis and a cold pack should be applied and the patient is warned of a possible "bruised" spot.

Blindly probing an area of diffuse tenderness where there is no palpable band or muscle attachment is futile. Such an area is most likely to be a pain reference zone, not TrPs. Injecting a local anesthetic in the reference zone may temporarily reduce the referred pain, but it does not eliminate the cause of the pain.

The importance of distinguishing between TrPs in the muscle belly, the myotendinous junction, or enthesis when TrPI or DN is applied was illustrated (Figure 72-4) by Fischer.[30] The precision required to penetrate the TrP with a needle is a skill that requires practice. When using flat palpation, as illustrated in Figures 72-1C and 72-3A and B, the needle is inserted between the fingers that have located the TrPs. The needle penetrates the skin 1 to 2 cm away from the TrP so that it can approach it at an acute angle of about 30° to the skin. Adequate tension of the muscle fibers is required to penetrate the TrP. The needle should explore both the deep and superficial fibers of the muscle. For

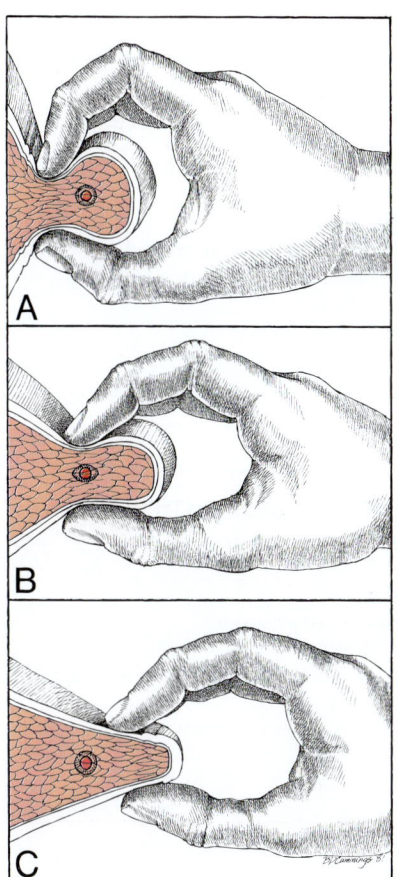
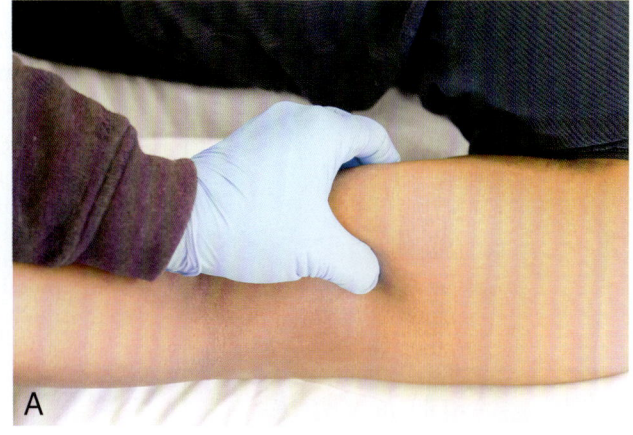

Figure 72-2. Cross-sectional schematic drawing showing cross-fiber pincer palpation of a taut band (black ring) at a TrP (red spot). Cross-fiber pincer palpation is used for muscles (light red) that can be picked up between the digits, such as the sternocleidomastoid, pectoralis major, and latissimus dorsi muscles. A, Muscle fibers surrounded by the thumb and fingers in a pincer grip. B, Hardness of the taut band felt clearly as it is rolled between the digits. The change in the angle of the distal phalanges produces a rocking motion that improves discrimination of fine detail. C, The palpable edge of the taut band is sharply defined, as it escapes from between the fingertips, often with a local twitch response.

TrPI, the syringe may be held between the fingers of the injecting hand, and thumb pressure used against the plunger, which is the method shown in most of the figures illustrating injection in this chapter. Thumb pressure on the plunger slowly introduces small amounts of 0.5% procaine solution as the needle advances within the muscle. This ensures that the procaine is present to relieve pain at the instant that the needle tip encounters an active locus of the TrP. The filiform needle can be easily redirected with the needling hand to induce and eradicate all the LTRs in the area.

The clinician should avoid inserting the needle to the hub where the needle is most likely to break off. Some additional depth of penetration can be safely obtained by compressing the skin and subcutaneous tissues with the palpating hand if needed. Once the skin and subcutaneous tissues have been compressed, the clinician should maintain the compression until the needle is withdrawn.

The dense contracture knots in TrPs often feel, to the practitioner, as if the needle tip has encountered hard rubber that is resistant to penetration and tends to slide to one side, as described by Gold and Travell many years ago. Using the needle as a probe, the TrP sometimes feels like a dense globule, 2 to 3 mm in diameter; resistance to penetration helps identify it.[31] Occasionally, when the needle makes contact with the TrP, it may feel "gritty." Adequate tension of the muscle helps stabilize the position of the TrP to permit precise penetration by the needle, especially for deep TrPs that cannot be easily fixed in position by manual palpation.

If an LTR and referred pain were elicited from the TrP prior to TrPI or DN, then both should be observed when the needle penetrates the TrP during the procedure. Hong[32] showed that when needle penetrations of a TrP produced LTRs, they were much more likely to result in subsequent pain relief than penetrations that did not elicit an LTR. Following effective needling, most TrP characteristics should have minimized or disappeared. The taut band is more relaxed following effective needling and may no longer be distinguishable by manual palpation. Nevertheless, the topic of the LTR during DN is currently under debate.[12]

Sometimes a cluster of TrPs are present in one part of the muscle. This fact is often recognized when the muscle is initially palpated for TrPs. When one of these TrPs has been inactivated, the area is peppered in a fan-like manner or in a full circle[32] in an effort to ensure that all remaining TrPs in the group are inactivated, as illustrated in Figure 72-3B. Following each probing movement, the needle tip must be withdrawn to the subcutaneous tissue and redirected before the next movement. When this probing search of the region is completed, the site is palpated for any remaining spots of tenderness. If another one is found, it is accurately localized with the fingers and needled. All potential tender spots in that region should be eliminated before withdrawing the needle through the skin, if possible. Box 72-1 describes a general guideline for TrPI or DN procedures. Boxes 72-2 and 72-3 identify absolute contraindications and precautions to TrPI or DN, respectively. Box 72-4 lists caveats from Travell and Simons regarding TrPI or DN.

Hong[32] introduced two needling techniques: one was a safer way to hold the syringe and the other was a different way to perform the injection itself, that is DN. When a clinician injects a TrP in locations that pose a hazard should the patient make a sudden unexpected movement (such as a startle reaction, sneeze, and/or cough), Hong[11,32] recommends a way to hold the syringe

Section 8: Treatment Considerations for Myofascial Pain and Dysfunction

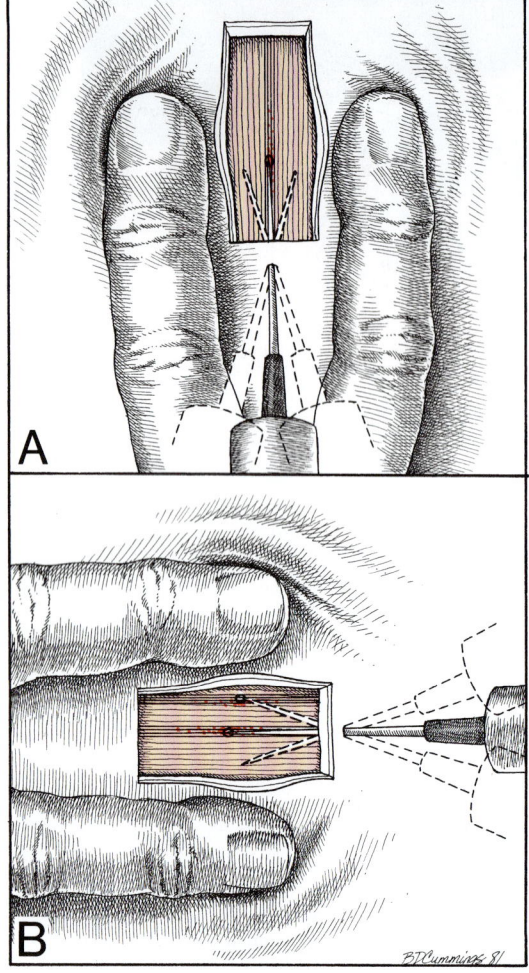

Figure 72-3. Schematic top view of two approaches to the flat needling of a TrP area (dark red spot) in a palpable taut band (closely spaced black lines). A, Needling away from fingers, which have pinned down the TrP so it cannot slide away from the needle. Dotted outline indicates additional probing to explore for additional adjacent TrPs. The fingers are pressing downward and apart to maintain pressure for hemostasis. B, Needling toward the fingers, with similar finger pressure. Additional TrPs are often found in the immediate vicinity by probing with the needle.

Box 72-1 General guidelines for TrP injection or dry needling

Palpate and identify anatomic landmarks
Palpate the taut band with cross-fiber flat or pincer palpation
Identify the TrP and fix with either a pincer grasp or flat palpation
Needle with straight in and out motions
Elicit a local twitch response (or referred pain)
Draw the needle back to the subcutaneous tissue and re-redirect the needle to treat other TrPs in the same or nearby areas
Provide hemostasis immediately upon withdrawal of the needle
Apply a postneedling intervention for reducing postneedle soreness

---

Box 72-2 Contraindications to TrP injection or dry needling

Inadequately trained practitioner
Needle phobia
Cognitive impairment
Patient's unwillingness to be treated
Patient's inability to give consent
Local skin lesions
Local or systemic infections
Needling directly over implants

Box 72-3 Precautions to TrP injection or dry needling

First trimester of pregnancy
Vascular disease
Abnormal bleeding tendency (anticoagulant therapy, thrombocytopenia)
Compromised immune system
Intercostal area
Needle aversion

---

that is safer than the usual way. His technique ensures that the syringe will move with the patient and not enter an unintended tissue, and that the finger on the plunger of the syringe will move with the syringe and not cause an accidental injection. The hand holding the syringe must be firmly supported by the patient's body; this is readily accomplished with his technique, as illustrated in Figure 72-5. The syringe is held between the thumb and lesser fingers, and the plunger is depressed with the index finger. This technique is particularly valuable when injecting over the lung or when the needle is directed toward major arteries or nerves.

6. NUMBER OF NEEDLING SESSIONS

Note the definition of one injection at the beginning of this chapter. The number of TrP sites that need to be injected per visit and the number of visits required are strongly dependent on the patient's condition and the practitioner's skill and judgment. To date, no medical specialty has adopted the diagnosis and treatment of myofascial TrPs as an official part of the training program, nor have *specialty* standards of training and practice been established for this diagnosis. The *International Association for the Study of Pain* has published recommended standards of TrP training.[33]

Active myofascial TrPs with no long-lasting perpetuating factors or additional tissue damage due to mechanical injury to other structures should resolve with one or two needling sessions. This estimate is especially true if the patient has been provided with adequate self-management techniques, which are discussed in Section 5 of each muscle chapter. When initial TrP therapy is delayed and symptoms have not subsided with time, the longer the period of delay before starting TrP therapy, the higher the number of TrPI or DN techniques that will be required over a longer period of time.[34] Some chronic TrP problems could involve several injections over a span of months of treatment. In this situation, the primary guideline is that the period of relief from TrP pain and dysfunction should become progressively longer

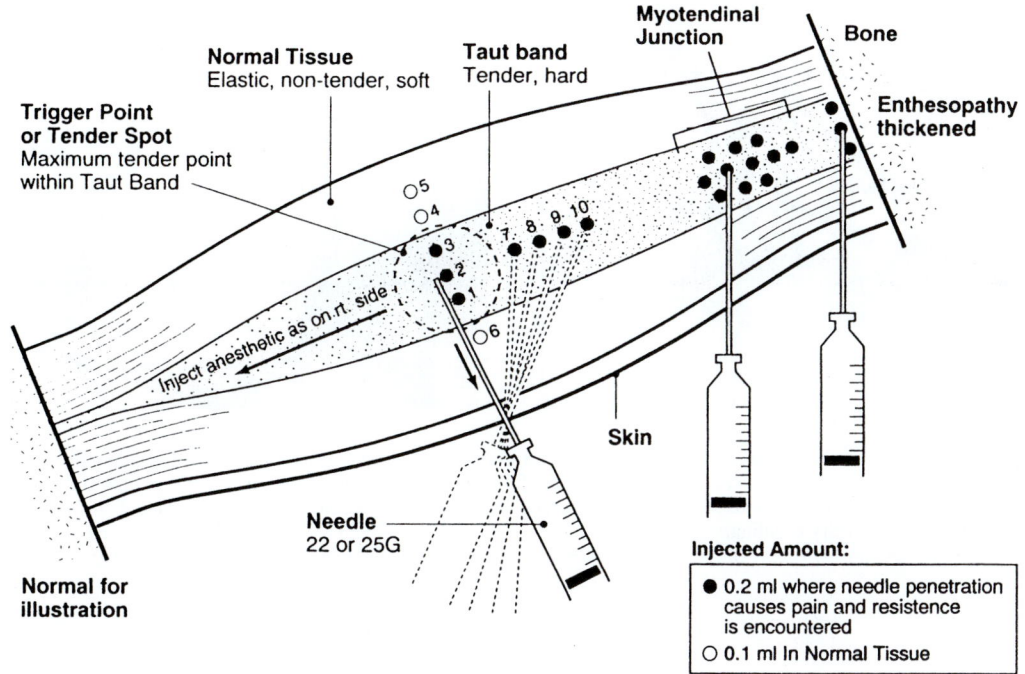

Figure 72-4. Diagrammatic representation of preneedling sites (open circles), and needling sites (solid circles) of local anesthetic in relation to the TrP (large broken circle). The taut band is represented by the enclosed stippled area. This diagram distinguishes the mid-muscle belly TrP within the broken circle from the myotendinous junction and at the attachment of the tendon to the bone. Each of these three TrP regions can be identified by the individual spot tenderness and anatomic locations. No rationale is apparent for needling the part of the taut band that lies between solid circles numbers 7 to 10. Reproduced with permission from Fischer AA. New approaches in treatment of myofascial pain: myofascial pain–update in diagnosis and treatment. *Phys Med Rehabil Clin North Am.* 1997;8(1):153-169.

with successive TrPI or DN treatments, and the patient should be performing a self-management program between sessions.

When a patient demonstrates multiple active TrPs in functionally related muscles, there is a distinct advantage to inactivating them as a group. Thus, 5 or even 10 needling treatments at one visit may be appropriate but could be more than tolerable. Because a properly performed and effective needling treatment produces an LTR that is often associated with considerable pain, there is a limit as to how many painful injections should be performed at one visit given the patient's emotional and autonomic distress level.

The presence of unrecognized perpetuating factors (see Chapter 4) will lead to unnecessary TrPI or DN. The presence of associated joint dysfunctions that need manipulation can cause poor response to needling and prompt recurrence of the TrP activity. After appropriate treatment of the joint(s), one or two more TrPI or DN sessions should resolve the problem. The presence of concurrent fibromyalgia will increase the number of needling sessions required and can justify recurrent TrPI or DN every 6 to 8 weeks because fibromyalgia acts as a perpetuating factor that has no cure. Inactivating TrPs can provide significant pain relief for many of these patients.

Box 72-4 Travell and Simons caveats for TrP injection or dry needling

By NEVER aiming the needle at an intercostal space, the clinician avoids the distressing complication of a *pneumothorax*. As a resident, Dr Travell found in her early experience of doing many pleural taps for pleural effusions, that patients consistently reported a salty taste in the mouth whenever the pleura was punctured. The patient might say, "Oh, I can taste the solution." When the lung is punctured and collapses, dyspnea, cough, and chest pain characteristic of a pneumothorax follow.

A needle is prone to break where it attaches to the hub. The needle should never be inserted solidly to its hub because of the difficult situation that would ensue should it break off at the hub and disappear under the skin. Recovering the needle can be a time-consuming, frustrating process for the clinician. A long enough needle should be used, or the skin compressed around it, to ensure that some of the needle projects above the skin surface.

The location of the needle tip can readily be misjudged when using a long slender needle. It is especially important to insert the needle straight and avoid any side pressure that might bend the needle.

When the tip of a needle contacts the bone, the impact frequently curls the tip to produce a "fishhook" burr that feels "scratchy" and drags as the needle is drawn through tissues; it causes unnecessary bleeding and pain and the needle should be replaced immediately. It is especially important to avoid using such a barbed needle for TrPI or DN TrPs in muscles like the scalene that lie near nerve trunks.

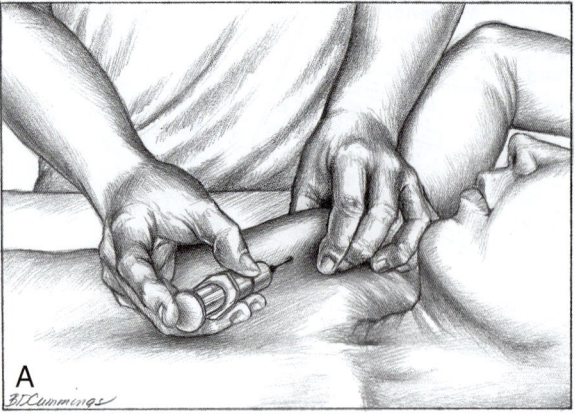 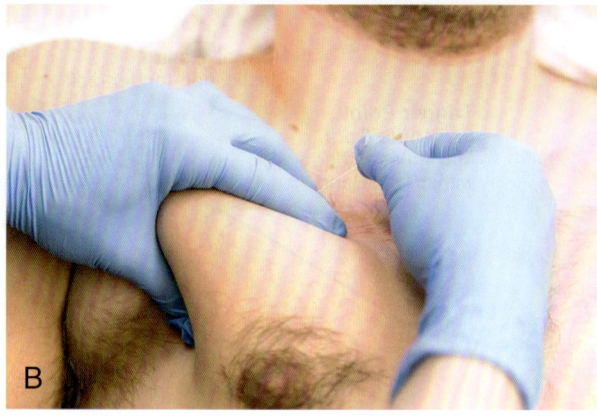

Figure 72-5. Trigger point injection using a technique for holding the syringe that minimizes the danger of accidentally inserting the needle farther than intended if the patient makes a sudden unexpected movement. A, Drawn from an original photograph, courtesy of John Hong, MD who first described this method. Hong C-Z. Myofascial trigger point injection. *Crit Rev Phys Med Rehabil.* 1993;5:203-217. B, Similar technique shown for dry needling.

7. POSTNEEDLING PROCEDURES

Postneedling-induced soreness is thought to be a consequence of the neuromuscular damage generated by needling insertions into the muscle.[35] The presence of postneedling soreness can be associated with a possible reluctance to receive further needling therapy by the patient, generating patient dissatisfaction and reduction in treatment adherence. In fact, it is highly recommended to advise the patient about the presence of soreness after any needling therapies.[36] Therefore, postneedling procedures should always be implemented into a multimodal treatment approach.

Postural education and positioning, activity modification, self-stretch, and neuromotor retraining following TrPI or DN is an integral part of that treatment. Immediately following TrPI or DN, hemostasis should be applied for a minimum of 30 seconds or longer, the patient should actively move each muscle needled through its full range of motion three to five times, reaching its fully tolerable shortened and fully tolerable lengthened position during each cycle. The muscle usually feels stiff toward the end of full stretch range of motion on the first cycle, less on the second, and begins to feel comfortable through its full range by the third to fifth cycle. It is important that the patient move the muscle slowly to explore the end range of motion for additional release. It is also vital that the patient is able to activate the muscles that have been needled volitionally to improve motor control. An ice pack immediately following the TrPI or DN procedure, stretch,[37] manual compression,[38] or low-load eccentric exercise[39] can be helpful in reducing postneedling soreness and enhancing recovery.

The postinjection stretch is important because it helps to again equalize sarcomere lengths throughout the length of the affected muscle fibers, which relieves the abnormal tension and can eliminate the palpable taut bands.[37] Voluntary movement also relieves residual stiffness at full range of motion, helps the patient appreciate the improved range of motion, and provides the patient stretches that will be incorporated in the home management program. Additionally, this range-of-motion activity establishes the patient's conscious awareness of normal function in that muscle, while reprogramming the cerebellum to incorporate the newly restored full-range capability of the muscle into the patient's daily activities. Establishing a home exercise prescription for the patient following TrPI or DN is vital for treatment success.

Lewit[40] noted muscle soreness after DN and after TrPI with a local anesthetic but made no mention of applying heat or cold as part of the treatment. The postinjection soreness, per se, is not unfavorable if the patient's related pattern of referred pain has been relieved. In fact, some clinicians consider postneedling soreness as a "natural" or "positive" effect indicating that TrP inactivation has been effectively achieved. However, it is wise to let the muscle recover completely from postinjection soreness, which ordinarily lasts at most 48 to 72 hours independent of the postneedling intervention used,[37-39] before needling its TrPs again. Soreness can also be caused by ineffectually needling close to, but not into, TrPs.

If two or three treatments of TrPI or DN fail to eradicate the TrPs in a muscle, repeated TrPI or DN is rarely the answer. The perpetuating factors that are causing recurrence of the TrPs must be identified and managed (see Chapter 4). Box 72-5 lists possible reasons for failure of TrPI or DN to effectively treat the myofascial pain and dysfunction caused by TrPs.

Box 72-5 Possible reasons for failure of TrP injection or dry needling

1. Disregarding perpetuating factors is probably the most important reason for failure
2. Needling a latent TrP, not an active TrP
3. Needling the area of referred pain and referred tenderness, not the TrPs, therefore providing incomplete or temporary relief
4. Failure to needle the TrP itself
5. Inappropriate needle gauge
6. Injecting a solution with an irritating or allergenic bacteriostatic preservative
7. Inadequate hemostasis followed by irritation of the TrP due to local bleeding
8. Overlooking other active or associated TrPs that are contributing to the patient's pain
9. Failure to provide postneedling care including hemostasis, full stretch range of motion, postural and positioning instruction, activity modification, and neuromotor retraining
10. Failure to establish a home exercise prescription that includes intensity, frequency, and duration of the home management program

WET NEEDLING: TRIGGER POINT INJECTIONS

1. LOCAL ANESTHETICS

This discussion is an overview summary in the use of the TrPI solutions for treatment of myofascial pain and TrP dysfunction. Certainly, more specific and extensive research, scientific detail, and clinical opinion are available than can be addressed within the confines of this chapter.

A variety of solutions and combinations have been utilized in TrPI. Local anesthetics have been the most common solution utilized. Lidocaine, bupivacaine, and procaine are most frequently used local anesthetics for TrPI. Simons et al[2] were of the opinion that DN is as effective, but it results in greater postneedling soreness than treatment with the injection of a local anesthetic.[2,11] In fact, Simons et al[2] recommended using small amounts of solution, a few 10ths of a mL at any single location.

Many patients have chronic pain and are candidates to receive serial injections in clinical practice. It is common to make alterations in treatment approach relative to needle and solution choice to identify the optimal response for an individual patient. Treatment approach may also be adjusted for changes in the patient's presentation, such as in episodes of exacerbation or alteration in pain distribution.

Local anesthetics have a favorable safety profile when appropriately administered, mostly in the doses and concentrations used in TrPI. Mechanism of action for local anesthetics involves blockade of nerve conduction by reversibly binding to sodium channels, thus preventing depolarization. Duration of action is determined by protein binding capacity to the sodium channel receptors. Onset, duration, and maximum doses are referenced within Table 72-1. For patients with multiple areas requiring treatment, a lower concentration of local anesthetic may allow more areas to be safely injected.

Local anesthetics fall in to the biochemical category of ester or amide, as determined by the linking bond of the substance. Lidocaine and bupivacaine are commonly used local anesthetics that fall under the amide group. Amide local anesthetics are metabolized in the liver. This mechanism may be a consideration in patients with impaired hepatic function, although the volumes and concentrations of local anesthetics used for TrPI are not large and can be adjusted for patient condition. Procaine is an ester local anesthetic. Ester local anesthetics are hydrolyzed and rapidly metabolized and, therefore, have lower toxicity. Rapid degradation reduces the potential for adverse reaction if inadvertently introduced intravascularly. Para-aminobenzoic acid is a metabolite that can act as an allergen in some patients, but rapid metabolization reduces the likelihood of reaction when used in TrPI. Metabolites of procaine are excreted in the urine.[7] The half-life of local anesthetics may be prolonged in the setting of renal failure,[41] but local anesthetics are routinely used for procedures in renal failure and patients requiring dialysis. The quantity and dilution of local anesthetics used in TrPI would generally not be a concern in patients with renal dysfunction.

True allergy to local anesthetics is rare, accounting for less than 1% of adverse reactions.[42,43] Some patients have sensitivity to the antimicrobial preservative methylparaben contained in multidose vials. Most allergic reactions to local anesthetic are type IV hypersensitivity and have small risk of anaphylaxis. Although allergy testing can be conducted to assess whether or not a specific patient is truly allergic to a local anesthetic, the lack of overwhelming data supporting superiority of wet needling may then predispose the clinician to opt for treatment with DN. A common adverse event that may occur with any injection is a vasovagal reaction, usually secondary to needle insertion rather than to the administration of local anesthetics.

Myotoxicity of local anesthetics is another factor that may influence treatment decisions regarding the type of solution used or the option to use DN technique. The review by Zink and Graf[44] found that the intramuscular injection of local anesthetics frequently results in local myonecrosis, although significant skeletal muscle toxicity is a rare side effect. Myonecrosis persists for 24 to 48 hours until phagocytes invade the area. Intracellular dysregulation of Ca^{2+} appears to be an important element in myocyte injury. This effect is reversible and muscular regeneration occurs within 3 to 4 weeks. Muscle injury is noted to be least with use of procaine and most with bupivacaine. This effect appears to be dose and volume dependent as well as related to serial use.[44] Clinically, myotoxicity and resultant inflammation may be a consideration in patients who experience exacerbation within a few days of TrPI.

Some authors have proposed that the use of a local anesthetic may impair palpatory evaluation of response and treatment of

Table 72-1 Classification and Uses of Local Anesthetics

	Clinical Uses	Usual Concentration (%)	Usual Onset	Usual Duration (h)	Maximum[a] Single Dose (mg)	Unique Characteristics
Aminoesters						
2-Chloroprocaine	Infiltration	1	Fast	0.5-1.0	1000 + EPI	Lowest systemic toxicity
	PNB	2	Fast	0.5-1.0	1000 + EPI	Intrathecal route may be neurotoxic
	Epidural	2-3	Fast	0.5-1.5	1000 + EPI	
Procaine	Infiltration	1	Fast	0.5-1.0	1000	Used for differential spinal
	PNB	1-2	Slow	0.5-1.0	1000	
	Spinal	10	Moderate	0.5-1.0	200	
Tetracaine	Topical	2	Slow	0.5-1.0	80	
	Spinal	0.5	Fast	2-4	20	
Aminoamides						
Lidocaine	Topical	4	Fast	0.5-1.0	500 + EPI	
	Infiltration	0.5-1.0	Fast	1-2	500 + EPI	
	IV regional	0.25-0.5	Fast	1-3	500	
	PNB	1.0-1.5	Fast	0.5-1.5	500 + EPI	
	Epidural	1-2	Fast		500 + EPI	
	Spinal	5			100	

Table 72-1 Classification and Uses of Local Anesthetics (continued)

	Clinical Uses	Usual Concentration (%)	Usual Onset	Usual Duration (h)	Maximum[a] Single Dose (mg)	Unique Characteristics
Prilocaine	IV regional PNB Epidural	4 1.5-2.0 1-3	Fast	1.5-3.0	600 600 600	Least toxic amide Methemoglobinemia possible when >600 mg
Mepivacaine	PNB Epidural	1.0-1.5 1-2	Fast Fast	2-3 1.0-2.5	500 + EPI 500 + EPI	Duration of plain solutions Longer than lidocaine with EPI, useful when EPI contraindicated
Bupivacaine	PNB Epidural Spinal	0.25-0.5 0.25-0.75 0.5-0.75	Slow Moderate Fast	4-12 2-4 2-4	200 + EPI 200 + EPI 20	Exaggerated cardiotoxicity With accidental IV injection Low doses produce sensory > motor blockade
Etidocaine	PNB Epidural	0.5-1.0 1.0-1.5	Fast Fast	3-12 2-4	300 + EPI 300 + EPI	Motor > sensory blockade

[a]Maximum single dose is affected by many factors; this is only a guide.
EPI, epinephrine; IV, intravenous; PNB, peripheral nerve block.
Modified from Barash PG, Cullen BF, Stoelting RK. *Handbook of Clinical Anesthesia*. 2nd ed. Philadelphia, PA: Lippincott; 1993:206-207; Dreyer S, Beckworth W. Commonly used medications in procedures. In: Lennard TA, Vivian D, Walkowski S, Singla A, eds. *Pain Procedures in Clinical Practice*. 3rd ed. Philadelphia, PA: Elsevier-Saunders; 2011:5-12.

remaining TrPs. Limiting volume and concentration of local anesthetic injected at each site is a consideration. Also, clinicians should seek to localize the site of injection through skilled palpation and elicit an LTR before injecting solution.

Lidocaine without the vasoconstricting agent epinephrine is the most common solution utilized in TrPI. It is readily available and is relatively inexpensive. Lidocaine toxicity may cause central nervous system and cardiovascular effects. Toxicity is rare and dose dependent. It has a relatively immediate onset and duration of action from 30 to 90 minutes. Lidocaine is a category B drug for pregnancy, but is excreted in breast milk.

When reviewing the literature, there is considerable variation in the dosing of lidocaine used for TrPI. Volumes studied may range from 0.2 to 2 mL and concentrations from 0.25% to 2%, factors that may limit comparison between these studies. Lidocaine may be diluted with sterile water to a concentration of 0.25%, and it has been shown to be equivocal or better in effect to concentrations of 0.50% or 1% in a single study.[45] Iwama and Akama[46] showed diluted lidocaine to be less painful and have a longer duration of relief in a study of comparative treatment of trapezius TrPs.

Lidocaine has a pH of 6.3 to 6.4. Some clinicians will buffer lidocaine using 8.4% bicarbonate solution at a ratio of 10:1, with the goal of reducing burning discomfort. Conflicting results are noted in the studies of intradermal lidocaine injection. Matsumoto et al[47] noted that buffered lidocaine significantly reduced discomfort when compared with 10:1 dilution with normal saline, whereas Zaiac[48] found lidocaine with epinephrine diluted at 10:1 ratio with normal saline to be less painful than buffering with lidocaine. These studies were intradermal rather than intramuscular.

A study of the tolerability of intramuscular injection using 1% lidocaine as a diluent for ceftriaxone administration versus buffered 1% lidocaine as a diluent demonstrated no difference in pain or discomfort associated with the injection.[49] If this information may be extrapolated to intramuscular TrPI, there would be little benefit to buffering lidocaine for TrPI. Additional comparisons specific to comfort during TrPI would be helpful.

Procaine, similar to lidocaine, has a rapid onset and short duration of action. Procaine may have a lower myotoxicity effect and was the preferred local anesthetics recommended by Janet Travell, MD. Dr Travell recommended the use of the short-acting local anesthetic diluted to 0.5%, because a higher concentration showed no greater anesthetic effect.[50,51]

Bupivacaine or ropivacaine are longer-acting local anesthetics that are sometimes used alone or in combination for TrPI. Duration of action may last several hours. A comparison of intramuscular injection showed pain related to injection to be less with ropivacaine when compared with bupivacaine; however, this application was not assessed specific to TrP location.[52] Bupivacaine is the more common product cited in clinical use and in research for TrPI. Ropivacaine is more frequently used for procedural anesthesia such as spinal anesthesia or nerve block. Although it may be tempting for patients and clinicians to view longer-acting anesthetics as more powerful or giving longer postinjection soreness relief, longer-acting anesthetics have not been shown to be clearly superior to shorter-acting products for TrPI. There is potential for longer postinjection sensory or motor block if injected closer to a nerve as well as increased myotoxicity.

Finally, clinicians have empirically made additions to TrPI solutions, sometimes on theoretic basis and anecdotal information. Therefore, demonstrated efficacy and potential risks should be assessed before including additives to TrPI solutions.

2. CORTICOSTEROIDS

Corticosteroids have both anti-inflammatory and immunosuppressive effects. They are probably the most common additive to TrPI, although no clear overall benefit has been observed.

Table 72-2	Comparison of Commonly Used Glucocorticoid Steroids[a]				
Agent	Anti-inflammatory Potency[a]	Salt Retention Property	Plasma Half-life (min)	Duration	Equivalent Oral Dose (mg)
Hydrocortisone (Cortisol)	1	2+	90	S	20
Cortisone	0.8	2+	30	S	25
Prednisone	4-5	1+	60	I	5
Prednisolone	4-5	1+	200	I	5
Methylprednisolone (Medrol, Depo-Medrol)	5	0	180	I	4
Triamcinolone (Aristocort, Kenalog)	5	0	300	I	4
Betamethasone (Celestone)	25-35	0	100-300	L	0.6
Dexamethasone (Decadron)	25-30	30	100-300	L	0.75

[a]Relative to hydrocortisone
I, intermediate; L, long; S, short.
Adapted from Lennard TA. Fundamentals of procedural care. In: Lennard TA, ed. *Physiatric Procedures in Clinical Practice*. Philadelphia, PA: Saunders; 1995; Dreyer S, Beckworth W. Commonly used medications in procedures. In: Lennard TA, Vivian D, Walkowski S, Singla A, eds. *Pain Procedures in Clinical Practice*. 3rd ed. Philadelphia, PA: Elsevier-Saunders; 2011:5-12.

Simons et al[2] advocated against the use of long-acting steroids for use in TrPI. Steroid preparations with predominantly glucocorticoid activity rather than mineralocorticoid activity are used in pain management procedures (Table 72-2). Adverse effects of corticosteroid injection include facial flushing, depigmentation, and muscle atrophy. Local administration may produce systemic effects such as hyperglycemia in patients with diabetes. Potential risks should be included when considering this option for TrPI. Generally, corticosteroids can be mixed in the same syringe with local anesthetics. Betamethasone should not be mixed with local anesthetics containing methylparaben as a preservative because flocculation of the solution may result[7] (Celestone Package insert).

Results regarding the addition of corticosteroid to TrPI solution are mixed, and therefore, studies should be assessed for the inclusion of a control group. For example, an ultrasound-guided TrPI for piriformis syndrome performed using lidocaine was equivalent to injection using a combination of lidocaine and steroid.[53] Some studies have suggested benefit from the addition of steroid. A study of patients with headache compared treatment with DN, use of 0.25% lidocaine, and 0.25% lidocaine with 0.2 mL decadron 4 mg/mL.[54] Less postinjection discomfort and ingestion of rescue medication was noted in the group injected with a combination of a local anesthetic and corticoid.[54] On the contrary, cortisone injection directed toward the bursa for the treatment of greater trochanteric pain syndrome is a common procedure and did not prove superior to a series of DN TrP treatments.[55]

A case report of treatment of serratus anterior muscle pain syndrome describes the use of 2% lidocaine and 0.5% bupivacaine and 1 mL (40 mg) triamcinolone with a total of 3 mL deposited at each site via ultrasound guidance to target muscle fibers at the TrPs, localized by palpation.[56] A small sample group was treated but showed a fairly robust response in seven of eight patients relative to medication use and pain scale at 3 months and beyond. This patient group was unique in that pain syndrome was triggered following surgical intervention. Also, no control group for treatment without steroid or with DN was involved.[56]

Additional research may show benefit in particular patient types or anatomic locations. Positive steroid response may also be a factor that is concomitant rather than specific to addition to TrPI solution. Steroids are used in nerve blocks such as intercostal or greater occipital neuralgia and TrPI in these areas may have overlapping effects. Steroids by oral or infusion route are often a component of headache exacerbation management. In reviewing the literature or case reports showing positive result from adding steroid to TrPI, consideration should be given to proximity of injections to nerve or systemic effects before concluding benefit from the addition to TrPI solution.

Serapin is a sterile aqueous solution of salts of the Pitcher plant (sarracenia purpurea). It has been used in injections for more than 50 years to treat pain of both muscular and neuropathic origin. Limited research is available on the use of serapin for myofascial pain, and most available information is old. A mechanism of action of selectively blocking C-fiber activity was proposed.[57] Bates[58] noted longer relief with injection of serapin when compared with novocaine or saline without sensory or motor block. No RCTs of its use in TrPI are noted at this time.

Clinically, serapin can be successfully used in a 50/50 combination with a local anesthetic to treat patients in exacerbation, with a significant component of aching pain or if limited response to local anesthetic alone. No adverse reactions to the addition of serapin to TrPI solution have been seen with this technique. Any improvement in response quality or duration is purely observational. Serapin in no longer available on the US market, and it is not certain when or if the product will be available.

Hyaluronate is a glycosaminoglycan found in the extracellular matrix, especially of soft connective tissues. Product forms are used for intraarticular viscosupplementation injections. Comparison was made of TrPI using 0.5% lidocaine with the same solution of lidocaine mixed with hyaluronidase 600 IU/mL. No significant differences at day 0, 4, 7, or 14 were reported. Patients receiving hyaluronidase showed less postinjection soreness on day 1.[59] Given the very limited benefit and associated cost, it would be difficult to recommend unless additional supportive data became available.

Dextrose solution has been used for proliferative injection techniques such as prolotherapy at concentrations ranging from 10% to 20% and in perineural injection treatment buffered at 0.5% in sterile water. A proposed mechanism for the use of dextrose in myofascial pain cites glycopenia as a potential trigger for C-fiber excitation, neurogenic inflammation, and neuropathic pain.[60] A single Korean study proposed dextrose as an energy supplement for impaired energy metabolism of the TrPs. In this study, comparison of the pain intensity and pressure pain thresholds showed lower scores indicating greater improvement at 7 days for the group treated with 5% dextrose water than for the one treated with 0.5% lidocaine or normal saline.[61] More research would be needed before recommending the addition of dextrose to TrPI solutions.

Clinicians have added intramuscular vitamin preparations such as Vitamin B_{12}, D, or C to TrPI solutions. Although the assessment of overall health and nutritional status is an important consideration when addressing perpetuating factors for myofascial pain, there is no evidence to recommend the addition of vitamins (see Chapter 4).

The anti-inflammatory ketorolac is a nonsteroidal anti-inflammatory drug in the family of propionic acids, often used as an analgesic and antipyretic. Ketorolac acts by inhibiting bodily synthesis of prostaglandins. Approved use includes both intramuscular and intravenous administration. Ketorolac may be utilized to treat pain exacerbations, including musculoskeletal pain. No RCT that is specific to the addition of ketorolac to TrPI solution is available.

Potential remains for other types of solution to be helpful additions to TrPI, such as 5-HT3 receptor antagonists,[62] tumor necrosis factor blockers,[63] or autologous serum conditioned for interleukin-1 receptor antagonists. Quality research would be needed before recommending additional solution components for routine clinical use.

3. NEUROTOXINS

The use of neurotoxins for the treatment of musculoskeletal pain has expanded[64] and requires mention, although a full review of this treatment intervention is beyond the scope of this text.

Botox is produced by *Clostridium botulinum*, an anerobic, gram-positive organism that can be found in soil and water. Botox, when injected, causes a degree of flaccid paralysis by blocking the release of acetylcholine at the presynaptic terminal of the neuromuscular junction. There are multiple neurotoxins designated as types A, B, C1, C2, D, E, F, and G. Table 72-3 is a summary of the neurotoxins that are Food and Drug Administration (FDA) approved. Botox is used to treat multiple painful conditions such as cervical dystonia and chronic daily migraine headaches. Its effects on the motor neurons are well known, causing a relaxation of hypertonic or spastic muscle. It has also been found to inhibit the release of neurotransmitters involved in pain transmission, such as glutamate and substance P.[65] A study performed on rats, showed significantly reduced glutamate release as well as reduced local edema and diminished signs of pain after peripheral injection of toxin. This may be the rationale for why Botox reduces pain in addition to its motor effects.[66]

Muscle weakness can begin to take effect in 2 to 5 days, with maximum effect at about 2 weeks. As a result of the toxin's effect on the neuromuscular junction, the motor endplate fails and the nerve ending dies back. A new nerve ending sprouts from the residual axon, eventually forming the new neuromuscular junction. The neuromuscular junction is usually reestablished in approximately 3 months. Thus, Botox injections last for 3 months on average.[67]

The results reported in studies comparing the efficacy of TrPI with that of Botox are mixed. In reviewing the literature, the treatment response window studied often compared relatively short postinjection intervals. Given the neurotoxin duration of action, differences in response should have been evaluated 2 to 3 months from treatment rather than postinjection and at intervals of a few weeks after injection.[67,68] The Cochrane review found only four trials comparing the effects of Botox A against placebo in individuals with myofascial pain. The results were controversial because three trials reported no statistically significant differences between Botox A and placebo for reducing pain.[68]

A subset of individuals with chronic myofascial pain will have TrP reactivation despite repeated TrPI. This group of patients may be considered for botulinum injections. The injections can reduce the electrical activity of the TrPs and provide longer lasting response.[67] The method of identifying a locus for treatment may be different when evaluating for neurotoxin injection. Trigger point injection is directed by palpation, whereas evaluation for neurotoxin injection may be performed by needle EMG to appropriately identify and map out the muscles to be targeted. EMG mapping is generally used in the cervical region given the complexity of the anatomy. Manual palpation and clinical judgment are generally used in other regions of the body. Studies have shown that patients who have mapping studies tend to have a greater response to injections than those who do not.[69] Mapping may also include the use of ultrasound to evaluate deeper muscles that would ordinarily be avoided because of proximity to sensitive structures such as nerves, vessels, or pleura. Clinically, patients who have elevated activity of the muscles on testing tend to have better outcomes with neurotoxin injection than patients with minimal to no activity.

Neurotoxin injection may offer longer duration of relief of myofascial pain and may also offer a window of opportunity for rehabilitation efforts such as muscle reeducation, effective stretching, and postural correction. Longer duration of effect may also have negative consequences. Clinically, there are patients who tolerated TrPI well who experience significant exacerbation after neurotoxin treatment. Patients with underlying segmental or generalized hypermobility may be further destabilized by the weakness resulting from Botox injection. For example, shoulder pain may be worsened by a compromise of scapular stabilization by neurotoxin administration to treat TrPs at the medial scapular border.

Patients should be educated on the potential side effects from neurotoxin injections. As stated previously, the injections take about 2 weeks to begin taking effect. After 2 weeks, patients may notice a flare in the pain. If injecting neck muscles, they may also notice weakness in the neck with difficulty lifting the head up. Mild flu-like symptoms may also be reported. These side effects are self-limiting and should not last more than 2 weeks.

If a patient responds positively to neurotoxin injection, repeat injections should be considered at 3 months. If TrPs are deactivated and do not reactivate, patients may be able to stop treatment. Others may notice a return of symptoms after 3 months, requiring subsequent injections. Patients should be monitored after each injection to assess the need for further treatment.

4. SUMMARY OF TRIGGER POINT INJECTIONS

There continues to be a significant degree of empirical evaluation regarding the practice and efficacy of TrPI. This area of study offers many potential research opportunities. Comparisons are needed of treatment in matched patient types, solutions, and additives, as well as optimal frequency and duration regimens.

As noted by Simons et al,[2] patients may report a history of treatment by TrPI without benefit. Patients may also report a history of significant pain or postinjection soreness with previous treatments. Clinicians who perform TrPI should be both

Table 72-3 Summary of FDA Approved Neurotoxins

Molecular Name	Pharmaceutical Name	Type
Onabotulinum	Botox	A
Abobotulinum	Dysport	A
Incobotulinum	Xeomin	A
Rimabotulinum	Myobloc	B

From Davids HR. Botulinum toxin in pain management. https://emedicine.medscape.com/article/325574-overview#a4. Accessed August 31, 2017.

well-trained and experienced. With more states and countries acknowledging that DN is within the scope of physical therapist practice, patients will have greater access to qualified clinicians for the treatment of myofascial pain and dysfunction.

As the available literature does not overwhelmingly demonstrate superiority of TrPI over DN or of a particular solution for injection, it ultimately falls to the clinician to choose the initial treatment approach and individualize to each patient. Concomitant health issues, body habitus, and anatomy of treatment target are all factors to be considered when determining needle choice, solution, and possibly guidance assistance such as ultrasound or EMG. A combination of wet needling and DN may also be used. Subsequent treatments may be adjusted pending the patient's response.

There may be some benefit in the use of local anesthetics relative to postinjection comfort and possibly several weeks to months out from treatment. Lidocaine or procaine may be used at 1% or diluted with normal saline or sterile water down to a 0.5% or even 0.25% concentration. Longer-duration local anesthetic such as bupivacaine may be used but has not shown greater effect and may increase the component of myotoxicity and potential for longer neural blockade. Higher-concentration solutions have generally not shown better effect. Volumes greater than a few 10th of a milliliter at each site are generally not indicated. Limiting concentration, volume, and delay in the injection of local anesthetic may better allow the practitioner to localize TrPs and elicit LTRs.

Additives to TrPI solutions have been used empirically by clinicians but have limited or no support in the literature. Corticosteroids may have benefit in some patient types, but there is insufficient research to outline recommendations for use. Steroids carry additional local and systemic risks, especially if the dosage is higher, with multiple injection sites or with repeated use. A trial may be reserved for patients not responding to TrPI using only local anesthetic.

The use of neurotoxins in the treatment of myofascial pain remains controversial. It is possible that we have not yet fully teased out which patients are most likely to respond to the use of neurotoxin administration or which individual's pain may be temporarily exacerbated by its use. Given the higher costs associated for neurotoxin solution and administration, the use of local anesthetic TrPI should likely remain the first choice of intervention.[54] Evaluation for the use of neurotoxin should be reserved for cases in which response to TrPI or DN is limited or not of adequate duration. Positive response to the use of neurotoxin can reduce the frequency or eliminate the need for TrPI. Some patients benefit from the availability of TrPI between neurotoxin sessions to address the residual areas of myofascial dysfunction.

DRY NEEDLING

It is important to consider that filiform needles are used in acupuncture and DN. A discussion of the differences between both approaches is beyond the scope of this text. The American Physical Therapy Association defines DN as a "skilled intervention using a thin filiform needle (usually an acupuncture needle) to penetrate the skin that stimulates myofascial TrPs, muscles, and connective tissue for the management of neuromusculoskeletal disorders."[70]

Some authors have described different DN techniques. Probably the most expanded needling intervention is the one described by Hong.[11] Hong[11] described his "fast in, fast out" method of needling of a TrP that has been precisely located by palpation. The palpating finger should stay over or straddle the taut band in order to guide the needle insertion directly to the TrP area. The needle is held by the other hand. With the thin (27-gauge) needle remaining deep to the subcutaneous tissue, the muscle fibers of the TrP are explored with multiple needle insertions. The needle movement is rapid, "fast in" and "fast out." Hong has modified the technique as originally described by including a pause of 2 or 3 seconds between insertions. The pause following each insertion permits time to consider the tissue textures traversed by the needle and where to redirect the needle, the time for the identification of an LTR, and the time to immediately inject anesthetic solution into the same needle track when a twitch occurs. The needle is inserted deep enough to fully penetrate the TrP and then is pulled back to the subcutaneous tissue layer but not out of the skin. If the clinician is performing TrPI, a drop of 0.5% procaine (or lidocaine) is injected into the taut band following every LTR that is detected by the feeling of needle tip movement (from the hand holding the syringe), by palpating the twitch contraction (with the palpating hand), or by seeing, if the muscle is superficial, the movement of a visible twitch. The local analgesic agent should be injected only if an LTR accompanies needle insertion.

This rapid technique avoids muscle fiber damage from LTRs. Experience during research studies showed that LTRs are elicited more frequently when the needle is moved quickly rather than slowly. The track of needle insertion is usually very straight and the needle is less likely to be deflected by the dense contracture knots when the needle is inserted at high speed. For this reason, this "fast in, fast out" technique is well suited to the use of filiform (acupuncture) needles. Hong[11] originally proposed that an LTR should be obtained during the application of the technique to be effective. However, how many LTRs are needed to obtain a positive outcome is still debatable. A recent study has found no clinical differences in pain depending on the number of LTRs obtained during DN in the upper trapezius muscle in patients with neck pain.[71] Similarly, another study suggests that the LTR may not be as necessary as Hong[11] described for a successful outcome because no difference at 1 week was observed between patients experiencing LTR and those not experiencing LTR.[72] Discrepancies in the published studies have lead some authors to question the need of LTR during DN.[12]

Gunn[73] recommends identifying TrPs by spot tenderness in a taut band and then using DN techniques. He first identifies the TrPs as a spot of localized tenderness in a taut band and then identifies the precise skin location through which to insert the needle using a dermometer (point finder or skin resistance detector). He then inserts the needle through this location to the TrP where he feels a "grabbing" sensation at the needle tip, which is often associated with aching pain, as the needle enters into the TrP area. Gunn[73] defined this TrP needling technique as Intramuscular Stimulation.

The effectiveness of DN in many conditions is supported by systematic reviews and meta-analysis. For instance, it has been concluded that TrP-DN is effective, at least in the short term, for the management of pain conditions in the upper[74] and lower[75] quadrants, neck-shoulder pain,[13] low back pain,[76] and plantar heel pain.[77] An interesting meta-analysis found evidence suggesting that DN applied by physical therapists was superior to no treatment or sham, but it has been found to be equally effective as other physical therapy treatments for short- and mid-term follow-ups in individuals with musculoskeletal pain.[78] No clear evidence of long-term effects of DN is available. Nevertheless, the Canadian Agency for Drugs and Technologies in Health has accepted the use of DN following an appropriate clinical reasoning in the public health system.[79]

The underlying mechanism by which DN exerts its therapeutic effects is not understood, and both mechanical and neurophysiologic mechanisms are proposed.[80,81] From a mechanical point of view, disruption of the integrity of dysfunctional endplates, increase of sarcomere length, and reduction of the overlap between actin and myosin filaments are proposed.[1] From a neurophysiologic point of view, DN may reduce both peripheral and central sensitization by removing the source of peripheral nociception (TrP), by modulating spinal efficacy in the dorsal horn, and by activating central inhibitory pain pathways. Likely, DN acts simultaneously at different levels in this process.[82]

TRIGGER POINT INJECTION AND DRY NEEDLING PROCEDURES

1. HEAD AND NECK PAIN (Section 2)

Trapezius Muscle (Chapter 6)

Trigger point injection or DN of the upper trapezius muscle may be performed with the patient positioned in supine, side-lying, or prone. The middle and lower trapezius TrPs are best approached with the patient positioned in prone or side-lying on the unaffected side, whereas the upper trapezius muscle can be needled in supine and prone, depending on the TrP location. Different systematic reviews suggest that DN of the upper trapezius muscle is effective for reducing pain in individuals with mechanical neck pain.[4,13] The results are also maintained at 6-month follow-up.[83] Further, the application of DN into an active TrP of the lower fibers of the trapezius muscle was also effective for reducing pain in individuals with mechanical neck pain.[84]

Upper Trapezius Fibers (Figure 72-6)

For TrPI or DN of the upper fibers of the trapezius muscle, the patient should be positioned in supine or prone. If the patient is unable to assume these positions, the side-lying position can be utilized. The TrP is identified with cross-fiber pincer palpation and held firmly in a pincer grasp to lift the muscle away from underlying cervical structures and the apex of the lung. The needle is directed in an anterior-posterior (Figure 72-6A) or posterior–anterior (Figure 72-6B) direction. When the needle penetrates a TrP, the LTRs are typically quite strong and numerous.

Middle Trapezius Fibers (Figure 72-7)

For TrPI or DN of the middle fibers of the trapezius muscle, the patient is positioned prone. The TrP is identified with cross-fiber flat palpation and fixed on the underlying rib. The clinician identifies and blocks the intercostal spaces over and under the corresponding rib with the index and middle fingers of the palpating hand to avoid entering the lung field (Figure 72-7). The needle is directed toward the TrP. If the intercostal space can't be identified, the needle can be inserted tangentially and superficially into the muscle from a lateral to medial direction.

Lower Trapezius Fibers (Figure 72-8)

For TrPI or DN of the lower fibers of the trapezius muscle, the patient is positioned prone. The TrP is identified with cross-fiber flat palpation and fixed on the underlying rib. The clinician identifies and blocks the intercostal spaces over and under the corresponding rib with the index and middle finger of the palpating hand to avoid entering the lung field (Figure 72-8). The needle is directed from a posterior to anterior direction toward the TrP. If the intercostal space can't be identified, the needle can be inserted tangentially and superficially into the muscle from a lateral to inferomedial direction.

Sternocleidomastoid Muscle (Chapter 7) Figure 72-9

Sternocleidomastoid TrPs often react to injection therapy with headache and more local soreness than do other muscles, perhaps because of the multiplicity of TrPs, some of which remain

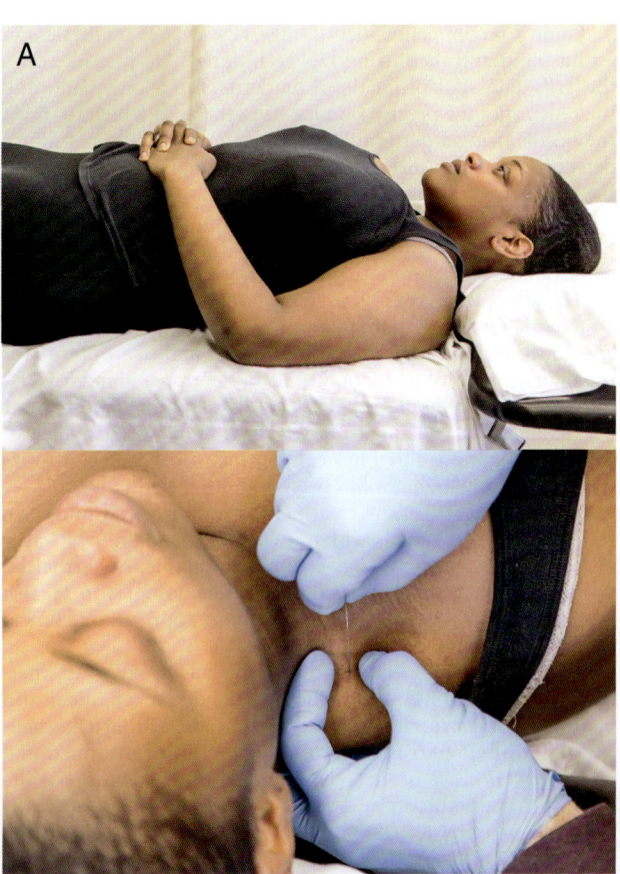
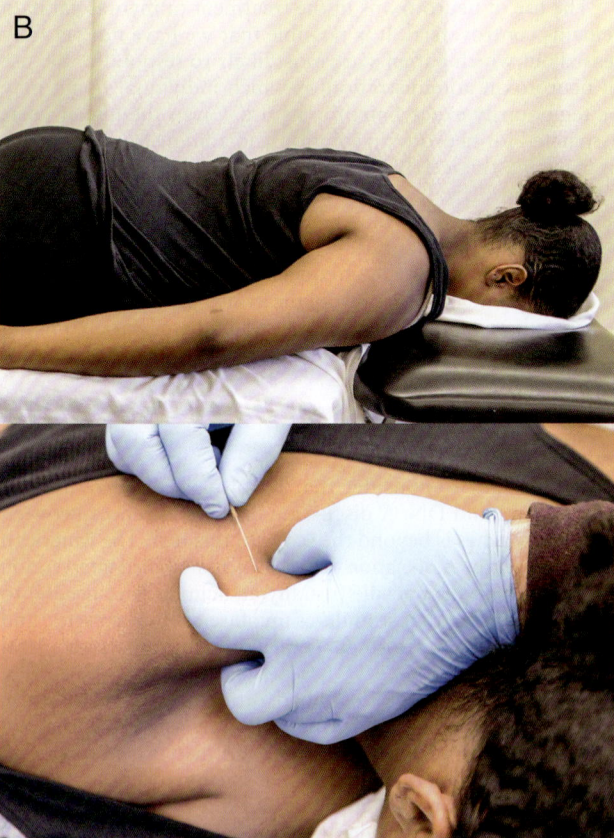

Figure 72-6. Trigger point injection or dry needling technique for **upper trapezius muscle fibers**. A, Supine. The needle is directed from anterior to posterior. B, Prone. The needle is directed from posterior to anterior. Note that the muscle is pulled away from the apex of the lung and other structures.

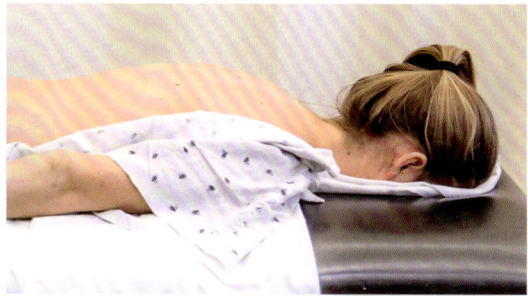

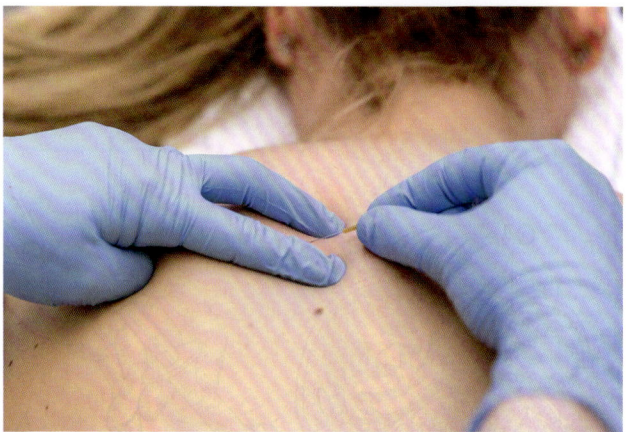

Figure 72-7. Trigger point injection or dry needling technique for the **middle trapezius muscle fibers**. Note the blocking of the intercostal space to avoid penetration of the lung field.

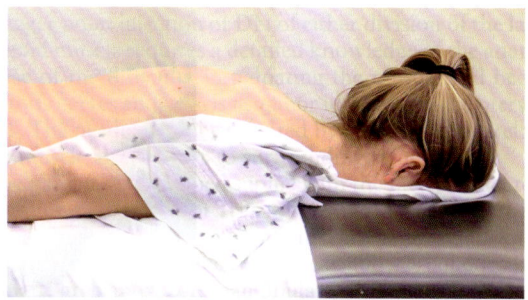

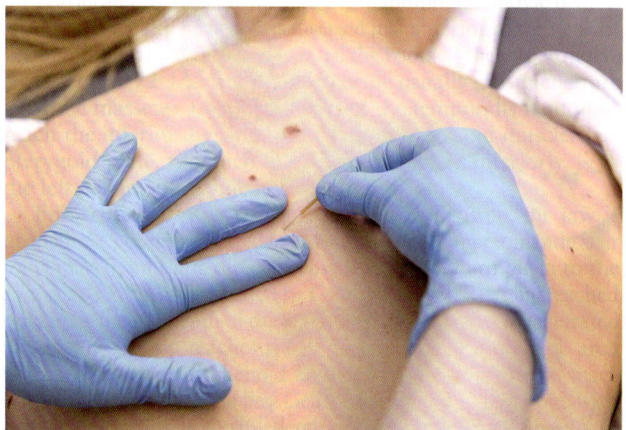

Figure 72-8. Trigger point injection or dry needling technique for the **lower trapezius muscle fibers**. Note the blocking of the intercostal space to avoid penetration of the lung field.

active in spite of treatment, or because of the strong autonomic influences of its TrPs. The muscle on only one side can be needled during the first session. Any TrPs on the contralateral side should be needled only after any reaction to the previous TrPI or after DN has subsided and if the injected TrP sites showed substantial improvement.

For TrPI or DN of either division, the patient is positioned supine (Figure 72-9A and B) and the TrP is identified with a cross-fiber pincer palpation and fixed with a pincer grasp between the clinician's thumb, index, and middle fingers. The muscle is slackened by tilting the ear toward the shoulder on the affected side with the face turned slightly upward and to the opposite side; a pillow may be placed under the shoulder of the affected side to lift the chest and further slacken the muscle. The course of the external jugular vein is outlined by blocking the vein with a finger just above the clavicle and the carotid artery is identified. When the mid-level of the muscle is being needled, the vein can be shifted either laterally or medially by the clinician's finger to avoid penetrating it.

For TrPI or DN of the sternal and clavicular heads (Figure 72-9B), the entire muscle should be encompassed by the clinician's thumb and fingers and lifted off the underlying blood vessels, nerves, and scalene muscles (Figure 72-9C). The needle is directed toward the clinician's finger on the posterior aspect of the muscle and the needle direction is from anterior to posterior. A TrP in the proximal portion of the muscle can be needled with the needle inserted and directed toward the clinician's finger and the mastoid process.

A 22- to 27-gauge hypodermic needle (preferably 25-gauge), that is 3.8 cm (1.5 in) long or a 0.30 × 30 mm filiform needle, should be selected. Penetration of the needle into the TrP at the precise point of maximal tenderness is confirmed by an LTR and/or by local pain with projection of the pattern of referred pain. Through a single skin puncture, multiple needling with a continuous injection of 1 or 2 mL of 0.5% procaine solution can be carried out until pain and LTR are no longer elicited

by the needle.[31,85] Usually, TrPs in the superficial, more medial sternal division are inactivated first (Figure 72-4A), followed by the TrPs in the deeper and more posterior clavicular division (Figure 72-9B).

Occasionally, during TrPI at or above the mid-level of the sternocleidomastoid muscle, the patient may describe numbness in the face, which involves tissue deeper than the skin. The patient can still feel light touch, heat, and cold, and may also feel a prickling pain in the angle of the jaw, cheek, and pinna of the ear. These symptoms may be due to anesthetic infiltration of the posterior branch of the greater auricular nerve that loops around and traverses the face from the sternocleidomastoid muscle. Depending on the solution, the sensation of numbness disappears in 15 or 20 minutes, as the local anesthetic effect dissipates.

Masseter Muscle (Chapter 8)
Figure 72-10

If the immediate treatment response of masseter TrPs to manual release techniques is not satisfactory, TrPI or DN of the masseter TrPs usually inactivates them. Trigger point injection or DN is most accurately performed with the patient positioned supine and the mouth slightly opened. Trigger points are typically located with cross-fiber flat palpation; however, cross-fiber pincer grasp may also be used with one digit localizing the TrP from inside the mouth against the thumb outside the mouth (Figure 72-10A). Needling of the posterior (deep) fibers requires awareness of the location of the facial nerve. The needle is directed into the muscle belly.

When the TrP is clearly identified and fixed between the clinician's index and middle fingers, the needle should be directed specifically into the muscle belly with multiple insertions (peppering) performed without withdrawing the needle (Figure 72-10B). The clinician should note any LTR and pain reactions indicating that the needle accurately encountered the TrPs.

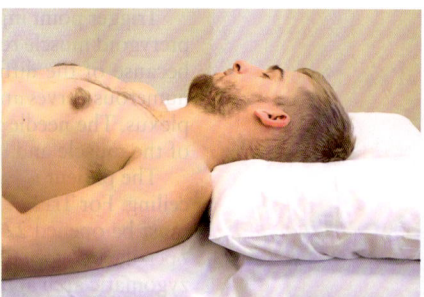
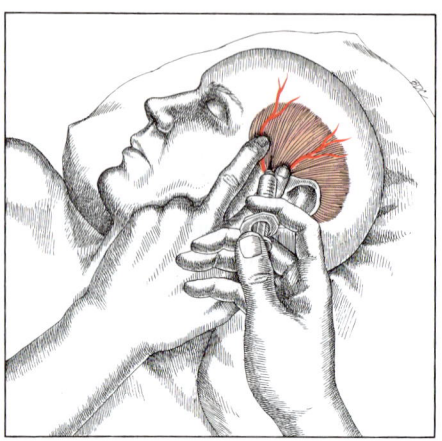
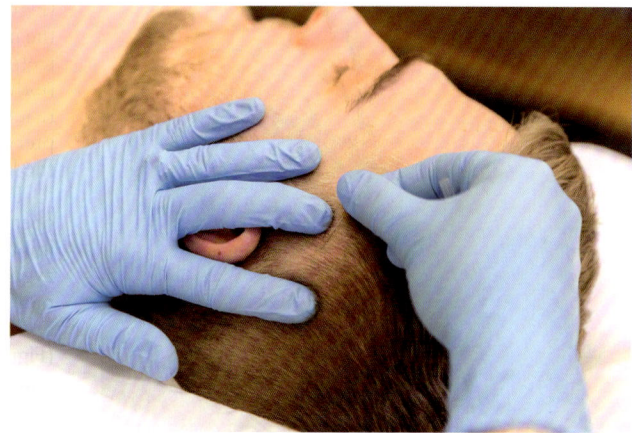

Figure 72-11. Trigger point injection or dry needling of the **temporalis muscle** (light red). The temporal artery (dark red) is avoided. A finger is placed on the artery to continuously monitor its location; other fingers localize a TrP.

program, TrPI or DN can be attempted in the anterior neck muscles. With the patient supine, either the posterior or anterior belly of the digastric TrPs may be fixed between the clinician's fingers and needled. When needling the posterior belly of the digastric muscle, it is wise not to penetrate the external jugular vein that is readily identified by blocking the vein lower in the neck (Figure 72-15A). During injection with a 3.8-cm (1½ in) 22-gauge hypodermic needle (Figure 72-10B) or a 0.30 × 30 mm filiform needle, one finger is used to displace the vein; the taut band containing the TrPs is localized between two fingers for tactile guidance of the needle. The internal carotid neurovascular bundle lies deep to the muscle.[87] It is avoided by determining the size of the muscle by palpation and then by needling within the confines of the muscle; the needle is directed posteriorly, as illustrated (Figure 72-15B). A 27-gauge needle can be used but only with the Hong technique.[11]

An LTR is an important indicator of a successful injection. When injecting posterior digastric TrPs, no effort is made to distinguish the posterior belly of the digastric muscle from the stylohyoid muscle. Needle penetration of these TrPs may cause a flash of pain over the occipital region, especially if that pain pattern is part of the patient's current pain report.

To needle the digastric anterior belly, the head and neck of the patient are extended, and the TrP spot tenderness in the taut subcutaneous muscle fibers is localized between two fingers of the palpating hand for needling (Figure 72-16).

If it is necessary to needle the other suprahyoid or infrahyoid muscles, a shorter (1 in, 27-gauge) hypodermic needle or 0.30 × 30 mm filiform needle is recommended with due consideration given to the local anatomy.

Trigger point injection or DN of the longus colli muscle is difficult and requires an advanced level of clinical experience and technique. The guide fingers are placed along a lateral border of the trachea and slowly advanced by separating the musculature from the adjacent trachea by gentle rocking and wiggling motions of the fingers. This palpatory advance stops when the fingertips reach the anterior portion of a vertebra, and the depth beneath the skin is carefully noted. Changes in the direction of pressure help locate the areas of maximum tenderness. The longus colli muscle can be a very thin muscle. The needle is advanced along the path identified by the fingers. It is advanced very slowly and gently as it approaches the depth

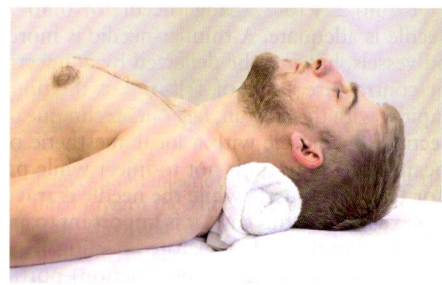
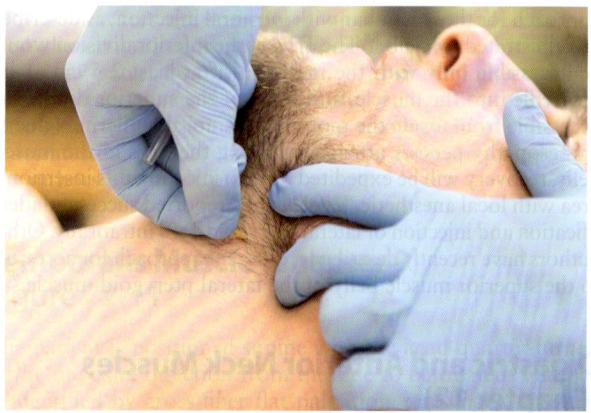

Figure 72-12. Trigger point injection or dry needling technique for the **medial pterygoid muscle**.

Chapter 72: Trigger Point Injection and Dry Needling   775

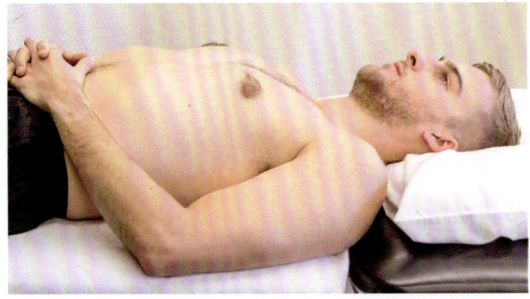

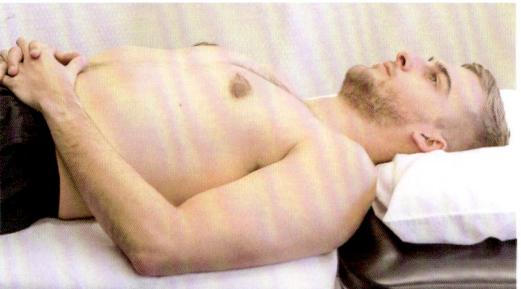

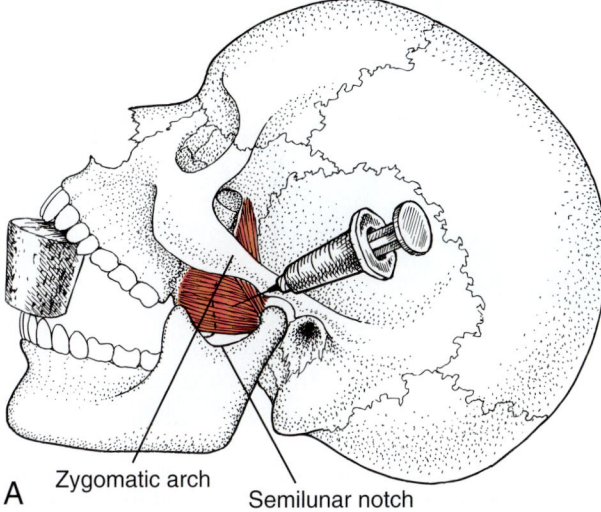

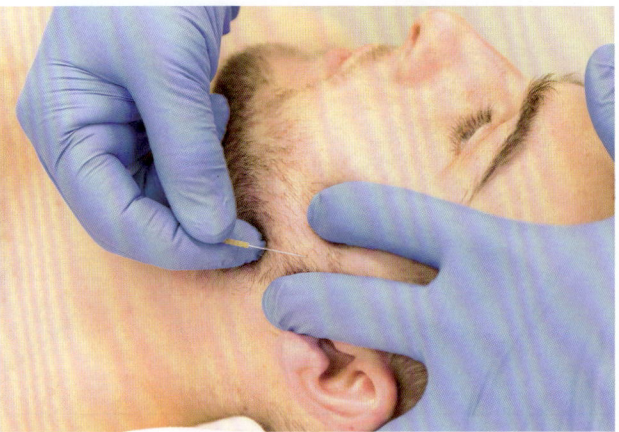

Figure 72-14. Trigger point injection or dry needling technique for the **superior division of the lateral pterygoid muscle**.

Facial Muscles (Chapter 13)
Figures 72-18 and 72-19A

Trigger point injection or DN of TrPs in the facial muscles is usually more effective than treatment by self-stretch alone. Refer to Chapter 13 for the specific anatomic location of each the facial muscles. The facial muscles are very superficial and typically a 0.15 × 15 mm filiform needle can be utilized.

Trigger point injection or DN of the zygomaticus major muscle is performed with the patient in the supine position, and the muscle is held in a pincer grasp between the digits for injection of the taut band at its TrP under tactile guidance. The needle is directed toward the zygomatic bone (Figure 72-18).

Trigger point injection or DN of the procerus muscle is performed with the patient in the supine position, and the TrP is located and fixed with pincer palpation. The needle is inserted superficially and directed in an inferior direction from the forehead toward the nose (Figure 72-19A).

The other facial muscles may be needled with a similar approach to the ones described above, taking account for the specific anatomy of each.

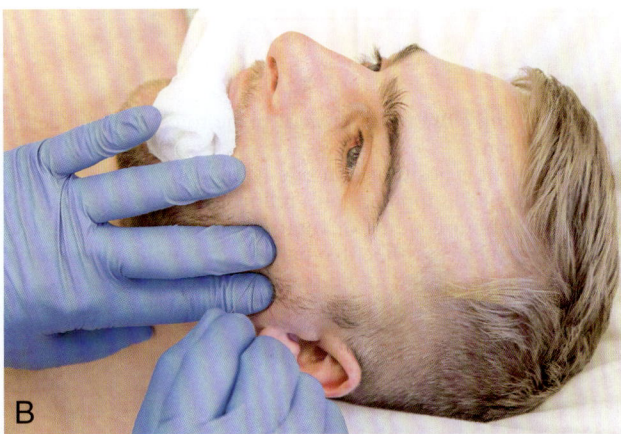

Figure 72-13. Trigger point injection or dry needling technique for the **inferior division of the left lateral pterygoid muscle** (dark red). A, Lateral view of its anatomic relationships when the jaw is propped open. The dotted line marks the posterior margin of the pterygoid plate to which the inferior division attaches. The needle reaches the inferior division through the bony aperture bounded by the zygomatic arch above, the semilunar (mandibular) notch below, the coronoid process in front, and the condyle of the mandible behind. B, Dry needling of the inferior division of the lateral pterygoid muscle.

Occipitofrontalis Muscle (Chapter 14)
Figure 72-19B

The frontalis muscle fibers are thin and very superficial, which makes its TrPs difficult to locate with the needle tip. To inject or DN it, a 2.5 cm (1 in), 24- or 25-gauge hypodermic needle or 0.15 × 15 mm filiform needle respectively is directed across the muscle fibers (parallel to the eyebrow), nearly tangential to the skin (Figure 72-19B).

The occipitalis muscle belly is thicker than the frontalis muscle and may require a longer needle. Needling of these posterior TrPs is technically more satisfactory because they seem to lie in a small hollow that holds sufficient muscle mass to receive the needle. However, considerable probing of the area may be necessary to locate them.

of the vertebral structures to minimize hard contact with the bony vertebra. Even gentle contact with the bone can bend the tip of the needle into a "fishhook" that feels "scratchy," especially whenever the needle is retracted. If this contact occurs, the needle should be immediately withdrawn and replaced. The anterior surface of the longus colli is very gently explored with the needle tip in the regions where palpation against the anterior surface of the vertebral column elicited the greatest tenderness. The clinician's palpating finger should remain in contact with the TrP during the entire needling technique (Figure 72-17).[91]

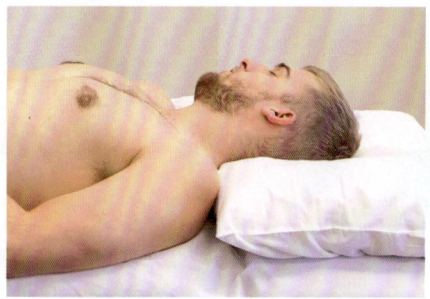
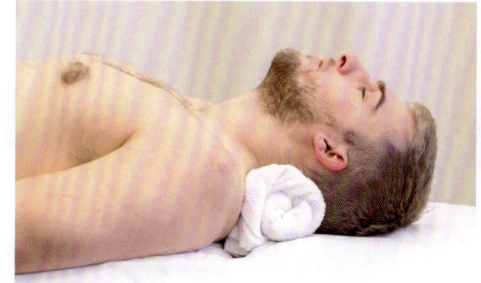

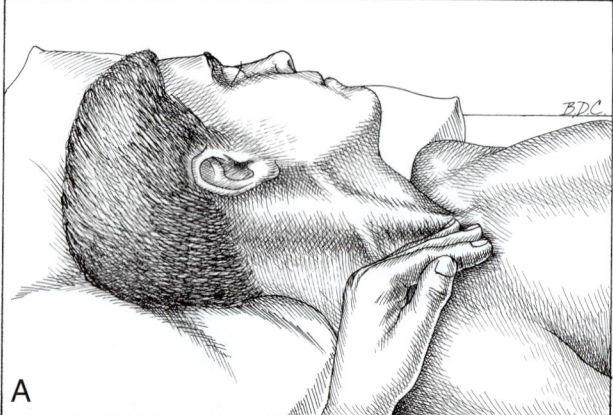
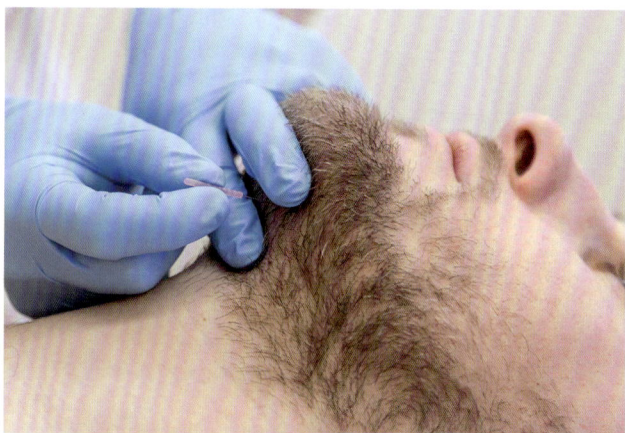

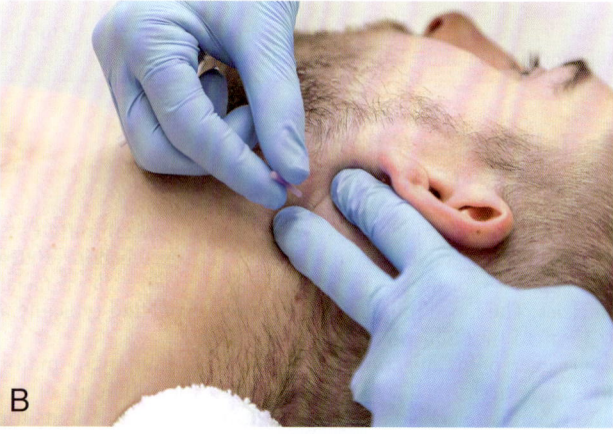

Figure 72-15. Trigger point injection or dry needling of the **posterior belly of the digastric muscle**. A, Manual occlusion of the external jugular vein to demonstrate its path near the angle of the jaw. B, Injection or DN of the muscle belly using the index finger to displace the external jugular vein to one side. The middle finger presses against the sternocleidomastoid muscle on the posterior aspect of the digastric muscle, and the posterior belly is fixed between the two fingers at the trigger point.

Figure 72-16. Trigger point injection or dry needling of the **anterior belly of the digastric muscle**. The patient's head is tilted upward to gain access to the muscle.

and remaining close to the frontal plane to control the depth of penetration.

The patient is positioned in side-lying with the affected side up, with the head supported on a pillow between the cheek and shoulder without bending or rotating the head and neck. The TrP is located by cross-fiber flat palpation. The clinician's finger identifies the taut band and directs the needle in a superior to inferior direction at a shallow angle toward the palpating finger.

Splenius Cervicis (Figure 72-20)

The patient is positioned the same as described for the splenius capitis muscle. Splenius cervicis TrPs are located mid-muscle belly[92] and are found by cross-fiber pincer palpation at approximately the level of the C7 spinous process. At this level, the splenius cervicis muscle lies medial and deep to the levator scapulae muscle and continues inferiorly, deep to the rhomboid and serratus posterior superior muscles. This muscle is located between the lower end of the splenius capitis and levator scapulae muscles, and it is best needled with the needle directed from anterior to posterior direction (Figure 72-20). The needle may be directed medially as the muscle is located away from the intervertebral foramen laterally. In this approach, the needle enters the splenius cervicis muscle either anterior to or through the anterior border of the upper fibers of the trapezius muscle. A palpated LTR confirms needle contact with the TrP.

During TrPI of splenius cervicis TrPs, Simons et al[2] noted that a few patients fainted as a result of the strong autonomic stimulus associated with the release of these TrPs. This fainting usually follows multiple large twitch responses with visible deviation of the head in the direction of the twitch. When the head moves, it is likely that the fibers of the splenius capitis and splenius cervicis muscles contract together. If the patient is being treated for a "stiff neck," any TrP in the levator scapulae should muscle be injected at the same time as those in the splenius cervicis muscle.

Splenius Capitis and Splenius Cervicis Muscles (Chapter 15)

Splenius Capitis (Figure 72-20)

The splenius capitis muscle can be injected safely at the level of C2-C3 with appropriate precautions. The semispinalis capitis muscle lies deep to the splenius capitis muscle (Figure 72-20) and provides a buffer between it and the unprotected portion of the vertebral artery (see Figure 16-3). Also, the exposed artery lies cephalad to the C1 spinous process (see Figure 17-1). Therefore, the splenius capitis muscle can be safely needled by directing the needle inferomedially, below the C2 vertebrae (Figure 72-20),

Chapter 72: Trigger Point Injection and Dry Needling 777

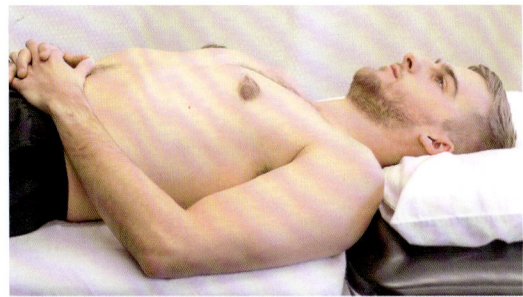

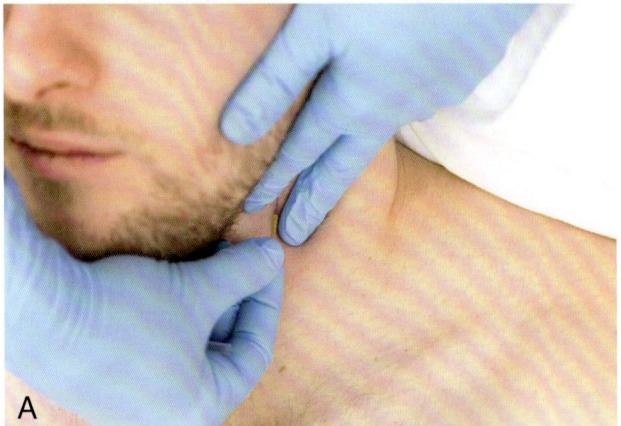

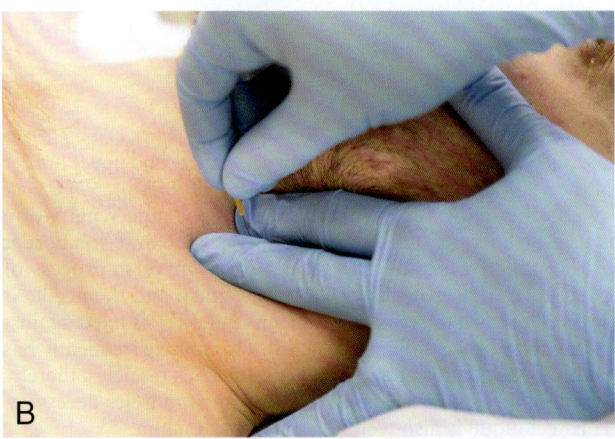

Figure 72-17. Trigger point injection or dry needling technique for the **longus colli muscle**. A, Frontal oblique view. B, Sagittal view. Note the middle finger holding the sternocleidomastoid muscle laterally to allow access to the longus colli muscle.

Posterior Cervical Muscles (Chapter 16)

Trigger point injection or DN is simplified by noting which segmental levels the TrPs typically occur for each of the posterior cervical muscles; although clinicians should remember that there is not a specific location of TrPs in any given muscle and the whole muscle must be examined. Injection or DN of TrPs in the upper portion of the semispinalis capitis muscle above the level of the second spinous process should be avoided because of the proximity of the unprotected vertebral artery; however, this muscle can be needled below that level if appropriate precautions are taken.

Trigger points in the posterior cervical muscles frequently occur bilaterally, so it is often necessary to treat both sides. A common mistake is the failure to needle deeply enough. The vertebral artery is avoided by carefully noting the spinal level and avoiding needling deep into the lateral posterior neck at, or above, the level of the C2 spinous process (Figure 16-3).

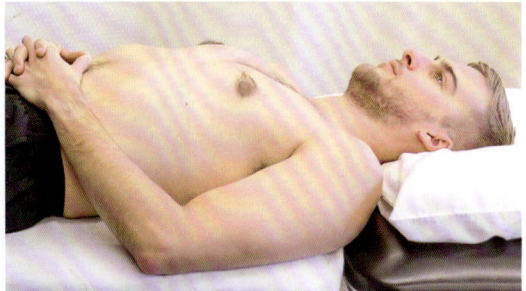

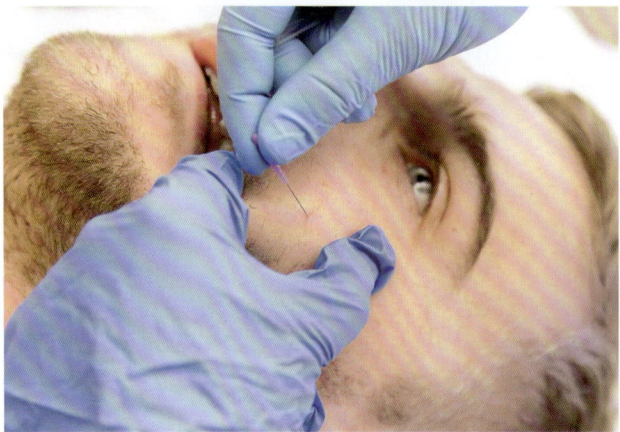

Figure 72-18. Trigger point injection or dry needling of the **right zygomaticus major muscle**, using pincer grasp to localize the trigger points between the digits.

Semispinalis Capitis and Cervicis (Figure 72-22)

For TrPI or DN of the semispinalis capitis and cervicis muscles, the patient is positioned side-lying with the affected side up and the taut band and TrPs are fixed by pincer grasp. The middle portion of the semispinalis capitis muscle lies deep to both the upper trapezius and splenius capitis muscles (see Figures 16-3 and 72-21), and therefore it requires relatively deep penetration. The needle is directed anterior to posterior at a shallow angle toward the clinician's finger and the posterior aspect of the cervical vertebrae (Figure 72-22).

Cervical Multifidus (Figure 72-23)

For TrPI or DN of the cervical multifidus muscle, the patient is positioned in prone. These muscles are not readily available for digital palpation; therefore, the needling can be diagnostic as well as therapeutic. The clinical decision to needle these muscles should be based on the deep pain referral and patient symptoms. The needle is inserted approximately 1 cm lateral to the cervical spinal process below C2 and above T1 vertebral levels (Figure 72-23). The needle is directed inferomedially toward the TrP and lamina of the cervical vertebrae. In a cadaveric study using ultrasound, Fernández-de-las-Peñas et al[93] have demonstrated that this DN approach is safe and effective to access the cervical multifidus muscle.

Suboccipital Muscles (Chapter 17)
Figure 72-24

If normal joint motion has been restored and other manual therapy techniques have failed to obtain expected results, and if the TrPs are resistant to noninvasive methods, it may be

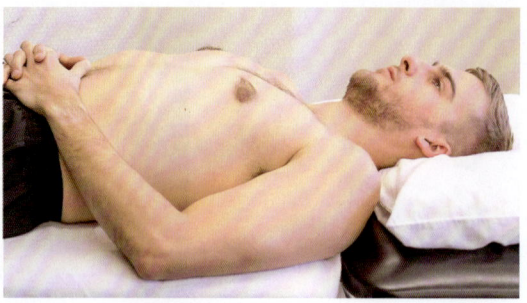
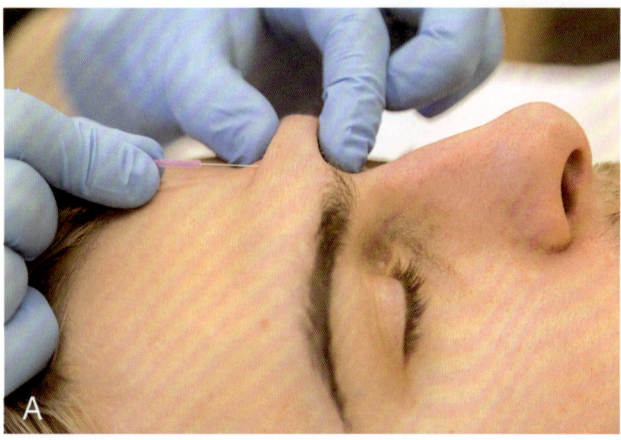
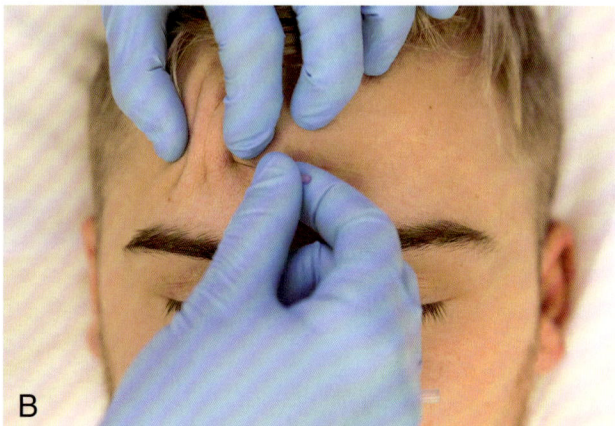

Figure 72-19. Trigger point injection or dry needling. A, **Procerus muscle**. B, **Frontalis muscle**. Note that both muscles can be needled with a pincer grasp.

necessary to consider needling of the suboccipital musculature with full precautions. Trigger point injection or DN requires a comprehensive anatomic knowledge, especially in terms of the location and relationship of the vertebral artery to the suboccipital muscles. The obliquus capitis inferior muscle is the suboccipital muscle that can be safely needled because of the vertebral artery's position above the arch of C1.

For TrPI or DN of the obliquus capitis inferior muscle, the patient is positioned in prone. This muscle is needled between the spinous process of C2 and the transverse process of C1. The needle is directed in a cranial and medial (oblique) direction toward the patient's opposite eye (Figure 72-24).

2. UPPER BACK, SHOULDER, AND ARM PAIN (Section 3)

Levator Scapula Muscle (Chapter 19)
Figure 72-25

For TrPI or DN of the levator scapula muscle (Figure 72-25), the patient is positioned in side-lying on the unaffected side with the back toward the clinician, and the patient's body is angled across the treatment table by placing the shoulder close to the edge of the table near the clinician. A pillow should support the head. The patient rests the uppermost arm on the body, with the elbow bent to balance it. If more tension is desired in the levator scapulae muscle, the uppermost arm can be placed in full internal rotation with the hand across the back to produce scapular winging. The clinician presses the free upper border of the trapezius muscle aside and palpates the levator scapulae muscle as it emerges from beneath the trapezius muscle (see Figure 20-7, Regional Anatomy, and Figure 72-21, Cross Section). The muscle is held in a pincer grasp for the needling technique. For the portion of the muscle that attaches to the superior angle of the scapula, the TrP is fixed between the clinician's index and middle fingers. The needle is inserted and directed toward the superior angle and upper border of the scapula at a shallow angle (Figure 72-25A).

For the mid-muscle portion, cross-fiber pincer palpation is used to identify TrPs laterally between the anterior border of the upper trapezius muscle and the transverse process of C1-C4. The TrP is fixed with a pincer grasp and the needle is directed toward the clinician's finger, or the TrP is fixed against a transverse process (Figure 72-25B). This muscle frequently has multiple taut bands and TrPs in its numerous fascicles, thereby making more extensive needling than most muscles necessary. This technique is also well illustrated by Rachlin.[92]

Scalene Muscles (Chapter 20)

Trigger point injection or DN may be necessary for complete relief of symptoms caused by the scalene muscles, but it must be done with a full understanding of, and respect for, the local anatomy (see Figure 20-7).

Anterior and Medium Scalenes (Figure 72-26)

For TrPI or DN in the anterior and middle scalene muscles, the patient is positioned supine and the head is turned slightly away from the side to be needled (Figure 72-26). In addition, it may help to elevate the head and shoulder slightly with a pillow to place the sternocleidomastoid and trapezius muscles in a slackened position.

The anterior scalene muscle is located in a triangle formed by the base of the clavicle, the external jugular vein, and the lateral edge of the clavicular head of the sternocleidomastoid muscle. The middle scalene muscle is located in a triangle formed by the base of the clavicle, the brachial plexus, and the scalenus posterior muscle. All scalene TrPI or DN is performed at least 3.8 cm (1½-in) above the clavicle.

For the anterior scalene muscle, the needle is directed toward the transverse processes of the cervical vertebrae about

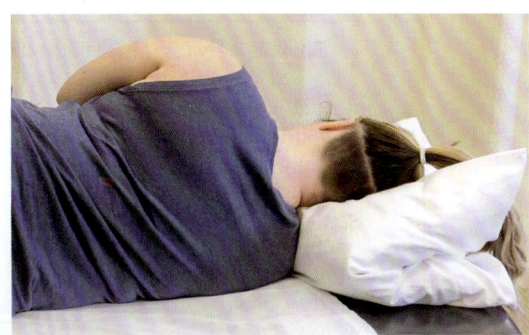
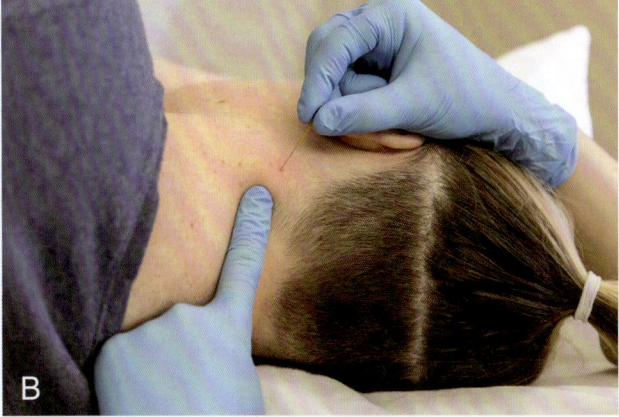
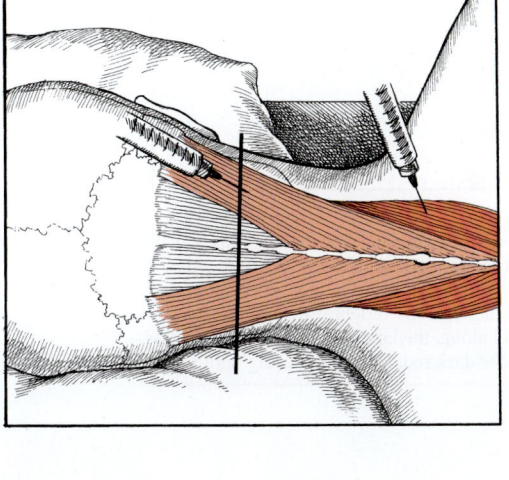
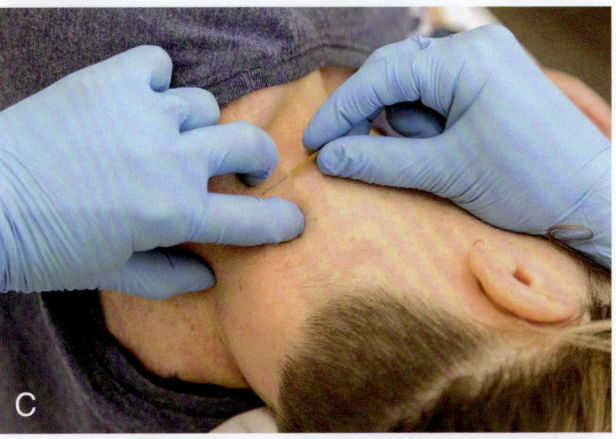

Figure 72-20. Trigger point injection or dry needling of the splenii muscles. A, **Mid-portion of the splenius capitis muscle** (light red), mid-portion of the splenius cervicis muscle (dark red). The semispinalis capitis muscle is shown without color. Needling of splenius capitis TrPs are safely performed below the thick black line below the level of C2. The exposed part of the vertebral artery lies superior to C1. B, Dry needling of the **splenius capitis muscle** with the needle directed inferomedially below C2. C, Dry needling of the **splenius cervicis muscle** with the pincer grasp in the lower cervical spine.

3 cm above the clavicle (Figure 72-26A). A taut band is fixed between the clinician's index and middle fingers to localize it for needling and to provide hemostasis during and after injection. The needle should be inserted well above the apex of the lung, which ordinarily extends about 2.5 cm (1 in) above the clavicle.[87]

When penetrated by the needle, scalene TrPs often refer sharp intense pain, strongly suggestive of neuropathic pain, to the arm and hand. This reproduction of the referred pain pattern is typical of scalene TrPs and does not necessarily indicate needle contact with brachial plexus nerve fibers. Effective penetration of a TrP consistently produces an LTR; penetration of a nerve does not. A 2.5-cm (1-in), 23- or 24-gauge hypodermic needle or a 0.30 × 30 mm filiform needle may be used. After TrPI or DN, pressure is maintained for hemostasis because bleeding within the scalene muscles causes local irritation.

For the middle scalene muscle, the needle should be inserted behind the brachial plexus, directed toward the posterior tubercle of the C2-C7 transverse processes of the cervical vertebra (Figure 72-26B).

Posterior Scalene

For needling of the posterior scalene muscle, the patient is positioned side-lying with the affected side up and the back toward the clinician; the head is tilted slightly toward the involved side to place the upper trapezius muscle on slack. The upper trapezius muscle will need to be pushed posteriorly to gain access to the posterior scalene muscle (see Figure 20-7). The needle is directed toward the posterior tubercle of the C4-C6 transverse processes of the cervical vertebra.

Section 8: Treatment Considerations for Myofascial Pain and Dysfunction

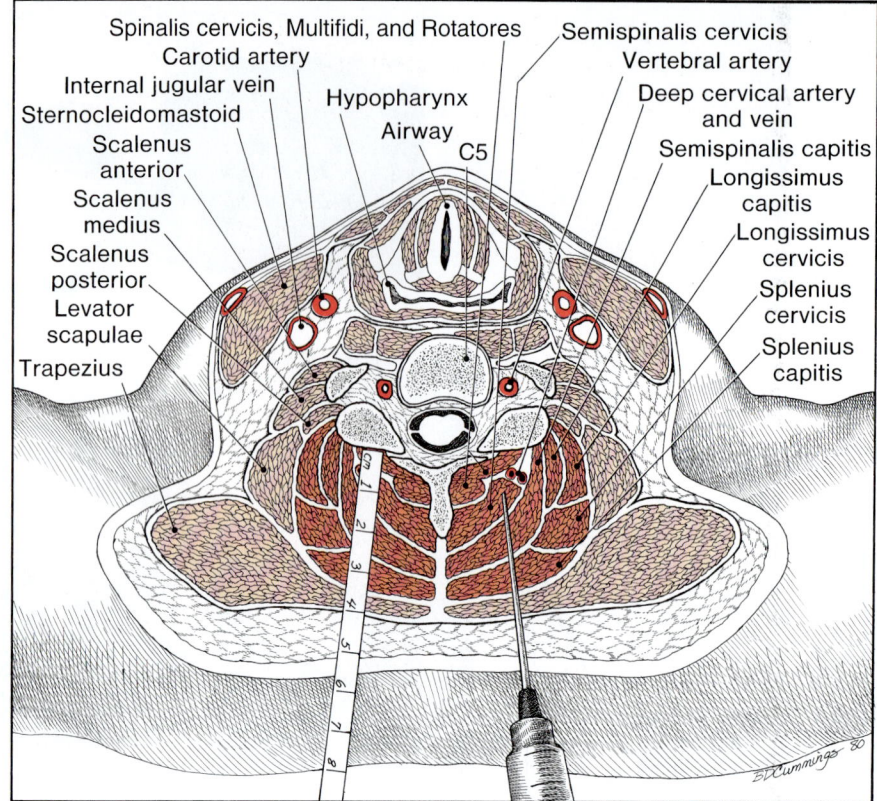

Figure 72-21. Cross-section of the neck through the C5 vertebra that corresponds to the mid-muscle belly of the semispinalis capitis muscle. The bony parts of the vertebra are stippled black and are outlined by a dark line surrounding black stipples. The ruler shows that the 5-cm (2-in) needle cannot penetrate the full depth of the posterior cervical muscles without compression of the skin. The vertebral artery is surrounded by the vertebral transverse processes. It travels anterior to, and along, the lateral border of the posterior cervical muscles. Paraspinal muscles and major blood vessels are dark red; other muscles are light red.

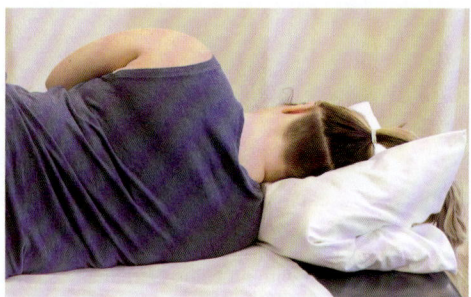

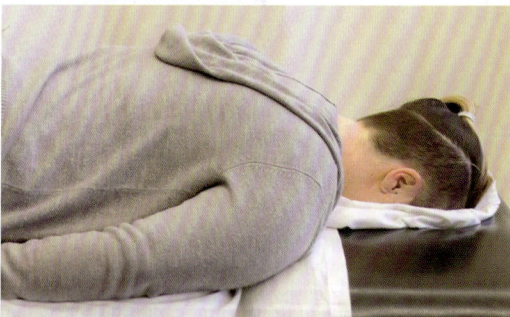

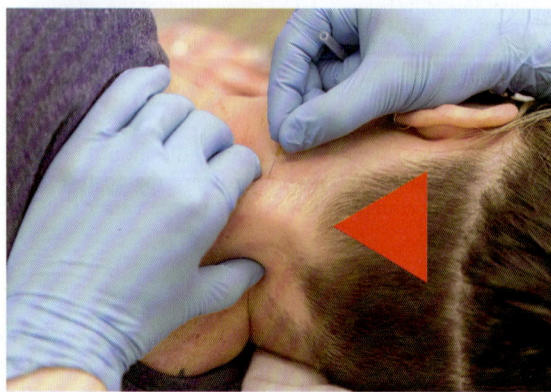

Figure 72-22. Trigger point injection or dry needling of the **left semispinalis muscles** (middle semispinalis capitis, semispinalis cervicis muscles) at approximately C4 level. The red color locates the suboccipital triangle that should not be needled, so as to avoid the unprotected vertebral artery.

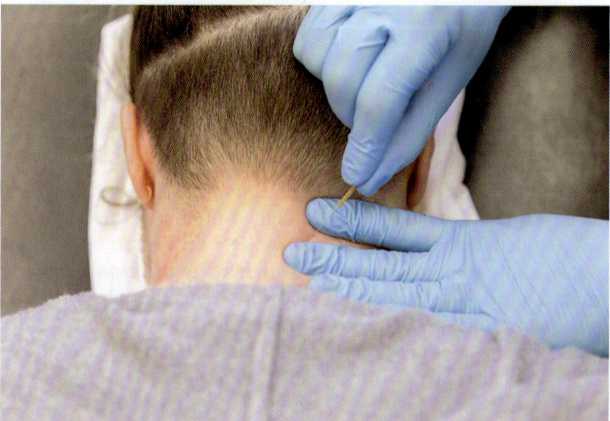

Figure 72-23. Trigger point injection or dry needling for the **cervical multifidus muscle.**

Suprapinatus Muscle (Chapter 21)
Figure 72-27

The inclusion of DN of the supraspinatus muscle, combined with an eccentric exercise program, in patients with subacromial pain syndrome has been demonstrated to be effective at long-term follow-up for improving related-disability.[94]

For TrPI or DN of the supraspinatus muscle, the patient is placed side-lying on the uninvolved side or prone, and the affected upper extremity is supported by a pillow. The TrPs are located by cross-fiber flat palpation and fixed between the clinician's index and middle fingers. A 3.2 to 3.8 cm (1.25-1.5 in) hypodermic needle or a 0.30 × 50 mm filiform needle is typically used. The needle is directed inferiorly and posteriorly toward the supraspinous fossa of the scapula just superior to the spine of the scapula (Figure 72-27B). The supraspinatus muscle is accessible only through the upper trapezius muscle, and the penetration of upper trapezius TrPs may produce a visible LTR and elicit referred pain to the neck. Continued movement of the needle deeper to penetrate the supraspinatus TrPs then elicits its referred pain pattern to the upper extremity. The clinician should probe the region with the needle to locate any additional supraspinatus TrPs.

If pressure on a well-localized spot deep in the lateral portion of the supraspinatus muscle refers pain in a pattern characteristic of the supraspinatus muscle, it is likely to be caused by an enthesopathy. The tenderness is elicited by applying pressure deep into the supraspinous fossa in the space between the spine of the scapula and the clavicle, just medial to the acromion. This location is beyond the reach of manual techniques and is marginal for the application of therapeutic pressure. The tenderness is usually best relieved by TrPI or DN of the tender spot using a needle that is long enough to reach it through the overlying upper trapezius muscle (Figure 72-27A). It is important to direct the needle precisely to the spot of deep tenderness. Needle contact with this sensitive region usually causes referred pain to the area of the deltoid muscle and down the arm.

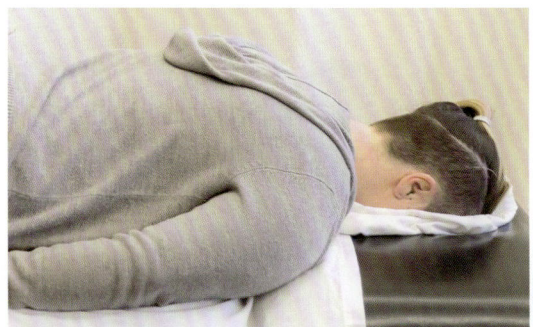

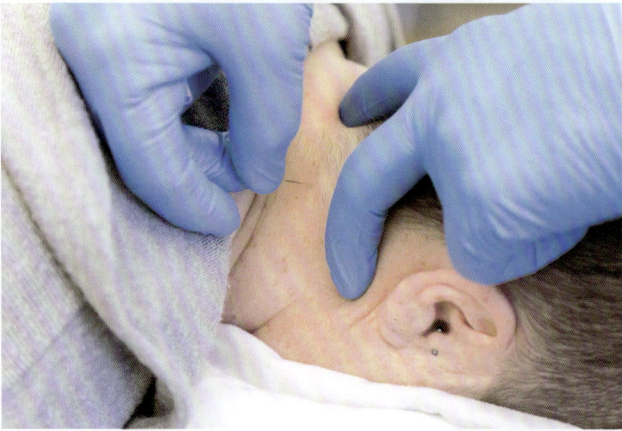

Figure 72-24. Trigger point injection or dry needling of the **obliquus capitis inferior muscle**. Note that the left index finger is palpating the C2 spinous process and the middle finger is palpating the transverse process of C1. The needle is directed toward the opposite eye.

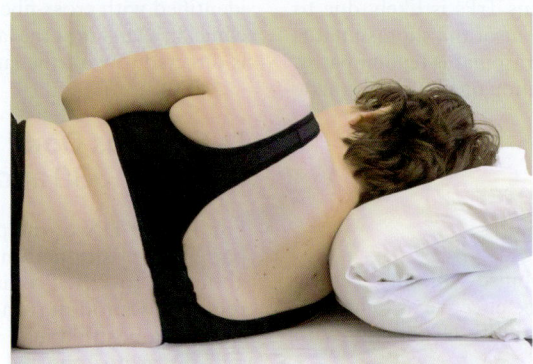

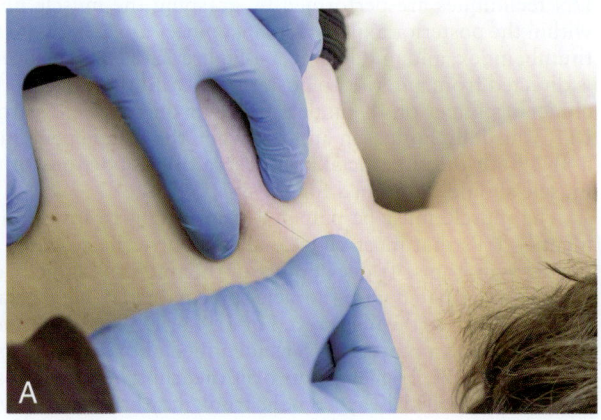

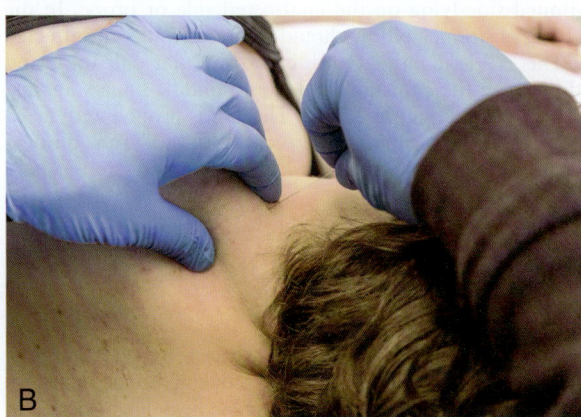

Figure 72-25. Trigger point injection or dry needling of the **levator scapulae muscle**. A, The needle directed toward the superior angle of the scapula. B, Mid-muscle belly between C2 and C4.

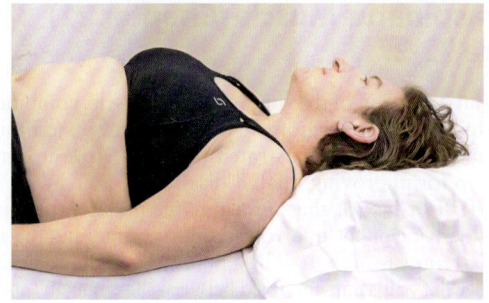
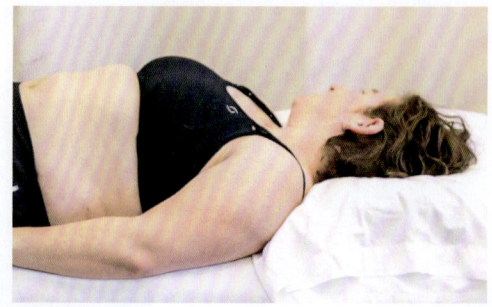
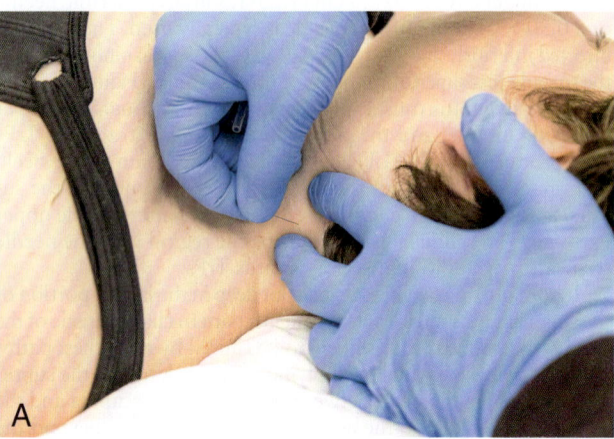
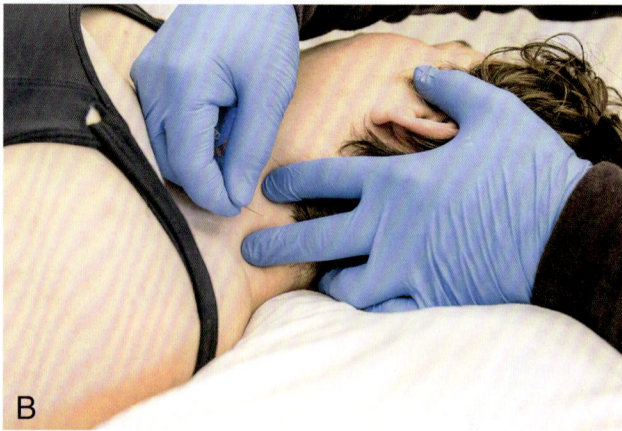

Figure 72-26. Trigger point injection or dry needling of the scalene muscles. A, **Scalenus anterior muscle**. B, **Scalenus medius muscle**. Fingers straddle the middle scalene muscle with the index finger in the groove between the scalenus anterior and medius muscles to locate the brachial plexus. The needle is directed posteriorly away from the groove to avoid the nerve fibers of the plexus.

Tenderness beneath the tip of the acromion that remains following inactivation of supraspinatus TrPs is likely due to enthesopathy of the humeral attachment of the supraspinatus tendon, which is often identified as supraspinatus tendinopathy. This tenderness should respond to injection of a local anesthetic or DN (Figure 72-27C).

Infraspinatus Muscle (Chapter 22)
Figure 72-28

DN of the infraspinatus muscle, combined with an eccentric exercise program, has been found to be effective at long-term follow-up for improving related-disability in patients with subacromial pain syndrome.[94]

For TrPI or DN of the infraspinatus muscle, the patient is positioned side-lying on the unaffected side or prone. In the side-lying position, a pillow should be placed under the affected arm. The TrP is identified with cross-fiber flat palpation and fixed between the clinician's index and middle fingers against the scapula bone (Figure 72-28). The TrP is probed with a 3.8 cm (1.5 in) hypodermic needle or a 0.30 × 50 mm filiform needle until the needle elicits an LTR and/or the referred pain pattern of the TrP.

Teres Minor Muscle (Chapter 23)
Figure 72-29

A recent case report described the effectiveness of DN of infraspinatus and teres minor muscles for reducing upper extremity symptoms in a patient with an unclear medical diagnosis.[95] For TrPI or DN of the teres minor muscle, the patient is positioned side-lying on the unaffected side or prone. In the side-lying position, a pillow should be placed under the affected arm (Figure 72-29A). In prone, the arm is positioned in 90° of glenohumeral abduction (Figure 72-29B). Trigger points are identified with cross-fiber flat palpation and fixed between the clinician's fingers at the lateral border of the scapula. The needle is directed toward the lateral border of the scapula.

Latissimus Dorsi Muscle (Chapter 24)
Figures 72-30 and 72-31

For TrPI or DN of the proximal latissimus dorsi muscle, the patient is positioned in prone or supine with the shoulder abducted to 90°. Proximal TrPs are typically more closely related to shoulder and upper extremity symptoms. The side-lying position may also be used with the affected side up and the arm supported on a pillow. The TrPs are identified with cross-fiber pincer palpation (Figure 72-30). The TrPI or DN techniques are performed by grasping the muscle fibers within the posterior axillary fold in a pincer grasp between the thumb, index, and middle fingers (Figure 72-31A). The needle is directed from anterior to posterior toward the TrPs and the clinician's finger on the undersurface of the muscle. A strong LTR is usually both seen and felt when the needle penetrates a TrP. Both the superficial and deep axillary portions of the muscle should be probed for TrPs.

The muscle must be palpated from origin to insertion to identify TrPs that must be treated to resolve the patient's reported symptoms. Trigger points in the mid-muscle belly are typically associated with thoracic spine pain and lateral trunk pain proximal to the iliac crest. For TrPI or DN, the same technique utilizing a pincer grasp as identified above may be used (Figure 72-31B). Trigger points over the trunk in muscle tissue that can't be pulled away from the trunk may be identified with cross-fiber flat palpation. The intercostal space is blocked above and below the rib where the TrP has been located, the TrP is fixed over a rib, and the needle is directed from a posterior to anterior direction tangentially toward the rib (Figure 72-31C).

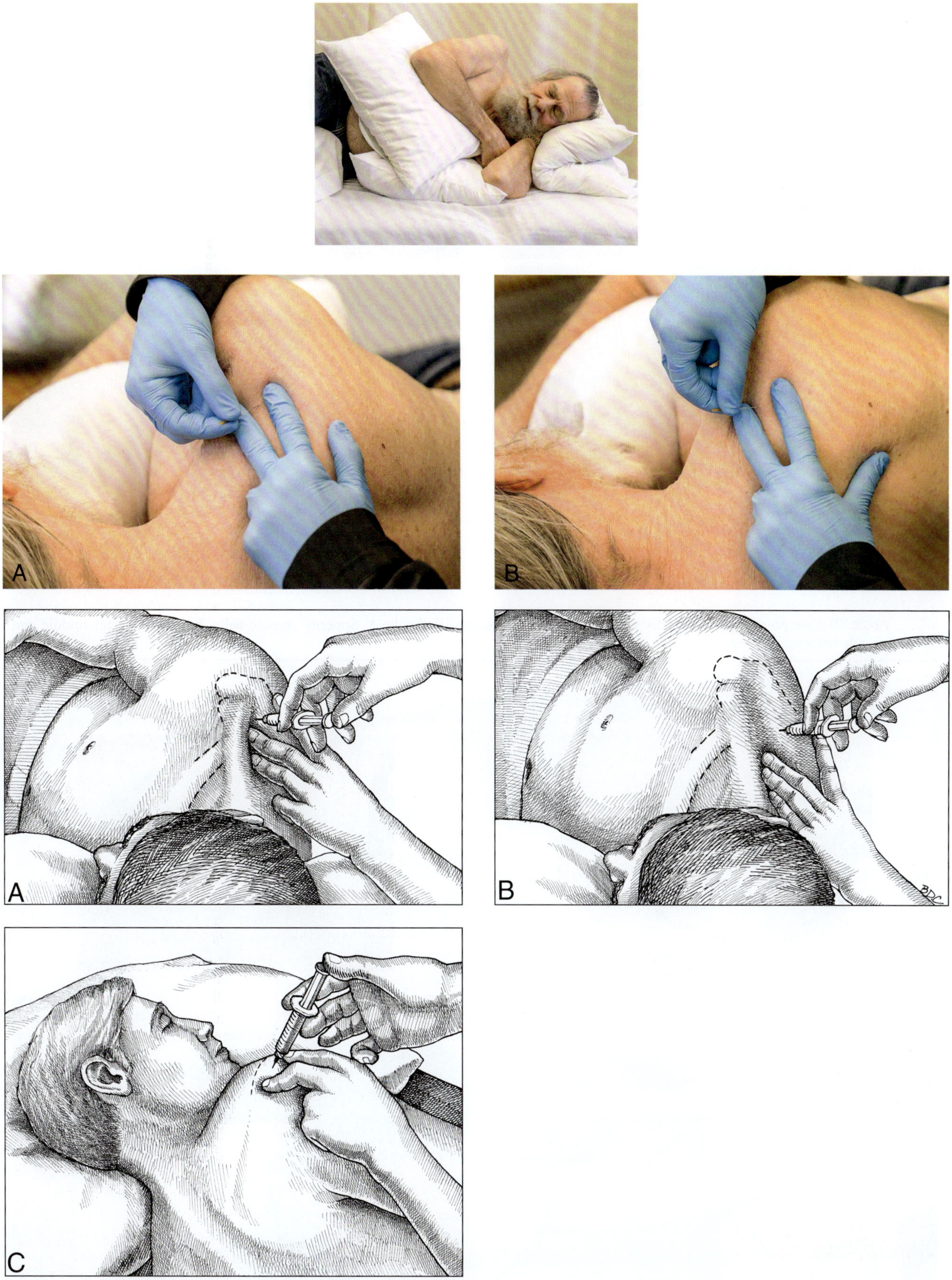

Chapter 72: Trigger Point Injection and Dry Needling 783

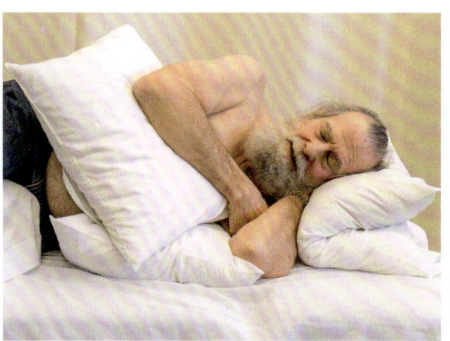

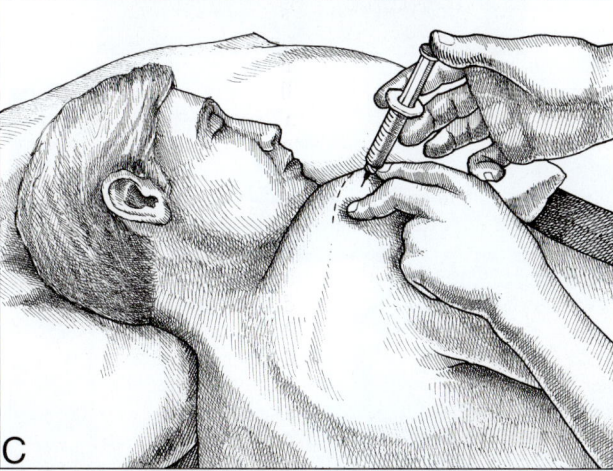

Figure 72-27. Trigger point injection or dry needling of the **right suprapinatus muscle** and tendon with the patient lying on the left side. A, Needling the lateral region of the musculotendinous junction. B, Mid-muscle belly. For A and B, the index finger of the palpating hand is on the spine of the scapula and the middle finger is on the superior border of the scapula. C, Injecting the region of attachment of the supraspinatus tendon beneath the acromion, viewed from behind.

Section 8: Treatment Considerations for Myofascial Pain and Dysfunction

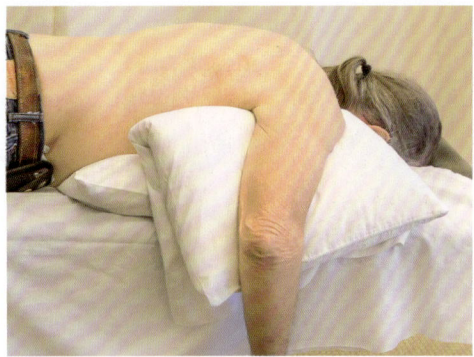

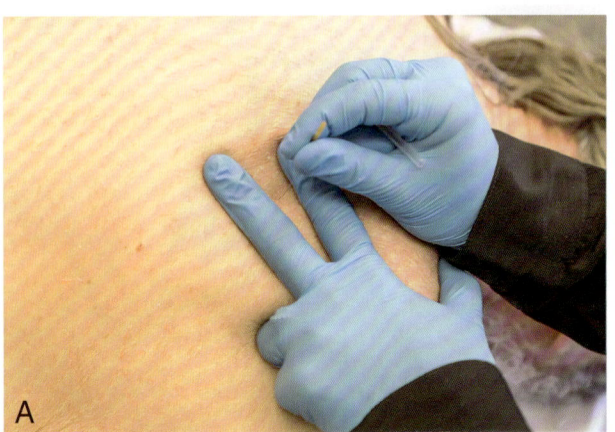
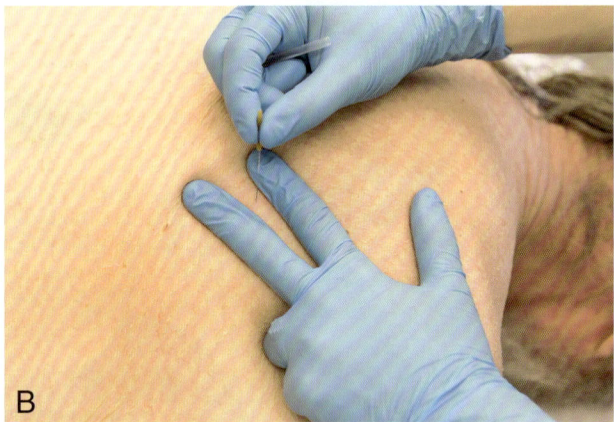

Figure 72-28. Trigger point injection or dry needling for the **infraspinatus muscle**. A, Superior muscle belly. B, Technique for middle and inferior muscle bellies.

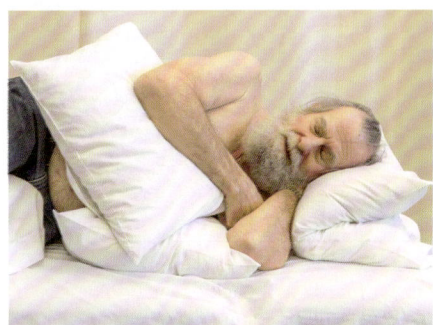
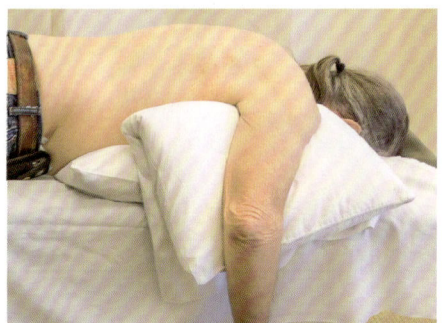

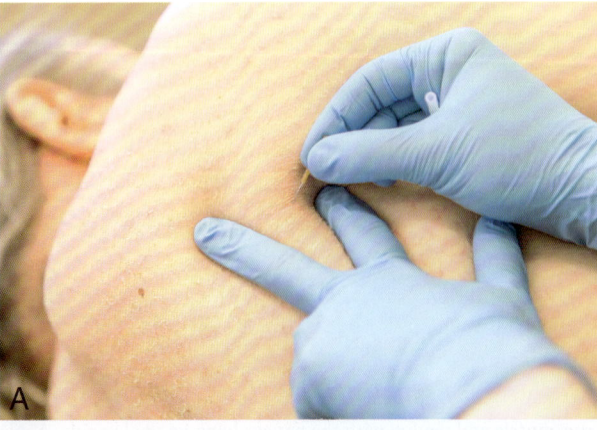
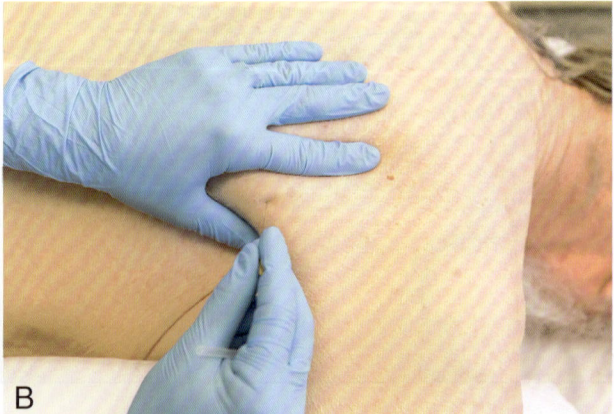

Figure 72-29. Trigger point injection or dry needling technique for the **teres minor muscle**. A, Side-lying with the affected arm positioned to take up slack in the muscle. The index finger of the palpating hand is on the lateral border of the scapula. B, Prone position with the thumb of the palpating hand on the lateral border of the scapula. The needle is angled toward the lateral border of the scapula between the teres major and infraspinatus muscles.

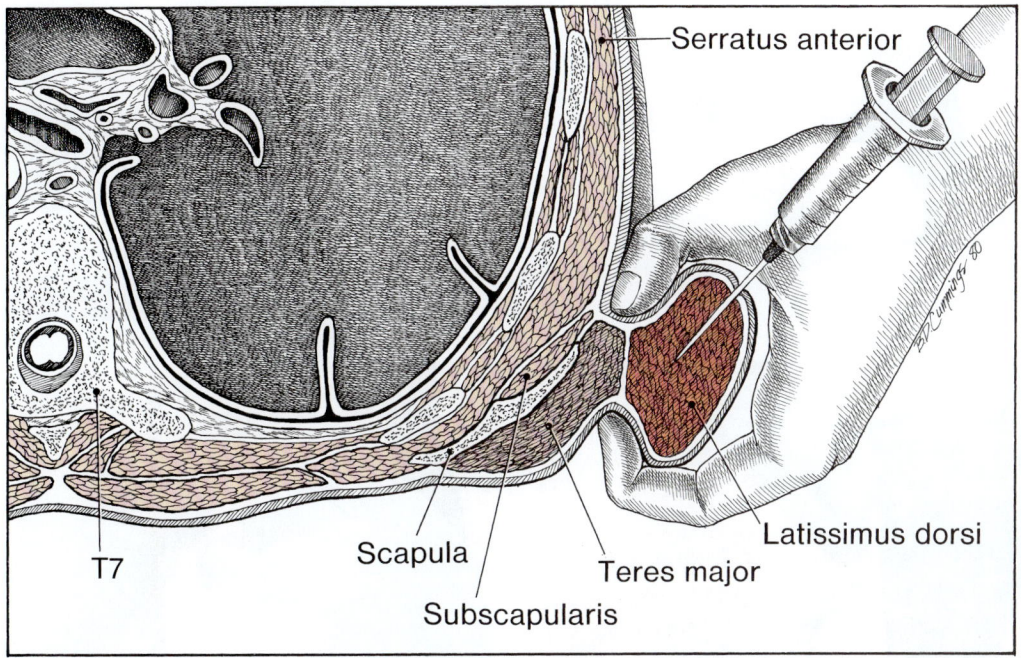

Figure 72-30. Cross-section view for TrP injection or dry needling technique of the right **latissimus dorsi muscle**, using pincer grasp.

Teres Major Muscle (Chapter 25)
Figure 72-32

For TrPI or DN of the teres major muscle, the patient is positioned prone with the upper extremity in 50° to 60° of glenohumeral abduction. The supine and side-lying positions can also be used to treat this muscle. The TrP is identified within the posterior axillary fold and localized between the thumb and fingers with cross-fiber pincer palpation (Figure 72-32). The TrPI or DN techniques are performed with a pincer grasp and the needle is directed anterolaterally in the prone position (Figure 72-32A) and posterolaterally in the supine position (Figure 72-32B). In side-lying, the needle is directed from a posterior to anterolateral direction, away from the rib cage (Figure 72-32C). LTRs are clearly felt when the needle penetrates the TrP. It is common to have multiple TrPs in the teres major muscle. It is also possible to needle TrPs in the adjacent latissimus dorsi muscle through the same skin puncture by directing the needle more laterally.

Subscapularis Muscle (Chapter 26)

Subscapularis TrPs can be treated from two different approaches: an axillary approach and a medial approach. Each of these techniques will be discussed separately.

Lateral (Axillary) Approach (Figure 72-33 A, B)

For TrPI or DN of the subscapularis muscle, the patient is positioned supine with the arm placed in 90° of glenohumeral abduction and full external rotation. The back of the patient's hand is placed on the forehead and a pillow can be placed under the upper arm if the patient can't tolerate the position (Figure 72-33A). The patient's body weight holds the scapula in position after it is pulled laterally (see Figure 26-4). If sufficient abduction and external rotation is not available to provide room for performing TrPI or DN, manual TrP release techniques should be applied to provide it. The TrPs are identified at the lateral margin of the anterior border of the scapula with cross-fiber flat palpation against the scapula. The TrPs are located and fixed between the fingers. A 6- or 7.5-cm (2½- or 3-in), 22-gauge hypodermic needle or 0.30 × 50 mm filiform needle is inserted between the clinician's fingers into the depth of the axillary fossa (Figure 72-33B). The needle is directed parallel to the rib cage and cephalad, toward the anterior surface of the scapula, directly into the TrP identified by palpation. The needle is inserted through the skin caudal to the TrPs being injected and directed cephalad to avoid encountering the rib cage, which can happen in this location.

Medial Approach (Figure 72-33C)

The medial approach requires a special consideration for TrPI or DN. The pain identified with cross-fiber flat palpation in this area could be a result of TrPs in the middle trapezius, lower trapezius, rhomboid, and/or serratus anterior muscles. Therefore, each of these muscles should be examined for TrPs, and if found, they should be inactivated. The subscapularis TrPs are needled with the patient lying prone with the glenohumeral joint in extension, adduction, and internal rotation so the back of the hand on the affected side is placed over the lumbar spine. This position, also known as the "hammerlock" position, will bring the medial border of the scapula away from the thorax. The needle is directed from medial to lateral toward the anterior surface of the scapula (Figure 72-33C).

Rhomboid Muscles (Chapter 27)
Figure 72-34

For TrPI or DN of the rhomboid muscles, the patient is positioned prone with a pillow or towel roll placed under the anterior aspect of the shoulder to put the rhomboid muscle in a neutral resting position. Trigger points are identified with cross-fiber flat palpation over the rib cage. The risk of pleural penetration by the needle can be essentially eliminated by placing the index and middle fingers into the intercostal spaces above and below the site to be needled (Figure 72-34). A study looking at the depth of needle insertion for TrP injections for the rhomboid major muscle determined that from 62 patients who visited a clinic with shoulder or upper back pain, subjects who had a body mass index (BMI) <23, the depth from the skin to the rhomboid minor was 1.2 ± 0.2 cm, 1.4 ± 0.2 cm for ≥23 BMI ≤25 and 1.8 ± 0.3 cm BMI ≥ 25.[96] Average thickness of the rhomboid major

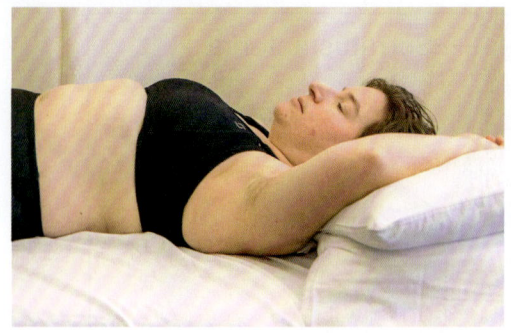
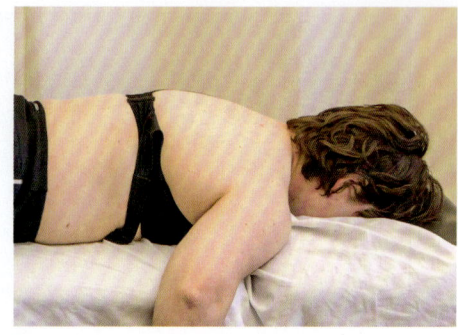
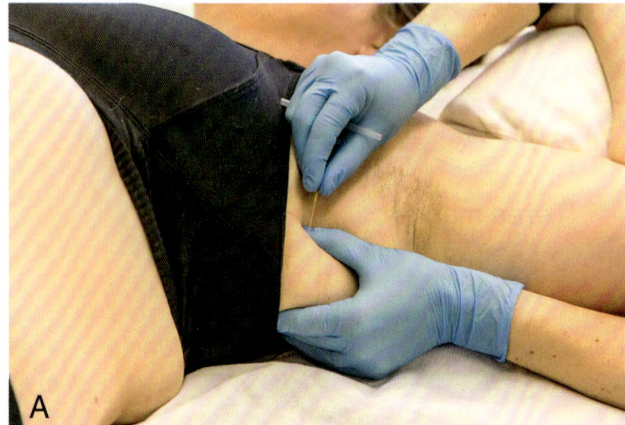
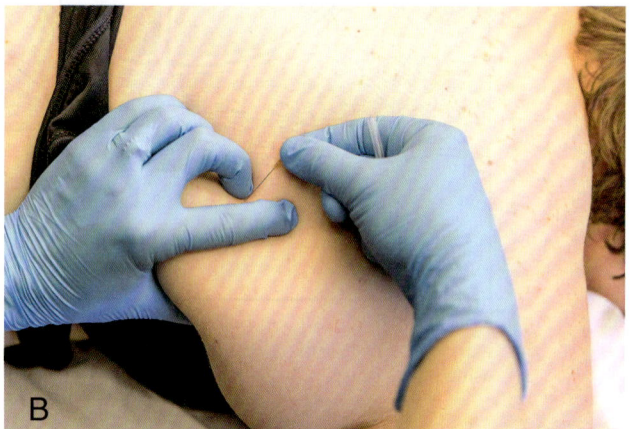
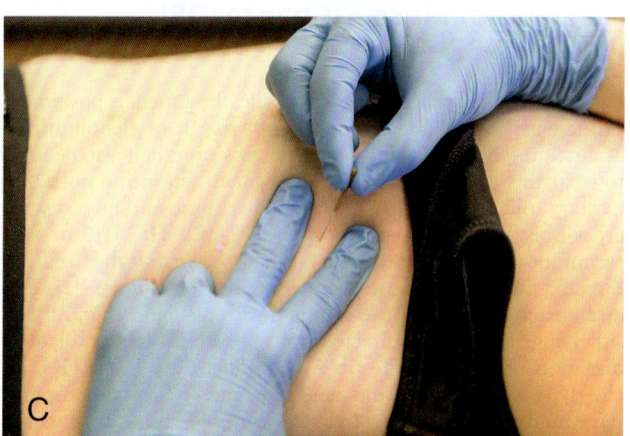

Figure 72-31. Trigger point injection or dry needling of the **latissimus dorsi muscle**. A, Supine position with the arm abducted to 90°. B, Prone position. C, Intercostal space blocking for lower TrPs in the latissimus dorsi muscle.

muscle for the underweight or normal BMI group (BMI < 23) was 0.9 ± 0.3 cm, for the overweight BMI (BMI ≥ 23, but ≤25) was 1.0 ± 0.2 cm, and for the obese group (BMI ≥ 25) muscle thickness was 0.8 ± 0.3 cm.[96] Therefore, for TrPI or DN of the TrP, a 3.8-cm (1½-in) hypodermic needle or 0.30 × 50 mm filiform needle is directed almost tangential to the surface toward a rib to avoid penetrating an intercostal space, and therefore reaching the lung. Injection of 0.5% procaine or 1% lidocaine reduces postinjection soreness compared with DN.[32]

Deltoid Muscle (Chapter 28)

Anterior Deltoid (Figure 72-35A)

For TrPI or DN of the anterior deltoid fibers, the patient is positioned supine with the affected shoulder approximately 45° at glenohumeral abduction. Trigger points in the anterior deltoid muscle are identified using cross-fiber flat palpation and are often close to the anterior border of the muscle where the cephalic vein lies subcutaneously between the deltoid and pectoralis major muscles. When needling (Figure 72-35A), the clinician can avoid the vein by placing one finger of the palpating hand on it, penetrating the skin with the needle close to it, and directing the needle away from the vein and into the muscle tissue.

Middle Deltoid (Figure 72-35B)

For TrPI or DN of the middle deltoid fibers, the patient is positioned supine, side-lying, or prone. Because the middle deltoid muscle has multiple interlaced digitations, its taut bands are shorter than in the anterior and posterior fibers, and TrPs are more scattered throughout the muscle. Trigger points are identified with cross-fiber flat or pincer palpation. The TrP is fixed between the clinician's fingers and the needle is directed toward the humerus (Figure 72-35B). The clinician can also use

Chapter 72: Trigger Point Injection and Dry Needling 787

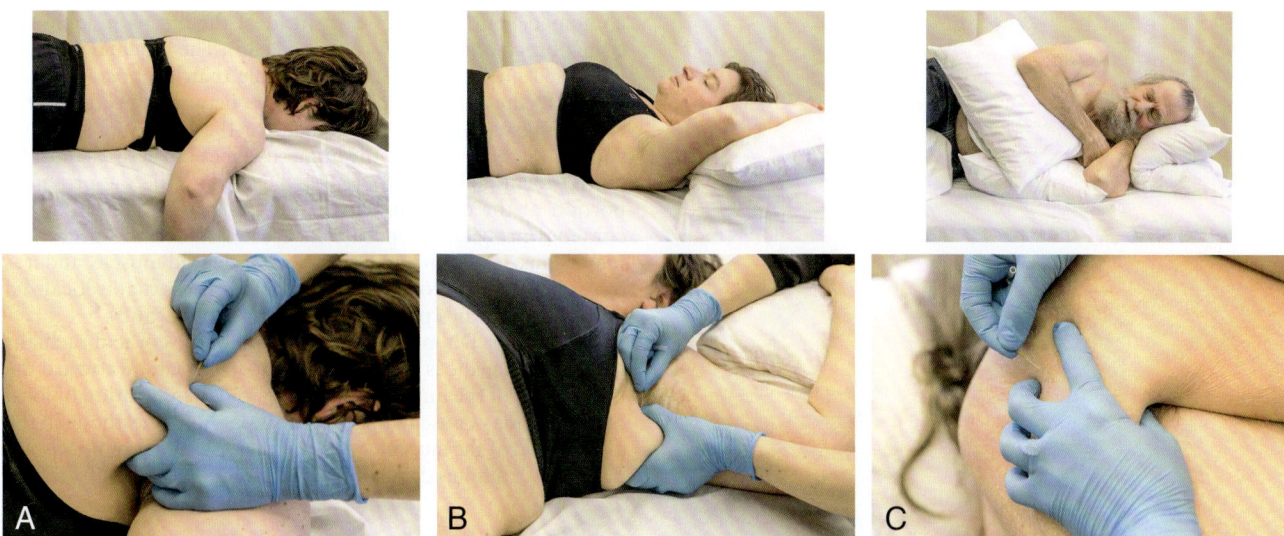

Figure 72-32. Trigger point injection or dry needling of the **teres major muscle**. A, Prone with pincer grasp. B, Supine with pincer grasp. C, Side-lying using pincer grasp with the upper extremity supported.

a pincer grasp to fix the TrPs, and the needle can be directed from posterior to anterior or vice versa toward the TrPs and the clinician's finger.

Posterior Deltoid (Figure 72-35C)

For TrPI or DN of the posterior deltoid fibers, the patient is positioned prone with the affected upper extremity in approximately 45° of glenohumeral abduction. Trigger points in the posterior deltoid are identified using cross-fiber flat palpation and fixed between the clinician's index and middle fingers. The needle is directed toward the humerus (Figure 72-35C).

Coracobrachialis Muscle (Chapter 29)
Figure 72-36

For TrPI or DN of the coracobrachialis muscle, the patient is positioned supine with the shoulder at approximately 60° of abduction and external rotation. The coracobrachialis muscle can be needled above or below the pectoralis major muscle because the musculocutaneous nerve is located beneath the pectoralis major muscle and over the coracobrachialis muscle.

The TrPs are identified with cross-fiber flat palpation deep in the axilla by reaching beneath the pectoralis major muscle and pressing against the humerus on the dorsal aspect of the

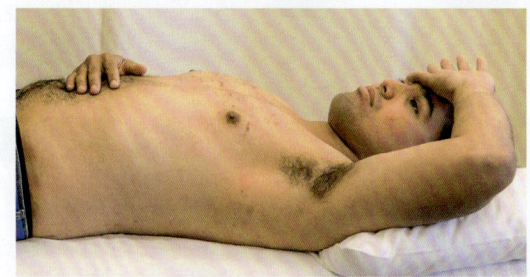

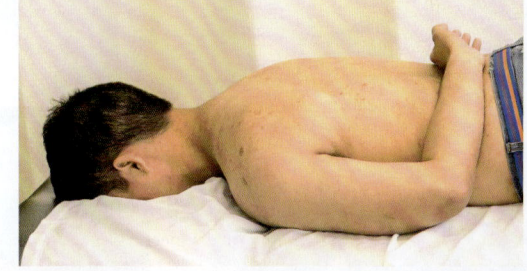

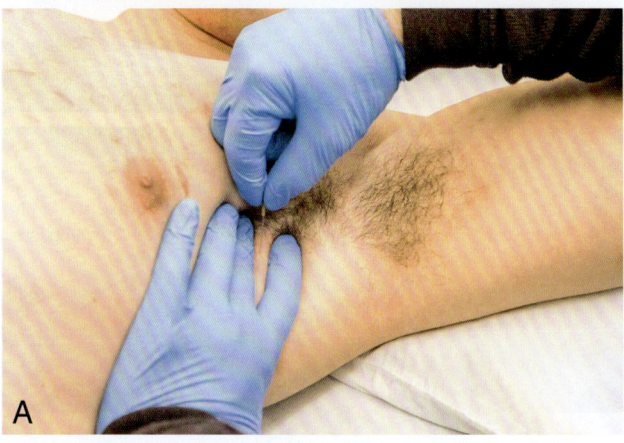

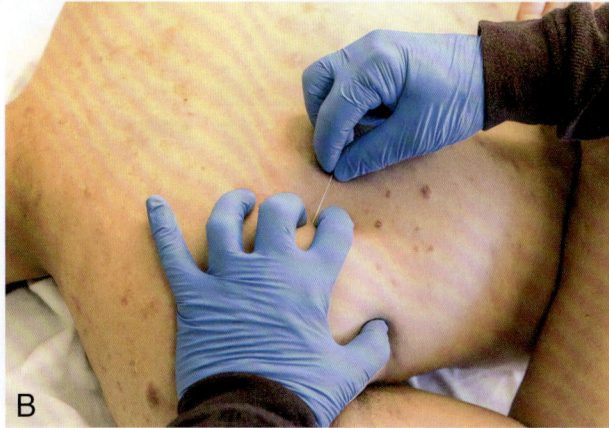

Figure 72-33. Trigger point injection or dry needling techniques for the **subscapularis muscle**. A, Supine position along the axillary border of the scapula. B, Medial approach in prone with the upper extremity of the affected side in the "hammerlock" position.

788 Section 8: Treatment Considerations for Myofascial Pain and Dysfunction

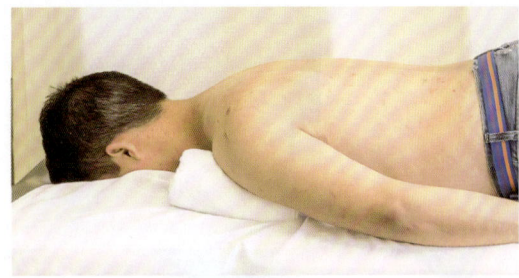

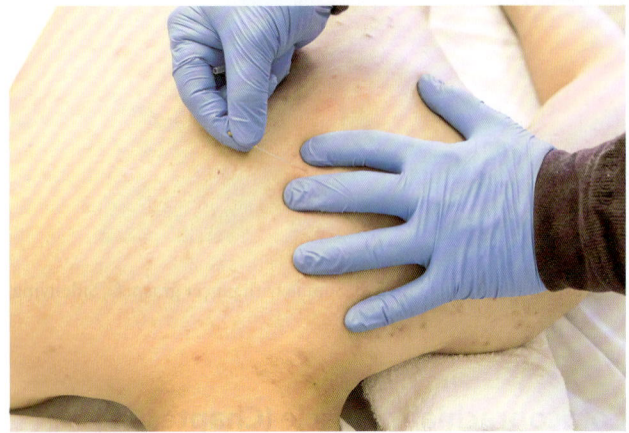

Figure 72-34. Trigger point injection or dry needling technique for the **rhomboid muscles**. Note the towel roll under the anterior shoulder to place the rhomboid muscle on slack allowing better access to the TrPs. The index and the middle finger of the palpating hand block the intercostal spaces.

combined bundle of the short head of the biceps brachii and coracobrachialis muscles (Figure 72-36). The brachial artery is identified in the neurovascular bundle that lies posterior and medial to the coracobrachialis muscle, between the coracobrachialis muscle and the attachment of the lateral head of the triceps brachii muscle to the humerus. These structures must be clearly identified prior to TrPI or DN. To needle the proximal portion of the coracobrachialis muscle near the origin at the coracoid process, the needle is inserted above the pectoralis major muscle and through the anterior deltoid muscle, and it is directed shallowly toward the coracoid process that is localized with the clinician's palpating finger (Figure 72-36B).

For TrPI or DN of the lower portion of the coracobrachialis muscle, the needle is directed from medial to lateral toward the upper third of the humerus (Figure 72-36C). Infiltration of local anesthetic may cause temporary weakness and anesthesia in the distribution of the musculocutaneous nerve with prompt recovery in 15 or 20 minutes depending on the solution used for injection.

Biceps Brachii Muscle (Chapter 30)
Figure 72-37

For TrPI or DN of the biceps brachii muscle, the patient is positioned supine with the arm slightly abducted, the elbow is flexed to about 45°, and the TrPs are identified with cross-fiber pincer palpation and held firmly in a pincer grasp between the clinician's thumb, index, and middle fingers. The TrPs are needled in the region within the pincer grasp and probed to ensure the penetration of all TrPs that can produce LTRs. This technique may be used for both the short head and long head of the biceps brachii muscle. The needle is directed from medial to lateral or lateral to medial toward the clinician's finger (Figure 72-37A). Needle penetrations may be aimed nearly tangential to the

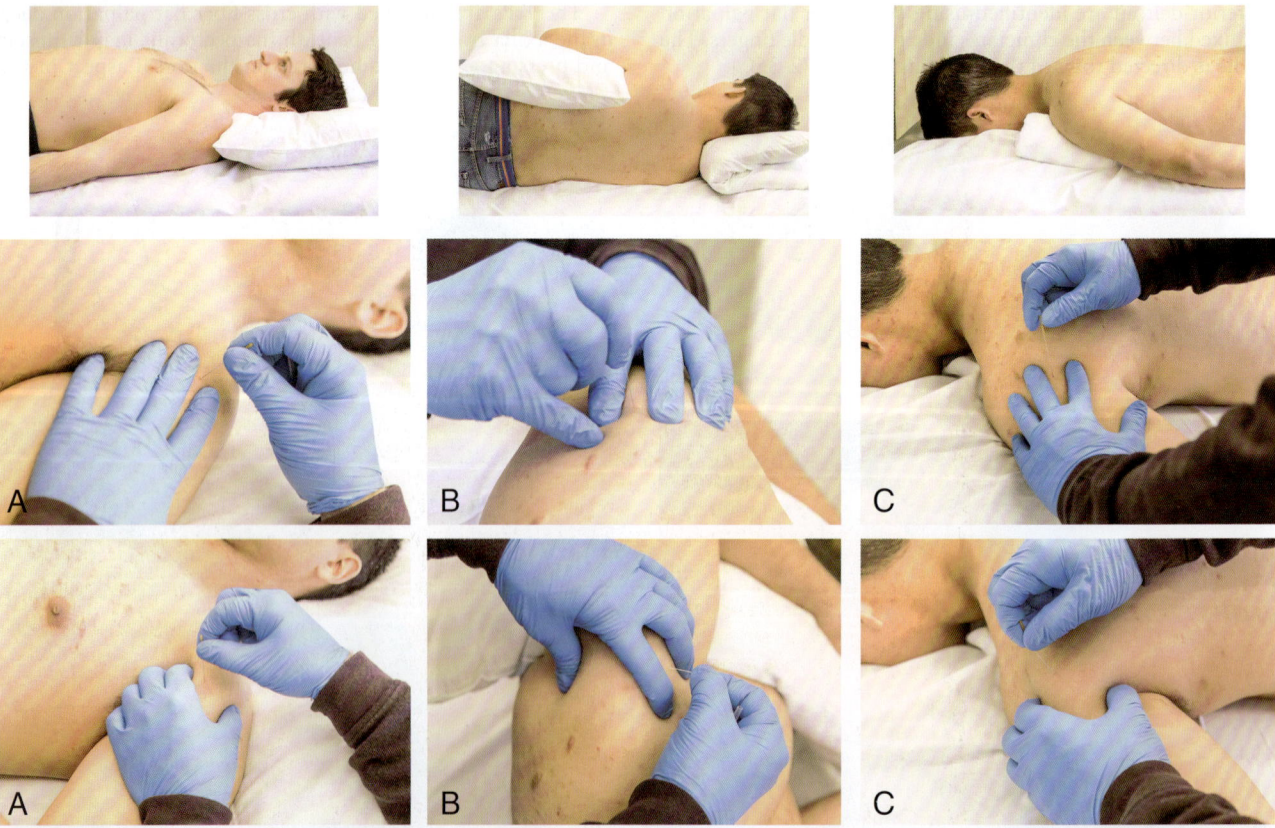

Figure 72-35. Trigger point injection or dry needling in the **right deltoid muscle**. A, **Anterior deltoid muscle**, with the patient supine (flat palpation and pincer grasp). B, **Middle deltoid muscle**, with the patient in side-lying (flat palpation and pincer grasp). C, **Posterior deltoid muscle**, with the patient lying prone (flat palpation and pincer grasp).

Chapter 72: Trigger Point Injection and Dry Needling 789

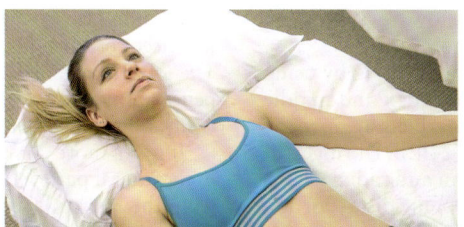

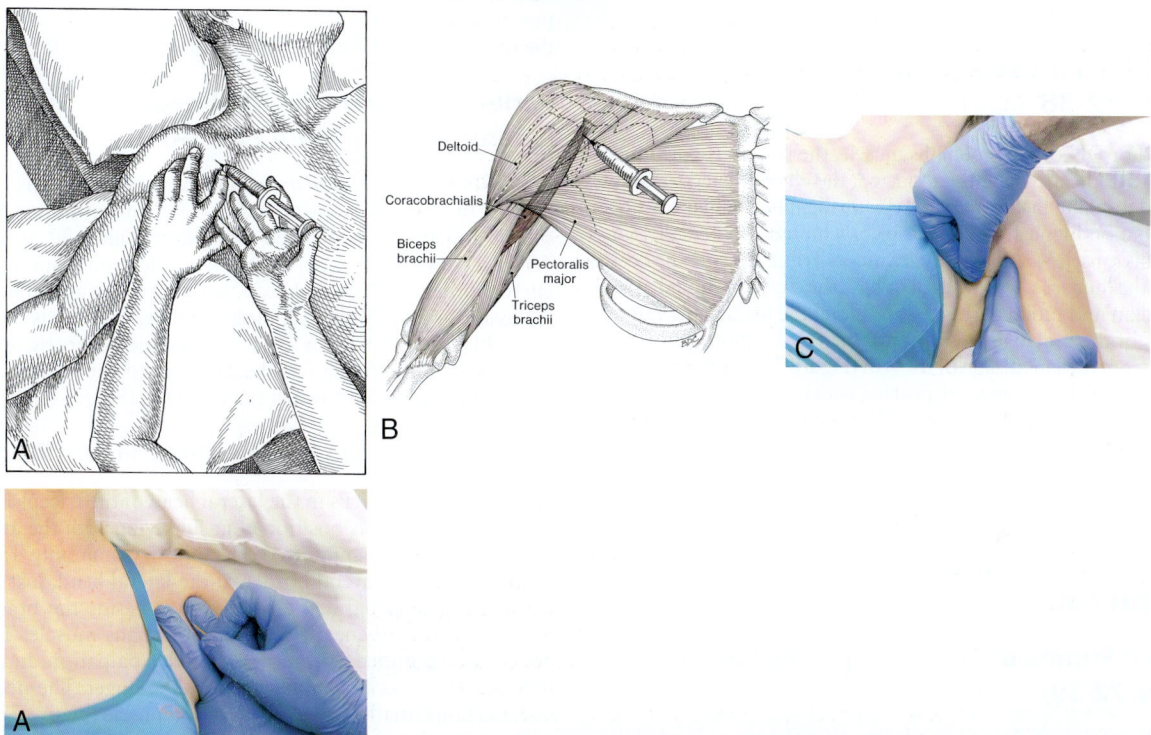

Figure 72-36. Trigger point injection or dry needling of the **coracobrachialis muscle**. The neurovascular bundle must be identified before TrPI or DN and avoided. A, Proximal portion. B, Schematic diagram showing injection of the coracobrachialis muscle (dark red) through the deltoid and pectoralis major muscles. C, DN technique just distal to the pectoralis major muscle.

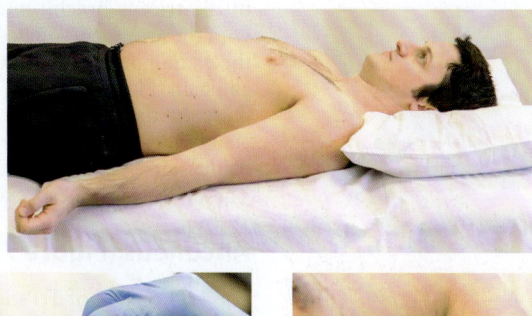

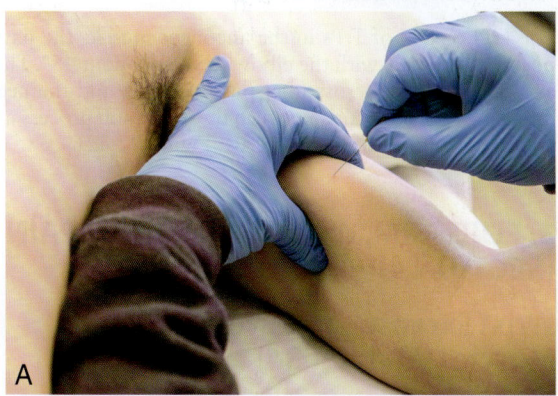
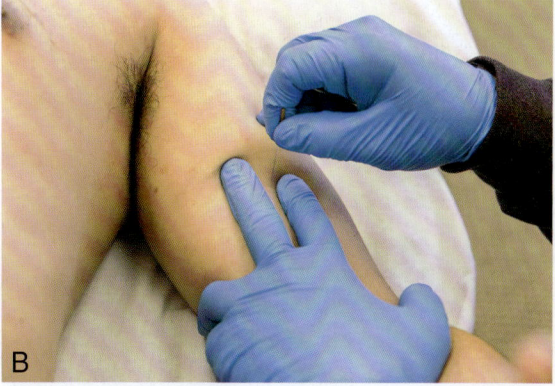

Figure 72-37. Trigger point injection or dry needling of the **biceps brachii muscle**. A, Short head using the pincer grasp. B, Long head with the TrP fixed between the clinician's fingers.

humerus, or may be directed perpendicularly toward it, avoiding the medial and lateral borders of the muscle.

Additionally, the TrPs may be located for needling by using flat palpation and straddling them with the index and middle fingers of the palpating hand. The TrPs are held against the underlying brachialis muscle, as in Figure 72-32B. During TrPI or DN, the clinician should avoid the median and radial nerves that lie along the medial and lateral borders of the distal portion of the biceps brachii and brachialis muscles, respectively.

Brachialis Muscle (Chapter 31)
Figure 72-38

For TrPI or DN of the brachialis muscle, the patient is positioned supine with the arm slightly abducted, the elbow flexed to about 45°, and the palm facing up. The TrPs are identified with cross-fiber flat palpation by pushing the biceps brachii muscle medially. The brachialis muscle is a thick muscle, and its TrPs frequently lie deep, next to the humerus. During TrPI or DN, the clinician should avoid the median and radial nerves that lie along the medial and lateral borders of the brachialis muscle, respectively.[87] Approaching the muscle from the lateral side of the arm (Figure 72-38), the needle is directed medially and upward, probing widely to explore the lateral and middle portions of the muscle. The needle may lightly contact the humerus, which ensures reaching the full depth of the muscle. If the needle contacts the bone, it should be replaced immediately.

Triceps Brachii and Anconeus Muscle (Chapter 32)

Patient Supine or Side-Lying (Long Head; Figure 72-39)

For TrPI or DN of TrPs in the medial portion of the long head of the triceps brachii muscle, the patient is positioned in supine with the shoulder abducted and externally rotated, so that the antecubital space faces up to place the long head on a slight stretch (Figure 72-39A). The clinician identifies TrPs using cross-fiber pincer palpation and lifts the muscle belly away from the underlying bone, the adjacent

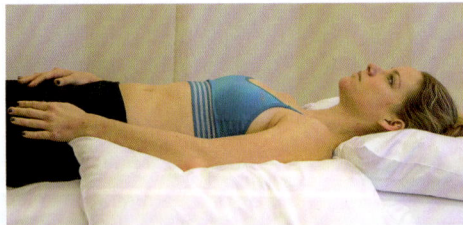

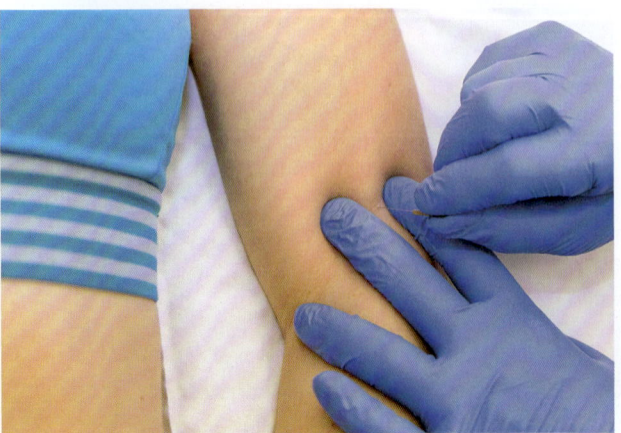

Figure 72-38. Trigger point injection or dry needling of the **brachialis muscle**, with the biceps brachii muscle pushed aside in a medial direction.

major blood vessels and nerve, and away from the lateral head of the triceps brachii muscle (beneath which the radial nerve courses). The TrP is fixed and needled between the tips of the digits. Effective penetration of these TrPs by the needle produces LTRs that are easily seen and can be felt by the palpating fingers and thumb.

If it is a more convenient position, or if the TrPs are located in the lateral part of the long head, this area can be approached from the lateral aspect of the arm. To do so, the patient is positioned side-lying with the affected side up, facing away from the clinician (Figure 72-39B), permitting the clinician to grasp the muscle and needle the TrPs as previously described.

Patient Side-Lying (Medial Head Lateral Border; Figure 72-40A)

For TrPI or DN of TrPs in the medial head of the triceps brachii muscle, the patient is positioned in side-lying with the affected side up and the arm supported on a pillow (Figure 72-40A). The TrP is identified using cross-fiber flat palpation distally in the lateral border of the medial head, adjacent to the attachments of the extensor carpi radialis longus and brachioradialis muscles. For TrPI or DN, the TrP is fixed between the fingers by pressing the muscle on both sides of the TrP against the humerus, and the needle is directed toward the humerus (Figure 72-40A).

Patient Side-Lying (Lateral Head; Figure 72-40B)

For TrPI or DN of TrPs in the lateral head of the triceps brachii muscle, the patient is positioned in side-lying with the affected side up and the arm supported on a pillow. Commonly, TrPs are located along the lateral border of the lateral head, just above the exit of the radial nerve that courses beside the brachialis muscle and then beneath the brachioradialis muscle. Trigger points are identified with cross-fiber flat palpation and fixed between the clinician's index and middle finger. The needle is inserted tangentially into a thin layer of muscle (Figure 72-40B) and may be directed either distally or proximally.

Patient Supine (Medial Head Medial Border; Figure 72-41)

For TrPI or DN of TrPs in the medial border of the medial head of the triceps brachii muscle, the patient is positioned prone with the arm in 90° of glenohumeral abduction with the arm off the examination table and resting on a pillow in the lap of the clinician (Figure 72-41). The TrPs are identified using cross-fiber flat palpation. The region of the TrPs is fixed between the clinician's index and middle fingers, with the needle directed parallel to the muscle fibers and usually upward toward the shoulder. These TrPs are not especially close to the neurovascular bundle.

Anconeus (Figure 72-42)

For TrPI or DN of TrPs in the anconeus muscle, the patient is positioned prone, with the elbow flexed to about 45°. The TrPs are identified with cross-fiber flat palpation and the needle is directed toward the ulna between the olecranon process and the lateral epicondyle of the humerus (Figure 72-42).

3. FOREARM, WRIST, AND HAND PAIN (SECTION 4)

Wrist Extensor and Brachioradialis Muscles (Chapter 34)

Wrist Extensors (Figure 72-43)

For TrPI or DN of the wrist extensor muscles, the patient is positioned supine with the forearm in full pronation resting on a pillow or other support. Because all three wrist extensor muscles

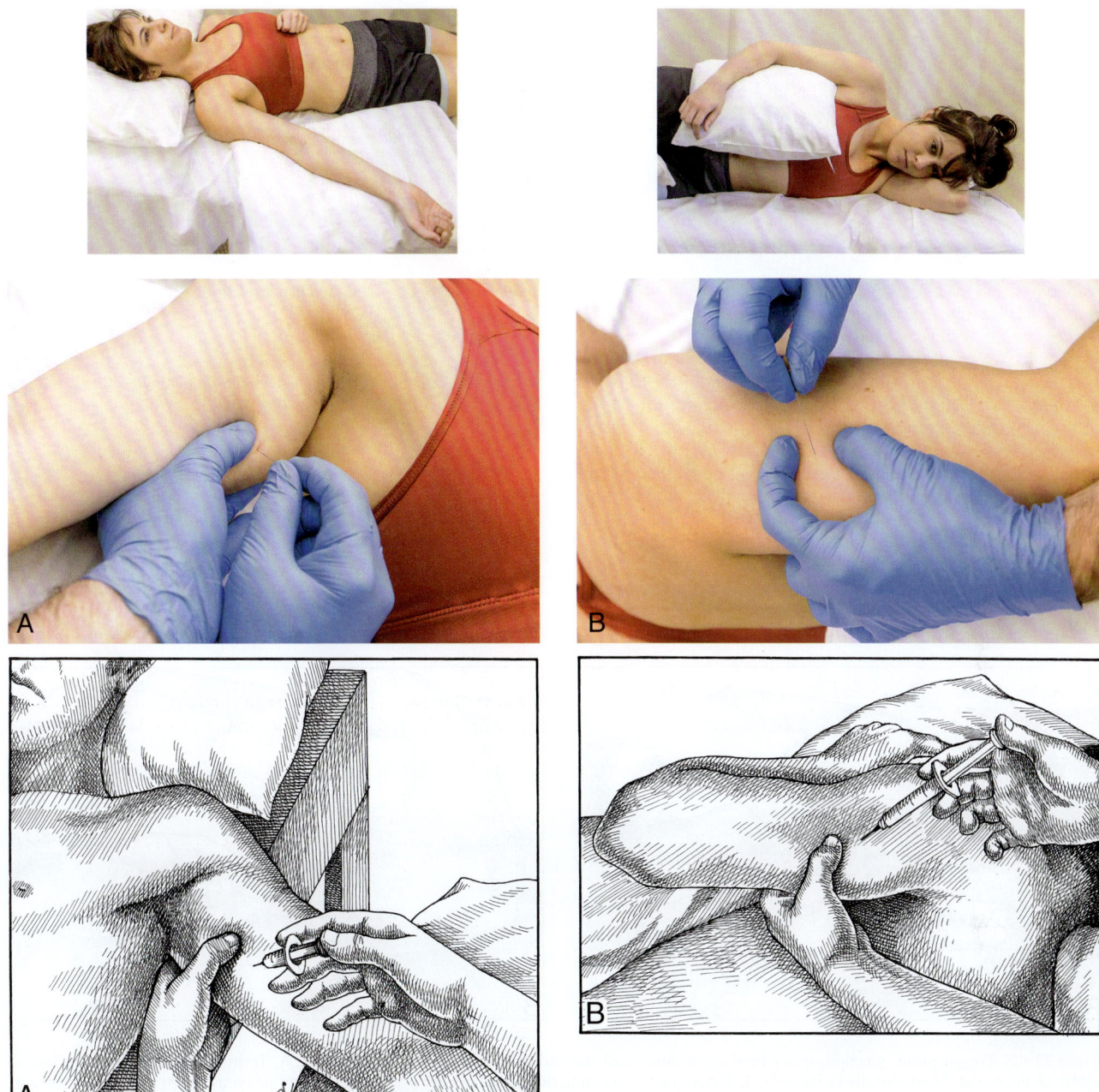

Figure 72-39. Trigger point injection or dry needling of the **triceps brachii muscle**. A, Anterior approach, with the patient supine. B, Posterior approach, with the patient lying on the uninvolved side.

are relatively superficial, palpation can precisely localize TrPs for needling. The extensor carpi radialis longus (ECRL) TrPs are identified with cross-fiber pincer palpation and then fixed with a pincer grasp between the clinician's thumb, index, and middle fingers. The needle is directed either medial to lateral or vice versa toward or between the clinician's fingers (Figure 72-43A). The ECRL muscle can also be needled with a flat palpation technique with the needle directed toward the radius. The extensor carpi radialis brevis (ECRB) muscle is medial to the ECRL muscle and its TrPs may be 3 or 4 cm (about 1½-in) more distal than ECRL TrPs. These TrPs are identified with cross-fiber flat palpation. The TrPs in the ECRB muscle are fixed between the clinician's index and middle finger and the needle is directed toward the radius (Figure 72-43B).

For TrPI or DN of the extensor carpi ulnaris muscle, TrPs are identified with cross-fiber flat palpation and fixed between the clinician's index and middle finger. The needle is directed toward the ulna (Figure 72-43C).

Brachioradialis (Figure 72-44)

For TrPI or DN of brachioradialis TrPs, the patient is positioned supine with the forearm in pronation resting on a pillow or other support. The brachioradialis TrPs are identified with cross-fiber pincer palpation and fixed with a pincer grasp between the clinician's thumb, index, and middle fingers. The needle is directed from medial to lateral or vice versa toward or between the clinician's fingers (Figure 72-44).

For the purposes of TrPI or DN, it is useful to distinguish TrPs that lie in the deepest brachioradialis fibers (which usually have no effect on wrist motion) from those in the underlying ECRL fibers that radially deviate and extend the wrist; the

792 Section 8: Treatment Considerations for Myofascial Pain and Dysfunction

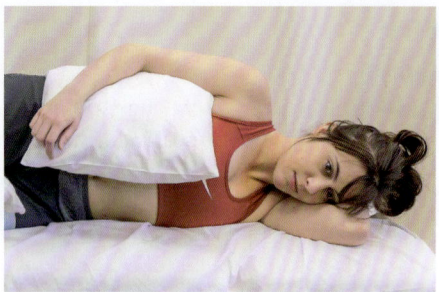

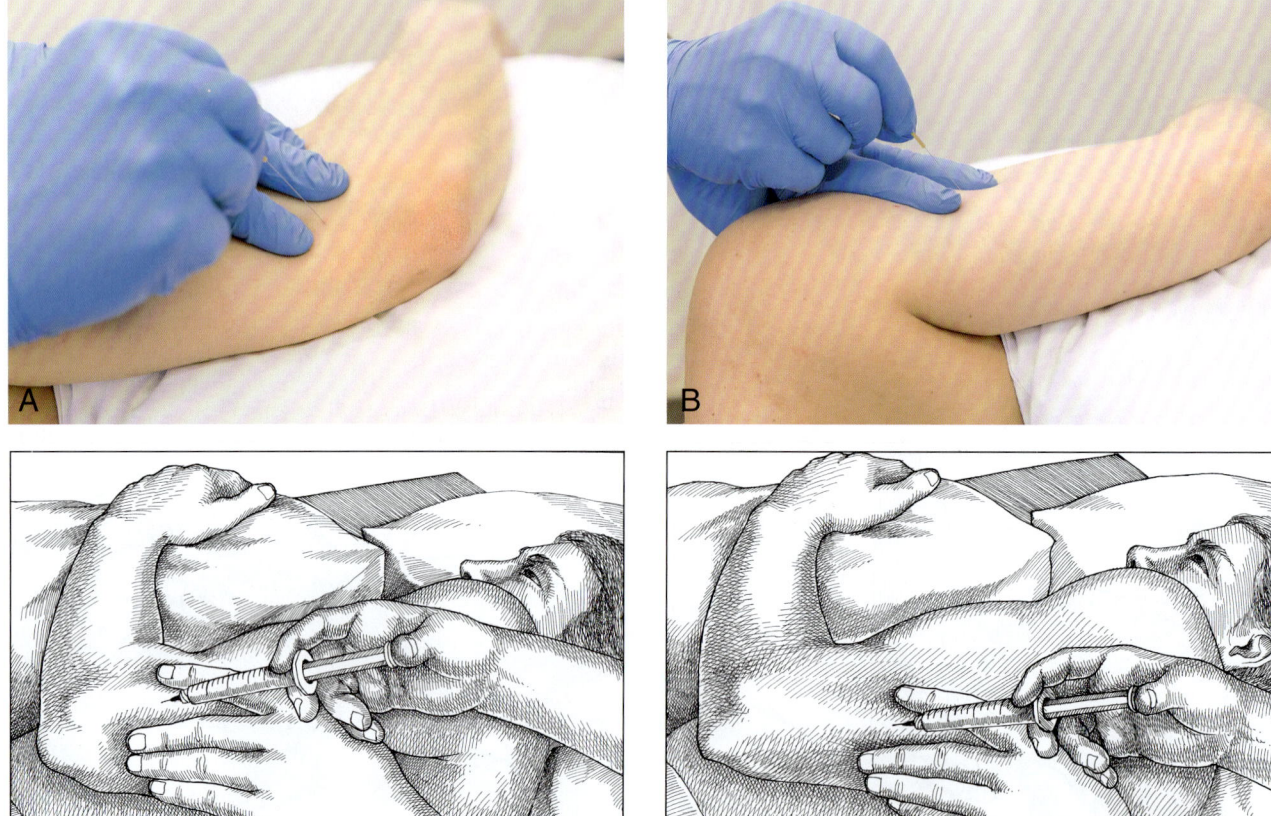

Figure 72-40. Trigger point injection or dry needling technique of the **triceps brachii muscle** in side-lying. A, Technique for needling the lateral border of the medial head, distally in the arm. B, Technique for needling the lateral border of the lateral head proximal (top) and distal (bottom) to the radial groove.

---

superficial (sensory) branch of the radial nerve passes between these two muscles.

When referred pain is evoked in the base of the thumb by a deep TrPI in the proximal forearm, the TrP may lie either in the brachioradialis muscle or in the underlying supinator muscle.

Extensor Digitorum and Extensor Indicis Muscles (Chapter 35)

Extensor Digitorum (Figure 72-45 A, B)

For TrPI or DN of the extensor digitorum muscle, the patient lies supine with the forearm in full pronation resting on a pillow or other support. Because this muscle is relatively superficial, palpation can precisely localize TrPs for TrPI or DN. The TrPs in the extensor digitorum muscle are identified with cross-fiber flat palpation, and the TrPs are fixed between the clinician's index and middle finger (Figure 72-45A). Because these are very flat muscles, it is best if the needle is inserted approximately 1 cm away and is directed toward the TrPs and the radius. Clinically, the middle finger extensor-muscle belly exhibits strong LTRs and clear pain patterns, as elicited by examination and needle penetration of the TrPs.

The TrPs in the 4th and 5th finger extensor muscles are located between those in the middle finger extensor fibers and the extensor carpi ulnaris muscle. The TrPs are identified with cross-fiber flat palpation and fixed between the clinician's index and middle fingers. The needle is inserted about 1 cm away from the TrP and directed toward the point of deep tenderness (Figure 72-45B).

Occasionally, a deep radial (dorsal interosseous) nerve block may inadvertently be produced during injection of these TrPs. The patient should be warned beforehand of possible temporary extensor-muscle weakness that resolves in 15 or 20 minutes depending on the solution that has been injected.

Extensor Indicis (Figure 72-45C)

For TrPI or DN of the extensor indicis muscle, the patient is in the same position as for the other wrist and finger extensor

Chapter 72: Trigger Point Injection and Dry Needling 793

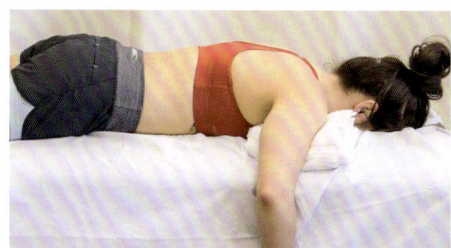
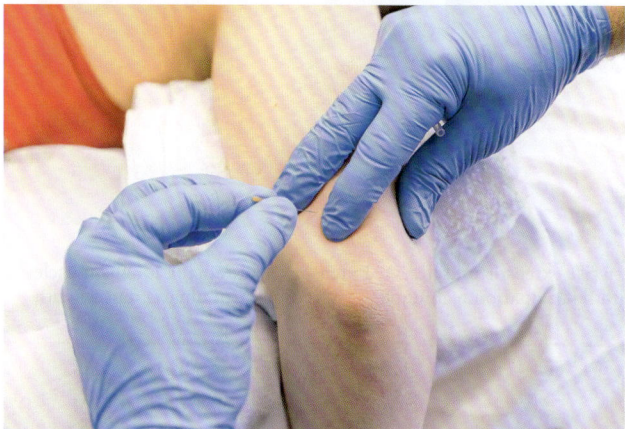

Figure 72-41. Trigger point injection or dry needling of the medial border of the **medial head of the triceps brachii muscle.**

Supinator Muscle (Chapter 36)
Figure 72-46

For TrPI or DN of TrPs in the supinator muscle, the patient is positioned supine with the upper extremity in slight abduction, elbow slightly flexed, and forearm supported and fully supinated. The brachioradialis muscle is pushed laterally so TrPs can be identified with cross-fiber flat palpation against the radius. For TrPI or DN, the needle is directed proximally into the TrP just lateral to the attachment of the biceps brachii tendon, where maximum tenderness was found on palpation (Figure 72-46). It is often difficult to see or feel an LTR in this muscle except through the needle. When the forearm is supinated, the deep radial nerve passes through the muscle lateral to this area (see Figure 36-1B and C) and thus is not usually encountered during TrPI or DN. The dorsal aspect of the muscle may also be treated with TrPI or DN in a similar manner.

Palmaris Longus Muscle (Chapter 37)
Figure 72-47

For TrPI or DN of the palmaris longus muscle, the patient lies supine with the arm slightly abducted, elbow extended, and the forearm fully supinated. The palmaris longus muscle, if present, is medial to the flexor carpi radialis muscle. Palmaris longus TrPs are identified by cross-fiber flat palpation and then fixed between the clinician's index and middle fingers. The needle is directed toward the TrPs and radius bone (Figure 72-47).

Wrist and Finger Flexor Muscles (Chapter 38)
Wrist Flexor Muscles (Figure 72-48A, B)

For TrPI or DN of TrPs in the flexor carpi radialis (FCR) muscle, the patient is positioned supine with the upper extremity in slight abduction, elbow slightly flexed, and forearm supported and

muscles. Extensor indicis TrPs are identified with cross-fiber flat palpation at the dorsal aspect of the middle third of the radius. The TrP is fixed between the clinician's index and middle finger and the needle is directed toward the radius (Figure 72-45C).

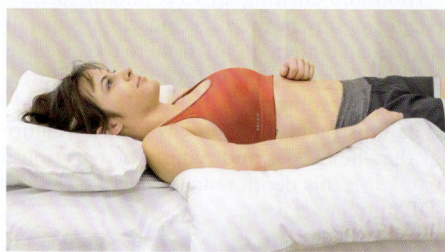
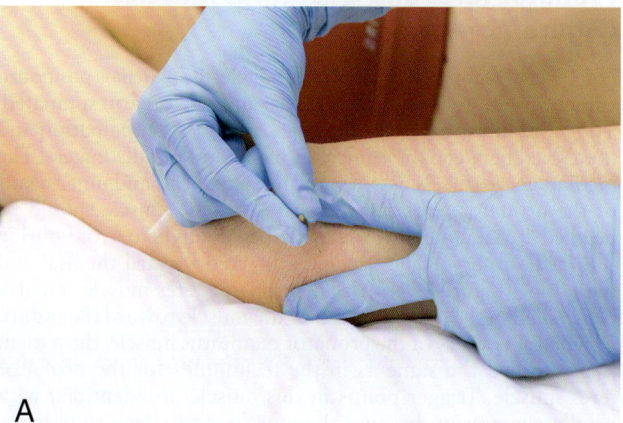

A

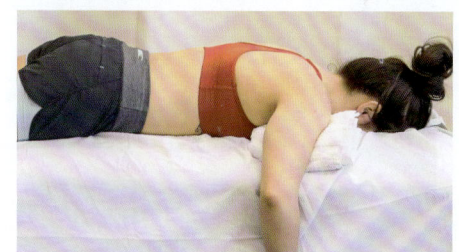
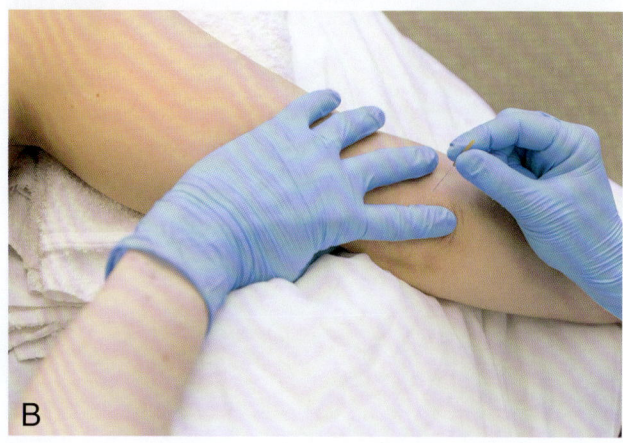

B

Figure 72-42. Trigger point injection or dry needling of the **anconeus muscle.** The index finger of the palpating hand is on the lateral epicondyle and the middle finger is on the olecranon process. A, Supine with the elbow flexed and arm supported on a pillow. B, Prone.

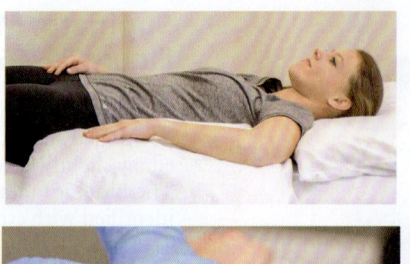
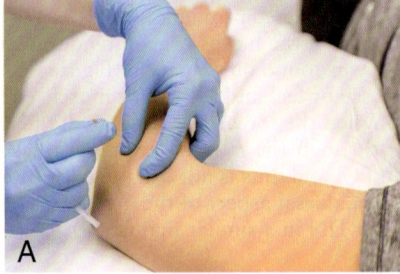 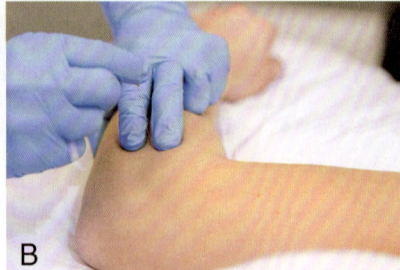 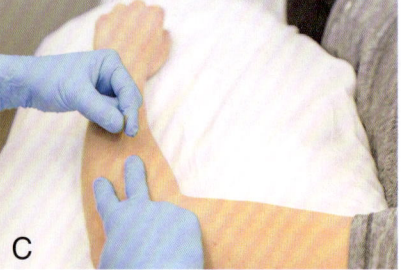

Figure 72-43. Trigger point injection or dry needling technique of the **wrist extensor muscles**. A, Extensor carpi radialis longus muscle with pincer grasp technique. B, **Extensor carpi radialis brevis muscle** with flat palpation technique. C, **Extensor carpi ulnaris muscle** with flat palpation technique.

fully supinated. Trigger points in the FCR muscle are identified using cross-fiber flat palpation and are then fixed between the clinician's index and middle fingers. The needle is directed toward the TrPs and the radius bone (Figure 72-48A).

For TrPI or DN of TrPs in the flexor carpi ulnaris (FCU) muscle, the patient is positioned supine with the glenohumeral joint in external rotation and the elbow in 90° flexion supported on a pillow to accommodate range-of-motion limitations (Figure 72-48B). The TrPs in the FCU muscle are identified by cross-fiber flat palpation and then fixed between the clinician's index and middle fingers. The needle is directed toward the TrP and the ulna bone (Figure 72-48B).

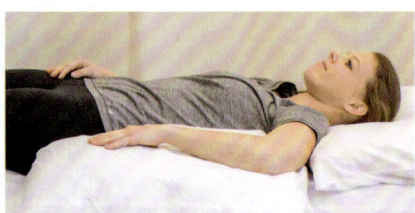

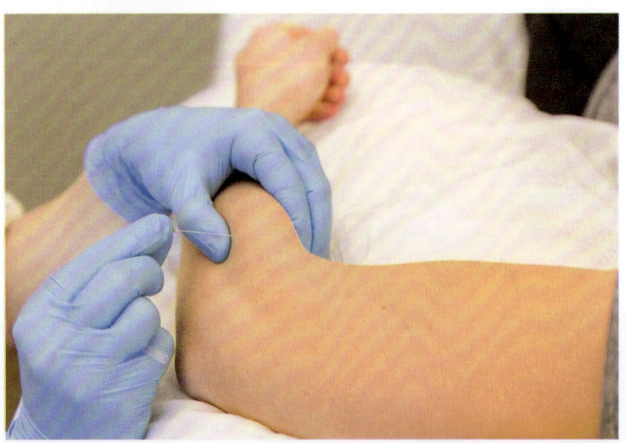

Figure 72-44. Trigger point injection or dry needling of the **brachioradialis muscle** using the pincer grasp technique. Note that the forearm is in a neutral position.

Finger Flexor Muscles (Figure 72-48C, D)

For TrPI or DN of the flexor digitorum superficialis (FDS) and flexor digitorum profundus (FDP) muscles, the patient is positioned supine with the elbow slightly flexed and the forearm in supination. Trigger points in the FDS muscle are identified by cross-fiber flat palpation and then fixed between the clinician's index and middle fingers. The needle is directed toward the interosseous membrane (Figure 72-48C). The median nerve runs between the FDS and FDP muscles, and the ulnar nerve runs between the FCU and FDP muscles. Both nerves should be avoided by directing the needle from midline toward the radius or ulna bones.

For TrPI or DN of the FDP muscle, TrPs are identified by needle insertion and eliciting an LTR and/or identifiable pain pattern. Trigger points in the FDP muscle are usually located approximately 3 cm (about 1½-in) distal to the medial epicondyle (Figure 72-48D). Trigger points in the FDP muscle are sometimes responsible for entrapment of the ulnar nerve and may also be needled as illustrated for the FCU muscle (Figure 72-48B) except that they lie deeper and require penetration to at least 2 cm (nearly 1 in); this depth reaches beyond the FCU muscle into the FDP muscle.

Pronator Teres and Quadratus Muscles (Figure 72-49)

For TrPI or DN of the pronator teres muscle, the patient is positioned supine with the elbow slightly flexed and the forearm supinated. Trigger points are identified using cross-fiber flat palpation and then fixed between the clinician's index and middle fingers. The median nerve travels between the humeral head and ulnar heads of the pronator teres muscle; therefore, the muscle should be needled 1 to 2 cm below the medial epicondyle to avoid hitting the median nerve. The needle is directed toward the TrP and ulna bone (Figure 72-49A). The pronator teres muscle can also be needled in the distal portion of the muscle toward the radius.

For TrPI or DN of the pronator quadratus muscle, the patient is positioned the same as in the techniques for the pronator teres muscle. Trigger points in this muscle are identified with needle penetration because the muscle is too deep to palpate. The anterior interosseous nerve runs in the center of the forearm between the transverse and oblique heads of the muscle. The needle is directed toward the radius or ulna bones in the distal third of the forearm (Figure 72-49B).

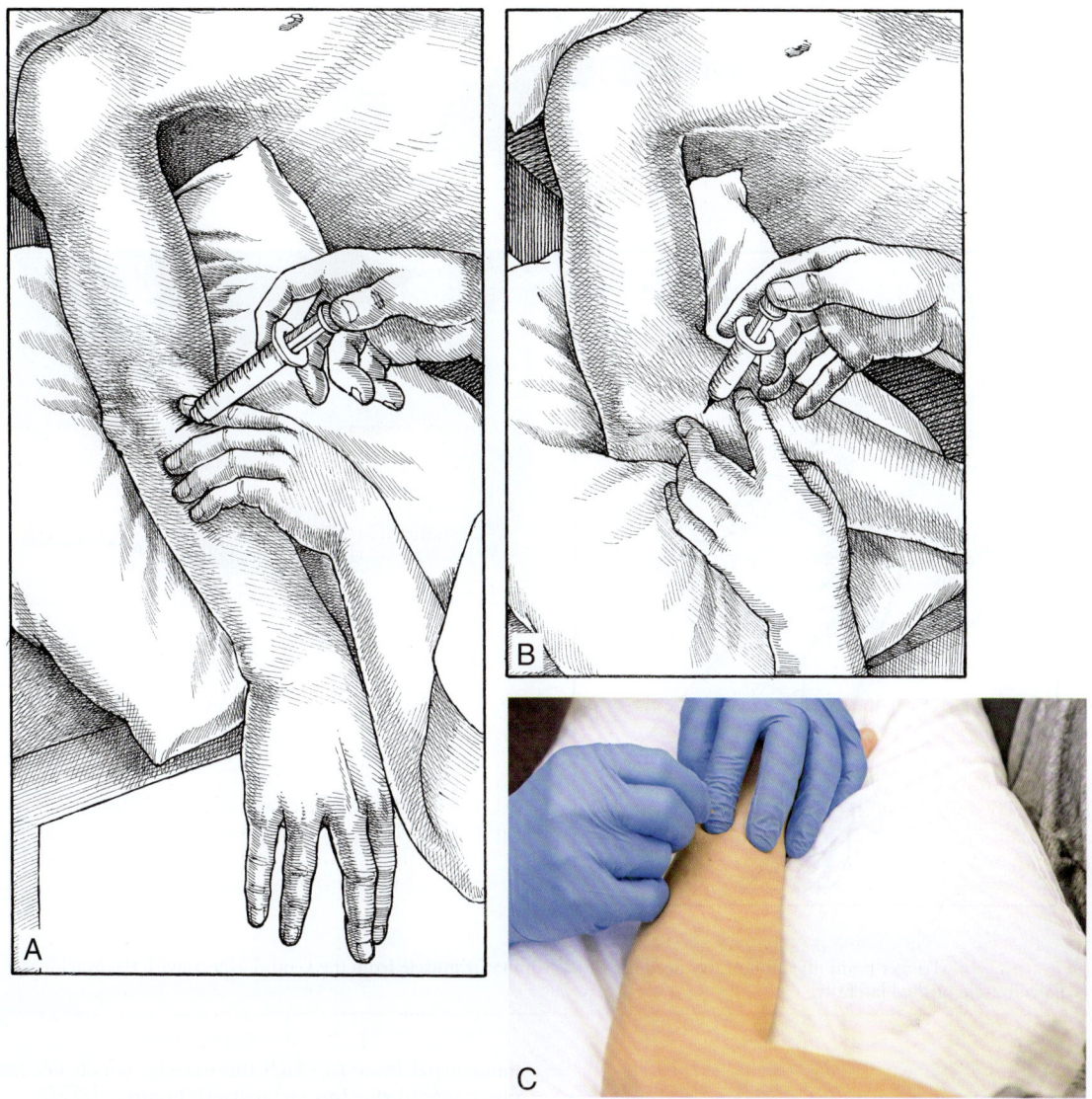

Figure 72-45. Trigger point injection or dry needling of the **finger extensor muscles**. A, **Middle finger extensor muscle**. B, **Ring and little finger extensor muscles**. Injection deep into the fourth and fifth finger extensor muscles sometimes also reaches a trigger point in the underlying supinator muscle, which refers pain to the lateral epicondyle. C, **Extensor indicis muscle**.

Adductor and Opponens Pollicis Muscle (Chapter 39)

Adductor Pollicis (Figure 72-50A)

For TrPI or DN of the adductor pollicis muscle, the patient is positioned supine with the forearm pronated or in mid-position. Trigger points are identified by cross-fiber pincer palpation and fixed with a pincer grasp between the clinician's thumb, index, and middle fingers (Figure 72-50A). The needle is directed from dorsal to ventral into the muscle and slightly toward the 2nd metacarpal. As the needle is directed toward this guiding finger, it should pass to the radial side of, or perhaps penetrate, the first dorsal interossei muscle.

Opponens Pollicis (Figure 72.50B)

For TrPI or DN of the opponens pollicis muscle, the patient is positioned supine with the forearm supinated. Trigger points are identified with either cross-fiber pincer or flat palpation. The needle is inserted from the radial aspect to avoid going through the palmar aspect of the thenar eminence (Figure 72-50B).

Interosseous, Lumbrical, and Abductor Digiti Minimi Muscles (Chapter 40)

Interossei and Lumbricals (Figures 72-51A and 72-52)

Trigger points in the palmar interosseous and lumbrical muscles are difficult to palpate; therefore, adequate exploration of the area with a needle is important. For TrPI or DN of the first dorsal interossei muscle, the patient is positioned supine with the hand in a mid-pronated or fully pronated position. Trigger points are identified with cross-fiber flat palpation, and the patient's index finger is fixed between the clinician's thumb and index fingers (Figure 72-51A). The needle is directed toward the TrP and the radial aspect of the 2nd metacarpal bone (Figure 72-51A).

For TrPI or DN of the second dorsal interossei muscle, the needle is aligned with the side of the 3rd metacarpal bone in the second interosseous space and is inserted into the center of the area (Figure 72-52A). If any tenderness remains, the needle is aligned with the 2nd metacarpal bone on the other side of the space, and the other head of the muscle is examined for TrPs.

For TrPI or DN of the first palmar interossei muscle (Figure 72-52A), the needle is directed away from the 3rd

796 Section 8: Treatment Considerations for Myofascial Pain and Dysfunction

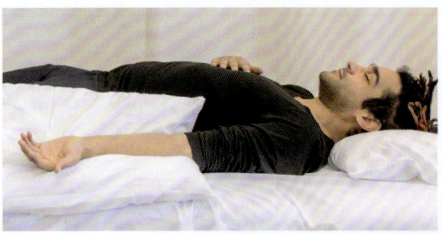

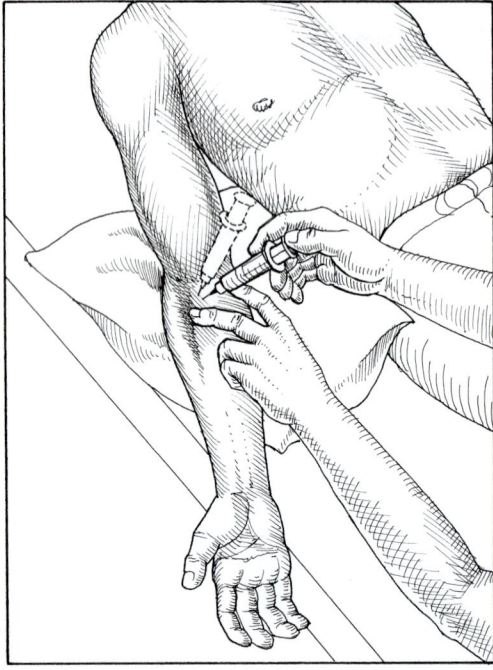

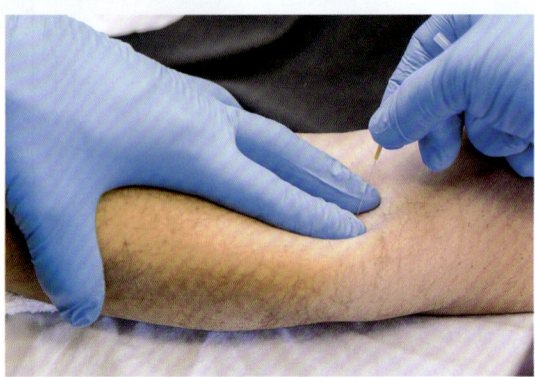

Figure 72-46. Trigger point injection or dry needling of the **supinator muscle** from the ventral aspect, with the brachioradialis muscle pushed laterally.

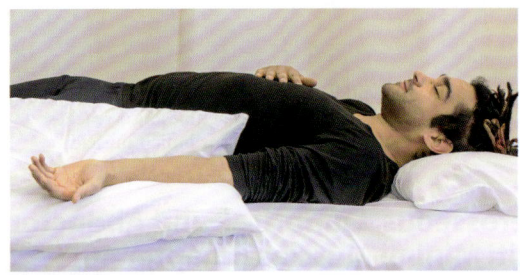

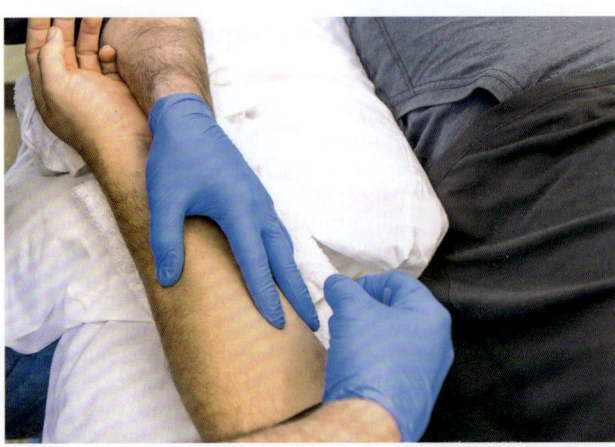

Figure 72-47. Trigger point injection or dry needling technique for the **palmaris longus muscle.**

metacarpal bone to reach the muscle, which lies beneath the ulnar side of the 2nd metacarpal (Figure 72-52B).

For TrPI or DN of the four lumbrical muscles, the needle is inserted between the metacarpal bones like the interosseous technique. The lumbrical muscles lie closer to the palmer aspect of the hand on the radial side of its perspective metacarpal bone.

Abductor Digiti Minimi (Figure 72-51B)

Trigger points in the abductor digiti minimi muscle are identified with either cross-fiber flat or pincer palpation and are fixed with a pincer grasp between the clinician's thumb and index fingers. The needle is directed toward the 5th metacarpal bone (Figure 72-51B).

4. TRUNK AND PELVIS PAIN (Section 5)

Pectoralis Major and Subclavius Muscles (Chapter 42)

Trigger point injection or DN requires care when injecting pectoral musculature given its location over the ventral surface of the ribcage. Therefore, the clinician must be mindful of the lung field and the depth of penetration of the needle to avoid entering the pleural cavity, possibly creating a pneumothorax. In the event that the clinician suspects that the needle violated the pleural cavity of the lung, the patient should be instructed to seek emergency care if he or she develops symptoms such as shortness of breath, persistent cough, or unusual chest or

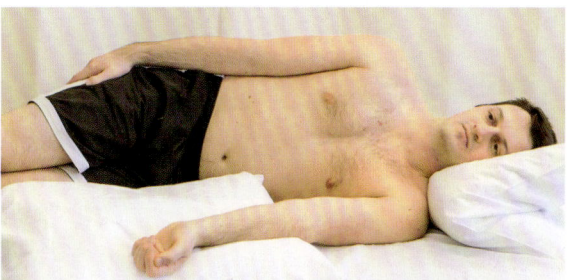

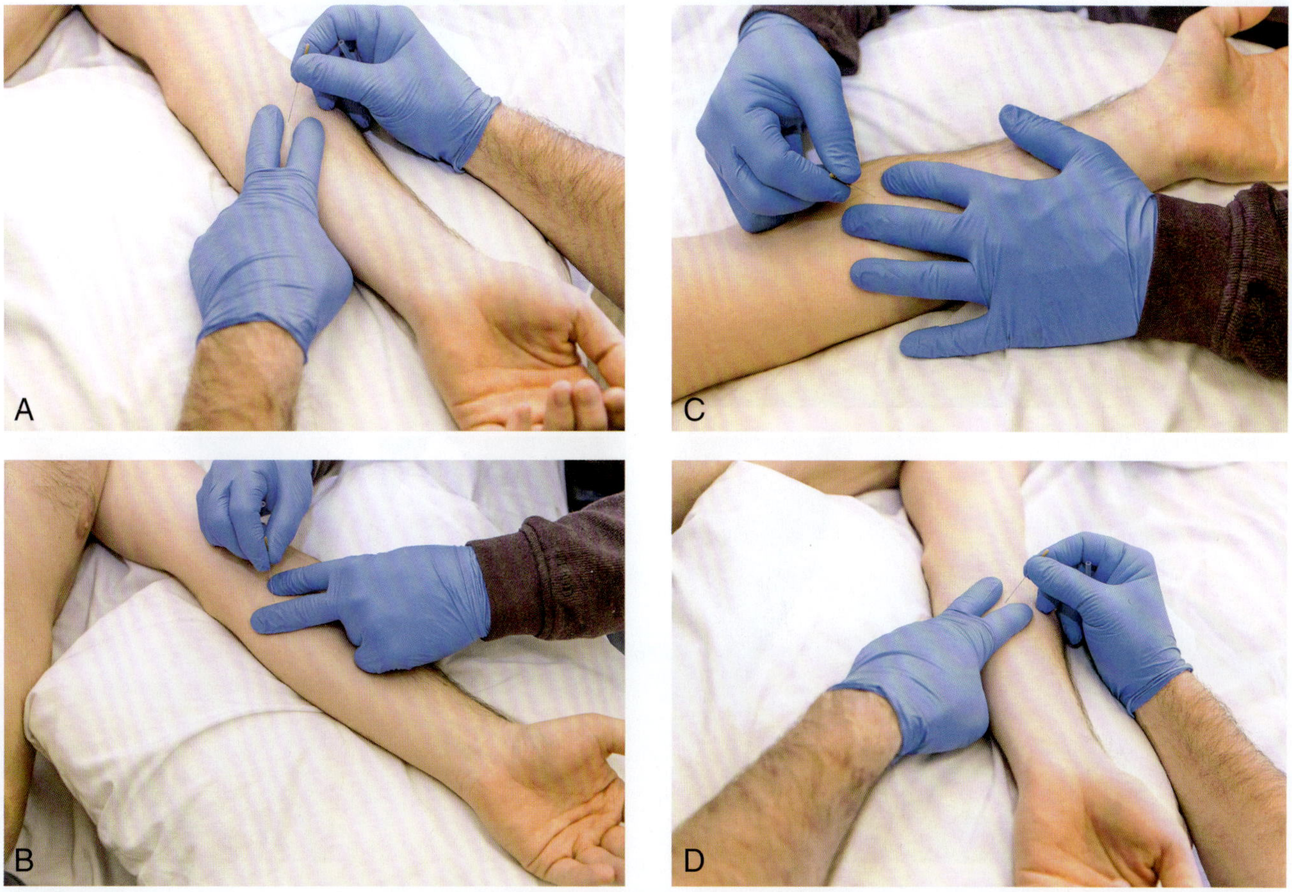

Figure 72-48. Trigger point injection or dry needling technique for the **wrist and finger flexor muscles**. A, Flexor carpi radialis muscle. B, Flexor carpi ulnaris muscle. C, Flexor digitorum superficialis muscle. D, Flexor digitorum profundus muscle.

rib cage pain. The patient should inform the emergency room staff that he or she received a TrPI or DN treatment over the chest wall. Radiographs of the chest are used to confirm a pneumothorax. Pleural penetration during a TrPI or DN technique typically causes a more severe pain than that of TrPs. While a pneumothorax is less likely to occur when using a filiform needle than when using a hypodermic needle, it has been reported.[97]

The clinician should be positioned comfortably and right-handed clinicians may have to perform the needling technique of the left pectoralis major muscle from the right side reaching across the patient, whereas the technique for the right pectoralis major muscle would be performed on the right side and vice versa for left-handed clinicians. Female patients should be asked to cover the breast with the hand and possibly move the breast tissue aside so TrPs may be needled effectively. For TrPs in the medial aspect of the sternal head, the patient's large breasts can be positioned on the ipsilateral side to move the breast tissue away from the medial aspect of the muscle.

Pectoralis Major Clavicular Head (Figure 72-53A)

For TrPI or DN of the clavicular head of the pectoralis major muscle, the patient is positioned prone with the upper extremity slightly abducted. Trigger points are identified with cross-fiber pincer palpation and fixed with a pincer grasp between the clinician's thumb, index, and middle fingers (Figure 72-53A). The needle is directed shallowly and tangentially toward the clinician's fingers to avoid penetration of the lung field and directed toward the clavicle or the shoulder (Figure 72-53A). Trigger point injection or DN may also be performed with a flat palpation; however, this technique increases the risk of penetration into the lung field.

Pectoralis Major Sternal and Abdominal Heads (Figure 72-53B-D)

About half of this most proximal portion of the pectoralis major's sternal section lies beneath the clavicular section (see Figure 42-2). Trigger points are identified with cross-fiber flat

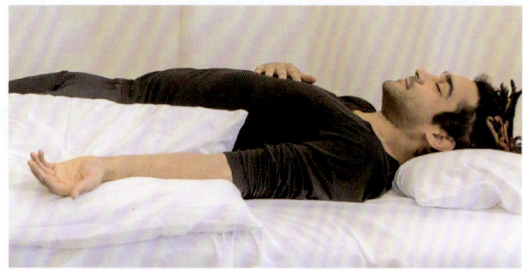

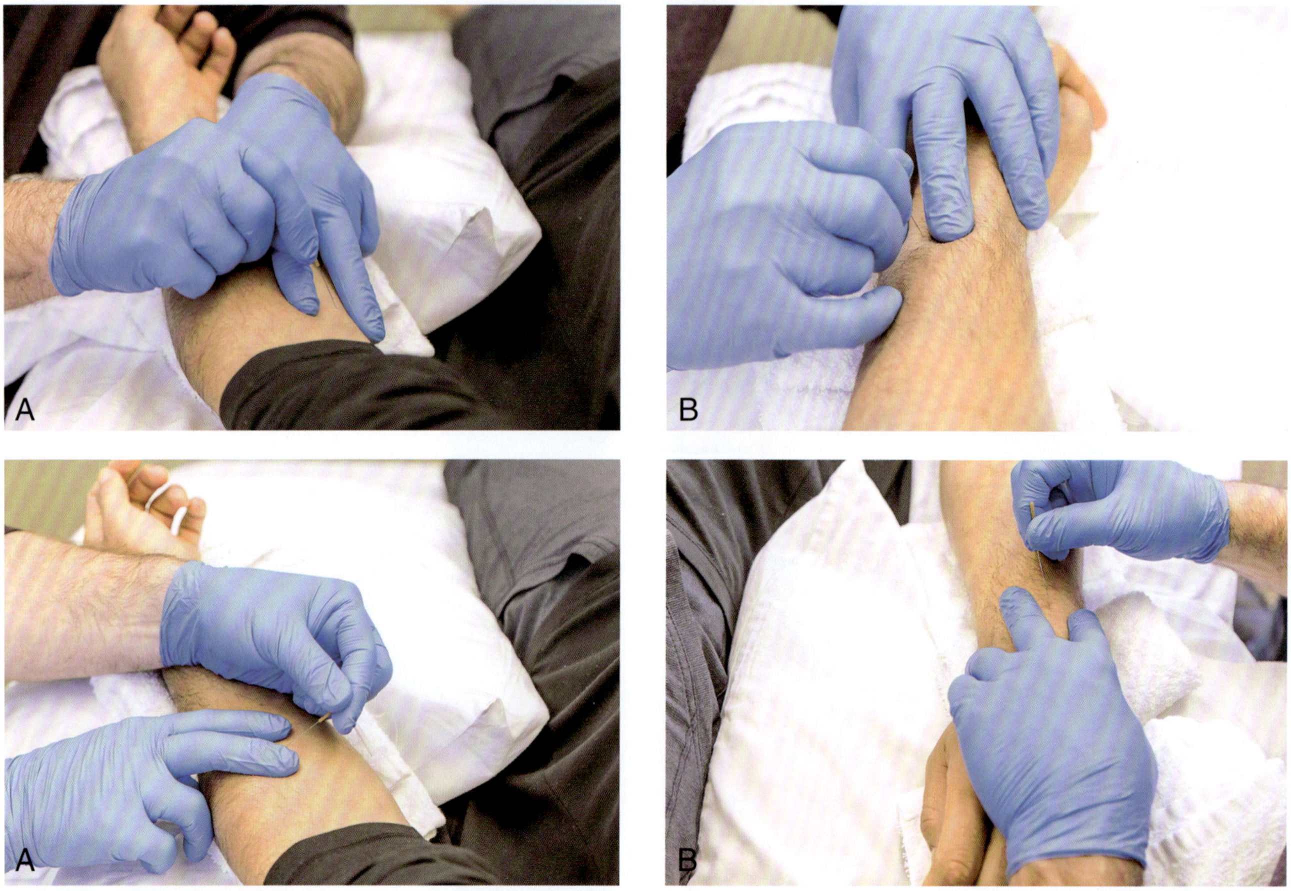

Figure 72-49. Trigger point injection or dry needling technique for the **pronator muscles**. A, **Pronator teres muscle**. Note that the needle is directed toward the ulna (top) or distally toward the radius (bottom) to prevent hitting the median nerve. B, **Pronator quadratus muscle** dorsal approach. Note that the needle is directed from midline either radially (top) or ulnarly (bottom) to avoid hitting the anterior interosseous nerve.

palpation and fixed over a rib between the clinician's index and middle fingers, which are placed in the intercostal spaces to prevent penetration into the lung field (Figure 72-53B). Trigger points in the upper, mid-sternal, and abdominal portion of the muscle are identified with cross-fiber pincer palpation and fixed with a pincer grasp between the clinician's thumb, index, and middle finger as in the technique for the clavicular head. The needle is directed tangentially and shallowly toward the clinician's finger and TrPs (Figure 72-53C).

Parasternal and costal pectoral TrPs are identified with cross-fiber flat palpation, and the TrPs are fixed over a rib. The clinician identifes and blocks the intercostal spaces over and under the corresponding rib with the index and middle fngers of the palpating hand to avoid entering the lung feld (Figure 72-53D). The needle is directed toward the rib tangentially and shallowly. If the rib can't be accurately identified, this technique should not be performed.

Subclavius Muscle (Figure 72-54)

Trigger points in the subclavius muscle can't be precisely identified with manual palpation; however, tenderness in the area of the muscle may be indicative of TrPs. For TrPI or DN, the patient is positioned supine. The needle is directed toward the point of maximum tenderness beneath the clavicle, usually in the middle of the muscle toward the junction of its medial and middle thirds (Figure 72-54).

Sternalis Muscle (Chapter 43)
Figure 72-53D

Trigger points in the sternalis muscle are identified using cross-fiber flat palpation, and the TrP is fixed over a rib or the sternum between the clinician's index and middle finger which blocks the intercostal space. For TrPI or DN of the sternalis muscle, the technique described for needling the parasternal fibers of the pectoralis major muscle would be utilized (Figure 72-53D). The needle is directed toward the rib, and when a TrP is penetrated, the patient typically reports a projection of pain under the sternum and sometimes across the upper pectoral region and down the ulnar aspect of the arm as far as the elbow. LTRs are not observed in this muscle.

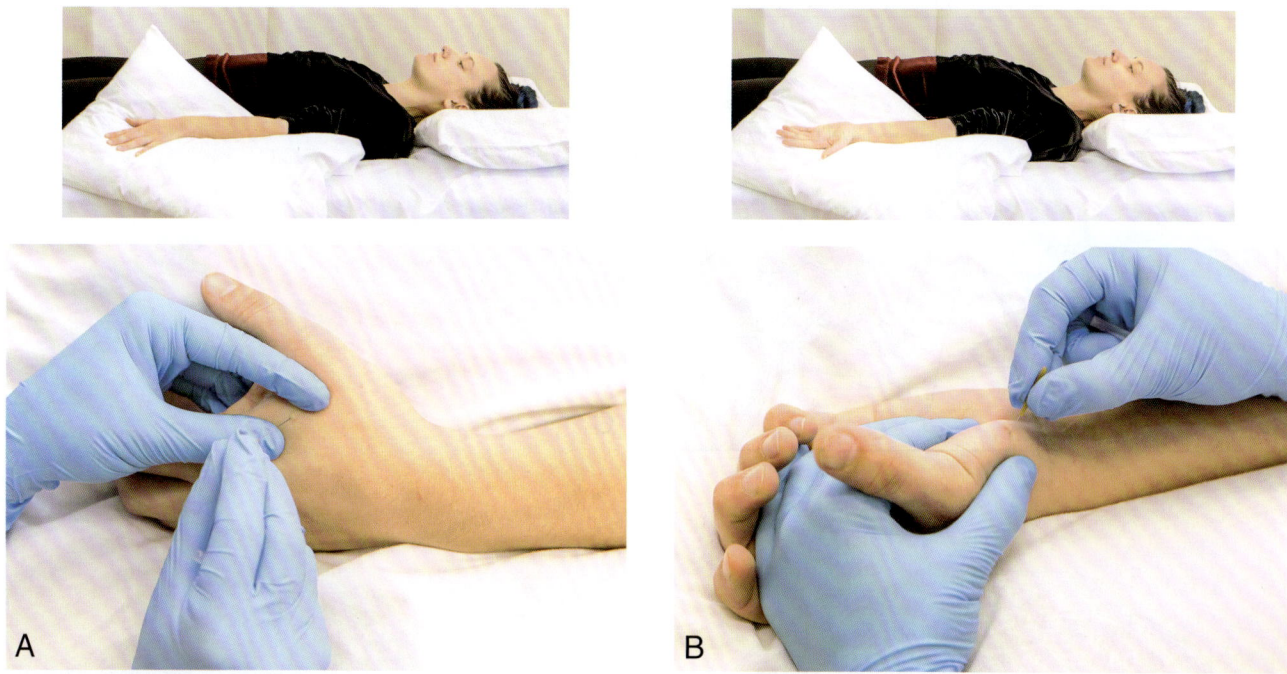

Figure 72-50. Trigger point injection or dry needling techniques for **thumb muscles**. A, Dorsal approach for the **adductor pollicis muscle**. B, Radial approach for the **opponens pollicis muscle**.

Pectoralis Minor Muscle (Chapter 44) Figure 72-55

Trigger point injection or DN requires care when injecting deeper pectoral musculature because the muscle is located over the ventral surface of the ribcage. Therefore, the clinician must be mindful of the lung field and the depth of penetration of the needle to avoid entering the pleural cavity, possibly creating a pneumothorax.

The patient is positioned supine with the upper extremity in a neutral position and supported with a pillow. Female patients should be asked to cover the breast with a hand and possibly move the breast tissue aside to allow the TrPs to be needled effectively. Trigger point injection or DN is performed by directing the needle nearly parallel to the chest wall and not toward the ribs, using pincer palpation wherever the patient's anatomy permits.

Trigger point injection or DN of pectoralis minor TrPs should be done after those in the pectoralis major muscle.

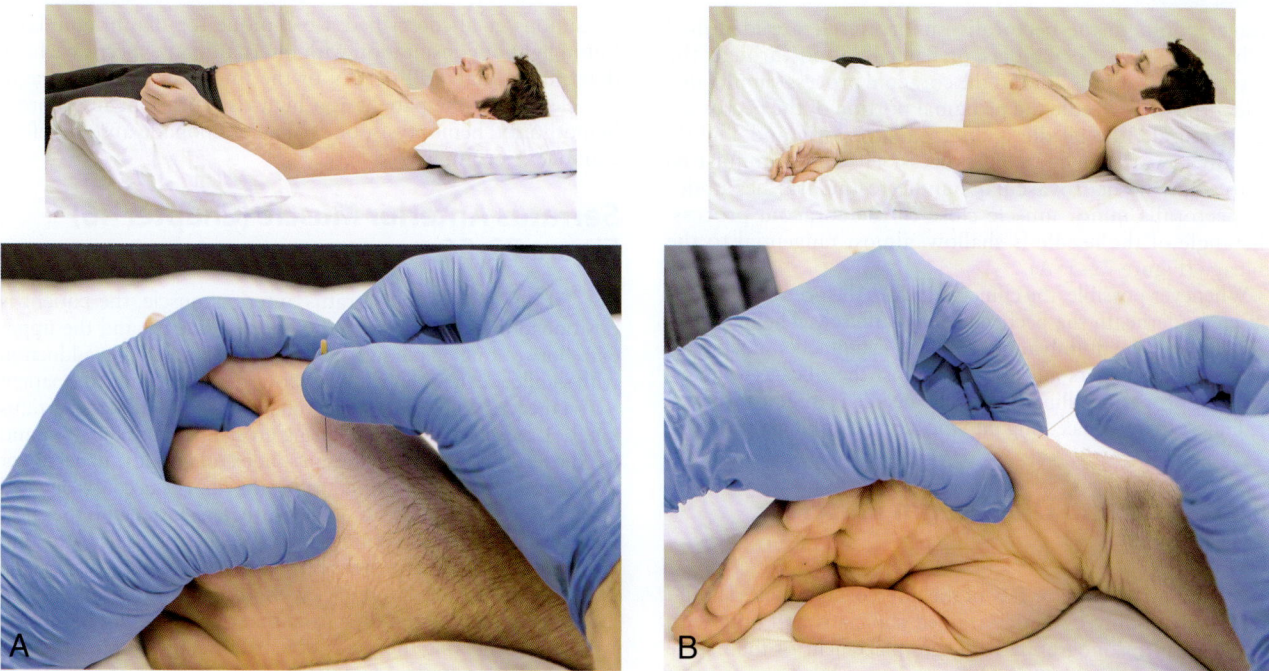

Figure 72-51. Trigger point injection or dry needling technique of the **intrinsic hand muscles**. A, **First dorsal interosseous** muscle approached from the dorsal aspect. B, The **abductor digiti minimi muscle,** approached from the ulnar aspect of the hand.

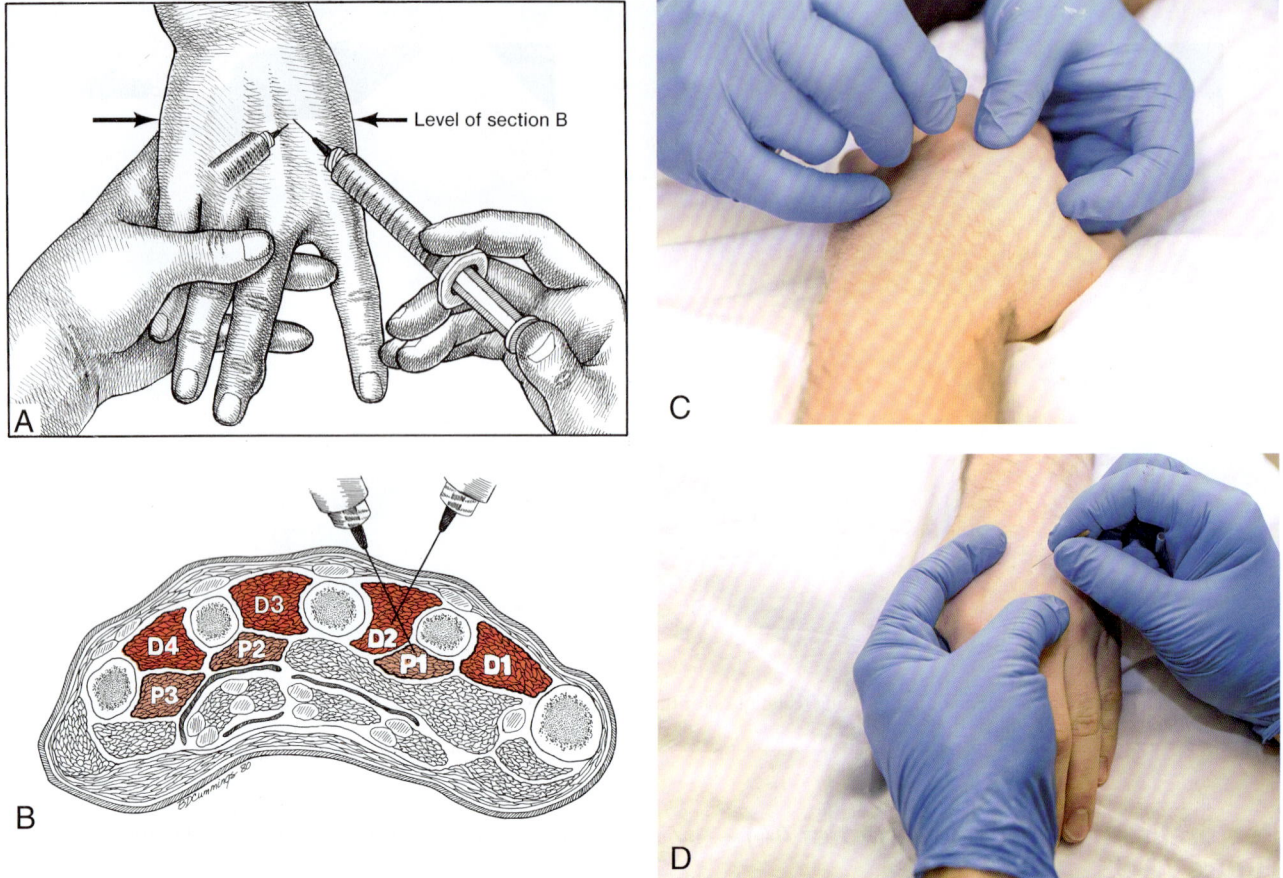

Figure 72-52. Trigger point injection or dry needling technique for the **interossei muscles**. A, The complete syringe is injecting a trigger point in the more ulnar penna of the second dorsal interosseous muscle; its corresponding Heberden's node is shown. The incomplete syringe is injecting the first palmar interosseous muscle that is reached as the needle penetrates deep to the 2nd metacarpal bone. B, Cross-section of A showing relation of the needles to the muscles being injected—dorsal interosseous muscles (dark red) and palmar interosseous muscles (light red). C, DN of the dorsal interosseous muscle. D, DN of the first palmar interosseous muscle.

Trigger points in the pectoralis minor muscle are identified with either cross-fiber pincer or flat palpation through the pectoralis major muscle, and the coracoid process should also be identified. To needle the proximal portion of the pectoralis minor muscle, the needle is directed superiorly and slightly laterally toward the coracoid process. The clinician must be aware that the neurovascular bundle to the arm lies under the pectoralis minor muscle close to the coracoid process. The angle of the needle is shallow, almost tangential to the rib cage (Figure 72-55A).

Whenever possible, the clinician locates the pectoralis minor muscle underneath the pectoralis major muscle. The muscle is held between the thumb and the fingers in a pincher grasp with the tips of the fingers and thumb against the ribcage to determine the proper needling angle. The needle is directed toward the fingers to avoid needling into the lung field (Figure 72-55B).

Intercostal and Diaphragm Muscles (Chapter 45)

Trigger point injection or DN of the intercostal muscles should be performed only by highly trained clinicians and only with the use of ultrasonography for exact placement of the needle in the intercostal muscles.[98] Although beyond the scope of this textbook, a more common intervention for chest wall pain is an ultrasound-guided intercostal nerve block. Both are high-risk procedures for a pneumothorax.

Simons et al[2] described a technique for diaphragm TrPI, but in light of consultation with international experts, we have determined that TrPI or DN of the intercostal or diaphragm muscles places the patient at a high risk for a pneumothorax, hemothorax, hemoptysis, or cardiac tamponade and therefore cannot be recommended here.[99]

Serratus Anterior Muscle (Chapter 46)
Figure 72-56

For TrPI or DN of the serratus anterior muscle, the patient is positioned in side-lying with the affected side up and the upper extremity resting on pillows in front, or the scapula is in adduction with shoulder extension with the elbow in flexion behind the patient to rest the wrist and hand on the trunk. Trigger points in the serratus anterior muscle are identified using cross-fiber flat palpation and fixed over a rib with the clinician's index and middle fingers over the intercostal space above and below the rib. The needle is directed toward the rib, at a shallow angle nearly tangential with the chest wall until the needle encounters the TrPs. These TrPs lie in the thin layer of the muscle between the rib and the skin (Figure 72-56). The pain reaction on needle contact with TrPs in this muscle is often less intense than the response from that of many other muscles.

Because the long thoracic nerve exclusively supplies the serratus anterior muscle, some degree of anesthesia of this motor nerve is to be expected when injecting an anesthetic. However, the patient is unlikely to notice only temporary weakness of a part of the serratus anterior muscle.

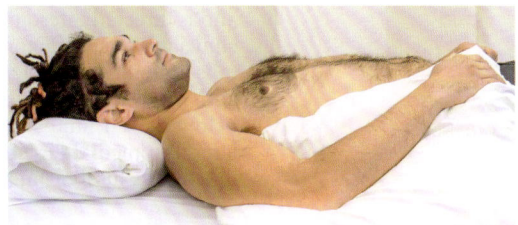
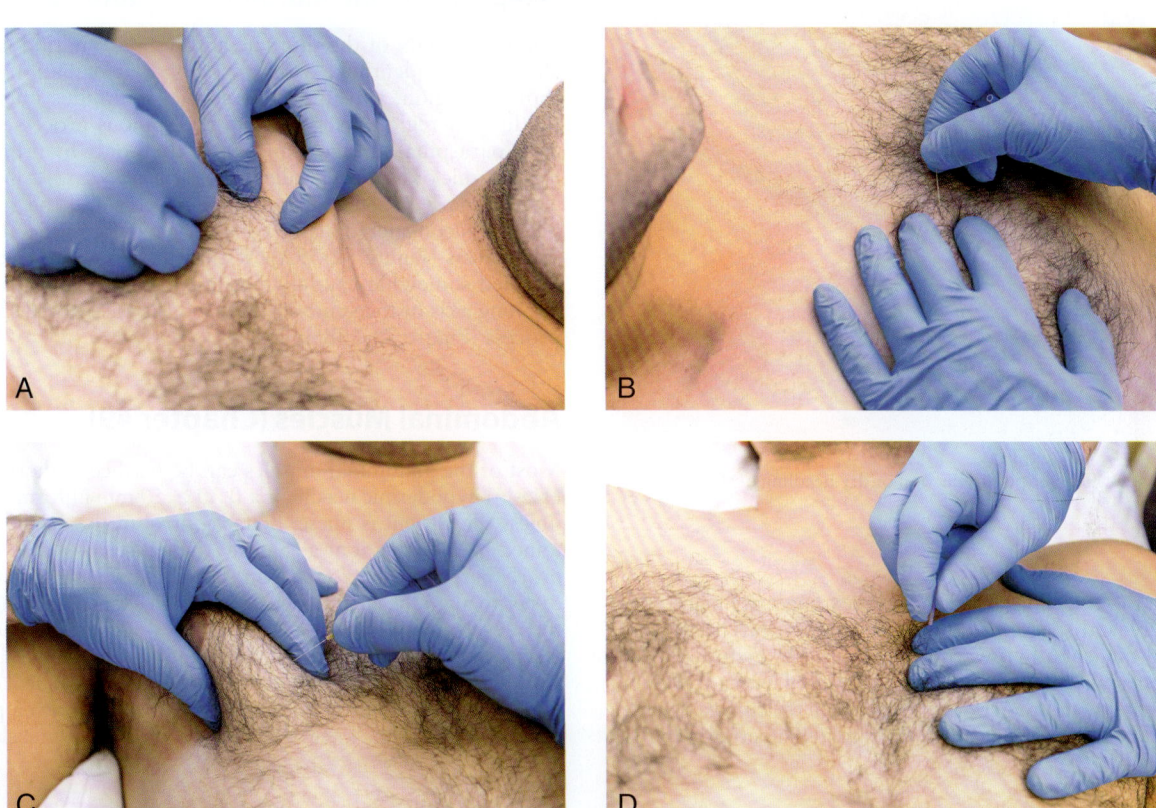

Figure 72-53. Trigger point injection or dry needling of the **pectoralis major muscle**. A, Clavicular head utilizing a pincer grasp. B, Flat palpation technique for upper sternal fibers. Note the index and middle finger over the intercostal space to protect the lung field. C, Mid-sternal and abdominal fibers using a pincer grasp. D, Parasternal fibers with flat palpation with the intercostal spaces blocked.

Serratus Posterior Superior and Inferior Muscles (Chapter 47)

Serratus Posterior Superior (Figure 72-57A)

For TrPI or DN of the serratus posterior superior muscle, the patient is positioned in prone with the scapula in full abduction and the arm hanging off the table, or the arm can be placed in extension, adduction, and internal rotation with the back of the hand resting on the low back (Hammerlock position). The TrPs are identified with cross-fiber flat palpation and fixed against an underlying rib, and the clinician's index and middle fingers are placed above and below the rib blocking the intercostal space (Figure 72-57A). The needle is directed nearly tangential to the thorax and is pointed toward a rib at all times.

Serratus Posterior Inferior (Figure 72-57B)

For TrPI or DN of the serratus posterior inferior muscle, the patient is positioned in prone or side-lying on the opposite side. Trigger points are identified with cross-fiber flat palpation and fixed against an underlying rib with the clinician's index and middle fingers placed above and below the rib, blocking the intercostal space. The needle is directed at a shallow angle toward the ninth, tenth, eleventh, or twelfth rib, depending on which digitations are involved (Figure 72-57B).

Thoracolumbar Paraspinal Muscles (Chapter 48)

For TrPI or DN of the thoracolumbar paraspinal muscles, the patient is positioned prone with a pillow under the abdomen to passively position the lumbar spine in a neutral position. If a patient has an increased thoracic kyphosis, additional pillows may be required so the patient is comfortable.

Superficial Paraspinal (Erector Spinae) (Figure 72-58)

For TrPI or DN of the longissimus thoracis muscle, a cross-fiber flat palpation technique is used and the needle is inserted slightly superior to the TrP and is directed tangentially at a shallow angle toward the clinician's fingers and the TrPs (Figure 72-58A). If possible, the TrP can be fixed against and underlying rib, and the clinician may block the intercostal spaces with the index and middle finger.

For TrPI or DN of the iliocostalis thoracis muscle, a cross-fiber flat palpation is used, and the TrP is fixed against an underlying

802 Section 8: Treatment Considerations for Myofascial Pain and Dysfunction

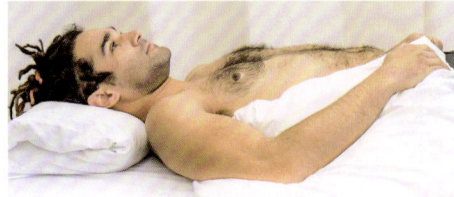

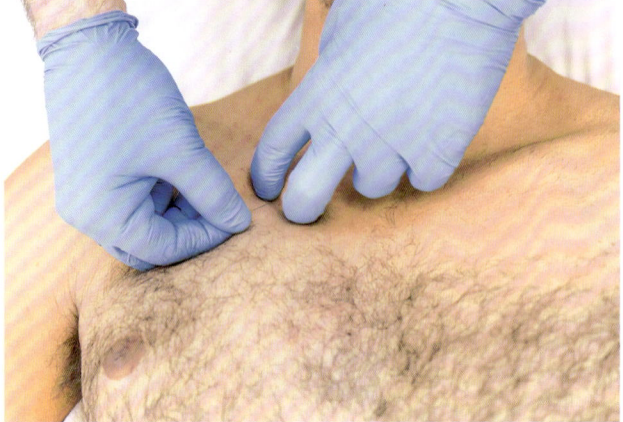

Figure 72-54. Trigger point injection or dry needling of the **subclavius muscle**.

rib, and the clinician's middle and index finger are placed over the intercostal spaces below and above the rib. The needle is directed tangentially toward the TrP and rib (Figure 72-58B). The iliocostalis lumborum TrPs are identified with a cross-fiber flat palpation, and the TrP is fixed between the clinician's index and middle finger. The needle is inserted just superior to the TrP

and is directed inferomedially toward the TrP and between the clinician's fingers (Figure 72-58C). Alternatively, for the iliocostalis lumborum muscle, the patient can be positioned side-lying with the affected side up, and a pincer grasp technique is utilized below the 1st lumbar vertebrae. The needle is directed from a lateral to medial direction toward the lumbar spine across the iliocostalis lumborum muscle (Figure 72-58D).

Deep Paraspinal (Multifidus) (Figure 72-59)

For TrPI or DN of the thoracic and lumbar multifidus muscle, TrPs are identified with cross-fiber flat palpation in the thoracic region, and in the superficial multifidus muscle of the lumbar region just lateral to the spinous processes. The deep paraspinal muscles can be palpated only by utilizing a hypodermic or filiform needle that is at least 5 cm (~2 in) long. The region between the transverse process and the spinous process is considered a safe zone for needling in the absence of scoliosis (Figure 72-59A). Within this zone, the needle is directed somewhat caudally and medially, nearly parallel to the long axis of the spine and toward the base of the spinous process (Figure 72-59B and C).

Abdominal Muscles (Chapter 49)

Most of the abdominal muscles can be reached with a 3.8-cm (1½-in) hypodermic needle or a 0.30 × 50 mm filiform needle, unless the patient is obese. Better control of the needle is obtained by inserting it at a shallow angle instead of inserting it nearly perpendicular to the skin. The shallower angle makes it easier to align the shaft of the needle with, or perpendicular to, the muscle fibers, and to feel the changes in consistency of fat, fascia, and muscle as the needle penetrates successive layers. Care should be taken to avoid penetrating the peritoneal cavity with the needle. The patient is positioned supine with a pillow or bolster under the knees to relax the abdominal muscles.

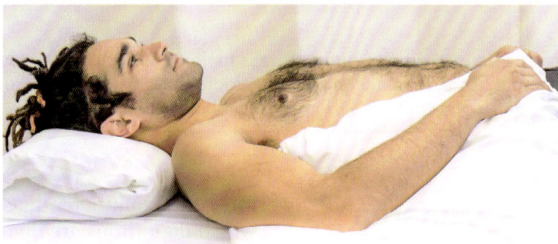

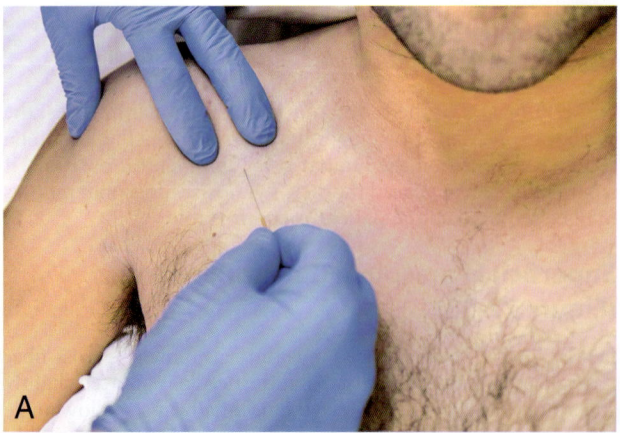

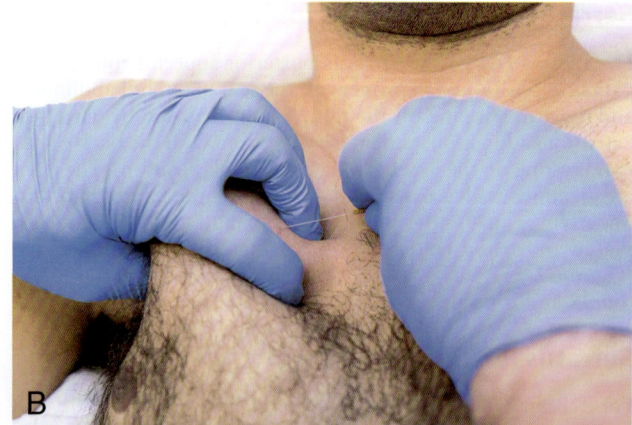

Figure 72-55. Trigger point injection or dry needling of the **pectoralis minor muscle**. A, Proximal portion using flat palpation. The needle is directed cranially, laterally, and shallowly toward the coracoid process. B, Mid-muscle belly using a pincer grasp. Finger tips are on the thoracic wall to avoid entering the thorax.

Chapter 72: Trigger Point Injection and Dry Needling   803

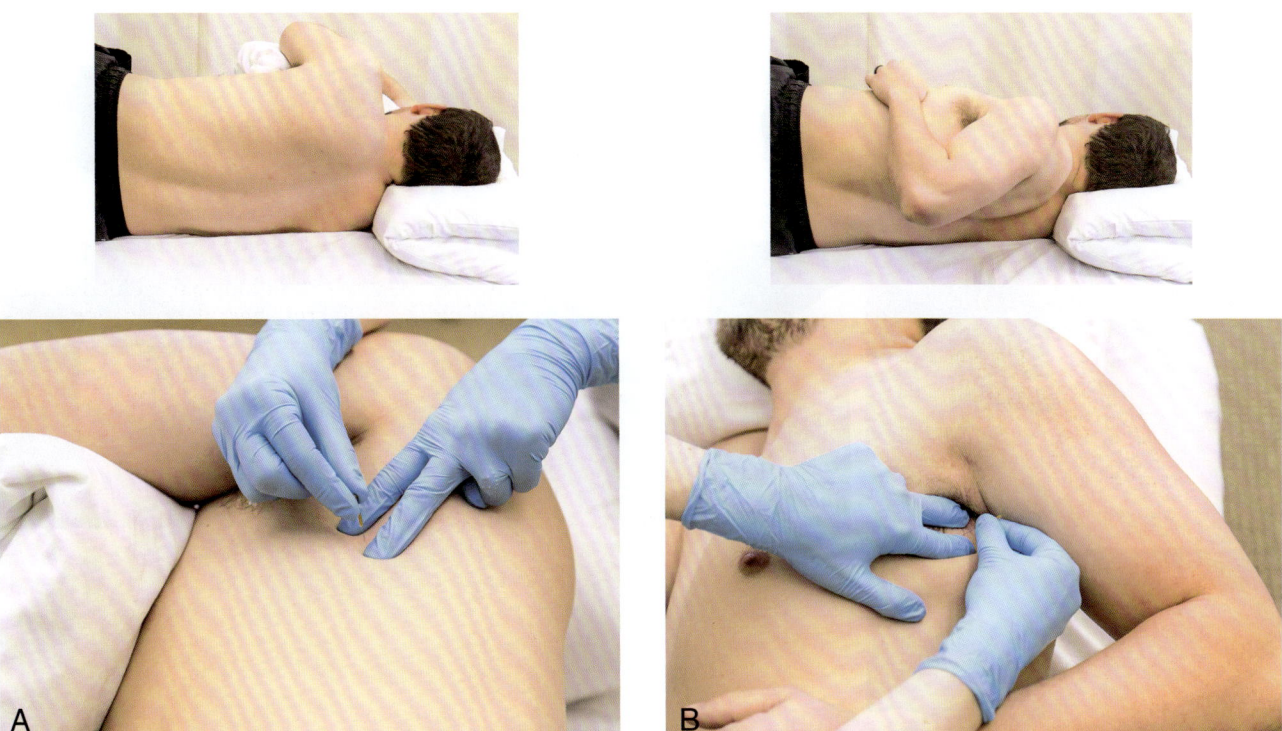

Figure 72-56. Trigger point injection or dry needling of the **serratus anterior muscle** with the patient side-lying on the opposite side. A, Arm in front supported on pillows over the sixth rib in the mid-axillary line. B, Adduction of the scapula and extension of the arm afford access to the muscle's upper portion. The needle is directed toward an underlying rib. Note that the clinician's fingers block the intercostal spaces.

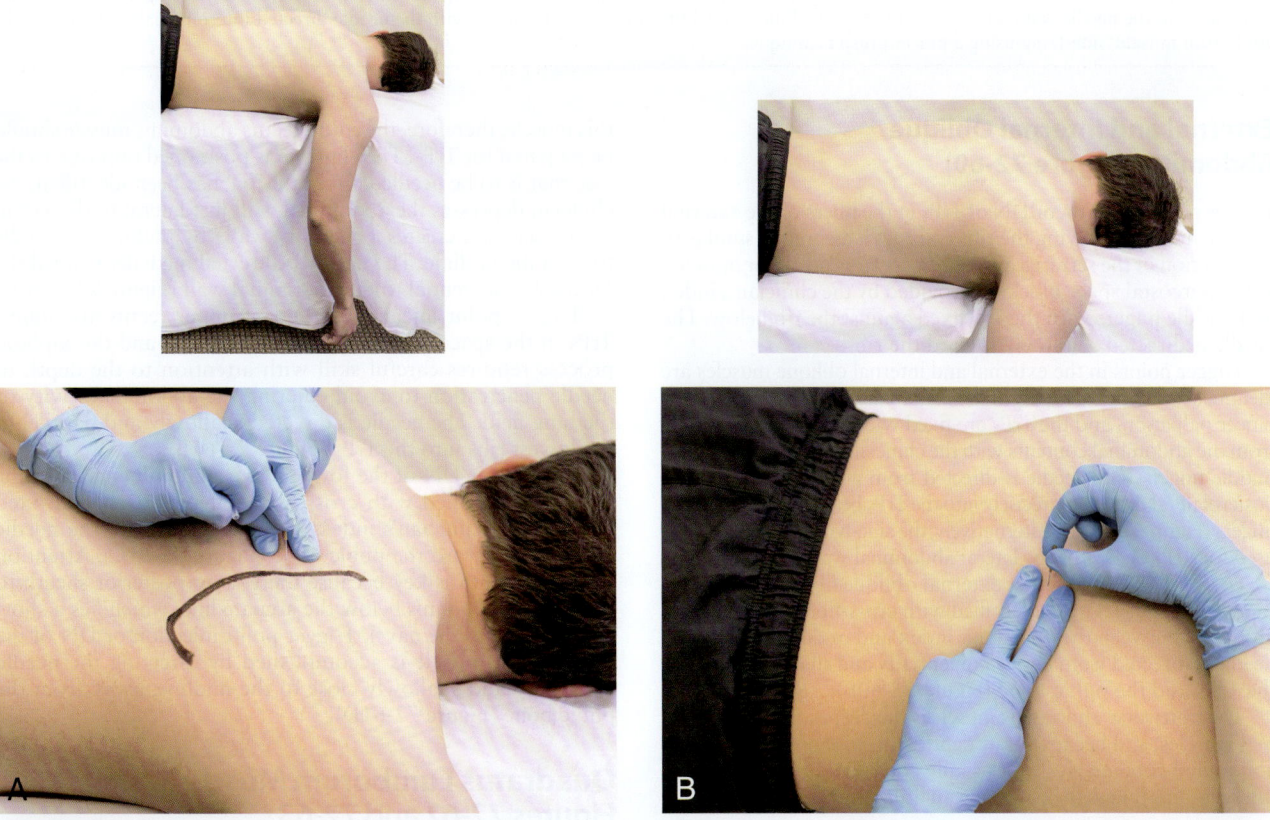

Figure 72-57. Trigger point injection or dry needling technique for **serratus posterior superior and inferior muscles.** A, **Serratus posterior superior muscle** in prone with the scapula fully abducted. The black line denotes the vertebral border of the scapula. The needle is directed nearly tangent to the chest wall and toward a rib; the clinician's fingers block the intercostal spaces. B, **Serratus posterior inferior muscle** in prone. The needle is directed at a shallow angle toward the ninth, tenth, eleventh, or twelfth rib, depending on the location of the TrPs, and the clinician's fingers block the intercostal spaces.

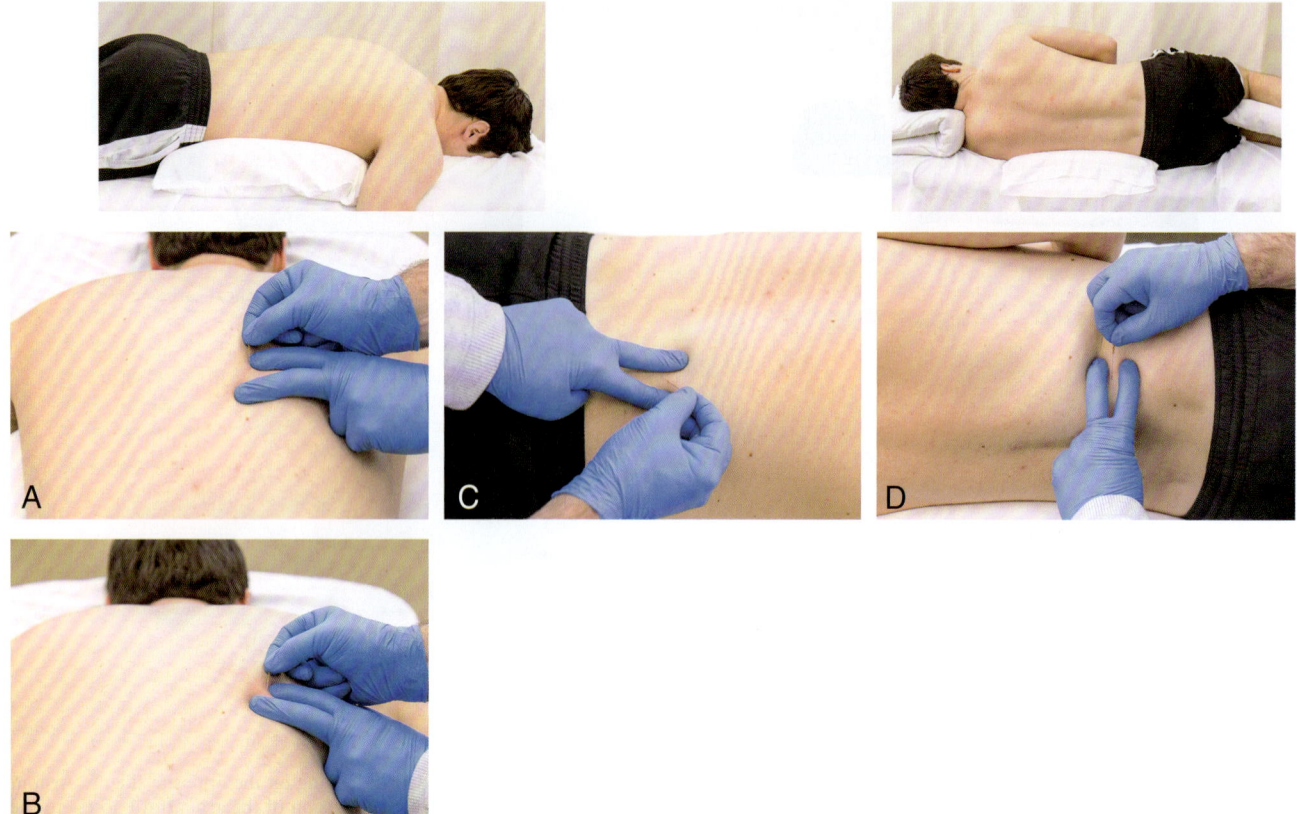

Figure 72-58. Trigger point injection or dry needling techniques for the **superficial thoracolumbar paraspinal muscles**. A, Longissimus thoracicis muscle using flat palpation and shallow needling technique with intercostal spaces blocked. B, Iiocostalis thoracicis muscle using intercostal space blocking, and the needle is directed toward the rib. C, Iliocostalis lumborum muscle, prone with the needle directed inferomedially. D, Iliocostalis lumborum muscle, side-lying using a pincer grasp technique.

External and Internal Oblique Abdominis (Figure 72-60)

Trigger point injection or DN of TrPs in the fibers of the external oblique muscle overlying the ribs employs a technique similar to the injection of the serratus anterior or serratus posterior muscles, with intercostal space blocking provided by the clinician's index and middle fingers with the TrP fixed against the rib below. The needle is directed shallowly toward the rib.

Trigger points in the external and internal oblique muscles are identified at the lateral aspect of the abdominal wall using cross-fiber pincer palpation, and the TrPs are fixed with a pincer grasp away from the abdominal contents with the clinician's thumb, index, and middle fingers. The needle is directed from an anteromedial to a posterolateral direction precisely into the TrPs between the clinician's fingers (Figure 72-60A). Alternatively, the side-lying position can be used for TrPI or DN of the lateral abdominal wall.

For TrPI or DN of lower external oblique fibers proximal to the pubic bone, TrPs are identified with cross-fiber flat palpation and fixed between the clinician's index and middle fingers. The needle is directed from above tangentially and shallowly toward the TrPs and the pubic bone (Figure 72-60B).

The transverse abdominis muscle is the deepest of the abdominal muscles, and because of its depth and close proximity to the abdominal contents, it is not usually considered for TrPI or DN interventions unless the clinician can utilize ultrasound guidance.

Rectus Abdominis and Pyramidalis (Figure 72-61)

For TrPI or DN of the rectus abdominis muscle, its TrPs are identified by cross-fiber flat palpation. There are several transcriptions in this muscle; therefore, the entire rectus abdominis muscle should be palpated for TrPs. The clinician is positioned opposite to the side that is to be needled. Once the TrP has been identified, the clinician depresses the abdominal wall just lateral to the TrP in the muscle and creates a shelf or "wall" by pulling the muscle toward the midline. The needle is directed medially toward the *linea alba*, tangential to the abdominal wall (Figure 72-61A).

Trigger point injection or DN of upper rectus abdominis TrPs in the space between the costal margin and the xiphoid process requires careful skill with attention to the depth of needle penetration to avoid entering the abdominal cavity or the lung field. The needle is directed shallowly and parallel to the lowest ribs into the TrPs (Figure 72-61B).

For TrPI or DN of the lower rectus abdominis muscle, the TrPs are identified with cross-fiber flat palpation and fixed between the clinician's index and middle fingers. The needle is directed toward the pubic bone (Figure 72-61C). Attention to needle depth is key because there is no posterior sheath to the rectus abdominis below the arcuate line, which lies a short distance below the navel. Trigger point injection or DN of the pyramidalis muscle is accomplished by directing the needle superiorly and shallowly close to the midline, away from the pubic bone (Figure 72-61D).

Quadratus Lumborum Muscle (Chapter 50) Figures 72-62 and 72-63

For TrPI or DN of the quadratus lumborum muscle, the patient is positioned in side-lying with the side to be treated facing up. If there is minimal space between the iliac crest and the twelfth rib, the patient can bring the ipsilateral arm overhead, and a bolster placed under the torso may improve access to the muscle.

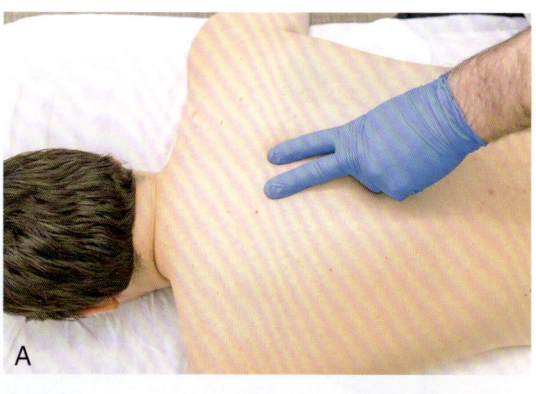
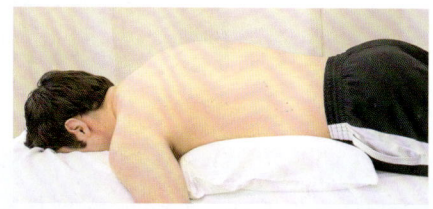
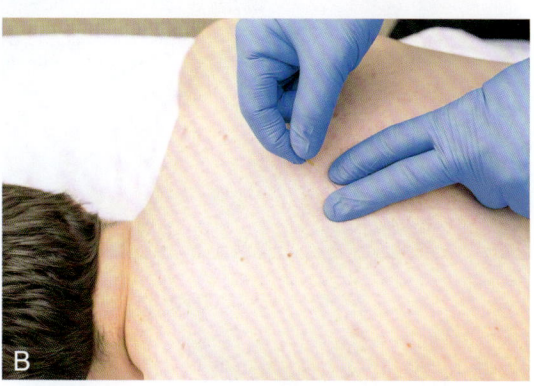
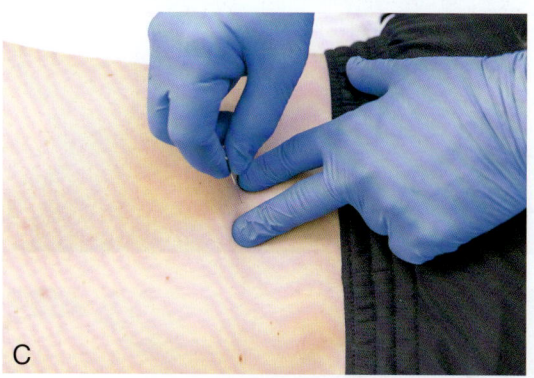

Figure 72-59. Trigger point injection or dry needling techniques for the **deep paraspinal (multifidus) muscles**. A, Safe needling zone in the valley next to the spinous process. B, **Thoracic multifidus muscle** with the needle directed inferomedially toward the lamina of the thoracic vertebra. C, **Lumbar multifidus muscle** with the needle directed in a slight medial and caudal direction toward the lamina of the lumbar vertebra. Both techniques are performed in the safe needling zone of the trunk.

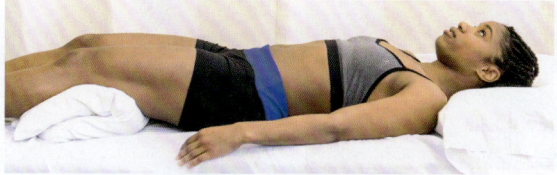
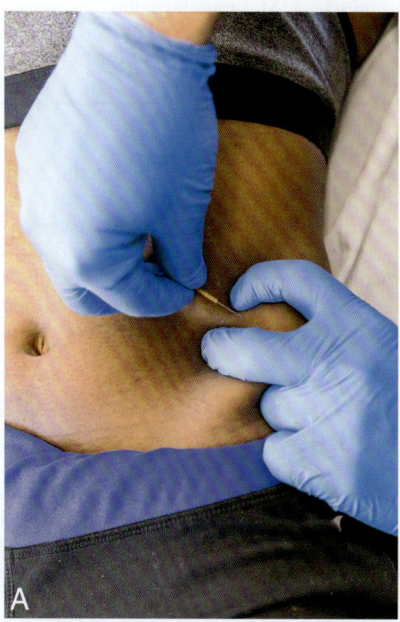
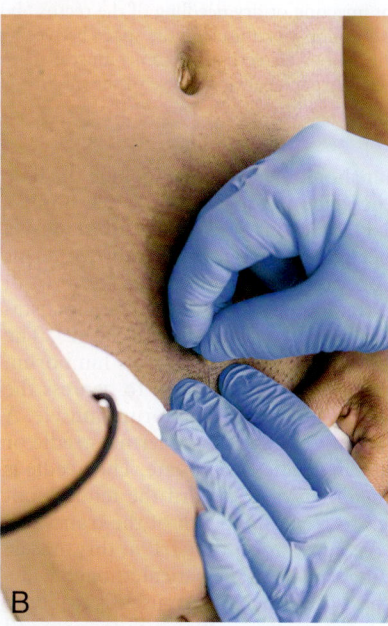

Figure 72-60. Trigger point injection or dry needling of the **external and internal abdominal oblique muscles**. A, Lateral abdominal wall using a pincer grasp pulling the muscles away from the abdominal contents. B, External oblique muscle proximal to the pubic arch.

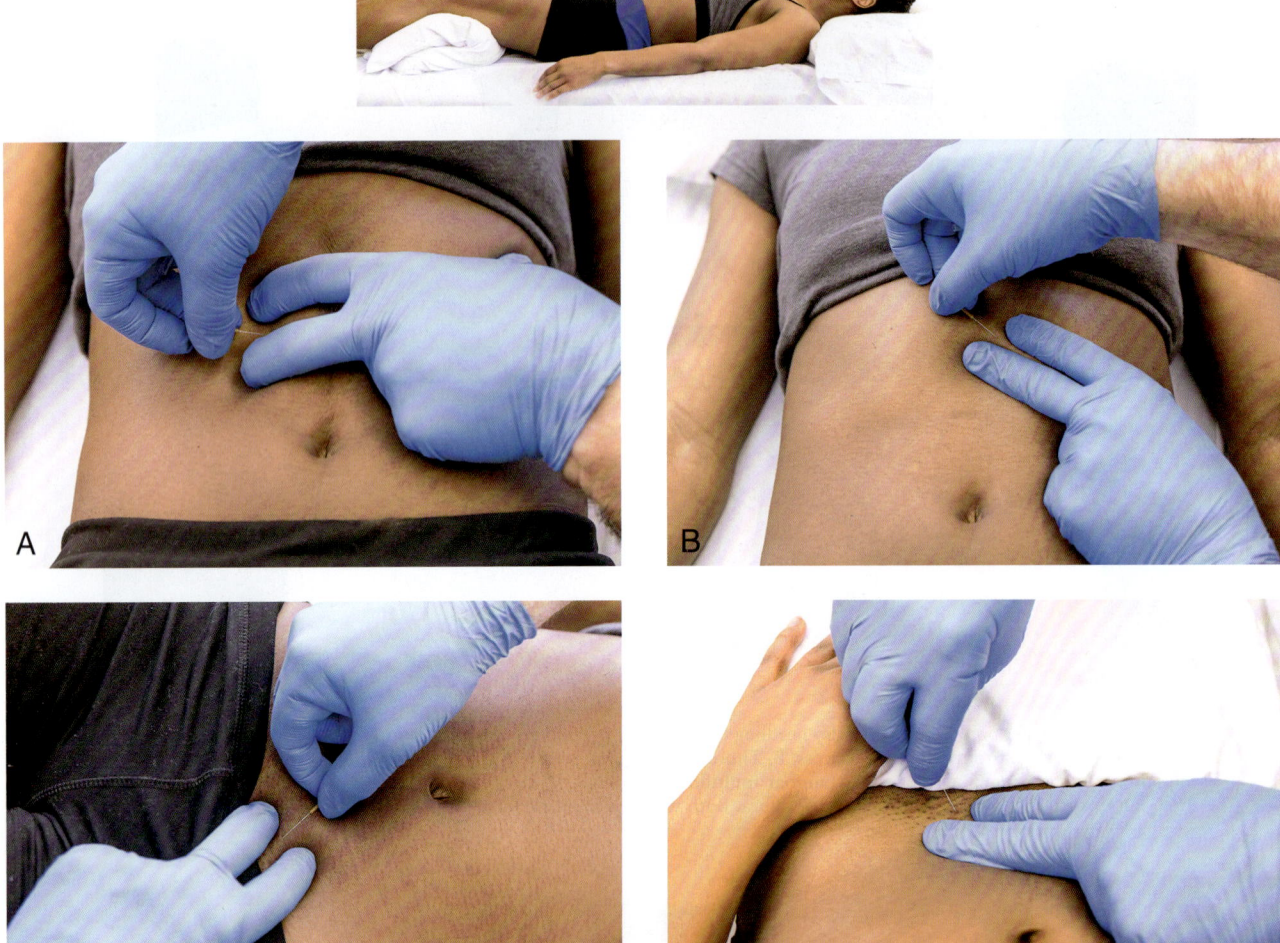

Figure 72-61. Trigger point injection or dry needling of the **rectus abdominis muscle**. A, Mid-muscle, pulling the muscle toward the clinician creating a shelf. B, Upper rectus abdominis muscle in the space between the costal margin and the xiphoid process. The needle is directed parallel to the lower ribs and shallowly. C, Lower rectus abdominis muscle. The needle is directed shallowly toward the pubic bone. D, Pyramidalis muscle. The needle is directing superiorly and shallowly close to the midline, away from the pubic bone.

Anatomic landmarks that should be identified include the iliac crest, twelfth rib, and the spinous process of the 4th lumbar vertebrae (see Figure 50-11). The quadratus lumborum muscle is identified by cross-fiber flat palpation in the more anterior fibers of the iliocostal portion of the quadratus lumborum muscle near the crest of the ilium just lateral to the iliocostalis lumborum muscle below the L3 level (Figure 72-62). The latissimus dorsi muscle lies between the quadratus lumborum muscle and the skin. Strong pressure is applied to depress the subcutaneous tissue over the quadratus lumborum muscle. A 62- to 87-mm (2½- to 3½-in) 22-gauge hypodermic needle or 0.30 × 60 to 75 mm filiform needle is adequate. The needle is aimed essentially straight downward toward the tender spot and must be long enough to reach the depth of the transverse processes (Figure 72-63A). Penetration of a TrP in this muscle usually elicits a strong pain response in the patient, though LTRs are difficult to detect in these deep fibers. The muscle is explored with the needle for TrPs by successive partial withdrawals and reinsertions, probing down to the transverse processes. Some of the needle shaft must always be left extending outside the skin for safety. Otherwise, if the needle is inserted fully to its hub and the patient sneezes or lateral pressure is accidentally exerted on the syringe, the needle could snap at the hub and disappear under the skin.

For TrPI or DN of the iliotransverse portion of the quadratus lumborum muscle, TrPs are identified with cross-fiber flat palpation just lateral to the edge of the iliocostalis lumborum muscle at the level of the 4th lumbar vertebrae. The needle is directed inferolaterally toward the anterior surface of the iliac crest (Figure 72-63B).

Iliopsoas Muscle Group (Chapter 51)
Figures 72-62 and 72-64

Generally, TrPI or DN of these muscles should be performed following inactivation of associated TrPs in the quadratus lumborum, rectus abdominis, rectus femoris, hamstring, and gluteal muscles. Iliopsoas TrPs can usually be inactivated by using manual therapy techniques, TrP self-pressure release, and self-stretching exercises. Occasionally, TrPs that remain require needling techniques. Iliopsoas muscle group TrPs can be identified with cross-fiber flat palpation in three areas with the patient in the supine position: (1) deep under the rectus abdominis muscle and abdominal contents for the psoas major

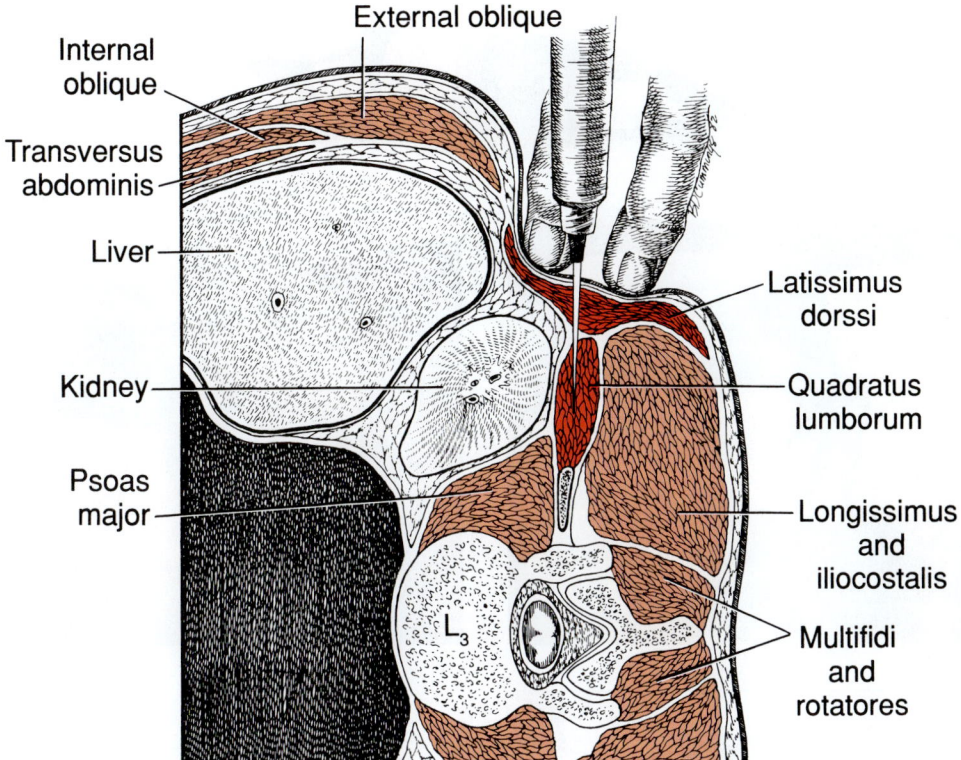

Figure 72-62. Trigger point injection or dry needling technique for the **quadratus lumborum muscle** (dark red) as seen in cross-section (patient side-lying). The compressed latissimus dorsi muscle, through which the needle usually must pass, is medium red, and the other neighboring muscles are light red. The cross-section passes through the body of the L3 vertebra.

muscle, (2) inside the brim of the pelvis on the anterior surface of the iliac crest just medial to the anterior superior iliac spine for the iliacus muscle, and (3) lateral to the femoral triangle above the combined insertion into the lesser trochanter (see Figure 51-4).

For TrPI or DN of the psoas major muscle, the patient is positioned in side-lying with the side to be treated facing up. If there is minimal space between the iliac crest and the twelfth rib, the patient can bring the ipsilateral arm overhead, and a bolster placed under the torso can improve access to the muscle. Anatomic landmarks that should be identified include the iliac crest, twelfth rib, and the spinous process of the 4th lumbar vertebrae (see Figure 50-11). Strong pressure is applied to depress the subcutaneous tissue over the lateral trunk wall. A 62- to 87-mm (2½- to 3½-in) 22-gauge hypodermic needle or 0.30 × 60 to 75 mm filiform needle is adequate. The needle is aimed slightly anteriorly downward toward the TrP and must be long enough to reach the depth of the transverse processes of L4 vertebrae (Figure 72-64A). If the needle touches the transverse process, it must be repositioned more anteriorly to penetrate the posterior fibers of the psoas muscle. The clinician will depend on symptom report from the patient because LTRs are quite difficult to determine because of the depth of the muscle.

For TrPI or DN of the iliacus muscle, the patient is positioned side-lying with the trunk and pelvis ¼ turned backward (semisupine) to allow better access to the muscle. The clinician identifies the tender area inside the brim of the pelvis behind the anterior superior iliac spine and uses the index and middle fingers to fix the TrP against the anterior surface of the iliac crest. The needle is directed inside the crest of the ilium between the clinician's fingers and directed to the TrPs (Figure 72-64B). The needle must travel close to the inner surface of the ilium and may occasionally contact the bone, which ensures that the needle is within the muscle. LTRs are rarely observed, and a pain response by the patient usually indicates that the needle encountered TrPs.

For TrPI or DN of the distal portion of the iliopsoas muscle group, the patient is positioned supine near the edge of the plinth with the thigh slightly extended, abducted, and externally rotated to separate the iliopsoas muscle as far as possible from the femoral nerve and artery (Figure 72-64C). The femoral artery is identified by palpation medial to the iliopsoas muscle; however, the clinician must be aware that the femoral nerve lies between the iliopsoas muscle and the femoral artery. The clinician maintains contact with one finger on the femoral artery, and the needle is directed laterally and away from the femoral artery and nerve toward the lesser trochanter (Figure 72-64C).

Pelvic Floor Muscles (Chapter 52)

Generally, only the perineal and sphincter ani muscles are accessible for TrPI or DN therapy. Needling treatment should be employed only if the TrP and its taut band are unmistakably palpable and precisely located. For TrPI or DN of the ischiocavernosus muscle in either sex, and of the bulbospongiosus muscle in the male patient, the clinician uses cross-fiber flat palpation to localize the TrPs. In a female patient, a TrP in the bulbospongiosus muscle is localized and held between a fingertip in the vagina and the tip of the thumb on the labium majus and then needled through the labium.

Needling of the sphincter ani muscle is performed bimanually. A 10-mL syringe with a 63-mm (2½-in) 21-gauge needle or a 0.30 × 50 mm filiform needle is used. A palpating finger localizes the taut band and its TrPs in the anal sphincter muscle. When the needle approaches the sphincter ani muscle, its tip is felt by the finger in the rectum, and that finger then directs the needle precisely to the TrP. Frequently, there is a cluster of TrPs to be inactivated. The muscle should be thoroughly palpated for any remaining TrPs, and these should be treated before the needle is withdrawn.

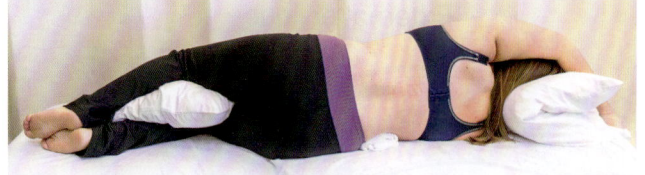
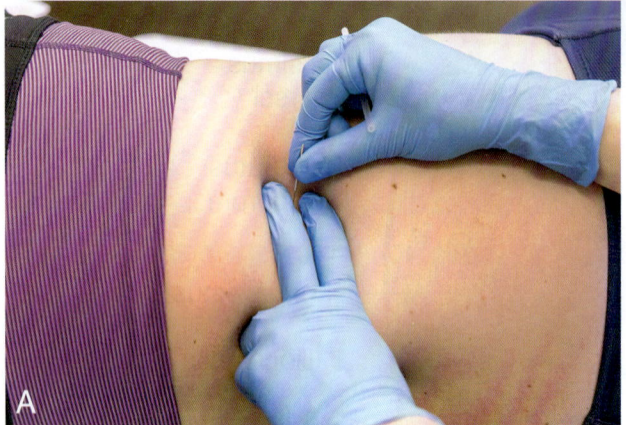
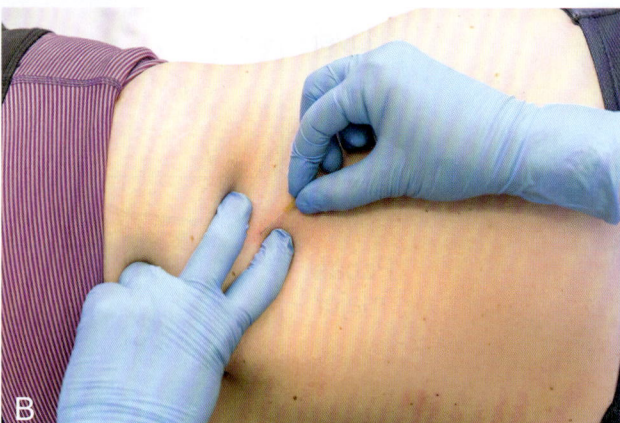
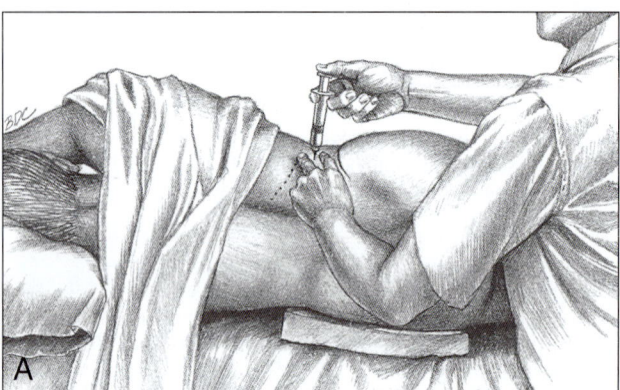

Figure 72-63. Trigger point injection or dry needling of the **quadratus lumborum muscle**. A, Deep quadratus lumborum muscle at L3. B, Iliotransverse fibers of the quadratus lumborum muscle.

Pubococcygeus Muscle of the Pelvic Diaphragm

For TrPI or DN of the pubococcygeus muscle, the patient is positioned in side-lying on the involved side with hips flexed to 90° and a pillow between the knees. The patient is asked to assist by lifting the gluteal muscles away from the anus. To approximate the muscle, the clinician places one finger on the perineal body and the other on the anal sphincter muscle. The other hand is used to palpate the pubococcygeus muscle through rectal palpation. The needle is angled at 45° toward the pubic bone, perpendicular to the muscle surface, and directly into the TrP identified by palpation. When the needle approaches the pubococcygeus muscle, its tip is felt by the finger in the rectum, and that finger then directs the needle precisely to the TrPs.

Iliococcygeus Muscle of the Pelvic Diaphragm

The patient is positioned in side-lying on the involved side with hips flexed to 90° and a pillow between the knees. The patient is asked to assist by lifting the gluteal muscles away from the anus. The clinician places the fingers slightly inferior and lateral to the anal sphincter muscle to approximate the muscle, lateral to the pubococcygeus muscle. The other hand palpates the iliococcygeus muscle through rectal palpation. The needle is directed at a 45° angle toward the pubic bone, perpendicular to the muscle surface and directly into the TrP identified by palpation. When the needle approaches the iliococcygeus muscle, its tip is felt by the finger in the rectum, and that finger then directs the needle precisely to the TrPs.

Coccygeus Muscle of the Pelvic Diaphragm

The patient is positioned in side-lying on the involved side with hips flexed to 90° and a pillow between the knees. The patient is asked to assist by lifting the gluteal muscles away from the anus. The clinician identifies the coccygeus muscle through rectal palpation. With the other hand, the clinician places one finger on the coccyx and the other on the inferior lateral angle of the sacrum to approximate the location of the muscle. The needle is angled away from the rectum, perpendicular to the muscle surface and directly into the TrP identified by palpation. When the needle approaches the coccygeus muscle, its tip is felt by the finger in the rectum, and that finger then directs the needle precisely to the TrPs.

Ischiocavernosus

The ischiocavernosus muscle runs parallel to the ischiopubic ramus in both women and men, inserting into the ischial tuberosity distally. In the lithotomy position, the length of the ischiopubic

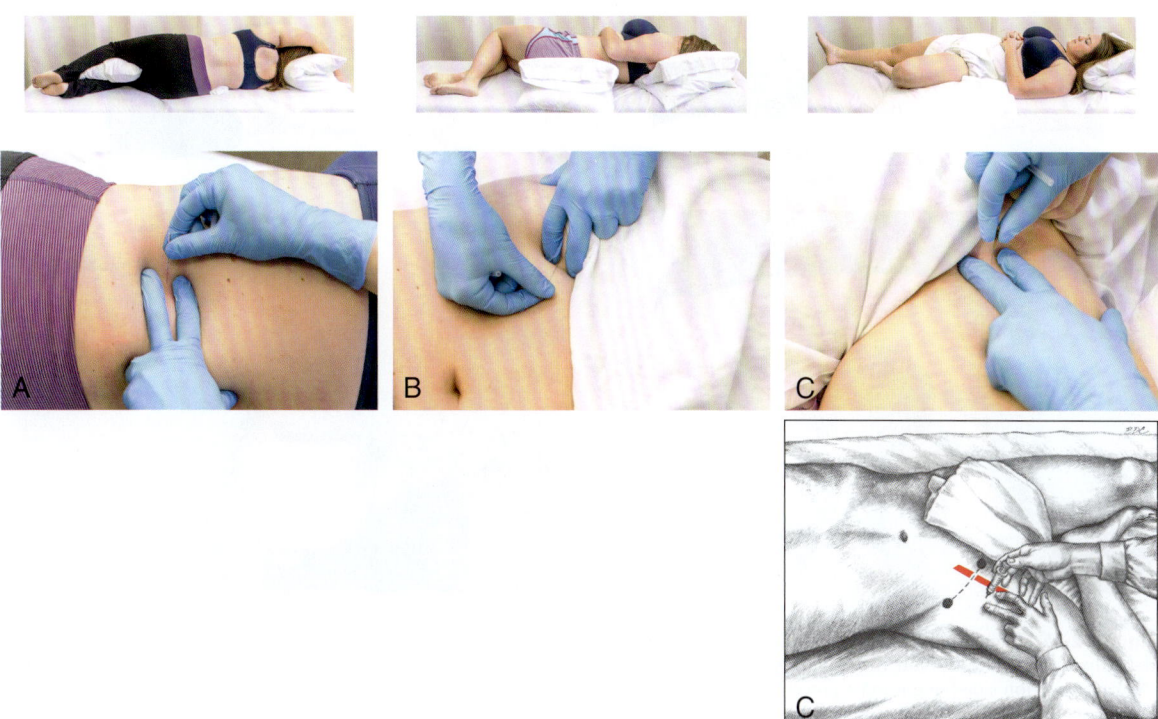

Figure 72-64. Trigger point injection or dry needling of the **iliopsoas muscle group**. A, **Psoas major muscle**, side-lying. B, **Iliacus muscle**, side-lying and ¼ turn backward (semisupine). C, Distal iliopsoas muscle group. The solid circles (lower illustration) cover the anterior superior iliac spine and the pubic tubercle. Between them, the inguinal ligament lies beneath the dashed line. The femoral artery is red. The thigh is abducted and externally rotated to separate the iliopsoas muscle and the femoral artery. The needle is directed toward the trigger point tenderness close to the lesser trochanter, laterally, away from the femoral artery.

---

ramus is examined to identify TrPs in the muscle belly through cross-fiber flat palpation. The needle is angled perpendicular to the muscle surface, directed toward the ischiopubic ramus and into the TrPs identified by internal or external palpation. In male patients, it is helpful to use a towel around the scrotum and have the patient move the scrotum out of the way. In female patients, the labia should be moved to the opposite side.

Bulbospongiosus (Bulbocavernosus)

In the lithotomy position, the muscle is identified with cross-fiber flat palpation. In the male patient, external palpation is sufficient. It is helpful to use a towel around the scrotum to help the patient move the scrotum out of the way. The clinician places one finger on the perineal body and the other superolaterally onto the muscle to brace the tissue. Muscle contraction can confirm placement. In the female patient, the same external technique may be used. Alternatively, the clinician can palpate the muscle using a cross-fiber pincer palpation with the index finger inserted into the vagina. The muscle attachments to the perineal body distally and the clitoral aponeurosis proximally should be noted. The needle is directed at an angle, perpendicular to the muscle surface and directly into the TrP identified by palpation.

For male and female patients, the muscle can also be treated by directing the needle at a slightly tangential angle that may be preferred for women in cases of hypersensitivity or when patients do not consent to vaginal insertion. In female patients, the labia should be moved to the opposite side and caution used when needling near the area of the clitoris.

Superficial and Deep Transverse Perinei

In the lithotomy position, the needle is directed perpendicular to the muscle surface and directly into the TrP. The needle may also be directed slightly tangential to the muscle surface to avoid needling through the muscle. Placing one finger on the perineal body and the other on the lateral border of the ischial tuberosity helps brace the tissue. Muscle contraction can confirm placement. In female patients, it may be preferential to utilize vaginal palpation of the transverse perineal muscle and to identify its TrPs by cross-fiber pincer palpation, holding the TrP in a firm pincer grasp prior to needle insertion. In male patients, it is helpful to use a towel around the scrotum and have the patient move the scrotum out of the way. In female patients, the labia should be moved to the opposite side.

5. HIP, THIGH, AND KNEE PAIN (Section 6)

Gluteus Maximus Muscle (Chapter 54)
Figure 72-65

For TrPI or DN of the upper portion of the gluteus maximus muscle, the patient is positioned prone with a pillow under the abdomen to place the lumbar spine in a neutral position. For TrPI or DN of the lower portion of the gluteus maximus muscle, the patient is positioned in side-lying; however, this position may also be used to needle the entire gluteus maximus muscle. Trigger points in the gluteus maximus muscle are identified using cross-fiber flat palpation for the entire muscle and cross-fiber pincer palpation in the lower portion.

In the prone position, the TrPs are identified and fixed between the clinician's index and middle finger with a strong compression of the subcutaneous tissue by the palpating hand to reduce the distance from the skin to the muscle, especially in those patients with a thick layer of subcutaneous fat. For thin individuals, a 21- or 22-gauge, 37-mm (1½-in) hypodermic needle or a 0.30 × 50 mm filiform needle is sufficient, but for some patients, a 21-gauge, 60-mm (2-in) or longer hypodermic or filiform needle may be necessary to penetrate the subcutaneous

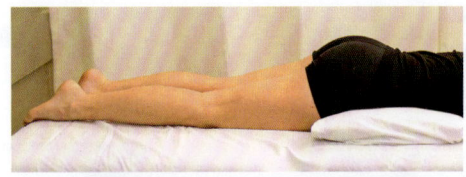
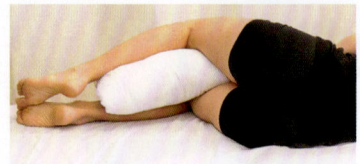
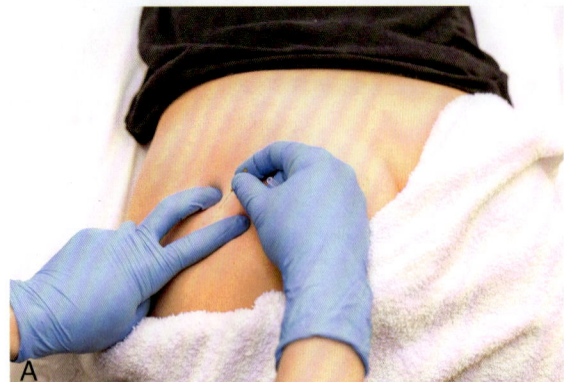
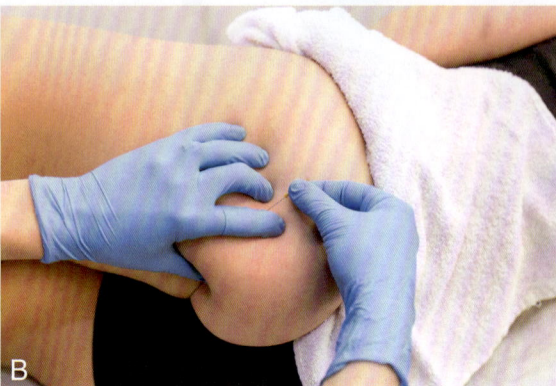

Figure 72-65. Trigger point injection or dry needling of the **gluteus maximus muscle**. A, Gluteus maximus muscle in prone using the flat palpation technique. Note the compression of tissue by the palpating hand to reduce the space between the skin and the muscle. B, Lower portion side-lying using a pincer grasp, the needle is directed toward the TrP and lower fingers.

fat and the full thickness of the gluteus maximus muscle. The needle is directed between the clinician's fingers toward the TrPs (Figure 72-65A). Localized twitch responses are readily observable for this muscle when the needle penetrates the TrPs. The clinician should be aware of the path of the sciatic nerve when performing deep TrPI or DN of the gluteus maximus muscle.

For TrPI or DN of the lower portion of the gluteus maximus muscle, TrPs are identified and fixed with a pincer grasp between the clinician's thumb, index, and middle fingers. The needle is directed toward the clinician's finger in the underside of the muscle (Figure 72-65B).

Gluteus Medius Muscle (Chapter 55)
Figure 72-66

For TrPI or DN of the gluteus medius muscle, the patient is positioned either in prone or side-lying. Trigger points are identified using cross-fiber flat palpation and fixed between the clinician's index and middle finger with a strong compression of the subcutaneous tissue by the palpating hand to reduce the distance from the skin to the muscle, especially in patients with a thick layer of subcutaneous fat. Similar needle sizes as described in the gluteus maximus techniques should be utilized. The needle is inserted and directed toward the TrPs and deep needling contact with periosteum of the iliac crest is common (Figure 72-66). It is sometimes possible to detect an LTR through the overlying thick gluteus maximus muscle.

Gluteus Minimus and Tensor Fasciae Latae Muscles (Chapter 56)

Gluteus Minimus (Figure 72-67)

Dry needling of lateral hip muscles has been found to be as effective as cortisone injections in patients with greater trochanteric pain syndrome.[55] For TrPI or DN of the gluteus minimus muscle, the preferred patient position is side-lying; however, the prone position may also be used. Trigger points are identified with cross-fiber flat palpation and fixed between the clinician's index and middle finger with a strong compression of the subcutaneous tissue by the palpating hand to reduce the distance from the skin to the muscle. Similar needle sizes as described in the gluteus maximus muscle techniques should be utilized. The needle is inserted and directed toward the TrP and with deep needling contact with periosteum of the iliac crest is very common (Figure 72-67A).

For TrPI or DN of the posterior fibers, the lower posterior border of the gluteus minimus muscle is located by defining the upper limit of the piriformis muscle. Directing the needle above this line and in an upward direction normally eliminates the risk of accidentally penetrating the sciatic nerve as it exits the pelvis through the sciatic foramen (Figure 72-67B).

Tensor Fasciae Latae (Figure 72-68)

For TrPI or DN of the tensor fasciae latae muscle, the preferred patient position is side-lying (Figure 72-68A); however, the supine position may also be used (Figure 72-68B). In either position, TrPs are identified using cross-fiber flat palpation and fixed between the clinician's index and middle finger. The needle is directed posteriorly and toward the TrP (Figure 72-68). If the tensor fasciae latae muscle has been accurately identified, no major nerves or vessels lie in the path of the needle.

Piriformis and External Rotator Muscles (Chapter 57)

Piriformis (Figure 72-69)

For TrPI or DN of the piriformis muscle, the patient is positioned in side-lying or prone. The piriformis muscle can be needled either laterally, near the greater trochanter, or medially, immediately lateral to the sacrum. The clinician should identify the piriformis muscle attachments at the medial border of the sacrum (S2-S4) and the greater trochanter of the femur.

To needle the lateral part of the piriformis muscle, the patient lies on the uninvolved side with the uppermost hip flexed to approximately 90°. The superior border of the piriformis muscle is located by visualizing a line that runs from just above the greater trochanter to the point where the palpable border of the sacrum encounters the ilium at the inferior border of the sacroiliac joint. This piriformis line, shown in Figure 72-69A, is divided into thirds, and the

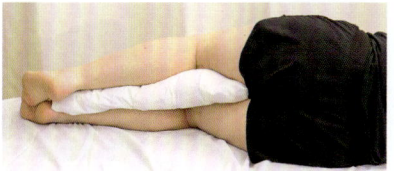

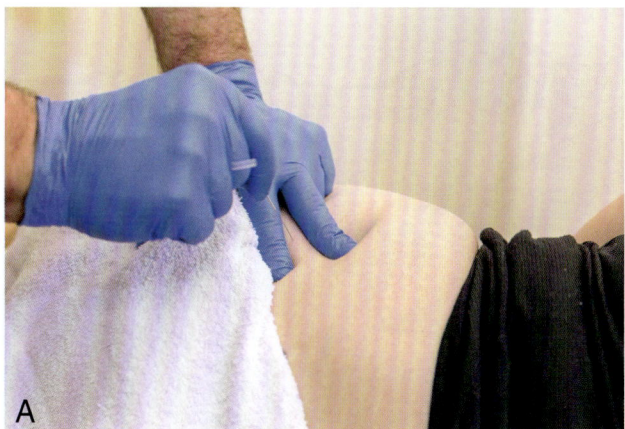
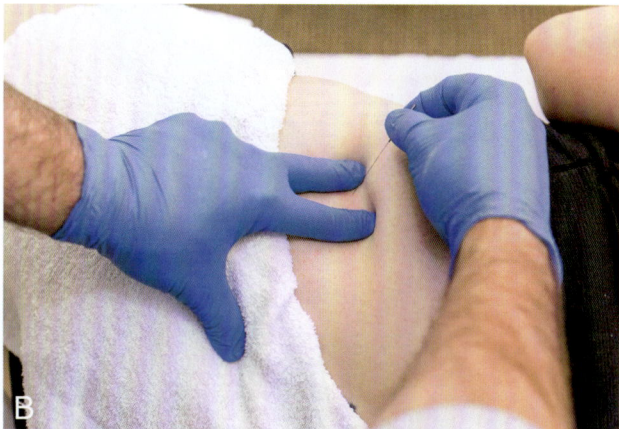

Figure 72-66. Trigger point injection or dry needling of the **gluteus medius muscle**. A, Posterior fibers. B, Anterior fibers.

piriformis muscle is palpated using cross-fiber flat palpation just inferior to it. The TrP is localized and fixed between the clinician's index and middle fingers.

Usually a 22-gauge, 50-mm (2-in) hypodermic needle is used on a 10-mL syringe, or a 0.30 × 50 mm filiform needle for lateral piriformis TrP location. The needle must be of sufficient length to reach through the skin, the gluteus maximus muscle, and the piriformis muscle to the hip joint capsule. This depth of penetration is necessary to ensure penetrating all of the TrPs in this portion of the piriformis muscle. Needle penetration of a TrP is recognized by the pain response of the patient, and particularly if it reproduces the patient's referred pain.

For TrPI or DN of the medial portion of the piriformis muscle, Simons and Travell[100] recommend that needling of TrPs in the medial region be accomplished bimanually. One finger palpates the inner surface of the medial third of the piriformis muscle using the rectal or vaginal route; the other hand inserts the needle externally, directing the needle toward the intrapelvic palpating fingertip (Figure 72-69B). With sufficient finger-reach, it is possible to palpate both the pelvic inner surface of the piriformis muscle and the pelvic sciatic nerve against the sacrum, as well as the area of the greater sciatic foramen.

The medial portion of the piriformis muscle can also be needled without internal palpation. The needle is inserted just lateral to

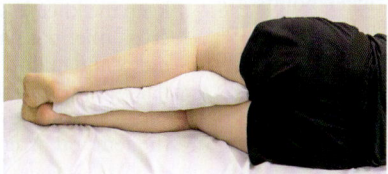

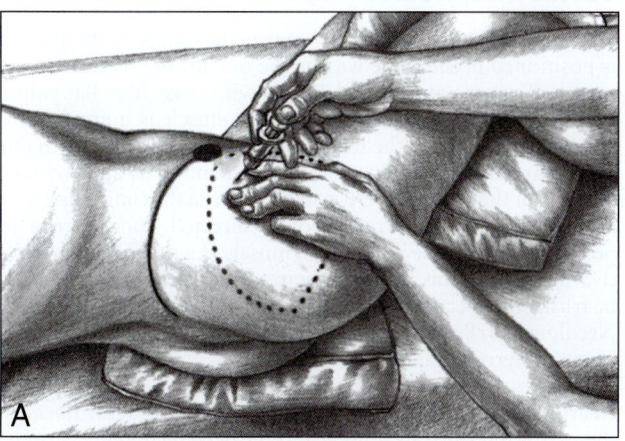
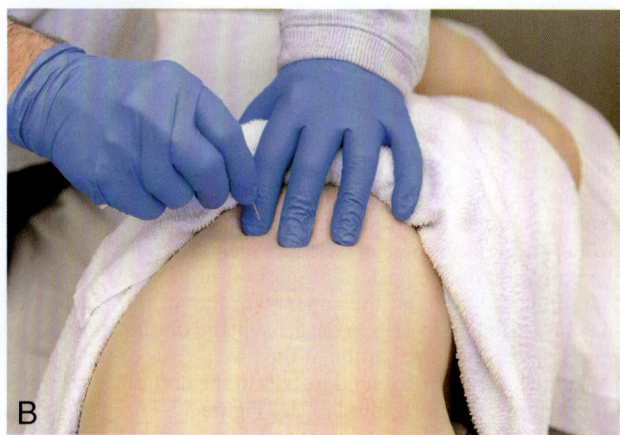

Figure 72-67. Trigger point injection or dry needling of the **gluteus minimus muscle**. A, Anterior fibers. B, Posterior fibers above the piriformis muscle to avoid the sciatic nerve.

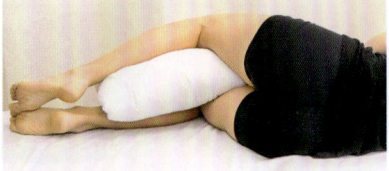

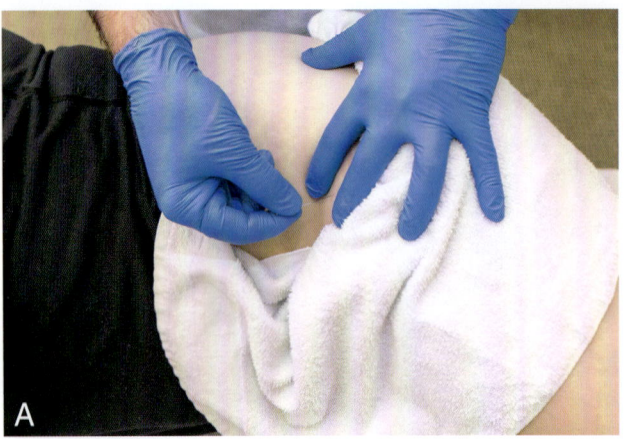
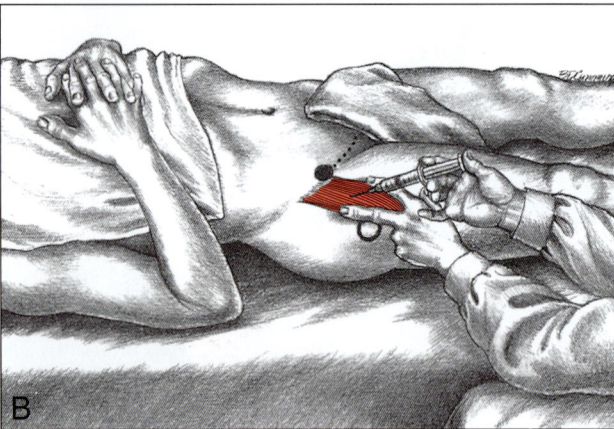

Figure 72-68. Trigger point injection or dry needling of the **tensor fasciae latae muscle**. A, Side-lying with flat palpation. B, Supine with flat palpation. The solid circle locates the anterior superior iliac spine. The dotted line identifies the inguinal ligament. The open circle marks the greater trochanter.

the sacrum and below the piriformis line and directed medially and inferiorly toward the TrPs and sacrum (Figure 72-69C).

Obturator Internus (Figure 72-70)

For TrPI or DN of the obturator internus muscle, the patient is positioned side-lying with the affected side down with the top hip and knee flexed (see Figure 57-8). Trigger points are identified at the insertion of the obturator internus muscle on the medial aspect of the ischial tuberosity. The needle is directed slightly anterior and toward the medial aspect of the ischial tuberosity into the TrP (Figure 72-70).

Alternatively, the obturator internus muscle can be needled with the patient in the lithotomy position. Trigger points are identified by cross-fiber flat palpation toward the obturator foramen, which is just lateral to the inferior border of the pubic ramus and the insertion of the adductor longus muscle tendon. The needle is directed laterally into the TrPs identified with either internal or external palpation.[1]

Obturator Externus, Gemelli, and Quadratus Femoris (Figure 72-71)

No literature describes the identification and injection of TrPs in the remaining four short external rotators. For practical purposes, localization to a specific muscle is not necessary and one need only distinguish two groups of muscles: the two gemelli muscles and lateral part of the obturator internus muscle constitute one group; the quadratus femoris and underlying obturator externus muscles constitute the other. The patient is positioned prone, and TrPs in these muscles are identified with cross-fiber flat palpation on the posterior aspect of the greater trochanter. Pain upon palpation at the upper ⅓ of the greater trochanter may be attributed to TrPs in the gemelli and obturator internus muscles. Pain upon palpation at the lower ⅔rds of the greater trochanter may be attributed to TrPs in the obturator externus and quadratus femoris muscles (see Figure 57-7).

When a TrP is identified in one of these groups and TrPI or DN is deemed necessary, the path of the sciatic nerve as it crosses over these muscles, usually midway between the ischial tuberosity and the greater trochanter, must be considered. The needle is directed toward the medial, posterior surface of the greater trochanter. The location at the posterior greater trochanter along with the patient's pain report can lead the clinician to determine which muscles are affected (Figure 72-71).

Quadriceps Femoris and Sartorius Muscles (Chapter 58)

Rectus Femoris (Figure 72-72A)

For TrPI or DN of the rectus femoris muscle, the patient is positioned supine with a small towel roll placed under the knee to keep the knee in slight flexion. Trigger points are identified with cross-fiber flat palpation and then fixed between the clinician's index and middle fingers (Figure 72-72A). If the involved muscle has been confirmed to be the rectus femoris muscle and not the sartorius muscle, there should be little likelihood of penetrating the femoral artery or nerve with the needle.

Vastus Intermedius (Figures 72-72B and 72-73)

For TrPI or DN of the vastus intermedius muscle, the patient is positioned in the same way as the one for the rectus femoris muscle. Trigger points are identified with cross-fiber flat palpation; however, direct palpation of this muscle is quite difficult because it lies deep to the rectus femoris muscle, and TrPs in this muscle are often located just above the femur. The approximate location of the suspected TrP is fixed between the clinician's index and middle finger and the needle is directed from anterior to posterior toward the TrPs in the muscle (Figure 72-72B). Inactivating TrPs in this muscle requires much persistence and can be frustrating because the true severity is easily underestimated. Needling of TrPs in the vastus intermedius muscle usually causes intense referred pain.

As shown in the cross-section in Figure 72-73, there is no clear anatomic delineation between the deep lateral fibers of the vastus intermedius muscle and the deep medial fibers of the vastus lateralis muscle. They are commonly involved together. Many of the difficulties experienced when injecting TrPs or DN in one muscle apply to the other. When one finds TrPs in either

Chapter 72: Trigger Point Injection and Dry Needling 813

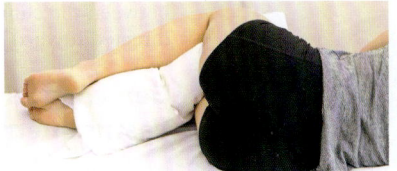

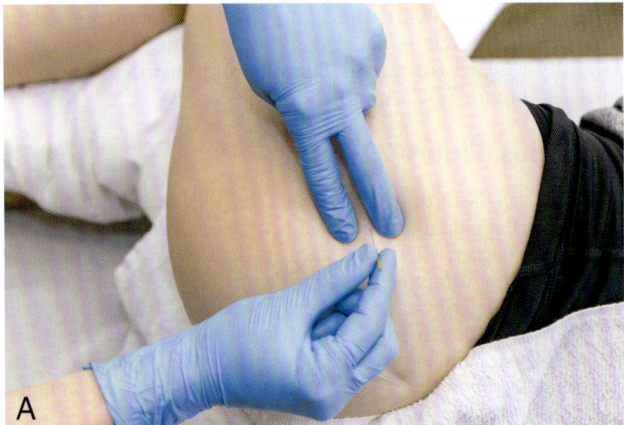

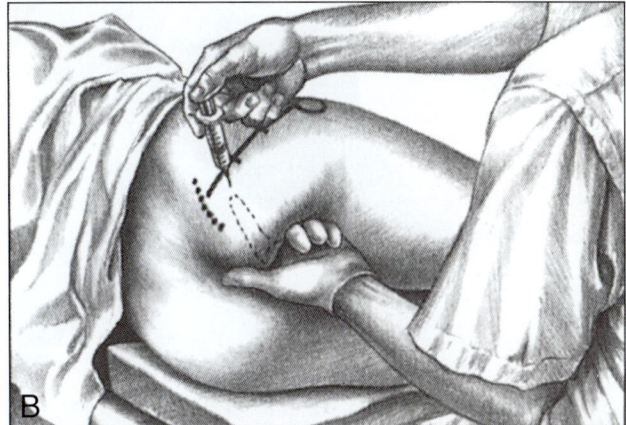

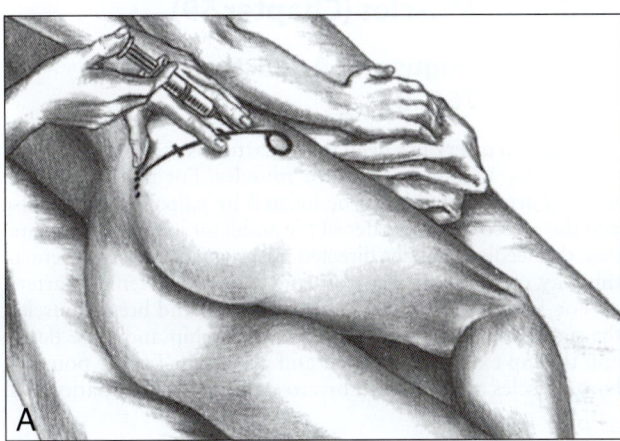

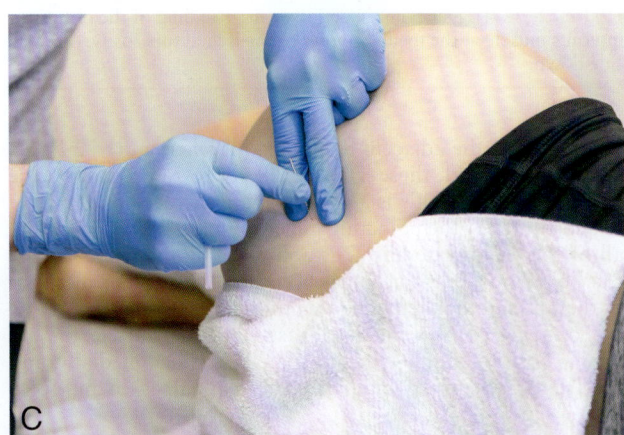

Figure 72-69. Trigger point injection or dry needling of the **piriformis muscle**. The open circle locates the greater trochanter; the dotted line, the palpable margin along the edge of the sacrum; and the solid line, marked in thirds, overlies the upper margin of the piriformis muscle. A, Technique for the lateral portion of the piriformis muscle. B, Bimanual technique for the medial piriformis muscle. The left hand locates the TrP tenderness via intrapelvic palpation, and the right hand directs the needle toward that fingertip. C, Medial piriformis muscle.

the vastus intermedius or vastus lateralis muscles that need TrPI or DN, it is prudent to explore for TrPs in the other muscle.

Vastus Medialis (Figure 72-72 C, D)

A recent study has demonstrated that DN of the vastus medialis muscle was effective for improving range of motion and related-disability in individuals who have undergone surgical reconstruction after complete anterior cruciate ligament rupture.[101]

For TrPI or DN of the vastus medialis muscle, the patient is positioned with the hip flexed and abducted and the knee flexed to approximately 90°, as illustrated in Figure 72-72C and D, to make the entire muscle accessible. Trigger points in the vastus medialis muscle are identified with cross-fiber flat palpation and fixed between the clinician's index and middle finger. For TrPI or DN in the proximal portion of the muscle, the femoral artery, which courses along that border, should be identified and the needle should be angled laterally away from the sartorius muscle and the artery (Figure 72-72C). For TrPI or DN of the distal portion of the muscle, the needle is directed toward the TrPs and femur, and it is very common to make contact with the femur with the needle (Figure 72-72D).

Vastus Lateralis (Figure 72-74)

For TrPI or DN of the large vastus lateralis muscle, the patient is positioned supine for the anterior portion and side-lying for the posterior portion. To access the posterior portion, it is often necessary to push the biceps femoris muscle aside to reach the posterior vastus lateralis muscle, which is located posteriorly against the posterior aspect of the femur. Trigger points in the vastus lateralis muscle are identified with cross-fiber flat palpation, and because of the size of this muscle, multiple TrPs are usually identified. The TrP is fixed between the clinician's index and middle finger, and the needle is directed in an anterior to posterior direction into the muscle belly and under the iliotibial band in the supine position (Figure 72-74A and B).

For TrPI or DN of the posterior portion of the vastus lateralis muscle in the average-sized individual, 63-mm (2½-in) hypodermic or 0.30 × 50 mm filiform needle may be required to reach the deepest part of the muscle posteriorly. The patient is positioned side-lying, and the TrPs are identified with cross-fiber pincer palpation and then fixed with a pincer grasp in between the clinician's thumb, index, and middle fingers. The needle is directed slightly anteriorly to stay in the vastus lateralis muscle

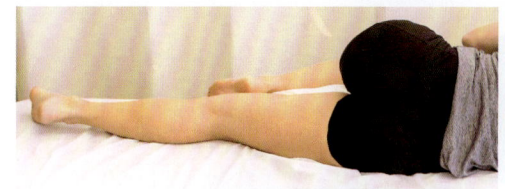

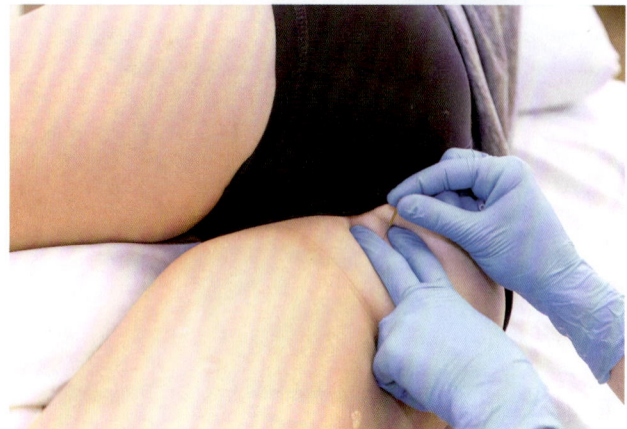

Figure 72-70. Trigger point injection or dry needling of the **obturator internus muscle** at the medial border of the ischial tuberosity. Affected side down.

and not enter the adjacent hamstring muscle (Figure 72-74C). When penetrated, these TrPs are likely to refer pain to the back of the knee. This is a region where the needle may have to substitute for the palpating finger to find the TrPs. Locating all of the vastus lateralis TrPs and needling them specifically can be tedious, but it becomes necessary when other methods of therapy fail to inactivate them fully.

For TrPI or DN of the distal vastus lateralis muscle, the patient is positioned side-lying, the patella is glided medially, and the TrPs are identified with cross-fiber flat palpation and fixed between the clinician's index and middle fingers. The needle is directed toward the TrP and femur (Figure 72-74D).

Genu Articularis and Tensor of the Vastus Intermedius (Figure 72-75A, B)

For TrPI or DN of the genu articularis muscle, the needle is directed through or underneath the tendon of the distal rectus femoris muscle toward the femur. The tensor of the vastus intermedius muscle is needled by angling the needle slightly laterally toward the vastus lateralis and vastus intermedius muscles (Figure 72-75A and B).

Sartorius (Figure 72-75C)

For TrPI or DN of the sartorius muscle, TrPs are identified with cross-fiber flat palpation and fixed in between the clinician's index and middle fingers, whereas the needle is directed tangentially, nearly parallel to the surface of the skin (Figure 72-75C). It is common that a sartorius TrP can be discovered serendipitously during TrPI or DN of a vastus medialis TrP deep to the sartorius muscle. When the needle encounters this superficial sartorius TrP, the patient reports a sharp or tingling pain felt diffusely over the adjacent thigh.

Adductor Muscles (Chapter 59)

Adductor Longus and Adductor Brevis (Figure 72-76A, B)

The femoral artery lies deep to the sartorius muscle and lateral to the long and short adductor muscles. For this reason, the femoral artery should first be located by palpating for a pulse and the anterolateral border of the adductor longus muscle, and then the needle should be directed posteromedially from there. In this way, one injects away from, not toward, the femoral artery.

For TrPI or DN of the adductor longus and brevis muscles, the patient is positioned supine with the hip and knee flexed and the hip externally rotated and abducted. Trigger points in both muscles are identified by cross-fiber pincer palpation and

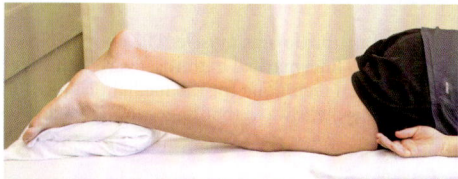

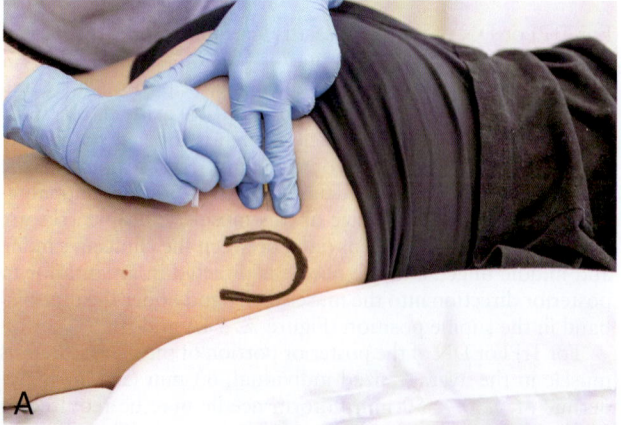
A

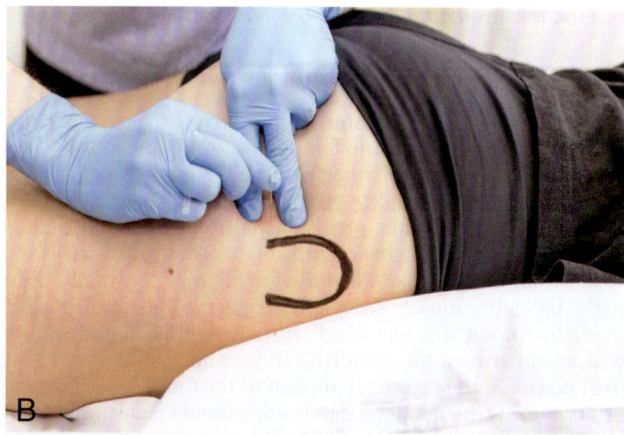
B

Figure 72-71. Trigger point injection or dry needling of the hip **external rotator muscles**. The black line depicts the greater trochanter of the femur. A, **Gemelli and obturator internus muscles** at the upper ⅓rd of the posterior greater trochanter. B, **Obturator externus and quadratus femoris muscles** at the lower ⅔rds of the posterior greater trochanter.

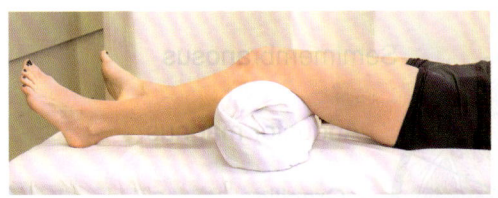
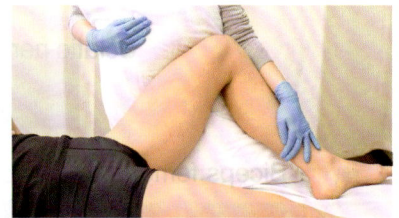
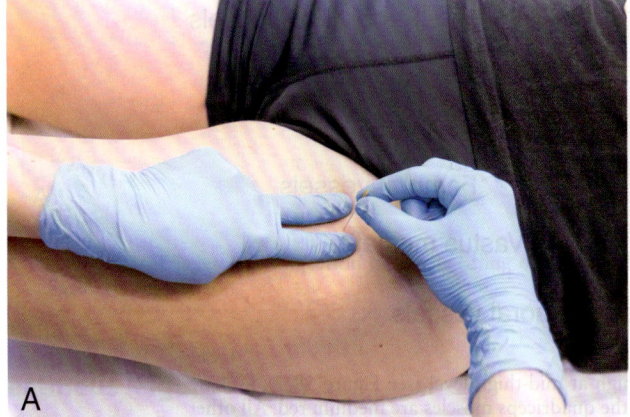
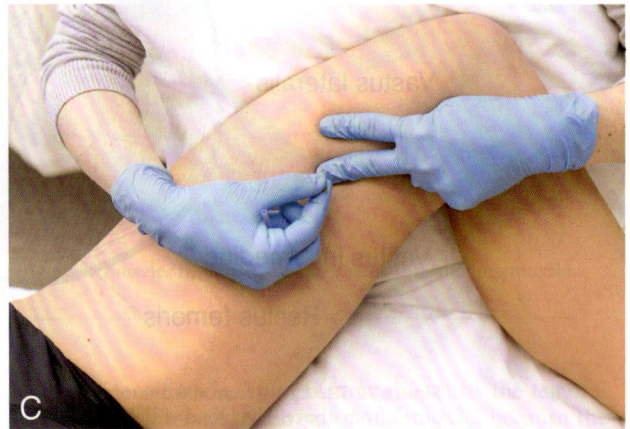
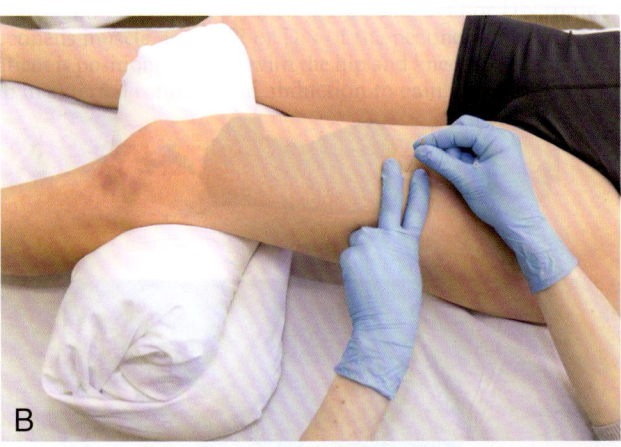
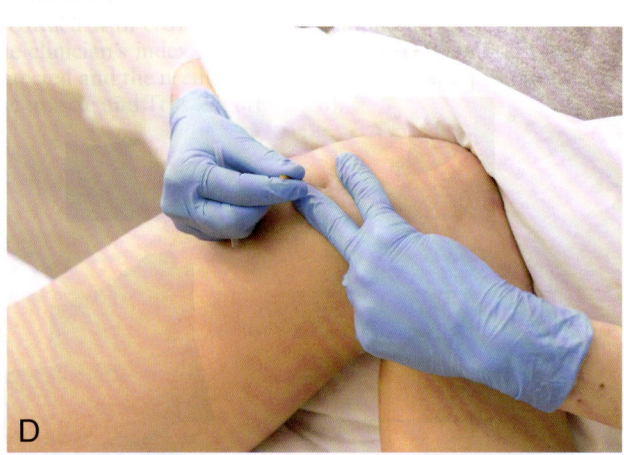

Figure 72-72. Trigger point injection or dry needling techniques for the **quadriceps femoris muscle group**. A, **Rectus femoris muscle**. B, **Vastus intermedius muscle**. C, **Vastus medialis proximal muscle**. Note that the needle is directed slightly anteriorly and laterally. D, **Vastus medialis muscle distal location**.

then fixed with a pincer grasp between the clinician's thumb, index, and middle fingers. For the adductor longus muscle, the needle is directed from an anterior to posterior direction into the TrPs of the muscle (Figure 72-76A).

For TrPI or DN of the adductor brevis muscle, TrPs are fixed with a pincer grasp and the needle is inserted between the pectineus and adductor longus muscle, perpendicular to the adductor brevis muscle, and directed posteriorly toward the clinician's fingers and into the TrPs of the muscle (Figure 72-76B). Oftentimes, the adductor longus and brevis muscles may be needled together with the same pincer grasp technique.

Adductor Magnus (Figures 72-76C, D and 72-77)

A review of cross-sectional anatomy (Figure 72-77) is recommended before injecting the deeper portions of the adductor magnus muscle. For TrPI or DN of the adductor magnus muscle, the patient is positioned supine, hip and knee flexed, and the hip in external rotation and abduction. Trigger points in the proximal ischiocondylar portion are identified with cross-fiber pincer palpation and fixed with a pincer grasp in between the clinician's thumb, index, and middle fingers.

The needle is directed form an anterior to posterior direction (Figure 72-76C).

For TrPI or DN in the mid-portion or proximal adductor magnus region, the femoral artery is unlikely to be encountered because the adductor longus muscle lies between the femoral artery and the anterior surface of the adductor magnus muscle. However, when needling from the medial aspect of the thigh (Figure 72-76D), the sciatic nerve, which passes against the adductor magnus muscle, between it and the hamstring musculature, should be avoided. The nerve passes deep to the ischiocondylar and middle parts of the adductor magnus muscle.

Gracilis (Figure 72-76C)

For TrPI or DN of the gracilis muscle, the patient is positioned as in the technique for the adductor magnus muscle. If more tension is needed on the muscle, the knee is extended. Trigger points are identified by either cross-fiber flat or pincer palpation of this superficial muscle, and they may be needled using either the pincer or flat palpation technique, depending on the flexibility of the subcutaneous tissue. The needle is directed perpendicular into the TrP which is fixed between the clinician's index and middle finger (Figure 72-76C).

818 Section 8: Treatment Considerations for Myofascial Pain and Dysfunction

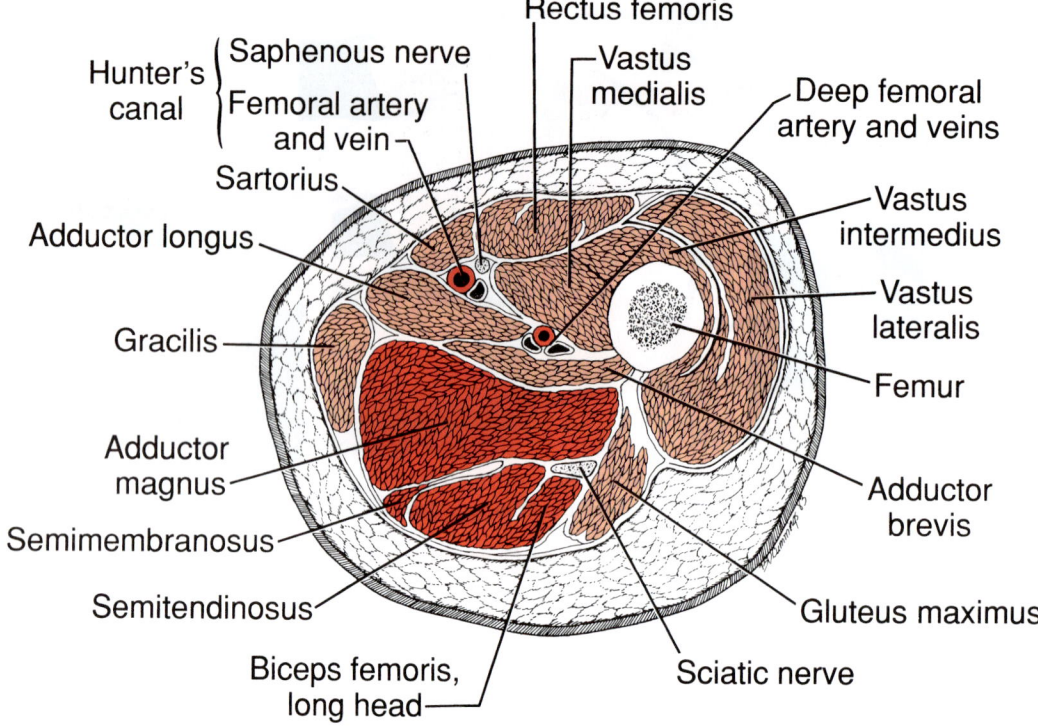

Figure 72-77. Cross-section of the thigh at the junction of its upper and middle thirds. See Figure 60-1 for the level of cross-section. Hamstring muscles, arteries, and veins are dark red. At this level, the adductor magnus muscle (intermediate red) is considerably larger than the hamstring muscle group. Other muscles of the thigh are light red. In this section, the semitendinosus and biceps femoris muscles appear to be fused. Redrawn with permission from Anderson JE. *Grant's Atlas of Anatomy*. 8th ed. Baltimore, MD: Williams and Wilkins; 1983.

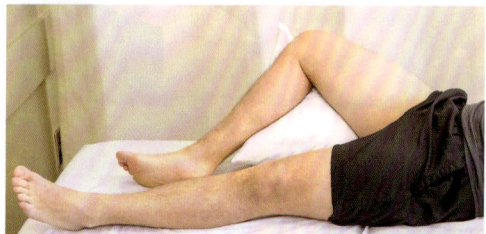

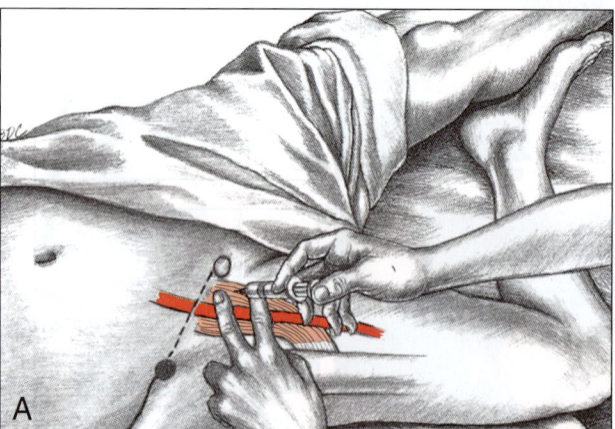
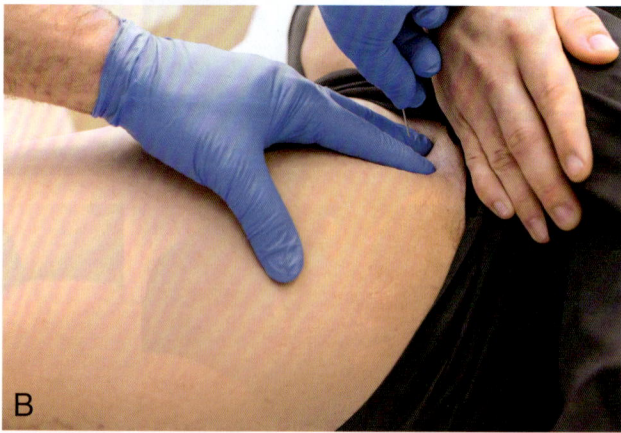

Figure 72-78. Trigger point injection or dry needling of the **pectineus muscle** (light red). The thigh of the patient is placed in abduction, external rotation, and slight flexion. A, The solid circle locates the anterior superior iliac spine; the dashed line, the inguinal ligament; and the open circle, the pubic tubercle. The femoral artery (dark red) is avoided by palpating its pulsations and directing the needle medially away from it. B, Dry needling with middle finger of the palpating hand on the femoral artery.

Hamstring Muscles (Chapter 60)
Figure 72-79

Prior to TrPI or DN of the hamstring muscles, one should review the course of the sciatic nerve. It passes down the posterior thigh underneath the long head of the biceps femoris muscle, which crosses over it about mid-thigh. Proximally, the nerve reaches the lateral border of the long head while still deep to the gluteus maximus muscle. Distally, at the popliteal space, the nerve's tibial portion emerges from under the medial border of the long head of the biceps femoris muscle about where the semimembranosus muscle and the long head part company. The femoral blood vessels join the sciatic nerve at about this same level by emerging posteriorly through the adductor canal from beneath the middle portion of the adductor magnus muscle. The tibial neurovascular bundle then lies deep to the semitendinosus muscle fibers and passes down the limb near the midline behind the knee. The fibular branch of the sciatic nerve follows beside or deep to the medial border of the short head of the biceps femoris muscle to the knee. When needling hamstring TrPs, it is wise to limit treatment to only one side of the body during every visit.

For TrPI or DN for both medial and lateral hamstring muscles, the patient is positioned prone with a pillow or bolster under the ankles to place the knee in slight flexion. Trigger points in the semimembranosus and semitendinosus muscles are identified with either cross-fiber flat or pincer palpation. For the flat palpation technique, the TrP is fixed between the clinician's index and middle fingers, and the needle is directed toward the ischial tuberosity (Figure 72-79A). Alternatively, the patient can be positioned supine with the hip in abduction and external rotation with the knee flexed. A pincer grasp is used to fix the TrPs and the needle is directed laterally through the muscle mass toward the clinician's fingers (Figure 72-79B).

For TrPI or DN of the long and short heads of the biceps femoris muscle, the patient is positioned prone with a pillow under the ankle. Trigger points in the long head of the biceps femoris muscle are identified with cross-fiber flat palpation and fixed between the clinician's index and middle finger. The needle is inserted close to the midline of the thigh and is directed laterally, away from the sciatic nerve and other major neurovascular structures (Figure 72-79C).

For TrPI or DN of the short head of the biceps femoris muscle, the TrPs are identified with cross-fiber flat palpation and fixed between the clinician's index and middle finger. The needle is directed from a lateral to medial direction and angled toward the femur. The fibular branch of the sciatic nerve travels along the medial aspect of the muscle and should be avoided (Figure 72-79D).

Popliteus Muscle (Chapter 61)
Figure 72.80

For TrPI or DN of the popliteus muscle, the clinician visualizes the course of the popliteal artery and vein and the tibial and fibular nerves in the posterior leg and popliteal fossa to avoid them. The muscle belly can be approached from either its lower medial part or its upper lateral part, depending on where the TrPs are located.

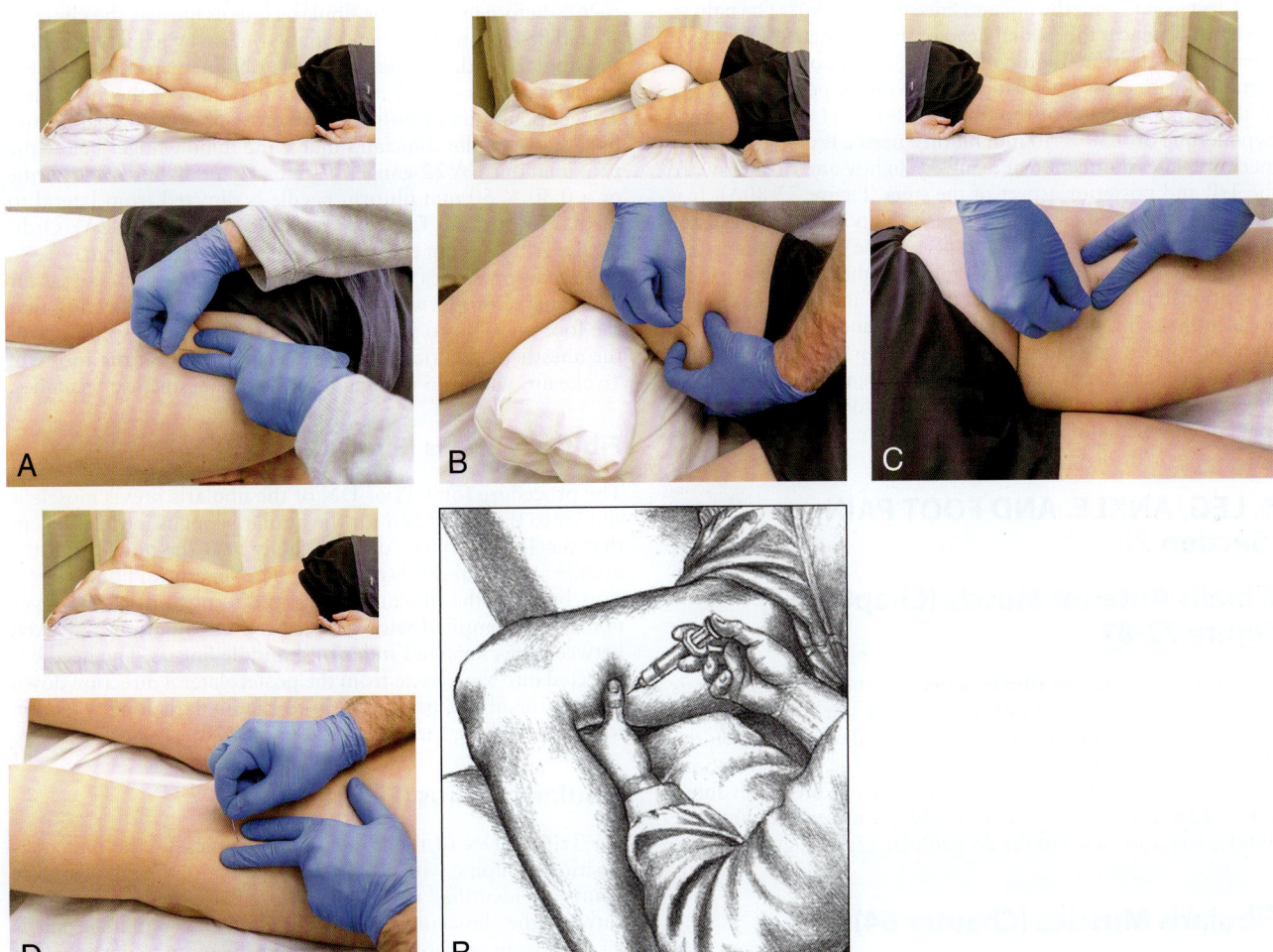

Figure 72-79. Trigger point injection and dry needling of the **hamstring muscles**. A, Proximal attachment of **semitendinosus and semimembranosus muscles** with the flat palpation technique. B, **Semitendinosus and semimembranosus** muscles, supine with hip in external rotation and abduction with a pincer grasp. C, **Biceps femoris muscle long head**. D, **Biceps femoris muscle short head**.

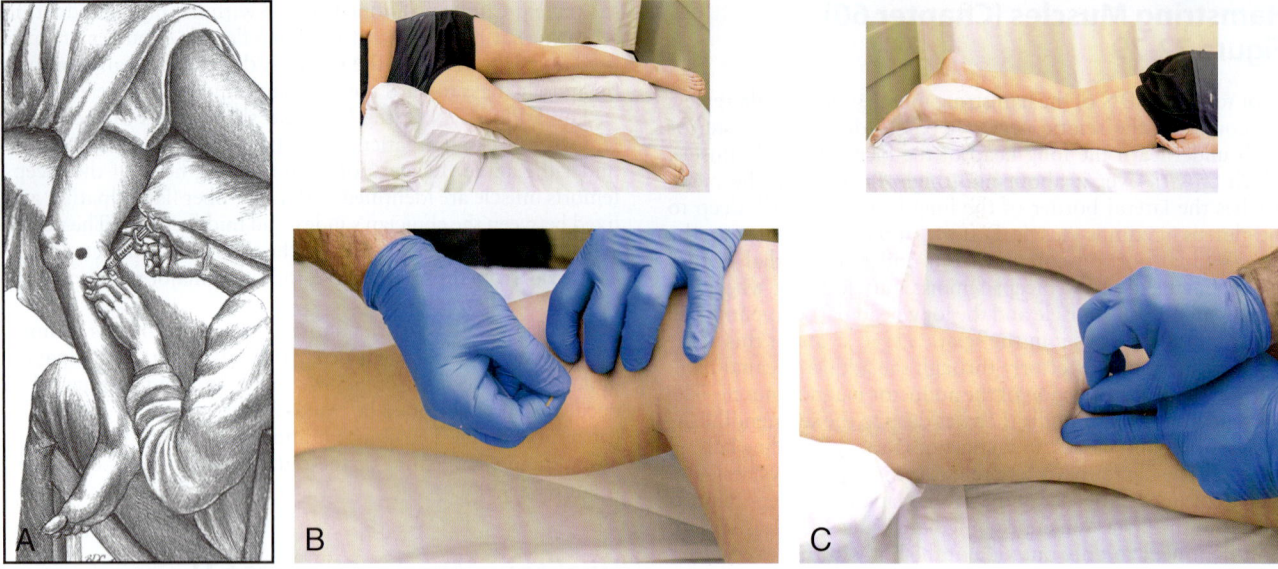

Figure 72-80. Trigger point injection or dry needling of the **popliteus muscle**. A, The solid circle locates the medial condyle of the tibia. The medial head of the gastrocnemius muscle is pressed aside posterolaterally to allow access to the popliteus muscle. B, The gastrocnemius muscle is partially slackened by plantar-flexing the foot at the ankle, whereas the knee is slightly flexed to permit slackening of popliteus muscle tension. A pillow is placed under the lateral aspect of the knee moving the gastrocnemius muscle laterally allowing better access to the popliteus muscle. C, Upper lateral portion, prone, medial to the biceps femoris muscle insertion. Note that the clinician's middle finger of the palpating hand is on the biceps femoris tendon.

For the medial portion, the patient is positioned in side-lying on the affected side with the hip and knee flexed to 90°. The palpating hand displaces the medial head of the gastrocnemius muscle laterally toward the middle of the leg, and popliteus TrPs are identified with cross-fiber flat palpation on the posterior surface of the proximal third of the tibia. A 38-mm (1½-in) 22-gauge hypodermic or 0.30 × 50 mm filiform needle is directed from a medial to lateral direction and angled slightly anteriorly toward the TrP and posterior aspect of the tibia (Figure 72-80A). It is very common for the needle to touch the posterior part of the tibia when needling the medial aspect of the popliteus muscle.

For TrPI or DN of the upper lateral end of the muscle, the patient is positioned prone with a bolster under the ankle. Trigger points are identified with cross-fiber flat palpation and fixed between the clinician's index and middle fingers. Caution is necessary when inserting the needle to keep the point of penetration medial to the biceps femoris muscle and tendon to avoid the fibular nerve that courses medial or deep to them (Figure 72-80B).

6. LEG, ANKLE, AND FOOT PAIN (Section 7)

Tibialis Anterior Muscle (Chapter 63) Figure 72-81

For TrPI or DN of the tibialis anterior muscle, the patient is positioned supine with a pillow under the knee. The TrPs are identified with cross-fiber flat palpation and fixed between the clinician's index and middle fingers. A 21-gauge, 38-mm (1½-in) hypodermic or a 0.30 × 50 mm filiform needle is directed at about a 45° angle toward the tibia to avoid the underlying anterior tibial artery and vein and the deep fibular nerve (Figure 72-81).

Fibularis Muscles (Chapter 64)

Fibularis Longus (Figure 72-82A)

For TrPI or DN of the fibularis longus muscle, the patient is positioned side-lying with the affected side up and a pillow placed under the leg and foot, and the hips and knees are flexed to 90°. Before needling the fibularis longus muscle, the clinician should first locate the common fibular nerve by palpation behind the fibular head. The nerve travels obliquely and deep to the fibularis longus muscle in the proximal third of the lateral leg. Trigger points are identified with a cross-fiber flat palpation and fixed between the clinician's index and middle finger below the proximal third. A 22-gauge, 37-mm (1½-in) hypodermic needle or a 0.30 × 50 mm filiform needle is directed from lateral to medial toward the TrPs and the fibula (Figure 72-82A). Ordinarily, TrPI does not cause a nerve block, but the TrP may be so close that sometimes the local anesthetic solution spreads as far as the nerve. It is wise to warn patients prior to injection that the foot may "go to sleep" briefly if there is any "spillover" of the anesthetic solution and to reassure them that the foot will "wake up" within 15 or 20 minutes as the anesthetic effect fades.

Fibularis Brevis (Figure 72-82B)

The procedure for TrPI or DN of the fibularis brevis muscle is similar to that described for the fibularis longus muscle, except that the TrPs are more distal, usually near the junction of the middle and distal thirds of the leg. The superficial fibular nerve runs between the fibularis brevis and tertius muscles. Trigger points are identified with cross-fiber flat palpation and fixed between the clinician's index and middle fingers. The needle is directed into the muscle from the posterolateral direction down toward the fibula, passing deep to the fibularis longus tendon to avoid needling the nerve (Figure 72-82B).

Fibularis Tertius (Figure 72-82C)

For TrPI or DN of the fibularis tertius muscle, the patient is positioned supine with a pillow placed under the knee. Trigger points are identified with a cross-fiber flat palpation and fixed between the clinician's index and middle fingers. The needle is directed from an anterior to posterior direction toward the TrP and the fibula (Figure 72-82C). This angle avoids the superficial fibular nerve overlying the fibularis brevis muscle and stays well clear of the deep fibular nerve and anterior tibial vessels on the interosseous membrane.

Gastrocnemius Muscle (Chapter 65)
Figures 72-83 and 72-84

For TrPI or DN of the gastrocnemius muscle, the clinician must be aware of the neurovascular structures, especially when considering needling the proximal medial or lateral heads of the gastrocnemius muscle. The proximal part of the medial head of the gastrocnemius muscle lies between the tibial nerve and the tendons of the semitendinosus and semimembranosus muscles, and the proximal portion of the lateral head of gastrocnemius muscle lies between the fibular nerve and the tibial nerve. The popliteal fossa must be thoroughly palpated to locate the nerves and tendons if needling of the proximal gastrocnemius muscle is indicated. Clinicians should identify the available safe needling zone between the semitendinosus muscle tendon and the tibial nerve, and the space between the fibular and tibial nerves and the relationship with the biceps femoris muscle tendon. Anatomic variations regarding a premature split of the two divisions of the common fibular nerve may be identified in the popliteal space and needling the proximal part of the lateral head of the gastrocnemius or plantaris muscles would not be indicated. The medial sural cutaneous nerve descends between the medial and lateral heads of the gastrocnemius muscle. When needling the central bellies of either head, the midline is avoided by angling the needle medially when needling the medial head and laterally when needling the lateral head.[1]

The patient is positioned prone for needling both the medial and lateral heads, and a pillow placed under the ankle and foot to position the knee in slight flexion. Trigger points in the medial head of the gastrocnemius muscle are identified with cross-fiber pincer palpation, and the TrPs are fixed with a pincer

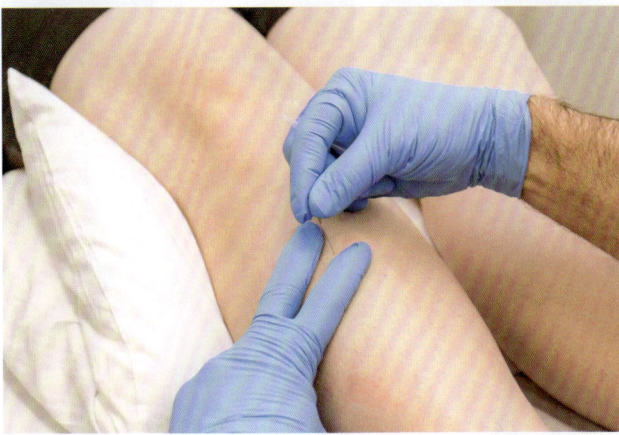

Figure 72-81. Trigger point injection or dry needling of the **tibialis anterior muscle**. Note that the needle is angled medially toward the tibia to avoid the deep fibular nerve.

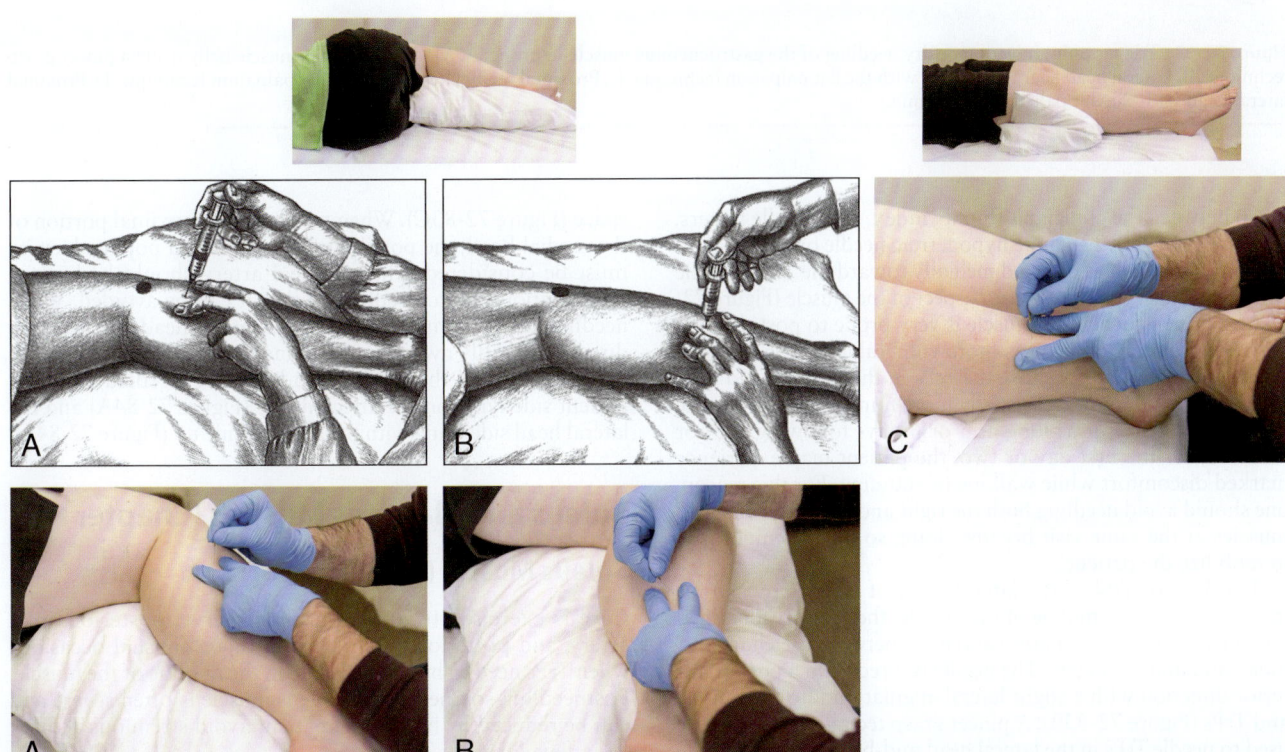

Figure 72-82. Trigger point injection or dry needling of TrPs in the **fibularis muscles**. The circle marks the head of the fibula. Note the pillow between the knees that extends to the ankles so that it supports the leg being injected. A, **Fibularis longus muscle** needling near, but distal, to the course of the common fibular nerve that crosses the fibula just below the fibular head. The needle is directed toward the underlying bone. B, **Fibularis brevis muscle**, posterolateral approach, near the junction of the middle and lower thirds of the leg on either side of, and deep to, the tendon of the fibularis longus muscle. C, **Fibularis tertius** TrP needling, anterior to posterior toward the fibula.

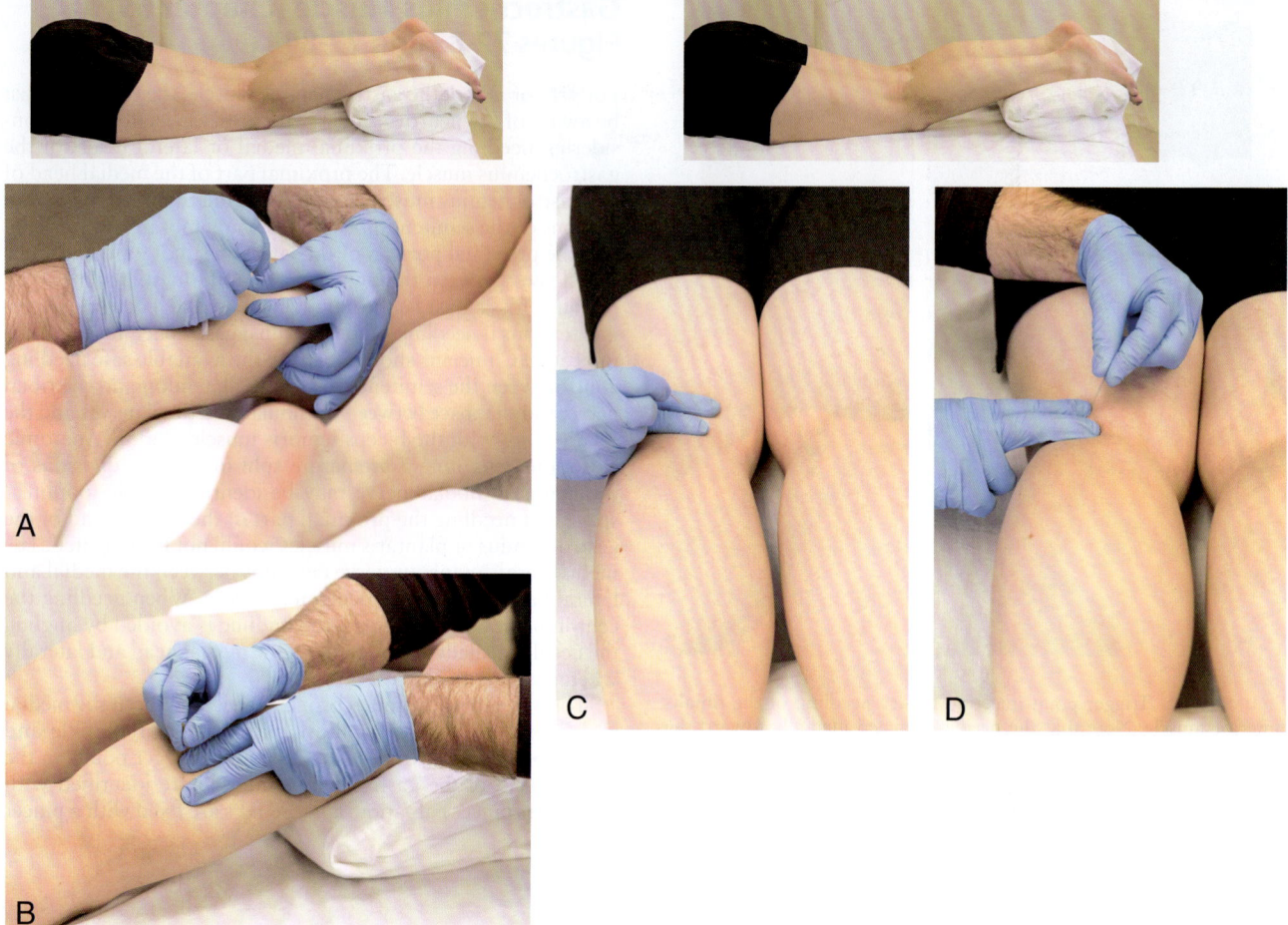

Figure 72-83. Trigger point injection or dry needling of the **gastrocnemius muscle** in prone. A, **Medial head** mid-muscle belly using a pincer grasp technique. B, **Lateral head** near the midline with the flat palpation technique. C, **Proximal medial head** with the flat palpation technique. D, **Proximal lateral head** with the flat palpation technique.

grasp between the clinician's thumb, index, and middle fingers. A 37-mm (1½-in), 22-gauge hypodermic needle or a 0.30 × 50 mm filiform needle is directed medially toward the TrPs and the clinician's fingers on the anterior aspect of the muscle (Figure 72-83A). The gastrocnemius muscle is very prone to postneedling soreness. The medial head is more vulnerable to this than the lateral head, perhaps because the TrPs in the medial head tend to be more tender and are usually more numerous. The muscle may remain sore for as long as 5 or 6 days following TrPI or DN and, for the first day or two, the patient may experience marked discomfort while walking or standing. For this reason, one should avoid needling both the right and left gastrocnemius muscles at the same visit because doing so might temporarily immobilize the patient.

For TrPI or DN in the lateral head of the gastrocnemius muscle toward the midline of the muscle, the TrPs are identified with cross-fiber flat palpation and fixed between the clinicians' index and middle fingers. The needle is directed in a posteroanterior direction with a slight lateral angulation into the muscle and TrPs (Figure 72-83B). A pincer grasp technique can also be used to needle TrPs in the lateral head mid-belly with the needle directed laterally toward the clinician's fingers on the opposite side of the muscle as described for the medial head.

For TrPI or DN of the proximal medial and lateral heads of the gastrocnemius muscle, the TrPs are identified with cross-fiber-flat palpation and fixed between the clinician's index and middle fingers. The needle should be directed away from the midline to avoid the neurovascular bundle that passes through the popliteal space (Figure 72-83C). When needling the proximal portion of the medial head, the possibility of a displaced popliteal artery must be considered. The popliteal artery should be located by palpation before needling so that it can be avoided. When needling the proximal portion of the lateral head, the needle is directed laterally away from midline (Figure 72-83D).

Alternatively, the medial head may be needled with the patient side-lying on the affected side (Figure 72-84A) and the lateral head side-lying with the affected side up (Figure 72-84B).

Soleus and Plantaris Muscles (Chapter 66)

Soleus Muscle (Figure 72-85)

Care is exercised to avoid the tibial nerve, posterior tibial artery, and posterior tibial veins on those unusual occasions when TrPs need to be needled deep in the midline of the muscle. Postneedling soreness of the soleus muscle is often severe and can be reduced by having the patient avoid strenuous activity for a few days.

For TrPI or DN of the soleus muscle, the patient is positioned in prone or side-lying depending on which aspect of the muscle needs to be treated. In many patients, a 37-mm (1½-in) 22-gauge hypodermic needle or a 0.30 × 50 mm filiform needle is sufficient depending on the size of the muscle. Trigger points in the muscle are identified by cross-fiber pincer palpation, and the TrPs are fixed with a pincer grasp between the clinician's thumb, index,

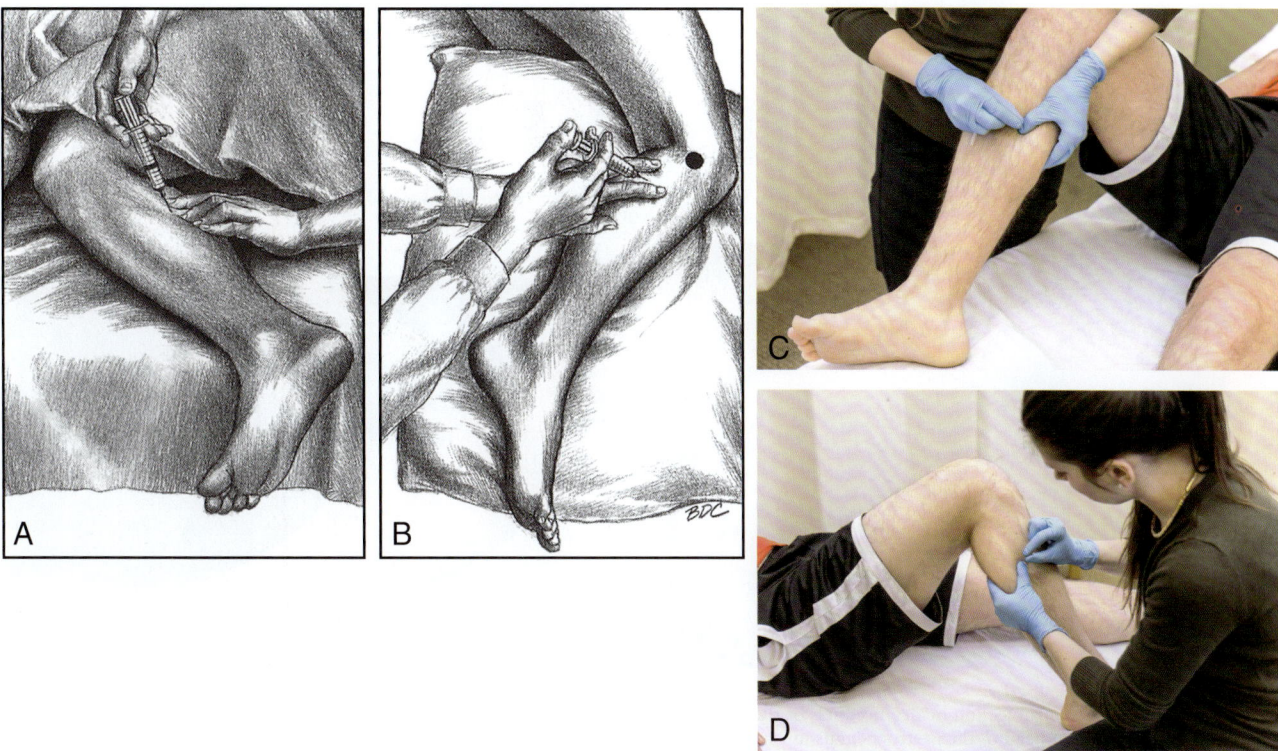

Figure 72-84. Trigger point injection or dry needling of **gastrocnemius muscle** alternate position. A, **Medial head** with the patient lying with the affected side down. B, **Lateral head** with the patient side-lying with the affected side up. C, Hook-lying **medial head**. D, Hook-lying **lateral head**.

and middle fingers. The needle is directed toward the clinician's finger on the opposite side (Figure 72-85A). In side-lying, the soleus muscle is easily approached from the medial side distal to the bulge that marks the lower end of the gastrocnemius muscle fibers. The patient lies on the right side for needling treatment of the right soleus muscle, with the uppermost (left) leg in front of the involved one (Figure 72-85B). The clinician applies counter pressure to the TrP with one finger pressing directly on the TrP

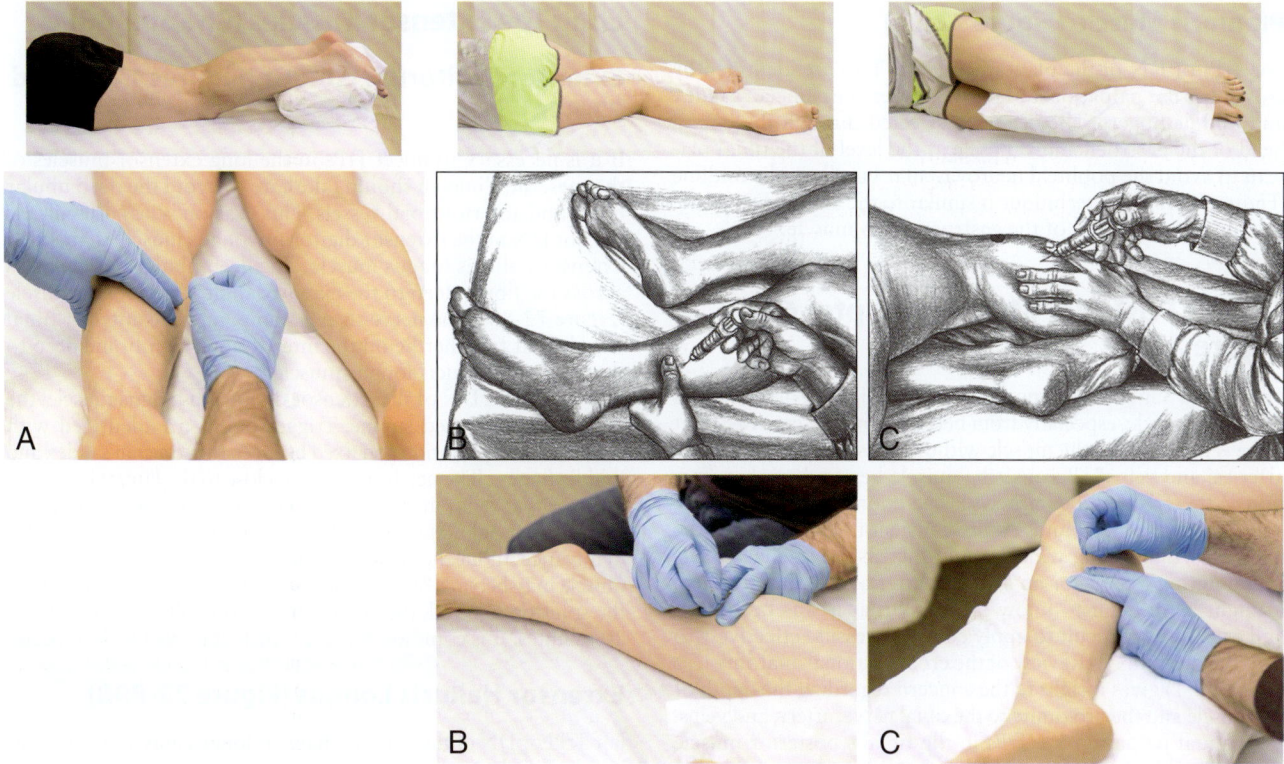

Figure 72-85. Trigger point injection or dry needling of the **soleus muscle**. A, Medial approach in prone position. B, Medial approach with the patient lying on the same (right) side. C, Lateral approach with the patient lying on the opposite side.

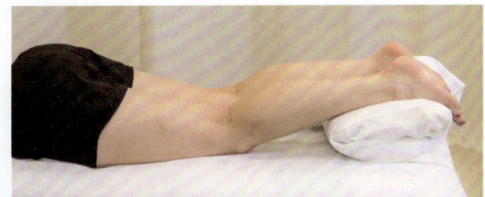
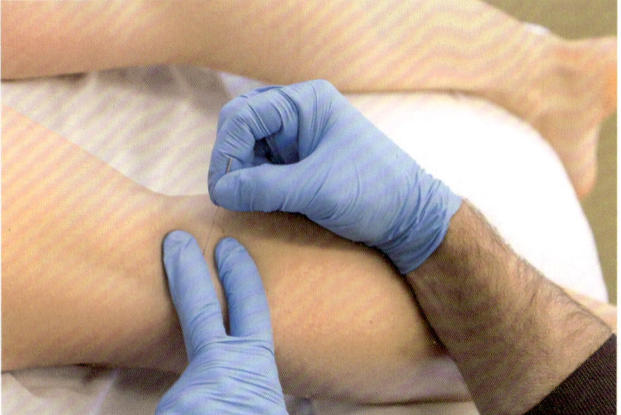

Figure 72-86. Trigger point injection or dry needling of the **plantaris muscle** through the lateral head of the gastrocnemius muscle.

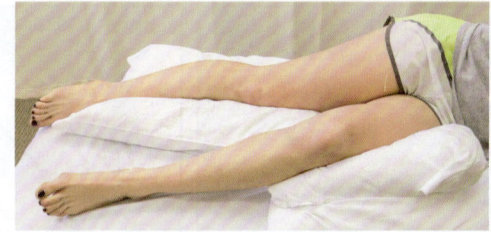
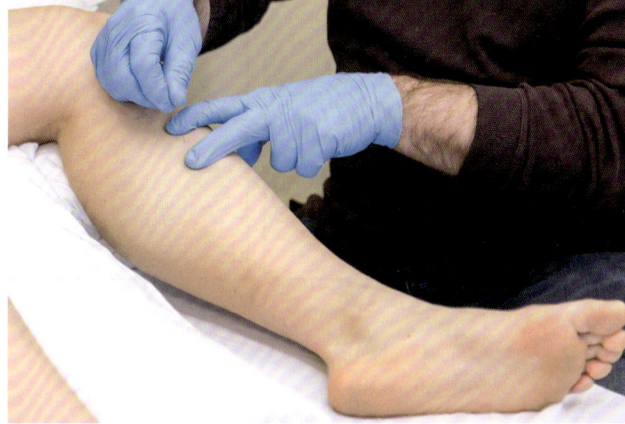

Figure 72-87. Trigger point injection or dry needling of the **tibialis posterior** muscle.

from the lateral side of the muscle, while the needle is inserted on the medial side and aimed directly at the center of that finger.

For TrPI or DN of the lateral aspect of the soleus muscle, the patient lies on the opposite side so that this muscle can be approached laterally. The needle is directed toward the fibula at the spot of maximum tenderness, which is encountered deep, close to the bone (Figure 72-85C).

Plantaris Muscle (Figure 72-86)

For TrPI or DN of the plantaris muscle, TrPs are identified by cross-fiber flat palpation and fixed between the clinician's index and middle fingers. The needle is directed through the lateral head of the gastrocnemius muscle at the level of the tibial plateau to avoid the popliteal neurovascular bundle in the midline (Figure 72-86). The technique is similar to the TrPI or DN of the proximal lateral head of the gastrocnemius muscle.

Tibialis Posterior Muscle (Chapter 67) Figure 72-87

Travell and Simons[100] did not recommend injection of the tibialis posterior muscle, especially from behind. The concern was "that there is no access to the muscle without passing close to nerves, arteries, and veins". Because the muscle lies so deep, localization of the TrPs will be imprecise. The poor localization of the TrPs in this muscle would require considerable probing for the TrPs with the needle, which would increase the danger of its encountering a nerve or an artery. If arterial bleeding resulted, it might be difficult to know promptly that it was occurring, and even more difficult to apply counter pressure effectively to stop the bleeding.[100] Review of the cross-sectional anatomy (see Figure 67-1) gives insight to the concern regarding the depth of the muscle and the proximity to the tibial nerve, artery, and veins.

Manual palpation for TrPs in the tibialis posterior muscle is not possible; however, tenderness to deep palpation may be indicative of TrPs in this muscle. For identification of TrPs in the tibialis posterior muscle, the needle is utilized both diagnostically and for treatment. The patient is positioned side-lying on the affected side with the hip and knee flexed to 90°. The needle is directed deeply in a lateral direction with slight anterior angulation. The needle is kept close to the posterior aspect of the tibia or even touching the bone with the tip of the needle as a reference of location (Figure 72-87).

Long Toe Extensor Muscles (Chapter 68)

Extensor Digitorum Longus (Figures 72-88 and 72-89A)

If it is necessary to inject TrPs in the long extensor muscles of the toes, the clinician should take care to avoid the deep fibular nerve and anterior tibial vessels. This evasion is less difficult for TrPI or DN in the extensor digitorum longus muscle than in the extensor hallucis longus muscle. The deep fibular nerve passes across the fibula deep to the extensor digitorum longus muscle (Figure 72-88). The nerve then accompanies the anterior tibial vessels that together lie on the interosseous membrane deep to the extensor hallucis longus muscle.

For TrPI or DN of the extensor digitorum longus muscle, the patient is positioned supine. Trigger points are identified with cross-fiber flat palpation and fixed between the clinician's index and middle fingers. The needle is inserted close to the lateral border of the tibialis anterior muscle and directed from anterior to posterior toward the fibula (Figure 72-89A). The patient should be warned in advance about the possibility of some numbness and that the muscle may become "lazy" following the injection. Depending on the solution injected, the nerve conduction will recover in 15 or 20 minutes. It is common for this transient nerve block to occur.

Extensor Hallucis Longus (Figure 72-89B)

For TrPI or DN of the extensor hallucis longus muscle, the patient is positioned supine, and the TrPs are identified with cross-fiber flat palpation and fixed between the clinician's index and middle fingers. The needle is inserted close to the lateral border of the tibialis anterior muscle in an anterior to posterior direction

Chapter 72: Trigger Point Injection and Dry Needling 825

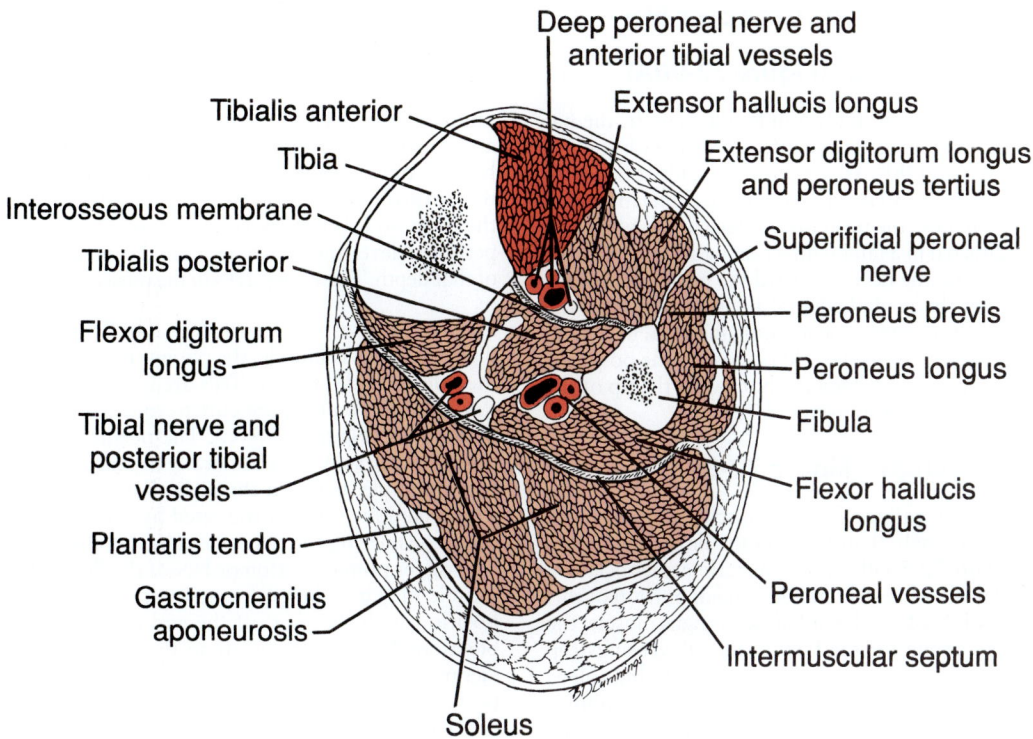

Figure 72-88. Cross-section through the lower part of the middle third of the right leg, viewed from above. Major blood vessels and the tibialis anterior muscle are dark red; other muscles are light red. Level of the cross-section, below the gastrocnemius muscle belly, is shown in Figure 63-1. From Anderson JE. *Grant's Atlas of Anatomy*. Baltimore, MD: Williams & Wilkins; 1983 (after Figure 4-73).

with a lateral angulation toward the fibula (Figure 72-89B). The clinician must be especially careful of the depth of needle penetration. One may have to pass the needle through the lateral portion of the tibialis anterior muscle to direct the needle toward the fibula at an angle deep enough to reach the TrPs in the extensor hallucis longus muscle, but one must be sufficiently superficial to avoid the underlying deep fibular nerve and anterior tibial vessels (Figure 72-88). The deep fibular nerve and the anterior tibial vessels are covered by the medial part of the extensor hallucis longus muscle and the tibialis anterior muscle. Angling the needle laterally toward the fibula helps avoid contact with the neurovascular bundle.

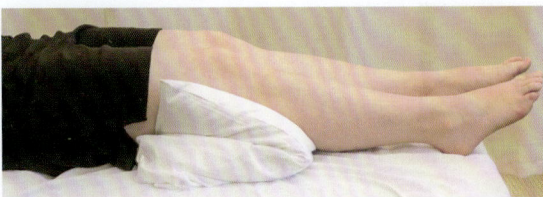

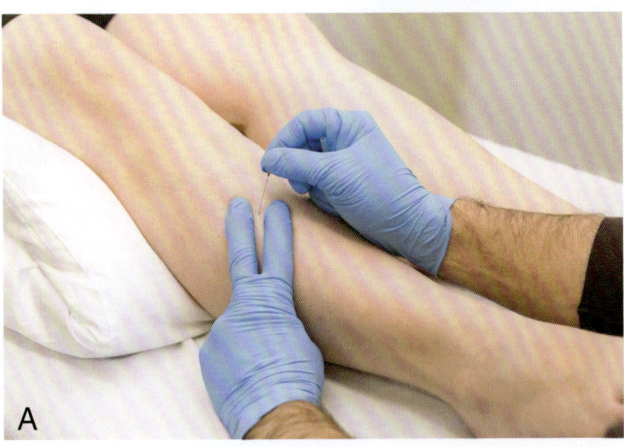
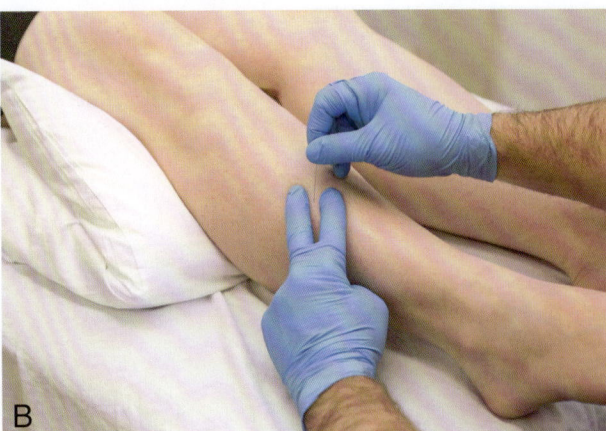

Figure 72-89. Trigger point injection or dry needling of the **long toe extensor muscles**. A, Extensor digitorum longus muscle. B, Extensor hallucis longus muscle.

Long Toe Flexor Muscles (Chapter 69)

Flexor Digitorum Longus (Figure 72-90A)

For TrPI or DN of the flexor digitorum longus muscle, the patient is positioned side-lying on the affected side with the hip and knee flexed to about 90°. Trigger points are identified with cross-fiber flat palpation and fixed between the clinician's index and middle finger against the posterior surface of the tibia. The needle is deeply directed in a lateral direction with slight anterior angulation. By angling the needle toward the posterior surface of the tibia through the medial edge of the soleus muscle, the clinician minimizes the danger of penetrating the tibial nerve and posterior tibial vessels. The needle is kept close to the posterior aspect of the tibia or even touching the bone with the tip of the needle as a reference of location (Figure 72-90A).

Flexor Hallucis Longus (Figure 72-90B)

The TrPs in the flexor hallucis longus muscle are even more difficult to needle precisely than those in the flexor digitorum longus muscle. Figure 72-88 illustrates the intimate association between the fibular blood vessels and the medial portion of this muscle. For TrPI or DN of the flexor hallucis longus muscle, the patient is positioned prone and the TrPs are identified using deep cross-fiber flat palpation through the gastrocnemius and soleus muscles. The needle is directed laterally away from the fibular vessels toward the posterior surface of the fibula. The posterior aspect of the fibula is used as an anatomic landmark to assure the proper position of the needle and to ensure sufficient depth of penetration to reach the TrPs in this muscle (Figure 72-90B).

Foot Intrinsic Muscles (Chapter 70)

Plantar Muscles—First Layer (Figure 72-91)

Abductor Hallucis Muscle. For TrPI or DN of the abductor hallucis muscle, the patient is positioned side-lying on the affected side with the knee flexed and the leg and foot supported on the table. The clinician stabilizes the leg to prevent any sudden or reflexive movements of the leg and foot (Figure 72-91A). Trigger points are identified with cross-fiber flat palpation and are fixed between the clinician's index and middle finger. The needle is directed laterally toward the underlying bone (Figure 72-91B). The neurovascular bundle passes deep to the muscle in the proximal third near its attachment. Although one might expect the TrPs in the abductor hallucis muscle to be close to the surface, they may be deep in this surprisingly thick muscle. The main TrPs often lie close to the bone, so it is usually necessary to advance the needle to the periosteal level and then to explore the muscle for TrPs just short of that depth. These deep TrPs in the muscle are easily overlooked.

Flexor Digitorum Brevis Muscle. For TrPI or DN of the flexor digitorum brevis muscle, the patient is positioned side-lying on the affected side, and the TrPs are identified by deep palpation through the plantar aponeurosis and from the medial border of the foot (Figure 72-91C). The needle enters at the medial border of the sole angled laterally to reach the flexor digitorum brevis muscle, between the medial and lateral plantar nerves. This technique is better tolerated by some patients and may be safer considering the neurovascular bundle.

Trigger point injection or DN of the flexor digitorum brevis muscle may also be performed with the patient in the prone position with the foot off the end of the table. The clinician positions himself or herself so that the leg can be stabilized against any reflexive movements during the technique. Trigger points are identified with cross-fiber flat palpation at an area of focal tenderness and fixed between the clinician's index and middle fingers. The focal area of tenderness could be caused by the plantar fascia, the flexor digitorum brevis, or the flexor accessorius (quadratus plantae) muscles or any combination thereof. The needle is guided from a plantar to dorsal direction toward the tender area down to bone (Figure 72-91D). The depth of penetration, tissue quality, and any referred pain will assist the clinician in identifying which structure is being needled.

Abductor Digiti Mini Muscle. For TrPI or DN of the abductor digiti minimi muscle, the patient is positioned in side-lying on the unaffected side. The clinician positions himself or herself so that the leg can be stabilized against any reflexive movements during the technique. Trigger points are identified using cross-fiber flat

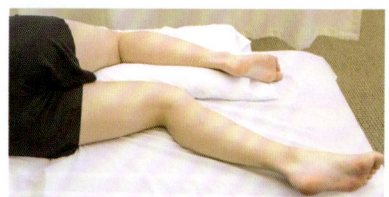

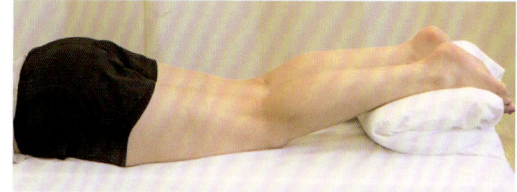

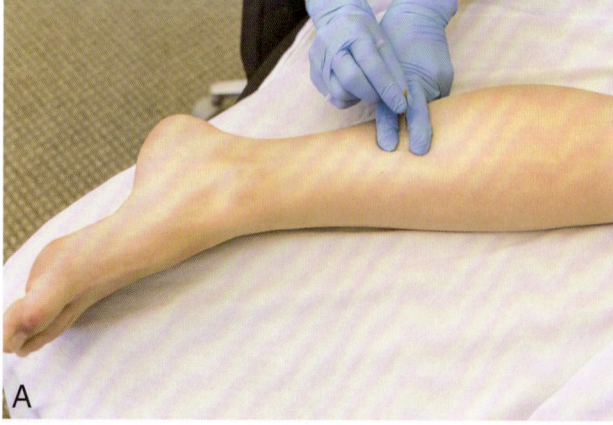

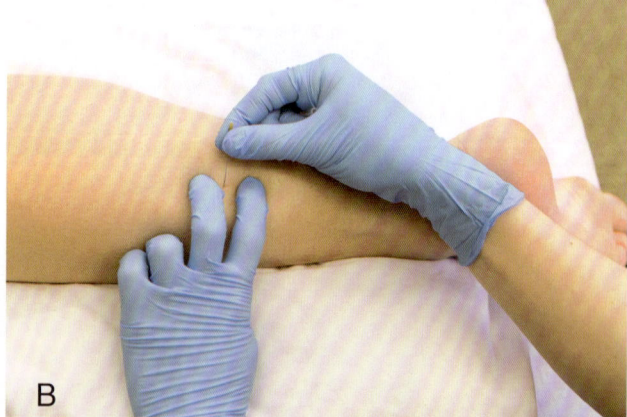

Figure 72-90. Trigger point injection or dry needling of the **long toe flexor muscles**. A, **Flexor digitorum longus muscle**, side-lying. B, **Flexor hallucis longus muscle**, prone.

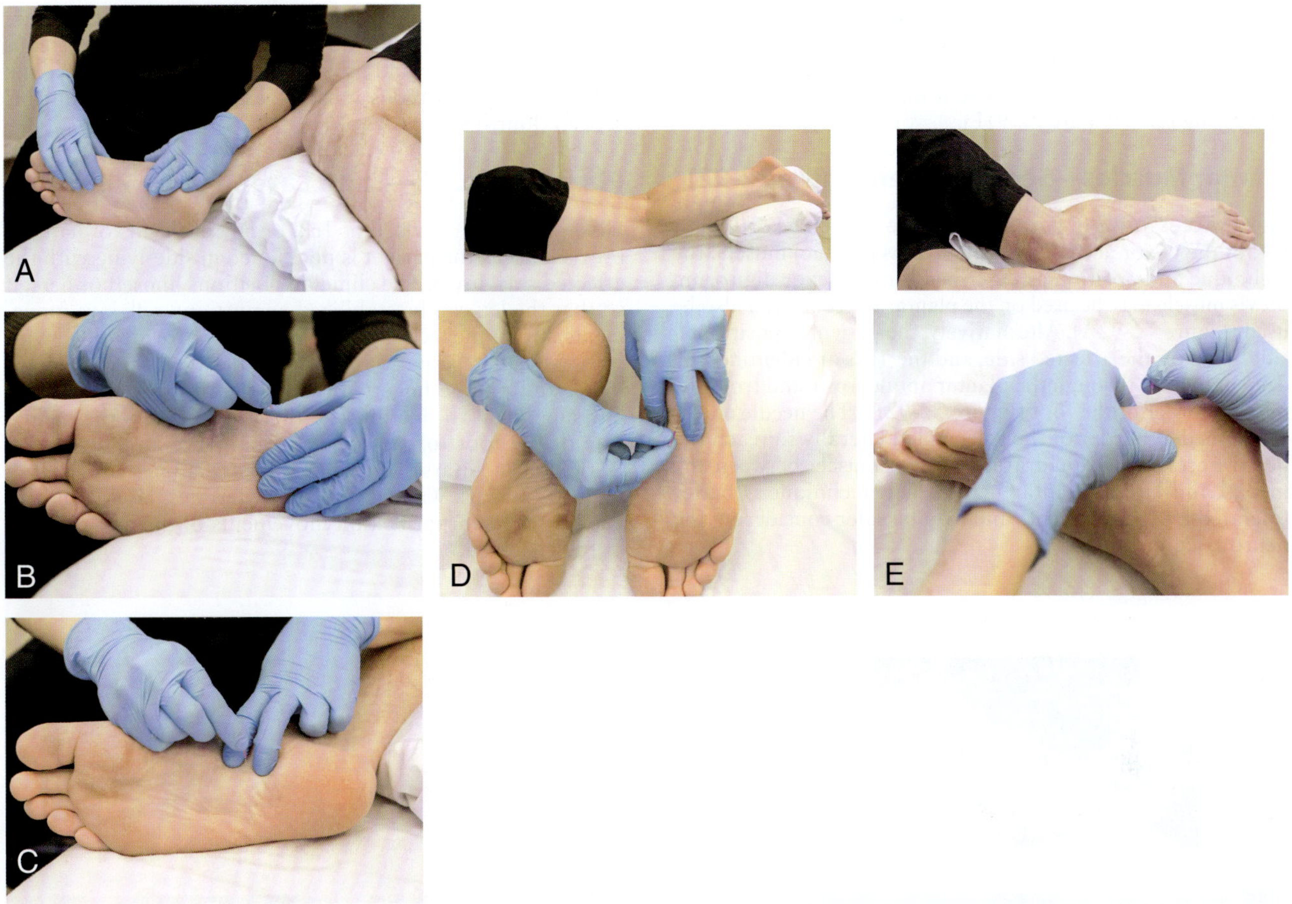

Chapter 72: Trigger Point Injection and Dry Needling   **827**

Figure 72-91. Trigger point injection or dry needling of the **plantar foot muscles' first layer**. A, Position for the clinician to stabilize the leg against reflexive movements. B, **Abductor hallucis muscle**. C, **Flexor digitorum brevis muscle**, medial approach. D, **Flexor digitorum brevis muscle**, plantar approach. E, **Abductor digiti minimi muscle**.

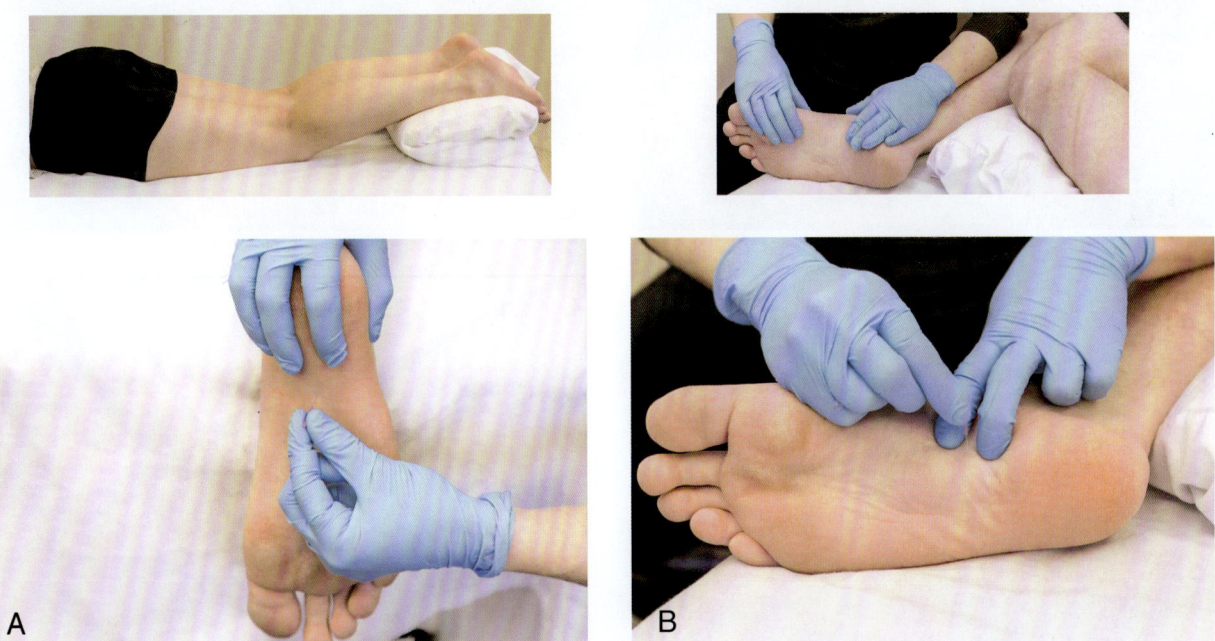

Figure 72-92. Trigger point injection or dry needling of **plantar foot muscles' second layer**. Flexor accessorius muscle (quadratus plantae) A, Plantar approach. B, Medial approach.

or pincer palpation and then fixed between the clinician's fingers. This muscle is not very thick, unlike the abductor hallucis muscle, and its taut bands and TrPs are generally easily localized. The needle is directed in a dorsomedial direction toward the underlying bone (Figure 72-91E).

Plantar Muscles—Second Layer (Figure 72-92)

Flexor Accessorius (Quadratus Plantae) Muscle. For TrPI or DN of the flexor accessorius (quadratus plantae) muscle, the technique and position as described for the flexor digitorum brevis muscle may be used or, the plantar approach can also be used (Figure 72-92A). Alternatively, the patient is positioned side-lying on the affected side, and the TrPs are identified by deep palpation through the plantar aponeurosis and from the medial border of the foot (Figure 72-92B). The needle enters at the medial border of the sole angled laterally to reach the flexor accessorius (quadratus plantae) muscle between the medial and lateral plantar nerves. This technique is better tolerated by some patients and may be safer considering the neurovascular bundle.

Lumbrical Muscles. The lumbricals are small muscles and are indistinguishable by palpation from the plantar interosseous muscles. The TrPs would probably be included when needling the plantar interosseous muscles, as described later in this section (fourth layer).

Plantar Muscles—Third Layer (Figure 72-93)

Flexor Hallucis Brevis. For TrPI or DN of the flexor hallucis brevis muscle, the patient is positioned in side-lying with the affected side down. The clinician positions himself or herself so that the leg can be stabilized against any reflexive movements during the technique. Trigger points are identified with cross-fiber flat palpation and fixed between the clinician's index and middle fingers. Because the proper digital nerve lies superficial to this muscle, the needle enters the medial side of the foot to pass deep to the nerve and superficial to the 1st metatarsal bone into flexor hallucis brevis TrPs (Figure 72-93A). When the needle penetrates the TrP, an LTR may produce abrupt flexion movements of the first phalanx of the great toe.

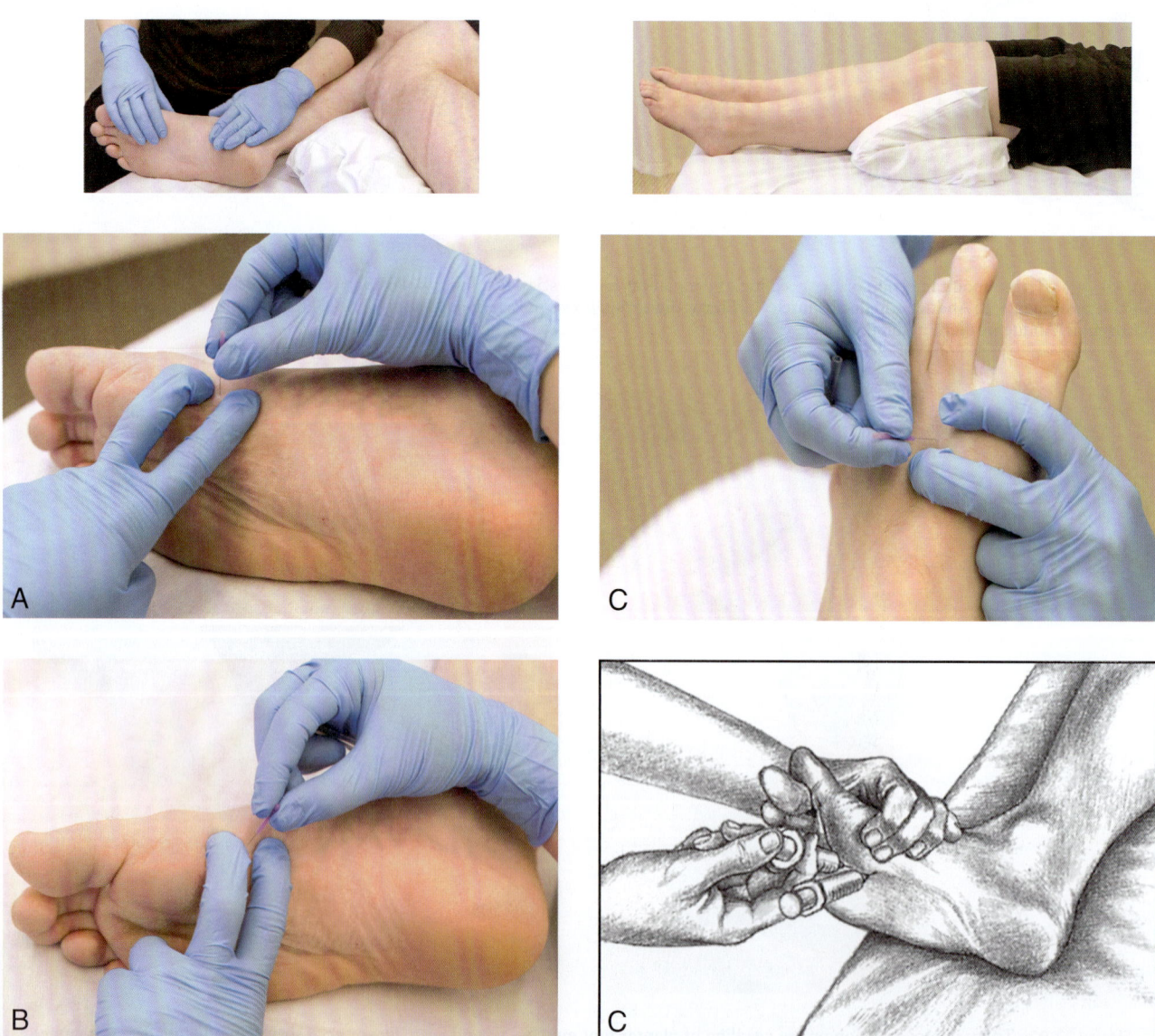

Figure 72-93. Trigger point injection or dry needling of the **plantar foot muscles' third layer**. A, **Flexor hallucis brevis muscle**. B, **Adductor hallucis muscle, oblique head**. C, **Adductor hallucis muscle, transverse head**, dorsal approach (top) and plantar approach (bottom).

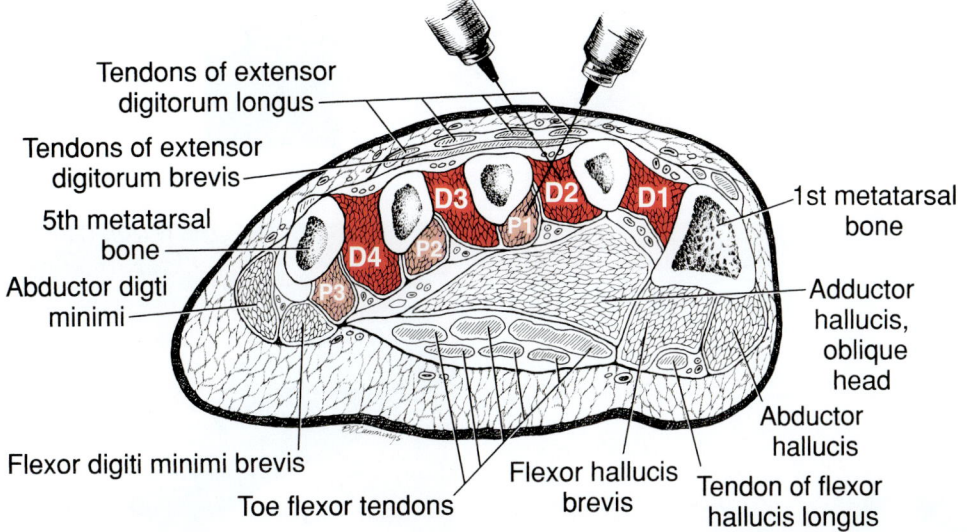

Figure 72-94. Cross-section through the foot just proximal to the metatarsal heads, viewed from the front. The dorsal interosseous muscles (D) are dark red; the plantar interossei muscles (P) are light red; other muscles, uncolored. Adapted from Ferner H, Staubesand J. *Sobotta Atlas of Human Anatomy.* 10th ed. Vol 2. Baltimore, MD: Urban and Schwarzenberg; 1983.

Adductor Hallucis Muscle. For TrPI or DN of the adductor hallucis muscle, the patient is positioned in side-lying on the affected side. The clinician positions himself or herself so that the leg can be stabilized against any reflexive movements during the technique. A focal area of tenderness is noted with deep cross-fiber flat palpation on the distal plantar aspect of the foot immediately behind the 2nd metatarsal head. The needle enters the medial side of the foot to pass deep to the digital nerve and superficial to the 1st metatarsal bone through the flexor hallucis brevis muscle into the oblique head of the adductor hallucis muscle (Figure 72-93B). LTRs may cause the great toe to move toward the second toe, confirming that the targeted TrP was needled.

For TrPI or DN of the transverse head of the adductor hallucis muscle, the patient is positioned supine. Trigger points are identified with deep cross-fiber flat palpation in the plantar aspect of the foot just proximal to the metatarsal heads and are fixed by the clinician with a modified pincer grasp with the thumb on the dorsal aspect of the foot and the index and middle fingers on the plantar aspect of the foot. The needle is inserted in the dorsum of the foot between the metatarsal bones and directed toward the clinician's fingers on the plantar aspect of the foot (Figure 72-93C). Needling of the transverse head of the adductor hallucis muscle is the same as the technique for the dorsal interossei muscle between the 1st and 2nd metatarsal bones.

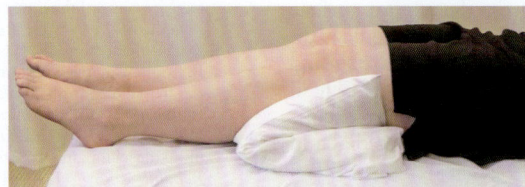

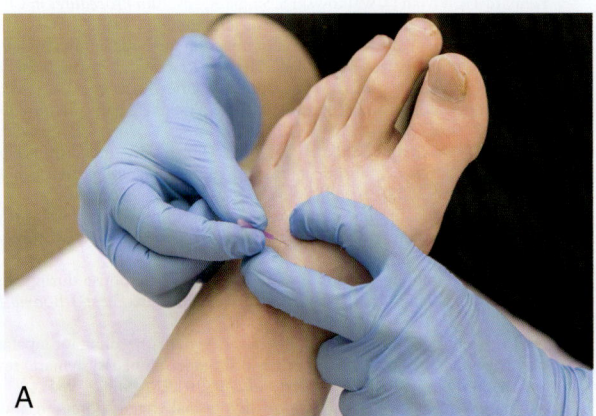
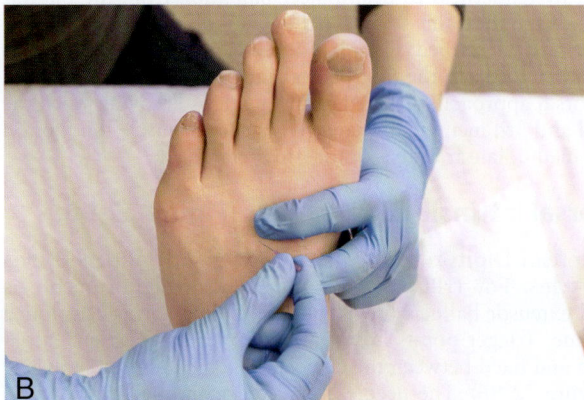

Figure 72-95. Trigger point injection or dry needling of the **plantar foot muscles' fourth layer.** A, Dorsal interosseous muscles. B, **Plantar interosseous muscles.**

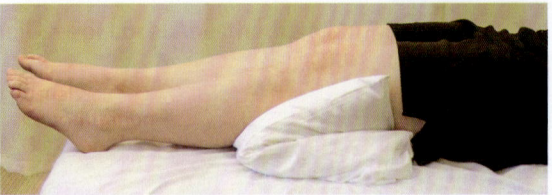

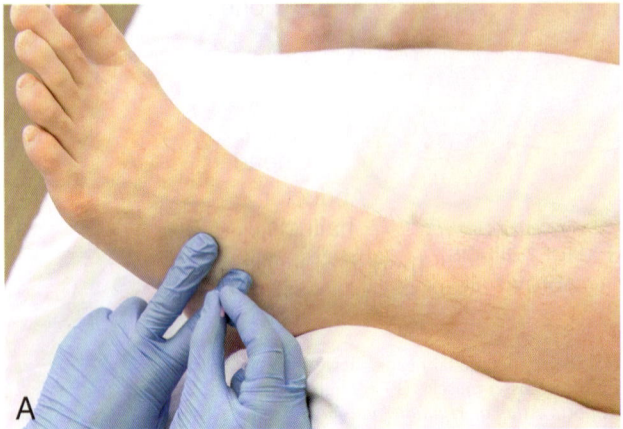
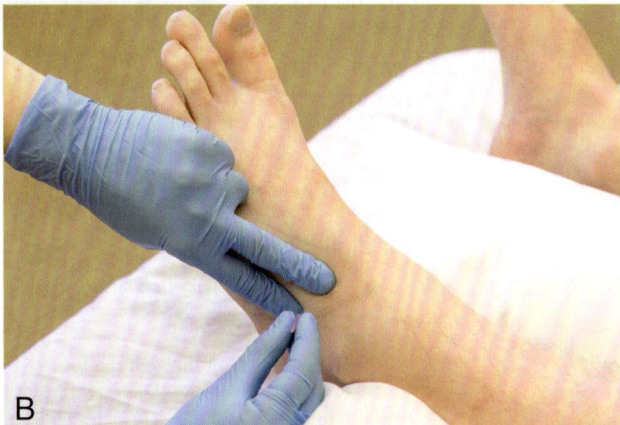

Figure 72-96. Trigger point injection or dry needling of the **dorsal intrinsic foot muscles**. A, Extensor digitorum brevis muscle. B, Extensor hallucis brevis muscle.

Fourth Layer (Dorsal and Plantar Interossei Muscles) (Figures 72-94 and 72-95)

For TrPI or DN of the dorsal and plantar interosseous muscles, they are approached from the dorsal surface of the foot. Figure 72-94 is an anatomic cross-section through the foot just proximal to the metatarsal heads showing the relationship of the dorsal and plantar interosseous muscles. The patient is positioned supine with a pillow under the knee. After localizing a TrP in the dorsal interosseous muscles by palpation, the clinician needles the muscle between the metatarsal bones. A modified pincer grasp is used, as described for the transverse head of the adductor hallucis muscle. The fingers of one hand press upward from the plantar surface of the foot into the interosseous space, whereas the needle is directed toward the clinician's finger (Figure 72-95A). Care should be taken to explore both bellies of a dorsal interossei muscle in order to locate all of the TrPs on each side of the interosseous space, and therefore, the needle must probe in both a medial and lateral direction as depicted in Figure 72-94.

For TrPI or DN of a plantar interossei muscle that is localized by tenderness to deep pincer palpation from the plantar side of the foot, the TrP is fixed by a modified pincer grasp as previously described (Figure 72-95B). Figure 72-94 shows why, in order to reach the first plantar interosseus muscle through a dorsal approach, the needle must angle laterally between the 2nd and 3rd metatarsal bones to probe the muscle that lies on the medioplantar aspect of the 3rd metatarsal.

Dorsal Intrinsic Foot Muscles (Figure 72-96)

Extensor Digitorum Brevis and Extensor Hallucis Brevis Muscles. For TrPI or DN of the extensor digitorum brevis and extensor hallucis brevis muscles, the patient is positioned supine. Trigger points are identified by cross-fiber flat palpation and fixed between the clinician's index and middle fingers (Figure 72-96). The needle is directed from medial to lateral into the muscle toward the underlying bone, which the needle typically contacts. The deep fibular nerve and vessels run medial to the extensor hallucis brevis muscle, and therefore, the needle should be directed laterally.

References

1. Dommerholt J, Fernandez-de-Las Penas C. *Trigger Point-dry Needling: An Evidence and Clinical-based Approach*. 1st ed. London, England: Churchill Livingstone; 2013.
2. Simons DG, Travell J, Simons L. *Travell & Simon's Myofascial Pain and Dysfunction: The Trigger Point Manual*. Vol 1. 2nd ed. Baltimore, MD: Williams & Wilkins; 1999.
3. Llamas-Ramos R, Pecos-Martin D, Gallego-Izquierdo T, et al. Comparison of the short-term outcomes between trigger point dry needling and trigger point manual therapy for the management of chronic mechanical neck pain: a randomized clinical trial. *J Orthop Sports Phys Ther*. 2014;44(11): 852-861.
4. Cagnie B, Castelein B, Pollie F, Steelant L, Verhoeyen H, Cools A. Evidence for the use of ischemic compression and dry needling in the management of trigger points of the upper trapezius in patients with neck pain: a systematic review. *Am J Phys Med Rehabil*. 2015;94(7):573-583.
5. De Meulemeester KE, Castelein B, Coppieters I, Barbe T, Cools A, Cagnie B. Comparing trigger point dry needling and manual pressure technique for the management of myofascial neck/shoulder pain: a randomized clinical trial. *J Manipulative Physiol Ther*. 2017;40(1):11-20.
6. Hong CZ, Hsueh TC. Difference in pain relief after trigger point injections in myofascial pain patients with and without fibromyalgia. *Arch Phys Med Rehabil*. 1996;77(11):1161-1166.
7. Dreyer S, Beckworth W. Commonly used medications in procedures. In: Lennard TA, Vivian D, Walkowski S, Singla A, eds. *Pain Procedures in Clinical Practice*. 3rd ed. Philadelphia, PA: Elsevier-Saunders; 2011:5-12.
8. Ay S, Evcik D, Tur BS. Comparison of injection methods in myofascial pain syndrome: a randomized controlled trial. *Clin Rheumatol*. 2010;29(1):19-23.
9. Botwin KP, Patel BC. Electromyographically guided trigger point injections in the cervicothoracic musculature of obese patients: a new and unreported technique. *Pain Physician*. 2007;10(6):753-756.
10. Botwin KP, Sharma K, Saliba R, Patel BC. Ultrasound-guided trigger point injections in the cervicothoracic musculature: a new and unreported technique. *Pain Physician*. 2008;11(6):885-889.
11. Hong CZ. Lidocaine injection versus dry needling to myofascial trigger point. The importance of the local twitch response. *Am J Phys Med Rehabil*. 1994;73(4):256-263.
12. Perreault T, Dunning J, Butts R. The local twitch response during trigger point dry needling: is it necessary for successful outcomes? *J Bodyw Mov Ther*. 2017;21(4):940-947.
13. Liu L, Huang QM, Liu QG, et al. Effectiveness of dry needling for myofascial trigger points associated with neck and shoulder pain: a systematic review and meta-analysis. *Arch Phys Med Rehabil*. 2015;96(5):944-955.
14. Huang QM, Liu L. Wet needling of myofascial trigger points in abdominal muscles for treatment of primary dysmenorrhoea. *Acupunct Med*. 2014;32(4):346-349.
15. Ong J, Claydon LS. The effect of dry needling for myofascial trigger points in the neck and shoulders: a systematic review and meta-analysis. *J Bodyw Mov Ther*. 2014;18(3):390-398.

16. Itoh K, Katsumi Y, Hirota S, Kitakoji H. Randomised trial of trigger point acupuncture compared with other acupuncture for treatment of chronic neck pain. *Complement Ther Med.* 2007;15(3):172-179.
17. Tekin L, Akarsu S, Durmus O, Cakar E, Dincer U, Kiralp MZ. The effect of dry needling in the treatment of myofascial pain syndrome: a randomized double-blinded placebo-controlled trial. *Clin Rheumatol.* 2013;32(3):309-315.
18. Hameroff SR, Crago BR, Blitt CD, Womble J, Kanel J. Comparison of bupivacaine, etidocaine, and saline for trigger-point therapy. *Anesth Analg.* 1981;60(10):752-755.
19. Karadas O, Gul HL, Inan LE. Lidocaine injection of pericranial myofascial trigger points in the treatment of frequent episodic tension-type headache. *J Headache Pain.* 2013;14:44.
20. Yoon SH, Rah UW, Sheen SS, Cho KH. Comparison of 3 needle sizes for trigger point injection in myofascial pain syndrome of upper- and middle-trapezius muscle: a randomized controlled trial. *Arch Phys Med Rehabil.* 2009;90(8):1332-1339.
21. Ga H, Choi JH, Park CH, Yoon HJ. Acupuncture needling versus lidocaine injection of trigger points in myofascial pain syndrome in elderly patients—a randomised trial. *Acupunct Med.* 2007;25(4):130-136.
22. Sola AE, Kuitert JH. Myofascial trigger point pain in the neck and shoulder girdle; report of 100 cases treated by injection of normal saline. *Northwest Med.* 1955;54(9):980-984.
23. Tizes R. Cardiac arrest following routine venipuncture. *JAMA.* 1976;236(16):1846-1847.
24. McEvoy J, Dommerholt J, Rice DA, Holmes L, Groblie C, Fernandez-de-las-Penas C. *Guidelines for Safe Dry Needling Practice.* Dublin, Ireland: Irish Society of Chartered Physiotherapists; 2012.
25. Bachmann S, Colla F, Grobli C, Mungo G, Grobli L, Reilich P. *Swiss Guidelines for Safe Dry Needling Association.* Winterthur, Switzerland: Dry Needling Verband Schweiz; 2014.
26. Travell J. Factors affecting pain of injection. *J Am Med Assoc.* 1955;158(5):368-371.
27. Travell J. Ethyl chloride spray for painful muscle spasm. *Arch Phys Med Rehabil.* 1952;33(5):291-298.
28. Kraus H. The use of surface anesthesia in the treatment of painful motion. *JAMA.* 1941;16:2582-2583.
29. Weeks VD, Travell J. *How to Give Painless Injections. AMA Scientific Exhibits.* New York, NY: Grune & Stratton; 1957:318-322.
30. Fischer AA. New Approaches in Treatment of Myofascial Pain. *Phys Med Rehabil Clin N Am.* 1997;8(1):153-169.
31. Kraus H. *Clinical Treatment of Back and Neck Pain.* New York, NY: McGraw-Hill; 1970.
32. Hong C-Z. Considerations and recommendations regarding myofascial trigger point injection. *J Musculoske Pain.* 1994;2(1):29-59.
33. Fields H. *Core Curriculum for Professional Education of the International Association for the Study of Pain.* Seattle, WA: IASP Press; 1995.
34. Hong C-Z. Myofascial trigger point injection. *Crit Rev Phys Med Rehabil.* 1993;5(2):203-217.
35. Domingo A, Mayoral O, Monterde S, Santafe MM. Neuromuscular damage and repair after dry needling in mice. *Evid Based Complement Alternat Med.* 2013;2013:260806.
36. American Physical Therapy Association. *Physical Therapists and the Performance of Dry Needling: An Educational Resource Paper.* Alexandria, VA: APTA Department of Practice and APTA State Government Affairs; 2012.
37. Martin-Pintado Zugasti A, Rodriguez-Fernandez AL, Garcia-Muro F, et al. Effects of spray and stretch on postneedling soreness and sensitivity after dry needling of a latent myofascial trigger point. *Arch Phys Med Rehabil.* 2014;95(10):1925.e1-1932.e1.
38. Martin-Pintado-Zugasti A, Pecos-Martin D, Rodriguez-Fernandez AL, et al. Ischemic compression after dry needling of a latent myofascial trigger point reduces postneedling soreness intensity and duration. *PM R.* 2015;7(10):1026-1034.
39. Salom-Moreno J, Jimenez-Gomez L, Gomez-Ahufinger V, et al. Effects of Low-Load Exercise on Postneedling-Induced Pain After Dry Needling of Active Trigger Point in Individuals With Subacromial Pain Syndrome. *PM R.* 2017;9(12):1208-1216.
40. Lewit K. The needle effect in the relief of myofascial pain. *Pain.* 1979;6(1):83-90.
41. Budenz AW. Local anesthetics and medically complex patients. *J Calif Dent Assoc.* 2000;28(8):611-619.
42. Giordano CN, Nelson J, Kohen LL, Nijhawan R, Srivastava D. Local anesthesia: evidence, strategies, and safety. *Curr Dermatol Rep.* 2015;4(3):97-104.
43. Eggleston ST, Lush LW. Understanding allergic reactions to local anesthetics. *Ann Pharmacother.* 1996;30(7-8):851-857.
44. Zink W, Graf BM. Local anesthetic myotoxicity. *Reg Anesth Pain Med.* 2004;29(4):333-340.
45. Raphael KG, Klausner JJ, Nayak S, Marbach JJ. Complementary and alternative therapy use by patients with myofascial temporomandibular disorders. *J Orofac Pain.* 2003;17(1):36-41.
46. Iwama H, Akama Y. The superiority of water-diluted 0.25% to neat 1% lidocaine for trigger-point injections in myofascial pain syndrome: a prospective, randomized, double-blinded trial. *Anesth Analg.* 2000;91(2):408-409.
47. Matsumoto AH, Reifsnyder AC, Hartwell GD, Angle JF, Selby JB Jr, Tegtmeyer CJ. Reducing the discomfort of lidocaine administration through pH buffering. *J Vasc Interv Radiol.* 1994;5(1):171-175.
48. Zaiac M, Aguilera SB, Zaulyanov-Scanlan L, Caperton C, Chimento S. Virtually painless local anesthesia: diluted lidocaine proves to be superior to buffered lidocaine for subcutaneous infiltration. *J Drugs Dermatol.* 2012;11(10):e39-e42.
49. Hayward CJ, Nafziger AN, Kohlhepp SJ, Bertino JS Jr. Investigation of bioequivalence and tolerability of intramuscular ceftriaxone injections by using 1% lidocaine, buffered lidocaine, and sterile water diluents. *Antimicrob Agents Chemother.* 1996;40(2):485-487.
50. Travell J. Temporomandibular joint pain referred from muscles of the head and neck. *J Prosthet Dent.* 1960;10:745-763.
51. McMillan AS, Nolan A, Kelly PJ. The efficacy of dry needling and procaine in the treatment of myofascial pain in the jaw muscles. *J Orofac Pain.* 1997;11(4):307-314.
52. Krishnan SK, Benzon HT, Siddiqui T, Canlas B. Pain on intramuscular injection of bupivacaine, ropivacaine, with and without dexamethasone. *Reg Anesth Pain Med.* 2000;25(6):615-619.
53. Misirlioglu TO, Akgun K, Palamar D, Erden MG, Erbilir T. Piriformis syndrome: comparison of the effectiveness of local anesthetic and corticosteroid injections: a double-blinded, randomized controlled study. *Pain Physician.* 2015;18(2):163-171.
54. Venancio Rde A, Alencar FG Jr, Zamperini C. Botulinum toxin, lidocaine, and dry-needling injections in patients with myofascial pain and headaches. *Cranio.* 2009;27(1):46-53.
55. Brennan KL, Allen BC, Maldonado YM. Dry needling versus cortisone injection in the treatment of greater trochanteric pain syndrome: a noninferiority randomized clinical trial. *J Orthop Sports Phys Ther.* 2017;47(4):232-239.
56. Vargas-Schaffer G, Nowakowsky M, Eghtesadi M, Cogan J. Ultrasound-guided trigger point injection for serratus anterior muscle pain syndrome: description of technique and case series. *A A Case Rep.* 2015;5(6):99-102.
57. Steward W, Hughes J, Judovich BD. Ammonium chloride in the relief of pain. *Am J Physiol.* 1940;129:474-475.
58. Bates W. Control of somatic pain. *Am J Surg.* 1943;59:83-86.
59. Choi TW, Park HJ, Lee AR, Kang YK. Referred pain patterns of the third and fourth dorsal interosseous muscles. *Pain Physician.* 2015;18(3):299-304.
60. MacIver MB, Tanelian DL. Activation of C fibers by metabolic perturbations associated with tourniquet ischemia. *Anesthesiology.* 1992;76(4):617-623.
61. Kim MY, Na YM, Moon JH. Comparison of treatment effects of dextrose water, saline, and lidocaine for trigger point injection. *J Korean Acad Rehab Med.* 1997;21(5):967-973.
62. Ettlin T. Trigger point injection treatment with the 5-HT3 receptor antagonist tropisetron in patients with late whiplash-associated disorder. First results of a multiple case study. *Scand J Rheumatol Suppl.* 2004;33(119):49-50.
63. Dahl E, Cohen SP. Perineural injection of etanercept as a treatment for postamputation pain. *Clin J Pain.* 2008;24(2):172-175.
64. Godoy IR, Donahue DM, Torriani M. Botulinum toxin injections in musculoskeletal disorders. *Semin Musculoskelet Radiol.* 2016;20(5):441-452.
65. Mauskop A. The use of botulinum toxin in the treatment of headaches. *Pain Physician.* 2004;7(3):377-387.
66. Davids HR. Botulinum toxin in pain management. https://emedicine.medscape.com/article/325574-overview#a4. Accessed August 31, 2017.
67. Gerwin R. Botulinum toxin treatment of myofascial pain: a critical review of the literature. *Curr Pain Headache Rep.* 2012;16(5):413-422.
68. Soares A, Andriolo RB, Atallah AN, da Silva EM. Botulinum toxin for myofascial pain syndromes in adults. *Cochrane Database Syst Rev.* 2014(7):CD007533.
69. Kilbane C, Ostrem J, Galifianakis N, Grace J, Markun L, Glass GA. Multichannel electromyographic mapping to optimize onabotulinumtoxina efficacy in cervical dystonia. *Tremor Other Hyperkinet Mov (N Y).* 2012;2.
70. American Physical Therapy Association. *Description of Dry Needling in Clinical Practice: An Educational Resource Paper.* In: APTA Public Policy Practice, and Professional Affairs Unit, ed. Alexandria, VA: American Physical Therapy Association; 2013.
71. Fernandez-Carnero J, Gilarranz-de-Frutos L, Leon-Hernandez JV, et al. Effectiveness of different deep dry needling dosages in the treatment of patients with cervical myofascial pain: a pilot RCT. *Am J Phys Med Rehabil.* 2017;96(10):726-733.
72. Koppenhaver SL, Walker MJ, Rettig C, et al. The association between dry needling-induced twitch response and change in pain and muscle function in patients with low back pain: a quasi-experimental study. *Physiotherapy.* 2017;103(2):131-137.
73. Gunn CC. *The Gunn Approach to the Treatment of Chronic Pain, Intramuscular Stimulation for Myofascial Pain of Radiculopathic Origin.* 2nd ed. New York, NY: Churchill Livingston; 1996.
74. Kietrys DM, Palombaro KM, Azzaretto E, et al. Effectiveness of dry needling for upper-quarter myofascial pain: a systematic review and meta-analysis. *J Orthop Sports Phys Ther.* 2013;43(9):620-634.
75. Morihisa R, Eskew J, McNamara A, Young J. Dry needling in subjects with muscular trigger points in the lower quarter: a systematic review. *Int J Sports Phys Ther.* 2016;11(1):1-14.
76. Liu L, Huang QM, Liu QG, et al. Evidence for dry needling in the management of myofascial trigger points associated with low back pain: a systematic review and meta-analysis. *Arch Phys Med Rehabil.* 2018;99(1):144.e2-152.e2.
77. He C, Ma H. Effectiveness of trigger point dry needling for plantar heel pain: a meta-analysis of seven randomized controlled trials. *J Pain Res.* 2017;10:1933-1942.
78. Gattie E, Cleland JA, Snodgrass S. The effectiveness of trigger point dry needling for musculoskeletal conditions by physical therapists: a systematic review and meta-analysis. *J Orthop Sports Phys Ther.* 2017;47(3):133-149.
79. *Dry Needling and Injection for Musculoskeletal and Joint Disorders: A Review of the Clinical Effectiveness, Cost-effectiveness, and Guidelines.* Ottawa, ON: Canadian Agency for Drugs and Technologies in Health; 2016.

80. Chou LW, Kao MJ, Lin JG. Probable mechanisms of needling therapies for myofascial pain control. *Evid Based Complement Alternat Med.* 2012;2012:705327.
81. Cagnie B, Dewitte V, Barbe T, Timmermans F, Delrue N, Meeus M. Physiologic effects of dry needling. *Curr Pain Headache Rep.* 2013;17(8):348.
82. Dommerholt J. Dry needling—peripheral and central considerations. *J Man Manip Ther.* 2011;19(4):223-227.
83. Cerezo-Tellez E, Torres-Lacomba M, Fuentes-Gallardo I, et al. Effectiveness of dry needling for chronic nonspecific neck pain: a randomized, single-blinded, clinical trial. *Pain.* 2016;157(9):1905-1917.
84. Pecos-Martin D, Montanez-Aguilera FJ, Gallego-Izquierdo T, et al. Effectiveness of dry needling on the lower trapezius in patients with mechanical neck pain: a randomized controlled trial. *Arch Phys Med Rehabil.* 2015;96(5):775-781.
85. Travell J. Symposium on mechanism and management of pain syndromes. *Proc Rudolf Virchow Med Soc.* 1957;16:126-136.
86. Cohen H, Pertes R. Chapter 11, Diagnosis and management of facial pain. In: Rachlin ES, ed. *Myofascial Pain and Fibromyalgia: Trigger Point Management.* St. Louis, MO: Mosby; 1994:361-382.
87. Standring S. *Gray's Anatomy: The Anatomical Basis of Clinical Practice.* 41st ed. London, UK: Elsevier; 2015.
88. Gelb H. Chapter 11, Effective management and treatment of the craniomandibular syndrome. In: Gelb H, ed. *Clinical Management of Head, Neck and TMJ Pain and Dysfunction.* Philadelphia, PA: W.B. Saunders; 1977 (pp. 299-314, Fig. 11-61).
89. Koole P, Beenhakker F, de Jongh HJ, Boering G. A standardized technique for the placement of electrodes in the two heads of the lateral pterygoid muscle. *Cranio.* 1990;8(2):154-162.
90. Mesa-Jimenez JA, Sanchez-Gutierrez J, de-la-Hoz-Aizpurua JL, Fernandez-de-las-Penas C. Cadaveric validation of dry needle placement in the lateral pterygoid muscle. *J Manipulative Physiol Ther.* 2015;38(2):145-150.
91. Minerbi A, Ratmansky M, Finestone A, Gerwin R, Vulfsons S. The local and referred pain patterns of the longus colli muscle. *J Bodyw Mov Ther.* 2017;21(2):267-273.
92. Rachlin ES. Chapter 10, Injection of specific trigger points. In: Rachlin ES, ed. *Myofascial Pain and Fibromyalgia.* St. Louis, MO: Mosby; 1994: 197-360.
93. Fernández-de-las-Peñas C, Mesa-Jimenez JA, Paredes-Mancilla JA, Koppenhaver SL, Fernandez-Carnero S. Cadaveric and ultrasonographic validation of needling placement in the cervical multifidus muscle. *J Manipulative Physiol Ther.* 2017;40(5):365-370.
94. Arias-Buria JL, Fernandez-de-Las-Penas C, Palacios-Cena M, Koppenhaver SL, Salom-Moreno J. Exercises and dry needling for subacromial pain syndrome: a randomized parallel-group trial. *J Pain.* 2017;18(1):11-18.
95. Lane E, Clewley D, Koppenhaver S. Complaints of upper extremity numbness and tingling relieved with dry needling of the teres minor and infraspinatus: a case report. *J Orthop Sports Phys Ther.* 2017;47(4):287-292.
96. Seol SJ, Cho H, Yoon DH, Jang SH. Appropriate depth of needle insertion during rhomboid major trigger point block. *Ann Rehabil Med.* 2014;38(1): 72-76.
97. Cummings M, Ross-Marrs R, Gerwin R. Pneumothorax complication of deep dry needling demonstration. *Acupunct Med.* 2014;32(6):517-519.
98. Retrouvey M, Chiodo T, Quidley-Nevares A, Strand J, Goodmurphy C. Use of ultrasound in needle placement in intercostal muscles: a method for increased accuracy in cadavers. *Arch Phys Med Rehabil.* 2013;94(7): 1256-1259.
99. Shanti CM, Carlin AM, Tyburski JG. Incidence of pneumothorax from intercostal nerve block for analgesia in rib fractures. *J Trauma.* 2001;51(3): 536-539.
100. Travell J, Simons DG. *Myofascial Pain and Dysfunction: The Trigger Point Manual.* Vol 2. Baltimore, MD: Williams & Wilkins; 1992.
101. Velazquez-Saornil J, Ruiz-Ruiz B, Rodriguez-Sanz D, Romero-Morales C, Lopez-Lopez D, Calvo-Lobo C. Efficacy of quadriceps vastus medialis dry needling in a rehabilitation protocol after surgical reconstruction of complete anterior cruciate ligament rupture. *Medicine (Baltimore).* 2017;96(17):e6726.

Chapter 73

Manual Therapy Considerations

Timothy J. McMahon, Derek Clewley, César Fernández de las Peñas, Timothy Flynn, Visnja King, and John Sharkey

1. INTRODUCTION

This chapter presents manual therapy techniques that can augment or complement the assessment and treatment of neuromusculoskeletal conditions, myofascial dysfunction, and, specifically, trigger points (TrPs). In no way exhaustive or comprehensive of the breadth of possible manual therapy techniques, this chapter provides an overview regarding the theoretical constructs of each technique and how these techniques may affect TrPs and myofascial dysfunction in regard to patient selection and application. Readers who are interested in an in-depth study of each technique are encouraged to explore more detailed description and application of techniques in other clinical textbooks and continuing education course work.

Manual therapy is defined as "a clinical approach utilizing skilled, specific hands-on techniques, including but not limited to soft-tissue mobilization, manipulation/mobilization, used by appropriate healthcare providers to diagnose and treat soft-tissue and joint structures for the purpose of modulating pain, increasing range of motion, reducing or eliminating soft-tissue inflammation, inducing relaxation, improving contractile and non-contractile tissue repair, extensibility and or stability, facilitating movement, and improving function".[1] Manual therapy is one of the oldest and most influential interventions in medicine dating back to ancient Thai cultures and described on Egyptian papyrus. The manual therapy techniques discussed in this chapter will include mobilization/manipulation, TrP pressure release, postisometric relaxation, strain counterstrain (SCS), neuromuscular therapy, and massage.

2. JOINT MOBILIZATION AND MANIPULATION

2.1. Overview

Joint mobilization is defined by the International Federation of Orthopaedic Manipulative Physical Therapists as "a manual therapy technique comprising a continuum of skilled passive movements to a joint complex that are applied at varying speeds and amplitudes, that may also include a small-amplitude/high-velocity therapeutic movement (manipulation) with the intent to restore optimal motion, function, and/or to reduce pain".[1,2] Manipulation is usually defined as a passive, high-velocity, low-amplitude thrust applied to a joint complex within its anatomic limit with the intent to restore optimal motion, function, and/or reduce pain (Figure 73-1), whereas mobilization is typically utilized to describe nonthrust techniques (Figure 73-2). Readers are referred to Mintken et al[3] for terminology.

Joint mobilization/manipulation has been, historically, an approach intended to resolve painful conditions thought to be related to the targeted joint. This direct pathoanatomic model influenced most of the clinical research, and thus, there is very little evidence for the direct effects of manual therapy on TrPs or myofascial dysfunction. Clinicians usually use joint-biased manual therapy interventions to treat conditions that are thought to be related to a myofascial dysfunction, such as fibromyalgia and other persistent (chronic) pain conditions. Mechanically, it is theorized that treating a joint can reduce the associated myofascial pain in the muscles around the joint, thereby, offering an explanation for the reduction in pain that may be experienced by the patient.[4] There is preliminary evidence supporting that a spinal manipulation can reduce TrP sensitivity in related innervated muscles[5]; however, this study included only latent TrPs.

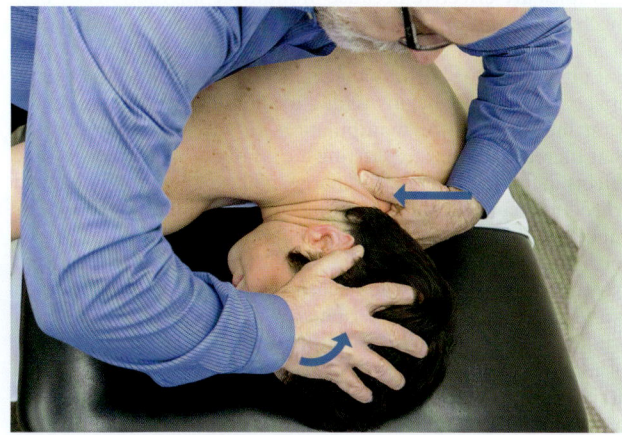

Figure 73-1. Thrust mobilization/manipulation of the cervicothoracic junction.

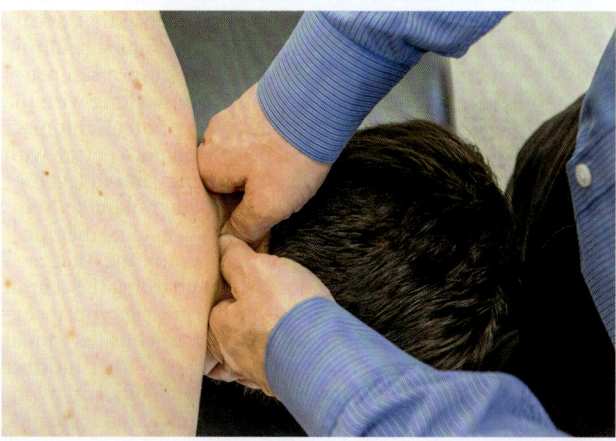

Figure 73-2. Nonthrust mobilization/manipulation of the cervical spine. Posterior-to-anterior-directed force in the mid-cervical spine.

2.2. Mechanisms of Joint-Biased Manual Therapy Interventions

The mechanisms of manual therapy have been a consistent topic researched over the last several years. In relation to high-velocity, low-amplitude manipulation techniques, two basic paradigms explaining their underlying effects have been suggested: biomechanical and neurophysiological.

Traditionally, biomechanical effects of manual therapies, based on palpation or manual identification for positional/movement faults and the choice of technique, were thought to be major determinants to effectiveness and positive therapeutic outcomes. However, because of poor reliability for assessment of the dysfunctional segment(s), demonstration of reduced specificity of the segment treated (including multiple popping sounds outside of the targeted area), and the ability to treat a distal area with positive effects, all help build the case for alternate underlying mechanisms aside from biomechanics.[6] Additionally, the fact that the ability to accurately locate the exact area of treatment is not directly associated to clinical outcomes[7,8] and that the vertebral motions and resulting neuromuscular reflex responses appear to be temporally related to the applied force during a manipulation[9] also reduce the relevance of biomechanical mechanisms as a sole explanation.

In the last decade, more authors have proposed that manual therapies are effective because of multiple interactions of biomechanical and/or neurophysiological responses.[7,10] Bialosky et al[8] described a comprehensive model proposing the potential interaction of both biomechanical and neurophysiological effects. The model begins with a mechanical stimulus, such as joint mobilization or manipulation, to the mechanoreceptors that increase discharge, starting a cascade of neurophysiologic effects including afferent discharge mediated by the spinal cord to reduce pain, alter range of motion, and improve muscular function. This model includes peripheral, spinal, and supraspinal mechanisms. The neurophysiologic mechanisms incorporate the patient's pain experience and beliefs with the complex interaction between the central and peripheral nervous systems.[10] Several studies support these potential neurophysiologic mechanisms of manual therapy. For instance, hypoalgesia and sympathetic activity responses succeeding after the application of different manual therapies are controlled by the periaqueductal gray substance.[11] Additionally, a lessening of temporal summation, which is mediated by the dorsal horn of the spinal cord, has been found when assessing immediate effects on thermal pain sensitivity following spinal manipulation in both healthy people and subjects with low back pain.[11,12]

Peripheral mechanisms may potentially be affected by manual therapy techniques because of the direct influence that occurs following a musculoskeletal injury. When an injury resulting in tissue damage occurs, an inflammatory response ensues that stimulates nociception and a pain response along with the healing process. Studies have demonstrated a potential impact on the inflammatory mediators and peripheral nociceptors with changes in blood and serum levels of cytokines, blood levels of beta-endorphin, anandamide, N-palmitoylethanolamide, serotonin, and endogenous cannabinoids following manual therapy.[13]

Pickar[14] also theorized that manual therapy may act as a counter irritant for pain modulation by "bombarding the central nervous system with sensory input from the muscle proprioceptors" which in turn demonstrates the need to consider spinal cord–mediated mechanism in manual therapy. Other indirect findings of spinal-mediated mechanisms include bilateral hypoalgesic effects, decreased afferent discharge in related segments, motor neuron pool activity, and changes in muscle activation.[10]

In addition to spinal-mediated mechanisms, supraspinal mechanisms have been also demonstrated to impact the pain experience.[15] The structures involved in the pain experience include the anterior cingulate cortex, amygdala, periaqueductal gray, and rostral ventromedial medulla. Current evidence supports that manual therapy is able to activate supraspinal mechanisms.[11] For instance, a significant decrease in the amplitude of somatosensory-evoked potentials following cervical spine manipulation has been reported.[16]

Other variables that may impact the supraspinal mechanisms may include patient expectation, placebo, and psychosocial factors (see Chapter 5). Patient expectation has been shown to influence spinal manipulation–induced hypoalgesia with similar responses to those presented to patients in either a positive, neutral, or negative expectation.[6]

2.3. Patient and Intervention Selection

Typically, manual therapy interventions, including joint mobilization/manipulation, have been applied for the correction of hypomobility or malalignment with the basis of biomechanical effects; however, current evidence provides information that manual therapy may in fact provide an effect on the nervous system and in the spinal cord directly for mediation of pain. Because the choice of technique does not correlate to clinical outcomes,[7] there may be a freedom to utilize manual therapy from a neurophysiological point of view rather than from a biomechanical point of view to provide a change in a patient's pain processing and in turn improve clinical outcomes and function. Nevertheless, the application of manual therapy interventions, such as spinal manipulation, should be integrated into a comprehensive clinical reasoning process on the basis of the neuroscience paradigm.

Impairments can take several forms, including, but not limited to, range of motion, strength, pain, and function. Any assessment should include palpation for TrPs along with the assessment of joint dysfunction.[4] These findings must be correlated to the patient's symptoms. By establishing baseline impairment values, a clinician can assess intervention effectiveness, both within session and between sessions. This assessment allows the clinician to better determine the effectiveness of an intervention, even if the theoretical construct does not explain the potential benefit. Additionally, pain associated with a musculoskeletal dysfunction may be caused by both muscle and joint tissue dysfunctions.[4] Managing a potential joint-related problem (ie, loss of range of motion due to a joint issue) with myofascial approaches may provide benefit. Likewise, muscular disturbances (ie, myofascial dysfunction) may respond to thrust manipulation.[5] Therefore, it is important to determine clinical features and physical musculoskeletal impairments in a patient before selecting a manual therapy approach. There is increasing evidence supporting that multimodal approaches including both joint-biased and muscle-biased interventions are more effective than either intervention alone.

A ritualistic aspect of manual therapy interventions exists that involves patient–therapist communication and the "laying on of hands." Furthermore, manual therapy is rarely provided in a vacuum, rather it is a component of a comprehensive treatment program that at a minimum includes patient education and exercise. Therefore, separating out the individual contributions of all of the factors in a patient encounter and finding out how each relates to patient outcomes is often a difficult task. Patients frequently have a positive view of manual therapy. Specifically, it has been shown that there is a significant relationship between patient expectations and outcomes, with more than 80% of patients with neck complaints expecting that manual therapy will provide relief from symptoms, prevent disability, and improve activity level and sleep.[17] Further, positive patient expectations toward manipulation demonstrated prognostic factors to predict patient outcomes.[18]

Ultimately, because of the paucity of research performed on joint-biased interventions for myofascial dysfunction, the decision to use joint mobilizations, including both thrust and nonthrust approaches, is mainly based on a clinical reasoning. Nonetheless, there is sufficient evidence for the selection of joint mobilization techniques for what is presumed to be a myofascial dysfunction including the identification of impairments that might be a factor in influencing the condition. These impairments have been identified in a thorough clinical examination that includes joint range of motion and the assessment of joint mobility. Furthermore, after performing a joint-directed intervention for a myofascial dysfunction, it is in the best interest of the patient for the clinician to reassess both the joint impairment and the presumed myofascial dysfunction.

2.4. Joint-Biased Interventions and Management of Myofascial Dysfunction

Scientific literature investigating joint-biased interventions for TrP dysfunction is limited, although the joint has been implicated in myofascial dysfunction.[4] The following section describes some of the research integrating joint-biased and muscle-biased interventions taking the head and the neck as an example.

Neck pain, a condition that is heterogeneous in nature, is often treated by clinicians utilizing a manual therapy approach. Recent clinical practice guidelines support the use of TrP or muscle-biased approaches for the management of neck pain.[19] Furthermore, there exists a large amount of literature advocating the use of joint-biased manual therapy approaches for a number of different types of neck disorders.[20] For instance, the upper cervical spine (ie, C0/C1, C1/C2, and C2/C3 joints) has been considered responsible for the development of significant impairment including neck pain, headaches, and orofacial pain. These joints have also been identified as possible causes of TrPs in the craniocervical region leading to some of the aforementioned regions that can be painful. In this scenario, the upper portion of the trapezius is a muscle that can easily develop active TrPs. Thrust manipulation of the upper and middle cervical spine has been shown to reduce pain pressure sensitivity in the upper fibers of the trapezius muscle and may be considered when targeting treatment of this muscle for neck pain and upper extremity dysfunction.[5] The use of thrust manipulation to the cervical spine has been shown to reduce pain pressure thresholds for individuals experiencing neck pain, further justifying the consideration of using thrust techniques for neck pain.[21] Therefore, a combined approach including both myofascial-directed approaches with joint mobilization may be effective, especially if the patient exhibits TrPs in some of the surrounding musculature of the neck.

Orofacial pain is also thought, to some extent, to be associated with both myofascial and joint dysfunctions. Joint range of motion associated with jaw pain may be improved with a myofascial treatment approach. A systematic review concluded that a onetime myofascial technique was shown to improve range of motion of the mandible; however, the quality of evidence was low with a high risk of bias.[22] Nevertheless, a onetime treatment of a myofascial technique is not a pragmatic approach for improving range of motion or any symptom, and typical clinical practice will incorporate a variety of treatments on the basis of the patient's impairments. A multimodal approach is, in fact, supported by different systematic reviews regarding this topic.[23,24] Therefore, it is worth considering both approaches, particularly because of the dual nature of temporomandibular pain disorders (eg, joint and myofascial). Additionally, clinicians are advised to treat patients using a regional interdependent approach, especially for both orofacial and neck pain. By treating the cervical spine with joint mobilizations (ie, nonthrust techniques), one may expect to have improved orofacial pain symptoms.[25] The evidence is supportive for incorporating both thrust and nonthrust techniques for the cervical and upper cervical spine for patients with orofacial pain to improve objective measures typically associated with jaw region myofascial dysfunction, eg, pain pressure threshold and the assessment of TrPs.[26]

It is important to consider that only a small number of musculoskeletal conditions have been presented here because of limited evidence related to the effectiveness of joint-biased interventions for myofascial dysfunction. Joint mobilization or manipulation is not a panacea treatment, and explanations for benefit are primarily theoretical. Even so, the evidence for joint-biased interventions can be conflicting for a number of conditions. Most studies investigating joint-biased approaches have used this intervention as part of a comprehensive treatment plan, similar to studies that investigate myofascial treatment approaches. In a clinical context, these interventions, ie, joint mobilizations and myofascial treatments, are often part of a multimodal treatment approach. However, a patient in the early phase of treatment may be best managed using one category of manual therapy interventions to enable the clinician to ascertain which approach was most effective.

3. TRIGGER POINT PRESSURE RELEASE

3.1. Overview

Several muscle-biased manual therapies are advocated for the management of TrPs. The term "TrP pressure release" has replaced the concept of ischemic compression used in the first edition of this book.[27] The first systematic review analyzing the available evidence was published in 2005 and found a few trials investigating muscle-biased manual therapy for the management of TrPs.[28] A more recent meta-analysis published concluded that muscle-biased manual therapies, mostly those focusing on TrPs, are effective for decreased pain sensitivity where there is a rationale for its use.[29,30] Clinical evidence and the nature of TrPs indicate that, when applying digital pressure to a TrP to inactivate it, there is no need to exert sufficient pressure to produce ischemia, as previously suggested.[31] Because the core of the TrP is already hypoxic surrounded by increased tissue oxygen tension, there is no reason to expect that additional ischemia as such would be helpful. Treatment needs to be directed at the release of the contracted sarcomeres of the TrPs. It is clinically important to consider that the term "ischemic" is associated with the presence of self-reported pain by the patient during the compression intervention.

Simons[31] proposed that compressing the sarcomeres by direct pressure in a vertical or perpendicular manner may equalize the length of the sarcomeres in the TrP and consequently decrease the pain; however, this notion has not been scientifically investigated. Other hypotheses suggest that pain relief from direct pressure may result from reactive hyperemia within the TrP or a spinal reflex mechanism for the relief of muscle tension.[32] It is almost sure that different mechanisms are involved concurrently in this process.

3.2. Patient and Intervention Selection

Different compression techniques have been described depending on the amount of pressure, the duration of application, the position of the muscle (shortened/lengthened), or the presence/absence of pain during the intervention. Trigger point pressure release techniques employ the barrier release concept in which tissue resistance is noted and released before more intense pressure is applied.[33] The pressure release approach seems to be equally effective clinically and is not likely to produce appreciable additional ischemia. In fact, Hou et al[32] found that low pressure below pain threshold for a prolonged period (90 seconds) or high pressure over pain threshold (pain tolerance) for a shorter period (30 seconds) was equally effective for decreasing pressure pain sensitivity over TrPs. Therefore, TrP pressure release is tailored to the needs of the individual's muscles, is less uncomfortable, and, therefore, is more likely to be preferred by the patient. The patient learns what optimal pressure feels like for subsequent self-pressure release treatment for home management. The barrier release approach, however, does require a higher-order skill of manual therapy.

Therefore, in clinical practice, the pressure level, duration of application, and position of the muscle are determined on the basis of the sensitizing mechanisms of the patient and the degree of irritability of the tissue. In a patient with a low degree of sensitization, more intense and/or painful techniques can be applied. Nevertheless, Gay et al[29] found that the intensity of pressure applied during muscle-biased techniques may be an important parameter for producing a positive effect in some patients. Therefore, a thorough clinical reasoning approach should be applied when deciding the amount and duration of the muscle-biased intervention on the basis of the findings of the physical examination.

Clinicians should also consider applying intentional consecutive sessions to the same patient instead of a single hard session. This hypothesis has been supported by a recent study suggesting that TrP manual therapy does not exhibit decreased tolerance to repetitive applications because both single and multiple applications decreased the sensitivity to pressure at the TrP.[34]

3.3. Clinical Application

To apply TrP pressure release, the clinician lengthens the muscle to the point of increasing resistance within the comfort zone of the patient and then applies gentle, gradually increasing pressure on the TrP until the finger encounters a definite increase in tissue resistance (engages the barrier) (Figure 73-3). At that point, the patient may feel a degree of discomfort but should not experience pain. This pressure is maintained (but not increased) until the clinician senses relief of tension under the palpating finger. The palpating finger increases pressure enough to take up the tissue slack and to engage a new barrier (the finger "follows" the releasing tissue). The clinician again maintains only light pressure until more of the muscle tension releases under the finger. During this period, the clinician may change the direction of pressure to achieve better results. This process of TrP pressure release can be repeated for each band of taut muscle fibers in that muscle. The virtue of this technique is that it is painless and imposes no additional strain on the TrP, and thereby avoids aggravating the symptoms.

In addition to simply taking up the slack in the muscle before beginning the procedure, the entire muscle can be maintained at a slack-free length throughout the process. Release of the TrP may be further enhanced by occasionally performing a contract-relax maneuver alternated with reciprocal inhibition. The goal is to release the contracture knots in the TrP and release the tension they cause in the muscle fibers comprising the taut band.

The barrier release approach may fail to afford relief because of several factors such as the following: (1) the TrP is too irritable to tolerate any additional mechanical stimulation; (2) the clinician misjudged the pressure required to reach the barrier; (3) the clinician pressed too hard, causing pain and autonomic responses with involuntary tensing by the patient; and (4) the patient has perpetuating factors that make the TrPs hyperirritable and resistant to manual treatment.

Obviously, the effectiveness of this passive approach can often be enhanced by including supplemental techniques. These additional techniques should not cause the patient any further discomfort. For instance, a recent meta-analysis has reported that exercise has small-to-moderate effects on pain intensity at short term in people with myofascial pain and that a combination of different types of exercises seems to achieve greater benefits.[35]

4. MUSCLE ENERGY TECHNIQUES AND STRETCHING INTERVENTIONS

4.1. Overview

There are many methods of applying a stretching procedure: passive stretching (where the clinician passively stretches the muscle without the patient participating), active stretching (where the patient actively stretches the muscle without participation of the clinician), spray and stretch, or postisometric relaxation.[27,33] The main differences between these procedures are the intensity of the stretching, the involvement or noninvolvement of the patient, and the inclusion or noninclusion of the muscle contraction. The muscle energy technique (MET) most commonly used in clinical practice is the postisometric relaxation.[33]

4.2. Patient and Intervention Selection

A stretching intervention can be applied to almost any muscle. Postisometric relaxation can be used for any muscle that can be lengthened and resisted isometrically, without pain if possible. Postisometric relaxation should be a gentle technique of lengthening of the muscle tissue and not an aggressive stretching. As it has been previously commented, the clinician should choose the application of a muscle energy intervention in any patient with a soft-tissue restriction in any part of the body.

4.3. Clinical Application

For a postisometric relaxation intervention, the muscle is brought to a position of submaximal length without stretch. The subject performs an isometric contraction with a force between 10% and 25% maximum voluntary contraction, with the clinician providing resistance for 6 to 10 seconds (Figure 73-4). It is hypothesized that if contractions performed with a strength greater than 30% of force is achieved, a recruitment of phasic muscle fibers (fast-twitch muscle fibers) occurs.

Once the muscle has relaxed, the clinician takes up slack in the muscle again to further lengthen the muscle without pain. The time for relaxation may vary from a few seconds to half a minute. Sensing the relaxation of muscle is essential for the clinician to maximize lengthening without causing reflex tightening of the muscle. Postisometric relaxation can be applied after other TrP interventions, such as dry needling or direct pressure release techniques, for augmenting the effects on the taut band and the TrP area.

Relaxation of the muscle can be enhanced with a variety of techniques. If relaxation of a muscle is unsatisfactory, the isometric contraction portion of the postisometric relaxation technique can be lengthened to 30 seconds.[36] Diaphragmatic

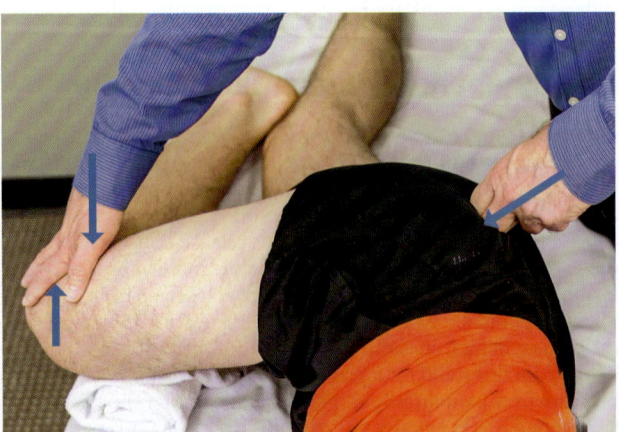

Figure 73-3. Gluteus maximus TrPs pressure release. The clinician applies gentle pressure to the TrPs in the gluteus maximus muscle. The patient is asked to gently lift the knee into the clinician's hand to activate the fibers in the gluteus maximus muscle below the clinician's knuckle.

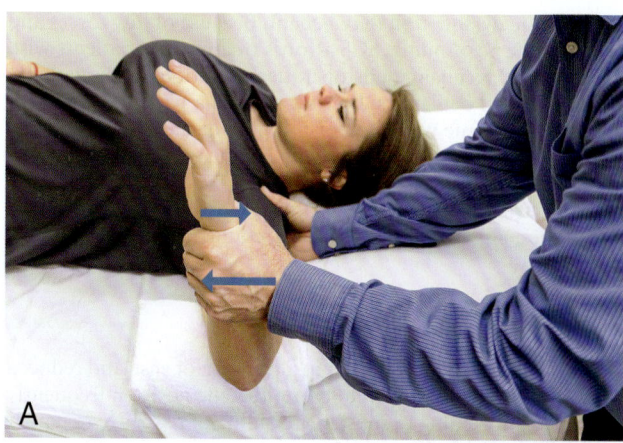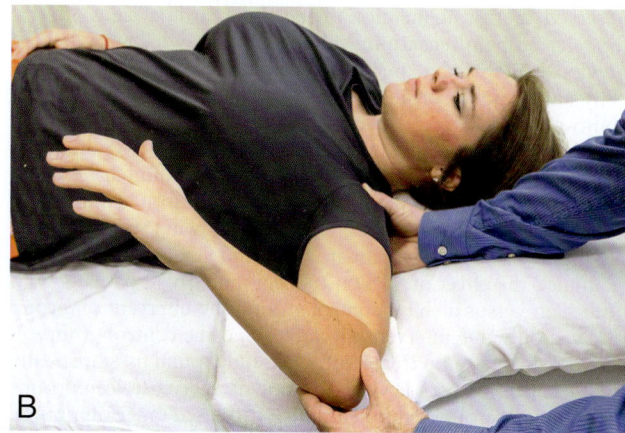

Figure 73-4. Postisometric relaxation for the infraspinatus muscle. A, Starting position. The clinician resists a gentle contraction by the patient in external rotation motion and holds for 6 seconds. B, Following the contraction, the patients slowly relaxes, letting the arm fall slowly into internal rotation until the barrier is reached. The process is repeated three to five times.

breathing, coupled with postisometric relaxation, can also be helpful. Combining postisometric relaxation with effective and relaxed breathing can enhance its effectiveness because inhalation facilitates contraction, whereas exhalation facilitates relaxation.[33] Lewit[33] referred to the phenomena as respiratory synkinesis: movement in one direction is coupled with inhalation and movement in opposite direction coupled with relaxation in exhalation. Refer to Chapter 45 for details regarding diaphragmatic breathing.

Eye movements can also be combined with postisometric relaxation because focusing vision in a specific direction can facilitate cervical movement in the same direction. Obviously, this will be most helpful on interventions applied to the cervical spine. Box 73-1 summarizes some key features for providing METs.

5. STRAIN COUNTERSTRAIN

5.1. Overview

Strain counterstrain (SCS) is a positional release technique that can be characterized as an indirect manual technique. Indirect techniques are manual therapy techniques that move the patient to a position of ease usually away from protective barriers. Jones et al[37] defined SCS as "a passive positional procedure that places the body in a position of greatest comfort, thereby relieving pain by reduction and arrest of inappropriate proprioceptive activity that maintains somatic dysfunction."

Proposed physiologic mechanisms for SCS have focused primarily on aberrant proprioceptive input from agonist and antagonistic muscle spindles and other sensory input as well as proposed changes in local circulation and inflammatory processes. The original theoretical construct of the neurophysiologic mechanism is referred to as proprioceptive theory, an osteopath paradigm.[38]

The proprioceptive theory postulates that strain activities around a joint or muscle cause agonist muscle spindles to fire rapidly, whereas antagonistic muscle spindles have a reduced output because of rapid shortening. The reduced output of antagonistic muscle spindles stimulates the nervous system through efferent output to cause the intrafusal fibers of muscle spindles to increase tension, thereby causing a resulting gain in gamma motor neuron output on return to a new resting position of the joint and muscle. The resulting effect is increased facilitative tension of agonist and antagonist muscles around a joint. The altered tension and sensitivity of muscle spindles can theoretically cause potential alterations in strength and motor control. Nevertheless, evidence of the proprioceptive theory is sometimes conflicting. Howell et al[39] investigated the effects of SCS on patients presenting with Achilles tendonitis compared with a control group who received sham SCS on stretch reflex and H-reflex (Hoffman reflex). This study identified a statistically significant reduction in the stretch reflex in the intervention group compared with matched controls, but the H-reflex did not demonstrate significant between-group changes. Additionally, those patients in the intervention group reported reduced soreness in the Achilles tendon, leaving open the possibility of reduction of pain response having a potential effect on the stretch reflex responses. In another study of foot and ankle application of SCS, Wynn et al[40] investigated the stretch and Hoffman reflexes and clinical outcomes of subjects with plantar fasciitis. The results of this study did not demonstrate differences in stretch or H-reflex responses, but did improve plantar flexion torque and reduced pain.

An important and common question from clinicians is what is the difference between a tender point, as described by Jones et al[37] in SCS, and myofascial TrPs. Jones et al[37] defined tender points as the area of hypersensitivity four times greater than normal. The tender point is approximately 1 cm in diameter and may be located on muscle, ligament, fascia, bone, or tendon. As it can be

---

Box 73-1 Standards and guidelines for muscle energy technique (MET)

- Assess range of motion before initiating the technique.
- Reiterate the importance of producing a mild contraction to the patient.
- No pain should be felt during or after an MET.
- Inform the patient of possible posttreatment symptoms—occasional soreness.
- Recommend the use of cryotherapy posttreatment, ie, coolant gels, cold sprays, cold water, etc.
- METs can be applied on pregnant women, but care should be taken, and muscles should be brought only through their functional range of motion.
- It is the therapist's responsibility to be aware of the contraindications and appropriate use of METs.

observed, there is no mention to one of the cardinal signs of TrPs, the referred pain sensation. Myofascial TrPs, which are defined previously in this text, are located within the taut band of muscle belly and may be considered active or latent depending on the ability of the TrP to reproduce the symptoms of the patient or not.

Lewis et al[41] examined the short-term effects of SCS on quantitative sensory measures at tender points of the lumbar region in subjects with low back pain. The results demonstrated immediate increase in pain pressure threshold (PPT) following SCS treatment, but the effect was not evident at 24, 48, and 96 hours. Klein et al[42] examined the effect of SCS on cervical mobility in patients with neck pain versus a sham control group. The intervention group received only one intervention of SCS and the control group received matched sham treatment. This study found no statistically significant differences in cervical spine mobility between groups because both groups exhibited similar increased range of motion. Similarly, the few studies that have investigated the reliability and validity of SCS tender points assessment have also shown conflicting results. Wong et al[43] examined the presence of tender points on the hip area in a sample of healthy subjects and found low levels of reliability and validity. The treatment group did demonstrate a reduced pain of tender points compared with a control group. McPartland and Goodridge[44] compared the reliability of both SCS tender points and traditional osteopathic examination procedures of the mid-to-upper cervical spine in patients with neck pain. The results demonstrated 72% agreement between examiners ($K = 0.45$) supporting moderate strength of agreement. The study included only posterior and anterior cervical tender points from C3 and above.

Additionally, some studies have also investigated the potential effects of SCS on identified myofascial TrPs despite separate theoretical constructs for SCS (mainly focused on tender points). Ibanez-Garcia et al[45] compared the effects of SCS versus a control group on latent TrPs in the masseter muscle in asymptomatic subjects. The intervention group experienced improved range of motion and increases in pain pressure thresholds compared with the control group. In a separate study by Rodríguez-Blanco et al[46] the SCS efficacy was compared with postisometric relaxation versus a control group in treating latent TrPs in the masseter muscle in asymptomatic subjects. The results of this study demonstrated that the postisometric relaxation technique showed significant improvement in active mouth opening, whereas the SCS group did not.

5.2. Patient and Intervention Selection

The advantage for SCS against other compression manual therapies is that it is pain-free and the technique does not involve lengthening of the affected muscle. In fact, patients in both acute and chronic dysfunction may benefit. Because of low forces and comfortable positioning, SCS affords treatment of patients with osteoporosis, pregnancy, postoperative conditions, hypermobility syndrome, and pediatrics. For instance, in a patient with fibromyalgia syndrome with high excitability of the central nervous system and the presence of allodynia, SCS may be a good first-line manual intervention for avoiding temporal summation of pain. Once the treatment sessions progress, more direct compression techniques, eg, TrP pressure release, could also be used.

5.3. Clinical Application

With SCS, the patient is placed in a position of ease and reduced tenderness of identifiable tender points. The position frequently requires a shortening of muscle or folding of tissues over tender points. This position is maintained for a minimum of 90 seconds (Figure 73-5). During the 90-second hold, the clinician monitors the tender points with gentle palpation. Small adjustments can be made to maximize the reduction in tenderness and tone of the tender points. The patient is returned to neutral positioning slowly so as not to stimulate protective muscle guarding.

In regard to the duration of SCS treatment, Dr Jones experimented with varying duration of the technique and was able to reduce the position of release to 90 seconds.[37] Less than 90 seconds resulted in some return to the prior level of hypersensitivity. When the position was held for at least 90 seconds, the hypersensitivity of the original point was significantly diminished. He defined a successful treatment as a reduction in tender point pain by 70% compared with initial palpation. Theoretically, the duration of sustained positioning may have significance with the latency involved to reduce aberrant input from proprioceptors, but this has not been scientifically confirmed.

6. NEUROMUSCULAR THERAPY

6.1. Overview

Neuromuscular techniques (NMTs) refer to the manual application of digital pressure or strokes, most commonly applied through finger, thumb, or elbow contact targeting soft tissues (Figure 73-6). These digital contacts can have either a diagnostic (assessment) or therapeutic objective, and the degree of pressure employed varies considerably between the therapist and the modes of application. The clinical reasoning for the application of NMT is based on a potential role of the fascia tissue in the development or perpetuation of TrPs. It seems that the complex nature of the

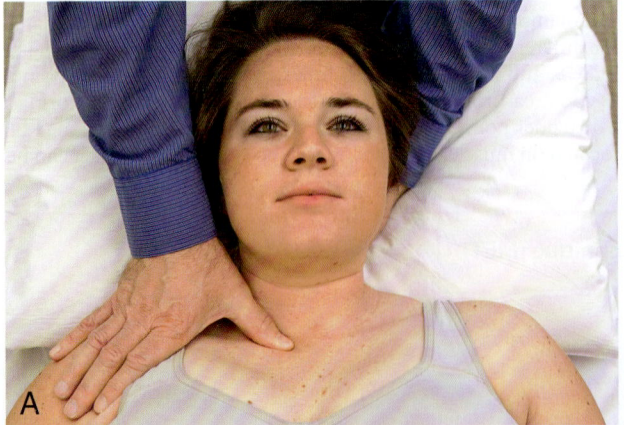 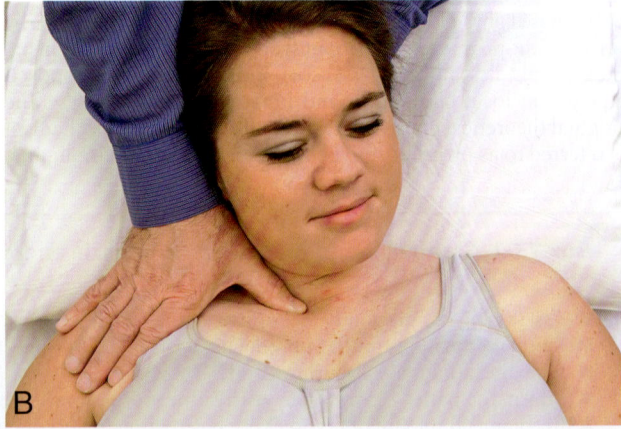

Figure 73-5. Strain counterstrain positional release technique for the right Anterior Cervical (AC7) (sternocleidomastoid muscle). A, Starting position with the clinicians thumb between the sternocleidomastoid clavicular and sternal heads at the clavicle. B, The head is moved into flexion, side bending toward and rotation away from the side to be treated.

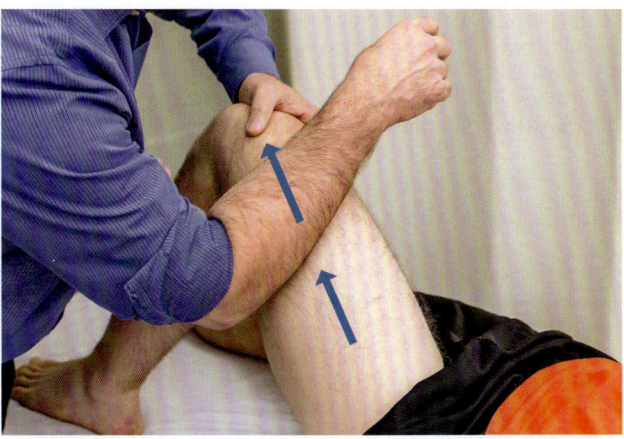

Figure 73-6. Neuromuscular therapy technique for the vastus lateralis muscle.

fascia serves to provide a helical medium for forces generated within muscle fibers. Such forces spread to neighboring muscles and are propagated to various fasciae more globally including the skin surface via specialized fascial thickenings called skin ligaments. Fascia is replete with a wide range of specialized mechanoreceptors, including spindle cells, which are activated by movement, no matter the intensity. The viscosity of the deep fascia can alter and influence the gliding potential and function of the associated muscles because of increased viscosity of the hyaluronic acid, creating friction and resistance to normal motion. This in turn inhibits proprioception and muscle function.[47] Therefore, in such a scenario, fascial restrictions can be perpetuating factors in the etiology and pathophysiology of TrPs. This hypothesis is consistent with a previous theory suggesting that muscle fibers should evolve from the term "protein of contraction" to a more complex and integrated biotensegrity model.[48]

The application of NMT over a TrP can provide a mechanical load leading to both a lowering of the viscosity of the hyaluronic acid and myofascial tension by returning normal gliding to thickened tissues overlying muscles.[47] These changes are relevant because it has been proposed that targeting the viscoelasticity of the connective tissues is important to modify specialized nociceptors within the fascia. As a result of increased thixotropic densification in myofascial tissues, mechanoreceptors change shape and consequentially lead to poorly coordinated muscle contractions, heightened spindle activation, reduced motor control, and myofascial pain.[47] Therefore, NMT can provide an indirect management technique to the surrounding structure of the TrP leading to successful outcomes without overtaxing the patient. In fact, preliminary evidence suggests that NMT applied to latent TrPs can be effective for increasing range of motion and decreasing pain sensitivity.[45]

6.2. Patient and Intervention Selection

Neuromuscular therapy (NMT) can be applied to any patient with either acute or chronic pain. Nevertheless, it is commonly accepted that NMT interventions should not be applied directly to the injured tissues within the first 72 hours following the injury, as this would tend to encourage increased blood flow to the already congested tissues, reducing the natural splinting that is required in this phase of recovery.[49] After 72 hours, NMT may be carefully applied to the injured tissues and applications to the supporting structures and muscles involved in possible compensating patterns. The same clinical reasoning approach should be applied when an active TrP is responsible or associated with the symptoms of the patient.

There is no specific rationale for applying an NMT before or after any other muscle-biased or joint-biased intervention. For instance, NMT could be applied before a pressure release or dry needling technique applied specifically for inactivating TrPs. It can also be applied after these interventions for reducing postneedling soreness. Similarly, in a patient with stiff cervical muscles, a spinal mobilization may be painful, and NMT could be applied first to reduce muscle tension, thus facilitating the application of a joint-biased intervention. The clinician should be able to determine the most proper application of the different manual therapy approaches for each particular patient on the basis of a sound clinical reasoning approach.

6.3. Clinical Application

The most important aspects to consider during an NMT technique are the pressure and the speed of the strokes. Clinically, it is proposed that the pressure should be adapted to the texture, stiffness, and character of the underlying tissue. Therefore, the pressure applied during an NMT is not consistent because the character and texture of tissue is always variable. The second aspect is the speed of the stroke. Speed should be adapted, similarly as with pressure, to the texture of the tissue and the presence or absence of pain. Unless the tissue being treated is excessively tender, the gliding stroke usually recommended covers 3 to 4 in (8-10 cm) per second. However, if the tissue is sensitive, a slower pace and reduced pressure is suggested. It is important to develop a moderate gliding speed in order to feel texture and resistance in the tissues. Movement that is too rapid may cause excessive pain or discomfort for the patient. A moderate speed will allow for numerous repetitions that will significantly increase blood flow and soften the fascia for further manipulation. Nevertheless, the speed should be adapted to each patient during each treatment session. Box 73-2 summarizes some practical aspects to consider during the application of NMT.

Some authors have proposed the application of NMT into a specific sequenced series of manual interventions.[49] In fact, these authors described the Integrated Neuromuscular Inhibition Technique consisting of a "logical" sequence, which incorporates

---

Box 73-2 General standards and guidelines during neuromuscular treatment

- Avoid treating too many muscles in a single treatment; limit treatment to between three and five muscles in one clinical session.
- Drag palpation: Fingers or a combination of fingers and thumb are used to locate the TrP and to identify key anatomic landmarks. Making light contact to the skin, without deformation, drag the digit over a 4-in area taking no more than 1 second per sweep. Drag the digit in all directions seeking out areas that feel tense or where sliding is restricted. Other tools, such as knuckles or elbow, can also be used if the sensitivity of the patient permits.
- Regular communication with the patient is advised during the treatment, ensuring that feedback and information is received from the patient.
- Look for nonverbal signs, such as facial expression, breath holding, and/or clenching.
- The most superficial tissues are usually treated before the deeper layers.
- The proximal portions of an extremity should be treated before the distal portions.
- When multiple areas of dysfunction and pain are present, treat the most proximal, most medial, and most painful tissue first avoiding overtreating the patient as a whole as well as the individual tissues.

SCS, together with pressure release, MET, and subsequent toning of inhibited myofascial structures. The application of all these techniques is specific to the myofascial structures targeted and involves finely tuned movement within motions of ease. Additional applications such as spray and stretch or the use of topical creams can be included if appropriate. This protocol has been found to be effective for decreasing pain in individuals with upper trapezius TrPs.[50] An example of the application of the Integrated Neuromuscular Inhibition Technique over the sternocleidomastoid muscle is described in Box 73-3 and Figure 73-7A to D.

Box 73-3 Integrated Neuromuscular Inhibition Technique application to the sternocleidomastoid muscle

Step 1: Identify TrPs in the sternocleidomastoid muscle utilizing cross-fiber pincer palpation (Figure 73-7A).
Step 2: Identify the current pain level caused by digital palpation of the TrP.
Step 3: Apply repeated cyclical pressure release for 5 seconds on and 2 seconds off until the patient reports a noticeable reduction in the pain. This can typically take five or more cycles.
Step 4: Apply sufficient digital pressure to warrant a score of 8 up to 10 on the pain scale used earlier.
Step 5: Position the targeted myofascial structure in a manner that significantly reduces the perceived pain reported by the patient between 0 and 3/10. This may involve fine-tuning the movements in the sagittal plane stacked on movement in the frontal plane stacked on movement in the transverse plane (in any order). Distraction or compression can be employed in addition to respiratory techniques (Figure 73-7B).
Step 6: Hold this position for up to one and half minutes, remembering to release the digital compression of the TrPs after 6 seconds. The fingers and thumb can remain in place to confirm a reduction in the tissue stiffness.
Step 7: Postisometric relaxation: The patient is asked to provide a mild contraction of the targeted tissues (Figure 73-7C). This is a crucial phase of the procedure. It is imperative to maintain the structures in place. Hold this contraction for approximately 10 to 12 seconds. The patient should avoid holding the breath. Stretching is not the objective but rather to reestablish normal physiologic pain-free range of motion.
Step 8: Repeat the procedure if required.
Step 9: Alternative to Step 7. If the patient reports that contraction of the targeted myofascial structures is too painful, the opposite structures can be used by having the patient "push" the head into the hands of the therapist (reciprocal inhibition) for 10 to 12 seconds (Figure 73-7D).
Step 10: Reassess to ensure all TrPs have been eradicated.

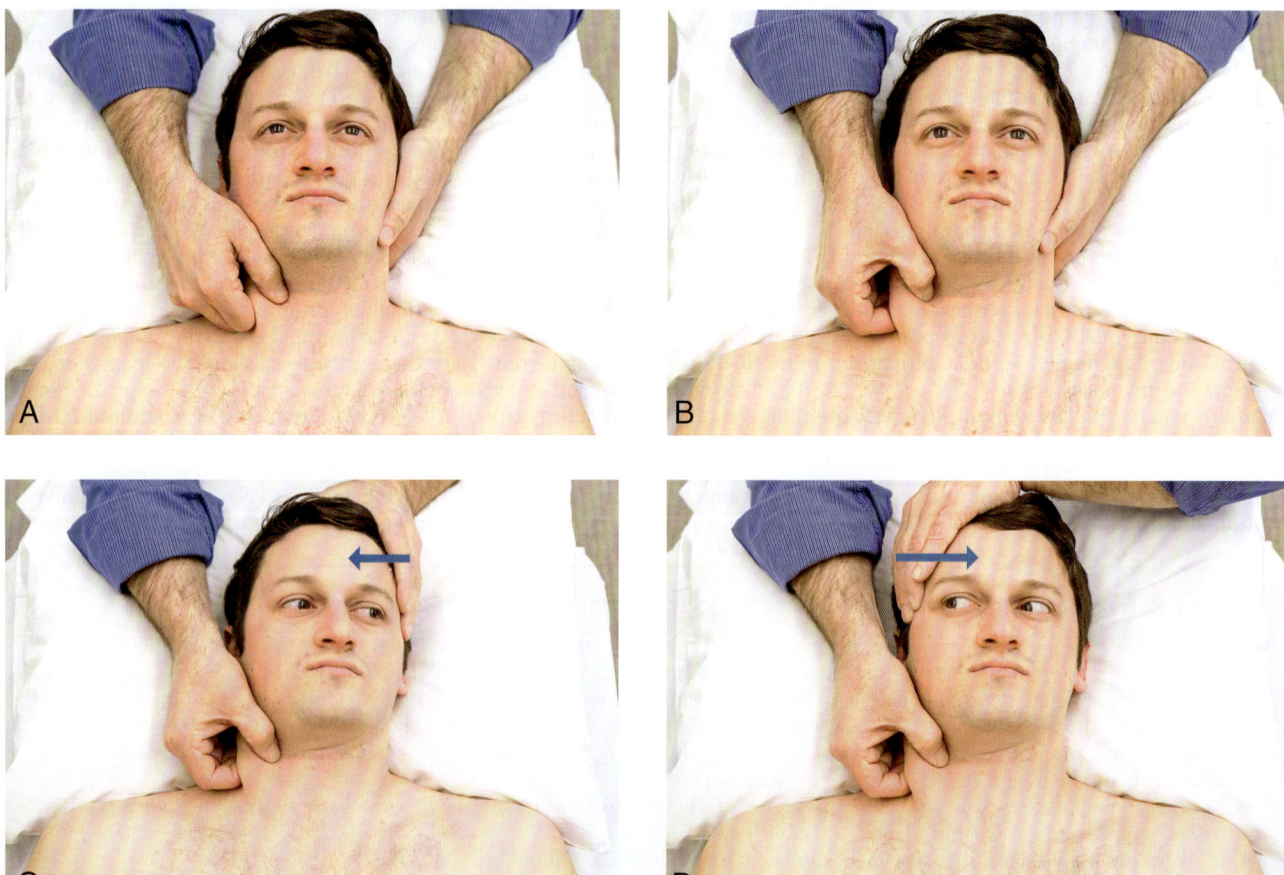

Figure 73-7. Integrated Neuromuscular Inhibition Technique application to the sternocleidomastoid (SCM) muscle. A, Cross-fiber pincer palpation to find TrPs. B, Distraction of SCM with respiratory technique. C, Postisometric relaxation. The clinician resists (arrow) gentle left rotation followed by relaxation. D, Reciprocal inhibition. The clinician resists (arrow) right rotation to achieve relaxation of the right sternocleidomastoid muscle.

7. DEEP-STROKING AND OTHER MASSAGE TECHNIQUES

7.1. Overview

The technique of deep-stroking massage (which is also called stripping massage) was historically the first widely accepted technique for treating fibrositis (many original descriptions of which fit myofascial TrPs)[27] and was widely practiced at the beginning of the 20th century. Danneskiold-Samsøe et al[51] found that application of deep massage to the "tender nodules" of "fibrositis" or of "myofascial pain" (which were consistent with the clinical characteristics of TrPs) relieved the signs and symptoms of most patients after 10 massage sessions. In this study, those patients experiencing pain relief had a transient elevation of serum myoglobin levels following the initial therapy sessions, but not after the final sessions when symptoms had been relieved and the tenderness and tension of the nodule being massaged had subsided. This finding suggests that the muscle fibers of TrPs and their contracture knots are more susceptible to mechanical trauma than uninvolved fibers and that local tissue manipulation can inactivate the symptoms produced by the TrPs.

This technique is not the same as deep friction massage as described by Cyriax, in which the clinician applies a deep massage across the long axis of the muscle fibers.[52] The Cyriax technique is more closely related to the strumming massage technique. Strumming is similar to deep-stroking massage except that the strumming finger runs across the taut bands at the level of the TrPs from one side of the muscle to the other. The clinician's finger pulls perpendicularly across the muscle fibers rather than along the length of the fibers. Fernández de las Peñas et al[53] found that the application of transverse friction massage (strumming massage) was similarly effective for reducing pain sensitivity over latent and active TrPs as pressure release.

7.2. Patient and Intervention Selection

Massage techniques like NMT can be applied to any patient with either acute or chronic pain. Nevertheless, it is commonly accepted that massage interventions should not be applied directly to the injured tissues within the first 72 hours following the injury, because this would tend to encourage increased blood flow to the already congested tissues and reduce the natural splinting that is required in this phase of recovery.[49] After 72 hours, massage techniques may be carefully applied to the injured tissues, supporting structures, and muscles involved. It may be necessary to perform quantitative sensory tests such as light touch, pain pressure threshold, or heat and cold sensitivity to determine the patient's tolerance to mechanical or thermal stimulation. Clinically, some patients with peripheral and/or centrally evoked pain states may have a delayed response of hyperalgesia if the technique is performed too vigorously.

7.3. Clinical Application

During any massage intervention, the therapist should pay close attention to restrictive barriers and their release. The patient must be positioned comfortably, so that the muscle to be treated is completely relaxed and lengthened without pain to the point that there is no residual slack in the muscle as a whole. The skin should be lubricated if the subcutaneous tissues are tense and immobile. For the deep-stroking massage, the thumbs or a finger of both hands are placed so they trap a taut band between them just beyond the band's TrPs. As the digits encounter the nodularity of the TrP caused by its contracture knots, pressure is exerted to engage the restrictive barrier (Figure 73-8). The digits progress no faster than tissue release occurs as the barrier "gives" to some extent. The purpose of the pressure directed along the length of the taut band is to maximally elongate the shortened sarcomeres to release their tension. The stroking massage should be continued along the length of the remaining taut band beyond the TrP toward the attachment of the muscle, helping restore the sarcomeres to normal length by

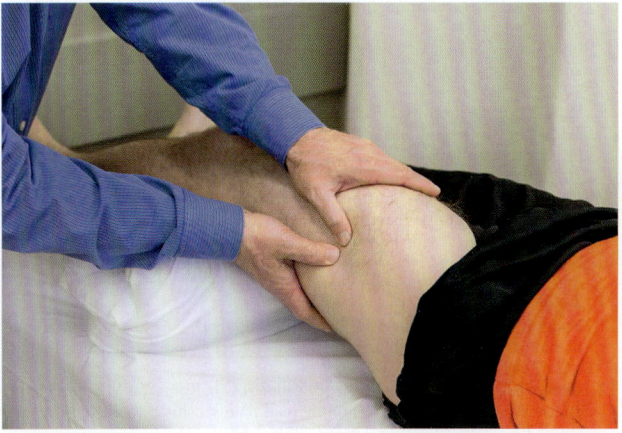

Figure 73-8. Deep-stroking massage technique for the vastus lateralis muscle and iliotibial band. Deep strokes from proximal to distal.

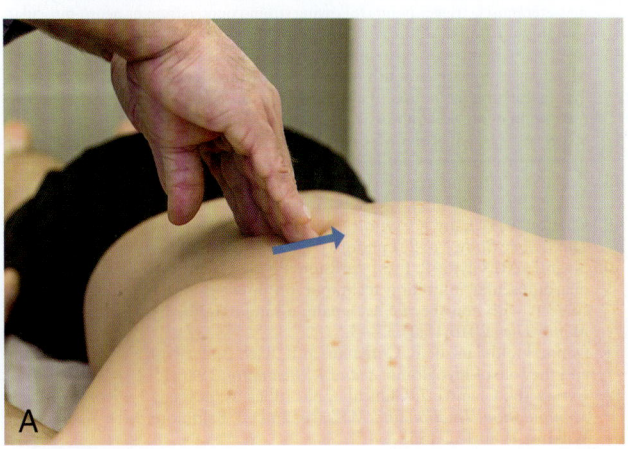

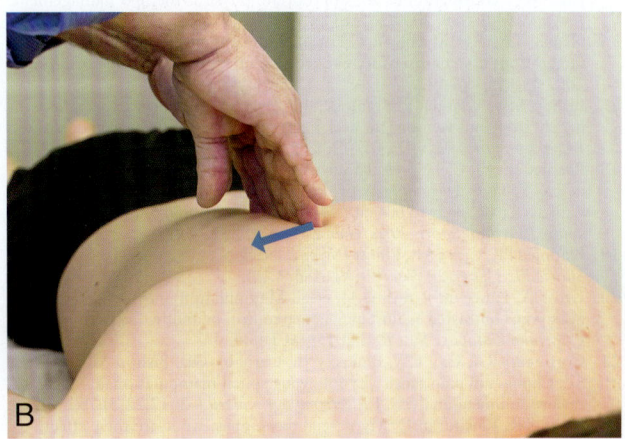

Figure 73-9. Strumming massage technique for a thoracic paraspinal muscle TrP. A, Starting position just lateral to the thoracic paraspinal musculature moving fingers medially (arrow). B, Ending position and reversing direction from medial to lateral (arrow).

continuing to exert traction on the contracture knots. The next massage stroke should go in the reverse direction starting on the same taut band but on the other side of the TrP to further release the contractured sarcomeres. This stroke now helps release the abnormal tension on the other half of the taut band and at the other muscle attachment.

Strumming consists of pulling the finger across the middle of the muscle fibers slowly until the TrP is encountered. Light contact is maintained at that point until the operator senses tissue release under the finger. The finger continues pulling across the TrPs in steps as tension releases, usually in a transverse direction of the taut band (Figure 73-9).

References

1. Paris SV. A history of manipulative therapy through the ages and up to the current controversy in the United States. *J Man Manip Ther.* 2000;8(2):66-77.
2. IFOMPT. International Federation of Orthopaedic Manipulative Physical Therapists. http://www.ifompt.org/About+IFOMPT.html.
3. Mintken PE, DeRosa C, Little T, Smith B; American Academy of Orthopaedic Manual Physical T. AAOMPT clinical guidelines: a model for standardizing manipulation terminology in physical therapy practice. *J Orthop Sports Phys Ther.* 2008;38(3):A1-A6.
4. Fernández-de-Las-Penas C, Fernandez-Carnero J, Miangolarra-Page J. Musculoskeletal disorders in mechanical neck pain: myofascial trigger points versus cervical joint dysfunction—a clinical study. *J Musculoske Pain.* 2005;13(1):27-35.
5. Ruiz-Saez M, Fernández-de-las-Penas C, Blanco CR, Martinez-Segura R, Garcia-Leon R. Changes in pressure pain sensitivity in latent myofascial trigger points in the upper trapezius muscle after a cervical spine manipulation in pain-free subjects. *J Manipulative Physiol Ther.* 2007;30(8):578-583.
6. Bialosky JE, Beneciuk JM, Bishop MD, et al. Unraveling the mechanisms of manual therapy: modeling an approach. *J Orthop Sports Phys Ther.* 2018;48(1):8-18.
7. Bialosky JE, Simon CB, Bishop MD, George SZ. Basis for spinal manipulative therapy: a physical therapist perspective. *J Electromyogr Kinesiol.* 2012;22(5):643-647.
8. Bialosky JE, Bishop MD, Robinson ME, Zeppieri G Jr, George SZ. Spinal manipulative therapy has an immediate effect on thermal pain sensitivity in people with low back pain: a randomized controlled trial. *Phys Ther.* 2009;89(12):1292-1303.
9. Colloca CJ, Keller TS, Gunzburg R. Neuromechanical characterization of in vivo lumbar spinal manipulation. Part II. Neurophysiological response. *J Manipulative Physiol Ther.* 2003;26(9):579-591.
10. Bialosky JE, Bishop MD, Price DD, Robinson ME, George SZ. The mechanisms of manual therapy in the treatment of musculoskeletal pain: a comprehensive model. *Man Ther.* 2009;14(5):531-538.
11. Voogt L, de Vries J, Meeus M, Struyf F, Meuffels D, Nijs J. Analgesic effects of manual therapy in patients with musculoskeletal pain: a systematic review. *Man Ther.* 2015;20(2):250-256.
12. George SZ, Bishop MD, Bialosky JE, Zeppieri G Jr, Robinson ME. Immediate effects of spinal manipulation on thermal pain sensitivity: an experimental study. *BMC Musculoskelet Disord.* 2006;7:68.
13. Kovanur-Sampath K, Mani R, Cotter J, Gisselman AS, Tumilty S. Changes in biochemical markers following spinal manipulation—a systematic review and meta-analysis. *Musculoskelet Sci Pract.* 2017;29:120-131.
14. Pickar JG. Neurophysiological effects of spinal manipulation. *Spine J.* 2002;2(5):357-371.
15. Courtney CA, Fernández-de-Las-Penas C, Bond S. Mechanisms of chronic pain—key considerations for appropriate physical therapy management. *J Man Manip Ther.* 2017;25(3):118-127.
16. Haavik-Taylor H, Murphy B. Cervical spine manipulation alters sensorimotor integration: a somatosensory evoked potential study. *Clin Neurophysiol.* 2007;118(2):391-402.
17. Bishop MD, Mintken PE, Bialosky JE, Cleland JA. Patient expectations of benefit from interventions for neck pain and resulting influence on outcomes. *J Orthop Sports Phys Ther.* 2013;43(7):457-465.
18. Puentedura EJ, Cleland JA, Landers MR, Mintken PE, Louw A, Fernández-de-Las-Penas C. Development of a clinical prediction rule to identify patients with neck pain likely to benefit from thrust joint manipulation to the cervical spine. *J Orthop Sports Phys Ther.* 2012;42(7):577-592.
19. Blanpied PR, Gross AR, Elliott JM, et al. Neck pain: revision 2017. *J Orthop Sports Phys Ther.* 2017;47(7):A1-A83.
20. Gross A, Langevin P, Burnie SJ, et al. Manipulation and mobilisation for neck pain contrasted against an inactive control or another active treatment. *Cochrane Database Syst Rev.* 2015;(9):CD004249.
21. Coronado RA, Gay CW, Bialosky JE, Carnaby GD, Bishop MD, George SZ. Changes in pain sensitivity following spinal manipulation: a systematic review and meta-analysis. *J Electromyogr Kinesiol.* 2012;22(5):752-767.
22. Webb TR, Rajendran D. Myofascial techniques: what are their effects on joint range of motion and pain?—a systematic review and meta-analysis of randomised controlled trials. *J Bodyw Mov Ther.* 2016;20(3):682-699.
23. Armijo-Olivo S, Pitance L, Singh V, Neto F, Thie N, Michelotti A. Effectiveness of manual therapy and therapeutic exercise for temporomandibular disorders: systematic review and meta-analysis. *Phys Ther.* 2016;96(1):9-25.
24. Calixtre LB, Moreira RF, Franchini GH, Alburquerque-Sendin F, Oliveira AB. Manual therapy for the management of pain and limited range of motion in subjects with signs and symptoms of temporomandibular disorder: a systematic review of randomised controlled trials. *J Oral Rehabil.* 2015;42(11):847-861.
25. La Touche R, Fernández-de-las-Penas C, Fernandez-Carnero J, et al. The effects of manual therapy and exercise directed at the cervical spine on pain and pressure pain sensitivity in patients with myofascial temporomandibular disorders. *J Oral Rehabil.* 2009;36(9):644-652.
26. Calixtre LB, Gruninger BL, Haik MN, Alburquerque-Sendin F, Oliveira AB. Effects of cervical mobilization and exercise on pain, movement and function in subjects with temporomandibular disorders: a single group pre-post test. *J Appl Oral Sci.* 2016;24(3):188-197.
27. Simons DG, Travell J, Simons L. *Travell & Simon's Myofascial Pain and Dysfunction: The Trigger Point Manual.* Vol 1. 2nd ed. Baltimore, MD: Williams & Wilkins; 1999.
28. Fernández-de-Las-Penas C, Campo MS, Carnero JF, Page M. Manual therapies in myofascial trigger point treatment: a systematic review. *J Bodyw Mov Ther.* 2005;9:27-34.
29. Gay CW, Alappattu MJ, Coronado RA, Horn ME, Bishop MD. Effect of a single session of muscle-biased therapy on pain sensitivity: a systematic review and meta-analysis of randomized controlled trials. *J Pain Res.* 2013;6:7-22.
30. Cagnie B, Castelein B, Pollie F, Steelant L, Verhoeyen H, Cools A. Evidence for the use of ischemic compression and dry needling in the management of trigger points of the upper trapezius in patients with neck pain: a systematic review. *Am J Phys Med Rehabil.* 2015;94(7):573-583.
31. Simons DG. Understanding effective treatments of myofascial trigger points. *J Bodyw Mov Ther.* 2002;6(2):81-88.
32. Hou CR, Tsai LC, Cheng KF, Chung KC, Hong CZ. Immediate effects of various physical therapeutic modalities on cervical myofascial pain and trigger-point sensitivity. *Arch Phys Med Rehabil.* 2002;83(10):1406-1414.
33. Lewit K. *Manipulative Therapy in Rehabilitation of the Locomotor System.* 3rd ed. Oxford, England: Butterworth Heinemann; 1999.
34. Moraska AF, Schmiege SJ, Mann JD, Butryn N, Krutsch JP. Responsiveness of myofascial trigger points to single and multiple trigger point release massages: a randomized, placebo controlled trial. *Am J Phys Med Rehabil.* 2017;96(9):639-645.
35. Mata Diz JB, de Souza JR, Leopoldino AA, Oliveira VC. Exercise, especially combined stretching and strengthening exercise, reduces myofascial pain: a systematic review. *J Physiother.* 2017;63(1):17-22.
36. Lewit K. Postisometric relaxation in combination with other methods of muscular facilitation and inhibition. *Manuelle Medizin.* 1986;2:101-104.
37. Jones LH, Kusunose RS, Goering EK. *Jones Strain-Counterstrain.* Boise, ID: Jones International; 1995.
38. Korr IM. Proprioceptors and somatic dysfunction. *J Am Osteopath Assoc.* 1975;74(7):638-650.
39. Howell JN, Cabell KS, Chila AG, Eland DC. Stretch reflex and Hoffmann reflex responses to osteopathic manipulative treatment in subjects with Achilles tendinitis. *J Am Osteopath Assoc.* 2006;106(9):537-545.
40. Wynne MM, Burns JM, Eland DC, Conatser RR, Howell JN. Effect of counterstrain on stretch reflexes, hoffmann reflexes, and clinical outcomes in subjects with plantar fasciitis. *J Am Osteopath Assoc.* 2006;106(9):547-556.
41. Lewis C, Khan A, Souvlis T, Sterling M. A randomised controlled study examining the short-term effects of Strain-Counterstrain treatment on quantitative sensory measures at digitally tender points in the low back. *Man Ther.* 2010;15(6):536-541.
42. Klein R, Bareis A, Schneider A, Linde K. Strain-counterstrain to treat restrictions of the mobility of the cervical spine in patients with neck pain: a sham-controlled randomized trial. *Complement Ther Med.* 2013;21(1):1-7.
43. Wong CK, Schauer CS. Reliability, validity, and effectiveness of strain counterstrain techniques. *J Man Manip Ther.* 2004;12(2):107-112.
44. McPartland JM, Goodridge JP. Counter-strain and traditional osteopathic examination of the cervical spine compared. *J Bodyw Mov Ther.* 1997;1(3):173-178.
45. Ibanez-Garcia J, Alburquerque-Sendin F, Rodriguez-Blanco C, et al. Changes in masseter muscle trigger points following strain-counterstrain or neuro-muscular technique. *J Bodyw Mov Ther.* 2009;13(1):2-10.
46. Rodríguez-Blanco C, Fernandez C, Xumet J, Algaba C, Rabadan M, Lillo M. Changes in active mouth opening following a single treatment of latent myofascial trigger points in the masseter muscle involving post-isometric relaxation or strain/counterstrain. *J Bodyw Mov Ther.* 2006;10(3):197-205.
47. Stecco A, Gesi M, Stecco C, Stern R. Fascial components of the myofascial pain syndrome. *Curr Pain Headache Rep.* 2013;17(8):352.
48. Levin SM. The importance of soft tissues for structural support of the body. *Spine.* 1995;9:357-363.
49. Chaitow L, DeLany J. *Clinical Applications of Neuromuscular Techniques: The Lower Body.* Vol 2. London, England: Churchill Livingston; 2002.
50. Nagrale AV, Glynn P, Joshi A, Ramteke G. The efficacy of an integrated neuromuscular inhibition technique on upper trapezius trigger points in subjects with non-specific neck pain: a randomized controlled trial. *J Man Manip Ther.* 2010;18(1):37-43.
51. Danneskiold-Samsøe B, Christiansen E, Bach Andersen R. Myofascial pain and the role of myoglobin. *Scand J Rheumatol.* 1986;15(2):174-178.
52. Cyriax JH. Chapter 7, Clinical applications of massage. In: Rogoff JB, ed. *Manipulation, Traction and Massage.* 2nd ed. Baltimore, MD: Williams & Wilkins; 1980:152-155.
53. Fernández-de-las-Peñas C, Alonso-Blanco C, Fernández-Carnero J, Miangolarra-Page JC. The immediate effect of ischemic compression technique and transverse friction massage on tenderness of active and latent myofascial trigger points: a pilot study. *J Bodyw Mov Ther.* 2006;10(1):3-9.

Chapter 74

Therapeutic Exercise Considerations

Blake A. Hampton, Joseph M. Donnelly, and César Fernández de las Peñas

1. INTRODUCTION

The physiologic basis of exercise is constructed from a cellular level to guide healthcare professionals in the design of exercise programs for individuals with myofascial pain syndrome or muscle dysfunction. When prescribing therapeutic exercise, enhancing muscular performance via nervous system efficiency, muscular strength, power, endurance, and flexibility are all essential considerations. Clinicians must also consider the effect trigger points (TrPs) have on the variables of therapeutic exercise. If these elements are all adequately addressed, a clinician can create an effective exercise prescription that will address activity limitations and participation restrictions and achieve functional goals.

2. MUSCLE FIBER TYPE

Muscle function is largely dependent on muscle fiber type ratio, which is generally related to an individual's genetic makeup. Fiber type must be considered to optimize results.

A motor unit comprises an individual motor neuron and all of the muscle fibers that it innervates.[1] The number of muscle fibers that a motor neuron innervates is dictated by the primary function of that muscle group. If a muscle group is primarily responsible for fine motor movements, the neuron to muscle fiber ratio may be low (ie, 1:10 for ocular muscles). If a muscle group is primarily responsible for gross motor movements, the neuron to muscle fiber ratio may be high (ie, 1:1000 for the gastrocnemius muscle). The primary reason for this variation in the neuron to muscle fiber ratio is that motor units operate in an "all or none" manner, and partial firing of a motor unit is not possible.

The recruitment of motor units or the muscle activation pattern is also specialized and task- or activity dependent. Smaller, type I motor units are recruited first because of their low threshold of excitation. They contain only a few terminal branches that innervate the muscle cells, and their activity can be maintained for prolonged periods of time on account of slow contraction velocity, high mitochondrial content, and oxidative capacity.[1] When greater force is required, type II motor units are subsequently recruited. With a greater number of neuronal terminal branches and larger muscle fibers, type II motor units increase the overall force production capacity.[1] Type II motor units have an increased demand for Myosin ATPase because of increased contraction velocity and greater expense of energy. They also fatigue much quicker than type I motor units. The de-recruitment of type II fibers must be considered as type I fibers are also the last to be "turned off" during the contraction cycle. This pattern is significant in that for higher-intensity activities requiring greater velocity and force, greater rest time is needed for adequate recovery. This principle has significant implications when designing aerobic and strengthening exercise prescriptions and for the progression of a therapeutic program.

A phenomenon referred to as "motor unit rotation" has been demonstrated in which newly recruited motor units replace previously active motor units. This substitution allows for improved motor control and sustainability with prolonged low-level contractions.[2] The phenomenon plays a key role in motor unit recruitment patterns in postural muscles that primarily function in maintaining prolonged low-level muscle contractions. One study suggests that muscle contraction failure may be related to changes in the motor unit recruitment pattern that more commonly occurs in muscles composed of a higher proportion of type II fibers.[3] This correlation may explain why speed and agility athletes tend to be more prone to muscle injuries than other athletes.

Although genetic makeup generally determines the ratio of type I to type II muscle fibers in an individual, muscle fiber plasticity allows for the conversion of one fiber type to another.[4] With training specificity, muscle fibers can adapt somewhat to meet demands. This adaptation progress is highly relevant for muscles, such as the lumbar multifidus, where structural changes (ie, fatty infiltration, atrophy, and muscle fiber distribution) in muscle fibers are often noted in patients with chronic pain.[5] Nevertheless, this training effect has limitations, and overall genetic makeup is the largest determinant of fiber type ratio in an individual.

3. EFFECTS OF TRIGGER POINTS IN MUSCLE FUNCTION

Evidence suggests that TrPs can have a negative impact on the aspects of muscular function, including fatigue, altered coordination, and altered intramuscular activity patterns.[6] The presence of pain has been shown to affect motor function of the affected, synergistic, and antagonist muscles by complex central and peripheral mechanisms.[7] Therefore, it would be expected that patients experiencing pain because of active TrPs would also exhibit altered motor control patterns. Yu and Kim[8] reported that muscles with active TrPs showed significantly higher median frequency and muscle fatigue than muscles with latent TrPs or no TrPs, suggesting an increased recruitment of motor unit action potential of type II fibers. Yassin et al[9] observed that patients with active TrPs in the neck-shoulder muscles need more time to react to stimulus (ie, delay in muscle activation) for moving the upper extremity when compared with those with latent or no TrPs in the same muscle. More recently, Florencio et al[10] found that the presence of active TrPs in the cervical muscles determined an altered activation of superficial neck flexor and extensor muscles during a low-load isometric task of the cervical spine in women with migraine headache.

It should be recognized that the literature related to TrPs and muscle function has been predominantly focused on the presence of latent TrPs. The effect of latent TrPs on muscle function, performance, and efficiency is profound. Supporting evidence has shown that latent TrPs affect pain, muscle activation patterns, rehabilitation, performance training, and the general function of the human body. Ge and Arendt-Nielsen[6] proposed that latent TrPs contribute to central sensitization mechanisms because of continuous low-level nociceptive inputs. These inputs lead to long-term potentiation causing a facilitated segment of the central nervous system and increasing the perception of pain as well as motor dysfunction. In another study, the same authors showed increased intramuscular electromyography (EMG) amplitude of the upper trapezius muscle when latent TrPs were present during isometric shoulder abduction.[11] These authors surmised that synergistic musculature with latent TrPs creates abnormal muscle activation patterns and may lead to synergistic muscle overload and pain propagation.[11] Studies by Lucas et al[12,13] showed variability in muscle activation times in the upward rotators of the shoulder when latent TrPs were present in the muscles of the shoulder girdle complex. Similarly, Bohlooli et al[14] found delayed activation and alteration in recruitment patterns of the upper trapezius muscle during rapid arm elevation in the presence of latent upper trapezius TrPs. Additionally, the synergistic shoulder muscles showed altered recruitment patterns, although these muscles did not exhibit TrPs.[14] The poor efficiency of the shoulder girdle musculature from TrPs leading to variance in muscle activation patterns will ultimately sacrifice performance. These results may have implications related to temporal summation for patients with musculoskeletal pain conditions secondary to the concept that TrPs are considered a neurophysiologic dysfunction that affects and is affected by the central nervous system.[12,13] Lucas et al[12] suggested that when there is dysfunction in a proximal body segment, distal segments must change workloads and muscle activation patterns to preserve the desired movement outcomes. This concept is important when treating patients with distal extremity dysfunctions when a TrP in a more proximal muscle may be a major contributing factor to pain and/or movement impairment.

Restricted joint range of motion, muscle inhibition, and accelerated muscle fatigue are commonly observed in patients with myofascial pain syndrome, and evidence supports that latent TrPs are contributing factors to these impairments.[6] In fact, the presence of latent TrPs is associated with overloading active motor units close to the TrP in addition to accelerated muscle fatigue.[15] Motor dysfunction can occur because of long-term potentiation of a nociceptive stimulus and the body's natural defense mechanism to reduce activation of the muscles where pain is perceived. This mechanical hyperalgesia may stem from ischemia associated with TrPs and a release of adenosine triphosphate that may facilitate acid-sensing ion channel number 3 by binding to P2X receptors.[6] This process may allow for reduced thresholds for nociception that would lead to increased action potentials causing the development of mechanical sensitivity. Substance P, calcitonin gene-related peptide, bradykinin, serotonin, norepinephrine, glutamate, nerve growth factor, and cytokines are also present in areas surrounding TrPs that lead to chemosensitivity related to inflammation. These inflammatory mediators can then be released by the dorsal root ganglion into the dorsal horn of the spinal cord, leading to spinal cord (central) sensitization. The facilitated segment then creates a feedback loop that can reduce efferent neuron excitability and ultimately cause the inhibition of all muscles associated with that segment, and with time, other agonistic and antagonistic muscles.[7]

All these motor disturbances can be particularly problematic when managing patients with pain and dysfunction related to a movement impairment (ie, subacromial pain syndrome). Failure to address TrPs, either latent or active, in synergistic and antagonist muscles surrounding the shoulder may result in poor outcomes. Therefore, increased intramuscular EMG activity is an important consideration for exercise prescription from both a performance and rehabilitation perspective. Importantly, and from a clinical point of view, latent TrPs can induce motor control disturbances that can have a significant impact on motor function; however, these latent TrPs are not always responsible for or associated with pain symptoms.

4. NEUROMUSCULAR REEDUCATION

The principles of neuromuscular reeducation are inextricable with muscle function and performance. It would be difficult to prescribe therapeutic exercise as it pertains to TrPs without discussing the principles of neuromuscular reeducation. It has been shown that for voluntary movement to occur, functionally active reflex arcs must be intact.[16] If these reflex arcs are impaired, muscle performance as it pertains to strength, power, and endurance will not be properly optimized. Dr Leonard Huddleston, one of the initial practitioners to pioneer neuromuscular reeducation, states that the strength of contraction of a given muscle is determined by the following factors presented in Box 74-1.[16]

There is an abundant arrangement of connections from the primary motor cortex, including the primary and secondary somatosensory cortices, the prefrontal cortex, and subcortical regions such as the thalamus, to cortical regions. These connections play a critical role in the recovery of normal effective motor function because of the system's dependence on sensory input.[17] Appropriate motor function is integrated with auditory, visual, and vestibular input along with proprioceptive input. Impaired sensory function results in poor and ineffectual motor control. The implication is that sensory stimulation plays an essential role in recovery from motor deficits that influence continued propagation of nociceptive input that causes weakness, among other impairments. Exercise prescription that focuses exclusively on motor function is not as effective as an exercise prescription that incorporates both sensory and motor function.[18] The goal of neuromuscular reeducation is to improve the efficiency and synergy in activation of the motor units, thus achieving greater muscle performance by improving organized synaptic facilitation of the motor neurons. Eccentric exercise may also be used to enhance neuromuscular control by addressing alterations in muscle morphology and affecting change in both the peripheral and central nervous systems.[19] Comprehensive exercise programs should include both concentric and eccentric training. Clinicians should be aware when designing exercises to include a greater eccentric emphasis and should consider where eccentric exercises fit in a systematic approach to postinjury retraining. Simons et al[20] says that lengthening contractions are safer for the patient to start with as the muscle is able to exert more force with less energy expenditure. These concepts are important in the facilitation of function in muscles with inhibition weakness due to TrPs. Following treatment of TrPs, especially needling therapies to regain optimal muscle performance and motor function, eccentric exercise may enhance neuromuscular control. In fact, it has been previously reported that low-load eccentric exercise provided protection against damage.[21]

Box 74-1 Factors that affect the strength of contraction of a muscle

1. Anatomic and physiologic status of the muscle fibers at the time of contraction
2. Number and synchrony of the contracting fibers
3. Number and frequency of nerve impulses reaching the muscle fibers
4. Functional status of the neuromuscular junctions
5. Structural and functional condition of the tissues surrounding the muscle fibers

5. MOTOR CONTROL TRAINING

Motor control training is a component of neuromuscular re-education. The foundation for motor control training is motor learning which consists of three phases as described by Fitts and Posner.[22] These phases are (1) cognitive phase, (2) associative phase, and (3) autonomous phase.[22] In the cognitive phase, the individual cognitively plans each action and is incapable of dual-tasking. In the associative phase, the individual is working to find a solution for the problem in their movement patterns. During the associative phase, it is important to allow the individual to make small errors while performing movement in an effective manner. In the autonomous phase, the individual is no longer having to cognitively work through movements or problem-solve, and he or she is able to automatically perform the movement or task and dual-task.[23]

Motor learning also pertains to declarative and procedural learning.[23] In declarative learning, every action and movement is analyzed, and repetitions are vital to this mode of learning. An individual requires approximately 3000 repetitions or more to master a skill.[23] In procedural learning, activities or tasks no longer require conscious thought, and skills are perfected through random practice in changing environments.[23]

Motor control can be defined as the ability to control and adjust postures and movements with central commands, spinal reflexes, and the organization of motor programs from activities and movements that the individual has already learned.[23] This process can be facilitated by a variety of activities such as developmental sequences and functional movement patterns that are similar to the desired movement pattern. There are four progressive phases of motor control, each with specific characteristics that should be manipulated within an exercise program. These characteristics are mobility, stability, controlled mobility/stability, and skill.[23]

Mobility is the ability to assume and maintain a posture or position while starting a movement.[23] As often observed clinically, the cause of reduced joint motion can be multifactorial. Joint restriction may be related to intrinsic articular hypomobility, a reflection of muscle imbalance, or a lack of muscle extensibility. In designing a therapeutic exercise program, clinical reasoning must be used to determine when it would be most appropriate to add mobility exercises including TrP management. In some cases, focusing on the impairments of muscle performance and motor control would be a priority, and this may actually reduce the dominance of some of the tight muscle groups.

Stability is the ability to stabilize a new position and control the forces of gravity acting on the body. Controlled mobility and stability occur when the movement can be controlled at any point from a stable foundation. Skill is when all movements are able to be performed, and all parts of the body can move in a controlled fashion in all directions.[23] The motor control phases are applied to specific exercises and positions that the individual cannot yet perform to assist in retraining. Tactile and verbal cueing may be necessary to further facilitate the desired movement patterns. External focus activities can be used to create an environment where functional retraining is goal specific, and the patient must progress through the phases of motor learning in order to achieve mastery of the desired movement pattern. This type of treatment requires a significant amount of time and can be tedious, but it is an extremely important aspect in the treatment of myofascial pain syndrome to avoid muscle overload.

6. PROPRIOCEPTIVE NEUROMUSCULAR FACILITATION

Proprioceptive Neuromuscular Facilitation (PNF) is a treatment concept for motor control and motor learning. It is utilized in many settings to address poor motor programming, deficient muscle activation patterns, and motor output dysfunctions that are commonly seen in individuals with myofascial pain syndrome. The tactile cues required during PNF integrate the sensory and motor systems to improve movement efficiency. The basic neurophysiologic principles of PNF are after discharge, temporal summation, spatial summation, irradiation, successive induction, and reciprocal (innervation) inhibition.[23]

After discharge is the effect a stimulus continues to have on the system after that stimulus is removed.[23] This concept is similar to the synaptic facilitation that occurs during neuromuscular reeducation as previously discussed. Temporal summation is the summation of several weaker stimuli in the same location that results in an increase in excitability of the motor neurons. The repetition of movement at lower amplitudes increases the excitability and effectiveness of the motor neurons. Spatial summation refers to weaker stimuli in multiple regions converging to effect greater activity.[23] Applying the concept of spatial summation allows for smaller, multijoint movements that may be less painful and may have a greater effect on the central nervous system than larger, single-joint movements. Irradiation is an increased response of the muscle that is related to the increase in number and/or strength of the stimuli provided, which may be either inhibitory or facilitatory depending on the desired outcome.[23] Successive induction is another neurophysiologic principle where there is an increase in excitation of the agonist muscle following a contraction of the antagonist muscle. This can be a powerful tool for retraining muscle activation patterns and for strength training. The neurophysiologic increase in the contraction force of the agonist muscle group affords the clinician the opportunity to apply the principle of overload more efficiently.

Reciprocal inhibition or innervation occurs when the contraction of an agonist muscle group results in a simultaneous inhibition of the antagonist muscle group.[23] Reciprocal inhibition is not only an involuntary spinal-level reflex but is effective when a contraction is initiated at the cortical level. When one muscle is activated, its antagonist is reflexively inhibited. The use of reciprocal inhibition is valuable for augmenting relaxation and release of muscle tension when stretching a muscle to inactivate TrPs. This concept is important because the presence of TrPs is associated with a reduced efficiency of reciprocal inhibition that can lead to an increased coactivation of the antagonist muscles following exercise, disordered fine movement control, and unbalanced muscle activation.[24] To invoke reciprocal inhibition, the muscles opposing the muscle being stretched are voluntarily contracted to actively assist the stretching movement. Thus, the muscle to be stretched is reciprocally inhibited. This method can be used alone to augment a simple stretch or it can be combined with other techniques such as spray and stretch or manual therapy.

The use of reciprocal inhibition as a neuromuscular mechanism for releasing tension involves more than inhibition of alpha motor neuron activity. The tension-release mechanisms may also be dependent on autonomic effects that are related to the inhibition of spontaneous electrical activity and spike activity of TrPs during exhalation and their augmentation by inhalation and mental stress. One clinical example is seen in an attempt to increase the stretch of the hamstring muscles. The patient or client activates the quadriceps muscle group at the point where the maximum hamstring muscle length is achieved, and upon relaxing the quadriceps muscle, the hamstring muscles are inhibited, thus allowing further stretch of these muscles. This is a technique that is commonly used across practice settings to improve flexibility.

The principle of contract-relax appears in various forms by differing names throughout the musculoskeletal treatment literature. The term contract-relax, as originally taught by Knott and Voss[25] and Voss et al,[26] was recommended for treatment of marked limitation of the range of passive motion with no active motion available in the muscle opposing the tight muscle. As they described this intervention, contract-relax employed maximum contraction in a pattern movement followed by relaxation of the tight muscle to permit active shortening of the opposing weak muscle. Release of tightness permitted improvement in the range of motion. Through the years, the exact meaning of the term has become somewhat diffuse. There are now numerous variations (and applications) of the basic principle that muscle tension is reduced immediately following voluntary contraction.

The contract-relax used for treating TrPs is a gentle, voluntary, minimally resisted contraction of the muscle. The intent is to activate the fibers of the TrP or surrounding muscle fibers. The contraction is followed by volitional relaxation to permit passive elongation of the muscle to a new stretch length. Contract-relax is the basic procedure in the postisometric relaxation method described by Lewit.[27]

Hold-relax is a variant of the contract-relax technique that is not commonly used for treating TrPs but may be employed when there is no joint movement desired during or after the procedure. It consists of isometric contraction of the tight muscle followed by relaxation but not via elongation of the tight muscle. When used in the treatment of muscles with TrPs, hold-relax is commonly combined with manual techniques applied directly to the targeted muscle, such as deep stroking massage and TrP pressure release.

7. STRENGTH TRAINING

An exercise prescription should be designed primarily for lengthening, strengthening, and/or conditioning specific muscles at the beginning of the program and for functional integration at the end of the program. Exercise to lengthen the involved muscles is key to sustained relief of myofascial pain. Improved conditioning (exercise tolerance or stamina) and increased strength of a group of muscles, achieved through exercise, reduces the likelihood of their developing TrPs. However, in most patients with active TrPs, conditioning and strengthening exercises can further activate these TrPs, encourage substitution by other muscles, and aggravate symptoms. On the contrary, the same exercises render latent TrPs less prone to reactivation if properly paced at a gradual rate of progression.

The kind of exercise prescribed depends largely on the irritability of the TrPs responsible for the pain. When the patient is experiencing pain at rest for a considerable part of the time, the TrPs should be inactivated with manual or, in some cases, needling therapies before beginning the exercise program. The object is to unload and restore normal range of motion to the overworked sore muscles; at that stage, active exercise that loads a contracting muscle is not indicated.

Strength training is often the main intention of therapeutic exercise programs and is an important intervention to assist the patient in achieving therapeutic and performance goals. There are seven variables that must be considered when developing a strengthening exercise prescription: needs analysis, exercise selection, training load, training frequency, exercise order, volume, and rest periods.[28]

The needs analysis is the most important design variable and is often times overlooked by practitioners. Prior to designing a strength program, a needs analysis is necessary to appropriately prescribe exercises that are tailored to the particular demands of the individual. A needs analysis includes the analysis of movement patterns, identification of key muscles required to perform the movement, and the examination of muscle imbalances between agonistic, synergistic, and antagonist muscle groups. In the muscle chapters, this group is referred to as the functional unit. This is highly important, because each particular individual will have specific demands for the muscles based on daily-life activities or sport practice. The exercise program should be adapted to these demands by using the same muscle groups and functional units.

Proper assessment of an individual's training experience requires evaluation of the current program, training age, frequency, and technique. These parameters are used to classify the individual as beginner, intermediate, or advanced in terms of initiating a strengthening program. A beginner classification includes an individual who is not currently training or just began a training program. This group consists of individuals with a training time of less than 2 months, frequency of training that is less than or equal to two to three times/week, and minimal to no training technique experience. Clinically, this is where a large population of patients with myofascial pain syndrome and TrPs can be classified, and these individuals are often times progressed too quickly. An intermediate classification includes those individuals who are currently training, have a training time period of 2 to 6 months, are training at a frequency of two to three times/week, and have basic technique experience. An advanced classification includes individuals who are currently training, have a training time period of at least 1 year, a training frequency of three to four times/week, and a high level of technique experience. Prior to placing an individual on a strength training program, these variables need to be identified to facilitate success.

Physiologic analysis is another aspect of the needs analysis that will help in the specificity of the exercise prescription, and it requires an assessment of the primary energy systems that are utilized during the daily activity or sport. Finally, an injury analysis must also be performed to evaluate common injuries associated with the specific activity or sport and to identify any contributing factors that may be involved with those particular injuries.

Exercise selection is the second design variable that needs to be incorporated into the exercise prescription, and it is determined by needs analysis. The specific adaptations to imposed demands principle is the key to expert selection of any particular exercise.[28] Specificity of exercise selection is important to ensure that the individual is trained in a specific manner to produce a particular adaptation or outcome. These adaptations are specific to the mode of training, the muscle group, and the movement pattern needed to perform a specific activity, joint range of motion, velocity of desired movement, type of muscle action, and activation of specific types of muscle fibers that are requirements of the sport or activity.[28] An example of specificity can be applied to the rotator cuff muscles. The rotator cuff muscles have a 1:1 ratio of type I and type II muscle fibers.[29] Therefore, it is necessary to establish an exercise prescription that includes both strength and endurance for the rotator cuff muscles.

Load is the third design variable, and often, where injuries in strength training occur, it is not managed properly. A study showed that to ensure safe loading, progressive overload should occur at a rate of 2.5% to 5% per week.[30] The same study showed that when the training load was increased by 5% to 10% from the previous week, there was less than 10% risk of injury. But when the training load was increased by greater than 15% from the previous week, there was a 21% to 64% risk of injury.[30] To apply overload, the program designer can increase the resistance, increase the training volume, alter rest periods, increase repetition velocity, or alter the sets and repetitions performed. It is important to note that when training with lighter loads, motor learning and coordination are improved.[28] Blanch and Gabbett[31] introduced the concept of acute to chronic workload ratio which has proven to be important when returning the patient or athlete back to function or sport. Acute workload is defined as the training that is performed in the current week.[31] Chronic workload is defined as the average training that is performed in the previous 4 weeks. An acute to chronic workload ratio of 0.5 would suggest that an individual trained half of the workload he or she prepared for in the previous 4 weeks. An acute to chronic workload ratio of 2.0 suggests that the individual performed twice the amount of work as he or she prepared for in the last 4 weeks. Blanch and Gabbett[31] concluded that the ideal acute to chronic ratio is less than 1.5 to keep injury risk below 5%.[31]

Frequency of training is the next variable of the exercise prescription that should be considered. Training load is directly related to frequency in that higher training loads require more recovery time. Therefore, the frequency should be reduced to allow for recovery. Lower-extremity exercises require greater recovery times than upper-extremity exercises, and frequency should reflect the regions of training. Multijoint exercises require greater recovery than single-joint exercises, and this should be reflected when prescribing frequency. Training status established from the needs analysis plays a key role in frequency prescription. For individuals with beginner training status, frequency guidelines recommend two to three sessions/week.[28] For individuals with intermediate training status, the guidelines recommend three to four training sessions/week.[28] And lastly, for individuals with advanced training status, training frequency guidelines recommend four to seven sessions/week.[28] A recent meta-analysis showed that major muscle groups should be trained two times/week to maximize hypertrophy and that there was no statistical difference between training two and three times/week.[32]

Volume is defined as the total amount lifted in a training session and is in an important variable of the exercise prescription. Volume can be based on repetitions or load, known as repetition volume and load volume, respectively. Repetition volume is the total number of repetitions performed for a single exercise.[28] For example, a repetition volume for 3 sets of 10 repetitions is 30. Load volume is the amount of weight lifted multiplied by the repetition volume. For the above example, if the individual was lifting 10 lb for each repetition, the load volume would be 300. A basic principle presented by the National Strength and Conditioning Association (NSCA) for load progression is the 2 for 2 rule that states a load should be increased when the individual being trained is able to perform two extra repetitions on the third set for two consecutive sessions.[28] Volume assignments for training goals are important for the specificity of training for different aspects such as strength, power, hypertrophy, or endurance.

When designing a strength program, it is vital to incorporate all seven design variables identified in Box 74-2 to ensure the safety of the individual while achieving optimal results. If any of these variables are excluded, the chance of injury increases at the expense of reduced performance required for specific activities. These exercise prescription design principles are essential when retraining muscles following treatment for TrPs and myofascial pain to enhance performance, return to function, and prevent recurrence of TrPs. For more detailed information regarding programming for strength training, refer to the NSCA's *Essentials of Strength Training and Conditioning* textbook.

8. FLEXIBILITY TRAINING

Flexibility training is an important aspect of muscle performance including strength, power, and endurance. In this manual, flexibility training (self-stretch exercises) is contained within the Corrective Actions section of each applicable muscle chapter.

Almost any method that gently stretches (lengthens) a muscle with TrPs and increases its pain-free range of motion is beneficial. However, a rapid, forceful stretch by itself causes pain, protective contraction, and reflex spasm of the muscles. All of these responses hurt the patient and obstruct further elongation of the muscle. Some method of suppressing these reactions must be added in order to release TrP tension. Rapid or "bouncing" stretches are to be avoided; they tend to irritate muscle tissue and TrPs, not release them. It is often possible, with a newly activated or a moderately irritable TrP, to inactivate it immediately by simply passively, slowly stretching the muscle. However, the release can be expedited and made less uncomfortable when stretch is combined with simple augmentation maneuvers such as coordinated exhalation, postisometric relaxation, contract-relax, and reciprocal inhibition.

Two approaches to stretching the muscle are available: elongating the muscle by moving the joint(s) it crosses or elongating it by direct manual traction applied to the muscle. Passive movement of the joint(s) crossed by the muscle is emphasized as a component that can be used for patient self-treatment and detailed on each of the muscle chapters in the Corrective Actions section. There are also numerous methods for augmenting stretch (usually called muscle energy techniques), including postisometric relaxation, reciprocal inhibition, exhalation, directed eye movement, and contract-relax. These various techniques can be used in many different combinations and integrated with augmentation techniques.

The contracture of the sarcomeres of a TrP must be released. Therefore, lengthening the contractured sarcomere by gentle sustained stretch with augmentation techniques induces gradual reduction in the overlap between actin and myosin molecules and reduces the energy being consumed. When the sarcomeres reach full stretch length, there is minimal overlap and greatly reduced energy consumption. This reduction breaks an essential link in the energy crisis vicious cycle related to TrPs. The sustained increased tension on contractured sarcomeres may cause tearing of the actin attachments to the Z lines as observed by Fassbender.[33]

Although there are several factors that affect flexibility and muscle lengthening, the main purpose of this section is to relate flexibility to connective tissue restrictions of the tendons and fascia as well as contractile restrictions in muscle. Fascial restrictions can occur in a response to trauma, inactivity/immobility, inflammation, or disease that results in increased viscosity of the extracellular matrix that causes a reduction in fascial mobility. Once mobility of the fascia has reduced, it can begin to bind to the surrounding soft tissue, impairing normal muscle mechanics and ultimately causing a reduction in soft-tissue extensibility.[34] Therefore, the fascia and contractile component of muscle and soft tissue share a close relationship when relating to flexibility. The best treatment for fascial restrictions is a controversial topic. In recent years, self-myofascial release techniques have become popular in rehabilitation settings and gyms alike. Fascia has a thixotropic property, and the extracellular matrix becomes viscous with immobility. Macdonald et al[34] suggest that friction generated by self-myofascial release techniques results in warming of the fascia that promotes a more fluid environment of the extracellular matrix, restoring soft-tissue extensibility. They showed, following a bout of foam rolling of 2 minutes, that there was a significant increase in joint range of motion for up to 10 minutes without significant differences in neuromuscular variables including force of contraction and fatigue.[34] Healey et al[35] found no significant differences in performance between planking and foam rolling for the same amount of time; however, fatigue relating to the activity was significantly less following a bout of foam rolling when compared with planking.

Stretching and flexibility training has long been considered to be the gold standard for improving range of motion and sport performance despite evidence that has suggested otherwise, specifically with preparticipation stretching activities. There is little evidence to support the notion that preparticipation stretching activities will result in a reduced risk of injury, and more studies suggest that static stretching has been shown to affect muscle performance.[28,36] Avela et al[36] showed that there is an immediate reduction in reflex sensitivity of the stretch reflex as well as a significant reduction in stretch-resisting force following a static stretching routine. Stretching should be done immediately

---

Box 74-2 Seven design variables for developing a strengthening exercise prescription

1. Needs assessment
2. Exercise selection
3. Training load
4. Frequency of training
5. Exercise order
6. Volume of load and repetition
7. Rest periods

following an activity within 5 to 10 minutes when the musculature temperatures are increased or as a separate session.[28]

9. AEROBIC TRAINING

Aerobic training can be a vital part of therapeutic exercise prescription depending on the patient's goals and medical needs. Aerobic training (conditioning exercise) is important for performance training, functional rehabilitation, and for the management of chronic pain syndromes. To condition both the cardiovascular system and a particular set of muscles, the exercise program should be continued at submaximal level to the point of fatigue. Walking, swimming, bicycling, tennis, treadmill, jogging, and jumping rope are examples of aerobic training exercises. Although not essential for recovery from TrPs, a regular conditioning exercise program is strongly recommended for optimal health and to minimize the chance of reactivating TrPs.

There are five design variables that are associated with aerobic training programs: exercise mode, training frequency, training intensity, exercise duration, and exercise prescription.[28]

Exercise mode is the specific activity performed by an individual. These activities should be specific to the subject to mimic the movement pattern that will be employed in the patient's desired activity or competition. The different modes of aerobic training are long- or slow-distance training, pace/tempo training, interval training, repetition training, and Fartlek training and can be seen in more detail in Table 74-1.

Optimizing training frequency influences positive adaptations in specific physiologic systems.[28] Training frequency is the number of training sessions conducted per day or per week and is dependent upon the interaction of exercise intensity and duration. For example, higher exercise intensities and longer durations may necessitate less frequency in training to allow sufficient recovery from sessions. Recovery is an important aspect of training frequency and is essential to an individual to obtain maximum benefits from the subsequent training session. Sufficient rest times between sessions, along with adequate rehydration, and a high-quality diet are required to ensure that metabolic resources are replenished.

Training intensity is the relative physical effort that is expended during a training session. High-intensity aerobic exercise increases cardiovascular and respiratory function that allows for improved oxygen delivery to working muscles.[28] Training intensity also lends itself to skeletal muscle adaptations; as intensity increases, greater recruitment of type II muscle fibers occurs to meet the increased power demand which helps increase aerobic capacity.[28] Intensity is specific to the individual's level of training. Slow walking may be considered high intensity for some. Others may need a greater level of challenge to reach an adequate level of intensity. Heart rate is the most frequently used method for prescribing exercise intensity because there is a close relationship between heart rate and oxygen consumption. Two equations are used to calculate target heart rate. The first option is to take the age-predicted maximum heart rate and multiply by the desired exercise intensity. The second method, which is more accurate but more difficult to derive, is the Karvonen formula. This method accounts for resting heart rate and heart rate reserve, giving a more accurate representation of the target heart rate than the maximal heart rate percentage formula. Rate of perceived exertion can also be used to regulate exercise intensity during aerobic training. For example, the 15-point Borg scale can be used to estimate intensity where light intensity would be equal to 9, moderate intensity is equal to 12 to 14, and high intensity can equate to 18 to 20 on the scale.

Exercise duration is the length of time for a given training session and is often influenced by the intensity of exercise. Exercise conducted at an intensity above the maximal lactate steady state, which is about 85% of VO_2max, will require a relatively short duration of about 20 to 30 minutes. Lower-intensity exercises performed at 70% VO_2max or less may be performed for several hours.[28]

Exercise prescription is the final variable that ties all the other aspects of aerobic program design together for the most important aspect: progression. It is important to note that research indicates that aerobic fitness does not decrease for up to 5 weeks when intensity is maintained and frequency decreases to as few as two times a week.[28] This is key when managing rehabilitation time frames for injuries to avoid a reduction in aerobic capacity for patients. When considering a progression in training, exercise frequency, intensity, or duration should not increase more than 10% to 15% each week.[28]

These program design variables should also be used in the management of patients with myofascial pain syndrome to begin a patient on a graded exercise program. A successful program accounts for the patient's subjective reports and allow him or her to select a starting point. The patient's goals should also be considered in choosing the best mode of exercise. For example, a patient's main goal may be to be able to walk 1 mile in order to navigate a large campus to see his or her daughter graduate from high school, but the patient is currently unable to walk to the mailbox and back without experiencing increased pain. The first short-term goal would be to walk to the mailbox and back without an increase in the pain report. To do so, the patient would be asked "how far do you think you can walk without absolute certainty that you will not experience or increase your pain?" The patient may say "half way to the mailbox and back." Then half the distance to the mailbox is the starting point for the graded exercise prescription. The clinician then increases the distance 10% to 15% per week until the patient has achieved his or her goal. If the patient experiences pain at any time in the continuum, then the clinician would revert to the previous

Table 74-1 Types of Aerobic Training and Required Frequency, Duration and Intensity

	Long, Slow Distance (LSD)	Pace/Tempo	Interval	Repetition	Fartlek
Frequency (sessions/week)	1-2	1-2	1-2	1	1
Duration	Race distance or longer (30-120 min)	20-30 min	3-5 min work followed by 3-5 min rest	30-90 s work followed by 2.5-7.5 min rest (1:5)	20-60 min
Intensity	70% VO_2max	At or slightly faster than race pace	Near VO_2max	Greater than VO_2max	Varies between LSD and pace/tempo training intensities

Adapted from Baechle TR, Earle RW. *Essentials of Strength Training and Conditioning*. 3rd ed. Champaign, IL: Human Kinetics; 2008.

distance that the patient was walking until he or she was able to have success. It can be a tedious process and may take a time to achieve goals, but it is highly effective for patients with chronic pain syndromes. This principle can be applied to reach any activity goal by adapting the method to the specific mode of exercise, which can require a little creativity.

Follow these guidelines, and always considering foundations of cardiopulmonary physiology when prescribing aerobic exercises is paramount. By doing so, the patient remains safe throughout the training program and obtains the physiologic adaptations required to achieve his or her goals. For more information on program design, refer to the NSCA's *Essentials of Strength Training and Conditioning* textbook.

10. FUNCTIONAL EXERCISES

Functional exercise utilizes all of the principles mentioned in the aforementioned sections to formulate an exercise prescription to achieve the patient's highest level of function. Functional exercises are designed to prepare muscles that work synergistically to achieve movements that are specific to an activity or sport. This preparation is accomplished through simulation of movements required for the specific activity or sport. Functional exercises should be incorporated following neuromuscular re-education to reinforce proper movement and muscle activation patterns. They should also be performed following strength or aerobic training to enhance and improve performance in the desired activity. Combined movements that incorporate both upper- and lower-extremity motions and simulate the functional task result in greater carryover to a functional activity. Squats, power cleans, and dead-lifts may also be considered functional exercises because they serve to prepare muscles to work together for common daily functional tasks. Yoga, Pilates, and tai chi may also be used as functional exercises. Innumerable options exist for patients with myofascial pain to perform functional exercise. In fact, patient preference should dictate the mode of functional exercise to improve adherence to the exercise prescription.

References

1. Magee DJ, Zachazewski JE, Quillen WS. *Scientific Foundations and Principles of Practice in Musculoskeletal Rehabilitation*. New York, NY: Elsevier Health Sciences; 2007.
2. Fallentin N, Jorgensen K, Simonsen EB. Motor unit recruitment during prolonged isometric contractions. *Eur J Appl Physiol Occup Physiol*. 1993;67(4):335-341.
3. Komi PV, Tesch P. EMG frequency spectrum, muscle structure, and fatigue during dynamic contractions in man. *Eur J Appl Physiol Occup Physiol*. 1979;42(1):41-50.
4. Scott W, Stevens J, Binder-Macleod SA. Human skeletal muscle fiber type classifications. *Phys Ther*. 2001;81(11):1810-1816.
5. Goubert D, Oosterwijck JV, Meeus M, Danneels L. Structural changes of lumbar muscles in non-specific low back pain: a systematic review. *Pain Physician*. 2016;19(7):E985-E1000.
6. Ge HY, Arendt-Nielsen L. Latent myofascial trigger points. *Curr Pain Headache Rep*. 2011;15(5):386-392.
7. Hodges PW. Pain and motor control: from the laboratory to rehabilitation. *J Electromyogr Kinesiol*. 2011;21(2):220-228.
8. Yu SH, Kim HJ. Electrophysiological characteristics according to activity level of myofascial trigger points. *J Phys Ther Sci*. 2015;27(9):2841-2843.
9. Yassin M, Talebian S, Ebrahimi Takamjani I, et al. The effects of arm movement on reaction time in patients with latent and active upper trapezius myofascial trigger point. *Med J Islam Repub Iran*. 2015;29:295.
10. Florencio LL, Ferracini GN, Chaves TC, et al. Active trigger points in the cervical musculature determine the altered activation of superficial neck and extensor muscles in women with migraine. *Clin J Pain*. 2017;33(3):238-245.
11. Ge HY, Monterde S, Graven-Nielsen T, Arendt-Nielsen L. Latent myofascial trigger points are associated with an increased intramuscular electromyographic activity during synergistic muscle activation. *J Pain*. 2014;15(2):181-187.
12. Lucas KR, Polus PA, Rich J. Latent myofascial trigger points: their effect on muscle activation and movement efficiency. *J Bodyw Mov Ther*. 2004;8:160-166.
13. Lucas KR, Rich PA, Polus BI. Muscle activation patterns in the scapular positioning muscles during loaded scapular plane elevation: the effects of Latent Myofascial Trigger Points. *Clin Biomech*. 2010;25(8):765-770.
14. Bohlooli N, Ahmadi A, Maroufi N, Sarrafzadeh J, Jaberzadeh S. Differential activation of scapular muscles, during arm elevation, with and without trigger points. *J Bodyw Mov Ther*. 2016;20(1):26-34.
15. Ge HY, Arendt-Nielsen L, Madeleine P. Accelerated muscle fatigability of latent myofascial trigger points in humans. *Pain Med*. 2012;13(7):957-964.
16. Huddleston OL. Principles of neuromuscular reeducation. *J Am Med Assoc*. 1954;156(15):1396-1398.
17. Silfies SP, Vendemia JMC, Beattie PF, Stewart JC, Jordon M. Changes in brain structure and activation may augment abnormal movement patterns: an emerging challenge in musculoskeletal rehabilitation. *Pain Med*. 2017;18(11):2051-2054.
18. Bolognini N, Russo C, Edwards DJ. The sensory side of post-stroke motor rehabilitation. *Restor Neurol Neurosci*. 2016;34(4):571-586.
19. Lepley LK, Lepley AS, Onate JA, Grooms DR. Eccentric exercise to enhance neuromuscular control. *Sports Health*. 2017;9(4):333-340.
20. Simons DG, Travell J, Simons L. *Travell & Simon's Myofascial Pain and Dysfunction: The Trigger Point Manual*. Vol 1. 2nd ed. Baltimore, MD: Williams & Wilkins; 1999.
21. Lin MJ, Chen TC, Chen HL, Wu BH, Nosaka K. Low-intensity eccentric contractions of the knee extensors and flexors protect against muscle damage. *Appl Physiol Nutr Metab*. 2015;40(10):1004-1011.
22. Fitts PM, Posner MI. *Human Performance*. Oxford, England: Brooks/Cole; 1967.
23. Adler SS, Beckers D, Buck M. *PNF in Practice: An Illustrated Guide*. 4th ed. Berlin, Germany: Springer Medizin; 2014.
24. Ibarra JM, Ge HY, Wang C, Martinez Vizcaino V, Graven-Nielsen T, Arendt-Nielsen L. Latent myofascial trigger points are associated with an increased antagonistic muscle activity during agonist muscle contraction. *J Pain*. 2011;12(12):1282-1288.
25. Knott M, Voss DE. *Proprioceptive Neuromuscular Facilitation: Patterns and Techniques*. 2nd ed. New York, NY: Hoeber Medical Division Harper & Row; 1968 (pp. 97-99).
26. Voss DE, Ionta MK, Myers BJ, Knott M. *Proprioceptive Neuromuscular Facilitation: Patterns and Techniques*. 3rd ed. Philadelphia, PA: Harper & Row; 1985.
27. Lewit K. *Manipulative Therapy in Rehabilitation of the Locomotor System*. 3rd ed. Oxford, England: Butterworth Heinemann; 1999 (pp. 151-210).
28. Baechle TR, Earle RW. *Essentials of Strength Training and Conditioning*. 3rd ed. Champaign, IL: Human Kinetics; 2008.
29. Lovering RM, Russ DW. Fiber type composition of cadaveric human rotator cuff muscles. *J Orthop Sports Phys Ther*. 2008;38(11):674-680.
30. Gabbett TJ, Hulin BT, Blanch P, Whiteley R. High training workloads alone do not cause sports injuries: how you get there is the real issue. *Br J Sports Med*. 2016;50(8):444-445.
31. Blanch P, Gabbett TJ. Has the athlete trained enough to return to play safely? The acute:chronic workload ratio permits clinicians to quantify a player's risk of subsequent injury. *Br J Sports Med*. 2016;50(8):471-475.
32. Schoenfeld BJ, Ogborn D, Krieger JW. Effects of resistance training frequency on measures of muscle hypertrophy: a systematic review and meta-analysis. *Sports Med*. 2016;46(11):1689-1697.
33. Fassbender H. Chapter 13, Non-articular rheumatism. *Pathology of Rheumatic Diseases*. New York, NY: Springer-Verlag; 1975:303-314.
34. MacDonald GZ, Penney MD, Mullaley ME, et al. An acute bout of self-myofascial release increases range of motion without a subsequent decrease in muscle activation or force. *J Strength Cond Res*. 2013;27(3):812-821.
35. Healey KC, Hatfield DL, Blanpied P, Dorfman LR, Riebe D. The effects of myofascial release with foam rolling on performance. *J Strength Cond Res*. 2014;28(1):61-68.
36. Avela J, Kyrolainen H, Komi PV. Altered reflex sensitivity after repeated and prolonged passive muscle stretching. *J Appl Physiol (1985)*. 1999;86(4):1283-1291.

Chapter 75

Therapeutic Modality Considerations

Thomas L. Christ, Joseph M. Donnelly, and Carolyn McMakin

1. INTRODUCTION

This chapter presents common therapeutic modalities the clinician can utilize as an adjunct to manual therapy, therapeutic exercise, and dry needling or trigger point (TrP) injection for patients with myofascial pain syndrome and TrPs. Thermal modalities include superficial heat, therapeutic ultrasound, cryotherapy, and vapocoolant spray. Electrotherapeutic modalities include transcutaneous electrical nerve stimulation (TENS), neuromuscular electrical stimulation (NMES), and biofeedback. An introduction to frequency-specific microcurrent (FSM) and its application is also presented. Thermal and electrotherapeutic modalities have a rich history and many therapeutic benefits for the treatment of various musculoskeletal conditions and for the treatment of myofascial pain syndrome and TrPs. The evidence of the effectiveness of the different modalities on impairments related to TrPs is discussed in detail when available, and recommendations for patient selection and the application of modalities are also provided. Clinicians should perform a full detailed history and consider each of the precautions and contraindications related to the modality being selected and applied. It is important to remember that modalities should never be considered a monotherapeutic intervention and should be performed in combination with other therapeutic interventions along with a home management program.

THERMAL MODALITIES

2. HEAT

Superficial heat has been used for years as a means of pain relief and relaxation. Heat alone is not an effective modality for the treatment of TrPs but can be a helpful adjunct to other interventions. Quantitative sensory testing is essential prior to administering or recommending heat to identify signs and symptoms of peripheral and/or central sensitization because heat may not be indicated in the presence of peripheral sensitization (see Chapter 1).

2.1. Background

Superficial moist heat with hydrocollator hot packs uses the principle of conduction to transfer heat from the hot pack to the individual. This transfer of heat increases circulation in the skin but does not increase circulation at the level of the muscle.[1] The increased circulation at the level of the skin may allow improved efficacy of other TrP interventions such as pressure release and stretching by reducing the tissue density. Benjaboonyanupap et al[2] showed that continuous ultrasound has been shown to be more effective in pain reduction and pain pressure threshold (PPT) following 20 minutes of superficial heating compared with continuous ultrasound before superficial heating. Similar results have been shown for other interventions that may be used to treat TrPs such as pressure release, TENS, and spray-and-stretch.[3]

Heat in the absence of peripheral sensitization can provide analgesia and reduce muscle tightness. Heat reduces the gamma efferent muscle activity within the muscle spindle, thereby reducing the afferent input from the intrafusal fibers to the alpha motor neuron pool.[1] This will inherently reduce the alpha motor neuron firing rate, thus causing relaxation.[1] Heat can also inhibit nociceptive signals and stimulate areas of the brain associated with comfort and relaxation.[4]

2.2. Patient Selection

Patients presenting with pain and tissue stiffness will often benefit from superficial heat prior to other interventions. Heat in the form of a shower is also readily available to most individuals as part of a home management program. Prior to the administration of heat, the clinician should review the precautions and contraindications to heat modalities and determine if it is safe for the patient.[5]

2.3. Application

The patient should be informed of the expected sensations such as mild-to-moderate warming that may take a few minutes after application to feel. A painful burning sensation is abnormal and the patient should be informed to avoid the same experience in the shower or bath.[1]

It is important to remember not to apply the hot pack directly to the patient's skin. Six to eight layers of towels or hot pack covering should interface between the patient and the hot pack. Additionally, the patient should not put his or her body weight on the hot pack or a home moist heat pad because this accelerates the heat transfer and could result in a burn to the patient.[1]

Heat is traditionally used as an adjunct to a treatment plan of care. Heat can be used intermittently at home through portable moist heating pads, a warm bath, or shower, but should only be an adjunct for the treatment of TrPs.

3. CRYOTHERAPY AND VAPOCOOLANT SPRAY

Cold has been used historically to treat acute musculoskeletal injuries and to manage edema. Cold has an analgesic effect that dampens the patient's perception of pain and slows local circulation. Cold therapy is commonly used following dry needling interventions and for pain management following treatment. Cold modalities include ice packs and gels, ice massage, and vapocoolant sprays. Vapocoolant sprays can be applied to the skin in the area of a TrP and its pain referral region with a "spray-and-stretch" technique. The essential therapeutic

850

component is the stretch. "Stretch is the action, spray is distraction." However, the expression "spray-and-stretch" is preferred to "stretch and spray" because it is important that the spray be applied before or concurrently with, but not after, the muscle is stretched. Stretch without some additional technique to release muscle tension and suppress pain is likely to aggravate TrPs.

3.1. Background

Cold therapy is traditionally used in the acute inflammatory phase of injury, but can be used for the treatment of active TrPs as well.[6] The use of cold therapy in the form of a cold pack can be applied after manual interventions such as pressure release or dry needling.[6] Ice massage can be used prior to manual treatments to reduce pain caused from TrPs and improve PPT.[7] Vapocoolant sprays can be a very effective means of deactivating symptomatic TrPs by utilizing a "spray-and-stretch" technique, which was introduced by Simons et al, 1983.[8] A single-muscle syndrome of recent onset frequently responds with a full return of pain-free function when two or three sweeps of spray are applied while the muscle is being extended gently to its full stretch length.[9] In addition, when many muscles in one region of the body, such as the shoulder, are involved and the TrPs are interacting strongly with one another, spray-and-stretch is a practical means of releasing an entire functional group of muscles together to make more rapid progress toward pain relief. The spray-and-stretch technique does not require the precise localization of the TrP that is needed for pressure release, dry needling, or injection. It only requires identification of where the taut bands are located in the muscle to ensure that those fibers are released.

The effectiveness of the vapocoolant spray (spray-and-stretch) is related to the analgesic properties of the chemical. The vapocoolant must be dispensed as a fine stream, rather than a dispersed spray as in products that are used for athletic injuries. The cooling effect of the vapocoolant spray occurs from the instant evaporation of the spray. Because of the rate of evaporation, it is pivotal that the clinician applies the spray from the appropriate distance (12-18 in from the skin). If applied too close to the skin, the liquid's temperature will be too warm at impact to produce much effect; if applied too far away, the liquid will contact the skin at subfreezing temperatures.

Ethyl chloride is too cold for optimum release of TrP tension as usually applied. It is a rapidly acting general anesthetic that has a dangerously low margin of safety, is flammable, and is explosive when 4% to 15% of the vapor is mixed with air.[10] If ethyl chloride spray is used, rigorous precautions must be observed. Fire hazards must be eliminated, and neither the patient nor the clinician should inhale the heavy vapor. Ethyl chloride should never be given to a patient for home use. There are other commercially available products that do not contain fluorocarbons or ethyl chloride that are safer for the patient and the environment.

There are multiple physiologic mechanisms for how the application of a cooling agent to the skin dampens nociception and pain perception. Trigger points can reduce the threshold of noxious stimulus required to generate nociception and a pain response. Cryotherapy can temporarily counteract the change in pain threshold. Decreasing the temperature of the surrounding tissues as well as the nerve will increase an individual's nociceptive threshold, thus requiring more noxious stimulus for the patient to perceive pain. Cryotherapy also reduces nerve conduction velocity, therefore slowing the rate of the noxious stimulus to the central nervous system.[11] Cryotherapy can help reduce inflammation in the tissue, reducing the influx of chemical mediators such as histamine, mast cells, substance P, calcitonin gene-related peptide, bradykinin, and others that can activate and sensitize peripheral receptors. This change can prevent worsening of symptoms and the potential progression to peripheral and central sensitization. The reduction in nociception and perception of the TrPs allows the muscles to be stretched without increasing the level of nociceptive input from the TrP.

3.2. Patient Selection

Patients presenting with acute pain or inflammation, as well as those receiving manual therapy, dry needling, or TrP injections may benefit from cryotherapy to reduce inflammation as well as posttreatment soreness. Prior to the administration of cryotherapy or vapocoolant spray, the clinician should determine if it is safe for the patient by considering the precautions and contraindications to this treatment.[5]

3.3. Application

Quantitative sensory testing (especially heat and cold tolerance) should be carried out prior to the application of cryotherapy. Cold packs can be applied over larger areas of the body. To prevent skin damage, towels should be used as an interface between the ice and skin; damp towels are preferred to dry towels to better facilitate the transfer of energy. Ice packs, gel packs, and bags of frozen vegetables can all be used as the cold pack, although true ice itself may be the most beneficial and safest because it will lose its cold properties over time.[12] Before the application of the ice pack, the patient should be informed of the expected sensations. The patient is likely to feel a cold sensation at first, followed by a warming sensation for a few minutes. This feeling gives way to an achy sensation and finally anesthesia. Some mild redness on the skin is expected. The application of cold packs should last no longer than 20 to 30 minutes with longer duration for larger areas.[12] Following treatment, pain should be temporarily lessened and patients should avoid activity that could aggravate their injury or TrPs. In each of the muscle chapters, corrective actions are presented with suggestions of a home management program.

Ice massage can be performed over smaller areas and applied directly onto the skin. Ice massage can be used directly on the muscle belly over the TrPs, along the referred pain area, on the tendon, bursa, and other tissues. Ice massage requires freezing water in a paper cup, or in the fingers of a nonlatex glove, allowing the clinician to peel off part of the cup to expose the ice or breaking off one of the glove fingers and using the exposed ice.[12] The ice is slowly massaged over the target region in small circles for 5 to 10 minutes. Expected sensations for ice massage are the same as with ice packs and it is important to communicate with patients about their experience. The ice from the finger of the glove can be used in place of the vapocoolant spray by starting at the identified TrP in a muscle and moving into the pain referral area three to five times, followed by immediate stretching.

Vapocoolant sprays are applied directly to the skin. The patient must be positioned comfortably and well supported to allow relaxation of the muscles of interest. The spray is applied in a fine stream from 12 to 18 in away from the skin, at a 30° angle.[13] Figure 75-1 depicts the spray-and-stretch technique for the upper fibers of the trapezius muscle and gluteus medius muscle. Clinicians should perform one spray of the entire muscle belly length and its pain referral area two to three times and then immediately place that muscle on stretch. While still on stretch, the clinician should follow up with two or three more full-length sprays (Spray-and-stretch).[13] Latent TrPs may be activated incidental to spray-and-stretch therapy. Although one group of muscles is being passively stretched, their antagonists are shortening much more than usual. Fortunately, if latent TrPs in the antagonists are painfully activated in this way, they can be inactivated quickly by then spraying and stretching them. After application, the skin needs time to warm up again before reapplication. During this time, the patient can gently actively stretch the muscle or a moist heat pad can be applied. Vapocoolant sprays may provide pain relief and increase range of motion after one session, or may require several sessions and other skilled therapeutic interventions such as manual therapy, pressure release, dry needling, or TrP injection.

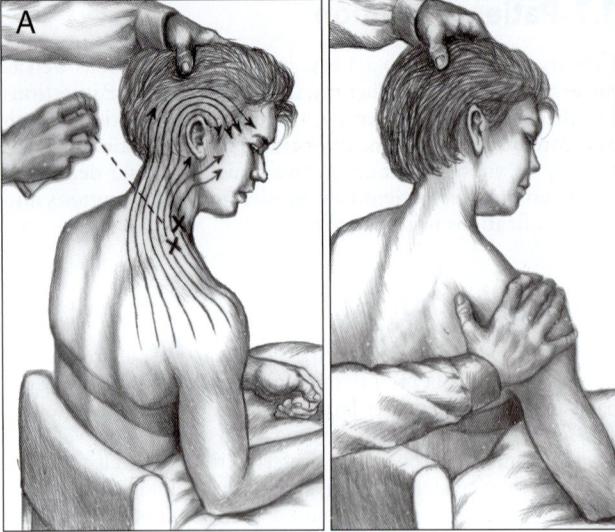
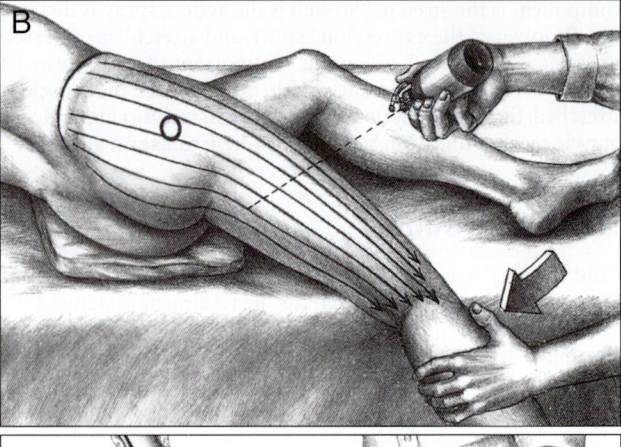
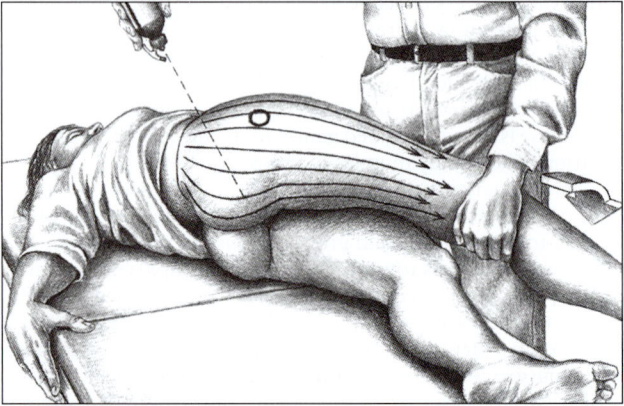

Figure 75-1. Application of vapocoolant spray for treatment of TrPs. A, Upper trapezius muscle. Note that the vapocoolant spray is applied over the muscle and pain referral pattern. B, Gluteus medius muscle. Note that the vapocoolant spray is applied from proximal to distal over the muscle through a full range of motion.

All forms of cryotherapy are performed in conjunction with other means of skilled therapeutic intervention for TrPs and are not considered stand-alone treatments. Clinicians should be mindful of their patient's responses to cryotherapy and make appropriate adjustments if necessary.

4. ULTRASOUND THERAPY

A large amount of literature on the efficacy of ultrasound therapy for patients with TrPs exists, although the effectiveness of the modality is still debated because of a lack of homogeneity in study designs. Ultrasound therapy has commonly been studied for its effects on pain (Visual Analog Score), PPT, and cervical range of motion.[2,14-23] The various available parameters for ultrasound therapy and success of placebo groups make for inconsistency in the research, although some trends in ultrasound efficacy for TrPs are beginning to emerge.

4.1. Background

Ultrasound therapy has been shown to be effective in reducing patients' pain associated with TrPs. Several studies have used a visual analog scale (VAS) for subjective pain reports and show a reduction in pain with the utilization of ultrasound therapy for the treatment of TrPs.[2,14-16,18,21-23]

Continuous ultrasound is the most commonly studied ultrasound parameter. Improvements in VAS scores with continuous ultrasound have been shown to occur immediately following treatment in some cases[2,18,23] or following several intervention sessions in other studies.[16,21,22] The results from nonthermal effects of pulsed ultrasound therapy, although far less researched, have also shown improvements in VAS pain scores in patients with TrPs, but not as effective when compared with continuous ultrasound.[15,22]

High-power pain threshold static ultrasound therapy is another method that has shown rapid improvements in VAS scores when compared with conventional continuous ultrasound therapy.[16] However, this mode has not been commonly studied and lacks additional support. In this method, the sound head is held statically over the TrP as the intensity is increased to the patient's pain threshold level (up to 1.5 W/cm^2) and is held in place for 4 to 5 seconds, and is reduced to half the intensity for 15 seconds. This procedure is repeated for 2 to 3 minutes.

The mechanisms for pain relief of performing ultrasound over TrPs are multifactorial. The application of the sound head and the deep heating excites the Aβ mechanoreceptors, thus exploiting the gate-control theory for pain modulation.[15] The thermal effects of continuous ultrasound generate local vasodilation and subsequent increased circulation, which filters out neurokines (pain-sensitizing substances) helping to reverse the hypoxic environment. The heating of the tissue reduces muscle spasm and allows sarcomeres to return to their normal length.[2,15] The increased blood supply to the TrP and resetting the sarcomere to its normal length are two important factors that need to be considered when treating TrPs.[15] Sarrafzadeh et al[15] suggest that with nonthermal ultrasound, rapid pressure changes within the tissue cause an increase in cell membrane permeability, allowing ions and molecules to be removed from the muscle tissue.

Pain pressure threshold, while subjective in nature, has been shown to be a reliable measure for muscle tenderness[21] and is commonly used as an outcome measure when studying the effectiveness of treatment on TrPs and myofascial pain syndrome.[2,14,15,20,21,23] Both continuous (thermal)[2,14,21,23] and pulsed (mechanical)[15] ultrasound therapy have been shown to be effective in the improvement of PPT. The mechanism of action to increase a patient's PPT is likely related to the reduction of neurokines in the local tissue environment, thus reducing nociceptive input and pain perception. This chemical change aids in the disruption of the local energy crisis caused by ischemia and hypoxic environment in the area of the TrP by the flushing of nociceptive-sensitizing substances out of the tissue.[15]

Ultrasound therapy of TrPs in the cervical spine region to improve cervical range of motion has been investigated with mixed results.[14-17,21,24] Improvements in range of motion are typically present with all modes of ultrasound, but the rate of improvement and reliability of the results are variable. High-powered ultrasound therapy has been shown to produce the fastest significant improvements in cervical range of motion[16]; however, as stated previously, the evidence is scant. Continuous ultrasound has also demonstrated good improvements in cervical range of motion,[16,21,24] although it often takes a frequency of 5 days a week for several weeks to see significant improvements. Pulsed ultrasound therapy is inconsistent in regard to improvements in cervical range of motion. Sarrafzadeh et al[15] showed improvements in cervical lateral flexion following six sessions of pulsed ultrasound therapy, while on the contrary, Aguilera et al[17] did not see significant improvements in cervical lateral flexion range of motion following only one treatment session with pulsed ultrasound. The reason for improvements in range of motion with thermal modes of ultrasound is likely due to its deep heating effects. Heat increases tissue extensibility, allowing the joint to go through further range of motion before being limited by the muscle containing TrPs.[14]

Overall, the literature suggests that ultrasound is an effective modality for reducing the pain perception and PPT, but is less conclusive with its effects on range of motion. The criticism with ultrasound therapy research is the lack of homogeneity and the observed improvements in placebo sham ultrasound groups. Outside of the differences in the effects of thermal and nonthermal ultrasound, there is no established parameters for treating TrPs. Placebo groups have been shown to improve significantly in pain scores,[21-23] PPT,[21,23] and cervical range of motion,[14,21,24] further questioning the true efficacy of ultrasound therapy. In some cases, improvement may result from the subsequent interventions incorporated in the treatment sessions,[14,22,24] but in other cases, no exercise treatment was provided and placebo groups still showed improvements comparable to the treatment groups.[21,23]

4.2. Patient Selection

Patients with TrPs or myofascial pain syndrome in muscles that are easily accessible by the ultrasound head are appropriate for ultrasound therapy. The application, procedures, precautions, and contraindications for ultrasound therapy are beyond the scope of this chapter, and the clinician is advised to review these parameters in other sources prior to the application of ultrasound for the treatment of TrPs and myofascial pain syndrome.

4.3. Application

The clinician should inform the patient of expected sensation such as heating, and to inform the clinician if the sound head is too hot and becomes painful. The clinician must consider the patient's medical history and should review all the precautions and contraindications prior to treatment.[5]

Continuous ultrasound therapy is the most commonly studied mode and should be used for patients who have pain or restricted mobility due to the presence of TrPs. Continuous ultrasound provides deep heating to the tissue that reduces nociception and improves muscle tissue extensibility.[2,18,23] Although it is more effective for the treatment of TrPs, continuous ultrasound has many more precautions and contraindications that must be considered before treatment.[5] Pulsed ultrasound therapy may be beneficial for reducing nociception associated with TrPs, but is not as effective for improving range of motion.[15,17] The main advantage that pulsed ultrasound therapy has over continuous ultrasound therapy is that it does not create a deep tissue heating; therefore, it may be used in the acute stages of healing[5] or when the patient presents with the signs and symptoms of peripheral sensitization. High-powered ultrasound therapy can be used for TrP-related nociception as well as range of motion, but there is a limited evidence of recommended dosage as well as precautions and contraindications to this mode of ultrasound.[16] The inconsistency in the specific parameters is one of the main reasons for the clinical controversy over ultrasound therapy effectiveness. Recommended settings for continuous and pulsed ultrasound are provided in Box 75-1. Because of the paucity in available research on high-powered ultrasound, a full recommendation on parameters is not listed.

Box 75-1 Recommendation for ultrasound therapy parameters for the treatment of TrPs

		Ultrasound Parameter Recommendations		
Mode	Intensity	Frequency	Duration	Applicator Diameter
Continuous[25]	■ Lowest intensity that still experiences desired effects. Deeper tissue will need greater intensity.	■ 1 MHz for deeper tissues up to 6 cm deep ■ 3 MHz for superficial tissues up to 2.5 cm deep	■ 5-10 min. Deeper tissue needs longer duration.	■ Sound head should be no less than half the size of the treatment area.
Pulsed[25]	■ Lowest intensity that still experiences desired effects.	■ 1 MHz for deeper tissues up to 6 cm deep ■ 3 MHz for superficial tissues up to 2.5 cm deep	■ 5-10 min. Deeper tissue needs longer duration.	■ Sound head should be no less than half the size of the treatment area.
High-power[a,16]	■ Gradually increased until level of maximum pain tolerance than reduced to half and repeated.	■ N/A	■ Held for 4-5 s at maximum pain tolerance than reduced for 15 s than repeated three times.	■ N/A

[a]High-power ultrasound recommendations are based off limited evidence.

TRANSDERMAL MEDICATION DELIVERY

5. PHONOPHORESIS

Phonophoresis is the utilization of ultrasound therapy to drive a topical medication into the subcutaneous tissue.[25] Various topical medications, most commonly hydrocortisone and local analgesics such as lidocaine, have been administered via phonophoresis.[25] Although an abundance of research exists on the efficacy of phonophoresis for various musculoskeletal conditions, there is limited literature available on its effectiveness for the treatment of myofascial pain syndrome or TrPs.

5.1. Background

The topical medications used in phonophoresis can be applied either directly onto the ultrasound head or mixed with the ultrasound gel.[25] Because phonophoresis requires the use of ultrasound therapy to drive the medication into the desired tissue, phonophoresis will provide many of the same positive effects as ultrasound therapy. The predominate effects on TrPs include reduction of pain intensity on VAS, improvement in PPT, and improvement in range of motion.[14,15,26] Many of the mechanisms of action are due to the ultrasound therapy as previously discussed in this chapter.

Some studies show significant differences between experimental phonophoresis groups compared with conventional ultrasound control groups on pain and PPT.[15,26] In one study, hydrocortisone 1% gel was used as the topical medication. Both the phonophoresis and ultrasound groups showed significant improvements in pain and PPT; however, the phonophoresis group showed significantly greater improvements when compared between groups.[15] Ustun et al[26] studied the effects of EMLA, a topical mixture of lidocaine (2.5%) and prilocaine (2.5%) used as the topical medication and compared with ultrasound therapy. Both groups showed significant reduction in pain after 15 sessions, but the eutectic mixture of local anesthetics (EMLA) phonophoresis group was significantly better when compared between groups.[26] In both of these studies, significant improvements were also found in cervical lateral flexion range of motion in both the phonophoresis and ultrasound groups, but no differences between groups existed.

Ay et al[14] used diclofenac gel as the topical medication and did not find significant differences in the reduction of pain, PPT, or range of motion between the phonophoresis and ultrasound groups.

The medication selection is an important factor in the therapeutic effects of phonophoresis. The literature does not show that phonophoresis is superior to ultrasound in improving range of motion,[14,15,26] which suggests that the improvements in range of motion are from the ultrasound therapy alone. Hydrocortisone is a powerful anti-inflammatory corticosteroid that was demonstrated to be significantly more effective than ultrasound alone in improving pain and PPT[15]; however, these results were not shown when diclofenac gel was used.[14]

5.2. Patient Selection

Patient selection for phonophoresis therapy is similar to ultrasound therapy. The patient must be prescribed the topical mediation by a physician in order to receive phonophoresis treatment. Clinicians must consider all of the precautions and contraindications to ultrasound as well as any allergies to the medication being applied before performing phonophoresis.[5]

5.3. Application

The setup and application for phonophoresis treatment is similar to that of ultrasound, with the addition of the topical medication. The medication may stand in as the coupling medium[14] or may be mixed with ultrasound gel. Both pulsed and continuous modes of ultrasound have been utilized to drive the topical medication into the desired tissue with the remaining parameters similar.[14,15,26]

Improvements in pain may occur right after treatment because of the effects of the medication but likely will take several sessions to become significant.[14,15,26] Improvements in range of motion may also occur following one session but will often take multiple intervention periods to become significant.[14,15,26] Phonophoresis is not a stand-alone treatment and should be performed in conjunction with therapeutic exercise and other skilled therapy.

6. IONTOPHORESIS

Iontophoresis is an electrical means for transcutaneous administration of drugs into the subcutaneous tissues. Iontophoresis is prescribed for a number of reasons, including pain, inflammation, and muscle spasm. Although these are all characteristics of TrPs, the literature is scarce on iontophoresis efficacy for the treatment of TrPs.

6.1. Background

Iontophoresis is a means of using charged molecules to drive topical medications past the largely impermeable stratum corneum layer of the skin into the subcutaneous tissue.[27] Negatively charged medications are repelled and directed into the skin by the cathode lead, and positively charged medications are repelled and directed into the skin by the anode lead.[28] Iontophoresis is a noninvasive, low-risk method of drug delivery that has beneficial pharmacokinetic properties such as faster release of the drug to its target tissue and easier control of dosage due to skipping the hepatic first-pass effect.[27]

Historically, iontophoresis has been used for conditions such as tendonitis, joint replacement, whiplash-associated disorder, and a variety of other musculoskeletal conditions. Iontophoresis can also be used for the treatment of TrPs, although the evidence is limited.

Lidocaine, a popular local anesthetic, has been used in the treatment of myofascial pain and TrPs on various posterior neck and back muscles.[29] Kaya et al[29] demonstrated that 10 days of lidocaine iontophoresis treatment significantly reduced PPT and VAS pain score, increased cervical range of motion, and improved a variety of other outcomes. The control group received 10 days of direct current electrical stimulation without lidocaine and also showed significant improvements in all outcomes, thus questioning if lidocaine was a significant variable in the patients' improvement.[29] Older research has shown significant success with the administration of a dexamethasone and lidocaine-mixed solution in improving active glenohumeral abduction.[30] Lidocaine is a commonly used amide local anesthetic that works by blocking the sodium channels, thus inhibiting neural transmission.[31] This physiologic effect makes it plausible that administration would reduce the pain associated with TrPs. Dexamethasone is a corticosteroid commonly prescribed for its anti-inflammatory effects, which could make it effective in flushing out the nociceptive substances present with TrPs.[31]

There is a need for more research on the efficacy of this mode of drug delivery for the treatment of TrPs.

6.2. Patient Selection

Patients dealing with pain related to TrPs are appropriate for iontophoresis as long as they do not have any precautions or contraindications to electrotherapeutic modalities or currents.[5] Additionally, clinicians should screen for any allergies to the medication being administered.

6.3. Application

The application of iontophoresis requires at least two electrodes to act as the medium for electrical conduction, the medication being administered, lead wires, and an electrical stimulation unit. The patient's skin should be cleaned with alcohol or soap and water, and excess hair should be removed before applying the electrodes. Negatively charged medications should be applied to the cathode electrode placed over the target tissue. Positively charged medications should be applied to the anode electrode placed over the target tissue.[28] Prior to initiating iontophoresis, the clinician should instruct the patient on expected sensations such as a low-level tingling or redness under the electrode, and adverse effects such as burning, stinging, blistering, or bright redness.[28]

There are no universally accepted parameters for the administration of iontophoresis. The dosage of drug to be administered along with the patient's tolerance to higher intensities (current mA) will dictate the electrical stimulation settings.[28] An example of the relationship between dosage and patient tolerance is shown in Box 75-2. Notice how when the current increases the duration of treatment reduces. Higher currents drive the medication into the target tissue at a faster rate than lower currents.[28]

Following treatment, the clinician should examine the patient's skin for signs of adverse effects such as blistering or bright redness that does not resolve within a few hours.[28] The patient may experience an improvement in symptoms, although this may be temporary as iontophoresis is not a stand-alone treatment and should be performed as an adjunct to other therapeutic interventions.

ELECTROTHERAPEUTIC MODALITIES

7. TRANSCUTANEOUS ELECTRICAL NERVE STIMULATION

TENS is an electrical modality commonly used for pain relief in addition to other therapeutic interventions. TENS can utilize a low- or high-frequency electrical current to activate internal antinociceptive mechanisms, either inhibiting nociceptive signaling or increasing the body's natural anti–nociceptive-relieving substances.[32,33] TENS is well established as a means of temporary pain relief, but limited evidence exists on the long-term effectiveness of this modality. Additionally, evidence on TENS impact on TrPs is inconclusive, largely due to the inconsistency in the methodology of the research as well as the inability to establish sound parameters for the effectiveness of TENS on TrP-related outcomes such as pain scores (VAS), PPT, and range of motion.

7.1. Background

A bulk of literature exists on TENS effectiveness on pain reduction in a variety of musculoskeletal disorders.[32,34-36] The local and referred pain generated by TrPs is signaled through small-diameter A-delta and C fibers carrying noxious stimulus from the periphery to the dorsal horn of the spinal cord where the noxious stimulus is encoded in the substantia gelatinosa.[32] Conventional high-frequency TENS exploits the "gate-control theory" to stimulate nonnoxious A-beta fibers that inhibit the transmission of the noxious A-delta and C fibers, thus inhibiting the transmission of noxious stimulus on the second-order neurons in the dorsal horn of the spinal cord.[32] The effects of high-frequency TENS (>80 Hz) are typically short-lived and do not persist more than a few hours after application.[32] Low-frequency TENS (<10 Hz) taps into the body's natural release of encephalin and β-endorphins, stimulated from the periaqueductal gray. This release activates the descending inhibitory pathways to the dorsal horn of the spinal cord, reducing nociceptive input, especially nociceptive input, from muscle nociceptors from forming effective synapses with second-order neurons in the spinal cord.[37] The effectiveness of TENS on patients with pain from TrPs follows the same pain science mechanisms as its use on any other musculoskeletal source of pain. Low-frequency TENS produces low-level muscle contractions and has been shown to improve blood flow within the muscle.[38] This effect may be beneficial in helping flush out nociceptive-sensitizing substances associated with TrPs such as substance P, bradykinine, prostaglandins, and serotonin.[33] A new study by Ferreira et al[34] examined the effects of combined high and low-frequency TENS by performing low-frequency TENS for 25 minutes followed immediately by high-frequency TENS for 25 minutes. Improvements in pain reports lasted up to 48 hours following intervention, far longer than effects typically last.

TENS effect on PPT is less conclusive as studies have produced mixed results. Ferreira et al[34] used low- and high-frequency TENS and found significant reductions in PPT lasting up to 48 hours. The muscle contraction from a low-frequency TENS may be beneficial in improving PPT by normalizing the endplate acetylcholine release and increasing blood flow to flush out the nociceptive-sensitizing substances within the TrPs,[33,34,38] although not all studies using low-frequency TENS have shown improvements in PPT.[39] High-frequency TENS has shown both positive[32] and no effect[35,40] on PPT. Burst TENS has shown to improve PPT in the short term[33] and may be an effective modality for patients experiencing pain from TrPs. The lack of homogeneity in the methods clouds the results and makes it difficult to state whether or not TENS is a beneficial modality for improving PPT in patients with myofascial pain syndrome or TrPs.

The effects of TENS on range of motion are also not clear. High-frequency TENS and burst TENS have shown to improve cervical range of motion.[32,33,35] The pain relief with TENS can induce relaxation of the muscle and deactivation of the taut band, allowing the sarcomere to lengthen, giving the patient less resistance with motion.[33] But increased range of motion does not always occur as evidenced by other researchers who have shown no improvement.[39,40]

Overall, both high-frequency and low-frequency TENS may be a beneficial intervention for reducing pain, and increasing PPT, and improving range of motion restrictions caused by TrPs. TENS should be considered an adjunct modality that could be used as an adjunct to a home management program in addition to other forms of skilled therapy including dry needling, manual therapy, and exercise (see Chapters 72 to 74). For patients experiencing higher levels of pain that may prevent them from participating in therapy, TENS can be beneficial in dampening nociceptive levels that may allow participation in therapy.

7.2. Patient Selection

Patients presenting with pain and impairments from TrPs may benefit from TENS to dampen pain and allow for function and participation during therapy. Clinicians should be always review the precautions and contraindications to electrotherapeutic modalities prior to administering TENS.[5]

Box 75-2 Iontophoresis parameters

Example of Iontophoresis Parameters		
Dosage (mA min)	Current (mA)	Duration (min)
40	1	40
40	2	20

7.3. Application

Prior to initiating TENS, the clinician should instruct the patient on expected sensations such as tingling and slight redness under the skin, and signs of adverse effects like burning, stinging, blistering, or bright redness.[41] There are various parameters for application of TENS in a patient with myofascial pain or TrPs. To date, there is no consensus on a TENS protocol for the treatment of myofascial pain syndrome or TrPs; however, there are parameters that may address peripheral and or central sensitization and/or neuropathic pain.[34] Therefore, the clinician should use sound clinical reasoning to evaluate the patient's associated mechanisms of symptoms when determining TENS parameters for the patient. Electrode size can influence the current density, and generally, smaller electrodes are indicated for TrPs because they are able to localize the current to a more distinct tissue.[41] Box 75-3 lists general guidelines for various settings of TENS.

The ability of TENS to modulate nociceptive input through gate-control and/or descending modulating systems activates the bodies' endogenous opiate release. This relief of pain is typically not long lasting. TENS may augment or allow therapeutic procedures to be implemented, be part of a home management program, and afford the patient to be productive at home and in society. TENS is typically not a stand-alone modality and should be part of a comprehensive pain management strategy. TENS is an affordable modality and should be considered as an alternative to opioid prescriptions.

8. NEURO-MUSCULAR ELECTRICAL STIMULATION

Electrical stimulation has long been applied by clinicians for treating a variety of musculoskeletal disorders. NMES is one method of electrical stimulation that has been utilized to stimulate motor units to improve the synchronization and efficacy of muscle contractions. NMES mimics function of the motor cortex through artificial depolarization of the peripheral nerves (motor end plate) and has been shown to increase motor performance, strength, and hypertrophy.[42,43] NMES is less likely to be used to deactivate TrPs, but may be effective in retraining muscle activation patterns, functional activities, and awkward postures that are contributing factors to the development of TrPs.

8.1. Background

The activation and perpetuation of TrPs can occur for many reasons, including unaccustomed eccentric loading, eccentric exercise in an unconditioned muscle, or maximal or submaximal concentric loading.[44] Muscles that are inhibited or untrained are, therefore, more prone to the development of TrPs and are often difficult for patients to volitionally contract and strengthen because of pain, fatigue, and inefficiency of muscle activation patterns.

Postural considerations are also important factors. Patients presenting with forward head posture, upper cross syndrome, or lower cross syndrome often have muscle groups that are overlengthened and inhibited, and are difficult to activate volitionally. NMES may enhance muscle activation to improve motor control of these inhibited muscles through artificial electrical stimulus to the motor end plate of the muscle. This stimulus mimics that generated by the motor cortex during volitional contraction by creating the same action potential propagation and subsequent release of the acetylcholine neurotransmitter.[42] NMES does not function the same as volitional contraction nor does it have the same physiologic and mechanical effects. With NMES, all motor units are recruited at once rather than type I slow-twitch fibers being depolarized and activated first followed by type II fast-twitch fibers as in Hanneman's size principle.[42,45] Additionally, in volitional contraction, the motor units have an opportunity to rotate their "on" and "off" time within a contraction, allowing brief periods of rest, which is not the case with NMES. With NMES, all motor units are turned "on" throughout the contraction, thus increasing the rate of muscle fatigue.[42]

There is a paucity of NMES research directly related to TrPs, but an extensive amount of literature supports its ability to strengthen weak muscles and improve motor performance.[42,43,46,47] There is a vast amount of research on NMES because it relates to postoperative rehabilitation following knee surgeries when the quadriceps femoris muscle group is inhibited or weakened and is associated with impairments in gait due to weakness and poor motor unit recruitment. NMES, combined with exercise, has been shown to be more effective than exercise alone in quadriceps strength and function.[43] There is limited evidence for NMES in other areas of the body, but the same principles can be applied. The posterior shoulder and scapular muscles are commonly either lengthened, weak, or inhibited and are typically a site of TrP development. NMES can be used as part of a neuromuscular reeducation program to retrain muscle function and muscle activation patterns, subsequently improving posture and function and preventing further TrP development.[48,49]

8.2. Patient Selection

Patients who show signs of muscular imbalance such as forward head posture, upper cross syndrome, or lower cross syndrome (see Chapter 76) are likely to have muscle groups that are lengthened, inhibited, or weak, creating muscle overload and altered movement patterns. Patients with these impairments are at risk for developing TrPs because of either the overactivity or underactivity of the functional unit. A combination of NMES with volitional

---

Box 75-3 TENS parameters

TENS Parameter Recommendations[41]

Mode	Pulse Frequency	Pulse Duration (μs)	Intensity (mA)	Duration (min)
Conventional (high-frequency)	>80 Hz	50-100	Sensory level, to patient tolerance	20-30
Conventional (low-frequency)	<10 Hz	>150	Motor level, to elicit a visible muscle twitch	20-45
Burst	~100 Hz, burst frequency 1-4 Hz	200	Motor level, to elicit a visible muscle twitch	N/A

Abbreviation: TENS, transcutaneous electrical stimulation.

muscle contraction as a means to retrain the underactive muscle groups may be beneficial for patients presenting with inhibition weakness due to TrPs. Prior to the application of NMES, the clinician should review the precautions and contraindications to determine if the patient is appropriate for NMES.[5]

8.3. Application

There are a number of different parameters clinicians can use for NMES. Burst-modulated (Russian) is common and generally promotes faster and greater gains, although it increases the rate of fatigue and is less tolerable. Pulsed biphasic is another common waveform that is generally effective and more tolerable. For strengthening effects, the pulse duration should be the highest level that the patient can tolerate,[45,47] with larger muscles able to tolerate longer durations than smaller muscles. A pulse frequency of at least 30 pulses/s is needed to generate a forceful contraction, but can be as high as 80 pulses/s.[45] As mentioned, NMES tends to lead to muscle fatigue faster than volitional isolated muscle contractions. Therefore, a work-to-rest ratio should be established.[45,47] A 1:5 work-to-rest ratio is recommended initially and can be progressed to 1:4 and 1:3 as muscle performance improves. The amplitude (intensity) is dependent on patient tolerance. For strength gains to occur, the intensity of the contraction should be near maximal levels, but pain and fatigue prevent reaching higher levels of intensity; therefore, the clinician should start at patient tolerance and slowly progress to greater amplitudes.[45,47] Electrodes should be placed over the motor end plate, and a minimum of 2 in apart. Larger muscles may require larger electrodes and an additional channel, four electrodes rather than two.[47]

Following NMES, the patient may experience delayed onset muscle soreness (DOMS) as well as some slight redness on the skin.[45] In this case the muscle should be examined for TrPs as the overload by the NMES may cause the formation of TrPs especially in the presence of DOMS. The clinician should be aware of signs and symptoms suggestive of rhabdomyolysis, because this has been reported in some cases with improper NMES prescription.[47] NMES can be used indirectly to treat TrPs by correcting postural and muscular overload. NMES is never a stand-alone therapy and should be used as an adjunct to a detailed clinical reasoning process and therapeutic exercise prescription. Once volitional activation can be achieved, NMES should be withdrawn to improve motor control during functional activities.

9. BIOFEEDBACK

Biofeedback is a way to monitor and attempt to modify a patient's autonomic functions. Biofeedback is often used to study a patient's muscle or brain activity through electromyography (EMG), functional MRI (fMRI), monitoring,[50] and other types of physiologic feedback. It can be an effective modality for patients with TrPs to help reduce their activity and modulate their perception of pain.

9.1. Background

Biofeedback utilizing EMG can help the clinician identify muscular dysfunctions caused by TrPs, or may be causing associated TrPs in other muscles leading to the patient's pain or movement impairments.[51,52] Electrodes can be placed on the skin over the muscle belly or inserted into the muscle belly (in-dwelling) recording the electrical activity occurring at the motor end plate.[45] The raw data collected is rectified into visual or audio feedback that the clinician can use to interpret the activity occurring in the muscle. These data help the clinician to identify muscles that may be underactive or overactive, asymmetries, faulty motor unit recruitment, and ineffective timing and synchronization. It may also help identify unwarranted muscle activity that may be contributing to the patient's symptoms. The auditory or visual feedback from the EMG data can be used to help retrain muscular dysfunctions, whether it be through recruitment of motor units or inhibition of overactive motor units. Although beneficial for any muscle group, EMG biofeedback has been predominately studied in the treatment of patients reporting temporomandibular joint (TMJ) pain by reducing muscular tension around the TMJ. These investigators found that muscle tension and pain scores remained reduced up to 6 months following conclusion of the intervention.[51-53]

Biofeedback using fMRI proposes potential ability to train patients to manipulate the activity of the rostral anterior cingulate cortex associated with conscious pain perception.[54] deCharms et al,[54] in a study using real-time functional MRI, showed that through training, when subjects were presented with a noxious stimulus, they were able to increase or decrease the perception of pain on command.[54] The same held true for patients with persistent pain. Myofascial TrPs can lead to peripheral and central sensitization, and this type of biofeedback may be beneficial in helping these patients self-modulate their pain perception. However, because of the cost of this equipment, this intervention may not be feasible for all patients. Less expensive options for biofeedback should be researched.

9.2. Patient Selection

Following the patient's subjective report, the clinician should hypothesize if certain muscles are over- or underactive, leading to TrP activation and pain. Psychosocial variables should also be assessed because many of these conditions lead to increased muscle tension. Individuals under stress often experience increased muscle tension and pain.[52] If the clinician feels that muscle tension or dysfunctional motor performance is a contributing factor in the patient's presentation, biofeedback may be indicated. Biofeedback is also indicated in patients with persistent pain caused by muscle pain and TrPs. Because biofeedback is strictly information gathering, and no stimulus is being applied to the patient, there are no precautions or contraindications other than allergies to the electrode, which makes biofeedback an appropriate intervention for most individuals.[45]

9.3. Application

The setup for EMG biofeedback requires recording electrodes, a recording device, computer software to rectify the raw data, and an auditory or visual mode to present the information to the clinician and patient.[45] The correct size and location of the electrode is important to study the desired muscle and to avoid cross-talk. Other forms of biofeedback will have individual technology requirements for use.

Biofeedback is not a treatment in itself, but it provides useful information about an individual's performance, and allows the clinician to select interventions appropriately and provides quantitative data to monitor progress.

10. FREQUENCY-SPECIFIC MICROCURRENT

By Carolyn McMakin

FSM was first used to treat TrPs in 1996. The technique uses manual therapy combined with frequencies thought to address certain pathologies in specific tissues delivered as square wave pulses by a standard two-channel microcurrent device. The frequencies were developed by physicians in the early 1900s and used on devices not seen since the 1930s. A 1922 frequency list was discovered with one of the old devices in 1946. The device was abandoned and the list was filed away until 1996 when it came to be used in the treatment of myofascial pain syndrome and TrPs on a two-channel microcurrent device.[55,56]

10.1. Background

The FSM technique uses a frequency on one channel described on the list as neutralizing a specific pathology combined and applied simultaneously with a frequency on a second channel described as addressing a specific tissue. The microcurrent device delivers the frequencies with ramped square wave pulses of subsensory current between 100 and 300 µA. Research shows that water in the body is organized into structures resembling a semiconductor matrix allowing the instantaneous transmission of current and information throughout the body. There is considerable evidence in the biophysics literature that cells, nerves, and organ systems communicate by way of frequencies and biologic resonance. Cell membrane receptors have the ability to reconfigure in response to information provided by chemical signaling from the environment and by coherent signals supplied to or by the system to those same receptors. Cell membrane receptors connect to internal cellular structures and modify transcription factors that alter genetic expression, allowing the cell to respond appropriately to the environment. This is the most reasonable model for the mechanism of action for frequency effects on biologic tissue.[57-61]

Microamperage current below 500 µA has been shown to increase adenosine triphosphate (ATP) production by 500% in three different tissue culture studies.[62-64] It is presumed, but not proven, that the increase in ATP production plays some role in the effectiveness of the therapy by providing the energy required to relax the sarcomeres.

The available data show that the frequency described as "reducing inflammation," 40 Hz, reduces all of the inflammatory cytokines by factors of 10 and 20 times in 90 minutes. All of the inflammatory cytokines responded and all stopped in the normal range.[65] In an unpublished blinded animal trial, this same frequency was shown to reduce lipoxygenase-mediated inflammation by 62% in 4 minutes and cyclooxygenase-mediated inflammation by 30% in 4 minutes in every animal tested. This was a time-dependent response with half of the effect present at 2 minutes and the full effect present at 4 minutes.[66] These data suggest that the frequencies have their effect by modifying cell signaling and changing epigenetic expression to reduce the production of inflammatory peptides. There is no other mechanism that explains the unprecedented rate and magnitude of cytokine reduction down to, but not below, the normal range. When treating TrPs with specific treatment protocols, the tissues begin to soften and change tone in seconds. This rapid response suggests, but doesn't confirm, the cell signaling mechanism model.

The frequency described as removing the scar tissue (13 Hz) appears to do so by way of resonance that loosens the cross-links holding the connective tissue in a shortened configuration. This particular frequency, when combined with the frequencies for various tissues, especially the nerve and fascia, anecdotally has a dramatic effect on increasing range of motion. It affects only the abnormal scar tissue and has not been observed to reduce normal repair tissue in a fully healed injury. If used before the repair tissue has matured, it can delay healing and should not be used when there is a new injury. There is only clinical observation for the effect of this frequency. Further research needs to be done to confirm its effects and mechanism.[67]

The frequencies and treatment protocols found to be effective for TrPs have been refined in the last 21 years and are currently being used by more than 3000 clinicians in 13 countries.[68] Collected case reports on the treatment of myofascial pain syndrome in the head, neck, and face and the low back were published in 1998 and 2004.[55,56]

10.2. Patient Selection

FSM uses subsensory current and the frequencies create fairly rapid tissue softening independent of manual pressure, making it an ideal technique for neurologically sensitized patients and for TrPs in muscles near sensitive vascular, visceral, or autonomic structures. The device contacts are placed at the nerve roots innervating the muscles in an entire biomechanical region as they exit the spine allowing for the treatment of multiple muscle-couples simultaneously. This makes FSM particularly useful for athletes and for patients with active, latent, and associated TrPs in multiple muscles and muscle functional units. The FSM myofascial protocols all begin with the frequencies to reduce nerve activity, making it particularly helpful in patients where nerve inflammation drives increased muscle tone and perpetuates TrP activity.

Patients with TrPs associated with the consumption of statins may not respond to this technique unless they take 200 to 400 mg of CoQ10 per day for a period of 2 weeks prior to treatment. Once the patient is taking CoQ10, he or she should respond as expected.

10.3. Precautions

Pacemaker

Microcurrent is classified as a TENS device, even though it delivers 1000 times less current than a TENS and has a completely different mechanism of action. TENS devices are contraindicated in patients with pacemakers; therefore, FSM should be used with caution in patients with a pacemaker, although no adverse events have been reported to date in this patient group.

Infection

The frequency to reduce inflammation, 40 Hz, will reduce inflammation even in the presence of active infection. The frequency appears to override the signaling from physical bacterial or viral lipopolysaccharides (LPS) fragments and will reduce inflammation for 2 to 6 hours. During the time when inflammation is reduced, active infection can and has been shown to proliferate. It is, therefore, inadvisable to use this frequency when the patient has an active infection anywhere unless the patient is on antibiotics.

New Injury

The frequency to remove the scar tissue, 13 Hz, should not be used when a patient has sustained a new injury in any place on the body. Because the body is a semiconductor, there is no place on the body where the frequency does not have an effect, and new injuries require the scar tissue to form in order to heal. Using the frequency to remove scarring within 6 weeks of a new injury will delay healing. Ninety-one hertz can be used safely to soften the tissue once the new injury is 4 weeks old, and 13 Hz can be used safely once the new injury is 6 weeks old.

Hydration

For FSM to be effective, the patient must be hydrated and should have consumed one quart of water in the 4 hours preceding treatment. This amount of water intake may be inappropriate for patients with compromised cardiac or renal function, and the clinician or patient should consult with the physician monitoring these conditions prior to the consumption of the recommended pretreatment water intake. Treatment may be attempted without the recommended water intake, but clinically we have found this to be less effective.

Detoxification Reactions

FSM treats multiple muscles in a short period of time, and patients who experience detoxification reactions such as fatigue or nausea after massage may find this detox reaction amplified when FSM is used in addition to manual therapy. Water intake immediately following treatment along with a meal that includes sulfur-bearing vegetables seems to ameliorate this detox reaction.

Stenosis

Some patients with central spinal or foraminal stenosis have been observed to experience increased pain when polarized positive DC current is used. In patients with known stenosis, alternating current should be used instead of polarized positive current.

Ligamentous Laxity

Because FSM can soften muscles and increase range of motion so dramatically in a short period of time, it may not be appropriate for patients with known ligamentous laxity, especially in the cervical spine. Therapeutic measures should be taken to repair the injured ligaments.

10.4. Contraindications

Pregnancy

Because the frequency 40 Hz reduces prostaglandins and certain prostaglandins are required to maintain pregnancy, FSM should not be used on a patient known to be pregnant. No known adverse effects have been reported, but once a woman is known to be pregnant, FSM should not be used for any indication.

10.5. Application

Preparation

The well-hydrated patient should have the treatment area skin exposed, while preserving modesty with a gown or drape. FSM can be used in any muscle or muscle group including the pelvis, scalp, and jaw as well as axial and extremity muscles. Box 75-4 outlines a pretreatment script for clinicians.

10.6. Equipment

FSM requires a two-channel microcurrent device that can provide accurate independent three-digit-specific frequencies on each channel using a ramped square wave. The device should be a constant current generator with the device automatically varying the voltage to maintain the current levels set for patient treatment. Current levels should be between 20 and 500 µA and

> **Box 75-4 Typical pretreatment script used by the clinician**
>
> 1. I am going to use FSM to treat your muscles. You will not be able to feel the current because it is the same kind of current your body produces on its own.
> 2. I am going to apply the current by wrapping these warm wet towels (or wraps) to the area to be treated. One contact will go at the spine where the nerves to the painful muscles leave the spine. We'll place the other contact so the current flows through the muscles we need to treat.
> 3. We can use conductive gel electrode pads instead of wet contacts if you prefer, as long as you are not sensitive to the adhesive.
> 4. Are you pregnant?
> 5. Do you have a pacemaker?
> 6. Do you have an active untreated infection anywhere?
> 7. Have you had any new physical injuries or wounds in the last 4 weeks?
> 8. Do you have any questions or concerns?

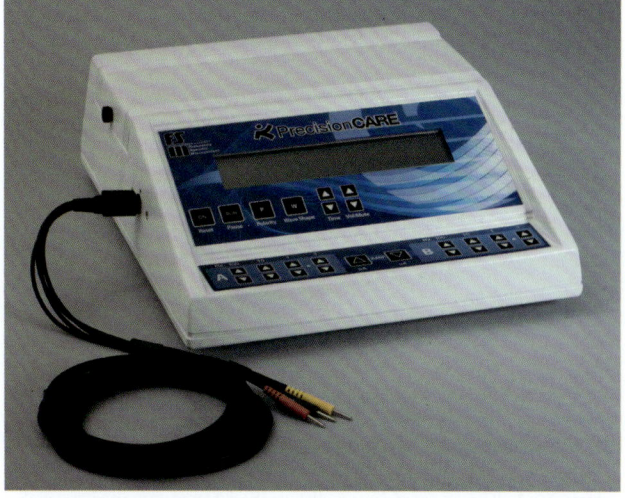

Figure 75-2. The Precision Care (Precision Distributing, Vancouver WA) allows the clinician to set independent frequencies, adjust amperage, current polarity, and wave slope quickly and manually.

able to be used polarized positive or alternating. The polarized positive current is more accurately described as pulsed positive direct current with the negative portion or the wave removed. A typical tabletop manual device and a small programmable device are show below, but there are a number of microcurrent devices on the market that fulfill the requirements, and any device can be used that meets the criteria above.

The device typically comes with six-foot leads. The leads end in pin-plug tips that will fit into graphite conducting gloves that can be wrapped in a warm wet hand towel or washcloth. The pins will also fit into alligator clips that can be attached to a warm wet fabric wrap or cloth. Tap water used to wet the towels or wraps serves as the conductive agent. Distilled water will not conduct current and should not be used. Some clinics use towel warmers to keep the wet fabric wraps warm. The contacts are sanitized in the warmer and by simple washing in a washing machine. Adhesive conductive electrode pads can be used multiple times by the same patient but cannot be transferred from one patient to another. Figures 75-2 through 75-9 show the FSM equipment and patient setup.

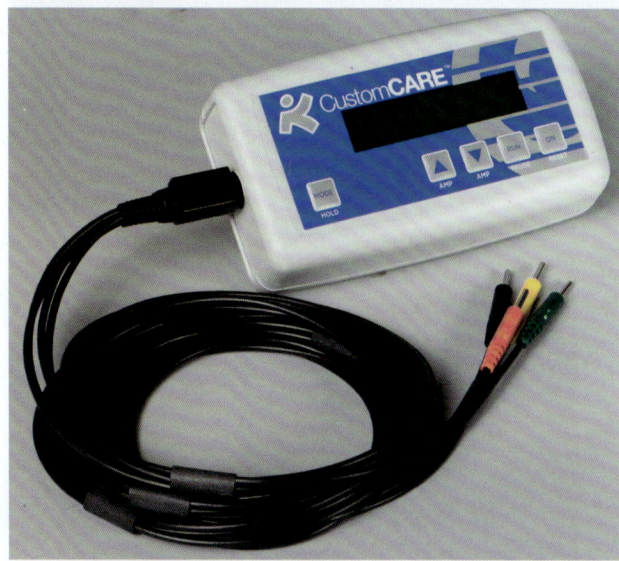

Figure 75-3. The CustomCare is a small handheld unit that can be programmed from a computer. Frequency protocols can be programmed into the small satellite unit for the times suggested in the tables. This device doesn't have a manual mode, and the frequency applications must be modified by the computer software and programmed on to the satellite.

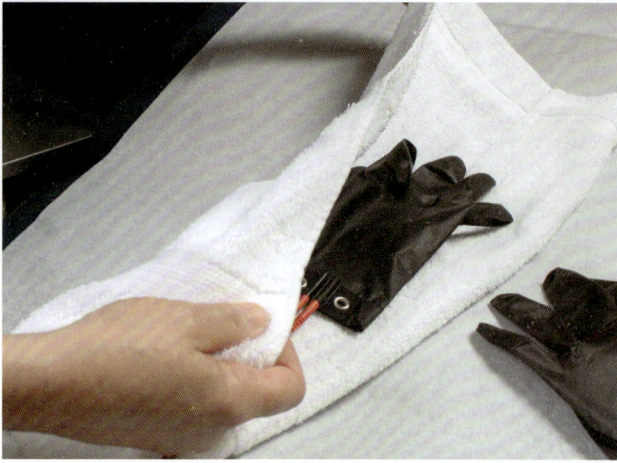

Figure 75-4. The current is usually applied for myofascial work by wrapping a graphite glove in a warm wet hand towel or by attaching alligator clips to a warm wet hand towel or wash cloth. The water conducts the current and the towel provides a large conductive surface area for treating muscle groups together.

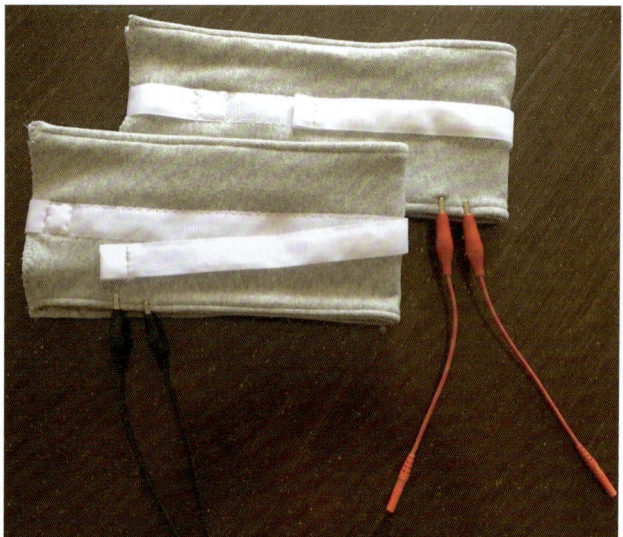

Figure 75-5. A wet fabric strip or "wrap" can attached to the device by way of alligator clips and secured to the patient with the Velcro strips. The wrap application allows treatment while the patient is seated or moving.

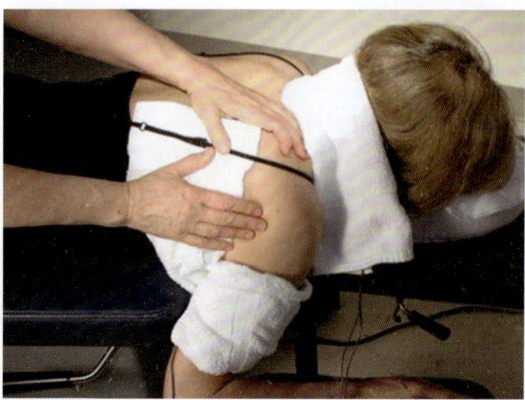

Figure 75-6. Setup for treatment of neck and shoulder complex.

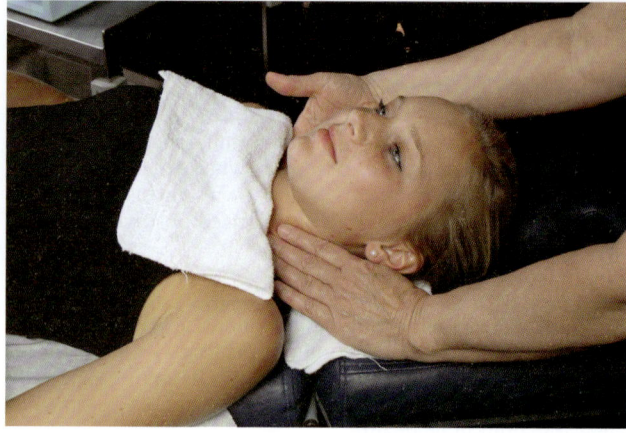

Figure 75-7. Setup for treatment of the cervical spine and suboccipital region.

The manual therapy technique performed while the current is running does not typically require massage lotion because the fingers are used to apply local pressure on the taut bands of TrPs similar to pressure release techniques rather than requiring long effleurage strokes or deep pressure. The frequencies soften the tissue, so minimal manual pressure is required.

10.7. Application Options

The treatment variables depend on the area or region to be treated and the perceived causes of or perpetuating factors for the TrPs. In general, the current is applied with the positive leads covering the nerve roots related to the treated muscles where they exit the spine and the negative leads are placed just distal to the muscles being treated so the current passes through the muscles in three dimensions. The frequencies used will vary depending on muscle location, function, innervation, and the factors causing or perpetuating the TrPs. As a general rule, frequencies for the nerve are used first.

Dosing

In general, patients are treated twice a week for 4 to 6 weeks. Patients with persistent chronic pain should be treated twice in the first week with treatment at least 2 days apart. Treatment can be discontinued as soon as pain and TrPs resolve. Data suggest chronic myofascial pain will resolve in approximately

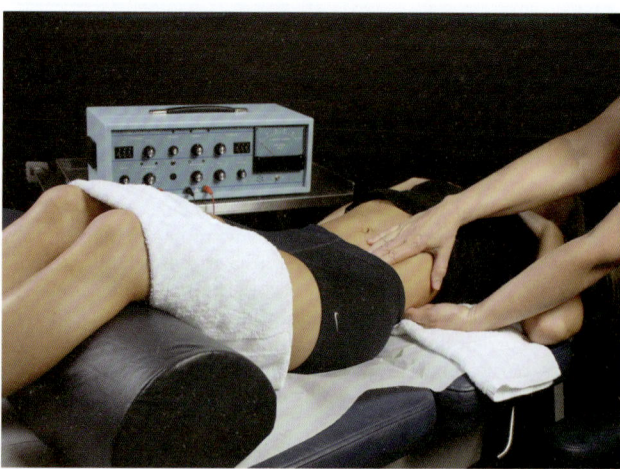

Figure 75-8. Setup for treatment of the lumbar spine, psoas, and abdominal muscle groups.

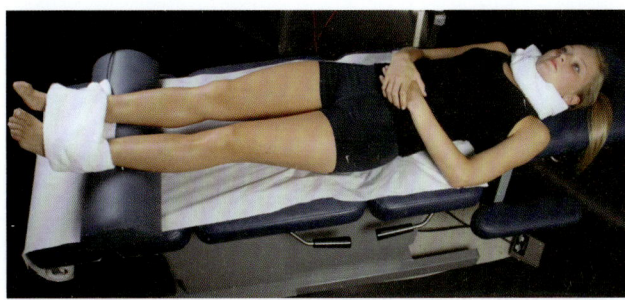

Figure 75-9. Setup for treatment of widespread myofascial pain syndrome.

six treatments administered in 6 weeks. Simple or uncomplicated myofascial pain may resolve in one session, but at least one follow-up session is recommended. If the patient has spinal ligamentous laxity creating increased translation of spinal vertebral segments, resolution of TrPs will take much longer and additional treatments will need to address the ligamentous laxity.

The following application suggestions are presented in more detail in the textbook *Frequency Specific Microcurrent in Pain Management*[69] or in a 4-day training course or in online training modules (www.frequencyspecific.com).

Treatment Application

Treatment of the cervical spine and the subscapularis and posterior shoulder muscles is displayed in Box 75-5.

Manual Technique

The placement of the contacts for treating the shoulder complex is depicted in Figure 75-6. This allows the current to address all of the shoulder muscles and any potential adhesions between the subscapular nerve and subscapularis muscle that might impact shoulder mechanics. Palpate the subscapularis evaluating for TrPs and tenderness. Use settings 40/396 until subscapularis muscle tenderness is significantly reduced, then change the frequency to 13/396 and begin to mobilize the subscapularis muscle and shoulder complex. The manual technique involves firm gentle pressure applied to all of the muscles in the area being treated in a gentle kneading motion. Use frequencies, in order, as shown in Box 75-5. Response to this protocol has been clinically predictable and consistent.

Treating Cervical Spine and Suboccipital Complex

Treatment parameters for the cervical spine, the cervical paraspinal muscles, and the suboccipital muscles are displayed in Box 75-6.

Manual Technique

Manual therapy with FSM differs from manual muscle therapy. Moderate manual pressure is used to palpate the treated muscles. Figure 75-7 shows the setup for treatment of the paraspinal muscles in the cervical region and the suboccipital muscles. The frequencies will soften the muscles and the manual pressure simply follows the muscle softening and assists the loosening of the scar tissue bonds. 40/94 will soften the upper trapezius muscle, and manual therapy senses and assists the upper trapezius muscle softening. Once the upper trapezius muscle softens, the suboccipital, the splenius, and the cervical paraspinal muscles become more apparent and the underlying tight muscles overlying the fact joints become apparent. The current 124/100 softens the suboccipital muscles, especially if the alar ligaments have ever been traumatized. Once the suboccipital muscles are softer, the rectus capitis posterior (RCP) minor muscle will stand out as tight in the midline of the suboccipital space. The RCP minor muscle has a connective tissue slip between it and the dura mater. The frequency to remove "scarring from the dura mater" 13/443 will soften the RCP minor where it attaches to the dura mater if it is gently rocked in 5 mm upward motions. Once the suboccipital muscles are softened, the

---

Box 75-5 Parameters for treating cervical spine, subscapularis and posterior shoulder muscles

Frequency Used	Description Condition/Tissue	Expected Action	Minutes
40/94	Inflammation/medulla	Reduce tone and TrPs in upper trapezius	2
40/10	Inflammation/spinal cord	Reduce tone in cervical paraspinal muscles	2
40/396	Inflammation/nerve	Should reduce tone and TrPs in cervical and shoulder muscles. Should reduce tone and tenderness in subscapularis	4
13/396	Scarring/nerve	Mobilize subscapularis and neck and shoulder muscles. Should increase shoulder mobility	4
13/142	Scarring/fascia	Mobilize subscapularis and neck and shoulder muscles. Should increase mobility, reduce tone and TrPs	4
40/710	Inflammation/disc	Should reduce tone and TrPs in medial scalenes and paraspinals	2-4
40/157	Inflammation/cartilage, facet	Should reduce tone and TrPs in cervical paraspinal muscles	2-4
40/480	Inflammation/joint capsule, facet	Should reduce tone and TrPs in posterior cervical paraspinal muscles	2-4
91/142	Hardening/fascia	Should reduce tone and TrPs in all muscles between occiput and shoulder	2
81/142	Increase secretions/Fascia	Should further soften muscles and support fascia recovery	2
[a]NOTE: 124/191 124/77	Repair disrupted/tendon Repair disrupted/connective tissue	If one of the rotator cuff tendons is disrupted, the TrPs will not resolve until these frequency pairs are used. These frequencies are time dependent. Repair may take extended time or multiple sessions. Use until TrPs resolve.	10-60

Box 75-6 Parameters for treating cervical spine and suboccipital complex

Frequency Used	Description Condition/Tissue	Expected Action	Minutes
40/94	Inflammation/medulla, accessory nerve	Should reduce tone and TrPs in SCM and upper trapezius and allow palpation of suboccipital muscles	2-4
40/10	Inflammation/spinal cord	Should reduce tone in cervical paraspinal muscles	2
40/396	Inflammation/nerve	Should soften all DRG-innervated muscles between contacts	4
124/100	Disruption/ligaments	Should reduce tone and TrPs in the suboccipital and cervical muscles associated with ligamentous injury	4
13/443	Scarring/dura	Should reduce tone and TrPs in rectus capitus posterior minor specifically. Rock suboccipital area during use	4
40/157	Inflammation/cartilage, facet	Should reduce tone and TrPs in upper cervical paraspinal muscles.	2-4
40/480	Inflammation/joint capsule, facet	Should reduce tone and TrPs in upper cervical paraspinal muscles	2-4
40/783	Inflammation/periosteum	Should reduce tone and TrPs in the cervical paraspinal muscles	2-4
91/480	Hardening/joint capsule	Should soften multifidi and paraspinal muscles overlying the facet joint capsule	2
40/710	Inflammation/disc	Should reduce tone and TrPs in lower cervical paraspinal muscles and anterior scalene muscles	2-4
13/396	Scarring/nerve	Should reduce adhesions between nerve and fascia and increase range of motion	2
91/142	Hardening/fascia	Should reduce tone, TrPs in cervical muscles between the contacts	2
91/62	Hardening/muscle belly	Should reduce tone, TrPs in cervical muscles between the contacts	2
81/142	Increase secretions/fascia	Should further soften muscles and fascia	2

DRG, dorsal root ganglion; SCM, sternocleidomastoid.

cervical paraspinal muscles will be palpably tight and the taut bands overlying the facet joints will be more noticeable. These muscles will soften when the frequencies to reduce inflammation in the cartilage, the periosteum, and the joint capsule are used. The muscles overlying the joint capsule may still be firm or hard at this point and should soften when the frequency for "hardening in the joint capsule" is used. The next muscles to become apparent will be the scalene muscles and lower cervical paraspinal muscles. These muscles seem to soften in response to the frequency to reduce inflammation in the disc annulus.

Treating Lumbar Spine, Psoas Muscle Group, Abdominal Muscle Group

Treatment parameters for the lumbar spine, the psoas muscle group, and the abdominal muscle group are displayed in Box 75-7.

Manual Technique

Manual therapy for muscles in the lumbar spine involves steady firm pressure to follow the muscle as it softens in response to the frequencies applied. Figure 75-8 shows the setup for treatment of the lumbar spine, psoas, and abdominal muscle groups.

When using the frequencies to modify adhesions between the nerve and any structure, it is necessary to move the tissue while running the frequencies to remove the scar tissue. For TrPs associated with disc inflammation, the patient may be more comfortable in slight lumbar extension whether prone or supine, and the lumbar paraspinal muscles should be mobilized with a broad flat finger contact and a slight kneading motion. For TrPs associated with facet inflammation, the patient should be treated while supine with the knees bent and the back flat. Mobilizing the lumbar muscles in these patients while using the frequencies to alleviate scarring between the nerve and fascia or nerve and joint capsule is simply a matter of gently rocking the knees gently from side to side within the pain-free range. This movement allows the nerves to glide between fascial layers and increases segmental range of motion in lumbar rotation.

The manual technique for treating the psoas and abdominal muscle groups requires some care to avoid deep vascular and visceral structures. The clinician should use a broad flat-fingered contact, avoid any circular scrubbing motions, and simply apply firm steady but sensitive downward pressure while the frequency response causes tissue softening. If slow muscle guarding is identified at any point, the clinician should pause and reduce pressure.

Treating Widespread Multiple Trigger Points

The following FSM protocol is used when the patient has widespread and numerous TrPs in the upper and lower body (Box 75-8), is not on any statin medication, and does not have any other genetic muscle pathology or deficiency that would explain their presence. The patient may or may not have the neuroendocrine component of fibromyalgia but may have been diagnosed as having fibromyalgia in addition to the diagnosis of myofascial pain syndrome. The contacts are placed at the neck and feet.

Manual Technique

There is no manual technique advised for this class of patient. The setup for treatment is shown in Figure 75-9. The data suggest that TrPs in this type of patient are neurologically driven by

Box 75-7 Treating lumbar spine, psoas muscle group, rectus abdominus muscles

Frequency Used	Description Condition/Tissue	Expected Action	Minutes
TrPs Associated With Disc Inflammation			
40/396	Inflammation/nerve	Should soften all DRG-innervated muscles between back and abdomen	4
40/710	Inflammation/disc annulus	Should reduce tone and TrPs in quadratus lumborum, rectus abdominus, psoas	4
40/630	Inflammation/disc as a whole	Should reduce tone and TrPs in quadratus lumborum, rectus abdominus, psoas	2
40/330	Inflammation/disc nucleus	Should reduce tone and TrPs in quadratus lumborum, rectus abdominus, psoas	4
13/396	Scarring/nerve Mobilize paraspinal muscles while using	Should reduce adhesions between nerve and fascia and increase range of motion	2
91/142	Hardening/fascia	Should reduce tone, TrPs in lumbar muscles	2
91/62	Hardening/muscle belly	Should reduce tone, TrPs in cervical muscles between the contacts	2
81/142	Increase secretions/fascia	Should further soften muscles and support fascia recovery	2
TrPs Associated With Facet Joints			
40/396	Inflammation/nerve	Should soften all DRG-innervated muscles between back and abdomen	4
40/783	Inflammation/periosteum	Should reduce tone and TrPs in the cervical paraspinal muscles	2-4
40/157	Inflammation/cartilage, facet	Should reduce tone and TrPs in lumbar paraspinal muscles	2-4
40/480	Inflammation/joint capsule, facet	Should reduce tone and TrPs in the cervical paraspinal muscles	2-4
91/480	Hardening/joint capsule	Should soften multifidi and paraspinal muscles overlying the facet joint capsule	2
13/396	Scarring/nerve Rock the knees to move the joints while using	Should reduce adhesions between nerve and fascia and increase range of motion	2
91/142	Hardening/fascia	Should reduce tone, TrPs in cervical muscles between the contacts	2
91/62	Hardening/muscle belly	Should reduce tone, TrPs in lumbar muscles	2
81/142	Increase secretions/fascia	Should further soften muscles and support fascia recovery	2
Psoas Muscle Group TrPs			
13/60[a], 142	Resolves psoas TrPs associated with scarring (13/) between the ureter (/60) and fascia (/142)	When prior kidney stone, infection or trauma is the cause, 13/60 reduces the pain, psoas tightness and resolves TrPs. Gentle rocking of abdominal muscles assists action. If psoas tightness is not associated with the ureter, this application will not have any effect on psoas TrPs.	10-20
Rectus Abdominus Muscle TrPs			
40/22[a]	Resolves TrPs caused or perpetuated by food sensitivities and inflammation (40/) in the small intestine (/22)	If the TrPs are associated with inflammation in the small intestine, this frequency will soften the taut bands and eliminate the TrPs. If there is no intestinal inflammation, this application will have no effect on tone or TrPs	10-20
Abdominal Oblique TrPs			
40/7[a]	Resolves TrPs associated with inflammation (40/) from ovarian cysts (/7[a])	If the TrPs are associated with inflammation from an ovarian cyst, this frequency will soften the taut bands and eliminate the TrPs. If there is no ovarian cyst, this application will have no effect on tone or TrPs.	10-20
40/65[a], 129[a]	Resolves TrPs associated with inflammation (40/) in the descending (/65[a]) and sigmoid (/129[a]) colon	If the TrPs are associated with inflammation in the descending or sigmoid colon, this frequency will soften the taut bands and eliminate the TrPs. If there is no intestinal inflammation, this application will have no effect on tone or TrPs.	

[a]These frequencies are described on the original frequency list as resonating with specific visceral organs; however, no claims for such effects can be made. Resolving TrPs in these specific muscles is the only clinical effect documented for these frequencies.

50. Pal US, Kumar L, Mehta G, et al. Trends in management of myofascial pain. *Natl J Maxillofac Surg.* 2014;5(2):109-116.
51. Dalen K, Ellertsen B, Espelid I, Gronningsaeter AG. EMG feedback in the treatment of myofascial pain dysfunction syndrome. *Acta Odontol Scand.* 1986;44(5):279-284.
52. Turk DC, Zaki HS, Rudy TE. Effects of intraoral appliance and biofeedback/stress management alone and in combination in treating pain and depression in patients with temporomandibular disorders. *J Prosthet Dent.* 1993;70(2):158-164.
53. Flor H, Birbaumer N. Comparison of the efficacy of electromyographic biofeedback, cognitive-behavioral therapy, and conservative medical interventions in the treatment of chronic musculoskeletal pain. *J Consult Clin Psychol.* 1993;61(4):653-658.
54. deCharms RC, Maeda F, Glover GH, et al. Control over brain activation and pain learned by using real-time functional MRI. *Proc Natl Acad Sci U S A.* 2005;102(51):18626-18631.
55. McMakin C. Microcurrent treatment of myofascial pain in the head, neck, and face. *Top Clin Chiropr.* 1998;5(1):29-35.
56. McMakin C. Microcurrent therapy: a novel treatment method for chronic low back myofascial pain. *J Bodyw Mov Ther.* 2004;8(2):143-153.
57. Oschman J. *Energy Medicine the Scientific Basis.* 2nd ed. New York, NY: Elsevier; 2015.
58. Becker RO, Selden G. *The Body Electric.* New York, NY: William Morrow and Company; 1985.
59. Szent-Gyorgyi A. Towards a new biochemistry? *Science.* 1941;93(2426):609-611.
60. Pollack GH. *Cells, Gels, and the Engines of Life: A New Unifying Approach to Cell Function.* Seattle, WA: Ebner & Sons; 2001.
61. Cosic I. Macromolecular bioactivity: is it resonant interaction between macromolecules?—Theory and applications. *IEEE Trans Biomed Eng.* 1994;41(12):1101-1114.
62. Cheng N, Van Hoof H, Bockx E, et al. The effects of electric currents on ATP generation, protein synthesis, and membrane transport of rat skin. *Clin Orthop Relat Res.* 1982(171):264-272.
63. Seegers JC, Engelbrecht CA, van Papendorp DH. Activation of signal-transduction mechanisms may underlie the therapeutic effects of an applied electric field. *Med Hypotheses.* 2001;57(2):224-230.
64. Seegers JC, Lottering ML, Joubert AM, et al. A pulsed DC electric field affects P2-purinergic receptor functions by altering the ATP levels in in vitro and in vivo systems. *Med Hypotheses.* 2002;58(2):171-176.
65. McMakin C, Gregory WM, Philips TM. Cytokine changes with microcurrent treatment of fibromyalgia associated with cervical spine trauma. *J Bodyw Mov Ther.* 2005;9(3):169-176.
66. Reilly WG, Reeve VE, McMakin CR. Anti-inflammatory effects of interferential frequency-specific applied microcurrent. Paper presented at: Proceedings of the National Health and Medical Research Council, 2004.
67. Huckfeldt R, Mikkelson D, Larson K, Hammond L, Flick B, McMakin C. The use of microcurrent and autocatalytic silver plated nylon dressings to reduce scarring in human burn patients: a feasibility study. Paper presented at: Proceedings of John Boswick Burn and Wound Symposium February 21, 2003; Maul, HI.
68. McMakin C. *The Resonance Effect: How Frequency Specific Microcurrent is Changing Medicine.* Berkeley, CA: North Atlantic Books; 2017.
69. McMakin C. *Frequency Specific Microcurrent in Pain Management.* Edinburgh, Scotland: Elsevier; 2010.

Chapter 76

Postural Considerations

"The Living Engine Light"

Joshua J. Lee, Robert D. Gerwin, Ryan Reed, Thomas Eberle, and Gabriel Somarriba

1. INTRODUCTION

Posture is the summative visual reflection of how the body has adapted to gravity and external forces in a particular position. In a sense, posture can be considered a theoretical construct, a view of the body as a constantly adapting framework, adjusting to the forces of gravity along with the stressors of habitually repeated movements. In its entirety, however, posture tells a story about the musculoskeletal system through both the alignment of posture and the capacity it holds for movement. Janda believed that the status of the central nervous system (CNS) and peripheral nervous system was reflected in the musculoskeletal system that provides the clinician with a wealth of information.[1] The musculoskeletal system provides the clinician with an opportunity to identify structural factors that can influence myofascial pain and dysfunction. It may also aid in the identification of musculature that has become dysfunctional based on visual observation and abnormal postural alignments. Through a thorough history; assessment of static, dynamic, and functional postures; and a sound clinical reasoning process, the clinician must determine how to utilize that information and organize the physical examination. Though a plethora of textbooks have been written solely on posture, this chapter primarily aims to highlight the components of posture related to muscle dysfunction and myofascial pain syndrome.

2. POSTURAL FACTORS

One of the most fascinating qualities of the human body is its incredible capacity to adapt. The body is never truly at rest, constantly working down to the cellular level to meet vital expectations and functional needs while resisting both intrinsic and extrinsic forces. Factors such as posture and muscle, posture and trigger points (TrPs), posture and pain, gravitational and biomechanical considerations, postural stability, posture development and genetics, and postures of occupation and recreation are briefly discussed in this chapter. The clinician should also consider psychosocial variables that can affect posture as presented in Chapter 5.

2.1. Posture and Muscle

Postural stability and control are achieved by the coordination of the peripheral nervous system and CNS along with the passive restraints of bone, joint, cartilage, tendon, and ligaments. When overloaded, these structures may cause nociception, potentially translating into an experience of pain. Poor alignment may result in abnormal compressive or tensile loads. Furthermore, a lack of mobility may cause excessive compressive loading of joints leading to faulty alignment. With this loss of mobility, the faulty alignment may remain constant because of the associated tissue stiffness.[2] This may also be the result of muscle tightness or inhibition weakness because of biomechanical inefficiencies and TrPs, resulting in the inability of muscles to move the joint through the desired motion. Muscle tightness can maintain the body in faulty alignment, whereas muscle inhibition weakness can alter the body position, affecting alignment. Muscles in a resting lengthened position may test weaker because of passive vweak because of active insufficiency. Trigger points can be involved in both muscle tightness and inhibition weakness.

2.2. Posture and Trigger Points

In a well-functioning system, the body will have normal compensations and adaptations to forces with mild changes in alignment and symmetry. However, abnormal or non-neutral alignment, as defined by Putz-Anderson,[3] can lead to a poorly functioning neuromusculoskeletal system with a decreased capacity to manage forces efficiently. This can lead to aberrant changes in alignment or a new framework on which the neuromuscular system must perform. The net result of a change in alignment leads to muscle overload. This dysfunctional framework can result in chronic structural and functional stressors that disrupt the body's homeostatic capacities for resisting external forces. This results in confounding effects on the body such as muscle imbalances that could further lead to postural imbalances, poor motor control, and poor postural control.[1] These compensations may place muscles in a prolonged lengthened or shortened position, precipitating the formation of TrPs. Janda[4] stated, "Postural muscles, structurally adapted to resist prolonged gravitational stress, generally resist fatigue. When overly stressed these same postural muscles become irritable, tight, and shortened," instigating the formation of TrPs. Conversely, the antagonists of these postural muscles can demonstrate inhibitory characteristics or TrPs with inhibition weakness secondary to overload.[5] The summative effects of TrPs and maladaptive alignments can result in impairing the function of posture, with visible telltale signs found during the postural assessment.

Although the visual representation of posture can be described as the alignment of the body, the intrinsic function and role of posture is primarily for movement. According to Sherrington, "posture follows movement like a shadow."[6] The main component required for movement is posture and not vice versa.[7] Though typically assessed in static positions, posture is an inherently dynamic concept. This dynamic process can be described as the continuous attainment of the desired static position or as the active holding of body segments against gravity and other external forces mediated by the CNS.[7,8] This active holding, or postural stabilization, is achieved through the positioning of joints via the coordinated muscular activity of agonists and antagonists (functional unit), allowing for an erect posture and locomotion of the body as a whole.[9] However, the inhibitory motor characteristics of TrPs can disrupt the coordinated muscular activity, resulting in poor postural stabilization and poor movement capacity. Furthermore, abnormal alignment may also lead to altered and maladaptive movement patterns that have consequences on the CNS feeding into the effects of myofascial pain syndrome. See Chapter 4 "Perpetuating Factors" for further information on maladaptive movement patterns and their effect on the nociceptive system.

2.3. Posture and Pain

Contemporary views regarding posture and pain refute theoretical constructs regarding postural alignment, dysfunction, and pain. Older research shows an absence of a generalized relationship between postural findings and identified impairments.[10,11] More recent research shows that there is no definitive relationship between postural abnormalities and pain.[12-14] However, these findings may be explained by the fact that the studies utilized static measures, and posture and movement are dynamic. One must be careful concluding that the assessment of posture is not an essential component of the functional examination as it is the starting point for all movement. Several studies have shown structural pathologies in asymptomatic individuals; therefore, dysfunctional postures do not necessarily predict the presence of pain as the human body is highly adaptable.[15-26] However, if the posture becomes pathologic, the movement system may become dysfunctional and signal for help through nociceptive mechanisms. As Lewit states, "The movement system is the most common source of pain in an organism and, in turn, pain is also the most common sign of a movement system dysfunction. The reason is obvious: the movement system is the largest system in the body, and moreover, it is the effector of our willpower. It does not possess any means of 'defense' other than to cause pain."[7,27]

It is essential to determine if the patient's current report of symptoms is related to tissue pathologies, pain mechanisms, impairments, or dysfunctional posture. Postural assessment must go beyond the static observation and incorporate movement and function to determine its relationship to the patient's symptoms.

2.4. Gravity and Biomechanical Considerations

Despite all of our individual variabilities, there is one major constant the body is subjected to at all times: the law of gravity. Though posture may be a theoretical construct, gravity is a known established law. The constant static force of gravity and how the body adapts to that force is what we have theorized to be posture. In an effort to capture the effects of posture, Sahrmann[28] categorized pain disorders into movement impairment categories based on the body's compensatory adaptations to favor movement in the path of least resistance. The line of gravity (LOG) as a static force has an effect on postural alignment and, therefore, movement. The static forces of gravity can contribute to the changes in the relationship between agonists and antagonists secondary to poor adaptations of postural alignment.[28]

For example, in an individual with swayback posture, due to the LOG shifting posteriorly relative to the hip joint, the demand on the gluteal musculature is decreased, allowing for atrophy, while increasing the demand on the hip flexor muscles. These static forces contribute to increased activity in some muscle groups and atrophy in others.[28]

Biomechanical concepts are the rules the body follows according to the law of gravity. These concepts are critical to consider when assessing and providing interventions for postural deviations that are being considered as a contributing factor to the patient's clinical presentation. The patient's body center of mass (BCOM) and body center of gravity (BCOG) are synonymous terms when the gravitational field is uniform. The BCOM essentially is the location in which the weight of the body may be considered to be concentrated.[29] The BCOM in a neutral standing erect position generally lies just in front of the S2 vertebra[30] and changes as a person moves. The BCOM in a person moving from sit to stand moves from a position anterior to the body to just below the S2 vertebra. The changing BCOM is important to understand and identify during the different sequences of a task when assessing dynamic postures. This affords the clinician the ability to identify both intrinsic and extrinsic forces on the musculoskeletal system and those forces that may be a contributing factor to muscle overload that can be modified.

The LOG is an invisible vertical line representing the force of gravity through the BCOG or BCOM in the downward direction toward the center of the earth. In normal posture, as seen in Figure 76-1, the LOG lies posterior to the cervical spine, anterior to the thoracic spine, posterior to the lumbar spine, and anterior to the sacrum.[30]

When the LOG is within a person's base of support (BOS) the person is said to be in a stable and balanced position. When the LOG falls outside the BOS the person is said to be unstable or off balance.[31] Identifying where the LOG falls in both the frontal and sagittal views is necessary to further evaluate movement impairments. From an anterior or posterior view, the LOG will assist the clinician to identify asymmetries within an individual. In the sagittal view, the LOG will assist the clinician in identifying the relationship between the LOG and the antigravity muscles.

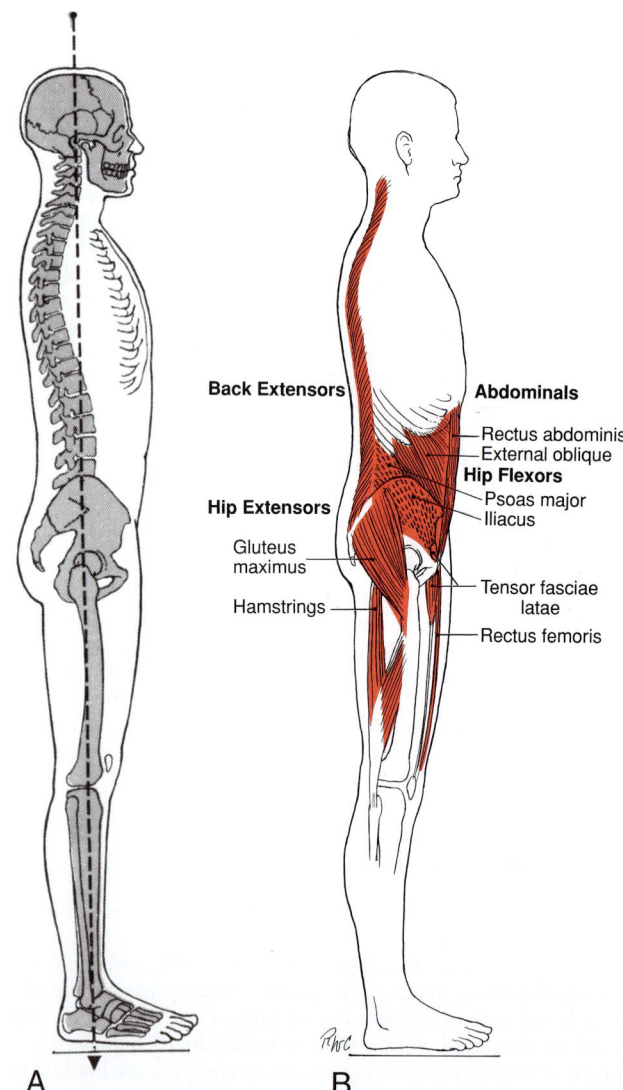

Figure 76-1. Static postural alignment sagittal view. A, Skeletal alignment with plumb line. B, Anterior and posterior postural muscles of the trunk.[2]

Antigravity muscles act to counterbalance the pull of gravity and keep the body in an upright position.[2] The main role of antigravity muscles is to generate torque across joints to resist the forces of gravity. These muscles help to keep limbs, joints, and the body in proper alignment or posture so that the BCOG falls within the BOS. This concept is the relationship between balance and posture. Efficient posture permits proficient movement patterns and allows joints to be loaded symmetrically. Efficient postures decrease or distribute loads on cartilage, bone, connective tissue, tendons, and ligaments, and they result in decreased stress and strain on structures of the musculoskeletal system.[32] Muscles are also required to work less in these inherently efficient postural positions.

2.5. Posture and Stability

Balance, or postural stability, is the ability of the body to maintain its center of gravity within the BOS. Postural stability is the culmination of the input, processing, and output of information from the peripheral nervous system to the CNS.[1] This information in particular comes from the vestibular, visual, and somatosensory systems, which can impact postural alignment over time. The visual system is responsible for the orientation of the eyes in the environment, which will affect the position of the head on the neck.[1] Visual perception also plays a role in purposeful movement and the facilitation of an appropriately coordinated motor response within our surroundings.[33]

The vestibular system provides the CNS with information regarding the position of the body and head and feedback from a moving BOS.[1] The vestibular system and vertical line perception have implications on postural dysfunctions such as scoliosis and its development. However, it is not clear whether the contributions to a scoliosis develop from abnormal vertical line perception or if vertical line perception is altered in people with scoliosis.[33]

Nonetheless, the CNS receives all peripheral input including proprioception, thermoreception, and nociception through the somatosensory system.[1] Proprioception or body perception plays a major role on movement in regard to its precision and efficiency. Relatedly, if the patient has clumsiness or poor coordination, this may be suggestive of abnormal proprioceptive control.[33] The patient's capacity for balance should also be considered in the clinician's examination as it will further delineate the patient's ability to stabilize posture against gravity.

2.6. Posture Development and Genetics

The development of posture, or postural ontogenesis, has a genetic component, whereas motor functions develop automatically and are dependent on the visual orientation and emotional needs of the infant.[7] With motor functions, the morphologic development of the skeletal structure and its joint positions (hip joint shape, spinal curvature, plantar arch, etc.)[34] is very much dependent on the stabilizing function of muscles[7] such as the diaphragm and the abdominal muscles.[34] Breathing and spinal stability in infants are related to development and genetically determined programs that influence the maturation of the CNS[35]; neither need to be taught except when adverse events affect natural development.

Genetics plays an essential role in posture and some genetic predispositions cannot be controlled (see Chapter 4). Conditions such as osteoporosis, osteoarthritis, or scoliosis, which may have genetic components, can lead to postural dysfunctions, particularly spinal malalignment. This results in some anatomic changes that may not be modified without surgery; however, the variation in genetics relating to tissue mobility also has implications on the magnitude of alignment change in regard to postural dysfunctions such as scoliosis.[36]

2.7. Posture and Occupation/Recreation

Habitual postures of occupation can be both static and repetitive and can lead to tissue adaptation, muscle overload, or degeneration.[37] Over time, these adaptive changes can result in observed postural deviations that will assist the clinician in directing the examination. Some of the more at-risk occupations include truck drivers, construction workers, administrative occupations, dentists, and dental hygienists, to name a few. These occupations require specific postural demands that contribute to abnormal and awkward postures, which may lead to prolonged shortening or lengthening of muscles and inefficiency of movement. Some common postural deviations include forward head posture (FHP), flat back, sway back, and scoliosis. Figure 76-22 illustrates common postural deviations and depicts muscles that may be shortened or elongated, possibly leading to overload and TrP formation.

Recreational or sporting activities with increased postural demands include weight-lifting, swimming, cycling, running, and gymnastics, which, over time, may lead to postural deviations. The repetitive nature of recreational activities or sports may lead to wear and tear on the active and passive structures involved with posture and may make some muscles tight or weak leading to muscular imbalances, TrP formation, and overload, as identified in Figure 76-2.

3. CONSIDERATIONS FOR POSTURAL ASSESSMENT AND EXAMINATION

Postural assessment is an essential component of the examination for patients presenting with activity limitations and participation restrictions as a result of myofascial pain and movement impairment. The posture examination assists clinicians in identifying contributing factors to the patient's presentation along with activating and perpetuating factors of TrPs. A thorough subjective and physical examination with the inclusion of postural assessment must be performed before treatment to avoid creating assumptions based solely on the location of the patient's pain, as pain oftentimes stems from other perpetuating factors and dysfunctions, with pain being the end result. There is a substantial amount of information that can be obtained from assessment of standing posture regarding the muscular system, and this should not be overlooked.[38] However, the clinician must consider what is considered "typical" posture and what is "dysfunctional" for each patient.

3.1. Postural Norms and Dysfunctions

Normative factors of postural function or alignment have always been difficult to establish because of the varied views of individual authors.[9] Vele[39] stated that it was impossible to establish one standard for correct body posture because of a varied correct postural alignment for every individual. It is more or less a construct to have correct posture. Kuchera and Kuchera[40] define optimal posture as follows:

> A balanced configuration of the body with respect to gravity. It depends on normal arches of the feet, vertical alignment of the ankles, and horizontal orientation (in the coronal plane) of the sacral base. The presence of an optimum posture suggests that there is perfect distribution of the body mass around the center of gravity. . . Structural and functional stressors on the body, however, may prevent achievement of optimum posture. In this case, homeostatic mechanisms provide for 'compensation' in an effort to provide maximum postural function within the existing structure of the individual. Compensation is the counterbalancing of any defect of structure or function.

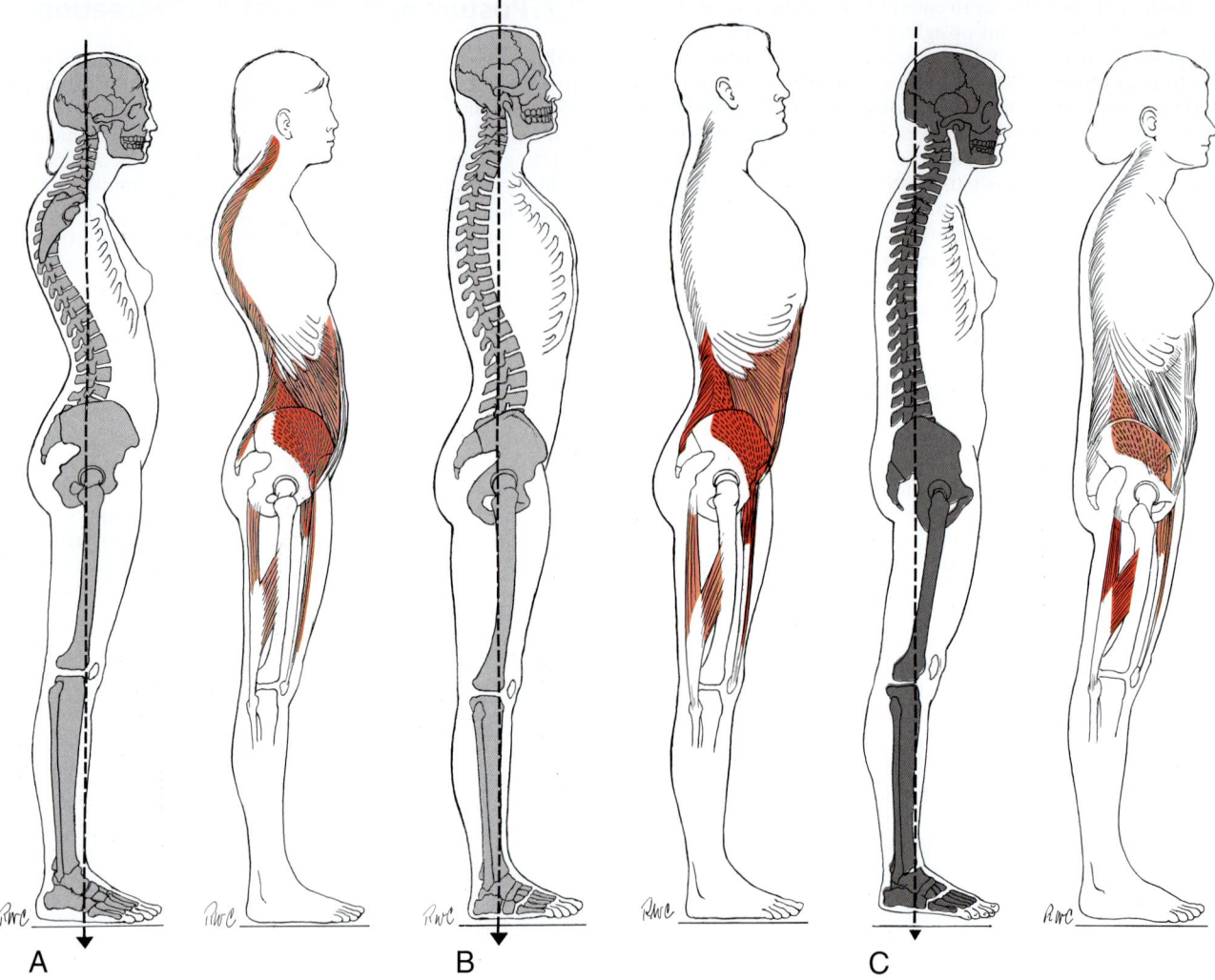

Figure 76-2. Common postural dysfunctions affecting muscle lengths and strength. A, Flat back posture. B, Lordotic posture. C, Kyphotic forward head posture.[2]

This description highlights the decreased likelihood of an example of optimal posture. Patients with persistent pain may present with mild asymmetries but so do many individuals who are asymptomatic.[12-26] Ideal posture then must be identified in the context of the individual patient and their environmental demands. It is important to keep these considerations in mind when referencing neutral alignment, as sometimes a slight deviation from neutral alignment may not necessarily be pathologic. Nevertheless, the focus should be on the more noticeable dysfunctions and aberrant deviations from neutral and how they contribute to the patient's current problem.

The source of postural dysfunctions and aberrant deviations is typically from postural disharmony or postural disturbances, which can be divided into the following deficits: anatomic, neurologic, and functional.[7] Neurologic deficits, such as cerebellar, vestibular, and extrapyramidal impairments, typically arise from a neurologic dysfunction, whereas anatomic dysfunctions, such as femoral anteversion, postinjury morphologic changes, and sacral dysplasia, are typically innate or acquired and difficult to change.[7] Postural dysfunctions related to neurologic deficits are beyond the scope of this chapter; however, the clinician should be discerning when the patient has neurologic deficits.

Functional deficits as defined by Kolar[7] are the impairments in postural muscles resulting in decreased postural stabilization and function of the postural muscles during static positions and movement. Kolar[7] describes functional deficits as a result of three main causes: central coordination disturbances during postural development; the manner in which stereotypical movements have been changed, strengthened, and modified, usually in the context of the individual's psychological state; and dysfunction due to nociceptive control. With dysfunction due to nociceptive control, when nociceptive information is transmitted secondary to a pathologic situation, the motor system will automatically make changes in motor function development, frequently resulting in the formation of TrPs in a muscle.

Postural impairments such as a slouched position are modifiable and respond well to cues to change alignment.[36] Structural or anatomic dysfunctions, on the other hand, are innate and difficult to change, regardless of the position of the individual, because of fixed alignments of the boney structures.[36]

3.2. Static Standing Assessment

The most common and practical assessment of posture is static standing, because of the wealth of information that can be obtained regarding the status of the muscular system. Upon initial observation of static standing posture, the clinician should obtain a general assessment of symmetry, spinal curvatures, structural or biomechanical variations, positioning of the pelvis in relation to the axis of the diaphragm muscle, and the extent and distribution of muscle tension.[1,7,41] The clinician should refer to

Figure 76-1 in regard to neutral standing posture. Figure 76-1 shows the sagittal view of neutral standing posture with a plumb line as a reference to the LOG through neutral alignment, as well as the trunk and thigh muscles responsible for maintaining it. Also of note in Figure 76-1 are the postural muscles of the trunk as they are oftentimes the first to be involved with postural deviations. There are several variations to the landmarks in relation to the plumb line depending on the source. O'Sullivan et al[42] showed disagreement among 295 physical therapists in four different European countries on what constituted seated neutral spine posture.

It is crucial to note the orientation of the eyes and facial features related to the position of the head as it is an important indicator, diagnostically, for chronic musculoskeletal pain. If the patient has facial asymmetry, or facial scoliosis (Figure 76-3A to D), where the bridge of the nose, eyes, and mouth are not parallel, this can indicate a severe issue with alignment affecting the entire body. Janda identified four points, or landmarks, on the face to be aligned: the bridge of the nose, the middle of the forehead, mid-mouth, and the mid-jaw (Figure 76-3E to F).[1]

To acquire an observation of breathing patterns, respiration patterns should also be assessed in the standing position while the patient is unaware. Respiration and posture are interdependent functionally,[43] a concept that will be discussed in depth later in this chapter.

The age of the patient being examined must be considered as development of structures changes the typical alignment. The cumulative effects of lifestyle and physical stressors may change anatomic structures accordingly and may impact the examiner's postural assessment in regard to seeking a relatively normative comparison.

3.3. Regional Assessments

In order for the clinician to get a summative view of posture, they should evaluate each region of the spine and the extremities and correlate observed asymmetries or non-neutral alignment to the patient's presentation. Further details on specific muscle function, assessment, and treatments are located in their respective chapters in this text as referenced throughout the following sections. The following information incorporates both Janda's approach to muscle imbalances[1,38] and the Sahrmann[28] postural component of movement impairment syndromes approach.[28,36] This section does not aim to fully cover either approach but rather focuses on a few common postural dysfunction findings based solely on their implications for muscles.

Pelvis and Hips

Because most chronic musculoskeletal pain is first evident in postural asymmetries of the pelvis, it is suggested by Page et al[1] to observe this area first, regardless of the area of primary symptoms. The pelvis can reflect deviations from the trunk as well as the extremities.[7] The pelvis should be assessed for any excessive tilting, torsion, shifting relative to the trunk, and rotation. Muscle tension distribution should be assessed around the hips and pelvis. Regarding alignment, from a lateral view the clinician should find minimal angular deviation, varying up to 12°, with a line drawn from the posterior superior iliac spine (PSIS) to the anterior superior iliac spine (ASIS) in comparison to horizontal.[28] Excessive anterior tilting of the pelvis (Figure 76-4A), or when the ASIS is 20° lower than the PSIS,[28] may have an associated increase in lumbar lordosis. In contrast to excessive anterior tilting, excessive posterior tilting (Figure 76-4B) occurs when the ASIS is roughly 20° higher than the PSIS.[28] Posterior tilt of the pelvis is commonly associated with a flat back or decreased lumbar lordosis.[28] The clinician should look for the ASIS to be in the same vertical plane as the pubic symphysis to assess for unilateral superior tilt of the pelvis (Figure 76-4C).[28] Excessive unilateral rotation of the pelvis can be denoted when the patient's unilateral ASIS is anterior to the contralateral ASIS.[1,28] Box 76-1 depicts pelvic asymmetries and their associated muscle dysfunctions.[7,28]

The excessive facilitation or inhibition of the muscles of the hip and pelvis often causes secondary dysfunctions by association with other muscles, so it is important to denote findings during observation of these muscles. Hypertrophy or dominance of the hamstrings (Figure 76-5A) can be observed particularly in the lower two-thirds of the belly of the hamstrings. Observation of hypertrophy of the one-joint adductor muscles, typically the pectineus muscle, may present as an increased or deeper "S" shape in the proximal groin. This is also known as an adductor notch (Figure 76-5B) or increased adductor bulk, which could suggest TrPs in the adductor muscles.[1] When observing the gluteus maximus muscles, they should be examined mostly for symmetry and muscle tension. If there is unilateral sagging or bulk, it may give information on the motor function

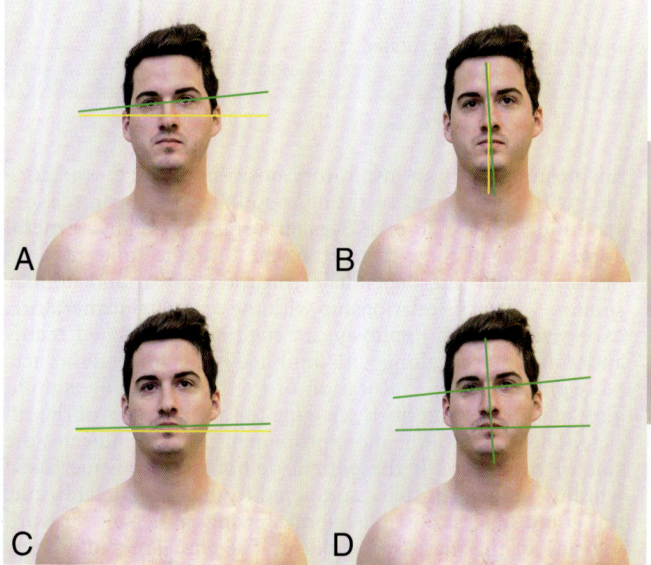
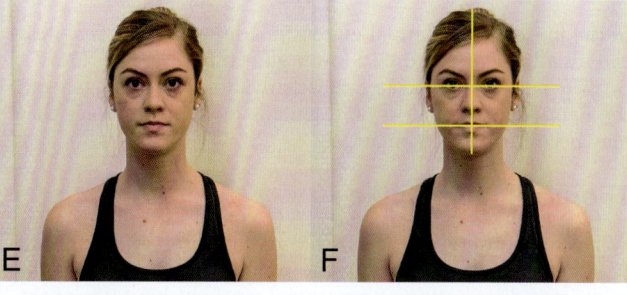

Figure 76-3. Facial scoliosis, with side by side comparison with lines (light green for actual position, yellow for 90° horizontal/vertical comparison). A, Eyes. B, Bridge of nose. C, Mouth line. D, All three combined. E, F, Example of normal facial alignment with comparison lines.

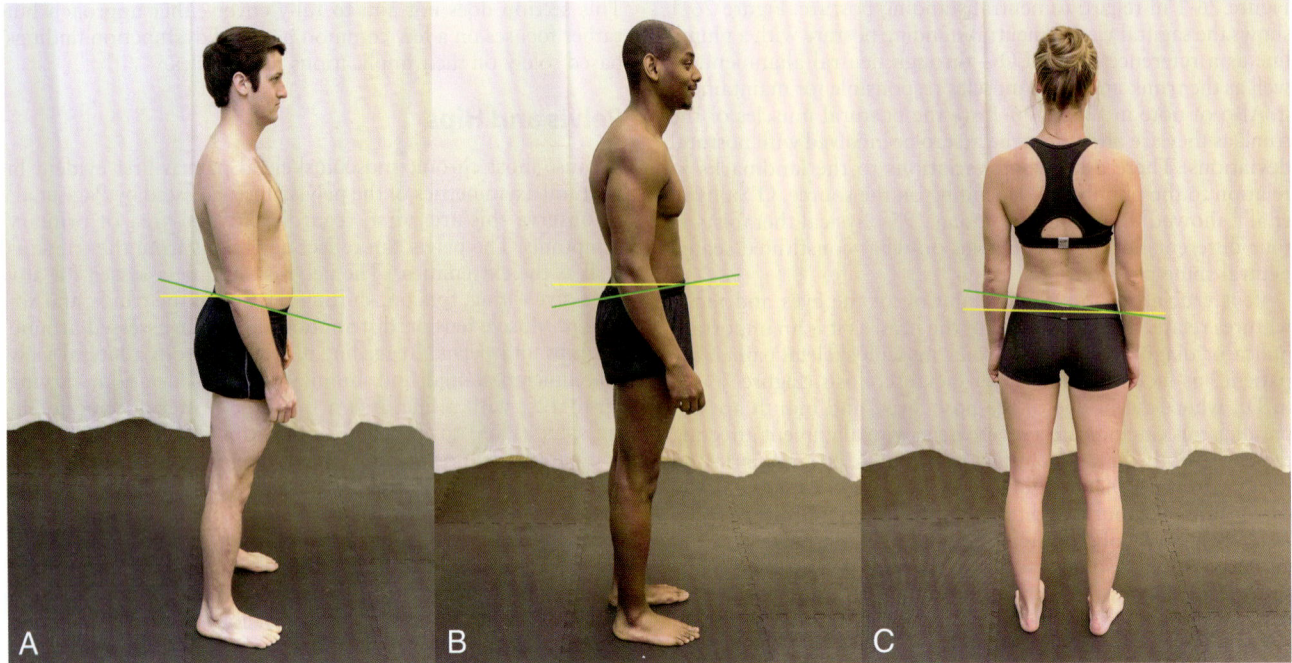

Figure 76-4. Pelvis and hip postural findings. A, Anterior pelvic tilt as denoted by the green line. B, Posterior pelvic tilt as denoted by the green line. C, Unilateral superior tilt of left pelvis as denoted by the green line.

Box 76-1 Postural non-neutral alignment

Examples of muscle dysfunction of the pelvis and hip.[7,28] Refer to identified chapters in this book for specific muscle assessment.

Pelvic Alignment	Shortened/Facilitated Muscles	Lengthened/Inhibited Muscles
Anterior tilt	Psoas muscle group (Chapter 51) Iliacus (Chapter 51) Erector spinae (Chapter 48)	Abdominal muscles Gluteus maximus
Posterior tilt	Hamstring muscles (Chapter 60) Abdominal muscles (Chapter 49)	Psoas muscle group
Superior lateral tilt	Ipsilateral quadratus lumborum (Chapter 50) Ipsilateral latissimus dorsi (Chapter 24) Ipsilateral hip abductor (Chapter 55,56)	Contralateral hip abductors
Unilateral rotation	Tensor fasciae latae (Chapter 56) on the side in which the pelvis is rotated	

---

of the muscle.[44] Ipsilateral gluteus maximus muscle weakness can usually be depicted by a lower gluteal fold (Figure 76-5C). Box 76-2 depicts associated muscle dysfunction findings from the hamstring, adductors, and gluteus maximus muscles that may need further examination.

Thoracolumbar Spine

When first observing the posture of the spine, there should be a general appreciation of the spinal curves, assessing for symmetry, distribution of paraspinal tension, skin folds of the trunk, and the position of the head and neck. Normal alignment of the lumbar spine is widely dictated by the positioning of the sacrum and pelvis but looking for an inward curve roughly of 20° to 30°.[28] In the thoracic spine, normal alignment has an even distribution of flexion, with a mild posterior convexity attributed to the slight wedging of the vertebrae.[36] The alignment of the rib cage should be assessed in regard to the position of the thorax above the pelvis.[7] A common deficit related to this positioning is an inspiratory position of the thorax coupled with pelvic anterior tilting, also known as open scissors syndrome (Figure 76-6A).[7] It is important to obtain a general appreciation of the curvature of the thoracic spine because of its regional interdependence on the cervical and lumbar spine as well as its relationship with the scapula. Furthermore, excessive thoracic kyphosis can suggest a shortened rectus abdominis muscle along with inhibited or lengthened thoracic paraspinal muscles.[28] Rotation of the thoracic spine should also be assessed anteriorly, viewing for asymmetries of the rib cage. The side with the more prominent rib cage indicates the side of rotation.[36] If the patient demonstrates an increased window in the arm space compared to the contralateral side, this could suggest possible lateral shifting of the spine toward the side of the increased window. The clinician should also assess for possible scoliotic curves, which inherently have asymmetric muscle lengths and areas of hypertrophy. Refer to Figure 76-7 for muscles that may be involved in a scoliotic thoracolumbar curve (Figure 76-6B). Excessive hypertrophy of

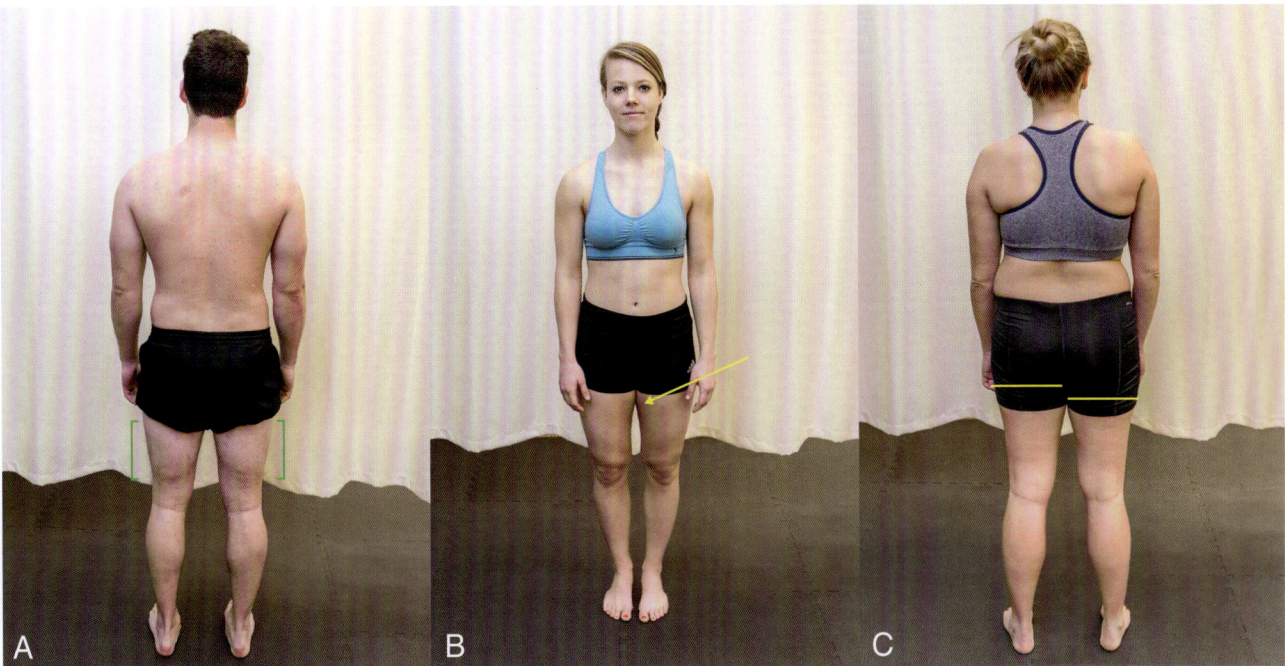

Figure 76-5. Myofascial dysfunction in the pelvis/hip. A, Bilateral hamstring hypertrophy in the lower two-thirds of the muscle belly. B, Adductor notch, more visible on the subject's right side (arrow). C, Lower gluteal fold on the subject's right side.

Box 76-2 Examples of dysfunction in the hamstrings, adductors, and gluteus maximus muscles and their associated muscle dysfunction[1]

Refer to identified chapters in this book for specific muscle assessment.

	Associated Muscle Dysfunction
Hamstring hypertrophy/dominance (Chapter 60)	Inhibited or weakened gluteus maximus (Chapter 54) Thoracolumbar paraspinal hypertrophy (compensations for gluteus maximus weakness/inhibition)
Adductor hypertrophy/dominance (Chapter 59)	Inhibited or weakened hip abductor Inhibited or weakened abdominal wall musculature
Ipsilateral gluteus maximus atrophy/weakness (lower gluteal fold) (Chapter 54)	Ipsilateral hamstring muscle tightness/shortness/facilitated Ipsilateral hip extension compensations at the thoracolumbar paraspinal muscles resulting in repetitive instability of the thoracolumbar spinal segments

---

thoracolumbar extensor muscles (Figure 76-6C) may indicate overactive compensations for poor stability of the deep spinal stabilizers of the lumbar spine, shortened or tight hip flexor muscles, or a weak or inhibited gluteus maximus muscle.[1] The clinician should also assess horizontal creases in the lumbar spine as this may suggest where excessive motion is occurring.

Abdominal Wall

The abdominal wall should be assessed because of its suggested role in stabilizing the spine. If the abdomen is sagging or protruding, this may be due to a generalized weakness of the abdominal muscles. A lateral bulging of the abdomen, just superior to the beltline (Figure 76-8A), may indicate weakness of the transverse abdominis muscle[1] or lack of space between the 12th rib and the iliac crest. The upper and lower quadrants of the abdomen should also be compared. If the rib cage is superiorly elevated with an increased tension of the upper quadrant compared to the lower quadrant, this could suggest a faulty respiratory pattern and generation, which are vital for intra-abdominal pressure (IAP) regulation and postural stabilization, respectively.[7,34,45] If a distinct groove lateral to the rectus abdominus muscle is observed (Figure 76-8B), it may indicate a decreased capacity for stabilization of the abdominal muscles in the anterior and posterior direction.[1] The abdominal wall should also be assessed for lateral hollowing or flaring of the ribs, which would demonstrate a poor function of the diaphragm muscle, abdominal oblique muscle weakness, or transverse abdominis muscle weakness. Furthermore, if the patient demonstrates a general drawing in of the abdominal wall with increased activity of the upper abdominal muscles (Figure 76-8B), this is referred to as an hourglass syndrome posture.[7] With this posture, there is typically an inspiratory breathing pattern, hypertrophy, or increased tension of the paravertebral muscles about the thoracolumbar junction (Figure 76-6C), as well as an increase in anterior pelvic tilt.[7] Refer to Chapters 45 and 49 regarding assessment and treatment of the diaphragm and abdominal musculature, respectively.

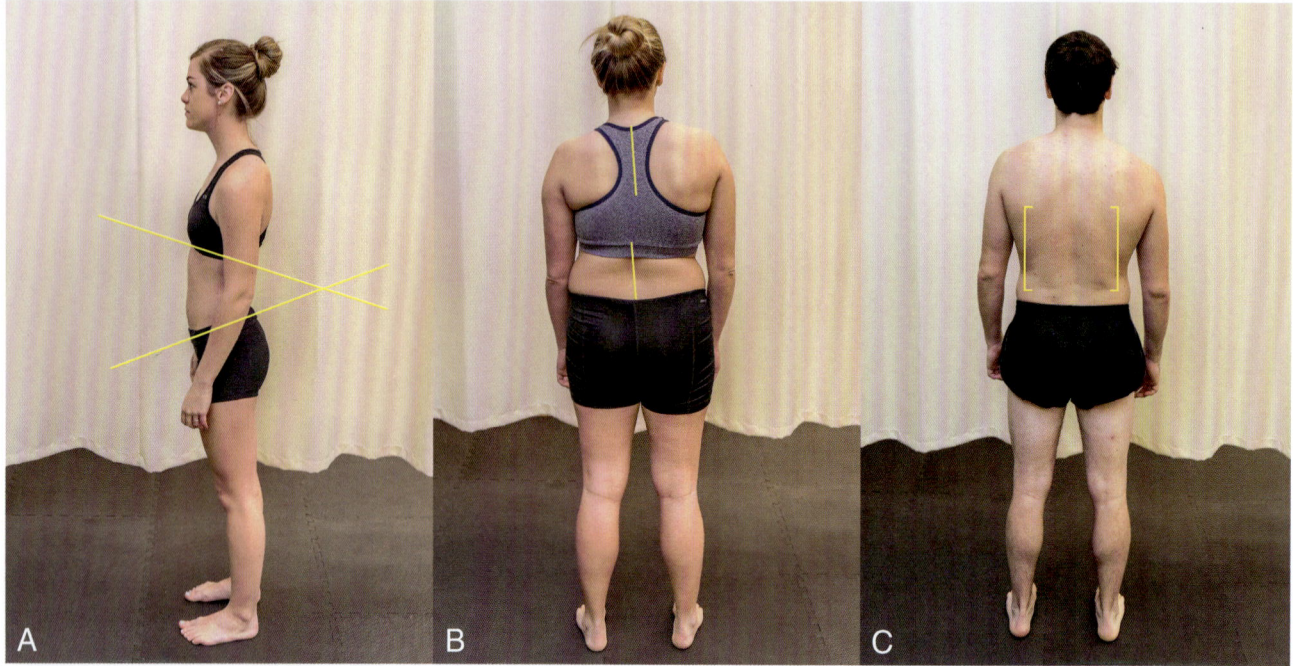

Figure 76-6. Postural dysfunction findings in the thoracolumbar region. A, Open scissors syndrome as denoted by the lines. B, Thoracolumbar scoliotic curve. C, Thoracolumbar paraspinal muscle hypertrophy as denoted by brackets.

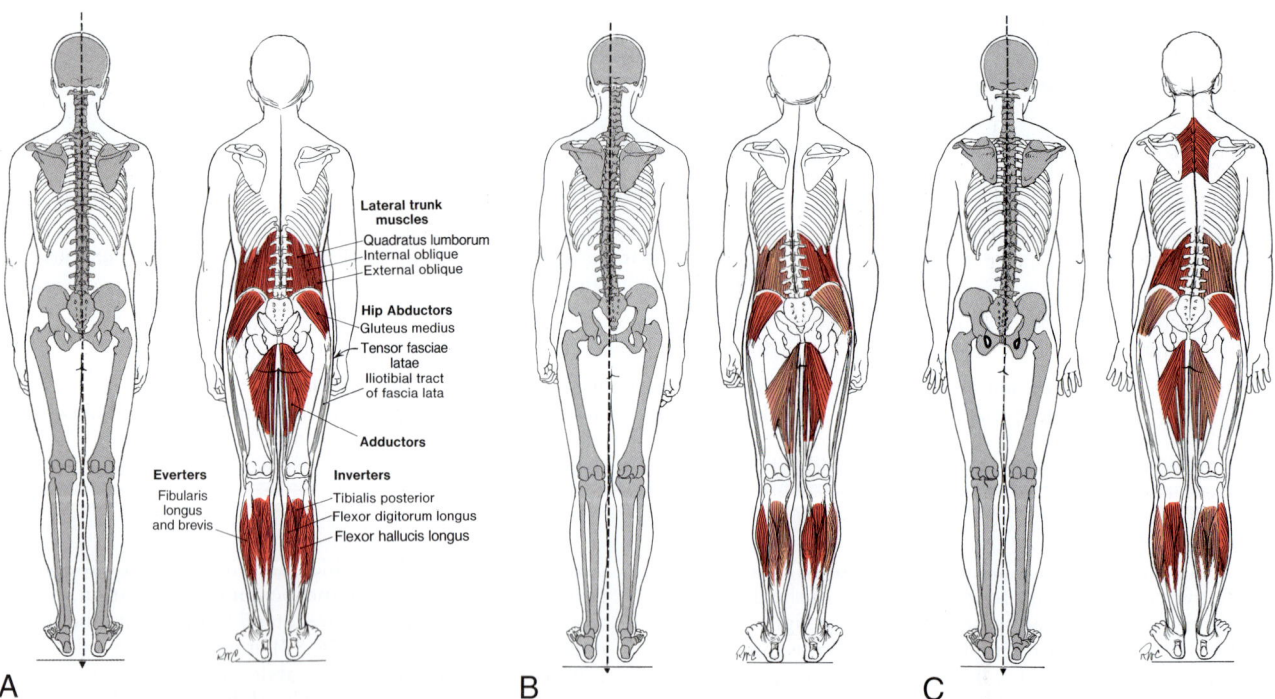

Figure 76-7. Effects of scoliosis on muscle length. A, Typical spinal alignment from a posterior view. B, Left thoracolumbar curve. C, Right slight thoracolumbar curve. Dark red depicts muscles that are shortened and light red are those that are typically elongated.[2]

Cervical Spine and Head

When assessing the posture of the cervical spine, initially a general assessment of curve, muscle tension, and symmetry is obtained. Then the clinician should assess the relationship of the head to the rest of the body in regard to gravity and the workload on the cervical spine, looking for a 90-degree angle between the chin and the neck, also known as the throat line.[38] Ideally, the acoustic meatus should line up with the acromion process. If there is straightening of the throat line or an increase in the chin-neck angle (Figure 76-9A), this suggests a sign of increased tension of the suprahyoid muscles, which may contribute to temporomandibular joint (TMJ) dysfunction and often is found with TrPs upon palpation.[38] The sternocleidomastoid

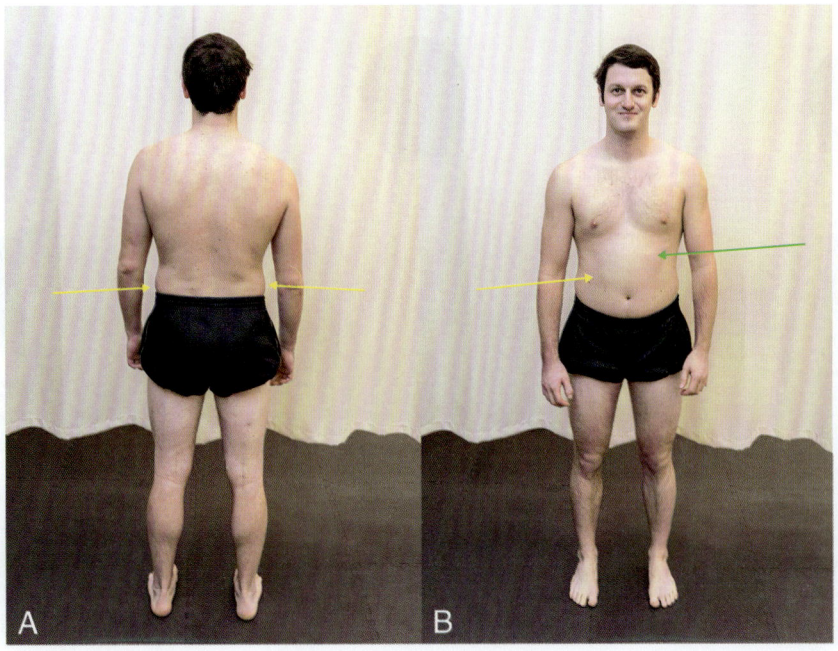

Figure 76-8. Postural dysfunction findings in the abdominal wall. A, Bilateral lateral bulging of the abdominal wall musculature. B, Lateral groove next to rectus abdominis muscle denoted by the yellow arrow, upper abdominal activity with hourglass posture denoted by the green arrow.

muscle should not be prominent; however, if there is a groove along the sternocleidomastoid (Figure 76-9B), this may suggest an early sign of weakness in the deep neck flexors.[38] Lastly, the clinician should assess the relationship of the scapulae with the neck, as many of the periscapular muscles have an inherent origin and insertion relationship with the cervical spine. The line of the neck and shoulder should be assessed for Gothic shoulders (Figure 76-9C), for upper trapezius muscle tightness, as well as a levator notch (Figure 76-9C). This is an upward bulge of the superior angle of the scapula as a result of levator scapulae muscle tightness.[1] Refer to Chapter 6 for further examination and treatment of the upper trapezius muscle and Chapter 19 for the levator scapulae muscle.

Scapulae

General postural assessment of the scapulae should include distribution of muscle tightness, symmetry of the scapula, presence of winging, and general position of the scapulae in relation to the thoracic spine. The medial border of the scapulae should be parallel to the thoracic spine at the levels of T2 through T7 and approximately 3 in away from the spinous processes.[28] The resting position of the scapulae can be widely affected by the alignment of the thoracic spine.

The scapulae position should be assessed for bilateral or unilateral excessive elevation, depression, winging, and anterior tilting (Figure 76-10A). The scapulae should also be assessed for rotation, such as a downwardly rotated scapula (ie, the superior angle is further from the spine than the inferior angle), and abduction (Figure 76-10B) (ie, the medial border of the scapula is more than 3 in from the thoracic spinous processes). Box 76-3 depicts scapulae postural asymmetries and their associated muscle dysfunctions.[1,28] The supraspinous or infraspinous fossa (Figure 76-10C) should also be assessed for hollowing, which could indicate possible inhibition and weakness of the posterior rotator cuff muscles. All of the muscles in Box 76-3 must be examined for TrPs. Please refer to Chapters 22, 23, 26, and 42 for further examination and treatment of the scapular musculature.

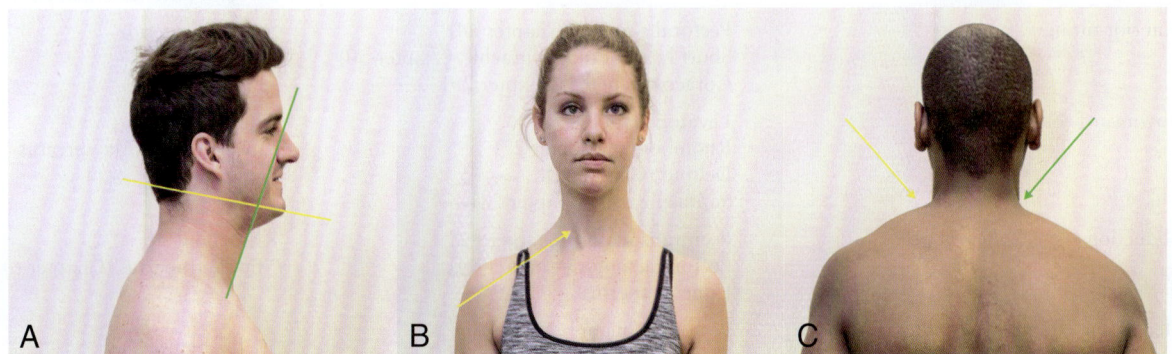

Figure 76-9. Postural dysfunction findings in the head and cervical region. A, Increased chin-neck angle. B, Groove along the sternocleidomastoid muscle (arrow). C, Levator notch denoted by the yellow arrow on the left side. Gothic shoulder denoted by the green arrow on the right side.

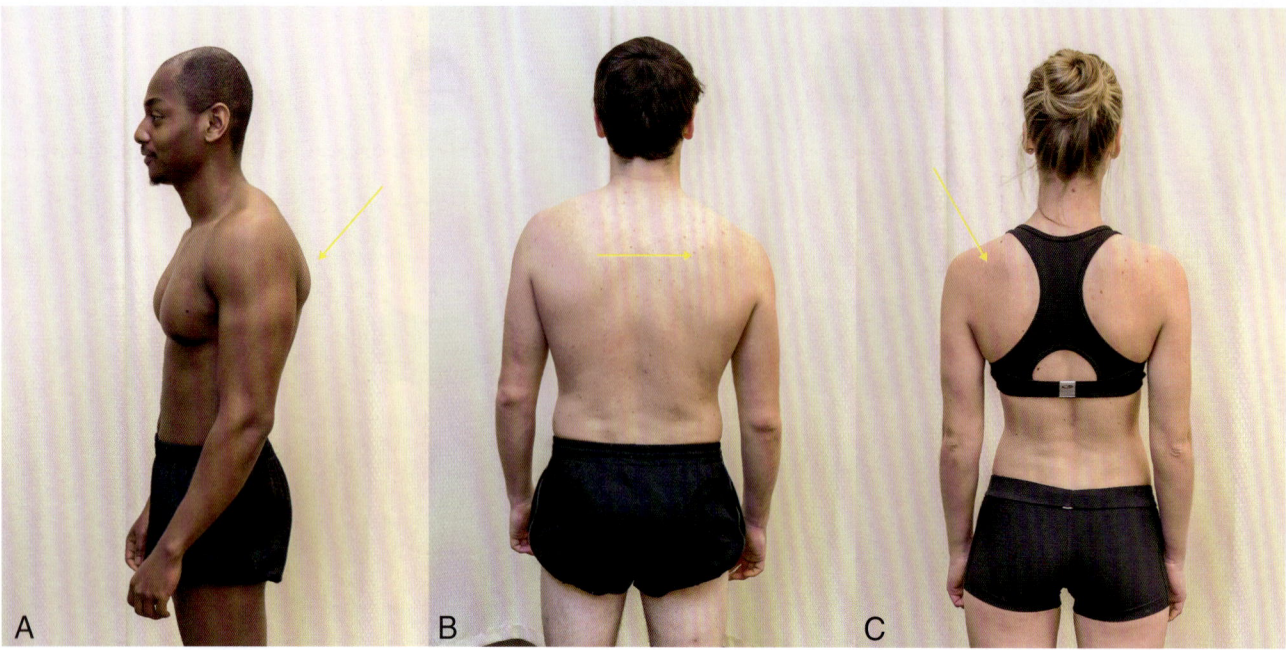

Figure 76-10. Postural dysfunction findings in the scapular region. A, Anterior tilting of the scapula. B, Scapular abduction. C, Hollowing of the infraspinous fossa.

Upper Extremity

General postural assessment of the upper extremities should include humeral head position relative to the acromion, general distribution of muscle tension, excessive pronation or supination of the antebrachium, and guarding, if present, of the shoulder or arm. The head of the humerus should be resting less than one-third anterior to the acromion, with the shaft of the humerus resting parallel to the thorax.[28] The antecubital fossa should be facing anteriorly, demonstrating neutral rotation of the shoulder and with the elbow in slight flexion.[36] Box 76-3 depicts an example of dysfunction of excessive anterior humeral head positioning and medial antecubital fossa/anterior elbow crease angle (Figure 76-11A) and associated muscle dysfunctions.[1,28]

Evaluation of the shoulder girdle is necessary when assessing for dysfunctions of the elbow and hand. If the alignment of the

Box 76-3 Postural non-neutral alignment

Examples of muscle dysfunction of the scapulae and upper extremity.[1,28] Refer to identified chapters in this book for specific muscle assessment.

Scapula Alignment	Shortened/Facilitated Muscles	Lengthened/Inhibited Muscles
Elevation	Upper trapezius (Chapter 6) Levator scapulae (Chapter 19)	
Depression		Upper trapezius Levator scapulae
Winging		Lower trapezius Serratus anterior (Chapter 46)
Anterior tilting	Pectoralis minor (Chapter 44) Short head of biceps brachii (Chapter 30) Coracobrachialis (Chapter 29)	Serratus anterior
Downward rotation	Levator scapula Rhomboids (Chapter 27) Deltoid (Chapter 28) Supraspinatus (Chapter 21)	Upper trapezius Lower fibers of the serratus anterior
Abduction	Pectoralis major (Chapter 42) Pectoralis minor (Chapter 44) Upper trapezius	Rhomboid Middle trapezius (Chapter 6)
Medial angle of antecubital fossa, oblique angle of anterior elbow crease	Pectoralis major Latissimus dorsi (Chapter 24)	
Head of humerus resting more than one-third anterior to acromion	Pectoralis major Infraspinatus (Chapter 22) Teres minor (Chapter 23)	Subscapularis (Chapter 26)

shoulder girdle is dysfunctional, it should be corrected before examining the alignment of the elbow and forearm for a more accurate assessment of the elbow and forearm alignment.[36] When examining the elbow, a general view of the patient's resting position should be considered along with the general assessment of the extensor and flexor muscle mass in comparison to the rest of the arm. The anterior creases in the elbow should be compared bilaterally and should be fairly horizontal. The carrying angle of the elbow is not easily accessible in resting standing position but should be measured during the physical examination. Excessive flexion of unilateral or bilateral elbows at rest (Figure 76-11B) may suggest loss of range of motion (ROM) from repeated eccentric loading of the elbow flexor muscles,[46] possibly resulting in the formation of TrPs.

The forearm at rest should demonstrate neutral rotation, with the thumb oriented anteriorly and the digits facing medially[36] with the fingers more progressively flexed from the radial to the ulnar aspect of the hand.[47] Both hands should rest at a relatively even level. If one hand is observed to rest lower than the other, it may be a result of scapular depression (Figure 76-11C). Please refer to Chapters 30 to 32 and 34 to 38 for further details on examination and treatments of the muscles of the elbow and wrist.

Thigh and Knee

Postural assessment of the lower extremity should include the distribution of muscle tension in the quadriceps muscle group, patella positioning, Q angle, angle of the popliteal crease, presence of genu recurvatum, and tibial torsion. The lower extremity commonly functions as a whole unit, and therefore, the alignment of the entire hip and leg must be taken into consideration.

Other observations include the bilateral comparison of the angle of the popliteal crease. The popliteal crease should be horizontal to the ground, and a deviation in angle (Figure 76-12A) can suggest a predilection of the hip to go into adduction/abduction or internal/external rotation, and/or can suggest foot and ankle torsions. Observation of a crease/groove near the distal lateral thigh may suggest a shorter tensor fascia latae, weak gluteus medius muscle, and a superolateral shift of the patella. If there is a superior positioning of the patella unilaterally, the rectus femoris muscle is likely in a shortened state. Observation of genu recurvatum often suggests vastus medialis muscle hypertrophy.[1] If the patient presents with genu varum (Figure 76-12B), it may suggest lengthened and/or weak lateral rotators of the hip.[36] All of these muscles must be examined for the presence of TrPs. Observation of knee flexion in standing may suggest an acute injury, excessive hamstring muscle shortness with an associated weakness of the quadriceps muscle group, or end-stage osteoarthritis, whereas unilateral knee flexion in standing may suggest a shorter lower limb on the contralateral side.[36] Please refer to Chapters 57 to 60 for further examination and treatment of the muscles of the hip and thigh.

Foot and Ankle

Evaluation of the ankle and foot should include examination of plantar arch height, angle of resting dorsiflexion, heel shape, a comparison of muscle tension bilaterally, tibial torsion, general tendency toward pronation or supination, and toe-out angle. It is relatively easy for the clinician to overanalyze the posture of the foot and make quick conclusions regarding arch heights, pronation, and supination without considering its role as a team player for the entire musculoskeletal system. Conversely, muscle imbalances of the lower kinetic chain can disrupt the precise balance of the foot, leading to tendon stress, muscle overload, or deformities.[1] The clinician should take into account whether or not the patient utilizes a foot or ankle orthotic, as foot and ankle posture may change standing posture accordingly when barefoot.

The ankle in standing should be in relative neutral dorsiflexion at 0°. The clinician should observe if the patient's body weight is shifted excessively anteriorly or posteriorly (Figure 76-13A). Excessive weight shifting can be observed in the heel shape from a posterior view. If weight bearing is normal into the heel and

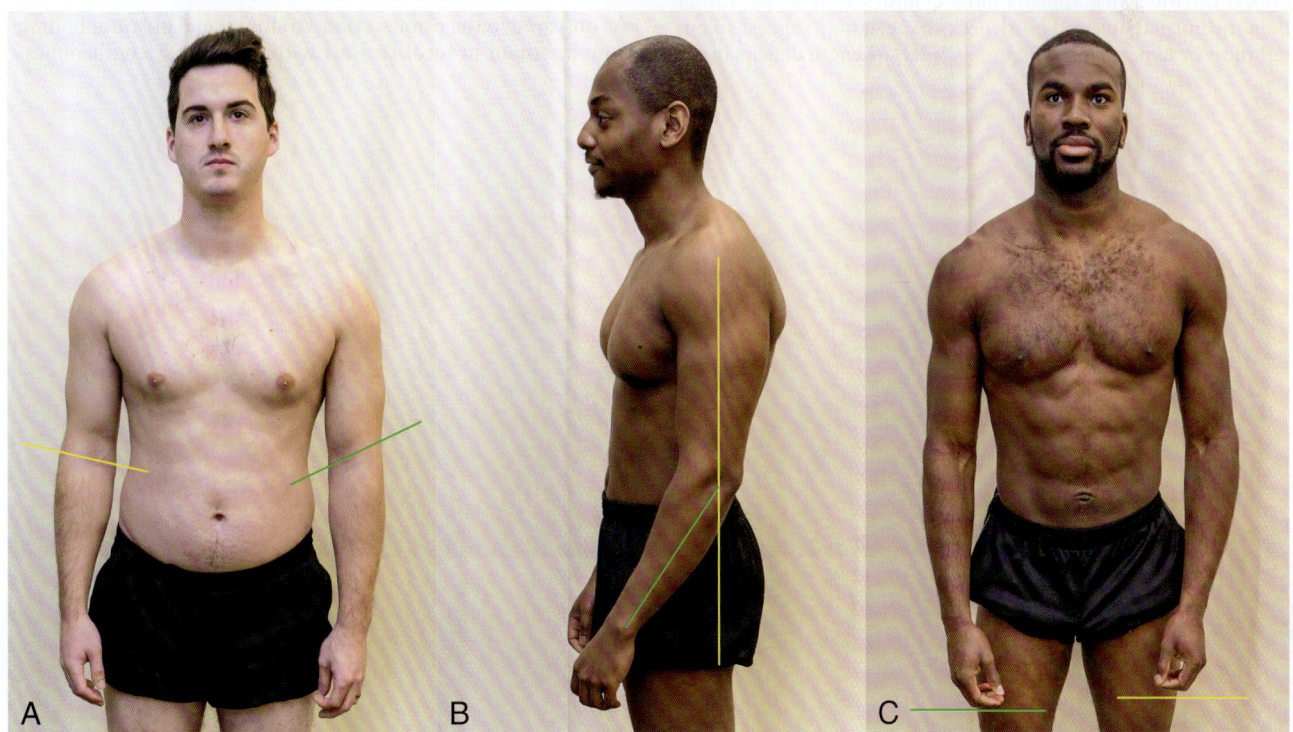

Figure 76-11. Postural dysfunction findings in the upper extremity region. A, Medial angle of antecubital fossa/elbow crease angle (more apparent on the subject's left elbow). B, Excessive elbow flexion at rest. C, Suggested right scapular depression based on the hand position (right hand being lower than the left).

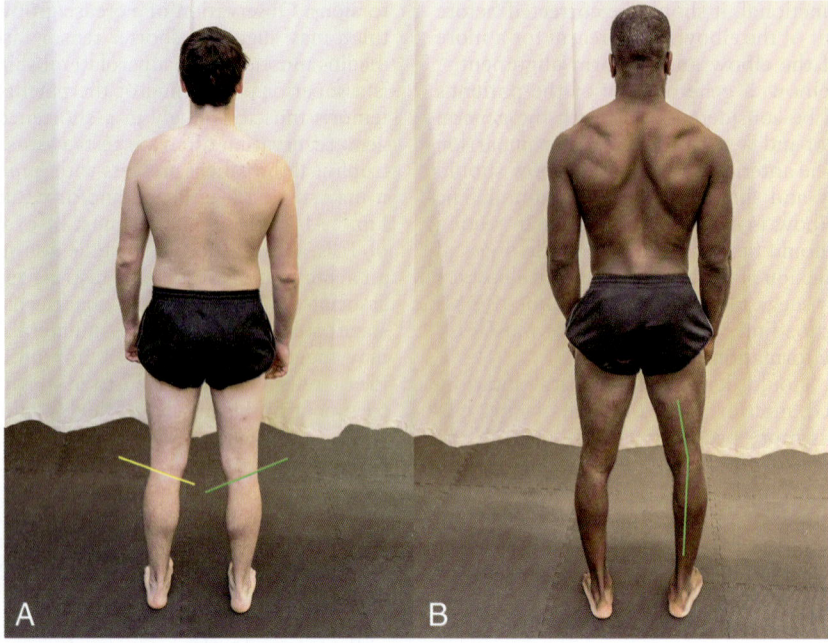

Figure 76-12. Postural dysfunction findings in the thigh and knee. A, Oblique angle of popliteal creases (deviating toward internal rotation of the femur bone/external rotation of the tibia bone [green line]). B, Genu varum depicted by green lines.

forefoot, the heel should be rounded in shape. With a center mass directed posteriorly, the patient may have a quadratic or square-shaped heel (Figure 76-13B), suggesting poor shock absorption with further possible dysfunctions at the knee, hip, and spine. Conversely, with an excessively anteriorly directed center of mass, the heel may appear more pointed in shape (Figure 76-13C), suggesting excessive forefoot stress during gait.[1]

In regard to general muscle appearance, a shorter and broader Achilles tendon may suggest a short or tight triceps surae. However, if the lower leg appears more cylindrical in shape, rather than the normal inverted bottleneck shape, it may suggest soleus tightness or hypertrophy (Figure 76-13D).[1] Length deficits in the soleus muscle may be a cause of back pain (see Chapter 66) and could suggest prior or current ankle or foot dysfunction. Refer to Chapters 63 to 69 for in-depth examination of the muscles of the foot and ankle that affect alignment.

4. JANDA'S CROSSED AND LAYER SYNDROMES

As observed in the prior section, dysfunctional postural findings may be found in local regions with associated lengthening or

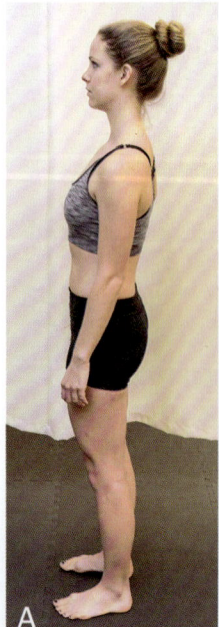
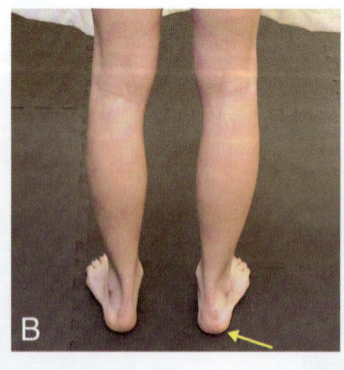
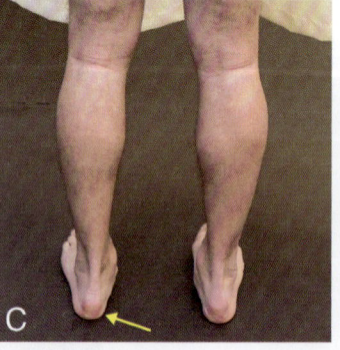
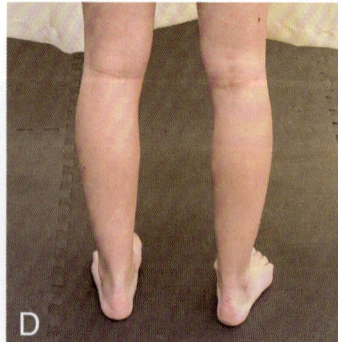

Figure 76-13. Postural dysfunction findings in the ankle and heel region. A, Posterior sway. B, Quadratic heel (more apparent on the subject's right heel). C, Pointed heel (more apparent on the subject's left heel). D, Cylindrical lower leg (demonstrating soleus tightness).

shortening, weakness, and/or tightness of muscles. However, the interplay between these impairments has the capacity to affect the entire musculoskeletal system, with a somewhat predictable pattern. With postural function, there are certain muscles with a predilection for being chronically inhibited and lengthened and other muscles with the opposite tendency of being hypertonic and shortened.[7] Kolar et al[9] through their observations and treatment of patients with chronic musculoskeletal pain and neurologic disorders, found that in response to joint dysfunction, the muscle responses were similar to patterns in lesions of the upper motor neurons, concluding that muscle imbalances originate and are controlled by the CNS.[4] Kolar[7] states the following:

> The fact that some muscles are posturally inclined toward inhibition while others toward hypertonia, shortening or even contractures has been known for a long time, but these predispositions for muscular imbalance were not systematically organized until Janda described these observations. The layout of muscle tone (muscle tension) deficits is so characteristic that Janda describes them as syndromes – the upper and lower crossed syndromes and the layer syndrome.[7]

These syndromes are defined by particular patterns of muscle tightness and weakness that cross between the posterior and anterior sides of the body.[1] These observable changes of shortening/tightness and/or inhibition/lengthening of muscles used for posture stabilization can predispose them to overload, leading to the formation of TrPs, thus resulting in pain and decreased function. It should be emphasized, however, that the crossed syndromes were an observation made by Janda of a combined tendency of certain muscle groups to become inhibited or facilitated in either the neck and shoulder girdle or the lumbopelvic girdle. This is not suggesting a direct association with pain per se, but an inefficiency of movement and decreased optimal function secondary to a postural dysfunction, which may result in a report of pain by an individual. The crossed syndromes are to assist the clinician in formulating a hypothesis of possible related structures that are currently contributing to the patient's symptoms. This then helps guide and shape the clinician's examination, which should include minimally the examination for the presence of both active and latent TrPs, muscle length, strength deficits, and movement impairments. These observations are consistent with the functional unit described in each of the muscle chapters.

4.1. Upper Crossed Syndrome

Often coinciding with the term "FHP," the upper crossed syndrome (UCS) (Figure 76-14) is evident when the position of the head, upper quarter, and cervicothoracic postural alignment is shifted from neutral, with the head moving forward relative to the shoulders. From a lateral view, the external acoustic meatus is positioned anterior to the acromion. The theory of UCS is that both the posterior cervical and the anterior thoracic musculature will become shortened over time, altering alignment and mobility.[48] More specifically, there is a shortening of the levator scapulae muscle, the upper portion of the trapezius, and the suboccipital muscles posteriorly, and shortening of the pectoralis major and minor and the sternocleidomastoid muscles anteriorly.[7] On the other hand, the deep cervical flexor muscles, rhomboids, and lower trapezius muscles often become inhibited and lengthened.[7]

The consequences of UCS are typically FHP with muscle length and strength deficits. Articular dysfunctions may be common at the occiput-C1, C4/C5, and T4/T5 segments, as these are transitional zones of curvature in the spine.[49] Janda noted that these transitional zones, in which there are focal areas of stress within the spine, correspond to areas where neighboring vertebrae change in morphology.[1]

In individuals with FHP, there is an associated rounded shoulder posture with inhibited scapular depressor muscles, leading to early shoulder elevation during shoulder abduction.[41] This has been correlated with a muscle imbalance between the upper trapezius muscles being overactive and the lower trapezius muscles being underactive,[50] leading to the glenohumeral joint being positioned higher secondary to the malalignment of the scapulae.[7] This may also lead to the protraction of the scapulae, impacting the supraspinatus muscle and its likely degeneration with concurrent overloading from the action caused by an overactive levator scapulae muscle (Chapters 19 and 21, respectively).[7] This could lead to associated TrPs in the upper trapezius and levator scapulae muscles, with individuals presenting with neck pain and associated FHP or the UCS.[51] This muscle imbalance is commonly associated with shoulder impingement syndromes.[52]

FHP alters body mechanics, predisposing the individual to develop TrPs by overloading muscles when compensatory efforts are made to overcome limitations imposed by FHP. Maximal voluntary isometric contraction is reduced in the cervical

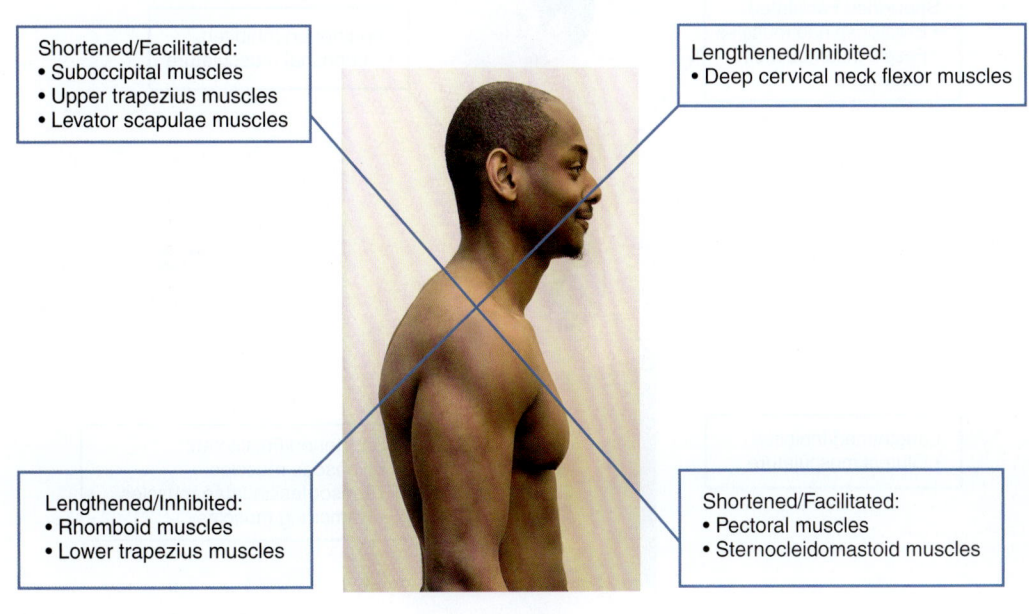

Figure 76-14. Upper cross syndrome.[1]

muscles, consistent with the effects of suboptimal muscle fiber length.[53] Neck pain secondary to FHP is also associated with decreased upper limb external rotation and weakness of shoulder abduction.[54] Respiratory function can also be compromised with FHP, with reduced vital capacity and decreased forced expiratory volume.[55] There is a general notion that FHP is associated with TMJ dysfunction, perhaps because the mandible is displaced posteriorly, a displacement commonly associated with TMJ-related pain.[56] However, opinions are conflicting in this regard as studies have been mixed in their reports of a relationship between head posture and TMJ disorders.[57-59] The problem is exacerbated by inconsistency in the criteria for the diagnosis of TMJ disorder, and the poor quality of the studies. Some studies only looked at intrinsic joint dysfunction, and few studies have looked at the relationship of FHP, orofacial TrPs, and TMJ pain. Perhaps unexpectedly, FHP was not associated with rounded (protracted) shoulder posture in young adults, although FHP was associated with neck pain and disability.[60] Laptop and smartphone use for an extended period of time is a risk factor for FHP-induced headache and neck and shoulder pain in young adults.[61,62] Similarly, studies of office workers show a correlation between FHP and neck pain.[63]

Consideration of postures during computer use has been a necessary part of head and neck pain assessment among students, often referred to as ergonomic assessment when applied to the workplace, but now should also be considered when assessing headache and neck pain in persons who use laptop computers. Wearing high heels is directly correlated with potentially harmful postural changes in adolescent girls, including FHP, lumbar hyperlordosis, and knee valgus.[64] The problem with these and similar studies is that they are very small in numbers of subjects, although they are consistent with other studies of the effect of ergonomic stress on muscle.

Backpacks can put young children at risk for neck and back pain later in life. Wearing a backpack weighing 7.5% of a child's body weight results in a significant decrease in the craniovertebral angle producing FHP,[65] which is likely to be an important risk factor for maintaining an FHP in adolescence and adulthood, although longitudinal studies have not been done yet. FHP is associated with moderate carpal tunnel syndrome, but no causal relationship can be implied.[66] Children who mouth breath are also more likely to have an FHP.[67]

Treatment of FHP is mostly accomplished through physical therapy programs that include posture corrective exercises. These have been shown in randomized controlled trials (RCTs) to decrease FHP.[68] A series of exercises that included McKenzie exercises, Kendall exercises, and self-stretches improved the craniovertebral angle and the scapular index,[69] and an RCT looking at Pilates decreased pain and neck disability.[70] A combination of upper thoracic spine mobilization and mobility exercises had better outcomes than upper cervical spine mobilization.[71] Suboccipital release improved the treatment outcome when added to craniocervical flexion exercises.[72] Cervical exercises also reduced FHP induced by smartphone use.[73] The difficulty with some of these studies, like some of the studies cited previously, is that the number of subjects is small.

4.2. Lower Crossed Syndrome

Lower crossed syndrome (LCS), also known as the distal or pelvic crossed syndrome, has been classified into two subtypes: type A posture and type B posture.[1] The more commonly known subtype, type A posture (Figure 76-15), occurs when there is a presentation of tight erector spinae muscles and fascia in the lumbosacral segments, tight rectus femoris, tensor fasciae latae, hamstrings, and iliopsoas muscles, and concomitant weakness of the abdominal and gluteal muscles.[7] As a result, theoretically, this leads to an anterior pelvic tilt with an increase in the lumbar lordosis.[7] Also in subtype A posture, there is a tendency to use more hip flexion and lumbar extension movement for mobility.[1] Subtype B posture (Figure 76-16) is more associated with FHP (Figure 76-14), with the same impairments as FHP, but with concomitant thoracic kyphosis, decreased lumbar lordosis, and the BCOG positioned posteriorly with secondary genu recurvatum.[1]

The evidence, perhaps not surprisingly, is varied and conflicted when it comes to musculoskeletal pain and certain components of the LCS and lumbopelvic posture. There is also a void of valid studies regarding the relationship of TrPs on LCS posture or lumbopelvic posture in general. However, it can be hypothesized that in the following studies, mentions of shortening or lengthening of muscles can precipitate the formation of TrPs and should be included in the examination.

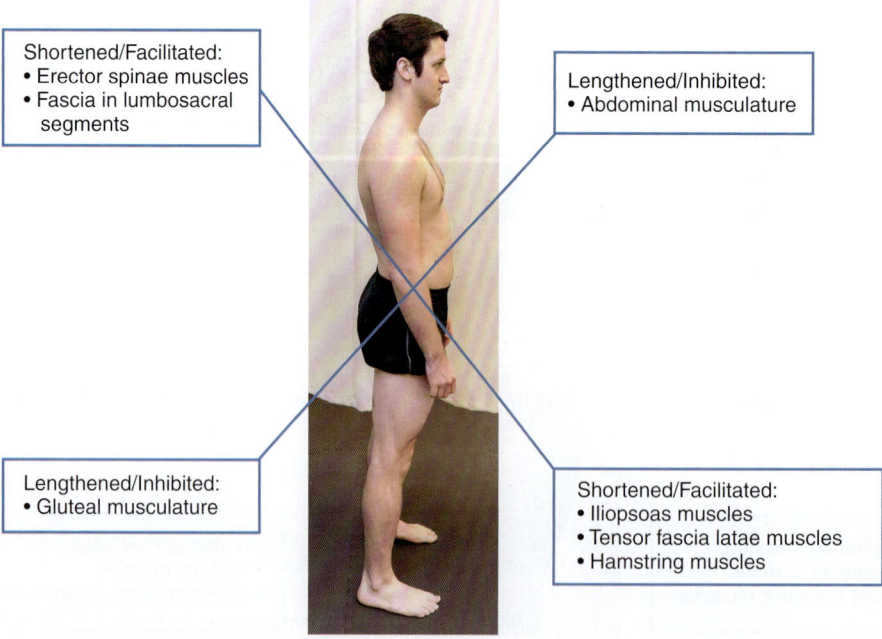

Figure 76-15. Lower cross syndrome (subtype A).[1]

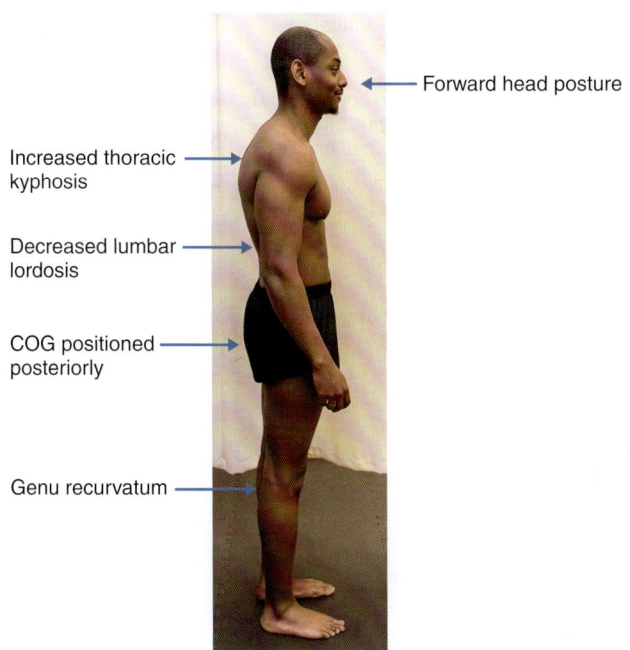

Figure 76-16. Lower cross syndrome (subtype B).[1]

There are studies in support of hip extension mobility deficits secondary to tight hip flexor muscles with an association of low back pain[74-77] and shorter iliopsoas muscle as contributing to low back pain,[78,79] characteristics found in LCS. A study performed by Ranger et al[80] suggested that shorter lumbar paraspinal fascia was associated with high-intensity low back pain via magnetic resonance imaging. Furthermore, a study performed by Malai et al[81] suggested that hold-relax stretching of the iliopsoas muscle in patients with chronic nonspecific lower back pain with lumbar hyperlordosis was significant for reducing pain, improving hip flexor muscle length, decreasing the lumbar lordosis angle, and enhancing transverse abdominus muscle activation. However, a study performed by Walker et al[11] found that there was no relationship between standing lumbar lordosis, pelvic tilt, and abdominal muscle performance. A study performed by Nourbakhsh and Arab[14] found that there was no strong association with low back pain (LBP) and structural factors such as size of lordosis, pelvic tilt, iliopsoas length, or lumbar paraspinal length.

Furthermore, Heino et al[10] found that there was no clear relationship between hip extension ROM and standing pelvic tilt, standing lumbar lordosis, or abdominal muscle performance and even suggested that clinicians should not base treatment from a visual inspection of postural malalignments, specifically stretching of the hip flexor myofascia, based on a view of posture alone. Heino et al[10] suggested that specific examination procedures should be the guiding factors for treatment. It should be noted, though, that the study performed by Heino et al[10] was performed on healthy younger individuals (ages 21-49) and the study by Walker et al[11] was performed on healthy younger individuals (ages 20-33) without lower back pain.

Gluteal muscle weakness or inhibition is one of the associated findings with LCS. Evidence has shown some key links between gluteal muscle weakness and other muscle dysfunctions, similar to the observations found in LCS. Lee and Oh[82] and Arab et al[83] found that there was a suggested association of gluteus maximus muscle weakness and hamstring muscle length deficits. Furthermore, in the study by Arab et al[83] it was suggested that in patients with sacroiliac joint dysfunction with gluteus maximus muscle weakness, there was a significant association with hamstring muscle length deficit. It was suggested by van Wingerden et al[84] that hamstring muscle tightness in patients with low back pain was a compensatory mechanism to adjust for pelvic instability. However, the study performed by Nourbakhsh and Arab[14] suggested that there was no association between hamstring muscle length, pelvic tilt, or low back pain. Lee et al[82] found that without normalization of gluteus maximus muscle strength, it demonstrated a nonsignificant negative correlation with hamstring muscle length; however, with normalization of the participant's gluteus maximus muscle strength by height and weight, there was a positive significant correlation with hamstring muscle length. This finding holds huge implications for prior studies and erroneous conclusions regarding strength variables and associations with postural variables, because of the high correlation of body size and strength. However, in this study by Lee et al,[82] it should be noted that participants were all healthy young males and the study did not include any participants with lower back pain.

Increased tension in the thoracic paraspinal muscles or hypertrophy of lumbar paraspinal muscles may be the result of abdominal muscle weakness[2] or, if accompanied by LBP as a compensatory mechanism to hip flexor muscle shortening, weak gluteal and abdominal muscles.[85] Hultman et al[86] and Lankhorst et al[87] also found a decrease in lumbar extensibility in patients with low back pain. The study performed by Nourbakhsh and Arab[14] found that subjects with low back pain had the highest association with lumbar extensor endurance deficits.

Inhibited or lengthened abdominal muscles and their relationship to the rest of the LCS characteristics have been under contention by several studies such as Youdas et al,[88] Walker,[11] and Levine et al,[89] suggesting that there was no association between abdominal muscle strength, pelvic tilt, and lumbar lordosis. Toppenberg and Bullock[90] and Youdas et al[88] suggested that there was no significant relationship between lumbar lordosis and abdominal muscle length. There are several studies, however, suggesting that abdominal muscle weakness is related to lower back pain.[78,91-94] Nonetheless, considering the varied and convoluted debate on abdominal or core strength and the testing methods to obtain these results, many of these studies will need to be read in detail for individual opinion.

The most common pathology resulting from components of LCS is typically persistent chronic lower back pain. However, treatment of persistent chronic lower back pain has been debated for decades by researchers, with limited consensus. What is lacking in the research is the postural considerations of TrPs, particularly in the lumbar region. Please refer to Sections 5 and 6 in this text for more details on the examination and treatment of TrPs in the trunk and hip musculature.

With the extreme variability of body types and postures, it might be expected that there is no specific relationship or correlation of certain aspects of posture with pain, based on current set norms for posture. For example, in a study by Laird et al[12] of 62 participants with and without low back pain, it was concluded that there were no significant differences with standing lordosis angles. However, this study did not define or describe low back pain other than having had LBP for 12 or more weeks with or without leg pain and scored more than a 2 out of 10 on the numeric pain rating scale. Based on similar studies, it would be easy for a clinician to interpret such findings as a reason to disregard certain variables, such as lordosis angles, during the postural examination.

4.3. Layer Syndrome

Also known as stratification syndrome, the layer syndrome as described by Janda is the combination of both the UCS and the LCS.[1] It essentially denotes the layering of muscular hypertrophy or shortening and hypotrophy or lengthening.[7] From a dorsal perspective (Figure 76-17), there is typically muscular hypertrophy or shortening of the hamstring muscles, erector spinae muscles in the thoracolumbar region, erector spinae muscles in the cervical region, upper trapezius, and levator scapulae muscles.[7] This is paired with muscular hypotrophy or lengthening of the gluteal muscles and lower stabilizers of the scapulae.[1] Ventrally, there

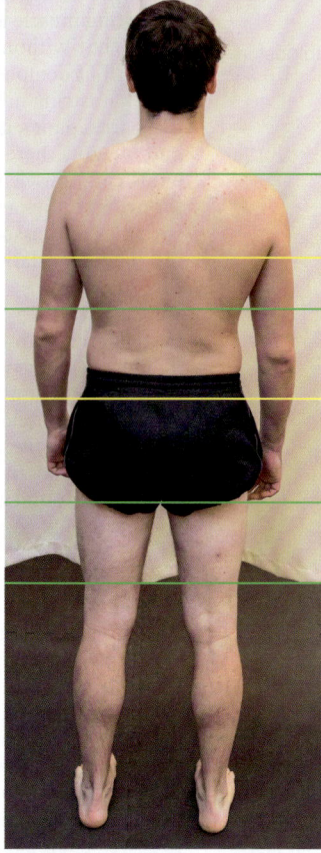

Figure 76-17. Layer syndrome (dorsal aspect).[1]

is typically muscular hypertrophy or shortening of pectoralis, sternocleidomastoid, iliopsoas, and rectus femoris muscles.[7] This is paired with muscular hypotrophy or lengthening of the abdominal muscles and deep cervical neck flexor muscles.[1]

4.4. Summary of the Janda Approach Regarding Postural Syndromes

In regard to treatment of the layer syndrome, UCS, or LCS, it is suggested to consider the Janda approach in managing these postures. In general, the Janda approach to the postural syndromes begins with a static postural assessment followed by observation of single-leg stance and gait.[1] Next, movement pattern characteristics are assessed as well as muscle length of suspect musculature for tightness or shortness.[1] Once muscle imbalances are evaluated, the clinician then hypothesizes on the cause of dysfunction based on the information gathered and selects interventions accordingly. Treatment begins with normalizing the periphery, which essentially involves normalizing the afferent input into the sensorimotor system via postural corrections and applying biomechanical corrections via manual therapy techniques to provide an optimal environment for healing. Once the peripheral structures are normalized, there must be a restoration of muscle balance. If there is no coordination between muscles, the strongest muscle in the chain cannot be functional. Likewise, in the presence of tight or short antagonistic muscles as described in the UCS, LCS, and layer syndrome, restoring normal muscle tension and length must be addressed before strengthening weak musculature.[1] Hypothetically, with those shortened and tight muscles, there is a predisposition for TrP formation; therefore, assessing these predictable muscle groups may be essential in regard to treating the TrPs to restore normal muscle tension and function. "Sensorimotor training"[1] follows the restoration of muscle balance, increasing proprioceptive input to facilitate automatic and appropriately timed muscle coordination in order to facilitate a reflexive joint and postural stabilization, rather than specific muscle strengthening. Finally, endurance of coordinated movement patterns with a focus on low-intensity exercises performed at high volume is emphasized because of fatigue being the predisposing factor to compensated movement patterns.[1] The home exercise prescription is absolutely vital as the patient must be practicing consistently in order to make changes at the CNS level. See Chapter 4 "Perpetuating Factors" for further information on maladaptive movement patterns and their effect on the nociceptive system. The clinician should seek the appropriate sources as referenced for further information on the Janda approach to treatment.[1,7,95]

5. POSTURAL CONSIDERATIONS OF BREATHING

The primary objective of respiration, the exchange of oxygen and carbon dioxide, is to meet the metabolic demands of the body.[96] This exchange is achieved through breathing, which is regulated and coordinated by the autonomic nervous system and influenced by physical, chemical, and emotional factors. However, with injury or pain, faulty respiration occurs at a subcortical level as compensation. This can lead to a faulty breathing pattern becoming perpetuated at the subcortical level, and eventually being an imbedded motor program, even when the initial trigger or threat is no longer present.[1] There is also the likelihood of the formation of TrPs in muscles that must compensate for the dysfunctional stabilization of the spine secondary to diaphragm muscle not fulfilling its role as a postural stabilizer.

Breathing, on a neural and mechanical level, extrinsically and intrinsically serves several purposes for posture and movement and can be seen through more obvious examples such as musicians sniffing to coordinate the initial note, martial artists breathing or yelling when they strike or flow into the next step, tennis players yelling before they hit the ball, or weight lifters grunting prior to exertion.

This section aims to focus on the role of breathing on posture and movement. See Chapter 45 for further details on the mechanics of normal respiration as illustrated in Figures 45-8 and 45-9.

5.1. The Postural Function of the Diaphragm Muscle

Lewit stated, "If breathing is not normalized—no other movement pattern can be."[97] Because of the inherent relationship of breathing with movement, breathing naturally has an influence on postural function as well.[8] Both posture and movement are linked by the diaphragm muscle.[5] Refer to Chapter 45 for the anatomy and function of the diaphragm muscle. The diaphragm muscle is often overlooked despite its known role in vital functions. However, the diaphragm muscle, when performing poorly, can be the underlying cause of dysfunctional stabilization of posture or uncoordinated movements because of its role in the IAP and the integrated spinal stability system (ISSS).[98]

The diaphragm muscle has a dual role as both a respiratory and postural muscle, which is essential for spinal stability and resultant movements.[98] With the involvement of the CNS, the diaphragm muscle assists with postural body control[8] through flattening or caudally descending the dome of the diaphragm muscle during either respiration or trunk postural stabilization.[8]

During its caudal descent during postural exertion, the diaphragm muscle works as a piston, building pressure on the abdominal viscera and increasing IAP against the pelvic floor and abdominal muscles.[8] This results in an eccentric expansion of the abdominal wall to an adequate abdominal and thoracic wall volume and then maintained isometrically. In an ideal scenario, such as lifting a heavy object, this "eccentric–isometric" muscle activity will match the degree of muscle exertion and work necessary to meet the demands of the motion.[8]

The regulation of IAP occurs via the diaphragm, pelvic floor, multifidi, and transversus abdominis muscles, providing anterior lumbopelvic postural stability.[98] As discussed by Frank et al,[98] there is a general consensus that an increase in IAP creates spinal stability[99-105] and is a parameter for influencing spinal mechanics and stiffness. Thus, IAP then coordinates with the ISSS for dynamic stability of the spine.

The ISSS, as described by Kolar et al,[8] is a balanced system of coactivation between spinal extensor muscles in the cervical and upper thoracic region, the deep cervical flexor muscles, as well as the diaphragm, pelvic floor, and all sections of the abdominal and spinal extensor muscles in the lower thoracic and lumbar region.[98] Coordinating with IAP, the ISSS creates spinal stiffness, contributing to dynamic stability of the spine.[98] The muscles of the ISSS constitute the "deep core" and, via a "feed forward control mechanism," their activation precedes most voluntary movements.[98]

ISSS provides the stable base or punctum fixum on which muscles can produce motion.[98] An example of this provided by Frank et al[98] occurs when the psoas major muscle relies on the thoracolumbar spine as a BOS to act as a hip flexor; however, if the ISSS is inefficient, the psoas major muscle may cause anterior shear stress on the lumbar spine from muscular forces and pull. Furthermore, a study performed by Kolar et al[106] demonstrated that IAP regulation and ISSS can be disturbed by a decreased capacity of the diaphragm's postural function, resulting in compensatory activity of the superficial spinal extensors. As a result, there are increased compressive forces on the spine.[106] The decreased capacity of the diaphragm's postural function also results in an imbalance between lower and upper chest musculature, leading to an abnormal position of the thoracic rib cage and chest.[106] Abnormal stabilization function of the diaphragm typically is paired with dysfunctional breathing patterns.[8]

5.2. Assessment of the Diaphragm Muscle

The evaluation of breathing patterns is crucial for the assessment of the stabilization function of the spine.[7] It demonstrates the functional interplay and relationship between the activation of the diaphragm and the abdominal muscles.[7]

Assessment of Breathing and the Diaphragm

Normal contraction of the diaphragm pushes the abdominal contents down toward the pelvis, causing protrusion of the abdomen and increased lung volume in the lower chest during inhalation. Normal resting inhalation involves coordinated contraction of the diaphragm with expansion of the *lower* thorax and elevation of the rib cage, all of which increase lung volume. With the caudal descent of the diaphragm, there should also be an increase in IAP if there is normal maintenance of abdominal wall and pelvic floor tension.[98] With tidal breathing there should be relaxation of the accessory breathing muscles with ventral movement of the sternum and without motion in the transverse plane.[7]

When assessing breathing, the clinician should first assess posture in static standing and assess for the patient's natural breathing patterns, the shape and size of the thoracic wall, natural muscle tension of the abdominal wall, shoulder position (for protraction or retraction), head position, and whether paradoxical breathing is present. With normal tidal breathing, there should be an observation of symmetrical expansion of the lower thoracic and abdominal cavities, particularly the lower aperture of the thorax with ventral movement of the sternum.[35] Following the observation of breathing and posture, it is suggested to follow this with the seated diaphragm test and the IAP test to further assess diaphragmatic activity with appropriate ability to generate and maintain IAP. It should be noted that these tests are for qualitative purposes as objective measures are limited.[98] Refer to the following sources on how to perform the seated diaphragm muscle test and the IAP test.[9,95,98]

The mechanics of normal respiration are presented in detail in Chapter 45 and illustrated in Figures 45-7 and 45-8.

Dysfunctional Breathing

If the patient demonstrates an hourglass syndrome posture, as described in the abdominal wall section of the static standing postural assessment, this would indicate the presence of inverse or paradoxical diaphragm function.[7] With paradoxical respiration, these chest and abdominal functions oppose each other. On inhalation, the chest expands (moves up and out) while the abdomen moves in, elevating the diaphragm and decreasing lung volume. On exhalation, the reverse occurs. Consequently, a normal effort produces inadequate tidal volume, and the muscles of the upper chest, especially the scalene muscles, overwork to exchange sufficient air via cranial pull on the upper ribs. This usually results in a nociceptive chain of the cervical region (Box 76-4) secondary to the scalene muscles along with the sternocleidomastoid muscles pulling the cervical spine forward, causing an FHP at the craniocervical junction.[51] This results in movement restrictions in the upper cervical spine, the cervicothoracic junction, and the upper ribs[51] secondary to poor coordination of the major components of the respiratory apparatus.

Respiratory function can also be compromised with FHP. This is due to a dominance of accessory inspiratory respiratory muscles versus utilizing the diaphragm, contributing to an inspiratory position of the rib cage with stiffness of the thoracic spine due.[51] A reduced vital capacity and decreased forced expiratory volume secondary to FHP have been reported.[55] Furthermore,

Kolnes[107] observed that chronic costal or upper chest patterns of breathing can lead to a constant excessive facilitation of the respiratory muscles, such as the scalenes and sternocleidomastoid muscles, perpetuating FHP and TrPs.

Dysfunctional Postural Function of the Diaphragm

In regard to the dysfunctional postural function of the diaphragm muscle, in the hourglass syndrome posture, the diaphragm flattens significantly less. The centrum tendineum of the diaphragm becomes the punctum fixum and pulls the intercostal spaces and lower ribs inward via the pull of the diaphragm attachments on the lower ribs. As a result of the nonproportional activation, the lumbar portions of the diaphragm contract more, and as a result of compensation for poor postural diaphragmatic function and coordinated IAP, the superficial paraspinal muscles near the thoracolumbar junction hypertrophy over time[7] and inhibit the abdominal wall muscles.[95] Furthermore, associated TrPs in the thoracic region typically occur in the diaphragm, pectoralis major, and dorsal erector spinae muscles with concomitant joint restriction of the thoracic spine and rib cage.[51] If an altered or dysfunctional respiratory postural pattern is identified, it suggests the presence of poor inter- and intramuscular coordination, which is mediated by the CNS.[108]

5.3. Treatment Considerations for the Diaphragm's Dual Role

In order to have physiologic stabilization of the spine, there must be normal physiologic breathing and vice versa.[108] However, without that physiologic stabilization of the spine, this can cause inappropriate or unstabilized muscle pull throughout the entire body, precipitating the formation of TrPs.

Trigger points in the kinetic chain muscles can have great influences on faulty breathing patterns, such as paradoxical breathing or faulty postural patterns.[51,97,109] Page et al also described nociceptive chains similar to the kinetic chain, with associated TrPs throughout the chain. It was observed that nociceptive chains were typically unilateral and are mostly present in patients with chronic pain.[1] Box 76-4 depicts the associated nociceptive chains that warrant examination for TrPs.

Because of the ability TrPs to alter firing sequences in the kinetic chains,[109] the TrPs in the nociceptive chains may need to be assessed and treated in order to restore balance of diaphragmatic breathing and function.

If the patient has poor mobility of the thoracic spine, abdominal wall, or the thoracic wall, it will likely be difficult to maintain or achieve physiologic breathing patterns and adequate trunk stabilization.[108] For improvement of independent thoracic wall movement, the mobility of the thoracic fascia, with emphasis on the lower intercostal spaces, should be improved.[108]

Once the diaphragm has improved capacity for function, the patient must then relearn appropriate diaphragmatic breathing. To learn normal diaphragmatic breathing, while in a recumbent position, the patient exhales fully with one hand on the chest and the other on the abdomen (Figure 20-15B). Diaphragmatic respiration alone is most easily learned if the patient holds the chest fixed in the collapsed position, rather than expanded (Figure 20-15C), and concentrates on breathing by alternately contracting the diaphragm and abdominal muscles (allowing the abdomen to move out during inhalation and move in during exhalation) without expanding the upper chest or elevating the sternum. When smooth easy diaphragmatic breathing is achieved, the patient then learns to coordinate costal and diaphragmatic respiration during inhalation (Figure 20-12) and exhalation (Figure 20-13). When respiration is coordinated, the chest and abdomen move in and out together. The patient should note the closeness of the hands during exhalation and their separation during inhalation; the hands move up and down together. It may help for the patient to then think of also expanding the "lateral bellows" or "bucket handles" (expanding the lower rib cage laterally) and elevating the sternum (the "pump handle") to expand the chest during full, normal, coordinated inhalation. Positional feedback from the hands is often helpful for a patient to learn this technique. If the patient has difficulty with this, manual pressure at the lower rib cage with a quick stretch upon full exhalation can stimulate activation of the diaphragm. The patient can be instructed to provide this pressure and stretch in supine.

The patient should practice coordinated breathing at intervals throughout the day and before bed each night. Taking each breath to the count of "4 in" and a count of "4 out," then a pause, "hold-and-relax" for a count of 4 improves pacing and provides rhythm. The patient should become aware of using this coordinated breathing throughout the day.

Having learned to breathe properly while recumbent, the patient must transfer this learning to the upright posture. The patient sits in a chair with a firm flat seat (Figure 20-13), tilts the front of the pelvis forward and down (exaggerating the lumbar lordosis), and draws in a slow deep breath. This anterior pelvic tilt separates the anterior chest from the symphysis pubis, making it easy and natural to contract the diaphragm and to protrude the abdomen while inhaling. Then, by rocking the pelvis backward (posterior pelvic tilt or abdominal curl movement) and leaning slightly forward during slow exhalation, the abdomen moves in and the increased IAP pushing up against the diaphragm assists elevation of the relaxed diaphragm.

Box 76-4 Associated muscles of the nociceptive chain to include for examination of TrPs to improve diaphragmatic breathing and function

Cervical Region	Thoracic Region	Lumbar/Abdominal Region	Shoulder Girdle
Sternocleidomastoid	Pectoralis major	Pelvic floor	Subscapularis
Scalenes	Pectoralis minor	Diaphragm	Infraspinatus
Posterior cervical	Diaphragm	Gluteus maximus	Supraspinatus
Splenii	Subscapularis	Gluteus medius	Deltoids
Upper trapezius	Serratus anterior	Piriformis	Teres major
Levator scapulae	Iliocostalis thoracis	Iliacus	Triceps brachii long head
		Short adductors	
		Hamstrings	
		Rectus femoris	
		Tensor fascia latae	

Adapted from Liebenson C. *Rehabilitation of the Spine a Practitioner's Manual.* 2nd ed. Baltimore, MD: Lippincott Williams & Wilkins; 2007 (p. 784).

6. COMMON POSTURES

Common statically held postures such as prolonged sitting, desk jobs and office work, driving, and sleeping can overload muscles and other structures. This section will discuss suggestions of ideal positions for these common postures; however, the clinician should accommodate for the individual patient when making suggestions for accommodations.

6.1. Sitting

Prolonged sitting has been regarded as the "new smoking" by many clinicians and researchers, because of the implications of sitting on all-cause mortality.[110,111] Wilmot et al[112] suggest that sedentary behavior in general had an association with diabetes, cardiovascular disease, and all-cause mortality. Frequent rest breaks are recommended by the Occupational Safety and Health Administration (OSHA). Although the OSHA recommends a 10-minute break every 2 hours for computer workers, frequent shorter rest breaks may be more beneficial, as it can allow the patient to recognize and adjust posture. With any activity or occupation that requires sitting for hours at a time, seated positioning is critical.

Sitting alignment is a widely debated topic with unclear parameters on how much lumbar flexion is appropriate, as increased lumbar flexion has some associations with LBP.[42]

Normal supported sitting alignment for most people is described by Sahrmann[36] as having the "spine erect and supported, the shoulders aligned over the hips, the feet supported, and the hips flexed to 90°," whereas in unsupported sitting, the pelvis will be in a slight posterior tilt resulting in a flatter lumbar spine with a relatively unchanged thoracic and cervical spinal alignment in comparison to standing. However, Sahrmann[36] states that "because of the variation in posture and anthropometrics among individuals, no chair or sitting surface is perfect for everyone." With variations in spinal curvatures, height, and limb proportions, each individual who does not meet the "ergonomic" norm is always at a disadvantage, having to sit in a chair that may not support them adequately. Chair modifications can be made, such as a lumbar roll or support for individuals with increased lumbar lordosis, making note that the support only fills the space of the lordosis and the chair, not pushing the lumbar spine into extension.

Another approach to correcting poor sitting posture would be Brugger's sitting posture, utilizing a postural cogwheel–like mechanism.[1] By changing the bottom cogwheel—the pelvis—the patient has control of the reversal of curves and assumes appropriate sitting posture by changing one region of the body.[1]

In the age of technologic advances in which cellphones and laptops are commonly used, prolonged use of such devices, as mentioned earlier in the chapter, can result in FHP-induced headache as well as neck and shoulder pain in younger adults.[61,62] As seen in Figure 76-6, the patient, in order to maintain his viewing angle, has to sit with an excessive posterior tilt of the pelvis, causing the abnormal reversal of curves as described in Brugger's sitting position.[1] Constant viewing of the device's screen results in FHP, and a lack of support under his elbows causes further protraction of the scapulae. With the correction of pillows and support under his elbows as seen in Figure 76-18, the patient now has improved reversal of curves, decreased FHP, and improved overall alignment.

6.2. Computer or Workstation Ergonomic Analysis

According to the Bureau of Labor Statistics,[113] over half of the workforce (~77 million Americans) uses a computer at work. This increasing number of employees using a computer for work has sparked interest in the ergonomics of the workstation. Additionally, musculoskeletal complaints have continued to increase and are reported to be from 20% to 75% of computer workers.[114] Laptop and smartphone use for an extended period of time is a risk factor for FHP-induced headache, neck pain, and shoulder pain in young adults.[61,62] Numerous companies have entered the market to provide equipment that is better suited for an ergonomic workstation.

Correction of the individual's workstation is often the most powerful intervention. For desk workers, a desktop computer or a laptop with a docking station should be used, with the keyboard allowing the elbows and shoulders to be relaxed at 90° (Figure 76-19A). The computer screen or laptop should be directly in front of the body and at an angle, two-thirds of the screen below eye level, that encourages erect posture while minimizing glare.

Documents should be placed on a stand at the same level as the computer screen (rather than flat on the desk to one side) for optimum viewing and to avoid excessive muscular strain.

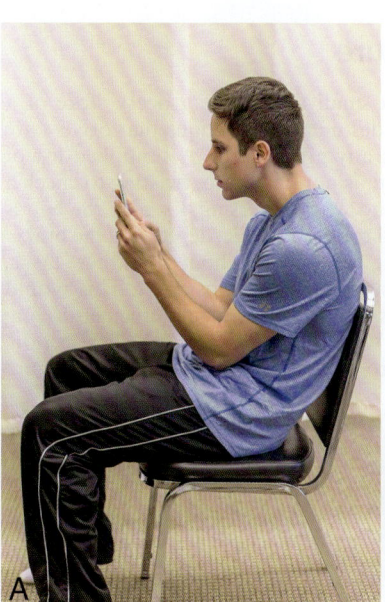
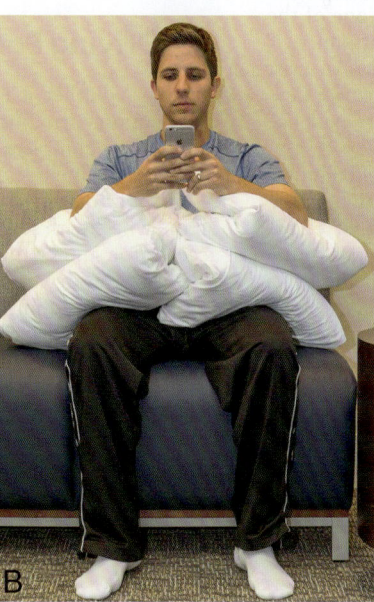
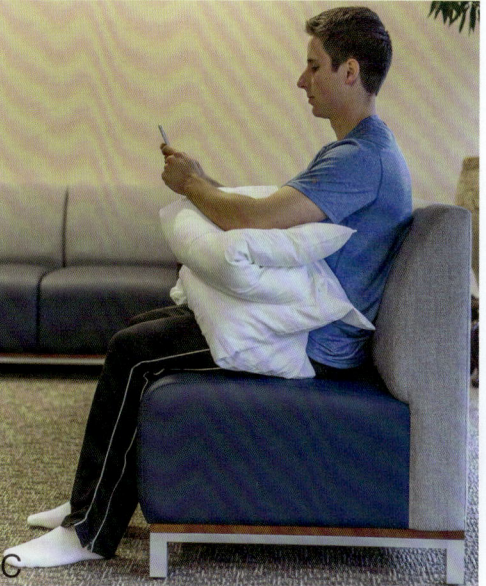

Figure 76-18. A, Poor sitting posture secondary to phone use. B and C, Corrected sitting posture with pillows.

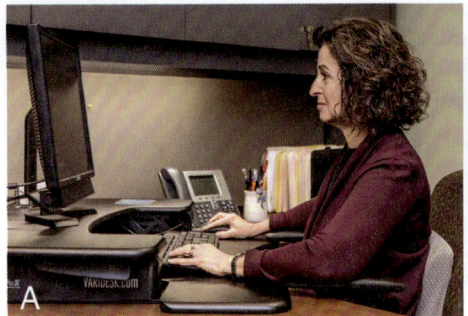 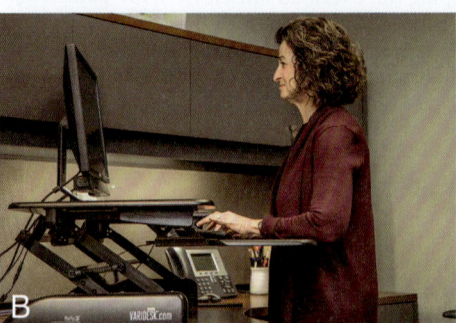 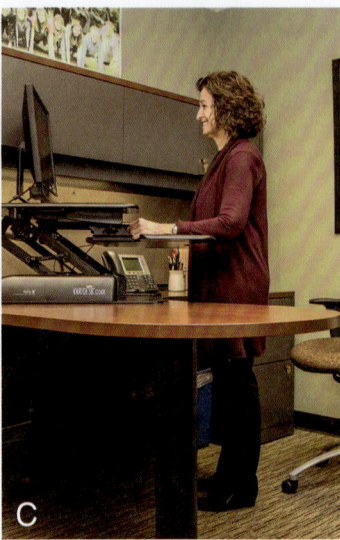

Figure 76-19. Workstation. A, Efficient sitting posture. B and C, Neutral standing posture with a standing desk.

Reflections on eyeglasses and contact lenses can be managed by changing the relative position of the light source or by using antiglare lenses. Nearsightedness should also be corrected, because it favors a head-forward posture, which shortens the sternocleidomastoid muscles. Patients who have recently received new progressive lenses should have their workstation reevaluated to ensure good ergonomics.

The computer mouse should be at the level of the keyboard, which may require the addition of a keyboard and/or mouse tray. The patient should consider alternating sides for mouse use. Although this discipline can take weeks or months to learn, it is possible to become ambidextrous with the mouse, which can halt the perpetuation of TrPs in many upper extremity and shoulder girdle muscles.

According to international standards, based on ergonomic principles,[115] the comfort zone for the wrist is defined as between 45° flexion, 45° extension, 20° ulnar deviation, or 15° radial deviation.[116] Decreasing the computer keyboard slope also decreases the wrist extension needed to use the keyboard.[117] The location of the mouse is also relevant in the overload of wrist extensor muscles and a central mouse position, with the mouse centered between the keyboard and the user's body one of the best choices regarding general stress in the upper extremity,[118] although the best recommended position to avoid excessive wrist extension was locating the mouse by the side of a narrower keyboard, without a number keypad.[118] There is moderate evidence for the use of vibratory feedback in the mouse.[119]

Interrupting prolonged typing or data entry every 30 minutes or so to do the finger-flutter exercise (Figure 35-6) can help the wrist extensor muscles recover from prolonged activity. This exercise is performed by dropping the hands to the sides of the body, completely relaxed, and moving the arms and elbows to cause passive relaxed shaking of the hands and fingers.

When considering office seating postures, the chair is important to assess. It is important to have seating with weight-bearing on the ischial tuberosities, so that diaphragmatic breathing is easier. If the chair has a headrest, it should not push the head forward. Lumbar rolls, as discussed earlier, must ensure that the lumbar lordosis is supported but not increased.[36] A wedge cushion that anteriorly tips the pelvis or an adjustable chair is an option if the patient presents with excessive posterior tilting of the pelvis as discussed earlier.[1] Lastly, consider the positioning of the hips on the chair. It is recommended that the hips attain 90° of flexion along with the knees, and the feet can be placed flat on the floor. This is the primary consideration of the seat height that is required. If the seat height is at its lowest point and hip flexion remains above 90°, then a raised flat surface may be placed on the floor to elevate the floor height but not the chair (Box 76-5).

Achieving the alignment as indicated above facilitates a position that is efficient and maintains the spine in a neutral position. The chairs that are available for purchase are endless, but having a chair that can adjust up and down and also has an adjustable back is of greatest value. Standing desks are also a viable option for active posture as depicted in Figure 76-19B and C.

6.3. Driving Posture

Driving, whether it is a small trip to the grocery store or a cross-country trip, includes numerous actions that drivers are required to complete at any given point. A simplified list of these actions includes, but is not limited to, twisting to check a blind spot, looking behind when reversing, keeping the hands on the wheel with several rotations made, depressing the brake/accelerator, and changing gears. Throughout all of these tasks, however, the driver is seated for the most part. This would call for increased importance of a neutral and efficient driving position for all drivers. With the increase in vehicle selection, from tiny compact cars to large trucks, the seating systems are

---

Box 76-5 Key points to a proper ergonomic workstation setup

1. The monitor height should be placed so that the eyes are in a horizontal plane.
2. The keyboard and mouse should be positioned so that the elbow is in 90° flexion.
3. The wrists should be in a slightly extended position.
4. The hips should be at a 90-degree angle and the feet placed flat on the floor.
5. The head, shoulder, and hips should be aligned, with the back supported by the chair.

relatively similar. What will matter most in regard to the vehicle is its capabilities of adjusting.

Sitting posture while operating a vehicle is demonstrated in Figure 76-20. This optimal position while driving is what should be achieved prior to operating a vehicle. This position will allow most driving tasks to occur without greater demand or physical strain on the body.

With seat height, the hips should be relatively flexed, with hips at the height of the knees. The driver must also have easy access to view the entire dashboard without the need to lean forward or sit up higher. Most new cars have the option of adjusting the seat height; however, in the event the seat height is not adjustable, a pad may be used to achieve the correct seat height. Seat depth, on the other hand, is a position that is at times difficult to adjust as most vehicles do not have this option. Normally, there should be an inch between the popliteal space and the chair to avoid excessive compression of the nerves and vessels in that location.

When a driver sits in the car for the first time, a common initial adjustment is typically the anterior/posterior positioning of the chair. Ideally, the chair should be positioned where the driver can manage to press the accelerator and brakes while the back maintains contact with the seat and the knees are able to maintain roughly 20° to 30° of flexion. If the steering wheel is adjustable, it is recommended that the elbows maintain a position of about 120° of flexion while the arms are in the normal position on the steering wheel. However, for safety purposes, per the National Highway Traffic Safety Administration (NHTSA),[120] the driver's chest should always remain at least 10 in away from the air bag. There are exceptions for different body types and medical conditions. Please refer to the NHTSA's website for further information on the subject, and if the reader is from a country other than the United States, please refer to the appropriate government website for up-to-date information.

The seat of the car should be used to provide support to the thoracic and lumbar spine. The suggested angle is 100° to 120°. This slightly extended posture decreases the stress on the spine. Regarding the cervical spine, it is important to consider the headrest. The design of the headrest is mostly considered in regard to safety. In the event of a motor vehicle accident, the headrest would support the head when a rear force makes contact with the vehicle. However, the headrest should also be positioned in such a way that the occiput makes contact with the center of the headrest. This helps to provide cervical support, as well as cue the driver to avoid FHP.

Once the main adjustments have been made, the driver should then proceed to adjust the rear view and side mirrors. The mirrors should be positioned in such a way that the driver does not have to excessively alter sitting position in order to view.

6.4. Sleeping Postures

Sleep is the human body's method for recovery and repair for maintenance of physical and mental health.[121] As individuals face their daily stressors of life, they must sleep to replenish for the next day. Roughly one-third of human life is spent sleeping, which means that a large portion of life is spent in a relatively static position. This unfortunately also has implications in regard to TrPs. Trigger points can impede sleep because of pain and because of the muscle being in a lengthened or shortened position. Trigger points can be activated and perpetuated during sleep. Sleep is also impeded in patients with pain in general, whether it is shoulder pain or LBP. Patients often report that they cannot find a comfortable position for sleep. However, modifying the patient's sleeping position can improve sleep quality, decrease strain on muscles with TrPs, and facilitate improved recovery.

Although many people have their own preferences for sleeping postures, the main objective for most sleep postures should be to find a neutral position or alignment while adjusting for the patient's anatomy. Starting with the cervical spine, it is important to consider the positioning of the pillow. Regardless of whether it is a supine, side-lying, or prone position, the head should remain in neutral rotation, with the nose in line with the sternum. In supine positioning, if the patient demonstrates a severe forward head, the clinician may need to accommodate for that with additional pillows but without creating excessive cervical flexion (Figure 76-21B). The end goal of pillow positioning in both supine and side-lying would be to provide enough support of the cervical spine to promote relaxation of cervical spine musculature. If the patient has an excessive lordotic curve in supine positioning, it may be necessary to place a few folded bedsheets under the lumbar spine to take up the space and provide adequate support. Another adjustment to this would be to place a pillow or two under the knees to decrease load on the

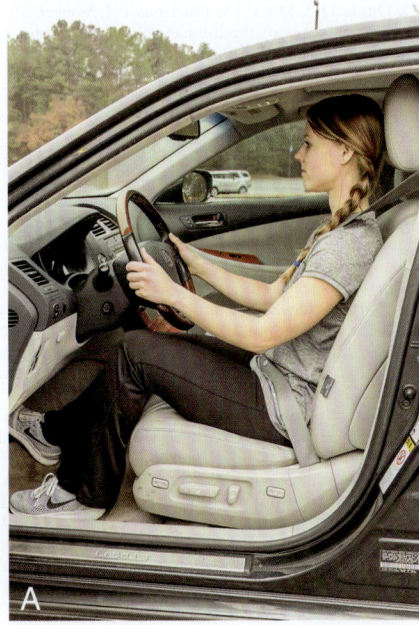
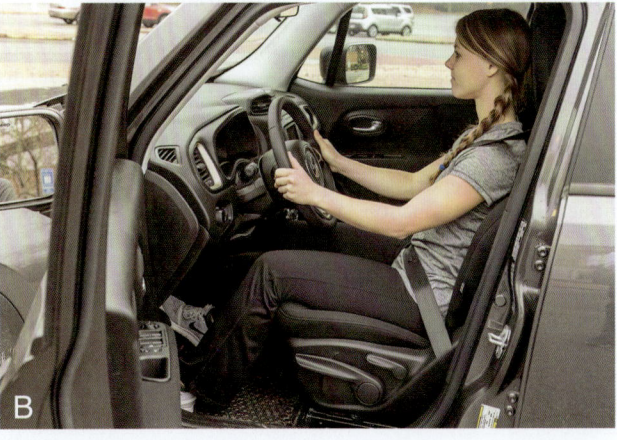

Figure 76-20. Driving posture showing the key joints considered while sitting in a vehicle. A, Sedan. B, Sport utility vehicle (SUV).

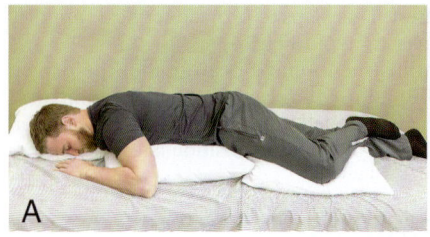 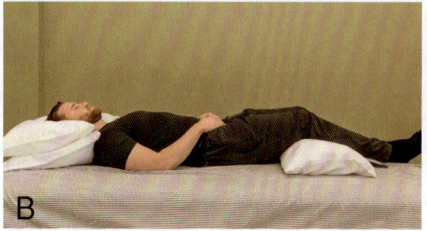 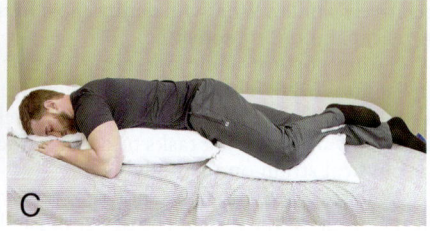

Figure 76-21. Recommended sleeping postures. A, Side-lying emphasizing a neutral spine. B, Supine. C, Prone with ¼ turn to decrease stress on cervical musculature.

lumbar spine. The firmness or softness of the mattress should also be taken into consideration.

In side-lying positioning, if the patient presents with slight side bending, it may again be necessary to place a few folded bedsheets under the lumbar spine to take up the space and provide adequate support. A pillow can be placed between the knees to promote a better positioning of the hips, as well as a pillow on the superior arm to provide support of the shoulder (Figure 76-21).

In prone positioning, it is important that the patient is placed in a relatively oblique position via pillow placements as seen in Figure 76-21C. The head should still be as neutral as possible even in this position, angling the head with the edge of the pillow. The superior leg should be flexed with a pillow underneath the knee for improved support. Modifications should be performed with the thought of decreasing strain on painful regions and placing muscles in a neutral resting position.

7. SUMMARY

Posture is very much like a map—it does not necessarily show any particular destination, but it shows the broad picture. However, without considering static or dynamic posture, treating myofascial pain is very much akin to journeying without any of the roads. Therefore, when a clinician chooses to disregard postural malalignments during the examination, then the examination must essentially be performed without any general direction of where to go. The argument can be made that viewing posture can skew or bias the clinician; however, it depends on the relative ability of the clinician to read the map. When assessing posture, the clinician is viewing a relatively still snapshot of an inherently dynamic system. Therefore, the clinician must consider the body as a whole functioning unit.

The clinician must ascertain if the patient's postural alignment is contributing to the medical history as gathered by the clinician or if the patient's postural adaptations are no longer functional and have the capacity to accept the forces of gravity and the patient's daily life stressors. With every postural assessment, the clinician should be looking at postural dysfunctions or poor adaptations that are currently contributing to the symptoms with which the patient is reporting and presenting.

As mentioned in the introduction of this chapter, posture is the summative visual reflection of how the body has adapted to gravity and external forces in a particular position. Posture may not conclude pain; rather, it maps it out for the clinician. It is up to the clinician to utilize clinical reasoning skills to interpret the map to plan a route to their intended destination. Then, the examination becomes like a well-planned journey, leading toward treatment or how to approach the next step.

References

1. Page P, Frank C, Lardner R. *Assessment and Treatment of Muscle Imbalance. The Janda Approach.* Champaign, IL: Human Kinetics; 2010 (pp. 65, 67, 70, chapter 22).
2. Kendall FP, McCreary EK. *Muscles: Testing and Function, with Posture and Pain.* 5th ed. Baltimore, MD: Lippincott Williams & Wilkins; 2005 (pp. 30-31, 65, 66-68).
3. Putz-Anderson V. *Cumulative Trauma Disorders: A Manual of Musculoskeletal Diseases of the Upper Limbs.* Bristol, PA: Taylor and Francis; 1988.
4. Jull GA, Janda V. Chapter 10, Muscles and motor control in low back pain: assessment and management. In: Twomey L, Taylor JR, eds. *Physical Therapy of the Low Back*. New York, NY: Churchill Livingstone; 1987:253-278.
5. Chaitow L, Bradley D, Gilbert C. The structure and function of breathing. In: Chaitow L, Bradley D, Gilbert CH, eds. *Recognizing and Treating Breathing Disorders: A Multidisciplinary Approach*. 2nd ed. London, England: Elsevier; 2014:23-43 (p. 30).
6. Sherrington C. Hughlings Jackson Lecture on quantitative management of contraction for "lowest-level" co-ordination. *Br Med J*. 1931;1(3657):207-211.
7. Kolar P. Examination of postural functions. In: Kolar P, Sulc J, Kyncl M, et al, eds. *Clinical Rehabilitation*. 1st ed. Praha 5: Alena Kobesova; 2013:36-59 (pp. 40, 42, 45, 69).
8. Kolar P, Kobesova A, Valouchova P, Bitnar P. Dynamic neuromuscular stabilization: developmental kinesiology breathing sterotypes and postural-locomotion function. In: Chaitow L, Bradley D, Gilbert CH, eds. *Recognizing and Treating Breathing Disorders: A Multidisciplinary Approach*. 2nd ed. London, England: Elsevier; 2014:11-22.
9. Kolar P, Sulc J, Kyncl M, et al. *Clinical Rehabilitation*. 1st ed. Praha 5: Alena Kobesova; 2013 (p. 37, 40).
10. Heino JG, Godges JJ, Carter CL. Relationship between hip extension range of motion and postural alignment. *J Orthop Sports Phys Ther*. 1990;12(6):243-247.
11. Walker ML, Rothstein JM, Finucane SD, Lamb RL. Relationships between lumbar lordosis, pelvic tilt, and abdominal muscle performance. *Phys Ther*. 1987;67(4):512-516.
12. Laird RA, Kent P, Keating JL. How consistent are lordosis, range of movement and lumbo-pelvic rhythm in people with and without back pain? *BMC Musculoskelet Disord*. 2016;17(1):403.
13. Laird RA, Gilbert J, Kent P, Keating JL. Comparing lumbo-pelvic kinematics in people with and without back pain: a systematic review and meta-analysis. *BMC Musculoskelet Disord*. 2014;15:229.
14. Nourbakhsh MR, Arab AM. Relationship between mechanical factors and incidence of low back pain. *J Orthop Sports Phys Ther*. 2002;32(9):447-460.
15. Fredericson M, Ho C, Waite B, et al. Magnetic resonance imaging abnormalities in the shoulder and wrist joints of asymptomatic elite athletes. *PM R*. 2009;1(2):107-116.
16. Boden SD, Davis DO, Dina TS, Patronas NJ, Wiesel SW. Abnormal magnetic-resonance scans of the lumbar spine in asymptomatic subjects. A prospective investigation. *J Bone Joint Surg Am*. 1990;72(3):403-408.
17. Brant-Zawadzki MN, Jensen MC, Obuchowski N, Ross JS, Modic MT. Interobserver and intraobserver variability in interpretation of lumbar disc abnormalities. A comparison of two nomenclatures. *Spine (Phila Pa 1976)*. 1995;20(11):1257-1263; discussion 1264.
18. Teresi LM, Lufkin RB, Reicher MA, et al. Asymptomatic degenerative disk disease and spondylosis of the cervical spine: MR imaging. *Radiology*. 1987;164(1):83-88.
19. Borenstein DG, O'Mara JW Jr, Boden SD, et al. The value of magnetic resonance imaging of the lumbar spine to predict low-back pain in asymptomatic subjects: a seven-year follow-up study. *J Bone Joint Surg Am*. 2001;83-A(9):1306-1311.
20. Hitselberger WE, Witten RM. Abnormal myelograms in asymptomatic patients. *J Neurosurg*. 1968;28(3):204-206.
21. Jensen MC, Brant-Zawadzki MN, Obuchowski N, Modic MT, Malkasian D, Ross JS. Magnetic resonance imaging of the lumbar spine in people without back pain. *N Engl J Med*. 1994;331(2):69-73.
22. De Smet AA, Nathan DH, Graf BK, Haaland BA, Fine JP. Clinical and MRI findings associated with false-positive knee MR diagnoses of medial meniscal tears. *AJR Am J Roentgenol*. 2008;191(1):93-99.
23. Wiesel SW, Tsourmas N, Feffer HL, Citrin CM, Patronas N. A study of computer-assisted tomography. I. The incidence of positive CAT scans in an asymptomatic group of patients. *Spine (Phila Pa 1976)*. 1984;9(6):549-551.
24. Sher JS, Uribe JW, Posada A, Murphy BJ, Zlatkin MB. Abnormal findings on magnetic resonance images of asymptomatic shoulders. *J Bone Joint Surg Am*. 1995;77(1):10-15.
25. Connor PM, Banks DM, Tyson AB, Coumas JS, D'Alessandro DF. Magnetic resonance imaging of the asymptomatic shoulder of overhead athletes: a 5-year follow-up study. *Am J Sports Med*. 2003;31(5):724-727.
26. Guten GN, Kohn HS, Zoltan DJ. 'False positive' MRI of the knee: a literature review study. *WMJ*. 2002;101(1):35-38.

27. Lewit K. *Manipulative Therapy in Rehabilitation of the Locomotor System*. 3rd ed. Oxford, England: Butterworth Heinemann; 1999 (pp. 2-10, 26-29).
28. Sahrmann S. *Diagnosis and Treatment of Movement Impairment Syndromes*. St. Louis, MO: Mosby; 2002 (pp. 42, 122, 139).
29. Gard SA, Miff SC, Kuo AD. Comparison of kinematic and kinetic methods for computing the vertical motion of the body center of mass during walking. *Hum Mov Sci*. 2004;22(6):597-610.
30. Magee DJ. *Orthopedic Physical Assessment*. 6th ed. St Louis, MO: Saunders Elsevier; 2014 (pp. 558-563, 1017-1020).
31. Le Huec JC, Saddiki R, Franke J, Rigal J, Aunoble S. Equilibrium of the human body and the gravity line: the basics. *Eur Spine J*. 2011;20 suppl 5:558-563.
32. Kisner C, Colby L. *Therapeutic Exercise: Foundations and Techniques*. 6th ed. Philadelphia, PA: FA Davis; 2012 (pp. 409-437).
33. Kobesova A, Kolar P. Developmental kinesiology: three levels of motor control in the assessment and treatment of the motor system. *J Bodyw Mov Ther*. 2014;18(1):23-33.
34. Kolar P. Facilitation of agonist antagonist coactivation by reflex stimulation methods. In: Liebenson C, ed. *Rehabilitation of the Spine*. 2nd ed. Philadelphia, PA: Lippincott Williams & Wilkins; 2007:203-225.
35. Kolar P, Kobesova A, Valouchova P, Bitnar P. Dynamic neuromuscular stabilization: assessment methods. In: Chaitow L, Bradley D, Gilbert CH, eds. *Recognizing and Treating Breathing Disorders: A Multidisciplinary Approach*. 2nd ed. London, England: Elsevier; 2014:93-98.
36. Sahrmann S. *Movement System Impairment Syndromes of the Extremities, Cervical and Thoracic Spines*. St Louis, MO: Elesevier; 2010 (pp. 104-105, 111).
37. Tardieu C, Tabary JC, Tardieu G, Tabary C. Adaptation of sarcomere numbers to the length imposed on muscle. In: Guba F, Marechal G, Takacs O, eds. *Mechanism of Muscle Adaptation to Functional Requirements*. Elmsford, NY: Pergamon Press; 1981:99-114.
38. Janda V, Frank C, Liebenson C. Evaluation of muscle imbalances. In: Liebenson C, ed. *Rehabilitation of the Spine*. 2nd ed. Philadelphia, PA: Lippincott Williams & Wilkins; 2007:203-225.
39. Vele F. *Kineziologie pro klinickou praxi*. Praha, Slovakia: Grada Publishing; 1997.
40. Kuchera M, Kuchera W. General postural considerations. In: Ward R, ed. *Foundations for Osteopathic Medicine*. Baltimore, MD: Williams and Wilkins; 1997.
41. Liebenson C, Brown J, Sermersheim NJ. Functional evaluation of faulty movement patterns. In: Liebenson C, ed. *Functional Training Handbook*. Hong Kong, China: Wolters Kluwer; 2014:59-92.
42. O'Sullivan K, O'Sullivan P, O'Sullivan L, Dankaerts W. What do physiotherapists consider to be the best sitting spinal posture? *Man Ther*. 2012;17(5):432-437.
43. Kobesova A, Valouchova P, Kolar P. Dynamic neuromuscular stabilization: exercises based on developmental kinesiology models. In: Liebenson C, ed. *Functional Training Handbook*. Hong Kong, China: Wolters Kluwer; 2014:25-52.
44. Janda V, Va'Vrova M, Herbenova A, Veverkova M. Sensory motor stimulation. In: Liebenson C, ed. *Rehabilitation of the Spine*. 2nd ed. Philadelphia, PA: Lippincott Williams & Wilkins; 2007:203-225.
45. Lewit K. *Manipulative Therapy in Rehabilitation of the Locomotor System*. 2nd ed. Oxford, England: Butterworth Heinemann; 1991.
46. Reinold MM, Wilk KE, Macrina LC, et al. Changes in shoulder and elbow passive range of motion after pitching in professional baseball players. *Am J Sports Med*. 2008;36(3):523-527.
47. Seftchick JL, Detullio LM, Fedorczyk JM, Aulicino PL. Clinical examination of the hand. In: Skirven TM, Osterman AL, Fedorczyk J, Amadio PC, eds. *Rehabilitation of the Hand and Upper Extremity: Expert Consult*. 6th ed. Philadelphia, PA: Mosby; 2011.
48. Silverthorn DU. *Human Physiology: An Integrated Approach*. 7th ed. San Francisco, CA: Pearson; 2016.
49. Soames RW, Atha J. The role of the antigravity musculature during quiet standing in man. *Eur J Appl Physiol Occup Physiol*. 1981;47(2):159-167.
50. McQuade KJ, Dawson J, Smidt GL. Scapulothoracic muscle fatigue associated with alterations in scapulohumeral rhythm kinematics during maximum resistive shoulder elevation. *J Orthop Sports Phys Ther*. 1998;28(2):74-80.
51. Lewit K. Managing common syndromes and finding the key link. In: Liebenson C, ed. *Rehabilitation of the Spine*. 2nd ed. Philadelphia, PA: Lippincott Williams & Wilkins; 2007:203-225.
52. Smith M, Sparkes V, Busse M, Enright S. Upper and lower trapezius muscle activity in subjects with subacromial impingement symptoms: is there imbalance and can taping change it? *Phys Ther Sport*. 2009;10(2):45-50.
53. Goodarzi F, Rahnama L, Karimi N, Baghi R, Jaberzadeh S. The effects of forward head posture on neck extensor muscle thickness: an ultrasonographic study. *J Manipulative Physiol Ther*. 2018;41(1):34-41.
54. Shin YJ, Kim WH, Kim SG. Correlations among visual analogue scale, neck disability index, shoulder joint range of motion, and muscle strength in young women with forward head posture. *J Exerc Rehabil*. 2017;13(4):413-417.
55. Kim MS, Cha YJ, Choi JD. Correlation between forward head posture, respiratory functions, and respiratory accessory muscles in young adults. *J Back Musculoskelet Rehabil*. 2017;30(4):711-715.
56. Ohmure H, Miyawaki S, Nagata J, Ikeda K, Yamasaki K, Al-Kalaly A. Influence of forward head posture on condylar position. *J Oral Rehabil*. 2008;35(11):795-800.
57. Olivo SA, Bravo J, Magee DJ, Thie NM, Major PW, Flores-Mir C. The association between head and cervical posture and temporomandibular disorders: a systematic review. *J Orofac Pain*. 2006;20(1):9-23.
58. Faulin EF, Guedes CG, Feltrin PP, Joffiley CM. Association between temporomandibular disorders and abnormal head postures. *Braz Oral Res*. 2015;29.
59. Cortese S, Mondello A, Galarza R, Biondi A. Postural alterations as a risk factor for temporomandibular disorders. *Acta Odontol Latinoam*. 2017;30(2):57-61.
60. Kim EK, Kim JS. Correlation between rounded shoulder posture, neck disability indices, and degree of forward head posture. *J Phys Ther Sci*. 2016;28(10):2929-2932.
61. Mingels S, Dankaerts W, van Etten L, Thijs H, Granitzer M. Comparative analysis of head-tilt and forward head position during laptop use between females with postural induced headache and healthy controls. *J Bodyw Mov Ther*. 2016;20(3):533-541.
62. Kim SY, Koo SJ. Effect of duration of smartphone use on muscle fatigue and pain caused by forward head posture in adults. *J Phys Ther Sci*. 2016;28(6):1669-1672.
63. Nejati P, Lotfian S, Moezy A, Nejati M. The study of correlation between forward head posture and neck pain in Iranian office workers. *Int J Occup Med Environ Health*. 2015;28(2):295-303.
64. Silva AM, de Siqueira GR, da Silva GA. Implications of high-heeled shoes on body posture of adolescents. *Rev Paul Pediatr*. 2013;31(2):265-271.
65. Mosaad DM, Abdel-Aziem AA. Backpack carriage effect on head posture and ground reaction forces in school children. *Work*. 2015;52(1):203-209.
66. De-la-Llave-Rincon AI, Fernandez-de-las-Penas C, Palacios-Cena D, Cleland JA. Increased forward head posture and restricted cervical range of motion in patients with carpal tunnel syndrome. *J Orthop Sports Phys Ther*. 2009;39(9):658-664.
67. Neiva PD, Kirkwood RN, Godinho R. Orientation and position of head posture, scapula and thoracic spine in mouth-breathing children. *Int J Pediatr Otorhinolaryngol*. 2009;73(2):227-236.
68. Ruivo RM, Pezarat-Correia P, Carita AI. Effects of a resistance and stretching training program on forward head and protracted shoulder posture in adolescents. *J Manipulative Physiol Ther*. 2017;40(1):1-10.
69. Lee DY, Nam CW, Sung YB, Kim K, Lee HY. Changes in rounded shoulder posture and forward head posture according to exercise methods. *J Phys Ther Sci*. 2017;29(10):1824-1827.
70. Lee SM, Lee CH, O'Sullivan D, Jung JH, Park JJ. Clinical effectiveness of a Pilates treatment for forward head posture. *J Phys Ther Sci*. 2016;28(7):2009-2013.
71. Cho J, Lee E, Lee S. Upper thoracic spine mobilization and mobility exercise versus upper cervical spine mobilization and stabilization exercise in individuals with forward head posture: a randomized clinical trial. *BMC Musculoskelet Disord*. 2017;18(1):525.
72. Kim BB, Lee JH, Jeong HJ, Cynn HS. Effects of suboccipital release with craniocervical flexion exercise on craniocervical alignment and extrinsic cervical muscle activity in subjects with forward head posture. *J Electromyogr Kinesiol*. 2016;30:31-37.
73. Kong YS, Kim YM, Shim JM. The effect of modified cervical exercise on smartphone users with forward head posture. *J Phys Ther Sci*. 2017;29(2):328-331.
74. McGill S, Grenier S, Bluhm M, Preuss R, Brown S, Russell C. Previous history of LBP with work loss is related to lingering deficits in biomechanical, physiological, personal, psychosocial and motor control characteristics. *Ergonomics*. 2003;46(7):731-746.
75. Kujala UM, Taimela S, Salminen JJ, Oksanen A. Baseline anthropometry, flexibility and strength characteristics and future low-back pain in adolescent athletes and nonathletes. A prospective, one-year follow-up study. *Scand J Med Sci Sports*. 1994;4:200-205.
76. Van Dillen LR, Sahrmann SA, Norton BJ, et al. Effect of active limb movements on symptoms in patients with low back pain. *J Orthop Sports Phys Ther*. 2001;31(8):402-413; discussion 414-408.
77. Van Dillen LR, Gombatto SP, Collins DR, Engsberg JR, Sahrmann SA. Symmetry of timing of hip and lumbopelvic rotation motion in 2 different subgroups of people with low back pain. *Arch Phys Med Rehabil*. 2007;88(3):351-360.
78. Ashmen KJ, Swanik CB, Lephart SM. Strength and flexibility characteristics of athletes with chronic low back pain. *J Sport Rehabil*. 1996;5(4):275-286.
79. Mellin G. Correlations of hip mobility with degree of back pain and lumbar spinal mobility in chronic low-back pain patients. *Spine (Phila Pa 1976)*. 1988;13(6):668-670.
80. Ranger TA, Teichtahl AJ, Cicuttini FM, et al. Shorter lumbar paraspinal fascia is associated with high intensity low back pain and disability. *Spine (Phila Pa 1976)*. 2016;41(8):E489-E493.
81. Malai S, Pichaiyongwongdee S, Sakulsriprasert P. Immediate effect of hold-relax stretching of iliopsoas muscle on transversus abdominis muscle activation in chronic non-specific low back pain with lumbar hyperlordosis. *J Med Assoc Thai*. 2015;98 suppl 5:S6-S11.
82. Lee DK, Oh JS. Relationship between hamstring length and gluteus maximus strength with and without normalization. *J Phys Ther Sci*. 2018;30(1):116-118.
83. Arab AM, Nourbakhsh MR, Mohammadifar A. The relationship between hamstring length and gluteal muscle strength in individuals with sacroiliac joint dysfunction. *J Man Manip Ther*. 2011;19(1):5-10.
84. van Wingerden JP, Vleeming A, Kleinrensink GJ, Stoeckart R. The role of the hamstring in pelvic and spinal function. In: Vleeming A, Mooney V, Dorman T, Snijders C, Stoeckart R, eds. *Movement Stability and Low Back Pain. The Essential Role of the Pelvis*. New York, NY: Churchill Livingstone; 1997:207-210.
85. Norris CM. Spinal stabilisation: 4. Muscle imbalance and the low back. *Physiotherapy*. 1995;81:127-138.
86. Hultman G, Saraste H, Ohlsen H. Anthropometry, spinal canal width, and flexibility of the spine and hamstring muscles in 45-55-year-old men with and without low back pain. *J Spinal Disord*. 1992;5(3):245-253.
87. Lankhorst GJ, Van de Stadt RJ, Van der Korst JK. The natural history of idiopathic low back pain. A three-year follow-up study of spinal motion, pain and functional capacity. *Scand J Rehabil Med*. 1985;17(1):1-4.
88. Youdas JW, Suman VJ, Garrett TR. Reliability of measurements of lumbar spine sagittal mobility obtained with the flexible curve. *J Orthop Sports Phys Ther*. 1995;21(1):13-20.

89. Levine D, Walker R, Tillman LJ. The effect of abdominal muscle strengthening on pelvic tilt and lumbar lordosis. *Physiother Theory Pract*. 1997;13(3):217-226.
90. Toppenberg RM, Bullock MI. The interrelation of spinal curves, pelvic tilt and muscle lengths in the adolescent female. *Aust J Physiother*. 1986;32(1):6-12.
91. Hemborg B, Moritz U. Intra-abdominal pressure and trunk muscle activity during lifting. II. Chronic low-back patients. *Scand J Rehabil Med*. 1985;17(1):5-13.
92. Lee JH, Ooi Y, Nakamura K. Measurement of muscle strength of the trunk and the lower extremities in subjects with history of low back pain. *Spine (Phila Pa 1976)*. 1995;20(18):1994-1996.
93. McNeill T, Warwick D, Andersson G, Schultz A. Trunk strengths in attempted flexion, extension, and lateral bending in healthy subjects and patients with low-back disorders. *Spine (Phila Pa 1976)*. 1980;5(6):529-538.
94. Nachemson A, Lindh M. Measurement of abdominal and back muscle strength with and without low back pain. *Scand J Rehabil Med*. 1969;1(2):60-63.
95. Liebenson C. *Rehabilitation of the Spine a Practitioner's Manual*. 2nd ed. Baltimore, MD: Lippincott Williams & Wilkins; 2007 (p. 784).
96. Hall J, Guyton A. *Guyton and Hall Textbook of Medical Physiology*. 12th ed. Philadelphia, PA: Saunders Elsevier; 2011.
97. Lewit K. Chain reactions in the locomotor system in the light of co-activation patterns based on developmental neurology. *J Orthop Med*. 1999;21(1):52-57.
98. Frank C, Kobesova A, Kolar P. Dynamic neuromuscular stabilization & sports rehabilitation. *Int J Sports Phys Ther*. 2013;8(1):62-73.
99. Cholewicki J, Juluru K, McGill SM. Intra-abdominal pressure mechanism for stabilizing the lumbar spine. *J Biomech*. 1999;32(1):13-17.
100. Cholewicki J, Juluru K, Radebold A, Panjabi MM, McGill SM. Lumbar spine stability can be augmented with an abdominal belt and/or increased intra-abdominal pressure. *Eur Spine J*. 1999;8(5):388-395.
101. Cresswell AG, Grundstrom H, Thorstensson A. Observations on intra-abdominal pressure and patterns of abdominal intra-muscular activity in man. *Acta Physiol Scand*. 1992;144(4):409-418.
102. Gardner-Morse MG, Stokes IA. The effects of abdominal muscle coactivation on lumbar spine stability. *Spine (Phila Pa 1976)*. 1998;23(1):86-91; discussion 91-82.
103. Hodges PW, Eriksson AE, Shirley D, Gandevia SC. Intra-abdominal pressure increases stiffness of the lumbar spine. *J Biomech*. 2005;38(9):1873-1880.
104. Hodges PW, Gandevia SC. Changes in intra-abdominal pressure during postural and respiratory activation of the human diaphragm. *J Appl Physiol (1985)*. 2000;89(3):967-976.
105. Shirley D, Hodges PW, Eriksson AE, Gandevia SC. Spinal stiffness changes throughout the respiratory cycle. *J Appl Physiol (1985)*. 2003;95(4):1467-1475.
106. Kolar P, Sulc J, Kyncl M, et al. Postural function of the diaphragm in persons with and without chronic low back pain. *J Orthop Sports Phys Ther*. 2012;42(4):352-362.
107. Kolnes LJ. Embodying the body in anorexia nervosa—a physiotherapeutic approach. *J Bodyw Mov Ther*. 2012;16(3):281-288.
108. Kolar P, Kobesova A, Valouchova P, Bitnar P. Dynamic neuromuscular stabilization: treatment methods. In: Chaitow L, Bradley D, Gilbert CH, eds. *Recognizing and Treating Breathing Disorders: A Multidisciplinary Approach*. 2nd ed. London, England: Elsevier; 2014:163-167.
109. Chaitow L. Osteopathic assessment of structural changes related to BPD. In: Chaitow L, Bradley D, Gilbert CH, eds. *Recognizing and Treating Breathing Disorders: A Multidisciplinary Approach*. 2nd ed. London, England: Elsevier; 2014:99-117.
110. Katzmarzyk PT, Church TS, Craig CL, Bouchard C. Sitting time and mortality from all causes, cardiovascular disease, and cancer. *Med Sci Sports Exerc*. 2009;41(5):998-1005.
111. van der Ploeg HP, Chey T, Korda RJ, Banks E, Bauman A. Sitting time and all-cause mortality risk in 222 497 Australian adults. *Arch Intern Med*. 2012;172(6):494-500.
112. Wilmot EG, Edwardson CL, Achana FA, et al. Sedentary time in adults and the association with diabetes, cardiovascular disease and death: systematic review and meta-analysis. *Diabetologia*. 2012;55(11):2895-2905.
113. NRC. *Musculoskeletal Disorders and the Workplace. Low Back and Upper Extremities*. Washington, DC: National Academy Press; 2001.
114. Hsu WH, Wang MJ. Physical discomfort among visual display terminal users in a semiconductor manufacturing company: a study of prevalence and relation to psychosocial and physical/ergonomic factors. *AIHA J (Fairfax, Va)*. 2003;64(2):276-282.
115. ANSI. Ergonomics-Manual handling-Part 1:Lifting and carrying. https://webstore.ansi.org/RecordDetail.aspx?sku=ISO+11228-1%3A2003&gclid=Cj0KCQjw7Z3VBRC-ARIsAEQifZQ4uMea-dGQhxIwOhOrNdHOSd7pGqpjYz-_pnY-oGHBTZU0lx8oErMaAv6EEALw_wcB. Accessed April 21, 2018.
116. Gaudez C, Cail F. Effects of mouse slant and desktop position on muscular and postural stresses, subject preference and performance in women aged 18-40 years. *Ergonomics*. 2016;59(11):1473-1486.
117. Simoneau GG, Marklin RW, Berman JE. Effect of computer keyboard slope on wrist position and forearm electromyography of typists without musculoskeletal disorders. *Phys Ther*. 2003;83(9):816-830.
118. Dennerlein JT, Johnson PW. Changes in upper extremity biomechanics across different mouse positions in a computer workstation. *Ergonomics*. 2006;49(14):1456-1469.
119. Van Eerd D, Munhall C, Irvin E, et al. Effectiveness of workplace interventions in the prevention of upper extremity musculoskeletal disorders and symptoms: an update of the evidence. *Occup Environ Med*. 2016;73(1):62-70.
120. Air Bags. National Highway Traffic Safety Administration. https://www.nhtsa.gov/equipment/air-bags. Accessed May 4, 2018.
121. Bradley D. Physiotherapy in rehabilitation of breathing disorders. In: Chaitow L, Bradley D, Gilbert CH, eds. *Recognizing and Treating Breathing Disorders: A Multidisciplinary Approach*. 2nd ed. London, England: Elsevier; 2014:185-196.

Chapter 77

Footwear Considerations

Deborah M. Wendland

1. INTRODUCTION

Footwear is a possible contributor to the overload of muscles of the lower extremity and can be a possible treatment for trigger points (TrPs) (Chapters 64, 65, 66, and 71). Footwear, along with foot orthotic devices and taping, should be assessed and addressed in patients with myofascial pain. Specifically, footwear is paramount for muscles around the ankle (eg, fibularis longus and brevis, tibialis posterior, soleus, and gastrocnemius) and in the foot. The recruitment and function of these muscles should be examined in light of their environment (ie, shoes, foot orthotic devices, and taping).

Trigger points have been associated with changes in muscle activity and recruitment patterns.[1-3] Pain itself can result in and from a change in movement patterns. When increased loading of a muscle occurs in the presence of TrPs, the movement pattern is uncoordinated and inconsistent.[4] Moreover, postural habits can also perpetuate pain.[5] As a case in point, gastrocnemius and soleus TrPs may cause calf, Achilles tendon, and heel pain along with decreased ankle range of motion (ROM).[6,7] Given these impairments, it is not surprising that function can be affected.[7] Addressing the TrPs improves ankle ROM[6] and function.[7] Changes can occur in the presence of TrPs and also be mitigated by the treatment of TrPs. Likewise, these changes may be improved, supported, or maintained by utilizing footwear, foot orthotic devices, and/or taping.

Certain foot postures, gait biomechanics, and even fatigue, all modifiable by footwear, can contribute to the development of TrPs and/or changes in muscle recruitment patterns.[8,9] Common foot types include pes planus (flat foot) and pes cavus (high-arched foot). These foot types are linked to the height of the medial longitudinal arch (MLA) and are associated with common physical (including gait) or injury presentations.

Pes planus is linked to a low MLA and exhibits an increased flexibility of the foot. Injuries typically associated with pes planus are those responding to increased or abnormal joint movement or muscle overuse. Specifically, excessive or abnormal pronation is a common movement pattern seen in people with pes planus. This movement pattern is associated with the altered function of the tibialis posterior and fibularis longus muscles.[10] Alterations in the function of the flexor digitorum longus and the flexor hallucis longus muscles should also be considered, given their role in the support of the longitudinal arch of the foot.[11] Associated problems may include muscle overuse or dysfunction (eg, tibialis posterior), proximal joint pain, plantar fasciitis, and foot/toe limitations or deformities.[12] Footwear, foot orthotic device selection, or taping can be useful in mitigating these associated complications.[12-17]

Pes cavus, on the other hand, is associated with a high MLA and tends to result in a foot with a stiffer structure.[18] Injuries associated with pes cavus are those that relate to the foot's inability to absorb shock or distribute load.[18,19] People with this foot type have a tendency to lack sufficient pronation, which helps to absorb ground reaction forces. These changes in foot mechanics are linked to changes in the muscle activation patterns during gait, contributing to muscle overuse, which can contribute to or perpetuate TrPs. Fortunately, the selection of footwear or the use of foot orthotic devices can be influential to minimize dysfunctions associated with cavus-related movement and muscle activation patterns.[19]

Fatigue must also be considered as a contributor for TrPs (Chapter 66). As a possible contributor, it is important to assess causes of fatigue that are modifiable. Modifiable factors like energy shielding techniques may include shoe selection and/or the use of foot orthoses. An increased metabolic cost has been associated with the increased muscle activity associated with high-heeled walking.[20] But Curran et al reported that when wearing high heels with foot orthoses, heart rate and energy consumption were both lowered.[21] These results demonstrate that footwear and its modification can affect metabolic cost. Understanding why metabolic cost is affected (eg, changing walking speed or heel height) can facilitate the ability to minimize a metabolic cost increase, especially when treating TrPs.

2. PHYSICAL STRESS

The Physical Stress Theory[22] was designed to guide practice and the selection of appropriate treatment interventions. At its core, the critical principle is that biologic tissue responds to stress in a predictable way.[22] With this insight, clinicians can modify stresses to improve tissue healing and then develop a program that progressively reloads tissue to improve stress tolerance.[22] To achieve this design, the clinician must recognize the origins of stress and how it may be affecting tissue loading responses and healing.

With injury and inflammation, tissue needs to be off-loaded to allow healing to occur.[22] Similarly, in the case of TrPs, muscle needs to be supported or off-loaded in a way that facilitates healing and the removal of conditions that may be contributing to the activation and perpetuation of the TrPs. Muscle activation changes with gait and can be altered by shoe type, foot orthotic device, or taping. Moreover, muscles are recruited differently depending on posture. Given the influence of posture and activity on muscle recruitment and function, clinicians should recognize that both posture and movement patterns can be modified by adjusting footwear selection and fit, including the use of foot orthotic devices or taping within footwear.

First, prior to modifying foot position or movement, stressors to biologic tissue should be assessed. Postures maintained over time can cause overuse of some muscle groups and underuse of others. With muscle imbalance, some muscles can become shortened and other muscles may become lengthened. As such, it is crucial to assess posture (see Chapter 76) so that muscle balance can be addressed. Furthermore, it is also important to assess how an individual moves to determine muscle balance in practice. Together, posture and gait assessment facilitate the understanding of muscle loading factors that contribute to the body's healing or lack thereof.[22]

Once stressors are determined, the clinician needs to consider how tissue can be off-loaded to allow for healing. Because stress results from movement or position, it is vital to learn and design various ways to minimize these abnormal or repetitive loads to tissues. Altered loading can occur with exercise, a modification in footwear design or fit, the use of foot orthotic devices, or taping. In the presence of injury, regardless of its origin, the tissue will be less responsive to stress and will therefore require off-loading to facilitate healing.[22]

Once tissue has healed, reloading needs to occur so the weakened tissue can return to its previous functional level and better tolerate stress.[22] This reloading can facilitate the balancing of muscles in a way that allows for improved patterns of motion and decreased continued stress (overuse) of muscle and other tissues. Reloading can occur by changing the fit of the shoe or by modifying the shoe itself; foot orthotic devices or taping can also facilitate reloading of the muscle tissue.

3. FOOTWEAR

Footwear is one means by which feet can be supported and the biomechanics of gait can be altered. Of primary concern with using footwear to address the mechanics of motion is shoe fit. Beyond shoe fit, shoe construction can impact foot posture and gait mechanics through the density of material, the positioning of material thickness, shoe design (eg, boot vs. low top; heel height), and even the mechanism of shoe closure (eg, lacing or straps). Together, shoe fit and construction should be selected based on the patient presentation as well as the patient response to the selected intervention.

Shoe fit is among the most critical components of footwear selection. With an inappropriate fit, a seemingly appropriate shoe selection will prove ineffective in accomplishing the intended task. In fact, a poorly fitting shoe may even cause blister or callus formation, an increased risk for falls,[23] and a change in movement patterns, including overrecruitment of muscles (eg, toe flexors to aid in keeping a shoe on). With well-fitted footwear, gait speed may increase along with the confidence of the wearer.[23]

Rarely are adults measured for footwear anymore. Even with measurement using a Brannock device, shoe size is dependent on the last around which the shoe is built. Thus, even with measurement, it is important that a shoe is actually assessed for fit. It is especially critical that shoe fit is assessed with whatever modifications may be made to footwear or with the inclusion of a foot orthotic device if one is to be used.

Proper Shoe Fitting

A major challenge to shoe fit assessment is that the shoe, a static object, needs to accommodate the foot, a dynamic tissue, that varies in size and shape as it moves, bears weight, and changes temperature.[24] Although shoe fit may be based on 15 or more individual assessments,[24] these assessments can be narrowed to a simple mnemonic to assist the fitting process. Figure 77-1 identifies the parts of a shoe to facilitate the assessment of shoe fit. To assess shoe fit, one should remember his or her **ABCS** (Box 77-1).

The upper part of the shoe (vamp) should be able to be pinched in a way that there is material that can be grasped, showing that room in the area of the toes and forefoot is sufficient (Figure 77-2). If the shoe is too snug, material will not be able to be grasped and lifted. Care should be taken to identify that even the lesser toes are not being pinched.[24] Some shoes come in various widths (A, B, C, etc.) but may also come in "extra wide." These distinctions are footwear brand specific. Similarly, shoes come in extra-depth sizes as well. Extra-depth shoes may be selected to accommodate for a foot deformity or a foot orthotic device if the removal of the shoe's insole is not enough. Finally, as size is assessed, it is important to identify that the heel fit is appropriate[24] and movement at the heel is minimal.

Shoe Design

Although fit is critical, it is also important to recognize that the actual design of a shoe will affect the mechanics of the body. Shoes come in various styles that can affect foot and gait biomechanics differently. By managing these biomechanics, movement patterns and muscle recruitment may be altered. This alteration in muscle recruitment and movement patterns may serve to off-load specific muscles, thus facilitating healing and appropriate loading and preventing the formation or perpetuation of TrPs. Footwear can be used to control motion or shift loading such that the gait pattern is affected. Furthermore, certain shoe style aspects, such as the high heel, are commonly worn and can have major ramifications on biomechanics.

One shoe purpose is control of motion. Motion can be controlled in footwear by a number of mechanisms. Many athletic shoes, for instance, are termed "motion control" because the medial midsole is thicker (rearfoot post or wedge) or more dense[13,14] compared to the lateral midsole. With the thicker or stiffer material in the location that has excessive motion, motion in that direction is restricted.[14,25] The heel counter can also be used as a means to control motion. The longer the heel counter, the more motion is controlled. Motion can be selectively controlled by having one side of the counter longer than the other. Motion toward the side of the longer counter will be more limited. The addition of a stabilizer at the back of the shoe can also lead to increased motion control. Likewise, a low heel can be lengthened either medially (Thomas heel) or laterally (reverse Thomas heel) to mitigate excessive motion medially or laterally, respectively.

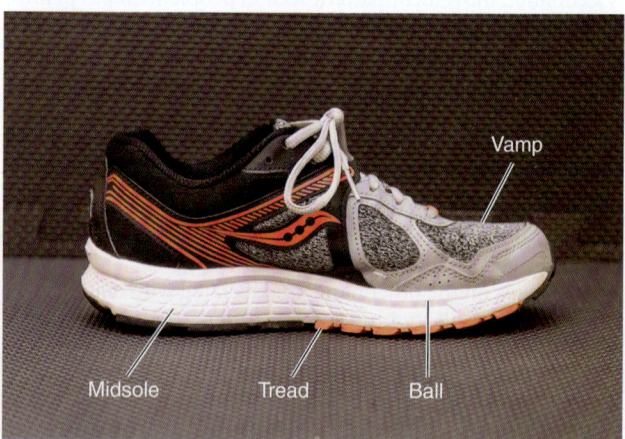

Figure 77-1. Important parts of the shoe to be considered by the clinician.

> **Box 77-1** Mnemonic for proper shoe fit: ABCS
>
> **A, Arch**
> The arch location and size are critical for shoe fit. The arch should be sized such that it snugly contacts the foot.[24] The arch of the shoe should be located at the same position as the arch of the foot and should be consistent in length.
>
> **B, Ball**
> The ball of the foot should be situated in the same spot as the widest part of the shoe. That is, the length from the heel to the ball of the foot should be equal to that from the heel to the "ball" of the shoe. This must be the case on both the medial and lateral sides of the shoe to allow for accurate bending of the shoe. Similarly, the ball should be appropriately placed from the end of the shoe such that the toe to ball lengths match.[24] The width of the shoe, including its tread, should also correspond to the width of the foot.
>
> **C, Cut**
> The shoe must be an appropriate cut such that the trim lines of the shoe or even the stitching does not impinge on the foot or apply undo pressures to any spot.[24] Special attention needs to be given to areas of bony landmarks such as the malleoli, navicular bone, or toes. The cut should also be such that gapping is not seen between the shoe and the foot. Rather, the foot should have sufficient space to move without allowing excessive shear movement.
>
> **S, Size**
> The size of the shoe, assessed in standing, includes the length, the width, and the depth. The length of the shoe should allow 1/2" to 5/8" beyond the longest toe,[24] which in many cases is the second toe. The width of the shoe can be assessed along with its depth using a simple standing test.

Shoe Modifications

Modifications can be made to the shoe itself to increase stability. Shoe modifications, including a flange or flare (material added to the sole of the shoe to make it wider and more stable) or stabilizer (material added to the side of the shoe), will limit motion toward the side on which the modification is placed.[12] Modifications that can be added to footwear are consistent with modifications that can be made to foot orthotic devices as well.

The literature reports shoes as being able to reduce rearfoot motion when comparing motion control shoes to neutral shoes[13,14] or cushion shoes,[25] whether the individual was fatigued or not.[13] Additionally, Lilley et al found that motion control shoes also limited medial rotation at the knee.[14] Furthermore, motion control shoes have been shown to reduce instantaneous loading rate, especially in those with a lower arch.[25] Despite Butler et al's findings that instantaneous loading rate was affected by arch height, they suggested that the choice of footwear should be matched to the foot mechanics rather than to the posture in which the foot presents.[25] With these opportunities for control of motion, it becomes apparent that footwear could decrease muscle activity in muscles that try to control motion in these ways (eg, tibialis posterior and fibularis muscles). It is important to note that when motion control is not needed, a motion control shoe should not be worn. Rather, a neutral shoe should be selected (eg, for people with pes cavus).[19]

The sole or tread of a shoe may affect gait mechanics. Appropriate flexibility of the shoe sole can decrease the overload to the plantar flexor muscles (Chapters 65 and 66). Likewise, a rocker bottom may affect the gait mechanics of an individual.[26] Depending on where the apex of the rocker lies, a rocker is typically used to off-load different areas of the forefoot.[26] A rocker bottom helps to return motion that was otherwise taken away, but may also result in reduced electromyography activity at the tibialis anterior muscle while producing increased gastrocnemius muscle activity.[26] Using a rocker bottom can result in kinematic changes at both the ankle and the hip.[26] These kinematic changes must be acknowledged so that shoe choices are appropriately made and total biomechanical changes are monitored.

The intensity of a modification affects the variability of the biomechanical response with gait. Thies et al reported that the degree of the rocker bottom has an effect on outcome. Specifically, toe clearance was better with 10° and 15° rockers, but with a further increase of the rocker to 20°, a decrease in gait speed was noted when walking on a decline.[27] Step variability, on the other hand, did not appear to be significantly affected by varying the degree of the rocker bottom.[27] Thus, the degree to which footwear is modified can affect the gait pattern and likely the muscle activity. Gait should be assessed on an individual basis to determine the individual response to the footwear.

Heel height is another footwear variable that should be considered when assessing how to modify the forces applied to tissue or the loading of muscle. With consideration of lower extremity posture alone, it is easy to see that wearing higher heels results in the shifting of body weight from the whole foot toward the forefoot. However, because an individual wants to be able to perceive his or her environment, he or she makes further modifications to his or her posture to enable the head to remain forward-looking. These postural changes, along with increased pressure born at the forefoot, should be considered because gait mechanics may also change in response to discomfort felt in the forefoot or further up the kinetic chain. The frequency of wearing this kind of shoe and possible impact of any pain report must also be considered.

A number of specific changes to muscle activity have been reported with heeled walking. Murley et al report that as heel height increases, muscle activity increases at the erector spinae,

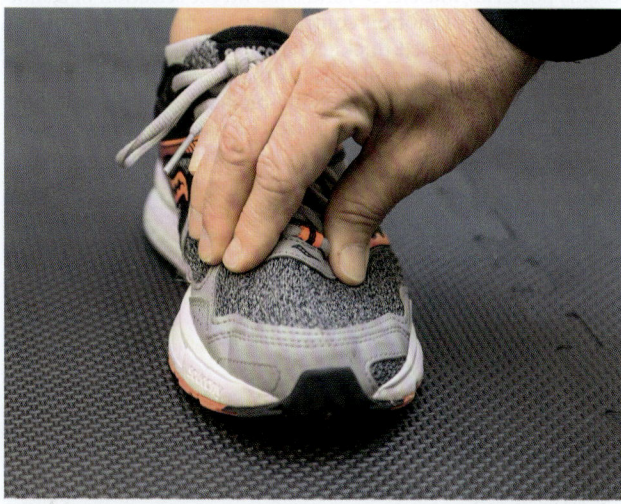

Figure 77-2. Assessment of vamp fit by grasping material to ensure adequate space. One should be able to grasp a small amount of material at the forefoot location.

rectus femoris, soleus, and fibularis longus muscles and decreases at both the medial gastrocnemius and tibialis anterior muscles.[28] Other investigators found an increase in peak amplitude with heeled walking versus barefoot walking in the tibialis anterior, soleus, vastus lateralis, rectus femoris, biceps femoris, and semimembranosus muscles.[20] The presence of variability between studies (eg, tibialis anterior) makes it important to explicitly assess the response of each individual to footwear or other foot interventions.

Like with a rocker shoe, the actual height (intensity) of the heel must also be considered. Stefanyshyn et al reported that muscle activation changes with the changing kinematics and kinetics of gait according to height of the heel.[29] Specifically, they reported increased activity in the soleus and rectus femoris muscles with increasing heel height. However, they did not find a graded increase in the hamstrings, vastus medialis, tibialis anterior, or gastrocnemius muscles with increasing heel height.[29] It is thus important to recognize that loading of the tissues can be modified by changing the height of the heel, even without eliminating the heel entirely.[29] Similarly, unlike high-heeled shoes, negative heeled shoes were shown to have increased muscle activity in the lateral hamstring, tibialis anterior, and lateral gastrocnemius muscles.[30] Moreover, the frequency with which a particular heel height is worn will also affect muscular activity response.[28]

Another component of the shoe construction itself, the closure mechanism (eg, lacing), affects the fit of the shoe. Associated with this component is the type of shoe, including its height (boot vs. low-top shoe). Shoe fit has been shown to affect gait mechanics.[31] Slippage of the foot within a shoe can contribute to muscle overload (see Chapter 66). The weight of a shoe or boot can also affect the muscle activation pattern. The heavier the shoe, the higher the muscle activity level (see Chapter 68).[32] Again, the gait mechanics and slippage must be assessed on a case-by-case basis.

Orthotic Devices

The use of foot orthotic devices is another method by which muscle loads or activity can be diminished and healing supported. Foot orthoses come in many varieties and can be customized by selection of material density and material thickness, including placement of thickness (posting or padding). As with footwear, higher density material and posting will tend to restrict motion.[12] Padding, on the other hand, may serve as a means to off-load particular areas (metatarsal pads).[12]

Specific foot orthotic devices can be considered as an approach to manage certain musculoskeletal conditions. In general, overpronation can be managed with medial posting at the forefoot, rearfoot, or both.[12,15] Like with the stabilizing shoe modifications to the medial side, medial posting will limit motion in the direction of the posting. More motion control is obtained when rearfoot posting is used, either alone or in combination.[15] Likewise, a foot orthotic device with a lateral bar has been shown to decrease the muscle activity of the fibularis longus muscle.[33] Again, lateral posting will limit motion in a way similar to modifications on the lateral side of the shoe.

Use of specific paddings or foot orthotic modifiers can be helpful for certain patient presentations.[12] Usage of a foot orthotic device has also been reported to change the activity of the plantar flexor muscles.[34,35] Specifically, Achilles tendon dysfunction can be off-loaded with the use of a heel lift.[12] A heel lift resulted in decreased activity in the gastrocnemius muscle across sexes[34,35] but resulted in variable effects on the activity of the tibialis anterior muscle.[34,35] Metatarsal pads, bars, or similar mechanisms of off-loading have been used to treat metatarsalgia, neuromas, sesamoiditis, and the like.[12,36] Decreasing pain complaints can alter gait mechanics and thus muscle activity. When semi-custom and custom foot orthotic devices in individuals with different arch heights were compared, it was reported that the semi-custom device was a suitable alternative to the custom device.[37] When changes are made using a foot orthotic device, it should be noted that the response is variable by individual and should therefore be individually assessed.[38]

Taping

Taping is one more method by which the load on a muscle or muscles can be modified to support healing as well as reloading. Taping has been shown to alter the activity of muscles in the leg in the case of people with low MLA or flat-arched feet.[16,17] Specifically, antipronation type of taping such as a low-Dye technique has been shown to decrease the maximal activity at the tibialis anterior and tibialis posterior muscles.[16,17] The fibularis longus muscle had variable results.[16,17] Similar results were seen for ankle bracing as well.[17] With this support for neuromuscular change with mechanical support to the foot, it should be considered that the use of such a technique could be helpful to reduce excessive forces experienced in the feet and assist in determining a more permanent solution (eg, foot orthotic device) to force management.

4. COMMON FOOT PRESENTATIONS

Pronatory Foot Type

In the case of an individual with a pronatory foot (Box 77-2), foot position and movement patterns could be contributory to TrPs or in response to TrPs. Several means can be used to mitigate the excess amounts of load placed on the muscles that are attempting to control the excessive motion, including the tibialis posterior muscle. Beyond shoe fit, the selection of a shoe with some type of motion control may be utilized (eg, medial midsole with increased thickness compared to the lateral midsole, increased material density to the medial shoe, increased bulk of the heel counter, especially medially, and the addition of some version of a heel stabilizer or flare). Beyond motion control, a good means to control excessive motion is the use of a foot orthotic device that may control excessive pronation

---

Box 77-2 Strategies for abnormal pronatory foot

Shoe[12]	Foot Orthotic Device	Taping
■ Midsole thicker medially ■ Midsole density higher medially ■ Counter longer medially ■ Medial flange or flare ■ Medial stabilizer ■ Thomas heel	■ Medial wedge (rearfoot or forefoot or both)[15] ■ Higher medial density or hardness[12]	■ Augmented low-Dye taping[16,17,39] ■ Antipronation taping[40] ■ Kinesiotaping does not correct pronation compared to sham[41]

Chapter 77: Footwear Considerations

Box 77-3 Strategies for abnormal supinatory foot

Shoe	Foot Orthotic Device	Taping
■ Neutral shoe[19] ■ Cushioned[12,19] ■ Counter longer laterally[12] ■ Lateral flange or flare[12] ■ Reverse Thomas heel[12]	■ Cushion/accommodative[12,19] ■ Lower medial density or hardness[12] ■ Lateral bar[33]	■ Heel lock or calcaneal eversion

insole are most appropriate. Motion control footwear should be avoided and a neutral shoe should be selected.[19] In severe cases, footwear with a lateral flange or longer lateral counter may be necessary to facilitate movement in the direction of pronation for a more efficient gait pattern. Additionally, a reverse Thomas heel could be an effective means to control excessive supinatory motion. A foot orthosis with a lateral bar could serve as a means to decrease activity at the fibularis longus.[33]

Although the pronatory and supinatory foot are among the most common foot types that are associated with specific muscle activation patterns, muscle activation associated with gait is variable. With such variability, it is important to assess each individual's gait along with his or her response to any adjustments made with his or her footwear, foot orthotic device, or taping. Certain adjustment can be expected to affect muscle activation in certain ways (Box 77-4).

by several different mechanisms including increased density or thickness on the medial side (medial posting). Depending on foot structure, the increase in thickness medially (medial post) could occur at the forefoot, the rearfoot, or both. As a more temporary control of excessive motion into pronation, taping or bracing can be utilized.[16,17,39] These more temporary means of controlling excessive motion may serve as a trial basis for a more permanent solution to control motion (eg, foot orthotic device or footwear modification).

Supinatory Foot Type

For people with a more supinatory or high-arched foot (Box 77-3), the natural tendency is to have decreased motion and a stiffer foot. With a stiffer foot, typically a more cushioned shoe and

5. SUMMARY

The impact of footwear, foot orthotic devices, and taping should be considered when assessing contributors and perpetuators of TrPs. Any of these factors can contribute to muscle activation dysfunction. Similarly, footwear, foot orthotic devices, and/or taping or their simple modification can also support the remediation of TrPs and promote improved muscle function.

Certain foot postures are both common and amenable to modification through the use of footwear, foot orthotic devices, and taping. Specifically, pes planus, which may influence the mechanical loading of the tibialis posterior, fibularis longus, flexor digitorum longus, and flexor hallucis longus muscles, can be supported through motion control. Motion control footwear, for example, can use an extended counter, medial posting, wider

Box 77-4 Considerations for loading and off-loading different muscles using footwear, foot orthotic devices, or taping strategies

Muscle	Shoes	Foot Orthotic Device (FO)	Taping Strategy
Tibialis anterior	■ Rocker: Decrease activation[26] ■ High heel: Decrease activation[28] or increase activation[20] ■ Negative heel: Increase activation[28]	■ FO: Decreased peak amplitude and activity[33] ■ FO with medial rearfoot wedge: Increased activation similar to that measured with shoe (responses variable)[38]	■ Antipronation (eg, low-Dye taping): Decrease max activation[16,17]
Fibularis longus	■ High heel: Increase activation[28] ■ Unstable shoe: Increase activation[42]	■ FO with lateral bar: Decreased peak amplitude and activity[33]	■ Antipronation (eg, low-Dye taping): Variable response of muscle activation[16,17] ■ Kinesio taping: No effect on muscle activation[43]
Gastrocnemius	■ High heel: Decrease activation[28] ■ Negative heel: Increase activation[28]	■ Heel lift: Decrease activation[34,35]	■ Kinesio taping: Shorten lateral gastroc activity during gait (healthy) but does not decrease activity amplitude[44]
Lateral hamstring	■ High heel: Increase activation[20] ■ Negative heel: Increase activation[28]		
Tibialis posterior	■ Motion control shoe: Control rearfoot motion in those who overpronate[20]	■ FO with medial wedge (custom and prefabricated): Decreased peak amplitude[45]	■ Antipronation (eg, low-Dye taping): Decrease max activation[36,37]
Soleus	■ High heel: Increase activation[20,28] ■ Increasing height of heel: Increase activation[29]		

base (medial flare), or the optimization of material density to accomplish the increased control of excessive pronation. Foot orthotic devices can similarly use medial posting to limit excessive motion.

Pes cavus, another common foot posture, can be addressed with footwear or foot orthotic devices that provide cushioning to absorb pressure. Furthermore, lateral control within footwear (lateral posting or lateral flare) or foot orthotic devices (lateral posting) can facilitate movement into normal pronation. Together, these work to address this more rigid foot type.

Other modifications can be applied to footwear or foot orthotic devices, such as a metatarsal pad, to off-load the metatarsal heads or the sesamoid bones. A heel lift can be used to off-load the Achilles tendon and the plantar flexor muscles. Additionally, taping techniques can be very useful to determine what more permanent solution may be effective in managing movement challenges of the lower extremity. All of these work as the means by which the clinician can facilitate both off-loading and reloading tissue so that healing can occur (Physical Stress Theory).

References

1. Lucas KR, Polus BI, Rich PA. Latent myofascial trigger points: their effects on muscle activation and movement efficiency. *J Bodyw Mov Ther.* 2004;8(3):160-166. doi:10.1016/j.jbmt.2003.12.002.
2. Ge H-Y, Monterde S, Graven-Nielsen T, Arendt-Nielsen L. Latent myofascial trigger points are associated with an increased intramuscular electromyographic activity during synergistic muscle activation. *J Pain.* 2014;15(2):181-187. doi:10.1016/j.jpain.2013.10.009.
3. Bohlooli N, Ahmadi A, Maroufi N, Sarrafzadeh J, Jaberzadeh S. Differential activation of scapular muscles, during arm elevation, with and without trigger points. *J Bodyw Mov Ther.* 2016;20(1):26-34. doi:10.1016/j.jbmt.2015.02.004.
4. Lucas KR, Rich PA, Polus BI. Muscle activation patterns in the scapular positioning muscles during loaded scapular plane elevation: the effects of latent myofascial trigger points. *Clin Biomech.* 2010;25(8):765-770. doi:10.1016/j.clinbiomech.2010.05.006.
5. Edwards J. The importance of postural habits in perpetuating myofascial trigger point pain. *Acupunct Med.* 2005;23(2):77-82.
6. Grieve R, Clark J, Pearson E, Bullock S, Boyer C, Jarrett A. The immediate effect of soleus trigger point pressure release on restricted ankle joint dorsiflexion: a pilot randomised controlled trial. *J Bodyw Mov Ther.* 2011;15:42-49.
7. Grieve R, Barnett S, Coghill N, Cramp F. Myofascial trigger point therapy for triceps surae dysfunction: a case series. *Man Ther.* 2013;18:519-525.
8. Gefen A. Biomechanical analysis of fatigue-related foot injury mechanisms in athletes and recruits during intensive marching. *Med Biol Eng Comput.* 2002;40(3):302-310.
9. Zuil-Escobar JC, Martinez-Cepa CB, Martin-Urrialde JA, Gomez-Conesa A. Prevalence of myofascial trigger points and diagnostic criteria of different muscles in function of the medial longitudinal arch. *Arch Phys Med Rehabil.* 2015;96:1123-1130.
10. Kokubo T, Hashimoto T, Nagura T, et al. Effect of the posterior tibial and peroneal longus on the mechanical properties of the foot arch. *Foot Ankle Int.* 2012;33(4):320-325. doi:10.3113/FAI.2012.0320.
11. Jacob HA. Forces acting in the forefoot during normal gait—an estimate. *Clin Biomech.* 2001;16(9):783-792. doi:10.1016/S0268-0033(01)00070-5.
12. Janisse D, Hultquist N. *Introduction to Pedorthics.* Columbia, MD: Pedorthic Footwear Association; 1998.
13. Cheung RT, Ng GY. Efficacy of motion control shoes for reducing excessive rearfoot motion in fatigued runners. *Phys Ther Sport.* 2007;8(2):75-81.
14. Lilley K, Stiles V, Dixon S. The influence of motion control shoes on the running gait of mature and young females. *Gait Posture.* 2013;37:331-335.
15. Johanson MA, Donatelli R, Wooden MJ, Andrew PD, Cummings GS. Effects of three different posting methods on controlling abnormal subtalar pronation. *Phys Ther.* 1994;74(2):149-158. doi:10.1093/ptj/74.2.149.
16. Franettovich M, Chapman A, Vicenzino B. Tape that increases medial longitudinal arch height also reduces leg muscle activity: a preliminary study. *Med Sci Sports Exerc.* 2008;40(4):593-600. doi:10.1249/MSS.0b013e318162134f.
17. Franettovich MM, Murley GS, David BS, Bird AR. A comparison of augmented low-Dye taping and ankle bracing on lower limb muscle activity during walking in adults with flat-arched foot posture. *J Sci Med Sport.* 2012;15(1):8-13. doi:10.1016/j.jsams.2011.05.009.
18. Burns J, Crosbie J, Hunt A, Ouvrier R. The effect of pes cavus on foot pain and plantar pressure. *Clin Biomech.* 2005;20(9):877-882. doi:10.1016/j.clinbiomech.2005.03.006.
19. Manoli A, Graham B. The subtle cavus foot, "the Underpronator," a review. *Foot Ankle Int.* 2005;26(3):256-263. doi:10.1177/107110070502600313.
20. Simonsen EB, Svendsen MB, Nørreslet A, et al. Walking on high heels changes muscle activity and the dynamics of human walking significantly. *J Appl Biomech.* 2012;28(1):20-28.
21. Curran SA, Holliday JL, Watkeys L. Influence of high heeled footwear and pre-fabricated foot orthoses on energy efficiency in ambulation. *Podiatry Rev.* 2010;67(3):16-22.
22. Mueller MJ, Maluf KS. Tissue adaptation to physical stress: a proposed "Physical Stress Theory" to guide physical therapist practice, education, and research. *Phys Ther.* 2002;82(4):383-403.
23. Davis AM, Galna B, Murphy AT, Williams CM, Haines TP. Effect of footwear on minimum foot clearance, heel slippage and spatiotemporal measures of gait in older women. *Gait Posture.* 2016;44:43-47.
24. Rossi WA, Tennant R. *Professional Shoe Fitting.* New York, NY: Pedorthic Footwear Association with Acknowledgement to the National Shoe Retailers Association; 2000.
25. Butler RJ, Davis I, Hamill J. Interaction of arch type and footwear on running mechanics. *Am J Sports Med.* 2006;34(12):1233-1240.
26. Hutchins S, Bowker P, Geary N, Richards J. The biomechanics and clinical efficacy of footwear adapted with rocker profiles—evidence in the literature. *Foot.* 2009;19:165-170.
27. Thies S, Price C, Kenney L, Baker R. Effects of shoe sole geometry on toe clearance and walking stability in older adults. *Gait Posture.* 2015;42:105-109.
28. Murley GS, Landorf KB, Menz HB, Bird AR. Effect of foot posture, foot orthoses and footwear on lower limb muscle activity during walking and running: a systematic review. *Gait Posture.* 2009;29:172-187.
29. Stefanyshyn DJ, Nigg BM, Fisher V, O'Flynn B, Liu W. The influence of high heeled shoes on kinematics, kinetics, and muscle EMG of the normal female gait. *J Appl Biomech.* 2000;16(3):309-319.
30. Li JX, Hong Y. Kinematic and electromyographic analysis of the trunk and lower limbs during walking in negative-heeled shoes. *J Am Podiatr Med Assoc.* 2007;97(6):447-456.
31. Doi T, Yamaguchi R, Asai T, et al. The effects of shoe fit on gait in community-dwelling older adults. *Gait Posture.* 2010;32:274-278.
32. Dobson JA, Riddiford-Harland DL, Bell AF, Steele JR. Work boot design affects the way workers walk: a systematic review of the literature. *Appl Ergon.* 2017;61:53-68. doi:10.1016/j.apergo.2017.01.003.
33. Moisan G, Cantin V. Effects of two types of foot orthoses on lower limb muscle activity before and after a one-month period of wear. *Gait Posture.* 2016;46:75-80. doi:10.1016/j.gaitpost.2016.02.014.
34. Lee KH, Shieh JC, Matteliano A, Smiehorowski T. Electromyographic changes of leg muscles with heel lifts in women: therapeutic implications. *Arch Phys Med Rehabil.* 1990;71(1):31-33.
35. Lee K, Matteliano A, Medige J, Smiehorowski T. Electromyographic changes of leg muscles with heel lift: therapeutic implications. *Arch Phys Med Rehabil.* 1987;68(5 Pt 1):298-301.
36. Hsi W-L, Kang J-H, Lee X-X. Optimum position of metatarsal pad in metatarsalgia for pressure relief. *Am J Phys Med Rehabil.* 2005;84(7):514-520. doi:10.1097/01.phm.0000167680.70092.29.
37. Zifchock RA, Davis I. A comparison of semi-custom and custom foot orthotic devices in high- and low-arched individuals during walking. *Clin Biomech.* 2008;23(10):1287-1293. doi:10.1016/j.clinbiomech.2008.07.008.
38. Murley GS, Bird AR. The effect of three levels of foot orthotic wedging on the surface electromyographic activity of selected lower limb muscles during gait. *Clin Biomech.* 2006;21(10):1074-1080. doi:10.1016/j.clinbiomech.2006.06.007.
39. Vicenzino B, Feilding J, Howard R, Moore R, Smith S. An investigation of the anti-pronation effect of two taping methods after application and exercise. *Gait Posture.* 1997;5(1):1-5.
40. Prusak KM. *A Comparison of Two Tape Techniques on Navicular Drop and Center of Pressure Measurements* [dissertation]. Provo, Utah: Brigham Young University; 2012.
41. Luque-Suarez A, Gijon-Nogueron G, Baron-Lopez FJ, Labajos-Manzanares MT, Hush J, Hancock MJ. Effects of kinesiotaping on foot posture in participants with pronated foot: a quasi-randomised, double-blind study. *Physiotherapy.* 2014;100(1):36-40. doi:10.1016/j.physio.2013.04.005.
42. Landry SC, Nigg BM, Tecante KE. Standing in an unstable shoe increases postural sway and muscle activity of selected smaller extrinsic foot muscles. *Gait Posture.* 2010;32(2):215-219. doi:10.1016/j.gaitpost.2010.04.018.
43. Briem K, Eythörsdóttir H, Magnúsdóttir RG, Pálmarsson R, Rúnarsdóttir T, Sveinsson T. Effects of kinesio tape compared with nonelastic sports tape and the untaped ankle during a sudden inversion perturbation in male athletes. *J Orthop Sports Phys Ther.* 2011;41(5):328-335. doi:10.2519/jospt.2011.3501.
44. Martinez-Gramage J, Merino-Ramirez M, Amer-Cuenca J, Lison J. Effect of Kinesio Taping on gastrocnemius activity and anlke range of movement during gait in healthy adults: a randomized controlled trial. *Phys Ther Sport.* 2016;18:56-61.
45. Murley GS, Landorf KB, Menz HB. Do foot orthoses change lower limb muscle activity in flat-arched feet towards a pattern observed in normal-arched feet? *Clin Biomech.* 2010;25:728-736.

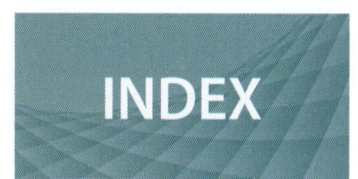

Note: Page numbers of definitive presentations are in boldface. Boxes, Figures and table are in italics.

A
ABCS mnemonic, *893*
Abdominal breathing. *See* Diaphragmatic breathing
Abdominal lamina, *408*, *408*
Abdominal muscle, **483**. *See also specific muscles*
  anatomic considerations, 483–484, *483*, *484*, *485*
    function, 486–487, *486*
    functional unit, 487–488, *487*
    innervation and vascularization, 484, *486*
  clinical presentation of
    patient examination, 491–492
    referred pain pattern, 488–489, *489*, *490*
    symptoms, 490–491, *491*
    trigger point examination, 492–493, *493*
  corrective actions for, 494–495, *495*
  differential diagnosis of
    associated pathology, 494
    associated trigger points, 494
    trigger points, activation and perpetuation of, 493–494
  group
    frequency-specific microcurrent, manual therapy with, *860*, *862*
    treatment parameters for, *863*
  testing, 487
Abdominal myofascial syndrome, 490
Abdominal oblique muscles
  external and internal, trigger point injection/dry needling of, *805*
  patient examination for, 492
  referred pain patterns of, 488, *489*
Abdominal tension test, 491, *492*
Abdominal visceral diseases, 549
Abdominal wall assessment, *873*, *875*
Abduction, **378**
Abductor digiti minimi muscle, **386**, **734**, *735*
  anatomic considerations of, 386, *387–388*
    function, 388–390, *737*
    functional unit, 390
    innervation and vascularization, 386, *388*, *736*
  clinical presentation of
    patient examination, 390, 739
    referred pain pattern, *389*, 390, *738*, *739*
    symptoms, 390, 738–739
    trigger point examination, 390–391, *391*, *741*, *742*
  corrective actions for, 392–393, *393*
  differential diagnosis of
    associated pathology, 392
    associated trigger points, 391–392, 744
    trigger points, activation and perpetuation of, 391
  trigger point injection/dry needling technique for, 796, 799, 826–828, *827*
Abductor hallucis muscle, 750, *751*
  anatomic considerations of, **734**, *735*
  associated pathology of, 744
  associated trigger points in, 744
  function of, 737
  innervation of, *736*
  patient examination for, 739
  referred pain pattern of, 738, *738*
  symptoms from, 738–739
  trigger point examination of, *741*, *742*
  trigger point injection/dry needling technique for, 826, *827*
A-beta fibers, 855
Aβ mechanoreceptors, 852
Abnormal accessory movement testing, 545
Abscess

  dental, 100
  psoas, 519
Academy of Orthopaedic Physical Therapy (APTA), 662
Acceptance and Commitment Therapy, 69
Acceptance of pain, 70
Accessory joint motion testing, 390
  for cervical joints, 191
  for coracobrachialis muscle, 287
  for elbow and shoulder joints, 313
  for headache and neck pain, 191
Accessory obturator nerve, 622, *624*
Accessory plantaris muscle, 699
Accessory soleus muscle, **698**
Acetabular labral tear, 656
Acetyl-coenzyme A (acetyl-CoA), 49
Acetylcholine (ACh), 17–18, *18*, 30–31
  effects at motor endplate, 33–34
  excessive, causes of, 35
  nonquantal release, 32–33
  release, regulation of, 34
Acetylcholinesterase (AChE), 36
Ach. *See* Acetylcholine (ACh)
AChE (acetylcholinesterase), 36
Achilles tendinitis, 705
Achilles tendinopathy, **692–693**, 705–706
  chronic, 693
  diagnosis of, 693
  insertional, 693
  noninsertional/mid-portion, 693
  risk factors for, 693
Achilles tendon, 687, 697, 698, 701, 705
Acid-sensing ion channels (ASICs) receptor, 10
ACL (citrate lyase), 49
ACL (anterior cruciate ligament), 660–661, 688
ACR (American College of Rheumatology), 655, 659
Actin, 31, 44, 46
Active infection, 858
Active stretching procedure, **836**
Active trigger points, **2**
Activity-based stresses, trigger points and, 166
Acupuncture, 51
Acute fibularis tendon dislocation/tearing, 683
Acute myocardial infarction, 416
Adduction, **378**
Adductor brevis muscle, **621**
  anatomic considerations of, 621, *623*
    function, 624–625
    functional unit, 625, *625*
    innervation and vascularization, 622
  clinical presentation of
    patient examination, 626–628, *628–629*
    referred pain pattern, 625–626, *626*
    symptoms, 626
    trigger point examination, 628–629, *629*
  corrective actions for, 631–633, *632–633*
  differential diagnosis of
    associated pathology, 630–632
    associated trigger points, 630
    trigger points, activation and perpetuation of, 630
  trigger point injection/dry needling technique for, 814–815, *817*
Adductor canal, 621
Adductor hallucis muscle
  anatomic considerations of, **734**, *735*
  corrective actions for, 744, *744*
  function, 737

897

Adductor hallucis muscle (*continued*)
  innervation and vascularization, 736
  referred pain pattern of, 738, *740*
  trigger point examination of, 741, *743*
  trigger point injection/dry needling technique for, *828*, 829
Adductor longus muscle, **621**
  anatomic considerations of, 621, *622*
    function, 624–625
    functional unit, 625, *625*
    innervation and vascularization, 622
  clinical presentation of
    patient examination, 626–628, 628–629
    referred pain pattern, 625–626, *626*
    symptoms, 626
    trigger point examination, 628–629, *629*
  corrective actions for, 631–*633*, 632–*633*
  differential diagnosis of
    associated pathology, 630–632
    associated trigger points, 630
    trigger points, activation and perpetuation of, 630
  trigger point injection/dry needling technique for, 814–815, *817*
Adductor magnus muscle, **621**
  anatomic considerations of, 621, *623*
    function, 624–625
    functional unit, 625, *625*
    innervation and vascularization, 622
  clinical presentation of
    patient examination, 626–628, 628–629
    referred pain pattern, 626, *627*
    symptoms, 626
    trigger point examination, 629, *629*
  corrective actions for, 631–*633*, 632–*633*
  differential diagnosis of
    associated pathology, 630–632
    associated trigger points, 630
    trigger points, activation and perpetuation of, 630
  trigger point injection/dry needling technique for, 815, *817*, *818*
Adductor minimus muscle, 621
Adductor notch, **871**, *873*
Adductor pollicis muscle, **378**
  anatomic considerations of, 378, *379*–*380*
    function, 378
    functional unit, 379–380, *379*
    innervation and vascularization, 378
  clinical presentation of
    patient examination, 381–382
    referred pain pattern, 380, *381*
    symptoms, 380–381
    trigger point examination, 382, *382*
  corrective actions for, 383–384, *384*, *385*
  differential diagnosis of
    associated pathology, 383, *383*
    associated trigger points, 383
    trigger points, activation and perpetuation of, 382–383
  trigger point injection/dry needling technique for, 795, *799*
Adductor tenoperiostitis, 630
A-delta fibers, 855
Aδ nociceptors, 5
Adenosine diphosphate (ADP), 49
Adenosine receptor activation effect, 34
Adenosine triphosphate (ATP), 32, 33, 36, 49
  acetylcholine release from motor nerve terminals by, 34
  muscle contractions and, 49
  role of, 40
  ultimate depletion of, 40
Adenylyl cyclase, stimulation and inhibition of, 11
Adhesive capsulitis, 228, 324. *See* Frozen shoulder syndrome
ADP (adenosine diphosphate), 49
Adson test, 320, 432
Aerobic exercises, 63
  duration, 848
  mode, 848
  prescription, 848
  training program, 848–849
    design variables for, 848
    frequency, 848
    intensity, 848

Afferent fiber, primary, 5
Agency for Health Care Policy and Research (AHCPR), 540
Agenesis, 360
Agonist–antagonist interaction, 345
AHCPR (Agency for Health Care Policy and Research), 540
Allergies, scalene TrPr and, 217
Allodynia, 16, 412
Alpha-1&2-adrenergic blocking agent, 39
Alpha-adrenergic effects on muscle function, 40
α-amino-3-hydroxy-5-methyl-4-isoxazolepropionic acid (AMPA), 5, 7
Alpha-motor neuron, *38*, 47
Altered muscle activation patterns, 63–64
American Academy of Neurology, 363
American Association of Electrodiagnosis, 363
American College of Rheumatology (ACR), 655, 659
American Physical Medicine and Rehabilitation Academy, 363
American Physical Therapy Association, 750–751, 769
Amide local anesthetics, 765
Anconeus epitrochlearis muscle, 315
Anconeus muscle, **307**
  anatomic considerations of, 307
    function, 309
    functional unit, 310, *310*
    innervation and vascularization, 307–308
  clinical presentation of
    patient examination, 310–313
    referred pain pattern, 310, *312*
    symptoms, 310
    trigger point examination, 314, *314*
  corrective actions for, *315*, 316
  differential diagnosis of
    associated pathology, 314–315
    associated trigger points, 314
    trigger points, activation and perpetuation of, 314
  trigger point injection/dry needling technique for, 790, *793*
Anesthesia. *See also* Local anesthetics
  cold, 759
  saddle, 544–545
Anger, pain and, 71
Angina pectoris, 416
Ankle
  dorsiflexion, 690, 703
  eversion, 674
  instability, 677, **748**
  neutral position, 683, 693, 706, 715, 723, 732
  plantar flexion, 706
  postural dysfunction findings in, 877–878, *878*
  pump exercise, 671
  sprain
    acute, 748
    overview of, 748
    patient evaluation with, 748
    trigger points and, 748–749
Ankylosing spondylitis (AS), 175, 546–547
Anomalous muscle, 709
Ansa cervicalis nerves, 137
Antagonistic iliopsoas, 562
Antagonists, 519
  gastrocnemius muscle as, 688
  to hamstring muscle, 641
Antecubital space, 302
Anterior abdominal wall syndrome, 491
Anterior circumflex humeral artery, 277
Anterior cruciate ligament (ACL), 660–661, 688
Anterior deltoid fibers, 264
  anatomic considerations of, 276, *276*
  function of, 277
  trigger point examination of, 280, *281*
Anterior drawer test, 141, 748
Anterior humeral circumflex artery, 285, 293
Anterior interosseous nerve, 368
  compression syndrome, 399
Anterior neck muscles, **135**
  anatomic considerations of, 135–137, *136*, *137*, *138*
    function, 138–139
    functional unit, 139, *139*
    innervation and vascularization, 137–138

clinical presentation of
  patient examination, 141
  referred pain pattern, 139–140, *140*
  symptoms, 140–141
  trigger point examination, 141–142, *142*
corrective actions for, 144–145, *144*, *145*
differential diagnosis of
  associated pathology, 143–144
  associated trigger points, 143
  trigger points, activation and perpetuation of, 142–143
Anterior scalene muscle block (ASMB), 217–218
Anterior superior iliac spine (ASIS), 503, 871
Anterior tibial artery, 667, 676–677
Anterior vertebral muscles. *See specific muscles*
Anterolateral shin splints, **670**
Anticoagulation therapy, 706
Antinociception, 55
Anxiety, pain and, 64
Apley's scratch test, 202, 226, *226*, 243, 323, 355
  of coracobrachialis muscle, 287
  deltoid muscle, 279
  infraspinatus muscle, 235
  subscapularis muscle, 262
Aponeurotic fascia, 50–51
Apparent leg length discrepancy, distortion of, 503, *503*
Appendicitis, 519
  pseudo-appendicitis, 489
Arcade of Frohse, 352
Arcade of Struthers, 399
Aristocort (triamcinolone), 767
Aromatase, 56, 57
Arteria lumbalis, 472
Arthralgia, acute, 189
Arthritis
  carpometacarpal, 400
  cervical, 264, 277
  of fingers, 346
  glenohumeral joint, 282
  hip, 562
  in humeroulnar joint, 398
  osteoarthritis, 400
  radiocapitellar, 396
  in radiocapitellar joint, 396
  reactive, 175
  trapeziometacarpal joint, 357
Articular dysfunction
  with abdominal muscle trigger points, 491
  adductor pollicis and opponens pollicis muscles, 382
  associated with pelvic floor muscle trigger points, 529
  in C4, C5, and C6, 218
  in glenohumeral joint, 287
  interosseous muscle, 392
  with interscapular pain, 89
  intra-articular dysfunction, 630
  for pectoralis major and subclavius muscles, 413
  posterior cervical muscles, 176
  psoas major muscle with, 519
  of sacroiliac joints, 533
  scalene muscles, 213
  serratus posterior superior muscle, 467
  thoracolumbar, 478, 508
AS (ankylosing spondylitis), 175, 546–547
ASICs (acid-sensing ion channels) receptor, 10
ASIS (anterior superior iliac spine), 503, 871
ASMB (anterior scalene muscle block), 217–218
Astigmatism, 154
Athletic pubalgia, 656
Atlantoaxial instability, 63
ATP. *See* Adenosine triphosphate (ATP)
Attention switching mechanism, 64
Attribution theory, 70
Atypical facial neuralgia, 96
Auscultation using stethoscope, 188
Autonomous phase, of motor control training, 845
Auxiliary heart, 487
Avoidant behaviors, defined, **71**
Axillary artery, 259, 285, 308, *428*
Axillary nerve, 241, 277
Axons, 6, 7

B
Back pain
  low. *See* Low back pain (LBP)
  and scalene muslce, 211
  and thoracolumbar paraspinal muscles, 473
Back pocket sciatica, 561, 598
Backpacks, 880
Baker cyst, 651–652, **693**
  rupture of, 652
Bamboo spine, 175, 547
Barrier release approach, and trigger points, 836
Base of support (BOS), 868–869
Baxter nerve, **744**
BCOG (body center of gravity), 868–869
BCOM (body center of mass), 868
Beevor's sign, 492
Behavioral learning theories, 68
Beighton criteria, 61, 62
Benign paroxysmal positional vertigo (BPPV), 99
Bent-knee fallouts, 632–633, *632*
Beta-adrenergic stimulation, 39–40
Betamethasone (Celestone), 767, *767*
Biceps brachii muscle, **292**, 302
  anatomic considerations of, 292–293, *292*
    function, 293–294
    functional unit, 294, *294*
    innervation and vascularization, 293
  clinical presentation of
    patient examination, 294–295, *296*
    referred pain pattern, 294, *295*
    symptoms, 294
    trigger point examination, 295–297, *296*
  corrective actions for, 298, 299, *299*
  differential diagnosis of
    associated pathology, 297–298
    associated trigger points, 297
    trigger points, activation and perpetuation of, 297
  proximal attachments of, 292
  supinator muscle and, 352
  trigger point injection/dry needling technique for, 788–790, *789*
Biceps brachii tendon instability, 298
Biceps-extension test, 295, *296*
Biceps femoris muscle, 636–637, 635–636. *See also* Hamstring muscles
Biceps pulley, 293
Biceps–labral complex dysfunction, 297–298
Bicipital aponeurosis, 297
Bicipital tendinitis, 282
Bicipital tendinopathy, 252, 432
Bilateral agenesis, 360
Bilateral hamstring hypertrophy, 871, *873*
Bilateral handgrip test, 346
Bilateral migraine, 192, *193*
Bilateral quadratus lumborum muscle, 499
Biochemical milieu of trigger points, 19
Biofeedback, 857
Biopsychosocial model, 67
  challenges to practicing within, 72
Bleeding, prevention of, 760, 762
Blepharospasm, 154
Blood vessel entrapment, 143
Body center of gravity (BCOG), 868–869
Body center of mass (BCOM), 868
Body's second heart, 700
BOS (base of support), 868–869
Botox (onabotulinum), 768, *768*
Botox A injection, 154, 757, 768
Botulinum toxin, 99
  A (Botox A), injection, 154, 757, 768
Bouchard nodes, 400
Boundaries, 73
Bowstringing, 329
Boxer's fractures, 391
BPPV (benign paroxysmal positional vertigo), 99
Brachial and antebrachial fascia, 297
Brachial artery, 293, 308
Brachial plexus, 259

Brachialis muscle, **301**, 349
  anatomic considerations of, 301–302, *301*
    function, 302
    functional unit, 302, *302*
    innervation and vascularization, 302
  clinical presentation of
    patient examination, 302–303
    referred pain pattern, 302, *303*
    symptoms, 302
    trigger point examination, 303, *304*
  corrective actions for, 304–305, *304*
  differential diagnosis of
    associated pathology, 304
    associated trigger points, 304
    trigger points, activation and perpetuation of, 303–304
  trigger point injection/dry needling technique for, 790, *790*
Brachioradialis muscle, **331**, 349
  anatomic considerations of, 331, *332*
    function, 333
    functional unit, 333, *333*
    innervation and vascularization, 332
  clinical presentation of
    patient examination, 334–336
    referred pain pattern, 334, *336*
    symptoms, 334
    trigger point examination, 337, *338*
  corrective actions for, 339–340, *339*, *340*
  differential diagnosis of
    associated pathology, 338–339
    associated trigger points, 338
    trigger points, activation and perpetuation of, 337–338
  trigger point injection/dry needling technique for, 791–792, *794*
Breast cancer surgery, 455
Breast soreness, 416
Breast surgery, 424
Breast tenderness. *See* Breast soreness
Breathing. *See also* Chest breathing; Diaphragmatic breathing; Mouth breathing; Nasal breathing
  diaphragm muscle
    assessment of, 883–884
    postural function of, 883
    treatment considerations for, 884
  dysfunctional, 883–884, *884*
  labored, 211
  mouth breathing *vs.*, 143
  postural considerations of, 882–884
  posture and, 882–883
  quiet, 442
Bridging maneuver, 558, *560*
Bronchitis, scalene TrPr and, 217
Brugger's sitting posture, 885
Bruxism, 125
Buccal nerve, 127
Buccinator muscle, 108, **148**
  anatomic considerations of, 148
    function, 150–151
    functional unit, 151
    innervation and vascularization, 150
  clinical presentation of
    patient examination, 151, 153
    referred pain pattern, 150, 151
    symptoms, 151
    trigger point examination, 153
  corrective actions for, 154–155, *155*
  differential diagnosis of
    associated pathology, 154
    associated trigger points, 154
    trigger points, activation and perpetuation of, 153–154
Buckling knee muscle. *See* Vastus medialis muscle
Bulbocavernosus muscle. *See* Bulbospongiosus muscle
Bulbospongiosus muscle
  anatomic considerations of
    in female, 525, *525*
    in male, 525
  function of, 526–527
  referred pain pattern, *528*
  trigger point examination of
    in female, 532
    in male, 533

trigger point injection/dry needling technique for, 809
Bunion. *See* Hallux valgus
Bupivacaine
  for serratus anterior muscle pain syndrome, 767
  in trigger point injection, 765, 766, *766*
Bursa
  iliopsoas, 514
  large subscapular, 259
  large trochanteric, 555
  painful, 242
  pes anserine, 622
  popliteal, 647
  subacromial, 322
  subdeltoid, 322
  subtendinous, 666
  trochanteric
    of gluteus medius muscle, 566
    of gluteus minimus muscle, 578
Bursitis, 322
  iliopsoas, 519
  ischiogluteal, 643
  olecranon, 314, 467
  pes anserine, 643
  psuedotrochanteric, 582
  scapulothoracic, 264
  subacromial, 228, 257, 264, 289
  subdeltoid, 224, 228, 257, 282, 297
  trochanteric, 501, 508, 585
    psuedotrochanteric, 582
    subacute, 563
B vitamins, 58–59

C

C4-C8 radicular pain/radiculopathy, 175
C5 radicular pain/radiculopathy, 264, 373
C5-C6 radicular pain/radiculopathy, 218, 233, 297, 357
C6 radicular pain/radiculopathy, 264, 392
C6-C7 radicular pain/radiculopathy, 257
C7 radicular pain/radiculopathy, 264, 282, 289, 349, 373
C7-C8 radicular pain/radiculopathy, 416, 432, 457, 467
Ca^{2+}-induced Ca^{2+} release process, 39
Ca^{2+} pump, 49
Calcaneal tendon, 687
Calcific tendinopathy, 322
Calcific tendonitis, of popliteus tendon, 651
Calcitonin gene-related peptide (CGRP), 5, 18, 32, 36
Canadian Agency for Drugs and Technologies in Health, 769
Cancer, 519
  treatment of, 143
Carbocaine (mepivacaine), 766, 773
Cardiac arrhythmia, *412*, 415, 445, 447
Cardiac diseases, 448
Cardiolipin, 49
Carnett's technique, 491
Carpal compression test, 403
Carpal tunnel syndrome (CTS), 304, 319, 399, 402–403
  adductor and opponens pollicis muscles, 383
  coracobrachialis muscle, 289
  infraspinatus muscle, 233
  interossei, lumbricals, and abductor digiti minimi muscles, 392
  palmaris longus muscle, 360, 363–364
  scalene muscle, 218
  wrist and finger flexors, 374
Carpometacarpal joint (CMCJ)
  arthritis, 400–401
  osteoarthritis, 383
Carpometacarpal thumb joint, 302, *303*
Catastrophizing, 62, 69
Catecholamine, 40
Caudal (abdominal) surface of diaphragm muscle, *440*
Celestone (betamethasone), 667, 767
Cell-surface receptors, 8–10
Central nervous system (CNS) function, altered, 63–64
Central neuropathic pain, 12–13
Central nociceptive sensitivity, 16
Central pain modulation (CPM), 55
Central sensitization, 4, *4*, 15
Cephalad, 94
Cephalobrachialgia, 217

Cervical arthritis, 227, 264
Cervical disc pathology, 211
Cervical distraction test, 318
Cervical dorsal rami, 161
Cervical dystonia, 143
Cervical exercises, 880
Cervical flexion-extension injury whiplash, 141. See also Whiplash
Cervical flexion–rotation test, 181, *182*
Cervical multifidus muscle
    anatomic considerations of, *168, 169, 170*
    function, 171
    referred pain pattern, 173
    trigger point examination of, 173, *174*
    trigger point injection/dry needling technique for, 777, *780*
Cervical paraspinal muscles
    frequency-specific microcurrent, manual therapy with, 860, 861–862
    treatment parameters for, *862*
Cervical post-laminectomy pain syndromes, 175
Cervical radicular pain/radiculopathy, **318**, 304, 338, 252. See also *specific nerves*
    characterized by, 397
    initial evaluation of, 318
    trigger points and, 318–319
Cervical rib, incidence of, 320
Cervical spine
    dysfunction, 325
    frequency-specific microcurrent, manual therapy with, 860, 861–862
    levator scapulae muscle attachments to, 199
    nonthrust mobilization/manipulation of, *833*
    postural dysfunction findings in, 874–875, *875*
    testing, 371
    thrust mobilization/manipulation of, *833*
    treatment parameters for, *862*
    zygapophyseal (facet) joints of, 168, 170
Cervical spondylosis, 211
Cervical zygapophyseal joints, 159, 175
Cervicogenic headache, 108–109, 117, 158, 175
    associated active scalene trigger points, 211
    associated with trigger points in SCM muscle, 99
    characteristics of, 190
    levator scapulae muscle, 204
    trigger points and, 193
C fibers, 5, 855
CGRP (calcitonin gene-related peptide), 5, 18, 32, 36
Chair and push-up tests, 396
Channelopathies, polymorphisms and, 41
Checkrein function, 171
Cheiralgia paresthetica, 357
Chest breathing, 213, 221, 447, 520, 884
    chronic cough, emphysema, or asthma, 98
    vs. diaphragmatic breathing, 217
Chest pain, 548–549
    anterolateral part of, 455
    atypical, 448
Chest wall
    movement of, 439, *440*
    syndrome, 416
"Child's pose" position, 253. See also Quadruped position
Chin-neck angle, 874–875, *875*
2-Chloroprocaine, in trigger point injection, 765
Cholinergic synaptic transmission, 17
Chronic obstructive pulmonary disease (COPD), 447, 461
Chronic Pain Acceptance Questionnaire, 70
Chronic pain syndromes, aerobic training for, 848
Chronic pelvic pain (CPP), 547–548, **547**, *548*
Chronic pelvic pain syndrome (CPPS), 490, 547
    chronic prostatitis and, 535
Cinderella Hypothesis, 17, 48
"Circle of concern/circle of influence" concept, 73
Circumflex scapular artery, 231, 241, 254
Citrate lyase (ACL), 49
Classic hammer toe, 722
Claviclar lamina, 408, *408*
Clavicle, 82
Clavicular division of sternocleidomastoid muscle
    anatomic considerations of, 95
    referred pain pattern, 96

Claw hand dysfunction, 389
Claw toe, 720, 722, 729, 730, 740
Clinical reasoning, **75**
    multimodal treatment strategies, 75–76
    referral, role of, 76
Clinicians
    challenges to practicing within biopsychosocial model, 72
    as educator, 74–75
    psychosocial strategies for clinical practice
        boundaries, 73
        effective therapeutic alliance, 73
        first impressions, 74
        intentional and therapeutic communication, 75
        self-care, 74
        sphere of influence, focusing on, 73
        unconditional positive regard, 73
        validation, 74
    self-awareness
        countertransference, 72
        discomfort with negative emotions, 73
Clostridium botulinum, 768
Closure mechanism, in shoe, 894
Coagulopathy, 758–759
Coccydynia, 473, 562
Coccygeus muscle, **523**
    anatomic considerations of, 524, *524, 525*
    function of, 526
    referred pain pattern, *528*
    trigger point examination of, 531
Coccygodynia, 527, **534**
Cocktail, 60
Cognitive-behavioral therapy (CBT), 63, 69, 74, 110
    meaning/beliefs/illness perceptions, 68–69
    self-efficacy and locus of control, 68
Cognitive distortions, 69
Cognitive phase, of motor control training, 845
COL5A1 gene, 62
COL5A2 gene, 62
Cold anesthesia, 759
Cold detection threshold, 14
Cold pack, 851
Cold, scalene trigger points and, 217
Cold therapy. See Cryotherapy
Collagens, 51
Colon inflammation, 519
Common-Sense Model of Self-Regulation, 68
Compartment syndrome, **670**, 706, 714
    acute, 682
    acute exertional, 682
    acute spontaneous, 349
    anterior, 706, 722
    chronic exertional, **670**, 682, **722**
    chronic exertional/exercise induced, **682**
    deep posterior, 715
    paraspinal, 479
    posterior, 706, 715
Complex regional pain syndrome, 12–13
Complex repetitive discharges (CRDs), 29
Compression test, 544
Computer/workstation ergonomic analysis, 885–886, *886, 886*
Congenital abnormalities, 320
Congestion, 133
Conjoined tendon tear. See Athletic pubalgia
Conservative management, for ankle sprains, 748
Constipation, psoas trigger points, 516
Continuous ultrasound therapy, 853
Contractile unit testing
    for humeroulnar joint pathology, 398
    for radiocapitellar joint pathology, 396
Contract–relax technique, 320, 845–846
    for adductor muscle stretch, 633, *633*
    for pectoralis major and subclavius muscles, 418
    principle of, 845–846
    for subscapularis muscle, 262
    for supraspinatus muscle, 229
Contracture knots, 42
Contralateral excursion, 128
Conventional therapy, 64
COPD (chronic obstructive pulmonary disease), 447, 461

Coracobrachialis muscle, **285**, 294
    anatomic considerations of, 285, *286*
        function, 285–286
        functional unit, 286
        innervation and vascularization, 285
    clinical presentation of
        patient examination, 287, *288*
        referred pain pattern, 286, *287*
        symptoms, 287
        trigger point examination, 287–289, *288*
    corrective actions for, 289, 290–291, *290*
    differential diagnosis of
        associated pathology, 289–290
        associated trigger points, 289
        trigger points, activation and perpetuation of, 289
    trigger point injection/dry needling technique for, 787–788, *789*
Coracoid pressure syndrome, 320
Corrugator supercilii muscle, 108
    anatomic considerations of, 149
        function, 151
        functional unit, 151
        innervation and vascularization, 150
    clinical presentation of
        patient examination, 151, 153
        referred pain pattern, 151
        symptoms, 151
        trigger point examination, 153, *154*
    corrective actions for, 154–155, *155*
    differential diagnosis of
        associated pathology, 154
        associated trigger points, 154
        trigger points, activation and perpetuation of, 153–154
Corticosteroids, 758, 766–768
    adverse effects of, 767
    commonly used glucocorticoid steroids, 767
Cortisol (hydrocortisone), 767
Cortisone, 767
    injections, 810
Costal lamina, 408, *408*
Costochondritis, 416, 424, 447, 448, 548, 549
Costoclavicular maneuver, 320
Costoclavicular space/first rib, 319–320
Costoclavicular syndrome, 319
Costotransverse diagonal fibers, 497, *498*
Coughing
    chronic, 447
    intercostal and diaphragm muscle and, 443, 445
Countertransference, 72
Cozen test, 336, 396
CP (creatine phosphate), 49
CPM (central pain modulation), 55
CPP (chronic pelvic pain), 547–548, *547*, *548*
CPPS (chronic pelvic pain syndrome), 490, 547
    chronic prostatitis and, 535
Cramp-type pain, 556
Cranial nerves, 137
Craniocervical flexion exercises, 880
CRDs (complex repetitive discharges), 29
Creatine phosphate (CP), 49
Crepitation, 188
Crepitus, 181
Crohn's disease, 488, 519
Cross-bridging, 42
Cross-fiber flat palpation, 86, *87*
    of abductor digiti minimi muscle, 741, 742, 796, 799, 826–828, 827
    of abductor hallucis muscle, 741, 742, 826, *827*
    of adductor brevis muscle, 629
    of adductor hallucis muscle, 741, *743*, 828, *829*
    of anconeus muscle, 314, *314*
    of anterior deltoid muscle, 280, *281*, 786, *788*
    of biceps femoris muscle, 640, *642*, 819, *819*
    of brachialis muscle, 790, *790*
    of bulbospongiosus (bulbocavernosus) muscle, 809
    of coracobrachialis muscle, 287–288, *288*, 787–788, *789*
    of corrugator supercilii muscle, 153, *154*
    of deep paraspinal (multifidus) muscles, 802, *805*
    of distal adductor magnus muscle, 629, *629*
    of distal medial hamstring muscles, 640, *641*
    of distal triceps brachii, *313*, 314
    of dorsal interosseous muscle, 390, *391*, 741–742, *743*
    of extensor carpi radialis brevis muscle, 336, *337*, 790–791, *794*
    of extensor carpi ulnaris muscle, 790–791, *794*
    of extensor digitorum brevis muscle, 742, *743*, 830, *830*
    of extensor digitorum longus muscle, 721–722, *721*, 824, *825*
    of extensor digitorum muscle, 792, *795*
    of extensor hallucis brevis muscle, 742, *743*, 830, *830*
    of extensor hallucis longus muscle, 721–722, *721*, 824–825, *825*
    of extensor indicis muscle, 792–793, *795*
    of fibularis brevis muscle, 680, *680*, 820, *821*
    of fibularis longus muscle, 679–680, *680*, 820, *821*
    of fibularis tertius muscle, 680, *680*, 820, *821*
    of finger extensor muscles, 348, *348*
    of finger flexor muscles, 794, 797
    of flexor accessorius (quadratus plantae) muscle, 741, 742, 827, 828
    of flexor digiti minimi brevis muscle, 741, 742
    of flexor digitorum brevis muscle, 741, 742, 826, *827*
    of flexor digitorum longus muscle, 729–730, *729*, 826, *826*
    of flexor hallucis brevis muscle, 741, *743*, 828, *828*
    of flexor hallucis longus muscle, 729–730, *729*, 826, *826*
    of gastrocnemius muscle, 690–691, *691*–*692*, 822, *822*–*823*
    of gemelli muscle, 596–597, *597*
    of gluteus maximus muscle, 559, *563*, 809, *810*
    of gluteus medius muscle, 571, *572*, 810, *811*
    of gluteus minimus muscle, 583, *583*, 810, *811*
    of gracilis muscle, *629*, 630, 815, *817*
    of hamstring muscles, 819, *819*
    for identifying trigger points, 759–760, *760*
    of iliacus muscle, 518, *518*
    of iliocostalis lumborum muscle, 802, *804*
    of iliocostalis thoracis muscle, 477, *477*, 801–802, *804*
    of iliopsoas muscle group, 806–807, *807*, 809
    of infraspinatus muscle, *236*, 782, *784*
    of intercostal and diaphragm muscles, 446, 447
    of ischiocavernosus muscle, 808–809
    of lateral head, of triceps brachii muscle, 790, 792
    of latissimus dorsi muscle, 251, *251*, 782, *786*
    of levator scapulae muscle, 203, *203*
    of longissimus thoracis muscle, 477, *477*, 801, *804*
    of longus colli muscle, 142, *142*
    of lower trapezius muscle fibers, 770, *771*
    of lumbar iliocostalis muscle, 477, *477*
    of lumbrical muscles, 741, *742*
    of masseter muscle, *107*, 108, 771–772, *773*
    of medial and lateral heads of triceps brachii muscle, 313, *313*
    of medial border, of medial head, of triceps brachii muscle, 790, *793*
    of medial head, of triceps brachii muscle, 790, 792
    of medial pterygoid muscle, 123–124, *123*, 772, *774*
    of middle deltoid muscle, 281, *281*, 786–787, *788*
    of middle trapezius muscle fibers, 770, *771*
    of obturator externus muscle, 597, *597*, 598
    of obturator internus muscle, 596–597, *597*, 812, *814*
    of opponens pollicis muscle, 382, *382*
    of orbicularis oculi muscle, 153
    of palmaris longus muscle, 363, *363*, 793, *796*
    of pectineus muscle, *629*, 630, 817, *818*
    of pectoralis major muscle, 414, *415*, 797–798, *801*
    of pectoralis minor muscle, 430, *431*, 799–800, *802*
    of piriformis muscle, 596, *597*
    of plantar interosseous muscles, 741–742, *743*
    of plantaris muscle, 703, *704*, 824, *824*
    of popliteus muscle, 650–651, *650*, 819–820, *820*
    of posterior deltoid muscle, 281, *281*, 787, *788*
    of procerus muscle, 153, *154*
    of pronator teres muscle, 372, *373*, 794, *798*
    of proximal medial hamstring muscles, 640, *641*
    of psoas major muscle, 518, *518*
    of quadratus femoris muscle, 597, *597*
    of quadratus lumborum muscle, 505, *505*, 804, 806, *807*, 808
    of rectus abdominis muscle, 492–493, *493*
    of rectus femoris muscle, 812, *815*
    of rhomboid minor and major muscles, 272, *272*
    of rhomboid muscles, 785–786, *788*
    of rotatores muscles, 478
    of sartorius muscle, 814, *817*
    of scalene muscle, 215, *216*

of serratus anterior muscle, 457, *457*, 800, *803*
of serratus posterior inferior muscle, 466, *466*, 801, *803*
of serratus posterior superior muscle, 466, *466*, 801, *803*
of soleus muscle, 703, *704*
of splenius capitis muscle, 776, *779*
of sternalis muscle, 423, *423*, 798, *801*
of suboccipital muscles, 182
of subscapularis muscle, 262, *263*, 785, *787*
of supinator muscle, 356, *356*, 793, *796*
of supraspinatus muscle, 227, 781, *783*
of temporalis muscle, 116, 772, *774*
of tensor fasciae latae muscle, 583–584, *584*, 810, *812*
of teres major muscle, 256, *256*
of teres minor muscle, 244, *244*, 782, *784*
of tibialis anterior muscle, 669, *669*, 820, *821*
of tibialis posterior muscle, 713, *713*, 824, *824*
of vastus intermedius muscle, 812, *815*
of vastus lateralis muscle, 813, *816*
of vastus medialis muscle, 813, *815*
of wrist and finger flexors in forearm, 372, *373*
of wrist flexor muscles, 372, *373*, 793–794, *797*
Cross-fiber pincer palpation
of abductor digiti minimi muscle, 391, *391*, 796, *799*
of adductor brevis muscle, 628–629, *629*, 814–815, *817*
of adductor longus muscle, 628–629, *629*, 814–815, *817*
of adductor magnus muscle, 815, *817*
of adductor pollicis muscle, 382, *382*, 795, *799*
of biceps brachii muscle, 295–296, *296*, 788–790, *789*
of brachioradialis muscle, 337, *338*, 791, *794*
of buccinator muscle, 153
of bulbospongiosus (bulbocavernosus) muscle, 809
of corrugator supercilii muscle, 153, *154*
of deep transverse perinei muscle, 809
of extensor carpi radialis longus muscle, 336, *337*, 790–791, *794*
of extensor carpi ulnaris muscle, 337, *337*
of external oblique muscle, 492, *493*, 804, *805*
of gastrocnemius muscle, 690–691, *691*–692, 821–822, *822*–823
of gluteus maximus muscle, 559, *563*
of gracilis muscle, 815, *817*
of hamstring muscles, 819, *819*
for identifying trigger points, 759–760, *761*
of internal oblique muscles, 804, *805*
of interossei muscle, 390–391, *391*, 795–796, *799–800*
of latissimus dorsi muscle, 251, *251*, 782, *785–786*
of levator scapula muscle, 203, *203*, 778, *781*
of long head of triceps brachii muscle, 313, *313*, 790, *791*
of lower portion, of gluteus maximus muscle, 810, *810*
of lumbrical muscles, 390–391, *391*
of masseter muscle, *107*, *108*, 771–772, *773*
of middle deltoid muscle, 786–787, *788*
of opponens pollicis muscle, 795, *799*
of pectoralis major muscle, 797–798, *801*
of pectoralis minor muscle, 430–431, *431*, 799–800, *802*
of platysma muscle, 153, *153*
of procerus muscle, 153, *154*
of proximal adductor magnus muscle, 629, *629*
of semimembranosus muscles, 640, *641*
of semitendinosus muscles, 640, *641*
of soleus muscle, 703, *704*, 822–824, *823*
of splenius cervicis muscle, 776, *779*
of sternocleidomastoid muscle, 98, *98*, 771, *772*
of superficial transverse perinei muscle, 809
of teres major muscle, 256, 785, *787*
of upper trapezius muscle fibers, 770, *770*
of vastus lateralis muscle, 813–814, *816*
of zygomaticus major muscle, 153, *153*
Crow's feet, 150
Cruciate, 94
Cryotherapy, 850–851
CTS. *See* Carpal tunnel syndrome (CTS)
Cubital tunnel syndrome, 315, 373, 399
Cupola, 209
Curriculum, 74
CustomCare, *859*
Cyamella, 647
Cyanocobalamin, 58–59
Cyclical swings in abdominal pressure, 487
Cyriax technique, 841
Cyst. *See specific cysts*

Cytoskeleton, 12, *13*
Cytosolic Ca^{2+} ($[Ca^{2+}]c$), 32
alpha-adrenergic effects on, 40
excessive, problem of, 40
ion channel polymorphisms as cause of increased, 40
requirement for muscle contraction, 31, *33*, *34*, *35*
second messenger system regulation of, 39

D
DAB mnemonic, 388
Dantrolene, 61
DASH (Disability of Arm, Shoulder, and Hand), 236
de Quervain's stenosing tenosynovitis, 304, 339, 349, 357, 383, 400
Deafness, 96
Decadron (dexamethasone), 767, 854
Deep cervical flexor impairment, 193
Deep circumflex artery, 514
Deep fibular nerve, 670, 676
Deep layer of masseter muscle, 105
Deep neck flexors, activation of, *144*, 145
Deep paraspinal muscle, 469
anatomic considerations of, 471–472, *471*
functions of, 472
patient examination of, 477
referred pain pattern of, 473
trigger point examination of, 477–478
trigger point injection/dry needling technique for, 802, *805*
Deep posterior chronic exertional compartment syndrome (dp-CECS), 706, 715
Deep-stroking massage technique
clinical application of, 841–842, *841*
overview of, 841
patient and intervention selection, 841
Deep temporal nerves, anterior and posterior, 113
Deep transverse perinei muscle, 809
Delayed onset muscle soreness (DOMS), 857
Deltoid muscle, 302. *See also specific muscles*
anatomic considerations of, 276–277, *276*
function, 277–278
functional unit, 278, *278*
innervation and vascularization, 277
clinical presentation of
patient examination, 278–279, *280*
referred pain pattern, 278, *279*
symptoms, 278
trigger point examination, 280–281, *281*
corrective actions for, 282–283, *283*
differential diagnosis of
associated pathology, 282
associated trigger points, 282
trigger points, activation and perpetuation of, 281–282
trigger point injection/dry needling technique for, 786–787, *788*
Dental abscess, 99
Depo-Medrol (methylprednisolone), 767
Depression
of diaphragm muscle, 439, *441*
pain and, 64, 70
of shoulder, 427
Depressor caudae lateralis, 526
Depressor caudae medialis, 526
Desmin, 46
Detoxification reactions, and FSM technique, 858–859, 864
Dexamethasone (Decadron), 767, 854
Dextrose solution, in proliferative injection techniques, 767
DHPR (dihydropyridine receptor), 31
Diagnostic Criteria for TMD (DC TMD), 189
Dialectical behavioral therapy, 63, 69
Diaphragm muscle, **436**
anatomic considerations of, 436, *438*, *439*, *440*
function, 438–443, *440*, *441*
functional unit, 443–444, *443*
innervation and vascularization, 437–438
assessment of
breathing and, 883
dysfunctional breathing, 883–884, *884*
clinical presentation of
patient examination, 445–446
referred pain pattern, *444*, 445

Diaphragm muscle (*continued*)
    symptoms, 445
    trigger point examination, *446*, 447
  corrective actions for, 448–450, *449*, *450*
  differential diagnosis of
    associated pathology, 448
    associated trigger points, 447–448
    trigger points, activation and perpetuation of, 447
  postural function of, 883
    dysfunctional, 884
    treatment considerations for, 884
  trigger point injection/dry needling technique for, 800
Diaphragmatic breathing, 101, 520
  for abdominal muscles, 494
  assessment of, 445
  chest breathing and, 217
  instruction in, 448, *449*
  with postisometric relaxation technique, 836–837
  scalene muscles, 213, *220*, 221
  for trigger points
    in serratus anterior muscle, 458
    in serratus posterior superior muscle, 467
Diaphragmatic dysfunction, 456
Diffuse noxious inhibitory control (DNIC), 13
Digastric muscle, **135**
  anatomic considerations of, 135, *136*
  functions of, 138
  innervation and vascularization of, 137–138
  referred pain pattern, 139, *140*
  trigger point examination of, 141, *142*
  trigger point injection/dry needling technique for, 773–774, *776*
Dihydropyridine receptor (DHPR), 31
Dimenhydrinate (Dramamine), 97
Disability of Arm, Shoulder, and Hand (DASH), 236
Disc extrusion, 541
Disc herniation, 318, 599
Disc prolapse, 541
Disc protrusion, 541
Disc sequestration, 541
Disc–capsule complex, 127
Discogenic lower back pain (DLBP), 541
Disease-modifying anti-rheumatic drugs (DMARDs), 547
Distal radial ulnar joint instability, 401
Distal triceps brachii muscle
  referred pain pattern of, 310, *311*
  trigger point examination of, *313*, 314
Distal/pelvic crossed syndrome. *See* Lower crossed syndrome
Distinctive clinical syndrome, 175
Distraction test, 544
Dizziness, vestibular disease, 99
DLBP (discogenic lower back pain), 541
DMARDs (disease-modifying anti-rheumatic drugs), 547
DN technique. *See* Dry needling (DN) technique
DNIC (diffuse noxious inhibitory control), 13
DOMS (delayed onset muscle soreness), 857
Dorsal forearm muscle, 343, *344*
Dorsal interosseous muscles, 386
  anatomic considerations of, 735–**736**, *736*
  function of, 737
  innervation and vascularization of, 736–737
  referred pain pattern of, 738, *740*
  strength examination of, 740
  trigger point examination of, 741–742, *743*
  trigger point injection/dry needling technique for, *829*, 830
Dorsal intrinsic foot muscles
  anatomic considerations of, 735, *736*
    function, 737
    functional unit, 737, *738*
    innervation and vascularization, 737
  clinical presentation of
    patient examination, 739–741
    referred pain pattern, 738, *741*
    symptoms, 738–739
    trigger point examination, 742, *743*
  corrective actions for, 744–746, *745–746*
  differential diagnosis of
    associated pathology, 744
    associated trigger points, 744
    trigger points, activation and perpetuation of, 742–744

Dorsal metacarpal artery, 386–387
Dorsal proximal forearm, pain in, 354
Dorsal scapular artery, 200, 222, 268
Dorsal scapular nerve, 89, 199–200, 268
Dorsalis pedis pulse, palpation of, 740
Dorsiflexion, 674
  fibularis tertius muscle in, 677
  of foot, 668, *678*
Dorsiflexor muscles, 671–672
Double- and single-leg squat, 582
Double crush phenomenon, 399
Double leg lowering test, 492
Double-leg squat, 557, *557*, 627, 639, 669, 679, 689, 702, 712, 720, 729
Downhill running/walking, popliteus muscle during, 649, 652
dp-CECS (deep posterior chronic exertional compartment syndrome), 706, 715
Dramamine (dimenhydrinate), 97
Driving posture, 886–887, *887*
Drop arm test, 322
Drop sign, 244
Dry needling (DN) technique, 19, 51, 758, 769
  for abductor digiti minimi muscle, 796, 799, 826–828, *827*
  for abductor hallucis muscle, 826, *827*
  for adductor brevis, 814–815, *817*
  for adductor hallucis muscle, *828*, 829
  for adductor longus, 814–815, *817*
  for adductor magnus muscle, 815, *817*, *818*
  for adductor pollicis muscle, 795, 799
  for anconeus muscle, 790, *793*
  for ankle sprain, 748–749
  for biceps brachii muscle, 788–790, *789*
  for brachialis muscle, 790, *790*
  for brachioradialis muscle, 791–792, *794*
  for bulbospongiosus (bulbocavernosus) muscle, 809
  for cervical multifidus muscle, 777, *780*
  clinical guideline for, 759–762, *760–763*, 762
  for coccygeus muscle, of pelvic diaphragm, 808
  contraindications to, 762
  for coracobrachialis muscle, 787–788, *789*
  for deep paraspinal (multifidus) muscles, 802, *805*
  for deep transverse perinei muscle, 809
  defined, **757**, **769**
  for deltoid muscle, 786–787, *788*
  for diaphragm muscle, 800
  for digastric muscle, 773–774, *776*
  for dorsal interosseous muscles, *829*, 830
  for extensor digitorum brevis, 830, *830*
  for extensor digitorum longus muscle, 824, *825*
  for extensor digitorum muscle, 792, *795*
  for extensor hallucis brevis muscle, 830, *830*
  for extensor hallucis longus muscle, 824–825, *825*
  for extensor indicis muscle, 792–793, *795*
  for external oblique muscle, 804, *805*
  "fast in, fast out" method, 769
  for fibularis brevis muscle, 820, *821*
  for fibularis longus muscle, 820, *821*
  for fibularis tertius muscle, 820, *821*
  for finger flexor muscles, 794, *797*
  for flexor accessorius (quadratus plantae) muscle, *827*, 828
  for flexor digitorum brevis muscle, 826, *827*
  for flexor digitorum longus muscle, 826, *826*
  for flexor hallucis brevis muscle, 828, *828*
  for flexor hallucis longus muscle, 826, *826*
  for gastrocnemius muscle, 821–822, *822–823*
  for gemelli muscle, 812, *814*
  for genu articularis muscle, 814, *817*
  for gluteus maximus muscle, 809–810, *810*
  for gluteus medius muscle, 810, *811*
  for gluteus minimus muscle, 810, *811*
  for gracilis muscle, 815, *817*
  for greater trochanteric pain syndrome, 658
  for hamstring muscles, 819, *819*
  for iliococcygeus muscle, of pelvic diaphragm, 808
  for iliocostalis lumborum muscle, 802, *804*
  for iliocostalis thoracis muscle, 801–802, *804*
  for iliopsoas muscle group, 806–807, *807*, *809*
  for infraspinatus muscle, 782, *784*
  for intercostal muscles, 800
  for internal oblique muscles, 804, *805*

for interossei muscle, 795–796, 799–800
for ischiocavernosus muscle, 808–809
for knee osteoarthritis, 659–660
for lateral pterygoid muscle, 773, 775
for latissimus dorsi muscle, 782, 785–786
for levator scapula muscle, 778, 781
for longissimus thoracis muscle, 801, 804
for longus colli muscle, 774–775, 777
for lower trapezius muscle fibers, 770, 771
for lumbrical muscles, 796, 828
for masseter muscle, 771–772, 773
for medial pterygoid muscle, 772–773, 774
for middle trapezius muscle fibers, 770, 771
needle gauge, selection of, 758–759
needling sessions, number of, 762–763
for obturator externus muscle, 812, 814
for obturator internus muscle, 812, 814
for occipitofrontalis muscle, 775, 778
for opponens pollicis muscle, 795, 799
for palmaris longus muscle, 793, 796
for pectineus muscle, 817, 818
for pectoralis major muscle, 796–798, 801
for pectoralis minor muscle, 799–800, 802
for piriformis muscle, 810–812, 813
for plantar fasciitis, 750
for plantar heel pain, 702, 713
for plantaris muscle, 824, 824
for popliteus muscle, 819–820, 820
postneedling procedures for, 764
precautions to, 762
for procerus muscle, 775, 778
for pronator quadratus muscle, 794, 798
for pronator teres muscle, 794, 798
for pubococcygeus muscle, of pelvic diaphragm, 808
for pyramidalis muscle, 804, 806
for quadratus femoris muscle, 812, 814
for quadratus lumborum muscle, 804, 806, 807, 808
reasons for failure of, 764
for rectus abdominis muscle, 804, 806
for rectus femoris muscle, 812, 815
for rhomboid muscles, 785–786, 788
for right zygomaticus major muscle, 775, 777
for sartorius muscle, 814, 817
for scalene muscles, 778–779, 782
for semispinalis capitis muscle, 777, 780
for semispinalis cervicis muscle, 777, 780
for serratus anterior muscle, 800, 803
for serratus posterior inferior muscle, 801, 803
for serratus posterior superior muscle, 801, 803
for soleus muscle, 822–824, 823
for splenius capitis muscle, 776, 779
for splenius cervicis muscle, 776, 779
for sternalis muscle, 798, 801
for sternocleidomastoid muscle, 770–771, 772
for subclavius muscle, 798, 802
for suboccipital muscles, 777–778, 781
for subscapularis muscle, 785, 787
for superficial transverse perinei muscle, 809
for supinator muscle, 793, 796
for supraspinatus muscle, 781–782, 783
for temporalis muscle, 772, 774
for tensor fasciae latae muscle, 810, 812
for teres major muscle, 785, 787
for teres minor muscle, 782, 784
for tibialis anterior muscle, 820, 821
for tibialis posterior muscle, 824, 824
Travell and Simons caveats for, 763
for triceps brachii muscle, 790, 791–793
for triceps surae muscles, 702
for upper trapezius muscle fibers, 770, 770
for vastus intermedius muscle, 812–814, 815–817
for vastus lateralis muscle, 660, 813–814, 816
for vastus medialis muscle, 813, 815
for wrist extensor muscle, 338, 790–791, 794
for wrist flexor muscles, 793–794, 797
Duloxetine, 13
Duodenal ulcer, 494
Dupuytren contracture, 364, 371, 374, 403–404
Dural headache, 183

Dutch Orthopaedic Association, 322, 661
Dysmenorrhea, 488, 490
   primary, 490
Dyspareunia, 527
Dysphagia, 123, 125, 131
Dysport (abobotulinum), 768
Dystonia, 143–144
   cervical dystonia, 143
   hyoid dystonia, 143
   jaw-closing dystonia, 125
   oromandibular, 124, 125, 133, 143

E

Eagle syndrome, 143, 144
ECC (excitation-contraction coupling), 35–36, 35, 36
Eccentric exercise, 844
ECM (extracellular matrix), 50–51, 63
ECRB (extensor carpi radialis brevis), 329, 338, 349
ECRL (extensor carpi radialis longus), 329, 349
ECU (extensor carpi ulnaris), 329, 349, 401
ED muscle. *See* Extensor digitorum (ED) muscle
Edema, 214
EDL muscle. *See* Extensor digitorum longus (EDL) muscle
EDS (Ehlers-Danlos syndrome), 61, 62, 349
   management of, 63
   pain in, 63
Effective therapeutic alliance, 73
EHL muscle. *See* Extensor hallucis longus (EHL) muscle
Ehlers-Danlos syndrome (EDS), 61, 62, 349
   management of, 63
   pain in, 63
EI muscle. *See* Extensor indicis (EI) muscle
Electrical activity of active trigger points, 38
Electrocardiogam analysis, serratus anterior muscle, 454
Electrodiagnostic tests, 399
   median nerve, 363
   for thoracic outlet syndrome, 320
Electromyography (EMG), 442, 844
   for adductor magnus muscle, 625
   for biceps femoris muscle, 637
   biofeedback using, 857
   for brachioradialis muscle, 333
   for deltoid muscle, 277
   for extensor hallucis longus muscle, 720
   for fibularis brevis muscle, 677
   for fibularis longus muscle, 677
   for gastrocnemius muscle, 693
   for gluteus medius muscle, 567
   for gracilis muscle, 625
   for infraspinatus muscle, 232
   for interosseous muscles, 388
   for lateral pterygoid muscle, 128
   for latissimus dorsi muscle, 247, 249
   for levator scapulae muscle, 201
   for masseter muscle, 104
   for occipitofrontalis muscle, 156
   peak activity, temporalis muscle, 113
   for pectoralis major muscle, 409–410
   for pectoralis minor muscle, 427
   for quadratus lumborum muscle, 498–499
   for rhomboid minor and major muscles, 269–270
   for rotator cuff muscles, 260
   for scalene muscles, 210
   for semimembranosus muscle, 637
   for semispinalis capitis, 171
   for semitendinosus muscle, 637
   for serratus anterior muscle, 454
   for short external rotators, 592–593
   for shoulder and upper extremity, 309
   for sphincter ani muscle, 526
   for subscapularis muscle, 259–261
   supinator muscle and, 352–353
   for supraspinatus muscle, 224
   for tarsal tunnel syndrome, 750
   for thoracic outlet syndrome, 320
   for tibialis anterior muscle, 667, 668
   for tibialis posterior muscle, 710
   for trigger point, 29
   for wrist extensors, 333

Electrotherapeutic modalities, for trigger points treatment
  biofeedback, 857
  frequency-specific microcurrent. See Frequency-specific microcurrent
  neuro-muscular electrical stimulation, 856–857
  transcutaneous electrical nerve stimulation, 855–856, *856*
EMG. See Electromyography (EMG)
EMLA (eutectic mixture of local anesthetics), 854
Emotional stressors, trigger points in masseter muscle, 108
Emphysema, 465
"Empty can" test, 224, 322
Endogenous stimuli, 5
Endoplasmic reticulum, 12, *13*
Endplate noise, 33, 39
Endplate spikes (EPS), 29
Energy crisis hypothesis, 17
Energy crisis theory of Simons, 33
Enthesopathy, 541
Environmental stress, splenius capitis/cervicis muscles trigger points, 166
Epicranial aponeurosis, 156
Epicranius muscle. See Occipitofrontalis muscle
Epinephrine, 40
Episacroiliac lipoma, 599
EPS (endplate spikes), 29
Erector clitoridis, 525
Erector spinae muscle. See Superficial paraspinal muscle
Ester local anesthetics, 765
Estradiol (17-β-estradiol), 55, 56
Estrogen, 55–56
Estrone, 55
Ethyl chloride, 851
Etidocaine, in trigger point injection, 766
Euphoria, 864
European association of urology, 491, 530, 548
The European League Against Rheumatism, 655
Eustachian tube, 123
Eutectic mixture of local anesthetics (EMLA), 854
Eversion, of foot, 678
Excessive lumbar lordosis, 557, *557*
Excitation-contraction coupling (ECC), 35–36, *35, 36*
Exercises
  aerobic. See Aerobic exercises
  cervical, 880
  craniocervical flexion, 880
  duration, in aerobic training program, 848, *848*
  eccentric, 844
  finger-flutter, 349, 374, 392, 886
  flexibility, 660
  "full can," 224
  functional, 849
  Kendall, 880
  McKenzie, 880
  middle trapezius fibers, 89–90, *90*
  mode, in aerobic training program, 848
  pelvic tilt, 495, *495*
  prescription, in aerobic training program, 848
  selection of, 846
  sit-back/abdominal-curl/sit-up, 486, 495
  to strengthen intrinsic foot muscles
    first-toe extension exercise, 746, *746*
    second-to-fifth-toe extension exercise, 746, *746*
    short-foot exercise, 746, *746*
    toe curling, 746, *746*
    toes-spread-out exercise, 746, *746*
  therapeutic. See Therapeutic exercise
  for triceps brachii and anconeus muscles, 316
  trigger points activation, 478
Exertional compartment syndromes, 670, 697, 698, 706, 714, 731
Exhalation, 438, 442
Existential-humanistic therapy
  nonpathologic approach, 69
  patient-centered care, 69
  values and meaning, 69
Exogenous stimuli, 5
Exostosis, **752**
Extensor carpi radialis accessorius muscle, 331
Extensor carpi radialis brevis (ECRB), 329, 338, 349

Extensor carpi radialis longus (ECRL), 329, 349
Extensor carpi ulnaris (ECU), 329, 349, 401
Extensor digitorum (ED) muscle, **343**
  anatomic considerations of, 343, *344*
    function, 345
    functional unit, 345–346, *345*
    innervation and vascularization, 345
  clinical presentation of
    patient examination, 346–347, *348*
    referred pain pattern, 346, *347*
    symptoms, 346
    trigger point examination, 347–348, *348*
  corrective actions for, 349–350, *350*
  differential diagnosis of
    associated pathology, 349
    associated trigger points, 349
    trigger points, activation and perpetuation of, 348–349
Extensor digitorum brevis muscle
  anatomic considerations of, 735, **736**
  associated trigger points in, 744
  function, 737
  innervation and vascularization, 737
  patient examination, 739
  referred pain pattern of, 738, *741*
  trigger point examination of, 742, *743*
  trigger point injection/dry needling technique for, 830, *830*
Extensor digitorum longus (EDL) muscle, 671–672, 675, **718**
  anatomic considerations of, 718, *719*
    function, 719–720
    functional unit, 720, *720*
    innervation and vascularization, 719
  clinical presentation of
    patient examination, 720–721
    referred pain pattern, 720, *721*
    symptoms, 720
    trigger point examination, 721–722, *721*
  corrective actions for, 718, 723–724, *723–724*
  differential diagnosis of, 718
    associated pathology, 722–723
    associated trigger points, 722
    trigger points, activation and perpetuation of, 722
  trigger point injection/dry needling technique for, 824, *825*
Extensor hallucis brevis muscle, **736**
  anatomic considerations of, *735*
  associated trigger points in, 744
  function of, 737
  innervation and vascularization of, 737
  patient examination of, 739
  referred pain pattern of, 738, *741*
  trigger point examination of, 742, *743*
  trigger point injection/dry needling technique for, 830, *830*
Extensor hallucis longus (EHL) muscle, 671–672, **718**
  anatomic considerations of, 718, *719*
    function, 719–720
    functional unit, 720, *720*
    innervation and vascularization, 719
  clinical presentation of
    patient examination, 720–721
    referred pain pattern, 720, *721*
    symptoms, 720
    trigger point examination, 721–722, *721*
  corrective actions for, 718, 723–724, *723–724*
  differential diagnosis of, 718
    associated pathology, 722–723
    associated trigger points, 722
    trigger points, activation and perpetuation of, 722
  trigger point injection/dry needling technique for, 824–825, *825*
Extensor indicis (EI) muscle, **343**
  anatomic considerations of, 343, *344*
    function, 345
    functional unit, 345–346, *345*
    innervation and vascularization, 345
  clinical presentation of
    patient examination, 346–347, *348*
    referred pain pattern, 346, *347*
    symptoms, 346
    trigger point examination, 347–348, *348*
  corrective actions for, 349–350, *350*
  differential diagnosis of

associated pathology, 349
  associated trigger points, 349
    trigger points, activation and perpetuation of, 348–349
  trigger point injection/dry needling technique for, 792–793, 795
External iliac artery, 514
External intercostal muscles, 435, 436, 437, 442
External oblique muscle
  anatomic considerations of, 483, 484
  functions of, 486–487
  innervation and vascularization of, 484, 486
  referred pain pattern of, 488, 489
  trigger point examination of, 492, 493
  trigger point injection/dry needling technique for, 804, 805
External pelvic examination, 533
External perineal muscle, 530
External rotation lag test, 244
External rotator fatigue, 323
Extracellular matrix (ECM), 50–51, 63
Extracellular milieu, 8–11, 9, 10, 11
Extracorporeal shock wave therapy, 702
Extraoral active release of masseter muscle, 110, 110
Eye movements, with postisometric relaxation technique, 837

F

FABER (Flexion Abduction External Rotation) test, 628, 628, 656
Facet joint mobility, 549
Facet syndrome, 599
Facet/zygapophyseal joint dysfunction, 204
Facial artery, 104
Facial asymmetry, 125
Facial muscles. *See specific muscles*
Facial nerve, 156
Facial scoliosis, 871, 871
FADIR (flexion, adduction, and internal rotation) test, 657
FAI (femoral acetabular impingement), 519, 656
FAIR (flexion adduction internal rotation) test, 595, 658
Falciform ligament, 293
Fall on an outstretched hand (FOOSH) injury, 297
Fascia, 50
  biomechanical considerations of, 50–51
  fascial connections to skin, muscles, and nerve, 50
  filiform needle in, 51
  sensory aspects of, 51
  tridimensional direction of, 50
Fascia Research Congress, 50
Fascial attachments, psoas major muscle, 514
Fascial pliability, changes in, 50
Fascial restrictions, 847
Fascicles muscle, 80–81, 515
Fatigue
  and Ehlers-Danlos syndrome, 63
  and trigger points, 891
FCR muscle. *See* Flexor carpi radialis (FCR) muscle
FCU muscle. *See* Flexor carpi ulnaris (FCU) muscle
FDA (Food and Drug Administration), 768, 768
FDL muscle. *See* Flexor digitorum longus (FDL) muscle
FDP muscle. *See* Flexor digitorum profundus (FDP) muscle
FDS muscle. *See* Flexor digitorum superficialis (FDS) muscle
Fear and anxiety, pain and, 71
Feet, flat-arched, 894
Femoral acetabular impingement (FAI), 519, 656
Femoral artery, 514, 606, 622, 624
Femoral nerve, 606
  entrapment, 520
  innervation, 514, 622, 624, 662
  slump test, 662
Femoroacetabular impingement syndrome, 64, 562
FHL muscle. *See* Flexor hallucis longus (FHL) muscle
FHP. *See* Forward head posture (FHP)
Fiber arrangement of gluteal muscles, 559, 562
Fibrin, 51
Fibroblasts, 51
Fibrodysplasia ossificans progressive, 479
Fibromyalgia Impact Questionnaire (FIQ), 60
Fibromyalgia syndrome (FMS), 12–13, 56, 173, 175, 180, 448, 479, 838
Fibronectin, 51
Fibrosis, 51
Fibrositic nodules, 491

Fibrositis, deep-stroking massage for, 841
Fibular artery, 709, 737
Fibular nerve, 719
Fibular neuropathy, 681
Fibularis brevis muscle, 585, **675**, 710
  anatomic considerations of, 675–**676**, 675–676
    function, 677
    functional unit, 678, 678
    innervation and vascularization, 676
  clinical presentation of
    patient examination, 678–679
    referred pain pattern, 678, 679
    symptoms, 678
    trigger point examination, 680, 680
  corrective actions for, 683–684, 684
  differential diagnosis of
    associated trigger points, 681
    pathology, 681–683, 682
    trigger points, activation and perpetuation of, 680–681
  trigger point injection/dry needling technique for, 820, 821
Fibularis longus muscle, 585, 710
  anatomic considerations of, 674–**675**, 675–676
    function, 677
    functional unit, 678, 678
    innervation and vascularization, 676
  clinical presentation of
    patient examination, 678–679
    referred pain pattern, 678, 679
    symptoms, 678
    trigger point examination, 679–680, 680
  corrective actions for, 683–684, 684
  differential diagnosis of
    associated pathology, 681–683, 682
    associated trigger points, 681
    trigger points, activation and perpetuation of, 680–681
  loading and off-loading considerations for, 895
  trigger point injection/dry needling technique for, 820, 821
Fibularis muscles, 748–749. *See also specific muscles*
Fibularis tendon subluxation, 683
Fibularis tertius muscle
  anatomic considerations of, **675**, 676
    function, 677–678
    functional unit, 678, 678
    innervation and vascularization, 676–677
  clinical presentation of
    patient examination, 678–679
    referred pain pattern, 678, 679
    symptoms, 678
    trigger point examination, 680, 680
  corrective actions for, 683–684, 684
  differential diagnosis of
    associated trigger points, 681
    pathology, 681–683, 682
    trigger points, activation and perpetuation of, 680–681
  trigger point injection/dry needling technique for, 820, 821
Filiform needle, 730, 757, 758–759, 769
Finger extension test, 371, 372
Finger flexion test, 213–214, 216, 346, 348, 414
Finger flexor muscles. *See also Specific muscles*
  trigger point injection/dry needling technique for, 794, 797
Finger-flutter exercise, 349, 374, 392, 886
Finkelstein test, 400
FIQ (Fibromyalgia Impact Questionnaire), 60
First impressions, 74
First-toe extension exercise, 746, 746
Flange, 893
Flank of trunk, 463
Flare. *See* Flange
Flat-arched feet, 894
Flat back posture, 869, 870
"Flat feet," 738–739
Flatfooted gait, 712
Flexibility exercises, 660
Flexibility training program, 847–848
Flexion, 378
Flexion Abduction External Rotation (FABER) test, 628, 628, 656
Flexion, adduction, and internal rotation (FADIR) test, 657
Flexion adduction internal rotation (FAIR) test, 595, 658
Flexion-extension injuries, 142

Flexion-internal rotation test, 657
Flexor accessorius muscle
  anatomic considerations of, **734**, *735*
  associated pathology of, 744
  function of, 737
  innervation and vascularization of, 736
  referred pain pattern of, 738, *739*
  trigger point examination of, 741, *742*
  trigger point injection/dry needling technique for, 827, *828*
Flexor carpi radialis (FCR) muscle, **366**
  anatomic considerations of, 366, *367*
    function, 368–369
    functional unit, 369, *369*
    innervation and vascularization, 368
  clinical presentation of
    patient examination, 371, *372*
    referred pain pattern, 369, *370*
    symptoms, 371
    trigger point examination, 371–372, *373*
  corrective actions for, 374–376, *376*
  differential diagnosis of
    associated pathology, 373–374, *374*, *375*
    associated trigger points, 373
    trigger points, activation and perpetuation of, 372–373
Flexor carpi ulnaris (FCU) muscle, **366**, 399
  anatomic considerations of, 366, *367*
    function, 368–369
    functional unit, 369, *369*
    innervation and vascularization, 368
  clinical presentation of
    patient examination, 371, *372*
    referred pain pattern, 369, *370*
    symptoms, 371
    trigger point examination, 371–372, *373*
  corrective actions for, 374–376, *376*
  differential diagnosis of
    associated pathology, 373–374, *374*, *375*
    associated trigger points, 373
    trigger points, activation and perpetuation of, 372–373
  tendinopathy, 401, 402
Flexor digiti minimi brevis muscle
  anatomic considerations of, **734–735**, *735*
  function of, 737
  innervation and vascularization of, 736
  referred pain pattern of, 738, *739*
  trigger point examination of, 741, *742*
Flexor digitorum brevis muscle, 726, 751
  anatomic considerations of, **734**, *735*
  associated pathology of, 744
  associated trigger points in, 744
  function of, 737
  innervation and vascularization of, 736
  patient examination of, 739
  referred pain pattern of, 738, *739*
  symptoms from, 738–739
  trigger point examination of, 741, *742*
  trigger point injection/dry needling technique for, 826, *827*
Flexor digitorum longus (FDL) muscle, 710, 712, **726**
  anatomic considerations of, 726, *727*
    function, 727
    functional unit, 727, *728*
    innervation and vascularization, 727
  clinical presentation of
    patient examination, 729
    referred pain pattern, 728, *728*
    symptoms, 728–729
    trigger point examination, 729–730, *729*
  corrective actions for, 726, 731–732, *731–732*
  differential diagnosis of, 726
    associated pathology, 730–731
    associated trigger points, 730
    trigger points, activation and perpetuation of, 730
  trigger point injection/dry needling technique for, 826, *826*
Flexor digitorum profundus (FDP) muscle, **366**, 399
  anatomic considerations of, 366, *367*
    function, 368–369
    functional unit, 369, *369*
    innervation and vascularization, 368
  clinical presentation of
    patient examination, 371, *372*
    referred pain pattern, 369, *370*
    symptoms, 371
    trigger point examination, 371–372, *373*
  corrective actions for, 374–376, *376*
  differential diagnosis of
    associated pathology, 373–374, *374*, *375*
    associated trigger points, 373
    trigger points, activation and perpetuation of, 372–373
Flexor digitorum superficialis (FDS) muscle, **366**
  anatomic considerations of, 366, *367*
    function, 368–369
    functional unit, 369, *369*
    innervation and vascularization, 368
  clinical presentation of
    patient examination, 371, *372*
    referred pain pattern, 369, *370*
    symptoms, 371
    trigger point examination, 371–372, *373*
  corrective actions for, 374–376, *376*
  differential diagnosis of
    associated pathology, 373–374, *374*, *375*
    associated trigger points, 373
    trigger points, activation and perpetuation of, 372–373
Flexor hallucis brevis muscle
  anatomic considerations of, **734**, *735*
  associated pathology of, 744
  function of, 737
  innervation and vascularization of, 736
  patient examination of, 740
  referred pain pattern of, 738, *740*
  trigger point examination of, 741, *743*
  trigger point injection/dry needling technique for, 828, *828*
Flexor hallucis longus (FHL) muscle, 712, **726**
  anatomic considerations of, 726–727, *727*
    function, 727
    functional unit, 727, *728*
    innervation and vascularization, 727
  clinical presentation of
    patient examination, 729
    referred pain pattern, 728, *728*
    symptoms, 728–729
    trigger point examination, 729–730, *729*
  corrective actions for, 726, 731–732, *731–732*
  differential diagnosis of, 726
    associated pathology, 730–731
    associated trigger points, 730
    trigger points, activation and perpetuation of, 730
  injury, 730
  trigger point injection/dry needling technique for, 826, *826*
Flexor pollicis longus (FPL) muscle, **366**
  anatomic considerations of, 366, *368*
    function, 369
    functional unit, 369, *369*
    innervation and vascularization, 368
  clinical presentation of
    patient examination, 371, *372*
    referred pain pattern, 370, *370*
    symptoms, 371
    trigger point examination, 371–372, *373*
  corrective actions for, 374–376, *376*
  differential diagnosis of
    associated pathology, 373–374, *374*, *375*
    associated trigger points, 373
    trigger points, activation and perpetuation of, 372–373
FMS (fibromyalgia syndrome), 12–13, 56, 173, 175, 180, 448, 479, 838
Foam roller, 563, 643–644
Food and Drug Administration (FDA), 768, *768*
FOOSH (fall on an outstretched hand) injury, 297
Foot
  drop, **669**
  orthoses, 891
  postural dysfunction findings in, 877–878, *878*
  posture, 891
  pronatory foot, 894–895, *894*
  slap, **669**
  sleeping posture with, 693, *694*
  squeeze test, 681
  supinatory foot, 895, *895*

Footballer hernia. *See* Athletic pubalgia
Footwear, 891, 892
    foot presentations
        pronatory foot, 894–895, *894*
        supinatory foot, 895, *895*
    heel height for, 893
    orthotic devices, 894
    physical stress theory, 891–892
    shoe
        design, 892
        modifications, 893–894
        parts of, *892*
        proper fitting of, 892, *893*, 893
    taping, 894
Forefoot varus/valgus, 740
Forward head posture (FHP), 61–62, 106–107, 166, 184, 869, 879–880
    for anterior neck muscles, 144
    excessive, 183
    -induced headache, 885
    lateral pterygoid muscle, 133
    mandibular position induced by, 117
    masseter muscle, 108, 109
    medial pterygoid muscle, 125
    of occipitofrontalis muscle, 159
    respiratory function and, 883–884
    suboccipital muscles, 180–181
    treatment of, 880
FPL muscle. *See* Flexor pollicis longus (FPL) muscle
Freiberg's sign, 595
Frequency-specific microcurrent (FSM), 850, 857–858
    application options for
        dosing, 860–861
        manual technique, 860–*861*, 861–864
        treatment, 861, *861*
    background of, 858
    contraindications of, 859
    equipment, 859–860, *859–861*
    patient
        preparation for, 859
        selection of, 858
        setup for, 860–*861*
    for persistent chronic myofascial pain, 864
    posttreatment care for, 864
    precautions for
        detoxification reactions, 858–859
        hydration, 858
        infection, 858
        ligamentous laxity, 859
        new injury, 858
        pacemaker, 858
        stenosis, 859
    pretreatment script, for clinicians, 859
    side effects of, *864*
        detoxification reactions, 864
        euphoria, 864
        increased joint pain, 864
        midscapular pain, from stenosis, 865
        radicular pain, 865
Froment sign, 402
Frontalis muscle, 156–157, *156*
    referred pain pattern, 157, *158*
Frozen shoulder, 257, 261, 282
    initial evaluation of, 324
    trigger points and, 324–325
Frozen shoulder syndrome (FSS), 264–265, **264**
Frustrator muscle. *See* Vastus intermedius muscle
FSM. *See* Frequency-specific microcurrent (FSM)
"Full can" exercise, 224
Functional ankle instability, defined, **748**
Functional Atlas of the Human Fascial System, 50
Functional exercises, 849
Functional heterogeneity, 128
Functional MRI (fMRI), biofeedback using, 857

G

Gaenslen test. *See* Torsional stress test
Gait
    analysis, 582
    cycle, 500, 555, 572, 580
    calf muscle activation, 711
    tibialis posterior muscle in, 711–712
    flatfooted, 712
    hamstrings muscles during, 637, 639
    mechanics
        rocker bottom and, 893
        shoe fit and, 894
        shoe sole and, 893
    push-off phase of, 727
    stance phase of, 727
    swing phase of, 727
Galea aponeurotica, 156
Gamma motor neurons, *38*
Ganglion cyst, 344, 349, 400–401
Gastrocnemius muscle, **687**
    anatomic considerations of, 687, *687*
        function, 688
        functional unit, 688, *688*
        innervation and vascularization, 688
    clinical presentation of
        patient examination, 689–690, *690*
        referred pain pattern, 688–689, *689*
        symptoms, 687, 689
        trigger point examination, 690, 691–692
    corrective actions for, 693–695, *694–695*
    differential diagnosis of, 687
        associated trigger points, 692
        pathology, 692–693
        trigger points, activation and perpetuation of, 691
    and hamstring muscle trigger points, 640–641
    loading and off-loading considerations for, 895
    trigger point injection/dry needling technique for, 821–822, *822–823*
Gate control theory, 3, 4, 67, 855
Gemelli muscle, **590**
    anatomic considerations of, 590, 592
        function of, 592–594
        functional unit, 594, *594*
        innervation and vascularization, 591
    clinical presentation of
        patient examination, 595–596
        referred pain pattern, 594–595
        symptoms, 595
        trigger point examination, 596–597, *597*
    corrective actions for, 599–600, *600*, *601*
    differential diagnosis of
        associated pathology, 598–599
        associated trigger points, 598
        trigger points, activation and perpetuation of, 597–598
    trigger point injection/dry needling technique for, 812, *814*
Gemellus superior muscle, 591
Genetics, and posture, 869
Genicular artery, 606, 622
Geniohyoid muscle
    anatomic considerations of, 135
    functions of, 138
    innervation and vascularization of, 137–138
Genitofemoral nerve, entrapment of, 631
Genu articularis muscle, 606, 814, *817*
Genu varum, 877, *878*
German Research Network on Neuropathic Pain (DFNS), 13
Giant cell arteritis. *See* Temporal tendinitis
Gilmore groin. *See* Athletic pubalgia
Glenohumeral Internal Rotation Deficit, 235, 243
Glenohumeral joint, 222, 259–260, 430
    arthritis, 282
    arthrokinematic forces at, 309
    assessment, 243
    posterior capsule tightness, 235, 238, 243
    role of, 323
    stability, 231–232
Glenoid fossa, angulation of, 232
Glial cells, 8
Global Burden of Disease, 190
Glucocorticoid steroids, 767
Glutamate injection, for gastrocnemius muscle TrP, 689
Gluteal fold, lower, 871–872, *873*
Gluteal muscle, 881
Gluteal skyline, assessment of, 557, *558*
Gluteal tendinopathy, 574, 657

Gluteus maximus muscle, 554
　anatomic considerations of, 554–555, *554*
　　function, *555*
　　functional unit, 555, *555*
　　innervation and vascularization, *555*
　clinical presentation of
　　patient examination, 557–558, *557*, *558*, *559*, *560*, *561*
　　referred pain pattern, 556, *556*
　　retraining program, 561
　　symptoms, 556
　　trigger point examination, 559, *562*, *563*
　corrective actions for, 563, *564*
　differential diagnosis of
　　associated pathology, 562–563
　　associated trigger points, 562
　　trigger points, activation and perpetuation of, 559, 561–562
　trigger point injection/dry needling technique for, 809–810, *810*
　trigger point pressure release for, 836, *836*
Gluteus medius muscle, 507, **566**
　anatomic considerations of, 566, *566*
　　function, 567
　　functional unit, 567, *568*
　　innervation and vascularization, 567
　clinical presentation of
　　patient examination, 569–571, *569*, *570*, *571*
　　referred pain pattern, 567–568, *568*
　　retraining, 572
　　symptoms, 568–569
　　trigger point examination, 571–572, *572*, *573*
　corrective actions for, 574–575, *574*, *575*
　differential diagnosis of
　　associated pathology, 573–574
　　associated trigger points, 572–573
　　trigger points, activation and perpetuation of, 572
　trigger point injection/dry needling technique for, 810, *811*
Gluteus minimus muscle, 507, 566, 573, **577**
　anatomic considerations of, 577–578, *577*, *578*
　　function, 579–580
　　functional unit, 580, *580*
　　innervation and vascularization, 579
　clinical presentation of
　　patient examination, 582
　　referred pain pattern, 580–581, *581*
　　symptoms, 582
　　trigger point examination, 583, *583*
　corrective actions for, 585–586, *586*
　differential diagnosis of
　　associated pathology, 585
　　associated trigger points, 584–585
　　trigger points, activation and perpetuation of, 572, 584
　function of, 567
　patient examination of, 569
　retraining, 571, 572
　self-stretching, 575, *575*
　single-leg squat assessment of, 569
　sleeping position for, 574
　trigger point injection/dry needling technique for, 810, *811*
　trigger points, 681
　weakness, 570, *570*
Glycolysis, 49
Golf hands, 391
Golfer's elbow, 310, 314, 363
Golgi apparatus, 12
Gonadal hormones. *See* Estrogen; Testosterone
Good test–retest reliability, 263
G-protein, 5, 11, *11*
　-coupled estrogen receptors (GPER), 56
Gracilis muscle, **622**
　anatomic considerations of, 622, *624*
　　function, 624–625
　　functional unit, 625, *625*
　　innervation and vascularization, 624
　clinical presentation of
　　patient examination, 626–628, *628–629*
　　referred pain pattern, 626, *628*
　　symptoms, 626
　　trigger point examination, 629, *630*
　corrective actions for, 631–633, *632–633*
　differential diagnosis of
　　associated pathology, 630–632
　　associated trigger points, 630
　　trigger points, activation and perpetuation of, 630
　trigger point injection/dry needling technique for, 815, *817*
Gravity
　-assisted stretching
　　of adductor muscles, 633, *633*
　　of gluteus medius muscle, 575, *575*
　　of gluteus minimus muscle, 586
　　of scalene muscles, 221
　and biomechanical considerations, 868–869, *868*
　-induced postisometric relaxation, 101, *101*
Greater occipital nerve, 80, 170, *170*, 173
　compression, 159
Greater sciatic foramen, 589
Greater trochanteric pain syndrome (GTPS), 574
　overview of, 657
　patient, initial evaluation of, 657
　trigger points and, 657–658
Groin pain, 625–626, 656
Gross joint trauma, 63
GTPS. *See* Greater trochanteric pain syndrome (GTPS)
Gum pain, 124
Guyon canal syndrome, 360, 383, 392
Guyon tunnel syndrome, 401, 402

H
HA (hyaluronan), 50
Haglund syndrome, **706**
Hallux trigger. *See* Claw toe
Hallux valgus, 681, 723, 729, **731**, 740, 744, **752**
　overview of, 752
　patient evaluation with, 752
　trigger points and, 752
Halsted's test, 432
Hammer toe, 720, 722, 729, 739, 740
Hamstring muscles, **635**. *See also specific muscles*
　anatomic considerations of, 635–637, *635–637*
　　function, 637
　　functional unit, 637–638, *638*
　　innervation and vascularization, 637
　clinical presentation of
　　patient examination, 638–639, *639–640*
　　referred pain pattern, 638, *638*
　　symptoms, 638
　　trigger point examination, 640, *641–642*
　corrective actions for, 643–645, *643–645*
　differential diagnosis of
　　associated pathology, 641–643
　　associated trigger points, 640–641
　　trigger points, activation and perpetuation of, 640
　injury, 693
　90/90 length test, 639, *639*, 642
　strains, defined, 641–642
　trigger point injection/dry needling technique for, 819, *819*
Hamstring syndrome, 638, 642
Hand-held dynamometer, 371
Hand-to-shoulder-blade test, 235
Hawkin's impingement test, 228, 265
Hawkins–Kennedy test, 322
Head and neck pain
　cervicogenic headache
　　characteristics of, 190
　　trigger points and, 193
　initial evaluation of, 191, *191*
　migraine headache
　　without aura, 190
　　trigger points and, 192, *193*
　neck pain
　　characteristics of, 190
　　mechanical, 194
　neuropathic pain syndromes, 195, *195*
　temporomandibular disorder, 187–189, *187*
　tension-type headache
　　characteristics of, 190
　　trigger points and, 193–194, *194*
　whiplash, 194–195
Headache. *See also specific headaches*
　dural, 183

levator scapulae muscle, 202, 204
    model, 191
    and suboccipital muscle trigger points, 180–181
Health-focused locus of control (HLOC), 68
Healthy behaviors, defined, **71**
Heart rate, for prescribing exercise intensity, 848
Heartburn, 488, *489*
Heberden's node, 383, *388*, 390, 392, 400
Heel counter, 892
Heel height, for footwear, 893
Heel lift, 894
Hematomas, of iliacus muscle, 519
Hemiparetic shoulder pain syndrome, 265
Hemipelvis, small, 474–475, 507, 519
Hemiplegia
    -related shoulder pain, 265
    shoulder girdle pain with, 235
Hemostasis, after TrPI/DN technique, 764
Henneman's size principle, 48
Hernia
    inguinal, 630
    lumbar, 491
    spigelian, 491
    sports, 519, 630
Herniation
    disk, 318, 599
    subcutaneous, 671
Herpes simplex (oral) recurrent infection, 99–100
Herpes zoster, 195, *195*, 448
High hamstring tendinopathy, 642
High-power pain threshold static ultrasound therapy, 852
High-powered ultrasound therapy, 853
High-stepping gait. *See* Swing-out gait
High-stepping/steppage gait, *721*
Hindfoot varus/valgus, 740
Hip
    abduction, 624
        muscle activation, 503, *504*
    arthritis, 562
    extension, 520, 579
    and external rotation strength testing, 595
    flexion, 579
        and stability, 514–515
    flexor length assessment, 558, *560*
    internal and external rotation, 515
    joint pathology/dysfunction, 569, 573–574
    and knee, nerve entrapment, 662
    muscle activation pattern, 570
    osteoarthritis
        overview of, 655
        patient, initial evaluation of, 655–656
        trigger points in, 656
    pain, 582
        overview of, 656
        patient, initial evaluation of, 656–657
        trigger points and, 657
    postural asymmetries of, 871–872, *872*, 872, *873*, 873
    strength testing, 570
    training, 570, *572*
HLOC (health-focused locus of control), 60
Hockey player's groin. *See* Athletic pubalgia
Hoffman reflex (H-reflex), 837
Hold-relax technique, 846
Hook-lying position
    diaphragmatic breathing in, *220*
    for trigger point examination
        in gastrocnemius muscle, 690–691, *691*–692
        in gluteus minimus muscle, 583, *583*
        in popliteus muscle, 650, *650*
        in soleus muscle, 703, *704*
Hooking maneuver, 491
Hormonal factors for myofascial pain syndrome
    estrogen, 55–56
    subclinical hypothyroidism, 57–58
    testosterone, 57
Hormone replacement therapy (HRT), 56
Horner's syndrome, 151
Hourglass syndrome posture, 873, *875*, 884
HRT (hormone replacement therapy), 56

5 HT (serotonin), 11, 32
Human glutamate receptors, 5
Humanist client-centered therapy model, 73
Humeroulnar arcade, 374
Humeroulnar arthritis, 398
Humeroulnar joint, 355, 398
Hunter's canal. *See* Adductor canal
Hyaluronan (HA), 50
Hyaluronate, 767
Hydrarthrosis, 651
Hydration, for FSM technique, 858
Hydrocortisone (Cortisol), 767, 854
Hyoglossus muscle
    anatomic considerations of, 135
    functions of, 138
    innervation and vascularization of, 137–138
Hyoid bone, 141
Hyoid dystonia, 143
Hyper-abduction syndrome, 320, 430
Hyper-abduction test. *See* Wright test
Hyperabduction test, 320
Hyperacusis, 130
Hyperalgesia
    mechanical, 51
    secondary. *See* Referred pain
Hyperalgesic priming, 12
Hypermobile feet ("flatfooted"), 677
Hyperparathyroidism, secondary, 60
Hypersensitive xiphoid syndrome, 416
Hypertonic saline injection, 51, 129, 278, 354, 390, 488, 491, 501, 668
    quadratus lumborum muscle, 501
    splenius capitis muscle, 162
Hypertrophy, of medial pterygoid muscle, 124–125
Hypoacusis, 130
Hypodermic needles
    needle gauge, selection of, 758–759
    of trigger point injection, 757, 758
Hypoesthesia, 373
    cutaneous, 391
Hypoglossal nerve, 95, 137
Hypomagnesemia, 60
Hypothyroid myopathy, 58
Hypothyroidism, 57–58, 60, 117

I

IAP (intra-abdominal pressure), 873, 883
Ice massage, 851
ICHD (International Classification of the Headache Disorders), 190
Idiopathic Heberden's node, 392
Idiopathic myalgia, 369
IH (intramuscular hemangiomas), 100, 109, 143
IHLP (inferior head of lateral pterygoid) muscle, 128
Iliac crest height, 503
Iliac fascia, 514
Iliacus muscle, **514**
    anatomic considerations of, 514
        function, 514–515
        functional unit, 515, *515*
        innervation and vascularization, 514
    clinical presentation of
        patient examination, 516–517, *517*
        referred pain pattern, 515–516, *516*
        symptoms, 516
        trigger point examination, 518, *518*
    corrective actions for, 520–521, *520*
    differential diagnosis of
        associated pathology, 519–520
        associated trigger points, 519
        trigger points, activation and perpetuation of, 518–519
Iliococcygeus muscle, 524
Iliocostal fibers, 497, *498*
Iliocostalis lumborum muscle, 469, *470*, 473, 474. *See also* Thoracolumbar paraspinal muscles
    trigger point injection/dry needling technique for, 802, *804*
Iliocostalis thoracis muscle, 473, 474, 549
    trigger point injection/dry needling technique for, 801–802, *804*
Iliohypogastric nerve entrapment, 520
Ilioinguinal nerve entrapment, 520

Iliolumbar artery, 486, 498, 514
Iliolumbar ligament, 497–498, 505, 506
Iliopsoas bursa, 514
Iliopsoas bursitis, 519
Iliopsoas common tendon, 517–518, 518
Iliopsoas muscle, 630. See also specific muscles
    myofascial trigger points in, 516, 516
    trigger point injection/dry needling technique for, 806–807, 807, 809
Iliotibial band syndrome (ITBS). See Iliotibial tract friction syndrome
Iliotibial tract friction syndrome, 585, 660
Iliotransverse diagonal fibers, 497–498, 498
Impaired 6-minute walking test, 58
Impingement test. See Flexion, adduction, and internal rotation (FADIR) test
Imploding migraine, 192
Incobotulinum (Xeomin), 768
Infection
    active, 858
    herpes simplex (oral) recurrent, 99–100
    precautions for, 858
    sinus, 97
Inferior calcaneal nerve. See Baxter nerve
Inferior gluteal artery, 555, 591, 637
Inferior gluteal nerve, 555, 592
Inferior head of lateral pterygoid (IHLP) muscle, 128
Inferior medial artery, 649
Inferior thyroid artery, 138, 209
Inferior ulnar collateral artery, 302
Infestation, protozoal, 64
Inflammatory lumbar pain, 547
Infliximab, 547
Infrahyoid muscle. See specific muscles
Infraspinatus muscle, 222–223, 223, **231**, 297
    anatomic considerations of, 231, 232
        function, 231–233
        functional unit, 233, 233
        innervation and vascularization, 231
    clinical presentation of
        patient examination, 235
        referred pain pattern, 233, 234
        symptoms, 233–235, 234
        trigger point examination, 235–236, 236
    corrective actions for, 237–238, 238, 239
    differential diagnosis of
        associated pathology, 237
        associated trigger points, 237
        trigger points, activation and perpetuation of, 236–237
    postisometric relaxation technique for, 836, 837
    trigger point injection/dry needling technique for, 782, 784
Infraspinous fossa, 875, 876
Inguinal hernia, 630
Inguinal insufficiency. See Athletic pubalgia
Inhalation, 435, 438
    movement of chest wall during, 439, 440
    muscles of, 440, 442
    quiet, 442
Innermost intercostal muscles, 435
Innervation. See under individual muscles
Innominate shear dysfunction, 529
Insertional tendinopathy, 693
Integrated Hypothesis, 29, 36–38, 37, 37
Integrated Neuromuscular Inhibition Technique, 839–840, 840, 840
Integrated spinal stability system (ISSS), 883
Integrins, 8
Intense preoccupation, 184
Intentional communication, 75
Intercostal muscles. See also External intercostal muscles; Innermost intercostal muscles
    anatomic considerations of, 435, 436, 437
        function, 438–443, 440, 441
        functional unit, 443–444, 443
        innervation and vascularization, 437
    clinical presentation of
        patient examination, 445–446
        referred pain pattern, 444, 444
        symptoms, 445
        trigger point examination, 446–447, 446
    corrective actions for, 448–450, 450, 451
    differential diagnosis of
        associated pathology, 448
        associated trigger points, 447–448
        trigger points, activation and perpetuation of, 447
    trigger point injection/dry needling technique for, 800
Internal iliac artery, 526
Internal oblique muscle, **484**
    anatomic considerations of, 483, 484
    functions of, 486–487
    innervation and vascularization of, 484, 486
    referred pain pattern, 488, 489
    trigger point
        examination of, 492
        injection/dry needling technique for, 804, 805
Internal pudendal artery, 591
International Association for the Study of Pain, 2, 3, 762
International Classification of Functioning, Disability and Health model, 73
International Classification of the Headache Disorders (ICHD), 190
International Federation of Orthopaedic Manipulative Physical Therapists, 833
International Headache Society, 99, 190
Interosseous muscle, 343, **386**
    anatomic considerations of, 386, 387–388
        function, 388–390
        functional unit, 390
        innervation and vascularization, 386, 388
    clinical presentation of
        patient examination, 390
        referred pain pattern, 389, 390
        symptoms, 390
        trigger point examination, 390–391, 391
    corrective actions for, 392–393, 393
    differential diagnosis of
        associated pathology, 392
        associated trigger points, 391–392
        trigger points, activation and perpetuation of, 391
    trigger point injection/dry needling technique for, 795–796, 799–800
Interphalangeal (IP) joint, 722
Interscalene triangle, entrapment at, 319
Intersection syndrome, 339, 400
Intertransversarii laterales muscle, 499
Intra-abdominal pressure (IAP), 873, 883
Intra-articular dysfunction, 630
Intracellular modulation, 11–12
Intractable benign pain, chronic, **183**
Intramuscular hemangiomas (IH), 100, 109, 143
Intramuscular lipomas, 143
Intrathecal Endomorphin 2 i(EM2)s, 56
Ion channel polymorphisms, 40
Ionotropic receptors, 5
Iontophoresis, 854–855, 855
Iron deficiency, 64
Irradiation, 845
Ischial bursitis. See Ischiogluteal bursitis
Ischiocavernosus muscle
    anatomic considerations of
        of female, 525, 525
        of male, 525
    function of, 526–527
    referred pain pattern, 528
    trigger point
        examination of, 532–533
        injection/dry needling technique for, 808–809
Ischiococcygeus muscle. See Coccygeus muscle
Ischiofemoral ligament impingement, 562–563, 599
Ischiogluteal bursitis, 643
ISSS (integrated spinal stability system), 883

J

Jackknife positioning, 314
Jafri's hypothesis, 40–41
Janda's crossed syndromes
    lower crossed syndrome, 880–881, 881
    upper crossed syndrome, 879–880, 879
Jaw-closing dystonia, 125

Jaw opening, 123, 125, *125*
Joint-biased manual therapy interventions. *See* Joint mobilization/manipulation technique
Joint capsule tenderness, 188
Joint clicking sounds, 188
Joint dysfunctions of elbow/wrist, 338
Joint hypermobility syndrome, 61, *62*
Joint inflammation, 188
Joint mobilization/manipulation technique
   for ankle instability, 748
   defined, 833
   intervention selection, patient and, 834–835
   management of, 835
   mechanisms of, 834
   overview of, 833, *833*
Joint pain, with FSM technique, 864
Joint stress, 88
Juncturae tendinae, 343

K

Kainate receptors, 5
Karvonen formula, 848
K_{ATP} receptor channel
   activation and trigger points, 41
   channel deficiency, 41
   polymorphisms, 41
Kenalog (triamcinolone), 767
Kendall exercises, forward head posture, 880
Ketorolac, for musculoskeletal pain, 768
Kidney disease, chronic, 599
Kienbock's disease, 339
Kinesiophobia, 62, 71
Knee
   abnormal, loading, 659
   flexion, *688*
      hamstring muscles and, 637
   and hip, nerve entrapment, 662
   injuries
      overview of, 660–661
      patient, initial evaluation of, 661
      trigger points and, 661
   osteoarthritis, 615
      overview of, 659
      patient, initial evaluation of, 659
      trigger points and, 659–660
   pain, 59
   postural dysfunction findings in, 877, *878*
Kyphotic forward head posture, 870

L

Labored breathing, 211
Lachman test, to identify ACL tear, 661
Lacrimation, excessive, 96
Lamellar fibroblasts, 51
Large subscapular bursa, 259
Large trochanteric bursa, 555
Lasegue sign, 595, 642
Latent tigger points, **2**
Lateral abdominal wall muscles. *See* External oblique muscle; Internal oblique muscle
Lateral common extensor tendinopathy, 373
Lateral elbow pain, 339
   trigger points and, 397–398
Lateral epicondylalgia. *See* Tennis elbow
Lateral epicondyle, 354, 357
Lateral epicondylitis, 314
Lateral femoral circumflex artery, 579
Lateral femoral cutaneous nerve entrapment, 520
Lateral genicular artery, 649
Lateral hamstring muscle, loading and off-loading considerations for, *895*
Lateral head of triceps brachii muscle, **306**
   anatomic considerations of, 306–307, *307*, *308*
   referred pain pattern, 310, 311–*312*
   trigger point examination of, 313–314, *313*
Lateral pectoral nerve, 426
Lateral pivot-shift test, 396
Lateral plantar nerve, 736–737

Lateral pterygoid muscle, **127**
   anatomic considerations of, 127, *128*, *129*
      function, 128–129
      functional unit, 129–130, *130*
      innervation and vascularization, 127–128
   clinical presentation of
      patient examination, 131
      referred pain pattern, 130, *130*
      symptoms, 130–131
      trigger point examination, 131, *132*
   corrective actions for, 133
   differential diagnosis of
      associated pathology, 132–133
      associated trigger points, 132
      trigger points, activation and perpetuation of, 132
   trigger point injection/dry needling technique for, 773, *775*
Lateral sacral artery, 472, 591
Latissimus dorsi muscle, **247**, 294, 320, 427
   anatomic considerations of, 247, *248*
      function, 247–249
      functional unit, 249, *249*
      innervation and vascularization, 247
   clinical presentation of
      patient examination, 251
      referred pain pattern, 249–250, *250*
      symptoms, 251
      trigger point examination, 251, *252*
   corrective actions for, 252–253, *252*, *253*
   differential diagnosis of
      associated pathology, 252
      associated trigger points, 252
      trigger points, activation and perpetuation of, 252
   surgical transfer of, 249
   and teres major muscle, 254, 256–257
   tightness, 271
   trigger point injection/dry needling technique for, 782, 785–786
Laughter exercise, for abdominal muscles, 495
Law of proportional activation, 277
Layer syndrome, 881–882, *882*
LBP. *See* Low back pain (LBP)
LEFS (Lower extremity functional scale), 690
Leg length discrepancy, 474, 507, 519
Levator ani muscles, **523**
   anatomic considerations of, 523–524, *524*, *525*
   function of, 526
   referred pain pattern, *528*
   trigger point examination of, 531, *532*
Levator ani syndrome, 527, 534
Levator notch, 875, *875*
Levator scapulae muscle, *162*, **199**, 215
   anatomic considerations of, 199, *200*
      function, 200–201
      functional unit, 201, *201*
      innervation and vascularization, 199–200
   clinical presentation of
      patient examination, 202
      referred pain pattern, *201*, 202
      symptoms, 202
      trigger point examination, 203, *203*
   corrective actions for, 205–206, *205*
   differential diagnosis of
      associated pathology, 204
      associated trigger points, 204
      trigger points, activation and perpetuation of, 203–204
   trigger point injection/dry needling technique for, 778, *781*
Levatores costarum muscles, 435, *437*, 442
Levothyroxine, 58
Lidocaine (Xylocaine), 773, 854
   with hyaluronidase, 767
   as local anesthetics, 765
   for pain reduction, 758
   for serratus anterior muscle pain syndrome, 767
   in trigger point injection, 765–766, *765*
Lift-off test, 322
Ligamentous laxity, and FSM technique, 859
Ligamentum nuchae, 182
Line of gravity (LOG), 868
Lingual nerve entrapment, 124

Lithotomy position
    for bulbospongiosus (bulbocavernosus) muscle, 809
    for deep transverse perinei muscle, 809
    for external pelvic examination, 533
    for ischiocavernosus muscle, 808–809
        for obturator internus muscle, 812, *814*
    for superficial transverse perinei muscle, 809
Load, and strength training program, 846
Load volume, 847
LOC (locus of control), 68
Local anesthetics
    allergic reactions to, 765
    benefits of, 765–766, 769
    classification of, 765–766
    mechanism of action for, 765
    myotoxicity of, 765
    in trigger point injections, 758, 765–766, 765–766
Local cardiac myocyte contraction, 32
Local twitch response (LTR), 235, 336, 757, 758, 760, 769
Locus of control (LOC), 68
LOG (line of gravity), 868
Long head of biceps brachii, 292–293, *292*
Long head of triceps brachii muscle, 306
    anatomic considerations of, 306, *307*
    referred pain pattern, 310, 311–312
    trigger point examination of, 313, *313*
Long sitting position
    for trigger point examination
        in dorsal muscles, 742, *743*
        in plantar muscles, 741–742, *742–743*
        in tibialis anterior muscle, 669, *669*
Long thoracic nerve damage, 458
Long toe extensor muscles. *See* Extensor digitorum longus (EDL) muscle; Extensor hallucis longus (EHL) muscle
Long toe flexor muscles. *See* Flexor digitorum longus (FDL) muscle; Flexor hallucis longus (FHL) muscle
Longissimus capitis muscle
    anatomic considerations of, *169*, 170
    function of, 171
    referred pain pattern of, 172
    trigger point examination of, 173
Longissimus thoracis muscle, 467, 469–470, 473
    trigger point injection/dry needling technique for, 801, *804*
Longus capitis muscle
    anatomic considerations of, 137
    functions of, 139
    innervation and vascularization of, 137–138
    referred pain pattern, 140
    symptoms, 140
Longus colli muscle
    anatomic considerations of, 137
    functions of, 139
    innervation and vascularization of, 137–138
    referred pain pattern, 139, *140*
    symptoms, 140
    trigger point examination of, 142, *142*
    trigger point injection/dry needling technique for, 774–775, 777
Lordotic posture, *870*
Low back pain (LBP), 479, 543, 544, 569, 573, 656
    classification systems, 540–541
    discogenic pain, 541–542
    guidelines for, 540
    initial evaluation of, 542
    prevalence of, 540
    by quadratus lumborum muscle, 502, 507, 508
    trigger points and, 542
Low-Dye taping technique, 894
Lower brachial plexus, *428*
Lower crossed syndrome, 880–881
    subtype A, 880, *880*
    subtype B, 880, *881*
Lower extremity functional scale (LEFS), 690
Lower rib release, 450, *451*
Lower subscapular nerves, 254
Lower trapezius fibers
    anatomic considerations of, 81
    associated pathology, 88
    functional unit of, 83
    functions of, 82
    patient examination for, 85–86
    referred pain pattern, 84, *85*
    symptoms from, 85
    trigger points
        activation and perpetuation of, 88
        corrective actions for, 90–91, *91*
        examination of, 86, *87*
        injection/dry needling technique for, 770, *771*
        self-pressure release of, *91*
LTR (local twitch response), 235, 336, 757, 758, 760, 769
Lumbago, 473
Lumbar artery, 472, 498, 514
Lumbar disc derangement, 508
Lumbar facet joint dysfunction, 562
Lumbar facet syndrome, 479
Lumbar hernia, 491
Lumbar joint dysfunction, 569
Lumbar ligament sprain, 545–546
Lumbar ligament strain, 545–546
Lumbar lordosis, 63, 467
Lumbar multifidus muscle, 562
    trigger points, 478
Lumbar plexus, roots of, 519–520
Lumbar radicular pain/radiculopathy, 562, 573, 584, 585, 662, 670, 692
Lumbar spinal nerve, 472, 514
Lumbar spine
    dysfunction, 562
    frequency-specific microcurrent, manual therapy with, *860*, *862*
    instability, 545
    spine active range of motion
        assessment of, 503
        paraspinal muscles, 474
    treatment parameters for, *863*
Lumbar stenosis, 544–545
Lumbar vertebrae, 503
Lumbo-pelvic girdle, 444
Lumborum muscles, 549
Lumbosacral plexus, 699, 719
Lumbosacral radicular pain/radiculopathy, 599
Lumbrical muscle, 343, **386**
    anatomic considerations of, 386, *387–388*, *734*, *735*
        function, 388–390, *737*
        functional unit, 390
        innervation and vascularization, 386, 388, *736*
    clinical presentation of
        patient examination, 390
        referred pain pattern, *389*, 390, *738*, *740*
        symptoms, 390
        trigger point examination, 390–391, *391*, *741*, *742*
    corrective actions for, 392–393, *393*
    differential diagnosis of
        associated pathology, 392
        associated trigger points, 391–392
        trigger points, activation and perpetuation of, 391
    strength examination of, *740*
    trigger point injection/dry needling technique for, 796, 828

M

Magnesium (Mg^{2+})
    role of, 60–61
    supplementation, 60
Magnesium citrate, 60
Magnetic resonance imaging (MRI), 698, 714
    for hamstring tendinopathy, 643
    hyperintense signals, detection of, 641
Maladaptive cognition, 63
Maladaptive movement patterns, 63–64
Malignant hyperthermia, 40, 61
Malignant tumors of iliopsoas muscles, 519
Mallet toe, 722
Mandible, 120, *121*
    movements of, 113
    range of motion, 188–189
Mandibular nerve, 103, 127
Manipulation, defined, 833, *833*
Manual palpation, of gastrocnemius muscle, 690–691, *691–692*
Manual pincer grasp for adductor pollicis muscle, *384*
Manual therapy

biomechanical effects of, 834
deep-stroking massage technique
  clinical application of, 841–842, *841*
  overview of, 841
  patient and intervention selection, 841
defined, **833**
joint mobilization/manipulation technique
  defined, **833**
  intervention selection, patient and, 834–835
  management of, 835
  mechanisms of, 834
  overview of, 833, *833*
muscle energy techniques
  clinical application of, 836–837, *837*
  overview of, 836
  patient and intervention selection, 836
  standards and guidelines for, *837*
neuromuscular therapy
  clinical application of, 839–840, *840, 840*
  overview of, 838–839, *839*
  patient and intervention selection, 839
  standards and guidelines for, *839*
strain counterstrain technique
  advantages of, 838
  clinical application of, 838, *838*
  defined, **837**
  overview of, 837–838
  patient and intervention selection, 838
stretching interventions
  clinical application of, 836–837, *837*
  overview of, 836
  patient and intervention selection, 836
trigger point pressure release technique
  clinical application of, 836, *836*
  overview of, 835
  patient and intervention selection, 835–836
for trigger points, 757–758
Massage
  deep, 520
  Thiele, 537–538
Masseter hypertrophy, 109
Masseter muscle, **103**, 124
  anatomic considerations of, 103, *104*
    function, 104–105
    functional unit, 105, *105*
    innervation and vascularization, 103–104
  clinical presentation of
    patient examination, 106–107, *107*
    referred pain pattern, 105, *106*
    symptoms, 105–106
    trigger point examination, 107–108, *107*
  corrective actions for, 109–110, *109, 110*
  differential diagnosis of
    associated pathology, 108–109
    associated trigger points, 108
    trigger points, activation and perpetuation of, 108
  trigger point injection/dry needling technique for, 771–772, *773*
Masseteric nerve, 103
Mastectomy, 455
Master emotion. *See* Shame
Mature organism model, 4
Maudsley's test, 329, 336, 346
Maxillary artery, 104, 113, 128
  pterygoid branches of, 120
Mcburney's point, 489, *490*
McGill Pain questionnaire, 61
McKenzie exercises, for forward head posture, 880
McKenzie mechanical diagnosis and therapy classification, 540
McMurray test, for meniscus tear, 661
Meaning/beliefs/illness perceptions, 68
Mechanical (radiographic) lumbar instability, 545
Mechanical pain threshold, 15–16, *16*
Mechanical perpetuating factors for myofascial pain syndrome
  Ehlers-Danlos syndrome, 61, *62*
  forward head posture, 61–62
  other mechanical stresses, 62–63
Mechanical/tactile detection threshold, 14, *16*
Medial circumflex femoral artery, 591, 622, 624, 637

Medial common flexor tendinopathy (golfer's elbow), 373
Medial elbow pain
  potential nerve entrapments causing, 398–400
  trigger points and, 399–400
Medial epicondylalgia, **398**, 432
Medial epicondyle, 360, 369
Medial head of triceps brachii muscle, **306**
  anatomic considerations of, 306, *307, 308*
  referred pain pattern of, 310, *311–312*
  trigger point examination of, 313, *313*
Medial intermuscular septum, 399
Medial longitudinal arch (MLA), 891, 894
Medial pectoral nerve, 426
Medial plantar nerve, 736
Medial pterygoid muscle, **120**
  anatomic considerations of, 120, *121*
    function, 120–121
    functional unit, 122, *122*
    innervation and vascularization, 120
  clinical presentation of
    patient examination, 123
    referred pain pattern, 122–123, *122*
    symptoms, 123
    trigger point examination, 123–124, *123*
  corrective actions for, 125, *125*
  differential diagnosis of
    associated pathology, 124–125
    associated trigger points, 124
    trigger points, activation and perpetuation of, 124
  trigger point injection/dry needling technique for, 772–773, *774*
Medial talar tilt test, 748
Medial tibial stress syndrome (MTSS), 731, **714**, 744. *See also* Achilles tendinopathy
Median nerve, 361, 368, 378, 386
  conduction, 374
  electrodiagnostic examination of, 363
  entrapment, 373–374
  neurodynamic testing, 371
Meditation, 69–70
  -overuse headaches, 195
Medrol (methylprednisolone), 767
Membrane ion channel, 10, *10*
Ménière disease, 99
Meniscal injuries, 660–661
Meniscus tears, 651
Mepivacaine (Carbocaine), 766, 773
MEPPs (miniature endplate potentials), 29, 33, 40
Meralgia paresthetica, 585
MERFF (Myoclonic Epilepsy with Ragged Red Fibers) syndrome, 49
Metabotropic receptors, 5
Metatarsal pads, for forefoot plantar pain, 744
Metatarsal stress fracture
  overview of, 751
  patient evaluation with, 751
  trigger points and, 751
Metatarsophalangeal (MP) joint, 722
Methylprednisolone (Medrol, Depo-Medrol), 767
Microglia, 59
Mid-portion tendinopathy. *See* Noninsertional tendinopathy
Mid-thoracic articular dysfunctions, 458
Middle deltoid fibers
  anatomic considerations of, 277
  function of, 277
  trigger point examination of, 281, *281*
Middle finger extensor, 346, *347*
Middle scalene muscle, 319
Middle-swing phase, semitendinosus muscle in, 637
Middle trapezius fibers
  anatomic considerations of, 81
  associated pathology of, 88
  functional unit of, 83
  functions of, 82
  patient examination for, 85
  referred pain pattern of, 84–85, *84*
  symptoms from, 85
  trigger points
    activation and perpetuation of, 88
    corrective actions for, 89, *90, 91*

Middle trapezius fibers (*continued*)
  examination of, 86, 87
  injection/dry needling technique for, 770, *771*
  self-pressure release of, *91*
Midscapular pain, from stenosis, 865
Migraine, 117, 132, 158, 180
  without aura, 190
  levator scapulae muscle, 204
  trigger points, 192, *193*
    in scalene muscle, 211
    in sternocleidomastoid muscle, 99
    in trapezius muscle and, 85
Military posture, 417, 432
Mill stretch maneuver, 396
Mindfulness, 69–70
Miniature endplate potentials (MEPPs), 29, 33, 40
Mitochondria, 12, 49
  role of, 12, *12*
Mitochondrial supercomplex activity, 49
MLA (Medial longitudinal arch), 891, 894
Mobility, **845**
Mobilization, defined, **833**, *833*
Modifications, shoe, 893–894
Modified Ober test, IT band, assessment of, 660
Modulation, nociception and, 11–13, *11*, *12*, *13*, *14*
Monofilament needle, identifying tibialis posterior trigger points, 713
Morgagni syndrome, 124
Morphine, 58–59
Morton foot structure, **681**, 744
Morton neuroma, **681**
  overview of, 751–752
  patient evaluation with, 752
  trigger points and, 752
"Motion control" shoes, 892
Motion palpation test, 543
Motor adaptation model, 3–4
Motor control
  assessment, *559*
  defined, **845**
  dysfunctions, 338
  training, 845
Motor dysfunction, 844
Motor endplate
  acetylcholine effects at, 33–34, *35*
  excitation-contraction coupling, 35–36, *36*
  neurotransmitter feedback control mechanisms, 36
  role of, 17–19, *17*, *18*
Motor learning, 845
Motor units
  recruitment of, 843
  rotation, **843**
  type I, 843
  type II, 843
Mouth breathing, 133
  anterior neck muscles, 145
  chronic, 124
  vs. nasal breathing, 143
  vs. naso-diaphragmatic breathing, 125
Movement-systems impairment model, 540
MRI (magnetic resonance imaging), 698, 714
  for hamstring tendinopathy, 643
  hyperintense signals, detection of, 641
MSA equipment, 14
MTSS (medial tibial stress syndrome), **714**, 731, 744
Multifidus muscle, 467, 472
Multimodal treatment strategies, 75–76
Muscle-biased manual therapy, for management of trigger points, 835–836
Muscle referred pain, 19
Muscle-specific resisted testing
  for biceps brachii muscle, 295
  for coracobrachialis muscle, 287
  for deltoid muscle, 279
  for infraspinatus muscle, 235
  for subscapularis muscle, 262
  for supraspinatus muscle, 226
  for triceps brachii muscle, 312–313
Muscles. *See also specific muscles*
  activation pattern testing, for gluteus minimus muscle, 582
  anatomy and physiology, 44–48, *45*, *46*, *47*, *48*
  approaches for stretching, 847
  classification of, 44
  contractions, 31, *33*, *34*, *35*, 48–49
    and adenosine triphosphate, 49
    mitochondria, and Ca^{2+} pump, 49
    molecular basis of, *47*
  cramps, 689
  dysfunction, reactive oxygen species and, 40–41
  energy techniques, 847
    clinical application of, 836–837, *837*
    overview of, 836
    patient and intervention selection, 836
    standards and guidelines for, *837*
  function, trigger points, effects of, 843–844
  imbalance, iliopsoas muscles, 517
  length assessment, 399, 558, *560*
  overload, 55
  and posture, 867
  spindle hypothesis, 38–39, *38*
  structure of, *47*
Muscular strain, 349
Musculocutaneous nerve, 285, 290, 293, 302
Myalgia, 63
Myalgic spots, 608
Mylohyoid muscle
  anatomic considerations of, 135
  functions of, 138
  innervation and vascularization of, 137–138
  referred pain pattern, 139
Myobloc (rimabotulinum), 768
Myocardial infarction, 448
Myoclonic Epilepsy with Ragged Red Fibers (MERFF) syndrome, 49
Myofascial dysfunction, management of, 835
Myofascial pain, 2
  disorders, 445
  historical review of, 17
  integrated hypothesis
    biochemical milieu of trigger points, 19
    motor endplate, role of, 17–19, *17*, *18*
    pain and trigger points, 19–20, *20*
  sympathetic nervous system in, 39–40
  taut bands and trigger points, identifying, 17
  in trapezius muscle, 88
Myofascial pain syndrome, 12–13, 44
  chronic pain, altered CNS function, and maladaptive movement patterns, 63–64
  hormonal factors for
    estrogen, 55–56
    subclinical hypothyroidism, 57–58
    testosterone, 57
  mechanical perpetuating factors for
    Ehlers-Danlos syndrome, 61, *62*
    forward head posture, 61–62
    other mechanical stresses, 62–63
  nutritional factors for
    B vitamins, 58–59
    magnesium, 60–61
    vitamin D, 59–60
  other perpetuating factors
    iron deficiency, 64
    protozoal infestation, 64
    sleep deprivation, 64
  and radial tunnel syndrome, 398
  role of fascia in. *See* Fascia
  role of muscles in. *See* Muscles
Myofascial pseudothoracic outlet syndrome, 257
Myofascial trigger points (MTrPs), 55, 837–838. *See also* Trigger points (TrPs)
Myofibrils, 44
Myogenic headaches, 190, 194
Myonecrosis, 765
Myopalladin, 46
Myosin, 31, 44
Myositis ossificans, 124, 125, 133, 143, 479

N

N-methyl-d-aspartate (NMDA), 5, 7, 58–59
NADH (nicotinamide adenine dinucleotide), 49
Nasal breathing, mouth breathing *vs.*, 143
Naso-diaphragmatic breathing, 133

National Health and Nutrition Examination Study, vitamin D deficiency, 59
National Highway Traffic Administration, 374
National Highway Traffic Safety Administration (NHTSA), 887
National Strength and Conditioning Association (NSCA), 847
Nausea, 97
Navicular drop test, 712, 729
NE (norepinephrine), *11*, 13, 40
Nebulin, 46
Neck pain, 325
    characteristics of, 190
    levator scapulae muscle, 202
    manual therapy for, 835
    mechanical, 194
    trigger points, in trapezius muscle and, 85
    from upper cervical joint dysfunction or trigger points, *193*
Neck retraction, active, 184, *184*
Neck rotation, scalene TrP activity and, 213
Needle gauge, selection of, 758–759
Needling therapy. *See also* Dry needling (DN) technique; Trigger point injection (TrPI) technique
    clinical guideline for, application of, 759–762
    for trigger points, 757–758
Needs analysis, and strength training program, 846
Neer impingement test, 228, 265
Neer's sign, 322
Negative emotions, discomfort with, 73
Nephrolithotomy, 314
Nerve conduction testing, for tarsal tunnel syndrome, 750
Nerve entrapment, 598–599
    hip and knee, 662
    lateral pterygoid muscle, 132
Nerve growth factor (NGF), 5
Neuralgia, 630
Neuro-muscular electrical stimulation (NMES), 850
    application of, 857
    background of, 856
    patient selection of, 856–857
    of soleus muscle, 703
Neurodynamic testing, 237, 399, 403, 582
    for gluteus minimus muscle, 582
    for mechanical nerve sensitivity, 658
Neurogenic thoracic outlet syndrome, 430
Neurologic testing, 662
Neuromatrix model, 4
Neuromuscular junction, *48*
    cytosolic Ca^{2+} requirement for muscle contraction, 31, *33*, *34*, *35*
    motor endplate and, 36
    orthodromic axon-stimulus-evoked release, 31, *31*, *32*
    subthreshold depolarization, 31–32
    trigger point taut band, 30
Neuromuscular reeducation, 844, *844*, 845
Neuromuscular therapy (NMT)
    clinical application of, 839–840, *840*, *840*
    overview of, 838–839, *839*
    patient and intervention selection, 839
    standards and guidelines for, *839*
    for vastus lateralis muscle, 838–839, *839*
Neuropathic pain, 4, 373
    syndromes, 195, *195*
Neurophysiological effects, of manual therapies, 834
Neurotoxins
    side effects from, 768
    for trigger point management, 758, 768
Neurotransmitters, 32–33
    feedback control mechanisms, 36
Neurotrophins, 5
Neutral standing posture, sagittal view of, *868*
NGF (nerve growth factor), 5
NHTSA (National Highway Traffic Safety Administration), 887
Nicotinamide adenine dinucleotide (NADH), 49
Nifedipine, 530
NMDA (N-methyl-d-aspartate), 7, 58–59
NMDAR channel, magnesium and, 60
NMES (neuro-muscular electrical stimulation), 850
    application of, 857
    background of, 856
    patient selection of, 856–857

NMT. *See* Neuromuscular therapy (NMT)
Noble compression test, for iliotibial band syndrome, 660
Nociception, 4–5, 5, 6, 7, 55–56
    and modulation, 11–13, *11*, *12*, *13*, *14*
    peripheral, stages of, 9
    and sex differences, 7–8
    stages of, 5
    and transduction, 5–6, 7
    and transmission, 6–7, *8*
Nociceptive pain, **4**
Nociceptors, 10, 51
Nocturnal (nighttime) calf cramps, **687**, 689, 693
Nonarthritic hip pain
    overview of, 656
    patient, initial evaluation of, 656–657
    trigger points and, 657
Noncontact injury, **661**
Noninsertional tendinopathy, 693
Nonpathologic approach, 69
Nonspecific arm pain, 338
Nonsteroidal anti-inflammatory drugs (NSAIDs)
    for ankle sprains, 748
    for ankylosing spondylitis, 547
    and plantar heel pain, 750
Nonthrust mobilization/manipulation, of cervical spine, *833*
Nontraumatic unilateral shoulder pain, chronic, 312
Norepinephrine (NE), *11*, 13, 40
Noxious stimuli, 5
NPRS (numeric pain rating scale), 502
NSAIDs (nonsteroidal anti-inflammatory drugs)
    for ankle sprains, 748
    for ankylosing spondylitis, 547
    and plantar heel pain, 750
NSCA (National Strength and Conditioning Association), 847
Numbness
    of thumb, 211
    and tingling, 212
Numeric pain rating scale (NPRS), 502
Nutritional factors for myofascial pain syndrome
    B vitamins, 58–59
    magnesium, 60–61
    vitamin D, 59–60
Nystagmus, 97

O

Ober test, 583, 660
Obliquus capitis inferior muscle
    anatomic considerations of, 178, *179*
    trigger point examination of, 182–183
Obliquus capitis superior muscle
    anatomic considerations of, 178, *179*
    trigger point examination of, 182
Obturator artery, 622, 624
Obturator externus muscle, **590**
    anatomic considerations of, 590, *592*
        function of, 592–594
        functional unit, 594, *594*
        innervation and vascularization, 591
    clinical presentation of
        patient examination, 595–596
        referred pain pattern, 594–595
        symptoms, 595
        trigger point examination, 597, *597*, 598
    corrective actions for, 599–600, *600*, *601*
    differential diagnosis of
        associated pathology, 598–599
        associated trigger points, 598
        trigger points, activation and perpetuation of, 597–598
    trigger point injection/dry needling technique for, 812, *814*
Obturator femoral artery, 591
Obturator foramen, 590
Obturator internus muscle, **523**, **590**, 591
    anatomic considerations of, 524, *525*, 590, *592*
        function of, 592–594
        functional unit, 594, *594*
        innervation and vascularization, 591
    clinical presentation of
        patient examination, 595–596
        referred pain pattern, 594–595

Obturator internus muscle (*continued*)
    symptoms, 595
    trigger point examination, 596–597, *597*
  corrective actions for, 599–600, *600, 601*
  differential diagnosis of
    associated pathology, 598–599
    associated trigger points, 598
    trigger points, activation and perpetuation of, 597–598
  function of, 526
  referred pain pattern, *528*
  trigger point examination of, 532
  trigger point injection/dry needling technique for, 812, *814*
Obturator nerve, 591, 622, 624
  entrapment, 520
Occipital neuralgia, 85, 163, 173, 195, *195*
Occipitalis muscle, 156–157, *157*
  referred pain pattern, 157, *158*
Occipitofrontalis muscle, **156**
  anatomic considerations of, 156, *157*
    function, 156–157
    functional unit, 157
    innervation and vascularization, 156
  clinical presentation of
    patient examination, 158–159
    referred pain pattern, 157, *158*
    symptoms, 158
    trigger point examination, 159
  corrective actions for, 159–160, *159, 160*
  differential diagnosis of
    associated pathology, 159
    associated trigger points, 159
    trigger points, activation and perpetuation of, 159
  trigger point injection/dry needling technique for, 775, *778*
Occlusal imbalance, 124
Occlusal splint, 110
Occupation, habitual postures of, 869
Occupational Safety and Health Administration (OSHA), 885
Occupational strain, chronic, 494
Ocular migraine, 192
Ocular torticollis, 99
Odynophagia, 131
Olecranon bursitis, 314, 467
Omohyoid muscle, 214, *215,* 217
  anatomic considerations of, 136–137
    functions of, 138–139
    innervation and vascularization of, 137–138
    symptoms, 140
    trigger point examination of, 141
Omohyoid muscle syndrome, 144
Onabotulinum (Botox), 768, *768*
Open heart surgery, 447
Open kinetic prone position, for gluteus maximus muscle, 557
Open scissors syndrome, 872, *874*
Opponens pollicis muscle, **378**
  anatomic considerations of, 378, *379–380*
    function, 379
    functional unit, 379–380, *379*
    innervation and vascularization, 378
  clinical presentation of
    patient examination, 381–382
    referred pain pattern, 380, *381*
    symptoms, 380–381
    trigger point examination, 382, *382*
  corrective actions for, 383–384, *384, 385*
  differential diagnosis of
    associated pathology, 383, *383*
    associated trigger points, 383
    trigger points, activation and perpetuation of, 382–383
  trigger point injection/dry needling technique for, 795, *799*
Optimal posture, defined, **869**
Orbicularis oculi muscle, *157*
  anatomic considerations of, 148, *149*
    function, 150
    functional unit, 151
    innervation and vascularization, 150
  clinical presentation of
    patient examination, 151, 153
    referred pain pattern, 151, *152*
    symptoms, 151
    trigger point examination, 153
  corrective actions for, 154–155, *155*
  differential diagnosis of
    associated pathology, 154
    associated trigger points, 154
    trigger points, activation and perpetuation of, 153–154
Orofacial pain, 835
Oromandibular dystonia, 124, 125, 133, 143
Orthodromic axon-stimulus-evoked release, 31, *31,* 32
Orthopaedic Section of the American Physical Therapy Association (APTA), 661
Orthotic devices, 894
  for pronatory foot, *894*
  for supinatory foot, *895*
Os peroneum, 674, 683
OSHA (Occupational Safety and Health Administration), 885
Osteoarthritis (OA), 315, 392, 400, 651
  carpometacarpal joint, 383
  hip, 574
    overview of, 655
    patient, initial evaluation of, 655–656
    trigger points in, 656
  knee, 615
    overview of, 659
    patient, initial evaluation of, 659
    trigger points and, 659–660
Osteoarthritis Research Society International, 655
Osteoarthrosis, 188
Ottawa Ankle Rules, 748
Outcome measures, use of, 75
Overt hypothyroidism, 58
Oxidative phosphorylation (OXPHOS), 49
Oxytocin, 10

P

Pace abduction test, 595
Pacemaker, and FSM technique, 858
Pacini receptors, 51
Pacinian receptors, 51
PAD mnemonic, 388
Padding, 894
PAG (periaqueductal gray matter), 12, *14*
Pain, 3, 67, 233, 488. *See also* Back pain; Psychosocial considerations
  -adaptation model, 3
  affective responses to, 70–71
  behavioral responses to, 71
  chronic, **2,** 63–64
    types of, 2
  complexity of psychosocial experience of, 70
  experience of living with, 71–72
  model, 3–4, 191–192
  myofascial. *See* Myofascial pain
  and posture, 868
  provocation tests, 543
  of scapula and shoulder, 318
  treatment and clinicians. *See* Clinicians
  and trigger points, 19–20, *20*
Pain-free grip test, 336
Painful arc sign test, **322**
Pain–spasm–pain cycle, 3
Palmar aponeurosis, 360
Palmar fascia, 361
Palmar interosseous muscle, 386
Palmar metacarpal artery, 386–387
Palmaris longus muscle, **360**
  anatomic considerations of, 360–361, *361*
    function, 361
    functional unit, 361–362, *362*
    innervation and vascularization, 361
  clinical presentation of
    patient examination, 362, *363*
    referred pain pattern, 362, *362*
    symptoms, 362
    trigger point examination, 362–363, *363*
  corrective actions for, 364, *364*
  differential diagnosis of
    associated pathology, 363–364
    associated trigger points, 363
    trigger points, activation and perpetuation of, 363

trigger point injection/dry needling technique for, 793, 796
Panniculosis, 474
Pain Catastrophizing Scale, 75
Pain neuroscience education (PNE), 74, 76
Pain pressure threshold (PPT), 690
    subscapularis muscle, 265
    of trigger points of the infraspinatus muscle, 235
Para-aminobenzoic acid, 765
Paradoxical breathing. *See* Chest breathing
Paradoxical nasal obstruction, 123
Paradoxical respiration, 442
Paraspinal compartment syndrome, 479
Passive stretching procedure, **836**
Patellofemoral pain syndrome (PFPS), 507, 571, 574, 614–615, 744
    overview of, 658
    patient, initial evaluation of, 658–659
    treatments for, 658
    trigger points and, 659
Patellar tendinopathy, 615
Patient-centered care, 69
Patient–therapist communication, of manual therapy, 834
Patte test, 244
Pectineus muscle, **621**
    anatomic considerations of, 621–622, *624*
        function, 624–625
        functional unit, 625, *625*
        innervation and vascularization, 622, *624*
    clinical presentation of
        patient examination, 626–628, *628–629*
        referred pain pattern, 626, *627*
        symptoms, 626
        trigger point examination, *629*, 630
    corrective actions for, 631–633, *632–633*
    differential diagnosis of
        associated pathology, 630–632
        associated trigger points, 630
        trigger points, activation and perpetuation of, 630
    trigger point injection/dry needling technique for, 817, *818*
Pectoralis major muscle, **407**, **427**
    anatomic considerations of, 407–409, *407, 408*
        function, 409–410
        functional unit, 410, *410*
        innervation/vascularization, 409
    clinical presentation of
        patient examination, 412–414, *414*
        referred pain pattern, 410–411, *411*
        symptoms, 411–412, *412*
        trigger point examination, 414–415, *415*
    corrective actions for, 417–419, *417, 418, 419*
    differential diagnosis of
        associated pathology, 416–417
        associated trigger points, 416
        trigger points, activation and perpetuation of, 415–416
    trigger point injection/dry needling technique for, 796–798, *801*
Pectoralis minimus muscle, 426
Pectoralis Minor Index (PMI), 430
Pectoralis minor muscle, **426**
    anatomic considerations of, 426, *427*
        function, 427–429
        functional unit, 429, *429*
        innervation and vascularization, 426–427, *428*
    clinical presentation of
        patient examination, 430
        referred pain pattern, 429, *429*
        symptoms, 429–430
        trigger point examination, 430–431, *431*
    corrective actions for, 432–433, *432–433*
    differential diagnosis of
        associated pathology, 432
        associated trigger points, 431–432
        trigger points, activation and perpetuation of, 431
    length assessment, 465
    trigger point injection/dry needling technique for, 799–800, *802*
Pectoralis minor syndrome, 430, 432
Pelvic diaphragm
    coccygeus muscle of, 808
    iliococcygeus muscle of, 808
    pubococcygeus muscle of, 808
Pelvic floor muscles, **523**. *See also specific muscles*

anatomic considerations of, *523–526, 524, 525*
    function, 526–527
    functional unit, 527
    innervation and vascularization, 526
clinical presentation of
    patient examination, 529, *529*
    referred pain pattern, 527, *528*
    symptoms, 527
    trigger point examination, 530–533, *531, 532*
corrective actions for, *534*, 536–538, *537*
differential diagnosis of
    associated pathology, 535
    associated trigger points, 533–535
    trigger points, activation and perpetuation of, 533
postural asymmetries of, 871–872, *872, 872, 873, 873*
Pelvic inflammatory disease, chronic, 598
Pelvic organ dysfunction, 729
Pelvic tilt
    anterior, 871, *872*
    exercise, 495, *495*
    posterior, 871, *872*
Perforating artery, 622, 637, 737
Periaqueductal gray matter (PAG), 12, *14*
Perimysium, 50
Peripheral nerve
    compression, 159
    compression syndrome, 398
    entrapment, 159
Peripheral nociception, stages of, *9*
Peripheral primary afferent nociceptors, 8
Peripheral sensitization, 4, *15*
Peritendinitis, 705
Peroneal muscles. *See* Fibularis muscles
Persistence behaviors, defined, **71**
Persistent sarcomere contractures theory, 37
Pes anserine bursa, 622
Pes anserine bursitis, 643
Pes anserinus, 635
Pes cavus, 740
    injuries with, 891
Pes equinus, 740
Pes planus, injuries with, 891
PFL (popliteofibular ligament), 647, 652
PFPS. *See* Patellofemoral pain syndrome (PFPS)
Phalen test, 402, 403
Phantom pain, **369**
Phentolamine, 40
    depressant effect of, 38
    on endplate noise, 39
Phonophoresis, for trigger points treatment, 854
Photophobia, 153
Physical stress theory, for footwear, 891–892
Physical therapy, treatment-based classification, 540, *541*
Piano key test. *See* Ulnomeniscotriquetral dorsal glide test
Piezo channels, 10, *11*
Pincer grasp sitting, *417*
PIP (proximal interphalangeal) joint, 346, 722
Piriformis muscle, **523**, **589**
    anatomic considerations of, *524–525*, 589, *590, 591, 592*
        function of, 526, 592–594
        functional unit, 594, *594*
        innervation and vascularization, 591
    clinical presentation of
        patient examination, 595–596
        referred pain pattern, 594–595, *594*
        symptoms, 595
        trigger point examination, 596, *596, 597*
    corrective actions for, 599–600, *600, 601*
    differential diagnosis of
        associated pathology, 598–599
        associated trigger points, 598
        trigger points, activation and perpetuation of, 597–598
    internal palpation of, *531*
    syndrome, 595, 598
    trigger point examination of, *532*
    trigger point injection/dry needling technique for, 810–812, *813*
Piriformis myofascial pain syndrome, 594, 598, 658
Pittsburgh Sleep Quality Index, 503
Pivot shift test, to identify ACL tear, 661

Plantar fasciitis. *See* Plantar heel pain
Plantar heel pain, 702, 744, **750**
    overview of, 750
    patient evaluation with, 750–751
    trigger points and, 751
Plantar interosseous muscles
    anatomic considerations of, **736**, *736*
    function, 737
    innervation and vascularization, 737
    referred pain pattern of, 738, *740*
    strength examination of, 740
    trigger point examination of, 741–742, *743*
Plantar intrinsic foot muscles, **734**
    anatomic considerations of, 734–736, *735–736*
        function, 737
        functional unit, 737, *737*
        innervation and vascularization, 736–737
    clinical presentation of
        patient examination, 739–741
        referred pain pattern, 738, *738–740*
        symptoms, 738–739
        trigger point examination, 741–742, *742–743*
    corrective actions for, 744–746, *745–746*
    differential diagnosis of
        associated pathology, 744
        associated trigger points, 744
        trigger points, activation and perpetuation of, 742–744
Plantaris muscle, **697**
    anatomic considerations of, *697*, 698–699
        function, 700
        functional unit, 700, *701*
        innervation and vascularization, 699
    clinical presentation of
        patient examination, 702–703
        referred pain pattern, 702, *702*
        symptoms, 702
        trigger point examination, 703, *704*
    corrective actions for, 706–708, *707*
    differential diagnosis of
        associated trigger points, 705
        pathology, 705–706
        trigger points, activation and perpetuation of, 704–705
    injury, 705
    trigger point injection/dry needling technique for, 824, *824*
Platysma muscle, 362
    anatomic considerations of, 148–149, *149*
        function, 151
        functional unit, 151
        innervation and vascularization, 150
    clinical presentation of
        patient examination, 151, 153
        referred pain pattern, 151, *152*
        symptoms, 151
        trigger point examination, 153, *153*
    corrective actions for, 154–155, *155*
    differential diagnosis of
        associated pathology, 154
        associated trigger points, 154
        trigger points, activation and perpetuation of, 153–154
Pleural dome, 209
Pleural effusion, 447, 448
PMI (Pectoralis Minor Index), 430
Pneumonia, 217
Pneumothorax, 447, 796
PNF (Proprioceptive Neuromuscular Facilitation), 845–846
Pointed heel, 878, *878*
Polarized positive current, 859
Polymodal receptors, 10
Polymorphisms
    and channelopathies, 41
    ion channel, 40
    K$_{ATP}$ receptor channel, 41
Polymyalgia rheumatica, 117
Popliteal artery, 622, 637, 649, 688, 699
Popliteal bursa, 647
Popliteal crease, 877, *878*
Popliteal cyst. *See* Baker cyst
Popliteal veins, 700
Popliteofibular ligament (PFL), 647, 652

Popliteus muscle, **647**
    anatomic considerations of, 647, *648*
        function, 649
        functional unit, 649, *649*
        innervation and vascularization, 649
    clinical presentation of
        patient examination, 650, *650*
        referred pain pattern, 649–650, *649*
        symptoms, 650
        trigger point examination, 650–651, *650*
    corrective actions for, 652–653, *652–653*
    differential diagnosis of
        associated pathology, 651–652
        associated trigger points, 651
        trigger points, activation and perpetuation of, 651
    rupture of, 693
    surgical treatment for, 652
    trigger point injection/dry needling technique for, 819–820, *820*
Popliteus tendinopathy, 651
Popliteus tenosynovitis, 651
Positron emission tomography, 241
Post-laminectomy syndrome, 598
Posterior auricular nerve, 156
Posterior cervical muscles, **168**. *See also specific muscles*
    anatomic considerations of, 168–170, *168, 169, 170*
        function, 171
        functional unit, 171–172, *171*
        innervation and vascularization, 171
    clinical presentation of
        patient examination, 173
        referred pain pattern, 172–173, *172*
        symptoms, 173
        trigger point examination, 173–174, *174*
    corrective actions for, 176–177, *176*
    differential diagnosis of
        associated cervical joint dysfunctions, 176
        associated pathology, 175
        associated trigger points, 175
        trigger points, activation and perpetuation of, 174–175
Posterior circumflex humeral artery, 277, 308
Posterior deltoid fibers
    anatomic considerations of, 277
    function of, 277–278
    trigger point examination of, 281, *281*
Posterior humeral circumflex artery, 241
Posterior intercostal artery, 437, 472
Posterior interosseous nerve, 332, 352
    compression, 397
    entrapment, 357
    nerve syndrome, 338
    neuropathy, 357
Posterior superior iliac spine (PSIS), 503, 597, 871
Posterior sway, 877–878, *878*
Posterior tibial artery, 649, 667, 688, 699, 709, 719, 727
Posterior tibial pulse, palpation of, 740
Posterolateral fibers, 580
Posterolateral rotatory drawer test, 396
Posterolateral rotatory instability, 338, 357, 396
Posteromedial shin splints, **671**
Posterosuperior internal impingement, 321
Postinjection stretch, after TrPI/DN technique, 764
Postisometric relaxation technique, 632
    for brachialis muscle, 305
    with diaphragmatic breathing, 836–837
    with eye movements, 837
    for infraspinatus muscle, 238, *239*, 836, *837*
    for levator scapulae muscle, 206
    for psoas muscles, 520–521
    for sternocleidomastoid muscle, 101, *101*
    for supraspinatus muscle, 229
Postsynaptic effects, 33–34, *35*
Postural education, 764
    for abdominal muscles, 494
    for extensor digitorum muscle, 349
    for extensor indicis muscle, 349
    for gastrocnemius muscle, 693
    for infraspinatus muscle, 237
    for intercostal and diaphragm muscles, 448

for paraspinal muscles, 479
for popliteus muscle, 652
for soleus and plantaris muscles, 706
for subscapularis muscle, 265
for supinator muscle, 357–358, *358*
for supraspinatus muscle, 228–229
for teres minor muscle, 245
Postural orthostatic tachycardia (POTS), 63
Postural stresses, 165, *165*
Posture, 867. *See also* Forward head posture; Postural education
for anterior neck muscles, 144
assessment and examination, considerations for
abdominal wall, 873, *875*
ankle, 877–878, *878*
cervical spine, 874–875, *875*
foot, 877–878, *878*
head, 874–875, *875*
hips, 871–872, *872*
knee, 877, *878*
pelvis, 871–872, *872*
postural dysfunctions, 869–870
postural norms, 869–870
scapulae, 875, *876*, 876
static standing, 870–871, *871*
thigh, 877, *878*
upper extremity region, 876–877, *876, 877*
biomechanical consideration, 868–869, *868*
and breathing, 882–883
diaphragm muscle, 883–884
computer/workstation ergonomic analysis, 885–886, *886*, 886
for coracobrachialis muscle, 290
development of, 869
driving, 886–887, *887*
and foot, 891
genetics, 869
for gluteus maximus muscle, 563
gravitational consideration, 868–869, *868*
for gravitational stress reduction, 176
Janda's crossed syndromes
lower crossed syndrome, 880–881, *881*
upper crossed syndrome, 879–880, *879*
layer syndrome, 881–882, *882*
for levator scapulae muscle, 205
medial pterygoid muscle, 125
and muscle, 867
observation of, 163, 473, 503, 516
and occupation/recreation, 869, *870*
and pain, 868
rhomboid minor and major muscles, 273
for scalene muscles, 219
sitting, 885, *885*
sleeping, 887–888, *888*
and stability, 869
and trigger points, 867–868
POTS (Postural orthostatic tachycardia), 63
PPT (pressure pain threshold), 156, 190, 228
Prayer stretch. *See* Quadruped position
Precision Care, 859
Precordial catch syndrome, 416, 448
Prednisolone, 767
Prednisone, 767
Pregnancy
FSM technique and, 859
hip pain during, 568
Preinjection block, for trigger point injection technique, 759
Pressure pain hypersensitivity, 116
Pressure pain threshold (PPT), 156, 190, 228
Presynaptic neurotransmitters, 32–33
Prickling sensation, 362, *362*
Prilocaine, of trigger point injection, 766
Primary motor cortex of brain, 63–64
Procaine, 761, 765, *765*, 766, 773
Procerus muscle
anatomic considerations of, 149
function, 151
functional unit, 151
innervation and vascularization, 150
clinical presentation of
patient examination, 151, 153
referred pain pattern, 151
symptoms, 151
trigger point examination, 153, *154*
corrective actions for, 154–155, *155*
differential diagnosis of
associated pathology, 154
associated trigger points, 154
trigger points, activation and perpetuation of, 153–154
trigger point injection/dry needling technique for, 775, 778
Procollagen, type V, 62
Proctalgia fugax, 534–535
Profunda artery, 622
Profunda brachii artery, 302, 308, 332
Profunda femoris artery, 622, 624
Pronator quadratus muscle, **367**
anatomic considerations of, 366–367
function, 368–369
functional unit, 369, *369*
innervation and vascularization, 368
clinical presentation of
patient examination, 371, *372*
referred pain pattern, 371, *371*
symptoms, 371
trigger point examination, 371–372, *373*
corrective actions for, 374–376, *376*
differential diagnosis of
associated pathology, 373–374, *374, 375*
associated trigger points, 373
trigger points, activation and perpetuation of, 372–373
trigger point injection/dry needling technique for, 794, 798
Pronator syndrome, 399
Pronator teres muscle, **366**
anatomic considerations of, 366
function, 369
functional unit, 369, *369*
innervation and vascularization, 368
clinical presentation of
patient examination, 371, *372*
referred pain pattern, 370–371, *370*
symptoms, 371
trigger point examination, 371–372, *373*
corrective actions for, 374–376, *376*
differential diagnosis of
associated pathology, 373–374, *374, 375*
associated trigger points, 373
trigger points, activation and perpetuation of, 372–373
trigger point injection/dry needling technique for, 794, 798
Pronator teres syndrome, 374
Pronatory foot, 894–895, *894*
Prone hip extension, *559*
Prone position
sleeping posture in, 888, *888*
for trigger point examination
in dorsal muscles, 742, *743*
in flexor digitorum longus muscle, 729, *729*
in flexor hallucis longus muscle, 729, *729*
in gastrocnemius muscle, 690–691, *691–692*
in gluteus maximus muscle, 559, *563*
in plantaris muscle, 703, *704*
in popliteus muscle, 653, *653*
in rhomboid muscles, 272, *272*
in semimembranosus muscle, 640
in semitendinosus muscle, 640
in soleus muscle, 703, *704*
in splantar muscles, 741–742, *742–743*
in trapezius fibers, 86, *87*
for trigger point injection/dry needling technique
of anconeus muscle, 790, *793*
of biceps femoris muscle, 819, *819*
of cervical multifidus muscle, 777, *780*
of deep paraspinal (multifidus) muscles, 802, *805*
of flexor hallucis longus muscle, 826, *826*
of gastrocnemius muscle, 821–822, *822–823*
of gemelli muscle, 812, *814*
of gluteus maximus muscle, 809–810, *810*
of gluteus medius muscle, 810, *811*
of gluteus minimus muscle, 810, *811*

Prone position (*continued*)
    of hamstring muscles, 819, *819*
    of iliocostalis lumborum muscle, 802, *804*
    of infraspinatus muscle, 782, *784*
    of latissimus dorsi muscle, 782, *786*
    of lower trapezius muscle fibers, 770, *771*
    of middle trapezius muscle fibers, 770, *771*
    of obturator externus muscle, 812, *814*
    of piriformis muscle, 810, *813*
    of plantaris muscle, 824, *824*
    of popliteus muscle, 819–820, *820*
    of posterior deltoid muscle, 787, *788*
    of quadratus femoris muscle, 812, *814*
    of rhomboid muscles, 785–786, *788*
    of serratus posterior inferior muscle, 801, *803*
    of serratus posterior superior muscle, 801, *803*
    of soleus muscle, 822–824, *823*
    of suboccipital muscles, 778, *781*
    of supraspinatus muscle, 781, *783*
    of teres minor muscle, 782, *784*
    of upper trapezius muscle fibers, 770, *770*
Proprioceptive Neuromuscular Facilitation (PNF), 845–846
Proprioceptive theory, 837
Prostatitis, 630
  chronic, 519, 535
Protozoal infestation, 64
Protrusion of mandible, 128
Proximal hamstring tendinopathy, 642–643
Proximal interphalangeal (PIP) joint, 346, 722
Proximal musculocutaneous nerve injury, 290
Pseudo-appendicitis, 489
PSIS (posterior superior iliac spine), 503, 597, 871
Psoas major muscle, **513**
  anatomic considerations of, 513–514, *513*
    function, 514–515
    functional unit, 515, *515*
    innervation and vascularization, 514
  clinical presentation of
    patient examination, 516–517, *517*
    referred pain pattern, 515–516, *516*
    symptoms, 516
    trigger point examination, 518, *518*
  corrective actions for, 520–521, *520*
  differential diagnosis of
    associated pathology, 519–520
    associated trigger points, 519
    trigger points, activation and perpetuation of, 518–519
Psoas minor muscle, **514**
  anatomic considerations of, 514
    function, 514–515
    functional unit, 515, *515*
    innervation and vascularization, 514
  clinical presentation of
    patient examination, 516–517, *517*
    referred pain pattern, 515–516, *516*
    symptoms, 516
    trigger point examination, 518
  corrective actions for, 520–521, *520*
  differential diagnosis of
    associated pathology, 519–520
    associated trigger points, 519
    trigger points, activation and perpetuation of, 518–519
Psoas muscle group. *See also* Psoas major muscle; Psoas minor muscle
  frequency-specific microcurrent, manual therapy with, *860*, 862
  treatment parameters for, *863*
Psoriasis, 175
Psuedotrochanteric bursitis, 582
Psychological acceptance, of pain, 70
Psychological theory of classical/respondent conditioning, 68
Psychosocial considerations
  behavioral learning theories
    classical conditioning, 68
    operant conditioning, 68
  clinical reasoning, 75
    multimodal treatment strategies, 75–76
    referral, role of, 76

cognitive-behavioral themes
  meaning/beliefs/illness perceptions, 68–69
  self-efficacy and locus of control, 68
existential-humanistic themes
  nonpathologic approach, 69
  patient-centered care, 69
  values and meaning, 69
pain
  affective responses to, 70–71
  behavioral responses to, 71
  complexity of psychosocial experience of, 70
  experience of living with, 71–72
  treatment and clinicians. *See* Clinicians
psychological and sociological frameworks, 67
sociologic theories
  attribution theory, 70
  stigma, 70
third-wave behavioral themes
  acceptance, 70
  mindfulness and meditation, 69–70
  validation, 70
Pterygoid fovea, 127
Pterygoideus proprius muscle, 127
Ptosis, 96, 97
P2Y receptor, 11
Pubococcygeus muscle, 523
Puborectalis muscle, 523
Pubovaginal muscle, 526
Pubovaginalis muscle, 523–524
Pudendal nerve, 526
Pudendal plexus, 526
Pulsed ultrasound therapy, 853
"Pump bump," 706
Pump-handle movement of inhalation, 439
Purigenic adenosine receptors, 34
Pyomyositis, 132–133
Pyothorax, 447, 448
Pyramidalis muscle, **484**
  anatomic considerations of, 484, *485*
  functions of, 487
  innervation and vascularization of, 486
  referred pain pattern, 489, *490*
  trigger point injection/dry needling technique for, 804, *806*
Pyridoxine, 58–59

Q

QST. *See* Quantitative sensory testing (QST)
Quadratic heel, 877–878, *878*
Quadratus femoris muscle, **590**
  anatomic considerations of, 590–591, *592*
    function of, 592–594
    functional unit, 594, *594*
    innervation and vascularization, 591
  clinical presentation of
    patient examination, 595–596
    referred pain pattern, 594–595
    symptoms, 595
    trigger point examination, 597, *597*
  corrective actions for, 599–600, *600, 601*
  differential diagnosis of
    associated pathology, 598–599
    associated trigger points, 598
    trigger points, activation and perpetuation of, 597–598
  trigger point injection/dry needling technique for, 812, *814*
Quadratus labii superioris muscle, zygomatic head of, 151
Quadratus lumborum muscle, **497**, 573, 585
  anatomic considerations of, 497–498, *497, 498, 499, 500*
    function, 498–499, *501*
    functional unit, 499–500, *500*
    innervation and vascularization, 498
  clinical presentation of
    patient examination, 503–504, *503, 504*
    referred pain pattern, 500–502, *502*
    symptoms, 502–503
    trigger point examination, 504–507, *505*
  corrective actions for, 508–511, *508, 509, 510, 511*
  differential diagnosis of
    associated pathology, 508

associated trigger points, 507–508
  trigger points, activation and perpetuation of, 507
  serial cross sections of, 506
  trigger point injection/dry needling technique for, 804, 806, 807, 808
Quadratus plantae muscle. *See* Flexor accessorius muscle
Quadriceps femoris muscles, **604**. *See also specific muscles*
  anatomic considerations of, 604–606, *604, 605*
    function, 606–607
    functional unit, 607, *607*
    innervation and vascularization, 606
  clinical presentation of
    patient examination, 610–611
    referred pain pattern, 607–608, *608, 609*
    symptoms, 610
    trigger point examination, 611–612, *612, 613*
  corrective actions for, 615–616, *616, 617, 618*
  differential diagnosis of
    associated pathology, 614–615
    associated trigger points, 614
    trigger points, activation and perpetuation of, 613
Quadrilateral space syndrome, 245, 257
Quadruped position
  self-stretch of right quadratus lumborum muscle in, 511, *511*
  for thoracolumbar paraspinal muscles, 479, *480*
  for trapezius muscle, 91, *91*
Quadruped rocking, 557, *558*
Quantitative sensory testing (QST), 13–14, **13**, *15*, 850, 851
  mechanical pain threshold, 15–16, *16*
  mechanical/tactile detection threshold, 14, *16*
  thermal detection and pain threshold, 14
  and trigger points, 16–17
  vibration detection threshold, 14, *16*
Quebec Task Force, 190
Quick awkward movement, 478

R
Radial nerve
  compression, 303
  entrapment, 302, 304, 315, 397–398
  innervation, 307–308, 345
  neurodynamic testing of, 355
Radial tunnel syndrome, 336, 338, 357, 397
Radicular pain/radiculopathy, 479, 692, 865, **692**. *See also* Cervical radicular pain/radiculopathy; Lumbar radicular pain/radiculopathy
Radiocapitellar arthritis, 396
Radiocapitellar joint pathology, 338, 357, 396
Radiohumeral joint, 355
Radioulnar joint, 355
Rapid/bouncing stretches, 847
Rational Emotive Behavior Therapy, 71
Raynaud phenomenon, 399
Reactive arthritis, 175
Reactive oxygen species (ROS), 40–41
Reciprocal click, 188
Reciprocal inhibition/innervation, 845
Recreation, and posture, 869, *870*
Rectus abdominis muscle, **484**, 562
  anatomic considerations of, 484, *485*
    functions of, 487
    innervation and vascularization of, 484, 486
  patient examination for, 492
  referred pain pattern, 488–489, *490*
  trigger point examination of, 492–493, *493*
  trigger point injection/dry needling technique for, 804, *806*
Rectus abdominis–diaphragmatic reflex inhibition, 492
Rectus capitis anterior muscle, **137**
  anatomic considerations of, 137
  functions of, 139
  innervation and vascularization of, 137–138
Rectus capitis lateralis muscle, **137**
  anatomic considerations of, 137
  functions of, 139
  innervation and vascularization of, 137–138
Rectus capitis posterior major muscle, **178**
  anatomic considerations of, 178, *179*
  trigger point examination of, 182

Rectus capitis posterior minor muscle, **178**
  anatomic considerations of, 178, *179*
  trigger point examination of, 182
Rectus femoris muscle, **604**
  anatomic considerations of, 604, *604*
  associated trigger points of, 614
  referred pain pattern of, 607, *608*
  symptoms from, 610
  tightness of, 519
  trigger point examination of, 611, *612*
  trigger point injection/dry needling technique for, 812, *815*
Referral, role of, 76
Referred pain, 2, 4, 19–20, 178. *See also under* individual muscles
Referred sensation, 4, 19
Reiter's syndrome, 175
Renal diseases, 467
Repetition volume, 847
Resisted jaw opening, 110, *110*, 125, *125*
Resisted movement testing of the wrist extensors, 336
Respirasomes, 49
Respiration, 882
Respiratory function, 883–884
Respiratory mechanics, 439, *441*
  assessment, 445–446
Respiratory synkinesis, **837**
Restless legs syndrome, 64
Retropharyngeal calcific tendinitis, 143
Reverse Phalen test, 403
Reverse Thomas heel, 892, 895
Revised FIQ SF-36v2, 61
Rheumatoid arthritis, 124, 349, 714
Rhomboid interdigitating, 268
Rhomboid minor and major muscles, **268**
  anatomic considerations of, 268, *269*
    function, 269–270
    functional unit, 270, *270*
    innervation and vascularization, 268–269
  clinical presentation of
    patient examination, 271–272
    referred pain pattern, 270, *271*
    symptoms, 270–271
    trigger point examination, 272, *272*
  corrective actions for, 273–274, *273, 274*
  differential diagnosis of
    associated pathology, 273
    associated trigger points, 273
    trigger points, activation and perpetuation of, 272
  trigger point injection/dry needling technique for, 785–786, *788*
Rhomboid tertius muscle, 268
Rib positions, change of, 439, *440*
Rib-tip syndrome, 416, 491
Right finger extensor muscle, 343, *344*
Right zygomaticus major muscle, 775, *777*
Rigor mortis, 40
Rimabotulinum (Myobloc), *768*
Ring finger extensor, 346, *347*
Rocker bottom shoe, 893–894
Roland-Morris Low Back Questionnaire, 503
Romberg sign, 97, 545
Roos' test, 314, 320, 432
Ropivacaine, 766
Rostral ventromedial medulla (RVM), 56
Rotator cuff muscles. *See salso* pecific muscles
  tears, 244, 282
Rotator cuff syndrome, 321–322
Rotatores muscles, 472
  anatomic considerations of, *168, 169,* 170
  function, 171
  referred pain pattern, 173
  trigger point examination of, 173, *174*
Rounded shoulder, 219
Rounded shoulder posture, 166, 273, 429, 455
  correction of, 432
Royal London Hospital Test, 693
Ruffini receptors, 51
RVM (rostral ventromedial medulla), 56
Ryanodine receptor (RyR) calcium channel, 31
Rydel–Seiffer tuning fork, 14

S

Sacral artery, 498, 591
Sacral multifidus trigger points, 478
Sacral nerve, 526, 591
Sacral plexus, 591, 666
Sacral stress test, 544
Sacrococcygeus ventralis muscle, **526**
    anatomic considerations of, 526
    trigger point examination of, 532
Sacroiliac arthritis. *See* Sacroiliitis
Sacroiliac joint (SIJ), 249
    dysfunction, 542–543, 562, 569, 573
        causes of pain, 543
        initial evaluation of, 543–544
        signs and symptoms, 543
        trigger points and, 544
    ipsilateral, 701, 702
    movement assessment, 503
    stability, 555
Sacroiliac syndrome, 479
Sacroiliitis, 598, 599
Sacrospinous ligament, 589
Saddle anesthesia, 544–545
Sarcomere, 42, *42*, 44, *46*
Sarcoplasmic/endoplasmic reticulum Ca^{2+} ATPase (SERCA) pump, 49
Sartorius muscle, **604**
    anatomic considerations of, 606, *606*
        function, 607
        functional unit, 607, *607*
        innervation and vascularization, 606
    clinical presentation of
        patient examination, 610–611
        referred pain pattern, 608, *610*
        symptoms, 610
        trigger point examination, 613, *614*
    corrective actions for, 615–616, *618*, *619*
    differential diagnosis of
        associated pathology, 615
        associated trigger points, 614
        trigger points, activation and perpetuation of, 614
    trigger point injection/dry needling technique for, 814, *817*
Satellite glial cells, 8
Scalene cramp test, 213, *213*
Scalene muscles, **208**, 441, 442, 466
    anatomic considerations of, 208–209, *209*, *210*
        function, 209–210
        functional unit, 210, *210*
        innervation and vascularization, 209
    clinical presentation of
        patient examination, 212–214, *213*, *214*
        referred pain pattern, 211, *212*
        symptoms, 211–212
        trigger point examination, 214–216, *215*, *216*
    corrective actions for, 219–221, *219*, *220*
    differential diagnosis of
        associated pathology, 217–219, *218*
        associated trigger points, 217
        trigger points, activation and perpetuation of, 216–217
    trigger point injection/dry needling technique for, 778–779, *782*
Scalene pain, 211
Scalene relief position, 213, *214*
Scalene syndrome, 392
Scalenotomy, 210
Scalenus anterior muscle, 208, **208**, *209*
Scalenus anticus (anterior scalene) syndrome, 217
Scalenus medius muscle, 208, **208**, *209*, 215
Scalenus minimus muscle, 208–209, **208**, *210*, 216
Scalenus posterior muscle, 208, **208**, *209*, 215
Scapula
    abduction of, 262
    anterior tilting of, 875, *876*
    coracoid process of, 426, *427*
    levator scapulae muscle attachments to, 199
    movements of, 81–82, *82*
    pain in, 455, 462
    position of, 465
    postural assessment of, 875, *876*, *876*

SICK, 204
    winged, 430, 465
Scapular abduction, 875, *876*
Scapular depression, 877, *877*
Scapular dyskinesia, **228**, **265**, **323**, 429, 465
    initial evaluation of, 323
    trigger points and, 323–324
Scapular posterior tilting, 91, *91*
Scapular protraction, 273
Scapular retractor, 82
Scapular rotation, loss of, 202
Scapular winging, 271, 458
Scapulocostal syndrome, 325, 464–465, 467
Scapulothoracic bursitis, 264
Scapulothoracic joint, 430
SCEBS model, 75
Sciatic nerve, 591, 593, *593*, 622, 637, 662
Sciatica, 508, **581**, 599, 638
    back pocket, 598
SCM muscle. *See* Sternocleidomastoid (SCM) muscle
Scoliosis, 869
Scotty dog collar fracture, 546
Scour test, 656
Scratch collapse test, 681
SCS technique. *See* Strain counterstrain (SCS) technique
SEA (spontaneous electrical activity), 29, *30*
Seated position
    activation of deep neck flexors in, 145, *145*
    for acutely painful shoulder, 265, *266*
    assessment of, 503
    differentiation of rhomboid muscles in, 272, *272*
    for pelvic floor muscles, 536
    trigger point self-pressure release
        of adductor muscles, *631*, 632
        of infraspinatus muscle, 238, *238*
        of levator scapulae muscle, 205–206, *205*
        of quadratus lumborum muscle, 510, *510*
        of quadriceps femoris muscles, 615, *616*
        of tibialis posterior muscle, 715, *715*
Second-to-fifth-toe extension exercise, 746, *746*
Secondary messenger, 5, 8, 39
Segmental joint dysfunction, 479
Segmental sarcomere contraction, 29, *30*
Self-audit, 72
Self-awareness
    countertransference, 72
    discomfort with negative emotions, 73
Self-care, 74
Self-efficacy, 68
Self-intraoral release, of masseter muscle, 109
Self-pressure release techniques
    for adductor muscles, *631*, 632
    for adductor pollicis muscle, 384, *384*
    for brachialis muscle, 304–305, *304*
    for coracobrachialis muscle, 289, *290*
    for deltoid muscle, 283, *283*
    for diaphragm muscle, 448–450, *449*, *450*
    for extensor digitorum muscle, 350, *350*
    for extensor indicis muscle, 350, *350*
    for fibularis muscles, 683, *684*
    for flexor digitorum longus muscle, *731*, 732
    for flexor hallucis longus muscle, *731*, 732
    for frontalis trigger points, 159, *159*
    for gastrocnemius muscle, 693–694, *694*
    for gluteus maximus muscle, 563, *564*
    for gluteus medius muscle, 574, *574*
    for gluteus minimus muscle, 585–586, *586*
    for hamstring muscles, 643–644, *643*
    for infraspinatus muscle, 238
    for intercostal muscle, 448, *449*, *450*
    for interosseous, lumbrical, and abductor digiti minimi muscles, 392, *393*
    for latissimus dorsi muscle, 252–253, *252*
    for levator scapulae muscle, 205, *206*
    for long toe extensor muscles, 723–724, *723*
    for occipitalis trigger points, 159, *160*
    for opponens pollicis muscle, 384, *384*
    for paraspinal muscles, 479, *480*
    for pectoralis major muscle, 417, *418*, *418*

for pectoralis minor muscle, 432, *432*
for piriformis and deep external rotator muscles of hip, 599, *600*
for plantar foot muscles, 745, *746*
for popliteus muscle, 652, *652*
for quadratus lumborum muscle, 510, *510*
for quadriceps femoris, 615–616, *617*
for rhomboid minor and major muscles, 273–274, *273*, *274*
for sartorius muscles, *616*, *618*
for serratus anterior muscle, 458, *458*
for serratus posterior superior muscle, 467, *467*
for soleus muscle, 706–707, *707*
for sternalis muscle, 424, *424*
for subscapularis muscle, 265, *266*
for supraspinatus muscle, 228, *229*
for tensor fasciae latae muscle, *586*, *587*
for teres major muscle, 257–258, *257*, *258*
for teres minor muscle, 246
therapeutic wand and instrument for, *534*
for tibialis anterior muscle, 671, *671*
for tibialis posterior muscle, 715–716, *715*
for triceps brachii muscle, *315*, 316
using pincer palpation technique, *298*, 299
for wrist extensor muscle, 339, *339*
for wrist flexor, finger flexor, and pronator muscles, 375, *376*
Self-reflection, 72
Self-regulation, 68
Self-Regulation Model of Illness. *See* Common-Sense Model of Self-Regulation
Self-stretching techniques. *See also* Flexibility training program
for adductor muscles, 633, *633*
for adductor pollicis muscle, *384*, 385
for biceps brachii muscle, 299, *299*
for brachialis muscle, 305
for brachioradialis muscle, 340, *340*
for buccinator muscle, 155, *155*
for coracobrachialis muscle, 290–291, *290*
for extensor digitorum longus muscle, 724, *724*
for extensor hallucis longus muscle, 724, *724*
for fibularis muscles, 683, *684*
for finger extensor muscles, 350, *350*
for flexor digitorum longus muscle, 732, *732*
for flexor hallucis longus muscle, 732, *732*
for gastrocnemius muscle, 694–695, *695*
for gluteus maximus muscle, *563*, *564*
for gluteus medius muscle, 574–575, *575*
for gluteus minimus muscle, 586
for hamstring muscles, 644–645, *644–645*
for iliopsoas muscles, 520, *520*
for infraspinatus muscle, 238, *239*
for intercostal and diaphragm muscles, 450
for interosseous, lumbrical, and abductor digiti minimi muscles, *392*, *393*
for lateral pterygoid muscle, 133
for latissimus dorsi muscle, 253, *253*
for levator scapulae muscle, *205*, 206
for opponens pollicis muscle, *384*, 385
for palmaris longus muscle, 364
for paraspinal muscles, 479, *480*
for pectoralis major muscle, 418–419, *418*, *419*
for pectoralis minor muscle, 432–433, *433*
for piriformis and deep external rotator muscles of hip, 599, *601*
for popliteus muscle, 652–653, *653*
for quadratus lumborum muscle, 510–511, *510*, *511*
for scalene muscles, 219, *219*, 221
for serratus anterior muscle, 458, *459*
for serratus posterior inferior muscle, 468, *468*
for soleus muscle, 707–708, *707*
for sternocleidomastoid muscle, 100–101, *101*
for suboccipital musculature, 184–185, *184*
for subscapularis muscle, 265–266, *266*
for supraspinatus muscle, 229, *229*
for temporalis muscle, 118, *118*
for tensor fasciae latae muscle, *587*, 587
for teres major muscle, 258, *258*
for teres minor muscle, 246
for tibialis anterior muscle, 671–672, *672*
for tibialis posterior muscle, 715, 716
for toe flexors, 745, *746*
for triceps brachii muscle, 316, *316*

for wrist extensors, 340, *340*
for wrist flexor, finger flexor, and pronator muscles, 375–376, *376*
for zygomaticus major muscle, 155, *155*
Semimembranosus muscle, 635–636, 636–637. *See also* Hamstring muscles
Semispinalis capitis muscle, **169**
anatomic considerations of, 169–170, *169*, *170*
function of, 171
referred pain pattern of, 172, *172*
trigger point examination of, 173
trigger point injection/dry needling technique for, 777, *780*
Semispinalis cervicis muscle, **170**
anatomic considerations of, *168*, 170
function of, 171
referred pain pattern of, 173
trigger point examination of, 173–174
trigger point injection/dry needling technique for, 777, *780*
Semitendinosus muscle, **635**, *635*. *See also* Hamstring muscles
Semmes Weinstein monofilaments, 14, 403, 740
Sensitization, characteristics of, 4
Sensorimotor training, 882
Sensory deficits, 392
cervical radicular pain, 318
Sensory fibers, 51
Serape effect, 453
Serapin, 767
SERCA (Sarcoplasmic/endoplasmic reticulum Ca^{2+} ATPase) pump, 49
Seronegative spondyloarthropathy disorders, 175
Serotonin (5 HT), 11, 32
Serratus anterior muscle, **453**
anatomic considerations of, *454*
function, 453–454
functional unit, 455, *455*
innervation and vascularization, 453
clinical presentation of
patient examination, 455–457
referred pain pattern, 455, *456*
symptoms, 455
trigger point examination, 457, *457*
corrective actions for, 458, *458–459*
differential diagnosis of
associated pathology, 457–458
associated trigger points, 457
trigger points, activation and perpetuation of, 457
trigger point injection/dry needling technique for, 800, *803*
Serratus posterior inferior muscle, **460**
anatomic considerations of, 460, *463*
function, 461
functional unit, 462
innervation and vascularization, 460
clinical presentation of
patient examination, 465–466
referred pain pattern, 463, *465*
symptoms, 465
trigger point examination, 466, *466*
corrective actions for, 467, 468, *468*
differential diagnosis of
associated pathology, 467
associated trigger points, 467
trigger points, activation and perpetuation of, 466
trigger point injection/dry needling technique for, 801, *803*
Serratus posterior superior muscle, **460**
anatomic considerations of, 460, *461*, *462*
function, 460
functional unit, 462
innervation and vascularization, 460
clinical presentation of
patient examination, 465
referred pain pattern, 462–463, *464*
symptoms, 463–465
trigger point examination, 466, *466*
corrective actions for, 467, *467*
differential diagnosis of
associated pathology, 467
associated trigger points, 466–467
trigger points, activation and perpetuation of, 466
trigger point injection/dry needling technique for, 801, *803*

Sesamoid bone, 647
Sesamoiditis, 752–753
    overview of, 752–753
    patient evaluation with, 753
    trigger points and, 753
Sex differences, nociception and, 7–8
Sexual dimorphism, 57
Shame, 71
SHLP (superior head of lateral pterygoid) muscle, 128
Shoe
    design, 892
    modifications, 893–894
    parts of, 892
    for pronatory foot, 894
    proper fitting of, 892, 893, 893
    rocker bottom, 893–894
    for supinatory foot, 895
Shin splints, **670**
    anterolateral, **670**
    posteromedial, **671**
    syndrome, 714
Short external rotators. *See specific muscles*
Short-foot exercise, 746, *746*
Short head of biceps brachii, 293
"Short of breath," 455
Short Physical Performance Battery, 61
Shoulder(s)
    abduction, 222–223
    depression function, 427
    frozen, 447, 257, 324. *See also* Subscapularis muscle
    impingement syndrome, 228, 237, 261, 295, 321–323, 879
    ipsilateral, 445
    muscular regional anatomy of, *288*
    musculature, activation of, 224
    pain, 228, 321
        chronic nontraumatic unilateral, 297, 312
        hemiplegia-related, 265
        levator scapulae muscle, 202
        scalene trigger points, 211, 217
Sibson's fascia, 209
SICK scapula, 204
Sick stomach, 97
Side-lying position
    hip abduction muscle activation, 503, *504*, 570, *571*
    sleeping posture in, 100, *100*, 888, *888*
    for trigger point examination
        in flexor digitorum longus muscle, 729, *729*
        in flexor hallucis longus muscle, 729, *729*
        in gastrocnemius muscle, 690–691, *691–692*
        in gluteus minimus muscle, 583, *583*
        in intercostal muscles, 446, *447*
        in latissimus dorsi muscle, 251, *251*
        in pectoralis major muscle, 414–415, *415*
        in right external oblique muscle, 492, *493*
        in serratus anterior muscle, 457, *457*
        in soleus muscle, 703, *704*
        in tensor fasciae latae muscle, 583, *584*
        in thoracolumbar paraspinal muscles, 477, *477*
        in tibialis posterior muscle, 713, *713*
        in vastus lateralis muscle, 612, *613*
        in wrist and finger flexors, 372, *373*
    for trigger point injection/dry needling technique
        of abductor digiti minimi muscle, 826–828, *827*
        of abductor hallucis muscle, 826, *827*
        of adductor hallucis muscle, 828, *829*
        of coccygeus muscle, of pelvic diaphragm, 808
        of fibularis brevis muscle, 820, *821*
        of fibularis longus muscle, 820, *821*
        of flexor accessorius (quadratus plantae) muscle, 827, 828
        of flexor digitorum brevis muscle, 826, *827*
        of flexor digitorum longus muscle, 826, *826*
        of flexor hallucis brevis muscle, 828, *828*
        of gluteus maximus muscle, 809–810, *810*
        of gluteus minimus muscle, 810, *811*
        of iliococcygeus muscle, of pelvic diaphragm, 808
        of iliocostalis lumborum muscle, 802, *804*
        of infraspinatus muscle, 782, *784*
        of lateral head, of triceps brachii muscle, 790, *792*
        of levator scapula muscle, 778, *781*
        of long head, of triceps brachii muscle, 790, *791*
        of medial head, of triceps brachii muscle, 790, *792*
        of middle deltoid muscle, 786–787, *788*
        of obturator internus muscle, 812, *814*
        of piriformis muscle, 810, *813*
        of popliteus muscle, 819–820, *820*
        of pubococcygeus muscle, of pelvic diaphragm, 808
        of quadratus lumborum muscle, 804, 806, *807*, 808
        of semispinalis capitis muscle, 777, *780*
        of semispinalis cervicis muscle, 777, *780*
        of serratus anterior muscle, 800, *803*
        of soleus muscle, 822–824, *823*
        of splenius capitis muscle, 776, *779*
        of splenius cervicis muscle, 776, *779*
        of supraspinatus muscle, 781, *783*
        of tensor fasciae latae muscle, 810, *812*
        of teres major muscle, 785, *787*
        of teres minor muscle, 782, *784*
        of tibialis posterior muscle, 824, *824*
        of vastus lateralis muscle, 813–814, *816*
    trigger point self-pressure release
        of adductor muscles, 631, *632*
        of diaphragm muscle, 448, *449*
        of gluteus maximus muscle, 563, *564*
        of gluteus medius muscle, 574, *574*
        of infraspinatus muscle, 238, *238*
        of pectoralis major muscle, 417, *418*
        of pelvic floor muscles, 536–537, *537*
Signalosome, 12
SIJ. *See* Sacroiliac joint (SIJ)
Silfverskiold sign, 690, *690*
Simons' Integrated Hypothesis, 29, 36–38, *37, 37*
Single-heel-rise test, 712, 714
Single-leg squat, 627, 669, 679, 689, 702, 712, 720, 729
Single-leg stance posture, 569, *569*
Single-muscle syndrome, 338, 584, 585, 744, 851
Sinus
    drainage, 98
    infection, 97
    pain, 123, 130
Sinusitis, 96, 99, 105, 123, 130, 133
SIS (Subacromial impingement syndrome), 204, 228, 237, 265, 282, 289, 429
Sit-back/abdominal-curl/sit-up exercise, 486, 495
Sit-to-stand technique, 509, *510*
    for paraspinal muscles, 479
Sitting position, 885, *885*
    for extensor digitorum and extensor indicis muscles, 350, *350*
    for gluteus maximus muscle, 563
    for hamstring muscle examination, 639
    for piriformis and deep external rotator muscles of hip, 599
    popliteus muscle, relaxation of, 653, *653*
    for psoas muscles, 520
Skeletal muscle. *See* Muscles
Skinner's theory of operant conditioning, 68
Sleep apnea, 64
Sleep deprivation, 64
Sleeping position, 204, 887–888, *888*
    for biceps brachii muscle, 298, *299*
    for brachialis muscle, 304
    for coracobrachialis muscle, 290
    of fetal position, 519
    with foot, 693, *694*
    for gluteus maximus muscle, 563
    for gluteus medius muscle, 574
    for gluteus minimus trigger points, 585
    for hamstring trigger points, 643
    for infraspinatus muscle, 237–238, *238*
    for latissimus dorsi muscle, 252
    for medial pterygoid muscle, 125
    for paraspinal muscles, 479
    for piriformis and deep external rotator muscles of hip, 599, *600*
    prone position, 888, *888*
    for psoas muscles, 520
    for quadratus lumborum muscle, 508–509, *508*
    for scalene muscles, 216, 219
    for serratus anterior muscle, 458
    for serratus posterior superior muscle, 467

side-lying position, 888, *888*
supine position, 887, *888*
for supporting finger extensors, 349, *350*
for supraspinatus muscle, 228
for tensor fasciae latae trigger points, 587
for teres major muscle, 257
for teres minor muscle, 245–246
for triceps brachii and anconeus muscles, 316
Sliding-filament mechanism, 34, *46*
of muscle contraction, *35*
Slipping rib syndrome, 416, 448, 491
SLR (straight leg raise), 542, 662, 692
for hamstring muscle length assessment, 639, *640*, 642
Slump test, 595, 658, 662
"Slumped" posture, 263
Social-learning theory of personality, 68
Sociologic theories
attribution theory, 70
stigma, 70
Sodium chloride injection, 211, 294
Soft collar, for relieving stress on posterior neck muscles, *176*, 177
Soleus enthesopathy, 714
Soleus muscle, 669, 671, 687, **697**, 729–730
anatomic considerations of, 697–698, *697–700*
function, 699–700
functional unit, 700, *701*
innervation and vascularization, 699
clinical presentation of
patient examination, 702–703, *703*
referred pain pattern, 701, *701*
symptoms, 697, 702
trigger point examination, 703, *704*
corrective actions for, 706–708, *707*
differential diagnosis of, 697
associated pathology, 705–706
associated trigger points, 705
trigger points, activation and perpetuation of, 704–705
fiber orientation of, 700
injury, 705
loading and off-loading considerations for, *895*
trigger point injection/dry needling technique for, 822–824, *823*
weakness testing, 703
Soleus tightness/hypertrophy, 878, *878*
Somatic Symptom Disorder, 72
Somaticizing tendency, 69
Somato-visceral effects, 490, 547–548, *548*
Somatosensory system, 869
"Sore feet," 718
Sore inflamed joint, 390
Sore throat, 96
Spasmodic torticollis (cervical dystonia), 204
Spatial summation, 845
Sphenoid bone, 120, *121*, 773
Sphere of influence, focusing on, 73
Sphincter ani muscle, **523**
anatomic considerations of, 523, *524*
function of, 526
needling of, 807
referred pain pattern, *528*
trigger point examination of, 530
Sphincter vaginae, 525
Spigelian hernias, 491
Spinal-mediated mechanisms, of manual therapy, 834
Spinal nerve, 209, 285, 332, 368, 514, 649
Spinal rotation and flexion, 488
Spinal stabilization program, 521
Spinal stenosis, 508
Spinalis muscle, 469
Spinotransverse muscle. *See* Deep paraspinal muscle
Spiralizer, 94
Splenius capitis muscle, **161**
anatomic considerations of, 161, *162*
function, 161
functional unit, 162, *163*
innervation and vascularization, 161
clinical presentation of
patient examination, 163
referred pain pattern, 162–163, *164*
symptoms, 163

trigger point examination, 163, *165*
corrective actions for, 166
differential diagnosis of
associated pathology, 166
associated trigger points, 166
trigger points, activation and perpetuation of, 165–166, *165*
trigger point injection/dry needling technique for, 776, 779
Splenius cervicis muscle, **161**
anatomic considerations of, 161, *162*
function, 161–162
functional unit, 162, *163*
innervation and vascularization, 161
clinical presentation of
patient examination, 163
referred pain pattern, 162–163, *164*
symptoms, 163
trigger point examination, 163–165, *165*
corrective actions for, 166
differential diagnosis of
associated pathology, 166
associated trigger points, 166
trigger points, activation and perpetuation of, 165–166, *165*
trigger point injection/dry needling technique for, 776, 779
Splinting, 392
Spondyloarthritides, 546
Spondylolisthesis, **546**
Spondylolysis, **546**
Spontaneous electrical activity (SEA), 29, *30*
Sports hernia, 630, 519. *See also* Athletic pubalgia
Sprain, ankle
overview of, 748
patient evaluation with, 748
trigger points and, 748–749
"Spray-and-stretch" technique, 850–851
Spurling sign, 237, 297, 371
Spurling's test, 318
Square-shaped heel. *See* Quadratic heel
Stability, **845**
and posture, 869
Stabilizer, 893
Stance phase
popliteus muscle during, 649
Stand-to-sit technique, *509*, 510
for paraspinal muscles, 479
Star Excursion Balance Test, 748
Static standing assessment, of posture, *868*, 870–871
Static stiffness, 42, *42*
Stenosing tenosynovitis, 730
Stenosis
frequency-specific microcurrent, for patients with, 859
midscapular pain from, 865
Steppage gait, **669**
Sternal division of sternocleidomastoid muscle
anatomic considerations of, 94, *94*
referred pain pattern, 96
Sternal lamina, 408, *408*
Sternalis muscle, **421**
anatomic considerations of, 421, *422*
function, 421
functional unit, 422
innervation and vascularization, 421
clinical presentation of
patient examination, 423
referred pain pattern, 422–423, *423*
symptoms, 423
trigger point examination, 423
corrective actions for, 424, *424*
differential diagnosis of
associated pathology, 424
associated trigger points, 424
trigger points, activation and perpetuation of, 423–424
trigger point injection/dry needling technique for, 798, *801*
Sternoclavicular joint, 430
Sternocleidomastoid (SCM) muscle, 62, **94**, 117, 124, 132, 140, *144*, 208, 215, *215*
anatomic considerations of, 94–95, *94*
function, 95
functional unit, 95–96, *95*
innervation and vascularization, 95

Sternalis muscle (*continued*)
    clinical presentation of
        patient examination, 97
        referred pain pattern, 96–97, *96*
        symptoms, 97
        trigger point examination, 97–98, *98*
    corrective actions for, 100–101, *100*, *101*
    differential diagnosis of
        associated pathology, 99–100
        associated trigger points, 99
        trigger points, activation and perpetuation of, 98–99
    groove along, 874–875, *875*
    Integrated Neuromuscular Inhibition Technique for, 839–840, *840*, *840*
    trigger point
        injection/dry needling technique for, 770–771, *772*
        of migraine, *193*
        of tension-type headache, *194*
Sternohyoid muscle, **135**
    anatomic considerations of, 135
    functions of, 138–139
    innervation and vascularization of, 137–138
    syndrome, 144
Sternothyroid muscle, **135**
    anatomic considerations of, 135
    functions of, 138–139
    innervation and vascularization of, 137–138
Sternum, change of position, 439, *440*
Steroids, for ankylosing spondylitis, 547
Stiff neck syndrome, 85, 97, 100, 163, 202, 325
Stigma, 70
Straight leg raise (SLR), 542, 662, 692
    for hamstring muscle length assessment, 639, *640*, 642
Strain counterstrain (SCS) technique
    advantages of, 838
    clinical application of, 838, *838*
    defined, **837**
    overview of, 837–838
    patient and intervention selection, 838
Stratification syndrome. *See* Layer syndrome
Strength training program, 846–847
    design variables for, 846, *847*
    exercise selection, 846
    load and repetition, volume of, 847
    needs analysis, 846
    training frequency, 846–847
    training load, 846
Stress
    abdominal wall trigger points and, 494
    activity-based, 166
    management, 125
    masseter muscle, 110
    testing, carpal tunnel syndrome and, 403
Stretch reflex, 837
Stretching interventions
    clinical application of, 836–837, *837*
    overview of, 836
    patient and intervention selection, 836
Stretching training program, 847–848
String models, 593
Stripping massage. *See* Deep-stroking massage technique
Strumming massage technique, 841–842, *841*
Stuck patella muscle, 608. *See also* Vastus lateralis muscle
Stylohyoid muscle
    anatomic considerations of, 135
    functions of, 138
    innervation and vascularization of, 137–138
    referred pain pattern, 139
Subacromial bursa, 322
Subacromial bursitis, 228, 257, 264, 289
Subacromial impingement syndrome (SIS), 204, 228, 237, 265, 282, 289, 429
Subacromial pain syndrome, 228, 264, 426, 429, 457
    initial evaluation of, 322
    rotator cuff syndrome and shoulder impingement, 321–322
    trigger points and, 322–323, *323*
Subclavian artery, 210, *210*
Subclavius muscle, **409**
    anatomic considerations of, 409

function, 410
functional unit, 410
innervation/vascularization, 409
clinical presentation of
    patient examination, 412–414, *414*
    referred pain pattern, 411
    symptoms, 411–412
    trigger point examination, 415, *415*
corrective actions for, 417–419
differential diagnosis of
    associated pathology, 417
    associated trigger points, 416
    trigger points, activation and perpetuation of, 415–416
trigger point injection/dry needling technique for, 798, *802*
Subcostal artery, 472, 498
Subcostales muscle, 436
Subcutaneous herniation, of tibialis anterior muscle, 671
Subdeltoid bursa, 322
Subdeltoid bursitis, 224, 228, 257, 282, 297
Suboccipital muscles, **178**. *See also* individual muscles
    anatomic considerations of, 178, *179*
        function, 179, *180*
        functional unit, 179–180, *180*
        innervation and vascularization, 179
    clinical presentation of
        patient examination, 180–181, *181*–*182*
        referred pain pattern, 180, *181*
        symptoms, 180
        trigger point examination, 182–183
    corrective actions for, 183–184, *184*
    differential diagnosis of
        associated pathology, 183
        associated trigger points, 183
        trigger points, activation and perpetuation of, 183
    frequency-specific microcurrent, manual therapy with, *860*, 861–862
    treatment parameters for, *862*
    trigger point
        injection/dry needling technique for, 777–778, *781*
        of migraine, *193*
        of tension-type headache, *194*
Subpectoralis minor space, 320
Subscapular artery, 247, 259
Subscapularis muscle, 222, 223, **259**, 294, 320
    anatomic considerations of, 259, *260*
        function, 259–261
        functional unit, 261, *261*
        innervation and vascularization, 259
    clinical presentation of
        patient examination, 262
        referred pain pattern, 261, *261*
        symptoms, 261–262
        trigger point examination, 262–263, *263*, *264*
    corrective actions for, 265–266, *266*
    differential diagnosis of
        associated pathology, 264–265
        associated trigger points, 264
        trigger points, activation and perpetuation of, 263
    trigger point injection/dry needling technique for, 785, *787*
Subscapularis myofascial dysfunction, 261
Subscapularis tendon, humeral attachment of, 325
Substance P, 5, 19, **864**
Subtalar inversion, *728*
Subtendinous bursa, 666
Subthreshold depolarization, 31–32
Successive induction, 845
Sulfasalazine, 547
Supercomplexes, 49
Superficial cervical artery, 209
Superficial fibular nerve, 670, 676
Superficial heat, for pain management, 850
Superficial layer of masseter muscle, 105
Superficial paraspinal muscle, **469**
    anatomic considerations of, 469, *470*
    functions of, 472
    patient examination of, 476
    referred pain pattern of, 473
    trigger point examination of, 477, *477*
Superficial temporal artery, 104
Superficial transverse perinei muscle, 809

Superior gluteal artery, 567, 579, 591
Superior gluteal nerve, 567, 579
Superior head of lateral pterygoid (SHLP) muscle, 128
Superior intercostal artery, 472
Superior oblique muscle
  trigger points
    of migraine, 193
    of tension-type headache, 194
Superior ulnar collateral artery, 302, 308
Supinator longus. See Brachioradialis muscle
Supinator muscle, 352
  anatomic considerations of, 353
    function, 352–353, 354
    functional unit, 353–354, 354
    innervation and vascularization, 352
  clinical presentation of
    patient examination, 354–355
    referred pain pattern, 354, 355
    symptoms, 354
    trigger point examination, 356, 356
  corrective actions for, 357–358, 358
  differential diagnosis of
    associated pathology, 357
    associated trigger points, 357
    trigger points, activation and perpetuation of, 356
  trigger point injection/dry needling technique for, 793, 796
Supinatory foot, 895, 895
Supine position
  for pectoralis major muscle length test, 413, 414
  sleeping posture in, 887, 888
  for trigger point examination
    in adductor brevis muscle, 628–629
    in adductor longus muscle, 628–629
    in coracobrachialis muscle, 287
    in dorsal muscles, 742, 743
    in extensor digitorum longus muscle, 721, 721
    in extensor hallucis longus muscle, 721, 721
    in masseter muscle, 107, 108
    in plantar muscles, 741–742, 742–743
    in popliteus muscle, 650, 650
    in quadriceps femoris and sartorius muscles, 612, 613
    in sternocleidomastoid muscle, 98, 98
    in subscapularis muscle, 262
    in teres major muscle, 256, 256
    in tibialis anterior muscle, 669, 669
    in trapezius fibers, 86, 87
  for trigger point injection/dry needling technique
    of abductor digiti minimi muscle, 796, 799
    of adductor brevis, 814–815, 817
    of adductor longus, 814–815, 817
    of adductor magnus muscle, 815, 817
    of adductor pollicis muscle, 795, 799
    of anterior deltoid muscle, 786, 788
    of biceps brachii muscle, 788–790, 789
    of brachialis muscle, 790, 790
    of brachioradialis muscle, 791, 794
    of coracobrachialis muscle, 787–788, 789
    of digastric muscle, 773–774, 776
    of dorsal interosseous muscles, 829, 830
    of extensor digitorum brevis, 830, 830
    of extensor digitorum longus muscle, 824, 825
    of extensor digitorum muscle, 792, 795
    of extensor hallucis brevis muscle, 830, 830
    of extensor hallucis longus muscle, 824–825, 825
    of extensor indicis muscle, 792–793, 795
    of fibularis tertius muscle, 820, 821
    of flexor carpi radialis muscle, 793–794, 797
    of flexor carpi ulnaris muscle, 794, 797
    of flexor digitorum profundus muscle, 794, 797
    of flexor digitorum superficialis muscle, 794, 797
    of gracilis muscle, 815, 817
    of hamstring muscles, 819, 819
    of iliopsoas muscle group, 806–807, 807, 809
    of lateral pterygoid muscle, 773, 775
    of latissimus dorsi muscle, 782, 786
    of long head, of triceps brachii muscle, 790, 791
    of longus colli muscle, 774–775, 777
    of masseter muscle, 771–772, 773
    of medial head medial border, of triceps brachii muscle, 790, 793
    of medial pterygoid muscle, 772, 774
    of opponens pollicis muscle, 795, 799
    of palmaris longus muscle, 793, 796
    of pectineus muscle, 817, 818
    of pectoralis minor muscle, 799, 802
    of procerus muscle, 775, 778
    of pronator quadratus muscle, 794, 798
    of pronator teres muscle, 794, 798
    of rectus femoris muscle, 812, 815
    of right zygomaticus major muscle, 775, 777
    of scalene muscles, 778–779, 782
    of sternocleidomastoid muscle, 771, 772
    of subclavius muscle, 798, 802
    of subscapularis muscle, 785, 787
    of supinator muscle, 793, 796
    of temporalis muscle, 772, 774
    of tensor fasciae latae muscle, 810, 812
    of teres major muscle, 785, 787
    of tibialis anterior muscle, 820, 821
    of upper trapezius muscle fibers, 770, 770
    of vastus intermedius muscle, 812, 815
    of vastus lateralis muscle, 813, 816
    of wrist extensor muscles, 790–791, 794
  for trigger point pressure release
    deep neck flexors, activation of, 144, 145
    diaphragm muscle, 448, 449
    infraspinatus muscle, 238, 238
    quadratus lumborum muscle, 510, 511
Supine/prone nonweight-bearing position, 690, 690
Supportive sleeping posture, 417
Suprahyoid aponeurosis, 135
Suprahyoid muscles. See specific muscles
Supraorbital nerve entrapment, 159
Supraorbital neuralgia, 195
Suprascapular artery, 231, 259
Suprascapular nerve, 222, 231
  entrapment, 228, 237, 252
  injury, 237
Supraspinatus muscle, **222**
  anatomic considerations of, 222, 223
    function, 222–224
    functional unit, 224, 224
    innervation and vascularization, 222
  clinical presentation of
    patient examination, 226–227, 226
    referred pain pattern, 224–225, 225
    symptoms, 225
    trigger point examination, 227, 227
  corrective actions for, 228–229, 228, 229
  differential diagnosis of
    associated pathology, 227–228
    associated trigger points, 227
    trigger points, activation and perpetuation of, 227
  trigger point injection/dry needling technique for, 781–782, 783
Supraspinatus tendinitis, 289
Supraspinatus tendinopathy, 257, 432, 782
Sural arteries, 688
Sural nerve, 688, **688**
Sway back posture, 639, 869
Swing-out gait, **669**, **721**
Sympathetic nervous system of myofascial pain, 39–40
Symphysitis, 630
Syndesmosis sprains, 722
Synkinesis, respiratory, **837**

T

Tactile vision, 760
Talocrural joint test, 669, 703
Tapentadol, 13
Taping, 894
  for pronatory foot, 894
  for supinatory foot, 895
Tarlov cyst, 63
Tarsal tunnel syndrome, **749**
  extrinsic factors for, 749–750
  intrinsic factors for, 749
  overview of, 749–750
  patient evaluation with, 750
  trigger points in, 750

Taut band, 679–681
   of fibularis longus muscle, 681, *682*
   palpation of, 760
   trigger point, 17, 30
Tegretol therapy, 448
Temporal arteritis, 117
Temporal bone, *104*
Temporal summation, 16, 845
Temporal tendinitis, 117
Temporalis muscle, **113**
   anatomic considerations of, 113, *114*
      function, 113–114
      functional unit, 114, *114*
      innervation and vascularization, 113
   clinical presentation of
      patient examination, 116
      referred pain pattern, 114–115, *115*
      symptoms, 116
      trigger point examination, 116, *116*
   corrective actions for, 117–118, *118*
   differential diagnosis of
      associated pathology, 117
      associated trigger points, 117
      trigger points, activation and perpetuation of, 116–117
   trigger point
      injection/dry needling technique for, 772, *774*
      of migraine, *193*
      of tension-type headache, *194*
Temporomandibular disorder (TMD), 109, **187**
   associated with trigger points of SCM muscle, 99
   clinical sign of, 187
   initial evaluation of patients with, 187–189, *187*
   lateral pterygoid muscle involvement, 132
   overview of, 187
   temporalis muscle in, 114–115
   trigger points and, 189
Temporomandibular joint (TMJ), 122, *122, 128,* 187, 773, 857, 880
   ankylosis, 124
   anteriorly displaced disc of, 117
   dysfunction, 874–875
   hypermobility of, 189
   internal derangements, 108, 132
   palpation of, 188
   screening examination of, 123
   stability, 113
Temporoparietalis muscle, *157*
Tenascin-C gene, 51
Tenascin X, 62
Tender points, 175, 837–**838**
Tendinopathy, **730**
Tendinous digitation, 103
Tendinous pectoralis major muscle, 408
Tendon fenestration, 658
Tendon rupture, spontaneous, 349
Tennis elbow, 303, 304, 310, *311,* 313, 314, 330, 334, 338, 346, 349, 354–357, 363, 395–396
Tennis leg, 693, **705**
TENS. *See* Transcutaneous electrical nerve stimulation (TENS)
Tension myalgia of pelvic floor, 535
Tension-type headache (TTH), 62
   characteristics of, 190
   chronic and episodic, 193–194, *194*
   episodic, 193–194, *194*
   trigger points, 193–194, *194*
      of levator scapulae muscle, 204
      of occipitofrontalis muscle, 158–159
      of sternocleidomastoid muscle, 99
      of temporalis muscle, 114–116
Tensor fasciae latae muscle, **577**
   anatomic considerations of, 578–579, *579*
      function, 580
      functional unit, 580, *581*
      innervation and vascularization, 579
   clinical presentation of
      patient examination, 582–583, *583*
      referred pain pattern, 581–582, *582*
      symptoms, 582
      trigger point examination, 583–584, *584*
   corrective actions for, *586,* 587, *587*
   differential diagnosis of
      associated pathology, 582
      associated trigger points, 585
      trigger points, activation and perpetuation of, 584
   trigger point injection/dry needling technique for, 810, *812*
Teres major muscle, 252, **254**, 294, 320
   anatomic considerations of, 254, *255*
      function, 254
      functional unit, 254–255, *255*
      innervation and vascularization, 254
   clinical presentation of
      patient examination, 255–256
      referred pain pattern, 255, *256*
      symptoms, 255
      trigger point examination, 256–257, *256*
   corrective actions for, 257–258, *257, 258*
   differential diagnosis of
      associated pathology, 257
      associated trigger points, 257
      trigger points, activation and perpetuation of, 257
   trigger point injection/dry needling technique for, 785, *787*
Teres minor muscle, 222, *223,* **241**
   anatomic considerations of, 241, *242*
      function, 241
      functional unit, 241–242, *242*
      innervation and vascularization, 241
   clinical presentation of
      patient examination, 243–244, *244*
      referred pain pattern, 242, *243*
      symptoms, 242–243
      trigger point examination, 244, *244, 245*
   corrective actions for, 245–246
   differential diagnosis of
      associated pathology, 244–245
      associated trigger points, 244
      trigger points, activation and perpetuation of, 244
   trigger point injection/dry needling technique for, 782, *784*
Testosterone, 55, 57
Tetanus, 109, 124
Tethered cord syndrome, 63
Tetracaine, of trigger point injection, 765
TFCC (triangular fibrocartilage complex), 401–402
TH (thyroid hormone), 57–58
THA (total hip arthroplasty), 585, 599
"The thumb," 334
Therapeutic communication, 75
Therapeutic exercise
   aerobic training, 848–849, *848*
   flexibility training, 847–848
   functional exercise, 849
   for lateral epicondylalgia, 396
   motor control training, 845
   muscle fiber type, 843
   muscle function, trigger points in, 843–844
   neuromuscular reeducation, 844, *844*
   proprioceptive neuromuscular facilitation, 845–846
   strength training, 846–847
Therapeutic modalities
   electrotherapeutic modalities
      biofeedback, 857
      frequency-specific microcurrent. *See* Frequency-specific microcurrent (FSM)
      neuro-muscular electrical stimulation, 856–857
      transcutaneous electrical nerve stimulation, 855–856, *856*
   thermal modalities
      cryotherapy, 850–852
      heat, 850
      ultrasound therapy, 852–853, *853*
      vapocoolant spray, 850–852, *852*
   transdermal medication delivery
      iontophoresis, 854–855, *855*
      phonophoresis, 854
Therapeutic neuroscience education (TNE), 74
Thermal detection and pain threshold, 14
Thermal modalities
   cryotherapy, 850–852
   heat, 850

ultrasound therapy, 852–853, *853*
vapocoolant spray, 850–852, *852*
Thessaly test, for meniscus tear, 661
Thiamine. *See* Vitamin B₁
Thiele massage, 537–538
Thigh
  pain, by quadratus lumborum muscle trigger points, 501
  postural dysfunction findings in, 877, *878*
  thrust test, 544
Third-wave behavioral therapy
  acceptance, 70
  mindfulness and meditation, 69–70
  validation, 70
Thomas heel, 892
Thomas plastic collar, 177
Thomas test, 516, *517*, *560*, *582*, *583*, 660
  for hip flexor length, 516, *517*
Thoracic and chest pain, 548–549
Thoracic multifidus muscle
  trigger point injection/dry needling techniques for, 805
  trigger points in, 478
Thoracic nerve, 453, 484
Thoracic outlet syndrome (TOS), 211, 214, **319**, 430, 437
  as cause of medial elbow pain, 398–399
  computed tomographic view of, *218*
  entrapment
    at costoclavicular space/first rib, 319–320
    due to congenital abnormalities, 320
    at interscalene triangle, 319
    at subpectoralis minor space, 320
  initial evaluation of, 320–321
  interosseous muscle and, 392
  latissimus dorsi muscle and, 252
  vs. pectoralis minor syndrome, 430, 432
  by scalene muscles, *216*
  subscapularis muscle and, 264
  teres major muscle and, 252
  trigger points and, 321
  wrist and finger flexors and, 373
Thoracic radiculopathy, 448
Thoracic surgery, 424
Thoracoacromial artery, 277, 285, 293, 409, 421, 426
Thoracodorsal artery, 247, 254, 453
Thoracodorsal nerve, 208, 247, 254
Thoracolumbar articular dysfunction, 508
Thoracolumbar paraspinal muscles, **469**. *See also specific paraspinal muscles*
  anatomic considerations of, 469–472, *470*, *471*
    function, 472
    functional unit, 472–473, *472*
    innervation and vascularization, 472
  clinical presentation of
    patient examination, 473–477, *476*
    referred pain pattern, 473, *474*, *475*
    symptoms, 473
    trigger point examination, 477–478, *477*
  corrective actions for, 479, *480*
  differential diagnosis of
    associated pathology, 478–479
    associated trigger points, 478
    trigger points, activation and perpetuation of, 478
  hypertrophy, 872–873, *874*
Thoracolumbar scoliotic curve, 872, *874*
Thoracolumbar spine
  postural assessment of, 465
  postural asymmetries of, 872–873, *874*
Three-knuckle test, 107
Thrust mobilization/manipulation, *833*, 835
Thumb muscles. *See also specific muscles*
  attachments of, 379–380
  palpation for trigger points in, *382*
  referred pain patterns for, *381*
  trigger point injection/dry needling techniques for, 799
Thyrohyoid muscle
  anatomic considerations of, 135
    functions of, 138–139
    innervation and vascularization of, 137–138
Thyroid hormone (TH), 57–58

Thyroid-stimulating hormone (TSH), 57–58
Tibial nerve, 592, 649, 688, 699, 709, 727
Tibial stress fracture, 722
Tibialis anterior muscle, **666**
  anatomic considerations of, 666, *666*, *667*
    function, 667
    functional unit, 668, *668*
    innervation and vascularization, 666–667
  clinical presentation of
    patient examination, 669
    referred pain pattern, 668, *668*
    symptoms, 669
    trigger point examination, 669, *669*
  corrective actions for, 671–672, *671*–*672*
  differential diagnosis of
    associated pathology, 670–671
    associated trigger points, 670
    trigger points, activation and perpetuation of, 669–670
  downslope walking and, 667
  loading and off-loading considerations for, *895*
  subcutaneous herniation of, 671
  trigger point injection/dry needling technique for, 820, *821*
Tibialis posterior muscle, **709**, 749
  anatomic considerations of, 709, *710*–*711*
    function, 710–711
    functional unit, 711, *711*
    innervation and vascularization, 709
  clinical presentation of
    patient examination, 712–713
    referred pain pattern, 712, *712*
    symptoms, 712
    trigger point examination, 713, *713*
  corrective actions for, 709, 715–716, *715*
  differential diagnosis of, 709
    associated pathology, 713–715
    associated trigger points, 713
    trigger points, activation and perpetuation of, 713
  dysfunction, 729
  loading and off-loading considerations for, *895*
  trigger point injection/dry needling technique for, 824, *824*
Tibialis posterior musculotendinous deficit, 714
Tibialis posterior tendinopathy. *See* Tibialis posterior tendon dysfunction
Tibialis posterior tendon dysfunction, 714, 744
  overview of, 749
  patient evaluation with, 749
  stage I, 714, 749
  stage II, 714, 749
  stage III, 714, 749
  stage IV, 714, 749
  trigger points in, 749
Tibialis secundus muscle, **709**
Tiered three-finger test, 107, *107*
Tietze's syndrome, 416, 424, 447, 448, 491, 548
Tilted shoulder girdle axis, 217, 218–219
Tinel sign, 175, 320, 401–403, 681
Tinnitus, **106**, 109
Tissue healing, 891–892
Titin, 42, 44, 46
TMD. *See* Temporomandibular disorder (TMD)
TMJ. *See* Temporomandibular joint (TMJ)
TNE (therapeutic neuroscience education), 74
TNX-B gene, 62
Toe curling, 730–731
  exercise, 746, *746*
Toe flexion, *728*
Toe flexor cramping, 729
Toes-spread-out exercise, 746, *746*
Tongue position
  for digastric muscle and anterior neck muscles, 144
  for lateral pterygoid muscle, 133
  for masseter muscle, 109–110
  for medial pterygoid muscle, 125
  for suboccipital muscles, 184
  for temporalis muscle, 118
Tonsillitis, 130, 133
"Too many toes" sign, 712
Tooth, diseased, 108

Toothache, 105
Top-down modulation, 12–13
Topographical mapping, 235
Torsional stress test, 544
Torticollis, 202
TOS. *See* Thoracic outlet syndrome (TOS)
Total hip arthroplasty (THA), 585, 599
Towel scrunches, for strengthening intrinsic muscles, 746, *746*
Training frequency
    of aerobic training program, 848
    of strength training program, 846–847
Training intensity, of aerobic training program, 848, *848*
Tramadol, 13
Transcutaneous electrical nerve stimulation (TENS), 850
    application of, 856
    background of, 855
    parameters for, 856
    patient selection of, 855
Transdermal magnesium chloride, 61
Transduction, nociception and, 5–6, *7*
Transient receptor potential (TRP) ion channels, 8, 10, *11*
Transmission, nociception and, 6–7, *8*
Transvaginal tape, 599
Transverse cervical artery, 268
Transversus abdominis muscle, **484**
    anatomic considerations of, 484, *485*
    functions of, 486–487
    innervation and vascularization of, 484, 486
    patient examination for, 492
    referred pain pattern, 488
Transversus perinei muscle
    anatomic considerations of
        of female, 525, *525*
        of male, 526
    function of, 526–527
    trigger point examination of, 533
Transversus thoracis muscle, 436
Trapeziometacarpal joint arthritis, 357
Trapezius muscle, **80**, 162. *See also specific muscles*
    anatomic considerations of, 80–81, *80, 81*
        function, 81–82, *82*
        functional unit, 82–83, *83*
        innervation and vascularization, 81
    clinical presentation of
        patient examination, 85–86
        referred pain pattern, 83–84, *84*
        symptoms, 85
        trigger point examination, 86, *87*
    corrective actions for, 89–91, *90, 91*
    differential diagnosis of
        associated pathology, 88–89
        associated trigger points, 88
        trigger points, activation and perpetuation of, 86–88
    sternocleidomastoid muscle and, 96
    upper, 117, 215, *215*
Trendelenburg sign, 569, *570,* 574, 595
Triamcinolone (Aristocort, Kenalog), 767, *767*
Triangular fibrocartilage complex (TFCC), 401–402
Triangular interval syndrome, 257
Triceps brachii muscle, 349, **306**. *See also specific muscles*
    anatomic considerations of, 306–307, *307, 308*
        function, 308–309
        functional unit, 310, *310*
        innervation and vascularization, 307–308
    clinical presentations of
        patient examination, 310–313
        referred pain pattern, 310, *311–312*
        symptoms, 310
        trigger point examination, 313, *313*
    corrective actions for, *315,* 316
    differential diagnosis of
        associated pathology, 314–315
        associated trigger points, 314
        trigger points, activation and perpetuation of, 314
    trigger point injection/dry needling technique for, 790, *791–793*
Triceps coxae, 590
Triceps surae muscles, **687**, 690, 697, **698**, 730
    dry needling to, 702
    dysfunction, 702

Trigeminal nerve, 103, 113, 120
Trigeminal neuralgia, 99, 132, 195, *195*
Trigeminocervical nucleus caudalis, 190–192
Trigger finger, 371, 374, 403–404
Trigger point injection (TrPI) technique
    for abductor digiti minimi muscle, 796, *799,* 826–828, *827*
    for abductor hallucis muscle, 826, *827*
    for adductor brevis, 814–815, *817*
    for adductor hallucis muscle, 828, *829*
    for adductor longus, 814–815, *817*
    for adductor magnus muscle, 815, *817, 818*
    for adductor pollicis muscle, 795, *799*
    for anconeus muscle, 790, *793*
    for biceps brachii muscle, 788–790, *789*
    for brachialis muscle, 790, *790*
    for brachioradialis muscle, 791–792, *794*
    for bulbospongiosus (bulbocavernosus) muscle, 809
    for cervical multifidus muscle, 777, *780*
    clinical guideline for, 759–762, *760–763,* 762
    for coccygeus muscle, of pelvic diaphragm, 808
    contraindications to, 762
    for coracobrachialis muscle, 787–788, *789*
    corticosteroids for, 766–768
        adverse effects of, 767
        commonly used glucocorticoid steroids, 767
    for deep paraspinal (multifidus) muscles, 802, *805*
    for deep transverse perinei muscle, 809
    defined, **757**, 758
    for deltoid muscle, 786–787, *788*
    for diaphragm muscle, 800
    for digastric muscle, 773–774, *776*
    for dorsal interosseous muscles, *829,* 830
    for extensor digitorum brevis, 830, *830*
    for extensor digitorum longus muscle, 824, *825*
    for extensor digitorum muscle, 792, *795*
    for extensor hallucis brevis muscle, 830, *830*
    for extensor hallucis longus muscle, 824–825, *825*
    for extensor indicis muscle, 792–793, *795*
    for external oblique muscle, 804, *805*
    for fibularis brevis muscle, 820, *821*
    for fibularis longus muscle, 820, *821*
    for fibularis tertius muscle, 820, *821*
    for finger flexor muscles, 794, *797*
    for flexor accessorius (quadratus plantae) muscle, *827,* 828
    for flexor digitorum brevis muscle, 826, *827*
    for flexor digitorum longus muscle, 826, *826*
    for flexor hallucis brevis muscle, 828, *828*
    for flexor hallucis longus muscle, 826, *826*
    for gastrocnemius muscle, 821–822, *822–823*
    for gemelli muscle, 812, *814*
    for genu articularis muscle, 814, *817*
    for gluteus maximus muscle, 809–810, *810*
    for gluteus medius muscle, 810, *811*
    for gluteus minimus muscle, 810, *811*
    for gracilis muscle, 815, *817*
    for hamstring muscles, 819, *819*
    for iliococcygeus muscle, of pelvic diaphragm, 808
    for iliocostalis lumborum muscle, 802, *804*
    for iliocostalis thoracis muscle, 801–802, *804*
    for iliopsoas muscle group, 806–807, *807, 809*
    for infraspinatus muscle, 782, *784*
    for intercostal muscles, 800
    for internal oblique muscles, 804, *805*
    for interossei muscle, 795–796, *799–800*
    for ischiocavernosus muscle, 808–809
    for lateral pterygoid muscle, 773, *775*
    for latissimus dorsi muscle, 782, *785–786*
    for levator scapula muscle, 778, *781*
    local anesthetics for, 765–766
        allergic reactions to, 765
        classification, and uses of, 765–766
        mechanism of action, 765
        myotoxicity of, 765
    for longissimus thoracis muscle, 801, *804*
    for longus colli muscle, 774–775, *777*
    for lower trapezius muscle fibers, 770, *771*
    for lumbrical muscles, 796, 828
    for masseter muscle, 771–772, *773*
    for medial pterygoid muscle, 772–773, *774*

for middle trapezius muscle fibers, 770, *771*
needle gauge, selection of, 758–759
needling sessions, number of, 762–763
neurotoxins for, 768, *768*
　side effects from, 768
for obturator externus muscle, 812, *814*
for obturator internus muscle, 812, *814*
for occipitofrontalis muscle, 775, *778*
for opponens pollicis muscle, 795, *799*
for palmaris longus muscle, 793, *796*
for pectineus muscle, 817, *818*
for pectoralis major muscle, 796–798, *801*
for pectoralis minor muscle, 799–800, *802*
for piriformis muscle, 810–812, *813*
for plantaris muscle, 824, *824*
for popliteus muscle, 819–820, *820*
postneedling procedures for, 764
precautions to, 762
for procerus muscle, 775, *778*
for pronator quadratus muscle, 794, *798*
for pronator teres muscle, 794, *798*
for pubococcygeus muscle, of pelvic diaphragm, 808
for pyramidalis muscle, 804, *806*
for quadratus femoris muscle, 812, *814*
for quadratus lumborum muscle, 804, 806, *807*, *808*
reasons for failure of, 764
for rectus abdominis muscle, 804, *806*
for rectus femoris muscle, 812, *815*
for rhomboid muscles, 785–786, *788*
for right zygomaticus major muscle, 775, *777*
for sartorius muscle, 814, *817*
for scalene muscles, 778–779, *782*
for semispinalis capitis muscle, 777, *780*
for semispinalis cervicis muscle, 777, *780*
for serratus anterior muscle, 800, *803*
for serratus posterior inferior muscle, 801, *803*
for serratus posterior superior muscle, 801, *803*
for soleus muscle, 822–824, *823*
for splenius capitis muscle, 776, *779*
for splenius cervicis muscle, 776, *779*
for sternalis muscle, 798, *801*
for sternocleidomastoid muscle, 770–771, *772*
for subclavius muscle, 798, *802*
for suboccipital muscles, 777–778, *781*
for subscapularis muscle, 785, *787*
for superficial transverse perinei muscle, 809
for supinator muscle, 793, *796*
for supraspinatus muscle, 781–782, *783*
for temporalis muscle, 772, *774*
for tensor fasciae latae muscle, 810, *812*
for teres major muscle, 785, *787*
for teres minor muscle, 782, *784*
for tibialis anterior muscle, 820, *821*
for tibialis posterior muscle, 824, *824*
Travell and Simons caveats for, *763*
for triceps brachii muscle, 790, 791–793
for upper trapezius muscle fibers, 770, *770*
for vastus intermedius muscle, 812–813, *815–816*
vastus intermedius muscle, tensor of, 814, *817*
for vastus lateralis muscle, 813–814, *816*
for vastus medialis muscle, 813, *815*
for wrist extensor muscles, 790–791, *794*
for wrist flexor muscles, 793–794, *797*
pain Trigger points (TrPs), 17, **44**, 178, **687**. *See also under individual muscles;* Self-pressure release techniques; Self-stretching techniques
　and ankle sprain, 748–749
　and ankylosing spondylitis, 547
　barrier release approach and, 836
　biochemical milieu of, 19
　and carpal tunnel syndrome, 403
　cervical radicular pain, 318–319
　and chronic pelvic pain, 547–548
　clinical characteristics of, 3
　defined, **2**
　electrophysiology, 29–30, *30*
　fatigue and, 891
　frozen shoulder, 324–325
　and greater trochanteric pain syndrome, 657–658
　and hallux valgus, 752
　and hand pain, 404
　headaches
　　cervicogenic, 193
　　contributing to, 191–192, *192*
　　migraine, 192, *193*
　　tension-type, 193–194, *194*
　of hip osteoarthritis, 656
　histopathology of, 36
　　acetylcholine release, regulation of, 34
　　adenosine receptor activation effect, 34
　　adenosine triphosphate and energy crisis theory of Simons, 33
　　neurotransmitters, 32–33
　　postsynaptic effects, 33–34, *35*
　hypotheses
　　integrated, 36–38, *37*, 37
　　muscle spindle, 38–39, *38*
　　sympathetic nervous system of myofascial pain, 39–40
　ion channel polymorphisms, 40
　K_{ATP} receptor channel polymorphisms, 41
　lateral elbow pain, 397–398
　low back pain, 542, *543*, *544*
　lumbar instability, 545
　lumbar ligament sprain, 546
　lumbar stenosis, 545
　manual therapy for, 757–758
　medial elbow pain, 399–400
　metatarsal stress fracture, 751
　Morton neuroma, 752
　motor endplate
　　excitation-contraction coupling, 35–36, *36*
　　neurotransmitter feedback control mechanisms, 36
　of muscle function, effects of, 843–844
　needling therapy for, 757–758
　neuromuscular junction
　　cytosolic Ca^{2+} requirement for muscle contraction, 31, *33*, *34*, *35*
　　orthodromic axon-stimulus-evoked release, 31, *31*, *32*
　　subthreshold depolarization, 31–32
　　trigger point taut band, 30
　and neuropathic pain syndromes, *195*
　and nonarthritic hip pain, 657
　pain and, 19–20, *20*, *187*
　and plantar heel pain, 751
　and posture, 867–868
　pressure release technique
　　clinical application of, 836, *836*
　　for deltoid muscle, 283
　　of gluteus maximus muscle, 836, *836*
　　overview of, 835
　　patient and intervention selection, 835–836
　　for scalene muscles, 221
　　for serratus anterior muscle, 458
　　quantitative sensory testing and, 16–17
　and radial wrist/thumb pain, 401
　reactive oxygen species and muscle dysfunction, 40–41
　and sacroiliac joint dysfunction, 544
　and scapular dyskinesia, 323–324
　segmental sarcomere contraction, 29, *30*
　and sesamoiditis, 753
　and sleeping postures, 887
　and spondylolysis and spondylolisthesis, 546
　static stiffness, 42, *42*
　and subacromial pain syndrome, 322–323, *323*
　of tarsal tunnel syndrome, 750
　taut bands and, 17
　and temporomandibular disorders, 189
　and thoracic and chest pain, 549
　thoracic outlet syndrome and, 321
　of tibialis posterior tendon dysfunction, 749
　treatment of
　　cryotherapy for, 850–852
　　ultrasound therapy for, 852–853, *853*
　　vapocoolant spray for, 850–852, *852*
　types of, 2
　and ulnar wrist pain, 402
　widespread multiple
　　frequency-specific microcurrent technique for, *861*, *862*, *864*
　　treatment parameters for, *864*

Trigger thumb, 383
Trismus, 109, 124
Trochanteric bursa
  of gluteus medius muscle, 566
  of gluteus minimus muscle, 578
Trochanteric bursitis, 501, 508, 585
  psuedotrochanteric bursitis, 582
  subacute, 563
Trochanteric pain syndrome, 810
Tropomodulin, 46, *47*
Tropomyosin, 46, *47*
Troponin, 46
TRP (transient receptor potential) ion channels, 8, 10, 11
TrPI technique. *See* Trigger point injection (TrPI) technique
Trunk and pelvic pain
  clinical considerations of
    ankylosing spondylitis, 546–547
    chronic pelvic pain, 547–548, *548*
    low back pain, 540–542, *543*, *544*
    lumbar instability, 545
    lumbar ligament sprain and strain, 545–546
    lumbar stenosis, 544–545
    sacroiliac joint dysfunction, 542–544
    spondylolysis and spondylolisthesis, 546
    thoracic and chest pain, 548–549
Trunk control, for gluteus medius muscle, *574*
Trunk movement and stability, 515
TSA-II, 14
TSH (thyroid-stimulating hormone), 57–58
TTH. *See* Tension-type headache (TTH)
T-tubule membrane, 31, *32*, 35
Tumoral calcinosis, **599**
Turf-toe, **744**
TVT ABBREVO tape, 599
Two-jointed puzzler. *See* Rectus femoris muscle
Two-knuckle test, 107, *107*, 116, 123
Two-point discrimination test, 403

U

UCS (upper crossed syndrome), 201, 879–880, *879*
Ulnar artery, 368, 388
Ulnar collateral ligament (UCL), 398
Ulnar impaction syndrome, 401, *402*
Ulnar nerve, 399
  entrapment, 315, 373–374, *374*
  and FCU muscle, 375, *375*
  innervation, 308, 363, 368, 378, 386
  neurodynamic testing, 371
Ulnar neuropathy, 392, 467
Ulnar wrist pain, 401–402
Ulnomeniscotriquetral dorsal glide test, 402
Ultrasonography
  application of, 853
  background of, 852–853
  for lateral epicondylalgia, 395
  for metatarsal stress fracture, 751
  patient selection of, 853
  recommendation for, 853
  for tenosynovitis, 651
ULTT (Upper Limb Tension Test), 318
Unconditional positive regard, 73
Unilateral migraine, 192, *193*
Unilateral superior tilt, of pelvis, 871, *872*
Upper crossed syndrome (UCS), 201, 879–880, *879*
Upper extremity, postural assessment of, 876–877, *876*, *877*
Upper Limb Tension Test (ULTT), 318
Upper trapezius muscle
  anatomic considerations of, 80–81, *80*, *81*
  associated pathology, 88
  functional unit of, 83
  functions of, 82
  patient examination for, 85
  referred pain pattern of, 83–84, *84*
  symptoms from, 85
  trigger points in
    activation and perpetuation of, 86–88
    corrective actions for, 89, *90*
    examination of, 86, *87*

injection/dry needling technique for, 770, *770*
of migraine, *193*
of tension-type headache, *194*

V

Vaginal examination
  of anal sphincter muscle, 530
  fo bulbospongiosus muscle, 532
  of ischiocavernosus muscle, 532–533
Vaginal pain, 527
Valgus extension overload syndrome, 398
Valgus stress test, 398
Validation, 70, 74
Valsalva, 219
Vamp, assessment of, 892, *893*
Vapocoolant spray, 759, 850–852, *852*
Variant axillary arch muscle, 247
VAS (visual analog scale), 852
Vascularization of muscles. *See under* individual muscles
Vastus intermedius muscle, **604**
  anatomic considerations of, 604, *605*
  associated trigger points of, 614
  referred pain pattern of, 607, *608*
  symptoms from, 610
  tensor of, 606
  trigger point examination of, 611, *612*
  trigger point injection/dry needling technique for, 812–814, *815–816*, *817*
Vastus lateralis muscle, **605**
  anatomic considerations of, 605–606, *605*
  associated trigger points of, 614
  neuromuscular therapy for, 838–839, *839*
  referred pain pattern of, 608, *609*
  symptoms from, 610
  trigger point examination of, 612, *612*
  trigger point injection/dry needling technique for, 813–814, *816*
Vastus medialis muscle, **605**, **621**
  anatomic considerations of, 605, *605*
  associated trigger points of, 614
  referred pain pattern of, 607–608, *609*
  symptoms from, 610
  trigger point examination of, 611–612, *612*
  trigger point injection/dry needling technique for, 813, *815*
Vastus medialis obliquus (VMO), 605
VDD (vitamin D deficiency), 58, 59–60
Venous sinuses, 700
Venous thrombosis, 599
Ventral rami nerve, 666
Vertigo, 99
Vestibular system, 869
Vibration detection threshold, 14, *16*
Vibration perception threshold, 14, *16*
Visceral disease, 490, 494
Viscero-somatic effect, 490, 548
Viscero-somatic reflex, 494
Visual analog scale (VAS), 852
Visual system, 869
Vitamin B$_1$, 58–59
Vitamin B$_{12}$, 58
Vitamin C, 64
Vitamin D, 59–60
  deficiency (VDD), 58, 59–60
  supplementation, 59–60
Vladimir Janda approach, 251
VMO (vastus medialis obliquus), 605
Volume, and strength training program, **847**
Vomiting, intercostal and diaphragm muscle and, 443
Von Frey hairs, 14

W

Waddling gait, **669**, **721**
Warm detection threshold, **14**
Wartenberg sign, 402
Wartenberg syndrome, 339, 357, 400–401
Watershed position, 228
Watershed zone, 709
Weeder's thumb syndrome, 372, 382

Wet needling, 757, 758
   Whiplash, 194–195
mechanism of injury, 478
   Whiplash-associated disorder (WAD), 142, 144, 194–195, 214
     neck pain associated with, 190
     scalene muscles trigger points, 217
Widespread multiple trigger points
   frequency-specific microcurrent technique for, *861*, 862, 864
   treatment parameters for, *864*
Windlass mechanism, 712, 729
Winged scapula, 430, 465
Work-to-rest ratio, 857
Workload ratio, acute to chronic, 846
Wright test (hyper-abduction test), 320, *428*, 430, 432
Wrist extensor muscles, **329**. *See also specific muscles*
   anatomic considerations of, 329–331, *330–331*
     function, 333
     functional unit, 333, *333*
     innervation and vascularization, 332
   clinical presentation of
     patient examination, 334–336
     referred pain pattern, 334, *335*
     symptoms, 334
     trigger point examination, 336–337, *337*
   corrective actions for, 339–340, *339*, *340*
   differential diagnosis of
     associated pathology, 338–339
     associated trigger points, 338
     trigger points, activation and perpetuation of, 337–338
   trigger point injection/dry needling technique for, 790–791, *794*
Wrist flexor muscles. *See also specific muscles*
   trigger point injection/dry needling technique for, 793–794, *797*

X

Xeomin (incobotulinum), *768*
Xiphoidalgia, 448
X-ROS signaling, 18
Xylocaine. *See* Lidocaine

Y

Yergason's sign, 322
Yoga strap–assisted stretching
   for gracilis muscle, 633, *633*
   for hamstring muscle, 645, *645*

Z

Zygapophyseal joint, 168, 170
   dysfunction, 325
   pain, role of, 166
Zygomatic arch, 103, *104*, 127, *128*
Zygomatic bone, *104*
Zygomaticus major muscle, **148**
   anatomic considerations of, 148, *149*
     function, 151
     functional unit, 151
     innervation and vascularization, 150
   clinical presentation of
     patient examination, 151, 153
     referred pain pattern, 151, *152*
     symptoms, 151
     trigger point examination, 153, *153*
   corrective actions for, 154–155, *155*
   differential diagnosis of
     associated pathology, 154
     associated trigger points, 154
     trigger points, activation and perpetuation of, 153–154